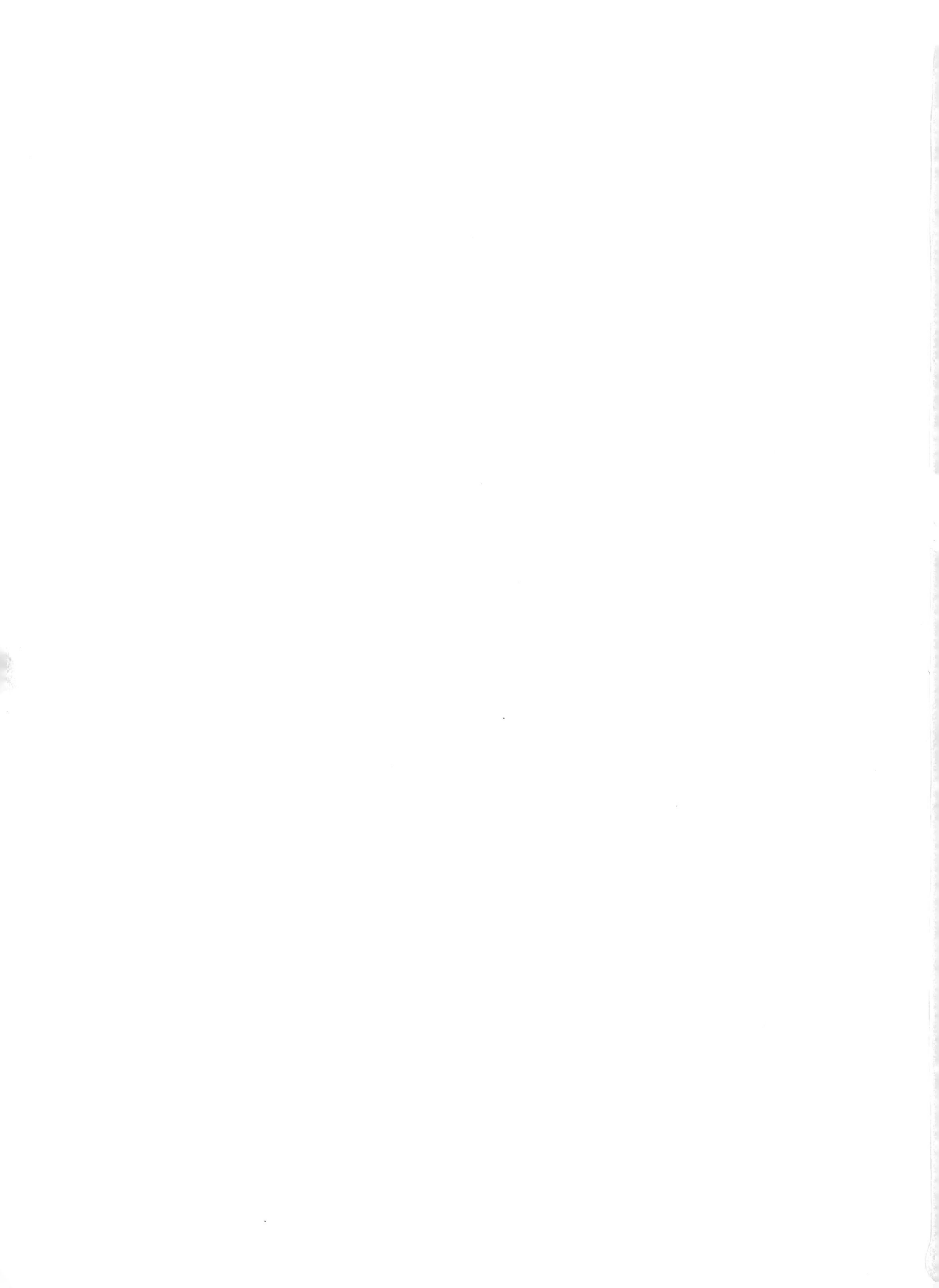

PRINCIPLES AND PRACTICE OF GASTROINTESTINAL ONCOLOGY

SECOND EDITION

Editors

David P. Kelsen, MD

Professor of Medicine
Weill Medical College of Cornell University
Chief, Gastrointestinal Oncology Service
Edward S. Gordon Chair in Medical Oncology
Department of Medicine
Memorial Sloan-Kettering Cancer Center
New York, New York

John M. Daly, MD

Harry C. Donahoo Professor of Surgery
Department of Surgery
Sections of General Surgery and Surgical Oncology
Dean, Temple University School of Medicine
Philadelphia, Pennsylvania

Scott E. Kern, MD

Professor of Oncology and Pathology
Departments of Oncology and Pathology
The Sidney Kimmel Comprehensive Cancer Center
The Johns Hopkins University School of Medicine
Baltimore, Maryland

Bernard Levin, MD

Professor of Gastrointestinal Medicine and Nutrition
Vice President for Cancer Prevention and Population Sciences
Betty B. Marcus Chair in Cancer Prevention
The University of Texas MD Anderson Cancer Center
Houston, Texas

Joel E. Tepper, MD

Professor and Chair
Hector MacLean Distinguished Professor of Cancer Research
Department of Radiation Oncology
University of North Carolina School of Medicine
North Carolina Clinical Cancer Center
Chapel Hill, North Carolina

Eric Van Cutsem, MD, PhD

Professor of Medicine
Gastroenterology Section
Department of Pathophysiology
University of Leuven
Head, Division of Digestive Oncology
University Hospital Gasthuisberg
Leuven, Belgium

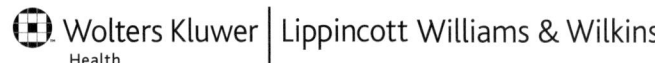

Wolters Kluwer | Lippincott Williams & Wilkins
Health

Philadelphia • Baltimore • New York • London
Buenos Aires • Hong Kong • Sydney • Tokyo

Senior Executive Editor: Jonathan W. Pine, Jr.
Senior Managing Editor: Anne E. Jacobs
Project Manager: Alicia Jackson
Senior Manufacturing Manager: Benjamin Rivera
Design Coordinator: Terry Mallon
Cover Designer: Larry Didona
Production Service: Aptara, Inc.

Library of Congress Cataloging-in-Publication Data

Principles and practice of gastrointestinal oncology / [edited by] David P.
Kelsen ... [et al.]. — 2nd ed.
   p. ; cm.
   Rev. ed. of: Gastrointestinal oncology. c2002.
   Includes bibliographical references and index.
   ISBN-13: 978-0-7817-7617-2
   ISBN-10: 0-7817-7617-1
   1. Digestive organs—Cancer. I. Kelsen, David. II. Gastrointestinal oncology.
  [DNLM: 1. Gastrointestinal Neoplasms. WI 149 P957 2008]
  RC280.D5G384 2008
  616.99′433—dc22

                                      2007034193

10 9 8 7 6 5 4 3 2 1

Susan C. Abraham, MD
Associate Professor of Pathology
University of Texas MD Anderson Cancer Center
Houston, Texas

N. Volkan Adsay, MD
Professor of Pathology
Emory University
Vice Chair and Director of Anatomic Pathology
Emory University Hospital
Atlanta, Georgia

Muyiwa A. Aremu, MB, FRCSI
Lecturer, Department of Surgery
University of Dublin
Trinity College Dublin
Adelaide and Meath Hospital
Tallaght, Dublin, Ireland

Timothy R. Asmis, MD, FRCPC
Assistant Professor
University of Ottawa
Medical Oncologist
Ottawa Hospital Cancer Center
Ottawa, Ontario, Canada

David L. Bartlett, MD
Bernard Fisher Professor of Surgery
University of Pittsburgh
Chief, Division of Surgical Oncology
University of Pittsburgh Medical Center
Pittsburgh, Pennsylvania

Monica M. Bertagnolli, MD
Associate Professor of Surgery
Department of Medical Oncology
Brigham and Women's Hospital
Boston, Massachusetts

Sheila A. Bingham, PhD, FMed Sci
Director of Centre for Nutritional Epidemiology in Cancer
Prevention and Survival
University of Cambridge
Cambridge, United Kingdom

Craig D. Blinderman, MD, MA
Instructor of Medicine
Harvard Medical School
Attending Physician
Palliative Care Service
Massachusetts General Hospital
Boston, Massachusetts

Heimer Boeing, Prof. Dr, MSPH
Head, Department of Epidemiology
Germany Institute of Human Nutrition Potsdam-Rehbruecke
Nuthetal, Germany

H. Bas Bueno-de-Mesquita, MD, MPH, PhD
Project Director, Nutrition and Chronic Diseases
Center for Nutrition and Health
National Institute for Public Health and the Environment
Bilthoven, the Netherlands

Marcia Irene Canto, MD, MHS
Associate Professor of Medicine and Oncology
John Hopkins University School of Medicine
Director of Clinical Research
Department of Medicine
Division of Gastroenterology and Hepatology
Johns Hopkins Medical Institutions
Baltimore, Maryland

Barrie R. Cassileth, MS, PhD
Chief, Integrative Medicine Service
Memorial Sloan-Kettering Cancer Center
New York, New York

Ian D. Chin, MD
Assistant Professor
Department of Surgery
Queen's University, Hotel Dieu Hospital
Kingston, Ontario, Canada
Staff Physician
Department of Surgery
Lakeridge Health Oshawa
Oshawa, Ontario, Canada

Steven J. Cohen, MD
Associate Member
Divisions of Medical and Population Science
Fox Chase Cancer Center
Philadelphia, Pennsylvania

Kevin C. Conlon, MD, FACS, FRCS, MBA
Professor
Department of Surgery
University of Dublin
Trinity College Dublin
Dublin, Ireland
Chair of Surgery
TCD Department of Surgery
Adelaide and Meath Hospital
Tallaght, Dublin, Ireland

Sean D. Curran, FFR, RCSI
Radiologist
Memorial Sloan-Kettering Cancer Center
Department of Radiology
New York, New York

Steven A. Curley, MD, FACS
Professor of Surgical Oncology
Department of Surgical Oncology
University of Texas M. D. Anderson Cancer Center
Houston, Texas

Kimberly Moore Dalal, MD
Assistant Clinical Professor (Volunteer)
Department of Surgery
University of California at San Francisco
Chief, Surgical Oncology
Major, United States Air Force
David Grant United States Air Force
    Medical Center
Travis Air Force Base, California

John M. Daly, MD
Harry C. Donahoo Professor of Surgery
Department of Surgery
Sections of General Surgery and Surgical
    Oncology
Dean, Temple University School of Medicine
Philadelphia, Pennsylvania

David A. Dean, MD
Director, Cardiothoracic Surgical Research
Chief, Section of Thoracic Transplantation
    and VAD's
Department of Thoracic & Cardiovascular
    Surgery
Allegheny General Hospital
Pittsburgh, Pennsylvania

Jochen Decaestecker, MD
Department of Pathology
University of Hospital Gasthuisberg
Leuven, Belgium

Evan S. Dellon, MD
Clinical Instructor in Medicine
Division of Gastroenterology and Hepatology
Center for Esophageal Diseases and Swallowing
University of North Carolina School
    of Medicine
Chapel Hill, North Carolina

George D. Demetri, MD, FACP
Assistant Professor of Medicine
Center for Sarcoma and Bone Oncology
Harvard Medical School
Dana-Farber Cancer Institute
Boston, Massachusetts

Caroline De Vleechouwer
University Hospital Gasthuisberg
Leuven, Belgium

Andre D'Hoore, MD, PhD
University of Hospital Gasthuisberg
Leuven, Belgium

Gary E. Deng, MD, PhD
Physician
Integrative Medicine Service
Memorial Sloan-Kettering Cancer Center
New York, New York

Vikram Deshpande, MD
Instructor in Pathology
Harvard Medical School
Massachusetts General Hospital
Boston, Massachusetts

Frank C. Detterbeck, MD, FACS, FCCP
Professor and Chief
Thoracic Surgery
Surgical Director
Yale Thoracic Oncology Program
Associate Director, Clinical Affairs, Yale Cancer Center
Yale University School of Medicine
New Haven, Connecticut

Cathy Eng, MD
Assistant Professor
Gastrointestinal Medical Oncology
University of Texas MD Anderson Cancer Center
Houston, Texas

Cecilia M. Fenoglio-Preiser, MD
Director of Gastrointestinal Pathology
Ameripath Arizona
Phoenix, AZ

Yuman Fong, MD
Professor of Surgery
Weill Cornell Medical Center
Murray F. Brennan Chair in Surgery
Memorial Sloan-Kettering Cancer Center
New York, New York

Eike Gallmeier, MD
Department of Medicine
University Hospital Grosshadern
Ludwig-Maximillians-University
Munich, Germany

Christopher J. Gannon, MD
Department of Surgical Oncology
University of Texas M. D. Anderson Cancer Center
Houston, Texas

Hans Gerdes, MD
Professor of Clinical Medicine
Weill Medical College of Cornell University
Attending Physician
Department of Medicine
Memorial Hospital for Cancer and Allied Disease
New York, New York

Michael Goggins, MD
Associate Professor
Department of Pathology, Medicine, Oncology
Johns Hopkins Medical Institute
Baltimore, Maryland

Carlos A. Gonzalez, MD
Chief
Group Nutrition, Environment and Cancer
Catalan Institute of Oncology
Barcelona, Spain

William M. Grady, MD
Associate Member
Clinical Research Division
Fred Hutchinson Cancer Research Center
Associate Professor and Section Chief
Division of Gastroenterology
University of Washington
Seattle, Washington

Mark L. Greaves, MD
Fellow in Medicine
Weill Medical College of Cornell University
Fellow in Gastroenterology
Department of Medicine
Memorial Hospital for Cancer and
    Allied Disease
New York, New York

F. Anthony Greco, MD
Centennial Medical Center
Sarah Cannon Cancer Center
Nashville, Tennessee

John D. Hainsworth, MD
Chief Scientific Officer
The Sarah Cannon Cancer Center
Nashville, Tennessee

James P. Hamilton, MD
Post-doctoral Fellow
Department of Medicine
Johns Hopkins University School of Medicine
Hepatology Fellow
Division of Gastroenterolgoy and Hepatology
Baltimore, Maryland

John P. Hoffman, MD
Professor
Department of Surgery
Temple University School of Medicine
Senior Member
Department of Surgical Oncology
Fox Chase Cancer Center
Philadelphia, Pennsylvania

Ralph H. Hruban, MD
Professor and Pathologist
Department of Pathology
Johns Hopkins Medical Institutions
Baltimore, Maryland

Elizabeth T. Jacobs, PhD
Assistant Professor
Department of Epidemiology and Biostatistics
Arizona Cancer Center
Tucson, Arizona

Jeremy R. Jass, MD, FRCPath
Professor
Division of Surgery, Oncology, Reproductive Biology
    and Anesthetics
Imperial College London
London, United Kingdom
Consultant Histopathologist
Department of Cellular Pathology
St. Mark's Hospital
Harrow, Middlesex, United Kingdom

Morton S. Kahlenberg, MD, FACS
Associate Professor
Chief, Surgical Oncology
Department of Surgery
University of Texas Health
    Science Center
San Antonio, Texas

Ellen Kampman, PhD
Associate Professor
Division of Human Nutrition
Wageningen University
Wageningen, the Netherlands

David P. Kelsen, MD
Professor of Medicine
Weill Medical College of Cornell University
Chief, Gastrointestinal Oncology Service
Edward S. Gordon Chair of Medical Oncology
Department of Medicine
Memorial Sloan-Kettering Cancer Center
New York, New York

Andrew S. Kennedy, MD
Co-Medical Director
Wake Radiology Oncology
Cary, North Carolina

Scott E. Kern, MD
Professor of Oncology and Pathology
Departments of Oncology and Pathology
The Sidney Kemmel Comprehensive Cancer Center
Johns Hopkins University School of Medicine
Baltimore, Maryland

Michael C. Kew, MD, DSc, FRCP
Dora Dart Professor of Medicine
Department of Medicine, Faculty of Health Sciences
University of the Witwatersrand
Senior Physician of Medicine
Johannesburg Academic Hospital, Parktown
Johannesburg, Ganteng, South Africa

David S. Klimstra, MD
Professor of Pathology and Laboratory Medicine
Weill Medical College of Cornell
Attending Pathologist and Chief of Surgical Pathology
Memorial Sloan-Kettering Cancer Center
New York, New York

Richard P. M. Koehler, MD
Thoracic Surgeon
Department of Surgery
Virginia Mason Medical Center
Seattle, Washington

Matthew H. Kulke, MD
Assistant Professor of Medicine
Department of Medical Oncology
Dana-Farber Cancer Institute
Harvard Medical School
Boston, Massachusetts

Rene Lambert, MD, FRCP
Visiting Scientist
Group of Screening
International Agency for Research on Cancer (IARC)
Lyon, France

Gregory Y. Lauwers, MD
Associate Professor of Pathology
Harvard Medical School
Director of Gastrointestinal Pathology
Massachusetts General Hospital
Boston, Massachusetts

Theodore Lawrence, MD, PhD
Isadore Lampe Professor and Chair
Department of Radiation Oncology
University of Michigan
University Hospital
Ann Arbor, Michigan

Bernard Levin, MD
Professor of Gastrointestinal Medicine and Nutrition
Vice President and Division Head
Betty B. Marcus Chair in Cancer Prevention
Cancer Prevention and Population Sciences
The University of Texas MD Anderson Cancer Center
Houston, Texas

Keith D. Lillemoe, MD
Jay L. Grosfeld Professor and Chairman
Department of Surgery
Indiana University School of Medicine
Surgeon-in-Chief
Indiana University Hospital
Indianapolis, Indiana

Steven Lipkin, MD, PhD
Associate Professor
Department of Medicine
University of California, Irvine
Director, Cancer Genetics Clinic
Chao Family NCI Designated Comprehensive Cancer Center
University of California, Irvine Medical Center
Irvine, California

Albert B. Lowenfels, MD
Professor of Surgery
New York Medical College
Valhalla, New York

Alessandro Lugli, MD
Attending Physician
Institute of Pathology
University Hospital Basel
Basel, Switzerland

Patrick Maisonneuve, Eng
Director Epidemiology
Division Epidemiology and Biostatistics
European Institute of Oncology
Milan, Italy

Arnold J. Markowitz, MD
Assistant Clinical Professor of Medicine
Weill Medical College of Cornell University
Memorial Hospital for Cancer and
    Allied Disease
New York, New York

Maria Elena Martinez, MD
Professor of Epidemiology and Nutrition
Arizona Cancer Center
University of Arizona
Tucson, Arizona

Joel B. Mason, MD
Associate Professor
Schools of Medicine and Nutritional Science
Tufts University
Staff Physician
Divisions of Gastroenterology and Clinical Nutrition
Tufts New England Medical Center
Boston, Massachusetts

Stephen J. Meltzer, MD
Professor and Director of GI Biomarker
    Research Laboratory
Department of Medicine
Johns Hopkins University School of Medicine
Division of Gastroenterology and Hepatology
Johns Hopkins Hospitals
Baltimore, Maryland

Bruce D. Minsky
Vice Chairman
Department of Radiation Oncology
Memorial Sloan-Kettering Cancer Center
New York, New York

Rajnish Mishra, MD
Fellow, Department of Medicine
Department of Gastroenterology
University of Virginia Health System
Charlottesville, Virginia

Michael Molls, MD
Professor
Technical University
Chief
Department of Radiotherapy and Radiation Oncology
Keinikumtechls der lsar
Munchen, Germany

Attila Nakeeb, MD
Associate Professor
Department of Surgery
Indiana University School of Medicine
Attending Surgeon
Indiana University Hospital
Indianapolis, Indiana

Bernard Nordlinger, MD
Department of Digestive and Oncologic Surgery
Ambroise Paré Hospital
Boulogne, France

Kenneth Offit, MD, MPH
Professor of Medicine
Weil Medical College, Cornell University
Chief, Clinical Genetics Service
Memorial Sloan-Kettering Cancer Center
New York, New York

Sam G. Pappas, MD
Assistant Professor
Department of Surgery
Medical College of Wisconsin
Assistant Professor
Department of Surgery
Froedtert Hospital
Milwaukee, Wisconsin

Donald Max Parkin, MD
Clinical Trials Service Unit and Epidemiological Studies
University of Oxford
Headington, Oxford, United Kingdom

Bogdan C. Paun, MD
Locum Tenens
Department of Surgery
Headerson General Hospital
Hamilton, Ontario, Canada

Freddy Penninckx, MD, PhD
Department of Abdominal Surgery
University Hospital Gasthuisberg
Leuven, Belgium

Nicholas Petrelli, MD
Professor of Surgery
Department of Surgery
Thomas Jefferson University
Philadelphia, Pennsylvania
Bank of America Endowed Medical Director
Deparment of Surgery
Helen F. Graham Cancer Center
Newark, Delaware

Joel Picus, MD
Associate Professor
Department of Medicine
Washington University School of Medicine
Barnes Hospital
St. Louis, Missouri

Henry A. Pitt, MD
Professor
Department of Surgery
Indiana University
Indianapolis, Indiana

Ronnie T-P Poon, MD, FRCS(Ed)
Professor
Department of Surgery
University of Hong Kong
Queen Mary Hospital
Hong Kong, China

Russell K. Portenroy, MD
Professor of Neurology
Albert Einstein College of Medicine
Bronx, New York
Chairman
Department of Pain Medicine and
    Palliative Care
Beth Israel Medical Center
New York, New York

Steven M. Powell, MD
Associate Professor
Department of Medicine
University of Virginia Health System
Charlottesville, Virginia

Adam Raben, MD
Attending
Department of Radiation Oncology
Christiana Care-Helen F. Graham Cancer Center
Newark, Delaware

Chandrajit P. Raut, MD, MSc
Instructor
Associate Surgeon
Department of Surgery
Harvard Medical School
Brigham and Women's Hospital
Boston, Massachusetts

Dennis L. Rousseau, Jr., MD, PhD
Director of Surgical Oncology
Department of Medical Education
Florida Hospital Cancer Institute
Orlando, FL

Brian P. Rubin, MD, PhD
Assistant Professor
Department of Pathology
University of Washington Medical Center
Seattle, Washington

Leonard B. Saltz, MD
Professor of Medicine
Weill Medical College of Comell University
Attending Physician and Member
Department of Medicine
Memorial Sloan-Kettering Cancer Center
New York, New York

Robert S. Sandler, MD, MPH
Distinguished Professor of Medicine
University of North Carolina
Chief, Division of Gastroenterology and Hepatology
University of North Carolina Hospitals
Chapel Hill, North Carolina

Hanna K. Sanoff, MD
Assistant Professor
Department of Medicine, Hematology-Oncology
University of North Carolina at Chapel Hill
Chapel Hill, North Carolina

Deborah Schrag, MD, MPH
Associate Attending Physician
Department of Health Outcome Research Group,
Epidemiology and Biostatistics
Memorial Sloan-Kettering Cancer Center
New York, New York

Richard D. Schulick, MD
John L. Cameron Endowed Chair Chief,
    Surgical Oncology
Department of Surgery, Oncology, Obstetrics,
    and Gynecology
Johns Hopkins Medical Institutions
Baltimore, Maryland

Lawrence H. Schwartz, MD
Radiologist
Memorial Sloan-Kettering Cancer Center
Department of Radiology
New York, New York

Manish A. Shah, MD
Assistant Member
Department of Medicine, Gastrointestinal Oncology
Memorial Sloan-Kettering Cancer Center
Assistant Attending Physician
Department of Medicine
Memorial Hospital
New York, New York

Nicholas J. Shaheen, MD, MPH
Associate Professor of Medicine and Epidemiology
Director, Center for Esophageal Diseases and
    Swallowing
University of North Carolina School of Medicine
Chapel Hill, North Carolina

Morris Sherman, MD
Associate Professor of Medicine
University of Toronto
Staff Gastroenterologist
University Health Network
Toronto, Ontario, Canada

J. Rudiger Siewert, MD
University Professor of Surgery
Chairman, Department of Surgery
Chirurgische Klinik und Poliklinik
Munchen, Germany

Thomas C. Smyrk, MD
Associate Professor
Department Pathology
Mayo Clinic
Rochester, Minnesota

Bianca Stam, MSc
Division of Human Nutrition
Wageningen University
Wageningen, Netherlands

Grant N. Stermmermann, MD, CM
Professor of Pathology
University of Cincinnati College of Medicine
Cincinnati, Ohio

Jon F. Strasser, MD
Attending Physician
Department of Radiation Oncology
Helen F. Graham Cancer Center
Christiana Care Health System
Newark, Delaware

Rachel Stolzenberg-Solomon, PhD, MPH, RD
Investigator
Nutritional Epidemiology Branch
Division of Cancer Epidemiology and Genetics
National Cancer Institute
Rockville, Maryland

Philippe Taleb, MD
Department of Digestive and Oncologic Surgery
Ambroise Paré Hospital
Boulogne, France

Joel E. Tepper, MD
Professor and Chair
Hector MacLean Distinguished Professor of Cancer Research
Department of Radiation Oncology
University of North Carolina School of Medicine
North Carolina Clinical Cancer Center
Chapel Hill, North Carolina

Patricia A. Thompson, PhD
Assistant Professor
Department of Pathology
University of Arizona
Tucson, Arizona

Hans F. A. Vasen, MD, PhD
Staff Member
Department of Gastroenterology
Leiden University Medical Centre
Leiden, Netherlands

Eric Van Cutsem, MD, PhD
Professor of Medicine
Gastroenterology Section
Department of Pathophysiology
University of Leuven
Head, Division of Digestive Oncology
University Hospital Gasthuisberg
Leuven, Belgium

Cornelius J. H. van de Velde, MD, PhD, FRCS (London), FRCS (Glasgow)
Professor of Surgery
Leiden University Medical Center
Leiden, Netherlands

Pieter van't Veer, PhD
Professor in Nutrition and Epidemiology
Division of Human Nutrition
Wageningen University
Wageningen, Netherlands

Alan P. Venook, MD
Professor
Department of Clinical Medicine
University of California, San Francisco
San Francisco, California

H. Rodney Withers, MD, DSc
Professor of Experimental Radiation
    Oncology
University of California at Los Angeles
Los Angeles, California

Christopher G. Willett, MD
Leonard R. Prosnitz Professor and Chair
Department of Radiation Oncology
Duke University Medical School
Durham, North Carolina

Derrick Wong, MD
Senior Clinical Fellow
Department of Medicine
Division of Hematology/Oncology
University of California, San Francisco
San Francisco, California

Tsung-Teh Wu, MD, PhD
Professor of Pathology and Laboratory
    Medicine
Division of Anatomic Pathology
Mayo Clinic College of Medicine
Rochester, Minnesota

Andrew D. Zelenetz, MD
Associate Professor
Department of Medicine
Weill Medical College of Cornell University
Chief, Lymphoma Service
Department of Medicine
Memorial Sloan-Kettering Cancer Center
New York, New York

As a group, gastrointestinal malignancies are the most common cause of cancer in the world. A recent review indicated that, of the 10.8 million people in the world each year who develop cancer, approximately 3.3 million have gastrointestinal malignancies, including esophagogastric cancer, colorectal, hepatocellular, and pancreatic malignancies. In comparison, lung cancer occurs in approximately 1.4 million people each year and breast cancer in 1.2 million women per year. Furthermore, gastrointestinal malignancies are one of the most lethal malignancies. Twenty-nine percent of cancer-related deaths are caused by gastrointestinal cancers. Particularly for esophagogastric cancer, hepatocellular, and pancreatic cancer, the annual incidence and annual mortality are very similar. Prevention, early diagnosis, and improved therapy are urgently needed in gastrointestinal malignancies.

Although the incidence of gastrointestinal cancers varies substantially between different regions of the world, there is considerable overlap in their cause and in the strategies pursued for improvement in outcome. Some gastrointestinal malignancies should be nearly totally preventable, such as hepatocellular carcinoma secondary to cirrhosis from viral hepatitis or alcohol abuse and anal canal cancer secondary to infection with human papilloma virus. In both of these diseases, the development of vaccines against the infectious agent that leads eventually to the malignancy should markedly decrease the incidence of cancer. Proof of principle has already been demonstrated for hepatocellular cancer using vaccines against hepatitis B. In the case of colorectal cancer, removal of a premalignant lesion should prevent the development of subsequent cancer.

If the tumor cannot be prevented, finding it at an earlier stage also improves outcome. This has been demonstrated for colorectal cancer as well as for upper gastrointestinal tract malignancies such as gastric cancer. On the other hand, for some tumors, including pancreatic cancer, the etiology of the disease is less clear, although some progress has been made. Screening and surveillance programs have not yet been adequately developed, and the majority of patients with gastrointestinal malignancies present with extensive and frequently metastatic cancers.

Since the publication of the first edition of this book, there have been important advances in understanding the cause and pathogenesis of gastrointestinal malignancies, a far better understanding of the molecular events leading to the development of these cancers, some improvements in surveillance and screening, and improvements in therapy. From the pathogenesis point of view, colorectal cancer is a model for understanding the neoplastic process from the development of an adenoma through increasing degrees of dysplasia and carcinoma. Better preclinical models, such as genetically engineered mouse models, hold promise for an improved understanding of gastrointestinal malignancies, including such difficult-to-access tumors as pancreatic cancer. Rapid advances in molecular biology (including the sequencing of the human genome) and the development of high through-put systems hold promise for the development of better prognostic and predictive markers in the individual patient.

This second edition of *Principles and Practices of Gastrointestinal Oncology* is a comprehensive, in-depth review of the commonest group of human cancers. The editors and the chapter authors represent an international group of experts who are leaders in their respective fields. They have helped develop current standards of care and direct many important research initiatives. The book features an introductory section that reviews the principles of modern oncology, including both basic and translational science points of view. The principles underlying individual disciplines—including surgery, radiation, medical oncology, diagnostic imaging, and epidemiology—are presented as they apply to gastrointestinal cancers.

The second portion of the book is an updated, in-depth review of gastrointestinal malignancies from the prospective of each individual organ. Each site-specific section features chapters that focus on epidemiology, molecular biology and pathology, prevention (including screening and surveillance), staging, and therapeutic options for that individual tumor site. The chapters are current and include the results of recent important clinical trials that may have either changed the standard of care or demonstrated that an important research initiative did not substantially change outcome. In general, the site-specific chapters dealing with clinical management are multi-authored by experts in appropriate disciplines, including medical, radiation, and surgical oncology.

We hope that this new edition of *Principles and Practices of Gastrointestinal Oncology* will be useful to all physicians, practitioners, and scientists who have an interest in gastrointestinal malignancies. Our understanding of gastrointestinal cancer is changing rapidly, and we hope that the book provides a readable and in-depth presentation of the most current information available to help our colleagues in the management of patients with cancer of the gastrointestinal tract.

David P. Kelsen, MD
John M. Daly, MD
Scott E. Kern, MD
Bernard Levin, MD
Joel E. Tepper, MD
Eric Van Cutsem, MD, PhD

Gastrointestinal (GI) cancers (i.e., malignancies of the esophagus, stomach, liver and the associated biliary tree, pancreas, colon, rectum, and anal canal, and GI neuroendocrine tumors) as a group are common diseases in developed and developing countries. World Health Organization statistics from 1999 (the most recent available) indicated that approximately 2,500,000 people died of esophageal, gastric, colorectal, hepatocellular, or pancreatic cancer worldwide. Although the incidence of cancer of the organs making up the GI tract varies between regions, overall they share some similar promises and problems. As we develop a better understanding of their etiology, some malignancies will prove to be preventable (e.g., hepatocellular carcinoma arising from cirrhosis secondary to viral hepatitis and colorectal cancer developing from adenomatous polyps that can be removed). In addition, when some cancers (e.g., colorectal cancers) are found at an early stage, many are curable. For other gastrointestinal tumors, the etiology is less clean screening and surveillance programs are poorly developed, and the majority of patients present with extensive, frequently metastatic, cancers.

Important advances have led to a better understanding of the cause and pathogenesis of certain gastrointestinal cancers, better surveillance and screening, and improved therapy over the last 5 years. For example, we now know a great deal about the molecular events leading to colon cancer, in which the neoplastic process moves from an adenomatous polyp through increasing degrees of dysplasia to intraepithelial neoplasia and then to carcinoma. In addition to helping define etiology, the breathtakingly rapid advances in molecular biology have led to important screening, surveillance, and therapeutic research efforts.

Gastrointestinal Oncology: Principles and Practice is a comprehensive and in-depth review of this important group of malignancies. The editors and authors are leaders in their fields who have helped develop current standards of care and who frequently chair the most important research initiatives. We have attempted to provide comprehensive coverage of the various issues of importance to allow a full understanding of the biology, development, prevention, diagnosis, and management of GI malignancies. Multimodality management is emphasized, because, to offer patients with GI tumors the best chance for a favorable outcome, new diagnostic staging, and therapeutic advances require collaboration between experts in several disciplines.

The first section of the text reviews the principles of oncologic topics as they relate to GI oncology. It offers an overview of epidemiology, molecular pathology, screening and surveillance, and imaging. Therapeutic principles of surgical, radiation, and medical oncology, as well as advances in biologic therapies, are presented.

The second portion of the text is devoted to an in-depth review of each organ-specific cancer. Each section is introduced by an editorial overview, which highlights recent advances and challenges for that particular tumor. This is followed by individual chapters covering the epidemiology, molecular biology, pathology, prevention (including screening and surveillance), staging, and therapeutic options for each tumor type. Up-to-date clinical trial results are integrated into each chapter. For the therapeutic sections, we have assembled teams of authors who are experts in medical, radiation, and surgical oncology.

Gastrointestinal Oncology: Principles and Practice is directed toward all physicians and scientists with an interest in GI malignancies, including medical, radiation, and surgical oncologists, gastroenterologists, internists, and general surgeons. Although the field of GI oncology is advancing rapidly, we hope that this text supplies an in-depth presentation of the most current information regarding patients with GI neoplasms.

David P. Kelsen, MD
John M. Daly, MD
Scott E. Kern, MD
Bernard Levin, MD
Joel E. Tepper, MD

With thanks to my wife, Suzanne, and my children, Benjamin, Judith, Tamar, Jonathan, Moshe, and Alex, and to Hannah, Ike, Joshua, and Elisheva for their support over many years; to my colleagues and patients who have taught me much about gastrointestinal malignancies; and to my coeditors and the many contributors who have given their time, effort, and enthusiasm to the second edition of this textbook.

D.P.K.

To my wife, Mary, who has shown by example the courage and tenacity to live with her gastrointestinal cancer for the past 10 years.

J.M.D.

With gratitude to my wife, Ronnie, and our children, Adam and Katie, for their love and support; to my assistants, Rosanne Lemon Evans and Nora Burkhalter, for their expert help; and to my many colleagues around the world and my patients from whom I have learned much.

B.L.

I want to thank my wife, Laurie, and my family, including Miriam, Abigail, Adam, Zekariah, and Zohar, for the love and support they have given me through the good times and the bad, and my many colleagues, who have inspired me and taught me to be a better physician.

J.E.T.

CONTENTS

SECTION I: PRINCIPLES OF GASTROINTESTINAL ONCOLOGY

SECTION II: ESOPHAGEAL CANCER

SECTION VII: COLORECTAL CANCER

SECTION VIII: UNCOMMON CANCERS OF THE GASTROINTESTINAL TRACT

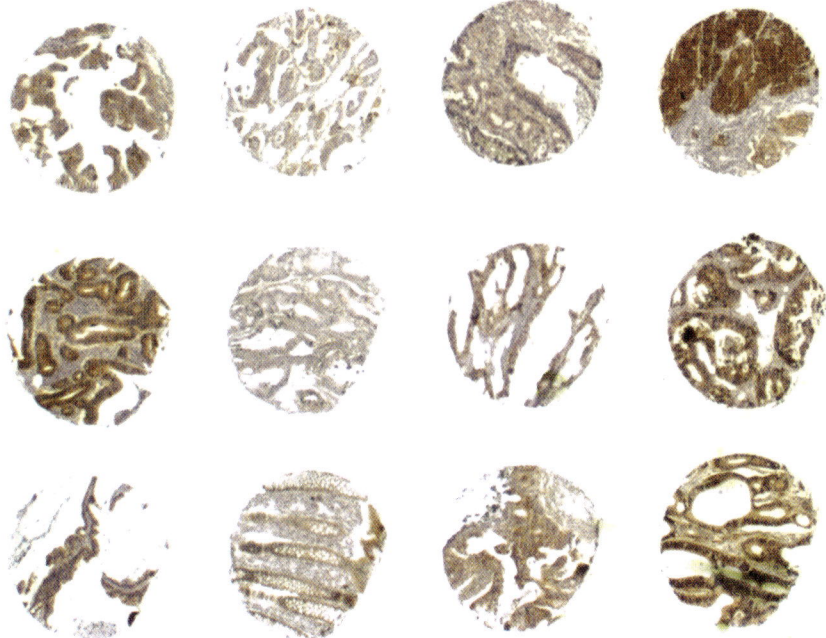

FIGURE 2.1. Tissue microarray showing differing intensity of epidermal growth factor receptor immunohistochemistry in multiple colorectal cancer punches (2×). *Source:* From the Archives of the Institute of Pathology, University Hospital Basel, Institute of Clinical Pathology, Basel and Institute of Pathology, Stadtspital Triemli, Zürich, Switzerland.

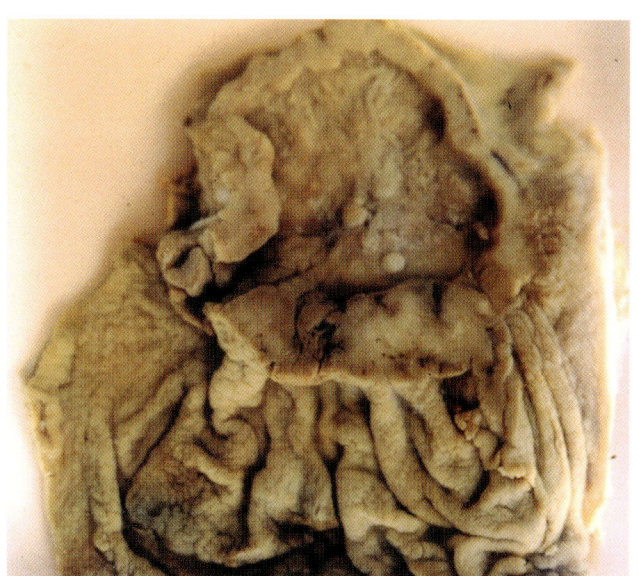

FIGURE 2.2. Gastric cancer, ulcerated type (Borrmann III). The ulcer base is necrotic, and the tumor borders are irregular and have been trimmed to show pale cancer tissue.

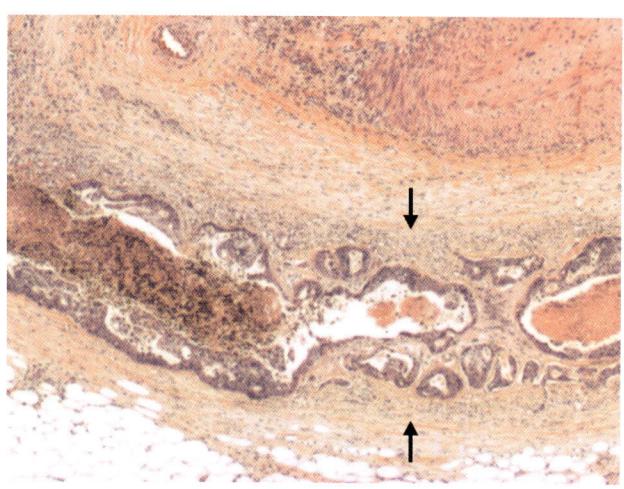

FIGURE 2.3. Invasion of large extramural vein in colorectal cancer. Note the smooth muscle in the vein wall (arrows).

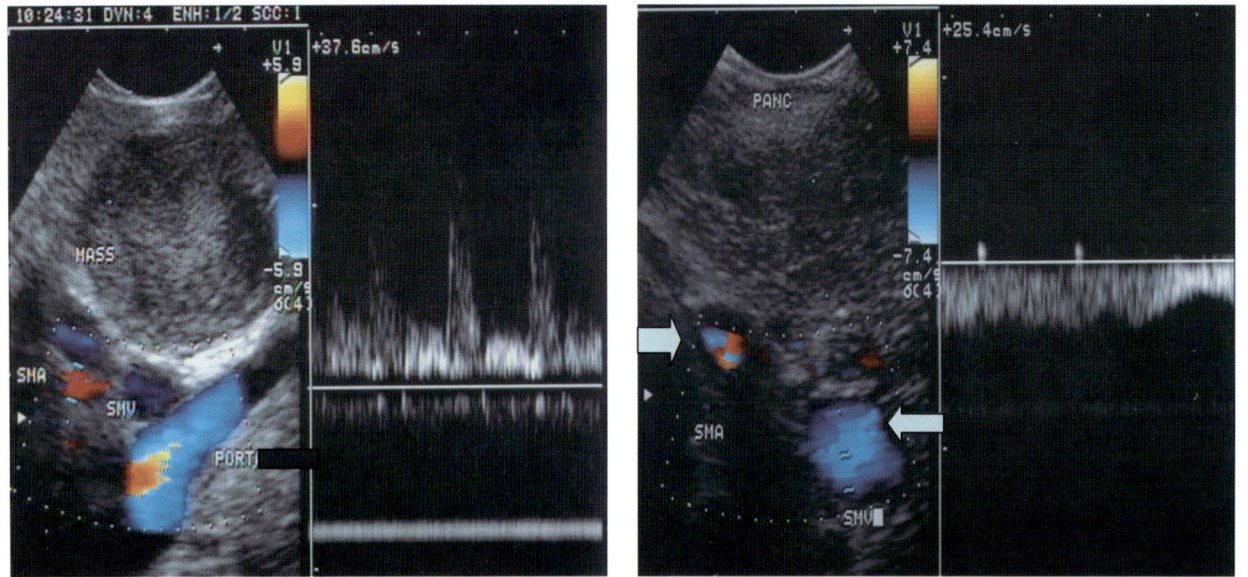

FIGURE 10.5. A: Endoscopic ultrasonography (EUS) image from a linear scanning ultrasound endoscope (Pentax Medical Systems, Montvale, New Jersey) showing a resectable pancreatic mass in the head. **B:** In contrast, this mass is clearly unresectable because of encasement of both the superior mesenteric artery and vein (*arrows*). At the same outpatient procedure, EUS-guided fine-needle aspiration obtained abundant cells consistent with adenocarcinoma, and celiac plexus neurolysis was performed to palliate cancer pain.

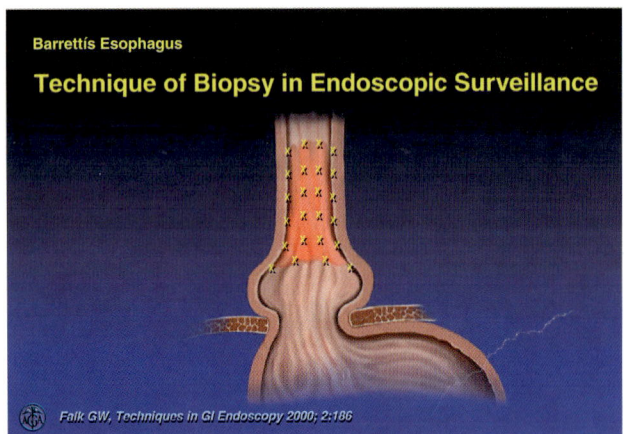

FIGURE 14.2. Surveillance biopsy protocol in Barrett esophagus (BE). Note that biopsies are obtained in each of the four quadrants at 2-cm intervals in the segment of esophagus with BE. Used with permission. Copyright American Gastroenterologic Association Institute, Bethesda, MD.

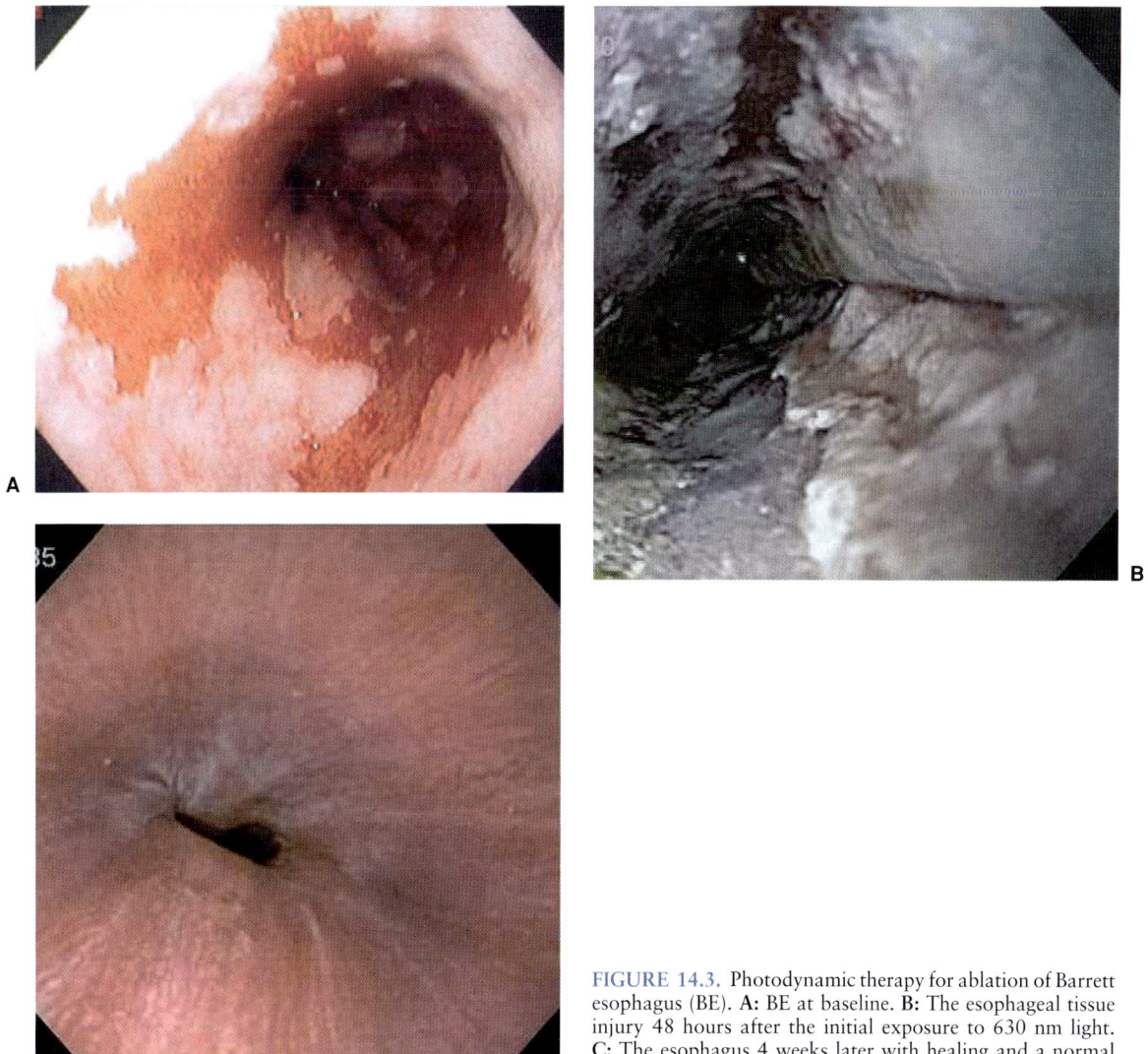

FIGURE 14.3. Photodynamic therapy for ablation of Barrett esophagus (BE). **A:** BE at baseline. **B:** The esophageal tissue injury 48 hours after the initial exposure to 630 nm light. **C:** The esophagus 4 weeks later with healing and a normal layer of esophageal squamous mucosa.

FIGURE 21.8. A: Hematoxylin-and-eosin−stained ulcer margin has a small area of dysplastic mucosa bordering a healing ulcer. **B:** This dysplastic mucosa has p53 overexpression shown by immunohistochemistry.

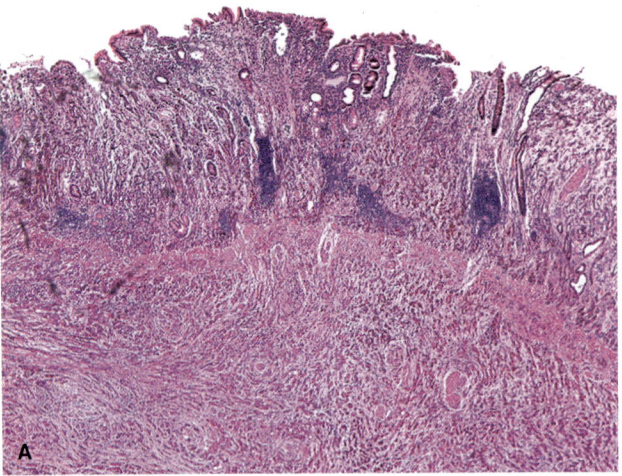

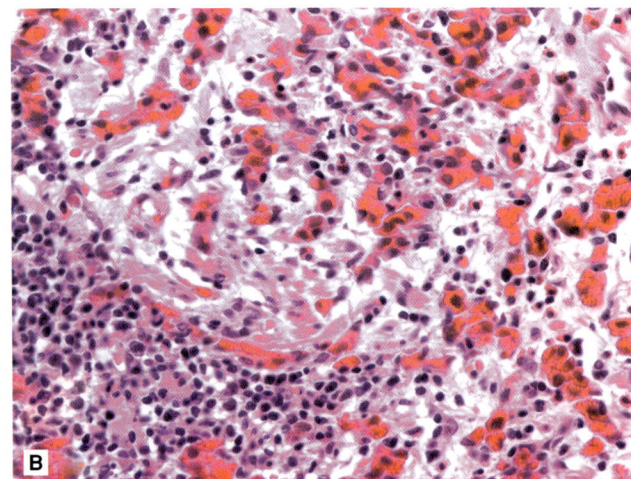

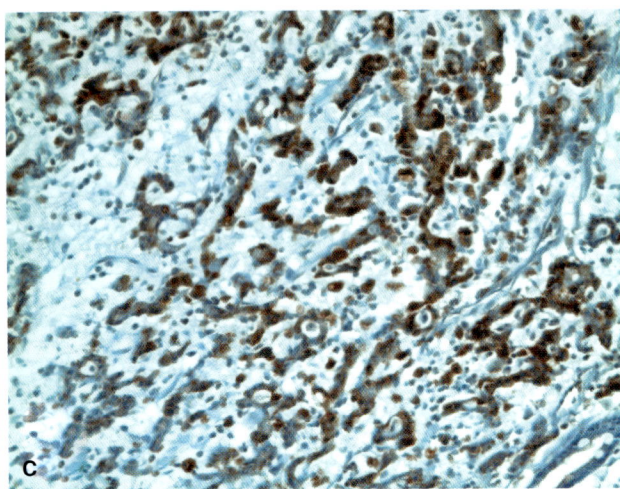

FIGURE 21.22. Paneth cell cancer arising in the setting of complete intestinal metaplasia. This flat, stage 1, infiltrating cancer (**A**) is composed of cells with bright red cytoplasmic granules (**B**). Immunohistochemistry for lysozomes (**C**) confirms the nature of these granules. This patient developed a peritoneal recurrence 7 years after subtotal resection.

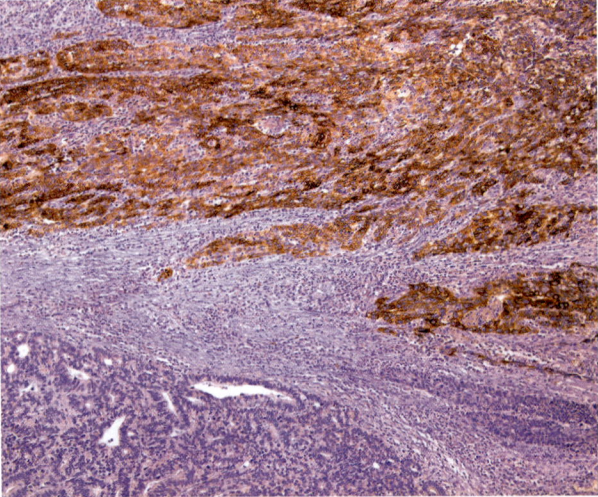

FIGURE 21.24. Heterogeneity of pepsinogen group II (PGII) expression. Immunohistochemistry for PGII labels a poorly differentiated portion of a stage 3, intestinal-type antral cancer. An adjacent, well-differentiated component of the cancer does not label for this product. This patient died 5 months after a palliative resection.

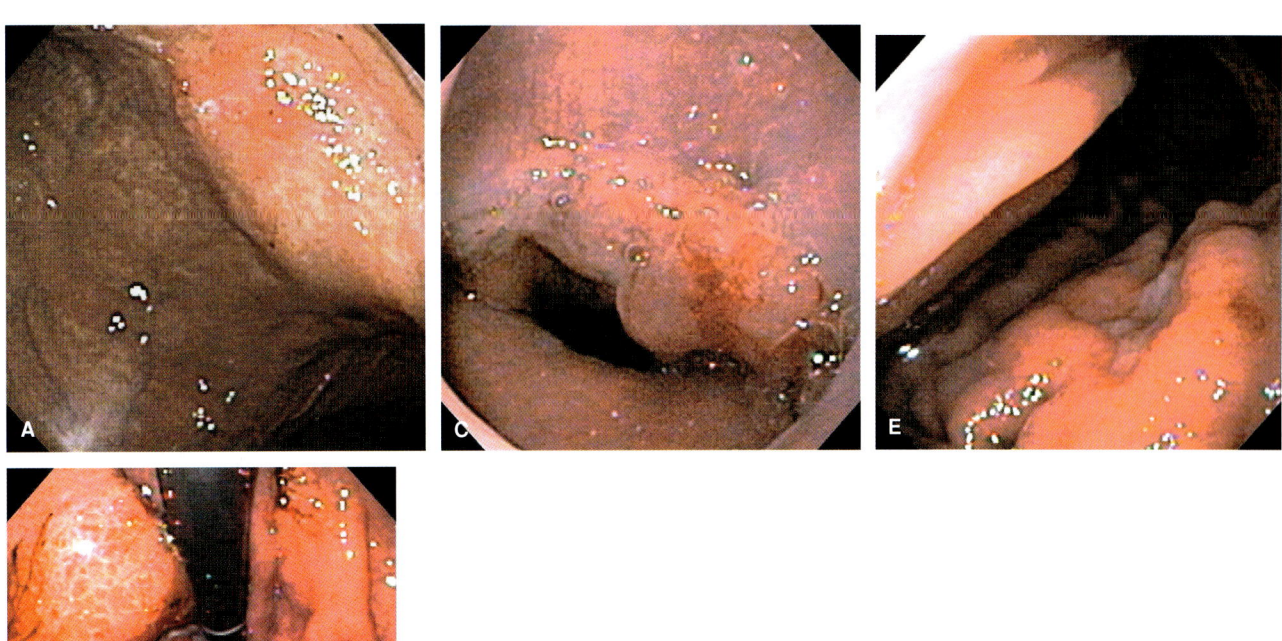

FIGURE 22.2. The endoscopic and corresponding endoscopic ultrasonography (EUS) images of different T-staged gastric cancers. **A:** T1 lesion. **C:** Another T1 lesion. **E:** T2 lesion. **G:** T3 lesion.

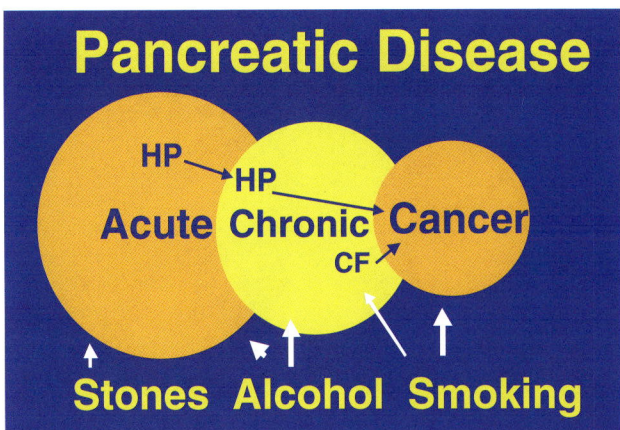

FIGURE 24.4. Possible relationship among acute pancreatitis, chronic pancreatitis, and pancreatic cancer. Shaded areas show extent of overlap between acute and chronic pancreatitis and between chronic pancreatitis and pancreatic cancer. Major risk factors are shown at the bottom of the diagram. Circle size approximates relative incidence of the three diseases. CF, cystic fibrosis; HP, hereditary pancreatitis. *Source:* From ref. 18.

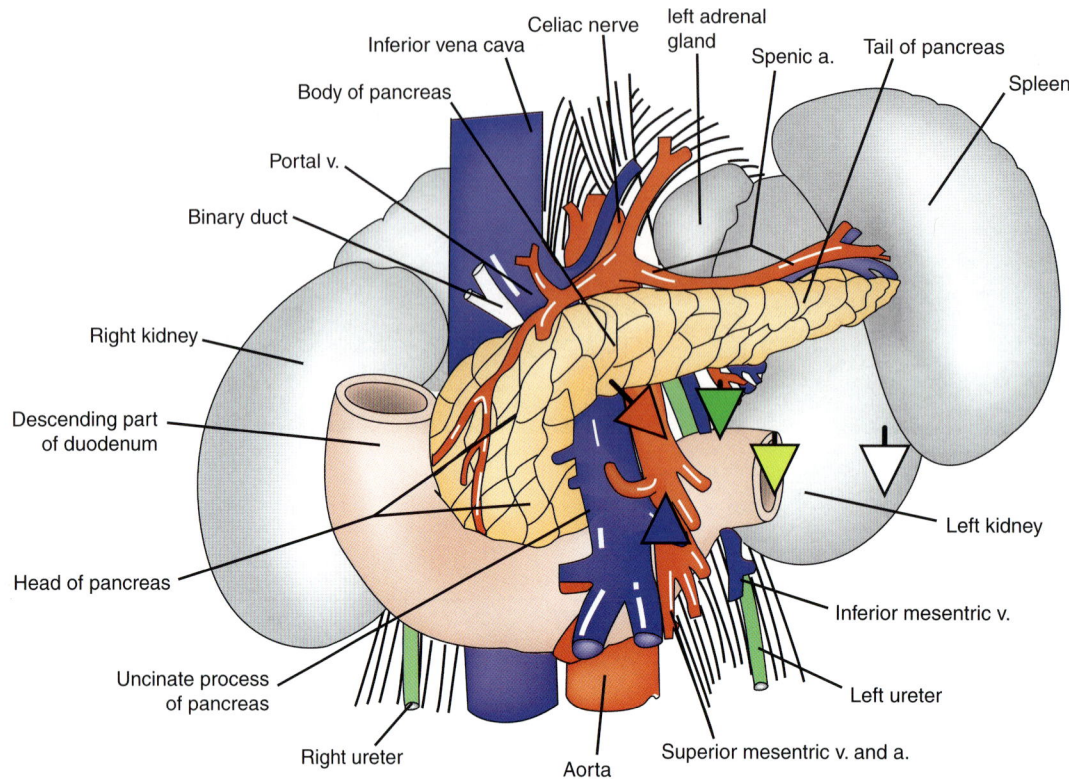

FIGURE 26.1. Anatomy of the pancreas and related structures. *Source:* Adapted from ref. 7.

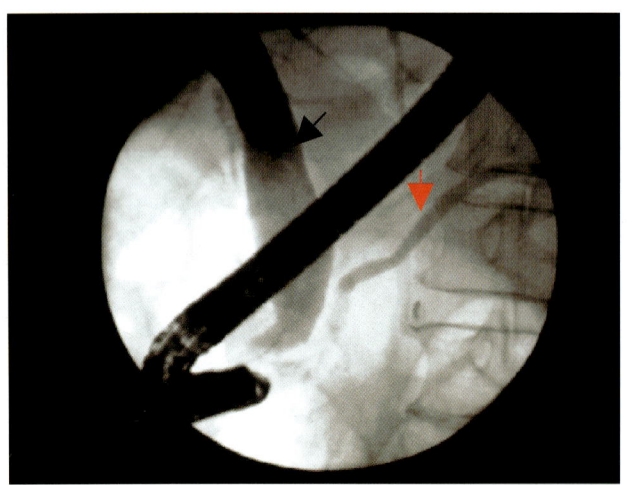

FIGURE 26.3. ERCP showing double duct sign—dilated pancreatic duct (*red arrow*) and dilated common bile duct (*black arrow*).

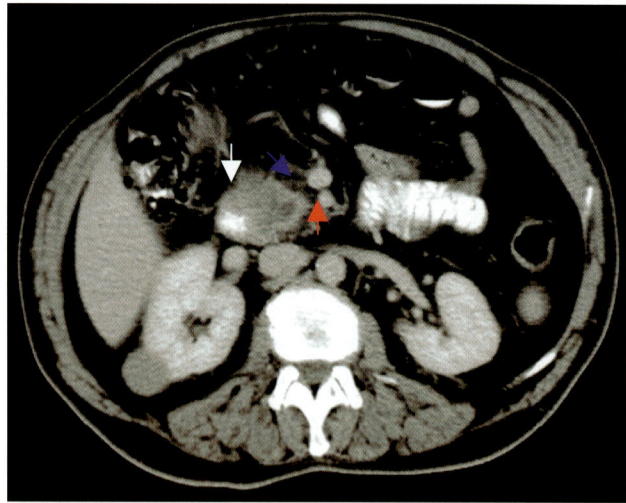

FIGURE 26.4. CT showing clear fat pad between head of pancreas tumor (*white arrow*) and the superior mesenteric vessels (*blue arrow*, superior mesenteric vein; *red arrow*, superior mesenteric artery).

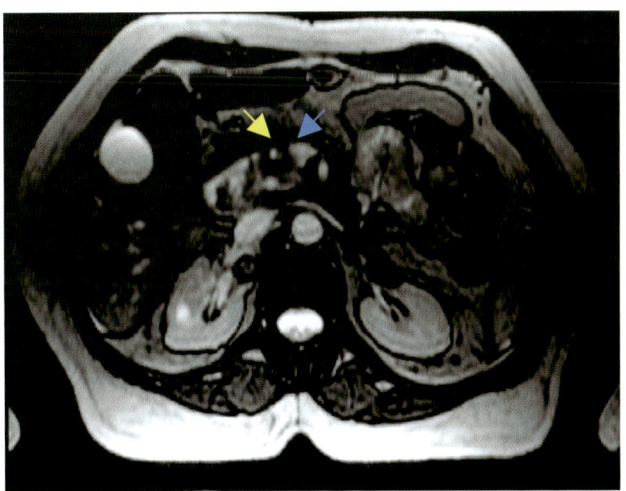

FIGURE 26.5. MRI–T$_1$-weighted image showing encroachment of the superior mesenteric vein (*blue arrow*) by pancreatic tumor (*yellow arrow*).

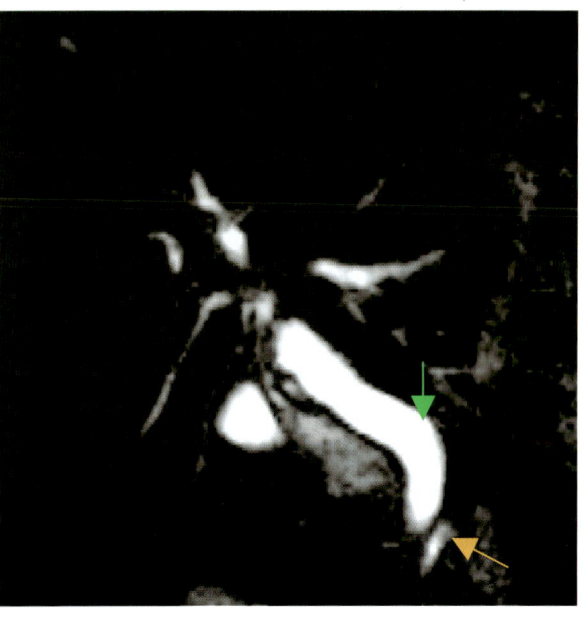

FIGURE 26.7. MRCP showing dilated common bile duct (*green arrow*) and obstructed pancreatic duct (*orange arrow*).

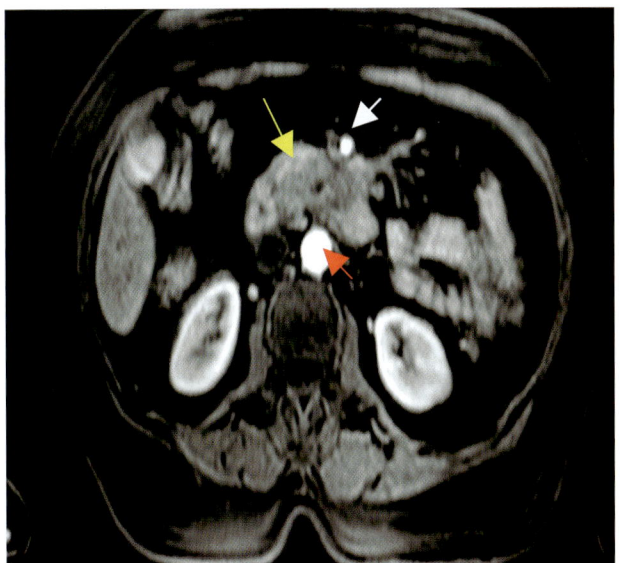

FIGURE 26.6. MRI–T$_2$-weighted image (*yellow arrow*, pancreatic tumor; *red arrow*, aorta; *black arrow*, superior mesenteric artery).

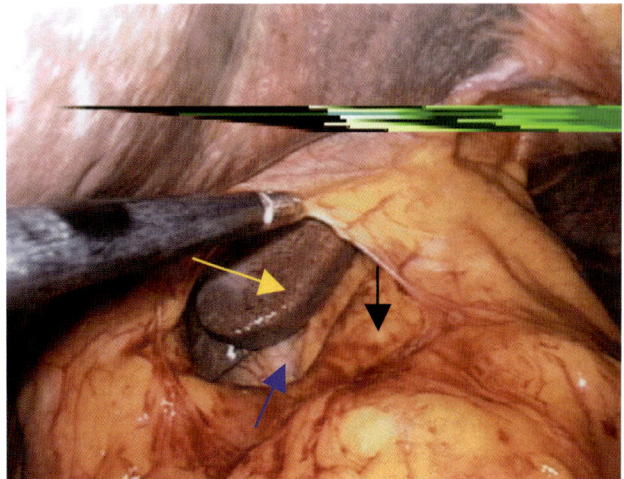

FIGURE 26.10. Laparoscopy showing the lesser sac via the lesser omentum (*yellow arrow*, caudate lobe; *blue arrow*, inferior vena cava; *black arrow*, celiac axis).

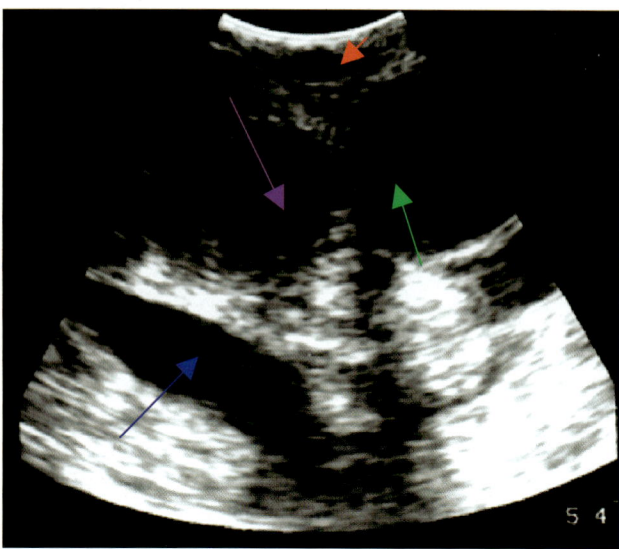

FIGURE 26.11. Laparoscopic ultrasound picture showing hepatic artery (*red arrow*), tumor inside the portal vein (*purple arrow*), common bile duct (*green arrow*), and inferior vena cava (*blue arrow*).

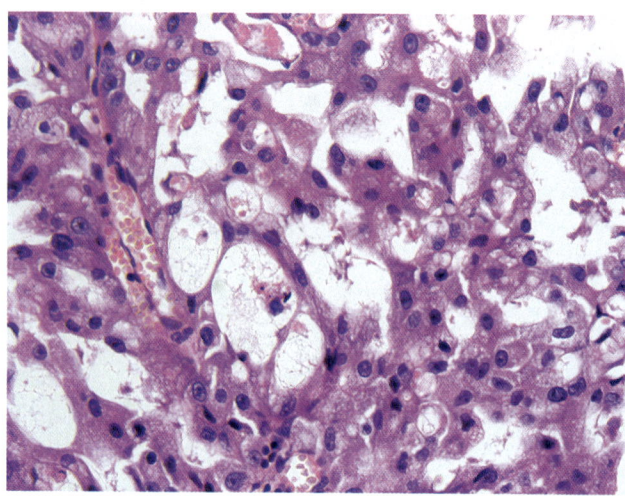

FIGURE 27.13. Intraductal oncocytic papillary neoplasm. Complex papillae are lined by large, eosinophilic cells. Intraepithelial lumina are present.

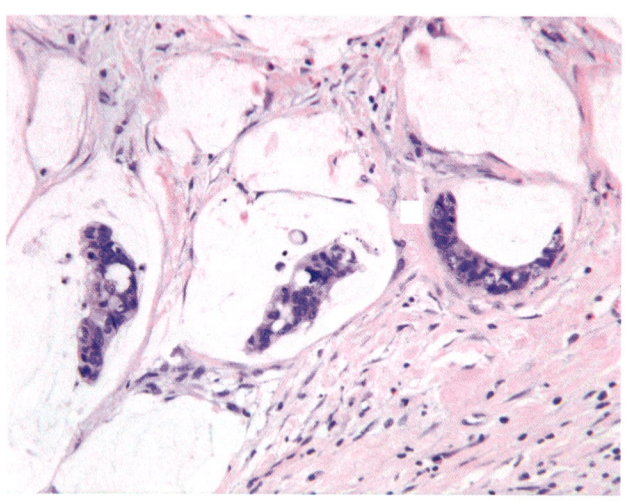

FIGURE 27.4. Colloid carcinoma. Strips of neoplastic glandular epithelium float in abundant extracellular pools of mucin.

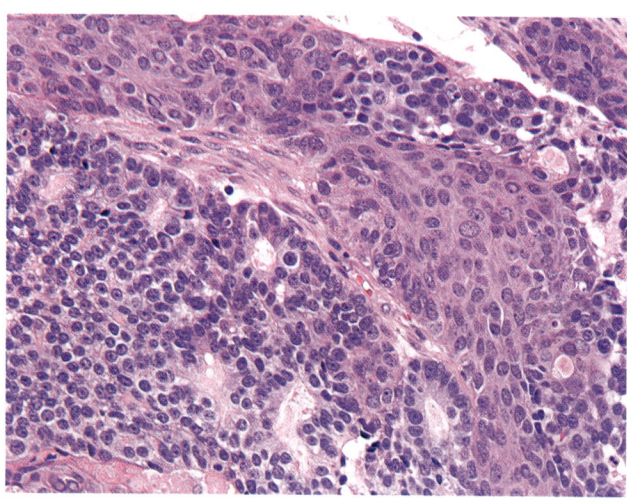

FIGURE 27.19. Pancreatoblastoma. Acinar formations and squamoid nests are present.

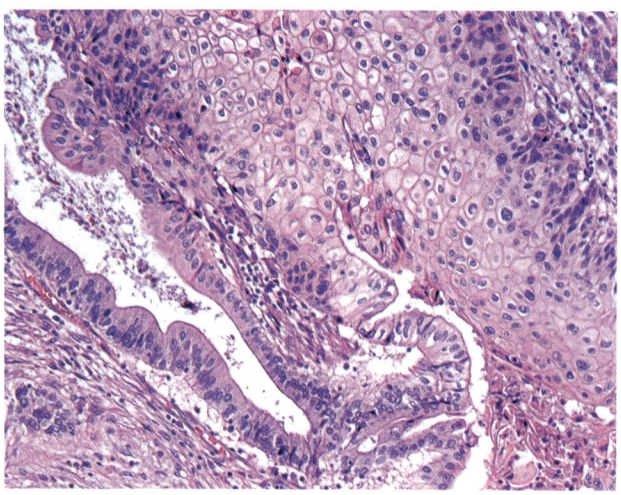

FIGURE 27.5. Adenosquamous carcinoma. Sheets of squamous cells (*right*) are juxtaposed to well-formed glands (*left*).

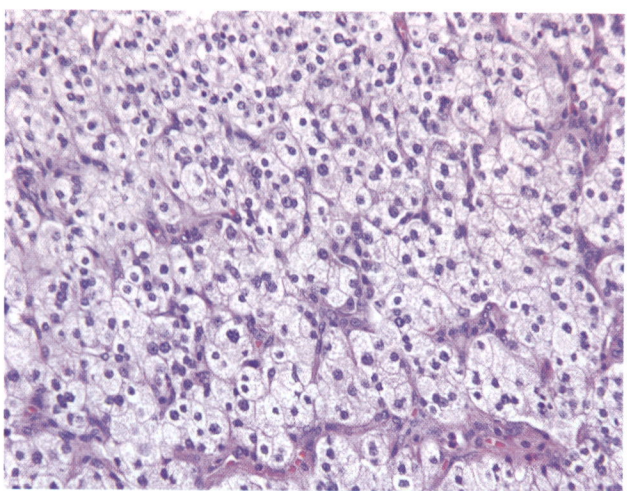

FIGURE 27.22. Clear cell pancreatic endocrine neoplasm. The cells have microvesicular, clear cytoplasm.

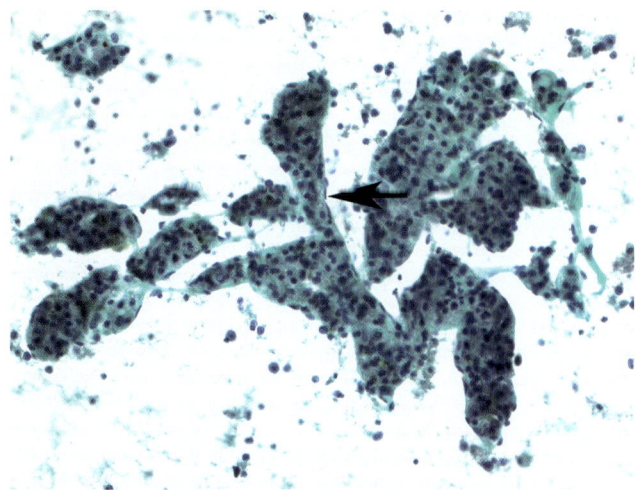

FIGURE 31.8. Cytomorphologic features of HCC with a macrotrabecular pattern encased by a rim of endothelial cells (*arrow*).

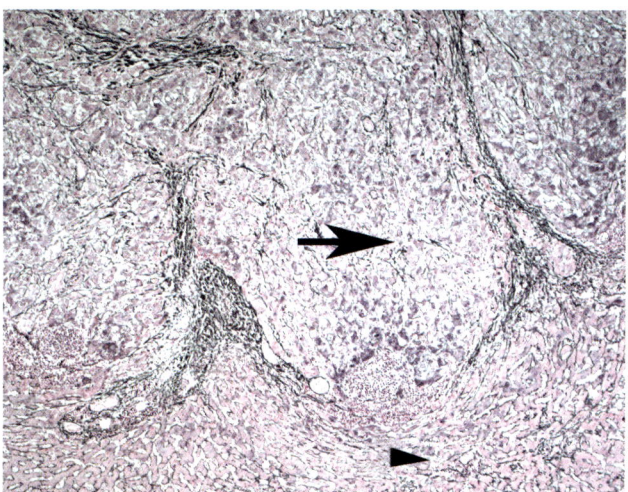

FIGURE 31.9. Reticulin stain demonstrating partial loss of reticulin fibers (*arrow*). The adjacent benign hepatic parenchyma shows a normal and preserved reticulin framework (*arrowhead*).

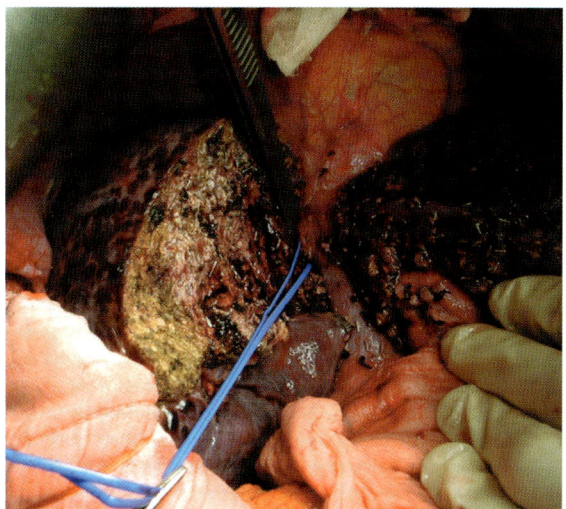

FIGURE 33.1. A cirrhotic patient with a large HCC (9 cm) (**B**). The patient has remained diseasefree for 3 years.

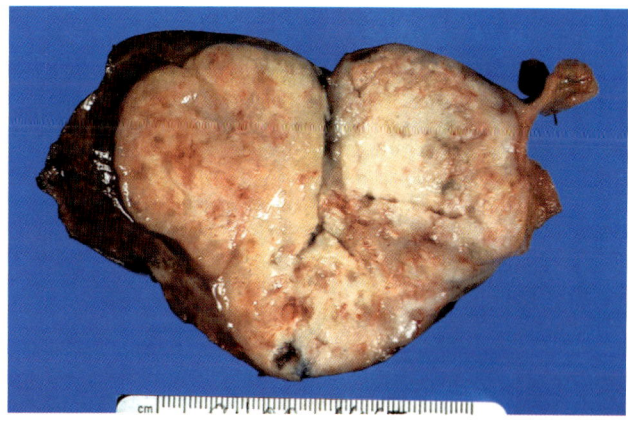

FIGURE 35.1. Adenocarcinomas of the biliary tract are usually characterized by a scirrhous, gray-white, firm cut surface. Extension into the liver, as seen here, may cause more sharply demarcated appearance.

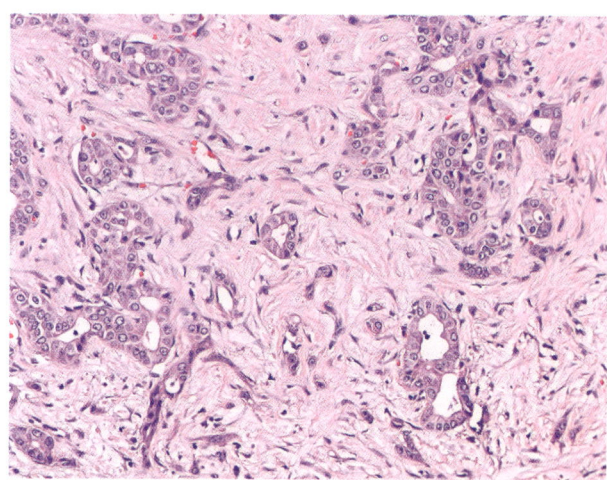

FIGURE 35.2. Adenocarcinoma (pancreatobiliary type). Small glandular units lined by cuboidal cells. They are often embedded in a dense, desmoplastic stroma.

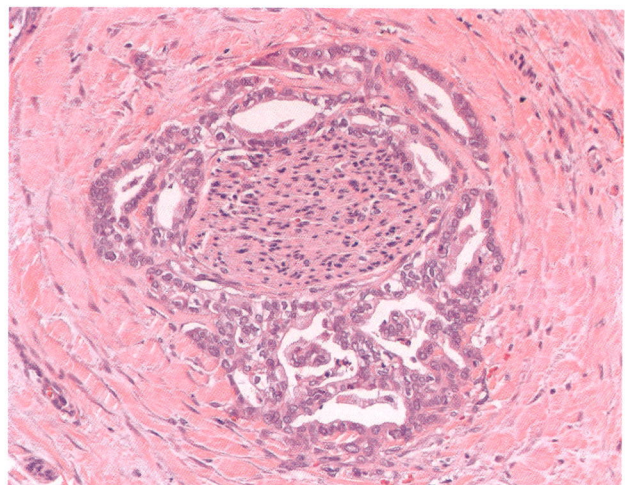

FIGURE 35.3. Adenocarcinoma, perineural invasion. Relatively well-differentiated adenocarcinoma wrapping around a nerve is a common finding in biliary adenocarcinomas.

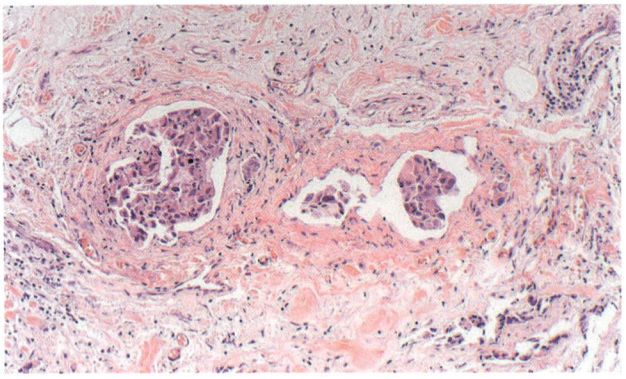

FIGURE 35.4. Adenocarcinoma, vascular invasion. Vascular invasion is commonly detected in adenocarcinomas of biliary tract.

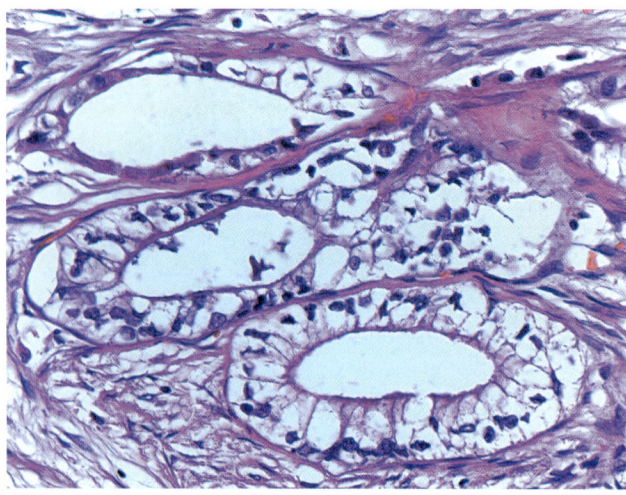

FIGURE 35.6. Adenocarcinoma, clear cell pattern. Variations that can be seen in the morphologic phenotype of adenocarcinomas include the clear cell pattern.

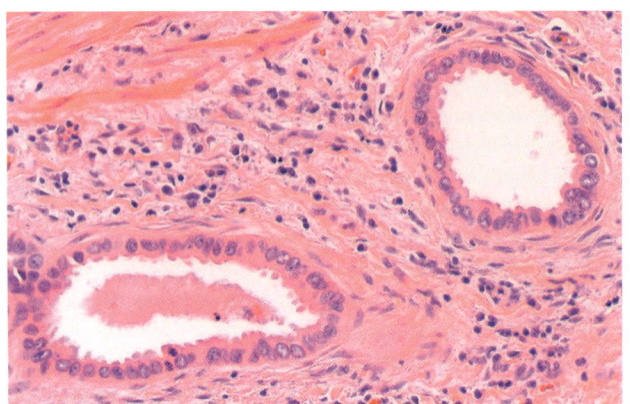

FIGURE 35.5. Adenocarcinoma, well differentiated. In many cases, neoplastic cells exhibit bland cytologic features and well-defined glandular structures, creating a deceptively benign appearance.

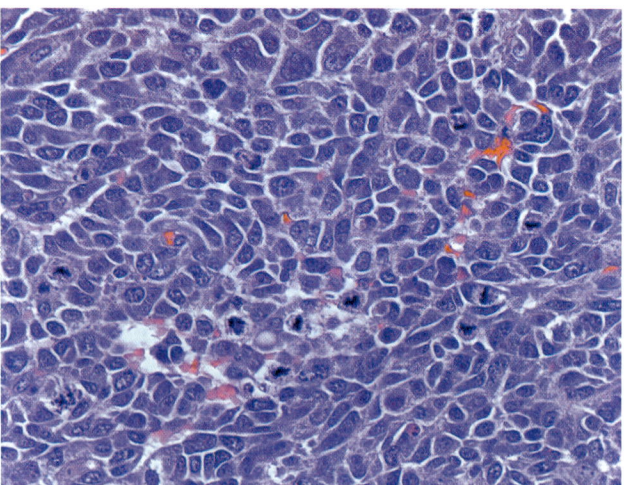

FIGURE 35.7. Adenocarcinoma, poorly differentiated. This carcinoma is characterized by a diffuse, sheetlike growth pattern of large cells. Characteristics of ordinary carcinomas such as gland formation or papillae are not evident.

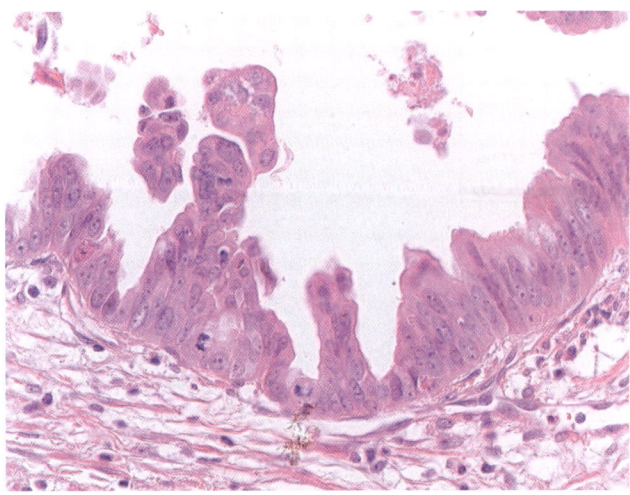

FIGURE 35.8. Dysplasia, high grade. There is nuclear stratification, marked nuclear enlargement, pleomorphism, and hyperchromasia. Mitotic figures are also present.

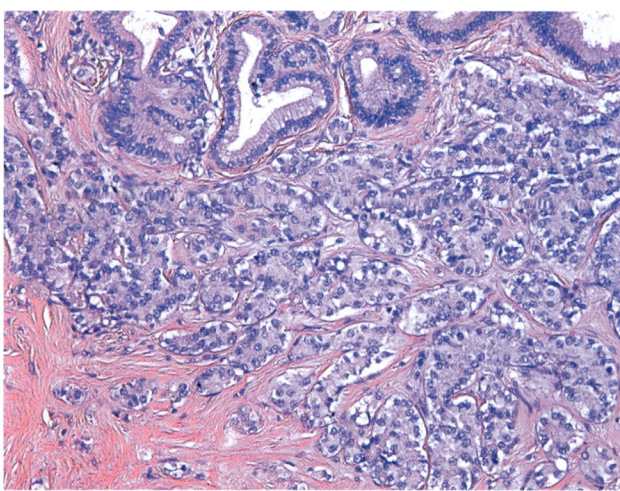

FIGURE 35.10. Carcinoids in the biliary tract have the typical morphologic characteristics of carcinoids elsewhere, exhibiting distinct nests of cells with round and uniform nuclei, endocrine chromatin pattern, and a fair amount of cytoplasm.

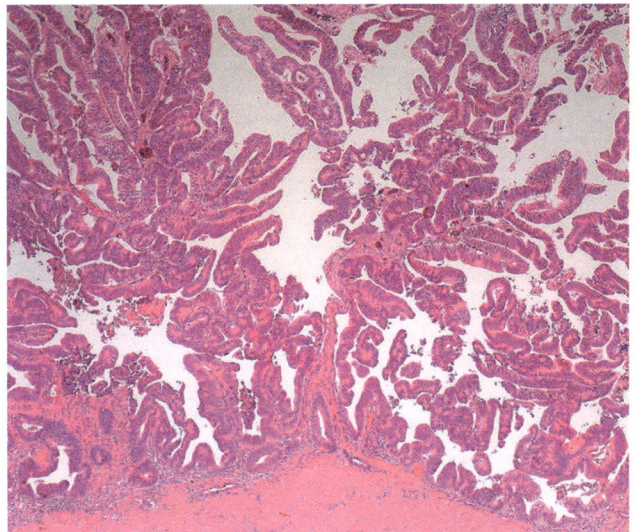

FIGURE 35.9. Adenoma, intestinal type. Just like in colonic villous adenomas, these have villous architecture with pseudostratified, cigar-shaped nuclei.

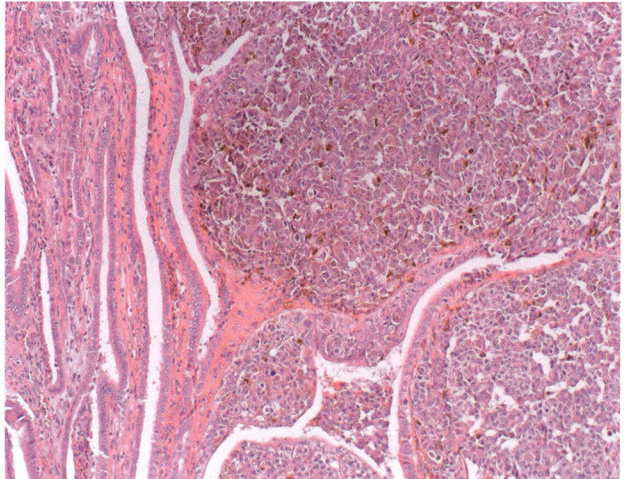

FIGURE 35.11. Sheets of pigmented melanoma cells filling the lamina propria.

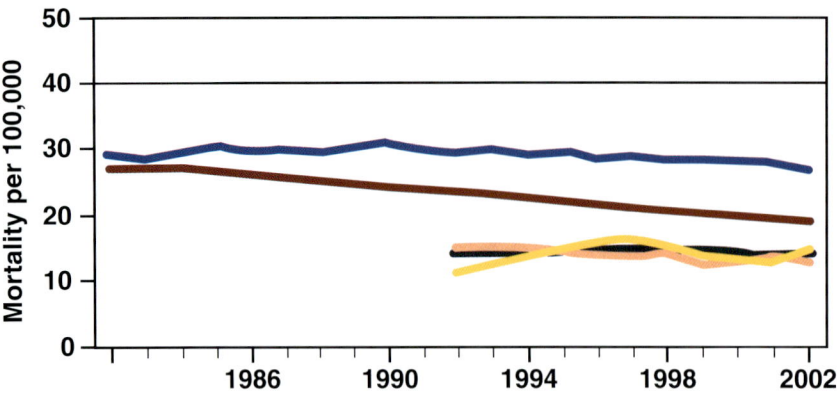

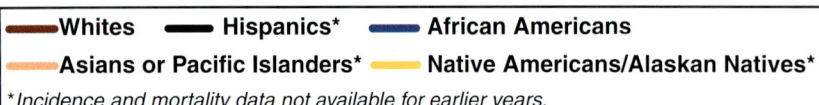

FIGURE 39.1. U.S. colorectal cancer mortality. *Source:* Adapted from Surveillance, Epidemiology, and End Results (SEER) Program and NCHS, 2006.

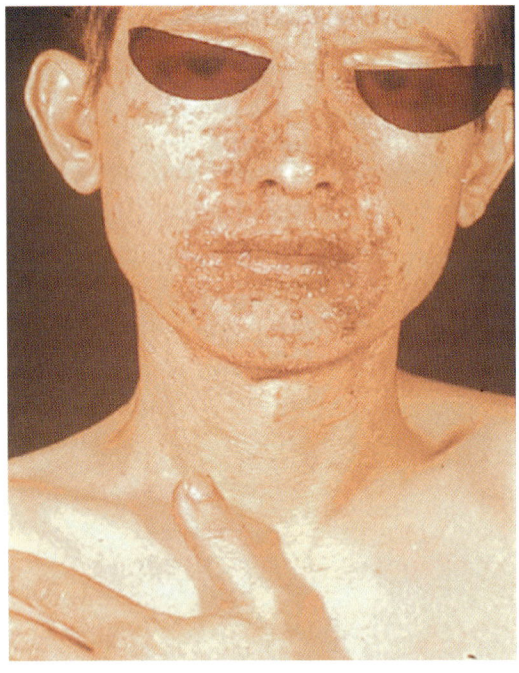

FIGURE 48.1. Necrolytic migratory erythema associated with glucagonoma syndrome.

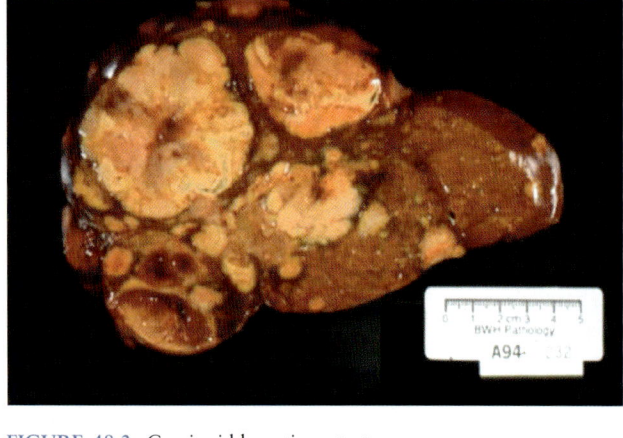

FIGURE 48.3. Carcinoid hepatic metastases.

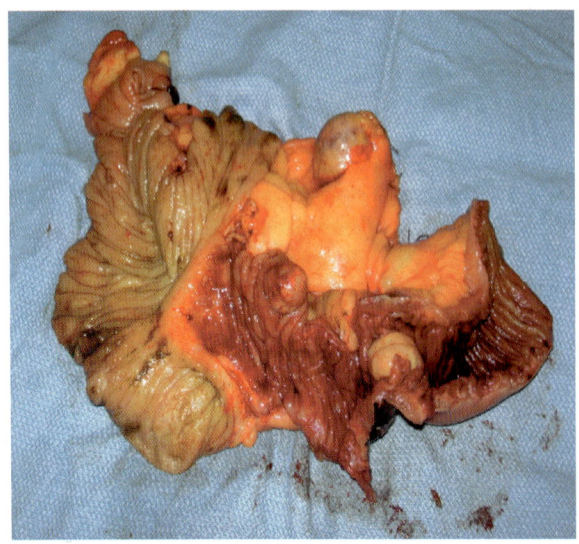

FIGURE 48.2. Multicentric carcinoids of the small intestine.

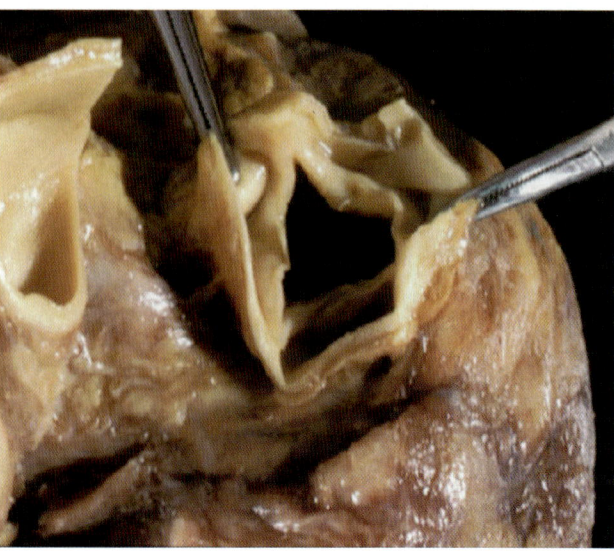

FIGURE 48.4. Carcinoid heart disease.

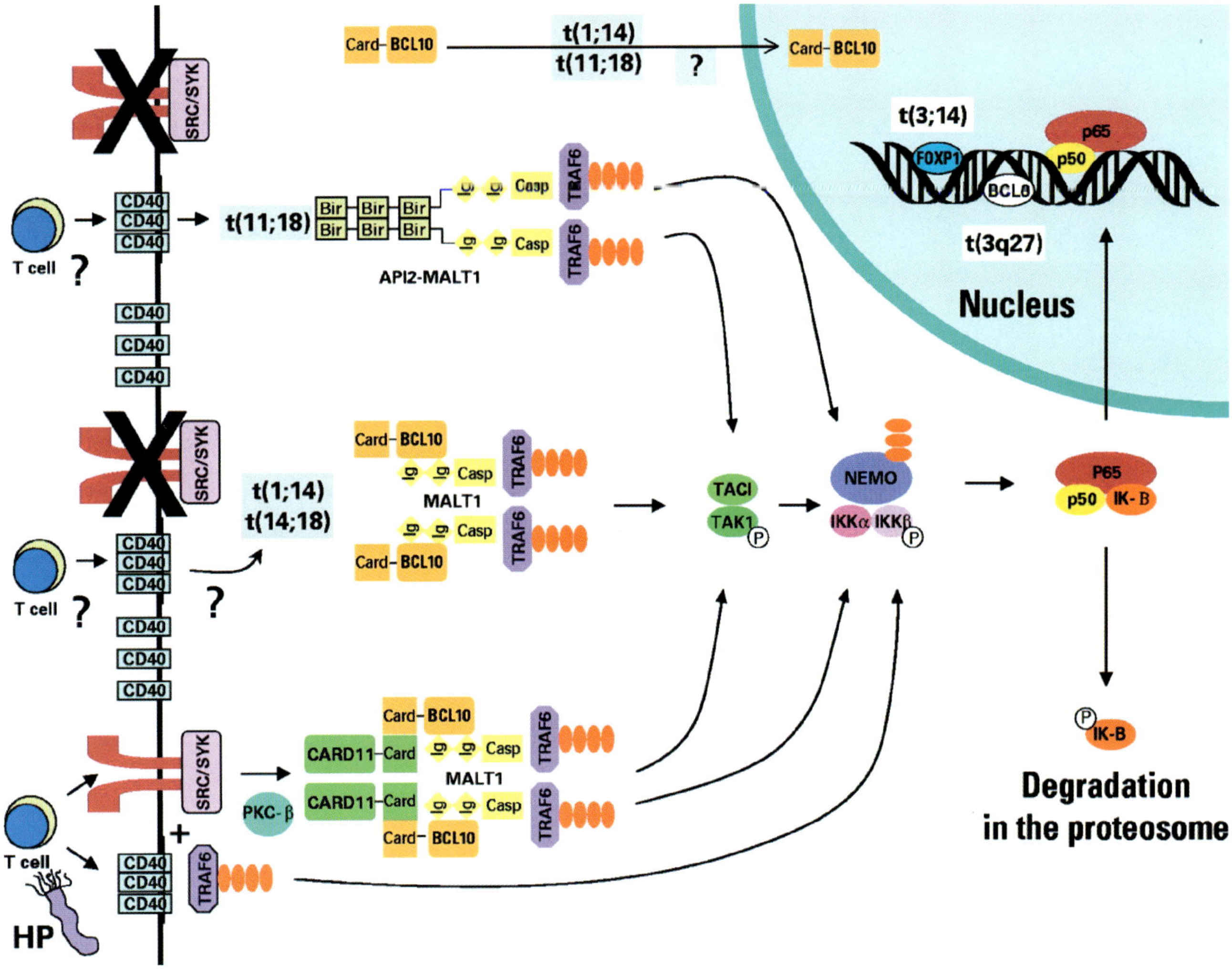

Card–BCL10   t(1;14) / t(11;18)   ?   Card–BCL10

t(3;14)

FOXP1   BCL6   p50   p65

t(3q27)

Nucleus

SRC/SYK

CD40 CD40 CD40

T cell ?

t(11;18)   Bir Bir Bir / Bir Bir Bir   Ig Ig Casp   TRAF6 / Ig Ig Casp   TRAF6

API2-MALT1

CD40 CD40 CD40

SRC/SYK

CD40 CD40 CD40

T cell ?

t(1;14) / t(14;18)   ?

Card–BCL10   Ig Ig Casp   TRAF6

MALT1

Card–BCL10   Ig Ig Casp   TRAF6

CD40 CD40 CD40

TACI / TAK1 (P)

NEMO / IKKα IKKβ (P)

P65 / p50 IK-B

SRC/SYK

CARD11–Card   Card–BCL10   Ig Ig Casp   TRAF6

PKC-β

CARD11–Card   Ig Ig Casp   TRAF6

MALT1

Card–BCL10

T cell

CD40 CD40 CD40   TRAF6

HP

+

(P) IK-B

Degradation in the proteosome

FIGURE 49.1. Molecular pathways in gastric mucosal-associated lymphoid tissue (MALT) lymphoma. T cells specific for *Helicobacter pylori* signal the B cell via CD40 and the immunoglobulin receptor (IGR). BCL10 interacts with CARD11 and MALT1-activating tumor necrosis factor (TNF) receptor activating factor 6 (TRAF6) promoting phosphorylation of IκB and thereby activation of NF-κB. The needs for IGR or CD40 activation is lost (or significantly diminished) with the t(1;14) translocation resulting in BCL10 overexpression or t(14;18) resulting in MALT1 overexpression. Similarly, the novel fusion protein API2-MALT1 produced as a consequence of the t(11;18) translocation bypasses the need for signaling via the IGR and CD40 and can interact with TRAF6 to activate NF-κB. Reprinted with permission from Farinha P, Gascoyne RD. Molecular pathogenesis of mucosa-associated lymphoid tissue lymphoma. *J Clin Oncol.* 2005;23:6370–6378.

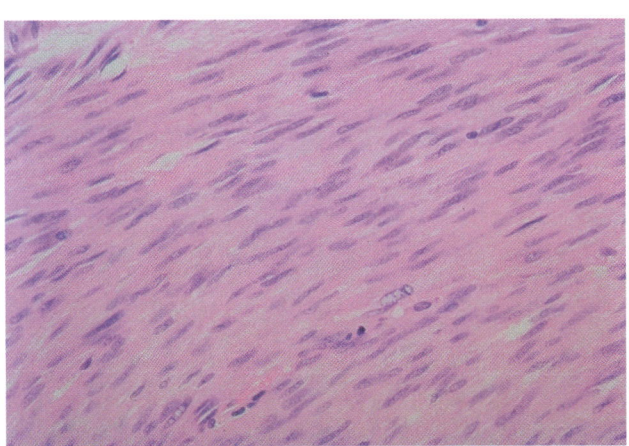

FIGURE 50.1. Hematoxylin-and-eosin section of a typical low-grade spindle cell gastrointestinal stromal tumor. (See also color Fig. 50.1.)

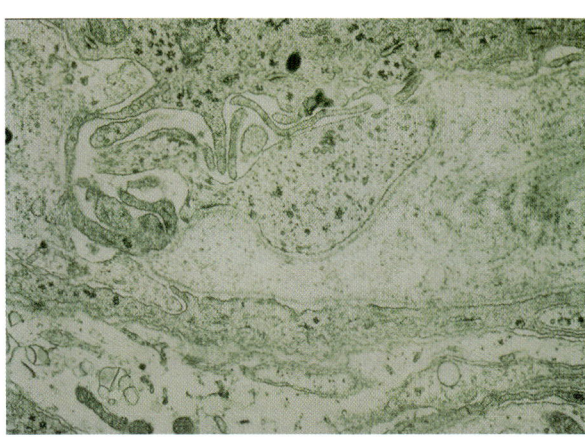

FIGURE 50.2. Gastrointestinal stromal tumor with a bulbous, synapselike structure containing dense core granules. (See also color Fig. 50.2.) *Source:* Courtesy of Dr. Christopher Fletcher, Brigham & Women's Hospital, Boston, MA.

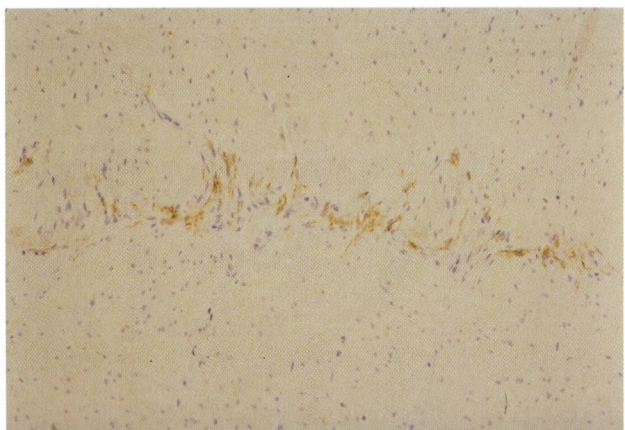

FIGURE 50.3. KIT immunostaining highlights the interstitial cells of Cajal in a section of small bowel. (See also color Fig. 50.3.)

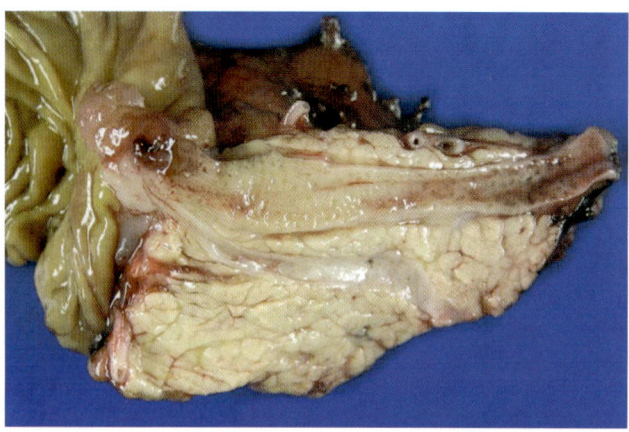

FIGURE 51.5. Gross photograph of an ampullary adenocarcinoma that demonstrates the longitudinal course of the pancreatic duct ending at the ampulla, which is obliterated by the adenocarcinoma. *Source:* Courtesy of Jinru Shia, MD, Gastrointestinal Pathology, Memorial Sloan-Kettering Cancer Center, New York, NY.

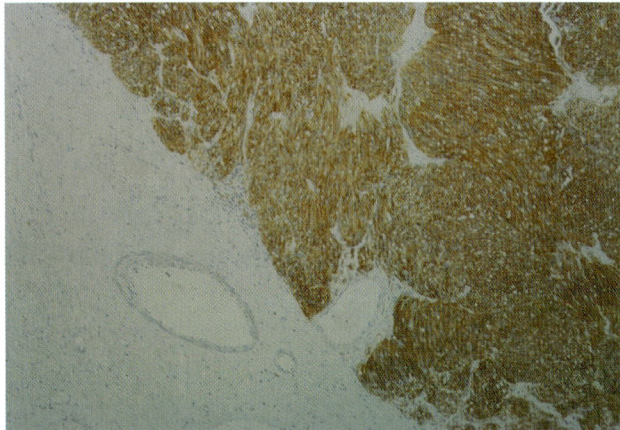

FIGURE 50.4. Strong and diffuse KIT immunoreactivity in a gastrointestinal stromal tumor. (See also color Fig. 50.4.)

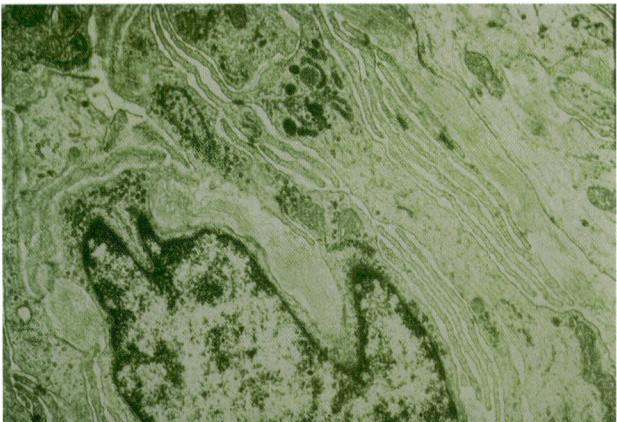

FIGURE 50.5. Gastrointestinal stromal tumor showing numerous interdigitating processes. (See also color Fig. 50.5.) *Source:* Courtesy of Dr. Christopher Fletcher, Brigham & Women's Hospital, Boston, MA.

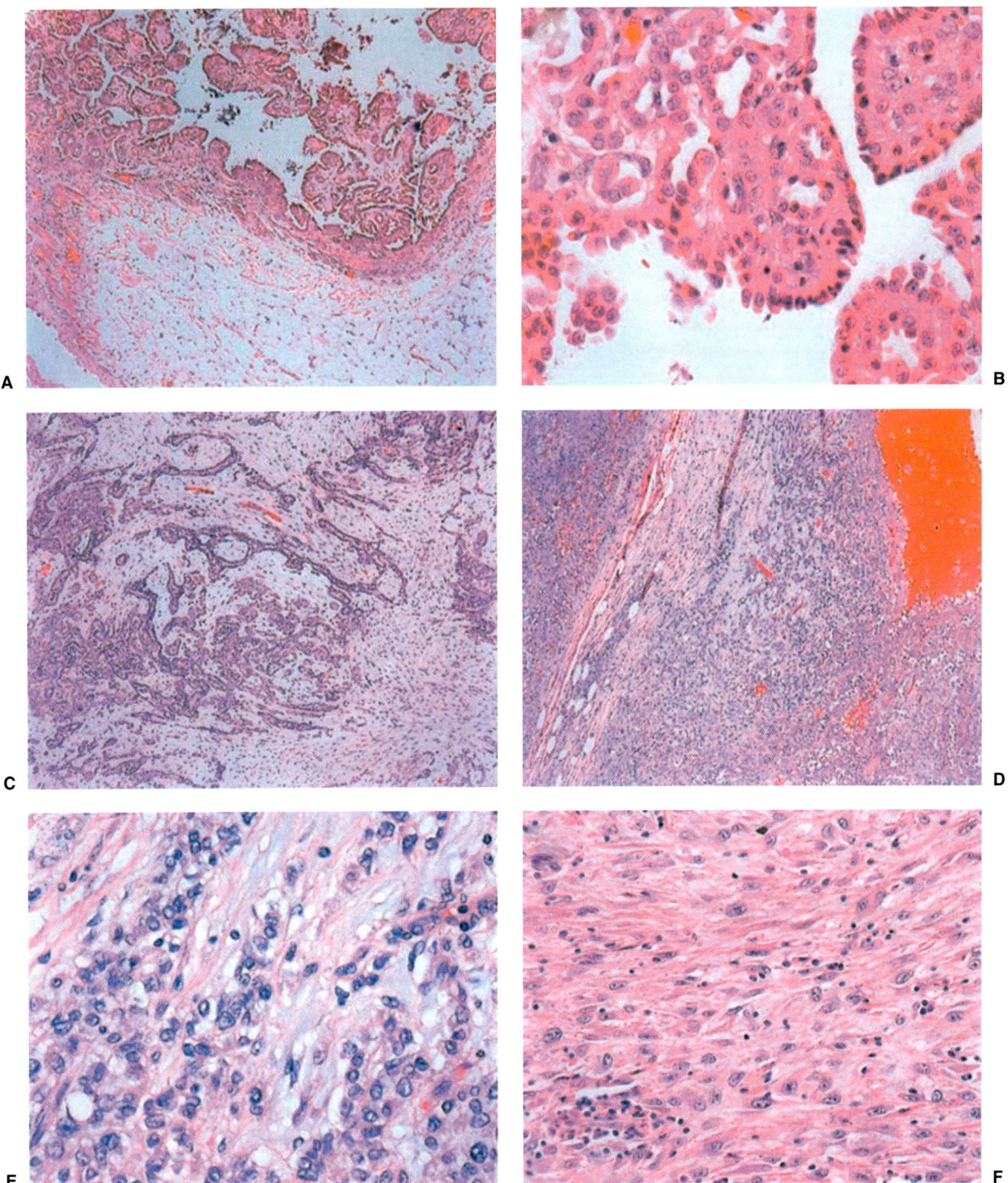

FIGURE 53.1. Histopathology of peritoneal mesothelioma. **A, B:** Low-grade, tubulopapillary type, without deep tissue invasion or desmoplasia. **C:** Low-grade, tubulopapillary type, with deep invasion and desmoplasias. **D, E:** High-grade, epithelioid type, with deep invasion and desmoplasia. **F:** High-grade, sarcomatoid type. [A, C, and D, 100×; B and E, 600×; F, 400×]. Permission for reprint pending from Feldman et al.

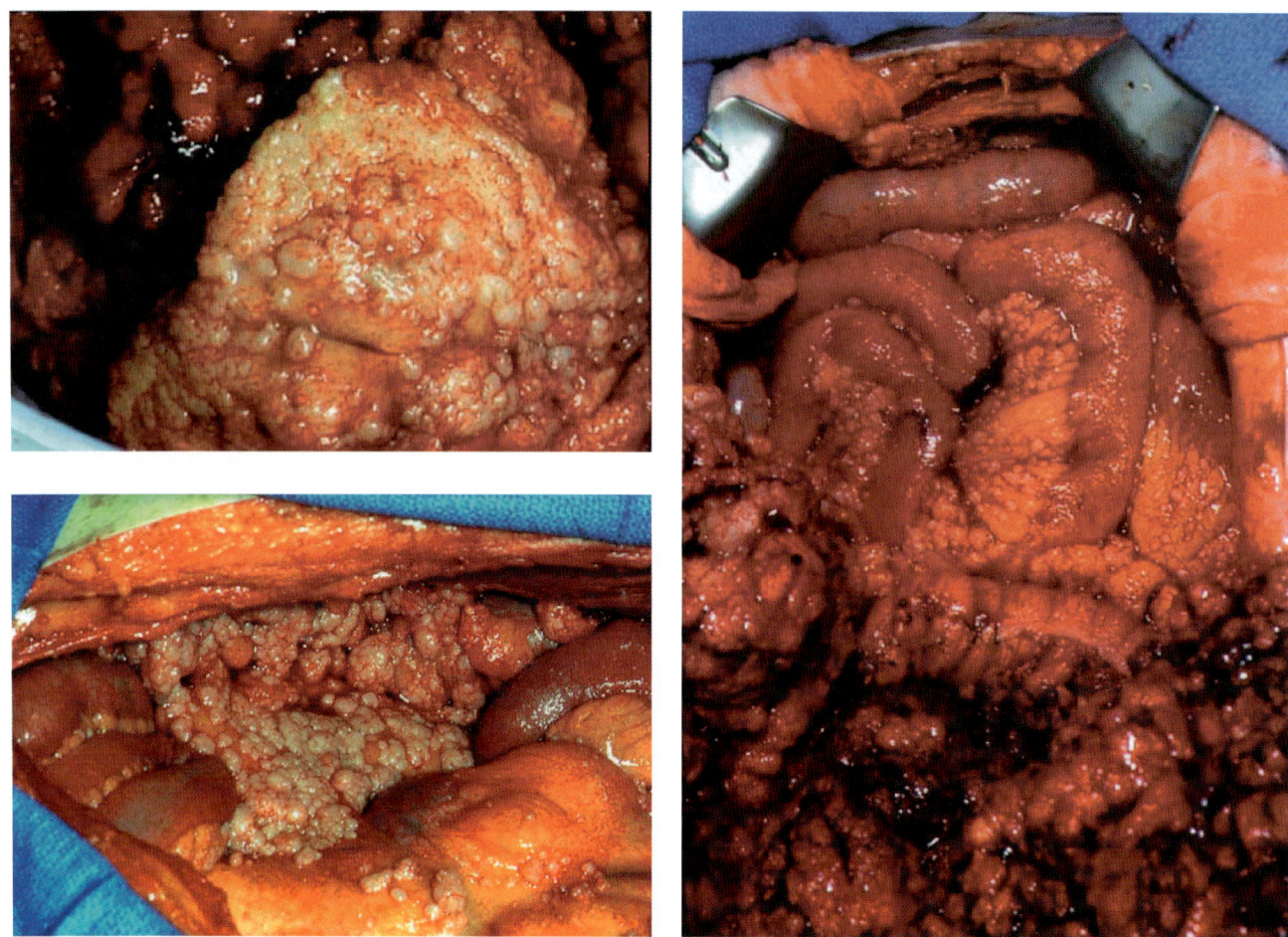

FIGURE 53.3. Malignant peritoneal mesothelioma involving the visceral surface of the intestine diffusely. Reprint permission pending.

PRINCIPLES OF GASTROINTESTINAL ONCOLOGY

CHAPTER 1 ■ GASTROINTESTINAL CANCER: EPIDEMIOLOGY

ELLEN KAMPMAN, H. BAS BUENO-DE-MESQUITA, HEINER BOEING, CARLOS A. GONZALEZ, BIANCA STAM, PIETER VAN'T VEER, RACHAEL STOLZENBERG-SOLOMON, SHEILA A. BINGHAM, AND HANS F. A. VASEN

Gastrointestinal (GI) cancers are among the most frequently occurring cancers worldwide. The incidence of these cancers varies markedly, with the United States, Europe, Australia, and Japan having the highest prevalence of colorectal cancer and Africa and Asia having a relatively high prevalence of stomach and liver cancer. Environmental and inherited factors may contribute to the etiology of these tumors. Besides smoking, other lifestyle factors—such as infectious exposures, alcohol consumption, physical activity, and dietary habits—may play an important role in the occurrence of these types of cancer. This chapter includes the descriptive epidemiology for each GI subsite separately, discusses several environmental exposures and lifestyle factors involved in the etiology of most GI tumors, and concludes with genetic syndromes contributing to a relatively small proportion of these tumors.

DESCRIPTIVE PATTERNS, RISK FACTORS, AND EARLY DETECTION

Cancer of the Oral Cavity

Cancer of the oral cavity is widespread in humans with about 275,000 (176,000 men and 99,000 women) new cases per year (1). About 127,000 subjects die as a result of this cancer each year. The age-standardized incidence is about 6.3 per 100,000 in men and 3.2 per 100,000 in women. Compared to other sites, the ratio of mortality and incidence of 0.46 is high. Such a high ratio points to the fact that we are currently not in a good position to cure this malignancy and that there is potential for new successful therapeutic and preventive strategies (2).

There are several areas with high incidence of cancer of the oral cavity. According to recent estimates from national cancer registries (1), in men, the highest age-adjusted rates are found in Papua New Guinea (40.9 per 100,000), Solomon Islands (34.1 per 100,000), Sri Lanka (24.5 per 100,000), and Botswana (23.1 per 100,000). Other regions with high incidence of about 12 per 100,000 are Southcentral Asia and Western Europe. More specific data from regional registries from the high incidence countries indicate that regional hot spots exist.

Overall, the time trend of cancer of the oral cavity was stable since the 1970s. In the United States, a decline in older whites was observed, whereas in African Americans and younger whites, an increase was seen (3). In some countries, the incidence of oral cancer is increasing (4). Most (95%) of the cancers are squamous cell carcinomas. Cancers appearing in the parotis and other salivary glands (C07, C08) of the mouth are mostly adenocarcinomas and should be considered as a separate entity in etiologic studies.

The low ratio of female-to-male incidence seems to be directly related to the gender-specific distribution of the major risk factors. Tobacco smoking and alcohol drinking are being consistently linked to this cancer site in observational epidemiologic studies that are almost uniformly of the case-control design. Both habits are positively interrelated, but more evidence is needed to conclude that they follow the multiplicative model (5). In other areas of the world, particularly Southeast Asia, chewing of tobacco and betel nuts is positively related to the occurrence of this malignancy (6). Furthermore, tobacco and betel chewing are often the main causative agents for this malignancy in countries with low alcohol consumption (7). However, low intake of fruits and vegetables has been related to increased risk, albeit mostly in case-control studies (8). Thus, the recent expert evaluation on fruit and vegetables by the International Agency of Research on Cancer (IARC) called for prospective studies to clarify the relation between diet and risk of this carcinoma due to the methodologic problems with the retrospective case-control design. Precancerous lesions such as oral leukoplakia are linked with the risk factors for oral cancer. It has been shown that smoking cessation decreases the prevalence of precancerous lesions (9). However, intervention with vitamin A and beta-carotene does not seem to be a successful treatment (10). Cancer of the lip seems to be caused in part by heavy sunlight exposure (11). This may be one of the factors that drive the occurrence of this cancer in countries such as Australia.

Cancer of the Pharynx

Cancer of the pharynx lining of the upper GI tract includes the oropharynx (C10) and the hypopharynx (C13). In the recent tabulation of incident cancer cases worldwide (1), about 130,000 new cases of incident pharynx cancer are reported, excluding the nasopharynx. The latter, with about 80,000 new cases per year, should be separated from the GI site of the pharynx due to another anatomic localization and different etiology, and thus is not considered further in this chapter. The ratio of mortality to incidence of cancer of the pharynx is 0.64. The age-standardized incidence of pharyngeal cancer worldwide was calculated to be 3.8 per 100,000 in men and 0.8 per 100,000 in women, with men having a distinct higher frequency in the more developed regions.

High incidence on the countrywide scale was seen in 2002 in men in Hungary (16.9 per 100,000), France (15.4 per 100,000), Luxembourg (13.1 per 100,000), and Slovakia (11.1

per 100,000), as well as in Bangladesh (12.5 per 100,000) and India (9.6 per 100,000) (1).

Reports on time trends give a mixed picture. Since the 1980s in the United States, a decrease in pharyngeal cancer has been observed (12,13), whereas in other areas of the world, such as Japan, pharyngeal cancer is increasing (14,15). The high incidence of this cancer in Europe is the result of past increases in incidence (16). Pharyngeal cancer seems to be high in India for a longer time period (17).

There is the common view that the incidence and mortality of pharyngeal cancer is going along with the degree and trend in alcohol and tobacco use in a population (12–14,18,19). Tobacco use includes chewing and smoking. However, the distribution and time trends of the two major risk factors also leave room for further hypotheses on how incidence of pharyngeal cancer can be influenced by dietary or occupational exposures.

Esophageal Cancer

Layers of epithelial cells originally line the esophagus. Thus, most of the cancers appearing in this organ are diagnosed as squamous cell carcinomas. However, over time the morphologic appearance of the cells can change and metaplastic tissues can appear, particularly in the lower part of the esophagus. The cancers appearing from these tissues are often adenomas that might have a different etiology and are therefore described separately.

The available worldwide statistics cover the whole organ, recording about 462,000 new cases of incidence esophageal cancers in 2002 (315,394 men and 146,723 women) (1). In the same year, about 386,000 deaths due to esophageal cancer were estimated. This results in a ratio of mortality to incidence of 0.84. Thus, esophageal cancer is by far the most deadly cancer in the upper GI tract. Cancer rates of more then 20 age-standardized incident cases per 100,000 on a country level can be found in Ethiopia, Kenya, South African Republic, China, Mongolia, Kazakhstan, Turkmenistan, and Fuji (1).

The time trends seem to differ in various parts of the world. In developed countries such as the United States, squamous cell carcinomas decrease while adenocarcinomas increase (20). Detailed data from the United States show that African Americans have twice the rates of esophageal cancer as whites and that squamous cell carcinoma was more prevalent in African Americans and women than in white men (21). In Africa, esophageal cancer rates appear to be remaining stable since the 1990s or are even increasing (22,23), and an often sharp decrease in incidence is reported from Southcentral and Southeast Asian countries since the 1970s and 1990s, respectively (24,25).

Tobacco and alcohol use are the major risk factors of this disease, followed by diet (26). In some areas, betel nut chewing contributes substantially to risk (27).

Adenocarcinoma of the esophagus is a malignant epithelial tumor with glandular differentiation, arising predominantly from Barrett's intestinal metaplasia of the mucosa in the lower third of the esophagus or the esophagus gastric junction. Because adenocarcinoma originating from the distal esophagus may infiltrate the gastric cardia and adenocarcinoma of the gastric cardia may grow into the distal esophagus, distinction between these entities, particularly in tumors involving the esophagus gastric junction is relatively difficult in clinical practice (28). During the healing process of chronic inflammatory injury typically associated with gastroesophageal reflux disease, in the Barrett's intestinal metaplasia, the normal esophagus epithelium is replaced by columnar epithelium.

Since the 1980s, incidence rates of adenocarcinoma of esophagus (ACE) have been increasing in both genders in developed countries. ACE is the fastest rising malignancy among white men in the United States, with a relative increase even higher than that observed for breast cancer, malignant melanoma, or prostate cancer. From 1975 to 2001, the incidence of ACE increased sixfold in the United States, from 4 to 23 cases per million (29). As a consequence of this increase and a parallel decrease of squamous cell carcinoma, ACE in whites is the most frequent type of esophageal cancer since 1990 in the United States (30). From 1996 to 2000, adenocarcinoma in white males represented 65.7% of total cases of esophageal cancer, whereas the rate was only 18% for Asian and Pacific Islanders and 9.4% for blacks (31). Similar increasing trends have been observed in Canada and several European countries (32). Although part of the large increase could be associated with improved case ascertainment due to a wider practice of endoscopy and/or reclassification of related cancers, it has been shown that the lower third of the esophagus is the only location with increased incidence and that a similar trend has been observed for mortality of esophageal adenocarcinoma that rose sevenfold from 2 to 15 deaths per million for the same period (29).

The incidence rate of ACE varies markedly among ethnicities and gender. In the United States, the incidence of ACE in white men was double of that in Hispanic men and over four times higher than in blacks, Asians, and Native Americans (33). Rates of women in all ethnicities are significantly lower than for men, although similar ethnic patterns persist by gender. The incidence rate of esophageal cancer in whites in the United States is seven times higher in men than in women (33). However, the increasing trends of ACE vary by age, being more pronounced among older rather than younger men (34). Although incidence of ACE is higher among whites than blacks, an inverse relation with socioeconomic status has been observed, even after adjusting for all recognized risk factors (35).

Reflux of acidic gastric juice is the most important etiologic factor for Barrett's esophagus and ACE (36), although reflux of bile and pancreatic juice may play also a role (37). Normally, gastroesophageal junctional anatomic structures, swallowing-induced peristalsis, and the esophageal sphincter serve as protective barriers against the retrograde escape of gastric acid. Another recognized risk factor of ACE is obesity. The rapidly increasing incidence rate of ACE in the United States coincides with the increasing incidence of obesity and gastroesophageal reflux disease in this population (30). Smoking and low consumption of fruit and vegetables seem to be modest risk factors, while alcohol consumption does not seem to be associated with risk or may be a weak risk factor (38). There is some evidence that *Helicobacter pylori* infection may protect against ACE (39).

Stomach Cancer

Despite a steady decline in the incidence of gastric cancer (GC) in the United States (30) and most other countries since the mid-1950s, GC remained in the year 2000 the fourth most frequent cancer and the second most common cause of cancer death in the world (40). It has been estimated that there are approximately 876,000 new cases (8.7% of the total) and 647,000 deaths (10.4% of cancer deaths) of GC each year. Almost two-thirds of them occur in developing countries (40). The highest incidence rates are observed in Japan, East Asia, the Andean regions of South America, and Eastern Europe, whereas the lowest rates are observed in North and East Africa, Northern Europe, and North America (40). In cancer deaths in the United States, GC ranks 10th among women and 11th among men (30), and approximately 90% are adenocarcinomas (31). It is now recognized that risk factors, time trends, and geographic distribution differ according to the anatomic localization of the tumor (proximal stomach or gastric cardia adenocarcinoma and distal stomach or noncardia adenocarcinoma) and the main histologic types of the Lauren classification (intestinal and diffuse).

Although the incidence of noncardia gastric cancer declined in most countries of the world during the past decades (40), the incidence of cardia cancer remained stable (41) or rose in several European countries (42), Japan (43), and the United States (30). Similar increasing trends have been observed for adenocarcinomas at the gastroesophageal junction (34). The increase in cardia cancer is less marked than that in esophageal adenocarcinoma and may even be stabilized in the United States after 1988. It is not clear whether there was a change in risk between generations (cohort effect) or whether the change affected all age groups simultaneously (period effect) (32).

The incidence rate of cardia and noncardia stomach cancer varied markedly according to race and gender group. In the United States between 1996 and 2000, cardia adenocarcinoma accounted for 37% of all GC in white men, while it represented only 11% of GC in black men and Asian/Pacific Islanders, with substantially lower percentages of cardia adenocarcinoma among women than men for all racial groups (31). The incidence rate of cardia GC in whites in the United States was five times higher in men than in women, while the incidence of noncardia GC was 1.8-fold (30). The increasing trends of cardia adenocarcinoma also vary by age, with a much greater upward trend among older rather than younger men (35). Low socioeconomic status, which is a surrogate of lifestyle and environmental factors, has been related to excess risk of both cardia and noncardia gastric cancer (30).

Intestinal adenocarcinoma is the most frequent histologic type, particularly in high-incidence areas, and is considered responsible for most of the large international variation of GC (44). However, since the 1950s, the decline of gastric cancer has primarily been of the intestinal type, and consequently, the diffuse type has become relatively more common. A decrease in incidence of the intestinal types has been observed in the United States and Japan, while the diffuse type has increased in the United States (45) or has shown a stable trend in Japan (46). As a consequence of these changes, in some countries such as Finland, in patients younger than 60 years, the diffuse type has become more common than the intestinal type (47).

Different trends in cardia and noncardia gastric cancer suggest, at least in part, different etiologic factors. In fact, *H. pylori* infection is a recognized causal factor for noncardia but not cardia gastric cancer (48). Obesity and gastroesophageal reflux disease are associated with cardia cancer (49). Tobacco smoking is associated with both cardia and noncardia cancer (50), and dietary factors are believed to play an important role, but differences according to anatomic subtypes are not yet well established.

Liver Cancer

Primary liver cancer includes hepatocellular carcinoma (HCC) as well as angiosarcoma, cholangiocarcinoma, and hepatoblastoma. HCC accounts for 90% of all cases (44). It is the fifth most common cancer throughout the world (44,51). In 2000, approximately 560,000 cases occurred, accounting for 5.6% of all cases of cancer. The incidence is highest in developing countries, where 80% of all patients are found (with 54% in China) (44,51). Liver cancer incidence is about three times higher among men than women (51,52). HCC is rarely detected in an early stage and is usually fatal within a few months (53). The disease has a 5-year survival rate of less than 5% (52).

The major risk factors for liver cancer are hepatitis B virus (HBV) and hepatitis C virus (HCV) (53–56). Excessive alcohol consumption, resulting in alcoholic cirrhosis, is also an important risk factor for liver cancer (53–56), as well as contamination of food with aflatoxins, a group of metabolites produced by the phylogenetically related *Aspergillus flavus* and *Aspergillus parasiticus* (54,56–58). In 1997, a World Cancer Research Fund International (WCRF International) expert panel concluded that contamination of food with aflatoxin probably increases risk (59) and that the evidence that regular high consumption of alcohol increases the risk of liver cancer, mediated by liver cirrhosis, was convincing. The panel noted that diets high in vegetables possibly decrease the risk of liver cancer. Evidence that selenium decreases and iron increases the risk of liver cancer was considered insufficient (59).

Apart from HBV and HCV, smoking is an established cause of liver cancer. The most effective means of preventing liver cancer is to avoid exposure to these viruses and not to use tobacco. The most effective dietary means of preventing liver cancer are limited consumption of alcohol and avoidance of food liable to be contaminated with aflatoxin (59).

Gallbladder Cancer

The gallbladder is a small pear-shaped organ on the distal side of the liver at the right side of the abdomen. The gallbladder is connected to the liver by the hepatic duct. It is approximately 8 to 10 cm long and 3 cm wide. The function of the gallbladder is to store and concentrate bile that is produced in the liver before it is secreted into the intestines. In the intestines, the bile acids are required for the digestion of fatty foods. Bile consists of three major components: cholesterol, bile salts, and bilirubin. When the gallbladder does not function properly, the composition of bile is unbalanced, which leads to the formation of gallstones. The majority of stones are composed of cholesterol, whereas the others consist of bilirubin.

Gallbladder cancer is a rare, highly malignant tumor with a poor 5-year survival rate (60). It is difficult to diagnose this malignancy at an early stage due to its nonspecific symptoms (60). Gallbladder cancer has the highest incidence in adult women and elderly men and women (60).

There is a prominent geographic variability of gallbladder cancer incidence. The populations with the highest incidences are Chileans, Bolivians, Native Americans, Mexican Americans, and Central Europeans. Gallbladder cancer occurs rarely in the rest of the world (60).

There is not much evidence in support of the hypothesis that food and nutrition affects the risk of gallbladder cancer (60–62). Because obesity is a risk factor for gallstones, which are associated with an increased risk of gallbladder cancer, a higher body mass may play a role—either direct or indirect—in gallbladder cancer (59).

Pancreatic Cancer

Pancreatic cancer is estimated to be the 12th most frequent incident cancer and cause of cancer death in the world (63). In Western European, it ranks 12th for cancer incidence and 7th for cancer mortality (63). In the United States, it ranks 11th for cancer incidence, but it is the 4th most common cause of cancer mortality for men and women (64). More than 9 out of 10 pancreatic cancers are ductal adenocarcinomas, with islet cell tumors constituting about 5% (65). There are no effective screening methods for pancreatic cancer; therefore, it is most often diagnosed at advanced stages, resulting in a 5-year relative survival rate of only 4.3%. The incidence of pancreatic cancer is generally higher in men compared with women (66). Internationally, rates of pancreatic cancer vary by 10- to 15-fold (66), with the highest rates in Northern and Eastern Europe and the lowest rates in Hong Kong (67). Rates have been increasing in Spain, Italy, and Japan, likely reflecting cigarette smoking patterns (67,68). Within the Untied States, this is a site often noted for its relevance to cancer disparities, with both black men and black women experiencing incidence rates 30 to 40% higher than their white counterparts (69). This disparity may be due to differences in the prevalence of risk factors (70).

Of the few risk factors that have been identified, cigarette smoking is the most consistent (65). Chronic pancreatitis also predisposes to the disease (71,72). Type 2 diabetes mellitus and glucose intolerance have been consistently associated with pancreatic cancer (73,74). However, whether diabetes is etiologically involved in pancreatic carcinogenesis or the result of subclinical malignancy has been controversial. A modest positive association with obesity has been reported in the majority of studies (75). One recent prospective study that showed a twofold increased risk with fasting insulin concentrations measured up to 16.7 years prior to cancer diagnosis (76) may support the hypothesis that insulin and insulin resistance may be a potential mechanism that explains the diabetes and obesity associations. However, the effect of physical activity and dietary factors is unclear. Inverse associations have been reported for fruit and vegetable intake (66). Genetic susceptibility plays a role, with some cases being familial or related to hereditary familial atypical melanoma, Peutz-Jeghers syndrome, hereditary breast or ovarian cancer (BRCA1 and BRCA2), familial pancreatitis, cystic fibrosis, and hereditary nonpolyposis colon cancer (HNPCC) (77).

Cancer of the Small Intestine

Although the small bowel comprises about 75% of the length of the GI tract and is exposed to a wide variety of potentially noxious endogenous and exogenous substances, malignant tumors of the small bowel are unusual and account for only 1% to 5% of all GI tract malignancies (78). Data from cancer registries participating in the Surveillance, Epidemiology, and End Results (SEER) program in the United States from 1973 to 1990 (79) showed that the average annual incidence rate was 9.9 per million people. Carcinoid tumors and adenocarcinomas were the most common histologic subtypes, with average annual incidence rates of 3.8 and 3.7 per million people, respectively, followed by lymphomas (1.1 per million people) and sarcomas (1.3 per million people). For all histologic subtypes, men had higher rates than women. Most tumors occurred in older adults; more than 90% of cases occurred in people older than 40 years (79). The incidence of small bowel tumors has risen slowly over time. Small intestinal adenocarcinoma resemble large bowel adenocarcinoma in that they both arise from adenomatous polyps, co-occur in the same individuals, and have a similar pattern of incidence rates by country.

An association of Crohn's disease and cholecystectomy with small intestine adenocarcinoma is hypothesized, but the analytic epidemiology of small intestine malignancies has not received much attention because of small numbers. One case-control study conducted among 36 cases with small intestinal cancer (19 adenocarcinoma and 17 malignant carcinoid tumors) and 52 controls with nonmalignant conditions showed a four- to fivefold increased risk with cigarette smoking and alcohol consumption (80).

Cancer of the Large Intestine

Colorectal cancer is one of the most common types of cancer in the world. Colon and rectal cancers accounted for about 1 million new cancer cases in 2002 (9.4% of the world total) (1). The age-standardized incidence rates for colorectal cancer ranges from around 60 in the Czech Republic and Hungary to less than 5 per 100,000 in Middle Africa and Southcentral Asia (1,40). In general, the incidence of colorectal cancer is increasing rapidly in countries where overall risk was formerly low (especially in Japan), whereas in high-risk countries, trends are either gradually increasing, stabilizing (Northern and Western Europe), or declining with time (81). Unlike most cancer sites, colorectal cancer incidence is not so different in men and women (ratio, 1.2:1). Colorectal cancer incidence ranks fourth in frequency in men and third in women (1). Survival estimates (in men) at 5 years are 65% in North America, 54% in Western Europe, 34% in Eastern Europe, and 30% in India (81). Given the overall relatively good prognosis, prevalence is second only to that of breast cancer worldwide, with an estimated 2.8 million persons living with colorectal cancer diagnosed in the past 5 years (81).

There is at least a 25-fold variation in occurrence of colorectal cancer worldwide. The highest incidence rates are in North America, Australia/New Zealand, Western and Eastern Europe, and affluent Asian countries (e.g., Japan). Incidence tends to be low in Africa and nonaffluent Asian countries and intermediate in southern parts of South America (40). The geographic distribution of colon and rectal cancer is similar, although the variation between countries is more striking for colon cancer. In high-risk populations, the ratio of colon to rectal cancer incidence is 2:1 or more. In low-risk countries, colon and rectal cancer rates are similar. Genetic differences, different environmental exposures, or both may explain the large geographic differences for colorectal cancer. Migrants' studies that evaluate tumor risk in populations moved from low- to high-risk areas show that the incidence of colorectal cancer increases rapidly within the first generation, implying that environmental factors constitute a major component of risk. Japanese individuals born in the United States now have higher rates than those of whites in the United States, and the rates in Japanese individuals living in Hawaii and Los Angeles are among the highest in the world (82). These rates may be attributable to interplay between Westernized dietary habits and genetic susceptibility to these dietary factors (83).

Although there is clear evidence of genetic predisposition to colorectal cancer, genetic syndromes such as familial adenomatous polyposis (FAP) and HNPCC may explain less than 10% to 15% of all colorectal cancer. It is estimated that dietary habits may account for 50% to 60% of all colorectal cancer cases (59). Epidemiologic studies find consistent evidence that physical inactivity and a body mass index (BMI) of more than 25 kg/m^2 may increase colon cancer risk. A relatively high intake of alcohol and high consumption of red and processed meat and low consumption of fruits and vegetables probably increases risk of colon and rectal cancer. High consumption of dairy products and a high intake of calcium and vitamin D may reduce risk (59,84,85). Regular use of aspirin and other nonsteroidal anti-inflammatory drugs as well as hormone replacement therapy tend to decrease risk, whereas longtime cigarette smoking increases risk of colorectal cancer (85).

Colorectal cancers are believed to arise from epithelial DNA alterations, which progressively facilitate uncontrolled cell growth, the so-called adenoma-carcinoma sequence (86). The early detection and removal of precancerous colorectal adenomas may have contributed to the decline in colorectal cancer incidence and mortality, particularly in the United States. The United States has been recommending annual fecal occult blood (FOB) screening starting at age 50 since the 1980s, and national surveys indicate that around 40% of the eligible population comply with this advice (87). In Europe, several countries have been or will be introducing colorectal cancer screening programs based on the FOB test. Other screening options include immunochemical FOB tests, flexible sigmoidoscopy, colonoscopy, virtual colonoscopy (colonography using computed tomography), and fecal DNA tests.

ENVIRONMENTAL RISK FACTORS

Alcohol Intake

Alcohol belongs to the risk factors that are of prime interest to the World Health Organization (WHO). Alcohol use can be estimated from global production statistics with the disadvantage of only having per capita information. The better resources of information are representative surveys that request data on use of alcoholic beverages from the individual. In contrast to many other nutrients, data on alcohol use can be requested with high validity and reliability (88). The international statistics on alcohol use sees Europe and North America as the leading regions, with about 10 and 7 L per capita consumption, respectively, and a decreasing trend (89). Additional characteristics of alcohol drinking habits in a population are the percentage of abstainers and heavy drinkers. The percentage of abstainers is about 3% in Denmark, but this percentage can rise to more than 90% in some of the Islamic states. Heavy drinkers can cover half of the male population, such as in Columbia or Georgia. "Binge drinking" defined as a risky single drinking occasion can be found in more than one-third of the male population in Belgium, Canada, the Czech Republic, Finland, Germany, Iceland, Japan, and the Netherlands, and in one-fifth of the female population in Iceland and Finland. In some countries, more than 10% of the male population and 5% of the female population are considered alcohol dependent (89). In Europe, alcohol from beer and wine prevails; in North America, from beer and spirits; and in many others, from spirits and beer. In Africa, locally brewed drinks dominate.

To investigate the role of alcohol for health properly, the two dimension of alcohol use, the pattern of drinking and the average volume drank, should be considered (90). There seems to be a difference as to whether someone drinks two glasses of wine for lunch every day or one or more bottles in the evening every few days. However, most of the available data refer to the average use per day. Thus, the majority of studies report on the impact of this dimension of alcohol use on health. A summary of the current knowledge on the role of alcohol for disease and health was recently published by WHO based on the Global Burden project (89). It was estimated that about 6.5% of the total disability adjusted life years lost in men and 1.3% in women can be attributed to alcohol use (89). The Global Burden project identified five different cancer sites for which a good data basis exists on the role of alcohol (mouth and oropharynx, esophagus, liver, and breast) (91). With the exception of breast, these sites are the subject of this chapter. In addition, publications of the IARC introduced the colon and rectum as specific cancer sites related to alcohol (92). The relation between alcohol use and cancer is less clear for the other cancer sites, although increasing amounts of data are becoming available.

There are several meta-analyses that evaluated the impact of alcohol consumption on the risk of GI cancer. The most complete data collections were available within the Global Burden project and from a group in Italy. This group recently published the results of a meta-analysis referring to the cancer sites identified in the Global Burden project plus colon and rectum. They calculated the relative risks for various consumption levels (25 g/d equals two drinks per day) derived from a risk function calculated from the studies included in the meta-analysis. In a previous meta-analysis of this group with less studies, further risk estimates for GI cancer sites were presented (93,94). The results regarding GI cancers are shown in Table 1.1.

In all cancer sites, risk increased with increasing consumption. This argues against a j-shaped relationship and for the notion that small intakes are associated with increased risk. The strongest effect per gram of alcohol was found for cancer of the oral cavity and pharynx, followed by esophageal cancer. The nonlinear approximation of the relationship for these cancer sites can be found in Polesel et al. (95). In another study, the proportion of cancer attributed to alcohol use was investigated (92). The results were as follows: 30.4% for oral cavity and pharynx, 18.5% for esophagus, 3.2% for colon and rectum, and 9.4% for liver. These figures highlight again that the cancers in the upper GI tract and liver are mostly related to alcohol use.

There seems to be a gender-specific effect regarding the relative risk of the same drinking unit. In Bagnardi et al. (94), the meta-analysis indicated a significant higher relative risk for esophageal and liver cancer in women for the same drinking units. In particular, the increased risk in women for liver cancer was striking (1.62 in men compared to 9.13 in women for 100 g alcohol per day) (94).

The role of genetic variation of the genes metabolizing alcohol such as alcohol dehydrogenases, acetaldehyde dehydrogenases, and cytochrome P450 E1 for risk of GI cancer in

TABLE 1.1

RELATIVE RISK OF GASTROINTESTINAL CANCER BY DEGREE OF ALCOHOL USE

Cancer site	Relative risk (95% confidence interval)			
	Nonalcohol	25 g alcohol/day	50 g alcohol/day	100 g alcohol/day
Oral cavity and pharynx[a]	1	1.86 (1.76–1.96)	3.11 (2.85–3.39)	6.45 (5.76–7.24)
Esophagus[a]	1	1.39 (1.36–1.42)	1.93 (1.85–2.00)	3.59 (3.34–3.87)
Stomach[b]	1	1.07 (1.04–1.10)	1.15 (1.09–1.22)	1.32 (1.18–1.49)
Small intestine[b]	1	1.02 (0.89–1.17)	1.04 (0.79–1.37)	1.08 (0.63–1.88)
Colon[a]	1	1.05 (1.01–1.09)	1.10 (1.03–1.18)	1.21 (1.05–1.39)
Rectum[a]	1	1.09 (1.08–1.12)	1.19 (1.14–1.24)	1.42 (1.30–1.55)
Liver[a]	1	1.19 (1.12–1.27)	1.40 (1.25–1.56)	1.81 (1.50–2.19)
Gallbladder[b]	1	1.17 (0.73–1.86)	1.36 (0.54–3.44)	No data
Pancreas[b]	1	0.98 (0.90–1.05)	1.05 (0.93–1.18)	1.18 (0.94–1.49)

[a]From ref. 93.
[b]From ref. 94.

conjunction with alcohol use is still unclear. Some studies provided already reasonable hints that risk differs with different genetic makeup (96,97).

The exact mechanisms by which chronic alcohol use stimulates carcinogenesis are not known (98). Ethanol does not seem to be a carcinogen, but under certain experimental conditions it is acting as a cocarcinogen and/or tumor promoter. However, the metabolism of ethanol leads to the generation of acetaldehyde and free radicals. Acetaldehyde is carcinogenic and mutagenic, binds to DNA and proteins, destructs folate, and results in secondary hyperproliferation. In addition, for some cancers of the GI tract, local mechanisms may be of particular importance.

Infectious Exposures

Human papillomaviruses (HPVs) are recognized causes of cancer of the anogenital tract. The HPV-mediated transformation of normal epithelial cells has been recognized as a multistep process resulting from deregulated transcription of the viral oncogenes E6 and E7 in the proliferating cells and interference of E6 and E7 in the cell cycle, inducing genetic instability and oncogenic alterations (99). There is epidemiologic evidence showing that HPV is also associated with the upper digestive tract, particularly with oral and oropharyngeal squamous cell carcinomas (OOSCCs) and *tonsil cancer* (100). In a review of 60 studies on OOSCC, overall HPV detected prevalence was 25.9%, with HPV16 being the most common type associated with these cancers, whereas HPV18 was rarely detected (101). HPV may be associated with precursor lesions of oral cavity cancer such as oral papillomas, focal epithelial hyperplasia, and erythroplakias (100). Oral sex and mother-to-child transmission are possible sources of infection (100).

Infection with HPV is also associated with the development of anal squamous cell carcinoma among both men and women (102). HPV16 is the most frequent HPV type, followed by HPV18, -31, and -33 (103). In both genders, high-risk sexual behaviors, HIV infection, and HPV-associated malignancy are associated with anal carcinoma.

Squamous cell carcinomas of the anal region in young men that are positive for HPV are often related to homosexual behavior and are associated with some types of anal intraepithelial neoplasia, a precursor of the anal cancer (103).

Hepatitis B virus and *hepatitis C virus* are the most important etiologic factors of HCC. Overall, 75% to 80% of HCC cases are related to hepatitis infection (104). Worldwide in 2002, 54.4% of HCC cases were attributable to HBV and 31.1% to HCV (104). In developing countries such as Africa and Asia, 58.8% of cases of HCC were related to persistent viral infection with HBV and 33.4% with infection with HCV. In developed countries, 23.3% of cases were attributable to persistent infection with HBV and 19.9% to HCV (104). The risk of HCC is greatly increased in chronic viral carriers exposed to other recognized cofactors, mainly alcoholic cirrhosis and possibly diabetes in the United States and Europe and aflatoxin B1 exposure in Africa and Asia. Among individuals infected with HBV, those who express HBV surface antigen (HBsAg carriers) are approximately 20 times more likely to develop HCC than those who do not (105).

Age at HBV infection is a key determinant of the HCC risk. In developed countries at low risk of HCC, most of the HBV infections are acquired during adolescence or adulthood, through sexual contacts, blood transfusions, or other contaminated invasive procedures. In these populations, HBV acquisition at birth or during childhood is rare. On the contrary, in most of the high-risk countries, the mother-to-child and child-to-child transmission of the HBV in the first years of life predominates. The higher incidences rates of HCC in China and Africa may be related with early age of the onset of viral infection.

In developed countries, the risk of HCV infection is mainly related to drug use, unsafe injections, and contaminated equipment used in health care–related procedures (106). Factors that predispose to HCC among HCV-infected persons include male gender, older age, HBV coinfection, heavy alcohol drinking, possible diabetes, and a transfusion-related source of HCV infections (107). It was estimated that among 1% to 3% of HCV-infected persons would develop HCC after 30 years (106). HCC in HIV-infected patients is mainly associated with underlying chronic hepatitis C and has a more aggressive clinical course.

There is an important international variation in the prevalence of specific viral genotypes. HBV genotype A is predominant in the United States and the Caribbean, type D in Europe and Middle East, and types B and C predominate in Asia, while types A, C, and D are equally prevalent in Africa. Within the United States, type A is more frequent in the South, types C and B in the West, and type D in the East (108). The importance of HBV genotypes remains incompletely understood, although it was suggested that genotype B may be associated with less serious clinical outcomes. A recent study in Taiwan (109) showed that genotype C HBV was associated with increased viral load and a higher risk of HCC compared with other genotypes.

The integration of hepatitis B vaccine into existing childhood vaccination schedules has the greatest likelihood of reducing HCC risk worldwide. However, by the year 2000, only 116 countries had established such a policy, representing only 31% of births of the world (110).

Helicobacter pylori, isolated from the human gastric mucosa for the first time in 1982, was classified as being carcinogenic for humans in 1994. *H. pylori* is a contributory cause of adenocarcinoma of stomach and gastric lymphoma (111). It has been estimated that 63.4% of gastric cancer in the world is associated with *H. pylori* infection (104). The most recent meta-analysis including 12 prospective studies has shown that *H. pylori* infection increases the risk of gastric cancer by two- to threefold (odds ratio: 2.36; 95% confidence interval: 1.98–2.81). No association was observed between *H. pylori* infection and the cancer of the gastric cardia (48). There is some evidence that *H. pylori* may even be inversely associated to cardia and esophageal adenocarcinoma (112).

H. pylori is one of the most common bacterial pathogens in humans, although prevalence of infections varies in different regions of the world. It was estimated (104) that in middle-age adults, 74% of populations in developing countries and 58% in developed countries are infected by *H. pylori*, but other authors think that the prevalence in developed countries is lower, around 40% or less (113). The most likely mode of transmission is from person to person, either by the oral–oral route or by the fecal–oral routes. Waterborne transmission due to fecal contamination may be a source of infection in developing populations receiving untreated water (114). Prevalence of *H. pylori* infection is similar by gender, directly associated with age, and inversely associated with socioeconomic status. The infection seems to be decreasing with improvement in hygiene practices. In the United States, prevalence of infection is substantially lower in whites than blacks or Hispanics (113). In general, infection is acquired during childhood, and the acquisition rate of *H. pylori* appears to be faster in developing countries than developed countries.

H. pylori colonizes and proliferates in the mucus layer over the epithelium. The ability to survive and grow in gastric acid is linked to its ability to maintain a tolerable pH by activation of internal urease production. In the majority of infected humans, there are no clinical consequences from *H. pylori* infection. Only 15% to 20% of those infected will develop severe gastroduodenal pathology (duodenal or gastric ulcer) and less than 1% will eventually develop a gastric tumor in their life (115). Gastric cancer is the result of a long multistage and multifactorial carcinogenic process involving interaction between *H. pylori* factors, dietary and other environmental factors, and host genetic susceptibility. An inflammatory gastritis in the antrum is believed to be the initial lesion that may progress toward a chronic atrophic gastritis in the corpus, followed by intestinal metaplasia, dysplasia, and finally adenocarcinoma (117). Local and systematic responses can be observed after *H. pylori* infection, including productions of proinflammatory and immunoregulatory cytokines and growth factors. Some cytokines are powerful inhibitors of gastric acid secretion. It is believed that low acid secretion, resulting from progressive destruction of gastric glands that are replaced by intestinal-type mucosa, together with inhibition of acid secretion by cytokines, allows the spread of inflammation from the antrum to the corpus and permits the growth of other bacteria that enhance the endogenous production of carcinogenic N-nitroso compounds (117). Genetic diversity of *H. pylori* and variability in virulence factors (e.g., cytotoxin CagA, vacuolating cytotoxin VacA, neutrophil-activating protein) of different strains may explain different outcomes of infection and could be useful in identification of persons for whom *H. pylori* eradication would be most important (116). However, the epidemiologic evidence showed that any marker could be used as predictor of specific outcomes (118). The first published randomized controlled trial on *H. pylori* eradication to prevent gastric cancer risk in a high-risk region of China (119) observed a reduction in the risk only in those without precancerous lesions. It seems that in patients with gastric atrophy, intestinal metaplasia, or dysplasia, eradication treatment does not modify the risk of gastric cancer.

Body Mass Index, Energy Balance, and Physical Activity

Since the mid-1980s, the proportion of people with obesity (BMI >30 kg/m^2) has increased by 66% in the United States (120), and has been increasing in most developed and many developing countries in the world (121). In the United States, approximately two-thirds of the adult population is overweight, with 30% being obese (122). The prevalence of overweight and obesity in European countries ranges from 10% to 50% and 2% to 40.9%, respectively (121). In particular, the increase in obesity in the United States has paralleled an increase in the incidence rates for adenocarcinoma of the esophagus, esophagogastric junction, gastric cardia (30), and liver and intrahepatic bile duct cancer (123). These ecologic associations may suggest that obesity contributes to these cancers. A generalized decrease in physical activity is considered the greatest contributor to the increase prevalence in overweight and obesity (124).

Accumulating evidence suggests that obesity may be associated with increased risk of many GI cancers, including esophageal adenocarcinoma and gastric cardia, and small intestine, gallbladder, liver, pancreas, colon, and rectum cancers, with colorectal cancer being the most studied (125–128). The obesity-associated risk for these cancer sites has been approximately 2-fold for esophagus, 1.4- to 4-fold for gastric and/or gastric cardia, 1.5- to 1.9-fold for small intestine, 2-fold for gallbladder, 1.4- to 4.5-fold for liver, 1.2- to 2.7-fold for pancreas, and 1.5-fold for colon and rectal (125–128). The IARC concluded that the evidence was "sufficient" to support a causal association for excess body weight with adenocarcinoma of the esophagus and colon. Evidence was also "sufficient" to support regular physical activity, thus reducing the risk for colon cancer (126). Overweight (BMI >25 kg/m^2) and lack of physical activity, respectively, account for 11% and 14%, or together 25%, of colon cancer, while overweight may be attributable for 37% of esophageal cancer (124). Lifestyle changes that promote weight control and increased physical activity may result in prevention and possibly reduction of many of these GI malignancies.

The proposed mechanisms that explain the associations between adiposity and GI malignancies differ across cancer sites. Obesity, specifically intra-abdominal adiposity, leads to metabolic changes, including higher insulin concentrations, insulin resistance, and potentially increases the bioavailability of other growth factors, particularly insulinlike growth factor-1 (IGF-1). Insulinlike growth factors (IGFs) are endocrine mediators of growth hormone that act in paracrine and autocrine fashion to regulate cell growth, differentiation, apoptosis, and transformation (129), and have been hypothesized to enhance the development of several GI malignancies, including adenocarcinoma of the colon, rectum, and pancreas (130–132). The IGF axis is complex and is comprised of growth factors (IGF-1, IGF-2, and insulin), cell surface receptors (IGF-1R and IGF-2R), six binding proteins (IGFBP-1–6), IGFBP proteases, and other IGFBP-interacting molecules that regulate the IGF axis' actions. Increased insulin concentrations increase the bioavailability of IGF-1 by increasing its synthesis and by decreasing IGFBP-1 and IGFBP-2 (133), thus linking the IGF-1 axis to glucose metabolism. Because type 2 diabetics are known to exhibit hyperinsulinemia during the early stages of their disease (134), the hyperinsulinemia hypothesis is further supported by the fact that positive associations for higher glucose concentrations and biochemical-defined diabetes with esophagus, stomach, liver, pancreas, and colorectal cancer have been reported in prospective studies (135–138). In addition, adiponectin, a peptide produced by the adipocytes that mediates insulin sensitivity (139), has been inversely associated with gastric, particularly gastric cardia cancer, and colon adenomas and colorectal cancer (140–142). Adiponectin has also been inversely associated with adiposity (141) and type 2 diabetes (143). Although the etiology of cancers arising in the small intestine is unclear, adenocarcinomas of the small and large intestine are believed to have similar risk factors (80).

In contrast, anatomic, nonmetabolic abnormalities that result from obesity may contribute to esophageal adenocarcinoma and gastric cardia, gall bladder, and liver cancers. Epidemiologic and molecular differences between esophageal adenocarcinoma and gastric cardia cancer suggest that these malignancies are biologically different (124); however, an increase in gastroesophageal reflux disease as a result of increased abdominal adiposity had been proposed as an underlying cause for both malignancies (30,144). This hypothesis is also supported by the observation that medications that lower esophageal sphincter pressure also increase reflux and have been associated with esophageal adenocarcinoma (145). Obesity and lack of physical activity is likely associated with gallbladder cancer indirectly by contributing to the development of cholesterol gallstones, which is a major risk factor for gallbladder cancer. The means by which stones predispose to gallbladder cancer are not entirely clear, but they appear to involve chronic inflammatory processes (146). Recent studies have also implicated obesity and diabetes mellitus as conditions predisposing to nonalcoholic steatohepatitis and to hepatocellular carcinoma (123). The chronic inflammation that results from obesity for these later sites may create a microenvironment that facilitates malignant transformation and tumor growth via endocrine and autocrine growth factors (147–149).

Vegetables and Fruits

The role of vegetables and fruits in reducing the risk of GI cancer has been known since the 1980s. In 1991, Steinmetz and Potter were the first to summarize all available epidemiologic data (mainly, case-control studies) (150), concluding that the evidence was consistent with higher consumption being associated with lower risk of many epithelial cancers. In 1997, the World Cancer Research Fund/American Institute for Cancer Research (WCRF/AICR) report reviewed all available epidemiologic literature up to 1996 (59). This report concluded that vegetables and fruits were probably or convincingly associated with lower risk of several GI cancers: cancers of mouth, larynx, esophagus, pancreas, stomach, and colorectum (vegetables only) (59).

In 2003, the Working Group of IARC on Vegetables, Fruits and Cancer (8) concluded that fruit consumption is associated with decreased risk of cancer of the oral cavity, pharynx, salivary gland/nasopharynx, larynx, esophagus, stomach, colon, and rectum in case-control studies, with reduction of risk ranging from nearly 60% (oral cavity, pharynx) to about 15% (colon/rectum) comparing high to low fruit consumption. For colorectal cancer, cohort studies did not show an association with fruit consumption. For vegetables, the Working Group also observed a decreased risk in case-control studies for these cancer sites, with risk reductions ranging from 50% (oral cavity, pharynx, larynx) to 33% (stomach) comparing high with low vegetable consumption. Cohort studies did not show significant associations between vegetable intake and these cancers (8). A quantitative meta-analysis of the epidemiologic literature on vegetables, fruits, and GI cancer did show that risk reductions may occur with an increase of 100 g of vegetables or fruits per day, taking smoking habits into account (151).

As pointed out by all reviews, in general, recent epidemiologic studies tend to show weaker associations or no results as compared to older studies. Previously, more case-control studies were conducted, whereas the results of prospective cohort studies with longer follow-up time have been published more recently. Associations observed in case-control studies were stronger than in cohort studies. Recall bias and the potential impact of prediagnostic symptoms on exposure measurement in case-control studies may explain this difference. In cohort studies, the observed associations may be underestimated by limited variation in dietary intakes within each cohort, imprecise measurement of intake, multivariate modeling in the presence of weak associations, and short follow-up (152). For gastric cancer, results of prospective studies were stronger for studies with longer follow-up time (153). Recent human intervention trials increasing the intake of vegetables and fruits did not show an effect on the recurrence of colorectal adenoma (154), biomarkers of proliferation in Barrett's esophagus (155), and colorectal cancer risk (156). In general, intervention trials increasing the intake of vegetables and fruits may be hindered for instance by the use of surrogate end points (markers of preclinical cancer or imminent recurrence), by relatively short intervention periods, and by relatively small differences between intervention and control groups, possibly because of compliance issues occurring during longer follow-up.

Besides methodologic issues, inconsistencies in epidemiologic studies may also be explained by not taking into account cooking methods that may influence associations observed between vegetable consumption and GI cancer risk. As reviewed by Link and Potter (157), raw vegetables were more often inversely associated with esophageal and gastric cancer than cooked vegetables. A protective effect of both raw and cooked vegetables was, however, observed in most studies on oral, pharyngeal, and laryngeal cancers (157).

As pointed out by Potter, we should take into account that cancer-preventing properties of plant foods may be reduced over time due to changes in food sources, plant breeding and harvesting, transport, and storage accounting for the differences between earlier and recent epidemiologic findings (158).

Based on a meta-analysis, Norat and Riboli (159) concluded that worldwide, increasing vegetable consumption could potentially prevent up to 50% of gastric cancer cases and up to 29% of colorectal cancer cases. Increasing fruit consumption could potentially prevent up to 45% of esophageal cancer cases and 50% of gastric cancer cases.

In 2007, WCRF International and AICR will publish an update of the 1997 report, which will include quantitative meta-analyses on vegetables, fruits, and GI cancers (160).

Until now, epidemiologic studies do not convincingly point to one type of vegetable or fruit that may be particularly beneficial. For some GI cancers, reduced risks were stronger for allium, cruciferous, and green vegetables or citrus fruits (59).

Vegetables and fruits contain a variety of components, including vitamins (e.g., vitamin C, carotenoids, folate), minerals (selenium, potassium, calcium, iron), dietary fiber, polyunsaturated fatty acids, plant sterols, protease inhibitors, phenols, and secondary metabolites such as glucosinolates (in cruciferous vegetables) and flavonoids, many of which can inhibit cell proliferation and induce apoptosis, and which may well act synergistically when combined in the human diet.

Meat

An association between red meat and colorectal cancer, as well as a protective effect of fish, have been suggested by a number of studies and recently confirmed by the European Prospective Investigation into Cancer and Nutrition (EPIC) study of 1,329 incident colorectal cancer cases (59,161–166). An intake of 160 g or more of red and processed meat (two or more portions per day) was associated with a 35% increase in colorectal cancer compared with less than one portion per week, whereas an intake of 80 g or more of fish was associated with a 30% reduction in risk. No association with poultry consumption was observed. Inclusion of folate did not affect results. The overall picture was consistent for red and processed meat and fiber across all European populations studied. The association with red and processed meat was particularly strong in individuals eating a low-fiber diet (167). This compelling evidence that red meat increases colorectal cancer risk has received some support from a study investigating mechanisms. Red meat contains heme, absent from white meat, and increases the endogenous formation of apparent N-nitrosocompounds (NOC), including direct-acting diazopeptides or N-nitrosopeptides, able to form alkylating DNA adducts in the colon. In colonic exfoliated cells, the percentage staining positive for the NOC-specific DNA adduct, O^6-carboxymethyl guanine (O^6CMG), was significantly ($p < 0.001$) higher on a high red meat diet. If these O^6CMG adducts are not repaired, and if other related adducts are formed and not repaired, this may explain the association of red meat with colorectal cancer (167).

Three cohort studies (168–170) observed no associations between total meat, beef, or pork intakes and gastric cancer risk, whereas one study found a weak but statistically nonsignificant association (171). Processed meat (e.g., bacon or sausage) was statistically significantly and positively associated with gastric cancer in two cohort studies (169,172). An association between total, red, and processed meat intakes and gastric noncardia cancer was recently confirmed by the EPIC study of 159 incident noncardia cancer cases, especially in *H. pylori* antibody-positive subjects, but not in cardia gastric cancer cases (173). Besides other plausible mechanisms of action, such as potential effects of heme in red meats, of fat and protein, of salt, and of heterocyclic amines and polycyclic aromatic hydrocarbons, as in colorectal cancer, endogenous formation of nitrosocompounds may also account for this association (174).

Genetic Syndromes

In a small proportion (1%–5%) of cases of colorectal, gastric, and pancreatic cancer, inborn genetic factors play a significant role. In this section, the most common hereditary GI cancers and the genes that are involved in their development are discussed.

Colorectal Cancer

A family history of colorectal cancer may be found in up to 15% of all patients with this cancer. In one-third of the cases with a positive family history, a hereditary colorectal cancer syndrome is involved. The most common dominant inherited colorectal cancer syndrome is Lynch syndrome or HNPCC, which is responsible for 3% to 5% of all colorectal cancer cases (175). Another well-described syndrome is familial adenomatous polyposis (FAP), which is responsible for 1% of the cases.

Lynch syndrome is characterized by the development of colorectal cancer, endometrial cancer, and cancer at several other sites at an unusually young age. The average age at diagnosis of colorectal cancer is 45 years. Other cancers associated with the syndrome are cancer of the small bowel, urinary tract (pelvis and ureter), brain, and ovaries. Colorectal cancers predominantly develop in the proximal part of the colon. There is an increased incidence of multiple, synchronous, or metachronous colorectal cancers (176).

Lynch syndrome is associated with germline mutations in four genes with so-called mismatch repair (MMR) function (i.e., *MSH2, MLH1, MSH6,* and *PMS2*). The protein products of MMR genes are key players in the correction of mismatches that arise during DNA replication. Loss of MMR function results in mutations in microsatellites (referred to as *microsatellite instability [MSI]*). Microsatellites are repetitive DNA sequences found throughout the genome. Because more than 90% of colorectal cancers from patients with Lynch syndrome express a high level of MSI, MSI may aid in the diagnosis of this syndrome. However, MSI is not specific to Lynch syndrome because it occurs in 15% of apparently sporadic colorectal cancers. Clinical criteria (the Bethesda criteria) have been developed for the identification of families suspected of this syndrome (Table 1.2) (177).

In all patients that meet these criteria, there is an indication for testing of the colon tumor for MSI. If MSI is found in the tumor, the following step is a search for a mutation in one of the MMR genes. In individuals that meet these criteria, a pathogenic mutation can be identified in about half of the cases.

FAP is another autosomal dominant inherited syndrome characterized by the development of a large number of adenomas in the colon. The natural history of the disease is well known: patients develop adenomas during adolescence, present with signs or symptoms around the age of 30 years, and due to the high number of adenomas they have a risk of almost 100% of developing colorectal cancer with a mean age at diagnosis of 40 years (178). The syndrome is also associated with various other extracolonic features, including upper GI polyps, desmoid tumors, and congenital hypertrophy of the retinal pigment epithelium, osteoma, dental abnormalities, and epidermal cysts (179). There is also an increased risk of developing thyroid cancer, duodenal cancer, and brain tumors. FAP is caused by mutations in the *APC* gene. This gene is involved in several cellular processes, including transcription, cell cycle control, migration, differentiation, and apoptosis.

A mutation can be identified in 50% to 60% of the families. Recently, another polyposis causing mutation was identified on chromosome 1, the *MUTYH* gene (180). Mutations in this base excision repair gene are associated with an autosomal recessive mode of inheritance. *MUTYH*-associated polyposis is usually characterized by a relatively low number of adenomas (between 15 and 100) and a more advanced age at diagnosis compared to polyposis caused by an *APC* gene defect (181).

Two other, rare, dominant inherited conditions with an increased colorectal cancer risk are Peutz-Jeghers syndrome and juvenile polyposis, both characterized by hamartomatous colorectal polyposis. The Peutz-Jeghers syndrome is also characterized by pigmentation in the face, lips, mouth, and anal region. Mutations have been identified in the *LKB1/STK11* gene in 50% of the patients (182). Juvenile polyposis is characterized by the development of hamartomatous polyposis before the age of 10 years (183). Mutations have been identified in *SMAD4* and *BMPR1A* genes.

Gastric Cancer

Studies have shown that familial clustering occurs in 10% of the gastric cancer cases. Inherited forms of gastric cancer are associated with two hereditary cancer syndromes (i.e., Lynch syndrome and a syndrome of hereditary gastric cancer caused by *E-cadherin* mutations).

The first family reported with Lynch syndrome was characterized by the combined occurrence of gastric cancer, colorectal cancer, and endometrial cancer (184). Currently, gastric cancer is rarely observed in Lynch syndrome families from Western countries and occurs only in the older generations. However, in families from the Far East (Japan, South Korea), hereditary gastric cancer is frequently reported (185). The type of gastric cancer found in Lynch syndrome is usually of the intestinal type. Families with inherited gastric cancer associated with *E-cadherin* mutations have diffuse type of gastric cancer with poor differentiation and an infiltrative growth pattern. This type of cancer is difficult to detect during gastroscopy. The only effective preventive measure in carriers of *E-cadherin* mutation is, therefore, a prophylactic gastrectomy (186).

Pancreatic Cancer

Epidemiologic studies have shown that 3% to 10% of pancreatic cancer patients have a positive family history for pancreatic cancer (187). Families with clustering of pancreatic cancer can be subdivided into families with pancreatic cancer without other malignancies (site-specific pancreatic cancer), families with a specific hereditary cancer syndrome and families with hereditary pancreatitis. The familial atypical multiple mole melanoma (FAMMM) syndrome is one of the syndromes associated with pancreatic cancer. This syndrome predisposes family members to develop dysplastic nevi and melanoma. In at least 25% of FAMMM families, the syndrome is caused by a mutation in the *P16* suppressor gene. It has been demonstrated that carriers of a *P16* mutation have a 15% to 20% lifetime risk of developing pancreatic cancer (188). Also, hereditary breast cancer syndrome associated with *BRCA2* mutations predisposes not only to the development of breast cancer but also pancreatic cancer; *BRCA2* mutation carriers are reported to have a three- to fourfold increased risk of pancreatic cancer

---

TABLE 1.2

BETHESDA CRITERIA

1. Colorectal cancer diagnosed in a patient younger than 50 y of age.
2. Presence of synchronous, metachronous colorectal, or other Lynch syndrome–related tumors,[a] regardless of age.
3. Colorectal cancer with microsatellite instability histology diagnosed in a patient younger than 60 y of age.
4. Patient with colorectal cancer and a first-degree relative with a Lynch syndrome–related tumor, with one of the cancers diagnosed younger than 50 y of age.
5. Patient with colorectal cancer with two or more first- or second-degree relatives with a Lynch syndrome–related tumor, regardless of age.

[a]Lynch syndrome–related tumors include colorectal, endometrial, stomach, ovarian, pancreas, ureter, renal pelvis, biliary tract, and brain tumors; sebaceous gland adenomas and keratoacanthomas; and carcinoma of the small bowel.

(189). Finally, Lynch syndrome, Peutz-Jeghers syndrome, and hereditary pancreatitis are associated with an increased risk of developing pancreatic cancer.

References

1. Ferlay J, Bray F, Pisani P, Parkin DM. *Globocan 2002: Cancer Incidence, Mortality and Prevalence Worldwide, Version 2.0.* IARC CancerBase No. 5. Lyon, France: IARC Press; 2004.
2. Mignogna MD, Fedele S, Lo Russo L. The World Cancer Report and the burden of oral cancer. *Eur J Cancer Prev* 2004;13:139–142.
3. Shiboski CH, Shiboski SC, Silverman S, Jr. Trends in oral cancer rates in the United States, 1973–1996. *Community Dent Oral Epidemiol* 2000;28:249–256.
4. Lin YS, Jen YM, Wang BB, Lee JC, Kang BH. Epidemiology of oral cavity cancer in Taiwan with emphasis on the role of betel nut chewing. *ORL J* 2005;67:230–236.
5. Boeing H. Alcohol and risk of cancer of the upper gastrointestinal tract: first analysis of the EPIC data. *IARC Sci Publ* 2002;156:151–154.
6. Nair U, Bartsch H, Nair J. Alert for an epidemic of oral cancer due to use of the betel quid substitutes gutkha and pan masala: a review of agents and causative mechanisms. *Mutagenesis* 2004;19:251–262.
7. Khawaja MI, Shafiq M, Nusrat R, Khawaja MR. Preventing the oral cavity cancer epidemic. *Asian Pac J Cancer Prev* 2005;6:420.
8. International Agency for Research on Cancer (IARC). *IARC Handbooks of Cancer Prevention Vol. 8: Fruit and Vegetables.* Lyon, France: IARC Press; 2003.
9. Gupta PC, Mehta FS, Pindborg JJ, et al. Primary prevention trial of oral cancer in India: a 10-year follow-up study. *J Oral Pathol Med* 1992;21:433–439.
10. Lodi G, Sardella A, Bez C, Demarosi F, Carrassi A. Interventions for treating oral leukoplakia. *Cochrane Database Syst Rev* 2004;3.
11. Busik TL, Uchida T, Wagner RFJ. Preventing ultraviolet light lip injury: beachgoer awareness about lip cancer risk factors and lip protein behavior. *Dermatol Surg* 2005;31:173–176.
12. Morse DE, Pendrys DG, Neely AL, Psoter WJ. Trends in the incidence of lip, oral, and pharyngeal cancer: Connecticut, 1935–94. *Oral Oncol* 1999;35:1–8.
13. Polednak AP. Recent trends in incidence rates for selected alcohol-related cancers in the United States. *Alcohol* 2005;40:234–238.
14. Kurumatani N, Kirita T, Zheng Y, Sugimura M, Yonemasu K. Time trends in the mortality rates for tobacco- and alcohol-related cancers within the oral cavity and pharynx in Japan, 1950–94. *J Epidemiol* 1999;46–52.
15. Su WZ, Tohnai I, Kuwamura T, et al. Trends in site-specific mortality from oral and pharyngeal cancer among Japanese males, 1950–94. *Oral Oncol* 1999;35:9–16.
16. La Vecchia C, Lucchini F, Negri E, Levi F. Trends in oral cancer mortality in Europe. *Oral Oncol* 2004;40:433–439.
17. Elango JK, Gangadharan P, Sumithra S, Kuriakose MA. Trends of head and neck cancers in urban and rural India. *Asian Pac J Cancer Prev* 2006;7:108–112.
18. Franceschi S, Bidoli E, Herrero R, Munoz N. Comparison of cancers of the oral cavity and pharynx worldwide: etiological clues. *Oral Oncol* 2000;36:106–115.
19. La Vecchia C, Lucchini F, Negri E, Levi F. Trends in oral cancer mortality in Europe. *Oral Oncol* 2004;40:433–439.
20. Brown LM, Devesa SS. Epidemiologic trends in esophageal and gastric cancer in the United States. *Surg Oncol Clin N Am* 2002;11:235–256.
21. Baquet CR, Commiskey P, Mack K, Meltzer S, Mishra SI. Esophageal cancer epidemiology in blacks and whites: racial and gender disparities in incidence, mortality, survival rates and histology. *J Natl Med Assoc* 2005;97:1471–1478.
22. Walker AR, Adam F, Walker J, Walker BF. Cancer of the oesophagus in Africans in sub-Saharan Africa: any hopes for its control? *Eur J Cancer Prev* 2002;11:413–418.
23. McGlashan ND, Harington JS, Chelkowska E. Changes in the geographical and temporal patterns of cancer incidence among black gold miners working in South Africa, 1964–1996. *Br J Cancer* 2003;88:1361–1369.
24. Sadjadi A, Nouraie M, Mahagheghi MA, Mousavi-Jarrahi A, Malekzadeh R, Parkin DM. Cancer occurrence in Iran in 2002, an international perspective. *Asian Pac J Cancer Prev* 2005;6:359–363.
25. Wang JM, Xu B, Hsieh CC, Jiang QW. Longitudinal trends of stomach cancer and esophageal cancer in Yangzhong County: a high-incidence rural area of China. *Eur J Gastroenterol Hepatol* 2005;17:1339–1344.
26. Stoner GD, Gupta A. Etiology and chemoprevention of esophageal squamous cell carcinoma. *Carcinogenesis* 2001;22:1737–1746.
27. Wu IC, Lu CY, Kuo FC, et al. Interaction between cigarette, alcohol and betel nut use on esophageal cancer risk in Taiwan. *Eur J Clin Invest* 2006;36:236–241.
28. Lindblad M, Ye W, Lindgren A, Lagergren J. Disparities in the classification of esophageal and cardia adenocarcinomas and their influence on reported incidence rates. *Ann Surg* 2006;243:479–485.
29. Pohl H, Welch HG. The role of overdiagnosis and reclassification in the marked increase of esophageal adenocarcinoma incidence. *J Natl Cancer Inst* 2005;97:142–146.
30. Brown LM, Devesa SS. Epidemiologic trends in esophageal and gastric cancer in the United States. *Surg Oncol Clin N Am* 2002;11:235–256.
31. Wu X, Chen VW, Ruiz B, Andrews P, Su LJ, Correa P. Incidence of esophageal and gastric carcinomas among American Asians/Pacific Islanders, whites, and blacks: subsite and histology differences. *Cancer* 2006;106:683–692.
32. Vizcaino AP, Moreno V, Lambert R, Parkin DM. Time trends incidence of both major histologic types of esophageal carcinomas in selected countries, 1973–1995. *Int J Cancer* 2002;99:860–868.
33. Kubo A, Corley DA. Marked multi-ethnic variation of esophageal and gastric cardia carcinomas within the United States. *Am J Gastroenterol* 2004;99:582–588.
34. Wijnhoven BP, Louwman MW, Tilanus HW, Coebergh JW. Increased incidence of adenocarcinomas at the gastro-oesophageal junction in Dutch males since the 1990s. *Eur J Gastroenterol Hepatol* 2002;14:115–122.
35. Devesa SS, Blot WJ, Fraumeni JF, Jr. Changing patterns in the incidence of esophageal and gastric carcinoma in the United States. *Cancer* 1998;83:2049–2053.
36. Shaheen N, Ransohoff DF. Gastroesophageal reflux, Barrett esophagus, and esophageal cancer: scientific review. *JAMA* 2002;287:1972–1981.
37. Lagergren J. Controversies surrounding body mass, reflux, and risk of oesophageal adenocarcinoma. *Lancet Oncol* 2006;7:347–349.
38. Engel LS, Chow WH, Vaughan TL, et al. Population attributable risks of esophageal and gastric cancers. *J Natl Cancer Inst* 2003;95:1404–1413.
39. Chow WH, Blaser MJ, Blot WJ, et al. An inverse relation between cagA+ strains of *Helicobacter pylori* infection and risk of esophageal and gastric cardia adenocarcinoma. *Cancer Res* 1998;58:588–590.
40. Parkin DM. International variation. *Oncogene* 2004;23:6329–6340.
41. Hansen S, Wiig JN, Giercksky KE, Tretli S. Esophageal and gastric carcinoma in Norway 1958–1992: incidence time trend variability according to morphological subtypes and organ subsites. *Int J Cancer* 1997;71:340–344.
42. Botterweck AA, Schouten LJ, Volovics A, Dorant E, Van den Brandt PA. Trends in incidence of adenocarcinoma of the oesophagus and gastric cardia in ten European countries. *Int J Epidemiol* 2000;29:645–654.
43. Liu Y, Kaneko S, Sobue T. Trends in reported incidences of gastric cancer by tumour location, from 1975 to 1989 in Japan. *Int J Epidemiol* 2004;33:808–815.
44. Parkin DM. Global cancer statistics in the year 2000. *Lancet Oncol* 2001;2:533–543.
45. Henson DE, Dittus C, Younes M, Nguyen H, Albores-Saavedra J. Differential trends in the intestinal and diffuse types of gastric carcinoma in the United States, 1973–2000: increase in the signet ring cell type. *Arch Pathol Lab Med* 2004;128:765–770.
46. Kaneko S, Yoshimura T. Time trend analysis of gastric cancer incidence in Japan by histological types, 1975–1989. *Br J Cancer* 2001;84:400–405.
47. Lauren PA, Nevalainen TJ. Epidemiology of intestinal and diffuse types of gastric carcinoma. A time-trend study in Finland with comparison between studies from high- and low-risk areas. *Cancer* 1993;71:2926–2933.
48. Helicobacter and Cancer Collaborative Group. Gastric cancer and *Helicobacter pylori*: a combined analysis of 12 case control studies nested within prospective cohorts. *Gut* 2001;49:347–353.
49. Mayne ST, Navarro SA. Diet, obesity and reflux in the etiology of adenocarcinomas of the esophagus and gastric cardia in humans. *J Nutr* 2002;132:3467S–3470S.
50. Gonzalez CA, Pera G, Agudo A, et al. Smoking and the risk of gastric cancer in the European Prospective Investigation into Cancer and Nutrition (EPIC). *Int J Cancer* 2003;107:629–634.
51. Kew MC. Epidemiology of hepatocellular carcinoma. *Toxicology* 2002;181/182:35–38.
52. El Serag HB, Mason AC. Risk factors for the rising rates of primary liver cancer in the United States. *Arch Intern Med* 2000;160:3227–3230.
53. Hassan MM, Hwang LY, Hatten CJ, et al. Risk factors for hepatocellular carcinoma: synergism of alcohol with viral hepatitis and diabetes mellitus. *Hepatology* 2002;36:1206–1213.
54. Braga C, La Vecchia C, Negri E, Franceschi S. Attributable risks for hepatocellular carcinoma in northern Italy. *Eur J Cancer* 1997;33:629–634.
55. Davila JA, Petersena NJ, Nelson HA, El Serag HB. Geographic variation within the United States in the incidence of hepatocellular carcinoma. *J Clin Epidemiol* 2003;56:487–493.
56. Kuper H, Tzonou A, Lagiou P, et al. Diet and hepatocellular carcinoma: a case-control study in Greece. *Nutr Cancer* 2000;38:6–12.
57. Romeo R, Colombo M. The natural history of hepatocellular carcinoma. *Toxicology* 2002;181/182:39–42.
58. Henry SH, Bosch FX, Troxell TC, Bolger PM. Policy forum: public health. Reducing liver cancer—global control of aflatoxin. *Science* 1999;288:2453–2454.
59. World Cancer Research Fund Panel. *Food, Nutrition and the Prevention of Cancer: A Global Perspective.* Washington, DC: American Institute for Cancer Research; 1997:148–175.
60. Randi G, Franceschi S, La Vecchia C. Gallbladder cancer worldwide: geographical distribution and risk factors. *Int J Cancer* 2006;118:1591–1602.
61. Chaurasia P, Thakur MK, Shukla HS. What causes cancer gallbladder? A review. *HPB Surg* 1999;11:217–224.

62. Zatonski WA, Lowenfels AB, Boyle P, et al. Epidemiologic aspects of gall-bladder cancer: a case-control study of the SEARCH Program of the International Agency for Research on Cancer. *J Natl Cancer Inst* 1997;89:1132–1138.

63. Shibuya K, Mathers CD, Boschi-Pinto C, Lopez AD, Murray CJ. Global and regional estimates of cancer mortality and incidence by site: II. Results for the global burden of disease 2000. *BMC Cancer* 2002;2:37.

64. Jemal A, Murray T, Ward E, et al. Cancer statistics, 2005. *CA Cancer J Clin* 2005;55:10 30.

65. Mayer RJ. Pancreatic cancer. In: Kasper DL, Braunwald E, Fauci AS, et al., eds. *Harrison's Principles of Internal Medicine*, 16th ed. http://www.harrisonsonline.com McGraw Hill; 2005.

66. Anderson KE, Mack TM, Silverman D. Pancreatic cancer. In: Schottenfeld D, Fraumeni JF, eds. *Cancer Epidemiology and Prevention*. New York: Oxford University Press; 2005.

67. Sahmoun AE, D'Agostino RA, Jr, Bell RA, Schwenke DC. International variation in pancreatic cancer mortality for the period 1955–1998. *Eur J Epidemiol* 2003;18:801–816.

68. Lowenfels AB, Maisonneuve P. Epidemiology and prevention of pancreatic cancer. *Jpn J Clin Oncol* 2004;34:238–244.

69. Edwards BK, Brown ML, Wingo PA, et al. Annual report to the nation on the status of cancer, 1975–2002, featuring population-based trends in cancer treatments. *J Natl Cancer Inst* 2005;97(19):1407–1427.

70. Silverman DT, Hoover RN, Brown LM, et al. Why do black Americans have a higher risk of pancreatic cancer than white Americans? *Epidemiology* 2003;14:45–54.

71. Lowenfels AB, Maisonneuve P, DiMagno EP, et al. Hereditary pancreatitis and the risk of pancreatic cancer. International Hereditary Pancreatitis Study Group. *J Natl Cancer Inst* 1997;89:442–446.

72. Lowenfels AB, Maisonneuve P, Cavallini G, et al. Pancreatitis and the risk of pancreatic cancer. International Pancreatitis Study Group. *N Engl J Med* 1993;328:1433–1437.

73. Huxley R, Ansary-Moghaddam A, Berrington DG, Barzi F, Woodward M. Type-II diabetes and pancreatic cancer: a meta-analysis of 36 studies. *Br J Cancer* 2005;92:2076–2083.

74. Silverman DT, Schiffman M, Everhart J, et al. Diabetes mellitus, other medical conditions and familial history of cancer as risk factors for pancreatic cancer. *Br J Cancer* 1999;80:1830–1837.

75. Berrington A, Sweetland S, Spencer E. A meta-analysis of obesity and the risk of pancreatic cancer. *Br J Cancer* 2003;89:519–523.

76. Stolzenberg-Solomon RZ, Graubard BI, Chari S, et al. Insulin, glucose, insulin resistance, and pancreatic cancer in male smokers. *JAMA* 2005; 294:2872–2878.

77. Hansel DE, Kern SE, Hruban RH. Molecular pathogenesis of pancreatic cancer. *Annu Rev Genomics Hum Genet* 2003;4:237–256.

78. Schottenfeld D, Islam SS. Cancers of the small intestine. In: Schottenfeld D, Fraumeni JF, eds. *Cancer Epidemiology and Prevention*. New York: Oxford University Press; 806–812.

79. Chow JS, Chen CC, Ahsan H, Neugut AI. A population-based study of the incidence of malignant small bowel tumours: SEER, 1973–1990. *Int J Epidemiol* 1996;25:722–728.

80. Neugut AI, Jacobson JS, Suh S, Mukherjee R, Arber N. The epidemiology of cancer of the small bowel. *Cancer Epidemiol Biomarkers Prev* 1998;7:243–251.

81. Parkin DM, Bray F, Ferlay J, Pisani P. Global cancer statistics 2002. *CA Cancer J Clin* 2005;55:74–108.

82. Parkin DM, Whelan SL, Ferlay J, et al., eds. *Cancer Incidence in Five Continents. Vol. VIII. IARC Scientific Publications No. 155.* Lyon, France: IARC Press; 2002.

83. Le Marchand L. Combined influence of genetic and dietary factors on colorectal cancer incidence in Japanese Americans. *J Natl Cancer Inst Monographs* 1999;26:101–105.

84. Potter JD. Nutrition and colorectal cancer. *Cancer Causes Control* 1996;7:127–146.

85. Giovannucci E. Modifiable risk factors for colon cancer. *Gastroenterol Clin North Am* 2002;31:925–943.

86. Fearon ER, Vogelstein B. A genetic model for colorectal tumorigenesis. *Cell* 1990;61:759–767.

87. Swan J, Breen N, Coates RJ, Rimer BK, Lee NC. Progress in cancer screening practices in the United States. Results from the 2000 National Health Interview Survey. *Cancer* 2003;97:1528–1540.

88. Kroke A, Klipstein-Grobusch K, Hoffmann K, Terbeck I, Boeing H, Helander A. Comparison of self-reported alcohol intake with the urinary excretion of 5-hydroxytryptophol:5-hydroxyindole-3-acetic acid, a biomarker of recent alcohol intake. *Br J Nutr* 2001;85:621–627.

89. World Health Organization (WHO). *Global Status Report on Alcohol*. Geneva: WHO; 2004.

90. Rehm J, Room R, Graham K, Monteiro M, Gmel G, Sempos CT. The relationship of average volume of alcohol consumption and patterns of drinking to burden of disease: an overview. *Addiction* 2003;98:1209–1228.

91. Danaei G, Vander Hoorn S, Lopez AD, Murray CJ, Ezzati M. Causes of cancer in the world: comparative risk assessment of nine behavioural and environmental risk factors. *Lancet* 2005;366:1784–1793.

92. Boffetta P, Hashibe M, La Vecchia C, Zatonski W, Rehm J. The burden of cancer attributable to alcohol drinking. *Int J Cancer* 2006;119:884–887.

93. Corrao G, Bagnardi V, Zambon A, La Vecchia C. A meta-analysis of alcohol consumption and the risk of 15 diseases. *Prev Med* 2004;38:613–619.

94. Bagnardi V, Blangiardo M, La Vecchia C, Corrao G. Alcohol consumption and the risk of cancer: a meta-analysis. *Alcohol Res Health* 2001;25:263–270.

95. Polesel J, Dal Maso L, Bagnardi V, et al. Estimating dose–response relationship between ethanol and risk of cancer using regression spline models. *Int J Cancer* 2005;114:836–841.

96. Lewis SJ, Smith GD. Alcohol, ALDH2, and esophageal cancer: a meta-analysis which illustrates the potentials and limitations of a Mendelian randomization approach. *Cancer Epidemiol Biomarkers Prev* 2005;14:1967–1971.

97. Hashibe M, Boffetta P, Zaridze D, et al. Evidence for an important role of alcohol- and aldehyde-metabolizing genes in cancers of the upper aerodigestive tract. *Cancer Epidemiol Biomarkers Prev* 2006;15:696–703.

98. Poschl G, Seitz HK. Alcohol and cancer. *Alcohol* 2004;39:155–165.

99. Steenbergen RD, de Wilde J, Wilting SM, Brink AA, Snijders PJ, Meijer CJ. HPV-mediated transformation of the anogenital tract. *J Clin Virol* 2005;32(suppl 1):S25–S33.

100. Herrero R. Chapter 7: human papillomavirus and cancer of the upper aerodigestive tract. *J Natl Cancer Inst Monogr* 2003;47–51.

101. Kreimer AR, Clifford GM, Boyle P, Franceschi S. Human papillomavirus types in head and neck squamous cell carcinomas worldwide: a systematic review. *Cancer Epidemiol Biomarkers Prev* 2005;14:467–475.

102. Daling JR, Madeleine MM, Johnson LG, et al. Human papillomavirus, smoking, and sexual practices in the etiology of anal cancer. *Cancer* 2004; 101:270–280.

103. Gillison ML, Shah KV. Chapter 9: role of mucosal human papillomavirus in nongenital cancers. *J Natl Cancer Inst Monogr* 2003;57–65.

104. Parkin DM. The global health burden of infection-associated cancers in the year 2002. *Int J Cancer* 2006;118:3030–3044.

105. Yu MW, Chen CJ. Hepatitis B and C viruses in the development of hepatocellular carcinoma. *Crit Rev Oncol Hematol* 1994;17:71–91.

106. Wasley A, Alter MJ. Epidemiology of hepatitis C: geographic differences and temporal trends. *Semin Liver Dis* 2000;20:1–16.

107. El-Serag HB. Hepatocellular carcinoma and hepatitis C in the United States. *Hepatology* 2002;36:S74–S83.

108. Bosch FX, Ribes J, Cleries R, Diaz M. Epidemiology of hepatocellular carcinoma. *Clin Liver Dis* 2005;9:191–211.

109. Yu MW, Yeh SH, Chen PJ, et al. Hepatitis B virus genotype and DNA level and hepatocellular carcinoma: a prospective study in men. *J Natl Cancer Inst* 2005;97:265–272.

110. Alter MJ. Epidemiology and prevention of hepatitis B. *Semin Liver Dis* 2003;23:39–46.

111. International Agency for Research on Cancer (IARC). *IARC Monographs on the Evaluation of Carcinogenic Risks to Humans. Vol. 61. Schistosomes, Liver Flukes and Helicobacter pylori.* Lyon, France: IARC Press; 1994.

112. Chow WH, Blaser MJ, Blot WJ, et al. An inverse relation between cagA+ strains of *Helicobacter pylori* infection and risk of esophageal and gastric cardia adenocarcinoma. *Cancer Res* 1998;58:588–590.

113. Brown LM. *Helicobacter pylori*: epidemiology and routes of transmission. *Epidemiol Rev* 2000;22:283–297.

114. Suerbaum S, Michetti P. *Helicobacter pylori* infection. *N Engl J Med* 2002; 347:1175–1186.

115. Montecucco C, Rappuoli R. Living dangerously: how *Helicobacter pylori* survives in the human stomach. *Nat Rev Mol Cell Biol* 2001;2:457–466.

116. Correa P, Schneider BG. Etiology of gastric cancer: what is new? *Cancer Epidemiol Biomarkers Prev* 2005;14:1865–1868.

117. El-Omar EM, Carrington M, Chow WH, et al. Interleukin-1 polymorphisms associated with increased risk of gastric cancer. *Nature* 2000;404: 398–402.

118. Gonzalez CA, Pena S, Capella G. Clinical usefulness of virulence factors of *Helicobacter pylori* as predictors of the outcomes of infection. What is the evidence? *Scand J Gastroenterol* 2003;38:905–915.

119. Wong BC, Lam SK, Wong WM, et al. *Helicobacter pylori* eradication to prevent gastric cancer in a high-risk region of China: a randomized controlled trial. *JAMA* 2004;291:187–194.

120. Flegal KM, Carroll MD, Kuczmarski RJ, Johnson CL. Overweight and obesity in the United States: prevalence and trends, 1960–1994. *Int J Obes Relat Metab Disord* 1998;22:39–47.

121. York DA, Rossner S, Caterson I, et al. Prevention conference VII: obesity, a worldwide epidemic related to heart disease and stroke: group I: worldwide demographics of obesity. *Circulation* 2004;110:e463–e470.

122. Ogden CL, Carroll MD, Curtin LR, McDowell MA, Tabak CJ, Flegal KM. Prevalence of overweight and obesity in the United States, 1999–2004. *JAMA* 2006;295:1549–1555.

123. El Serag HB. Hepatocellular carcinoma: recent trends in the United States. *Gastroenterology* 2004;127:S27–S34.

124. International Agency for Research on Cancer (IARC). *IARC Handbook of Cancer Prevention. Weight Control and Physical Activity.* Lyon, France: IARC Press; 2002.

125. Wolk A, Gridley G, Svensson M, et al. A prospective study of obesity and cancer risk (Sweden). *Cancer Causes Control* 2001;12:13–21.

126. Samanic C, Gridley G, Chow WH, Lubin J, Hoover RN, Fraumeni JF, Jr. Obesity and cancer risk among white and black United States veterans. *Cancer Causes Control* 2004;15:35–43.

127. Calle EE, Rodriguez C, Walker-Thurmond K, Thun MJ. Overweight, obesity, and mortality from cancer in a prospectively studied cohort of U.S. adults. *N Engl J Med* 2003;348:1625–1638.
128. Lukanova A, Bjor O, Kaaks R, et al. Body mass index and cancer: results from the Northern Sweden Health and Disease Cohort. *Int J Cancer* 2006;118:458–466.
129. Moschos SJ, Mantzoros CS. The role of the IGF system in cancer: from basic to clinical studies and clinical applications. *Oncology* 2002;63:317–332.
130. Calle EE, Thun MJ. Obesity and cancer. *Oncogene* 2004;23:6365–6378.
131. Wei EK, Ma J, Pollak MN, et al. A prospective study of C-peptide, insulin-like growth factor-I, insulin-like growth factor binding protein-1, and the risk of colorectal cancer in women. *Cancer Epidemiol Biomarkers Prev* 2005;14:850–855.
132. Kaaks R, Toniolo P, Akhmedkhanov A, et al. Serum C-peptide, insulin-like growth factor (IGF)-I, IGF-binding proteins, and colorectal cancer risk in women. *J Natl Cancer Inst* 2000;92:1592–1600.
133. Kaaks R, Lukanova A. Energy balance and cancer: the role of insulin and insulin growth factor-I. *Proc Nutr Soc* 2001;60:91–106.
134. Wang Y, Herrington M, Larsson J, Permert J. The relationship between diabetes and pancreatic cancer. *Mol Cancer* 2003;2:4.
135. Jee SH, Ohrr H, Sull JW, Yun JE, Ji M, Samet JM. Fasting serum glucose level and cancer risk in Korean men and women. *JAMA* 2005;293:194–202.
136. Gapstur SM, Gann PH, Lowe W, Liu K, Colangelo L, Dyer A. Abnormal glucose metabolism and pancreatic cancer mortality. *JAMA* 2000;283:2552–2558.
137. Batty GD, Shipley MJ, Marmot M, Smith GD. Diabetes status and post-load plasma glucose concentration in relation to site-specific cancer mortality: findings from the original Whitehall study. *Cancer Causes Control* 2004;15:873–881.
138. Stolzenberg-Solomon RZ, Graubard BI, Chari S, et al. Insulin, glucose, insulin resistance, and pancreatic cancer in male smokers. *JAMA* 2005;294:2872–2878.
139. Weyer C, Funahashi T, Tanaka S, et al. Hypoadiponectinemia in obesity and type 2 diabetes: close association with insulin resistance and hyperinsulinemia. *J Clin Endocrinol Metab* 2001;86:1930–1935.
140. Ishikawa M, Kitayama J, Kazama S, Hiramatsu T, Hatano K, Nagawa H. Plasma adiponectin and gastric cancer. *Clin Cancer Res* 2005;11:466–472.
141. Otake S, Takeda H, Suzuki Y, et al. Association of visceral fat accumulation and plasma adiponectin with colorectal adenoma: evidence for participation of insulin resistance. *Clin Cancer Res* 2005;11:3642–3646.
142. Wei EK, Giovannucci E, Fuchs CS, Willett WC, Mantzoros CS. Low plasma adiponectin levels and risk of colorectal cancer in men: a prospective study. *J Natl Cancer Inst* 2005;97:1688–1694.
143. Lihn AS, Pedersen SB, Richelsen B. Adiponectin: action, regulation and association to insulin sensitivity. *Obes Rev* 2005;6:13–21.
144. Engel LS, Chow WH, Vaughan TL, et al. Population attributable risks of esophageal and gastric cancers. *J Natl Cancer Inst* 2003;95:1404–1413.
145. Lagergren J, Bergstrom R, Adami HO, Nyren O. Association between medications that relax the lower esophageal sphincter and risk for esophageal adenocarcinoma. *Ann Intern Med* 2000;133:165–175.
146. Misra S, Chaturvedi A, Misra NC, Sharma ID. Carcinoma of the gallbladder. *Lancet Oncol* 2003;4:167–176.
147. Wellen KE, Hotamisligil GS. Inflammation, stress, and diabetes. *J Clin Invest* 2005;115:1111–1119.
148. Balkwill F, Coussens LM. Cancer: an inflammatory link. *Nature* 2004;431:405–406.
149. Coussens LM, Werb Z. Inflammation and cancer. *Nature* 2002;420:860–867.
150. Steinmetz KA, Potter JD. Vegetables, fruit, and cancer. I. Epidemiology. *Cancer Causes Control* 1991;2:325–357.
151. Riboli E, Norat T. Epidemiologic evidence of the protective effect of fruit and vegetable consumption on cancer risk. *Am J Clin Nutr* 2003;78:559–569.
152. Schatzkin A, Kipnis V. Could exposure assessment problems give us wrong answers to nutrition and cancer questions? *J Natl Cancer Inst* 2004;96:1564–1565.
153. Lunet N, Lacerda-Vieira A, Barros H. Fruit and vegetables consumption and gastric cancer: a systematic review and meta-analysis of cohort studies. *Nutr Cancer* 2005;53:1–10.
154. Schatzkin A, Lanza E, Corle D, et al. Lack of effect of a low-fat, high-fiber diet on the recurrence of colorectal adenomas. Polyp Prevention Trial Study Group. *N Engl J Med* 2000;342:1149–1155.
155. Kristal AR, Blount PL, Schenk JM, et al. Low-fat, high fruit and vegetable diets and weight loss do not affect biomarkers of cellular proliferation in Barrett esophagus. *Cancer Epidemiol Biomarkers Prev* 2005;14:2377–2383.
156. Beresford SA, Johnson KC, Ritenbaugh C, et al. Low-fat dietary pattern and risk of colorectal cancer: the Women's Health Initiative Randomized Controlled Dietary Modification Trial. *JAMA* 2006;295:643–654.
157. Link LB, Potter JD. Raw versus cooked vegetables and cancer risk. *Cancer Epidemiol Biomarkers Prev* 2004;13:1422–1435.
158. Potter JD. Vegetables, fruit, and cancer. *Lancet* 2005;366:527–530.
159. Norat T, Riboli E. Fruit and vegetable consumption and risk of cancer of the digestive tract: meta-analysis of published case-control and cohort studies. *IARC Sci Publ* 2002;156:123–125.
160. http://www.wcrf.org/research/fnatpoc.lasso.
161. Norat T, Lukanova A, Ferrari P, Riboli E. Meat consumption and colorectal cancer risk: dose–response meta-analysis of epidemiological studies. *Int J Cancer* 2002;98:241–256.
162. Willett WC, Stampfer MJ, Colditz GA, Rosner BA, Speizer FE. Relation of meat, fat, and fiber intake to the risk of colon cancer in a prospective study among women [see comments]. *N Engl J Med* 1990;323:1664–1672.
163. Giovannucci E, Rimm EB, Stampfer MJ, Colditz GA, Ascherio A, Willett WC. Intake of fat, meat, and fiber in relation to risk of colon cancer in men. *Cancer Res* 1994;54:2390–2397.
164. Goldbohm RA, van den Brandt PA, van't Veer P, et al. A prospective cohort study on the relation between meat consumption and the risk of colon cancer. *Cancer Res* 1994;54:718–723.
165. Singh PN, Fraser GE. Dietary risk factors for colon cancer in a low-risk population. *Am J Epidemiol* 1998;148:761–774.
166. Norat T, Bingham S, Ferrari P, et al. Meat, fish, and colorectal cancer risk: the European Prospective Investigation into Cancer and Nutrition. *J Natl Cancer Inst* 2005;97:906–916.
167. Lewin ML, Bailey N, Bandaletova T, et al. Red meat enhances the colonic formation of the DNA adduct O^6-carboxymethyl guanine: implications for colorectal cancer risk. *Cancer Res* 2006;66:1859–1865.
168. Ito LS, Inoue M, Tajima K, et al. Dietary factors and the risk of gastric cancer among Japanese women: a comparison between the differentiated and non-differentiated subtypes. *Ann Epidemiol* 2003;13:24–31.
169. Ngoan LT, Mizoue T, Fujino Y, Tokui N, Yoshimura T. Dietary factors and stomach cancer mortality. *Br J Cancer* 2002;87:37–42.
170. Kneller RW, McLaughlin JK, Bjelke E, et al. A cohort study of stomach cancer in a high-risk American population. *Cancer* 1991;68:672–678.
171. Inoue M, Tajima K, Kobayashi S, et al. Protective factor against progression from atrophic gastritis to gastric cancer—data from a cohort study in Japan. *Int J Cancer* 1996;66:309–314.
172. Van den Brandt PA, Botterweck AA, Goldbohm RA. Salt intake, cured meat consumption, refrigerator use and stomach cancer incidence: a prospective cohort study (Netherlands). *Cancer Causes Control* 2003;14:427–438.
173. Gonzalez CA, Jakszyn P, Pera G, et al. Meat intake and risk of stomach and esophageal adenocarcinoma within the European Prospective Investigation into Cancer and Nutrition (EPIC). *J Natl Cancer Inst* 2006;98:345–354.
174. Jakszyn P, Bingham S, Pera G, et al. Endogenous versus exogenous exposure to N-nitroso compounds and gastric cancer risk in the European Prospective Investigation into Cancer and Nutrition (EPIC-EURGAST) study. *Carcinogenesis* 2006;27:1497–1501.
175. Hampel H, Frankel WL, Martin E, et al. Screening for the Lynch syndrome (hereditary nonpolyposis colorectal cancer). *N Engl J Med* 2005;352:1851–1860.
176. Vasen HF. Clinical description of the Lynch syndrome [hereditary nonpolyposis colorectal cancer (HNPCC)]. *Fam Cancer* 2005;4:219–225.
177. Umar A, Boland CR, Terdiman JP, et al. Revised Bethesda guidelines for hereditary nonpolyposis colorectal cancer (Lynch syndrome) and microsatellite instability. *J Natl Cancer Inst* 2004;96:261–268.
178. Vasen HF. Clinical diagnosis and management of hereditary colorectal cancer syndromes. *J Clin Oncol* 2000;18:81S–92S.
179. Doxey BW, Kuwada SK, Burt RW. Inherited polyposis syndromes: molecular mechanisms, clinicopathology, and genetic testing. *Clin Gastroenterol Hepatol* 2005;3:633–641.
180. Al Tassan N, Chmiel NH, Maynard J, et al. Inherited variants of MYH associated with somatic G:C→T:A mutations in colorectal tumors. *Nat Genet* 2002;30:227–232.
181. Nielsen M, Franken PF, Reinards TH, et al. Multiplicity in polyp count and extracolonic manifestations in 40 Dutch patients with MYH associated polyposis coli (MAP). *J Med Genet* 2005;42:e54.
182. Lim W, Hearle N, Shah B, et al. Further observations on LKB1/STK11 status and cancer risk in Peutz-Jeghers syndrome. *Br J Cancer* 2003;89:308–313.
183. Chow E, Macrae F. A review of juvenile polyposis syndrome. *J Gastroenterol Hepatol* 2005;20:1634–1640.
184. Warthin AS. Heredity with reference to carcinoma. *Arch Int Med* 2006;12:546–555.
185. Park JG, Park YJ, Wijnen JT, Vasen HF. Gene–environment interaction in hereditary nonpolyposis colorectal cancer with implications for diagnosis and genetic testing. *Int J Cancer* 1999;82:516–519.
186. Fitzgerald RC, Caldas C. Clinical implications of E-cadherin associated hereditary diffuse gastric cancer. *Gut* 2004;53:775–778.
187. Schenk M, Schwartz AG, O'Neal E, et al. Familial risk of pancreatic cancer. *J Natl Cancer Inst* 2001;93:640–644.
188. Vasen HF, Gruis NA, Frants RR, Der Velden PA, Hille ET, Bergman W. Risk of developing pancreatic cancer in families with familial atypical multiple mole melanoma associated with a specific 19 deletion of p16 (p16-Leiden). *Int J Cancer* 2000;87:809–811.
189. van Asperen CJ, Brohet RM, Meijers-Heijboer EJ, et al. Cancer risks in BRCA2 families: estimates for sites other than breast and ovary. *J Med Genet* 2005;42:711–719.

CHAPTER 2 ■ GASTROINTESTINAL CANCER: PATHOLOGY AND MOLECULAR PATHOLOGY

ALESSANDRO LUGLI AND JEREMY R. JASS

INTRODUCTION

"Frequently consider the connection of all things in the universe and their relation to one another" wrote the Roman Emperor Marcus Aurelius (121–180 AD) in his *Meditations* (1). This quotation can be applied to the current management of human cancer, whereby practitioners from different disciplines work together to ensure the highest quality of treatment for their patients. Because pathology is the branch of medicine that studies the mechanisms of cell, tissue, and organ injury that underlie a disease process, the pathological evaluation of tumor tissue is an essential component of the management of patients with gastrointestinal cancer, from initial diagnosis through the various stages of treatment.

The pathologist's tumor diagnosis is generally based on classification schemes that encompass reproducible clinical, morphologic, and molecular criteria. These features provide the diagnostic signatures of human cancers. Tumor classifications are by their nature artificial because biological processes occur as continua. They are also provisional and susceptible to change in the face of new information and evidence. Nevertheless, highly successful and widely accepted classifications of human tumors have been published in a series by the World Health Organization (WHO) and in a systemic series of fascicles by the U.S. Armed Forces Institute of Pathology. The typing of neoplasia is based on histogenesis or comparison with a normal tissue counterpart.

The diagnosis of cancer may be suspected on the basis of a patient's symptoms, the findings on clinical examination, and imaging modalities such as computed tomography, ultrasound scanning, magnetic resonance imaging, and barium studies. However, a tissue diagnosis based on the morphologic evaluation of a tissue section stained with hematoxylin and eosin (H&E) is the gold standard for the diagnosis of malignancy. The first task of the pathologist is to differentiate a reactive process from neoplasia. Second, benign neoplasia must be distinguished from a malignant process that is characterized by the invasion and destruction of local tissues as well as the potential for metastasis. Sometimes, the differentiation between a primary tumor and a metastasis is not possible with an H&E stain. Ancillary studies using special stains, immunohistochemistry, or molecular analysis may assist in this fundamental distinction, and may contribute clinically useful information on the type, grade, and potential behavior of a tumor.

A uniform and standardized system for classifying the extent of malignancy (staging) is essential to compare therapeutic intervention and estimate outcome. The American Joint Committee on Cancer (AJCC), in cooperation with the TNM (tumor, node, metastasis) Committee of the International Union Against Cancer (UICC), has incorporated factors in relation to tumor spread into a comprehensive TNM staging system (2,3). For most organs, the size of the tumor at its primary site and/or the involvement of local structures describe the tumor topography (T). The presence and extent of regional lymph node (N) involvement and whether there is evidence of distant metastasis (M) indicate the tumor spread. The categories for T, N, and M are condensed into stages 0 to IV, which are the most important determinants of prognosis (2). For example, the prognosis of advanced gastric cancer (spread beyond submucosa or at least T2) is poor, and even after curative resection, the 5-year survival rate ranges from 26% to 35% (4).

The emerging knowledge on the molecular pathogenesis of gastrointestinal neoplasias has lead to the exploration of molecular alterations that could be used to improve diagnosis and management. For example, *KIT* alterations distinguish gastrointestinal stromal tumor (GIST) from other benign or malignant types of stromal tumors, whereas the immunohistochemical detection of proteins encoded by the mismatch repair genes, notably *MSH2*, *MLH1*, and *MSH6*, have been linked with hereditary forms of colorectal cancer.

Clinical symptoms are often forgotten tumor-related prognostic factors. The presence of tumor-related symptoms such as weight loss, obstruction, and perforation fever are important prognostic factors in most patients with cancer (5–8). Napoleon Bonaparte (1769–1821), who was afflicted with an advanced gastric cancer, presented with weight loss, fever, and night sweats (9,10).

This chapter introduces the reader to the general principles of gross pathology, histopathology, and molecular concepts that are essential for the diagnosis, classification, and prognostication of gastrointestinal neoplasms.

PATHOLOGY OF GASTROINTESTINAL MALIGNANCIES

Diagnosis of Malignant Gastrointestinal Tumors

The diagnosis of cancer includes the examination of cytologic and tissue specimens for features that differentiate a reactive process from benign or malignant neoplasia. Aspiration or core needle biopsy, biopsy, cell brushing, or tumor resection are procedures for obtaining samples of cells and tissues. The diagnosis of tumors as benign or malignant is primarily based on cytologic and histologic criteria. Nevertheless, immunocytochemistry (performed on cytologic preparations) and immunohistochemistry are complementary and useful tools, not only in the diagnosis of cancer but also in the differentiation between a primary malignant tumor and a metastatic process.

Cytologic Assessment of Gastrointestinal Malignancy

The use of cytology for diagnosis of gastrointestinal tumors varies according to institutional practice and available expertise. The location and type of malignancy may also determine the relative appropriateness of cytologic examination. In general, cytologic specimens may be acquired via brushing or lavage from luminal tumors approached endoscopically, via aspiration of fluid from cystic tumors (e.g., in the pancreas or liver), or via fine-needle biopsy. Tumors of the tubal gut (except the jejunum and most of the ileum), papilla of Vater, and pancreaticobiliary ducts may be approached endoscopically from the lumen and brushed to collect cells from a broad surface area. This technique may be especially useful when luminal stricturing limits access to the tumor for forceps biopsy. Acquisition of cytologic specimens from pancreatic and hepatic tumors often requires the use of ultrasonic or other radiologic guidance techniques. Overall, cytologic approaches may allow for preoperative diagnosis of tumors that are otherwise inaccessible to standard biopsy or that pose particular risks of biopsy-associated complications.

Cytologic diagnosis is limited almost exclusively to identification of tumor and determination of tumor type. Preservation of tissue architecture is limited in cytologic specimens; therefore, assessment for invasion is not possible. In addition to aiding the initial diagnosis, cytologic approaches may be useful in staging of gastrointestinal malignancy. For example, in the TNM staging system for colon cancer of the AJCC and UICC, tumor cells in peritoneal fluid are classified as distant metastasis by convention (2). Thus, positive peritoneal cytology would establish a tumor as stage IV.

Histologic Assessment of Gastrointestinal Malignancy

Masses discovered by clinical examination, imaging, or endoscopic studies that are suspicious for malignancy typically require biopsy confirmation before treatment is initiated. The role of the biopsy is twofold: (a) to exclude the presence of benign lesions that may mimic malignancy clinically, and (b) if malignant tumor is present, to determine the histologic type. The majority of gastrointestinal tumors are carcinomas, and outside the esophagus and anus, they are mainly adenocarcinomas. A large number of other malignant tumors, however, may clinically resemble gastrointestinal carcinomas. These include lymphomas, neuroendocrine tumors, mesenchymal tumors (e.g., GIST), metastatic tumors that exhibit tropism for the gastrointestinal tract (e.g., melanomas), and malignancies of adjacent organs that directly invade the gastrointestinal tract (e.g., cancers of the ovary, endometrium, urinary bladder, or prostate). Benign lesions that may mimic gastrointestinal carcinomas include adenomas, hamartomas, benign ulceration (usually due to ischemia or inflammatory processes, such as *Helicobacter pylori* infection in the stomach or cytomegalovirus infection in the colon), endometriosis, inflammatory conditions such as inflammatory bowel disease (Crohn's disease or ulcerative colitis), solitary rectal ulcer syndrome, and diverticular disease with mural stricturing.

Multiple biopsy specimens taken from the edges and base of an ulcerating lesion or from the surface of a polypoid mass typically reveal the correct diagnosis. When an obstructing mass is present, however, passage of an endoscope to obtain diagnostic tissue may be difficult; thus, brush cytology may be useful to confirm the diagnosis in this situation. Even when direct access to the tumor is possible, biopsy specimens may fail to yield a definitive diagnosis if the lesion is extensively ulcerated or otherwise necrotic and viable tumor tissue is not obtained on sampling. The diagnostic yield is improved when multiple biopsy samples are taken, and for ulcerated lesions, when samples are obtained from the ulcer edge at all four quadrants and from the ulcer center. For ulcerated carcinomas, biopsy specimens obtained from the periphery of the ulcer are likely to contain viable tumor. In contrast, for ulcerated lymphomas and sarcomas, biopsy samples obtained from the center of the lesion are likely to contain diagnostic tissue.

Even when incisional biopsies (i.e., diagnostic needle or endoscopic forceps biopsies) are successful, the type and amount of information that can be derived from the specimen is limited. Pathological confirmation of the presence of malignancy and its histologic type may be unequivocally established with an adequate biopsy, but the tumor grade and presence of invasion (of carcinomas) may be difficult or even impossible to determine. Even for carcinomas in which stromal invasion is identified with certainty, the deepest extent of invasion cannot be determined from incisional biopsy material. Furthermore, luminal biopsies from the tubal gut or the papilla of Vater, extrahepatic bile ducts, and pancreatic ducts are typically limited in depth to the superficial mucosa or deep lamina propria, respectively. Thus, tumors with primarily submucosal or mural growth, such as lymphomas, neuroendocrine tumors, and sarcomas, may be missed on luminal biopsy unless a single biopsy site is sampled repeatedly to obtain deeper tissue.

Immunohistochemical Assessment of Gastrointestinal Malignancy

Morphologic assessment may not be diagnostic in the case of poorly differentiated tumors. Additional techniques, including special histochemical stains, immunohistochemical stains, or electron microscopy, may be required to detect specific features of cell lineage or differentiation. Because electron microscopy is labor intensive, several days may be required to obtain results. It also requires tissue fixation in glutaraldehyde rather than 10% formalin for optimal preservation of ultrastructural features. For these reasons, electron microscopy is rarely adopted as the technique of choice for additional studies on diagnostic biopsy specimens. In contrast, special histochemical stains can be performed within hours on fixed tissue. For example, neutral and acidic mucins (adenocarcinoma), glycoproteins (adenocarcinoma or hepatocellular carcinoma), neurosecretory granules (neuroendocrine tumors), melanin (primary or metastatic melanoma), and other tumor cell products or associated proteins can be identified by special stains.

Immunohistochemical stains are now in common use and constitute the most powerful tools in the diagnostic armamentarium of the surgical pathologist. Compared with electron microscopy and special stains, immunohistochemistry is both more sensitive and more specific for revealing differentiation markers. Because the standard procedure in most institutions is to fix diagnostic biopsy specimens immediately in 10% formalin, antibodies that can be used on paraffin-embedded, formalin-fixed tissue are the most useful and widely used. Some antigens, however, are altered by fixation or heat (required for paraffin embedding), and fresh tissue may be required for their immunolocalization. Gastrointestinal lymphomas, for example, may require fresh tissue for immunolabeling of light chains to demonstrate clonality. There is increasing availability, however, of commercially available monoclonal antibodies that give excellent results with formalin-fixed tissues. It is absolutely essential that immunohistochemical analysis of a tumor is used in the context of a carefully selected differential diagnosis based on clinical data and morphologic features of the tumor.

TABLE 2.1

IMMUNOHISTOCHEMICAL STAINS USED IN THE DIAGNOSIS AND DIFFERENTIAL DIAGNOSIS OF GASTROINTESTINAL TUMORS

Antigen	Tumor type
CARCINOMAS	
Cytokeratin 22	Carcinomas
Cytokeratin 20+, Cytokeratin 7–	Adenocarcinoma of colon
Cytokeratin 7+, Cytokeratin 20–	Carcinoma of the ovary, stomach, pancreas
CDX2	Primary gastrointestinal carcinomas
Alpha-fetoprotein, hepatocyte paraffin 1 (Hep Par1), polyclonal carcinoembryonic antigen (pCEA)	Hepatocellular carcinoma
Amylase, trypsin, chymotrypsin, lipase	Pancreatic acinar cell carcinoma
Estrogen receptor (ER) and progesterone receptor (PR)	Breast cancer
RCC	Renal cell carcinoma
Prostatic-specific antigen (PSA)	Carcinoma of the prostate
Thyroid transcription factor (TTF)	Carcinoma of the lung
SARCOMAS	
Vimentin	Mesenchymal tumors
Actin, smooth muscle actin (SMA), desmin	Smooth muscle tumors
CD31, CD34	Angiosarcomas
HMB45, MelanA, S-100	Malignant melanoma
Calretinin	Mesothelioma
LYMPHOMAS	
Leukocyte common antigen (LCA; CD45)	Lymphoma
Antigens of B- and T-cell lineage	Hematologic malignancies
GENERAL MARKERS	
Ki-67 (MIB-1)	Cell proliferation marker in all tumors

One of the most challenging problems for a surgical pathologist is the diagnosis of a poorly differentiated tumor when no primary site is clinically evident. Fortunately, malignant cells, even when poorly differentiated, continue to express antigens that characterize the cell or tissue of origin. Lineage-dependent expression of proteins is therefore maintained in most poorly differentiated cancers. Immunohistochemical analysis with appropriate antibodies can usefully differentiate, for example, epithelial, mesenchymal tumors, neuroendocrine tumors, lymphomas, and melanomas. Pancytokeratin markers such as LU5 or CK22 can distinguish carcinomas (positive) from other poorly differentiated tumors (negative). The latter group includes the differential diagnosis of neuroendocrine tumors (positive for synaptophysin-, chromogranin-, and neuron-specific enolase), melanomas (positive for HMB45, S-100, and MelanA), and lymphomas (positive for CD45). Sarcomas of the gastrointestinal tract are recognized with antibodies to desmin (positive in smooth and skeletal muscle tissue), actin (smooth muscle tissue), and vimentin. GIST are typically positive for CD117 (KIT) and CD34.

In addition, cytokeratins (CKs) have a diverse and lineage-specific expression pattern that has been shown to identify the site of origin of many epithelial tumors. The CKs include at least 20 different polypeptide chains, and two-dimensional gel electrophoresis studies have shown that these are distributed in a relatively tissue-specific manner. The CK profile of the epithelial tissue of origin is retained by the tumor. For example, more than 95% of adenocarcinomas of the colon are CK20 positive but CK7 negative. This may assist with the distinction from ovar-

ian cancer, which is usually CK7 positive and CK20 negative. CDX2 is a homeobox domain-containing transcription factor important in the development and differentiation of the intestine. It serves as a sensitive and specific marker for colorectal adenocarcinoma and is also helpful in distinguishing adenocarcinomas of the papilla from those arising in the pancreas and biliary tree (11). Metastatic prostate cancer can be recognized by positivity for prostatic-specific antigen, and metastases of breast cancers are often positive for estrogen and/or progesteron receptors. In addition, but more rarely, metastasis from lung cancers (TTF positive), renal cancers (RCC positive), and mesothelioma (calretinin positive) have to be considered in the differential diagnosis. Some of the more commonly used antibodies in gastrointestinal tumor diagnosis are summarized in Table 2.1.

Unfortunately, the initial impression of high specificity for a particular marker of differentiation is frequently tempered by the test of time. In light of the inevitable limitation of a particular antibody with respect to its final utility as a diagnostic marker for a specific tumor type, there is a clear need for early and comprehensive analysis of novel diagnostic markers in both normal and neoplastic tissues. If traditional methods are used, such an evaluation would require the immunohistochemical interpretation of thousands of samples, a task that could not be completed by one laboratory in a reasonable time frame. Tissue microarray (TMA) technology is ideal for the standardized and high-throughput molecular analysis of new monoclonal antibodies (12–15). To analyze the specificity of an antibody in different normal and neoplastic tissue types, a set of TMAs

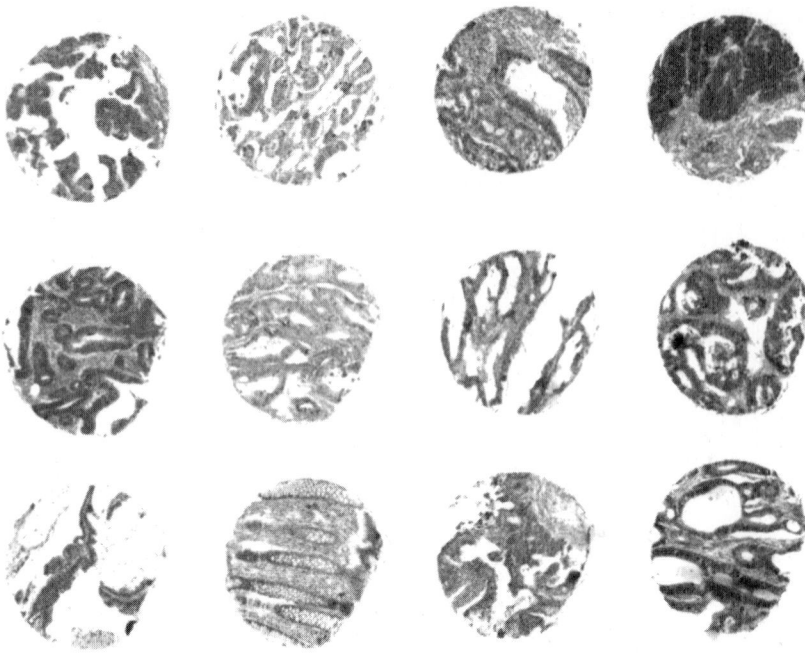

FIGURE 2.1. Tissue microarray showing differing intensity of epidermal growth factor receptor immunohistochemistry in multiple colorectal cancer punches (2×). *Source:* From the Archives of the Institute of Pathology, University Hospital Basel, Institute of Clinical Pathology, Basel and Institute of Pathology, Stadtspital Triemli, Zürich, Switzerland (See also color Figure 2.1).

containing either different tumor types or numerous examples of the same tumor type, as well as normal tissue samples, are prepared (16,17) (Figure 2.1). Beginning with archival specimens of formalin-fixed, paraffin-embedded tissue blocks, tissue cylinders with a diameter of 0.6 mm are punched from representative areas of each "donor" tissue block. These are then incorporated into a recipient paraffin block (3 × 2.5 cm) using, for example, a semiautomated tissue arrayer. The immunohistochemical results obtained by this method can be correlated with clinicopathological patient data to establish whether the marker is prognostic or predictive (18). In addition, the diagnostic utility of an antibody can be analyzed and characterized with respect to its immunohistochemical patterns. In a recent study, expression of hepatocyte paraffin 1 was found not only in hepatocellular carcinoma but also in gastric, small intestine, gallbladder, and adrenal gland carcinoma (19). Therefore, other markers would be required to distinguish these tumors: AFP, CD10, and p-CEA in hepatocellular carcinoma; CK7, CK13, and BerEp4 in gastric cancer; CK7, CK17, and BerEp4 in gallbladder carcinoma; CK13 and CK20 in small intestine carcinoma and vimentin; and MelanA and synaptophysin in adrenal gland carcinoma (19).

Apart from its application to immunohistochemistry, microarray technology allows the expression of thousands of genes within sets of tumors to be analyzed simultaneously. The first example of this revolution introducing a molecular as opposed to morphologic classification of tumors is seen in the analysis of lymphomas by Alizadeh et al. (20). Particular patterns of gene expression clusters may be correlated with morphologic, prognostic, or predictive outcomes to provide novel types of classification. However, it is likely that morphologic classifications will remain the gold standard for some time.

Classification of Malignant Gastrointestinal Tumors

The morphologic classification of tumors has evolved with the increased understanding of tumorigenesis. The classification of malignant gastrointestinal neoplasias has traditionally occurred at two levels: Macroscopic and microscopic.

Macroscopic Classification of Malignant Gastrointestinal Tumors

Despite the modern dominance of histologic features in achieving a final diagnosis, the macroscopic description of tumors on the basis of configuration, size, and anatomic site remains the first step in pathological examination. Classically, malignant tumors are solid, nonencapsulated, and characterized by large size, irregular and infiltrative borders, and presence of necrotic areas. An early example of a macroscopic classification is that of Borrmann. This subdivides advanced gastric cancer into four types: type I (polypoid), type II (fungating), type III (ulcerated), and type IV (infiltrative) (21). Types I and III occur commonly in the body, mainly the greater curvature, and account for about 25% of gastric carcinomas, whereas type II is frequently found in the antrum, along the lesser curvature, and represents approximately 35% of cases (22). Type IV is also known as linitis plastica. Macroscopic features have been used to distinguish a benign gastric ulcer from an ulcerated gastric carcinoma (type III). Gastric ulcers are usually small, well-circumscribed, punched-out lesions with a clean base and smooth, oedematosus margins. In contrast, ulcerated carcinomas have irregular borders, which are firm, fixed, and often raised, and the ulcer base is typically necrotic and hemorrhagic (23) (Figure 2.2). As stated by Ming and Goldman, careful inspection usually allows the observer to distinguish a malignant from a benign ulcer (24). A more contemporary contribution is the endoscopic classification of early gastric cancer (EGC) proposed by the Japan Gastroenterological Endoscopic Society (25). This system was developed in parallel with improving technology and increasing use of upper endoscopy, first in Japan and then worldwide (26–29). EGC is defined as invasive adenocarcinoma confined to the mucosa or submucosa with or without lymph node metastasis. EGC is subdivided into three types: Protruded (type I), superficial (type II), and excavated (type III). Type II is further subdivided into an elevated type IIa, flat type IIb, and depressed type IIc. The importance of recognizing an EGC lies in the fact that gastric surgery is then indicated and is usually curative (30).

The macroscopic classification of colorectal cancer (CRC) is similar to gastric cancer (31). (a) Exophytic, polypoid tumors typically occur in the cecum, rarely result in obstruction,

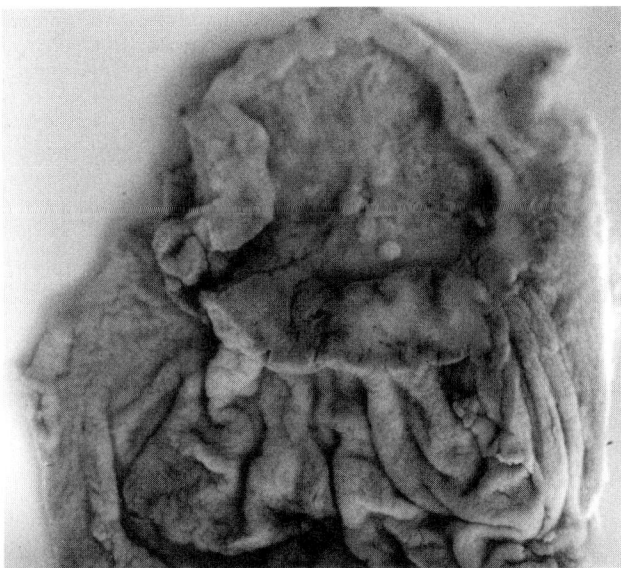

FIGURE 2.2. Gastric cancer, ulcerated type (Borrmann III). The ulcer base is necrotic, and the tumor borders are irregular and have been trimmed to show pale cancer tissue (See also color Figure 2.2).

and often achieve a large size before clinical presentation. (b) Ulcerating and infiltrative tumors are characterized by raised, irregular edges and a central ulcer. (c) Annular and constricting tumors often result in desmoplasia, which results in a firm consistency, proximal dilatation due to a functional obstruction and a characteristic double-contrast "apple-core" lesion. (d) Diffuse tumors infiltrate the entire bowel wall and are analogous to linitis plastica of the stomach. Although the gross appearance is variable, the cut section of all macroscopic types is normally homogenous, comprising firm pale tissue admixed with necrotic areas. There is no evidence that gross configuration is a prognostic indicator independent of the underlying histologic subtype (32). In contrast, anatomic site has been linked to prognosis. Tumors located in the cecum, ascending hepatic flexure, and transverse colon may be termed *right sided*, whereas tumors in the splenic flexure, descending, or sigmoid colon are grouped as *left sided*. Right-sided colon carcinomas have a better prognosis than left-sided ones (33). The main reason is probably related to the molecular pathogenesis rather than site per se because CRCs with microsatellite instability (MSI) tend to occur in the right colon.

Overall, the diagnostic, predictive, and prognostic importance of the macroscopic features of gastrointestinal cancers is limited, and histologic examination is mandatory in every case. Nevertheless, although the final classification is based on histologic characteristics, the absolute dependence of staging on meticulous dissection of surgical specimens should not be overlooked.

Histologic Classification of Malignant Gastrointestinal Tumors

For consistency and uniformity in pathological reporting of gastrointesinal malignancies, the use of internationally accepted terminology and diagnostic criteria is encouraged by the College of American Pathologists (CAP) and other professional bodies. On this basis, the standardized tumor classification for intestinal, hepatic, biliary, and pancreatic neoplasms established by the WHO is recommended (34). Tumors are classified on the basis of the tissues generated by the cancer. This approach is a histogenetic classification that may be ad-

dressed at four levels: (a) tissue of origin, (b) histologic subtype, (c) growth pattern, and (d) tumor grade.

Tissue of Origin. Two major classes of tissue are distinguished: Epithelium and connective tissue. Malignant tumors that arise from the epithelial cells are carcinomas, whereas those from the supporting tissues derived from the embryonic mesodermal layer are sarcomas. Cancers arising in connective tissue, fat, smooth muscle, skeletal muscle, vessels, cartilagenous tissue, and bone tissue are termed *fibrosarcomas, liposarcomas, leiomyosarcomas, rhabdomyosarcomas, angiosarcomas, chondrosarcomas,* and *osteosarcomas,* respectively. Haematopoietic and lymphoid cells give rise to leukemias and lymphomas. Most gastrointestinal cancers are carcinomas, followed by lymphomas and sarcomas.

Histologic Subtype. Carcinomas with a glandular growth pattern are adenocarcinomas, whereas those with squamous differentiation are squamous cell carcinomas. Adenocarcinomas comprise various histologic subtypes that may be illustrated with reference to the WHO classification of colorectal tumors. The *usual type* is characterized by medium to large glands, with moderate variability in gland size and configuration, and only moderate amounts of stroma. *Mucinous adenocarcinoma* is defined by the presence of abundant secretory mucin accounting for ≥50% of the tumor. The term "adenocarcinoma with mucinous differentiation" applies to tumors that show a significant mucinous component (>10% but <50%). *Signet ring cell adenocarcinoma* is composed of at least 50% signet ring cells. Histologically, tumor cells show a characteristic mucin vacuole that pushes the nucleus to the periphery of the cytoplasm. Although there is usually good concordance between types of normal epithelium and types of carcinoma, squamous cell carcinoma, adenosquamous carcinoma, and carcinoma with squamous metaplasia may occasionally occcur in the colon.

Growth Pattern. Malignant tumors within a given category display characteristic microscopic architectural patterns that can serve as clues to their histogenesis. The architectural pattern is often documented in the histologic pathological examination of tumor biopsies or tumor resection specimens. A *tubular pattern* refers to distended or anastomosing branching tubules of various sizes, whereas a *papillary pattern* shows epithelial projections with central fibrovascular cores. These two variants are encountered in the WHO classification of gastric adenocarcinoma. Tumors that grow in either *solid* or *trabecular* patterns include medullary carcinoma of the colon, neuroendocrine tumors, and hepatocellular carcinoma. *Cystic* growth is distinctive but relatively uncommon in gastrointestinal tumors, occurring in some mucinous carcinomas and endothelial (i.e., lymphangiomatous or hemangiomatous) tumors. In the pancreas, epithelial tumors with a cystic configuration occur relatively frequently. Solid tumors of any histologic type, however, including stromal tumors, lymphomas, and carcinomas, may undergo secondary cystification due to central necrosis, an occurence that may lead to misdiagnosis as a primary cystic neoplasm on imaging studies. Recently, colorectal carcinomas with a serrated glandular architecture have been linked with serrated polyp precursor lesions (35).

In general, the tumor growth pattern has little independent prognostic value in gastrointestinal malignancies (36,37). However, histologic subtype, growth pattern, and gross tumor configuration may be grouped together to give a useful global classification. With the Lauren classification, for example, gastric cancer is subdivided into three types: Intestinal, diffuse, and indeterminate/unclassified (38). The macroscopic appearance described as linitis plastica equates with the diffuse type of carcinoma that often shows signet ring cells and has a highly unfavorable prognosis (39). In CRC, tumor budding (single cells or clusters of up to four cells at the invasive tumor margin) has be shown to be associated with a diffuse pattern of infiltration and to confer a worse prognosis (40–45). These examples show that architectural patterns and growth characteristics may be merged to give complex but useful histologic classifications.

Tumor Grade. Tumor grade refers to the microscopic appearance of a malignancy of a given class and histologic type and the extent to which it resembles the tissue of origin. Although it is usually a purely morphologic parameter, grade is widely considered to reflect the biological properties of the tumor. In general, the higher the grade, the more aggressive the biological behavior. The microscopic features defining grade usually depend on several factors: The anatomic site of origin of the tumor, the class of the tumor (i.e., carcinoma, sarcoma, or lymphoma), and the histologic subtype within the class. In carcinomas, for example, grade is a semiquantitative measure of the degree of differentiation of the tumor and implies the maintenance or loss of of tissue-specific features reflecting specialization and function (e.g., gland formation in adenocarcinomas or degree of keratinization in squamous cell carcinomas). Within this general context, however, some histologic subtypes of carcinoma are either best left ungraded (e.g., medullary carcinoma of colon) or always assigned a given grade (e.g., signet ring carcinoma is defined as poorly differentiated or high-grade). Additional features such as highly infiltrative growth pattern or marked nuclear pleomorphism may contribute to the impression of a high-grade malignancy. For gastrointestinal lymphomas, the grade of the tumor is defined by the histologic subtype, and the anatomic site of origin is irrelevant to grading. The clinical implications of grade also differ according to the tumor class. For example, low-grade carcinoma or sarcomas are typically less biologically aggressive and more easily cured (by surgical excision) than their high-grade counterparts. In contrast, although low-grade lymphomas are indeed more slow growing than high-grade lymphomas, they are harder to cure (by medical therapy).

Historically, grading schemes for carcinomas or sarcomas (e.g., GIST) have varied as to the particular microscopic feature or features to be used as the basis for evaluation, the specific criteria for distinguishing among different grades, and even the number of grading subdivisions to be used. In some systems, grading of a given tumor is defined on the basis of a principal microscopic feature (e.g., the degree of gland formation in an adenocarcinoma), and in other systems, a large number of features are included in the evaluation (e.g., hepatocellular carcinoma or GIST) (37). Some systems base grade assignment on the least differentiated area of the tumor, whereas others reflect an average of the overall proportions of different degrees of differentiation. Despite these problems, histologic grade has been shown to be prognostically significant for most gastrointestinal malignancies, including carcinomas of the colorectum, anus, extrahepatic bile ducts, gallbladder, and exocrine pancreas (36,37).

One reason why the grading of gastrointestinal carcinomas and sarcomas is problematic is the lack of standardization. Among the various grading systems for carcinomas that have been described in the literature, few are universally accepted and uniformly used. In the absence of standardized guidelines with objective criteria for grading, the assignment of grade depends on the judgment of the observer. Even with adherence to a specific set of grading criteria, histologic variation among tumors of the same type and site may be wide enough to make implementation of even the simplest grading systems problematic and subjective. Therefore, it is not surprising that a significant degree of interobserver variability in the grading of the rectal carcinoma, for example, has been documented (46). Many pathologists stratify carcinomas of the gastrointestinal tract into four grades of differentiation: Well differentiated (grade 1), moderately differentiated (grade 2), poorly differentiated (grade 3), and undifferentiated (grade 4).

With ill-defined criteria for grade separation, discrepancies arise most often at the interfaces between grades. To avoid misrepresenting a complex tumor by assigning it a single grade, pathologists may indicate a range of differentiation (i.e., x% moderately and y% poorly differentiated). This approach is limited by the fact that each grade category may vary widely, and the clinical significance of small foci of poor differentiation is unknown. In an effort to simplify and standardize the grading of adenocarcinomas of the gastrointestinal tract (except the colorectum), pancreas, and biliary tree (including the gall bladder), the CAP has suggested a semiquantitative grading system based entirely on the proportions of gland formation by the tumor as shown in the following (37): Grade X (grade can not be assessed), grade 1 (well differentiated, >95% of tumor composed of glands), grade 2 (moderately differentiated, 50%–95% of tumor composed of glands), grade 3 (poorly differentiated, 5%–49% of tumor composed of glands), and grade 4 (undifferentiated, <5% of tumor composed of glands).

The CAP has also suggested a simplification of colorectal carcinoma grading, specifically, the use of a two-tiered system derived from published data (32). In multivariate analyses demonstrating the prognostic significance of tumor grade in colorectal cancer, the traditional grading scale has been collapsed for data analysis as follows: Low grade (well and moderately differentiated) and high grade (poorly differentiated and undifferentiated). Through this approach, high tumor grade has been demonstrated to be a stage-independent adverse prognostic factor. This two-tiered system is recommended not only because it preserves the proven prognostic import of grade in colon cancer but also because it may be expected to reduce the interobserver variability. The greatest discrepancies are associated with the stratification of low-grade tumors into well- or moderately differentiated categories, whereas diagnosis of poorly differentiated or undifferentiated tumors is more consistent. Thus, a relatively simple two-tiered system would be expected both to simplify the assessment of grade and to increase reproducibility of grade assignment. It should be cautioned, however, that some types of poorly differentiated adenocarcinoma may have a good prognosis. This applies to colorectal cancers with DNA microsatellite instability (47).

Staging of Malignant Gastrointestinal Tumors

For virtually all malignant tumors of the gastrointestinal tract, the best estimation of prognosis is related to the pathological staging. To promote uniformity and consistency of reporting of pathological stage, the CAP recommends the use of the TNM staging system of the AJCC and the UICC (2,3). The TNM system is widely used by national, regional, and local tumor registries in the United States, and it is internationally accepted. The TNM system, however, applies primarily to gastrointestinal carcinomas. For gastrointestinal lymphomas (48), GIST (49), and other mesenchymal (50) and neuroendocrine tumors (51), for instance, unique staging criteria based on the specific biological behavior of tumors in those classes have been devised.

General Principles of the TNM Staging of Gastrointestinal Carcinomas

In the TNM classification system, the designation T refers to the local extent of the primary tumor at the time of first diagnostic assessment, the designation N refers to the status of the regional lymph nodes, and M refers to distant metastatic disease. The symbol p used as a prefix refers to the pathological classification of the TNM, as opposed to the clinical classification, designated by the prefix c. Tumor remaining in a patient after primary therapy (e.g., surgical resection for cure) is categorized by a system known as the R classification. The designation R0 indicates complete excision of the tumor on surgical resection or complete remission of tumor treated by nonsurgical therapy (i.e., residual tumor cannot be detected by any diagnostic means) (3). A tumor involving any resection margin on pathological examination may be assumed to correspond to residual tumor in the patient and classified as to whether the involvement is macroscopic (R2) or microscopic (R1). Most pathologists do not use the R classification but comment on the clearance at the resection margins based on microscopic examination. A recurrent tumor after curative therapy is defined as a tumor that is recurrent after curative therapy, and the achievement of R0 status is classified according to the TNM categories but modified with the prefix r. For classification of tumor as "recurrent," a diseasefree interval must be documented (3). By convention, the recurrent tumor is topographically assigned to the proximal segment of the anastomosis unless the segment is another organ (e.g., a right colon cancer recurring at the anastomosis with the small bowel).

T Category

The staging category designated *carcinoma in situ* (pTis) refers to malignant cells that have not invaded the basement membrane of the epithelium in which they have arisen. In other words, the carcinoma that has not yet invaded the connective tissue underlying the organ's epithelial layer. Many pathologists (particularly in the West) do not use the terms *carcinoma in situ* or *intramucosal carcinoma* in most organs, preferring to equate pTis with the term *high-grade dysplasia* (or *intraepithelial neoplasia*). In contrast, all hepatocellular carcinomas are, by definition, considered invasive.

Direct extension of tumor into an adjacent organ (e.g., gastric carcinoma directly invading the liver) is not classified as a distant metastasis; rather, it is classified with the T category of the tumor (3). In contrast, direct extension of tumor into a regional lymph node via capsular penetration is classified as nodal metastasis within the N category. For most gastrointestinal carcinomas, direct invasion of other organs or structures constitutes the highest T category. This includes invasion of other segments of the same organ by way of the serosa or mesentery (e.g., invasion of the sigmoid colon by carcinoma of the cecum). Intramural extension of tumor from one subsite (segment) of a tubal organ into an adjacent subsite or organ, however, does not affect the pT classification (e.g., a cecal carcinoma with lateral spread into the right colon and the ileum) (3).

For all gastrointestinal sites except the liver, multiple simultaneous primary carcinomas of the same organ are codified according to the tumor with the highest T category. Multiplicity in a single organ may refer to multiple noninvasive tumors, invasive tumors, or a combination of both. In the liver, however, multiplicity is a criterion of the T category (3).

N Category

TNM stage–related outcome data have been derived from studies in which the pathological evaluation of the regional lymph nodes has been performed by conventional histologic staining of lymph nodes identified in the resection specimen. Typically, all lymph nodes found are submitted for microscopic examination. The actual number of lymph nodes present in any given resection specimen may be limited by anatomic variation, surgical technique, or preoperative radiotherapy, but the number found also depends on the diligence of the pathologist in examining the specimen. The CAP recommends that all grossly negative or equivocal lymph nodes be submitted entirely for microscopic examination (32). For grossly positive lymph nodes, microscopic examination of a representative sample for confirmation is considered adequate (32). In most circumstances, all lymph nodes in a resection specimen are within the regional drainage of the tumor and would be included in the determination of pN. In the event that the resection specimen includes nonregional lymph nodes, however, these must be examined separately because metastases in nonregional lymph nodes are classified as pM1 (2,3).

M Category

As stated, metastasis to any nonregional lymph node or to any distant organ or tissue is categorized as M1 disease. Peritoneal seeding of abdominal organs is also considered M1 disease, as are positive results of peritoneal fluid cytologic analysis (3). Isolated tumor cells found in the bone marrow are classified as distant metastasis. In contrast, multiple tumor foci in the mucosa or submucosa of adjacent bowel ("satellite lesions" or "skip metastasis") are not considered distant metastasis (3). Satellite lesions, however, must be distinguished from additional primary tumors.

Lymphatic Invasion by Tumor

Tumor seen microscopically within lymphatics is classified by the L (L0 indicates no lymphatic invasion and L1 indicates lymphatic invasion) category of the TNM classification (2,3). However, most pathologists will describe the finding without using the L category. Small vessel (usually interpreted as lymphatics) invasion has been implicated as an adverse prognostic factor for almost all gastrointestinal carcinomas, including those of the stomach, papilla of Vater, colorectum, exocrine pancreas, and gallbladder (32,36,37,52).

Venous Invasion by Tumor

The TNM classification classifies tumor detected in veins as V0 for no invasion, V1 for microscopic invasion, and V2 for macroscopic invasion (2,3). For many gastrointestinal malignancies, especially for hepatocellular carcinomas, colorectal carcinomas, pancreatic carcinomas, gastric carcinomas, and gastrointestinal sarcomas, large vessel invasion by tumor is an adverse prognostic factor (36). The likelihood of finding venous invasion is also determined, in part, by the number of tissue samples submitted for microscopic evaluation. A study has shown that the reproducibility of detecting extramural venous invasion in colorectal cancer increases proportionally from 59% with examination of two blocks of tissue at the tumor periphery to 96% with examination of five blocks (53) (Figure 2.3). Therefore, for colorectal cancer, the CAP recommends

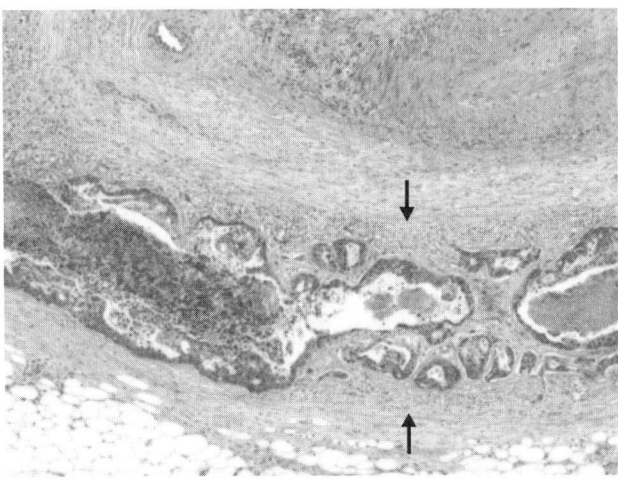

FIGURE 2.3. Invasion of large extramural vein in colorectal cancer. Note the smooth muscle in the vein wall (arrows) (See also color Figure 2.3).

that at least three blocks (optimally, five blocks) of tumor from its point of deepest extent be submitted for microscopic examination (32).

Tumor Border Configuration

For colorectal cancer, the growth pattern of the tumor at the advancing edge (tumor border) has been shown to have prognostic significance that is independent of stage and may predict tumor progression (32,52). Specifically, an irregular, infiltrating pattern of growth as opposed to a pushing border has been demonstrated to be an independent adverse prognostic factor by several univariate and multivariate analyses (46,54). Tumor budding has been defined as the presence of isolated single cells or small cell clusters (up to four) scattered in the stroma at the invasive tumor margin (41,45) and is an adverse prognostic factor in CRC (41). Tumor budding has been established as a practical prognostic indicator, and there are several recent reports highlighting the clinical value of tumor budding (40,42–45).

Perineural Invasion

Perineural invasion is a feature that has been suggested to be a stage-independent adverse prognostic factor for some gastrointestinal malignancies, particularly pancreatic and colorectal carcinomas (52). In general, however, the amount and quality of data on this feature and its relation to outcome are limited.

MOLECULAR PATHOLOGY IN GASTROINTESTINAL MALIGNANCIES

Integration of Molecular Pathology into the Management of Gastrointestinal Tumors

For many years, the prognosis of patients with gastrointesinal malignancies has been determined largely on the basis of disease stage. Among prognostic factors for gastrointestinal tumors, staging systems such as the TNM classification still remain the gold standard. The demonstration of extent of spread in continuity, lymph node metastasis, and distant metastasis are the key components for the anatomic description of tumor spread from which the clinicopathological stages I to IV are derived. However, the prognosis for the individual patient cannot be predicted with certainty by this system. For instance, some CRC patients with stage II disease will have an adverse outcome, whereas approximately 50% of stage III patients can be cured by surgery alone. It is in the subclassification of these indeterminant stages that newer prognostic markers offer the most promise.

Studies in different gastrointestinal tumors (e.g., gastric and colon cancer) have shown that histologic features such as tumor grade, architectural pattern, character of invasive margin, and lymphocytic infiltration may add further prognostic information (46,54). However, subjectivity and consequent interobserver variability may adversely impact the sensitivity and specificity of these features. Several studies have indicated that in gastrointestinal tumors, particular molecular findings could have a significant association with prognosis, independent of the stage of the disease. In addition, molecular features may indicate enhanced sensitivity for particular forms of adjuvant chemotherapy, allowing such treatment to be targeted more effectively. However, because a particular molecular finding that is linked to survival (prognostic marker) can also be implicated in the response to adjuvant therapy (predictive marker), it may be difficult to disentangle prognostic from predictive ef-

fects. For example, when markers indicate a good prognosis to the extent that the patient is likely to be cured, the patient will have no benefit from adjuvant therapy, regardless of the predictive marker findings. In contrast, in situations in which adjuvant therapy is the standard of care, predictive markers have a prognostic value in the treated group of patients. In other words, it may be difficult to determine if a good outcome marker in a treated group of patients is predictive or prognostic. To overcome this problem, retrospective studies using subjects from the preadjuvant era or prospective studies, including patients without adjuvant therapy, have been performed. Numerous biases such as patient age or general health often influence the decision to offer adjuvant therapy, and may confound a study even when treatment and nontreatment groups are matched by stage. In this section, we highlight the general principles of molecular advances that may provide clinically useful prognostic information beyond traditional pathological staging. In addition, we consider molecular technologies that facilitate pathological staging by increasing sensitivity beyond the capacity of microscopic examination.

Molecular Technologies in Gastrointestinal Pathology

The various facets of recombinant DNA technology have revolutionized the investigation of gastrointestinal neoplasia. Beneficial outcomes have included an improved understanding of etiology and pathogenesis; the development of clinically relevant classifications; and the characterization of novel markers of diagnostic, prognostic, or predictive importance. In addition, the underlying gene has been cloned in multiple hereditary forms of gastrointestinal neoplasia, allowing affected patients to be identified by germline mutation analysis. Methods that can be applied directly to tissue sections, such as *in situ hybridization (ISH)/fluorescence in situ hybridization (FISH)*, and methods that use DNA, mRNA, or proteins extracted from tissue samples (*polymerase chain reaction (PCR)* and *Southern, Northern,* or *Western blotting*) have all contributed to the advancement of gastrointestinal pathology. Additional powerful methodologies include *comparative genomic hybridization, DNA microarrays,* and *laser capture microdissection.* The principles and practical uses of the more frequently used technologies are briefly described as follows:

1. *Southern blotting*—This technique is rarely used because it requires large amounts of DNA; however, it provided the initial important breakthrough in linking recombinant DNA technology with the study of genetic disorders (of which cancer is a key example). Briefly, double-stranded DNA is cut by restriction endonuclease treatment and separated according to length by electrophoresis. A sheet of nitrocellulose paper is laid over the gel, and the separated DNA fragments are transferred to the sheet by blotting. The fragments of special interest are rendered single stranded and probed with radiolabeled markers of complementary DNA. Because this technique was invented by Southern in 1975, it is called *Southern blot.* There are also Northern blots for RNA and Western blots for proteins (a sort of biochemical joke). Southern blot may be used for detecting mutations (particularly, large deletions) or loss of heterozygosity (LOH) (55,56) but has been largely superseded by the PCR methodology discussed next.

2. *PCR*—The amount and quality of the extractable DNA is the limiting factor of the molecular biological analysis of DNA derived from tissue specimen. Relatively large amounts of DNA of particular quality are required to detect subtle mutations within oncogenes and loss of

tumor-suppressor genes, and for the demonstration of DNA MSI. Nevertheless, if the structure of the DNA sequence is known, single-stranded DNA can be replicated by a pair of primers and DNA polymerase. By using reverse transcriptase PCR, which generates cDNA, it is possible to analyze trace amounts of mRNA in the same way. The designation PCR is derived from the fact that the biochemical process is repeated until the DNA has been replicated, say, a millionfold (57). Because DNA can be extracted from formalin-fixed, paraffin-embedded tissues, this technique represents an important link between histopathology and molecular pathology. The PCR technique has been modified and adapted repeatedly. For example, it can provide quantitative data or distinguish methylated from nonmethylated DNA.

3. *ISH/FISH*—These techniques use nucleic acid probes in much the same way as labeled antibodies to locate specific nucleic acid sequences in situ termed *ISH*. This technique can be used for DNA in chromosomes and RNA in cells. Chromosomes are briefly exposed to a very high pH to disrupt the DNA base pairs and are hybridized by labeled nucleic acid probes. Originally, this technique was developed with highly radioactive DNA probes, but its spacial resolution was increased by labeling the DNA probes chemically (FISH). To detect a specific RNA sequence within cells or tissue sections, the tissue is not exposed to a high pH and gently fixed. The RNA can hybridize with labeled probes consisting of complementary DNA or RNA. One of the main diagnostic uses of this technique is the detection of viral DNA.

4. *Comparative genomic hybridization*—This technique is used to compare the ability of tumor DNA labeled with one fluorophore (i.e., green) and normal DNA labeled with another fluorophore (i.e., red) to hybridize to a chromosome spread from a given tissue specimen. Loss or gain of chromosomal material in a tumor can be determined by the color of the fluorophore hybridized to the region on the chromosome. In this way, a complete genomic map of genetic changes that occur in a tumor cell can be obtained. Tumorigenesis in different gastrointestinal tumors has been studied by this method (58–63). The technique is extremely powerful with respect to finding regions of interest but not specific genes.

5. *Laser-capture microdissection*—One of the challenges presented by molecular technology is the difficulty of obtaining pure tumor samples for analysis. In contrast to lymphomas and many sarcomas, which grow as relatively pure tumor masses, in most epithelial cancers the neoplastic cell population is intimately admixed with stromal tissues and inflammatory cells. The malignant cell population may be isolated for molecular analysis by laser-capture microdissection (64,65). Neverthless, this technique depends on the correct morphologic recognition of the malignant cells, which is very labor intensive. Its use is therefore limited in routine diagnostic work but finds an important application in DNA microarray analysis (discussed next).

6. *DNA microarray*—Microchip array of many thousands of genes (cDNA) that are expressed in normal tissues provides the baseline for the analysis of reduced or increased expression of mRNA derived from counterpart neoplastic tissues. This technique can accelerate the understanding of the role of known genes in carcinogenesis (66). In addition, it may be possible to use expression analysis as a means of prognostic classification by associating particular signatures of gene expression with stage and clinical outcome. Recently published studies highlight the potential for molecular staging (67,68). Neverthless, one of the limiting factors of this approach is the fact that key cancer genes whose effects are amplified by signaling pathways may be expressed at very low levels and therefore show only subtle differences in expression levels across normal versus malignant tumors. In addition, this technique depends heavily on bioinformatics support.

Principles in Gastrointestinal Oncogenesis

"There is nothing hidden under the sun," one quote of Lenoardo da Vinci (1452–1519), might presage the understanding of carcinogenesis as a molecular disorder. Although the existence of tumors has been known for centuries, evidence that cancer is in fact a genetic disease only began to accumulate in the 1980s. The term "genetic" refers not so much to hereditary influences, but to the somatic alterations of genes responsible for the regulation of growth, apoptosis, differentiation, cell-to-cell communication, and motility. By the 1990s, three major classes of cancer genes had been identified: Oncogenes, tumor-suppressor genes, and DNA repair genes.

Oncogenes

Proto-oncogenes are responsible for the regulation of cell division and can be classified as either cytoplasmic or nuclear, depending on where in the cell they are located. To cause cancer, these genes need to be activated by a genetic alteration. These alterations take the form of subtle mutations (e.g., base pair substitutions, insertions, or deletions), amplifications, or translocations. The net result is a protein product that no longer responds normally to growth regulatory cues. Only one allele of the gene needs to be altered for the oncogenic effect. Thus, oncogenes are mutated proto-oncogenes that carry dominant mutations and may cause excessive cell division, one of the fundamental characteristics of a cancer cell.

Nuclear oncogenes such as *MYC* regulate gene transcription. In hepatocellular carcinoma, for example, *MYC* is upregulated by hypomethylation of the *MYC* promoter and gene amplification (69,70). Many of the cytoplasmic proto-oncogenes, for example *ABL* which is activated by chromosomal translocation (71), code for tyrosine kinases. These enzymes phophorylate tyrosine residues of substrate proteins that control the various signaling cascades that regulate mitosis and other fundamental functions relating to cell growth and differentiation. Others, such as *RAS*, transmit cellular growth signals by binding guanine nucleotides. *RAS* is often mutated at a single amino acid residue, and this occurs in approximately 30% of human cancers (72). *KRAS* plays a key role in colorectal and pancreatic tumorigenesis and has also been identified as a potential prognostic marker in CRC (73–75). It should be stressed, however, that the activation of a single oncogene may not result in neoplastic transformation. The oncogenic effects need to be magnified by the loss of tumor-suppressor genes.

Tumor-Suppressor Genes

Tumor-suppressor genes act recessively insofar as a tumorigenic effect occurs when both copies are inactivated. This implies that one normal allele of a tumor-suppressor gene is sufficient for normal cell function. Patients with hereditary cancers frequently inherit one normal and one abnormal allele of a particular tumor-suppressor gene. If the normal allele is then lost at the somatic level, the protective effect of the gene product is compromised.

The *RB1* gene was the first tumor-suppressor gene identified and associated causatively with retinoblastoma, a rare hereditary cancer arising in the retina of children (76). The fundamental principle provided by *RB1* was then shown to apply to other tumor-suppressor genes. Among these, *TP53*, *APC* (adenomatous polyposis coli), *p16*, and *DPC4 (SMAD4)* play an important role in gastrointestinal carcinogenesis.

In normal cells, *TP53* serves to monitor DNA damage. When DNA damage occurs, the cell cycle is arrested by *TP53* to permit DNA repair. If DNA is damaged beyond repair, *TP53* initiates the process of apoptosis or programmed cell death. *TP53* is inactivated in approximately 70% of human cancers. In CRC, a systematic review of *TP53* abnormalities by IHC and mutation analysis was performed by Munro et al. (77). Generally, patients with abnormal *TP53* findings in CRC have an increased risk of death. However, IHC and mutation analysis can give different results with respect to predictive and prognostic value. For instance, *TP53* mutation in rectal cancer patients treated by radiotherapy or chemoradiation predicted treatment failure, whereas abnormal immunohistochemical results had no predictive value. Conceivably, truncating mutations of *TP53* might lead to complete loss of expression rather than nuclear accumulation of *TP53*, but these are uncommon in the case of CRC (73,77). Nevertheless, complete absence of *TP53* expression was found to be an adverse prognostic factor in one study (78). Another IHC study found that nuclear expression of *TP53* was an independent prognostic factor only in left-sided colon tumors and that at least some right-sided colon tumors evolve through a *TP53*-independent pathway (79). These findings indicate the existence of considerable genetic heterogeneity among CRCs (and other gastrointestinal malignancies) and emphasize the importance of molecular classifications. For example, Smyth et al. suggested that the adverse effect of *TP53* detected immunohistochemically in right-sided colon tumors was explained by the existence of a molecular subtype of CRC that lacks *TP53* alterations and has a good prognosis (80). This group corresponds to the subset of sporadic MSI-high (MSI-H) CRC that shows methylation and loss of expression of the mismatch repair gene MLH1.

APC may be regarded as the prototype tumor-suppressor gene in colorectal neoplasia. There is a clear parallel with *RB1* insofar as *APC* is linked to the initiation of CRC and is mutated in the germline of patients with the hereditary type colon cancer known as familial adenomatous polyposis. *APC* maps to 5q21 and codes for a multifunctional protein that is involved in the regulation of proliferation and differentiation in normal cells through the Wnt signaling pathway. As in the case of *TP53*, inactivation of the first copy of *APC* is usually by mutation, while the second allele may be either lost or mutated. The loss of a tumor-suppressor gene can be demonstrated by LOH. In CRC, LOH occurs frequently in chromosome 18q, where there are several candidate tumor-suppressor genes, including *DCC*, *SMAD4*, and *SMAD2*. LOH at 18q has been linked to poor prognosis in CRC, but, as in the case of *TP53*, data relating to the prognostic significance of loss at this locus are conflicting. Anwar et al. suggested multiple possible reasons for the different results in the studies: Use of different microsatellite markers, the fact that loss of a chromosomal region can implicate several different genes, and inadequate group matching by stage and suboptimal staging (73). Other tumor supressor genes include *p16-INK4A* on chromosome 9p21 that negatively regulates the cell cycle in a wide range of cancers (81) and *DPC4* (deleted in pancreatic cancer)/*SMAD4* on chromosome 18q that is lost in both pancreatic and colon cancer (82).

DNA Repair Genes

Mutations can inactivate the very genes that detect and repair mutations in other genes. This would allow mutations in cancer-causing genes to accumulate, thereby generating a state of hypermutability. The DNA mismatch repair genes *MLH1*, *MSH2*, *MSH3*, *MSH6*, and *PMS2* maintain genomic integrity by repairing mismatched base pairs that arise spontaneously and with a stable frequency during DNA replication (83). Mis-mach repair enzymes recognize and excise mismatched base pairs that are then replaced by new and correctly matched bases. Without such repair, mutations may be introduced into newly synthesized DNA. The inactivation of mismatch repair genes is a key event in specific subtypes of gastrointestinal cancers, notably in gastric and colon cancers (84).

Loss of mismatch repair in CRC occurs in (a) hereditary nonpolyposis CRC (HNPCC), in which there is a germline mutation in a DNA mismatch repair gene (usually *MLH1* or *MSH2*), and (b) sporadic MSI-positive CRCs, in which there is an acquired methylation of the *MLH1* promoter region leading to silencing of the gene. There is strong evidence that abnormal methylation of DNA at islands rich in CpG sequences plays a critical epigenetic role in the evolution of cancer. Hypermethylation of the promoter region therefore joins mutation and LOH as mechanism for inactivating tumor-suppressor genes (e.g., *E-cadherin*, *p16*, *p14*, *APC*, *RB1*, *VHL*, *WT1*). Hypomethylation has been associated with chromosomal instability.

Loss of DNA mismatch repair proficiency results in a phenotype characterized by mutation in microsatellite regions and known as MSI. CRCs with MSI can be subdivided into two groups, namely, MSI-H and MSI-low (MSI-L). However, only MSI-H is linked with loss of function of DNA mismatch repair genes. The anatomical pathologist can recognize subtle but discriminatory differences between CRCs with and without MSI-H at the light microscopic level. CRCs with MSI-H are more likely to be right-sided, poorly differentiated, or mucinous; well circumscribed; and infiltrated by intraepithelial lymphocytes. The list of clinicopathological features associated with MSI-H status in CRC has been comprehensively reviewed (85). Although HNPCC and sporadic MSI-positive CRC share multiple morphologic and molecular features, they must nevertheless be distinguished for the purpose of patient management. There is now evidence that the MSI-H CRCs that arise through these two backgrounds (hereditary vs. sporadic) are biologically distinct and should be separated not only for clinical management but also when assessing the prognostic and predictive value of markers (86–88).

Mismatch repair deficiency is determined either by the demonstration of MSI (Figure 2.4) or by the loss of expresssion of DNA mismatch repair proteins in IHC. A recent review and meta-analysis showed an improved prognosis in MSI-positive CRCs (47). Nevertheless, only 10% to 15% of CRCs are MSI positive; therefore, small studies may be underpowered and a source of erroneous negative findings.

Although the concept of MSI-L remains controversial, two studies have suggested that MSI-L CRCs have a poor prognosis (89,90). These studies illustrate the potential importance of tumor classification that is based on genetic features, particularly when analyzing the predictive or prognostic value of markers.

PERSPECTIVES

Advances in the understanding of molecular biology in gastrointestinal malignancies are now leading to an era in which traditional tumor classifications based exclusively on histogenesis and morphology will be strongly challenged. Nevertheless, in the immediate future, morphology supported by special stains and immunohistochemistry will continue as the cornerstone of tumor diagnosis. Time will be required to assess the increasing knowledge of DNA and gene expression alterations, and to establish the utility of this information in tumor classification, diagnosis, prognosis, and chemoresponsiveness. New biomarkers must be shown to be objective, reproducible, and independent with respect to clinically important end points. Although molecular approaches continue to show great promise,

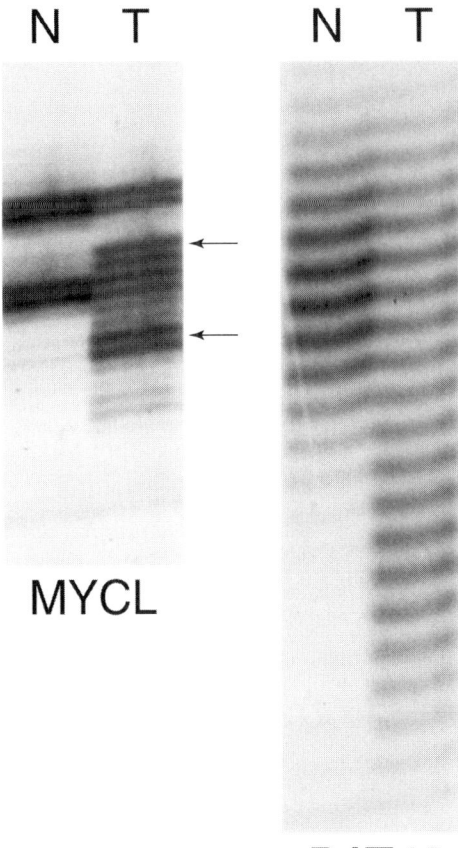

FIGURE 2.4. Examples of microsatellite instability in the markers MYCL and BAT40. With normal DNA (N), two MYCL alleles are evident (maternally and paternally derived). This pattern is typical of highly polymorphic markers in which the alleles generally have different lengths and can therefore be separated in a gel. In the tumor DNA (T), two additional sets of bands are seen (arrows), suggesting that both alleles have mutated. MYCL is a compound microsatellite marker that is sensitive but not highly specific for mismatch repair deficiency. BAT40 is a relatively monomorphic marker giving a typical ladder pattern in which maternal and paternal alleles are identical and not resolved into separate bands. Mutation is indicated by the additional bands in tumor DNA (T). BAT40, like the other mononucleotide markers BAT25 and BAT26, is both sensitive and specific for DNA mismatch repair deficiency.

their routine and widespread adoption cannot be justified until there is general agreement that the findings have had a clear impact on clinical management. This will probably lead to the combined use of conventional and new molecular approaches rather than complete replacement by the latter. Therapeutic decisions will therefore be based on all available evidence and not merely on the limited prognostic information provided by anatomical staging. The ultimate goal in the management of cancer patients is to develop treatment options that are individualized for each patient and that make full use of the clinical, morphologic, and molecular characteristics of the tumor.

References

1. Hays G. *Marcus Aurelius. Meditations.* A new translation, with an introduction by Gregory Hays. New York: Modern Library; 2003.
2. American Joint Committee on Cancer (AJCC). *AJCC Cancer Staging Manual.* 6th ed. New York: Springer Verlag; 2002.
3. Wittekind C, Hutter R, Greene FL, Klimpfinger M, Sobin LH, International Union Against Cancer. *TNM Atlas: Illustrated Guide to the TNM Classification of Malignant Tumours.* 5th ed. New York: Wiley-Liss; 2005.
4. Karpeh MS, Jr, Brennan MF. Gastric carcinoma. *Ann Surg Oncol* 1998;(5): 650–656.
5. Feinstein AR, Wells CK. A clinical-severity staging system for patients with lung cancer. *Medicine (Baltimore)* 1990;69(1):1–33.
6. Feldman JG, Saunders M, Carter AC, Gardner B. The effects of patient delay and symptoms other than a lump on survival in breast cancer. *Cancer* 1983;51(7):1226–1229.
7. Piccirillo JF, Feinstein AR. Clinical symptoms and comorbidity: significance for the prognostic classification of cancer. *Cancer* 1996;77(5):834–842.
8. Pugliano FA, Piccirillo JF, Zequeira MR, et al. Clinical-severity staging system for oral cavity cancer: five-year survival rates. *Otolaryngol Head Neck Surg* 1999;120(1):38–45.
9. Lugli A, Kopp Lugli A, Horcic M. Napoleon's autopsy: new perspectives. *Hum Pathol* 2005;36:320–324.
10. Lugli A, Zlobec I, Singer G, et al. Napoleon Bonapartes Gastric Cancer: a clinicopathologic approach to staging, pathogenisis and etiology. *Nat Clin Pract Gastroenterol Hepatol* 2007;4(1):52–57.
11. Kaimaktchiev V, Terracciano L, Tornillo L, Spichtin H. The homeobox intestinal differentiation factor CDX2 is selectively expressed in gastrointestinal adenocarcinomas. *Mod Pathol* 2004;17(11):1392–1399.
12. Bubendorf L, Nocito A, Moch H, et al. Tissue microarray (TMA) technology: miniaturized pathology archives for high-throughput in situ studies. *J Pathol* 2001;195(1):72–79.
13. Kallioniemi OP, Wagner U, Kononen J, et al. Tissue microarray technology for high-throughput molecular profiling of cancer. *Hum Mol Genet* 2001; 10(7):657–662.
14. Kononen J, Bubendorf L, Kallioniemi A, Barlund M. Tissue microarrays for high-throughput molecular profiling of tumor specimens. *Nat Med* 1998; 4(7):844–847.
15. Sauter G, Simon R. Predictive molecular pathology. *N Engl J Med* 2002;347 (25):1995–1996.
16. Lugli A, Forster Y, Haas P, Nocito A. Calretinin expression in human normal and neoplastic tissues: a tissue microarray analysis on 5233 tissue samples. *Hum Pathol* 2003;34(10):994–1000.
17. Huusko P, Ponciano-Jackson D, Wolf M, Kiefer JA. Nonsense-mediated decay microarray analysis identifies mutations of EPHB2 in human prostate cancer. *Nat Genet* 2004;36(9):979–983.
18. Lugli A, Spichtin H, Maurer R, Mirlacher M. EphB2 expression across 138 human tumor types in a tissue microarray: high levels of expression in gastrointestinal cancers. *Clin Cancer Res* 2005;11(18):6450–6458.
19. Lugli A, Tornillo L, Mirlacher M, et al. Hepatocyte paraffin 1 expression in human normal and neoplastic tissues: tissue microarray analysis on 3,940 tissue samples. *Am J Clin Pathol* 2004;122(5):721–727.
20. Alizadeh AA, Eisen MB, Davis RE, Ma C. Distinct types of diffuse large B-cell lymphoma identified by gene expression profiling. *Nature* 2000;403 (6769):503–511.
21. Borrmann R. *Geschwuelste des Magens und des Duodenums.* Berlin: Springer Verlag; 1926.
22. Lauwers GY. Epithelial neoplasms of the stomach. In: Odze RD, Goldblum JR, Crawford JM, eds. *Surgical Pathology of the GI Tract, Liver, Biliary Tract, and Pancreas.* Philadelphia, Pa.: WB Saunders; 2004;415.
23. Lewin KJ, Appelman HD. *Tumors of the Esophagus and Stomach.* Washington, DC: AFIP; 1996.
24. Ming SC, Goldman H. *Pathology of the Gastrointestinal Tract.* 2nd ed. Baltimore, Md.: Williams & Wilkins; 1998.
25. Murakami T. Pathomorphological diagnosis: definition and gross classification of early gastric cancer. *Gann Monogr Cancer Res* 1971;11:53–55.
26. Folli S, Dente M, Dell'Amore D, Gaudio M. Early gastric cancer: prognostic factors in 223 patients. *Br J Surg* 1995;82(7):952–956.
27. Sue-Ling HM, Martin I, Griffith J, Ward DC. Early gastric cancer: 46 cases treated in one surgical department. *Gut* 1992;33(10):1318–1322.
28. Hisamichi S. Screening for gastric cancer. *World J Surg* 1989;13(1):31–37.
29. Everett SM, Axon AT. Early gastric cancer in Europe. *Gut* 1997;41(2):142–150.
30. Morson BC, Sobin LH, Grundmann E, et al. Precancerous conditions and epithelial dysplasia in the stomach. *J Clin Pathol* 1980;33(8):711–721.
31. Redston M. Epithelial neoplasms of the large intestine. In: Odze RD, Goldblum JR, Crawford JM, eds. *Surgical Pathology of the GI Tract, Liver, Biliary Tract, and Pancreas.* Philadelphia, Pa.: WB Saunders; 2004;444–445.
32. Compton CC, Fielding LP, Burgart LJ, Conley B. Prognostic factors in colorectal cancer. College of American Pathologists Consensus Statement 1999. *Arch Pathol Lab Med* 2000;124(7):979–994.
33. Eisenberg B, Decosse JJ, Harford F, et al. Carcinoma of the colon and rectum: the natural history reviewed in 1704 patients. *Cancer* 1982;49(6): 1131–1134.
34. Hamilton SR, Aaltonen LA. *Pathology and Genetics of Tumours of the Digestive System.* Lyon, France: IARC Press; 2000.
35. Tuppurainen K, Makinen JM, Junttila O, Liakka A. Morphology and microsatellite instability in sporadic serrated and non-serrated colorectal cancer. *J Pathol* 2005;207(3):285–294.
36. Gospodarowicz MK, Henson DE, Hutter RVP, et al. *Prognostic Factors in Cancer.* 2nd ed. New York: Wiley-Liss; 2001.

37. Compton CC, College of American Pathologists. *Practice Protocols for the Examination of Specimens Removed from Patients with Cancer*. Northfield, Ill.: College of American Pathologists 1999.

38. Lauren P. The two histological main types of gastric carcinoma: diffuse and so-called intestinal-type carcinoma. An attempt at a histo-clinical classification. *Acta Pathol Microbiol Scand* 1965;64:31–49.

39. Fuchs CS, Mayer RJ. Gastric carcinoma. *N Engl J Med* 1995;333(1):32–41.

40. Hase K, Shatney C, Johnson D, et al. Prognostic value of tumor "budding" in patients with colorectal cancer. *Dis Colon Rectum* 1993;36(7):627–635.

41. Hase K, Shatney CH, Mochizuki H, Johnson DL. Long-term results of curative resection of "minimally invasive" colorectal cancer. *Dis Colon Rectum* 1995;38(1):19–26.

42. Shinto E, Mochizuki H, Ueno H, et al. A novel classification of tumour budding in colorectal cancer based on the presence of cytoplasmic pseudo-fragments around budding foci. *Histopathology* 2005;47(1):25–31.

43. Tanaka M, Hashiguchi Y, Ueno H, et al. Tumor budding at the invasive margin can predict patients at high risk of recurrence after curative surgery for stage II, T3 colon cancer. *Dis Colon Rectum* 2003;46(8):1054–1059.

44. Ueno H, Mochizuki H, Hatsuse K, et al. Indicators for treatment strategies of colorectal liver metastases. *Ann Surg* 2000;231(1):59–66.

45. Ueno H, Murphy J, Jass JR, et al. Tumour 'budding' as an index to estimate the potential of aggressiveness in rectal cancer. *Histopathology* 2002;40(2):127–132.

46. Jass JR, Atkin WS, Cuzick J, Bussey HJ. The grading of rectal cancer: historical perspectives and a multivariate analysis of 447 cases. *Histopathology* 1986;10(5):437–459.

47. Popat S, Hubner R, Houlston RS. Systematic review of microsatellite instability and colorectal cancer prognosis. *J Clin Oncol* 2005;23(3):609–618.

48. Jaffe ES, Harris NL, Stein H, Vardiman JW. *Pathology and Genetics of Tumours of Haematopoietic and Lymphoid Tissues*. Lyon, France: IARC Press; 2001.

49. Miettinen M, El-Rifai W, Sobin LH, et al. Evaluation of malignancy and prognosis of gastrointestinal stromal tumors: a review. *Hum Pathol* 2002;33(5):478–483.

50. Fletcher CDM, Unni K. *Pathology and Genetics of Tumours of Soft Tissue and Bone*. Lyon, France: IARC Press; 2002.

51. Lloyd R, DeLellis R, Heitz P, Eng C. *Pathology and Genetics of Tumours of the Endocrine Organs*. Lyon, France: IARC Press; 2004.

52. Compton CC. Pathology report in colon cancer: what is prognostically important? *Dig Dis* 1999;17(2):67–79.

53. Blenkinsopp WK, Stewart-Brown S, Blesovsky L, et al. Histopathology reporting in large bowel cancer. *J Clin Pathol* 1981;34(5):509–513.

54. Alexander J, Watanabe T, Wu TT, et al. Histopathological identification of colon cancer with microsatellite instability. *Am J Pathol* 2001;158(2):527–535.

55. Solomon E, Voss R, Hall V, Bodmer WF. Chromosome 5 allele loss in human colorectal carcinomas. *Nature* 1987;328(6131):616–619.

56. Bodmer WF, Bailey CJ, Bodmer J, Bussey HJ. Localization of the gene for familial adenomatous polyposis on chromosome 5. *Nature* 1987;328(6131):614–616.

57. Saiki RK, Gelfand DH, Stoffel S, Scharf SJ. Primer-directed enzymatic amplification of DNA with a thermostable DNA polymerase. *Science* 1988;239(4839):487–491.

58. Kimura Y, Noguchi T, Kawahara K, et al. Genetic alterations in 102 primary gastric cancers by comparative genomic hybridization: gain of 20q and loss of 18q are associated with tumor progression. *Mod Pathol* 2004;17(11):1328–1337.

59. Schlegel J, Stumm G, Scherthan H, Bocker T. Comparative genomic in situ hybridization of colon carcinomas with replication error. *Cancer Res* 1995;55(24):6002–6005.

60. Tay ST, Leong SH, Yu K, Aggarwal A. A combined comparative genomic hybridization and expression microarray analysis of gastric cancer reveals novel molecular subtypes. *Cancer Res* 2003;63(12):3309–3316.

61. Terracciano LM, Bernasconi B, Ruck P, Stallmach T. Comparative genomic hybridization analysis of hepatoblastoma reveals high frequency of X-chromosome gains and similarities between epithelial and stromal components. *Hum Pathol* 2003;34(9):864–871.

62. Terracciano LM, Glatz K, Mhawech P, Vasei M. Hepatoid adenocarcinoma with liver metastasis mimicking hepatocellular carcinoma: an immunohistochemical and molecular study of eight cases. *Am J Surg Pathol* 2003;27(10):1302–1312.

63. van Dekken H, Geelen E, Dinjens WN, Wijnhoven BP. Comparative genomic hybridization of cancer of the gastroesophageal junction: deletion of 14Q31–32.1 discriminates between esophageal (Barrett's) and gastric cardia adenocarcinomas. *Cancer Res* 1999;59(3):748–752.

64. Simone NL, Bonner RF, Gillespie JW, et al. Laser-capture microdissection: opening the microscopic frontier to molecular analysis. *Trends Genet* 1998;14(7):272–276.

65. Sirivatanauksorn Y, Drury R, Crnogorac-Jurcevic T, et al. Laser-assisted microdissection: applications in molecular pathology. *J Pathol* 1999;189(2):150–154.

66. Schena M, Shalon D, Davis RW, et al. Quantitative monitoring of gene expression patterns with a complementary DNA microarray. *Science* 1995;270(5235):467–470.

67. Bertucci F, Salas S, Eysteries S, Nasser V. Gene expression profiling of colon cancer by DNA microarrays and correlation with histoclinical parameters. *Oncogene* 2004;23(7):1377–1391.

68. Koehler A, Bataille F, Schmid C, Ruemmele P. Gene expression profiling of colorectal cancer and metastases divides tumours according to their clinico-pathological stage. *J Pathol* 2004;204(1):65–74.

69. Kaneko Y, Shibuya M, Nakayama T, Hayashida N. Hypomethylation of c-myc and epidermal growth factor receptor genes in human hepatocellular carcinoma and fetal liver. *Jpn J Cancer Res* 1985;76(12):1136–1140.

70. Nambu S, Inoue K, Saski H. Site-specific hypomethylation of the c-myc oncogene in human hepatocellular carcinoma. *Jpn J Cancer Res* 1987;78(7):695–704.

71. Heisterkamp N, Stam K, Groffen J, et al. Structural organization of the bcr gene and its role in the Ph' translocation. *Nature* 1985;315(6022):758–761.

72. Wittinghofer F. Ras signalling. Caught in the act of the switch-on. *Nature* 1998;394(6691):317, 319–320.

73. Anwar S, Frayling IM, Scott NA, et al. Systematic review of genetic influences on the prognosis of colorectal cancer. *Br J Surg* 2004;91(10):1275–1291.

74. Conlin A, Smith G, Carey FA, et al. The prognostic significance of K-ras, p53, and APC mutations in colorectal carcinoma. *Gut* 2005;54(9):1283–1286.

75. Gonzalez-Aguilera JJ, Oliart S, Azcoita MM, et al. Simultaneous mutations in K-ras and TP53 are indicative of poor prognosis in sporadic colorectal cancer. *Am J Clin Oncol* 2004;27(1):39–45.

76. Knudson AG, Jr. Mutation and cancer: statistical study of retinoblastoma. *Proc Natl Acad Sci U S A* 1971;68(4):820–823.

77. Munro AJ, Lain S, Lane DP. P53 abnormalities and outcomes in colorectal cancer: a systematic review. *Br J Cancer* 2005;92(3):434–444.

78. Prall F, Ostwald C, Nizze H, et al. Expression profiling of colorectal carcinomas using tissue microarrays: cell cycle regulatory proteins p21, p27, and p53 as immunohistochemical prognostic markers in univariate and multivariate analysis. *Appl Immunohistochem Mol Morphol* 2004;12(2):111–121.

79. Paluszkiewicz P, Berbec H, Pawlowska-Wakowicz B, et al. P53 Protein accumulation in colorectal cancer tissue has prognostic value only in left-sided colon tumours. *Cancer Detect Prev* 2004;28(4):252–259.

80. Smyth EF, Sharma A, Sivarajasingham N, et al. Prognostic implications of MLH1 and p53 immunohistochemical status in right-sided colon cancer. *Dis Colon Rectum* 2004;47(12):2086–2091; discussion 2091–2092.

81. Kamb A, Shattuck-Eidens D, Eeles R, Liu Q. Analysis of the p16 gene (CDKN2) as a candidate for the chromosome 9p melanoma susceptibility locus. *Nat Genet* 1994;8(1):23–26.

82. Hahn SA, Schutte M, Hoque AT, Moskaluk CA. DPC4, a candidate tumor suppressor gene at human chromosome 18q21.1. *Science* 1996;271(5247):350–353.

83. Kolodner RD, Marsischky GT. Eukaryotic DNA mismatch repair. *Curr Opin Genet Dev* 1999;9(1):89–96.

84. Alison MR. *The Cancer Handbook*. London: Nature; 2002.

85. Raut CP, Pawlik TM, Rodriguez-Bigas MA. Clinicopathologic features in colorectal cancer patients with microsatellite instability. *Mutat Res* 2004;568(2):275–282.

86. Jass JR. HNPCC and sporadic MSI-H colorectal cancer: a review of the morphological similarities and differences. *Fam Cancer* 2004;3(2):93–100.

87. McGivern A, Wynter CV, Whitehall VL, Kambara T. Promoter hypermethylation frequency and BRAF mutations distinguish hereditary non-polyposis colon cancer from sporadic MSI-H colon cancer. *Fam Cancer* 2004;3(2):101–107.

88. Clark AJ, Barnetson R, Farrington SM, et al. Prognosis in DNA mismatch repair deficient colorectal cancer: are all MSI tumours equivalent? *Fam Cancer* 2004;3(2):85–91.

89. Wright CM, Dent OF, Newland RC, Barker M. Low level microsatellite instability may be associated with reduced cancer specific survival in sporadic stage C colorectal carcinoma. *Gut* 2005;54(1):103–108.

90. Kohonen-Corish MR, Daniel JJ, Chan C, Lin BP. Low microsatellite instability is associated with poor prognosis in stage C colon cancer. *J Clin Oncol* 2005;23(10):2318–2324.

CHAPTER 3 ■ GASTROINTESTINAL CANCER: CANCER GENETICS

STEVEN M. LIPKIN AND KENNETH OFFIT

INTRODUCTION

Clinical genetic services for gastrointestinal (GI) cancer help the medical community effectively identify families with genetic syndromes. When properly diagnosed, these patients and their relatives can benefit from early detection through frequent cancer surveillance, risk modification, chemoprevention, and participation in screening and treatment clinical trials. The goal is to detect tumors early and improve survival and quality of life of families carrying these genetic mutations. At the same time, a related goal is to spare their relatives who are not at increased cancer risk the discomfort and expense of frequent cancer screening surveillance, or even unnecessary surgical resection of the relevant organs. By providing more precise and personalized prediction of cancer risk, clinical genetics can prevent cancer in patients and their families affected with genetic syndromes and more effectively can manage medical resources.

Germline mutations in genes that predispose to colorectal, small bowel, biliary tract, and pancreatic adenocarcinomas have been identified. Genetics has had a significant impact in identifying individuals who can be targeted for intensive screening surveillance and, when indicated, surgery. The contribution of germline mutations in known susceptibility genes, as described in this chapter, is generally believed to be 25% or less for GI malignancies. However, with each year more atypical presentations of the known syndromes appear that extends their spectrum. The contribution of hypomorphic (i.e., partial loss of function) mutations causing cancers at lower rates of penetrance, perhaps clinically indistinguishable from sporadic forms, is likely to be more common than currently appreciated, and the total contribution of GI cancer attributable to germline mutations revised upward.

Because many of these GI cancer genetic risk–related deaths are preventable with early detection, it is a critical ethical (and increasingly legal) imperative for primary care physicians to be familiar with and recognize cancer-related genetic syndromes. Eliciting the existence of early onset cancers in the personal or family medical history, constellations of cancers in a family that fit known syndromes, or tumor pathology associated with known syndromes, as described here, can be a lifesaving intervention. Similarly, a basic familiarity for the primary care provider during the physical exam of the physical stigmata associated with some of these syndromes (e.g., pigmented mucocutaneous lesions or extranumerary teeth) can help identify the individuals at risk. If the primary care physician were uncertain about the significance of patient history and physical exam findings, or associated pathological findings such as rare tumor subtypes (e.g., hamartomatous polyps), it would be important to refer the patient to qualified genetic professionals. These professionals include certified genetic counselors, medical geneticists, oncologists, and gastroenterologists, among others. If not available readily in the community practice setting, it is the responsibility of the primary care provider to refer to providers of these services. With reference to the interpretation of genetic tests, and indeed how to distinguish genetic variants from bona fide deleterious mutations, if the physician ordering the test were to be in doubt, consultation with genetic professionals should be performed. In terms of patient surveillance and management post identification of a genetic mutation related to tumors of the GI tract and related sites, these patients can be managed by the GI specialist, qualified genetic professionals, or a thoughtful and motivated primary care physician. Useful resources about specific genetic tests and the clinical presentations of genetic syndromes can be found on the Genetests and Online Mendelian Inheritance in Man Web sites.

Diagnosis of a genetic syndrome is made by mutation analysis of germline genomic DNA for specific candidate genes. In the United States, these tests currently cost about $200 to $3,000, depending on the analysis performed. A 5- to 10-cc blood sample provides ample DNA for testing. On occasion, other tissue sources, such as skin fibroblast biopsies, are used. Typically, all the exons in the coding region of the gene(s) to be analyzed are polymerase chain reaction (PCR) amplified and sequenced. If a gene variant were to truncate the candidate protein prematurely, such as by the creation of a new stop codon or an insertion/deletion causing a frameshift, it would be interpreted as a mutation. Deleterious changes in mRNA consensus splice donor and acceptor sites that bracket the exons are also interpreted as mutations. If a missense variant were evolutionarily well conserved and in a critical domain of a protein, it would also usually be diagnosed as a mutation. If no variant were identified by direct sequencing of the coding region, the test should be considered noninformative. In this situation, large genomic rearrangements such as whole exon deletions or insertions must be analyzed by techniques such as Southern blotting or multiplex quantitative PCR of all exons. If no mutations were identified, for certain diseases, immunohistochemistry of formalin-fixed, paraffin-embedded tissue is employed to detect the tumor-specific absence of the protein in question. On rare occasion, a balanced translocation missed by multiplex quantitative PCR is identified with a high-resolution karyotype or by fluorescent in situ hybridization.

Inactivation of specific genes can cause related molecular signatures that can be used to predict individuals who might benefit from genetic testing. A classic example is DNA mismatch repair (MMR) gene mutations in colorectal cancer (CRC), which causes a phenotype of microsatellite instability (MSI) (1–3). MSI refers to the contraction or expansion of short DNA sequences within the tumor DNA that arises due to defective repair of DNA polymerase slippage during replication. These expansions and contractions are directly visible when DNA from a tumor is compared by gel or capillary electrophoresis with DNA from normal epithelium. Defects in the insertion/deletion repair function create a phenotype that is largely believed to be unique to MMR. Tumors lacking MSI are referred to as microsatellite stable (MSS). MSS cancers are generally believed to have greater segmental aneuploidy and gross chromosomal arrangements, perhaps reflecting greater epigenetic abnormalities of DNA methylation and histone modification. It is anticipated that genomic technologies analyzing GI cancers at the levels of genomic DNA, allele-specific expression (allelotyping), mRNA levels, epigenetic modifications, and proteomics will permit recognition of additional molecular signatures of GI cancer subtypes, helping dictate management and therapy. When these molecular signatures of tumor subtypes are defined more precisely, it is anticipated that therapies can be developed that are finely targeted at the pathways affected by specific combinations of mutations in susceptibility genes. With the development of ultra high-throughput DNA sequencing technologies in the coming decade that aim to sequence an entire human genome for $1,000, it is anticipated that "personalized" tumor signatures and signature-directed therapies will begin to emerge.

BASIC CANCER GENETICS

Advances in molecular genetics since 1990 have indicated that cancer is a "disease of DNA" (4–6). Mutations in genes passed onto progeny occur in all cells in the body. These mutations are called *germline mutations*. A mutation present in all cells in a body that is not inherited from a parent is referred to as a *de novo mutation*. When mutations occur in individual cells, such as during DNA genomic replication or through DNA damage, this type of mutation is referred to as *somatic*. When a somatic mutation occurs shortly after fertilization and is present in many but not all cells in the body, it is called *mosaic*.

Germline mutations can be inherited with both chromosome alleles affected (recessive inheritance) or only one chromosome (dominant inheritance). Most GI cancer syndromes have *incomplete penetrance*. This term refers to the concept that an individual can inherit a mutated gene but not develop any features of the related syndrome in their lifetime. Incomplete penetrance is a common feature of all adult genetic disorders. *Expressivity* refers to the way in which a gene mutation manifests. For example, a brother and a sister from a family with a Lynch syndrome gene mutation could develop colon or endometrial cancer, respectively. Although they are both affected with Lynch syndrome, the gene mutation *expressivity* is different for each. *Somatic inactivation* refers to the situation where a gene either is mutated or has no mutation but has its mRNA transcription repressed by other mechanisms, such as DNA or histone modification or whole gene deletion (6). With reference to GI cancer genetics, almost all syndromes are caused by dominant mutations. Typically, the first mutation is inactivated through a germline inherited or de novo mutation, and the second allele is inactivated through somatic inactivation in individual cells. The classic description of this phenomenon was popularized by Knudson et al. with regard to the retinoblastoma syndrome (4). Somatic mutation and inactivation is believed to play a widespread role in many cancers that normally appear to be sporadic (i.e., without a family history). For example, while germline mutations of the *MLH1* gene cause Lynch syndrome, somatic inactivation of

MLH1 in both alleles causes an estimated 7.5% of sporadic CRC (7). Therefore, the same gene can be inactivated in hereditary and sporadic CRC, but through different mechanisms.

The three major classes of genes mutated are oncogenes, tumor-suppressor genes, and genes involved in the maintenance of genetic stability. For an in-depth discussion of this topic, the reader is referred to the excellent texts *The Genetic Basis of Human Cancer* (8) and *The Biology of Cancer* (6). Briefly, oncogenes and tumor suppressors are mutated genes that directly regulate the growth of cancer cells by inhibiting their growth and progression through the cell cycle or by promoting programmed cell death (apoptosis). Classically, oncogenes are "activated." A prime example is a somatically acquired missense mutation causing a constitutively active form of *KRAS* that inappropriately transduces growth-promoting signals commonly in colorectal and pancreatic cancers (7). Tumor-suppressor genes prevent cell cycle progression. Classic examples are *SMAD4 (DPC4)* inactivation through somatic deletion in pancreatic cancer and *APC* inactivating mutations in CRC (7,8).

Genes involved in the maintenance of genomic stability include the MMR genes. When these genes are inactivated, somatic mutation rates increase, with the subsequent appearance of oncogene and tumor-suppressor gene mutations. However, there can be some overlap in these categories. For example, the MMR genes play roles both in maintaining genomic integrity and in initiating apoptosis in response to DNA damage (6). The pathogenesis of CRC and other GI neoplasms results from a series of discrete genetic changes that include mutational inactivation of tumor-suppressor genes and activation of oncogenes (reviewed in 7,8). Briefly, mutations in an estimated 5 to 11 genes (9–11) are believed to be required for the development of a malignant tumor. These mutations follow a progression from normal epithelium to benign tumors and eventually to cancer by accumulating genetic alterations. Early mutations that confer a selective growth advantage lead to clonal proliferation and accumulation of additional mutations. The order of these mutations may be important because later genetic changes such as mutated *TP53* are not sufficient to initiate tumor development as singular early events. In addition, the activation of oncogenes in adult animals can have different consequences than activation during embryogenesis (12). In individuals with genome stability-maintenance genes such as MMR, oncogene and tumor-suppressor mutations accumulate at a faster rate. Recent studies suggest that oncogenes and tumor-suppressor mutations have particularly deleterious consequences when they occur in a small number of cancer-initiating cells with properties of self-renewal analogous to stem cells (13,14).

COLORECTAL CANCER

CRC is the second leading cause of cancer death in the United States (15). Approximately 10% to 15% of adults in the United States have a family history of CRC in a first-degree relative (16,17). A large proportion of CRC is preventable if detected early, usually with colonoscopic screening (18). Early detection is particularly important in high-risk subjects. Molecular genetics has made a significant impact in decreasing CRC mortality through the identification of genetic syndromes. Therefore, it is important to understand and recognize these syndromes. Since 1990, there have been significant advances in the understanding of the genes that underlie hereditary susceptibility to CRC. It is now well established that mutations in DNA repair genes (*MLH1, MSH2, MSH6, MYH, BLM*) and genes involved in signal transduction (*APC*, *LBK1*, *STK11*, *SMAD4*) underlie a significant percentage of hereditary CRC susceptibility. This section addresses the most important CRC genetic syndromes.

Lynch Syndrome and DNA Mismatch Repair

The phenotypic spectrum of Lynch syndrome includes cancer of the colorectum, endometrium, stomach, upper urinary tract, small bowel, ovary, and bile ducts. Although usually recognized by clinical criteria (e.g., the revised Bethesda guidelines) (19), colorectal adenocarcinoma arising in Lynch syndrome may often have several recognizable histopathological features, including a poorly differentiated, mucinous appearance, characteristic lymphocytic infiltrate, histologic heterogeneity, and signet ring features (20–22). Clinically, approximately two-thirds of colon cancers are right sided, compared to approximately one-third in sporadic cancer. Linkage analyses originally led to the identification of *MLH1* and *MSH2* mutations in highly penetrant Lynch syndrome pedigrees (23,24). These genes are estimated to cause >90% of Lynch syndrome. Subsequently, identifiable *MSH6* mutations have been shown to underlie less penetrant aggregations of CRC (25–27). In addition, rare atypical Lynch syndrome pedigrees with identifiable *PMS2* or *MLH3* mutations have also been described (28–30). An algorithm (31) for the clinical evaluation of Lynch syndrome is summarized in Figure 3.1.

Patients with Lynch syndrome mutations have significantly improved survival with intensive cancer surveillance, and family members who do not inherit a mutation are spared the discomfort, expense, and iatrogenic complications of cancer surveillance (32–35). Because the clinical management and prognosis of mutation versus nonmutation carriers differ so drastically, it is imperative that deleterious mutations be identified, and their clinical impact correctly interpreted. Overall, societal health care costs are decreased with Lynch syndrome diagnosis and subsequent management if the costs of subsequent hospitalization for metastatic disease are included (32–35). There is significant variation with regard to age of onset, clinical phenotypes, and tumor spectrum among families with Lynch syndrome mutations. The clinical phenotype ranges from families satisfying the highly specific Amsterdam criteria (36) to familial CRC (defined as proband plus either one affected first-degree relative or two affected second-degree relatives), isolated early onset disease, and even sporadic CRC (37). The wide range of clinical phenotypes complicates genetic counseling, and the implementation of individualized medical-surgical management for patients and their relatives carrying these mutations. There is no consensus on how to classify them as deleterious mutations or benign polymorphisms. They are often referred to as variants of uncertain significance. Part of the large variation in the *MLH1/MSH2* mutant cancer susceptibility is due to the frequent occurrence of missense mutations. Including all types of mutations (e.g., truncating, genomic deletion, duplication, rearrangement), 24% of hereditary nonpolyposis colon cancer (HNPCC) mutations cited in the International Society for Gastrointestinal Hereditary Tumor database are missense. Missense mutations cause a broad range of clinical phenotypes. Although some cause complete loss of protein function and result in a phenotype similar to mutations that truncate the protein prematurely, many create proteins that retain partial function. There is widespread agreement in the cancer genetics community that correct interpretation of the clinical significance of specific missense mutations is extremely challenging and is a limiting factor in the medical management of the families involved.

Lynch Syndrome Mutation Risk Prediction Clinical Models

The revised Bethesda guidelines were developed to identify screening criteria to identify subjects who are at high risk of having a germline MMR gene mutation (36). More recently, multivariate logistic regression risk models using personal and family medical history have been created to predict more precisely the probability that an individual carries a Lynch syndrome mutation. The results of MSI/IHC studies can also be included with the other information to assess risk. Barnetson et al. (38) and Chen et al. (39) independently developed and validated logistic regression models that predict an individual's risk of carrying a mutation in *MLH1/MSH2/MSH6* (referred to here, respectively, as Barnetson and MMRPro models). Balmana et al. similarly developed a logistic regression model to predict risk of carrying a mutation in *MLH1/MSH2* (PREMM$_{1,2}$) (40). These models, which employ either logistic regression or Bayesian analytic approaches to predict risk, outperform the revised Bethesda guidelines in accuracy of identifying MMR mutation high-risk individuals. At present, it has not been well defined if one model is preferred over the others, and future studies will be required to resolve this issue.

DNA Mismatch Repair and Mechanisms of Cancer Prevention

More than 1 billion years old, MMR plays critical roles in the maintenance of genomic stability in prokaryotes, simple eukaryotes, and metazoan organisms such as humans and rodents (41–43). Interest in DNA MMR and its mechanisms of action exploded in the early 1990s with the observation that germline mutations in MMR genes cause HNPCC (23,24,44,45). The biology of MMR has been extensively characterized in model organisms, and these studies have given tremendous insights into the function of specific proteins in humans. The model organisms in which MMR has been most extensively studied are *Escherichia coli* and *Saccharomyces cerevisiae*. Other systems in which MMR genes have been rigorously characterized include *Caenorhabditis elegans* and *Arabidopsis thaliana*. The precise mechanistic functions that each MMR protein performs in these model organisms, as well as humans and mice, has been covered in detail in numerous excellent reviews (43,46–53). Therefore, this subject is summarized only succinctly here, focusing on mechanisms most likely to be relevant to the discussion of tissue-specific carcinogenesis.

Briefly, there are nine mammalian MMR genes (*MLH1*, *MLH3*, *PMS1-2*, *MSH2-6*) (43,46). The MMR proteins interact with each other to create a combinatorial code of complexes that mediate distinct functions. The mammalian *E. coli* MutS homologues (MSH proteins) are believed to directly contact double-stranded DNA, scanning along the genomic DNA for mismatches analogous to a "sliding clamp" until they encounter a base pair containing a mismatch (54,55). The MSH proteins interact with multiple proteins including the mammalian *E. coli* MutL homologues (MLH) and yeast postmeiotic segregation (PMS) homologue proteins (which have significant amino acid identify and structural similarity to the MLH proteins), as well as RPA, EXO1, RFC, possibly HMGB1, and other less well-characterized proteins (reviewed in 43,46; also see 56–58, which discuss this topic in excellent detail). With respect to the mutator function, the MSH2-MSH6 heterodimer is believed to primarily repair single-base substitutions and 1 base pair insertion-deletion mutations, while MSH2-MSH3 is

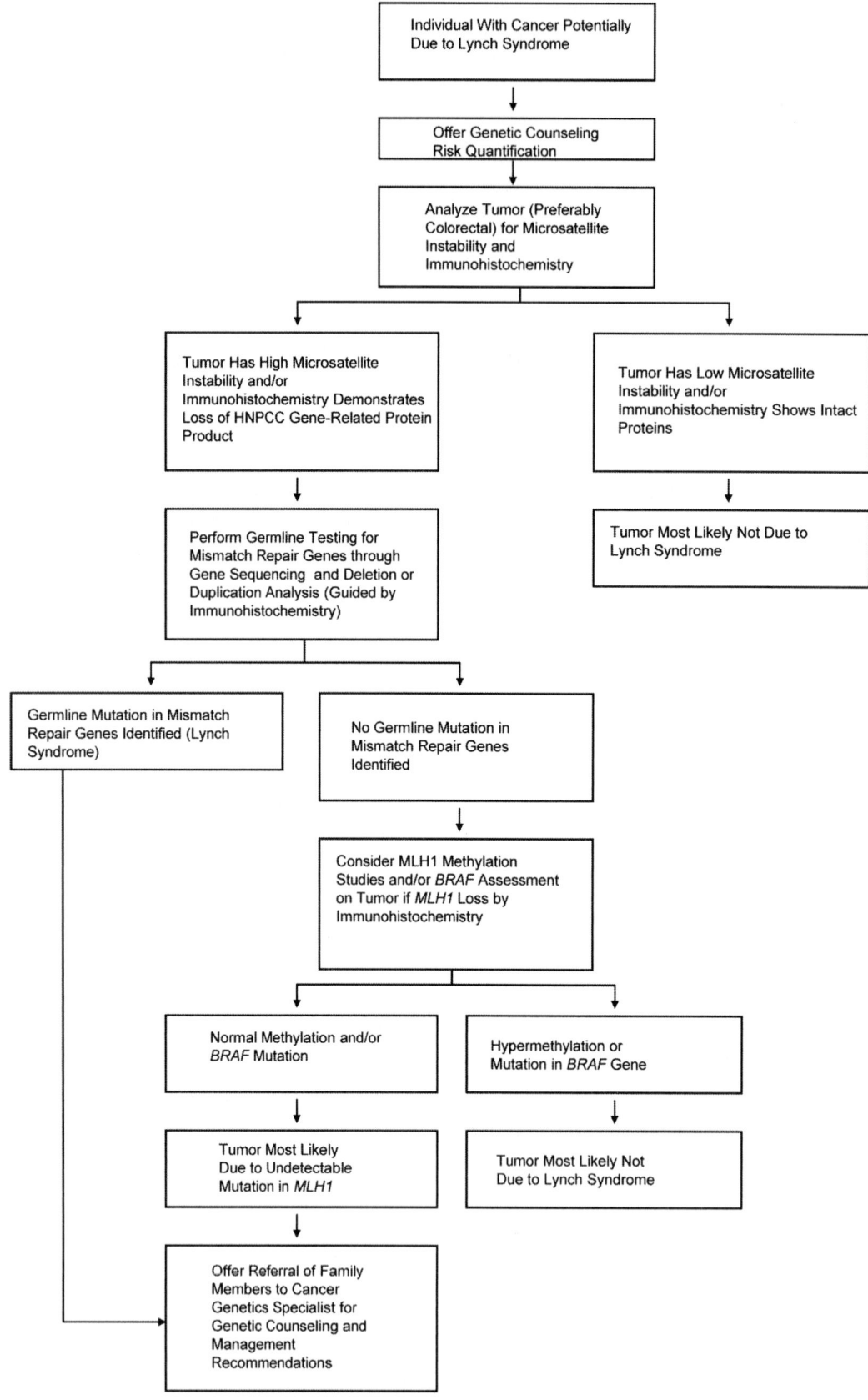

FIGURE 3.1. Algorithm for molecular diagnosis of Lynch syndrome. A consensus approach to the molecular diagnosis of Lynch syndrome in at-risk individuals. Individuals to be evaluated have a thorough personal medical and family history and physical exam. Revised Bethesda guidelines and risk prediction models quantify the likelihood of identifying a mutation in the genes underlying the Lynch syndrome. Molecular analyses are performed on tumor tissue, if available. The molecular phenotype of the tumor guides subsequent genetic testing. *Source:* Adapted from ref. 257.

believed primarily to repair 1 to 4 base pair insertion-deletion mutations (43,46). The *E. coli* MLH and yeast PMS proteins interact with heterodimers of MSH proteins to help catalyze their different functions. *MLH1-PMS2* is the primary MutL complex that interacts with both MSH2/6 and MSH3 complexes in mechanisms believed to be relevant to cancer prevention. Recent studies suggest that mammalian *MLH1-MLH3* also contributes to some of these processes, but in all mechanisms tested to a lesser degree than *MLH1-PMS2* (29,30,59,60). *MLH1-PMS1* clearly exists in mammalian cells, but it currently has no clearly defined role in processes relevant to cancer susceptibility (61,62). *MSH4* and *MSH5* are believed to play roles exclusively in meiosis and are currently not believed to contribute to mechanisms of cancer prevention (63).

A mutator phenotype causing increased mutation rates for single-base substitution and insertion-deletion mismatches have traditionally been believed to be the main functions in MMR cancer prevention. Defects in the insertion-deletion repair function create a phenotype that is largely believed to be unique to MMR. Because this function was originally characterized on short repetitive DNA microsatellite sequences, it is often referred to as MSI (1–3). MSI is divided into MSI-Low and MSI-High (MSI-H) subtypes, depending on the percentage of microsatellite markers that are mutated, but only the MSI-High subtype is clearly associated with defective MMR. Tumors with no MSI are referred to as MSS. (Consensus thinking on the topic of MSI was recently covered in detail by Umar et al. [19].) The precise mechanisms whereby MSI causes cancer are hypothesized to include a genomewide increased mutation rate that causes mutations not only in microsatellites, but also in exonic coding sequences of genes important in cancer suppression. MSI mutation rates in these short repetitive sequences in *MLH1-* or *MSH2*-deficient cells are estimated to be more than 100 times higher than that seen in MMR-proficient cells and used to test directly whether MMR deficiency is involved in specific tumor types. Almost all described *MLH1/MSH2* mutations cause MSI-H tumors, although recently MSS *MLH1* nonsynonymous amino acid substitutions causing deleterious mutations have been described (64,65). Current thinking is that MMR mutations are recessive (i.e., require two hits under the Knudson hypothesis) before cells become susceptible to cancer. However, it has been suggested that cells from subjects carrying heterozygous germline mutations may have detectable MSI using a more sensitive assay referred to as single-molecule or small pool PCR (66,67) that can detect approximately 5- to 10-fold elevations in MSI rates. These new findings are intriguing but require further investigation before the role of MMR haploinsufficiency in cancer susceptibility is clearly established.

In addition to its essential roles in insertion-deletion and single-base substitution repair, MMR proteins also participate in additional mechanisms that could contribute to carcinogenesis, most notably initiation of apoptosis in response to DNA damage (54,68). Recent studies using mouse models of single amino acid substitutions causing separation of function mutations have clearly demonstrated that decreased apoptosis plays an important role in MMR-deficient tumorigenesis (69,70). The precise mechanism by which MMR contributes to the initiation of programmed cell death remains unclear, with both futile cycles of repair causing high levels of double-strand breaks and direct signaling proposed (71,72). MMR mutant cells fail to activate a p73-dependent cell death activation pathway (73), which may explain the absence of a critical requirement for p53-mediated apoptosis (74). This failure impairs cell cycle and DNA damage checkpoint recognition (43).

In summary, the current models suggest that MMR mutations cause cancer primarily through the contribution of both mechanisms: (a) cells acquire mutations in components of critical tumor-suppressor gene pathways that allow them to proliferate, and (b) cells do not initiate apoptosis appropriately. It is unclear whether these mechanisms operate sequentially or concurrently in different cell types. MMR proteins also contribute to suppress homoeologous recombination (71,75), which could in principle contribute as an important mechanism of carcinogenesis. However, the contribution of increased rates of homoeologous recombination from MMR mutations to carcinogenesis is not well defined at this point in time.

Genetic Modifiers of HNPCC

HNPCC is known to have reduced penetrance and variable expressivity. Identifying the major determinants of this phenotypic heterogeneity is critical in tailoring cancer prevention strategies for individual high-risk patients, for example, which families require intensive surveillance for ovarian cancer, and which families can be spared the expense, iatrogenic complications, and inconvenience of this surveillance. Marked interfamily variation in risk of HNPCC spectrum cancer is clearly documented (76–83). The variance is in both (a) age of presentation of CRC in HNPCC, and (b) the distribution of different tumor types that develops in different HNPCC families (76–83). However, the reasons for these phenotypic variances are poorly understood. CRC presentation ranges from the early 20s to no disease in the early 90s for germline mutation carriers (82–84). Three population-based studies from Europe and the United States (82–84) have studied estimated lifetime CRC penetrance in HNPCC. A meta-analysis of these studies estimates lifetime CRC risk as approximating 74% for males and 39% for females (79).

Variants in the *Cyclin D1* gene have been proposed to be a genetic modifier of HNPCC penetrance. Cyclin D1 reaches maximal activity during the G1 phase, in which it plays an important role in the transition from the G1 phase to the S phase of the cell cycle. The *Cyclin D1* gene has a G to A variant at codon 242 in exon 4 that increases alternate splicing, creating a protein with significantly increased protein stability. HNPCC patients who are homozygous or heterozygous for the mutant allele developed CRC an average of 11 years earlier than patients who were homozygous for the normal alleles (85). However, this putative association has only been reported in one group of patients, and no validation in additional cohorts of HNPCC patients has been performed. Thus, it is unclear whether this putative modifier effect on HNPCC CRC onset is a true or chance association.

NAT2 is a highly polymorphic isozyme of *N*-acetyltransferase and is found in a variety of tissues, including the colorectal mucosa. It catalyzes the metabolism of xenobiotics and carcinogens by transferring an acetyl group to these agents, and has been suggested as a potential modifier of CRC risk. Frazier et al. (86) found HNPCC patients heterozygous for the variant allele NAT2*7 after adjustment for the *NAT2* mutant loci NAT2*5, and NAT2*6 had a significantly higher risk of CRC (hazard ratio, 2.96; $P < 0.012$) than individuals homozygous for the wild-type allele. However, without this adjustment, NAT2*7 allele carriers were not at increased CRC risk. Therefore, it is unclear whether this modifier effect is true or was ascertained only through multiple hypothesis testing.

Recently, this relationship has been clarified by several demonstrations that cigarette smoking selectively increases the subset of CRC that manifests MSI-High (77,87). The environmental component of this interaction can be incorporated through a quantitative assessment of lifetime smoking exposure, and quantitative estimates of smoking risk performed (79). However, it is likely that genetic factors impact the effect of smoking as well. For example, genetic factors have been described that significantly influence the ability of individuals to quit smoking (88,89), which likely has an important impact on lifetime smoking exposure.

Management

Individuals with known Lynch syndrome *MLH1/MSH2* mutations have colonoscopic surveillance every 1 to 2 years (31). Surveillance should start at ages 20 to 25. *MSH6* mutation carrier surveillance is not as well defined, but age 30 is often used for these patients (31). In women with Lynch syndrome mutations, there are no adequately powered studies that evaluated whether endometrial cancer screening improves survival. Nonetheless, as a high-risk population, endometrial cancer screening in these patients is reasonable. *MSH6* mutation carriers in particular may have greater endometrial cancer than CRC risk. Transvaginal ultrasound has been used, but there is a high false-positive rate (31). Endometrial biopsy is used in women who are symptomatic, such as presenting with pelvic pain and/or irregular pre- or postmenopausal vaginal bleeding. Endometrial biopsy beginning at ages 30 to 35 can be used every 1 to 2 years for surveillance. The absolute risk of Lynch syndrome carriers for other sites (e.g., ovary, brain, renal, stomach, bladder, biliary tract) is greater than the general population but is clearly less than colorectum and endometrium. Screening for these sites is therefore not well defined. Many clinicians will perform annual urinalysis with cytology and transvaginal ultrasound for ovarian cancer every 1 to 2 years as a reasonable surveillance strategy. A baseline upper endoscopy should be performed, but the optimal subsequent screening interval has yet to be established. An important general rule is that when families have a particular tumor type that is prominent, increased surveillance should be instituted for the tissue site. So, families that have gastric cancer should have endoscopy at 1- to 2-year intervals.

In terms of surgical management, prophylactic colectomy before the identification of colon cancer is typically not performed. However, once a first malignancy is identified, a subtotal colectomy with retention of the rectum (which preserves fecal continence) is performed. This management is in contrast to the segmental colectomy typically performed for sporadic colon cancer. After surgery, the rectum can be monitored with proctoscopy, sigmoidoscopy, or limited colonoscopy. Because there are no studies formally comparing subtotal colectomy versus segmental colectomy with frequent colonoscopic surveillance, patient preference is important to integrate into the surgical management strategy. For ovarian and endometrial cancer surgical management, a retrospective study of prophylactic bilateral oophorectomy and hysterectomy in 315 women with Lynch syndrome showed that after 10 years of follow-up, 0% of uterine/endometrial cancer developed in the women who had surgery, but 5.5% of the women who did not have surgery developed ovarian cancer, and 33% of these women developed endometrial cancer (90). Based on these data, prophylactic bilateral oophorectomy and hysterectomy is considered a reasonable option for women with Lynch syndrome. Women who do consider this option typically wait until after childbearing. Often, subtotal colectomy, oophorectomy, and hysterectomy are performed at the same time.

In addition to Lynch syndrome, there are at least three other relatively common forms of hereditary predisposition to colorectal neoplasia: familial adenomatous polyposis (FAP), attenuated FAP, and Peutz-Jeghers syndrome (PJS).

Familial Adenomatous Polyposis

Originally described in the late 19th century, FAP is a rare (1 in 7,000–8,000) syndrome characterized by presentation with hundreds or even thousands of colonic polyps in the late teens or early 20s and progression to colon cancer in virtually every case. A minimum of 100 polyps is generally necessary to make the diagnosis, whereas HNPCC families rarely have more than 50 polyps. Median age of adenomas is 16 (91), with 95% affected by 35 (92). Onset of CRC is 100% by age 40 (93), with average age of 36 (91). Benign hamartomas are seen in the fundus and body in about 50% of patients, and duodenal polyps in about 90%, with a 4% to 12% risk for duodenal/ampullary carcinoma. There is also an increased risk for small bowel cancer and thyroid cancer (follicular or papillary), mostly in women. Children are at risk for hepatoblastoma, and CNS tumors (medulloblastomas) can be seen in the Turcot variant. *Gardner syndrome* (94) is characterized by cutaneous soft tissue tumors; lipomas; fibromas; epidermoid/sebaceous cysts on legs, face, scalp, and arms; osteomas (skull and mandible); supernumerary teeth; congenital hypertrophy of the retinal pigment epithelium (CHRPE); and desmoid tumors and mesenteric fibromatosis (95–99). There is an association between FAP and juvenile nasopharyngeal angiofibroma, which is 25-fold more prevalent in men with FAP than in the general population (100–107).

An Israeli study documented extracolonic manifestations among 38 of 50 FAP patients, or 76%. Two of the 50 patients died, 1 from a mesenteric desmoid tumor and 1 of mesenteric malignant fibrous histiocytoma (108).

APC

The APC gene (5q21) encodes a large protein that acts in the Wnt pathway via several domains: to regulate cell cycle and apoptosis, to stabilize the cytoskeleton, and to mediate intercellular adhesion (109). The protein product of the APC gene was shown to associate with proteins (catenins) that bind to a cell surface molecule (cadherin), which is essential for cellular adhesion. These studies suggest that the APC protein may be a vital communications link between the cell surface and the microtubules necessary for cell division (110–112). An important region binds with ß-catenin, inhibiting it from interacting with T-cell factor/lymphoid enhancer factor (Tcf/Lef) to form a proliferative DNA transcription complex (113,114). About 30% of APC mutations are de novo, and 98% are truncating (115). Interstitial deletions of 5q22, which includes the APC gene, have been reported in individuals with adenomatous polyposis and mental retardation.

Severe polyposis is associated with APC mutations in codons 1250 to 1464, sparser polyps with mutations in codons 213 to 1249 and 1465 to 1597, CHRPE with mutations in codons 311 to 1444, and Gardner syndrome with mutations in codons 1395 to 1578. There is no clear relationship for duodenal, periampullar, and gastric adenomas (91,116–125).

In 205 kindreds, no extracolonic manifestations were associated with APC mutations between codons 177 and 452, more extracolonic manifestations with mutations from codons 457 to 1309, and nearly 90% with extracolonic manifestations were associated with mutations between codons 1395 and 1493 (126). Variable expressivity was also noted in a study of 31 members of four kindreds with 3' mutations at either codon 1979 or codon 2644, including cases with less than 100 polyps to classic FAP. These individuals did tend to have a later age of onset, averaging 50 years of age (127). Gastric adenocarcinoma associated with fundic gland polyps were reported in more than one kindred with known APC mutations and the attenuated FAP phenotype (128). Periampullary adenocarcinomas have also been reported in patients from kindreds with the attenuated FAP phenotype (129).

Of 24 cases of FAP-associated papillary thyroid cancers, 21 had mutations in exon 15, 22, one-third of which resulted in a specific protein truncation, and 17 of 18 examined were found to have CHRPE. Therefore, it has been suggested that FAP kindreds with CHRPE or with mutations in the 5' region of exon 15 should be screened for thyroid nodules starting at 15 years of age (130).

Among patients with no detectable APC mutation, exon 14 deletions were found in 7 of 60 FAP patients using a quantitative multiplex PCR assay. Of these 7 deletions, 6 encompassed the entire APC locus (131). Patients with truncating APC mutations proximal to exon 9 had fewer duodenal adenomas.

Because of variable phenotype with identical μs (132), clinical management should be based on degree of colonic polyposis (133). There is evidence of intrafamilial variation in expression of FAP in patients with identical APC mutations. In addition, there is more similarity of expression between first-degree relatives than between second-degree relatives, leading to strong suspicion that modifier genes play a role (134,135).

A hypermutable region exists at codon 1307 in the APC gene. This mutation does not lead to classic FAP with hundreds to thousands of polyps but does cause an increased risk of colon cancer (136). About 6% to 8% of Ashkenazi Jews have the I1309K, resulting in a ~10% to 20% lifetime risk of colon cancer (137). Of Ashkenazi Jews with CRC, 8% to 15% have this mutation, so targeted testing may be appropriate.

Management

Many gastroenterologists and surgeons consider it unnecessary to test for mutations in patients with FAP because diagnosis by sigmoidoscopy is clear, and the prognosis remains unchanged (100% penetrance). However, determination of family members actually at risk can reduce unnecessary screening of adolescents and young adults (138). Given the 100% penetrance for colon cancer, prophylactic colectomy is part of basic management of this syndrome (91). Guidelines for the management of patients with FAP have been promulgated by the American Gastroenterology Association and the National Comprehensive Cancer Network (NCCN) and should be consulted because they are updated regularly (139). In general, patients with APC mutations should undergo flexible sigmoidoscopy annually starting at ages 10 to 12, with colonoscopy once polyps are detected, and colectomy for dense polyposis (>~20–30) or during the midteens. Surgical options include colectomy and ileorectal anastomosis, proctocolectomy with ileostomy, and proctocolectomy with ileal pouch-anal anastomosis. The goal of colectomy is to preserve rectal function mutations (140). Postsurgical flexible sigmoidoscopy surveillance of the rectum with endoscopy snare polypectomy and argon coagulation endoscopy ablation is suggested at 6-month intervals (141). A large analysis of the Danish, Swedish, Finish, and Dutch polyposis registries revealed 47 rectal carcinoma diagnoses among 659 patients who had ileorectal anastomosis surgery. Of 167 individuals harboring known APC mutations, 7 had rectal cancer diagnoses. The 5-year median survival rate after rectal carcinoma diagnosis was 60% (140).

Upper GI endoscopy should be performed in FAP patients every 1 to 3 years, with baseline exam by ages 25 to 30 years. FAP and patients' thyroids should also be palpated. At-risk children should be screened for hepatoblastoma with abdominal palpation and abdominal ultrasound twice per year until age 6 years.

Presymptomatic individuals with a family history of FAP, but for whom mutation status is unknown, should have annual flexible sigmoidoscopy, beginning at ages 10 to 12 years until 24 years, every 2 years until 34 years, every 3 years until 44 years, and every 3 to 5 years thereafter; consider colonoscopy at 10-year intervals starting at age 20 years.

Interestingly, in FAP patients, regression of rectal polyps has been noted after ileorectal anastomosis, suggesting possible environmental modulators of the phenotype. As noted, careful surveillance of the upper GI tract is recommended every 3 years in FAP patients post colectomy, as are frequent rectal examinations.

Reduction in the number of polyps in patients with FAP has been demonstrated after treatment with the nonsteroidal anti-inflammatory drug (NSAID) sulindac (142). Postmenopausal hormone replacement therapy has been suggested as a chemoprevention for colon cancer, and during a 1 year chemoprevention study, an FAP patient assigned to the placebo group developed colorectal polyps, which subsequently regressed following oral contraceptive administration (143). Furthermore, in a large study of APC variants and their interactions with lifestyle and dietary factors, an APC polymorphism, Asp 1822Val, was found to be associated with a statistically significant decrease in CRC risk for postmenopausal hormone use compared to wild-type individuals who were not currently taking hormone replacement, although hormone replacement also had a chemopreventive effect for nonpolymorphism carriers (144).

A few case reports of polyp regression following cytotoxic chemotherapy have been published; further studies are required to determine if cytotoxic chemotherapy may be an alternative for FAP patients for whom colectomy is not an option, or for duodenal, ampullary, or papillary duct polyps that may be less amenable to surgery or treatment with NSAIDs (145).

NSAIDs will not prevent colorectal neoplasia in FAP patients. In a patient with an ileorectal anastomosis who was also on sulindac therapy, carcinoma of the rectum was diagnosed 51 months after surgery, and case reports of three rectal carcinomas in patients on sulindac following colectomy with ileorectal anastomosis illustrate that residual risk for rectal carcinoma remains (146). Of 19 FAP patients treated with 300 mg of sulindac daily for 6 months, 6 patients harboring two FMO3 polymorphisms, E158K and E308G, had more favorable regression of polyp size and number compared to those without the two polymorphisms. These polymorphisms confer a greater response to sulindac (147,148). Desmoid tumors are usually responsive to treatment with combined celecoxib and tamoxifen citrate therapy (108).

Attenuated FAP

A form of attenuated polyposis is characterized by later onset polyposis, average age 44 years, and CRC by average age 56 years (113). There are fewer colonic adenomas <100 and no associated CHRPE, but patients can have upper GI and other extracolonic features similar to FAP.

An even more attenuated form of FAP, characterized by familial desmoid tumor in the absence of the usual colonic or extracolonic features, has been described (149). In this syndrome, termed hereditary desmoid disease, mutations in the 3' end of APC were observed, consistent with the trend for desmoid tumors noted in FAP patients with 3' APC mutations (149). In one kindred, a germline mutation in codons 2643 to 2644 in the extreme 3' of APC was associated with the phenotype of a florid proliferation of desmoid tumors, with nearly 100% penetrance, but with variable expressivity, including cutaneous cysts, but no GI polyps, and few colon polyps (150).

In general, attenuated FAP is associated with mutations at 5' and 3' ends of APC gene, giving rise to hypomorphic alleles that do not completely inactivate the protein product. Mutations upstream of codon 169 are believed to be mild because downstream, at codon 184, there is an in-frame ATG amino acid sequence that can reinitiate protein translation. Mutations in exon 9 have been described (151). Germline μs in AXIN1 and CTNNB1 also appear to lead to multiple polyps (152). Axin is a scaffold protein that binds multiple proteins in the

Wnt pathway (153). Mutations in different binding regions may have varied phenotypic consequences. Somatic Axin mutations in tumor cell lines have demonstrated its effect on ß-catenin concentrations and association with hepatoblastomas and hepatocellular cancers (154–156). All elements involved in the Wnt signaling pathway are considered putative candidate genes that can cause CRC because mutations in any Wnt signalling pathway genes may impact degradation of the key effector molecule of the pathway, ß-catenin (153).

Mutations resulting in alternate splicing of exon 9 and mutations in the 3′ half of the coding region have also been associated with attenuated FAP (157,158). The exon 9 mutation, resulting in alternative splicing, downregulates ß-catenin–regulated transcription, APC's tumor-suppressor mechanism. Both the alternatively spliced and the wild-type copies of APC must be inactivated for tumorigenesis to occur. This may explain the attenuated phenotype compared to mutations resulting in a nonfunctional protein, which require somatic loss of only one copy of the APC gene. However, a common somatic mutation in colorectal tumors, 4666insA was found to inactivate the alternatively spliced exon 9 allele, but did not disrupt the wild-type allele (159). Another report of a large kindred with an exon 9 mutation noted marked variable expressivity, ranging from a complete lack of clinical or endoscopic findings for four individuals to classic FAP or colorectal neoplasia in 16 of 22 members with a truncating exon 9 mutation caused by an 11 base pair insertion with possible alternative splicing or unknown modifying factors (160). A Canadian genotype-phenotype study of 11 attenuated FAP kindreds found that those with mutations in the 5′ region had more severe upper GI manifestations and more variability in the number of adenomas. Mutations in the 3′ and exon 9 regions resulted in fewer adenomas that were more distally located. All attenuated familial adenomatous polyposis cases in this series had more right-sided adenomas, no desmoids and rectal sparing (161). Attenuated FAP may exhibit adenomas with a serrated morphology, according to a Japanese report (162). However, a British report noted that serrated lesions were present in eight individuals from the St. Mark's polyposis registry, all of whom had classic FAP with exon 15 mutations (141). The flat adenoma subtype of HNPCC is also believed to be a form of attenuated FAP because, in the index family, an APC mutation proximal to 5′ was described (163,164). As is discussed later in this chapter, the attenuated FAP phenotype has also been associated with mutations in MYH, the E. coli mutY human homolog (see MYH section) (165,166).

Management

For attenuated FAP, NCCN (167) generally recommends colonoscopy to be performed in the late teen years, and as long as no polyps are detected, colonoscopies may be repeated every 2 to 3 years. Once adenomatous polyp is detected, more frequent colonoscopies are recommended (e.g., every 1 to 2 years). Upper GI screening should also begin at age 25 to 30 years, and surveillance for skin, soft tissue, eye, and other manifestations of FAP are also appropriate. The role of prophylactic colectomy is less well established; however, NCCN guidelines call for strong consideration of this procedure at around age 40 years. Post colectomy, endoscopic rectal exam is performed annually.

MYH-Associated Polyposis

A proportion of FAP probands who test negative for germline APC mutations may harbor biallelic truncating or missense mutations in the base excision repair gene, MYH, the human homolog of the E. coli mutY gene. The phenotype is often indistinguishable from either FAP or AFAP. Microadenomas in the background colorectal mucosa in biallelic MYH mutation carriers was once considered pathognomic of FAP (168,169). MYH-associated polyposis is most commonly recessive because parents of affected homozygote or compound heterozygote mutation carriers have been reported to be unaffected (170). However, both monoallelic and biallelic germline mutations in MYH have been associated with multiple adenomas (170,171). Biallelic carriers have higher frequency of CRC than monoallelic patients (172). Patients with multiple adenomas (>15 without APC mutations) are more likely to have either homozygous or biallelic MYH μs than controls (169,173).

Duodenal adenomas have been reported, and one case of possible CHRPE has also been seen (174). Families with biallelic MYH mutations are comparable to patients with AFAP; they develop smaller numbers of adenomas. (175) found that CRC patients with monoallelic or biallelic MYH mutations have more first- and second-degree relatives with CRC than do CRC patients without MYH mutations, suggesting that even the monoallelic mutant MYH genotype may confer a predisposition for CRC.

Genetic testing for FAP that included MYH sequencing in addition to testing for APC mutations increased the positive yield of from 34.4% to 41.3% (176). Of 107 classic FAP patients with more than 100 adenomas, as well as 152 multiple adenoma probands with between 3 and 100 colorectal adenomas, 14 patients had biallelic MYH mutations, including 8 polyposis patients and 6 multiple adenoma patients. All MYH-positive probands expressed somatic APC G:C to T:A transversions, and all had family histories consistent with autosomal recessive inheritance patterns. No cases with germline MYH mutations had severe expression of more than 1,000 adenomas in this series, but three cases exhibited extracolonic manifestations, including two patients with duodenal polyps and one with CHRPE (177).

The mutations Y165C and G382D appear to be mutational hot spots, especially in white Europeans, comprising 86% of biallelic mutations in the Jones, Sieber, and Al-Tassan series (178,179), with an estimated carrier frequency of about 2% (180). Biallelic inheritance of the Y165C and G382D mutations were associated with the presence of ≥20 colonic polyps, and an age of CRC onset of 50 years or younger among 984 subjects (178,179). However, Y165C and G382D mutations were not identified in any of 266 Jewish CRC patients or in 450 Jewish controls (181).

Studies worldwide have revealed the population genetics of MYH mutations. The mutations Y90X and E466X were more prevalent in individuals of Pakistani and Indian origin, respectively (181). In a British study of 614 polyposis registry kindreds, 111 of whom were negative for an APC mutation, 25 were found to harbor biallelic MYH mutations (182). In an Italian series, about 20% of APC-negative FAP cases had autosomal recessive MYH mutations, predominantly Y165C, G382D, or a three base pair exon 14 deletion (466delE) that was identified in three unrelated subjects (183). In a Portuguese series, 21 MYH cases with biallelic mutations were identified among 53 APC mutation-negative individuals with classic FAP or multiple colorectal adenomas, almost twice as many as in the British and Italian series (184). In Australia, recessive MYH mutations accounted for 16% of 120 APC-negative polyposis (185). The Y165C, G382D mutations were not identified in 35 Japanese multiple adenomatous polyposis patients who tested negative for APC mutations. However, three unrelated patients in the Japanese cohort harbored an MYH exon 11 splice site mutation, IVS10-2 A to G, and one patient was homozygous for the mutation R231C (186). An additional MYH mutation, A459D in exon 14, was identified in three Finish CRC patients, and was shown to confer reduced DNA repair in in vitro experiments (187). In a series of 219 North Americans in whom no APC mutations were identified, 13 biallelic, common Y165C and G382D were found. Of 15 Y165C or G382D heterozygotes identified in this series, sequencing revealed additional mutations in 9 individuals, and 2 patients harbored homozygous mutations other than Y165C and G382D (the 466delF and 1395delGGA), suggesting that MYH sequencing may uncover additional deleterious mutations and could increase sensitivity (176). Autosomal recessive Y165 and G382D mutations accounted for 0.4% of 1,042 CRC cases in Finland, about equal to the percentage attributable to APC mutations. As few as five polyps were associated with recessive inheritance of MYH mutations at the time of cancer diagnosis (188). A separate, smaller Italian study found as many as 36% (5 of 14) of attenuated FAP cases were Y165C/G382D homozygotes or compound heterozygotes, compared to only 14% (2 of 14) in whom an APC mutation was detected (189). In 358 early onset polyposis cases unselected for APC mutation status, 2 cases were found to harbor biallelic MYH mutations, and 8 MYH mutation heterozygotes were identified. No MYH mutations were detected in 354 controls, leading authors to conclude that biallelic MYH mutations may account for up to 3% of early onset CRC. Patients in this series did not exhibit profuse polyposis, consistent with previous reports, and there was a prevalence of distally located tumors (165,166). MYH mutations were found in 15.6% of 45 patients with more than 15 polyps, although 2 of 122 patients with fewer than 15 polyps did harbor biallelic MYH mutations and had relatively early onset CRC at 50 years of age or younger. Furthermore, in this same series, 9 patients had family histories consistent with HNPCC, 7 meeting Bethesda guidelines and 2 meeting Amsterdam II criteria, and 22% of biallelic MYH mutation carriers would be missed if testing were offered based on multiple polyposis alone (190). A Dutch study of 40 biallelic MYH mutation carriers out of 170 APC-negative polyposis patients found no difference in the proportion of mutation carriers among patients with 10 to 99 polyps versus 100 to 1,000 polyps, so this genotype is equally prevalent among FAP and attenuated FAP cases. Of the 40 MYH carriers, 26 were diagnosed with CRC, with the age of onset ranging from 21 to 70 years and a median age of onset of 45 years. Duodenal polyps were diagnosed in 31% (5 of 16 for whom endoscopy reports were available), and breast cancer was diagnosed in 18% of females with biallelic MYH mutations (165,166). In one Italian, consanguineous kindred with homozygous frameshift MYH mutations, pilomatricomas, or tumors of the hair follicles, were observed in two siblings, in addition to early onset CRC (191).

A Canadian analysis of 1,238 colorectal cases and 1,250 healthy controls found an increased risk of CRC in first-degree relatives of both biallelic and monoallelic MYH Y165C and G382D carriers, with a relative risk of 1.54 and a 95% confidence interval of 1.10 to 2.16 (192). However, the association of an increased risk of CRC with heterozygous MYH mutation carrier status was not of statistical significance (193). In a separate series, 4 monoallelic and 2 biallelic Y165C and G382D MYH mutation carriers were identified among 555 colorectal cases, 255 of whom were non-Jewish white or white Hispanic. Among 918 healthy controls, 7 individuals harbored monoalleic Y165C and G382D MYH mutations. The 7 mutations in the control group were found exclusively among 392 non-Jewish whites and white Hispanics, suggesting a combined allele frequency of 0.9% (population frequency of 1.8%) for Y165C and G382D mutations in this population. Homozygosity for these two loci would be expected to be approximately 8 per 100,000, so the finding of 2 biallelic Y165C/G382D carriers among 255 non-Jewish white and white Hispanic CRC cases is supportive of Hardy-Weinberg disequilibrium in this population. This study is consistent with previous reports that suggest discrepancies in MYH mutation carrier frequencies based on the ethnicity of the population analyzed. The total monoallelic MYH mutation carrier frequency was 0.7% in CRC cases and 0.8% in controls in this series. However, carrier frequencies in cases and controls were 1.6% and 1.8%, respectively, when only the non-Jewish white and white Hispanic individuals were analyzed. There was no statistically significant increase in CRC associated with monoallelic MYH mutation carrier status (181). The question of heterozygous MYH mutation-associated CRC risk was further addressed in a population-based study of 2,239 cases and 1,845 controls. In this comparison, biallelic MYH mutation status conferred a 93-fold increased risk of CRC, with almost complete penetrance by age 60 years. Monoallelic MYH mutation carriers had a 1.68-fold increased risk of CRC, especially later in life, after age 55 years. The authors of this study also reported that 36% of those harboring biallelic MYH mutations did not exhibit multiple adenomatous polyps (194).

Management

For MYH-associated FAP, prophylactic colectomy is recommended, and given that more than one-third of biallelic MYH mutation carriers may not develop multiple polyps but remain at elevated risk for CRC, colonoscopy with polypectomies is not sufficiently preventative for this population (195). In general, management for biallelic MYH mutation carriers is identical to that of APC mutation-bearing FAP cases. Surgical options for mutant gene carriers include (a) ileorectal anastomosis for younger patients with few rectal adenomas and a milder family history, or with attenuated FAP, or (b) total proctocolectomy with the creation of an ileal pouch-anal anastomosis for more aggressive FAP.

Peutz-Jeghers Syndrome

PJS is a rare syndrome that is familial 75% of the time. It is characterized by hamartomatous polyposis of the GI tract and melanin pigmentation (oral and anal mucous membranes; palms of hands and feet), and has variable penetrance within families (196). Histologic examination of hamartomas is considered conclusive: connective tissue core with characteristic smooth muscle component (197). The most common associated malignancies are small intestine, stomach, pancreatic carcinoadenomas, and CRC. There is also increased risk of breast and uterine cancer, testicular and ovarian sex chord tumors, and lung cancer. Cumulative risk for all cancer types was 93% from ages 15 to 64 years (198). Risks of breast cancer are 54%; colon cancer, 39%; pancreatic cancer, 36%; stomach cancer, 29%; and ovarian cancer, 21%.

The syndrome is due to germline mutations in STK11/LKB1 on 19p13.3 (199). STK11 mutations are inactivating, and wild-type alleles are lost in hamartomas, suggesting a two-hit mechanism (197). Due to distinctive phenotype, molecular studies are often unnecessary to make the diagnosis (197). Mutations are detected in 70% of those with family history and in 20% to 30% of those without a family history (200). Mutations in LKB1/STK11 are believed to account for a maximum of 75% of PJS cases (201).

Some groups (202) found evidence suggestive of locus heterogeneity, and PJS families unlinked to 19p13.3 have been reported (203). A recent article casts doubt on promoter region harboring causative μs (204). Finally, in one study of patients with unexplained hamartomatous polyps, a mutation in PTEN was found in a patient classified as PJS (205).

Management

Stomach, large bowel, and small bowel are generally screened with upper and lower endoscopy, with removal of polyps as possible. Upper endoscopy should start at age 10 years, and colonoscopy by age 25 years, repeated at 2-year intervals. Breasts are examined by clinician examinations annually starting at age 20 years. Mammography should start at age 20 years and be repeated at 2- to 3-year intervals. Testicular exam is performed annually, starting at age 10 years. Gynecologic screening includes pelvic exam annually starting at age 20 years, and pelvic ultrasound also at around the same time. Pancreas screening can include endoscopic or abdominal ultrasound starting at age 30 years and be repeated every 1 to 2 years (196,197,202,206–210).

A recent advance in screening for this syndrome has been the development of wireless capsule endoscopy (WCE). It is clinically vital to visualize the small bowel in patients with PJS. With push enteroscopy, advancement into the small bowel is limited due to instrument size and discomfort. The disposable capsule is small enough to be swallowed and contains a video camera that transmits UHF signals of up to 50,000 bowel images per examination. Nonvigorous ambulation does not interfere with image transmission to a harness assembly worn by the patient. Bowel inflation is unnecessary, and the capsule is advanced via peristalsis. The disadvantage is that there is no therapeutic capability; lesion removal requires endoscopy. Also, less of the bowel may be seen when it is in uninflated and in a semicollapsed state. The instrument may cause obstruction. The battery may not last long enough for the capsule to reach the cecum, and evaluation of the images is time consuming (211,212). Some comparative studies between WCE and push enteroscopy in patients with occult bleeding indicate higher sensitivity but lower specificity with WCE. Diagnostic yield, especially in small bowel, was better with WCE (213–215).

FAMILIAL GASTRIC CANCER

The International Gastric Linkage Consortium specifies criteria for a clinical diagnosis of familial diffuse gastric cancer. These criteria consist of either (a) two or more documented cases of diffuse gastric cancer in first- or second-degree relatives, with at least one diagnosed before the age of 50 years, or (b) three or more cases of documented diffuse gastric cancer in first- and second-degree relatives, independently of age of onset (216). Approximately 30% of familial diffuse gastric cancer kindreds have mutations in the E-cadherin (CDH1) gene (217). The lifetime penetrance of CHD1 mutations is estimated to be 70% to 80% (217). However, diffuse gastric cancer has been diagnosed in affected individuals as young as 14 years, and the majority of mutation carriers die younger than 40 years (218,219). The clinical consensus is that individuals with diffuse gastric cancer younger than 35 years should be considered for CHD1 testing (219). Because of the early age of onset, similar to FAP, and the estimated 10% 5-year survival rate after diffuse gastric cancer diagnosis, individuals who are as young as 13 years and able to provide informed consent should be considered for genetic counseling.

The management options are surveillance upper GI endoscopy or prophylactic gastrectomy. Gastrectomy has a significant effect on the quality of life and should only be undertaken after extensive genetic counseling. The long-term morbidity that may result from gastrectomy includes weight loss, lactose intolerance, fat malabsorption and steatorrhea, dumping syndrome, bacterial overgrowth, postprandial fullness, and vitamin deficiencies. Based on the experience of Japan, which has population-based upper endoscopy screening programs to detect gastric cancer, early detection of gastric cancer can lead to 5-year survival rates greater than 90% (219). Therefore, upper endoscopy surveillance may be a viable approach to management. The clinical consensus is for a 30-minute endoscopy exam every 6 months, to be performed by experienced practi-

tioners (218). Because of the diffuse distribution of the lesions, chromoendoscopy may be more sensitive for early detection, and ultrasound is less likely to be effective in this setting. It is currently not well established whether any other sites develop cancer with increased frequency with CHD1 mutations, and there are no clear guidelines for additional surveillance.

It is of note that the GI cancer susceptibility of Asian, African, and Caribbean Lynch syndrome families generally have greater incidence of stomach cancer compared to North America, South America, and Europe, where CRC predominates (80,81,220). An important clue in this clinical presentation will be the existence of both endometrial and stomach cancer in the same family. It has been speculated that the shift in the GI cancer susceptibility relative to the rostral-caudal axis has reflected changes in food preparation and content. In particular, the decreased use of "smoked" and cured meats resulting from refrigeration and the high fat content of the modern European-American diet have been proposed as important factors (220). The smoking process of meats is believed to introduce heterocyclic amine by-products into the food, and the curing process involves nitrate salts that cause nitrosocompounds, which may act as mutagens. Epidemiologic and animal model studies provide evidence for this model (221,222). The first HNPCC family identified was described in 1913 by Alfred Warthin, a pathologist, and is referred to as Family G (220,223). In the early 20th century, the GI tumors in Family G and other similar kindreds were distinguished largely by an excess of stomach adenocarcinoma (224). In mid- and late 20th and early 21st centuries, the GI cancer susceptibility has shifted to include mostly CRCs.

FAMILIAL PANCREATIC CANCER

In the United States, familial pancreatic cancer (FPC), defined as kindreds containing at least two affected first-degree relatives, is observed in 2% to 5% of individuals with pancreatic adenocarcinoma (225–227). In the experience of many clinicians, some of the nonsyndromic FPC resemble classic Lynch syndrome or FAP in their Mendelian presentation (228,229). Therefore, it is likely that pure FPC genes exist, although they have yet to be identified. Efforts using linkage analyses to date have not been effective. It is anticipated that whole genome association studies will likely be conducted in the next several years to address this problem.

In the syndromic context of associated tumors, mutations in several genes are known to increase pancreatic cancer risk. These associations include breast and ovarian cancer, where FPC is observed in families with BRCA2 mutations (230,231) at rates that may be as high as 19% (231,232). Pancreatic cancer can also be observed in the syndromic context of melanoma, which is termed the *familial atypical multiple mole melanoma* (FAMMM) syndrome. Mutations in CDKN2A/p16 underlie ~10% of FAMMM (233). PJS, a previously discussed rare syndrome including GI hamartomatous polyps caused by mutations in STK11/LKB1, is also associated with pancreatic adenocarcinoma (234,235). Other distinctive syndromes include hereditary relapsing acute pancreatitis (caused by PRSS1/cationic trypsinogen mutations) and cystic fibrosis (caused by CFTR mutations), which lead to chronic inflammation. This chronic inflammation increases the risk of pancreatic cancer (236,237). Rarely, inherited mutations in MMR genes cause an unusual subtype referred to as medullary pancreatic cancer (238).

INFLAMMATORY BOWEL DISEASE

The inflammatory bowel diseases (IBDs), Crohn disease and ulcerative colitis, are common, chronic disorders that cause abdominal pain, diarrhea, bleeding, and increased cancer risk. Missense mutations in (a) the *CARD15* gene or (b) a risk haplotype (a block of DNA inherited together) containing multiple variants in the organic cation transporters *SLC22A4* and *SLC22A5* inherited together have been identified to cause inherited forms of IBD. These mutations are believed to trigger an overactive mucosal immune response to intestinal bacteria that causes chronic inflammation that subsequently increases CRC risk. Recently, a rare missense change in the IL-23 receptor (*IL-23R* Arg381Gln) was identified that confers strong protection against Crohn disease. It is hoped that this discovery will lead to novel therapies for IBD that antagonize IL23R signaling.

WHAT IS FAMILIAL COLORECTAL CANCER SYNDROME X?

Studies over the past several years have begun to frame the question of what characteristics are associated with families meeting Amsterdam I criteria who do not have identifiable mutations in the known susceptibility genes in more detail. In 1995, Jass et al. described clinical characteristics of families that were not consistent with HNPCC, although such families fully met Amsterdam I criteria (239). In 2003, a study by Renkonen et al. described 15 families identified through population-based ascertainment. (This chapter refers to this cohort as Finnish syndrome X.) All met Amsterdam I criteria. The mean age of CRC onset (54 years) in affected family members was later than in HNPCC or attenuated FAP, and more occurred in the distal colon and rectum than in HNPCC (240). The tumors in this group were all MSS (19). Overall, compared to that seen in HNPCC, the tumors were less poorly differentiated, more often aneuploid, and had less mucinous pathology than MSI families (240). Abdel-Rahman et al. performed a follow-up study on these families, plus 9 additional ones meeting Amsterdam I criteria (24 families total), analyzing molecular characteristics. There were no pathognomonic molecular or clinical features that distinguished these families from HNPCC families that were *MLH1/MSH2/MSH6* mutation positive or from sporadic CRC (240). However, comparing Finnish syndrome X to *MLH1/MSH2/MSH6* gene mutation-positive families, Finnish syndrome X families had statistically significantly more CRCs with aberrant CTNNB1 localization, p53 mutations, and other features associated with sporadic MSS colorectal tumors (240,241).

In families meeting Amsterdam I criteria that did not have mutations in the known susceptibility genes, Young et al. proposed an alternative pathway of colorectal carcinogenesis (242). This proposed new pathway associated with serrated adenoma precursor lesions, a tendency toward proximal colon location. Pathology features further showed less lymphocytic infiltration, "dirty necrosis" (granular eosinophilic extracellular material with nuclear debris), variable levels of MSI (referred to as MSI-V), including MSS tumors, high rates of somatic *BRAF*-activating mutations and *MINT31* locus promoter hypermethylation. Probands came from 11 families, of which all met Bethesda criteria and 55% met AC-I criteria. Mean age of CRC onset was 58 years of age. The authors concluded that these families represent a novel syndrome of hereditary CRC through a different pathway. This chapter refers to these families as serrated adenoma syndrome X.

Lindor et al. ascertained a large cohort of Amsterdam I criteria families from which HNPCC was excluded (243). From 11 large clinic-based studies (the vast majority being Colon CFR Consortium members) and population-based studies, they examined 173 families in total. Strict Amsterdam I criteria were used to select these families, all of which had CRCs that were MSS or MSI-L (19), expressed MLH1/MSH2/MSH6 proteins in tumor immunohistochemistry, and lacked clearly deleterious mutations in *MLH1/MSH2* coding regions as defined by sequencing. Notably, these families are clinically distinct from FAP/aFAP patients with dominant APC and recessive *MYH* mutations, which have scores to hundreds and thousands of polyps. (This chapter refers to this cohort as American syndrome X.) In total, 71 extended families (46 of which were identified through population based ascertainment) with 1,567 family members were studied. A stunning 45% of all families meeting Amsterdam I criteria qualified for American syndrome X, making American syndrome X approximately as frequent as HNPCC, the most common known cancer genetic syndrome. American syndrome X was characterized by later mean age of CRC onset (61 years) than HNPCC, and no increased extracolonic site risk (including stomach, small bowel, and endometrium).

Llor et al. described a cohort of families similar to American syndrome X, which this chapter refers to as Spanish syndrome X (244). Of 1,309 CRC subjects from a Spanish population-based ascertainment study, 15 (1.1% of all CRC probands) fulfilled Amsterdam I criteria but had tumors that were MSS and had normal MLH1/MSH2/MSH6 immunohistochemistry staining. Remarkably, these families constituted 60% of all Amsterdam I criteria fulfilling pedigrees, making Spanish syndrome X more common than HNPCC. Compared to HNPCC, the clinical characteristics of these families showed more left-sided tumors without lymphocytic infiltration, a later mean age of onset (68 years), lower overall penetrance, and, interestingly, were associated with non-CRC tumors of the HNPCC spectrum. *BRAF* mutations were excluded. Differences between American and Spanish syndrome X include similar proportions of relative percentages of colorectal tumor pathology as undifferentiated, and a perplexing increase in endometrial carcinomas in Spanish syndrome X.

Fearnhead et al. described probands with multiple polyps but less than criteria for aFAP. Interestingly, in these subjects, multiple putative deleterious germline variants from MMR and Wnt pathway genes were present. However, many of these 124 subjects did not meet Amsterdam I criteria (152,245). So, the inheritance pattern of multiple complex trait deleterious variants independently segregating does not fit well with the putative autosomal dominant segregation pattern of syndrome X, although pseudodominant inheritance of common variants with low penetrance cannot be ruled out completely.

Comparing these different studies, there is no one clinical or molecular feature that is common to all Amsterdam I criteria meeting families without identifiable mutations in the known genes, except later mean onset of CRC compared to HNPCC. For these studies, *APC* was not sequenced. So, low penetrance alleles analogous to *APC I1307K* (246) are difficult to exclude.

Given the inherent complexity and heterogeneity of CRC, it is unlikely that there is one answer that universally addresses this question to define syndrome X. With the exception of serrated adenoma syndrome X, it is difficult to distinguish these different syndrome Xs from the tail end of the expected statistical distribution of population-based CRC (Table 3.1).

There have recently been a number of studies analyzing significant numbers of CRCs with RNA microarrays (247–254). Consistently, these studies show the ability of expression profiling to distinguish MSI from MSS tumors. However, molecular signatures of additional CRC subtypes that might define syndrome X (or any other subtype of sporadic CRC) have not clearly been demonstrated by this approach. It is anticipated that more precise molecular and histopathological studies of CRC tumors will need to be performed to define more precisely whether mutations in specific genes exist to define syndrome X, whether specific shared dietary or environmental exposures are responsible, or whether these aggregations are attributable to chance in the hundreds of thousands of cases of CRC that unfortunately occur every year on this planet.

TABLE 3.1

CLINICAL CRITERIA FOR IDENTIFYING HEREDITARY NONPOLYPOSIS COLORECTAL CANCER

Classic ICG-HNPCC (Amsterdam I) Criteria	Revised ICG-HNPCC (Amsterdam II) Criteria	Bethesda Guidelines (for MSI Testing)
Three relatives (or more) with CRC (at least one of whom is a first-degree relative of the other two)	Three relatives (or more) with an HNPCC-associated cancer[a] (at least one of whom is a first-degree relative of the other two)	Individuals with cancer in families that meet the Amsterdam criteria
Two successive generations (or more) with CRC	Two successive generations (or more) with an HNPCC-associated cancer	Individuals with two HNPCC-associated cancers,[a] including synchronous and metachronous CRC or associated extracolonic cancers
One family member with CRC diagnosed before age 50	One family member with an HNPCC-associated cancer diagnosed before age 50 years	Individuals with CRC and a first-degree relative with CRC and/or HNPCC-associated extracolonic cancer and/or a colorectal adenoma; one of the cancers diagnosed before age 45 years, and adenoma diagnosed before age 40 years
FAP should be excluded	FAP should be excluded in the CRC case(s), if any	Individuals with CRC or endometrial cancer diagnosed before age 45 years
Tumors should be verified by pathological examination	Tumors should be verified by pathological examination	Individuals with right-sided CRC with an undifferentiated pattern (solid/cribriform) on histopathological analysis diagnosed before age 45 years Individuals with signet ring cell CRC diagnosed before age 45 years Individuals with adenomas diagnosed before age 40 years

ICG-HNPCC, International Collaborative Group on Hereditary Nonpolyposis Colorectal Cancer; MSI, microsatellite instability; CRC, colorectal cancer; HNPCC, hereditary nonpolyposis colorectal cancer; FAP, familial adenomatous polyposis.
[a] *HNPCC-associated cancer* refers to cancer of the colon or rectum, endometrium, small bowel, ureter, or renal pelvis.

CHEMOPREVENTION OF HEREDITARY COLORECTAL SYNDROMES

Because the progression from initiation of adenoma to carcinoma can take several years, prevention can have a major impact on morbidity and mortality. NSAIDs and the more selective cycloxygenase-2 (COX-2) inhibitors have demonstrated significant chemopreventative benefits in FAP. Four multiarm randomized, placebo-controlled trials have demonstrated that sulindac 300 to 400 mg/day and celecoxib 800 mg/day significantly reduce both the number and the size of rectal adenomas in FAP patients (reviewed in 255). When combined, these data suggest the benefits for 4 to 6 months of sulindac 300 to 400 mg/day treatment (21 subjects total) causes a ~70% drop in the rectal adenoma rate, and ~25% drop in patients treated with celecoxib 800 mg orally every day for 6 months (27 patients total). In contrast, sulindac doses of 150 to 200 mg/day appear ineffective. For primary prevention of adenomas in young (<age 18 years) patients who have yet to develop adenomas, sulindac did not prevent their development. It has been suggested that rectal mucosal prostaglandin levels and serum proteomic profiling might serve as potential biomarkers to identify NSAID responders versus nonresponders. However, these findings require more detailed studies before adoption.

There are currently ongoing trials evaluating new chemoprevention strategies for FAP, including a two-arm phase II prevention trial in adult FAP patients treated with celecoxib and an ornithine decarboxylase enzymatic inhibitor DFMO, and a phase I trial of celecoxib for primary polyp prevention in FAP patients from ages 10 to 14 years. It is important to note that surgery (subtotal colectomy) is reluctantly still the primary treatment for FAP and that NSAID/COX-2 chemoprevention in FAP is an adjunct to surgery, particularly in the postsurgery setting of remaining rectal tissue.

For HNPCC, the role of NSAIDs and COX-2 inhibitors in chemoprevention is less clear. This difference from FAP does not appear to reflect a bias of statistical underpowering because of the lower numbers of adenomas and carcinomas that occur in HNPCC versus FAP, but more likely it reflects the mechanistic differences between these two diseases. For example, it is intriguing that preclinical studies in mouse models are unclear for these drug classes in prevention of MMR defective GI epithelial cancers versus Apc/Wnt-mediated cancers. One study showed that NSAID treatment in *Msh2* knockout mice actually increased adenomas and that COX-2 inhibitors did not decrease colon adenomas (although they did decrease the rate of small bowel adenomas, which are more common in this model). NSAID/COX-2 adenoma prevention has been proposed to require BAX-mediated signal transduction. This observation is relevant to HNPCC because of the presence of a 9 adenine repeat in the BAX coding sequence, and its frequent inactivation by MSI. Mice do not have the 9 adenine repeat, and maintain in-frame Bax mRNAs, with Bax-mediated signaling intact.

There are currently several ongoing chemoprevention trials for HNPCC. There is a celecoxib study that is a randomized, placebo-controlled phase I/II multicenter trial evaluating the safety and efficacy of celecoxib in ~80 HNPCC subjects (256). This study compares three proposed interventions: celecoxib at 200 mg orally twice a day for 12 months, 400 mg orally twice a day for 12 months, and placebo orally twice a day for 12 months (256). The effects of these treatment arms on a number of endoscopic and tissue-based biomarker end points will be evaluated at baseline and 12 months. The CAPP2 (Concerted Action Polyp Prevention) study evaluates the preventative effects of aspirin and resistant starch in HNPCC carriers. In this study, carriers of HNPCC are randomized to received 600 mg enteric-coated aspirin or placebo and 30 g treatment starch or placebo. The primary end point of the study will be the number, size, and histologic stage of CRC found after 2 years on treatment or placebo (256).

There has recently been great concern over the safety of COX-2 inhibitors in the wake of the finding that rofecoxib (Vioxx) (and perhaps valdecoxib [Bexxar]) increases the rate of cardiovascular side effects such as stroke or myocardial infarction. This concern is timely because of the ongoing HNPCC chemoprevention trials using celecoxib. However, it is worth noting that even after extensive celecoxib use in many thousands of human subjects, there is currently no compelling evidence that these increased cardiovascular side effects are also induced by celecoxib. Pharmacologically, rofecoxib is a more selective COX-2 inhibitor than celecoxib, which has more pronounced effects on other pathways, including leukotriene production.

Chemoprevention for the hamartomatous polyposis syndromes, PJS and juvenile polyposis syndrome (JPS), is less well developed. A case report has described one JPS patient with polyp regression from sulindac treatment (255), and COX-2 expression has also been reported in JPS polyps, which is encouraging for the potential of NSAID/COX-2 inhibitor chemoprevention for these inherited syndromes. However, the rarity of these diseases makes it challenging to accrue the patients necessary for adequately powered studies with clinical end points.

ACKNOWLEDGMENTS

The authors want to thank Peter Thom, MS, and Donna Bernstein, MS, of Memorial Sloan-Kettering Cancer Center for their input on this chapter.

References

1. Thibodeau SN, Bren G, Schaid D. Microsatellite instability in cancer of the proximal colon. *Science* 1993;260:816–819.
2. Shibata D, Peinado MA, Ionov Y, et al. Genomic instability in repeated sequences is an early somatic event in colorectal tumorigenesis that persists after transformation. *Nat Genet* 1994;6:273–281.
3. Dietmaier W, Wallinger S, Bocker T, et al. Diagnostic microsatellite instability: definition and correlation with mismatch repair protein expression. *Cancer Res* 1997;57:4749–4756.
4. Offit K. *Clinical Cancer Genetics*. New York, NY: Wiley-Liss; 1998.
5. Varmus H. The new era in Cancer Res earch. *Science* 2006;312:1162–1165.
6. Weinberg R. *The Biology of Cancer*. New York, NY: Garland Science; 2006.
7. Herman JG, Umar A, Polyak K, et al. Incidence and functional consequences of hMLH1 promoter hypermethylation in colorectal carcinoma. *Proc Natl Acad Sci U S A* 1998;95:6870–6875.
8. Vogelstein B, Kinzler K. *The Genetic Basis of Human Cancer*. Baltimore, Md.: McGraw-Hill; 1998.
9. Armitage P, Doll R. The age distribution of cancer and a multi-stage theory of carcinogenesis. *Br J Cancer* 1954;8:1–12.
10. Armitage P, Doll R. The age distribution of cancer and a multi-stage theory of carcinogenesis. *Br J Cancer* 2004;91:1983–1989.
11. Sjoblom T, Jones S, Wood LD, et al. The consensus coding sequences of human breast and colorectal cancers. *Science* 2006;314:268–274.
12. Jackson EL, Willis N, Mercer K, et al. Analysis of lung tumor initiation and progression using conditional expression of oncogenic K-ras. *Genes Dev* 2001;15:3243–3248.
13. O'Brien C, Pollett A, Gallinger S, et al. A human colon cancer cell capable of initiating tumour growth in immunodeficient mice. *Nature* 2007; 445(7123):106–110.
14. Ricci-Vitiani L, Lombardi DG, Pilozzi E, et al. Identification and expansion of human colon-cancer-initiating cells. *Nature* 2007;445(7123): 111–115.
15. Levin B, Barthel JS, Burt RW, et al. Colorectal cancer screening clinical practice guidelines. *J Natl Compr Cancer Netw* 2006;4:384–420.
16. Fuchs CS, Giovannucci EL, Colditz GA, Hunter DJ, Speizer FE, Willett WC. A prospective study of family history and the risk of colorectal cancer. *N Engl J Med* 1994;331(25):1669–1674.
17. Burt RW. Familial association. *Adv Exp Med Biol* 1999;470:99–104.
18. Winawer S, Fletcher R, Rex D, et al. Colorectal cancer screening and surveillance: clinical guidelines and rationale—update based on new evidence. *Gastroenterology* 2003;124:544–560.
19. Umar A, Boland CR, Terdiman JP, et al. Revised Bethesda guidelines for hereditary nonpolyposis colorectal cancer (Lynch syndrome) and microsatellite instability. *J Natl Cancer Inst* 2004;96:261–268.
20. Jass JR. Familial colorectal cancer: pathology and molecular characteristics. *Lancet Oncol* 2000;1:220–226.
21. Jass JR. Pathology of hereditary nonpolyposis colorectal cancer. *Ann N Y Acad Sci* 2000;910:62–73; discussion 73–74.
22. Young J, Simms LA, Biden KG, et al. Features of colorectal cancers with high-level microsatellite instability occurring in familial and sporadic settings: parallel pathways of tumorigenesis. *Am J Pathol* 2001;159:2107–2116.
23. Bronner CE, Baker SM, Morrison PT, et al. Mutation in the DNA mismatch repair gene homologue hMLH1 is associated with hereditary non-polyposis colon cancer. *Nature* 1994;368:258–261.
24. Leach FS, Nicolaides NC, Papadopoulos N, et al. Mutations of a mutS homolog in hereditary nonpolyposis colorectal cancer. *Cell* 1993;75:1215–1225.
25. Akiyama Y, Sato H, Yamada T, et al. Germ-line mutation of the hMSH6/GTBP gene in an atypical hereditary nonpolyposis colorectal cancer kindred. *Cancer Res* 1997;57:3920–3923.
26. Kolodner R, De A. Germline MSH6 mutation in colorectal cancer families. *Cancer Res* 1999;59:5068–5074.
27. Miyaki M, Konishi M, Tanaka K, et al. Germline mutation of MSH6 as the cause of hereditary nonpolyposis colorectal cancer [letter]. *Nat Genet* 1997;17:271–272.
28. Nicolaides NC, Papadopoulos N, Liu B, et al. Mutations of two PMS homologues in hereditary nonpolyposis colon cancer. *Nature* 1994;371:75–80.
29. Liu HX, Zhou XL, Liu T, et al. The role of hMLH3 in familial colorectal cancer. *Cancer Res* 2003;63:1894–1899.
30. Wu Y, Berends MJ, Sijmons RH, et al. A role for MLH3 in hereditary nonpolyposis colorectal cancer. *Nat Genet* 2001;29:137–138.
31. Lindor, NM, Petersen, GM, Hadley, DW, et al. Recommendations for the care of individuals with an inherited predisposition to Lynch syndrome: a systematic review. *JAMA* 2006;296:1507–1517.
32. Jarvinen HJ, Aarnio M. Surveillance on mutation carriers of DNA mismatch repair genes. *Ann Chir Gynaecol* 2000;89:207–210.
33. Renkonen-Sinisalo L, Aarnio M, Mecklin JP, et al. Surveillance improves survival of colorectal cancer in patients with hereditary nonpolyposis colorectal cancer. *Cancer Detect Prev* 2000;24:137–142.
34. Syngal S, Weeks JC, Schrag D, et al. Benefits of colonoscopic surveillance and prophylactic colectomy in patients with hereditary nonpolyposis colorectal cancer mutations. *Ann Intern Med* 1998;129:787–796.
35. Vasen HF, van Ballegooijen M, Buskens E, et al. A cost-effectiveness analysis of colorectal screening of hereditary nonpolyposis colorectal carcinoma gene carriers. *Cancer* 1998;82:1632–1637.
36. Umar A, Risinger JI, Hawk ET, et al. Testing guidelines for hereditary nonpolyposis colorectal cancer. *Nat Rev Cancer* 2004;4:153–158.
37. Peltomaki P, Vasen H. Mutations associated with HNPCC predisposition—update of ICG-HNPCC/InSIGHT mutation database. *Dis Markers* 2004; 20:269–276.
38. Barnetson RA, Tenesa A, Farrington SM, et al. Identification and survival of carriers of mutations in DNA mismatch-repair genes in colon cancer. *N Engl J Med* 2006;354:2751–2763.
39. Chen S, Wang W, Lee S, et al. Prediction of germline mutations and cancer risk in hereditary nonpolyposis colorectal cancer. *JAMA* 2007; 296(12):1479–1487.
40. Balmana J, Stockwell DH, Steyerberg EW, et al. Prediction of MLH1 and MSH2 mutations in Lynch syndrome. *JAMA* 2006;296:1469–1478.
41. Eisen, JA. A phylogenomic study of the MutS family of proteins. *Nucleic Acids Res* 1998;26:4291–4300.
42. Kolodner RD, Marsischky GT. Eukaryotic DNA mismatch repair. *Curr Opin Genet Dev* 1999;9:89–96.
43. Muller A, Fishel R. Mismatch repair and the hereditary non-polyposis colorectal cancer syndrome (HNPCC). *Cancer Invest* 2002;20:102–109.
44. Fishel R, Lescoe MK, Rao MR, et al. The human mutator gene homolog MSH2 and its association with hereditary nonpolyposis colon cancer. *Cell* 1993;75:1027–1038. [Erratum appears in *Cell* 1994;77(1):167]
45. Papadopoulos N, Nicolaides NC, Wei YF, et al. Mutation of a mutL homolog in hereditary colon cancer. *Science* 1994;263:1625–1629.
46. Kunkel TA, Erie DA. DNA mismatch repair. *Annu Rev Biochem* 2005;74: 681–710.

47. de la Chapelle A. Genetic predisposition to colorectal cancer. *Nat Rev Cancer* 2004;4(10):769–780.

48. Edelmann L, Edelmann W. Loss of DNA mismatch repair function and cancer predisposition in the mouse: animal models for human hereditary nonpolyposis colorectal cancer. *Am J Med Genet C Semin Med Genet* 2004;129:91–99.

49. Marcon E, Moens PB. The evolution of meiosis: recruitment and modification of somatic DNA-repair proteins. *Bioessays* 2005;27:795–808.

50. Neuberger MS, Di Noia JM, Beale RC, et al. Somatic hypermutation at A.T pairs: polymerase error versus dUTP incorporation. *Nat Rev Immunol* 2005;5:171–178.

51. Kunz C, Schar P. Meiotic recombination: sealing the partnership at the junction. *Curr Biol* 2004;14:R962–R964.

52. Stojic L, Brun R, Jiricny J. Mismatch repair and DNA damage signalling. *DNA Repair (Amst)* 2004;3:1091–1101.

53. Kolodner RD, Putnam CD, Myung K. Maintenance of genome stability in *Saccharomyces cerevisiae. Science* 2002;297:552–557.

54. Fishel, R. The selection for mismatch repair defects in hereditary nonpolyposis colorectal cancer: revising the mutator hypothesis. *Cancer Res* 2001;61:7369–7374.

55. Acharya S, Foster PL, Brooks P, et al. The coordinated functions of the *E. coli* MutS and MutL proteins in mismatch repair. *Mol Cell* 2003;12:233–246.

56. Zhang Y, Yuan F, Presnell SR, et al. Reconstitution of 5′-directed human mismatch repair in a purified system. *Cell* 2005;122:693–705.

57. Constantin N, Dzantiev L, Kadyrov FA, et al. Human mismatch repair: reconstitution of a nick-directed bidirectional reaction. *J Biol Chem* 2005;280(48):39752–39761.

58. Dzantiev L, Constantin N, Genschel J, et al. A defined human system that supports bidirectional mismatch-provoked excision. *Mol Cell* 2004;15:31–41.

59. Chen P, Dudley S, Hagen W, et al. Contributions by MutL homologs Mlh3 and Pms2 to DNA mismatch repair and tumor suppression in the mouse. *Cancer Res* 2005;65:8662–8670.

60. Cannavo E, Marra G, Sabatés-Bellver J, et al. Expression of the MutL homologue hMLH3 in human cells and its role in DNA mismatch repair. *Cancer Res* 2005;65(23):10759–10766.

61. Prolla TA, Baker SM, Harris AC, et al. Tumour susceptibility and spontaneous mutation in mice deficient in Mlh1, Pms1 and Pms2 DNA mismatch repair. *Nat Genet* 1998;18:276–279.

62. Raschle M, Marra G, Nystrom-Lahti M, et al. Identification of hMutLbeta, a heterodimer of hMLH1 and hPMS1. *J Biol Chem* 1999;274:32368–32375.

63. Svetlanov A, Cohen PE. Mismatch repair proteins, meiosis, and mice: understanding the complexities of mammalian meiosis. *Exp Cell Res* 2004;296:71–79.

64. Liu T, Tannergard P, Hackman P, et al. Missense mutations in hMLH1 associated with colorectal cancer. *Hum Genet* 1999;105:437–441.

65. Lipkin SM, Rozek LS, Rennert G, et al. The MLH1 D132H variant is associated with susceptibility to sporadic colorectal cancer. *Nat Genet* 2004;36:694–699.

66. Coolbaugh-Murphy M, Maleki A, Ramagli L, et al. Estimating mutant microsatellite allele frequencies in somatic cells by small-pool PCR. *Genomics* 2004;84:419–430.

67. Alazzouzi H, Domingo E, Gonzalez S, et al. Low levels of microsatellite instability characterize MLH1 and MSH2 HNPCC carriers before tumor diagnosis. *Hum Mol Genet* 2005;14:235–239.

68. Li GM. The role of mismatch repair in DNA damage-induced apoptosis. *Oncol Res* 1999;11:393–400.

69. Lin DP, Wang Y, Scherer SJ, et al. An Msh2 point mutation uncouples DNA mismatch repair and apoptosis. *Cancer Res* 2004;64:517–522.

70. Yang G, Scherer SJ, Shell SS, et al. Dominant effects of an Msh6 missense mutation on DNA repair and cancer susceptibility. *Cancer Cell* 2004;6:139–510.

71. de Wind N, Dekker M, Berns A, et al. Inactivation of the mouse Msh2 gene results in mismatch repair deficiency, methylation tolerance, hyperrecombination, and predisposition to cancer. *Cell* 1995;82:321–330.

72. Fishel R. Signaling mismatch repair in cancer. *Nat Med* 1999;5:1239–1241.

73. Gong JG, Costanzo A, Yang HQ, et al. The tyrosine kinase c-Abl regulates p73 in apoptotic response to cisplatin-induced DNA damage. *Nature* 1999;399:806–809.

74. Zabkiewicz J, Clarke AR. DNA damage-induced apoptosis: insights from the mouse. *Biochim Biophys Acta* 2004;1705:17–25.

75. de Wind N, Dekker M, Claij N, et al. HNPCC-like cancer predisposition in mice through simultaneous loss of Msh3 and Msh6 mismatch-repair protein functions. *Nature Genet* 1999;23:359–362.

76. Lynch HT, de la Chapelle A. Hereditary colorectal cancer. *N Engl J Med* 2003;348:919–932.

77. Neugut AI, Terry MB. Cigarette smoking and microsatellite instability: causal pathway or marker-defined subset of colon tumors? *J Natl Cancer Inst* 2000;92:1791–1793.

78. Watson P, Lynch HT. Extracolonic cancer in hereditary nonpolyposis colorectal cancer. *Cancer* 1993;71:677–685.

79. Watson P, Lynch HT. Cancer risk in mismatch repair gene mutation carriers. *Fam Cancer* 2001;1:57–60.

80. Lynch HT, Watson P, Lanspa S, et al. Clinical nuances of Lynch syndromes I and II. *Prog Clin Biol Res* 1988;279:177–188.

81. Lynch HT, Watson P, Lanspa SJ, et al. Natural history of colorectal cancer in hereditary nonpolyposis colorectal cancer (Lynch syndromes I and II). *Dis Colon Rectum* 1988;31:439–444.

82. Vasen HF, Wijnen JT, Menko FH, et al. Cancer risk in families with hereditary nonpolyposis colorectal cancer diagnosed by mutation analysis. *Gastroenterology* 1996;110:1020–1027.

83. Aarnio M, Sankila R, Pukkala E, et al. Cancer risk in mutation carriers of DNA-mismatch-repair genes. *Int J Cancer* 1999;81:214–218.

84. Dunlop MG, Farrington SM, Carothers AD, et al. Cancer risk associated with germline DNA mismatch repair gene mutations. *Hum Mol Genet* 1997;6:105–110.

85. Kong S, Amos CI, Luthra R, et al. Effects of cyclin D1 polymorphism on age of onset of hereditary nonpolyposis colorectal cancer. *Cancer Res* 2000;60:249–252.

86. Frazier ML, O'Donnell FT, Kong S, et al. Age-associated risk of cancer among individuals with N-acetyltransferase 2 (NAT2) mutations and mutations in DNA mismatch repair genes. *Cancer Res* 2001;61:1269–1271.

87. Yang P, Cunningham JM, Halling KC, et al. Higher risk of mismatch repair-deficient colorectal cancer in alpha(1)-antitrypsin deficiency carriers and cigarette smokers. *Mol Genet Metab* 2000;71:639–645.

88. Erblich J, Lerman C, Self DW, et al. Stress-induced cigarette craving: effects of the DRD2 TaqI RFLP and SLC6A3 VNTR polymorphisms. *Pharmacogenomics J* 2004;4:102–109.

89. Lerman C, Shields PG, Wileyto EP, et al. Effects of dopamine transporter and receptor polymorphisms on smoking cessation in a bupropion clinical trial. *Health Psychol* 2003;22:541–548.

90. Schmeler KM, Lynch HT, Chen LM, et al. Prophylactic surgery to reduce the risk of gynecologic cancers in the Lynch syndrome. *N Engl J Med* 2006;354:261–269.

91. Merg A, Lynch HT, Lynch JF, et al. Hereditary colon cancer—part I. *Curr Probl Surg* 2005;42:195–256.

92. Solomon CH, Pho LN, Burt RW. Current status of genetic testing for colorectal cancer susceptibility. *Oncology* 2002;16:161–171; discussion 176, 179–180.

93. Aretz S, Uhlhaas S, Caspari R, Mangold E, et al. Frequency and parental origin of de novo APC mutations in familial adenomatous polyposis. *Eur J Hum Genet* 2004;12:52–58.

94. Gardner EJ. A genetic and clinical study of intestinal polyposis, a predisposing factor for carcinoma of the colon and rectum. *Am J Hum Genet* 1951;3:167–176.

95. Li FP, Thurber WA, Seddon J, Holmes GE. Hepatoblastoma in families with polyposis coli. *JAMA* 1987;257:2475–2477.

96. Krush AJ, Traboulsi EI, Offerhaus GJA, et al. Hepatoblastoma, pigmented ocular fundus lesions and jaw lesions in Gardner syndrome. *Am J Med Genet* 1988;29:323–332.

97. Garber JE, Li FP, Kingston JE, Krush AJ, et al. Hepatoblastoma and familial adenomatous polyposis. *J Nat Cancer Inst* 1988;80:1626–1628.

98. Giardiello FM, Offerhaus GJ, Krush AJ, Booker SV, et al. Risk of hepatoblastoma in familial adenomatous polyposis. *J Pediatr* 1991;119:766–767.

99. Hirschman BA, Pollock BH, Tomlinson GE. The spectrum of APC mutations in children with hepatoblastoma from familial adenomatous polyposis kindreds. *J Pediatr* 2005;147:263–266.

100. Giardiello FM, Hamilton SR, Krush AJ, et al. Nasopharyngeal angiofibroma in patients with familial adenomatous polyposis. *Gastroenterology* 1993b;105:1550–1552.

101. Ferouz AS, Mohr RM, Paul P. Juvenile nasopharyngeal angiofibroma and familial adenomatous polyposis: an association? *Otolaryngol Head Neck Surg* 1995;113:435–439.

102. Valanzano R, Curia MC, Aceto G, Veschi S, et al. Genetic evidence that juvenile nasopharyngeal angiofibroma is an integral FAP tumour. *Gut* 2005;54:1046–1047.

103. Soravia C, Sugg SL, Berk T, Mitri A, et al. Familial adenomatous polyposis-associated thyroid cancer: a clinical, pathological, and molecular genetics study. *Am J Pathol* 1999;154:127–135.

104. Xu B, Yoshimoto K, Miyauchi A, Kuma S, et al. Cribriform-morular variant of papillary thyroid carcinoma: a pathological and molecular genetic study with evidence of frequent somatic mutations in exon 3 of the beta-catenin gene. *J Pathol* 2003;199:58–67.

105. Chikkamuniyappa S, Jagirdar K. Cribriform-morular variant of papillary carcinoma: association with familial adenomatous polyposis—report of three cases and review of literature. *Int J Med Sci* 2004;1:43–49.

106. Lee S, Hong SW, Shin SJ, Kim YM, et al. Papillary thyroid carcinoma associated with familial adenomatous polyposis: molecular analysis of pathogenesis in a family and review of the literature. *Endocr J* 2004;51:317–323.

107. Chuah KL, Hwang JS, Ng SB, Tan PH, et al. Cytologic features of cribriform-morular variant of papillary carcinoma of the thyroid: a case report. *Acta Cytol* 2005;49:75–80.

108. Tulchinsky H, Keidar A, Strul H, Goldman G, et al. Extracolonic manifestations of familial adenomatous polyposis after proctocolectomy. *Arch Surg* 2005;140:159–163; discussion 164.

109. Fearnhead NS, Britton MP, Bodmer WF. The ABC of APC. *Hum Mol Genet* 2001;10:721–733.

110. Rubinfeld B, Souza B, Albert I, et al. Association of the APC gene product with ll-catenin. *Science* 1993;262:1731–1734.

111. Rubinfeld B, Albert I, Porfiri F, Fiol C, et al. Binding of GSK3—beta to the APC-beta-catenin complex and regulation of complex assembly. *Science* 1996;262:1023–1025.

112. Kinzler KW, Volgelstein B. Lessons from hereditary colorectal cancer. *Cell* 1996;87:159–170.

113. Hernegger GS, Moore HG, Guillem JG. Attenuated familial adenomatous polyposis: an evolving and poorly understood entity. *Dis Colon Rectum* 2002;45:127–134; discussion 134–136.

114. Shih IM, Yu J, He TC, et al. The beta-catenin binding domain of adenomatous polyposis coli is sufficient for tumor suppression. *Cancer Res* 2000;60:1671–1676.

115. Laurent-Puig P, Beroud C, Soussi T. APC gene: database of germline and somatic mutations in human tumors and cell lines. *Nucleic Acids Res* 1998; 26:269–270.

116. Gayther SA, Wells D, SenGupta SB, et al. Regionally clustered APC mutations are associated with a severe phenotype and occur at a high frequency in new mutation cases of adenomatous polyposis coli. *Hum Mol Genet* 1994; 3:53–56.

117. Nagase H, Miyoshi Y, Horii A, et al. Correlation between the location of germ-line mutations in the APC gene and the number of colorectal polyps in familial adenomatous polyposis patients. *Cancer Res* 1992;52:4055–4057.

118. Powell SM, Zilz N, Beazer-Barclay Y, et al. APC mutations occur early during colorectal tumorigenesis. *Nature* 1992;359:235–237.

119. Nugent KP, Phillips RK, Hodgson SV, et al. Phenotypic expression in familial adenomatous polyposis: partial prediction by mutation analysis. *Gut* 1994;35:1622–1623.

120. Caspari R, Friedl W, Mandl M, et al. Familial adenomatous polyposis: mutation at codon 1309 and early onset of colon cancer. *Lancet* 1994;343:629–632.

121. Olschwang S, Tiret A, Laurent-Puig P, et al. Restriction of ocular fundus lesions to a specific subgroup of APC mutations in adenomatous polyposis coli patients. *Cell* 1993;75:959–968.

122. van der Luijt RB, Vasen HF, Tops CM, et al. APC mutation in the alternatively spliced region of exon 9 associated with late onset familial adenomatous polyposis. *Hum Genet* 1995;96:705–710.

123. Caspari R, Olschwang S, Friedl W, et al. Familial adenomatous polyposis: desmoid tumours and lack of ophthalmic lesions (CHRPE) associated with APC mutations beyond codon 1444. *Hum Mol Genet* 1995;4:337–340.

124. Wallis YL, Morton DG, McKeown CM, et al. Molecular analysis of the APC gene in 205 families: extended genotype-phenotype correlations in FAP and evidence for the role of APC amino acid changes in colorectal cancer predisposition. *J Med Genet* 1999;36:14–20.

125. Davies DR, Armstrong JG, Thakker N, et al. Severe Gardner syndrome in families with mutations restricted to a specific region of the APC gene. *Am J Hum Genet* 1995;57:1151–1158.

126. Wallis YL, Morton DG, McKeown CM, Macdonald F. Molecular analysis of the APC gene in 205 families: extended genotype-phenotype correlations in FAP and evidence for the role of APC amino acid changes in colorectal cancer predisposition. *J Med Genet* 1999;36:14–20.

127. Brensinger JD, Laken SJ, Luce MC, Powell SM, et al. Variable phenotype of familial adenomatous polyposis in pedigrees with 3' mutation in the APC gene. *Gut* 1998;43:548–552.

128. Hofgartner WT, Thorp M, Ramus MW, Delorefice G, et al. Gastric adenocarcinoma associated with fundic gland polyps in a patient with attenuated familial adenomatous polyposis. *Am J Gastroenterol* 1999;94:2275–2281.

129. Trimbath JD, Griffin C, Romans K, Giardiello FM. Attenuated familial adenomatous polyposis presenting as ampullary adenocarcinoma. *Gut* 2003;52:903–904.

130. Cetta F, Montalto G, Gori M, Curia MC, Cama A, Olschwang S. Germline mutations of the APC gene in patients with familial adenomatous polyposis-associated thyroid carcinoma: results from a European cooperative study. *J Clin Endocrinol Metab* 2000;85:286–292.

131. Sieber OM, Lamlum H, Crabtree MD, Rowan AJ, et al. Whole-gene APC deletions cause classical familial adenomatous polyposis, but not attenuated polyposis or "multiple" colorectal adenomas. *Proc Natl Acad Sci U S A* 2002;99:2954–2958.

132. Giardiello FM, Krush AJ, Petersen GM, et al. Phenotypic variability of familial adenomatous polyposis in 11 unrelated families with identical APC gene mutation. *Gastroenterology* 1994;106:1542–1547.

133. Friedl W, Caspari R, Sengteller M, et al. Can APC mutation analysis contribute to therapeutic decisions in familial adenomatous polyposis? Experience from 680 FAP families. *Gut* 2001;48:515–521.

134. Crabtree MD, Tomlinson IP, Hodgson SV, et al. Explaining variation in familial adenomatous polyposis: relationship between genotype and phenotype and evidence for modifier genes. *Gut* 2002;51:420–423.

135. Houlston R, Crabtree M, Phillips R, et al. Explaining differences in the severity of familial adenomatous polyposis and the search for modifier genes. *Gut* 2001;48:1–5.

136. Laken SJ, Petersen GM, Gruber SB, et al. Familial colorectal cancer in Ashkenazim due to a hypermutable tract in APC. *Nat Genet* 1997;17:79–83.

137. Gryfe R, Di Nicola N, Lal G, et al. Inherited colorectal polyposis and cancer risk of the APC I1307K polymorphism. *Am J Hum Genet* 1999;64:378–384.

138. de la Chapelle A Genetic predisposition to colorectal cancer. *Nat Rev Cancer* 2004;4:769–780.

139. Winawer S, Fletcher R, Rex D, et al. Colorectal cancer screening and surveillance: clinical guidelines and rationale-Update based on new evidence. *Gastroenterology* 2003;124:544–560.

140. Bulow C, Vasen H, Jarvinen H, Bjork J, Bisgaard ML, Bulow S. Ileorectal anastomosis is appropriate for a subset of patients with familial adenomatous polyposis. *Gastroenterology* 2000;119:1454–1460.

141. Gallagher MC, Phillips RK. Serrated adenomas in FAP. *Gut* 2002;51:895–896.

142. Giardiello FM, Hamilton SR, Krush AJ, et al. Treatment of colonic and rectal adenomas with sulindac in familial adenomatous polyposis. *N Engl J Med* 1993;328:1313–1316.

143. Giardiello FM, Hylind LM, Trimbath JD, et al. Oral contraceptives and polyp regression in familial adenomatous polyposis. *Gastroenterology* 2005;128:1077–1080.

144. Tranah GJ, Giovannucci E, Ma J, et al. APC Asp1822Val and Gly2502Ser polymorphisms and risk of colorectal cancer and adenoma. *Cancer Epidemiol Biomarkers Prev* 2005;14:863–870.

145. Jones DH, Silberstein PT, Lynch H, Ternet C. Regression of colorectal adenomas with intravenous cytotoxic chemotherapy in a patient with familial adenomatous polyposis. *J Clin Oncol* 2005;23:6278–6280.

146. Utech M, Brewer M, Buerger H, Tubergen D, Senninger N. Rectal carcinoma in a patient with familial adenomatous polyposis coli after colectomy with ileorectal anastomosis and consecutive chemoprevention with sulindac suppositories. *Chirurg* 2002;73:855–858.

147. Hisamuddin IM, Wehbi MA, Chao A, Wyre HW, et al. Genetic polymorphisms of human flavin monooxygenase 3 in sulindac-mediated primary chemoprevention of familial adenomatous polyposis. *Clin Cancer Res* 2004;10:8357–8362.

148. Hisamuddin IM, Wehbi MA, Schmotzer B, Easley KA, et al. Genetic polymorphisms of flavin monooxygenase 3 in sulindac-induced regression of colorectal adenomas in familial adenomatous polyposis. *Cancer Epidemiol Biomarkers Prev* 2005;14:2366–2369.

149. Eceles DM, van der Luijt R, Breukel C, et al. Hereditary desmoid disease due to a frameshift mutation at codon 1924 of the APC gene. *Am J Hum Genet* 1996;59:1193–1201.

150. Couture J, Mitri A, Lagace R, Smits R, et al. A germline mutation at the extreme 3' end of the APC gene results in a severe desmoid phenotype and is associated with overexpression of beta-catenin in the desmoid tumor. *Clin Genet* 2000;57:205–212.

151. Spirio L, Olschwang S, Groden J, et al. Alleles of the APC gene: an attenuated form of familial polyposis. *Cell* 1993;75:951–957.

152. Fearnhead NS, Wilding JL, Winney B, et al. Multiple rare variants in different genes account for multifactorial inherited susceptibility to colorectal adenomas. *Proc Natl Acad Sci U S A* 2004;101:15992–15997.

153. Salahshor S, Woodgett JR. The links between axin and carcinogenesis. *J Clin Pathol* 2005;58:225–236.

154. Hsu W, Zeng L, Costantini F. Identification of a domain of Axin that binds to the serine/threonine protein phosphatase 2A and a self-binding domain. *J Biol Chem* 1999;274:3439–3445.

155. Kishida S, Yamamoto H, Hino S, et al. DIX domains of Dvl and axin are necessary for protein interactions and their ability to regulate beta-catenin stability. *Mol Cell Biol* 1999;19:4414–4422.

156. Taniguchi K, Roberts LR, Aderca IN, et al. Mutational spectrum of beta-catenin, AXIN1, and AXIN2 in hepatocellular carcinomas and hepatoblastomas. *Oncogene* 2002;21:4863–4871.

157. Soravia C, Berk T, Madlensky L, Mitri A, et al. Genotype-phenotype correlations in attenuated adenomatous polyposis coli. *Am J Hum Genet* 1998;62:1290–1301.

158. Su LK, Kohlmann W, Ward PA, Lynch PM. Different familial adenomatous polyposis phenotypes resulting from deletions of the entire APC exon 15. *Hum Genet* 2002;111:88–95.

159. Su LK, Barnes CJ, Yao W, Qi Y, Lynch PM, Steinbach G. Inactivation of germline mutant APC alleles by attenuated somatic mutations: a molecular genetic mechanism for attenuated familial adenomatous polyposis. *Am J Hum Genet* 2000;67:582–590.

160. Rozen P, Samuel Z, Shomrat R, Legum C. Notable intrafamilial phenotypic variability in a kindred with familial adenomatous polyposis and an APC mutation in exon 9. *Gut* 1999;45:829–833.

161. Ficari F, Cama A, Valanzano R, Curia MC, et al. APC gene mutations and colorectal adenomatosis in familial adenomatous polyposis. *Br J Cancer* 2000;82:348–353.

162. Matsumoto T, Iida M, Kobori Y, Mizuno M, et al. Serrated adenoma in familial adenomatous polyposis: relation to germline APC gene mutation. *Gut* 2002;50:402–404.

163. Lynch HT, Smyrk T, McGinn T, et al. Attenuated familial adenomatous polyposis (AFAP): a phenotypically and genotypically distinctive variant of FAP. *Cancer Epidemiol Biomarkers Prev* 1995;76:2427–2433.

164. Spirio L, Olschwang S, Groden J, Robertson M, et al. Alleles of the APC gene: an attenuated form of familial polyposis. *Cell* 1993;75:951–957.

165. Fleischmann C, Peto J, Cheadle J, Shah B, Sampson J, Houlston RS. Comprehensive analysis of the contribution of germline MYH variation to early-onset colorectal cancer. *Int J Cancer* 2004;109:554–558.

166. Nielsen M, Franken PF, Reinards TH, Weiss MM, et al. Multiplicity in

polyp count and extracolonic manifestations in 40 Dutch patients with MYH associated polyposis coli (MAP). *J Med Genet* 2005;42:e54.

167. Levin B, Barthel JS, Burt RW, David DS, Giardiello FM, Gruber SB. National Comprehensive Cancer Network. 2005.

168. Bussey HJ. Familial polyposis coli. *Pathol Annu* 1979;14(1):61–81.

169. Sieber OM, Lipton L, Crabtree M, et al. Multiple colorectal adenomas, classic adenomatous polyposis, and germ-line mutations in MYH. *N Engl J Med* 2003;348:791–979.

170. Jones S, Emmerson P, Maynard J, et al. Biallelic germline mutations in MYH predispose to multiple colorectal adenoma and somatic G:C→T:A mutations. *Hum Mol Genet* 2002;11:2961–2967.

171. Al-Tassan N, Chmiel NH, Maynard J, et al. Inherited variants of MYH associated with somatic G:C-->T:A mutations in colorectal tumors. *Nat Genet* 2002;30:227–232.

172. Russell AM, Zhang J, Luz J, et al. Prevalence of MYH germline mutations in Swiss APC mutation-negative polyposis patients. *Int J Cancer* 2005.

173. Jo WS, Bandipalliam P, Shannon KM, et al. Correlation of polyp number and family history of colon cancer with germline MYH mutations. *Clin Gastroenterol Hepatol* 2005;3:1022–1028.

174. Cheadle JP, Sampson JR. Exposing the MYtH about base excision repair and human inherited disease. *Hum Mol Genet* 2003;12(2):R159–R165.

175. Croitoru ME, Cleary SP, Di Nicola N, et al. Association between biallelic and monoallelic germline MYH gene mutations and colorectal cancer risk. *J Natl Cancer Inst* 2004;96:1631–1634.

176. Eliason K, Hendrickson BC, Judkins T, Norton M, et al. The potential for increased clinical sensitivity in genetic testing for polyposis colorectal cancer through the analysis of MYH mutations in North American patients. *J Med Genet* 2005;42:95–96.

177. Sieber OM, Lipton L, Crabtree M, Heinimann K, et al. Multiple colorectal adenomas, classic adenomatous polyposis, and germ-line mutations in MYH. *N Engl J Med* 2003;348:791–799.

178. Marra G, Jiricny J. Multiple colorectal adenomas—is their number up? [editorial]. *N Engl J Med* 2003;348:845–847.

179. Wang L, Baudhuin LM, Boardman LA, Steenblock KJ, et al. MYH mutations in patients with attenuated and classic polyposis and with young-onset colorectal cancer without polyps. *Gastroenterology* 2004;127:9–16.

180. Jones S, Emmerson P, Maynard J, Best JM, et al. Biallelic germline mutations in MYH predispose to multiple colorectal adenoma and somatic G:C→T:A mutations. *Hum Mol Genet* 2002;11:2961–2967.

181. Peterlongo P, Mitra N, Chuai S, Kirchhoff T, et al. Colorectal cancer risk in individuals with biallelic or monoallelic mutations of MYH. *Int J Cancer* 2005;114:505–507.

182. Sampson JR, Dolwani S, Jones S, Eccles D, et al. Autosomal recessive colorectal adenomatous polyposis due to inherited mutations of MYH. *Lancet* 2003;362:39–41.

183. Gismondi V, Meta M, Bonelli L, Radice P, et al. Prevalence of the Y165C, G382D and 1395delGGA germline mutations of the MYH gene in Italian patients with adenomatous polyposis coli and colorectal adenomas. *Int J Cancer* 2004;109:680–684.

184. Isidro G, Laranjeira F, Pires A, Leite J, et al. Germline MUTYH (MYH) mutations in Portuguese individuals with multiple colorectal adenomas. *Hum Mutat* 2004;24:353–354.

185. Kairupan CF, Meldrum CJ, Crooks R, Milward EA, et al. Mutation analysis of the MYH gene in an Australian series of colorectal polyposis patients with or without germline APC mutations. *Int J Cancer* 2005;116:73–77.

186. Miyaki M, Iijima T, Yamaguchi T, Hishima T, Tamura K, Utsunomiya J, Mori T. Germline mutations of the MYH gene in Japanese patients with multiple colorectal adenomas. *Mutat Res* 2005;578:430–433.

187. Alhopuro P, Parker AR, Lehtonen R, Enholm S, et al. A novel functionally deficient MYH variant in individuals with colorectal adenomatous polyposis. *Hum Mutat* 2005;26:393.

188. Enholm S, Heinonen T, Suomalainen A, Lipton L, et al. Proportion and phenotype of MYH-associated colorectal neoplasia in a population-based series of Finnish colorectal cancer patients. *Am J Pathol* 2003;163:827–832.

189. Venesio T, Malatore S, Cattaneo F, Arrigoni A, Risio M, Ranzani GN. High frequency of MYH gene mutations in a subset of patients with familial adenomatous polyposis. *Gastroenterology* 2004;126:1681–1685.

190. Jo WS, Bandipalliam P, Shannon KM, Niendorf KB, et al. Correlation of polyp number and family history of colon cancer with germline MYH mutations. *Clin Gastroenterol Hepatol* 2005;3:1022–1028.

191. Baglioni S, Melean G, Gensini F, Santucci M, et al. A kindred with MYH-associated polyposis and pilomatricomas. *Am J Med Genet* 2005;134:212–214.

192. Croitoru ME, Cleary SP, Di Nicola N, Manno M, et al. Association between biallelic and monoallelic germline MYH gene mutations and colorectal cancer risk. *J Natl Cancer Inst* 2004;96:1631–1634.

193. Tenesa A, Farrington SM, Dunlop MG. Re: Association between biallelic and monoallelic germline MYH gene mutations and colorectal cancer risk. *J Natl Cancer Inst* 2005;97:320–321; author reply 321–322.

194. Farrington S, Tenesa A, Barnetson R, et al. Germline susceptibility to colorectal cancer due to base-excision repair gene defects. *Am J Hum Genet* 2005;77:112–119.

195. Leite JS, Martins M, Martins M, Regateiro F, et al. Is prophylactic colectomy indicated in patients with MYH-associated polyposis? *Colorectal Dis* 2005;7:327–331.

196. Boardman LA. Heritable colorectal cancer syndromes: recognition and preventive management. *Gastroenterol Clin North Am* 2002;31:1107–1131.

197. Hemminki A. The molecular basis and clinical aspects of Peutz-Jeghers syndrome. *Cell Mol Life Sci* 1999;55:735–750.

198. Giardiello FM, Brensinger JD, Tersmette AC, et al. Very high risk of cancer in familial Peutz-Jeghers syndrome. *Gastroenterology* 2000;119:1447–1453.

199. Hemminki A, Tomlinson I, Markie D, et al. Localization of a susceptibility locus for Peutz-Jeghers syndrome to 19p using comparative genomic hybridization and targeted linkage analysis. *Nat Genet* 1997;15:87–90.

200. Abdel-Rahman WM, Peltomaki P. Molecular basis and diagnostics of hereditary colorectal cancers. *Ann Med* 2004;36:379–388.

201. Lim W, Hearle N, Shah B, et al. Further observations on LKB1/STK11 status and cancer risk in Peutz-Jeghers syndrome. *Br J Cancer* 2003;89:308–313.

202. Boardman LA, Couch FJ, Burgart LJ, et al. Genetic heterogeneity in Peutz-Jeghers syndrome. *Hum Mutat* 2000;16:23–30.

203. Mehenni H, Blouin JL, Radhakrishna U, et al. Peutz-Jeghers syndrome: confirmation of linkage to chromosome 19p13.3 and identification of a potential second locus, on 19q13.4. *Am J Hum Genet* 1997;61:1327–1334.

204. Hearle NC, Tomlinson I, Lim W, et al. Sequence changes in predicted promoter elements of STK11/LKB1 are unlikely to contribute to Peutz-Jeghers syndrome BMC. *Genomics* 2005;6:38.

205. Sweet K, Willis J, Zhou XP, et al. Molecular classification of patients with unexplained hamartomatous and hyperplastic polyposis. *JAMA* 2005;294:2465–2473.

206. Dunlop MG. Guidance on gastrointestinal surveillance for hereditary non-polyposis colorectal cancer, familial adenomatous polyposis, juvenile polyposis, and Peutz-Jeghers syndrome. *Gut* 2002;51(suppl 5):V21–V27.

207. Edwards DP, Khosraviani K, Stafferton R, et al. Long-term results of polyp clearance by intraoperative enteroscopy in the Peutz-Jeghers syndrome. *Dis Colon Rectum* 2003;46:48–50.

208. McGarrity TJ, Kulin HE, Zaino RJ. Peutz-Jeghers syndrome. *Am J Gastroenterol* 2000;95:596–604.

209. Pennazio M, Rossini FP. Small bowel polyps in Peutz-Jeghers syndrome: management by combined push enteroscopy and intraoperative enteroscopy. *Gastrointest Endosc* 2000;51:304–308.

210. Boardman LA, Thibodeau SN, Schaid DJ, et al. Increased risk for cancer in patients with the Peutz-Jeghers syndrome. *Ann Intern Med* 1998;128:896–899.

211. Adler DG, Gostout CJ. Wireless capsule endoscopy. *Hosp Physician* 2003;39:14–22.

212. Soares J, Lopes L, Vilas Boas G, Pinho C. Wireless capsule endoscopy for evaluation of phenotypic expression of small-bowel polyps in patients with Peutz-Jeghers syndrome and in symptomatic first-degree relatives. *Endoscopy* 2004;36:1060–1066.

213. Saurin JC, Delvaux M, Gaudin JL, et al. Diagnostic value of endoscopic capsule in patients with obscure digestive bleeding: blinded comparison with video push-enteroscopy. *Endoscopy* 2003;35:576–584.

214. Saurin JC, Delvaux M, Vahedi K, et al. Clinical impact of capsule endoscopy compared to push enteroscopy: 1-year follow-up study. *Endoscopy* 2005;37:318–323.

215. Soares J, Lopes L, Vilas Boas G, et al. Wireless capsule endoscopy for evaluation of phenotypic expression of small-bowel polyps in patients with Peutz-Jeghers syndrome and in symptomatic first-degree relatives. *Endoscopy* 2004;36:1060–1066.

216. Park JG, Yang HK, Kim WH, et al. Report on the first meeting of the International Collaborative Group on Hereditary Gastric Cancer. *J Natl Cancer Inst* 2000;92:1781–1782.

217. Pharoah PD, Guilford P, Caldas C. Incidence of gastric cancer and breast cancer in CDH1 (E-cadherin) mutation carriers from hereditary diffuse gastric cancer families. *Gastroenterology* 2001;121:1348–1353.

218. Barber M, Fitzgerald RC, Caldas C. Familial gastric cancer—aetiology and pathogenesis. *Best Pract Res Clin Gastroenterol* 2006;20:721–734.

219. Fitzgerald RC, Caldas C. Familial gastric cancer—clinical management. *Best Pract Res Clin Gastroenterol* 2006;20:735–743.

220. Lynch HT, Smyrk T, Lynch JF. Molecular genetics and clinical-pathology features of hereditary nonpolyposis colorectal carcinoma (Lynch syndrome): historical journey from pedigree anecdote to molecular genetic confirmation. *Oncology* 1998;55:103–108.

221. Reddy BS. The Fourth DeWitt S. Goodman lecture. Novel approaches to the prevention of colon cancer by nutritional manipulation and chemoprevention. *Cancer Epidemiol Biomarkers Prev* 2000;9:239–247.

222. Watson P, Ashwathnarayan R, Lynch HT, et al. Tobacco use and increased colorectal cancer risk in patients with hereditary nonpolyposis colorectal cancer (Lynch syndrome). *Arch Intern Med* 2004;164:2429–2431.

223. Lynch HT, Smyrk TC. Identifying hereditary nonpolyposis colorectal cancer. *N Engl J Med* 1998;338:1537–1538.

224. Douglas JA, Gruber SB, Meister KA, et al. History and molecular genetics of Lynch syndrome in family G: a century later. *JAMA* 2005;294:2195–2202.

225. Li D, Xie K, Wolff R, et al. Pancreatic cancer. *Lancet* 2004;363:1049–1057.

226. McWilliams RR, Bamlet WR, Rabe KG, et al. Association of family history of specific cancers with a younger age of onset of pancreatic adenocarcinoma. *Clin Gastroenterol Hepatol* 2006;4:1143–1147.

227. Petersen GM, de Andrade M, Goggins M, et al. Pancreatic cancer genetic epidemiology consortium. *Cancer Epidemiol Biomarkers Prev* 2006; 15:704–710.

228. Lynch HT, Deters CA, Lynch JF, et al. Familial pancreatic carcinoma in Jews. *Fam Cancer* 2004;3:233–240.

229. Eberle MA, Pfutzer R, Pogue-Gelle KL, et al. A new susceptibility locus for autosomal dominant pancreatic cancer maps to chromosome 4q32-34. *Am J Hum Genet* 2002;70:1044–1048.

230. Habbe N, Langer P, Sina-Frey M, et al. Familial pancreatic cancer syndromes. *Endocrinol Metab Clin North Am* 2006;35:417–430, xi.

231. Hahn SA, Greenhalf B, Ellis I, et al. BRCA2 germline mutations in familial pancreatic carcinoma. *J Natl Cancer Inst* 2003;95:214–221.

232. Xin W, Yun KJ, Ricci F, et al. MAP2K4/MKK4 expression in pancreatic cancer: genetic validation of immunohistochemistry and relationship to disease course. *Clin Cancer Res* 2004;10:8516–8520.

233. Lynch HT, Brand RE, Hogg D, et al. Phenotypic variation in eight extended CDKN2A germline mutation familial atypical multiple mole melanoma-pancreatic carcinoma-prone families: the familial atypical mole melanoma-pancreatic carcinoma syndrome. *Cancer* 2002;94:84–96.

234. Su GH, Hruban RH, Bansal RK, et al. Germline and somatic mutations of the STK11/LKB1 Peutz-Jeghers gene in pancreatic and biliary cancers. *Am J Pathol* 1999;154:1835–1840.

235. Westerman AM, Entius MM, Boor PP, et al. Novel mutations in the LKB1/STK11 gene in Dutch Peutz-Jeghers families. *Hum Mutat* 1999;13: 476–481.

236. Whitcomb DC, Gorry MC, Preston RA, et al. Hereditary pancreatitis is caused by a mutation in the cationic trypsinogen gene. *Nat Genet* 1996;14: 141–145.

237. McWilliams R, Highsmith WE, Rabe KG, et al. Cystic fibrosis transmembrane regulator gene carrier status is a risk factor for young onset pancreatic adenocarcinoma. *Gut* 2005;54:1661–1662.

238. Wilentz RE, Goggins M, Redston M, et al. Genetic, immunohistochemical, and clinical features of medullary carcinoma of the pancreas: a newly described and characterized entity. *Am J Pathol* 2000;156:1641–1651.

239. Jass JR, Cottier DS, Jeevaratnam P, et al. Diagnostic use of microsatellite instability in hereditary non-polyposis colorectal cancer. *Lancet* 1995; 346:1200–1201.

240. Renkonen E, Zhang Y, Lohi H, et al. Altered expression of MLH1, MSH2, and MSH6 in predisposition to hereditary nonpolyposis colorectal cancer. *J Clin Oncol* 2003;21:3629–3637.

241. Abdel-Rahman WM, Ollikainen M, Kariola R, et al. Comprehensive characterization of HNPCC-related colorectal cancers reveals striking molecular features in families with no germline mismatch repair gene mutations. *Oncogene* 2005;24:1542–1551.

242. Young J, Barker MA, Simms LA, et al. Evidence for BRAF mutation and variable levels of microsatellite instability in a syndrome of familial colorectal cancer. *Clin Gastroenterol Hepatol* 2005;3:254–263.

243. Lindor NM, Rabe K, Petersen GM, et al. Lower cancer incidence in Amsterdam-I criteria families without mismatch repair deficiency: familial colorectal cancer type X. *JAMA* 2005;293:1979–1985.

244. Llor X, Pons E, Xicola RM et al. Differential features of colorectal cancers fulfilling Amsterdam criteria without involvement of the mutator pathway. *Clin Cancer Res* 2005;11:7304–7310,

245. Fearnhead NS, Winney B, Bodmer WF. Rare variant hypothesis for multifactorial inheritance: susceptibility to colorectal adenomas as a model. *Cell Cycle* 2005;4:521–525.

246. Rennert G, Almog R, Tomsho LP, et al. Colorectal polyps in carriers of the APC I1307K polymorphism. *Dis Colon Rectum* 2005;48:2317–2321.

247. di Pietro M, Bellver JS, Menigatti M, et al. Defective DNA mismatch repair determines a characteristic transcriptional profile in proximal colon cancers. *Gastroenterology* 2005;129:1047–1059.

248. Banerjea A, Ahmed S, Hands RE, et al. Colorectal cancers with microsatellite instability display mRNA expression signatures characteristic of increased immunogenicity. *Mol Cancer* 2004;3:21.

249. Li SR, Ng CF, Banerjea A, et al. Differential expression patterns of the insulin-like growth factor 2 gene in human colorectal cancer. *Tumour Biol* 2004;25:62–68.

250. Mori Y, Yin J, Sato F, et al. Identification of genes uniquely involved in frequent microsatellite instability colon carcinogenesis by expression profiling combined with epigenetic scanning. *Cancer Res* 2004;64:2434–2438.

251. Shedden KA, Taylor JM, Giordano TJ, et al. Accurate molecular classification of human cancers based on gene expression using a simple classifier with a pathological tree-based framework. *Am J Pathol* 2003;163:1985–1995.

252. Giacomini CP, Leung SY, Chen X, et al. A gene expression signature of genetic instability in colon cancer. *Cancer Res* 2005;65:9200–9205.

253. Kruhoffer M, Jensen JL, Laiho P, et al. Gene expression signatures for colorectal cancer microsatellite status and HNPCC. *Br J Cancer* 2005;92: 2240–2248.

254. Kim H, Nam SW, Rhee H, Shan LL, et al. Different gene expression profiles between microsatellite instability-high and microsatellite stable colorectal carcinomas. *Oncogene* 2004;23:6218–6225.

255. Keller JJ, Giardiello FM. Chemoprevention strategies using NSAIDs and COX-2 inhibitors. *Cancer Biol Ther* 2003;2:S140–S149.

256. Annie Yu HJ, Lin KM, Ota DM, et al. Hereditary nonpolyposis colorectal cancer: preventive management. *Cancer Treat Rev* 2003;29:461–470.

257. Hampel H, Frankel WL, Martin E, et al. Screening for the Lynch syndrome (hereditary nonpolyposis colorectal cancer). *N Engl J Med* 2005;352:1851–1860.

CHAPTER 4 ■ GASTROINTESTINAL CANCER: SCREENING AND SURVEILLANCE

ROBERT S. SANDLER

Screening can be defined as the application of a test to detect a potential disease or condition in a person who has no known signs or symptoms (1). A screening test need not provide a definitive diagnosis, and most screening tests are not definitive. Instead, they help stratify screened subjects into those who are likely and those who are unlikely to have disease. Those at higher risk are then candidates for further diagnostic testing. Screening can be conducted by asking questions (e.g., about family history of cancer), by performing a physical examination (e.g., digital rectal examination), by obtaining a laboratory test (e.g., α-fetoprotein), or by performing an imaging or endoscopic examination. Ideally, a screening test should be cheap, safe, quick, well accepted, and well tolerated.

Surveillance is a special case of screening. It involves periodic reapplication of a screening or diagnostic test. Surveillance, too, may be restricted to those at highest risk, but it does not have to be. In contrast to screening, which detects existing or prevalent cases, surveillance is designed to detect new or incident cases.

This chapter reviews the general principles of screening and surveillance for gastrointestinal (GI) cancers. These principles are illustrated with specific examples, but detailed discussions of screening for individual cancers can be found in other chapters.

GENERAL PRINCIPLES OF SCREENING

Disease Must Have Serious Consequences

The first general principle of screening is that the disease must have serious consequences (2). Diseases that have significant morbidity and mortality would be candidates for screening. Importantly, the disease must also be recognized as serious by potential screenees for them to agree to participate in a screening program. Some conditions that demand screening are not themselves serious but lead to serious diseases. Barrett's esophagus, for example, is a benign condition that predisposes to adenocarcinoma of the esophagus. Routine surveillance of patients with Barrett's esophagus may decrease mortality from esophageal carcinoma. To achieve success, a Barrett's esophagus screening program requires that patients recognize the connection to cancer and embrace regular surveillance.

Disease Must Be an Important Health Problem

The disease must be an important health problem (3) to justify screening. This requirement has both societal and practical implications. From a public health or population perspective, allocating resources for population screening is not justified unless the disease is relatively common. In practical terms, if the disease is uncommon, large numbers of asymptomatic individuals will be subjected to screening with a very small yield. Thus, a highly fatal disease such as cholangiocarcinoma would not be a candidate for screening in the general population because it is too rare.

The "importance" requirement is dynamic and may vary with geography. Gastric cancer screening has been promoted in Japan, where disease incidence is high, but screening does not appear to be effective in Venezuela (4). High-risk subpopulations who would be candidates for screening for gastric cancer may also exist. Individuals who have had previous gastric resection for benign peptic ulcer disease are at higher risk of developing cancer in the gastric remnant after a 15- to 20-year latency (5). Such individuals might be candidates for screening in Germany, where the baseline risk of gastric cancer in the general population is moderate, but not in the United States, where the baseline risk is low.

The disease may be important to special populations. Although screening of the entire population might not be appropriate, screening might be very appropriate in a high-risk subgroup. An example would be screening for hepatocellular carcinoma. Screening is not recommended for the general population in the United States but may be appropriate for certain patients with cirrhosis.

Disease Must Have a Detectable Preclinical Phase

The purpose of screening is to detect cancer before symptoms develop. This means that the cancer must have a presymptomatic or preclinical phase during which it is potentially detectable by a screening test (3). For benefit to be derived from screening, it must be possible not only to detect the cancer during the preclinical phase but also, more importantly, to alter the natural history. The natural history of cancer is represented in Figure 4.1.

The biological onset of cancer occurs at point *A* in Figure 4.1. No units of measure are given in the figure, and the intervals are all relative. The age of development of cancer varies by cancer and may be modified by environmental and familial risks. For example, cancers secondary to radiation or gene mutations (e.g., familial polyposis) occur at a younger age than sporadic cancers.

At the time of onset (*A*), the tumor is too small to be detected. The point at which the disease is first potentially detectable by screening is shown as point *B*. The location of *B* depends on the tumor type and growth potential. For tumors

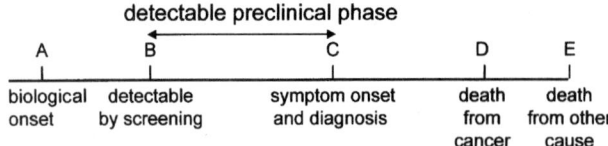

FIGURE 4.1. Natural history of cancer. A screening test must be able to detect cancer during the preclinical phase of disease.

that grow rapidly, the interval between A and B is short. The interval between B, the point at which the tumor is first potentially detectable by screening, and C, the point at which symptoms become apparent, is termed the *detectable preclinical phase* (6). Unless a preclinical phase exists during which the cancer is potentially detectable, no rationale exists for screening. The point in the detectable preclinical phase when the cancer is detected depends on the screening test; a more sensitive screening test has the potential to detect disease earlier in its natural history. An endoscopic procedure, for example, has the potential to detect a colorectal adenoma earlier than a fecal occult blood test. The detectable point also depends on characteristics of the disease. Colorectal cancers that do not bleed cannot be detected by fecal occult blood tests.

Symptom onset is depicted in Figure 4.1 at point C. The point of symptom onset represents the point of usual diagnosis in the absence of screening. For simplicity, the time of symptom onset and the time of usual diagnosis are represented as a single point in Figure 4.1, but the time of symptom onset and time of diagnosis are not always identical. A delay may occur before the individual first seeks medical attention after the onset of symptoms (*patient delay*). For example, patients may ignore rectal bleeding and thereby delay the diagnosis of rectal cancer. Even after the patient presents to the physician with symptoms, further delay may occur before the diagnosis is made (*physician delay*). The interval between presentation and diagnosis may be very brief if definitive tests are scheduled promptly or may be longer if symptoms are dismissed by patients or physicians. If the presenting symptoms are nonspecific or vague, such as nausea, fatigue, or weight loss, diagnosis may be substantially delayed.

After disease diagnosis and therapy, the patient may die from disease (D) or may be cured to later die from some other cause (E).

Treatment Must Exist That Is More Effective When Applied to Presymptomatic Cancer

An effective treatment for the disease must exist to justify screening. Moreover, the treatment must be more effective when it is applied during the presymptomatic interval than when it is applied to cancers detected at the usual time of symptom onset. Otherwise, there is no point in attempting to detect the cancer earlier. Determining whether early detection has a real impact in prolonging life is also important.

As shown in Figure 4.1, if a lesion is discovered during the preclinical phase, then the interval between diagnosis by screening and death (B→D) is longer than the interval between diagnosis after symptom onset and death (C→D). Death occurs at the same point, however. This apparent increase in survival is termed *lead-time bias*. Early detection has simply advanced the date of diagnosis without postponing death. A screening test is useful only if detection during the preclinical phase postpones death and prolongs life.

The survival advantage from early detection is D→E, the interval between the time of death from the cancer that was averted and the time of death from another cause. The age

at death from competing cause is variable and unpredictable. Clearly, the potential years of life saved by screening are greater for a 40-year-old than for an 80-year-old because of the longer life expectancy of a 40-year-old. The years of life saved are also fewer for individuals with significant comorbidity. Because death from competing cause is unpredictable, specifying when not to screen has been difficult for guideline developers. Clinicians often exercise their judgment by not screening the very elderly or those with substantial comorbidity. The overall effectiveness of a screening program depends on the number of life-years gained by screenees.

The point of death from other cause (E) can precede the point of death from cancer. Some patients die with their cancer but not from their cancer. If the cancer is not likely to be fatal, then detecting the cancer by screening incurs costs without prolonging life.

Test Must Be Safe

Screening tests are generally applied to individuals at low risk for cancer. Colorectal cancer screening, for example, is recommended for asymptomatic individuals older than 50 years. Because the risk of the disease is low, the screening test must be exceptionally safe. Otherwise, the risk of the screening test outweighs the benefits. The mortality from complications of the test must certainly be lower than the mortality from the disease.

Some authorities have recommended periodic colonoscopy to screen for colorectal cancer (7). Data from prospective studies of colonoscopy suggest that approximately 1 per 1,000 persons undergoing colonoscopy have perforations, 3 per 1,000 have major hemorrhage, and 1 to 3 per 10,000 die as a result of the procedure (8). Although these risk estimates probably overstate the risk in asymptomatic 50-year-old screenees, the risks of the procedure must be balanced against the potential gains.

The acceptable risk from screening depends on the population. It may be reasonable to adopt a riskier screening test if the risk for disease in a particular group is very high with the expectation that the risk–benefit ratio will remain favorable. Thus, although colonoscopy might be viewed as possibly less safe for asymptomatic 50-year-olds, the test would be quite appropriate for a member of a family with hereditary non-polyposis colorectal cancer in whom the risk for colon cancer is substantial (8).

The issue of safety must extend beyond the specific screening test to the more definitive diagnostic tests that are applied to individuals for whom screen results are positive. Individuals who are found to have positive results on a fecal occult blood test are referred for colonoscopy, a more definitive but riskier test (9). The risk for colonoscopy must be incorporated into risk estimates for a fecal occult blood test program. To do otherwise would falsely inflate the safety of the fecal occult blood test. For example, in the Minnesota fecal occult blood trial, 12,246 colonoscopies were performed at the university hospital in subjects with positive fecal occult blood test results (10). The colonoscopies resulted in 4 colonic perforations requiring surgery and 11 serious bleeds, 3 of which required surgery. Decision and cost-effectiveness models must incorporate these downstream risks when they evaluate a screening program.

Test Must Be Acceptable to Patients and Providers

To be effective, a screening test must be acceptable not only to potential screenees but also to their health care providers.

Lack of acceptance by either of these groups compromises the effectiveness of a screening program.

Acceptability to potential screenees is highly personal and largely unstudied (11). Fecal occult blood testing is touted as a simple method for mass screening, yet compliance in European controlled trials ranged from 53% to 67%. Fecal occult blood testing has been offered in Germany since 1977, but only 21% of women and 10% of men take advantage of the screening (12). Flexible sigmoidoscopy, a test that many believe to be more effective than mammography, is vastly underused. Lack of acceptance of sigmoidoscopy is largely due to the failure of patients to embrace the technique, either because they perceive that the test is uncomfortable or because they believe that they are not at risk. Providers share part of the responsibility, however. Many do not have the time, training, or equipment to provide flexible sigmoidoscopy. The use of nurse practitioners may help make the test acceptable to health care providers and thereby more available to patients (13,14). New technology, such as a sheathed endoscope that does not require time-consuming disinfection between uses, may also make a test more acceptable to providers by decreasing the time necessary to perform the test, although this technology has not become popular (15).

Test Must Be Available

The screening test must be available to potential screenees to have an impact. As noted previously, flexible sigmoidoscopy is not always available. Availability must also extend beyond the screening test to diagnostic tests for those who have positive results on the screening test. If colonoscopy is not available to evaluate individuals with positive fecal occult blood tests, then the program (screening test plus diagnostic test) is not available. Virtual colonoscopy is a radiologic technique that holds great promise for large bowel screening (16). It may take some time before the technology is widely available.

Test Must Be Affordable

The screening test must be reasonably inexpensive in both direct costs (dollars) and indirect costs (time missed from usual activities, discomfort, and inconvenience). The cost of the test to potential screenees depends, in part, on whether the test is covered by insurance. In 1998, Medicare began to cover the cost of screening with fecal occult blood tests every year and with flexible sigmoidoscopy every 2 years for individuals older than 50 years. Coverage by Medicare made the test more affordable, but it is probably too soon to determine whether any impact on use has occurred.

The cost of a test includes the cost of the test itself and any downstream costs for more definitive tests that are necessary to evaluate a positive test result. For example, fecal occult blood test kits are inexpensive (<$10), but the cost to evaluate a positive test may be $1,000. The cost of a screening program also includes the cost of treatment for lesions that are discovered as a consequence of screening. The cost of a colorectal cancer screening program includes the costs of screening (endoscopy and pathology) and the costs of treatment (surgery, oncology, radiation). The costs of the screening program must be balanced against the gains (17). Early detection should prolong life. An affordable program should have a reasonable cost per life-year gained when compared with other commonly accepted medical interventions (18).

The affordability criterion depends on perspective. Policy makers typically take the population perspective in deciding whether a screening test should be offered. To reach a decision, they evaluate the overall costs to society of the screening test and the opportunity costs of not spending the money on a different program. The population perspective is often at odds with the perspective of the individual patient, who may have the interest in and the funds to purchase the test, and the perspective of the physician, who has the obligation to serve as the advocate for the individual patient.

Test Must Be Accurate

Perhaps the most important requirement for a screening test is accuracy. To have an impact, the test must have high sensitivity and specificity to avoid misclassification. These concepts are discussed in the next section.

CHARACTERISTICS OF THE SCREENING TEST

Sensitivity

The fundamental purpose of screening is to distinguish people who potentially have the disease of interest from those who do not. The ability of a screening test to designate those with disease as positive is referred to as the *sensitivity* of the test (19). Sensitivity is defined as the proportion of diseased individuals with a positive test result (Fig. 4.2). A sensitive test has few false-negative results. Therefore, when a sensitive test is negative, it helps to rule out disease. That is because a sensitive test rarely gives negative results in the presence of disease (few false negatives) (20). A sensitive test should be used if an important penalty exists for missing disease.

The sensitivity of a test to detect disease may vary with the stage of disease. For example, an upper GI tract radiograph is more sensitive for a 10-cm mass than for a 1-cm mass. When tests are first developed, they are often used to evaluate patients with symptomatic or advanced disease. A test that is highly sensitive under these circumstances may perform more poorly for asymptomatic early-stage cancer (21). For a screening test to be effective, it must detect the disease in the preclinical phase and must have an impact on survival. A test that is only sensitive when the disease is advanced is not useful.

For tests such as fecal occult blood testing, a family of test sensitivities may exist. Each fecal occult blood card consists of two testing windows, and testing generally involves three cards (six windows). Testing may be repeated yearly. Thus, there is the sensitivity of each slide, the sensitivity of the set of three slides, and the sensitivity of the program repeated over years. These sensitivities are distinct but related (22). Different authors have reached different conclusions about the sensitivity

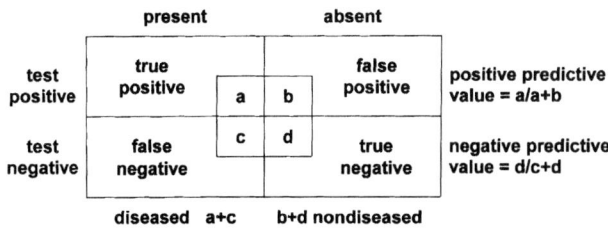

FIGURE 4.2. Characteristics of a screening test. Sensitivity and specificity are fixed characteristics of the screening test, whereas predictive value depends on disease prevalence. See text for details.

of fecal occult blood testing because they used different definitions of sensitivity (22,23).

The apparent sensitivity of a test may be influenced by *serendipity* (24,25). A screen-positive participant in a fecal occult blood screening program might be found to have a small adenoma on colonoscopy. Because the purpose of the screening program is to detect early disease, and because some adenomas progress to cancer, the program would take credit for an adenoma discovered following colonoscopy for a positive fecal occult blood test. The likelihood, however, is that the adenoma was not really responsible for the bleeding that led to the colonoscopy, and the positive fecal occult blood test result was really a false positive. Serendipitous findings of this type inflate the apparent sensitivity of the test.

A sensitive test may also uncover lesions that would never progress to advanced cancer. These findings have been termed *pseudodisease* (6). The problem with pseudodisease is that it leads to the expense and possible complications associated with treatment. For example, the natural history of Barrett's esophagus is poorly understood. Barrett's esophagus patients with dysplasia may be subjected to ablative therapy using heat probes, lasers, or photodynamic therapy. Ablative therapy may result in strictures or perforation. Perhaps such therapy is justified for dysplasia, but it is difficult to make decisions about the value of ablative therapy because our understanding of the natural history of Barrett's esophagus is incomplete.

Specificity

Specificity is the ability to designate those without the disease as negative. Specificity is defined as the proportion of nondiseased individuals with a negative test result (Fig. 4.2). A specific test has few false-positive results. When a specific test gives positive results, it helps rule in disease. This is because a specific test is rarely positive in the absence of disease (few false positives) (20). Using a specific test is important if a treatment based on a positive test result or the evaluation of a positive test result could harm the patient. For GI cancer, one would rely on a very specific test such as a biopsy before subjecting a patient to surgery or chemotherapy.

As shown in Figure 4.3, a trade-off exists between sensitivity and specificity. For a continuous measure, such as fecal

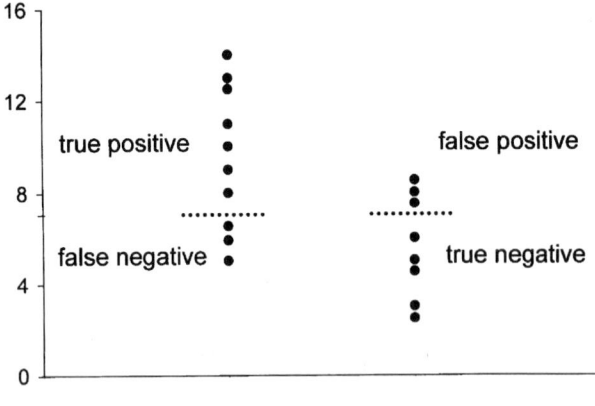

FIGURE 4.3. Trade-off between sensitivity and specificity. When the cut point for disease is set at 7 units (*dotted line*), three diseased individuals are falsely classified as having negative test results, and three nondiseased individuals are falsely classified as having positive test results. If the cut point were decreased to 4 units, the number of false negatives would decrease (improved sensitivity), but the number of false positives would increase (lower specificity).

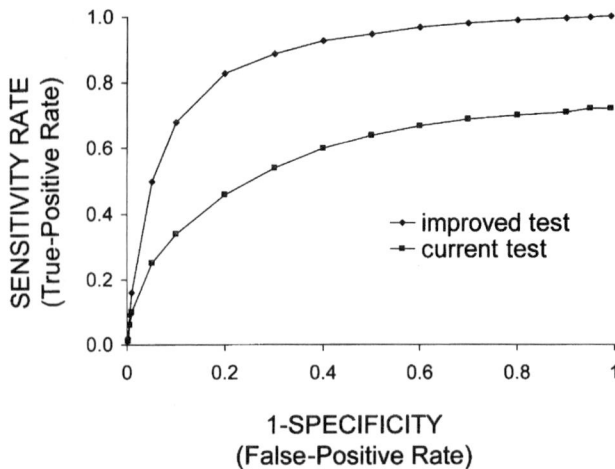

FIGURE 4.4. Receiver operating characteristic curve. For any given cut point for disease (represented by the ■ and ◆ symbols), a trade-off exists between the rate of true-positive results and the rate of false-positive results for each test. The optimal cut point is generally closest to the left upper corner, where the rate of true positives is highest and the rate of false positives is lowest. An improved test may have better sensitivity and specificity.

hemoglobin detected by a fecal occult blood test, the criterion for positivity or the cut point between a positive and a negative test result is somewhat arbitrary. If the cut point is set very low (a small amount of bleeding is called *positive*), then the number of screenees with a positive test result increases. Although the sensitivity increases when the cut point is lowered, so does the false-positive rate (1 – specificity). In the Minnesota randomized controlled trial of fecal occult blood testing to detect colorectal cancer, the samples were rehydrated before they were developed (10). Rehydration increased the sensitivity. An increase in true positives was achieved at the expense of an increase in false positives.

Because evaluating a positive result on a fecal occult blood test can be time consuming, expensive, uncomfortable, and sometimes dangerous, one might select a higher cut point for a positive test. Doing so decreases the number of positive test results—more blood is required for the test to give a positive result. The number of false positives would decrease (higher specificity), as would the number of true positives (lower sensitivity).

One way to represent the trade-off between sensitivity and specificity is as a *receiver operating characteristic* (ROC) curve (Fig. 4.4). The ROC curve plots the true-positive rate (sensitivity) against the false-positive rate (1 – specificity). The ROC curve can be useful to help set the cut point for a continuous measure such as fecal hemoglobin. As a general strategy, the optimal cut point would be located in the upper left corner of the ROC curve, where the number of true positives is highest and the number of false positives is lowest. The specific cut point chosen depends on the penalty for missing disease or the difficulty of evaluating a positive test. If a substantial penalty exists for missed disease, the policy maker might select a point farther to the right of the curve. This point would assure more true-positive results at the cost of more false-positive results.

An ROC curve generally cannot be applied to a test with a dichotomous (yes/no) outcome such as sigmoidoscopy, in which an adenoma is either present or not. The presence or absence of an adenoma is not precisely dichotomous, however. The detection of an adenoma depends on the visual resolution of the endoscope and on arbitrary decisions about whether to perform a biopsy on lesions below a certain size (9).

Although an inevitable trade-off exists between sensitivity and specificity for any given test, it may be possible to improve performance by using a different test. For example, a different type of fecal occult blood test might have both higher sensitivity and higher specificity than the test that is currently in widespread use. The improved test would have a different ROC curve. This is shown by the upper curve in Figure 4.4.

Predictive Value

Sensitivity and specificity describe properties of the screening test. They indicate how the test performs in evaluating individuals who either have or do not have the disease. For practical purposes, the sensitivity and specificity of a given test are considered "fixed" properties of the test. That is, the sensitivity and the specificity remain the same no matter where the test is applied.

When a screening test is administered, however, the examiner does not know whether the disease is present or absent. The examiner simply knows whether the test result is positive or negative. The relevant question is whether an individual with a positive test result has the disease, or whether one with a negative test result is disease-free. The answers to these questions are provided by the *predictive value* of the test. Positive predictive value is the proportion of cases in which persons with a positive screening test result have the disease in question (Fig. 4.2). Negative predictive value is the proportion of cases in which people with a negative test result do not have the disease in question.

In contrast to sensitivity and specificity, the predictive value of a test is not fixed. Predictive value varies with *prevalence*. Prevalence is the proportion of individuals in the population with a given disease, and prevalence is, in turn, proportional to the incidence (the development of new cancers) and the duration of cancer. When the prevalence of the disease is very low, most of the positive test results are false positives, and the positive predictive value (probability of disease after a positive test result, or posterior probability) is low. The opposite is true for negative predictive value—when the disease is rare, most of the negative test results are true negatives, and the negative predictive value is high. Conversely, when the prevalence of disease is high, most of the positive results are true positives, and the positive predictive value is high. When the prevalence is high, most of the negative results are false negatives, and the negative predictive value is low.

For example, if fecal occult blood tests were performed in a pediatric clinic, some positive test results would occur, but none of the patients with positive results would have colorectal cancer because children do not get colorectal cancer. Because the prevalence of the disease is low in children, the predictive value of a positive test in this setting is low. Similarly, if fecal occult blood tests were given to individuals with mass lesions of the colon seen on barium enema radiograph, the prevalence of cancer would be very high, and most of the positive results would be true positives. The positive predictive value in this setting would be high.

Table 4.1 shows the effect of disease prevalence on the predictive value of an excellent test (95% sensitivity and 95% specificity). When the prevalence of disease is 0.1% (about the prevalence of colorectal cancer in asymptomatic 50-year-olds), the predictive value of a positive test is only 2%. The positive predictive value increases to 50% when the prevalence is 5% and increases to 68% when the prevalence is 10%. Table 4.1 indicates that the predictive value of an excellent test is low when the disease is uncommon. The predictive value would be even worse if either the test sensitivity or specificity were lower.

The results of a test have little impact on clinical decision making when the prevalence of the disease is either very high or very low. Figure 4.5 graphs the posterior probability of

TABLE 4.1

EFFECT OF DISEASE PREVALENCE ON POSITIVE AND NEGATIVE PREDICTIVE VALUE FOR A TEST WITH 95% SENSITIVITY AND 95% SPECIFICITY

Prevalence (%)	Positive predictive value (%)	Negative predictive value (%)
0.1	2	99
1	19	99
5	50	99
10	68	99
50	95	95

disease after a positive or negative test result and illustrates the diagnostic gain compared to doing no test. The diagnostic gain is greater when the prior probability is in the midrange than when the prior probability is at the extremes. When the prior probability is 50%, a positive test result makes the disease highly likely (95%), and a negative test result makes the disease highly unlikely (5%). In the case of GI cancers, which are generally rare, a screening test is designed to identify individuals in whom the probability of disease is increased. These individuals would be candidates for more definitive diagnostic tests. Another strategy to increase the impact of screening is to focus on subgroups of patients with increased prevalence of disease. Screening tests perform better in high-risk groups because the higher prevalence increases predictive value of a positive test. Combining tests, as described in the next section, can also identify groups with increased prevalence and improve test performance.

Serial Testing

Combining tests to improve their performance may be helpful. Because a disease such as colorectal cancer is relatively

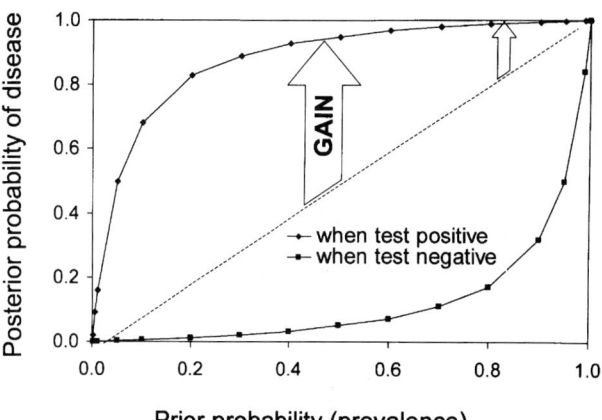

FIGURE 4.5. Relationship between prevalence and predictive value. This figure demonstrates the performance of a test with 95% sensitivity and 95% specificity. Compared to no testing (*dotted line*), the maximum gain from a positive test result occurs when the prevalence is in the midrange (*large arrow*). When the disease prevalence is very high, a positive test result makes less difference (*smaller arrow*). When the prior probability is 50%, a positive test result makes the target disease very likely, and a negative test result makes the target disease very unlikely. *Source:* Adapted form ref. 20.

TABLE 4.2

EFFECT OF SERIAL TESTING ON SENSITIVITY, SPECIFICITY, AND POSITIVE PREDICTIVE VALUE

Test	Sensitivity	Specificity	Positive predictive value[a]
Test 1	80	60	18
Test 2	90	90	50
Tests 1 and 2	72	96	67

[a] Assuming 10% prevalence.

uncommon in asymptomatic individuals older than 50 years, one might use a sensitive test with few false negatives to increase the odds of detecting the disease. As noted previously, however, because of the low prevalence, the predictive value of a positive test would be low. Most of the positive test results would be false positives. When individuals with positive test results are subsequently screened with a more specific second test, a higher proportion of the positive test results will be true positives. Individuals who had positive results on both tests would then be subjected to more definitive testing. As shown in Table 4.2, when tests are used in series, the overall sensitivity is lower than that of either of the individual tests. Importantly, the positive predictive value of the serial testing strategy is higher. The target disease is found in a higher proportion of individuals with a positive result on serial testing than in individuals with a positive result on either of the tests alone.

Such a strategy has been suggested for colorectal cancer screening (26). Testing is first conducted using a more sensitive stool guaiac test (Hemoccult Sensa, Blackman Coulter, Fullerton, CA), and the individuals with positive results are tested with an immunologic test that is more expensive but is more specific because it tests for human hemoglobin. Cost-effectiveness analysis has demonstrated that this kind of serial testing strategy can find more cancers at a lower cost than simply using the standard fecal occult blood test strategy (27).

Quality Control

The quality of a given screening test may vary. With fecal occult blood testing, for example, some variability and subjectivity exist in the way tests are scored. A high-quality screening program employs individuals who are carefully trained, monitored, and re-evaluated. The quality extends beyond the specific test to the program itself. A mechanism should exist to identify those with a positive test result and to assure that they are conscientiously followed up and that those who are diagnosed with disease comply with appropriate therapeutic procedures (28). If follow-up involves colonoscopy, an examiner who is experienced and meticulous should perform the procedure.

IMPROVEMENT OF SCREENING EFFICIENCY

Based on the previous discussion, several strategies can be suggested to improve the efficiency of a screening program:

1. *Change the criterion for positivity cut point.* Lowering the cut point increases the number of test results classified as positive and increases the number of true-positive results. If evaluation of positive test results is expensive, however, lowering the cut point might not make sense because of the increased cost to evaluate false-positive results.

2. *Change the interval between examinations.* If testing is expensive, one might increase the interval between examinations and thereby lower the cost of the program. For example, the National Polyp Study found that the interval between colonoscopy surveillance examinations could be safely increased to 3 years (29). The European fecal occult blood studies have shown a survival benefit from biannual testing (30,31).

3. *Change the number of tests.* Fecal occult blood testing customarily involves testing three pairs of samples (six tests). The number of slide windows has implications for cost. Much of the benefit from fecal occult blood screening possibly could be achieved at lower cost by testing fewer samples.

4. *Limit testing to high-risk groups.* Screening persons at high risk is more cost effective than screening a low-risk group because more lesions are discovered. The overall impact on cancer in the population may be modest using this approach, however, because high-risk individuals account for a small proportion of the overall cancers. For example, the hereditary colorectal cancers are believed to be responsible for only approximately 25% of cases of colorectal cancer (8). The majority of cancers would be missed if efforts were focused exclusively on high-risk individuals.

5. *Serial testing.* As noted previously, serial testing strategies improve the positive predictive value and therefore the efficiency of a screening program.

BIAS

Individuals whose cancer is detected during a screening program have better survival than individuals with cancers that are detected after symptoms develop. Although one might logically conclude that the survival advantage is due to detection of cancer at an early and curable stage, several forms of bias can inflate the apparent benefit of screening.

Lead-Time Bias

As described previously, the survival interval is always longer for screen-detected cancers than for symptom-detected cancers simply because the time of diagnosis has been advanced (Fig. 4.1). Unless the early detection actually extends survival, the benefit of the screening program will be overstated. Lead-time bias can be particularly troublesome in comparing different screening modalities.

Methods are available to estimate lead time. These techniques require information on unscreened controls for comparison (32).

Length Bias

The purpose of screening is to discover cancer during the detectable preclinical phase of disease and either prevent or postpone death from cancer. When screening programs are evaluated, one strategy is to compare the survival of patients with screen-detected cancers to that of patients with cancers that are discovered after symptoms develop. In addition to lead-time bias, *length bias* may inflate the apparent benefit of the screening program.

Length bias is illustrated in Figure 4.6. If cancers are assumed to have different growth characteristics, a slowly

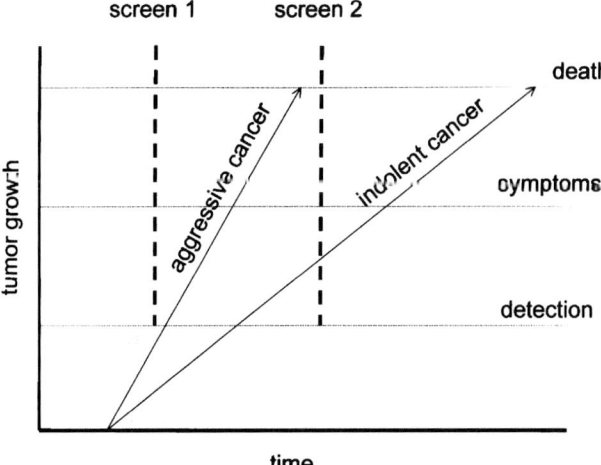

FIGURE 4.6. Length bias. Screening tests are more likely to detect indolent cancers that have a better prognosis. In a program with repeated screening, both aggressive and indolent cancers would be below the threshold for detection at the time of screen 1. The aggressive cancer would cause symptoms and result in death before the time of the second screen. Screen 2 would discover the indolent cancer during its presymptomatic phase. Although the indolent cancer also proves fatal, the time of death is later. The prolonged survival would be credited to the screening program even though the screening did not change the natural history.

growing cancer is more likely to be detected by a screening test simply because the slow growth creates more opportunities for detection. The detectable preclinical phase is longer. This is true either for a single screen or for repeated screens. A more aggressive cancer would elude detection by screening because its rapid growth would result in symptoms before the subject had a chance to be screened (shorter detectable preclinical phase). The rapidly growing cancer more quickly leads to cancer death. Therefore, the overall survival for patients with screen-detected cancer is larger because screening always selects more indolent, less aggressive cancers.

Selection Bias

Individuals who participate in screening programs are volunteers, and these volunteers tend to be healthier and more health conscious than members of the general population. As a consequence, they develop fewer cancers and have better survival. An example can be seen in the large, randomized fecal occult blood screening study conducted in Minnesota (10). The number of cancers that developed in the trial was lower than expected in both the cases and the controls. Some of the improved outcome in typical randomized trials results from the exclusion of individuals with significant comorbid disease.

Pseudodisease

Some cancers never cause death. When these lesions are discovered, the screening program is credited with detecting the cancer and preventing death from cancer, when, in truth, the cancer would not have killed the patient. Prostate cancer is a good example. Many elderly men are found to have prostate cancer at the times of their deaths from other causes. Screening programs that detect GI cancer precursors such as colorectal adenomas may be susceptible to this form of bias. Although most colorectal cancers arise from adenomas, most adenomas do not progress to cancer. Screening programs that detect ade-

nomas receive credit for the adenomas, yet most of them would remain harmless.

EVALUATION OF SCREENING PROGRAMS

Randomized Controlled Trials

The most reliable strategy to evaluate a potential screening program would be to conduct a *randomized controlled trial*. The strength of the randomized controlled trial derives from the fact that exposure to screening is assigned by the investigator. As a consequence, the screened and unscreened groups should be similar in all respects except for screening. Differences in outcomes can more confidently be attributed to the screening test.

Conducting a randomized trial of screening is neither cheap nor easy. Because GI cancer is relatively rare in the population, a study would have to be very large. Randomized controlled trials of fecal occult blood testing for colorectal cancer have enrolled between 46,000 and 152,000 individuals (10,30,31). The study would also have to be long enough to fully evaluate the impact of the screening program on cancer mortality. More than 20 years were required to evaluate the impact of the screening program on cancer mortality in the Minnesota fecal occult blood study (33).

Despite the strong scientific rationale for the randomized trial, threats to validity still exist. For example, some individuals who are assigned to screening may withdraw, and some in the control group may obtain screening. This type of contamination diminishes the apparent benefit of screening. The ability to generalize the results of a trial to other populations may be limited. Individuals who volunteer for screening are often healthier and more health conscious. Their survival may exceed that of the general population of potential screenees. Compliance in a screening trial may be better in a trial than in the community because of the zeal of the investigators and the motivation of trial participants. Quality control is generally better in randomized trials. In the Minnesota fecal occult blood trial, the investigators established a high-quality central laboratory to develop and evaluate the slides (10). In the general community, staff with minimal training and supervision often read the slides. Trials are sometimes conducted in high-risk individuals. High-risk individuals have more outcome events because of their high-risk status, so study power is improved. Findings from such a trial may be impossible to extrapolate to the general population. The findings of a trial may also be impossible to extrapolate to different populations. The results of a gastric cancer screening trial conducted in Japan may not be applicable in the United States, where the disease rates are lower. Results of a screening trial conducted among individuals older than 50 years cannot be extrapolated to 40-year-olds. Finally, because a long time may be required to complete a trial, the results may be obsolete by the time the study results are published. New and better tests may be available to replace the ones tested in the trial.

Case-Control Studies

Because of the difficulty in conducting randomized trials, investigators may resort to nonexperimental studies to investigate whether screened individuals are less likely to die from cancer. One such design is the case-control study in which the screening practices of individuals with cancer are compared with the practices of noncancer controls. The case-control study has some attractive advantages. Because of its retrospective design, a case-control study is quicker and cheaper to conduct than a randomized controlled trial. The retrospective nature creates the opportunity for several forms of bias, however (34,35). For example, determining prior screening history with accuracy (avoiding misclassification) and discerning whether the screening test was applied for early symptoms and not for screening may be difficult. There may be concern about whether the screened and the unscreened groups have comparable underlying risk of disease. Screenees may be the healthy conscious and healthier (healthy screenee bias). One must also estimate the detectable preclinical stage of disease and determine the screening activity of cases and controls during this period (36).

In the absence of a randomized trial, a well-conducted case-control study may provide reasonably convincing evidence. Selby et al. (37) conducted an elegant case-control study that provided compelling evidence for the benefit of screening sigmoidoscopy. A similar study by the same group demonstrated no benefit for digital rectal examination (38).

Uncontrolled Studies

Several types of uncontrolled or nonrandomized approaches exist to evaluate cancer screening. For example, one might compare the outcomes in a community in which screening was offered to outcomes in an adjacent community that was not screened. The individuals included in such a study would be more representative of the general population and less highly selected than participants in a randomized trial. Obviously, the validity would rest on whether the communities were comparable with respect to factors other than screening. Another nonrandomized approach might evaluate outcomes before and after a policy change. This is termed the *interrupted time series approach* (39). For example, one might look at colorectal cancer screening rates and mortality before and after 1998, when Medicare began reimbursing screening. Again, the validity of such a comparison depends on whether other secular trends have occurred that might impact mortality.

A common approach is simply to offer screening and report the results. This typically happens when a new test or procedure is developed. The approach is easy and relatively cheap. Information can be obtained about side effects, false-positive rates, costs, and number of cancers detected. Importantly, benefits cannot be determined. Policy decisions cannot be made based on the results of such studies.

With an uncontrolled study, finding an appropriate comparison group may be difficult. The National Polyp Study was a randomized trial of different surveillance intervals for adenoma patients. Because no control group existed, the authors compared their colorectal cancer incidence data to expected numbers from several other sources (40). The populations represented in these other sources were not precisely comparable, however.

SCREENING POLICY MAKING

To develop screening policy, one must estimate the health and economic outcomes—the benefits, harms, and costs. Then one must determine whether the benefits outweigh the harms and justify the costs. The health and economic outcomes can be measured with some precision, but decisions about whether the benefits justify the cost reflect personal preferences and values (1).

Outcomes

The outcome of screening includes both long- and short-term effects. The most important long-term outcome of screening is the length and quality of life. An effective cancer screening test detects disease early in the preclinical phase when treatment has an important impact on survival. The immediate effects of screening include the inconvenience, anxiety, discomfort, and occasional complications of the test. In contrast to the survival advantage, which is limited to a small number of screened subjects, the inconvenience and potential hazard of the test are suffered by all who are screened.

Screening is intuitively appealing—detecting disease early ought to be better than finding it later (41). However, as discussed, disease is rarely discovered, and only a small proportion of the screened population derives any benefit.

When the test result is a *true positive*, the screened individual benefits to the extent that early detection prolongs survival. If the disease is indolent and would not have progressed (pseudodisease), or if the disease is too far advanced for a difference to be made, then no benefit exists. If the disease is rare, only a small number of cases will be detected in a screening program.

Those with a *true-negative* test result benefit from the reassurance that they do not have the disease within the limits of the test. The benefits of reassurance come at the cost of the screening test (usually modest) and the potential harms and inconvenience of screening. If the disease is very rare, subjects could simply be told that they are unlikely to have the disease and not be screened.

Subjects with *false-negative* test results receive false reassurance that they are disease-free. In addition to the harms of the test, they fail to receive any benefit from early detection. The false-negative test results may actually delay proper evaluation, and those with false-negative test results may be significantly harmed.

Subjects with *false-positive* test results must endure the anxiety and expense of additional tests to demonstrate that they are diseasefree. Even when disease has been excluded, anxieties about the disease may persist. Several types of false-positive results exist (6). The case of individuals not found to have any disease is the most obvious. Some individuals will be found to have some other condition that resulted in a positive test result. For example, participants in a screening program for colorectal cancer using fecal occult blood testing may have a positive test result from an upper GI lesion (42). In subjects who are found to have a cancer that will never progress (pseudodisease), results are essentially false positive because detection of their cancer does not impact their life expectancy.

Recommendations

Making decisions about screening, either for the individual patient or for the population, is complex (41). The decision is easier if evidence of benefit has been found in randomized controlled trials, but this level of evidence is rarely available. Even when randomized controlled trial data are available, unanswered questions may lead different authorities to reach different recommendations (43,44). Evidence of benefit must be combined with estimates of costs and quality of life. Decisions may also be necessary about how frequently to repeat tests and whether to combine tests. The performance of a repeated test is different from the performance of the first test. The risk for an individual also changes over time—he or she is older, which increases the risk, but he or she has been screened previously, which lowers the risk.

The quality of the evidence can be incorporated into the recommendation. When evidence is available from one or more randomized controlled trials, the guideline may "strongly recommend" screening. If the evidence is weaker, the recommendation may state that "insufficient evidence" exists to make policy. Some organizations that make policy actually grade the evidence. With such a grading system, an "A recommendation" may be made when strong evidence is available from a controlled trial, and a "C recommendation" may be made when the evidence is more ambiguous.

Even when guidelines exist, they must be applied with flexibility; that is, why they are called guidelines and not laws. Circumstances of the individual patient may require more aggressive screening or none. For patients with significant comorbidity, screening would be optional or perhaps contraindicated.

Ethics

The screening encounter poses unique ethical concerns (45). In the usual medical encounter, individuals present to health care providers with symptoms. The provider has the obligation to exercise skill and expertise to cure disease and alleviate suffering (3).

The screening encounter is different. Subjects who qualify for screening have no symptoms. If they undergo screening, only the small minority with latent disease benefits. Some are harmed, and all are inconvenienced. The provider must be reasonably confident that the screening program will have a net overall benefit to the community, if not to the individual patient. Importantly, potential screenees must understand and accept the potential limitations and harms of the screening test.

THE FUTURE

This chapter has largely focused on the principles of screening for disease. Screening may also be conducted to detect risk markers that predispose to disease. For example, screening can be conducted to determine whether an individual harbors one of the mismatch repair genes that predisposes to hereditary nonpolyposis colorectal cancer (46). Those with the genetic abnormality are candidates for aggressive screening, and those without the genetic abnormality are candidates for conventional screening. When disease susceptibility and metabolizing gene abnormalities are fully understood, much more success may be achieved in determining risk and planning risk-appropriate screening and surveillance. Mutated genes might also be sought as disease markers, with the expectation that they will be more specific than current techniques. The feasibility of such an approach has already been demonstrated for colorectal cancer in which mutated genes have been detected in the stool (47).

The conventional disease screening tests can also be expected to improve. Development of new radiologic and endoscopic techniques should increase the ability to detect GI cancer early enough in the preclinical phase to make a difference in survival. When these tests are developed, however, they will need to undergo rigorous testing using the criteria that have been described in the preceding paragraphs.

The greatest challenge for the future is to develop strategies to increase screening compliance. The tests currently available have the potential to substantially lower the incidence and mortality from GI cancer, yet these tests are underused. The expertise of behavioral researchers and system scientists must be exploited to develop programs to increase exposure to screening.

ACKNOWLEDGMENT

The writing of this chapter was supported in part by grants from the National Institutes of Health (R01 CA44684, P30 DK034987, R01 CA66635).

References

1. Eddy DM. *Common Screening Tests*. Philadelphia, Pa.: American College of Physicians; 1994.
2. Hulka BS. Cancer screening. Degrees of proof and practical application. *Cancer* 1988;62:1776–1780.
3. Miller AB. Fundamental issues in screening for cancer. In: Schottenfeld D, Fraumeni JF, eds. *Cancer Epidemiology and Prevention*. 2nd ed. New York, NY: Oxford University Press; 1996:1433–1452.
4. Miller AB. Screening for gastrointestinal cancer. *Curr Opin Oncol* 1995;7: 373–376.
5. Sandler RS, Johnson MD, Holland KL. Risk of stomach cancer after gastric surgery for benign conditions. A case-control study. *Dig Dis Sci* 1984; 29:703–708.
6. Morrison AS. *Screening in Chronic Disease*. New York, NY: Oxford University Press; 1985.
7. Lieberman D. Cost-effectiveness of colon cancer screening. *Am J Gastroenterol* 1991;86:1789–1794.
8. Winawer SJ, Fletcher RH, Miller L, et al. Colorectal cancer screening: clinical guidelines and rationale. *Gastroenterology* 1997;112:594–642.
9. Lieberman DA. Colon cancer screening. The dilemma of positive screening tests. *Arch Intern Med* 1990;150:740–744.
10. Mandel JS, Bond JH, Church TR, et al. Reducing mortality from colorectal cancer by screening for fecal occult blood. Minnesota Colon Cancer Control Study. *N Engl J Med* 1993;328:1365–1371.
11. Blalock SJ, DeVellis BM, Sandler RS. Participation in fecal occult blood screening: a critical review. *Prev Med* 1987;16:9–18.
12. Mulcahy HE, Farthing MJ, O'Donoghue DP. Screening for asymptomatic colorectal cancer. *BMJ* 1997;314:285–291.
13. Maule WF. Screening for colorectal cancer by nurse endoscopists. *N Engl J Med* 1994;330:183–187.
14. Schoenfeld P, Lipscomb S, Crook J, et al. Accuracy of polyp detection by gastroenterologists and nurse endoscopists during flexible sigmoidoscopy: a randomized trial. *Gastroenterology* 1999;117:312–318.
15. Schroy PC III, Wilson S, Afdhal N. Feasibility of high-volume screening sigmoidoscopy using a flexible fiberoptic endoscope and a disposable sheath system. *Am J Gastroenterol* 1996;91:1331–1337.
16. Fenlon HM, Nunes DP, Schroy PC, et al. A comparison of virtual and conventional colonoscopy for the detection of colorectal polyps. *N Engl J Med* 1999; 341:1496–1503.
17. Eddy DM. Comparing benefits and harms: the balance sheet. *JAMA* 1990; 263:2493–2498, 2501.
18. Gold MR, Siegel JE, Russell LB, et al. *Cost effectiveness in health and medicine*. New York, NY: Oxford University Press; 1996.
19. Fletcher RH, Fletcher SW, Wagner EH. *Clinical Epidemiology: The Essentials*. 2nd ed. Baltimore, Md.: Williams & Wilkins; 1988.
20. Sackett DL, Haynes RB, Tugwell P. *Clinical Epidemiology: A Basic Science for Clinical Medicine*. Boston, Mass.: Little, Brown and Company; 1985.
21. Ransohoff DF, Feinstein AR. Problems of spectrum and bias in evaluating the efficacy of diagnostic tests. *N Engl J Med* 1978;299:926–930.
22. Church TR, Ederer F, Mandel JS. Fecal occult blood screening in the Minnesota study: sensitivity of the screening test. *J Natl Cancer Inst* 1997;89: 1440–1448.
23. Ahlquist DA, Wieand HS, Moertel CG, et al. Accuracy of fecal occult blood screening for colorectal neoplasia. A prospective study using Hemoccult and HemoQuant tests. *JAMA* 1993;269:1262–1267.
24. Ederer F, Church TR, Mandel JS. Fecal occult blood screening in the Minnesota study: role of chance detection of lesions. *J Natl Cancer Inst* 1997;89: 1423–1428.
25. Ransohoff DF, Lang CA. Small adenomas detected during fecal occult blood test screening for colorectal cancer. The impact of serendipity. *JAMA* 1990; 264:76–78.
26. Allison JE, Tekawa IS, Ransom LJ, et al. A comparison of fecal occult-blood tests for colorectal-cancer screening. *N Engl J Med* 1996;334:155–159.
27. Russo MW, Helm JF, Biddle AK, et al. Serial fecal occult blood testing detects more cancers at a lower cost [abstract]. *Gastroenterology* 1997;112:A648.
28. Prorok PC, Kramer BS, Gohagan JK. Screening theory and study design: the basics. In: Kramer BS, Gohagan JK, Prorok PC, eds. *Cancer Screening: Theory and Practice*. New York, NY: Marcel Dekker; 1999:29–53.
29. Winawer SJ, Zauber AG, OBrien MJ, et al. Randomized comparison of surveillance intervals after colonoscopic removal of newly diagnosed adenomatous polyps. The National Polyp Study Workgroup. *N Engl J Med* 1993; 328:901–906.
30. Hardcastle JD, Chamberlain JO, Robinson MH, et al. Randomised controlled trial of faecal-occult-blood screening for colorectal cancer. *Lancet* 1996;348:1472–1477.
31. Kronborg O, Fenger C, Olsen J, et al. Randomised study of screening for colorectal cancer with faecal-occult-blood test. *Lancet* 1996;348:1467–1471.
32. Walter SD, Day NE. Estimation of the duration of a pre-clinical disease state using screening data. *Am J Epidemiol* 1983;118:865–886.
33. Mandel JS, Church TR, Ederer F, et al. Colorectal cancer mortality: effectiveness of biennial screening for fecal occult blood. *J Natl Cancer Inst* 1999; 91:434–437.
34. Hosek RS, Flanders WD, Sasco AJ. Bias in case-control studies of screening effectiveness. *Am J Epidemiol* 1996;143:193–201.

35. Gill TM, Horwitz RI. Evaluating the efficacy of cancer screening: clinical distinctions and case-control studies. *J Clin Epidemiol* 1995;48:281–292.
36. Weiss NS, McKnight B, Stevens NG. Approaches to the analysis of case-control studies of the efficacy of screening for cancer. *Am J Epidemiol* 1992;135:817–823.
37. Selby JV, Friedman GD, Quesenberry CP, Jr, et al. A case-control study of screening sigmoidoscopy and mortality from colorectal cancer. *N Engl J Med* 1992;326:653–657.
38. Herrinton LJ, Selby JV, Friedman GD, et al. Case-control study of digital-rectal screening in relation to mortality from cancer of the distal rectum. *Am J Epidemiol* 1995;142:961–964.
39. Ray WA. Policy and program analysis using administrative databases. *Ann Intern Med* 1997;127:712–718.
40. Winawer SJ, Zauber AG, Ho MN, et al. Prevention of colorectal cancer by colonoscopic polypectomy. The National Polyp Study Workgroup. *N Engl J Med* 1993;329:1977–1981.
41. Harris R. Decision-making about screening: individual and policy levels. In: Kramer BS, Gohagan JK, Prorok PC, eds. *Cancer Screening: Theory and Practice*. New York, NY: Marcel Dekker; 1999:55–75.
42. Rockey DC, Koch J, Cello JP, et al. Relative frequency of upper gastrointestinal and colonic lesions in patients with positive fecal occult-blood tests. *N Engl J Med* 1998;339:153–159.
43. Simon JB. Should all people over the age of 50 have regular fecal occult-blood tests? Postpone population screening until problems are solved. *N Engl J Med* 1998;338:1151–1152.
44. Fletcher RH. Should all people over the age of 50 have regular fecal occult-blood tests? If it works, why not do it? *N Engl J Med* 1998;338:1153–1154.
45. Weed DL. Ethics and consent. In: Kramer BS, Gohagan JK, Prorok PC, eds. *Cancer Screening: Theory and Practice*. New York, NY: Marcel Dekker; 1999:89–118.
46. Wijnen JT, Vasen HF, Khan PM, et al. Clinical findings with implications for genetic testing in families with clustering of colorectal cancer. *N Engl J Med* 1998;339:511–518.
47. Osborn NK, Ahlquist DA. Stool screening for colorectal cancer: molecular approaches. *Gastroenterology* 2005;128:192–206.

CHAPTER 5 ■ GASTROINTESTINAL CANCER: SURGICAL ONCOLOGY

MONICA M. BERTAGNOLLI

Hippocrates had this to say about intestinal cancer: "It is better not to treat deep cancers, for those so treated die rapidly whereas the nontreated live for a longer time" (1). This statement held true until the advent of safe anesthesia and surgery, advancements that were not fully developed until the mid-20th century. The earliest successful surgical treatment of a gastrointestinal cancer was probably accomplished by Pillore of Rouen, who performed a cecostomy for an obstructing colon cancer in 1776. Unfortunately, in a disastrous attempt to relieve the obstruction, the patient ingested 2 lb of mercury before surgery. The patient died 28 days after surgery, and an autopsy showed that the cause of death was obstruction of the distal small intestine by the mercury (2). In 1844, Reybard reported a survival after resection and anastomosis for cancer of the colon. This is a remarkable accomplishment, considering that it antedates general anesthesia. The most significant of the many problems encountered during early intestinal surgery was the extremely high rate of fatal infection in the era before wide acceptance of aseptic technique and availability of antibiotics. In 1879, Christian Billroth resected a sigmoid cancer and exteriorized the proximal bowel as a permanent colostomy. This operation had a much lower incidence of infection and mortality than earlier attempts at resection and anastomosis. Billroth's technique was later modified by Bloch (1892), Paul (1895), and von Mikulicz-Radecki (1895–1905) to what became known as an *"obstructive"* resection for colon cancer. During these procedures, the loop of bowel containing the tumor was brought outside the abdominal cavity, and the incision was closed. Approximately 1 week after the initial surgery, the bowel was divided with a cautery, removing the segment containing the tumor and creating a loop colostomy. Because the abdominal cavity was closed several days before the bowel was opened, peritoneal contamination was less, and mortality from infection was significantly reduced. This technique was widely used by American surgeons as recently as 1940 (2).

The first successful surgery for gastric carcinoma is attributed to Billroth in 1881. During this procedure, the antrum and pylorus were removed and the duodenum was sutured to the gastric cardia, an operation that later became known as a *Billroth I gastrectomy*. W.C. Roentgen discovered x-rays in 1895, and by 1910, contrast-enhanced radiography was used to diagnose intestinal cancers, which allowed somewhat earlier diagnosis and better preoperative planning. The first cancer operation to meet present-day standards of adequate primary tumor resection and complete lymphadenectomy was performed by Miles, who developed the combined abdominoperineal resection in 1926. In 1938, Whipple successfully resected a tumor in the region of the pancreatic head, a complex procedure that involved removal of the distal stomach, duodenum, and pancreatic head, and required reanastomosis of the pancreatic duct, distal common bile duct, and stomach to the proximal jejunum. After World War II, advances in blood transfusion, antibiotics, metabolic support, and anesthesia substantially reduced the mortality from radical cancer resections such as these.

In 1958, Hirschowitz developed the first flexible fiberoptic instrument for endoscopy, and instruments allowing routine evaluation of the upper and lower gastrointestinal tract became widely available in the 1970s. These advances allowed the earlier detection of neoplastic lesions and endoscopic removal of premalignant adenomas, the first intervention shown to decrease colon cancer incidence. During the 1970s, the distinct natural histories of different tumors were recognized. For most solid tissue tumors, clinicians developed the view that tumor involvement of regional lymph nodes was an indicator of systemic disease unlikely to respond to more aggressive local surgery. In the late 20th century, contributions from radiation and chemotherapy produced modest improvements in survival when used as adjuvant therapy for patients with stage III colorectal cancer. Comparative gains are still lacking for the other primary gastrointestinal cancers.

This book contains sections that provide a comprehensive review of surgery for specific gastrointestinal cancers. This introductory chapter focuses on the general approach to surgical management of gastrointestinal cancer patients and also describes some of the less understood therapeutic approaches, such as intraoperative radiation therapy and intraperitoneal chemotherapy. In addition, this section outlines several new areas of investigation in management of gastrointestinal cancers that may improve patient care in the future.

SURGICAL EVALUATION

Preoperative Risk Assessment

Although minimal access surgery and early postoperative feeding have decreased the physiological impact of intestinal surgery, such surgery still requires general anesthesia and is frequently performed on patients with comorbid conditions and nutritional compromise. It is worthwhile, therefore, to consider a few issues in the preoperative evaluation and preparation of these patients. Decision making in major cancer surgery requires balancing of surgical risks and benefits, and the first step in this process involves assessing the patient's physiological reserves. This is particularly important in cancer patients of advanced age because age alone is not an accurate predictor of surgical risk. Physical classification systems to identify patients with increased risk of adverse outcomes after major

TABLE 5.1

FUNCTIONAL CLASSIFICATION OF PHYSICAL STATUS

Risk category	American Society of Anesthesiologists classification	Goldman classification
Class I	No physiological, biochemical, or psychiatric disturbance; the pathological process for which surgery is to be performed is localized and not conducive to systemic disturbance	Ordinary physical activity, such as walking and climbing stairs, does not cause angina. Angina occurs with strenuous, rapid, or prolonged exertion at work or recreation.
Class II	Mild to moderate systemic disturbance caused either by the condition to be treated surgically or by other pathophysiological processes	Slight limitation of ordinary activity. Angina occurs with walking or climbing stairs rapidly; walking uphill; walking or climbing stairs after meals or in cold, in wind, or under emotional stress; or during the first few hours after awakening. Angina occurs when walking more than two blocks on the level or climbing more than one flight of stairs at a normal pace and in normal conditions.
Class III	Severe systemic disturbance or pathology	Marked limitation of ordinary physical activity. Angina occurs when walking one to two blocks on the level or climbing one flight of stairs at a normal pace and in normal conditions.
Class IV	Severe systemic disorder that is immediately life threatening and not always correctable by the operative procedure	Inability to carry on any physical activity without discomfort. Angina may be present at rest.
Class V	Moribund condition; little chance of surviving surgery	
Emergency (E)	Any patient in one of the classes listed in this table operated on in an emergency situation	

surgery include those developed by the American Society of Anesthesiologists and by Goldman et al. (3) (Table 5.1).

It is particularly important to identify significant cardiac risk factors present before surgery because more than 50% of all major perioperative complications or deaths are related to cardiovascular disease. In addition, optimal perioperative physiological support can decrease surgical morbidity and mortality in patients with cardiac disease. The most commonly used method of assigning cardiac risk for patients undergoing major surgery was developed by Goldman et al. (3) (Tables 5.2 and 5.3). Based on this classification, patients whose preoperative state places them in risk category III or IV should be considered for invasive perioperative monitoring to allow optimal physiological support. Patients with evidence of potentially treatable cardiovascular disease, such as unstable angina or transient ischemic attacks, should undergo complete evaluation and treatment of these conditions before tumor resection. For patients with good functional status and no signs of cardiovascular disease, the risk and cost of noninvasive preoperative cardiac evaluation are not warranted because these individuals have a low risk of perioperative myocardial infarction or death from cardiac causes.

Nutrition

Most patients undergoing cancer surgery can withstand the associated brief period of nutritional deficit and catabolism without difficulty. It is not unusual, however, to encounter a patient whose nutrition has been compromised by his or her underlying condition. The degree of compromise can range from mild, with no adverse effect on treatment outcome, to cancer cachexia, a paraneoplastic syndrome characterized by anorexia, weight loss, and progression to multiple-organ dys-

function. For many patients with intestinal tumors, anorexia and the resulting malnutrition are exacerbated by tumor-associated changes in gastrointestinal function and by the surgery, chemotherapy, and radiation therapy used to treat the tumor. It is essential, therefore, to assess the nutritional status of cancer patients before therapy and provide optimal nutritional support during treatment and recovery.

Nutritional assessment for patients with cancer includes taking a dietary history, with documentation of recent weight change, anorexia, early satiety, or dysphagia. Findings on physical examination that suggest malnutrition include evidence of muscle wasting; dry, flaky skin texture; brittle hair or unusual hair loss; and ridging or spooning of the nails. Important laboratory tests for nutritional evaluation include serum albumin and transferrin levels. These assessments allow patients to be classified into clinically relevant categories that indicate the extent of their nutritional reserves (Table 5.4).

Maintenance of adequate preoperative oral nutrition should be a high priority for all patients undergoing major surgery. This imperative is sometimes overlooked when gastrointestinal cancer patients receive multiple preoperative endoscopic or radiologic evaluations requiring fasting or have tumor-associated anorexia or nausea. Controversy remains over the clinical benefits of nutritional intervention in cancer patients. In the most extreme case of patients with severe malnutrition, most studies support the use of perioperative total parenteral nutrition (TPN) (4). Aggressive nutritional support is also necessary for patients whose treatment results in prolonged periods (10–14 days) of inadequate nutritional intake (4). The benefits to these patients, including decreased operative morbidity and mortality, exceed the increased risk due to TPN-related infections. Patients with severe malnutrition should receive a minimum of 7 days of nutritional therapy before a major surgical procedure and should continue to receive adequate nutrition via TPN

TABLE 5.2

GOLDMAN'S CARDIAC RISK INDEX

Risk factor	Points
Jugular venous distension/S_3 gallop	11
Myocardial infarction in the previous 6 mo	10
Any rhythm other than sinus or PACs on preoperative ECG	7
More than 5 PVCs/min on preoperative ECG	7
Age older than 70 yr	5
Emergency procedure	4
Intrathoracic, intraperitoneal, or aortic operation	3
Poor general medical condition (Po_2 <60 mm Hg or Pco_2 >50 mm Hg; K^+ <3 mEq/L or BUN >50 mg/dL; abnormal SGOT; signs of chronic liver disease)	3
Hemodynamically significant aortic stenosis	3

Class	Point total	Minor complications	Life-threatening complications	Cardiac deaths
I ($n = 537$)	0–5	532 (99%)	4 (0.7%)	1 (0.2%)
II ($n = 316$)	6–12	295 (93%)	12 (5%)	5 (2%)
III ($n = 130$)	13–25	112 (86%)	15 (11%)	3 (2%)
IV ($n = 18$)	≥26	4 (22%)	4 (22%)	10 (56%)

PAC, premature atrial contraction; ECG, electrocardiogram; PVC, premature ventricular contraction; Po_2, partial pressure of oxygen; Pco_2, partial pressure of carbon dioxide; BUN, blood urea nitrogen; SGOT, serum glutamic-oxaloacetic transaminase.

or feeding jejunostomy, if necessary, as soon as possible after surgery. For all other patients, the risk of TPN-related complications is probably greater than the benefits of decreased recovery time and marginally improved survival. It is clear, however, that maximizing enteral nutrition by early postoperative feeding or nasogastric or jejunostomy feedings when necessary is an effective, safe, and sometimes overlooked way to speed patient recovery.

Staging

Accurate staging enhances the care of gastrointestinal cancer patients and becomes even more important as new therapeutic modalities emerge. Patients known to have localized disease can avoid extensive surgery or toxic adjuvant therapies, and identification of clinically significant micrometastatic disease selects a group of patients who are likely to benefit from adjuvant therapy. The wide range of treatment responses observed within the present staging categories for gastrointestinal cancers suggests that these categories are too large and that, particularly for stage II disease, more specific distinctions are needed. A number of different approaches to improved gastrointestinal cancer staging are under investigation. These include surgical methods, such as staging laparoscopy and sentinel node excision, as well as new techniques for examining tissue using immunohistochemical and molecular markers. A brief description of several promising staging modalities is presented here.

TABLE 5.3

REDUCTION OF PERIOPERATIVE CARDIAC RISK

Risk	Recommended preoperative cardiac evaluation	Recommended action
Low: Class I and <12 points	None	Proceed with surgery with usual monitoring
Medium: Class II or III, 12–26 points or cannot assess by history	Exercise testing, or if patient is unable to exercise, dipyridamole thallium or stress echo testing	Consider invasive perioperative monitoring
High: Class IV or >26 points	Cardiac catheterization	Coronary artery revascularization, if possible, before surgery

PREOPERATIVE NUTRITIONAL ASSESSMENT

	Normal nutritional reserves	Mild to moderate nutritional deficit	Severe malnutrition
Weight	Normal or recent loss of <6% of body weight	Recent loss of 6%–12% of body weight	Recent loss of ≥12% of body weight
Physical examination	Normal	Normal	Muscle wasting, skin, hair, or nail changes
Serum albumin level	≥3.5 g/dL	2.6–3.4 g/dL	≤2.5 g/dL
Serum transferrin level	≥200 mg/dL	151–199 mg/dL	≤150 mg/dL

Staging Laparoscopy

The application of minimally invasive technology to intestinal surgery has decreased staging and treatment morbidity for gastrointestinal cancer patients. The best example of this is avoidance of laparotomy by the use of staging laparoscopy, an approach that is particularly effective for cancers of the gastroesophageal junction, stomach, liver, and pancreas. Because laparoscopy is best used to examine the visible surfaces of the peritoneum and the abdominal organs, the sensitivity of laparoscopy for detection of unresectable disease is significantly increased by the application of endoscopic or laparoscopic ultrasonography.

In a study of 76 patients with upper gastrointestinal malignancies, including lower esophageal, gastric, and pancreatic cancers, laparoscopy alone provided more staging information than conventional imaging in 17 of 39 patients. Fourteen patients were upstaged through detection of peritoneal deposits and liver metastases, and three patients were downstaged and subsequently underwent successful resection. The addition of laparoscopic ultrasonography changed the clinical management of 13 of 37 patients by supplying more detailed information than that obtained with conventional imaging. These additional findings included portal vein invasion in three patients and liver metastases in three patients (5). In a prospective study comparing laparoscopy, ultrasonography, and computed tomography (CT) for staging of gastric cancer, 103 consecutively examined patients with gastric adenocarcinoma were assessed. Laparoscopy with ultrasonography was the most sensitive method for detection of hepatic, nodal, and peritoneal metastases, with an accuracy rate of 99% compared to 76% for ultrasonography and 79% for CT (6). In a study of 114 patients with pancreatic cancer and no evidence of distant disease by CT, laparoscopy confirmed intraabdominal disease extension in 27 (24%) (7). Of the remaining 87 patients without metastatic disease, 42 were shown to have vascular invasion by angiography, a determination that could have also been made by laparoscopic or endoscopic ultrasonography. Forty patients proceeded to laparotomy, and in 30 of these, the tumors were resectable (8).

The gold standard for evaluation of liver tumors is careful intraoperative palpation and intraoperative liver ultrasonography (9). Because patients with resectable hepatic metastases from colorectal cancer can achieve 25% to 30% long-term survival after hepatic resection, detection of small localized liver lesions is important (10). In one study, the combination of laparoscopy with laparoscopic ultrasonography was used to evaluate 15 patients undergoing elective laparotomy for colorectal cancer. Complete inspection and ultrasonography of the liver was possible in 13 patients, and liver metastases were identified in four patients. All patients proceeded to laparotomy with complete palpation and open ultrasonography of the liver, and one additional 0.8-cm lesion was detected; however, this was found to be benign by biopsy (11). In a study of 50 patients with liver tumors, laparoscopy with laparoscopic ultrasonography detected disease that precluded curative resection in 23 patients (46%). These included new lesions not seen by magnetic resonance imaging or CT in 14 patients (28%). Fourteen patients of this cohort were selected for resection, which was accomplished successfully in 13 patients. A historical control group had 58% resectability (12). Laparoscopy with laparoscopic ultrasonography may therefore be most useful in determining unresectability in patients with hepatic tumors without the need for open laparotomy.

Laparoscopy also provides the opportunity to perform peritoneal lavage for cytologic study. The use of peritoneal cytologic analysis for staging of gastrointestinal malignancies, however, is controversial. In patients with pancreatic cancer, the presence of positive peritoneal cytologic results is an ominous sign. In a report of 32 consecutively presenting pancreatic patients with positive results on peritoneal cytologic analysis, only two had disease amenable to resection, and the median survival in those with and without visible intraabdominal metastases was 7.8 and 8.6 months, respectively (13). At Academic Medical Center in Amsterdam, laparoscopic staging with peritoneal cytologic analysis was performed on 449 patients from 1992 to 1997. The indication was a variety of gastrointestinal tumors, including 87 esophageal cancers, 72 proximal bile duct tumors, 236 periampullary tumors, 17 tumors of the pancreatic body or tail, and 7 primary and 32 metastatic liver tumors. Lavage changed the assessment of stage and accurately predicted unresectable disease in only 6 of 449 patients (1.3%). In addition, of the 28 patients with positive lavage findings, 19 (68%) also had metastatic disease identifiable at laparoscopy, and three had false-positive results on peritoneal cytologic analysis and were found to have resectable disease on exploration. The authors conclude that the technique is not effective (14).

In summary, therefore, staging laparoscopy is best used to document unresectability in patients who would otherwise require laparotomy to reach this conclusion. This technique is most often useful for upper gastrointestinal malignancies that tend to exhibit peritoneal spread missed by noninvasive imaging techniques.

Significance of Micrometastatic Disease

One population for which staging could be improved includes patients with node-negative (N0) disease by conventional histopathology. For example, in patients undergoing potentially curative surgery for colon cancer, 35% to 45% will have N0 nodal status (15). Approximately 25% of these stage II patients will experience posttreatment disease recurrence, suggesting that for one in four patients with N0 disease, current histopathological staging methods fail to identify those destined to manifest tumor progression. The application of better techniques to detect these high-risk cases would identify patients who may benefit from adjuvant chemotherapy. These patients are also an important population for evaluating new treatments to target minimal residual disease.

"Micrometastasis" is a term used to describe evidence of tumor cell spread beyond a primary tumor that does not meet histologic criteria for N1 or M1 disease. Examples include tumor deposits in regional lymph nodes of $<200 \mu m$ in diameter, or single cells identified only following immunohistochemical stains for tumor-associated proteins such as cytokeratins or carcinoembryonic antigen. For solid tissue malignancies, the clinical significance of tumor cells discovered in lymph nodes, bone marrow, or circulating blood is unclear. Tumors readily shed individual cells into the circulation, and even individual tumor cells can be detected in tissue samples by immunohistochemical stains or polymerase chain reaction–based methods. The clinical importance of circulating tumor cells resides in their ability to lodge in host tissues and form an independent metastatic colony. Such micrometastases likely represent a small fraction of the cells shed from a tumor. To date, numerous studies have failed to correlate the presence of small numbers of tumor cells in lymph nodes, bone marrow, or circulating blood with clinical behavior of tumors (16–19). This distinction is obviously most important for tumors that are responsive to adjuvant therapies, such as colorectal or gastric cancers.

At present, the most important obstacles to understanding the clinical significance of micrometastatic disease are technical in nature. Techniques for detecting micrometastatic disease are difficult to standardize due to differences in antibodies, staining techniques, and scoring systems. The presence of tumor cells in the circulation and in lymphatics may also be affected by surgical manipulation of a tumor during resection (20,21). Perhaps for these reasons, most of the available retrospective studies failed to find prognostic significance for metastases detected by immunohistochemistry only (16–19).

Although micrometastatic disease has yet to be assigned clinical significance in gastrointestinal malignancies, research designed to investigate this issue is proceeding in parallel with work to improve early disease detection. In addition to benefit achieved by improvements in clinical staging, understanding the differences in character between micrometastatic disease and nonmetastasizing precursors would provide important targets for improved diagnostic and therapeutic agents. In the future, it is possible that imaging techniques, such as preoperative magnetic resonance or intravenously administered near-infrared fluorescence probes, will accurately detect small volume metastases from gastrointestinal solid tumors (22).

Sentinel Nodes in Gastrointestinal Cancer

Sentinel lymph node sampling (SLNS) identifies a small number of regional lymph nodes that accurately predict the status of all regional nodes in a patient undergoing cancer surgery. SLNS is based on the assumption that lymphatic flow drains sequentially from peripheral to central tissue locations, with limited functional collaterals outside the dominant vascular supply. Consequently, tracer substances injected at a tumor site must follow the same pathway by which metastatic tumor cells traverse lymphatic channels. If these conditions are met, the first lymph node encountered, termed the sentinel node, is a reliable indicator of the tumor status of the entire nodal basin. To a high degree, these principles hold true for the integumentary system because SNLS is a clinically validated indicator of nodal status for both breast cancer and melanoma (23,24).

SLNS has been evaluated for colon, gastric, and esophageal malignancies. The staging issues addressed by SLNS differ significantly among these three diseases. For esophageal and gastric cancer, assessment of nodal status prior to resection of the primary tumor can aid surgical decision making. For example, by identifying patients with stage III disease, SLNS is a minimally invasive method to select patients with advanced esophageal or gastric cancer that may benefit from preoperative chemoradiation. At the other end of the disease spectrum, studies are investigating the efficacy of minimally invasive surgery for resection of superficial gastric cancer. This procedure requires confirmation of node-negative status prior to definitive surgery, and single-institution studies indicate that the SLNS technique may achieve this goal (25). The development of minimally invasive surgery for early gastric cancer is therefore proceeding in close association with studies to confirm the accuracy of SLNS for this disease.

Unlike surgery for breast cancer or melanoma, the anatomy of the colon permits wide lymphadenectomy without significantly increasing the difficulty or morbidity of tumor resection. SLNS for colon cancer would be useful if it is therapeutic or if it improved the accuracy of pathological staging (26–28). Although proponents of SNLS for colon cancer report that this technique is highly accurate, with values ranging from 89% to 97% for the detection of node-positive disease (27,29–31), most of the studies that reached this conclusion applied different diagnostic criteria to the sentinel node than those used for nonsentinel nodes. For example, it was common for sentinel nodes but not nonsentinel nodes to be scored positive based on immunohistochemical results rather than standard histopathological criteria. In a recent prospective study performed by the Cancer and Leukemia Group B, sentinel nodes were sampled in 66 patients with respectable colon cancer (32). Examination of these nodes using standard histopathology failed to predict the presence of nodal disease in 13/24 (54%) of node-positive cases. Immunostains were then performed on both sentinel and nonsentinel nodes for cases whose lymph nodes were negative by standard histopathology. Depending on the immunohistochemical criteria used to assign lymph node positivity, sentinel node exam resulted in either an unacceptably high false-positive rate (20%), or a low sensitivity for detection of micrometastatic disease (40%). By examining both sentinel and nonsentinel nodes, this multiinstitutional study showed that sentinel nodes did not accurately predict the presence of either conventionally defined nodal metastases or micrometastatic disease (32). At the present time, therefore, SLNS is not used for staging of resectable colon cancer.

Radioimmunoguided Surgery

Radioimmunoguided surgery (RIGS) is a technique for intraoperative localization of tumor in tissues that would not ordinarily be removed as part of a standard cancer resection. This is done so additional tumor sites can be treated by extended resection, intraoperative radiation therapy, or adjuvant postoperative chemotherapy or radiation therapy. A radiolabeled monoclonal antibody (MAb) is injected into the patient 3 to 4 weeks before surgery. The antibody used most often for defining the extent of gastrointestinal cancers by RIGS is CC49, an MAb against the epithelial tumor antigen, tumor-associated glycoprotein-72 (TAG-72). This MAb is generally labeled with iodine 125 and therefore must be administered with a thyroid-blocking agent such as potassium iodide. The MAb is cleared from the bloodstream and concentrated in the tumor, and the patient is taken to surgery when a 2-second measurement of the precordial area with a gamma probe yields counts of <30 (33). During exploratory laparotomy, in addition to the usual inspection and palpation, the abdomen is scanned with a hand-held gamma probe, taking as background the count corresponding to that of circulating blood, obtained at the bifurcation of the aorta. The local tumor field and associated nodal basins are then scanned for increased signal, which indicates residual disease. Complete survey of the abdomen with the gamma probe also includes the liver, stomach, duodenum, posterior retroperitoneum including kidneys, and pelvis. In some studies of recurrent colorectal cancer, use of this technique altered surgical decisions as much as 30% of the time, generally by extending the resection to adjacent tissues to obtain a RIGS-negative field. Problems with the technique include low specificity in lymph node tissue, possibly due to clearance of the antibody by the reticuloendothelial system.

RIGS findings may have prognostic value. In a multicenter phase III trial for recurrent or metastatic intraabdominal cancer, surgical decision making was altered by RIGS analysis 20% of the time (34). In the patients with liver metastasis, RIGS identified occult metastasis in the periportal lymph nodes in 28.5% and identified those patients who were not likely to be cured by liver resection (35). Studies of the use of RIGS have not yet demonstrated an impact on patient treatment morbidity or survival, and this technique is costly and fairly cumbersome. Further study is required to determine both how accurate RIGS staging is and whether this method can be applied effectively in routine clinical care.

Molecular Characterization of Tumors

Research since the mid-1990s has provided an improved understanding of the molecular nature of gastrointestinal carcinogenesis. These observations are beginning to be translated into clinically useful predictors of tumor behavior. Tumor-associated genotypic or phenotypic markers add to conventional assessment of histologic grade or degree of invasion by measuring cell cycle control, angiogenic potential, or genomic stability, to name a few functional categories by which various markers are classified (Table 5.5).

One example of how a tumor-associated marker can provide useful clinical information is provided by thymidylate synthase (TS) measurement. TS is an enzyme required for DNA synthesis, as it converts 2'-deoxyuridine 5'-monophosphate to thymidine 5'-monophosphate. TS is a critical target for 5-fluorouracil (5-FU), the most common chemotherapeutic agent for gastrointestinal malignancies. DNA synthesis is inhibited by 5-FU through formation of a ternary complex between TS, the 5-FU metabolite fluorodeoxyuridylate, and CH_2FH_4, a folic acid derivative (36,37). Overexpression of TS protein in colorectal and gastric tumors is associated with resistance to 5-FU and may also indicate loss of p53 function (38–40). Increased expression of TS in tumors predicts a poor response to chemotherapy regimens using 5-FU in multiple clinical studies (41,42).

Most reports linking genotypic or phenotypic characteristics of tumors to clinical outcome are single-marker studies, performed either retrospectively or prospectively with small numbers of patients. Although some of these markers, like TS, appear to have important independent prognostic value, their clinical utility is still in question because of variability in laboratory methods, differences in treatment within the study cohort, and insufficient clinical follow-up. At the present time, however, several promising clinical trials are underway within the cancer cooperative groups to determine the association between multiple tumor markers and clinical outcome for colorectal, gastric, and pancreatic malignancies.

ADVANCING SURGICAL TECHNIQUES

Extent of Resection of Primary Tumor

Surgeons have always been highly critical of operative technique, and as a result, several uniformly accepted characteristics of an optimal operation for intestinal cancer evolved during the 20th century. These include sharp, rather than blunt dissection of the tissue planes; *en bloc* tumor resection with avoidance of tumor entry or spillage; complete regional lymphadenectomy; and achievement of as wide a tumor margin as possible without undue morbidity to the patient. Beyond a clear recognition of the importance of tumorfree excision margins, however, it is extremely difficult to objectively measure the impact of differences in surgical technique on treatment outcome. Even major points of technique such as total mesorectal excision versus "standard" resection for rectal cancer, or the D1 versus D2 lymphadenectomy for gastric cancer, have defied the standardization necessary to allow a definitive

---

TABLE 5.5

PUTATIVE MARKERS OF PROGNOSIS OR TREATMENT RESPONSE

Carcinoembryonic antigen	PCNA	p53
Thymidylate synthase	Ki67	p21
Thymidylate phosphorylase	Cyclin D1	p27
Matrix metalloproteinases	Ploidy	Myc
Cathepsin D	Apoptotic index	Bcl-2/Bax
Sialyl Lewis A/sialyl Lewis X	Microvascular density	17pLOH
CD44 v6, v8–10	VEGF	18qLOH
Plasminogen activator	Sucrase-isomaltase	DCC
uPA receptor	Prolactin receptor	Ki-ras
HER-2/neu	Vitamin D receptor	Microsatellite instability

PCNA, proliferating cell nuclear antigen; LOH, loss of heterozygosity; VEGF, vascular endothelial growth factor; DCC, deleted in colon cancer; uPA, urokinase plasminogen activator; HER-2, human epidermal growth factor receptor 2.

randomized, prospective trial. These disease-specific controversies over surgical technique are discussed in other chapters. Thus, it is useful here to consider a few basic principles that apply to all gastrointestinal cancer surgery.

As understanding of tumor biology has progressed, the surgical techniques used to remove cancers have evolved. Early cancer surgery was limited to daring resections in premorbid patients, with a dismal success rate in the preanesthetic, preantibiotic era. Advances in endoscopy, radiology, and perioperative support led to earlier diagnosis and more long-term survival among cancer patients. The "more is better" approach to cancer surgery was challenged by the observation that advanced cancer is a systemic disease. As outlined in the previous section, we are still struggling to understand the nature of clinically significant residual or micrometastatic disease. An interesting fashion in gastrointestinal cancer surgery came about in the 1960s, when the "no-touch" technique was championed by Turnbull et al. (43). An increased rate of shedding of tumor cells into the circulation was observed at the time of operative tumor manipulation. This was believed to predispose the patient to recurrence; therefore, a meticulous effort was made to isolate and ligate all vascular channels surrounding the tumor before its manipulation or removal, hence the term *no touch*. The no-touch approach has been shown to decrease the volume of tumor cells disseminated during surgery for colorectal cancer (21,44). Tumor cells are shed into the circulation from cancers at all stages, but the clinical significance of this is unknown and likely depends on whether the tumor cells themselves have the capacity to form an independent metastatic colony and whether they traverse a favorable target tissue. It is now believed that the shedding of cells into the bloodstream that is associated with tumor resection is not likely to contribute to tumor spread, and it may be the persistence of circulating tumor cells after potentially curative resection that has real prognostic significance (20,45,46).

Accurate measurements of the extent of surgical resection may be one of the most important pieces of clinical information for a gastrointestinal cancer patient. Frequently, this assessment occurs at the time of surgery, when intraoperative consultation with a surgical pathologist sometimes dictates the extent of the operation. In 1889, Friedrich von Esmarch, a professor of surgery at Kiel, had to convince the German Surgical Congress that a microscopic diagnosis of cancer should be established before a patient was subjected to extensive, disfiguring surgery (47). William S. Halsted was the first American surgeon to establish a division of surgical pathology, and from that time onward, the surgical pathologist became an integral part of the multidisciplinary cancer treatment team (48). The importance of proper handling of operative specimens before and during examination by the surgical pathologist cannot be overestimated. Complicated specimens demand a significant degree of experience and knowledge to be properly examined, and a microscopic diagnosis is of limited value unless it is interpreted in the context of essential clinical data. Only the operative surgeon fully understands the relationship of the tumor to the remaining tissues and the method or thoroughness of the resection. The addition of molecular and micrometastatic tumor analyses as complements to standard histopathology makes collaboration between the surgical pathologist and the cancer surgeon all the more critical to optimal cancer treatment.

Laparoscopic Cancer Resections

Minimally invasive surgical techniques have gained widespread application in general surgery since the mid-1990s. Laparoscopic resections of the gallbladder and spleen have become preferred operations because they provide a significant reduction in patient morbidity compared with open procedures. The laparoscopic approach is also frequently used in treating benign diseases of the stomach and large bowel such as gastroesophageal reflux, diverticulitis, or inflammatory bowel disease. As mentioned previously, laparoscopic staging of selected patients with gastrointestinal tumors is helpful in determining whether advanced disease in the abdomen makes laparotomy inadvisable. The use of minimally invasive techniques for potentially curative resection of gastrointestinal cancers, however, has been approached with caution by the surgical oncology community. The short-term benefits of decreased hospital stay and earlier return to activities cannot be gained at the expense of a decreased cure rate, an end point that takes many years to measure.

Since the mid-1990s, advances in minimally invasive surgery have allowed surgeons to adapt laparoscopic techniques that respond to the challenges of cancer surgery. In addition to using instruments introduced via 5- and 10-mm operative ports, an operative port large enough to admit the surgeon's hand can be inserted, thereby allowing "hand-assisted" laparoscopic surgery. This hand port allows a surgeon to overcome significant technical challenges during tumor mobilization, such as difficult tumor localization, dense adhesions, or significant amounts of mesenteric fat. Stapling devices inserted via standard laparoscopic ports facilitate high ligation of the mesenteric vasculature and permit wide lymphadenectomy. Anastomoses can be accomplished either intraabdominally or via small incisions through which the bowel segments can be exteriorized.

Major concerns facing laparoscopic oncologic surgery are whether these procedures allow an adequate regional lymphadenectomy and whether these techniques are associated with a higher rate of local or distant recurrence. Few studies have examined the effect of these techniques on the ultimate standard for treatment, overall survival. These issues have been best addressed for colon cancer (49–52). A large multiinstitutional prospective, randomized trial comparing laparoscopically assisted to open colectomy for colon cancer—the Clinical Outcomes of Surgical Therapy (COST) Study—was reported in 2004 (52). This study confirmed a small but significant decrease in use of intravenous postoperative narcotics (4 vs. 3.2 days) and length of hospital stay (5 vs. 6 days) for the group treated with minimally invasive surgery. This study confirmed equivalence of tumor margins and extent and adequacy of en bloc lymph node resections. Importantly, this study confirmed acceptably low rates of wound recurrence (0.5% vs. 0.2%) and local recurrence (17% vs. 27%) for laparoscopic versus open procedures, respectively. Overall survival at 3 years was similar in the laparoscopic and open groups at any stage of cancer treated. At least two other large prospective randomized trials of laparoscopic approaches for colon cancer are underway in Europe, with data expected in the near future.

Minimally invasive approaches are also under investigation for management of early cancers of the esophagus, stomach, and rectum (53–56). The challenges of these laparoscopic procedures vary considerably from those presented by colon surgery. In both instances, it can be difficult to precisely define the required margins at the time of resection. In addition, lymphatic drainage may be more variable in these sites, and it is unclear whether sentinel lymph node sampling can facilitate a laparoscopic approach. Decisions concerning the risk and benefit of minimally invasive procedures for these diseases await results from randomized trials in high-volume centers.

Intraoperative Radiation Therapy

Another promising addition to the surgical management of gastrointestinal tumors is the delivery of radiation to the tissues at the time of surgery, or intraoperative radiation therapy (IORT).

The combination of IORT with pre- or postoperative external beam radiation and chemotherapy theoretically allows delivery of a maximal dose of radiation therapy because dose-limiting structures such as small bowel or bladder can be excluded from the IORT field. The currently available methods of delivering IORT include electron beam IORT and IORT with high-dose brachytherapy. This latter method involves application of radiation through a flexible catheter system that can conform to complicated areas of anatomy such as the deep pelvis. Single-dose electron beam IORT delivers two to three times the equivalent dose of external beam radiation in terms of antitumor effect (57). This treatment is best applied in cases in which the risk of local recurrence without systemic metastases is relatively high. For this reason, IORT has been used for management of locally advanced rectal cancer, in which from 15% to 30% of patients develop isolated locoregional recurrence (58,59). IORT may also be appropriate in cases in which dose-limiting structures permit limited delivery of external beam radiation, even though the chance of systemic recurrence is high. These cases include selected patients with gastric (60), esophageal (61), pancreatic (62), or bile duct malignancies (63).

Results from randomized, controlled trials comparing IORT to regimens using standard external beam radiation alone are not yet available; however, comparison of results in patients receiving IORT with that of historical controls suggests a benefit to this treatment in certain clinical situations. Addition of IORT to management of locally advanced rectal cancer may significantly improve local control and 5-year actuarial survival, and may be particularly effective for patients who undergo complete tumor resection (64). In patients with advanced or locally recurrent rectal cancer, 2-year local relapse rates of 18% to 33% are reported following IORT, compared to rates of 73% to 76% in control groups (65–69). Similar improvements were seen in patients treated with intraoperative brachytherapy, a technique that may be more generally applicable because it does not require special operating suites equipped with lead shielding (70). IORT has also been applied to management of both locally advanced and resectable pancreatic cancer and gastric cancer (71–73). In these diseases, however, the limited studies available failed to demonstrate an advantage to adding IORT to external beam radiation therapy.

Although results in rectal cancer are promising, the reported series are still relatively small and contain heterogeneous patient populations. Several potentially important differences exist between patients treated with IORT and historical controls. These include heterogeneity with respect to operative or radiation therapy techniques and differences in operative or anesthesia time. Comparisons of morbidity are also lacking. These issues make it important for oncologists to continue to pursue this method of radiation delivery via prospective, randomized trials.

Cytoreductive Surgery and Peritoneal Chemotherapy/Brachytherapy

A small number of patients with gastrointestinal malignancies develop involvement of the peritoneal surfaces without evidence of disease in other organs such as the liver or lungs. Primary tumors that classically give rise to this condition are mucinous adenocarcinoma of the colorectum and adenocarcinoma of the stomach, small bowel, or appendix. In some cases, particularly for low-grade malignancies such as grade I mucinous adenocarcinoma or malignant pseudomyxoma peritonei, significant local disease control can be achieved by cytoreductive surgery, often with the addition of intraperitoneal chemotherapy (74,75). Cytoreductive surgery involves stripping the peritoneum from the surfaces of the diaphragm, an-

terior abdominal wall, and pelvis, in addition to performing an omentectomy and perhaps splenectomy, cholecystectomy, or antrectomy. Intraperitoneal chemotherapy is generally administered via catheters positioned in the abdominal cavity at the time of cytoreductive surgery. The theoretical advantage of intraperitoneal chemotherapy is that maximal doses can be delivered to the tumor-bearing peritoneal surface by this approach because a 10-fold higher concentration is tolerated by intraperitoneal administration than can be administered systemically (76).

Cytoreductive surgery and perioperative chemotherapy for peritoneal carcinomatosis arising from colorectal cancer has been evaluated in several multicenter phase II and a single phase III trial (77,78). The extent of tumor reduction achieved by cytoreductive surgery is the most important prognostic indicator for patients treated with this procedure (79). A prospective, randomized study of patients with metastatic colorectal cancer compared intraperitoneal and systemic chemotherapy to systemic chemotherapy alone following cytoreductive surgery (78). The median survival for the group for whom intraperitoneal chemotherapy was added was 22.3 months, compared to 12.6 months for the systemic only arm ($p = 0.032$) (78).

There are some data to suggest that intraperitoneal administration of chemotherapy may be effective in the adjuvant setting. In a study of patients with resected gastric and colon cancer, the intraperitoneal fluid distribution remained adequate in 94% of patients at 6 months, and combined intravenous and intraperitoneal dosing of 5-FU produced a peritoneal fluid-to-plasma drug concentration ratio of 100:1, with intraperitoneal 5-FU detected at 20 hours after dosing (80). Intraperitoneal administration concentrates chemotherapeutic agents in the hepatic parenchyma. Because local and hepatic metastases are the most common pattern of recurrence for patients with stage II and III colorectal cancer, the effectiveness of adjuvant intraperitoneal chemotherapy was assessed. In a randomized trial of 241 patients with resected stage III colon cancer, Scheithauer et al. demonstrated significantly longer diseasefree and overall survival after 6 months (six courses) of 5-FU plus leucovorin calcium were given both systemically and intraperitoneally, compared to the same agents given only systemically (81). Vaillant et al. extended this observation to patients with stage II colon cancer (82). The role of intraperitoneal chemotherapy for routine adjuvant therapy of colorectal and other intraabdominal malignancies, such as gastric or pancreatic tumors, has yet to be defined.

The cytostatic effect of some chemotherapeutic agents is potentiated by hyperthermia, perhaps through improved tissue penetration. In addition, application of chemotherapy to the abdominal cavity at the time of surgery offers the theoretical advantages of access of the chemotherapeutic agent to all tissue surfaces before the tumor cells are isolated by the healing process. Residual tumor cells that are freely mobile in the abdominal cavity at the completion of the cytoreductive surgery are also potentially treated before closure of the operative field. Intraperitoneal hyperthermic chemotherapy entails aggressive surgical debulking followed by heated intraperitoneal perfusion of chemotherapeutic agents, such as mitomycin C or cisplatin (83). Single-arm studies and some randomized clinical studies suggest that this treatment reduces local recurrence of gastric cancer and may increase diseasefree survival of patients with disseminated spread of appendiceal, colorectal, and pancreatic cancers (84,85). Responding patients are generally limited to those with minimal peritoneal spread or those at high risk due to the presence of bulky locoregional disease. In a series of 200 patients treated with this modality, complications, including pancreatitis, fistula formation, bleeding, and hematologic toxicity, occurred in approximately 27% of patients, and treatment-related mortality was 1.5% (86). In the absence of other effective but less morbidity-inducing treatments, intraperitoneal chemotherapy alone or with intraoperative hyperthermia remains an option for management of this patient population with an overall dismal prognosis.

Hepatic Artery Infusion

More than one-half of all patients with metastatic colorectal cancer develop liver metastases, and in many of these, the liver is the only or the predominant site of disease. Resection of limited disease in the liver clearly increases survival and offers the possibility of cure (10,87). Cryotherapy can also successfully ablate limited liver disease, and this technique has been added to the options available both in the operating room and via percutaneous access (88). Other nonoperative ablative techniques include percutaneous injection of lesions with ethanol or application of radiofrequency energy via probes (89,90). These procedures are useful for patients with limited physical reserves, but their use is limited to patients with small lesions that are relatively few in number. Unfortunately, many patients with colorectal cancer present with liver-only disease that is not amenable to resection or ablation. Because tumor metastases derive their blood supply from the hepatic artery, whereas hepatocytes are supplied by the portal vein, intraarterial administration of the 5-FU metabolite floxuridine (FUDR) produces significant intratumoral drug levels while theoretically limiting hepatic toxicity. A high first-pass extraction of FUDR (approximately 95%) limits the systemic effect of hepatic artery infusion. Despite the favorable drug ratio between tumor and hepatocytes, hepatic artery infusion is associated with the potentially fatal complications of drug-induced hepatitis and sclerosing cholangitis (91).

Hepatic artery infusional chemotherapy has been assessed both for treatment of patients with recurrent disease and as a means of preventing recurrence after potentially curative resection of hepatic metastases. For unresectable hepatic metastases, the effects of hepatic artery infusion added to standard intravenous chemotherapy have been difficult to assess. The available studies include fairly small patient numbers and have problems resulting from crossover between treatment arms and inability to establish adequate hepatic artery perfusion in some patients randomized to this treatment. Meta-analyses of the randomized trials reported to date, however, suggest that hepatic artery infusional therapy may increase short-term survival by 10% to 15% (92,93).

Hepatic artery infusional chemotherapy may also have an adjuvant role. Patients who undergo successful resection of hepatic colorectal metastasis still have a 70% to 80% incidence of disease recurrence, and in approximately 50% of these recurrences, the liver is the only site of disease (10,94). Understanding the contribution of hepatic artery infusional chemotherapy to recurrence or survival for these patients is hampered by several factors. First, no good data exist on the use of either standard 5-FU–based infusional chemotherapy alone or hepatic artery infusion alone after resection of hepatic metastases. Data from existing trials with small numbers of patients, however, do suggest a benefit to systemic chemotherapy plus hepatic artery infusional therapy for patients with resected liver metastases. In one study, coordinated by the Eastern Cooperative Oncology Group, 109 patients with liver-only colorectal cancer metastases were preoperatively randomized to receive either surgery alone or surgery plus hepatic artery infusional chemotherapy with FUDR, followed by infusional 5-FU (95). At a median follow-up of 4 years, the 3-year recurrencefree survival was 34% for the surgery-alone group and 58% for the patients receiving surgery plus both hepatic artery and intravenous chemotherapy ($p = 0.039$). A second randomized, prospective study compared hepatic artery infusion of FUDR plus dexamethasone combined with systemic 5-FU plus leucov-

orin with systemic 5-FU plus leucovorin alone in this same patient population (96). The 2-year diseasefree survival was 85% in the group receiving hepatic artery infusional chemotherapy versus 69% in the group receiving only systemic treatment. Taken together, these two studies suggest that chemotherapy, including hepatic artery infusional chemotherapy, may increase survival after resection of isolated hepatic metastases from colorectal cancer. In conclusion, a sound anatomical and pharmacologic rationale exists for hepatic artery infusional therapy, and the results of preliminary trials are promising. Because this treatment modality carries significant morbidity and its impact on overall survival is not yet proven, it is still considered investigational at this point.

SURGICAL SUPPORT OF GASTROINTESTINAL CANCER PATIENTS

Management of Malignant Bowel Obstruction

Bowel obstruction is relatively common in gastrointestinal cancer patients, whether it is the initial presentation of an intestinal malignancy, is produced by recurrent or metastatic disease, or is associated with benign causes such as postoperative adhesion formation. Approximately 15% of patients with intestinal cancer exhibit some degree of obstruction on initial presentation, and another 3% to 8% present with perforation of the carcinoma (97). Patients with these complications are generally older and have more advanced disease at the time of surgery, resulting in a crude 5-year survival of 25% to 34% (98). Prompt surgical intervention is essential for patients with acute intestinal obstruction or perforation. Even when distal colonic lesions are present, most patients with good physiological status and a relatively brief duration of preoperative symptoms can be treated by resection of the tumor with primary anastomosis, without diverting ileostomy or colostomy (99). For colorectal tumors, although the presence of obstruction or perforation is generally associated with advanced disease, 30% to 50% of these cases prove to be stage II (100,101). The 5-year survival for these "high-risk" stage II patients is less than that for patients presenting without complications, particularly among those with perforated tumors, for whom 5-year survival approaches that of patients with stage III disease (100).

One of the more difficult problems faced by a surgeon is the management of bowel obstruction in a patient with a past history of abdominal cancer. Of patients presenting with a bowel obstruction within 5 years of treatment for a primary gastrointestinal cancer, one-third have a benign cause for their obstruction (102). Of the remaining two-thirds, approximately half have carcinomatosis that can be identified by CT or by physical examination. In this setting, the goal is to identify patients with benign or localized disease whose obstruction can be treated or palliated surgically. All too often, however, patients with recurrent intestinal tumors and bowel obstruction have diffuse intraperitoneal disease for which attempted surgical treatment is at best ineffective and at worst may contribute substantially to disease morbidity. It is not surprising, therefore, that the hospital mortality of patients with bowel obstruction from recurrent intraabdominal tumor is 20% to 40% (45,102–105).

The operative approach to intestinal obstruction in patients with a history of intraabdominal malignancy is dictated by the extent of tumor and the location of the obstruction. Preoperative imaging is essential for these complicated cases because the presence of extensive tumor can make full surgical exploration difficult or impossible. Spiral CT scanning is an excellent method for determining the extent of disease and, frequently, the point of obstruction. Care must be taken to preserve the physiological reserves of patients who are potential surgical candidates, including the use of TPN if a trial of nonoperative management is attempted. Surgical exploration is clearly indicated for patients with a history of intraabdominal malignancy whose physical examination and imaging studies suggest a localized intestinal obstruction. Not only is benign disease the cause of the obstruction in a significant proportion of these patients, but for patients with good performance status, surgery to relieve localized malignant obstructions can improve the patient's quality of life by relieving nausea, vomiting, and abdominal pain. The most common procedures performed for palliation of malignant intestinal obstruction are lysis of adhesions, placement of self-expandable stents, small bowel bypass, decompressive colostomy, and gastrostomy. Complete resection of recurrent disease is possible only in rare instances.

It is unusual for a patient with diffuse carcinomatosis to present with an acute complete intestinal obstruction. Instead, these patients usually have a protracted course of nausea, vomiting, and crampy abdominal pain, and abdominal films are consistent with partial bowel obstruction. These patients are generally managed nonoperatively with nasogastric decompression, intravenous hydration or TPN, antiemetic treatment, and judicious use of pain medications. Stenting may be particularly helpful in cases where an isolated obstructed segment can be reached endoscopically. Nonoperative management is often only a temporary solution because approximately 50% of these patients eventually progress to complete obstruction (103). In addition, patients whose obstructions resolve after nonoperative management often continue to have obstructive symptoms after discharge. For patients with a significant disease burden, these symptoms also persist after palliative surgery for gastrointestinal cancer.

In patients with complete bowel obstruction due to diffuse intraabdominal tumor spread, surgery to relieve the obstruction is rarely successful. In this case, surgery is generally reserved for patients with good performance status because those with widespread visceral metastases whose activities are constrained are particularly unlikely to benefit from surgery (104). Survival in this patient population is extremely limited, particularly for patients whose nutritional status is compromised. Here, the focus is palliation of symptoms by use of antiemetics and pain medication. Anecdotal reports suggest that use of octreotide acetate alleviates the symptoms of malignant bowel obstruction, providing palliation of nausea and pain in patients with advanced disease (106,107).

Surgical Management of Complications of Radiation Therapy

Radiation injury to the intestine is characterized by both acute and chronic phases. Acute radiation enteritis is experienced by almost all patients receiving pelvic or abdominal radiation therapy. This complication is due to radiation-induced injury to the actively dividing cells of the intestinal mucosa and presents clinically as nausea, vomiting, abdominal pain, diarrhea, or tenesmus. The symptoms of acute radiation enteritis generally resolve within a few weeks of completion of therapy. The management of acute radiation enteritis is supportive and includes administration of antiemetics and pain medication, and maintenance of hydration.

Chronic radiation injury to the intestine is a progressive condition characterized histologically by fibrosis and obliterative endarteritis. The period between radiation exposure and clinical manifestations of a chronic radiation-associated injury averages 2 years, with a range of 3 months to 43 years reported in the literature (108,109). Chronic radiation-associated destruction of the intestine can progress to become a transmural injury, leading to obstruction, bleeding, perforation, fistulas, and stricture formation. The incidence and clinical consequences of treatment-related bowel injury were reviewed for 386 patients undergoing radiation therapy with or without chemotherapy for rectal cancer from 1981 to 1990. In this series, the overall incidence of chronic proctitis was 12.5%, and 5% of patients developed chronic enteritis. Reoperation for chronic treatment-related enteritis was required in 5% of the patients in this large cohort (110). Other studies also indicate that, due to the progressive nature of this disease, approximately 50% of the patients receiving surgical treatment will develop further symptoms related to radiation injury (111).

When chronic radiation enteritis presents with complications requiring operation, the treatment of choice is resection of the involved intestine with reanastomosis. For friable segments of strictured small intestine that are adherent deep in the pelvis or cannot be resected for other reasons, an intestinal bypass procedure is the treatment of choice, with diversion or exclusion reserved for the most recalcitrant cases. Because the remaining diseased segment is still subject to ulceration, bleeding, and fistula formation, a significant portion of patients will require a second operation after any procedure that leaves diseased bowel behind. Perioperative mortality from severe complications of radiation enteritis, such as obstruction and perforation, may be as high as 40% to 50% (112).

Obviously, chronic or acute radiation enteritis should be avoided whenever possible. The methods used include surgical exclusion of the small intestine from the pelvis, careful treatment delivery with three-dimensional planning after small bowel contrast studies, positioning strategies to minimize bowel entry into radiation fields, and systemic or regional administration of a radioprotectant such as amifostine. The efficacy of these methods has been examined primarily in small, single-institution studies. For this reason, the optimal method for protecting against radiation enteritis remains controversial (113).

Surgical technique may be an important factor in the development of radiation enteritis. A history of previous pelvic surgery is a significant risk factor in the development of this disease because the adhesions formed in the postoperative healing period entrap small intestine in the radiation fields. Careful closure of the peritoneum in the pelvis partially prevents this problem, but this tissue is rarely sufficient to allow adequate exclusion of small bowel from the pelvis. Omental flaps can be brought into the pelvic brim to serve an occluding role, but this tissue is also often lacking in cancer patients, either because of deliberate removal as part of the cancer operation or because of multiple previous abdominal procedures. Cancer surgeons have used a variety of prosthetic materials to elevate the small bowel out of the pelvis, the most useful of which is a sling constructed of absorbable mesh (114). Application of this technique significantly decreased the incidence of radiation enteritis in several small single-arm series with mean follow-up intervals of 18 to 36 months, and the technique has an acceptably low complication rate in experienced hands (113). Despite this, the procedure may add to the duration of surgery and increase postoperative ileus, and instances of intestinal obstruction caused by herniation of small bowel through the mesh have been described (115). For these reasons, and due to a lack of supportive evidence from randomized trials, this technique is not widely used.

The practice of preoperative radiation and chemotherapy for rectal cancer may also decrease the incidence of chronic radiation enteritis. The preoperative pelvis is free of adhesions, which allows the application of techniques such as prone positioning, maintenance of a full bladder, and use of a "belly board" to move the small intestine out of the radiation field more effectively. In addition, improved general mobility of the intestine prevents repeated delivery of radiation to a single area of intestine (116,117). Despite the theoretical advantages to preoperative radiation, the long-term complication rate associated with this approach remains unclear. In a Swedish study in which 1,168 patients were randomly assigned to receive either surgery alone or 1 week of radiation at 500 cGy/day with surgery shortly afterward, patients receiving radiation had a significantly increased 5-year survival (48% vs. 58%; $p = 0.004$). The incidence of postoperative morbidity, however, was higher in the irradiated group (44% vs. 34%; $p = 0.001$) (116). This study may not reflect the results obtained from standard treatment regimens used in the United States, in which the radiation is delivered in lower fractions over a longer period and in combination with 5-FU–based chemotherapy. Preliminary studies using this regimen suggest that the treatment-related toxicity is the same for the patients treated preoperatively as it is for those receiving postoperative adjuvant therapy (117). None of the available studies, however, is mature enough to evaluate differences in late sequelae.

PROPHYLACTIC CANCER SURGERY: SURGICAL MANAGEMENT OF FAMILIAL ADENOMATOUS POLYPOSIS, HEREDITARY NONPOLYPOSIS COLORECTAL CANCER, AND ULCERATIVE COLITIS

For the lower gastrointestinal tract, cancer prevention is effectively achieved by endoscopic surveillance with removal of premalignant adenomas from the intestinal tract (118). In three clinical disorders, however, colorectal cancer develops either with extremely high frequency or by acceleration of the adenoma-carcinoma sequence to the extent that prophylactic colectomy or proctocolectomy becomes an appropriate option for consideration. These conditions include familial adenomatous polyposis (FAP), hereditary nonpolyposis colorectal cancer (HNPCC), and ulcerative colitis (UC).

FAP is an autosomal dominant cancer predisposition syndrome characterized by the development of hundreds to thousands of colorectal adenomas and the inevitable progression to colorectal cancer by the third to fourth decades of life. FAP is now recognized as a systemic disease caused by germ-line mutation of the *APC* gene (119,120), and the phenotype can include desmoid tumors, duodenal adenomas and carcinomas, mandibular osteomas, congenital hypertrophy of the retinal pigmented epithelium, and cutaneous epidermoid tumors. The intestinal adenoma-carcinoma sequence was first described in FAP patients by Lockhart-Mummery in 1925. Until the 1940s, however, patients with this disease continued to die of colon or rectal cancer in the fourth or fifth decade of life. Prevention of death from colorectal cancer in FAP patients became possible during the 1940s, with the development of safe procedures for total colectomy. Although treatment with nonsteroidal antiinflammatory medications such as sulindac or celecoxib reduces tumor number and size in patients with FAP (121,122), total proctocolectomy is the only safe method of cancer prevention. Because 8% to 12% of these patients also develop duodenal carcinomas, lifetime surveillance of the upper gastrointestinal tract is also crucial.

Prophylactic surgery for patients with FAP involves either total proctocolectomy, generally with J-pouch ileoanal reconstruction, or total colectomy with ileorectal anastomosis, followed by lifetime surveillance of the remaining rectal segment.

The choice of operation requires balancing the higher rate of complications of a mucosal proctectomy with ileorectal anastomosis with the long-term cancer risk of a retained rectal segment. Before age 50, the cumulative risk of rectal carcinoma in FAP patients receiving an ileorectal anastomosis is 10% (123), but the risk likely increases significantly after this age (124). Even in patient populations receiving careful screening of the remaining rectum, as many as 10% develop a carcinoma (125). In addition, data from centers experienced with ileoanal procedures suggest a low complication rate with this operation when performed in young adulthood. In a series of 48 teenagers who underwent ileal pouch-anal anastomosis for FAP, the mean daytime and nighttime stool frequencies were 4 ± 1.5 and 1 ± 1, respectively, with only one patient reporting daytime incontinence. None of these patients experienced impotence or retrograde ejaculation, and 87% reported unchanged sexual function (126). For these reasons, most patients with FAP choose total proctocolectomy with J-pouch ileoanal reconstruction as prophylaxis for colorectal cancer.

HNPCC was first identified in kindreds with a high incidence of colorectal cancer but no overabundance of precursor adenomas. These families also had a high incidence of endometrial, gastric, and urothelial carcinomas (127), and an autosomal dominant pattern of inheritance. In the 1990s, DNA repair defects were identified in tumors from patients with this clinical syndrome. It is now known that HNPCC is caused by germline defects in genes encoding DNA mismatch repair enzymes. Faulty mismatch repair produces an enhanced potential for malignant transformation in the intestinal epithelium, a finding that is also present as a somatic event in 12% to 20% of sporadic colorectal cancers. Because of the associated DNA repair defects, the adenoma-carcinoma progression time may be accelerated in patients with HNPCC. Compared to patients with FAP, fewer individuals with the HNPCC genetic defect develop colorectal cancer, and the natural history of HNPCC is difficult to predict. Because of this uncertainty, the practice of prophylactic subtotal colectomy for germ-line carriers of mismatch repair mutations is controversial (128). For HNPCC patients presenting with a cancer at a young age, particularly those with multiple colonic adenomas, most surgeons agree that subtotal colectomy is appropriate.

Chronic UC is an autoimmune disorder of the large intestine characterized by abdominal pain, bleeding, and persistent inflammation associated with an increased incidence of colorectal cancer. Ten percent to 25% of patients with active UC for 25 or more years develop colorectal cancer, and colorectal cancer is the cause of death in up to 15% of patients with UC (129). The management of patients with UC consists of either lifelong frequent surveillance colonoscopy with biopsy to detect precancerous dysplasia, or prophylactic total proctocolectomy (130). The option chosen depends on the age of onset and the severity of the disease.

TRENDS FOR THE FUTURE

Since the 1970s, major improvements in the care of gastrointestinal cancer patients occurred. Better anesthesia, antibiotics, and metabolic and nutritional support have substantially increased the percentage of patients receiving potentially curative therapies and have increased the options for effective surgical palliation. Compared with the 1980s, cancer surgery patients now experience dramatically shorter hospital stays, fewer encounters with drains and nasogastric tubes, earlier return to normal activities such as eating and exercising, and fewer stomas. Multimodality therapy has produced significant increases in long-term survival. The management of gastrointestinal cancer continues to evolve as physicians acquire a greater understanding of the biological nature of this diverse group of diseases.

At the beginning of the 21st century, intestinal cancer is still primarily a surgical disease. However, one can be optimistic that chemopreventive agents will decrease overall cancer incidence, and that earlier detection and improved staging will be achieved through advances in imaging techniques and molecular diagnostics. The future will also bring new cancer therapeutics, such as biological response modifiers, that will improve the success rate of treatments for more advanced disease. In parallel with the development of new agents, progress in the molecular characterization of carcinogenesis will allow improved staging and individualization of treatment. For example, it will be increasingly important to understand the nature and clinical relevance of micrometastatic disease to optimize selection of both patients and agents for adjuvant therapy. Finally, continued development of minimally invasive surgical approaches to decrease treatment morbidity can be expected. Although it is unlikely that surgery will cease to play a role in the management of gastrointestinal cancer in the foreseeable future, shifting the prevalent patient population to one of earlier-stage, curable, disease is within our grasp.

References

1. Warren R. Tumors. In: Warren R, Cope O, et al., eds. *Surgery*. Philadelphia, Pa.: WB Saunders; 1963: 251.
2. Wangensteen OH, Wangensteen SD. *The Rise of Surgery*. Minneapolis: University of Minnesota Press; 1978.
3. Goldman L, Caldera DL, Nussbaum SR, et al. Multifactorial index of cardiac risk in noncardiac surgical procedures. *N Engl J Med* 1977;297(16): 845–850.
4. Buzby GB, Veterans Affairs TPN Cooperative Study Group. Perioperative TPN in surgical patients. *N Engl J Med* 1991;325:525–532.
5. Abbasakoor F, Senapati PSP, Brown TH, et al. Laparoscopy and laparoscopic ultrasonography in upper gastrointestinal cancer: do they improve staging [abstract]. *Br J Surg* 1998;85:412.
6. Stell DA, Carter CR, Stewart I, Anderson JR. Prospective comparison of laparoscopy, ultrasonography and computed tomography in the staging of gastric cancer. *Br J Surg* 1996;83(9):1260–1262.
7. Fernandez-del Castillo C, Rattner DW, Warshaw AL. Further experience with laparoscopy and peritoneal cytology in the staging of gastric cancer. *Br J Surg* 1995;82(8):1127–1129.
8. Midwinter MJ, Charnley RM. The current role of laparoscopic ultrasonography in the staging of pancreatic cancer. *Gut* 1997;41(4S):29E.
9. Clarke MP, Kane RA, Steele G, Jr., et al. Prospective comparison of perioperative imaging and intraoperative ultrasonography in the detection of liver tumors. *Surgery* 1989;106(6):849–855.
10. Fong Y, Cohen AM, Fortner JG, et al. Liver resection for colorectal metastases. *J Clin Oncol* 1997;15(3):938–946.
11. Foley EF, Kolecki RV, Schirmer BD. The accuracy of laparoscopic ultrasound in the detection of colorectal cancer liver metastases. *Am J Surg* 1998;176:262–264.
12. John TG, Gried JD, Crosbie JL, Miles WF, Garden OJ. Superior staging of liver tumors with laparoscopy and laparoscopic ultrasonography. *Ann Surg* 1994;220:711–719.
13. Makary MA, Warshaw AL, Centeno BA, Willet CG, Rattner DW, Fernandez-del Castillo C. Implications of peritoneal cytology for pancreatic cancer management. *Arch Surg* 1998;133:361–365.
14. Van Dijkum N, Els JM, Sturm PD, et al. Cytology of peritoneal lavage performed during staging laparoscopy for gastrointestinal malignancies: is it useful? *Ann Surg* 1998;228:728–733.
15. Jemal A, Murray T, Ward E, et al. Cancer statistics, 2005. *CA Cancer J Clin* 2005;55:10–30.
16. Soeth E, Vogel I, Roder C, et al. Comparative analysis of bone marrow and venous blood isolates from gastrointestinal cancer patients for the detection of disseminated tumor cells using reverse transcription PCR. *Cancer Res* 1997;57:3106–3110.
17. O'Sullivan GC, Collins JK, O'Brien F, et al. Micrometastases in bone marrow of patients undergoing "curative" surgery for gastrointestinal cancer. *Gastroenterology* 1995;109:1535–1540.
18. Litle AR, Warren RS, Moore D, Pallavicini MG. Molecular cytogenetic analysis of cytokeratin 20-labeled cells in primary tumors and bone marrow aspirates from colorectal carcinoma patients. *Cancer* 1997;79:1664–1670.
19. Calaluce R, Miedema BW, Yesus YW. Micrometastasis in colorectal carcinoma: a review. *J Surg Oncol* 1998;67:194–202.
20. O'Sullivan GC, Collins JK, Kelly J, Morgan J, Maden M, Shanahan F. Micrometastases: marker of metastatic potential or evidence of residual disease? *Gut* 1997;40:512–515.
21. Sales J-P, Wind P, Douard R, Cugnenc PH, Loric S. Blood dissemination of colonic epithelial cells during no-touch surgery for rectosigmoid cancer. *Lancet* 1999;354:392–394.
22. Harisinghani MG, Barentsz J, Hahn PF, et al. Noninvasive detection of clinically occult lymph-node metastases in prostate cancer. *N Engl J Med* 2003;348(25):2491–2499.
23. Giuliano AE, Dale PS, Turner RR, Morton DL, Evans SW, Krasne DL. Improved axillary staging of breast cancer with sentinel lymphadenectomy. *Ann Surg* 1995;222(3):394–399.
24. Morton DL, Thompson JF, Essner R, et al. Validation of the accuracy of intraoperative lymphatic mapping and sentinel lymphadenectomy for early-stage melanoma: a multicenter trial. Multicenter Selective Lymphadenectomy Trial Group. *Ann Surg* 1999;230(4):453–463.
25. Kitagawa Y, Fujii H, Kumai K, et al. Recent advances in sentinel node navigation for gastric cancer: a paradigm shift of surgical management. *J Surg Oncol* 2005;90(3):147–151.
26. Merrie AEH, van Rij AM, Phillips LV, Rossaak JI, Yun K, McCall JL. Diagnostic use of the sentinel node in colon cancer. *Dis Colon Rectum* 2001;44:410–417.
27. Saha S, Wiese D, Badin J, et al. Technical details of sentinel lymph node mapping in colorectal cancer and its impact on staging. *Ann Surg Oncol* 2000;7(2):120–124.
28. Tschmelitsch J, Klimstra DS, Cohen AM. Lymph node micrometastases do not predict relapse in stage II colon cancer. *Ann Surg Oncol* 2000;7:601–608.
29. Paramo JC, Summerall J, Poppiti R, Mesko TW. Validation of sentinel node mapping in patients with colon cancer. *Ann Surg Oncol* 2002;9:550–554.
30. Saha S, Bilchik A, Wiese D, et al. Ultrastaging of colorectal cancer by sentinel lymph node mapping techniques: a multicenter trial. *Ann Surg Oncol* 2001;8(9 suppl):94S–98S.
31. Bilchik AJ, Saha S, Tsioulias GJ, Wood TF, Morton DL. Aberrant drainage and missed micrometastases: the value of lymphatic mapping and focused analysis of sentinel lymph nodes in gastrointestinal neoplasms. *Ann Surg Oncol* 2001;8:82–85.
32. Redston M, Compton CC, Miedema BW, et al. Analysis of micrometastatic disease in sentinel lymph nodes from resectable colon cancer: results of Cancer and Leukemia Group B trial 80001. *J Clin Oncol* 2006;24(6): 841–842.
33. Arnold MW, Young DC, Hitchcock CL, Schneebaum S, Martin EW, Jr. Radioimmunoguided surgery in primary colorectal carcinoma: an intraoperative prognostic tool and adjuvant to traditional staging. *Am J Surg* 1995;170:315–518.
34. Daly JM, Burak W, Jr., Chevinsky A, et al. Radioimmunoguided surgery for large bowel cancer: results of prospective multi-institutional trials. American College of Surgeons, 82nd Congress; 1996.
35. Schneebaum S, Daly JM, Burak W, et al. RIGS efficacy in patients with colorectal cancer liver metastasis. *Eur J Surg Oncol* 1998;24:215.
36. Johnson PG, Lenz HJ, Leichman CG, et al. Thymidylate synthase gene and protein expression correlate and are associated with response to 5-fluorouracil in human colorectal and gastric tumors. *Cancer Res* 1995; 55:1407–1412.
37. Drake JC, Voeller DM, Allegra CJ, Johnston PG. The effect of dose and interval between 5-fluorouracil and leucovorin on the formation of thymidylate synthase ternary complex in human cancer cells. *Br J Cancer* 1995;71:1145–1150.
38. Leichman CG, Lenz HJ, Leichman L, et al. Quantitation of intratumoral thymidylate synthase expression predicts for disseminated colorectal cancer response and resistance to protracted-infusion fluorouracil and weekly leucovorin. *J Clin Oncol* 1997;15:3223–3229.
39. Lenz JG, Danenberg KD, Leichman CG, et al. p53 and Thymidylate synthase expression in untreated stage II colon cancer: associations with recurrence, survival and site. *Clin Cancer Res* 1998;4:1227–1234.
40. Yeh KH, Shun CT, Chen CL, et al. High expression of thymidylate synthase is associated with the drug resistance of gastric carcinoma to high dose 5-fluorouracil-based systemic chemotherapy. *Cancer* 1998;82:1626–1631.
41. Salonga D, Danenberg KD, Johnson M, et al. Colorectal tumors responding to 5-fluorouracil have low gene expression levels of dihydropyrimidine dehydrogenase, thymidylate synthase, and thymidine phosphorylase. *Clin Cancer Res* 2000;6:1322–1327.
42. Paradiso A, Simone G, Petroni S, et al. Thymidylate synthase and p53 primary tumor expression as predictive factors for advanced colorectal cancer patients. *Br J Cancer* 2000;82:560–567.
43. Turnbull RB, Kyle K, Watson FR, Spratt J. Cancer of the colon: the influence of the no-touch isolation technique on survival rates. *Ann Surg* 1967;166:420–427.
44. Hyashi N, Egami H, Kai M, Kurusu Y, Takano S, Ogawa M. No-touch isolation technique reduced intraoperative shedding of tumor cells into the portal vein during resection of colorectal cancer. *Surgery* 1999;125:369–374.
45. Turnbull ADM, Guerra J, Starnes HF. Results of surgery for obstructing carcinomatosis of GI, pancreatic, or biliary origin. *J Clin Oncol* 1989;1989:381–386.
46. Wiggers T, Jeekel J, Arrends JW, et al. No-touch isolation technique in colon cancer: a controlled prospective trial. *Br J Surg* 1988;75:409–415.
47. Rosai J. Gross techniques in surgical pathology. In: *Ackerman's Surgical Pathology*. St. Louis, Mo.: Mosby; 1989: 13–29.

48. Rosen G. Beginnings of surgical biopsy. *Am J Surg Pathol* 1977;1:361–364.
49. Stocchi L, Nelson H. Laparoscopic colectomy for colon cancer: trial update. *J Surg Oncol* 1998;68:255–267.
50. Wexner SD, Cohen SM, Johensen OB, Nogueras JJ, Jagelman DJ. Laparoscopic colorectal surgery: a prospective assessment and current perspective. *Br J Surg* 1993;80:1602–1605.
51. Tate JJT, Kwok S, Dawson JW, Lau WY, Li AK. Prospective comparison of laparoscopic and conventional anterior resection. *Br J Surg* 1993;80:1396–1398.
52. The Clinical Outcomes of Surgical Therapy Study Group. A comparison of laparoscopically assisted and open colectomy for colon cancer. *N Engl J Med* 2004;350:2050–2059.
53. Abe N, Mori T, Takeuchi H, et al. Laparoscopic lymph node dissection after endoscopic submucosal dissection: a novel and minimally invasive approach to treating early-stage gastric cancer. *Am J Surg* 2005;190(3):496–505.
54. Kitagawa Y, Kitano S, Kubota T, et al. Minimally invasive surgery for gastric cancer—toward a confluence of two major streams: a review. *Gastric Cancer* 2005;8(2):103–110.
55. Collins G, Johnson E, Kroshus T, et al. Experience with minimally invasive esophagectomy. *Surg Endosc* 2005;20:298–301.
56. Morino M, Allaix ME, Giraudo G, Corno F, Garrone C. Laparoscopic versus open surgery for extraperitoneal rectal cancer: a prospective comparative study. *Surg Endosc* 2005;19(11):1460–1467.
57. Gunderson LL, Martin JK, Beart RW, et al. Intraoperative and external beam irradiation for locally advanced colorectal cancer. *Ann Surg* 1988;207:52–60.
58. McDermott FT, Hughes ESR, Pihl E, Johnson WR, Price AB. Local recurrence after potentially curative resection for rectal cancer in a series of 1008 patients. *Br J Surg* 1985;72:34–37.
59. Galandiuk S, Weiland HS, Moertel CG, et al. Patterns of recurrence after curative resection of carcinoma of the colon and rectum. *Surg Gynecol Obstet* 1992;174:27–32.
60. Henning GT, Schild SE, Stafford SL, et al. Results of irradiation or chemoirradiation for primary unresectable, locally recurrent, or grossly incomplete resection of gastric adenocarcinoma. *Int J Radiat Oncol Biol Phys* 2000;46:109–118.
61. Wilson LD, Chung JY, Haffty BG, Cahow EC, Sasaki CT, Son YH. Intraoperative brachytherapy, laryngopharyngoesophagectomy, and gastric transposition for patients with recurrent hypopharyngeal and cervical esophageal carcinoma. *Laryngoscope* 1998;108:1504–1508.
62. Bodner WR, Hilaris BS, Mastoras DA. Radiation therapy in pancreatic cancer: current practice and future trends. *J Clin Gastroenterol.* 2000;30:230–233.
63. Willett CG. Intraoperative radiation therapy in resected bile duct cancer. *Int J Radiat Oncol Biol Phys* 2000;46:523–524.
64. Gunderson LL, Nelson H, Martenson J, et al. Locally advanced primary and recurrent colorectal cancer—disease control and survival with IOERT containing regimens. *Int J Radiat Oncol Biol Phys* 1995;32(suppl 1):267.
65. Schild SE, Martenson JA, Jr., Gunderson LL, Dozois RR. Long-term survival and patterns of failure after postoperative radiation therapy for subtotal resected rectal adenocarcinoma. *Int J Radiat Oncol Biol Phys* 1989;16:459–463.
66. Willett CG, Shellito PC, Tepper JE, Elisio R, Convery K, Wood WC. Intraoperative electron beam therapy for primary locally advanced rectal and rectosigmoid carcinoma. *J Clin Oncol* 1991;9(5):843–849.
67. Harrison LB, Enker WE, Anderson LL. High-dose-rate intraoperative radiation therapy for colorectal cancer. *Oncology* 1995;9:737–741.
68. Farouk R, Nelson H, Gunderson LL. Aggressive multimodality treatment for locally advanced irresectable rectal cancer. *Br J Surg* 1997;84:741–749.
69. Idrees K, Minsky B, Alektiar K, et al. Surgical resection and high dose rate intraoperative radiation therapy for locally recurrent rectal cancer. *Acta Chir Iugosl* 2004;51(3):11–18.
70. Sofo L, Ratto C, Doglietto GB, et al. Intraoperative radiation therapy in treatment of rectal cancers: results of phase II study. *Dis Colon Rectum* 1996;39(12):1396–1403.
71. Ihse I, Andersson R, Ask A, Ewers SB, Lindell G, Tranberg KG. Intraoperative radiotherapy for patients with carcinoma of the pancreas. *Pancreatology* 2005;5:438–442.
72. Willett CG, Czito BG, Bendell JC, Ryan DP. Locally advanced pancreatic cancer. *J Clin Oncol* 2005;23(20):4538–4544.
73. Silberman H. Perioperative adjunctive treatment in the management of operable gastric cancer. *J Surg Oncol* 2005;90(3):174–186.
74. Moran BJ, Cecil TD. The etiology, clinical presentation, and management of pseudomyxoma peritonei. *Surg Oncol Clin N Am* 2003;12:585–603.
75. Sugarbaker PH, Jablonski KA. Prognostic features of 51 colorectal and 130 appendiceal cancer patients with peritoneal carcinomatosis treated by cytoreductive surgery and intraperitoneal chemotherapy. *Ann Surg* 1995;221:124–132.
76. Speyer JL, Collins JM, Dedrick RL, et al. Phase I and pharmacologic studies of 5-fluorouracil administered intraperitoneally. *Cancer Res* 1980;40:567–572.
77. Glehen O, Kwiatkowski F, Sugarbaker PH, et al. Cytoreductive surgery combined with perioperative intraperitoneal chemotherapy for the management of peritoneal carcinomatosis from colorectal cancer: a multi-institutional study. *J Clin Oncol* 2004;22:3284–3292.
78. Verwaal VJ, van Ruth S, de Bree E, et al. Randomized trial of cytoreduction and hyperthermic intraperitoneal chemotherapy versus systemic chemotherapy and palliative surgery in patients with peritoneal carcinomatosis of colorectal cancer. *J Clin Oncol* 2003;21:3737–3743.
79. Harmon RL, Sugarbaker PH. Prognostic indicators in peritoneal carcinomatosis from gastrointestinal cancer. *Int Semin Surg Oncol* 2005;2(1):3.
80. Seymour MT, Halstead FR, Joel SP, et al. Intravenous (IV) plus intraperitoneal (IP) adjuvant chemotherapy for colorectal cancer: a pilot study. *Proc Am Soc Clin Oncol* 2000;19:282a.
81. Scheithauer W, Kornek GV, Marczell A, et al. Combined intravenous and intraperitoneal chemotherapy with fluorouracil + leucovorin vs. fluorouracil + levamisole for adjuvant therapy of resected colon carcinoma. *Br J Cancer* 1998;77:1349–1354.
82. Vaillant J-C, Nordlinger B, Deuffic S, et al. Adjuvant intraperitoneal 5-fluorouracil in high-risk colon cancer: a multicenter phase III trial. *Ann Surg* 2000;231:449–456.
83. Loggie BW, Fleming RA, McQuellon RP, Russell GB, Griesinger KR. Cytoreductive surgery with intraperitoneal hyperthermic chemotherapy for disseminated peritoneal cancer of gastrointestinal origin. *Am Surg* 2000;66:561–568.
84. Hirose K, Katayama K, Lida A, et al. Efficacy of continuous hyperthermic peritoneal perfusion for the prophylaxis and treatment of peritoneal metastasis of advanced gastric cancer: evaluation by multivariate regression analysis. *Oncology* 1999;57:106–114.
85. Bozzetti F, Vaglini M, Deraco M. Intraperitoneal hyperthermic chemotherapy in gastric cancer: rational for a new approach. *Tumori* 1998;84:483–488.
86. Stephens AD, Alderman R, Chang D, et al. Morbidity and mortality analysis of 200 treatments with cytoreductive surgery and hyperthermic intraoperative intraperitoneal chemotherapy using the coliseum technique. *Ann Surg Oncol* 1999;6:790–796.
87. Goldberg RM, Fleming TR, Tangen CM, et al. Surgery for recurrent colon cancer: strategies for identifying resectable recurrence and success rates after resection. *Ann Intern Med* 1998;129:27–35.
88. Ravikumar TS, Steele G, Jr., Kane R, King V. Experimental and clinical observations on hepatic cryosurgery for colorectal metastases. *Cancer Res* 1991;51:6323–6327.
89. Solbiati L, Goldberg SN, Ierace T, et al. Hepatic metastases: percutaneous radiofrequency ablation with cooled-tip electrodes. *Radiology* 1997;205:367–373.
90. Livraghi T, Lazzaroni S, Pellicano S, Ravasi S, Torzilli G, Vettori C. Percutaneous ethanol injection of hepatic tumors: single session therapy with general anesthesia. *AJR Am J Roentgenol* 1993;161:1065–1069.
91. Kemeny N, Daly J, Reichman B, Geller N, Botet J, Oderman P. Intrahepatic or systemic infusion of fluorodeoxyuridine in patients with liver metastases from colorectal carcinoma. *Ann Intern Med* 1987;107:459–465.
92. Harmantas A, Rotstein LE, Langer B. Regional versus systemic chemotherapy in the treatment of colorectal carcinoma metastatic to the liver. *Cancer* 1996;78:1639–1645.
93. Meta-Analysis Group in Cancer. Reappraisal of hepatic arterial infusion in the treatment of nonresectable liver metastases from colorectal cancer. *J Natl Cancer Inst* 1996;88:252–258.
94. Bozzetti F, Bignami P, Morabito A, et al. Patterns of failure following surgical resection of colorectal cancer liver metastases. *Ann Surg* 1988;155:264–270.
95. Kemeny MM, Adak S, Lipsitz S, et al. Results of the intergroup Eastern Cooperative Oncology (ECOG) and Southwest Oncology Group (SWOG) prospective randomized study of surgery alone versus continuous hepatic artery infusion of FUDR and continuous systemic infusion of 5-FU after hepatic resection for colorectal liver metastases. *Proc Am Soc Clin Oncol* 1999;18:264a.
96. Kemeny N, Cohen A, Huang Y, et al. Randomized study of hepatic arterial infusion (HAI) and systemic chemotherapy (SYS) versus SYS alone as adjuvant therapy after resection of hepatic metastases from colorectal cancer. *Proc Am Soc Clin Oncol* 1999;18:263a.
97. Runkel NS, Schlag P, Schwarz V, Herfarth C. Outcome after emergency surgery for cancer of the large intestine. *Br J Surg* 1991;78:183–188.
98. Kelly WE, Jr., Brown PW, Lawrence W, Jr., Terz JJ. Penetrating, obstructing, and perforating carcinomas of the colon and rectum. *Arch Surg* 1981;116:381–384.
99. White CM, Macfie J. Immediate colectomy and primary anastomosis for acute obstruction of the left colon and rectum. *Dis Colon Rectum* 1985;28:155–157.
100. Mulcahy HE, Skelly MM, Husain A, O'Donoghue DP. Long-term outcome following curative surgery for malignant large bowel obstruction. *Br J Surg* 1996;83:46–50.
101. Fielding LP, Phillips RKS, Fry JS, et al. Prediction of outcome after curative resection for large bowel cancer. *Lancet.* 1986;11:904–907.
102. Woolfson RG, Jennings K, Whalen GF. Management of bowel obstruction in patients with abdominal cancer. *Arch Surg* 1997;132:1093–1097.
103. Osteen RT, Guyton S, Steele G, Jr., Wilson RE. Malignant intestinal obstruction. *Surgery* 1980;87:611–616.
104. Weiss SM, Skibber JM, Rosato FE. Bowel obstruction in cancer patients: performance status as a predictor of survival. *J Surg Oncol* 1984;25:15–17.

105. Baines M, Oliver DJ, Carter RL. Medical management of intestinal obstruction in patients with advanced malignant disease: a clinical and pathological study. *Lancet* 1985;2:990–993.
106. Steadman K, Franks A. A woman with malignant bowel obstruction who did not want to die with tubes. *Lancet* 1996;347:944.
107. Mercadante S, Ripamonti C, Casuccio A, Zecca E, Groff L. Comparison of octreotide and hyoscine butylbromide in controlling gastrointestinal symptoms due to malignant inoperable bowel obstruction. *Support Care Cancer* 2000;8:188–191.
108. Mann WJ. Surgical management of radiation enteropathy. *Surg Clin North Am* 1991;71:977–990.
109. Fischer L, Kimose HH, Spjeldnaes N, Wara P. Late radiation injuries of the small intestine-management and outcome. *Acta Chir Scand* 1989;155: 47–51.
110. Miller AR, Martenson JA, Nelson H, et al. The incidence and clinical consequences of treatment-related bowel injury. *Int J Radiat Oncol Biol Phys* 1999;43:817–825.
111. Galland RB, Spencer J. The natural history of clinically established radiation enteritis. *Lancet* 1985;8440:1257–1258.
112. Deitel M, To TB. Major intestinal complications of radiotherapy. *Arch Surg* 1987;122:1421–1424.
113. Waddell BE, Rodriguez-Bigas MA, Lee RJ, Weber TK, Petrelli NJ. Prevention of chronic radiation enteritis. *J Am Coll Surg* 1999;189:611–624.
114. Devereux DF, Chandler JJ, Eisenstat T, Zinkin L. Efficacy of an absorbable mesh in keeping the small bowel out of the human pelvis following surgery. *Dis Colon Rectum* 1988;31:17–21.
115. Rodier J, Janser J, Rodier D, et al. Prevention of radiation enteritis by an absorbable polyglycolic acid mesh sling: a 60-case multicentric study. *Cancer* 1991;68:2545–2549.
116. Swedish Rectal Cancer Trial. Improved survival with preoperative radiotherapy in resectable rectal cancer. *N Engl J Med* 1997;336(9):980–987.
117. Hyams DM, Mamounas EP, Petrelli N, et al. A clinical trial to evaluate the worth of preoperative multimodality therapy in patients with operable carcinoma of the rectum: a progress report of National Surgical Breast and Bowel Project Protocol R-03. *Dis Colon Rectum* 1997;40:131–139.
118. Winawer SJ, Zauber AG, Ho MN, et al. Prevention of colorectal cancer by colonoscopic polypectomy. *N Engl J Med* 1993;329:1977–1981.
119. Groden J, Thliveris A, Samowitz W, et al. Identification and characterization of the familial adenomatous polyposis coli gene. *Cell* 1991;66:589–600.
120. Kinzler KW, Nilbert MC, Su L-K, et al. Identification of FAP locus genes from chromosome 5Q21. *Science* 1991;253:661–665.
121. Giardiello FM, Hamilton SR, Krush AJ, et al. Treatment of colonic and rectal adenomas with sulindac in familial adenomatous polyposis. *N Engl J Med* 1993;328:1313–1316.
122. Steinbach G, Lynch PM, Phillips RK, et al. The effect of celecoxib, a cyclooxygenase-2 inhibitor, in familial adenomatous polyposis. *N Engl J Med* 2000;342:1946–1952.
123. Nugent KP, Phillips RK. Rectal cancer risk in older patients with familial adenomatous polyposis. *Br J Surg* 1992;79:1204–1206.
124. Penna D, Karthueser A, Parc R, et al. Secondary proctectomy and ileal pouch-anal anastomosis after ileorectal anastomosis for familial adenomatous polyposis. *Br J Surg* 1993;80:1621–1623.
125. Heiskanen I, Jarvinen H. Fate of the rectal stump after colectomy and ileorectal anastomosis for familial adenomatous polyposis. *Int J Colorectal Dis* 1997;12:9–13.
126. Parc YR, Moslein G, Dozois RR, Pemberton JH, Wolff BG, King JE. Familial adenomatous polyposis: results after ileal pouch-anal anastomosis in teenagers. *Dis Colon Rectum* 2000;43:893–898.
127. Lynch HT, Smyrk T. Hereditary nonpolyposis colorectal cancer (Lynch syndrome): an updated review. *Cancer* 1996;78:1149–1167.
128. Rodriguez-Bigas MA. Prophylactic colectomy for gene carriers in hereditary nonpolyposis colorectal cancer: has the time come?. *Cancer* 1996;78:199–201.
129. Lennard-Jones JE, Melville DM, Morson BC, Ritchie JK, Williams CB. Precancer and cancer in extensive ulcerative colitis: findings among 401 patients over 22 years. *Gut* 1990;31:800–806.
130. Lasher BA. Recommendations for colorectal cancer screening in ulcerative colitis: a review of research from a single university-based surveillance program. *Am J Gastroenterol* 1992;87:168–175.

CHAPTER 6 ■ GASTROINTESTINAL CANCER MANAGEMENT: BIOLOGICAL ASPECTS OF RADIATION THERAPY

H. RODNEY WITHERS

KINETICS OF RESPONSE TO IRRADIATION OF MUCOSAL TISSUES

Most of the killing of cells by irradiation results from unrepaired or misrepaired injury to their genome, causing a loss of reproductive integrity among clonogenic cells. The rate of cell death is therefore related to the turnover rate of clonogenic cells. Overt injury in rapidly proliferating tissues such as gastrointestinal mucosa, bone marrow, hair, and skin appears early after irradiation, whereas such tissue as fibrovasculature, bones, kidney, and nervous system may not manifest overt injury for months or years. However, the response of a tissue to irradiation is not only a function of rate of turnover of the clonogenic (stem) cell population but is also influenced by the lifetime of the terminally differentiated cells derived from the steady-state proliferation/differentiation activity of the clonogenic cells. For example, when irradiation or drugs sterilize clonogenic cells in the bone marrow, the supply of differentiating functional cells is suppressed, causing a fall in peripheral blood counts. Because the terminally differentiated and nondividing platelets and granulocytes have a short half-life (days), their counts drop quickly, whereas anemia develops slowly (months), reflecting the long half-life of erythrocytes.

Another factor in the development of the radiation response of a tissue is the number of mitotic divisions a lethally injured cell can negotiate before it dies. After the relatively low daily dose of about 2 Gy used in radiation therapy a lethally injured cell may undergo several antemortem divisions, slowing the rate of overt manifestation of injury.

Normal Gastrointestinal Mucosa

Clonogenic cells in the gastrointestinal mucosa are located in the crypts, the site of the most intensive cell turnover in the body. In contrast, the cells lining the villi of the small intestine are terminally differentiated and no longer divide. The mean turnover time of clonogenic cells in the crypts of the small intestine is <24 hours, while the mucosal cells spend about 4 to 7 days on the villus. Therefore, cells in the crypts die fairly rapidly after irradiation, whereas villi shrink at the slower rate determined by the rate at which differentiated cells are shed or otherwise lost (e.g., by apoptosis) from the villous surface (Fig. 6.1).

At the usual rate of dose delivery in radiation therapy to the abdomen (e.g., 1.2–2.0 Gy/session), the development of mucosal injury is slowed or completely counterbalanced by a rapid and effective regenerative response by residual (surviving) clonogenic cells (Fig. 6.1). If small bowel mucosal injury becomes evident (e.g., as diarrhea), it usually begins after about 2 weeks of treatment. Continuation of therapy is possible because of the vigorous repopulation response by surviving clonogens in the crypts. The side effect of mucosal injury to the rectum in the treatment of genitourinary and rectal cancer is proctitis, which develops during the first few weeks of treatment and subsides in a few weeks after the end of treatment, provided injury (especially ulceration) is not excessive.

The kinetics of regeneration of jejunal and colonic mucosae has been measured in experimental mice. After a brief lag period (hours or days), the surviving clonogenic crypt cells regenerate rapidly, although at the expense of a reduced output of functional cells to the luminal surface of the mucosa. Without this vigorous repopulation, the intestinal mucosa would tolerate doses less than half of those used in clinical practice. Conversely, if the effectiveness of this response is compromised, it is easily possible to exceed tolerance of the bowel (e.g., by intensifying treatment), either by increasing the rate of accumulation of radiation dose or by adding drug cytotoxicity to that of the radiation. The most common cause of increased mucosal injury in current practice is from combining radiation and chemotherapy.

Tumors

Contrary to a common perception that tumor cells are more actively dividing than their normal counterparts, the average mitotic turnover rate in gastrointestinal tumors is less than in normal mucosa. Hence, their response to radiation therapy is slower. Most tumors require many weeks for significant regression. Exophytic papillary tumors are an exception and show a much faster rate of regression than the less proliferative ulcerating tumors because they consist of a high proportion of differentiating cells with a relatively rapid rate of turnover, that is, a high rate of "natural" cell loss by differentiation.

Apoptosis occurs extensively in normal tissues and tumors, contributing to the steady-state condition of normal mucosa and slowing the growth rate of tumors. It also increases soon after irradiation and accelerates the rate of response relative to that which would characterize a tissue or tumor without evidence of apoptosis. Agents that promote apoptosis may enhance radiation responses. To be useful clinically, they should influence tumor responses more than those of normal tissues. This may not be possible in the case of the mucosa, but

69

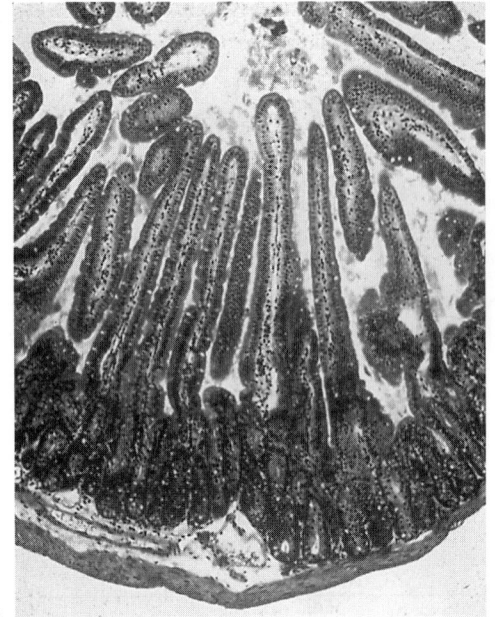

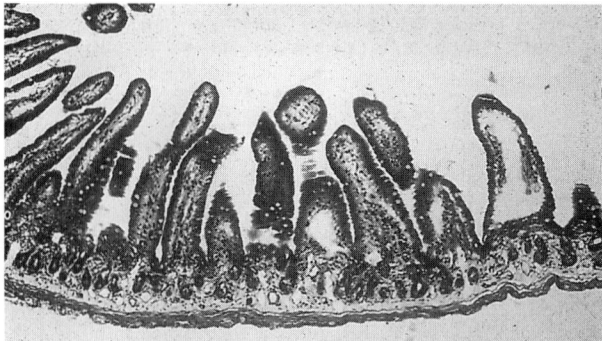

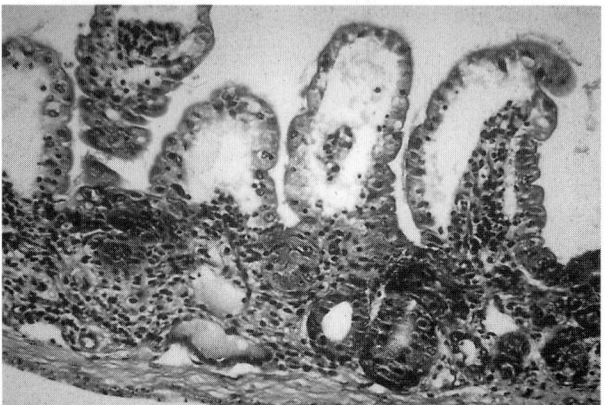

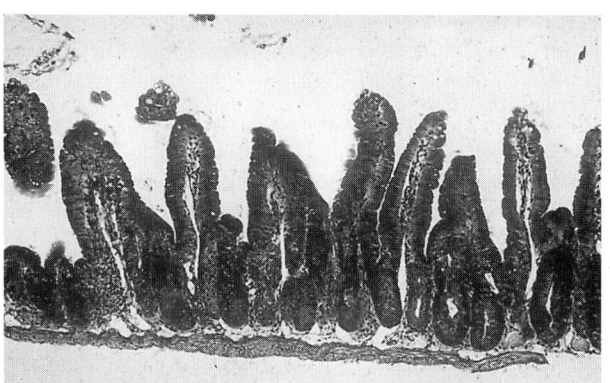

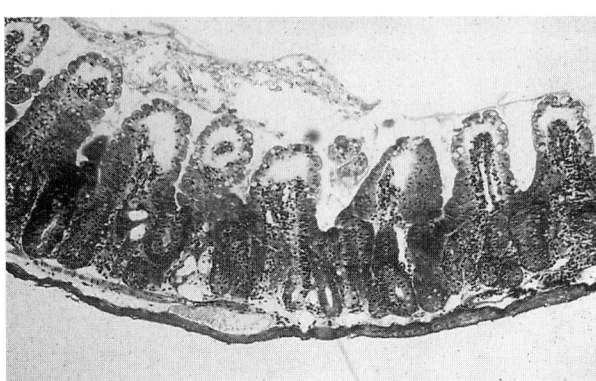

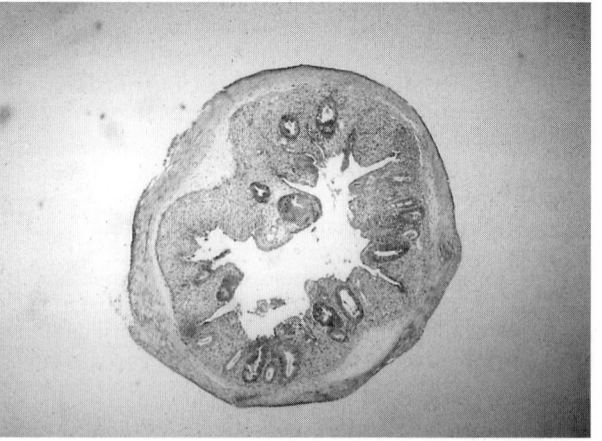

FIGURE 6.1. Histopathology of irradiated jejunum of the mouse. **A:** 0 dose, but after 4 hours of colcemid-induced mitotic blockade (in metaphase) of proliferating crypt cells Metaphases are identified by hyperchromatic nuclei raised off the basement membrane. **B:** 24 hours after a large single dose (10 Gy). Note the rapid depletion of crypt cells but little change in the number of nonproliferating cells of the villus. **C:** 72 hours after 12 Gy. The villi have shortened because of a cessation of supply of new cells from the crypt. Some crypts have been lost (no surviving clonogens), whereas others have regenerated rapidly from usually one but sometimes two or more cells that survived the irradiation. With increase in dose, there is a progressive decrease in the number of crypts in which a clonogenic cell survives. The rate of decline in the number of crypts regenerating from surviving clonogenic cells as a function of dose provides a measure of their radiosensitivity (2). **D:** 96 hours after 10 Gy. The crypts are completely regenerated and have even "overshot" their preradiation size. Migration of new cells to the villus has begun. **E:** 120 hours after 10 Gy. The villi are being reformed. **F:** Mouse descending colon 5.5 days after a high dose (13 Gy) showing regeneration of a proportion of the original 120 crypts visible within one cross-section. Each surviving crypt is derived from a single surviving clonogenic cell, providing an end point for quantifying the dose—survival relationship (radiosensitivity) and for quantifying the rate of regeneration of clonogenic cells (Fig. 6.8).

differentials in response should be achieved between a tumor undergoing extensive apoptosis and a slowly responding normal tissue in which cell turnover is slow or nonexistent and in which apoptosis is not observed.

REGENERATION AND THERAPEUTIC RATIO

The doubling times of surviving clonogenic cells in normal mucosa after a dose of 600 cGy have been measured to be as short as 8 to 12 hours in the jejunum and colon of experimental mice (1–3), and they are probably not much longer in humans. Because tumor clonogens surviving during a course of radiation therapy regrow less quickly than those of normal mucosa (4,5), a therapeutic gain is achieved by protracting treatment over several weeks. However, the small numbers of tumor clonogens surviving during the latter part of a course of radiation therapy can grow quickly. From consideration of the relative kinetics of early- and late-responding normal tissues and the average tumor, the optimal extent of protraction of treatment is the shortest in which the dose tolerated by late-responding tissues can be delivered without causing unacceptable mucosal injury. This principle applies to radiation therapy for all cancers and is also relevant to chemotherapy.

Late Injury

Bowel Wall

High doses of radiation can injure muscle and fibrovasculature of bowel wall, leading to narrowing and rigidity. These changes may reflect direct injury to connective tissue and muscle elements of the bowel wall or may be caused by scarring and contraction as a consequence of severe and/or protracted mucosal ulceration (6). In mice, complete ulceration of a 4-cm length of jejunal mucosa leads to stricture and death within 3 weeks of irradiation. This type of stricture develops too quickly to be a direct effect on muscle or fibrovasculature, and is a consequence of contraction during the healing of acute mucosal injury. More slowly developing changes in the muscle and fibrovasculature of the wall (e.g., a stricture or fistula) could be the direct result of radiation injury to the wall or could also reflect the end result of an inflammatory response to mucosal ulceration, or both.

Peritoneal Adhesions

Irradiating healthy undisturbed peritoneal surfaces does not result in the development of adhesions. However, in the presence of inflammatory processes, such as persist for weeks or months after laparotomy, or as can be induced in experimental animals by physical or chemical irritants or cytokines, irradiation has the capacity to increase the probability of small bowel obstruction from adhesions between loops of bowel (7).

The probability of this complication occurring is low until total doses exceed about 40 Gy (in 1.6–2.0 Gy fractions) but increases steeply with further escalation of dose. It also is increased when the volume of peritonealized bowel exposed to irradiation is increased (8). This "volume effect" is not an indication of increased radiosensitivity but merely reflects the greater likelihood of an obstruction occurring with the greater the length of bowel surface put at risk for adhesions (9).

Irradiated small bowel that has become entangled and restricted in its movements by adhesions becomes edematous, and its associated fragility can be of major clinical importance in surgery to relieve obstruction. Such changes are not prominent in the absence of adhesions or in the absence of irradiation.

Thus, it seems likely, although not established by investigations, that the edema in the wall of irradiated small bowel obstructed by adhesions can be caused both by radiation injury and hemo- and lymphodynamic disturbances.

Cell Killing by Radiation

Most of the cytotoxic effect of irradiation results from more pair of double-strand breaks in DNA and a consequent loss of capacity for indefinite replication. Presumably as an evolutionary requirement, cells have a great capacity to repair DNA injury, whether from radiation or chemical insult. After a dose of about 2 Gy, as used daily in a course of standard radiation therapy, about 50% of the exposed cells successfully repair sufficient damage to survive (about 2,000 single-strand DNA breaks and about 40 double-strand breaks per cell).

Some of the radiation injury to the genome results from ionizations that injure the DNA directly, but mostly it is induced by free radicals produced in the water of the cell that then damage the DNA. These events occur randomly throughout the cell and do not specifically target DNA. Structures other than DNA are also subject to injury but have greater redundancy and are less critical to the replication and survival of the cell.

Cell survival from radiation decreases geometrically (logarithmically), reflecting the random nature of the distribution of lethal ionization injury throughout a population of cells. Thus, each daily dose of 1.8 to 2.0 Gy, as commonly given in clinical practice, reduces survival of clonogenic cells by the same proportion, not the same number. For example, if 2.0 Gy reduced cell survival to 50% on day 1 of a series of treatments, it would further reduce it by 50% (i.e., to 25% of the initial number on day 2, to 12.5% of the initial number on day 3, etc.). The same sort of dose–response relationship characterizes most cytotoxic biological processes (e.g., sterilization of bacteria by antibiotics or heat, killing of cells by chemotherapy agents).

The quantitative relationship between radiation dose and cell killing has been determined in vitro and in vivo for a wide variety of normal and malignant mammalian cells. In general, the dose–survival curve reflects the addition of two types of injury. Nonrepairable or α-type injury can be envisaged as an instantaneous nonrepairable double-strand break reflecting contemporaneous and complementary single-strand breaks.

Repairable sublethal (β-type) injury reflects the accumulation and ultimately a lethal interaction between multiple individually nonlethal events (e.g., two complementary but sequential unrepaired single-strand breaks that result in a double-strand break). With nonrepairable injury, the probability of cell killing is a linear function of dose (i.e., if a dose, d, reduces survival to 50%, $2d$ would reduce it to 25%). If the coefficient for sensitivity to nonrepairable injury is α, cell survival plotted on a logarithmic ordinate as a function of dose on a linear abscissa would be described by a straight line defined by $e^{-\alpha d}$, as shown in Fig. 6.2. The curve for cell killing through the accumulation of individually sublethal injurious events (β-type injury) is continuously bending because the more sublethal radiation injury (dose) already accumulated in the cell, the greater the likelihood that an increment in sublethal injury will interact with existing injury to become lethal. As shown in Fig. 6.2, the logarithmic plot of cell survival for this type of injury bends downward with increasing dose. Over the dose range of clinical interest, this curve can be described in terms of the square of the dose–surviving fraction = $e^{-\beta d2}$, where β is the coefficient for radiosensitivity to accumulative sublethal injury. Thus, the composite curve that results from inflicting both types of cell killing is the lowermost curve in Fig. 6.2 and is described by

$$\text{Survival} = e^{-(\alpha d + \beta d2)}$$

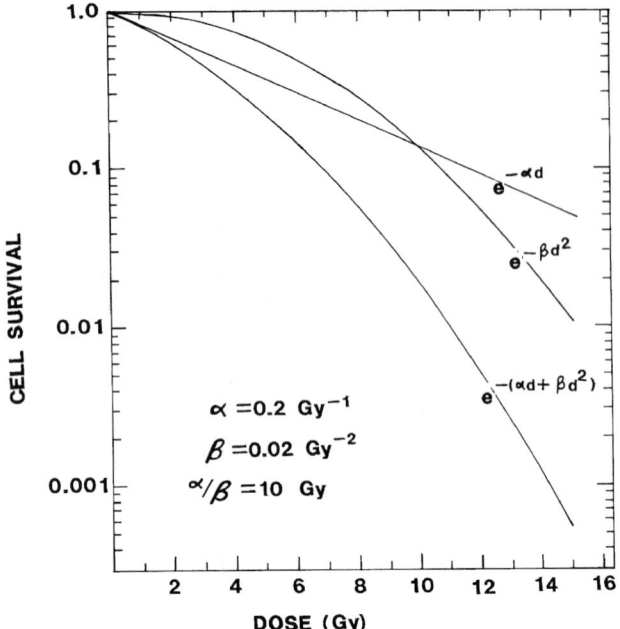

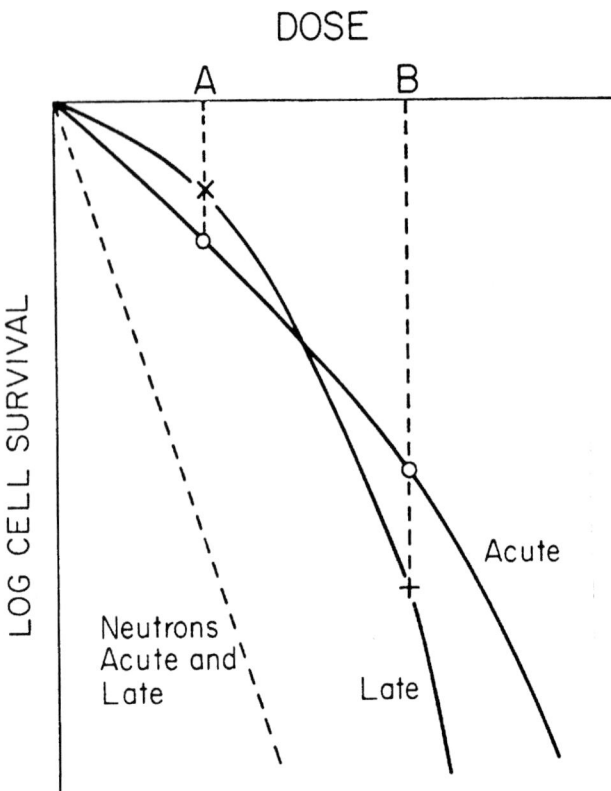

FIGURE 6.2. Dose–survival curves for x-irradiation of cells showing that the experimentally determined curve for acute exposures (lowermost) is the product of two mechanisms, single-hit nonrepairable injury described by a straight line ($e^{-\alpha d}$) with a coefficient for radiosensitivity of α, and multihit, or accumulative injury described by a continuously bending curve related by a coefficient β, to the square of the dose. The curve for single-hit killing can be measured experimentally by eliminating lethality from β-type accumulative injury through administration of doses in multiple small fractions or at a very low dose rate. The curve for multihit killing (βd^2) can be determined only indirectly from the parameters of the other two.

The higher the proportion of α- to β-type injury, the less the survival curve bends downward. For x-irradiation, acutely responding tissues exhibit a higher α/β ratio than slowly responding tissues (10,11). Exposure to densely ionizing beams such as neutrons results in a high proportion of nonrepairable injury, and the survival curve is essentially linear (i.e., the $<\alpha/\beta$ ratio is high) (Fig. 6.3).

FIGURE 6.3. Hypothetical survival curves for the target cells for acute and late effects in normal tissues exposed to x-rays or neutrons. The α/β ratio is lower for late effects than for acute effects in x-irradiated tissues, resulting in a greater change in effect in late-responding tissues with change in dose. At dose A, survival of target cells is higher in late effects than in acute effect tissues; at dose B, the reverse is true. Increasing the dose per fraction from A to B results in a relatively greater increase in late than acute injury. This is a characteristic of X-irradiation which is exploited by giving treatment as multiple small doses over several weeks. For neutrons, the α/β ratio is high with no detectable influence of the quadratic function (βd^2) over the first two decades of reduction in cell survival, implying that accumulation of sublethal injury plays a negligible role in cell killing by doses of neutrons of clinical interest.

Kinetics of Repair of Sublethal Injury

Injury which remains sublethal can be accumulated because multiple single-strand DNA breaks can be repaired rapidly by repair enzymes already existing within the cell or induced by radiation injury. The half-time for repair of sublethal injury varies among tissues. In some, it appears to be essentially complete in 3 to 4 hours, whereas in others the process may require more than 12 hours (10,12). In general, slowly dividing, late-responding tissues continue to repair sublethal injury longer than acutely responding tissues. This is important when a patient is being treated more than once per day in a "hyperfractionated" or accelerated regimen because to achieve the maximal differential in response between late-responding normal tissues and a tumor, it is necessary that repair in the normal tissue be complete before the next dose. Otherwise, incompletely repaired lesions in DNA are available for interaction with new injury from the subsequent dose (10). Because repair is generally slower in slowly or nonproliferating tissues, the effect of spacing dose fractions too closely (e.g., <6 hours) can be to selectively increase damage to the slowly repairing, late-responding normal tissues, which would then produce increased late toxicity (12).

Cell Killing by Multiple-Dose Fractions

Radiation therapy has evolved to using multiple-dose "fractions" rather than large single doses for most clinical applications. Initially, this approach was based on the observation that irradiation of the testes of experimental animals with multiple daily doses could render them infertile without evidence of desquamation of scrotal skin, whereas this was not possible with a single dose. Subsequent refinements in dose fractionation were based on empirical modifications and careful clinical evaluation of results until, more recently, an emerging body of knowledge of radiation biology has facilitated further refinements. The biological bases and the advantages of dose fractionation are discussed later in this chapter, but one of them relates to repair of sublethal injury, which is more effective, although slower, in slowly responding normal tissues than in proliferative tumors (10–13).

Provided the time interval between successive dose fractions is long enough for sublethal (β-type) injury to be completely repaired, there is no interaction of sublethal events from the two doses. Thus, the response to a subsequent dose is independent of the previous dose, and a series of equal doses each

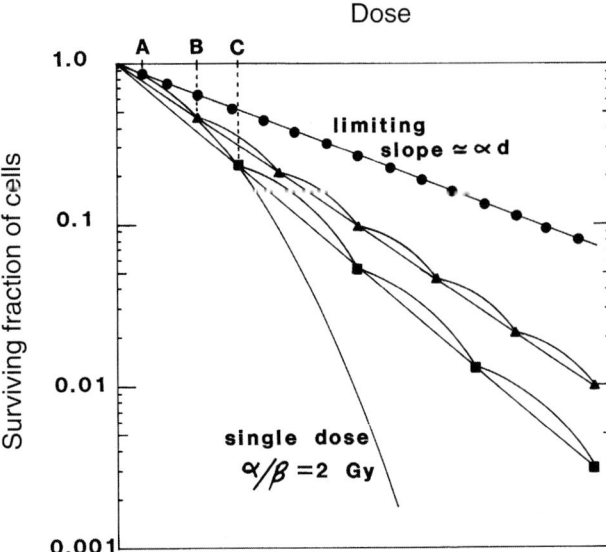

FIGURE 6.4. Multifraction dose–survival curves compared with a single-dose curve. Effective survival curves for multifraction regimens that produce an equal (proportionate) decrement in survival from each dose are linear, with shallower slopes than the single-dose curve. Slopes of the multifraction curves become less steep with decrease in fraction size until the dose per fraction is so low that multihit killing contributes negligibly and the slope is the limiting one determined by single-hit killing. The dose per fraction below which the effective survival curve becomes no shallower is a function of the efficiency of repair of sublethal injury and the curvedness of the single dose–survival curve, and, for convenience, it can be assumed to be approximately one-tenth of the α/β value. *Source:* Reprinted from ref. 27, with permission.

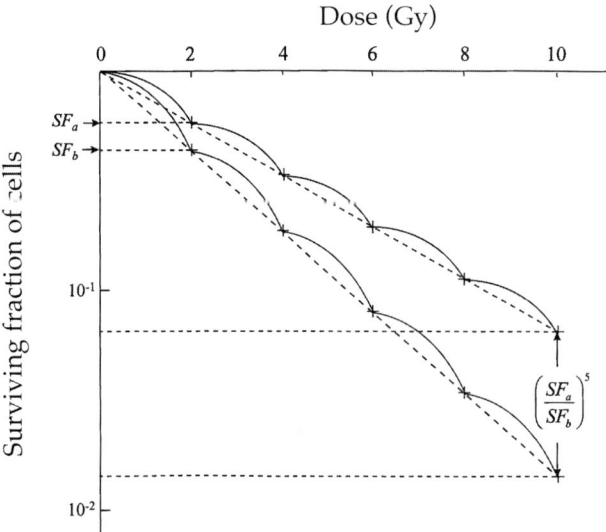

FIGURE 6.5. If the ratio of surviving fractions (*SF*) in two populations exposed to 2 Gy is SF_a/SF_b, then it is $(SF_a/SF_b)^5$ after five fractions.

produces an equal proportionate reduction in cell survival. Consequently, the "effective" survival curve for a series of equally effective dose fractions is linear with dose (Fig. 6.4). The slope of the effective survival curve reflects the shape of the shoulder of the survival curve. If it is very curvy (a low α/β ratio), there is a much greater change in survival with change in size of dose per fraction. This is illustrated by the large effect on the relative responses of the two theoretical cell populations (acute and late) shown in Fig. 6.3. If the dose per fraction is halved, from B to A, the killing of cells in the late-responding cell population changes from being greater to being less relative to that in acutely responding tissues. As a result, the reduction in severity of response, or the "sparing" effect from fractionating a dose, is much greater in tissues with a low α/β ratio. This effect is important in achieving a favorable differential between late-responding tissues, which characteristically have low α/β ratios, and tumors, the more proliferative of which have high α/β ratios (10,11,13).

The potential value from dividing a total dose into multiple smaller fractions (as shown by the curves in Fig. 6.4) is greater than it first appears from the single dose–survival curves. Although the difference in cell survival within the shoulder may be relatively small, it is amplified exponentially, as a power function of the number of dose fractions delivered (Fig. 6.5). In practice, the amplification of small differences continues beyond that from 5 fractions because curative treatments commonly involve 30 to 35 fractions, or even as many as 70 in a hyperfractionated regimen. For example, if survival from a daily dose of 2 Gy were 55% in one population of cells and 45% in another, then the ratio of survival after 35 fractions of 2 Gy (a common prescription in attempting curative treatment by x-irradiation alone) would be $(55/45)^{35} = 1,122$, that is, more than three decades on a logarithmic scale.

DOSE FRACTIONATION AND THERAPEUTIC INDEX

Radiation therapy given for cure is almost always delivered in multiple small-dose fractions, not single doses. The advantages of this in widening the therapeutic index are ascribed to the four Rs: *r*epair of sublethal injury, *r*edistribution of cells within the division cycle between dose fractions, *r*epopulation by surviving cells over the course of treatment, and *r*eoxygenation of tumor cells during fractionation intervals.

Repair

When β-type injury makes a relatively large contribution to the killing of relevant "target" cells, then repair of sublethal injury plays a large role in modifying the fractionated dose radiation response. Therefore, late-responding normal tissues, with their low α/β ratios, exhibit a relatively greater increase in radioresistance with reduction in dose per fraction than observed in proliferative tumors with a predominantly α-type response in which accumulation and repair of sublethal injury plays a relatively minor role in the dose fractionation response. This is illustrated by Figs. 6.3 to 6.5.

In general, tumors manifest an early response to irradiation and the change in total dose for an isoeffect as a function of change in size of each dose fraction resembles that in acutely responding normal tissues (13). Although this is well established for squamous cell carcinomas (14,15), it may not be true for more slowly growing tumors (e.g., prostate adenocarcinoma), which show a slow response to treatment and may characteristically have a low α/β ratio (16,17). However, for most tumors, decreasing the size of dose fractions would be expected to have little effect on their response but would permit the slowly responding normal tissues to tolerate a higher total dose. The extent of the increase in the "tolerance" dose for a certain late effect depends on the α/β ratio characterizing the fractionation response of that tissue. The lower the α/β ratio of the critical normal tissue, the greater the potential favorable differential to be gained by using smaller doses per fraction, that is, by hyperfractionation.

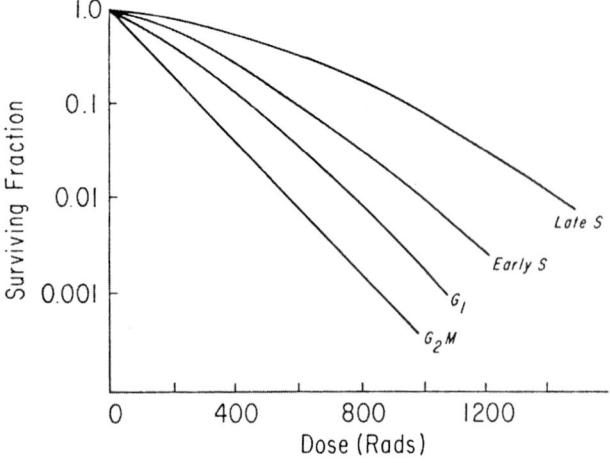

FIGURE 6.6. Radiation dose–survival curves for one line of mammalian cells (V-79 Chinese hamster) synchronized in four positions in the division cycle. Significant differences occur in the survival of cells at different stages of the mitotic cycle, with the ratios of survival being greatest at lower doses. The survival ratio between late S and G_2M cells after 2 Gy is approximately 5.

Redistribution Within the Mitotic Cycle

The radiosensitivity of cells to doses of about 2 Gy can vary by a factor of 5 or more (18) as they progress through the division cycle (Fig. 6.6). Division cycle-related fluctuations in radiosensitivity have also been demonstrated in jejunal crypt cells (19) (Fig. 6.7), which may be an important consideration in treatments combining cycle-active chemotherapy agents with radiation therapy. As the dose to an asynchronous population of cells is escalated, radiosensitive cells are rapidly and preferentially depleted, and the response to higher doses becomes

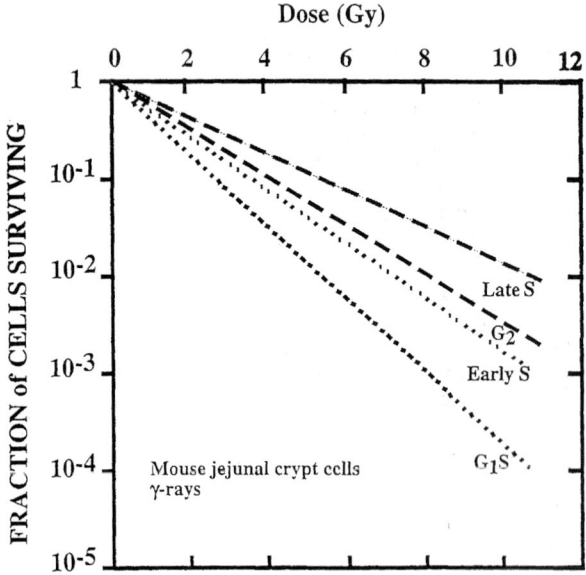

FIGURE 6.7. Curves for the "effective" radiosensitivity of jejunal crypt cells exposed to a large dose (11 Gy) of x-rays at various phases of the division cycle. The twofold range of radiosensitivities is not much less than that for the radioprotective effect of severe hypoxia and is also probably an underestimate of the ratios of survival after 2 Gy because the "true" survival curves for resistant subpopulations are more curved. *Source:* Reprinted from ref. 19, with permission.

determined by the radiosensitivity of surviving (and, therefore, relatively radioresistant) cells. If the exposure is stopped and a sufficient time interval (hours) is allowed for a proportion of the surviving, relatively radioresistant cells to progress into more sensitive phases of the mitotic cycle, a second dose can, once again, selectively eliminate cells in radiosensitive phases of the cycle without "wasting" a dose on relatively resistant subpopulations. This phenomenon of self-sensitization of a population of tumor cells through progression through the division cycle can be exploited for therapeutic gain because it will occur in tumors that are actively proliferative, but not in the slowly responding normal tissues that are commonly dose-limiting. This is another biological basis for expecting a gain from dose fractionation and additional gain from hyperfractionation.

Repopulation

Acutely responding normal tissues have a formidable capacity to regenerate themselves from surviving clonogenic cells (Fig. 6.1). The signal to initiate a regenerative response is triggered by a deficit of cells and, hence, will occur at a time after irradiation that varies with the rate of development of injury. Jejunal crypt cells are quickly depleted, in a dose-dependent manner, and a regenerative response may be initiated within 24 to 48 hours, or even sooner (Fig. 6.1). Early regeneration is also evident in colonic (Fig. 6.8) and gastric crypts, although not as promptly as in jejunum (1–3,9).

Once initiated, regeneration of clonogenic (stem) cells is rapid, reflecting a total, or near-total, shutdown of differentiation. Thus, the mean division cycle time of a regenerating crypt cell, measured by radiolabeling cell kinetics methods, is

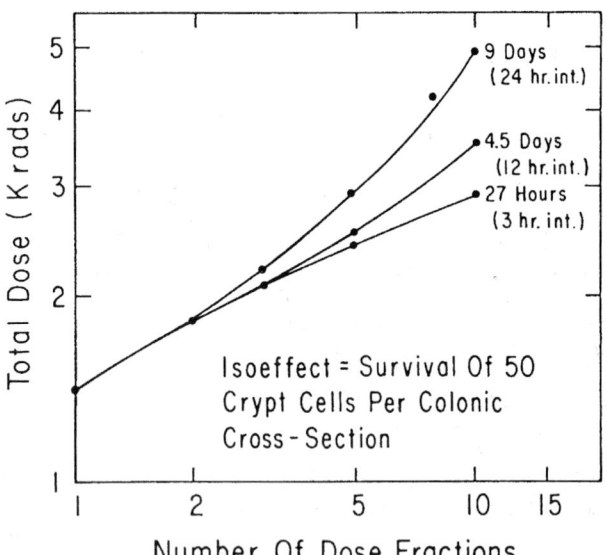

FIGURE 6.8. Total dose necessary to reduce colonic crypt cell survival to 50 per circumference of descending colon in the mouse as a function of dose fractionation. Compared with a single dose, fractionated doses given at 3-hour intervals over a period of up to 27 hours must be increased to be equally effective because of repair of sublethal damage between fractions. Increasing the interfraction interval to 12 or 24 hours introduces an additional effect from regeneration of surviving clonogenic cells within the overall treatment duration (of up to 9 days). An effect of regeneration was barely detectable when either 3 or 5 fractions were delivered over 48 hours, but when the overall time to deliver 10 fractions was extended from 27 hours to 9 days, the increment on the isoeffective dose attributable to repopulation exceeded that resulting from repair of sublethal injury.

essentially the same as the doubling time of clonogenic cells measured by clonogenic cell survival assays (i.e., about 7 to 8 hours in the mouse jejunal crypt) (1,2). This indicates that during regeneration all daughter cells retain the capacity for further mitotic divisions. These measurements of regeneration rates are also consistent with the histopathology of radiation injury, which shows that there is no migration of cells from crypt to villus until the crypt is completely regenerated, or actually regrown to a size larger than in unirradiated mucosa (Fig. 6.1).

Regeneration of colonic crypt cells is a little slower than jejunal crypt cells but is still a major factor contributing to the tolerance of the gastrointestinal tract to fractionated radiation therapy. This is illustrated for colonic mucosa in Fig. 6.8. The graph shows that when the overall duration of a 10-fraction regimen is extended to 9 days, the increment in total dose required to achieve a constant degree of crypt cell depletion is increased by about 20 Gy (2 Krads) above the increase already required from repair of sublethal injury occurring when a single dose is replaced by 10 fractions over 27 hours. Fig. 6.8 also indicates that repopulation only begins about 48 hours after the first dose and that, therefore, the regeneration that added 20 Gy to the isoeffect dose occurred during 7 days, from the second to ninth days of irradiation. This increase by almost 3 Gy/day in the dose for an isoeffect is thus more than sufficient to counterbalance the cell depletion from a daily dose fraction of 2 Gy. Although the rate of regeneration in humans is almost certainly slower than in mice, it is still a potent factor determining the tolerance of mucosa for fractionated irradiation.

Tumors also initiate a repopulation response to cytotoxic injury. In human oncology, this phenomenon has been best studied in head and neck cancer (20). After an average lag time of about 3 to 4 weeks from the start of radiation therapy, surviving tumor clonogens begin a rapid regrowth, doubling, on average, about every 3 days (Fig. 6.9). The median volume doubling time of an unirradiated head and neck tumor is 45 to 60 days (4). The 15- to 20-fold faster growth rate of clonogenic tumor cells beginning after 3 to 4 weeks of treatment is occurring in most cases when the primary tumor can still be seen to be regressing. The reason for this apparent disparity between rapid clonogen growth and a regressing tumor mass is that the repopulating clonogens are relatively few in absolute number and are scattered widely apart in a sea of sterilized but not yet resorbed tumor cells. Their growth is at the microscopic level and has no early impact on tumor volume. Rapid repopulation must occur before the end of treatment if it is to compromise the outcome of radiation and/or chemotherapy. The initiation of regeneration may be too late to influence the outcome of treatment in some more indolent tumors, such as those of prostate or breast but is likely to be a factor in most gastrointestinal cancers. The "natural" growth rate of subclinical deposits of rectal cancer is also rapid and is discussed later in this chapter.

Reoxygenation

Severe hypoxia reduces the radiosensitivity of cells by a factor of up to 3 for radiochemical, not metabolic, reasons (21) (Fig. 6.10).

The blood supply to tumors is provided by a rapidly developed system of new blood vessels, which not only provide an insufficient vascular surface area for optimal metabolite transfer but are also functionally defective in controlling blood flow. Fluctuating rates of blood flow, including stasis and insufficient capillary surface area, ensure fluctuating levels of oxygenation of tumor cells. Levels of hypoxia that reduce radiosensitivity sufficiently to pose an obstacle to eradication of tumor by irra-

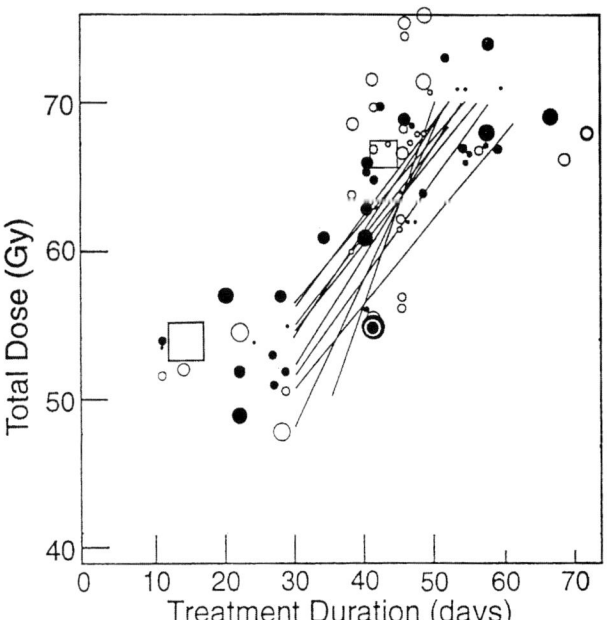

FIGURE 6.9. Doses to yield a tumor control rate of 50% (TCD$_{50}$) as a function of reported overall treatment duration estimated from results in the literature for radiation therapy of mostly T$_3$ squamous cell carcinomas of head and neck. The regression lines trace the increase in TCD$_{50}$ with time from a large series in which individual outcomes (control or failure) were known (13). The data are consistent with an average lag time of 3 to 4 weeks before the onset of regrowth of surviving tumor clonogens at an accelerated rate. The average doubling time can be calculated to be about 3 days, resulting in a loss equivalent to ~60 cGy/day in efficiency of treatment. *Source:* Reprinted from ref. 19, with permission.

diation are easily compatible with prolonged survival of tumor cells, and certainly may not always be evidenced by necrosis within the tumor.

In a manner analogous to using multiple small-dose fractions to exploit cell cycle redistribution, the threat to tumor control from fluctuating levels of oxygenation can also be circumvented by the use of multiple small-dose fractions. It is

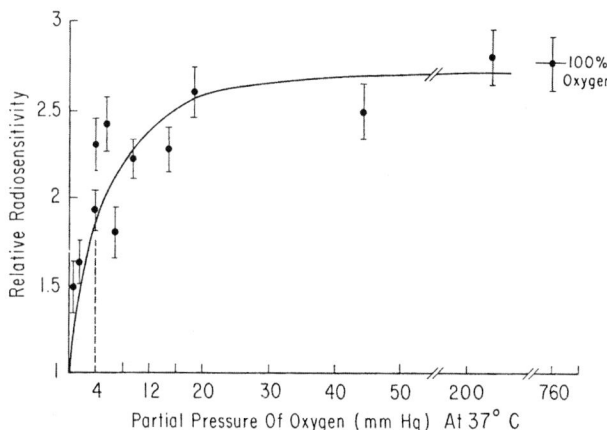

FIGURE 6.10. Curve relating cellular radiation sensitivity to partial pressure of oxygen at the time of irradiation. About one-half of the euoxic radiosensitivity (measured by the slope of a dose–survival curve) is lost at a partial pressure of 4 mm Hg, a level easily consistent with continued viability of tumor cells.

unusual for more than 10% to 30% of tumor cells to be hypoxic, even in rapidly growing mouse tumors. By using dose fractions that kill only about 50% of tumor cells (or even fewer with hyperfractionation) and interfraction intervals long enough (hours) for extensive reoxygenation of surviving cells, the elimination of the tumor can be achieved by repeatedly eroding the population of euoxic cells without the necessity for attempting to sterilize hypoxic cells (22).

Although reoxygenation during a course of fractionated radiation therapy may commonly circumvent the cure-limiting potential of hypoxic cells, there is evidence that cure rates may be enhanced by other strategies aimed at reducing the extent of hypoxia (e.g., by eliminating anemia, breathing elevated levels of oxygen, administering drugs that have the same radiochemical action as oxygen or that selectively kill hypoxic cells) (22).

TUMOR CONTROL PROBABILITY

Cure of a tumor by radiation therapy requires that no tumor clonogen survive. Cure only becomes likely when enough radiation has been delivered to sterilize a huge number of cells. For example, if a tumor contained 10^{10} (10 billion) cells, then reducing the average cell survival low enough to achieve a 90% probability of cure would require that the dose be sufficient to reduce survival to 10^{-11} (i.e., to 1 surviving cell in every 10 such tumors, with no surviving clonogenic cells in the other 9). For this reason, the curve relating tumor cure to dose, the tumor control probability (TCP) curve, has a large threshold (Fig. 6.10), its magnitude being greater the larger the number of clonogens in the tumor.

The detailed relationship of probability of cure to dose is also dictated by the random nature of cell killing. Thus, a dose that results in an average of 1 cell surviving per tumor leaves 100 surviving cells in 100 tumors, but, because of random chance, some (37%) would contain 0 surviving clonogens, the total of 100 surviving cells being distributed among the remaining 63 tumors, some with 1 cell, progressively fewer with 2, 3, 4, or even, occasionally, 5 cells. Because of the statistics of random cell killing, the rate of increase in tumor control is not abrupt but is traced by a sigmoid curve that approaches 100% asymptotically (Fig. 6.11).

Normal tissue dose responses are also described by a threshold sigmoid curve. The relative positions of the curves for tumor cure and normal tissue sequelae determine the therapeutic ratio. If the curve for normal tissue responses lies to the right of that for tumor control, as shown in Fig. 6.11, the therapeutic ratio is favorable, with tumors being cured at doses that do not result in complications, or at least with a higher rate of cure than of complications.

Determining the best trade-off between cure and complications is the art of radiation therapy. The potential gains in tumor control must be weighed against the risks of normal tissue injury. For example, the choices of A, B, or C for dose in the risk–benefit comparison illustrated in Fig. 6.11 involve consideration of many factors. Considerations that enter into the risk–benefit analysis include, but are not limited to, the historical cure rates for the particular stage of cancer, the likely incidence of distant metastases, the consequences of a complication (e.g., permanent transverse myelitis vs. temporary mucositis), and, importantly, the tolerance of the patient for complications or failure to cure. The "tolerance" for normal tissue injury depends on many variables that must be assessed by both the physician and the patient. The aim of research is to widen the separation of the curves for tumor control and normal tissue sequelae, increasing the rate of tumor control for an acceptable incidence of normal tissue sequelae.

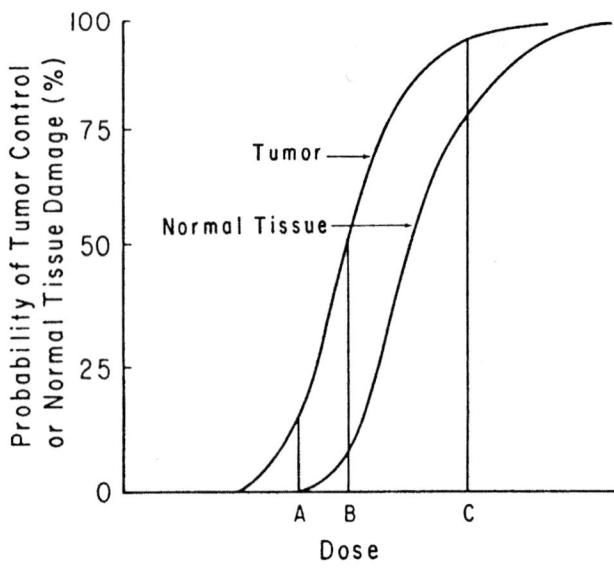

FIGURE 6.11. Tumor control probability (TCP) and the probability of normal tissue injury as a function of radiation dose in a hypothetical case in which the therapeutic ratio is "favorable" (i.e., the curve for tumor control is displaced to the left of that for normal tissue damage). Note, however, that if normal tissue injury is to be avoided altogether, the radiation dose cannot exceed A, and the TCP is low. By accepting a relatively small probability of normal tissue injury, the radiation dose can be increased to B, and the TCP is significantly improved. Further increase of radiation dose above C, when the TCP is ~90%, results in an increased complication rate with little improvement in TCP. In clinical practice, the choice among doses A, B, and C would rest on the acceptability of the normal tissue injury. As examples, dose A would be appropriate when considering radiation myelitis, dose B for soft tissue necrosis, and dose C for localized lung fibrosis. Although the curves in this figure for the probabilities of tumor control and normal tissue damage have been drawn parallel, they may vary in slope, but the general sigmoid shape is the same. *Source:* Reprinted from ref. 27, with permission.

Modification of Tumor Control Probability Curves

The dose–response curves derived from clinical data are less steep than those predicted using reasonable radiobiology parameters (23). This results from the considerable heterogeneity in biological characteristics among a series of tumors and in the biological effectiveness of physical dose prescriptions. Such heterogeneity increases the variation in the responses of both normal tissues and tumors, which leads to shallower dose–response curves. Characteristically, the curves for tumor control probability are less steep than those for sequelae in normal tissues.

Clonogen Number

A major source of uncertainty in predicting tumor responses is the uncertainty in the number of tumor clonogens requiring sterilization. If the tumor burden is large, the curves will be shifted to the right, if small, to the left, and for a mixture of large and small tumor cell burdens, the curve will be shallow, the measured curve beginning to rise at the threshold of the curve for small volume tumors but not approaching 100% until the upper end of the curve relevant to large-volume tumors. (An extreme example of this is shown in Fig. 6.13 and is discussed later in this chapter.) The extent of the variability in clonogen number per tumor is evident when, within one T stage, tumor volumes can vary by a factor of 10 or more. Another example is that a 2-cm diameter nodal deposit contains 64 times as many cells as a 0.5-cm deposit. (Volume of a sphere is a function of r^3.) In addition to variability in tumor volume, which for any one type of tumor is a reasonable surrogate for tumor cell number, there is variability in the proportion of tumor cells that have clonogenic capacity. Many cells in a tumor may be on a pathway to terminal differentiation and "natural" death, and do not require sterilization. Finally, a proportion of the tumor volume is composed of normal host cells and stroma, and this may vary.

Radiosensitivity

There is mounting evidence for variations in tumor cell radiosensitivity between tumor types and for tumors of the same histology in different individuals (13,16,17,24–26). As discussed previously, small differences in sensitivity to low doses (within the shoulder of the survival curve) can be amplified to rather large differences after treatment with repeated dose fractions. Thus, even small variability in radiosensitivity among tumors has a significant effect on the total doses required for tumor control. This variability in total dose required for cure contributes to a shallow dose–response curve for tumor control.

Regeneration

Accelerated tumor growth during a protracted course of treatment increases the number of tumor clonogens requiring sterilization. If the surviving tumor clonogens doubled every 3 days during the latter 3 weeks of treatment, as they do, for example, in irradiated squamous cell carcinomas of head and neck (14,15,20), the effective number of cells to be eradicated would increase by a factor 2^7 (as the result of seven doublings). This roughly 100-fold increase in cell number is equivalent, for example, to about a 2- or even 3-unit increase in T stage.

Other Causes for Variability in Dose–Response

Many other factors can affect the outcome of a course of radiotherapy. Each will influence the threshold and/or slope of the TCP curve. Examples of tumor-related phenomena are heterogeneity of oxygenation and reoxygenation kinetics. Treatment-related influences include the dose fractionation pattern, inhomogeneity of dose distribution within the tumor, and adjuvant chemotherapy.

As a result of the addition and interaction of these potential variables, the slopes of TCP curves determined from analysis of clinical data are relatively shallow (10,23). In the idealized situation, where all variables were strictly controlled, the probability of tumor cure would increase by about 10% per Gy over the range of 10% to 90% probability of tumor control. In fact, the steepest rate of increase in clinical studies is about 3% per Gy, and commonly, it is as low as about 1% to 2% per Gy (23,27–30).

TREATMENT OF SUBCLINICAL DISEASE

The aim of curative treatment is to achieve a constant high probability of tumor elimination throughout the whole target volume. This does not require that the dose be homogeneously distributed in that volume because the density of clonogenic infestation is variable. Higher doses are required to eliminate the primary tumor bulk than to sterilize microscopic subclinical extensions along tissue planes or lymphatics.

The aims of treatment are achieved by one of two basic approaches. The shrinking field or boost dose technique is used when radiation therapy is not used in conjunction with surgery.

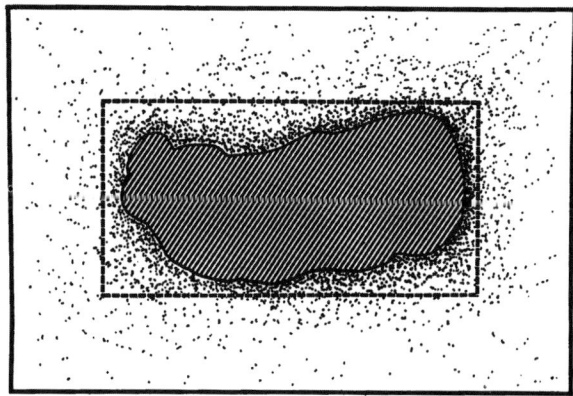

- - - - **Plane of excision**
——— **Radiotherapy field widely around gross tumor**

FIGURE 6.12. Diagram illustrating the advantages of combining surgery with radiation therapy and also of the shrinking field technique for radiation therapy alone. Conservative surgery can remove primary tumors while subclinical spread can be controlled by relatively low doses of radiation. If surgery is not performed, the large radiation treatment field can be reduced after a dose sufficient to control subclinical disease and a higher dose concentrated in the larger number of cells in the primary mass. If a tumor extends to the proposed surgical margins (e.g. a T_4 rectal cancer attached to a pelvic wall), a preoperative field covering the lymphatic drainage can be shrunk to boost the dose to the region at risk of recurrence following "cut-through". But if the primary is likely to be easily removed (e.g. T_3N_+ rectal cancer), the aim of preoperative radiation concentrates on sterilizing subclinical tumor infiltrates in tissues and lymphatics beyond the proposed surgical margins, contraindicating the use of a shrinking field (35). In the postoperative setting, centripetal contraction of surgical margins may justify the use of a boost dose through a shrunken field. *Source:* Reprinted from ref. 27, with permission.

Subclinical extensions receive, say, 50 Gy in 2-Gy fractions, after which the volume being irradiated is reduced in one or two stages to deliver higher doses to the primary tumor, the latter part of treatment being "conformal," as accurately as possible, to the primary tumor (Fig. 6.12). This maximizes dose to the densest mass of tumor cells and minimizes the volume of normal tissue exposed to high doses. In principle, the doses for the large treatment volume (subclinical disease) and the boost volumes (primary tumor) should be tailored to yield a constant probability of tumor control. For example, if there were 10^7 cells in the volume of subclinical spread and 10^{10} cells in the primary tumor bulk, the dose distribution required to yield a constant 90% probability of control throughout the whole irradiated volume would be that which reduced tumor clonogen survival to 10^{-8} and 10^{-11} in the subclinical disease volume and primary tumor, respectively. Because the effective survival curve for a regimen of multiple equal-dose fractions is linear for a logarithmic reduction in cell number, the isoeffective doses for the primary and subclinical disease (i.e., the doses to achieve a certain constant probability of tumor eradication throughout the total irradiated volume) should be in the ratio of 11/8 in this example.

The second generic technique is to remove the primary tumor surgically using less than radical methods, leaving only subclinical disease that can be eliminated by lower doses of radiation than would be necessary to control the primary if it were still in place. This eliminates the need for a high radiation dose to sterilize the primary tumor, the total dose to be administered being adjusted to achieve a high rate of elimination of the smaller (subclinical) burden of clonogenic tumor cells. This paradigm needs to be modified if surgery only "debulked" the tumor, leaving a macroscopically detectable residuum. For example, removal of 50% of the primary tumor only reduces the necessary dose by about 2 Gy, the dose that would kill approximately 50% of the cells in the original primary tumor. If it is assumed that 7 Gy of a 2 Gy per fraction regimen reduces tumor clonogen survival to 10%, then a 90% debulking reduces the needed dose by about 7 Gy and a 99% debulking by about 14 Gy.

Radiobiologically, surgical removal of abdominal or pelvic tumors is better performed after radiation therapy to avoid delay in irradiating subclinical tumor deposits, which may grow quickly, and to permit treatment of peritoneum and small bowel before a peritoneal inflammatory response is initiated by surgery.

The concern that metastases may be shed during preoperative radiation therapy is unfounded. Most metastases arise only when tumors are relatively large, as evidenced by the low incidence of metastases from small primary tumors. Within 1 week of the start of a regimen of 2-Gy fractions, clonogenic tumor cell survival is <5% of the starting number (even though the tumor volume may have shown little regression). Thus, the risk that new metastases will arise from a primary tumor during preoperative irradiation is markedly decreased by each successive dose of radiation, beginning on the first day, and being negligible from a 20-fold lower number of clonogenic cells, as would be the case after the first 5 days of treatment.

Dose−Response for Subclinical Metastases

A major role of radiation therapy in gastrointestinal oncology is as an adjuvant to surgery and the therapy is aimed at eliminating residual subclinical tumor deposits. For purposes of considering the treatment of subclinical regional metastases, there are three groups of patients:

- Those in whom removal of the primary tumor is curative (i.e., they harbor no subclinical metastases) and adjuvant therapy is of no value (even though it is usually given because of the lack of means to positively establish freedom from subclinical metastases).
- Those who present with established, clinically detectable metastases. Assuming the lower limit of detectability to be 10^9 tumor clonogens, the metastatic cell burden is this group exceeds 10^9. (Choosing values different from 10^9 by factors of 10 or 100 has little effect on the conclusions to be drawn.) In most cases, adjuvant therapy tolerated by abdominal organs is of no lasting value.
- Those without evidence of metastases but who will develop regional metastases later. Logically, if these metastases grow exponentially, the metastatic cell burden (measured logarithmically) should be evenly distributed between 1 and 10^9 cells. The simplest initial assumption is that 11% of patients in this category harbor between 1 and 10 cells, another 11% harbor between 10 and 100 cells, and so forth, the final 11% harboring between 10^8 and 10^9 cells. In this scenario, the first 11% would be cured of their metastases by a dose that would reduce metastatic cell numbers by a factor of 10 (i.e., by one common logarithm) to 10^{-1}. A second 11% would be cured by reducing metastatic cell burden to 10^{-2} (1%) and so forth; the final cohort requiring that metastatic cell survival be reduced to 10^{-9} to have a chance of cure. Thus, the tumor control probability curve for subclinical metastases is the sum of the TCP curves for each of the nine cohorts discussed previously and would rise linearly with dose with no significant threshold (Fig. 6.13) (31,32).

The clinical implications of a nonthreshold linear dose response are completely different from those of the threshold-sigmoid curve relevant to macroscopic tumors (32). For ex-

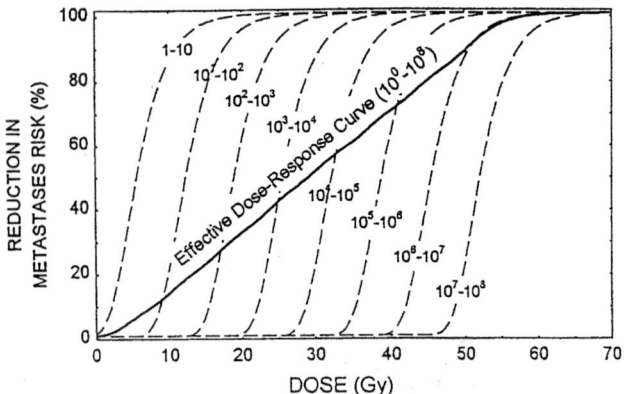

FIGURE 6.13. If there is an even distribution of the logarithm of metastatic cell burden of between 1 and 10^n, the effective dose−response curve shows a minimal threshold and is essentially linear with dose. In this figure, 10^n is assumed to be 10^8, and a series of dose−response curves are depicted to illustrate how the effective dose−response curve is a composite derived from assuming equal numbers of patients having the specified metastatic cell burdens (e.g., 1–10^8). This figure also illustrates how the assumed value of 10^n would not significantly affect the analysis if values for n ranged over even three decades (e.g., 10^7–10^{10}). *Source:* Reprinted from ref. 31, with permission.

ample, although fairly high doses are required to achieve high rates of control of subclinical deposits, the use of a lower dose, if necessary, would still reduce the incidence of metastases. In contrast, reducing the dose used to treat macroscopic tumors quickly leads to certain failure at doses below the threshold. For example, it is common to use a dose of 50 to 60 Gy in 2-Gy fractions for treating areas at risk for harboring subclinical metastases (27), but such a high dose could not be given in total abdominal irradiation as an adjunct to surgery for ovarian cancer because it would lead to a high rate of small bowel obstruction. A more tolerable dose of 30 Gy reduced the incidence of upper abdominal metastases by about 40% (33).

Growth of Subclinical Metastases and Tumor Control Probability

The linear, nonthreshold dose−response curve postulated for cure of subclinical disease will be lost if such deposits grow in the interval between surgery and the start of postoperative radiation therapy, or during the course of a fractionated regimen of treatment. Growth of microscopic deposits after removal of the primary tumor will result in a shift in the distribution of metastatic cell burden to higher values and the proportions of patients with small numbers of cells will decrease at a rate depending on the average growth rate of micrometastases. Such growth before or during treatment shifts the dose−response curve to the right and introduces a threshold. Conversely, the shift of the dose−response curve and the size of the threshold can be used to measure the growth rate of micrometastatic disease.

TCP curves from an analysis of the literature on pelvic recurrence rates following preoperative radiation therapy for rectal cancer (5) provide evidence on the growth rates of subclinical tumor deposits outside the subsequent surgical margins (Fig. 6.14). Although there are limitations in the conclusions to be drawn from retrospective analysis of literature reports, the rate of increase in pelvic recurrence rates with extension of the overall duration of preoperative radiation therapy is consistent with a fast growth rate of pelvic micrometastases. The best estimate of a doubling time is about 4 days (5). This growth

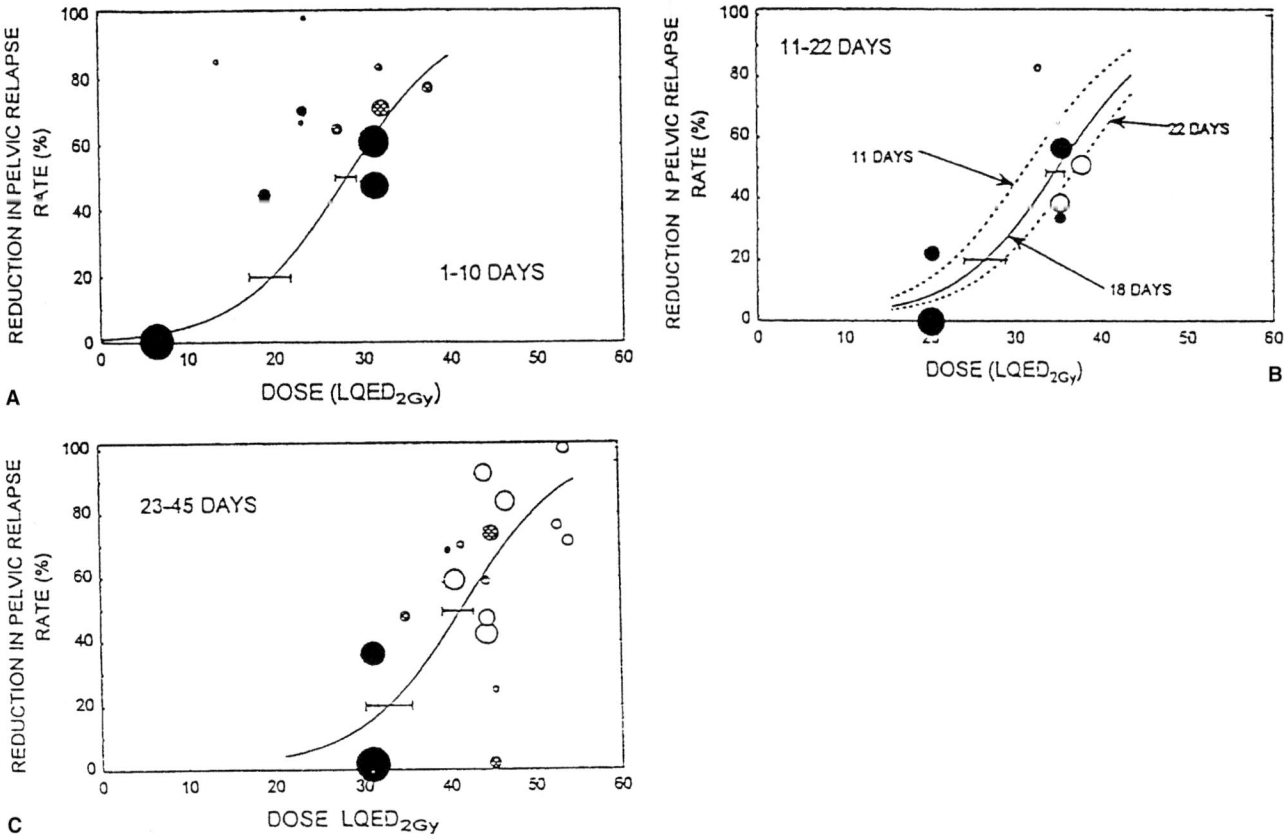

FIGURE 6.14. Reduction in pelvic relapse rate after preoperative radiotherapy for rectal cancer as a function of $LQED_{2Gy}$ (total dose normalized to its equivalent in 2-Gy fractions using an α/β value of 10 Gy). Open circles indicate studies lacking control groups (without XRT). Circles with a grid indicate studies with historical controls. Black circles indicate randomized trials. The area of the circle is proportional to the number of patients in the combined XRT and surgery groups. The curves are predicted by a statistical model fit to the entire data set. The horizontal bars indicate estimated $LQED_{2Gy}20\%$ and $LQED_{2Gy}50\%$ values with 95% confidence interval. **A:** Data for overall radiation treatment time shorter than 11 days, the curve being that predicted for an overall radiation treatment time of 5 days. **B:** Data for overall radiation treatment between 11 and 24 days. Curves are shown for 18 days and for both extremes of the grouping time (11 and 22 days) to illustrate that the choice of treatment days at which curves are shown is unimportant, all results being derived from the whole data set. **C:** Data for overall radiation treatment time longer than 24 days, the curve being that predicted for an overall radiation treatment time of 30 days. *Source:* Adapted from ref. 5.

rate is similar to the doubling rate of surviving clonogenic cells in squamous cell carcinomas of the head and neck (14,15,20) or cervix (34) late in a course of radiation therapy. In both instances, the growth rate is that characteristic of deposits of small numbers of tumor cells. In the pelvis, the residual rectal cancer cells presumably exist in small aggregates in lymphatics, lymph nodes, or fat, whereas in irradiated head and neck or cervix cancer, the surviving squamous cell clonogens are scattered as single cells in a sea of lethally injured cells undergoing lysis in a regressing primary tumor.

The clinical implications of such a rapid growth rate of micrometastatic tumor deposits are not widely appreciated. Clearly, delays in initiating adjuvant radiation or chemotherapy for subclinical tumor extension should be avoided, and the intensity of treatment should be as high as tolerated by normal tissues. Contrary to the urgency to initiate and complete neoadjuvant therapy (to minimize the probability of pelvic recurrence) is the lack of urgency for postradiation surgery. The lack of urgency reflects the inevitability of recurrence if the surgical excision does not encompass all residual tumor clonogens, regardless of whether there is just a single clonogenic surviving cell immediately after the last dose of chemoradiation or a larger regrown focus a few weeks later. Furthermore, there is the potential benefit from a better chance of sphincter

preservation by allowing a few weeks for cytotoxicity-induced regression of low-lying primary tumors (35). (These advantages are not available in postoperative chemoradiation because regrowth of residual tumor in the gap between surgery and irradiation will clearly render control more difficult, and the sphincter is already gone if it needed to be.)

ACKNOWLEDGMENTS

The authors thank Drs. Bill McBride, Steve Lee, Karin Haustermans, and Rafael Suwinski for their input, and Ms. Jan Haas for her help in preparing the manuscript.

References

1. Withers HR, Chu AM, Reid BO, Hussey DH. Response of mouse jejunum to multifraction radiation. *Int J Radiat Oncol Biol Phys* 1975;1:41–52.
2. Withers HR, Elkind MM. Radiosensitivity and fractionation response of crypt cells of mouse jejunum. *Radiat Res* 1969;38:598–613.
3. Withers HR, Mason KA. The kinetics of recovery in irradiated colonic mucosa of the mouse. *Cancer* 1974;34:896–903.
4. Steel GG. *Growth Kinetics of Tumours.* New York, NY: Oxford University Press; 1977.

5. Suwinski R, Taylor JMG, Withers HR. Rapid growth of microscopic rectal cancer as a determinant of response to preoperative adjuvant therapy. *Int J Radiat Oncol Biol Phys* 1998;42:943–951.

6. Bourne RG, Kearsley J, Groves WD, Roberts SJ. The relationship of early and late gastrointestinal complications of radiation for carcinoma of the cervix. *Int J Radiat Oncol Biol Phys* 1983;9:1445–1450.

7. McBride WH, Mason, KA, Davis CA, Withers HR, Smathers JB. Adhesion formation in experimental chronic radiation enteropathy. *Int J Radiat Oncol Biol Phys* 1989;16:737–743.

8. Gallagher MJ, Brereton HD, Rostock RA, et al. A prospective study of treatment techniques to minimize the volume of pelvic small bowel with reduction of acute and late effects associated with pelvic irradiation. *Int J Radiat Oncol Biol Phys* 1986;12:1565–1573.

9. Withers HR, McBride WH. Biologic basis of radiation therapy. In: Perez C, Brady L, eds. *Principles and Practice of Radiation Oncology*. Lippincott & Raven; 1997:79–118.

10. Thames HD, Hendry JH. *Fractionation in Radiotherapy*. London: Taylor & Francis; 1987.

11. Thames HD, Jr., Withers HR, Peters LJ, Fletcher GH. Changes in early and late radiation responses with altered dose fractionation: implications for dose–survival relationships. *Int J Radiat Oncol Biol Phys* 1982;8:219–226.

12. Ang KK, Jiang GL, Guttenberger R, et al. Impact of spinal cord repair kinetics on the practice of altered fractionation schedules. *Radiother Oncol* 1992;25:287.

13. Williams MV, Denekamp J, Fowler, JF. A review of $\alpha\beta$ ratios for experimental tumors. *Int J Radiat Biol Phys* 1985;11:87–96.

14. Maciejewski B, Withers HR, Taylor JMG, Hliniak A. Dose fractionation and regeneration in radiotherapy for cancer of the oral cavity and oropharynx. Part I. Tumor dose–response and repopulation. *Int J Radiat Oncol Biol Phys* 1989;16:831–843.

15. Withers HR, Peters LJ, Taylor JMG, et al. Local control of carcinoma of the tonsil by radiation therapy: an analysis of patterns of fractionation in nine institutions. *Int J Radiat Oncol Biol Phys* 1995;33:549–562.

16. Brenner D, Hall EJ. Fractionation and protraction for radiotherapy of prostate carcinoma. *Int J Radiat Oncol Biol Phys* 1999;43:1095–1101.

17. Duchesne GM, Peters LJ. What is the alpha/beta ratio for prostate cancer? Rationale for hypofractionated high-dose-rate brachytherapy [editorial]. *Int J Radiat Oncol Biol Phys* 1999;44:747–748.

18. Sinclair WK. Dependence of radiosensitivities upon cell age. In: *Time and Dose Relationships in Radiation Biology as Applied to Radiotherapy*. Brookhaven National Lab Report 50203 (C-57). 1969;97.

19. Withers HR. Radiation biology and treatment options in radiation oncology. *Cancer Res* 1999;59(suppl):1676s–1684s.

20. Withers HR, Taylor JMG, Maciejewski B. The hazard of accelerated tumor clonogen repopulation during radiotherapy. *Acta Oncol* 1988;27:131–146.

21. Deschner EE, Gray LH. Influence of oxygen tension on x-ray-induced chromosomal damage in Ehrlich ascites tumor cells irradiated in vitro and in vivo. *Radiat Res* 1959;11:115–122.

22. Brown JM, Giaccia AJ. The unique physiology of solid tumors: opportunities (and problems) for cancer therapy. *Cancer Res* 1998;58:1408–1416.

23. Okunieff P, Morgan D, Niemierko A, Suit HD. Radiation dose—response of human tumors. *Intl J Radiat Oncol Biol Phys* 1995;32:1227–1237.

24. Brock WA, Baker SL, Peters LJ. Radiosensitivity of human head and neck squamous cell carcinomas in primary cultures and its potential as a predictive assay of tumor radiocurability. *Int J Radiat Biol* 1989;56:751–760.

25. Deacon J, Peckham MJ, Steel GG. The radioresponsiveness of human tumors and the initial slope of the cell survival curve. *Radiother Oncol* 1984;2:317–323.

26. Peters LJ, Brock WA. Cellular radiosensitivity as predictors of treatment outcome: where do we start? [editorial; comment]. *Intl J Radiat Oncol Biol Phys* 1993;25(1):147–148; discussion 153.

27. Fletcher GH. *Textbook of Radiotherapy*. Philadelphia, Pa.: Lea & Febiger; 1980.

28. Fu KF, Pajak TF, Trotti A, et al. A Radiation Therapy Oncology Group (RTOG) phase III randomized study to compare hyperfractionation and two variants of accelerated fractionation to standard fractionation radiotherapy for head and neck and squamous cell carcinomas. *Intl J Radiat Oncol Biol Phys* In press.

29. Horiot JC, LeFur R, Nguyen T, et al. Hyperfractionation versus conventional fractionation in oropharyngeal carcinoma: final analysis of a randomized trial of the EORTC cooperative group of radiotherapy. *Radiother Oncol* 1992;25:231–240.

30. Zelefsky MJ, Leibel SA, Gaudin PB, et al. Dose escalation with three-dimensional conformal radiation therapy affects the outcome in prostate cancer. *Int J Radiat Oncol Biol Phys* 1998;41:491–500.

31. Withers HR, Suwinski R. Radiation dose response for subclinical metastases. *Semin Radiat Oncol* 1998;8:224–228.

32. Withers HR, Peters LJ, Taylor JMG. Dose response relationships for radiation therapy of subclinical disease. *Int J Radiat Oncol Biol Phys* 1995;31:353–359.

33. Dembo AJ, Davy M, Stenwig AE, Berle EJ, Bush RS, Kjorstad K. Prognostic factors in patients with stage I epithelial ovarian cancer. *Obstet Gynecol* 1990;75:263–273.

34. Fyles A, Keane TJ, Barton M, Simm J. The effect of treatment duration in the local control of cervix cancer. *Radiother Oncol* 1992;25:273–279.

35. Withers HR, Haustermans K. Where next with preoperative radiation therapy for rectal cancer? *Int J Radiat Oncol Biol Phys* 2004;58:597–602.

CHAPTER 7 ■ GASTROINTESTINAL CANCER: MEDICAL ONCOLOGY

TIMOTHY ASMIS AND MANISH A. SHAH

INTRODUCTION

A medical oncologist is a physician who uses medicines to treat cancer. Because the medical therapy of cancer is still a relatively modern occurrence, the field of medical oncology is a relatively new subspecialty of internal medicine. With increasing treatment options and increased complexity of care, the treatment of solid tumor malignancies has evolved into a team approach involving surgical, radiation, and medical oncologists, as well as diagnostic colleagues in radiology and pathology. Often, the medical oncologist will be responsible for the coordination of this care. In this chapter, the role of medical oncology as it pertains to gastrointestinal (GI) malignancies is reviewed.

HISTORY OF MEDICAL ONCOLOGY

Before the mid-20th century, the curative treatment of cancer was primarily carried out by the surgeon and the radiation oncologist. Indeed, the first cancer operations were performed several hundred years ago and expanded greatly with the development of ether anesthesia in the 19th century. However, following World War II, the therapeutic options expanded when two pharmacists (Goodman and Gilman) commissioned by the U.S. Department of Defense identified potential antineoplastic uses of nitrogen mustard (1). Specifically, from autopsies of people exposed to mustard gas during the First World War, physicians noted severe myeloid and lymphoid suppression. This led to their initial hypothesis that this chemical class may be active to treat myeloid and lymphoid malignancies, which they then tested in a mouse model of lymphoma. This ultimately led to the first treatment of a patient with non-Hodgkin lymphoma in 1946, where they observed a dramatic but transient reduction in size of the patient's tumor masses (1). This proof-of-principal clinical experiment introduced the concept of the pharmacologic therapy of malignancy. In 1958, the seminal publication by Hertz et al. first described the curative benefit of chemotherapy in the treatment of trophoblastic tumors in women (2). Even in this early report, the tenets that define medical oncology today were readily apparent. Specifically, these first medical oncologists were required to balance the potential benefits of medical therapy with its toxic side effects. They concluded that the curative effects of cytotoxic chemotherapy in solid tumors outweighed the risks, stating that "although the chemotherapeutic regimen is somewhat hazardous, the morbidity and mortality may be regarded as acceptable" (2). This publication marks the inauguration of the field of medical oncology. Over the past several decades, in parallel to the improvements in understanding the biology of malignancy, there has been an explosion in the discovery of new chemotherapy, hormonal, and targeted therapies, and an expansion of the role of the medical oncologist in the medical therapy of malignancy.

In 1972, medical oncology was designated as a specialty by the American Board of Internal Medicine, 7 years after the formation of the American Society of Clinical Oncology (ASCO) (3). The creation of medical oncology as a specialty largely resulted from the efforts of the society, which first coined the term "medical oncologist." Many credit the leadership of Arnoldus Goudsmit, MD, PhD, whose vision and leadership mobilized internists to take an active role in the treatment of cancer. Dr. Goudsmit and his colleagues sought to create an organization dedicated to expanding the knowledge of ways to improve survival with cancer chemotherapy, educating physicians in the safe uses of chemotherapy, and improving access of patients to quality cancer care. At the time of its creation in 1965, ASCO was comprised of 7 founding members (4). The society has since grown into an international organization of more than 20,000 members devoted to all aspects of cancer care.

Medical oncology is a subspecialty of internal medicine. Physicians who are pursuing a career in medical oncology first train and certify in internal medicine (5). On completion of an internal medicine residency, an aspiring medical oncologist will then complete a 2- to 3-year fellowship (6). In the early 1970 s, the scope of medical oncology, as defined by the American Board of Internal Medicine, included several areas of cancer: etiology, diagnosis, prevention, patient management, epidemiology, host effects, tumor biology, investigation, orientation, detection, and gerontology (7). Even a cursory glance of this list reveals that the medical oncologist is concerned with the total management of the cancer patient. Over the past several decades, there has been a rapid increase in the armamentarium of treatments that medical oncologists have in their arsenal. This unprecedented upsurge in new therapies and the increased complexity of multidisciplinary care has necessitated the further subspecialization of medical oncology to several disease types. This chapter focuses on the implications of the total management of the cancer patient in the modern era of subspecialized care focusing on the role of medical oncology for GI malignancies.

SCOPE AND SIGNIFICANCE

GI malignancies include a wide variety of cancers throughout the GI tract, with varying epidemiology, tumor biology, and treatments. Together, these cancers are the most common group of cancers worldwide, accounting for more than 30% of the global burden of cancer, surpassing lung, prostate, and breast cancer (8). Table 7.1 provides summary statistics of the common GI malignancies. In terms of new cancer diagnoses,

TABLE 7.1

WORLDWIDE SUMMARY STATISTICS OF THE COMMON GASTROINTESTINAL MALIGNANCIES

| | Incidence | | | | |
	Males	Females	Total	Worldwide rank	Median survival[a]
Colon/rectum	550,465	472,687	1,023,152	3	18–24 mo
Stomach	603,419	330,518	933,937	4	8–10 mo
Liver	442,119	184,043	626,162	6	4–6 mo
Esophagus	315,394	146,723	462,117	8	8–10 mo
Pancreas	124,841	107,465	232,306	13	4–6 mo
GI Total	2,036,238	1,241,436	3,277,674		
Total (all sites but skin)	5,801,839	5,060,657	10,862,496		

[a]Various sources—see text.
From ref. 8.

4 of the top 10 cancers worldwide are GI malignancies (8). As discussed later in this book, the epidemiologies of these cancers vary greatly. For example, liver cancer is associated with a significant male predominance of almost 3:1, whereas for colorectal and pancreatic cancers, females are almost as likely to develop the disease as males (1.16:1). Two-thirds of new cases of stomach cancer occur in developing countries, although the incidence is among the highest in an industrialized nation—Japan (8). GI malignancies affect people without regard to age, gender, race, or health status and together, unfortunately, have the highest case mortality. Except for colorectal cancer and squamous cell carcinoma of the anus, median survival for advanced disease for most GI malignancies is <1 year. Thus, the treatment of GI malignancies poses several challenges: They are prevalent, aggressive, and nondiscriminatory. The unique challenge of GI medical oncology is that the physician must become familiar with a wide range of malignant disease processes, each with its own unique epidemiology, biology, and treatment.

INITIAL EVALUATION

The medical oncologist must confirm and document whether a patient has a cancer, define the organ/tissue of origin, determine the extent of spread of the disease (staging), and assess the patient's therapeutic options. A patient will meet with a medical oncologist as a result of a referral: (a) for a cancer documented by biopsy or surgical procedure, (b) for the suspicion of malignant disease given clinical or laboratory abnormalities, and (c) because the patient has an increased risk of developing a specific neoplasm as a result of genetic or familial factors. In all three scenarios, the medical oncologist must decide whether he or she has sufficient information to adequately assign stage, determine an estimate of curability or ability to palliate, assess the patient's fitness to tolerate therapy, and design the optimal course of therapy.

Cancer Staging and Localized Disease

The primary function of staging a malignancy is to coordinate optimal care in the context of the prognostic information implied by the stage. For GI malignancies, localized disease is often treated with surgery as the primary modality in order to achieve maximum cytoreduction with the goal of long-term survival. The addition of chemotherapy or chemoradi-

ation is often used to treat microscopic disease to reduce the chance of recurrence. The GI medical oncologist often coordinates this additional "adjuvant" therapy. In GI oncology, there are two notable exceptions where chemotherapy and radiation are used as the primary curative treatment modality: the treatment of localized squamous cell carcinoma of the anus (9) and esophageal carcinoma (10). In the case of anal cancer, the use of chemotherapy with radiation as the primary treatment results in long-term survival in more than 90% of patients and the avoidance of a colostomy in approximately 85% of patients. In the case of esophageal cancer, which is a highly lethal malignancy, the surgical treatment carries a high morbidity and mortality, and patients often develop recurrent disease despite optimal surgery. Definitive chemoradiation is a standard care treatment option. This is an attractive option because chemotherapy augments the antitumor effects of the radiation while treating micrometastatic disease. In the seminal randomized trial performed by the Radiation Therapy Oncology Group, patients with locally advanced esophageal cancer not amenable to surgery were randomly assigned to receive radiation or chemotherapy with radiation. The combination of chemotherapy with radiation resulted in a 5-year survival of 27% as compared to 0% in those who received only radiation (11). These promising results rival those seen with treatment that involves surgery, as discussed later in this book.

In summary, on staging a malignancy, localized GI cancers will often undergo surgical resection, but a multidisciplinary approach is essential to providing the maximum chance of long-term survival and minimizing treatment mortality and morbidity. This multidisciplinary team is often coordinated by the GI medical oncologist—the physician who is perhaps most familiar with the morbidity and mortality of the surgical care, radiation, and medical care of the disease in the context of the individual patient with his or her specific comorbidities.

Advanced Disease

Conversely, when GI malignancies have metastasized, treatment is considered "palliative" because the goal of therapy may not be curative but rather to improve quality and length of life (12). When a patient has a very low chance of eradication of the cancer, both the physician and the patient must be confident that the benefits of treatment outweigh its risk and toxicity. In tailoring therapy to an individual patient, a medical oncologist must be an expert in medical health and disease. The presence of comorbid conditions will affect cancer risk, detection, progression, and treatment (13). For example, the metabolic syndrome of obesity and glucose intolerance is associated with increased mortality of GI cancers (14). Because there is often a choice of effective systemic therapy for GI cancers, comorbid conditions can influence the treatment selection in order to minimize serious toxicity. For example, oxaliplatin and docetaxel are associated with a severe sensory neuropathy in 10% to 15% of patients (15,16), and would therefore be contraindicated in a patient with a preexisting severe neuropathy. Certain comorbid conditions are specific to GI malignancies. Hepatocellular carcinoma usually arises in the presence of liver cirrhosis, and as discussed in later chapters, the severity of the cirrhosis relates closely to their morbidity and mortality, as well as the patient's ability to tolerate therapy (17). The medical oncologist must be able to identify comorbid conditions and customize therapy to minimize toxicity and maximize benefit to the patient.

Thus, the medical oncologist must be familiar with the nature and extent of the patient's disease, its estimated natural history and progression, the risks and benefits of proposed therapies, the possibility of participating in clinical trials, and the potential impact of cancer treatment on the patient's family. When a patient begins a course of systemic therapy, he or she forms a close partnership with the medical oncologist. This partnership is necessary to effectively care for the patient both physically and emotionally. From coping with the initial diagnosis to understanding the treatment plan to the highs and lows of treatment success and failure, a medical oncologist is uniquely positioned to assist the patient on his or her journey with cancer.

Another important role of the medical oncologist is as a communicator with patients and their families. A cancer diagnosis is often overwhelming for patients. Accordingly, when an individual is diagnosed with a GI malignancy, the medical oncologist must discuss many issues with the patient in an effective and compassionate manner. As mentioned previously, the medical oncologist must obtain essential information in order to select the best therapy for the patient as an individual. This information includes the patient's burden of other chronic illnesses, extent of disease, familial risk of cancer, and general fitness to determine whether he or she can tolerate systemic therapy. In turn, the medical oncologist must convey crucial information to the patient that will allow him or her to make an informed decision about treatment and to be prepared for the journey that lies ahead.

COORDINATION OF THERAPY

The medical oncologist must balance many factors in deciding the type, dose, and timing of systemic therapy for patients with curative GI malignancies. For example, medical comorbidities and recovery from surgery as measured by wound healing, maintenance of adequate caloric intake, and normal bowel function are all considered prior to initiation of adjuvant chemotherapy for colorectal cancer. There are few data on the optimal timing of the initiation of adjuvant therapy, although some studies observe that patients who initiate adjuvant therapy more than 2 to 3 months following surgery have a worse prognosis than initiating adjuvant therapy earlier (18,19). In one study, for example, increased age and more medical comorbid conditions increased the interval from surgery to initiation of adjuvant chemotherapy for colorectal cancer, and this was in turn associated with shorter duration of therapy and worse prognosis (18).

Coordination of treatment may be best illustrated for patients with localized gastroesophageal junction (GEJ) cancer, in which overlapping data support at least three different standard care options. One option involves neoadjuvant chemotherapy followed by surgery and then postoperative chemotherapy, with the chemotherapy combination of epirubicin, cisplatin, and fluorouracil infusion in patients with resectable gastric/GEJ cancer (20). One of the most important benefits of initiating therapy prior to surgery is that most patients will be able to receive systemic therapy initially. Following surgery, a significant number of patients are unable to receive adjuvant therapy (20). A principal disadvantage of neoadjuvant therapy is the possibility that the patient may not respond to systemic therapy or may progress prior to resection. Identifying response early in the treatment plan by functional imaging, or predicting response to therapy prior to initiation of therapy (e.g., by expression analysis), is an active area of research.

An alternative approach for the treatment of locally advanced gastric and GEJ cancers is surgical resection of the malignancy followed by adjuvant chemoradiation (21). By using this strategy, patients with locally advanced disease who are fit enough following resection, as measured by maintaining their weight and returning to an adequate performance status, will undergo a 4-month course of combined chemotherapy with radiation. Adjuvant therapy is associated with an approximate equivalent benefit in improvement of 3-year survival as compared to perioperative chemotherapy per the MAGIC study. A significant proportion of patients may not be able to receive therapy due to surgical morbidity. Moreover, chemoradiation is associated with moderate toxicity of nausea, vomiting, dehydration, and myelosuppression. An important consideration is also the irreversible kidney damage, with external beam radiation of approximately 80% of the left and 20% of the right kidney when delivered in a standard fashion (22).

A third standard care option in the treatment of GEJ cancers is definitive concurrent use of chemotherapy with radiation (10). With this approach, there may be increased localized toxicity (i.e., esophagitis, dysphagia in the GEJ example) and an inability to eradicate the localized disease (i.e., approximately 50% in the GEJ example) (23).

The medical oncologist considers many factors when deciding the preferred approach. Neoadjuvant chemotherapy involves the use of a more intensive chemotherapy regimen, including epirubicin, cisplatin, and fluorouracil, as compared to the 5-FU/LV administered in the adjuvant setting. A patient may have underlying comorbidity that precludes the use of cisplatin. For example, patients with hearing difficulty at diagnosis are more likely to develop severe hearing loss with moderate to high-dose cisplatin use (24). Thus, these patients may be better served by directly undergoing surgical resection followed by adjuvant chemoradiation, which does not require cisplatin. Another example in which the use of cisplatin would result in unacceptable toxicity would be in a patient with preexisting diabetic neuropathy, whereby the cisplatin would likely exacerbate the neurotoxicity (25). Alternatively, postoperative radiation may not be the preferred approach when a patient's kidney function is marginal or relies heavily on the left kidney.

There are many examples where the medical oncologist must weigh many factors of the patient's health when designing the most appropriate treatment strategy to treat a specific cancer.

MANAGEMENT OF SIDE EFFECTS OF THERAPY

Once a patient has initiated systemic therapy, the medical oncologist must prescribe appropriate supportive medications, including antiemetics, antidiarrheals, and possibly hematologic support factors. Supportive medications decrease side effects and improve the patient's quality of life while receiving systemic therapy, thereby allowing patients to receive therapy as an outpatient in a timely manner. Other than the use of supportive medications, treatment strategies to reduce the cumulative toxicity have also been developed. For example, the treatment of metastatic colorectal cancer (mCRC) with oxaliplatin is often complicated by severe neuropathy. This often leads to the discontinuation of the oxaliplatin while the patient is still responding to therapy. The Optimox 1 study was performed in order to establish the efficacy of intermittent administration of oxaliplatin and to attempt to reduce the severe neuropathy (26). This consisted of randomizing patients with mCRC to receiving either 5-FU/LV or oxaliplatin (FOLFOX) chemotherapy until evidence of disease progression/unacceptable toxicity or FOLFOX for 6 cycles, followed by 12 cycles of 5-FU/LV, and then reintroducing the oxaliplatin. The investigators found that intermittent dosing of oxaliplatin could be administered with similar efficacy in terms of overall survival and progression-free survival, while greatly reducing the extent of neurotoxicity. This demonstrated that a strategy of limiting the use of oxaliplatin can result in obtaining the same palliative benefit, while improving the patient's quality of life in terms of a reduction in distressing toxicity.

PALLIATIVE THERAPY

Management of the Symptoms of the Cancer

The medical oncologist also plays a crucial role in the management of the symptoms of cancer and end-of-life care. At least 50% of patients who are diagnosed with a GI malignancy will eventually die as a direct result of their cancer (27). Patients with GI malignancies have unique palliative care issues given the anatomical location of the disease and pattern of spread. For example, patients with advanced GI cancers often experience nausea, weight loss, pain, and bowel obstruction (28). Nutritional support with total parenteral nutrition may be an appropriate palliative measure in patients with a failure of the GI tract, but this benefit may not outweigh the risks of this intervention (29). The gastroenterologist will also perform palliative stenting procedures when a patient has a large bowel (30) or esophageal obstruction (31). Furthermore, approximately 90% of patients with advanced pancreatic cancer will experience intense abdominal discomfort. The medical oncologist must be able to recognize these symptoms and request the assistance of an anesthetist to perform a neurolytic celiac plexus block that decreases pain, thereby reducing narcotic requirements (32). In the setting of metastatic carcinoid tumor, hepatic arterial embolization is an effective palliative intervention (33). Once again, the medical oncologist must decide when this therapy is appropriate on a case-by-case basis. In summary, although the medical oncologist does not perform these procedures, he or she must be familiar with palliative interventions specific to GI malignancies and be able to coordinate these with allied medical specialists in order to improve the patient's quality and length of life.

The medical oncologist may also be charged with the task of the commencement of palliative care. Palliative care is defined as interdisciplinary care that is focused on the relief of suffering (34). One aspect of palliative care is the management of cancer-related pain in which the medical oncologist will prescribe appropriate analgesic medication and anxiolytics. The medical oncologist is also responsible for the transition from active therapy with systemic therapy to best supportive care. For a patient to benefit from hospice care, the referral must be made at least a few weeks prior to the patient's death. Most experts recommend 2 months (35). Many have observed that hospice care has been underutilized because cancer treatment has become more aggressive over time (36). This may be because patients are reluctant to "give up" or because the medical oncologist has overestimated the prognosis (37). The debate about when hospice care is appropriate is ongoing and illustrates that cancer treatment is both an "art" and a "science."

CLINICAL RESEARCH

The field of medical oncology is still in its infancy. With the improvements in our understanding of disease biology and with the concomitant explosion of new drugs, an ever-increasing role of the medical oncologist will be in clinical research. All medical oncologists, regardless of their practice setting, must be familiar with the interpretation of clinical trial results. This is essential to daily practice because the clinician must be able to rapidly incorporate the vast amount of new trial results into his or her daily practice in order to provide optimal care.

The development of new systemic therapies begins with pre-clinical evaluation, usually in culture and in animal models (38). The clinical evaluation of a new chemotherapeutic is initiated in phases. Each phase of clinical development is distinct with respect to its goals, required number of patients, and randomization. The primary end point of a phase I study is usually to determine the maximum dose that an agent can be safely administered in a limited number of patients with a diverse group of cancers. In phase II trials, patients with the same malignancy are evaluated with the primary goal of determining clinical efficacy and to further evaluate the safety of the study agent. The phase III trial is the largest of the three phases and is where patients with a defined malignancy are randomized between two groups—usually, one group receiving a standard treatment and the other receiving the new investigational treatment. The primary objective of a phase III clinical trial is to determine the superiority of one treatment over the other. Often, phase III studies can establish a new standard of care and are necessary for the registration of a new agent with regulatory agencies, such as the U.S. Food and Drug Administration or the European Union. The ethics of performing a random assignment study require clinical equipoise—the belief that the best treatment option for the patient is not clear and that it is reasonably possible that the investigational arm is as good as or superior to the current standard of care. If the research question is feasible, the results of the trial will provide a clinically meaningful benefit to patients and move the field forward. Although challenging to complete (39), a randomized controlled trial is the best way to establish the standard of care.

GLOBAL HEALTH CARE

As the complexity of cancer care continues to increase, so do the costs associated with the care (40). Between 1990 and 2004, the national cancer treatment expenditures rose from $27.1 to $72.1 billion in the United States, with an estimated $10 to $15 billion spent on screening in 2004 (41). As the indications for systemic therapy have expanded widely since the late 1990s, the costs associated with standard of care systemic therapy have also increased dramatically (42). For example, the cost for adjuvant FOLFOX 4 compared to 5-FU/LV for the treatment of stage III CRC is $29,000 versus $6,500 US, respectively. Although new discoveries and the use of new systemic therapy have undoubtedly improved both a patient's chance for survival and his or her quality of life with malignancy, they have come with an increase in financial cost. Besides the clinical benefits of new, higher-priced therapy, it may prove to be cost effective if it is able to prevent the use of possibly more expensive therapy at relapse or progression of disease. The medical oncologist will be called on in the future to balance patients' needs, as well as patients' and insurers' ability and willingness to fund increasingly more expensive cancer therapy (43).

The medical oncologist acts as a coordinator. As discussed previously, the effective treatment of GI malignancies depends on a multidisciplinary approach. This is particularly true of GI malignancies, where both curative and palliative treatments involve multiple disciplines, including medical, radiation, surgical oncology, pathology, radiology, and palliative care. The coordination of this team has become a de facto role of the medical oncologist, in part because of their clinical experience as internists and because of the frequency of their interaction with the patient. Optimally, the GI medical oncologist enjoys a close, collegial relationship with other allied consultants and meets with them regularly in multidisciplinary tumor board conferences. As new technologies emerge, the coordination is often the role of the medical oncologist. Examples of these include the timing of radiofrequency ablation of metastatic liver lesions, the use of positron emission tomography scans, and the use of microarray DNA analysis.

The medical oncologist is an educator. Educating physicians, surgeons, medical students, and residents about the diagnosis and treatment of cancer, as well as the special issues of cancer survivors, is extremely important. Not only is there a need for more clinical practitioners of medical oncology, but the next generation of researchers also needs to be trained. Both trainees and those in the allied health fields must be involved in the diagnosis, management, and treatment of GI cancers. GI malignancies are complex diseases, and the standard of care is constantly evolving. Despite published guidelines, there remain large gaps between community "real world" practice and the standard of care/routine practice (44). This can only improve as more members of the treatment team become involved in education and collaboration. Medical oncologists must also participate in the continued medical education of fellow clinicians because of the ongoing difficulties in coordinating care, even when national guidelines are instituted.

CONCLUSION

The role of the GI medical oncologist is evolving. As systemic therapy becomes more effective, more agents are being approved for an ever-expanding number of indications in patients with GI malignancies. As a result, the role of the GI medical oncologist continues to expand. For example, prior to 1990 and the adoption of routine adjuvant systemic therapy in the treatment of colon cancer (45), a medical oncologist would only offer palliative systemic therapy to patients with metastatic disease. There is now compelling evidence that adjuvant chemotherapy increases survival in colon, rectal, gastric, esophageal, and pancreatic cancers. Thus, most of these patients should be referred to a medical oncologist either prior to, or closely after, the surgical treatment.

The clinical demands of medical oncologists have significantly increased. There are now multiple effective systemic therapies in the metastatic setting that has increased the life expectancy of patients. Patients need to be followed closely by medical oncologists, and undergo intensive monitoring of their quality of life and of the disease response to therapy. The increase in the complexity of care, coupled with the expected rise in GI cancer incidence among the aging population (46), may compromise the ability to provide quality cancer care without a concomitant increase in GI medical oncologists (47).

With the rapid expansion of therapeutic options that have translated into improved patient outcomes, there has never been a more exciting time to be involved in GI medical on-

cology. But this optimism is tempered by the reality that the achievements outlined in this text have been modest, and much more work is required in the development of effective multidisciplinary treatments for GI cancers.

References

1. Goodman LS, Wintrobe MM, Dameshek W, et al. Nitrogen mustard therapy. Use of of methyl-bis (beta-chloroethyl)amine hydrochloride and tris(beta-chloroethyl)amine hydrochloride for Hodgkin's disease, lymphosarcoma, leukemia, and certain allied miscellaneous disorders. *JAMA* 1946;105:475–476. (Reprinted in JAMA 1984;1251:2255–1961)
2. Hertz R, Bergenstal DM, Lipsett MB, et al. Chemotherapy of choriocarcinoma and related trophoblastic tumors in women. *JAMA* 1958;168:845–854.
3. Kennedy BJ. Origin and evolution of medical oncology. *Lancet* 1999;354 Suppl:SIV41.
4. Krueger GM, Alexander LL, Whippen DA, et al. Arnoldus Goudsmit, MD, PhD: chemotherapist, visionary, founder of the American Society of Clinical Oncology, 1909–2005. *J Clin Oncol* 2006;24:4033–4036.
5. Muss HB, Von Roenn J, Damon LE, et al. ACCO: ASCO core curriculum outline. *J Clin Oncol* 2005;23:2049–2077.
6. Hansen HH, Bajorin DF, Muss HB, et al. Recommendations for a global core curriculum in medical oncology. *J Clin Oncol* 2004;22:4616–4625.
7. Kennedy BJ, Calabresi P, Carbone P, et al. Training program in medical oncology. *Ann Intern Med* 1973;78:127–130.
8. Parkin DM, Bray F, Ferlay J, et al. Global cancer statistics, 2002. *CA Cancer J Clin* 2005;55:74–108.
9. Nigro ND, Vaitkevicius VK, Considine B, Jr. Combined therapy for cancer of the anal canal: a preliminary report. *Dis Colon Rectum* 1974;17:354–356.
10. Herskovic A, Martz K, al-Sarraf M, et al. Combined chemotherapy and radiotherapy compared with radiotherapy alone in patients with cancer of the esophagus. *N Engl J Med* 1992;326:1593–1598.
11. Cooper JS, Guo MD, Herskovic A, et al. Chemoradiotherapy of locally advanced esophageal cancer: long-term follow-up of a prospective randomized trial (RTOG 85-01). Radiation Therapy Oncology Group. *JAMA* 1999;281:1623–1627.
12. Porzsolt F, Tannock I. Goals of palliative cancer therapy. *J Clin Oncol* 1993;11:378–381.
13. Extermann M. Interaction between comorbidity and cancer. *Cancer Control* 2007;14:13–22.
14. Calle EE, Rodriguez C, Walker-Thurmond K, et al. Overweight, obesity, and mortality from cancer in a prospectively studied cohort of U.S. adults. *N Engl J Med* 2003;348:1625–1638.
15. Andre T, Boni C, Mounedji-Boudiaf L, et al. Oxaliplatin, Fluorouracil, and Leucovorin as Adjuvant Treatment for Colon Cancer. *N Engl J Med* 2004;350:2343–2351.
16. Van Cutsem E, Moiseyenko VM, Tjulandin S, et al. Phase III Study of Docetaxel and Cisplatin Plus Fluorouracil Compared With Cisplatin and Fluorouracil As First-Line Therapy for Advanced Gastric Cancer: A Report of the V325 Study Group. *J Clin Oncol* 2006;24:4991–4997.
17. Burroughs A, Hochhauser D, Meyer T. Systemic treatment and liver transplantation for hepatocellular carcinoma: two ends of the therapeutic spectrum. *Lancet Oncol* 2004;5:409–418.
18. Hershman D, Hall MJ, Wang X, et al. Timing of adjuvant chemotherapy initiation after surgery for stage III colon cancer. *Cancer* 2006;107:2581–2588.
19. Chau I, Cunningham D. Adjuvant therapy in colon cancer—what, when, and how? *Ann Oncol* 2006;17:1347–1359.
20. Cunningham D, Allum WH, Stenning SP, et al. Perioperative chemotherapy versus surgery alone for resectable gastroesophageal cancer. *N Engl J Med* 2006;355:11–20.
21. Macdonald JS, Smalley SR, Benedetti J, et al. Chemoradiotherapy after surgery compared with surgery alone for adenocarcinoma of the stomach or gastroesophageal junction. *N Engl J Med* 2001;345:725–730.
22. Wieland P, Dobler B, Mai S, et al. IMRT for postoperative treatment of gastric cancer: covering large target volumes in the upper abdomen: a comparison of a step-and-shoot and an arc therapy approach. *Int J Radiat Oncol Biol Phys* 2004;59:1236–1244.
23. Minsky BD, Pajak TF, Ginsberg RJ, et al. INT 0123 (Radiation Therapy Oncology Group 94-05) phase III trial of combined-modality therapy for esophageal cancer: high-dose versus standard-dose radiation therapy. *J Clin Oncol* 2002;20:1167–1174.
24. Nagy JL, Adelstein DJ, Newman CW, et al. Cisplatin ototoxicity: the importance of baseline audiometry. *Am J Clin Oncol* 1999;22:305–308.
25. von Schlippe M, Fowler CJ, Harland SJ. Cisplatin neurotoxicity in the treatment of metastatic germ cell tumour: time course and prognosis. *Br J Cancer* 2001;85:823–826.
26. Tournigand C, Cervantes A, Figer A, et al. OPTIMOX1: a randomized study of FOLFOX4 or FOLFOX7 with oxaliplatin in a stop-and-Go fashion in advanced colorectal cancer—a GERCOR study. *J Clin Oncol* 2006;24:394–400.

27. Jemal A, Siegel R, Ward E, et al. Cancer statistics, 2007. *CA Cancer J Clin* 2007;57:43–66.
28. Maguire P, Walsh S, Jeacock J, et al. Physical and psychological needs of patients dying from colo-rectal cancer. *Palliat Med* 1999;13:45–50.
29. Abrahm J. *Nutritional Support in Patients with Esophageal and Gastric Cancers: Defining Appropriate Management and Intervention Gastrointestinal Cancers Symposium.* Orlando, FL: ASCO; 2007.
30. Harris GJ, Senagore AJ, Lavery IC, et al. The management of neoplastic colorectal obstruction with colonic endolumenal stenting devices. *Am J Surg* 2001;181:499–506.
31. Lambert R. Treatment of esophagogastric tumors. *Endoscopy* 2003;35:118–126.
32. Yan BM, Myers RP. Neurolytic Celiac Plexus Block for Pain Control in Unresectable Pancreatic Cancer. *Am J Gastroenterol* 2007;102:430–438.
33. Gupta S, Johnson MM, Murthy R, et al. Hepatic arterial embolization and chemoembolization for the treatment of patients with metastatic neuroendocrine tumors: variables affecting response rates and survival. *Cancer* 2005;104:1590–1602.
34. Abrahm JL. Update in palliative medicine and end-of-life care. *Ann Rev Med* 2003;54:53–72.
35. McCarthy EP, Burns RB, Ngo-Metzger Q, et al. Hospice use among Medicare managed care and fee-for-service patients dying with cancer. *JAMA* 2003;289:2238–2245.
36. Earle CC, Neville BA, Landrum MB, et al. Trends in the aggressiveness of cancer care near the end of life. *J Clin Oncol* 2004;22:315–321.
37. Christakis NA, Lamont EB. Extent and determinants of error in doctors' prognoses in terminally ill patients: prospective cohort study. *BMJ (Clin Res Ed)* 2000;320:469–472.
38. Dent SF, Eisenhauer EA. Phase I trial design: are new methodologies being put into practice? *Ann Oncol* 1996;7:561–566.
39. Ross S, Grant A, Counsell C, et al. Barriers to Participation in Randomised Controlled Trials: A Systematic Review. *J Clin Epidemiol* 1999;52:1143–1156.
40. Brown ML, Riley GF, Schussler N, et al. Estimating health care costs related to cancer treatment from SEER-Medicare data. *Med Care* 2002;40:IV–104–117.
41. National Cancer Institute. Cancer Trends Progress Report, 2005 update. http://progressreport.cancer.gov/doc_detail.asp?pid=1&did=2005&chid=25&coid=226&mid= 2005.
42. Meropol NJ, Schulman KA. Cost of cancer care: issues and implications. *J Clin Oncol* 2007;25:180–186.
43. Schrag D. The price tag on progress—chemotherapy for colorectal cancer. *N Engl J Med* 2004;351:317–319.
44. Cronin DP, Harlan LC, Potosky AL, et al. Patterns of care for adjuvant therapy in a random population-based sample of patients diagnosed with colorectal cancer. *Am J Gastroenterol* 2006;101:2308–2318.
45. NIH consensus conference. Adjuvant therapy for patients with colon and rectal cancer. *JAMA* 1990;264:1444–1450.
46. Hayat MJ, Howlader N, Reichman ME, et al. Cancer statistics, trends, and multiple primary cancer analyses from the Surveillance, Epidemiology, and End Results (SEER) Program. *Oncologist* 2007;12:20–37.
47. Erikson C, Salsberg E, Forte G, et al. Future supply and demand for oncologists: Challenges to assuring access to oncology services. *JOP* 2007;3:79–86.

CHAPTER 8 ■ GASTROINTESTINAL CANCER: NUTRITIONAL SUPPORT

JOEL B. MASON

Protein-calorie malnutrition, typically referred to simply as malnutrition, is a common but not invariable feature of cancer, the most frequent manifestation of which is weight loss. A large, multicenter survey of more than 3,000 patients awaiting the initiation of chemotherapy, for instance, observed weight losses exceeding 4% in one-third of the patients and, in one-half of these, the magnitude of loss exceeded 10% (1). Weight losses exceeding 10% are of particular significance because there is considerable evidence that weight loss of this magnitude in the setting of illness leads to significant increases in morbidity and mortality (2).

The likelihood that a particular individual will sustain substantial weight loss is related to many factors: the type of cancer is important, as is the presence of metastases, physical impedance of normal food intake by the cancer, and the presence of intervening emotional issues such as depression. In the aforementioned survey (1), only 4% to 7% of individuals with leukemias, sarcomas, and breast cancer experienced more than 10% weight loss, whereas individuals with gastrointestinal tract cancers had a much higher likelihood of this degree of weight loss: 14% of patients with colon cancer and 25% to 40% of individuals with pancreatic and gastric cancers showed such a loss. Not surprisingly, carcinoma of the oropharynx, which frequently interferes with the processes of chewing and swallowing, results in more than 10% weight loss in more than 40% of patients (3).

Nevertheless, arriving at precise figures for the prevalence of significant protein-calorie malnutrition among cancer patients is a frustrating task because it depends on the particular assessment tool that is used to define malnutrition. For instance, another survey that used creatinine-height index (a measure of muscle mass) as the criterion for protein-calorie malnutrition observed that 90% of hospitalized cancer patients are significantly malnourished (4). Ultimately, it is perhaps more constructive merely to be aware that malnutrition of a degree that is associated with worse clinical outcomes is a common phenomenon among cancer patients, that it is particularly common in cancers of the gastrointestinal tract, and that physicians need to be cognizant of this reality in their assessment and management of the patient.

Unequivocal proof that malnutrition independently contributes to the morbidity, mortality, and diminished quality of life among cancer patients does not exist, but this contention is almost certainly true. A plethora of case-control and prospective cohort studies in cancer patients indicate that a substantial degree of malnutrition diminishes tolerance of and responsiveness to chemotherapy (1,5) and radiotherapy (6), increases perioperative morbidity (7), worsens the quality of life (5), and diminishes the likelihood of survival (1,5,8–10). Most important, clinicians should realize that appropriate and prompt attention

to meeting the nutritional needs of malnourished patients improves the clinical outcome of many types of ill patients, as has been shown repeatedly in prospective, randomized trials (reviewed in 11). Improvements in clinical outcome as a result of aggressive nutritional support have been more difficult to demonstrate in the cancer patient, probably because other factors have such a major impact on the clinical course. Nevertheless, aggressive nutritional support has genuine benefits to offer the cancer patient in selected circumstances. A detailed discussion of these circumstances appears later in this chapter.

MALNUTRITION IN THE CANCER PATIENT: MECHANISMS

The development of malnutrition in the cancer patient is usually multifactorial, and an appreciation of such multiplicity in etiology is necessary if one is to design an effective approach to treatment. Table 8.1 outlines factors that are often observed to contribute to this problem.

Body Compartment Perspective

The type of tissue that is lost when an individual loses weight is critical in determining the pathological ramifications of the weight loss. The vast majority of the metabolic machinery that maintains normal homeostasis resides in the lean body mass, and maintenance of this body compartment is most critical for health. The lean body mass can be further subdivided into skeletal muscle mass; visceral lean mass (which includes the major organs); and extracellular lean mass, such as the interstitial fluid, blood serum, and the mineral matrix of the skeleton (Fig. 8.1). These are useful distinctions because the body draws on each of these compartments in a different fashion in the setting of weight loss. In the cancer patient, there is usually a disproportionately large contraction of the skeletal muscle mass and fat mass with relative sparing of the visceral mass, and in this respect, the weight loss is similar to that seen in many acute illnesses of a nonmalignant nature (12). For example, in one study of cancer patients who had lost, on average, one fourth of their preillness weight, fat mass and skeletal muscle mass each decreased by 75% to 80% of control values, whereas visceral lean mass was spared and did not decrease to a significant degree (13). By comparison, the weight loss in simple starvation is less detrimental because the body preferentially uses adipose tissue for energy needs; therefore, the percentage loss in skeletal muscle mass is considerably less than the proportional loss of fat mass. For example, in healthy volunteers fed a calorically

TABLE 8.1

FACTORS THAT CONTRIBUTE TO THE DEVELOPMENT OF PROTEIN-CALORIE MALNUTRITION IN THE CANCER PATIENT

Insufficient dietary intake
  Suppression of appetite
    Mediated by cytokines, other humoral factors
    Mediated by emotional depression
    Mediated by loss of taste sensation (neural destruction, drug effects, paraneoplastic syndrome)
    Learned aversion to eating due to adverse symptoms
    Nausea, vomiting, other symptoms due to surgery, radiation, or chemotherapy
  Physical impairment of deglutition
    Effects on chewing or swallowing mechanisms
      Reduction in saliva production (tumor invasion, effects due to surgery, radiation, or drugs)
      Mass effect of tumor
      Radiation- or chemotherapy-induced mucositis
      Surgical interruption of swallowing mechanism
Alterations in physiology and metabolism
  Malabsorption/maldigestion due to tumor or due to therapy
  Constipation/gastrointestinal dysmotility due to surgical ablation of autonomic innervation of gut or due to narcotics and sedatives
  Increases in protein catabolism
  Inefficiency in energy metabolism/increases in overall caloric expenditure

TABLE 8.2

COMPARISON OF BODY COMPARTMENT LOSSES IN STARVATION AND CANCER WASTING

	Skeletal muscle wasting	Visceral wasting	Loss of fat mass
Starvation	+	±[a]	+++
Wasting in cancer	+++	±[a]	+++

The number of + signs indicates the relative magnitude of loss. A ± sign indicates that loss may or may not be present.
[a]Viscera relatively spared early in the process but can become pronounced with extended starvation or wasting.

MECHANISMS OF WASTING IN CANCER

Anorexia

Anorexia commonly contributes to wasting in cancer. Particularly with cancers of the gastrointestinal tract, the act of eating may incite a variety of adverse symptoms (including pain, vomiting, and diarrhea); anorexia may therefore evolve as a learned means of avoiding such symptoms. The tumor mass may also preclude adequate ingestion of food, a factor that is particularly prevalent in cancers of the oropharynx, esophagus, and stomach. In addition, therapeutic modalities involving drugs, radiation, or surgery can directly induce anorexia or deter the patient from eating to avoid the gastrointestinal side effects of therapy. A prime example of this is chemotherapy-induced mucositis. The emotional adjustment associated with dealing with a major cancer continues to be a common precipitant of depression and anxiety (17), and these emotional states can also be important in producing a state of anorexia.

Nevertheless, anorexia is commonly present, even in the absence of any of the previously mentioned factors, and may even be the presenting symptom of the cancer. Anorexia in such a setting is believed to be due largely to the effects of tumor-associated cytokines that are known to induce anorexia (Table 8.3) and that are believed to chiefly originate from host cells that are descendants of the white blood cell lineage (macrophages and lymphocytes), which are responding to the presence of the neoplasm. A highly reproducible and remarkable degree of anorexia is observed with administration of tumor necrosis factor-α (TNF-α) (18), interleukin (IL)-1 (19), and interferon-γ (20).

inadequate diet for 3 months, approximately one fourth of the initial body weight was lost; this was accompanied by a 70% decline in fat mass but only a 24% drop in lean mass (14). Table 8.2 summarizes the relative losses in these body compartments observed in simple starvation versus those observed in the wasting associated with cancer.

The weight loss and muscle dissolution (the combination of which is now referred to as *wasting* [15]) that one sees in cancer can be perceived as a physiological adaptation to stress; that is, the body sacrifices large portions of the muscle mass to spare more immediately critical functions in the visceral mass. However, there are clear limitations to this adaptive response. First, contraction of the skeletal muscle mass leads to muscle weakness, decreased work tolerance, and measurable decreases in functional status (16). Second, sparing of the visceral mass is only relative, and sustained weight loss will eventually lead to contractions of this compartment as well.

Alterations in Metabolism

A wide spectrum of alterations in protein, lipid, and carbohydrate metabolism are commonly observed in patients bearing cancers (Table 8.3). In concert with the other factors outlined in Table 8.1, these factors contribute to the development of malnutrition. Although much of the work pertaining to mechanisms has been performed in models other than the intact human (human and nonhuman cell culture and animal models), studies in humans have been in general accord with the nonhuman models.

Effects on Protein Metabolism and Lean Body Mass

The skeletal muscle is where most of the initial contraction of lean body mass occurs in the wasting associated with cancer

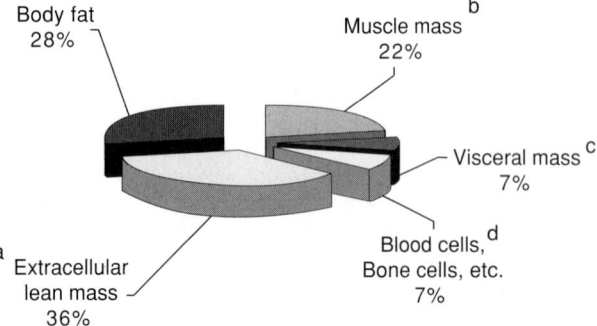

FIGURE 8.1. Typical body composition analysis by weight in a healthy adult. Segments a through d collectively represent lean body mass; segments b through d alone represent body cell mass.

TABLE 8.3

MAJOR CYTOKINES BELIEVED TO BE INVOLVED IN CANCER ANOREXIA AND WASTING

Cytokine	Production	Effects related to anorexia or cachexia
Tumor necrosis factor-α (TNF-α)	Levels do not correlate with malnutrition Produced by macrophages	Injection induces anorexia, weight loss, and cachexia May increase resting energy expenditure Has hypothalamic effects in inducing anorexia May have local gastrointestinal effects such as delay of gastric emptying Inhibits lipoprotein lipase Causes hypertriglyceridemia Depletes total body fat stores Increases skeletal protein breakdown Increases synthesis of acute-phase reactants Increases hepatic glucose output and gluconeogenesis
Interleukin (IL)-1 (IL-1)	Serum levels do not correlate with malnutrition Produced by macrophages	Injection induces anorexia, weight loss, and cachexia, more so than does TNF-α May increase resting energy expenditure Has hypothalamic effects in inducing anorexia Causes similar effects on fat metabolism as does TNF-α Causes similar effects on protein metabolism as does TNF-α
IL-6	Production induced by TNF-α and IL-1 Levels correlate with extent of tumor burden in animal models Produced by macrophages and fibroblasts Produced by activated T lymphocytes	Induces hepatic gluconeogenesis Increases production of acute-phase reactants Increases lipolysis Augments effects of TNF-α on lipid metabolism Inhibits lipoprotein lipase Inhibition by antibodies in tumor-bearing animals reduces weight loss Increases anorexia

Adapted from Mutlu EA, Mobarhan S. *Nutr Clin Care* 2000;3(1):6, with permission.

(13). The extent to which this compartment is diminished inversely correlates with the likelihood of survival, underscoring the import of this phenomenon (21). The contraction of skeletal muscle mass appears to be due to both a reduction in protein synthesis and an increase in protein degradation (22). Total body protein turnover is usually observed to be increased in this setting, and this increase is often present even before clinically evident wasting has occurred (23,24).

TNF-α and IL-6 appear to play major roles in mediating the dissolution of skeletal muscle in the wasting associated with cancer, and IL-1 and interferon-γ probably also play significant roles. Exogenous administration of TNF-α and IL-6 has these effects on skeletal muscle or its components (25,26), an effect that is overcome by specific antibodies directed against TNF-α (27). TNF-α and IL-6 are likely not the direct effectors of the response; rather, they probably act by stimulating the secretion or expression of more "downstream" mediators. In some instances, the neoplasm itself appears to be the source of the factor that mediates cachexia; proteolysis-inducing factor (PIF), a complex glycoprotein, promptly induces proteolysis in isolated muscle preparations and a reduction in lean mass in intact animals (28). It has been found in the urine of cancer patients with weight loss but not in that of those without loss of weight (29). It is not found in the urine of patients who have lost weight due to nonneoplastic illnesses. Thus, this factor appears to be highly specific for muscle wasting in cancer. Existing evidence suggests that PIF predominantly originates in the cells of the neoplasm, and among patients with gastrointestinal cancers, PIF expression in the tumor correlates with weight loss (30). Furthermore, in human prostate cancer, messenger RNA for PIF is localized solely to the epithelial cells of

the cancer and not in the stromal cells or normal prostate tissue (31). Nevertheless, observations regarding PIF have been somewhat difficult to reproduce; thus, its role in cancer wasting remains a matter of debate.

Effects on Lipid Metabolism and Adipose Tissue

In the wasting associated with cancer, the body continues to use adipose tissue as a major source of energy (although not as predominantly as in simple starvation), and therefore, a decrease in fat mass is usually seen. The net efflux of glycerol and fatty acids from the adipose tissue associated with use of this tissue appears to be due to at least three factors: (i) an increased rate of lipolysis in adipose tissue, which is apparently mediated through TNF-α, leukemia inhibitory factor, and lipid-mobilizing factor (32–34); (ii) a decrease in de novo lipogenesis in the adipose tissue, mediated largely by TNF-α and IL-1 (35); and (iii) diminished activity of lipoprotein lipase, which is necessary for the uptake of fatty acids from circulating lipoproteins and which appears to be mediated by TNF-α, IL-6, interferon-γ, and leukemia inhibitory factor (36,37). The decrease in lipoprotein lipase, in particular, explains why cancer patients have a diminished ability to clear an exogenous lipid load (38) and often have elevated plasma glycerol and triglyceride levels (39). Hypertriglyceridemia in cancer patients may also be related to increased rates of hepatic lipogenesis because several of the cytokines implicated in cancer wasting, including TNF-α, IL-1, and interferon-α, each stimulate hepatic lipogenesis (40). Like proteolysis-inducing factor, lipid-mobilizing factor is produced by cells of the neoplasm, although it differs in that its expression can also be induced in normal adipose tissue of animals on implantation of a cachexia-inducing tumor (41). Table 8.3 lists the mediators of these alterations in fat metabolism in the cancer patient afflicted with wasting.

Effects on Carbohydrate and Energy Metabolism

Cancer frequently produces a state in which the host expends more calories per kilogram of lean mass than is normal. This state of hypermetabolism is inherently less energy efficient and, therefore, predisposes to weight loss.

The Cori cycle, whereby lactate produced by the cancer or by peripheral tissues is converted back to glucose in the liver, is an inefficient means of salvaging glucose, consuming six molecules of adenosine triphosphate per cycle. If the cancer or other tissue is producing significant quantities of lactate by anaerobic glycolysis, which yields only two molecules of adenosine triphosphate per molecule of glucose substrate, substantial net loss of energy occurs (a so-called "futile cycle"). Increased activity of the Cori cycle has been reported to exist in individuals with cancer and, more specifically, in those cancer patients with weight loss (42). Nevertheless, the quantitative contribution to cancer wasting made by excessive activity of the Cori cycle is not known.

Other commonly altered aspects of carbohydrate metabolism include increased rates of gluconeogenesis and glucose flux, and the development of impaired insulin secretion as well as a modest degree of insulin insensitivity. The latter produces impaired use of glucose in peripheral tissues and glucose intolerance (43). Similar alterations in glucose metabolism are observed in any condition associated with a systemic inflammatory response and are largely believed to be due to TNF-α (44). These changes contrast considerably with those associated with weight loss unrelated to illness or cancer, in which insulin sensitivity is maintained (43).

ASSESSMENT OF NUTRITIONAL STATUS: A BRIEF INTRODUCTION

Providing nutritional support in a rational manner requires that the clinician acquire an objective means of systematically categorizing patients into those who are either well nourished or mildly malnourished versus those who have a moderate to severe degree of malnutrition. It is the patients in the latter category who will benefit from an aggressive approach to nutritional support. Patients with moderate to severe malnutrition have demonstrable impairments in many physiologic processes due to the malnutrition and suffer significantly greater morbidity and mortality as a result. Most important, the added morbidity and mortality can be attenuated or eliminated by diligent attention to their nutritional needs (reviewed in 11). Similar salutary benefits of aggressive nutritional support usually cannot be demonstrated in well-nourished or mildly malnourished patients.

A comprehensive assessment of protein-energy status involves taking a history (including a diet history), conducting a physical examination, taking anthropometric measures of nutritional status (e.g., weight, midarm muscle circumference, triceps fat fold), performing biochemical tests such as the measurement of serum albumin or prealbumin, and taking objective measurements of body compartments with tools such as body impedance analysis or dual-photon absorptiometry. The means of performing this type of comprehensive assessment is reviewed elsewhere (45–48) and is beyond the scope of this chapter. Far simpler algorithms, which are surprisingly accurate, can be used by the clinician if the primary purpose is merely to categorize patients either as well-

or mildly malnourished versus moderately to severely malnourished.

Perhaps the most straightforward means is to determine the percentage of unintentional weight loss that the patient has suffered as a result of disease. Because disproportionately large degrees of protein catabolism accompany acute inflammatory illnesses and cancer wasting, an unintentional weight loss of 10% or more of premorbid weight due to disease translates into a contraction of 15% to 20% of the critical protein-containing compartment of the body, and beyond this threshold, impaired physiologic functions, as well as increased morbidity and mortality, are observed (2). Clinical trials have repeatedly demonstrated that patients who exceed this threshold benefit from aggressive nutritional support (49,50).

Body weight can, however, be misleading. A common example in gastrointestinal/hepatobiliary malignancies is the patient with cirrhosis and ascites, in whom the weight of the ascites masks the loss in lean body mass. Studies that have used sophisticated means of assessing total body protein have demonstrated that nearly all patients who are categorized into Childs-Pugh class B or class C have lost more than 20% of total body protein; more surprising is the fact that half of patients with Childs-Pugh A classification have also lost this degree of total body protein (51).

Two other commonly used means of assessing protein-calorie status are the creatinine-height index and the prognostic nutritional index (PNI). The creatinine-height index, which is the amount of urinary creatinine excreted in 24 hours corrected for the patient's height, is an accurate reflection of muscle mass because a constant percentage (approximately 2%) of muscle creatine is converted to creatinine each day. However, incomplete urine collections, excessive meat ingestion, corticosteroid therapy, and abnormal or unstable renal function can each alter apparent or actual creatinine excretion independent of muscle mass. Gender-specific tables exist for normative values, and a patient whose index is 80% or less of the normative value can be considered to have a moderate to severe degree of malnutrition (Table 8.4). The PNI is one of several nutritional indices that represent a weighted regression of nutritional and physiological measures. The PNI has been shown to be a valid predictor of postoperative complications and mortality among inpatient cancer patients who are about to undergo surgery (52). The disadvantage of the PNI is that it requires the measurement of serum albumin and transferrin, triceps skinfold (the accurate measure of which is highly operator dependent), and delayed skin hypersensitivity. Although in reality the PNI is a reflection of both nutritional status and severity of illness, a value greater than 40% suggests moderate to severe malnutrition.

EFFICACY OF NUTRITIONAL SUPPORT

Aggressive nutritional support, defined here as the use of whatever means is necessary and practical to meet the nutritional needs of the patient, does not benefit every patient with cancer. Understanding on the part of the clinician as to what can reasonably be expected from a course of aggressive nutritional support is therefore of paramount importance so that an appropriate decision can be made about whether its use is warranted in a particular case.

First, one must recognize that the alterations in metabolism that accompany wasting in cancer make it exceedingly difficult in most patients to correct the existing nutritional deficits. In a patient with an untreated cancer, there is typically little accrual in the critical protein-containing compartment of the body in response to nutritional support; a gain in weight may not occur and, when it does, much of the weight that is

TABLE 8.4

NORMATIVE VALUES FOR CREATININE EXCRETION BASED ON HEIGHT

Men[a]		Women[b]	
Height (cm)	Ideal creatinine (mg)	Height (cm)	Ideal creatinine (mg)
157.5	1,288	147.3	830
160.0	1,325	149.9	851
162.6	1,359	152.4	875
165.1	1,386	154.9	900
167.6	1,426	157.9	925
170.2	1,467	160.0	949
172.7	1,513	162.6	977
175.3	1,555	165.1	1,006
177.8	1,596	167.6	1,044
180.3	1,642	170.2	1,076
182.9	1,691	172.7	1,109
185.4	1,739	175.3	1,141
188.0	1,785	177.8	1,174
190.5	1,831	180.3	1,206
193.0	1,891	182.9	1,240

[a]Creatinine coefficient (men) = 23 mg per kg of ideal body weight.
[b]Creatinine coefficient (women) = 18 mg per kg of ideal body weight.
Creatinine-height index = actual 24-hr urinary creatinine excretion divided by the normative value for height and gender.
From Blackburn GL, Bistrian BR, Maini BS, et al. Nutritional and metabolic assessment of the hospitalized patient. *JPEN J Parenter Enteral Nutr* 1977;1(1):11–22, with permission.

gained is due to water and to an expanded fat mass (53). It is nevertheless true that *even in the absence of weight gain, or demonstrable increases in the levels of serum proteins that reflect protein-energy status (e.g., albumin, prealbumin, retinol-binding protein), providing a course of nutritional support to an appropriate patient can improve physiologic functions and clinical outcome.* Once a tumor mass has been eliminated or shrunken by treatment, many of these metabolic aberrations disappear (54), and therefore, the expectation that aggressive nutritional support might help replete lean body mass is reasonable.

The next several subsections review common clinical scenarios in which substantial evidence exists that aggressive nutritional support provides benefit to the patient. Contained in the text accompanying each scenario are qualifications that describe the particular circumstances under which an aggressive approach is indicated.

Cancer Patient Undergoing Major Surgery

The setting in which nutritional support for the cancer patient has been most reproducibly demonstrated as beneficial is that of moderate to severe malnourishment in patients who are scheduled to undergo major surgery. Aggressive nutritional support for 7 or more days before surgery reproducibly reduces perioperative complications, and sometimes mortality, in malnourished patients when examined in a prospective and controlled fashion (49,55–57). The Veterans Administration Cooperative Trial (49), a multicenter trial encompassing nearly 500 subjects of whom two-thirds had cancer, demonstrated an important qualification to this benefit. Patients who were categorized as "severely" malnourished and who were ran-

domly assigned to receive preoperative total parenteral nutrition (TPN) experienced a nearly 90% decline in noninfectious perioperative complications, whereas no benefits were observed in mildly malnourished or well-nourished individuals. Consequently, in those trials that are confined to moderately to severely malnourished patients, preoperative nutritional support conveys large benefits. One trial that enrolled 90 patients with gastric or colorectal cancers undergoing surgery demonstrated a 35% decline in overall complications and a significant reduction in mortality (57). The fact that the benefits of preoperative nutritional support are limited to those with a substantial degree of malnutrition is not terribly surprising and is an observation that recapitulates the results of trials that have included only patients with nonneoplastic disease. The same conclusion has been reached by meta-analyses (58,59). Thus, the clinician must establish an objective and practical means of stratifying patients into those who are moderately to severely malnourished, using algorithms such as those discussed in the previous section. Another critical point is that the ability of aggressive nutritional support to diminish perioperative complications is probably lost if it is deferred until after surgery. This has been observed in many trials, including those encompassing patients with gastric, pancreatic, and colorectal cancers (57,60).

The benefits of aggressive nutritional support in the preoperative period are not confined to TPN; provision of nutrients via an enteral approach is also of substantial benefit. The number of trials done with preoperative enteral support are far fewer and less compelling than those with TPN, but the existing studies indicate that preoperative enteral support conveys the same nutritional (61) and clinical (62) benefits to the malnourished patient as TPN. As was the case with TPN, in the absence of aggressive preoperative support, postoperative enteral nutrition seems to convey little advantage to the patient in the perioperative period (63), although individuals who receive a specialized immunomodulatory enteral formula appear to be an exception to this rule, an issue that is discussed in detail in the following section.

If feasible, the preferred course is always to provide nutritional support via an enteral, rather than parenteral, route. Enteral feeding is accompanied by fewer metabolic complications, avoids the complications associated with placement of a central intravenous line, and is generally less expensive. At least one well-performed prospective, randomized trial indicates that serious infectious complications are significantly less frequent in enterally fed patients (even if one ignores infections of the central venous catheter) (64), although this point remains a matter of controversy (65). Increased rates of serious infections with parenteral nutrition are probably a consequence of hyperglycemia, which occurs more frequently with a parenteral route and even modest levels of which (115–215 mg/dL) seem to markedly increase infection risk in critically ill surgical patients (66). In the past, an enteral approach was frequently not considered in the setting of major abdominal surgery, but it is now evident that postoperative ileus is largely a function of gastroparesis; therefore, intraoperative placement of an nasojejunal tube or jejunostomy allows rapid institution of enteral feeds within 24 hours after surgery in most instances. This approach has been shown to be as effective as TPN in delivering nutrients in liver transplantation patients (67).

Patients Undergoing Chemotherapy or Radiation Therapy

Prospective cohort analyses certainly suggest that malnutrition is a risk factor for diminished responsiveness to chemotherapy, increased toxicity of the drugs, poorer quality of life, and shorter survival (68). Nevertheless, early intervention trials that examined the efficacy of nutritional support in chemotherapy were largely negative and culminated in a meta-analysis that concluded that routine nutritional support in this setting was not indicated (69). Subsequent intervention trials, which have stratified the patients by nutritional status, have generally shown that gains in nutritional status can be realized in malnourished patients undergoing chemotherapy, although a reduction in toxicity still has not been reproducibly demonstrable (70,71). If such patients subsequently proceed to surgery, the nutritional support appears to improve their perioperative course (71). Whether similar benefits are conveyed to individuals who solely receive chemotherapy is unknown.

The use of aggressive nutritional support for a cancer patient has frequently raised the concern of whether an acceleration of tumor growth might occur. This concern is generally supported by animal models of cancer. Both intravenous and enteral repletion in malnourished tumor-bearing animals stimulate tumor growth (72). Human data regarding this issue are scarce, although there is some suggestion that nutritional repletion in malnourished cancer patients may stimulate DNA synthesis in the tumor (71). Nevertheless, reports indicating any clinically significant acceleration of tumor growth with aggressive nutritional support are conspicuously lacking, and this is therefore not a concern that should discourage the use of aggressive support in an otherwise appropriate setting. This issue should be of even less concern in individuals who are embarking on chemotherapy because aggressive nutritional support does not enhance DNA synthesis in the tumor if chemotherapy is being concurrently administered (71). Indeed, there is some speculation that by providing nutritional support and placing more tumor cells in the vulnerable DNA synthesis phase of the cell cycle, sensitivity to cycle-specific chemotherapeutic agents is enhanced (71). This is an attractive hypothesis but one that has yet to be proven.

The use of aggressive nutritional support in patients undergoing radiation therapy has been most extensively studied in individuals who have head and neck and esophageal cancers because (a) such patients tend to have mechanical difficulties with deglutition, (b) they have a high prevalence of substantial malnutrition (3), and (c) radiation therapy is a commonly used modality of treatment. For such individuals, there is now reasonable evidence that placement of a percutaneous endoscopic gastrostomy tube and administration of supplemental tube feedings during and after the course of radiation therapy prevents further deterioration of nutritional status (73,74). In patients with head and neck cancers, nutritional support has also been shown to significantly improve objective indicators of the quality of life (73). Although no improvements in survival or decreased morbidity have yet been demonstrated, the improved quality of life alone may warrant its use in this setting.

Patients Undergoing Bone Marrow Transplantation

One situation in which the routine prophylactic use of TPN has been shown to be of benefit, even in well-nourished individuals, is bone marrow transplantation (75). Well-nourished individuals presumably benefit in this setting because the cytoreductive chemotherapy and radiation usually causes prolonged and severe gastrointestinal dysfunction, which limits oral intake for weeks at a time when physiologic stresses give rise to substantially increased energy and protein requirements. In the past, there was some concern that administration of conventional doses of intravenous lipids might increase the risk of bacteremias and fungemias, but prospective, randomized trials have largely eliminated this concern (76,77). In fact, what little immunosuppression might arise from the use of conventional lipid emulsions containing n-6 fatty acids may even diminish the likelihood of significant morbidity and mortality from graft-versus-host disease (77).

Clinicians have shown considerable reluctance to use enteral tube feeding regimens in these patients because of the presumed injury induced by the feeding tube to a mucosa whose integrity is already impaired by mucositis. Whether this should be a genuine concern is not yet clear. Nevertheless, when compared to TPN in prospective, controlled studies, tube feeding regimens have not been observed to increase diarrhea, impair nutritional restitution, increase the duration of hospitalization, or influence survival rate (78,79). The observed advantages of the enteral approach have included fewer episodes of hyperglycemia and a cost reduction of >50% for the nutritional support (79).

The use of TPN supplemented with glutamine in bone marrow transplantation patients is discussed in a later section.

USE OF AGENTS THAT COMBAT ANOREXIA IN NUTRITIONAL SUPPORT

Aggressive nutritional support does not invariably require tube feeding or TPN. If inadequate oral intake is largely related to anorexia, pharmacologic management of the anorexia is an excellent starting point for therapy. Resorting to enteric tube feeding or TPN can then be reserved only for those for whom such an approach fails.

Loss of appetite can be a result of both tumor- and host-derived substances, as well as of altered taste, dysphagia and other gastrointestinal symptoms, emotional depression, and the therapeutic modalities used to treat cancer, as discussed previously. The prevalence of anorexia is quite high: 15% to 40% of cases at diagnosis and 65% in advanced disease (80).

Several pharmacologic agents have been evaluated for their potential use in the treatment and symptomatic improvement of cancer anorexia and cancer wasting.

Progestational Agents

Both megestrol acetate (MA) and medroxyprogesterone acetate (MPA) are synthetic derivatives of progesterone for oral use. MPA is also available as an intramuscular depot injection. Both are well tolerated, although they are relatively contraindicated in individuals who have sustained prior thromboembolic events because agents in this class appear to enhance thrombotic potential.

Clinical trials using progesterone derivatives to treat hormone-responsive breast cancers initially reported increased appetite and weight gain as a side effect of MA therapy (81). Several randomized, controlled trials of MA subsequently confirmed a positive effect on appetite and weight gain in patients with a wide variety of cancers (82–84). Systematic reviews of existing trials have confirmed such benefits (85,86) and, in some instances, have demonstrated an improved health-related quality of life (86). Typical weight gains over several months have been in the range of 3 to 6 kg, compared to what are usually weight losses in the placebo group. The data have shown a very strong dose–response effect on appetite and food intake as the daily dose is increased from 160 to 800 mg, whereas doses in excess of 800 mg daily do not seem to provide any additional advantage (82). Significant increases in subcutaneous fat accompany the weight gain (84). Accrual of muscle mass or lean body mass has not yet been convincingly shown in cancer patients, although results of a parallel trial in patients with AIDS who had wasting showed a significant increase in lean mass (87). Although an increase in appetite usually occurs promptly, the median response time to achieve maximal weight gain has been found to be 6 to 10 weeks (87). A not insignificant benefit of MA therapy is a psychological one: Patients report an increase in "energy" (84). Similarly, in the trials involving patients with AIDS, a significant increase in "sense of well-being" was often observed (87,88).

Side effects of MA therapy include male impotence, vaginal spotting, mild pitting edema, and thromboembolic phenomena. Thromboembolic events tend to occur in approximately 5% of patients in most trials, but the fact that this figure is usually not significantly greater than the incidence in the placebo group suggests that the increase in risk is very minor.

MPA is a similar progestational agent used in Europe. Two randomized, placebo-controlled trials in cancer patients (89,90) demonstrated effects that were quite similar to those of MA: 500 mg twice daily for 12 weeks significantly increased food intake, arrested weight loss, and increased the fat mass. As was true of MA, no increase in fatfree mass was observed. Although MPA is well tolerated, contraindications are the same as for MA.

Cannabinoids

Cannabinoids are derivatives of the *Cannabis sativa* plant. Dronabinol is the most commonly used pharmacologic form, a synthetic and orally bioavailable form of tetrahydrocannabinol. It is approved by the U.S. Food and Drug Administration for chemotherapy-induced nausea and vomiting, as well as for AIDS- and cancer-associated anorexia. Dronabinol has been shown to be an effective antiemetic agent for cancer patients suffering chemotherapy-induced nausea (91), and its appetite-stimulating effects have been known for some time. A regimen of 2.5 mg orally twice a day has been used safely for appetite stimulation for up to 1 year in AIDS patients (92). Significant increases in appetite are uniformly observed in trials with both AIDS and cancer patients, although beneficial effects against weight loss have not yet been convincingly demonstrated. When compared directly with MA in cancer patients, appetite stimulation and weight gain were significantly superior with MA (93). Side effects are euphoria, dizziness, somnolence, and confusion, which result in dosage reduction or discontinuation in approximately 25% of patients.

Prokinetic Agents

Many patients with advanced cancer have symptoms related to gastroparesis, which arises from surgical or pharmacologic interruption of the autonomic innervation of the stomach. The prokinetic agents metoclopramide (adults: 10 mg orally four times a day), cisapride (10 mg orally four times a day), and domperidone (10 mg three times a day) are beneficial in the relief of anorexia, nausea, and early satiety when caused by poor gastrointestinal motility. Cisapride causes greater colonic motility, a potentially useful side effect in patients on opioids, strong anticholinergic agents, or other drugs that precipitate constipation.

A common limiting side effect of metoclopramide is sedation, although dose reduction is often sufficient to correct this problem. The alternative agents, cisapride and domperidone, do not tend to have this side effect but are no longer available in the United States due to rare but life-threatening prolongation of the QT interval and subsequent dysrhythmias.

TARGETED NUTRIENT THERAPY

Particular nutrients are sometimes administered in quantities that exceed what is needed to meet basal metabolic requirements to elicit specific physiological responses that might benefit the patient. This is sometimes referred to as a *targeted nutrient therapy*, and the nutrient in this circumstance is often referred to as a "nutriceutical" because it is being used as a pharmacologic agent rather than just as a substance to meet the nutritional needs of the individual. Examples of nutrients that have been used in this manner in cancer patients include omega-3 fatty acids, glutamine, arginine, vitamin E, and RNA.

Omega-3 Polyunsaturated Fatty Acids

The source of fat in conventional enteral and parenteral nutritional formulas is typically a vegetable oil rich in omega-6 polyunsaturated fatty acids. Replacing those fatty acids with one or both of the two major omega-3 polyunsaturated fatty acids, eicosapentaenoic acid and docosahexaenoic acid, has been examined for its potential to improve patient outcome, particularly the attenuation or reversal of cancer wasting.

Exchanging dietary n-3 fatty acids for n-6 fatty acids, or even just supplementing with n-3 fatty acids, is known to change the fatty acid composition of immune cell membranes and alter the immune response (94), although the nature of the altered immune response is not consistent among studies. In healthy volunteers, ingestion of supplemental n-3 fatty acids generally downregulates the systemic reaction to inflammatory mediators and diminishes immunoresponsiveness in general, probably through their inhibition of TNF-α, IL-1, IL-2, and IL-6 release (94–96). Interestingly, a paradoxical effect has sometimes been observed in malnourished cancer patients or those stressed by major surgery. Levels of mediators such as TNF-α may increase with the administration of n-3 fatty acids, and lymphocyte responsiveness has been shown to be enhanced (97,98). Thus, the direction of the immunomodulation induced by n-3 fatty acids may depend on several factors, including the health status of the individual taking the fatty acids.

Some observations also suggest that n-3 fatty acids may negatively impact the viability of an existing cancer in ways other than modulation of the immune response. In cell cultures of pancreatic or colon cancer cells, eicosapentaenoic acid induced apoptosis (99,100), and in other studies, n-3 fatty acids seemed to interfere with the microcirculation of a neoplasm, limiting its ability to enlarge (101).

Regardless of the mechanism(s) by which they operate, it has been speculated that administration of supplemental n-3 fatty acids might ameliorate the wasting associated with cancer or improve other clinical outcomes. The evidence from clinical trials, however, has been rather inconsistent, perhaps due to the wide range of doses used because trials using higher doses seem to be those that have observed significant improvements. Although existing observations suggest benefits are realized only at higher doses (>5 g/day of EPA), supplementation at these levels is problematic because symptoms of nausea, bloating, and frequent eructations with a "fishy taste" often interfere with patient compliance. When examined in a prospective controlled fashion, improved survival was observed among 60 cancer patients harboring a variety of solid neoplasms who received 18 g of n-3 fatty acids per day (97); moreover, among those patients who were malnourished, improved performance scores were observed despite the fact that no apparent benefit in protein-calorie status resulted from n-3 supplementation. Similarly, results of an uncontrolled study of patients with pancreatic cancer who were steadily losing weight suggested that the administration of n-3 fatty acids in conjunction with supplemental calories and protein enables such patients to gain weight and improve performance scores, (102) and, in a similar uncontrolled study in cancer patients who were losing a median of 4% of their weight per month before entry into the study, more than 80% had arrests in weight loss if they were able to consume approximately 7 g or more of EPA per day (103). In contrast, in two controlled trials in which 2 to 3 g of EPA were administered daily, there were no demonstrable improvements in weight or other clinical end points (104,105). An observed decrease in caloric expenditure per kilogram of lean mass in one of the positive studies provides a plausible mechanism for the anabolic potential of n-3 fatty acids (102), as do the observations indicating that these fatty acids can inhibit the release of the protein catabolic cytokines TNF-α and IL-6 (94–96).

More consistently positive clinical benefits are observed with multimodality supplements that contain, in addition to n-3 fatty acids other nutriceuticals that are also believed to have immunomodulatory activity, including arginine, RNA, and glutamine. This is described in the following section.

Arginine, RNA, Glutamine, and Multimodality "Immunomodulatory" Formulas

Many studies in tumor-bearing or otherwise stressed animals support the concept that supplementation with arginine, RNA, or glutamine as single-agent supplements can enhance cell-mediated immunoresponsiveness and, in some cases, improve survival (106–108). However, human trials have not consistently demonstrated comparable enhancements of immunoresponsiveness or improvements in clinical end points when these nutrients have been used individually.

The most extensively examined of these nutraceuticals as a single additive is glutamine. Initially, two prospective, controlled, intervention trials demonstrated significant improvements in clinical end points with the use of glutamine-supplemented TPN compared with the use of TPN not containing the amino acid, although it is important to note that this apparent benefit of glutamine was demonstrated only in bone marrow transplantation patients and, specifically, among those who were exclusively reliant on parenteral nutrition. In the first of these two positive studies (109), transplantation patients with malignancies demonstrated significantly improved nitrogen balance, a diminished incidence of clinically significant infections, lower rates of microbial colonization, and a mean reduction in hospitalization of approximately 1 week. The second study (110) observed a mean decrease in the duration of hospitalization of approximately 1 week but no decrease in infections or other indicators of morbidity. In both instances, 30% to 45% of the total amino acids delivered were glutamine. However, subsequent randomized trials of comparable size have observed either no benefits or marginal benefits with parenteral glutamine in this setting (111,112). Moreover, it is worth emphasizing that clinical benefits of glutamine have not been shown in enterally fed bone marrow transplantation patients or in cancer patients receiving other types of therapies. For instance, a follow-up study by Schloerb et al. (113) examined whether any benefits of glutamine supplementation in bone marrow transplantation patients could be demonstrated in those who were initially supported by enteral nutrition (and who therefore received oral glutamine) and who only then resorted to parenteral nutrition (containing glutamine) when necessary. No improvements in any clinical end points were seen in this setting. Thus, it remains controversial as to whether glutamine supplementation in the immediate posttransplantation period improves the clinical outcome for bone marrow transplantation patients. If it is used, it should only be among those who are reliant solely on parenteral nutrition. Although gastrointestinal tumors are not typically treated with bone marrow transplantation, the two studies by Schloerb et al. (110,113) included a substantial proportion of individuals receiving bone marrow transplants for solid tumors.

In contrast to the equivocal benefits conveyed by single agent n-3 fatty acids or glutamine, consensus continues to grow that the use of specialized enteral formulas containing a combination of RNA, n-3 fatty acids, arginine, and glutamine (in addition to "conventional" nutrients) improves clinical outcomes in patients undergoing surgery for gastrointestinal malignancies (114–117). In those studies in which immunologic and biochemical parameters were examined, the administration of these formulas demonstrated significant decreases in the levels of mediators of systemic inflammation, concurrent increases in cell-mediated immunity and, in some instances, an improvement in net protein balance (114,118–120). In the majority of the trials, this translated into a remarkable decrease in perioperative infections (114–117) and the duration of hospitalization (114,115,117). Two meta-analyses, the larger of which incorporated 22 trials, conclude that use of these formulas results in a 35% to 50% reduction in perioperative infections in elective cancer surgery (121,122). It is important to recognize that the trials demonstrating the most clear-cut benefits are those in which administration of these formulas is begun several days before surgery (as a supplement delivered orally or through an enteral tube); clinical benefits are not as predictably realized when feeding is begun in the 24-hour period following surgery (e.g., 123), and benefits are not generally observed if feedings are begun even later. In contrast to other strategies in nutrition support, clinical benefits are even realized in some trials among cancer patients who are not significantly malnourished (124). In conclusion, there is substantial evidence to indicate that the clinical course of patients with gastrointestinal malignancies can be significantly improved by the use of multimodality immunoenhancing formulas in situations involving a high degree of physiological stress, such as major surgery. In those instances in which these formulas were also compared with conventional TPN, they were found to convey a significant advantage (114,120). Whether they will also be shown to be efficacious in other settings, such as during courses of intensive chemotherapy, is not known.

Treatment of Oral Mucositis With Vitamin E or Glutamine

A prospective, randomized clinical trial, albeit of limited size, indicated that topical vitamin E (125) can provide significant healing and improvement of the oral mucositis associated with cytotoxic therapy. Similarly, glutamine suspensions that are swished in the mouth several times per day have been reported to improve radiation- or cytotoxin-induced mucositis (126–128), although one trial showed negative results (129). Although not proven in a definitive sense, these therapies offer essentially no risk of toxicity and are worth considering in patients suffering from this condition.

VITAMIN AND MINERAL DEFICIENCIES ASSOCIATED WITH SPECIFIC CIRCUMSTANCES

It is wise to anticipate the risk of select vitamin or mineral deficiencies specific to certain circumstances that arise in patients with gastrointestinal and hepatobiliary malignancies. The intent of this discussion is not to describe in detail the treatment of each of these deficiency states; this information can be found elsewhere. Rather, it is to point out those circumstances in which these deficiencies occur. The examples given here are only a few representative examples of the many that could be discussed.

High-Grade Biliary Obstruction or Biliary Diversion/Ileal Damage

Biliary obstruction of a high-grade nature, biliary diversion, or extensive loss of ileal function due to resection or radiation causes fat malabsorption. In the case of biliary disease, insufficient bile to emulsify fat reaches the lumen of the intestine, and in the case of ileal dysfunction, insufficient bile acids are recycled by the ileum, which overwhelms the liver's ability to upregulate bile acid synthesis and secretion. Ileal disease or resection exceeding 100 cm is usually associated with steatorrhea; less extensive involvement can usually be compensated for by increased hepatic biliary synthesis.

Compensation for the calories lost in malabsorbed fat and the attendant diarrhea are usually the focus of treatment. One should keep in mind, however, that fat-soluble vitamins as well as the divalent cationic minerals calcium, magnesium, zinc, and copper are also malabsorbed. Deficiencies of vitamins A, D, and K are common in patients with long-standing cholestasis, and the likelihood of this occurring is proportional to the magnitude of the elevation in serum bilirubin (130). Chronic total bilirubin elevations above 5 mg/dL should definitely raise a suspicion. Many of the deficiency states in this setting are too subtle to be evident clinically, so the diagnosis is made only when the index of suspicion is high and appropriate blood tests are obtained (130). Deficiency of vitamin E is observed less commonly but is certainly known to occur in association with other causes of chronic cholestasis such as biliary atresia. Losses of calcium, magnesium, zinc, and copper apparently occur because these cations bind to the unabsorbed fatty acids present in the stool; these losses are similarly proportional to the degree of cholestasis (131). Symptomatic hypocalcemia or hypomagnesemia and metabolic bone disease can occur.

Vitamin B_{12} Deficiency Due to Ileal or Gastric Insults

Age is one of the primary risk factors for the major gastrointestinal cancers such as cancer of the stomach, pancreas, and colorectum. This is pertinent to the phenomenon of atrophic gastritis, which also increases with age and reaches a prevalence in the general population of nearly 40% by the eighth decade of life (132). Elderly individuals with atrophic gastritis have lower vitamin B_{12} levels than elderly controls without the condition due to diminished bioavailability of protein-bound B_{12} in food. Furthermore, the clinical manifestations of B_{12} deficiency can occur with only modest reductions in the plasma B_{12} concentration, within what has traditionally been considered the normal range, a condition that is best identified by the presence of elevated methylmalonic acid levels in the blood (133). Up to 4% to 10% of elderly individuals whose plasma B_{12} levels are in the low-normal range of 180 to 400 pg/mL are now believed to actually have cellular deficiency of the vitamin. Neurologic degeneration due to this subtle form of B_{12} deficiency can arise without any hematologic manifestations, further obscuring the diagnosis (134).

Further compromises in B_{12} absorption can occur due to pharmacologic suppression of gastric acid secretion (135), surgical ablation of a portion of the stomach or ileum, or radiation damage to those organs. The risk of B_{12} deficiency goes up rapidly when more than 90 cm of ileum are lost or involved with disease (136). The clinician therefore needs to remain cognizant that either neurologic or hematologic manifestations of B_{12} deficiency may superimpose themselves on the myriad other reasons that cancer patients develop abnormalities of the nervous system and bone marrow, and that a "normal" plasma B_{12} level may not suffice to exclude the diagnosis.

Niacin Deficiency Due to Carcinoid Tumors

The pigmented dermatitis, mucositis, and central nervous system manifestations of pellagra, or niacin deficiency, have occasionally been reported to arise in carcinoid syndrome (137), presumably because the tumor preferentially uses tryptophan for serotonin synthesis and thereby diverts it away from nicotinic acid synthesis. In these instances, supplementation with nicotinamide has corrected the manifestations.

ALTERNATIVE NUTRITION FOR THE TREATMENT OF CANCER

The major cancers, including those of the gastrointestinal and hepatobiliary systems, carry with them substantial morbidity and mortality. To date, conventional medicine can provide only modest opportunities for treatment and palliation, particularly for the latter stages of disease. It is therefore not surprising that a significant portion of cancer patients pursue unproven natural remedies during the course of their illness in conjunction with traditional treatment. For example, in a cohort study (138) that examined 480 patients with newly diagnosed breast cancer, 10.6% of the women had used alternative medicine before they were given a diagnosis of breast cancer, and 28.1% started using some type of alternative medicine after the diagnosis was established. Alternative and complementary medicine in gastrointestinal malignancies is discussed at length in Chapter 12.

The majority of patients using alternative therapy do not discuss this therapy with their medical doctors unless specifically asked about it. This lack of communication is not in the best interest of the patient for a number of reasons. First, alternative therapies may contain harmful substances or substances that interact with conventional therapies. Second, the physician is often better equipped to manage the patient's care and make appropriate clinical decisions if he or she has a comprehensive understanding of the patient's perspectives on treatment options. Medical doctors should therefore ask their patients about their use of unconventional therapy and should be reasonably informed about the types of therapies available (139).

Table 8.5 shows several alternative nutritional remedies that are frequently used by cancer patients for the purpose of treatment. None has been demonstrated to be efficacious in a compelling fashion, although several of them are presently being studied in scientifically rigorous trials.

PRACTICAL CONCLUSIONS

1. Wasting—a form of protein-calorie malnutrition that involves loss of weight and lean mass—is common in patients with gastrointestinal and hepatobiliary cancers and carries with it negative consequences in regard to morbid events, ability to withstand therapy, and survival. An unintentional loss of 10% or more of usual body weight constitutes a convenient and surprisingly accurate

TABLE 8.5

ALTERNATIVE NUTRITIONAL REMEDIES USED BY CANCER PATIENTS

Treatment	Active agent	Purported activity	Side effects	References	Efficacy[a]
Bromelain	Protease, peroxidase, acid phosphatase	Reduces metastasis	Decreased platelet activity, gastrointestinal allergic reaction	140,141	−
Green tea	Polyphenol	Reduces recurrence of breast cancer	Safe, but no long-term studies	142,143	+
Shark cartilage	Sphyrnastatin 1 and 2	Inhibits angiogenesis	Nausea, vomiting, constipation, hepatitis	144,145	−
Laetrile	Amygdalin, vitamin B_{17}	Acts as tumoricidal	Cyanide toxicity	146,147	−
Macrobiotic diet	Cereal grain, vegetables, seaweed, beans	Corrects cancer cachexia	Low vitamin D and B_{12}, iron, and calcium; relatively low calories	148,149	−
Gerson diet	Raw vegetarian diet, vegetable and fruit juice, calf's liver, coffee enema	Detoxifies harmful substances	Very low fat content	149,150	−
Livingstone therapy	Vegetarian whole-food diet, blood transfusion, supplemental vitamins, autologous vaccination, enema	Enhances immune function	Worse quality of life	151,152	−

+ indicates there is evidence for a beneficial effect; − indicates no evidence for a beneficial effect.
[a] Defined as evidence of a beneficial effect in at least one prospective controlled trial in humans.

means of identifying those patients whose malnutrition is moderate to severe.

2. Routine identification of those cancer patients with moderate to severe malnutrition is important because these patients are the ones who will most clearly benefit from aggressive nutritional support in the preoperative setting and during chemotherapy and radiation. Providing aggressive nutritional support to well-nourished or mildly malnourished patients is nevertheless worthwhile if it is projected that they will fall far short of meeting their nutritional needs for a period of 7 days or more. An oral or enteral approach to aggressive nutritional support is more physiological than a parenteral approach, is less expensive, and appears to be associated with fewer instances of serious morbidity.

3. All cancer patients undergoing allogeneic bone marrow transplantation appear to benefit from aggressive prophylactic nutritional support. TPN has most often been used in this setting. Some evidence exists that when the parenteral approach is taken, supplementing the TPN with glutamine conveys nutritional and immunologic benefits that translate into fewer infections and shorter hospitalizations.

4. When aggressive nutritional support is undertaken in cancer patients who are about to undergo major surgery, a reduction in the risk of perioperative infections is realized by using immunoenhancing enteral formulas in the pre- and postoperative periods compared to using conventional tube feeds or TPN. Beginning these formulas several days before surgery appears to be important in attaining improved outcomes. Such benefits may occur even among patients who are not substantially malnourished.

5. Certain circumstances that arise in these patients are likely to produce select vitamin and mineral deficiencies. Diligent attention to these situations, with a proactive approach to prevention, will avert morbidity associated with these deficiencies.

6. A large proportion of patients with gastrointestinal cancers use alternative medical treatments in conjunction with conventional treatments and often do not mention such treatments unless specifically requested to do so. Thorough and sensible management of the patient dictates an awareness of all treatments being used.

ACKNOWLEDGMENTS

This writing of this chapter was supported in part by the National Cancer Institute (K05 CA100048) and by the U.S. Department of Agriculture, Agricultural Research Service Agreement 58-1950-9-001. The contents of this chapter do not necessarily reflect the policies or views of the U.S. Department of Agriculture nor does mention of trade names, commercial products, or organizations imply endorsement by the U.S. government.

References

1. Dewys WD, Begg C, Lavin P, et al. Prognostic effect of weight loss prior to chemotherapy in cancer patients. *Am J Med* 1980;69:491–497.
2. Hill G. Body composition research: implications for the practice of clinical nutrition. *JPEN J Parenter Enteral Nutr* 1992;16:197–218.
3. Mick R, Vokes E, Weichselbaum RR, et al. Prognostic factors in advanced head and neck cancer patient undergoing multimodality therapy. *Otolaryngol Head Neck Surg* 1991;105:62–73.
4. Nixon DW, Heymsfield SB, Cohen AE, et al. Protein-calorie undernutrition in hospitalized cancer patients. *Am J Med* 1980;68:683–690.
5. Andreyev H, Norman A, Oates J, et al. Why do patients with weight loss have a worse outcome when undergoing chemotherapy for gastrointestinal malignancies? *Eur J Cancer* 1998;34:503–509.
6. Lee JH, Machtay M, Unger LD, et al. Prophylactic gastrostomy tubes in patients undergoing intensive irradiation for cancer of the head and neck. *Arch Otolaryngol Head Neck Surg* 1998;124:871–875.
7. Patil PK, Patel SG, Mistry RC, et al. Cancer of the esophagus; esophagogastric anastomotic leak—a retrospective study of predisposing factors. *J Surg Oncol* 1992;49:163–167.

8. Van Bokhorst-de van der Schuer MA, Van Leeuwen PA, Kuik DJ, et al. The impact of nutritional status on the prognoses of patients with advanced head and neck cancer. *Cancer* 1999;86:519–527.

9. Lanzotti VJ, Thomas DR, Boyle LE, et al. Survival with inoperable lung cancer. *Cancer* 1977;39:303–313.

10. Kama NA, Coskun T, Yuksek YN, et al. Factors affecting post-operative mortality in malignant biliary tract obstruction. *Hepatogastroenterology* 1999;46:103–107.

11. Mason JB. A clinical nutritionist's search for meaning: why should we bother to feed the acutely ill, hospitalized patient? *Nutrition* 1996;12.279–281.

12. Wilmore DW. Catabolic illness. Strategies for enhancing recovery. *N Engl J Med* 1991;325:695–702.

13. Fearon KCH, Preston T. Body composition in cancer cachexia. *Infusionstherapie* 1990;17(Suppl 3):63–66.

14. Keys A, Brozek J, Henschel A, et al. *The Biology of Human Starvation.* Minneapolis: University of Minnesota Press; 1950.

15. Roubenoff R, Heymsfield SB, Kehayias JJ, et al. Standardization of nomenclature of body composition in weight loss. *Am J Clin Nutr* 1998;67:492–493.

16. Fiatarone MA, O'Neill EF, Ryan ND, et al. Exercise training and nutritional supplementation for physical frailty in very elderly people. *N Engl J Med* 1994;23:1769–1775.

17. Nordin K, Glimelius B. Psychological reactions in newly diagnosed gastrointestinal cancer patients. *Acta Oncol* 1997;36:803–810.

18. Stovroff M, Fraker D, Swedenborg J, et al. Cachectin/tumor necrosis factor, a possible mediator of cancer anorexia in the rat. *Cancer Res* 1988;48:920–925.

19. Opara E, Laviano A, Meguid M, et al. Correlation between food intake and CSF IL-1 in anorectic tumor bearing rats. *Neuroreport* 1995;6:750–752.

20. Langstein H, Doherty G, Fraker D, et al. The roles of gamma-interferon and tumor necrosis factor alpha in an experimental rat model of cancer cachexia. *Cancer Res* 1991;51:2302–2306.

21. Nixon DW, Heymsfield SB, Cohen AE, et al. Protein-calorie undernutrition in hospitalized cancer patients. *Am J Med* 1980;68:683–690.

22. Lundholm K, Bylund A, Holm J, et al. Skeletal muscle metabolism in patients with malignant tumor. *Eur J Cancer* 1976;12:465–473.

23. Fearon K, Hansell D, Preston T, et al. Influence of whole body protein turnover rate on resting energy expenditure in patients with cancer. *Cancer Res* 1988;48:2590–2595.

24. Heber D, Chlebowski R, Ishibashi D, et al. Abnormalities in glucose and protein metabolism in non-cachectic lung cancer patients. *Cancer Res* 1982;42:4815–4819.

25. Ebisui C, Tsujinaka T, Morimoto T, et al. Interleukin-6 induces proteolysis by activating intracellular proteases in C2C12 myotubes. *Clin Sci (Colch)* 1995;89:431–439.

26. Llovera M, Lopez-Soriano F, Argiles J. Effects of tumor necrosis factor-alpha on muscle protein turnover in female Wistar rats. *J Natl Cancer Inst* 1993;85:1334–1339.

27. Costelli P, Carbo N, Tessitore L, et al. Tumor necrosis factor-alpha mediates changes in tissue protein turnover in a rat cachexia model. *J Clin Invest* 1993;92:2783–2789.

28. Todorov P, McDevitt T, Cariuk P, et al. Induction of muscle protein degradation and weight loss by a tumor product. *Cancer Res* 1996;56:1256–1261.

29. Todorov P, Cariuk P, McDevitt T, et al. Characterization of a cancer cachectic factor. *Nature* 1996;379:739–742.

30. Cabal-Manzano R, Bhargava, Torres-Duarte A, et al. Proteolysis-inducing factor is expressed in tumors of patients with gastrointestinal cancers and correlates with weight loss. *Br J Cancer* 2001;84:1599–1601.

31. Wang Z, Corey E, Hass GM, et al. Expression of the human cachexia-associated protein (HCAP) in prostate cancer and in a prostate cancer animal model of cachexia. *Int J Cancer* 2003;105:123–129.

32. Hauner H, Petruschke T, Russ M, et al. Effects of TNF-alpha on glucose transport and lipid metabolism of newly-differentiated human fat cells in culture. *Diabetologica* 1995;38:764–771.

33. Marshall M, Doerrler W, Feingold K, et al. Leukemia inhibitory factor induces changes in lipid metabolism in cultured adipocytes. *Endocrinology* 1994;135:141–147.

34. Beck S, Tisdale M. Production of lipolytic and proteolytic factors by a murine tumor-producing cachexia in the host. *Cancer Res* 1987;47:5919–5923.

35. Valverde A, Teruel T, Navarro P, et al. Tumor necrosis factor-alpha causes insulin receptor substrate-2-mediated insulin resistance and inhibits insulin-induced adipogenesis in fetal brown adipocytes. *Endocrinology* 1998;139:1229–1238.

36. Fried S, Zechner R. Cachectin/tumor necrosis factor decreases human adipose tissue lipoprotein lipase mRNA levels, synthesis, and activity. *J Lipid Res* 1989;30:1917–1923.

37. Strassman G, Kambayashi T. Inhibition of experimental cancer cachexia by anti-cytokine and anti-cytokine receptor therapy. *Cytokines Mol Ther* 1995;1:107–113.

38. Muscaritoli M, Cangiano C, Cascino A, et al. Plasma clearance of exogenous lipids in patients with malignant disease. *Nutrition* 1990;6:147–151.

39. Rofe A, Bourgeois C, Coyle P, et al. Altered insulin response to glucose in weight-losing cancer patients. *Anticancer Res* 1994;14:647–650.

40. Grunfeld C, Dinarello C, Feingold K. Tumor necrosis factor-alpha, interleukin-1, and interferon-alpha stimulate triglyceride synthesis in HepG2 cells. *Metabolism* 1991;40:894–898.

41. Bing C, Bao Y, Jenkins J, et al. Zinc-α2-glycoprotein, a lipid mobilizing factor, is expressed in adipocytes and is up-regulated in mice with cancer cachexia. *Proc Natl Acad Sci USA* 2004;101:2500–2505.

42. Holyrode C, Babuzda T, Putnam R, et al. Altered glucose metabolism in metastatic carcinoma. *Cancer Res* 1975;35:3710–3714.

43. Tayek J, Manglik S, Abemayor E. Insulin secretion, glucose production and insulin sensitivity in underweight and normal-weight volunteers, and in underweight and normal-weight cancer patients: a clinical research center study. *Metabolism* 1997;46:140–145.

44. Qi C, Pekala P. Tumor necrosis factor-alpha-induced insulin resistance in adipocytes. *Proc Soc Exp Biol Med* 2000;223:128–135.

45. Newton J, Halsted C. Clinical and functional assessment of adults. In: Shils M, Olson J, Shike M, et al., eds. *Modern Nutrition in Health and Disease,* 9th ed. Baltimore: Williams & Wilkins; 1999: 895.

46. Heymsfield S, Baumgartner R, Pan S-F. Nutritional assessment of malnutrition by anthropometric methods. In: Shils M, Olson J, Shike M, et al., eds. *Modern Nutrition in Health and Disease,* 9th ed. Baltimore: Williams & Wilkins; 1999: 903–921.

47. Alcock N. Laboratory test for assessing nutritional status. In: Shils M, Olson J, Shike M, et al., eds. *Modern Nutrition in Health and Disease,* 9th ed. Baltimore: Williams & Wilkins; 1999: 923–935.

48. Dwyer J. Dietary assessment. In: Shils M, Olson J, Shike M, et al., eds. *Modern nutrition in health and disease,* 9th ed. Baltimore: Williams & Wilkins; 1999: 962.

49. The Veterans Administration TPN Cooperative Study Group. Perioperative total parenteral nutrition in surgical patients. *N Engl J Med* 1991;325:525–532.

50. Bastow M, Rawlings J, Allison S. Benefits of supplementary tube feeding after fractured neck of femur. *BMJ* 1983;287:1589–1594.

51. Prijatmoko D, Strauss B, Lambert J, et al. Early detection of protein depletion in alcoholic cirrhosis: role of body composition analysis. *Gastroenterology* 1993;105:1839–1845.

52. Nozoe T, Kimura Y, Ishida M, Saeki H, Korenaga D, Sugimachi K. Correlation of pre-operative nutritional condition with post-operative complications in surgical treatment for oesophageal carcinoma. *Eur J Surg Oncol* 2002;28:396–400.

53. Shike M, Russell D, Detsky A, et al. Changes in body composition in patients with small-cell lung cancer. *Ann Intern Med* 1984;101:303–309.

54. Russell D, Shike M, Marliss E, et al. Effects of total parenteral nutrition and chemotherapy on the metabolic derangements in small cell lung cancer. *Cancer Res* 1984;44:1706–1711.

55. Muller J, Brenner U, Dienst C, et al. Preoperative parenteral feeding in patients with gastrointestinal carcinoma. *Lancet* 1982;1:68–71.

56. Fan S, Lo C, Lai E, et al. Perioperative nutritional support in patient undergoing hepatectomy for hepatocellular carcinoma. *N Engl J Med* 1994;331:1547–1552.

57. Bozzetti F, Bavazzi C, Miceli R, et al. Perioperative TPN in malnourished, GI cancer patients: a randomized, clinical trial. *JPEN J Parenter Enteral Nutr* 2000;24:7–14.

58. Detsky A, Baker J, O'Rourke K, et al. Perioperative parenteral nutrition: a meta-analysis. *Ann Intern Med* 1987;107:195–203.

59. Heyland D, MacDonald S, Keefe L, et al. Total parenteral nutrition in the critically ill patient: a meta-analysis. *JAMA* 1998;16:2013–2019.

60. Brennan M, Pisters P, Posner M, et al. A prospective randomized trial of total parenteral nutrition after major pancreatic resection for malignancy. *Ann Surg* 1994;220:436–441.

61. Shirabe K, Matsumata T, Shimada M, et al. A comparison of parenteral hyperalimentation and early enteral feeding regarding systemic immunity after major hepatic resection—a randomized, prospective study. *Hepatogastroenterology* 1997;44:205–209.

62. Flynn M, Leightty F. Preoperative outpatient nutritional support of patient with squamous cancer of the upper aerodigestive tract. *Am J Surg* 1987;154:359–362.

63. Smith R, Hartemink R, Hollinshead J, et al. Fine bore jejunostomy feeding following major abdominal surgery: a controlled randomized clinical trial. *Br J Surg* 1985;72:458–461.

64. Kudsk K, Croce M, Fabian T, et al. Enteral versus parenteral feeding: effects on septic morbidity after blunt and penetrating abdominal trauma. *Ann Surg* 1992;215:503–511.

65. Lipman T. Grains or veins: is enteral nutrition really better than parenteral nutrition? A look at the evidence. *JPEN J Parenter Enteral Nutr* 1998;22:167–182.

66. van den Berghe G, Wouters P, Weekers F, et al. Intensive insulin therapy in the critically ill patients. *N Engl J Med* 2001;345:1359.

67. Wicks C, Somasundaram S, Bjarnason I, et al. Comparison of enteral feeding and TPN after liver transplantation. *Lancet* 1994;344:837–840.

68. Andreyev H, Norman A, Oates J, et al. Why do patients with weight loss have a worse outcome when undergoing chemotherapy for gastrointestinal malignancies? *Eur J Cancer* 1998;34:503–509.

69. McGeer A, Detsky A, O'Rourke K. Parenteral nutrition in cancer patients undergoing chemotherapy: a meta-analysis. *Nutrition* 1990;6:233–240.

70. De Cicco M, Panarello G, Fantin D, et al. Parenteral nutrition in cancer patients receiving chemotherapy: effects on toxicity and nutritional status. *JPEN J Parenter Enteral Nutr* 1993;17:513–518.

71. Jin D, Phillips M, Byles J. Effects of parenteral nutrition support and chemotherapy on the phasic composition of tumor cells in gastrointestinal cancer. *JPEN J Parenter Enteral Nutr* 1999;23:237–241.

72. Popp M, Morrision S, Brennan M. Total parenteral nutrition in a methylchloranthrene-induced rat sarcoma model. *Cancer Treat Rep* 1981;65(Suppl 5):137–143.

73. Senft M, Fietkau R, Iro H, et al. The influence of supportive nutritional therapy via percutaneous endoscopically guided gastrostomy on the quality of life of cancer patients. *Support Care Cancer* 1993;1:272–275.

74. Bozzetti F, Cozzaglio L, Gavazzi C, et al. Nutritional support in patients with cancer of the esophagus: impact on nutritional status, patient compliance, and survival. *Tumori* 1998;84:681–686.

75. Weisdorf S, Lysne J, Wind D, et al. Positive effect of prophylactic TPN on long-term outcome of bone marrow transplantation. *Transplantation* 1987;43:833–838.

76. Lenssen P, Bruemmer B, Bowden R, et al. Intravenous lipid dose and incidence of bacteremias and fungemia in patients undergoing bone marrow transplantation. *Am J Clin Nutr* 1998;67:927–933.

77. Muscaritoli M, Conversano L, Torelli G, et al. Clinical and metabolic effects of different parenteral regimens in patients undergoing allogeneic bone marrow transplantation. *Transplantation* 1998;66:610–616.

78. Mulder P, Bouman J, Gietema J, et al. Hyperalimentation in autologous bone marrow transplantation for solid tumors. *Cancer* 1989;64:2045–2052.

79. Szeluga D, Stuart R, Brookmeyer R, et al. Nutritional support of bone marrow transplant recipients: a prospective, randomized clinical trial comparing TPN to an enteral feeding program. *Cancer Res* 1987;47:3309–3316.

80. Donnelly S, Walsh D. The symptoms of advanced cancer. *Semin Oncol* 1995;22(Suppl 3):67–72.

81. Tchekmedyian NS, Tait N, Abrams J, et al. High-dose megestrol acetate in the treatment of advanced breast cancer. *Semin Oncol* 1986;113:37–43.

82. Loprinzi J, Michalak J, Schaid D, et al. Phase III evaluation of four doses of megestrol acetate as therapy for patients with cancer anorexia and/or cachexia. *J Clin Oncol* 1993;11:762–767.

83. Loprinzi J, Ellison N, Schaid D, et al. Controlled trial of megestrol acetate for the treatment of cancer anorexia and cachexia. *J Natl Cancer Inst* 1990;82:1127–1132.

84. Bruera E, Macmillan K, Kuehn N, et al. A controlled trial of megestrol acetate on appetite, caloric intake, nutritional status, and other symptoms in patients with advanced cancer. *Cancer* 1990;66:1279–1282.

85. Berenstein E, Ortiz Z. Megestrol acetate for the treatment of anorexia-cachexia syndrome. *Cochrane Databse Syst Rev* 2005: CD004310.

86. Pascual Lopez A, Roque I, Figuls M, Urrutia Cuchi G, et al. Systematic review of megestrol acetate in the treatment of anorexia-cachexia syndrome. *J Pain Symptom Manage* 2004;27:360–369.

87. Von Roenn J, Armstrong D, Kotler D, et al. Megestrol acetate in patients with AIDS-related cachexia. *Ann Intern Med* 1994;121:393–399.

88. Oster M, Enders S, Samuels S, et al. Megestrol acetate in patients with AIDS and cachexia. *Ann Intern Med* 1994;121:400–408.

89. Simons J, Aaronson N, Vansteenkiste J, et al. Effects of medroxyprogesterone acetate on appetite, weight, and quality of life in advanced stage non-hormone sensitive cancer: a placebo controlled multicenter trial. *J Clin Oncol* 1996;14:1077–1084.

90. Simons J, Schols A, Hoefnagels J, et al. Effects of medroxyprogesterone acetate on food intake, body composition, and resting energy expenditure in patients with advanced, nonhormone-sensitive cancer. *Cancer* 1998;82:553–560.

91. Sallan S, Cronin C, Zelen M, et al. Antiemetics in patients receiving chemotherapy for cancer. *N Engl J Med* 1980;302:135–138.

92. Beal J, Olson R, Lefkowitz L, et al. Long term efficacy and safety of dronabinol for acquired immunodeficiency syndrome-associated anorexia. *J Pain Symptom Manage* 1997;14:7–14.

93. Jatoi A, Windschitl H, Loprinzi C, et al. Dronabinol versus megestrol acetate versus combination therapy for cancer-associated anorexia: a North Central Cancer Treatment Group study. *J Clin Oncol* 2002;20:567–573.

94. Endres S, Ghorbani R, Kelley V, et al. The effect of dietary supplementation with n-3 polyunsaturated fatty acids on the synthesis of IL-1, and TNF by mononuclear cells. *N Engl J Med* 1989;320:265–271.

95. Wigmore S, Fearon K, Maingay J, et al. Down-regulation of the acute-phase response in patients with pancreatic cancer cachexia receiving oral EPA is mediated via suppression of interleukin-6. *Clin Sci (Colch)* 1997;92:215–221.

96. Endres S, Meydani S, Ghorbani R, et al. Dietary supplementation with n-3 fatty acids suppresses IL-2 production and mononuclear cell proliferation. *J Leukoc Biol* 1993;54:599–603.

97. Gogos C, Ginopoulos P, Salsa B, et al. Dietary omega-3 polyunsaturated fatty acids plus vitamin E restore immunodeficiency and prolong survival for severely ill patients with generalized malignancy. *Cancer* 1998;82:395–402.

98. Furukawa K, Tashiro T, Yamamori H, et al. Effects of soybean oil emulsion and eicosapentaenoic acid on stress response and immune function after a severely stressful operation. *Ann Surg* 1999;229:255–261.

99. Clarke R, Lund E, Latham P, et al. Effect of EPA on the proliferation and incidence of apoptosis in the colorectal cell line HT29. *Lipids* 1999;34:1287–1295.

100. Lai P, Ross J, Fearon K, et al. Cell cycle arrest and induction of apoptosis in pancreatic cancer cells exposed to EPA in vitro. *Br J Cancer* 1996;74:1375–1383.

101. Baronzio G, Galante F, Gramaglia A, et al. Tumor microcirculation and its significance in therapy: possible role of omega-3 fatty acids as rheological modifiers. *Med Hypotheses* 1998;50:175–182.

102. Barber M, Ross J, Voss Tisdale M, et al. The effect of an oral nutritional supplement enriched with fish oil on weight loss in patients with pancreatic cancer. *Br J Cancer* 1999;81:80–86.

103. Burns CP, Halabi S, Clamon G, et al. Phase II study of high-dose fish oil capsules for patients with cancer-related cachexia. *Cancer* 2004;101:370–378.

104. Bruera E, Strasser F, Palmer J, et al. Effect of fish oil on appetite and other symptoms in patients with advanced cacner and anorexia/cachexia: a double-blind, placebo-controlled trial. *J Clin Oncol* 2003;21:129–134.

105. Jatoi A, Rowland K, Loprinzi C, et al. An EPA supplement versus megestrol acetate versu both for patient with cancer-associated wasting: an NCCTG and NCI of Canada collaborative effort. *J Clin Oncol* 2004;22:2469–2476.

106. Saito H, Trocki O, Wang S, et al. Metabolic and immune effects of dietary arginine supplementation after burn. *Arch Surg* 1987;122:784–789.

107. Fanslow W, Kulkarni A, Van Buren C, et al. Effect of nucleotide restriction and supplementation on resistance to experimental murine candidiasis. *JPEN J Parenter Enteral Nutr* 1988;12:49–52.

108. Fox A, Kripke S, DePaula J, et al. Effect of glutamine-supplemented enteral diet on methotrexate induced enterocolitis. *JPEN J Parenter Enteral Nutr* 1988;12:325–331.

109. Ziegler T, Young L, Benfell K, et al. Clinical and metabolic efficacy of glutamine-supplemented parenteral nutrition after bone marrow transplantation. *Ann Intern Med* 1992;116:821–828.

110. Schloerb P, Amare M. Total parenteral nutrition with glutamine in bone marrow transplantation and other clinical applications. *JPEN J Parenter Enteral Nutr* 1993;17:407–413.

111. Scheid C, Hermann K, Kremere G, et al. Randomizeed, double-blind controlled study of glycyl-glutamine-dipeptide in the parenteral nutrition of patients with acute leukemia undergoing intensive chemotherapy. *Nutrition* 2004;20:249–254.

112. Blijlevens N, Donnelly J, Naber A, et al. A randomized, double-blinded, placebo-controlled pilot study of parenteral nutrition containing glutamine for allogeneic stem cell transplant patients. *Support Care Cancer* 2005;13:790–796.

113. Schloerb P, Skikne B. Oral and parenteral glutamine in bone marrow transplantation: a randomized, double blind study. *JPEN J Parenter Enteral Nutr* 1999;23:117–122.

114. Gianotti L, Braga M, Vignali A, et al. Effect of route of delivery and formulation of postoperative nutrition support in patients undergoing major operations for malignant neoplasms. *Arch Surg* 1997;132:1222–1230.

115. Braga M, Gianotti L, Radeelli G, et al. Perioperative immunonutrition in patients undergoing cancer surgery: results of a randomized double-blind phase 3 trial. *Arch Surg* 1999;134:428–433.

116. Senkal M, Zumtobel V, Vauer K-H, et al. Outcome and cost-effectiveness of perioperative enteral immunonutrition in patients undergoing elective upper gastrointestinal tract surgery: a prospective, randomized trial. *Arch Surg* 1999;134:1309–1316.

117. Daly J, Weintraub F, Shou J, et al. Enteral nutrition during multimodality therapy in upper gastrointestinal cancer patients. *Ann Surg* 1995;221:327–338.

118. Braga M, Gianotti L, Cestari A, et al. Gut function and immune and inflammatory responses in patients perioperatively fed with supplemented enteral formulas. *Arch Surg* 1996;131:1257–1265.

119. Gianotti L, Braga M, Fortis C, et al. A prospective, randomized clinical trial on perioperative feeding with an arginine-, n-3 fatty acid-, and RNA-enriched enteral diet: effect on host response and nutritional status. *JPEN J Parenter Enteral Nutr* 1999;23:314–320.

120. Hochwald S, Harrison L, Heslin M, et al. Early postoperative enteral feeding improves whole body protein kinetics in upper gastrointestinal cancer patients. *Am J Surg* 1997;174:325–330.

121. Heys S, Walker L, Smith I, et al. Enteral nutritional supplementation with key nutrients in patients with critical illness and cancer: a meta-analysis of randomized controlled clinical trials. *Ann Surg* 1999;229:467–477.

122. Heyland D, Novak F, Drover J, et al. Should immunonutrition become routine in critically ill patients? A systematic review of the evidence. *JAMA* 2001;286:944–953.

123. Heslin M, Latkany L, Leung D, et al. A prospective, randomized trial of early enteral feeding after resection of upper gastrointestinal malignancy. *Ann Surg* 1997;226:567–580.

124. Gianotti L, Braga M, Nespoli L, et al. A randomized controlled trial of preoperative oral supplementation with a specialized diet in patients with gi cancer. *Gastroenterology* 2002;122:1763–1770.

125. Wadleigh R, Redman R, Graham M, et al. Vitamin E in the treatment of chemotherapy-induced mucositis. *Am J Med* 1992;92:481–484.

126. Anderson P, Schroeder G, Skubitz K. Oral glutamine reduces the duration and severity of stomatitis after cytotoxic cancer chemotherapy. *Cancer* 1998;83:1433–1439.

127. Anderson P, Ramsay N, Shu X, et al. Effect of low-dose oral glutamine on painful stomatitis during bone marrow transplantation. *Bone Marrow Transplant* 1998;22:339–344.

128. Huang E, Leung S, Wang C, et al. Oral glutamine to alleviate radiation-induced oral mucositis: a pilot randomized trial. *Int J Radiat Oncol Biol Phys* 2000;46:535–539.

129. Okuno S, Woodhouse C, Loprinzi C, et al. Phase III controlled evaluation of glutamine for decreasing stomatitis in patients receiving 5-FU-based chemotherapy. *Am J Clin Oncol* 1999;22:258–261.

130. Kaplan M, Elta G, Furie B, et al. Fat-soluble vitamin nutriture in primary biliary cirrhosis. *Gastroenterology* 1988;95:787–792.

131. Whelton M, Kehayoglou A, Agnew J, et al. Calcium absorption in parenchymatous and biliary liver disease. *Gut* 1971;12:978–983.

132. Krasinski S, Russell R, Samloff I, et al. Fundic atrophic gastritis in an elderly population: effect on hemoglobin and several nutritional indicators. *J Am Geriatr Soc* 1986;34:800–806.

133. Lindenbaum J, Savage D, Stabler S, et al. Diagnosis of cobalamin deficiency: relative sensitivities of serum cobalamin, methylmalonic acid, and total homocysteine levels. *Am J Hematol* 1990;34:99–107.

134. Lindenbaum J, Savage D, Stabler S, et al. Neuropsychiatric disorders caused by cobalamin deficiency in the absence of anemia or macrocytosis. *N Engl J Med* 1988;318:1720–1728.

135. Marcuard S, Albernaz I, Khazanie P. Omeprazole therapy causes malabsorption of cyanocobalamin. *Ann Intern Med* 1994;120:211–215.

136. Filipsson S, Hulten L, Lindstedt G. Malabsorption of fat and vitamin B_{12} before and after intestinal resection for Crohn's disease. *Scand J Gastroenterol* 1978;13:529–536.

137. Swain C, Tavill A, Neale G. Studies of tryptophan and albumin metabolism in a patient with carcinoid syndrome, pellagra, and hypoproteinemia. *Gastroenterology* 1976;71:484–489.

138. Burstein HJ, Gelber S, Guadagnoli E, et al. Use of alternative medicine by women with early-stage breast cancer. *N Engl J Med* 1999;340:1733–1739.

139. Eisenberg DM, Kessler RC, Foster C, et al. Unconventional medicine in the United States—prevalence, costs, and patterns of use. *N Engl J Med* 1993;328:246–252.

140. Batkin S, Taussig S, Szekerczes J. Modulation of pulmonary metastasis (Lewis lung carcinoma) by bromelain, an extract of the pineapple stem (*Ananas comosus*). *Cancer Invest* 1988;6(2):241–242.

141. Batkin S, Taussig SJ, Szekerezes J. Antimetastatic effect of bromelain with or without its proteolytic and anticoagulant activity. *J Cancer Res Clin Oncol* 1988;114(5):507–508.

142. Nakachi K, Suemasu K, Suga K, et al. Influence of drinking green tea on breast cancer malignancy among Japanese patients. *Jpn J Cancer Res* 1998;89(3):254–261.

143. Komori A, Yatsunami J, Okabe S, et al. Anticarcinogenic activity of green tea polyphenols. *Jpn J Clin Oncol* 1993;23(3):186–190.

144. Sheu JR, Fu CC, Tsai ML, et al. Effect of U-995, a potent shark cartilage-derived angiogenesis inhibitor, on anti-angiogenesis and anti-tumor activities. *Anticancer Res* 1998;18:4435–4441.

145. Miller DR, Anderson GT, Stark JJ, et al. Phase I/II trial of the safety and efficacy of shark cartilage in the treatment of advanced cancer. *J Clin Oncol* 1998;16(11):3649–3655.

146. Unproven methods of cancer management. Laetrile. *CA Cancer J Clin* 1991;41(3):187–192.

147. Dorr RT, Paxinos J. The current status of laetrile. *Ann Intern Med* 1978;89(3):389–397.

148. Dwyer JT. Unproven nutritional remedies and cancer. *Nutr Rev* 1992;50(4 Pt 1):106–109.

149. Weitzman S. Alternative nutritional cancer therapies. *Int J Cancer* 1998;11(Suppl):69–72.

150. Gerson method. *CA Cancer J Clin* 1990;40(4):252–256.

151. Phillips DP, Kanter EJ, Bednarczyk B, et al. Importance of the lay press in the transmission of medical knowledge to the scientific community. *N Engl J Med* 1991;325(16):1180–1183.

152. Livingston-Wheeler therapy. *CA Cancer J Clin* 1990;40(2):103–108.

CHAPTER 9 ■ IMAGING OF GASTROINTESTINAL MALIGNANCIES

SEAN D. CURRAN AND LAWRENCE H. SCHWARTZ

INTRODUCTION

The imaging of gastrointestinal (GI) malignancies continues to evolve and improve. Several different imaging modalities are often required in the workup once a cancer is suspected or identified. Barium studies remain useful for assessment of luminal tumors and their extent. Cross-sectional studies such as computed tomography (CT), magnetic resonance imaging (MRI), and ultrasonography (US) remain the main modalities for diagnosis and staging of most cancers (1,2). Endoscopic ultrasound (EUS) is a powerful tool in experienced hands for diagnosis and intervention in selected patients with esophageal, rectal, and pancreatic cancer. The emergence of the combination of fluorodeoxy glucose positron emission tomography (FDG-PET) and positron emission tomography CT (PET-CT) in a single scanner has overshadowed PET in recent years due to its increased ability to fuse the functional information of PET with the accurate anatomical localization of CT, showing excellent results in detection and recurrence of colorectal cancer (CRC) and esophageal cancer, as well as treatment response of gastrointestinal stromal tumors (GISTs) and lymphoma. Significant improvement in the spatial resolution of CT with the introduction of 16- and 64-slice scanners has enabled the generation of clear images in the sagittal and coronal planes, rendering CT arteriography (CTA) an adequate replacement for invasive arteriography for assessment of hepatic vessels prior to surgery. In the future, functional imaging in the form of PET-CT and MRI will likely become an essential tool in the detection and monitoring of treatment response for many of these malignancies (3).

Imaging of cancers once diagnosed often determines and directs appropriate therapies that are stage dependent (Fig. 9.1). Determination of involvement of locoregional lymph nodes is critical, and imaging by CT or MRI can determine this by size (>1 cm on short axis diameter). However, it is well known that normal-size lymph nodes can harbor cancer cells and that enlarged nodes may not represent cancer (4).

Barium studies still remain the initial radiologic workup for suspected luminal cancers (5). The location and extent of the tumor may be shown to help direct biopsy or stent placement when required. Double-contrast barium enema (DCBE) can detect polyps and small tumors in those able to tolerate the procedure. Virtual colonoscopy (computed tomography colonography [CTC]) has not been proven accurate enough to be used as a screening method and is limited due to its inability to sample lesions.

Many GI cancers require several imaging modalities to direct further management, and test selection is based on availability of equipment and expertise, as well as the pretest probability of a positive result. Algorithms for test selection are given in Figs. 9.2 and 9.3.

PHYSICS OF IMAGING

There are significant differences in the physical principles on which the major imaging modalities are based. Although a detailed description of the physics of medical imaging is beyond the scope of this chapter, the essential points are briefly covered in this section.

Ultrasonography

High-frequency sound waves are transmitted through the body by a transducer. The transducer converts electric pulses into sound waves using a piezoelectric material. Transducer frequencies range from 2 to 16 MHz. The time of flight of the sound wave to be received back to the transducer is used to determine the depth of an object. The speed of sound in tissue is more than five times that in air; ultrasound functions only when there is no air between the probe and the target. Sound waves are reflected back in varying degrees, depending on the reflectivity of the tissues at interfaces. The amount reflected is based on both the angle of incidence and the difference between the acoustic impedances of the tissues on either side of the interface. The received echo signals are detected and translated into luminance to form an image with depth perception.

Spatial resolution in ultrasonography has two distinct components: an axial component and a lateral component. The axial resolution is defined as the ability to discern two objects that lie on top of one another. It is dependent on the length of the transmitted ultrasonographic signal. The lateral resolution, the ability to discriminate between two adjacent objects, is determined by the transducer beam width.

Tissue harmonic imaging refers to use of the second and greater fundamental frequencies to generate an image, thus reducing artefact and scatter at least in the near field. This technique has been shown to improve visualization of many structures, especially in the "difficult to scan" or obese patient.

Computed Tomography

CT uses conventional x-rays to generate two- and three-dimensional images with the help of a computer. The technology has continued to improve as scanners become faster each year. Early CT scanners used an incremental technology in which images were produced at a given table position. Each slice of the patient's anatomy was obtained by moving the x-ray tube in a circle around the patient, with the table remaining stationary. Image reconstruction started during the scan and was completed shortly after the scan was done. The table was

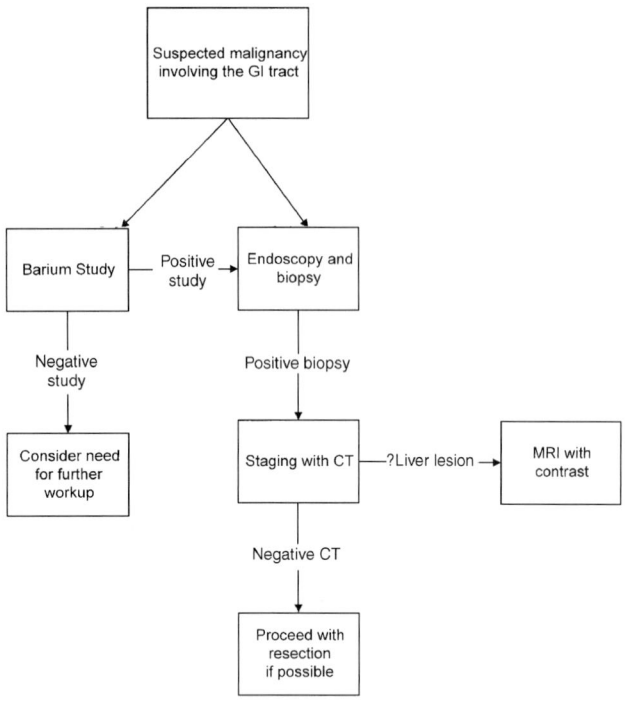

FIGURE 9.1. Algorithm for the investigation of a suspected malignancy involving the lumen of the gastrointestinal (GI) tract. CT, computed tomography; MRI, magnetic resonance imaging.

then moved and the process completed for each slice until the predetermined field of view (FOV) was covered.

All newer generation CT scanners are spiral, in which the tube (x-ray source) continuously rotates around the patient who is continuously moved (translated) at a certain speed defined by the pitch. There is continuous data acquisition, which allows for superior temporal resolution. The computer then generates true axial slice data from the oblique spiral data. Since 2002, CT scanners are now multidetector (4, 8, 16, or

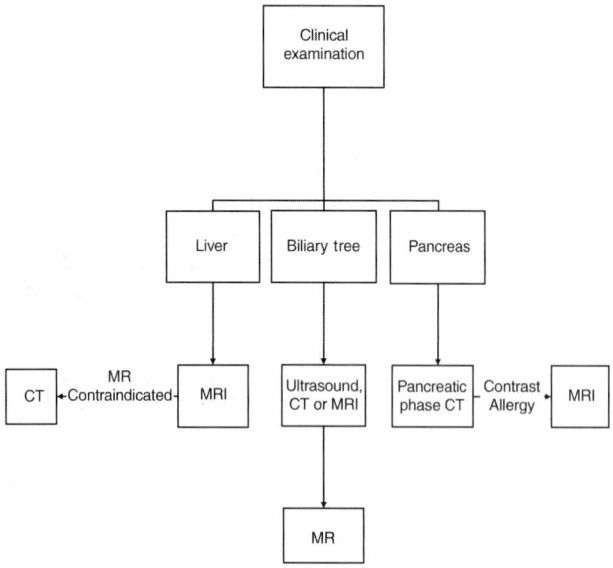

FIGURE 9.2. Workup of a suspected solid organ malignancy. CT, computed tomography; MRI, magnetic resonance imaging.

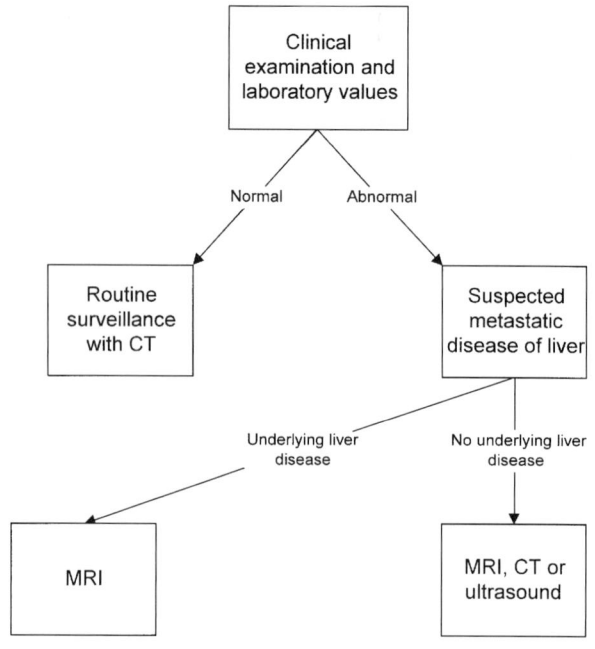

FIGURE 9.3. Workup of suspected metastatic disease to the liver. CT, computed tomography; MRI, magnetic resonance imaging.

64), meaning that instead of using a single detector, they use a row of detectors called a *detector array*. The detector array enables simultaneous acquisition of 4 or 16 slices during one gantry rotation. Subsecond gantry rotation speeds have enabled chest abdomen and pelvis to be fully scanned in a single breath-hold.

Because data are acquired as a volume, this volume can be reconstructed even retrospectively to obtain slices of different thickness from the raw data (as long as it has not been deleted). Thin reconstructed image slices of ≤1 mm can then be stacked together to generate a volume for three-dimensional reconstruction for angiography and "virtual" endoscopy. These newer generation multidetector (16- and 64-detector or "slice") CT scanners can generate isotropic volume data sets that can generate clear images in any plane similar to MRI.

CT images are considered high-resolution images (compared to MRI and ultrasonography) at a matrix of 512×512 pixels. The FOV divided by the number of pixels determines the resolution or pixel size (or voxel size when discussing three-dimensional volume). For example, if a 51.2-cm FOV is chosen, then each pixel is 1 mm; if a 25.6-cm FOV is chosen, then each pixel is 0.5 mm. Slice thickness plays a role in the voxel size; for example, if the slice thickness is 5 mm, then the voxel is $1 \text{ mm} \times 1 \text{ mm} \times 5 \text{ mm}$. The thinner the slice, the smaller is the volume of the imaging voxel, and this decreases volume averaging.

Magnetic Resonance Imaging

MRI is a technique that uses strong magnetic fields and multiple radiofrequency pulses to generate an image with outstanding spatial resolution and tissue contrast. Certain nuclei have a magnetic moment because they are composed of an odd number of protons and neutrons. When placed in a strong magnetic field, these nuclei attempt to align with the field and rotate or spin (precess) about the axis of the magnetic field. The frequency of precession (the Larmor frequency) depends on the specific nuclei and the field strength of the magnet.

The most commonly imaged nucleus is that of hydrogen 1 because of its abundance in the body and its high gyromagnetic ratio compared with other nuclei, such as those of other commonly found nuclei in the body (e.g., phosphorus 31, sodium 23, carbon 13). When hydrogen nuclei in a strong magnetic field are excited by the addition of a radiofrequency pulse, these nuclei gain energy. When the radiofrequency pulse is turned off, the nuclei return to their resting state and emit the previously absorbed energy at the same frequency. The magnitude of the emitted signal and the time it takes for the nuclei to return to the resting state depend on certain intrinsic properties of the nuclei, which include nuclear spin density (or proton density), longitudinal relaxation, transverse relaxation, and flow.

Spin density (proton density) refers to the density of nuclei potentially available to be imaged. The net signal measured in a given volume is the sum of the hydrogen protons. Therefore, tissues that have few or no hydrogen protons have no MRI signal, such as the air in the lungs or bowel and cortical bone (composed of calcium). The longitudinal (or T1) relaxation time is a measure of the time it takes the precessing nuclei to return to their baseline state (i.e., oriented parallel to the magnetic field) after the radiofrequency pulse has been turned off. The energy released during this process is absorbed by the surrounding molecular environment or lattice; hence, longitudinal or T1 relaxation is also known as *spin-lattice relaxation*. T1 is the time for the MRI signal to rise to 63% of its maximum equilibrium value. T1 varies between 200 and 800 milliseconds for most tissues. Tissues with a short T1 appear bright on T1-weighted images, and tissues with long T1 (those containing water) are dark.

The transverse (or T2) relaxation time is a measure of the loss of signal in the plane orthogonal to the long axis of the magnetic field due to the loss of phase coherence between the protons. The loss of phase coherence is due to the minute changes in the magnetic field caused by the spinning protons. For this reason, transverse or T2 relaxation is also known as *spin-spin relaxation*. T2 is the time it takes for the MRI signal to decrease to 63% of its original value. T2 varies between 50 and 200 milliseconds for most tissues. Tissues with a long T2 (those containing water) appear bright on a T2-weighted image.

A number of extrinsic parameters or variables may be manipulated to change the tissue contrast and thus the appearance of an image. The spin echo pulse sequence begins with a 90-degree radiofrequency pulse followed by a 180-degree refocusing radiofrequency pulse. A coherent signal is emitted from the nuclei at the echo time (TE). The complete image data set is produced by repeating this spin echo pulse sequence many times. The time between each successive 90-degree radiofrequency pulse is the repetition time (TR). By varying the TR and TE, one can change the image contrast to produce an image that is either T1 or T2 weighted. Images with a short TE and short TR tend to be T1 weighted, whereas images with a long TE and long TR tend to be T2 weighted. Image matrix size (number of pixels), FOV, and slice thickness may be varied according to the area being imaged, the required detail, and the time available to acquire the image.

Positron Emission Tomography

PET generates images by detecting energy given off by decaying radioactive isotopes. As they decay, radioactive isotopes emit positrons that collide with electrons and produce gamma rays that shoot off in opposite directions. PET systems use the information from the paths of these two gamma rays to determine the original collision point. The scanners have a circular array of gamma ray detectors similar to the arrangement in a CT scanner. The signals are then processed and converted into two- and three-dimensional images.

PET (superseded now by combination PET-CT) is a relatively new technique for use in the staging of GI malignancies (6). The most commonly used compound in clinical practice is FDG-PET scanning, whereby a glucose derivative is tagged with a radioactive label (fluorine 18). This tagged molecule is transported across the cell membrane, and because it is not suitable for complete glycolysis, it accumulates in the metabolically hyperactive cell. Because accumulation occurs at a greater rate than in most normal tissues, a measure of uptake, called the *standard uptake value* (SUV), may be calculated. Malignant processes tend to have a higher metabolic rate than benign processes, with the notable exception of inflammation or infection. Combination scanners now fuse the functional (PET) images onto anatomical images (CT), which has increased the accuracy of PET (7). Combination PET-CT is also up to 30% faster due to synergies using CT data for registration. Spatial resolution of PET images is currently limited to 5 mm.

Conventional Barium Studies (Fluoroscopy)

Barium studies remain an excellent way of diagnosing GI malignancies, particularly tumors involving lumens. They are obtained using conventional x-rays with the addition of a fluoroscopy unit. Fluoroscopy allows real time x-ray visualization of the patient with the help of variable amounts of barium and air (hence, "double" contrast). X-rays are continuously transmitted onto a fluorescent screen, and with the help of an image intensifier, are projected onto a television monitor for the radiologist. Other contrast agents such as nonionic intravenous contrast can be given in certain situations. Double-contrast examinations can show mucosal detail to a greater extent than single-contrast (barium only) examinations and more readily reveal early lesions (8–10). Barium examinations are an efficient way to evaluate the GI tract from the esophagus to the rectum and give useful dynamic information that cannot be achieved with cross-sectional imaging. Discussion of the relative roles of barium examinations and endoscopy is beyond the scope of this chapter. Numerous studies have addressed this issue (11–17). Barium examination and endoscopy each have advantages and disadvantages. The principal advantage of endoscopy is biopsy capability. In patients who are known to have a malignant polyp in the rectosigmoid region, the remainder of the colon should be examined endoscopically (15).

GASTROINTESTINAL MALIGNANCIES INVOLVING THE LUMEN OF THE GASTROINTESTINAL TRACT

Contrast studies of the GI tract can be performed with either barium or water-soluble contrast agents. If there is any risk of aspiration, it is best to use a nonionic contrast agent such as iopromide.

The imaging of suspected neoplasms of the GI tract lumen generally begins with a barium study for the evaluation of nonspecific GI complaints. Evaluation of the esophagus, stomach, and duodenum is best accomplished with an upper GI study. Suspected small bowel pathology may be evaluated with a small bowel follow-through after an upper GI study or with enteroclysis. Small bowel follow-through has poor sensitivity and may become a historical investigation if advances in both CT enteroclysis (18) and wireless capsule endoscopy continue (19). Enteroclysis is usually reserved for specific evaluation of small bowel pathology when a routine small bowel series is negative and disease is still clinically suspected. Enteroclysis requires small bowel intubation with the passage of a 10-French Maglite tube or similar under fluoroscopic guidance past the ligament of Treitz. Subsequently, a mixture of barium and methylcellulose is injected under pressure via a pump. The double-contrast enteroclysis gives exquisite detail of the small bowel mucosa. Coronal and curved CT reconstructions of the small bowel are likely to help in the diagnosis of small bowel lesions.

DCBE and CTC are used for detection (screening) of colonic polyps or masses in healthy individuals, as well as to exclude (synchronous) second primary lesions preoperatively. In certain circumstances, single-contrast studies, if performed carefully, can adequately evaluate for masses or constricting lesions (9). Double-contrast examinations have the added ability to evaluate the underlying mucosal detail.

Specific diagnosis is not always possible based on imaging findings. Criteria exist to allow for lesion stratification for likelihood of malignancy. Malignant and benign lesions have certain characteristics, depending on their location. Malignant lesions tend to have irregular margins and overhanging edges, which is termed *shouldering*. Esophageal lesions may also appear as strictures, and differentiating benign from malignant lesions may be difficult because there is overlap in the appearances (20). Benign strictures tend to be long with smooth, tapered edges. However, biopsy of any esophageal stricture seen on barium examination is prudent.

Esophagus

Primary radiographic evaluation of the esophagus usually entails a barium study (Fig. 9.4), although the esophagogram may be prompted by the appearance of abnormalities on images obtained using other modalities. Double-contrast esophagography has 95% sensitivity for detecting esophageal or gastroesophageal junction carcinoma (21). Several methods are available for staging esophageal carcinoma once diagnosed (22–24). However, no single imaging modality is ideal, and imaging assessment of esophageal cancer both preoperatively and post resection remains a difficult challenge. The current evidence

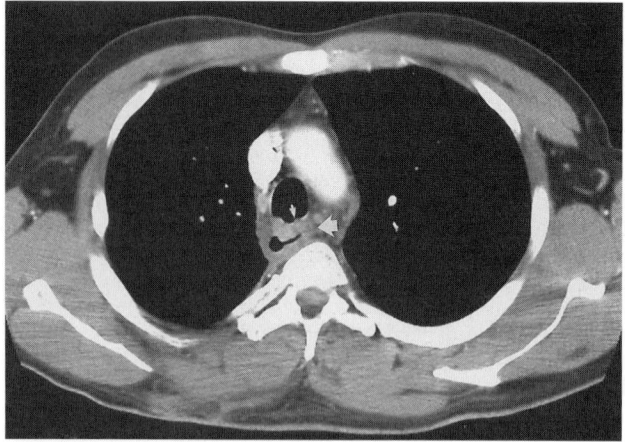

FIGURE 9.5. Esophageal carcinoma. Computed tomography image through the upper thorax demonstrating asymmetric soft tissue thickening of the esophagus (*large arrow*) in a patient with esophageal carcinoma. Note irregularity of the posterior wall of the trachea representing invasion by the carcinoma (*small arrow*).

shows that PET is more accurate than CT in the detection of occult metastatic disease, prediction of the response to therapy, and detection of recurrent disease (25,26). A combination of CT and EUS has been used until recently for locoregional staging (Fig. 9.5). PET has been shown to be more accurate than CT for detecting metastatic esophageal cancer, and so where available, it should be used to avoid unnecessary major surgery (27). PET-CT is now part of the routine workup of esophageal cancer (Fig. 9.6). Recent studies have shown hybrid PET-CT fused images have incremental value over PET and CT in staging (28). Work has also shown that changes in SUV uptake after treatment with combined chemoradiation correlates with progressionfree survival (29). EUS is the superior modality for

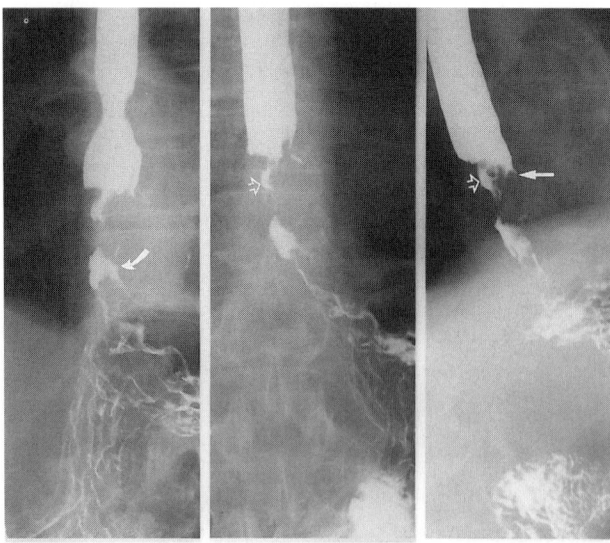

FIGURE 9.4. Esophageal carcinoma. Three images from a barium esophagram. A mass is present at the gastroesophageal junction with irregular margins (*curved arrows*), ulceration (*arrowhead*), and overhanging edges (*arrow*).

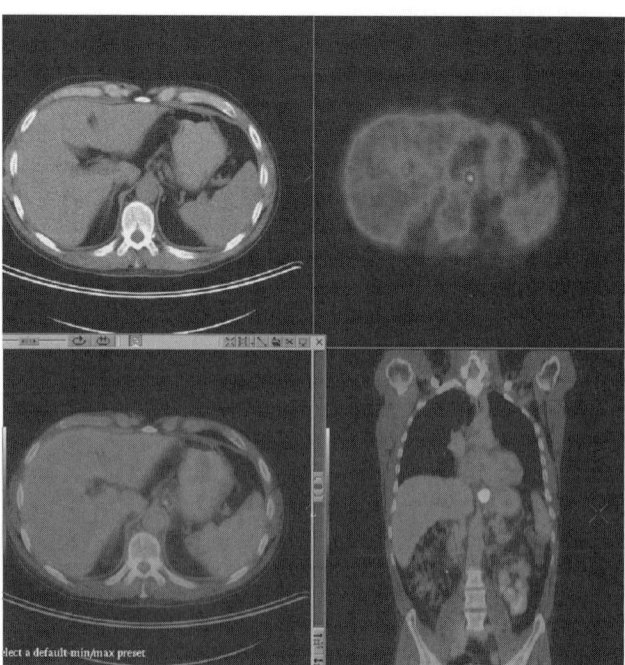

FIGURE 9.6. A 56-year-old man with lower esophageal fusion positron emission tomography computed tomography staging images showing a tumor at the gastroesophageal junction.

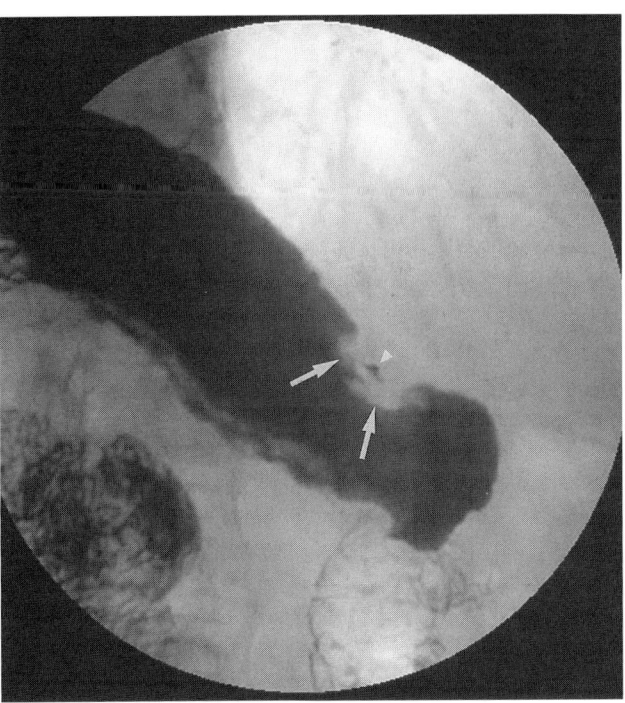

FIGURE 9.7. Gastric cancer. Image from an upper gastrointestinal examination demonstrates a mass (*arrows*) with central ulceration (*arrowhead*). Note that the mass projects into the gastric lumen, not beyond the expected location of the gastric wall as would be seen in a benign ulcer.

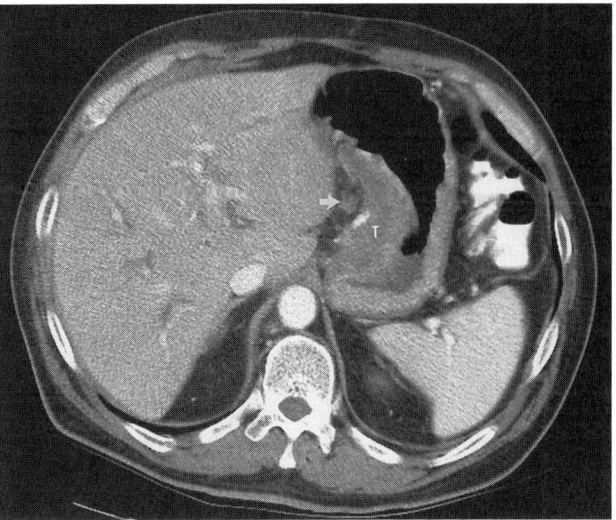

FIGURE 9.8. Gastric cancer. Computed tomography demonstrates a soft tissue tumor (T) in the gastric wall. Note the presence of a lymph node in the gastrohepatic ligament (*arrow*).

T staging (30). CT has limitations in detecting local invasion of the aorta and other adjacent structures, but virtual CT airway bronchoscopy may obviate fiber-optic bronchoscopy to detect invasion of the bronchial system (31). All modalities may either understage or overstage esophageal carcinoma, and the imaging strategy needs to be tailored for each individual patient.

Stomach and Small Bowel

Gastric carcinoma may present in several ways. Malignancies may appear as ulcers or linitis plastica, or as metastatic disease (32). Linitis plastica has a typical appearance in which the stomach is rigid, narrow, and tubular. Malignant gastric masses may also manifest as ulcers. These ulcerated masses may have characteristic appearances on barium studies (Fig. 9.7). Differentiating between benign and malignant ulcers is not always possible. Certain classic findings, however, are associated with both benign and malignant ulcers and are summarized in Table 9.1. Location in the stomach does not differentiate between benign and malignant ulcers. Although benign ulcers are more common on the lesser curvature and in the gastric antrum, malignant ulcers may appear there as well. The appearance of the gastric rugae near the ulcer crater may aid in differentiation. The folds of a benign ulcer extend to the edge of the ulcer crater, whereas the folds of a malignant ulcer end at a distance from the margin of the ulcer. The latter occurs because a mass is usually associated with a malignant ulceration. On a high-quality double-contrast barium study, classic benign ulcers with the features discussed previously may be followed to resolution. A large percentage of ulcers are indeterminate and require biopsy.

Once the diagnosis of a malignant lesion is made, the patient generally undergoes a CT examination for appropriate staging (33). CT is useful both for assessing local extent of gastric cancer and for identifying metastatic disease (Fig. 9.8). Occasionally, patients with gastric carcinoma present with extragastric symptoms such as jaundice, the cause of which may be seen on CT. The wall thickness of a well-distended stomach is variable but should always be <1 cm; additional enhancement patterns may aid in the diagnosis of gastric cancer (34). Water is used as a low attenuation oral contrast agent for several reasons. First, adequate distension of the stomach is essential

TABLE 9.1

IMAGING FINDINGS THAT AID IN DISTINGUISHING BETWEEN BENIGN AND MALIGNANT GASTRIC LESIONS

	Benign	Malignant
Location	75% lesser curvature, mostly antrum	Mostly antrum
Therapeutic response	Usually in 4–6 weeks	No response
Projection with respect to expected location of gastric wall	Projects beyond gastric wall	Mass projecting

for depiction of lesions, and enhancement of the stomach wall by intravenous contrast would be obscured by high-density oral contrast agents. Second, the use of traditional oral contrast agents would complicate two- and three-dimensional visualization of gastric vessels with CT angiography (35,36). The presence of a focal mass or focal thickening in a well-distended stomach should alert the physician to the possibility of a gastric malignancy. CT is a good modality for the identification of regional and distant spread; however, it is relatively insensitive for determining resectability. However, most prior studies used slice thicknesses of 5 to 10 mm, which have partial volume averaging with adjacent structures. The problem of partial volume averaging is greatly reduced by using section thicknesses of 1.25 mm with superior multiplanar reconstruction images due to the high speed of multidetector scanners, which also overcome breathing artefacts (37). Criteria used to assess resectability, such as irregularity of the tumor or loss of the fat plane between the mass and the adjacent organs, are not sensitive for invasion (38). When these findings are identified, they should alert one to the possibility of unresectability. It has been shown that PET can demonstrate response to treatment of GISTs by a reduction in SUU (39). This is particularly powerful in the setting of little or no change in tumor size.

Malignant processes may also involve small bowel. A barium examination of the small bowel may reveal an apple core–type lesion with an appearance similar to that of primary adenocarcinoma of the colon. Small lesions may be difficult to detect on a routine small bowel follow-through. If a primary small bowel tumor is suspected, enteroclysis is the preferred imaging modality. Recent advances in CT enteroclysis and wireless capsule endoscopy suggest that these will play a significant role in the future of small bowel tumor visualization (40).

The most common primary small bowel malignancy is carcinoid. The primary carcinoid tumor is frequently overlooked on CT scans, but the desmoplastic reaction produced by the tumor is easily recognizable. Frequently, small bowel carcinoids can be seen either on small bowel series or on enteroclysis. Again, the primary tumor may not be visualized, but the mesenteric metastasis tends to cause both mass effect and angulation with a stellate or sunburst pattern of bowel loops. Mesenteric carcinoids often calcify, and liver metastases are characteristically hypervascular. This constellation of findings suggests a probable diagnosis of carcinoid (Table 9.1).

Colon

An apple core–shaped lesion is the classic appearance of a primary adenocarcinoma of the colon on barium studies (Fig. 9.9). Some colonic carcinomas arise in polyps, and any filling defect on a barium study requires further evaluation with endoscopy.

Barium Enema

Barium enemas (BEs) can be performed with either barium alone (single-contrast) or barium and air (double-contrast) techniques. DCBE has a higher sensitivity for polyps <1 cm compared to single-contrast barium enema; however, there is no difference in sensitivity for clinically significant polyps >1 cm. DCBE is generally well tolerated, and serious complications such as colonic rupture are rare (1 in 30,000 examinations). A good rule of thumb is that if the patient requires more than one arm held while getting on the table, they are likely too frail to go ahead with the examination. Other contraindications to BE are recent colonic biopsy and toxic megacolon.

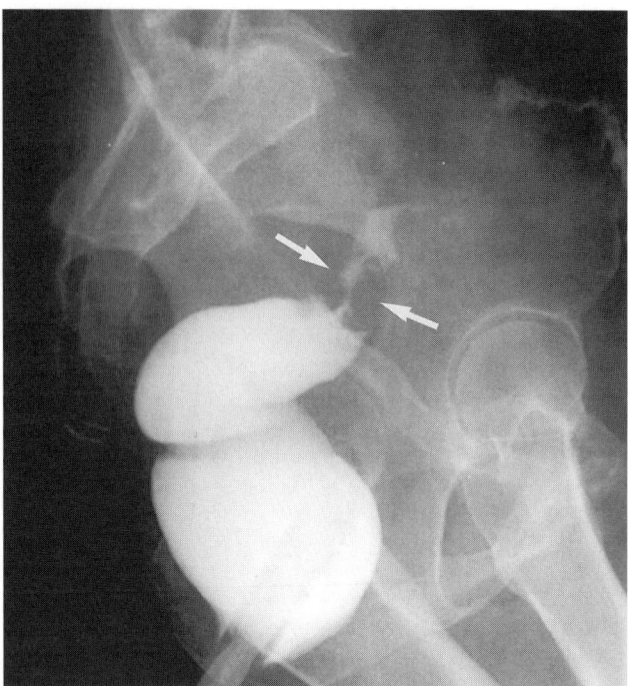

FIGURE 9.9. Adenocarcinoma of the colon presenting as an apple core lesion. Image from a barium enema study demonstrates a circumferential mass (*arrows*). This mass has disrupted the normal mucosal pattern and has irregular overhanging edges.

Several imaging techniques that complement endoscopic colonoscopy, such as DCBE, minimal preparation CT, and CTC, can be used to screen for CRC. However, no single imaging test has been approved for routine screening of an asymptomatic population. The use of BE has decreased dramatically since the mid-1990s, and many radiology residents have little or no experience with this technique. The decline in use of BE is due to the rise in popularity and sophistication of colonoscopy and CTC, which have been shown to have specificities and specificities approaching 100% for polyps >9 mm (41,42). Minimal preparation CT may be useful in an older population in centers where CTC is not available and BE is unsuitable (43).

Compared with other techniques, dynamic contrast-enhanced CT has the advantage of being fast and less invasive. The latest generation 16-slice CT scanners take 5-mm images, completing the full abdomen and pelvis in seconds.

Colon carcinomas usually appear as single or multiple lobulated masses on both CT and MRI (Figs. 9.10 and 9.11). Colon carcinoma may be found incidentally during a workup for nonspecific abdominal complaints, and their detection may be completely fortuitous. Frequently, an imaging study will identify an asymmetric soft tissue mass in the colon.

Computed Tomography Colonoscopy

Initially called virtual colonoscopy, CTC is a rapidly evolving technique that focuses on the colon and is being increasingly employed to detect polyps and cancer. CTC is noninvasive and has the advantage of detecting extracolonic lesions. Currently, CTC may be used as an alternative to conventional colonoscopy in cases of difficulty with sedation or incomplete colonography. As needed, the two examinations may be performed on the same day. Magnetic resonance colonography is

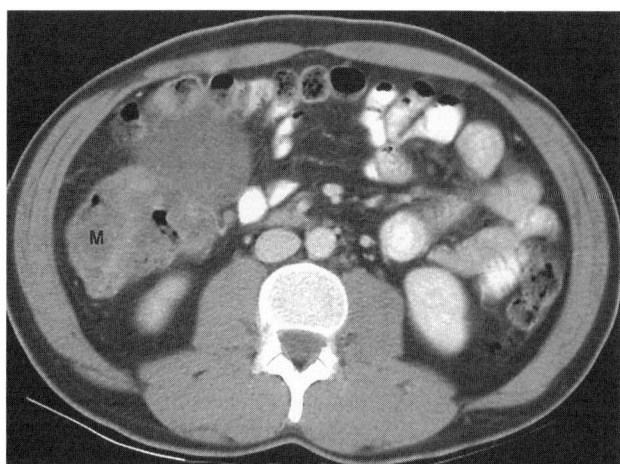

FIGURE 9.10. Adenocarcinoma of the ascending colon. A computed tomography image of a patient with vague abdominal complaints demonstrates a large nonobstructing mass (M) in the ascending colon.

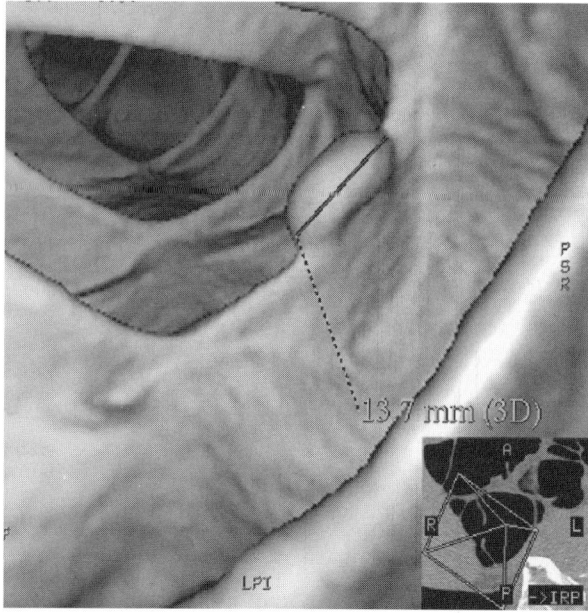

FIGURE 9.12. Computed tomography colonographic multiplanar reformatted three-dimensional endoluminal image (generated on a GE Advantage 4.2 workstation) showing a 1.4-cm polyp in the hepatic flexure.

a promising new technique that has the advantage of lacking ionizing radiation (44).

Because the reader learning curve is steep in CTC, it is recommended that radiologists review at least 25 to 50 studies and attend a dedicated training course. Computer-aided detection will likely play a major role in the future as an aid to interpretation. Dedicated reformatting workstations generate an endoluminal three-dimensional fly-through for optimal measurement of lesions.

Controversy exists among the large studies due to discrepancies in results that may be due to lack of reader experience and standardization of technique that varied widely across the studies. In particular, the study design may have contributed to an underestimation of the accuracy of CTC (45,46). Two particular problems with CTC are inadequate bowel preparation

and retained fluid causing difficulty in interpretation and lack of standardization of reporting. A recent consensus proposal has issued a new "C-RADS" classification of reporting (47). Fecal tagging is helping with inadequate preparation and is being used in the newer trials. Two large prospective multicenter American College of Radiology Imaging Network trials investigating the accuracy of CTC and its possible role in screening are near completion (48). The combination of faster CT scanners, better computer software, and fecal tagging, along with greater reader experience, indicates that CTC will likely become a key investigation for CRC screening in the future (Fig. 9.12).

Technique

In select patients, CTC is a promising technique for the detection of colonic polyps or masses. The technique is not entirely noninvasive because the colon must first be well cleansed. Bowel preparation is usually undertaken with a double-dose oral sodium phosphate solution. Fecal tagging can use iodine alone or iodine in combination with barium to subtract the tagged stool and fluid from images. Although the use of spasmolytics is not routine, they may be used if the patient poorly tolerates the air. Either room air or carbon dioxide may be insufflated to patient discomfort or early spasm with the use of a rectal tube. Intravenous contrast is optional. Patients are scanned in both prone and supine positions after the insufflation of air showing adequate bowel distension. Slice thickness of 3 mm is standard. Colonoscopy is recommended for all polyps >1 cm.

Rectal carcinoma is imaged differently from colon carcinoma, not only because of its different routes of spread but also because different imaging modalities are available that improve local staging of rectal cancer such as MRI and EUS (49–52). Sonography requires insertion of a probe into the rectum to obtain high-resolution images of the rectal wall and of any masses. EUS can be used to accurately demonstrate rectal tumors. However, it has several limitations, such as intolerance by the patient, a limited FOV, and operator dependence. MRI has

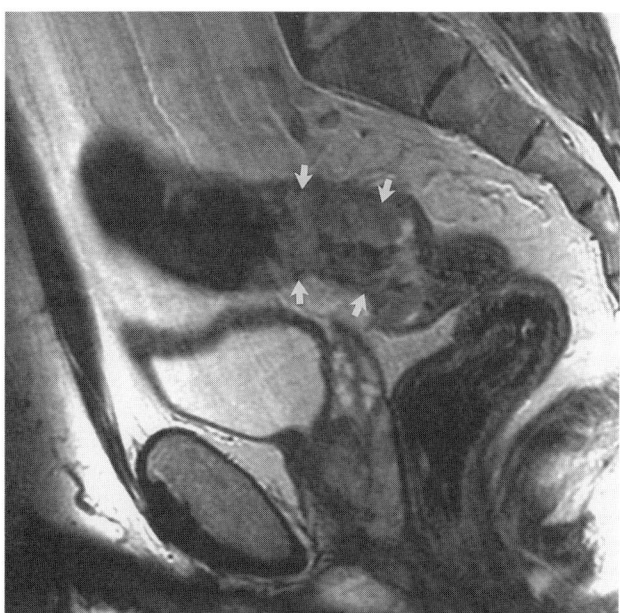

FIGURE 9.11. Adenocarcinoma of the colon. Sagittal T2-weighted magnetic resonance image demonstrates a mass in the sigmoid colon (*arrows*), proven adenocarcinoma.

TABLE 9.2

NORMAL APPEARANCE OF THE LAYERS OF THE RECTUM ON ENDORECTAL SONOGRAPHY AND T2-WEIGHTED MAGNETIC RESONANCE IMAGING (MRI) SCANS

Layer	Ultrasonography	T2-weighted MRI scans
Superficial mucosa	Echogenic	Hyperintense
Deep mucosa, including muscularis mucosae	Hypoechoic	Hypointense
Submucosa	Echogenic	Hyperintense
Muscularis propria	Hypoechoic	Hypointense
Serosa/perirectal fat	Echogenic	Hyperintense

the advantage of clearly demonstrating the mesorectal fascia, which should be the circumferential resection margin (CRM) in a well-done operation. High-spatial resolution MRI has been shown to be useful for staging of primary rectal tumors with a high positive predictive value for prediction of histologic status of the CRM, which allows stratification of therapy (53). When a clear margin of 5 mm or more is detected on MRI, there is a high degree of accuracy when correlated with histology (54). The mesorectal fascia and perirectal lymph nodes are well seen on MRI. T2-weighted images are most useful in detecting local spread (Table 9.2, Fig. 9.13).

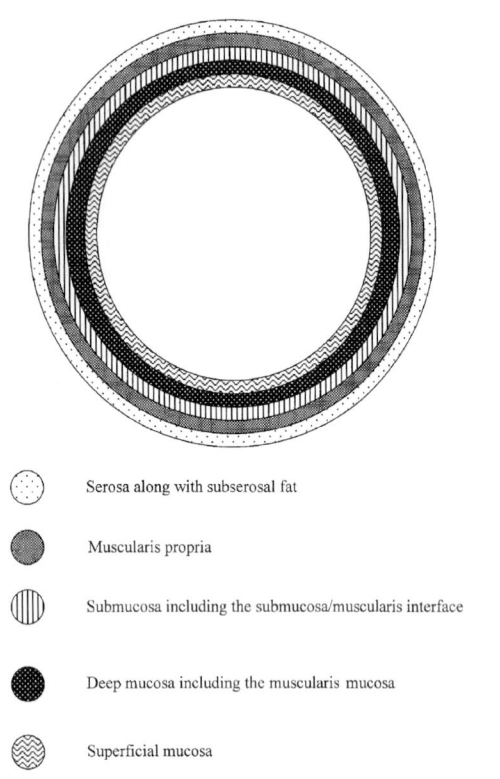

○ Serosa along with subserosal fat

● Muscularis propria

◫ Submucosa including the submucosa/muscularis interface

● Deep mucosa including the muscularis mucosa

◉ Superficial mucosa

FIGURE 9.13. Schematic representation of the rectal layers. See Table 19.2 for the associated findings on magnetic resonance imaging and ultrasonography.

SOLID ORGAN DISEASE

Hepatic Neoplasms

The liver is a common site of metastatic disease from GI malignancies (Fig. 9.14). In addition, primary neoplasms arise from the liver. In general, if ultrasound is negative, CT or MRI should be performed. Cross-sectional imaging is used to define the extent and number of lesions, the vascular anatomy, and the presence of extrahepatic disease (55). Hepatic metastases receive their blood supply from the hepatic artery. The normal hepatic parenchyma is supplied primarily by the portal vein. These divergent blood supplies have major implications for imaging of the liver. Because of the arterial blood supply of metastatic lesions, the majority are seen on the portal phase or equilibrium phase of contrast-enhanced CT or MRI. MRI has a higher sensitivity in detection of focal hepatic lesions than CT and ultrasonography (56–61).

Evaluation of liver metastases prior to possible liver resection has become more relevant now that ablation and embolization techniques may render some tumors resectable. CT is the mainstay for detection of liver metastases. In recent years, the introduction of multislice CT allows CTA to depict the vascular anatomy more clearly. Three-dimensional curved formats and volumetry are very helpful for surgical planning. The aim is to define the relation of the lesion(s) to segmental and vascular anatomy within the liver. Multiphase CT, including hepatic arterial and portal venous phases, can accurately depict the vascular anatomy preoperatively. A multimodality approach may be required in difficult cases to ascertain whether an adequate resection margin is likely. Both ultrasound and MRI will help problem solve in select cases. Intraoperative ultrasound is used in some centers to detect "occult" lesions not seen on preoperative imaging.

Benign liver lesions such as cysts and hemangiomas are commonly seen on all cross-sectional imaging modalities and are frequently encountered in patients who are being studied for a multitude of cancers (62). Simple hepatic cysts, which are four times more common in women, are easily diagnosed on ultrasonography as hypoechoic masses with thin walls (sometimes also with thin septations) and increased sound transmission. Hemangiomas are uniformly hyperechoic without a surrounding halo on ultrasonography. These findings are not specific, so CT or MRI is required to exclude metastases. MRI has the highest specificity for the diagnosis of hemangioma. MRI using iron oxide contrast agents is superior to CT arterial portography for the detection of malignant lesions (56,57,59). Other studies have demonstrated that multiphase MRI is superior to single-phase CT in the evaluation of liver metastases (58). However, CT remains the mainstay of staging and follow-up of patients because it provides coverage of the chest, abdomen, and pelvis (if required) in one session.

Primary malignancies of the liver are encountered less commonly than metastatic disease. Predisposing factors that may be seen on cross-sectional imaging include cirrhosis and chronic hepatitis. The method used for screening the liver for a primary hepatic neoplasm depends on the patient population, incidence of disease, and availability of imaging tests. Ultrasound is operator dependent but still has a role in evaluation of liver cancer and has been shown to identify as many lesions as CT or MRI (63). Hepatocellular carcinoma, the most common primary malignant neoplasm of the liver, tends to enhance on arterial phase images (hypervascular) and wash out on subsequent phases (64). Hemangiomas will not wash out on delayed imaging post contrast. MRI has been shown to be superior to CT in the detection of hypervascular masses in cirrhotic livers (65,66). Identifying hypervascular masses in cirrhotic patients

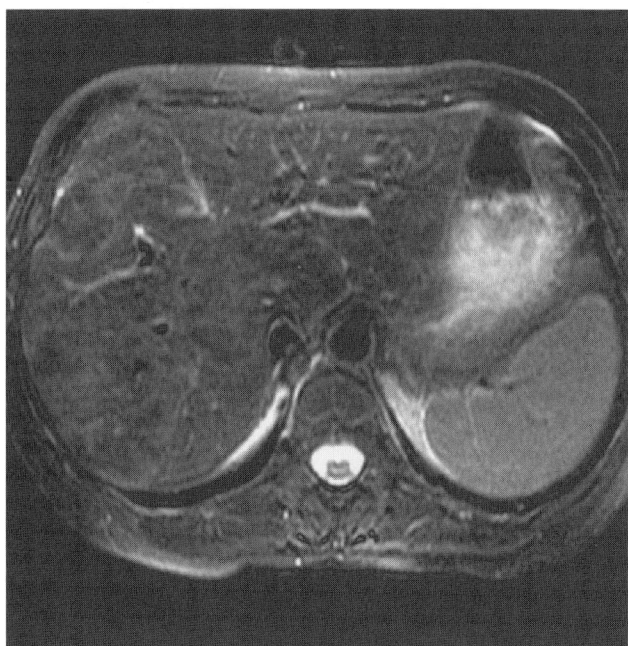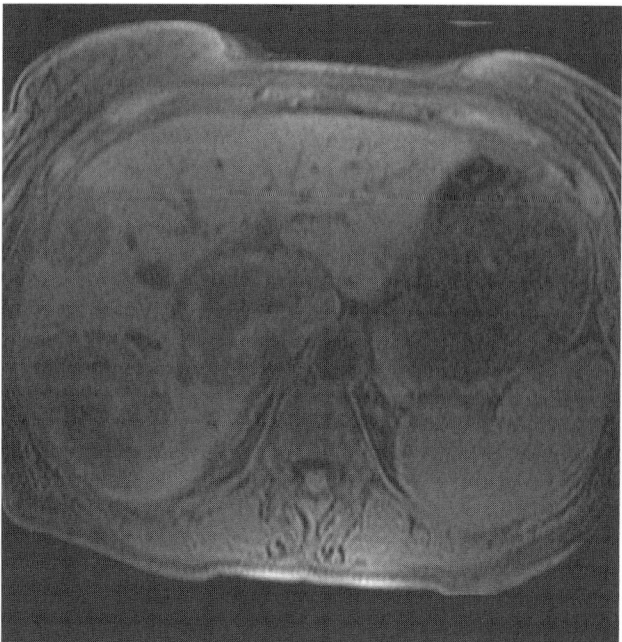

FIGURE 9.14. Hepatic metastases from colon carcinoma. *Left*: A fat-suppressed T2-weighted magnetic resonance imaging (MRI) scan of the liver demonstrates innumerable hepatic masses, which are only mildly hyperintense compared with hepatic parenchyma. These lesions are consistent with metastases. *Right*: Postcontrast MRI scan in the same patient demonstrates irregular enhancement. This feature is also characteristic of metastatic disease.

does not obviate the need to biopsy and correlate with laboratory values such as alpha-fetoprotein.

Hepatocellular carcinoma has a variable appearance on imaging studies (66–69). Some hepatocellular carcinomas have a pseudocapsule of compressed parenchyma that enhances on delayed images. Arterial venous shunting may also be associated with hepatocellular carcinomas. CT scanning protocols in patients with suspected hepatocellular carcinoma should include a precontrast study. Images should also be obtained during the arterial and portal venous phases of enhancement (70). On MRI, T2-weighted images generally demonstrate a hyperintense lesion that is inhomogeneous. The degree of hyperintensity is variable (68,69). Hepatocellular carcinomas enhance during arterial phase imaging on MRI (Fig. 9.15) and vascular invasion is common (Fig. 9.16). This feature may help differentiate hepatocellular carcinoma from other lesions in the liver. PET scanning has shown promise in evaluation of hepatocellular carcinoma (71).

The imaging appearance of intrahepatic cholangiocarcinoma overlaps with other primary malignancies of the liver. Tumors involving the bile duct may appear in three distinct patterns: (a) infiltrative mass with stenosis, (b) bulky exophytic mass, or (c) papillary or polypoid mass within the duct. The infiltrative mass subtype is most commonly seen on imaging studies. CT, magnetic resonance cholangiopancreatography (MRCP), and ultrasonography are useful tools for identifying and staging extrahepatic cholangiocarcinoma (72). Infiltrative masses at the hilum may be identified with these modalities. Vascular occlusions and vascular encasement can also be diagnosed. Dilatation of the intrahepatic bile ducts, which almost never happens in metastatic disease, occurs frequently in cholangiocarcinoma, and this is easily depicted on CT or MRI. Cholangiocarcinomas tend to demonstrate delayed contrast enhancement because of their high fibrous content (73). This enhancement pattern is useful in differentiating intrahepatic cholangiocarcinoma from other malignant lesions of hepatic parenchyma.

Pancreatic Neoplasms

Most pancreatic cancers are located in the head of the pancreas. Classically, pancreatic cancers appear as hypovascular masses after the administration of intravenous contrast (Fig. 9.17). They are often associated with biliary ductal dilatation and biliary stasis. The primary role of imaging in pancreatic cancer is for presurgical staging (74,75). CT is the modality of choice in assessing a pancreatic mass and evaluating for the potential for surgical resection (76). Contrast-enhanced CT performed during the pancreatic phase of enhancement (approximately 40 to 70 seconds after infusion of intravenous contrast material) increases visualization of most pancreatic lesions (75). Secondary signs of pancreatic masses may be present without an obvious pancreatic mass. In the normal aging process, fatty replacement of the pancreas occurs, which creates a feathery type of appearance on imaging studies. A focal area of nonfatty replaced pancreatic parenchyma in an otherwise fatty replaced pancreas raises suspicion for a mass.

Interruption of the pancreatic duct is a useful sign for identifying a potential mass. If the duct is interrupted or a change in caliber has occurred with more proximal dilatation, a mass should be suspected. A dilated pancreatic duct may be seen in a variety of conditions, including chronic pancreatitis, and is not specific for malignant lesions. The head of the pancreas normally has a somewhat rounded configuration, whereas the uncinate process generally has a beaked appearance. Rounding of the uncinate process should alert the examiner to the possibility of a mass.

A patient for whom the CT or ultrasonographic image of the pancreas raises suspicion should be referred for an MRI because of its superior contrast resolution (77,78). On fat-suppressed T1-weighted MRI images, the normal pancreas is hyperintense compared with normal liver. An adenocarcinoma of the pancreas usually appears as a hypointense lesion surrounded by normal pancreatic tissue. T2-weighted images are

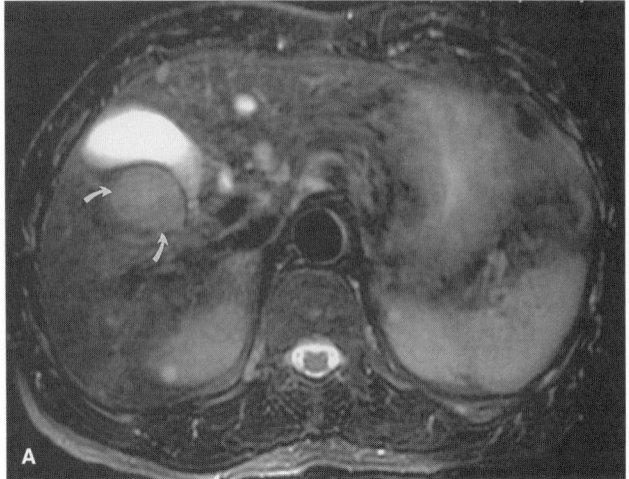

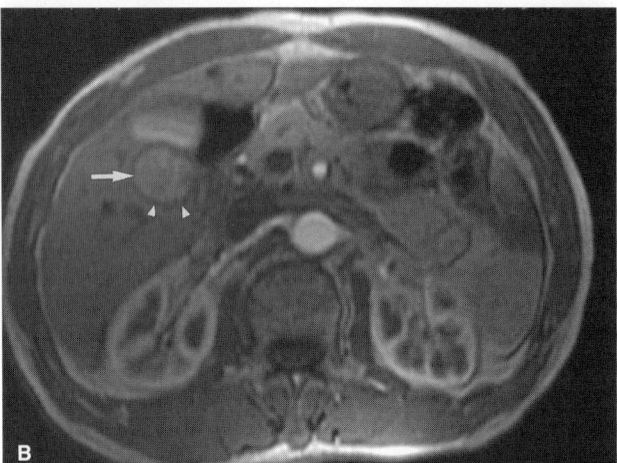

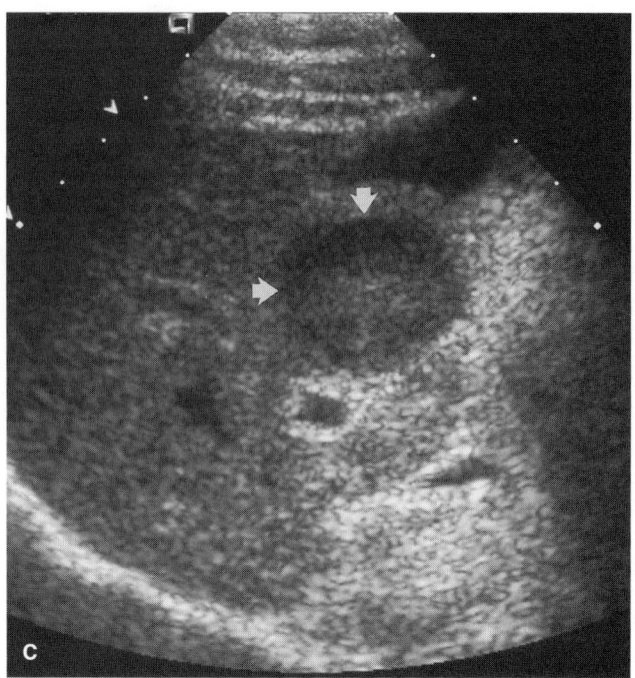

FIGURE 9.15. Hepatocellular carcinoma. **A:** Fat-suppressed T2-weighted magnetic resonance image demonstrates a well-circumscribed mass (*curved arrows*) mildly hyperintense relative to hepatic parenchyma. **B:** Arterial dominant phase images demonstrate that the mass enhances early (hypervascular) (*arrow*). Note the hypointense rim around the lesion (pseudocapsule) (*arrowheads*). On delayed images, the rim enhances, which is characteristic of a pseudocapsule (not shown). **C:** Same patient also had ultrasonography, which demonstrated the mass (*arrows*) to be heterogeneous with respect to hepatic parenchyma.

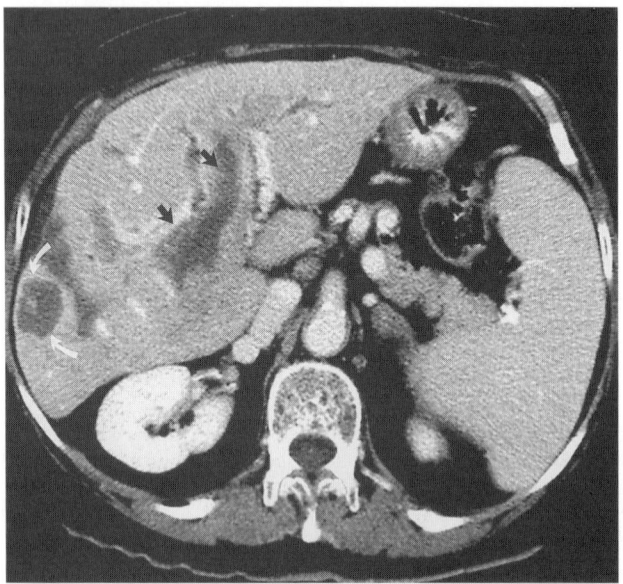

FIGURE 9.16. Hepatocellular carcinoma with portal venous thrombosis. Computed tomography image demonstrates portal vein thrombus (*black arrows* on thrombosed right and left portal veins). A mass (*curved white arrows*) is present in the right lobe of the liver.

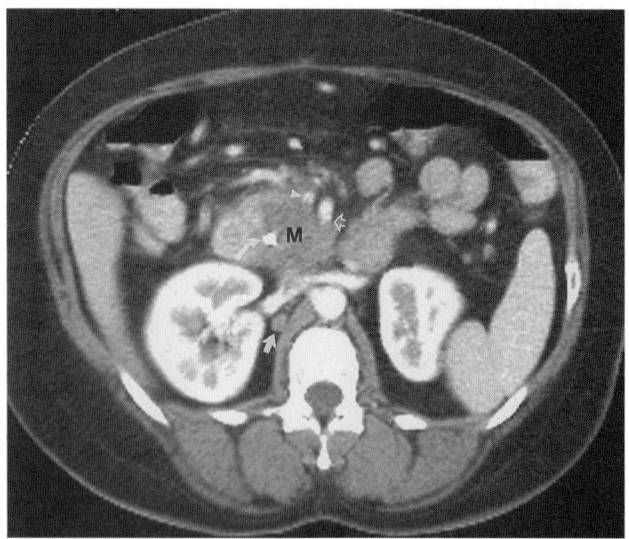

FIGURE 9.17. Pancreatic adenocarcinoma. Computed tomography image demonstrates an endoscopically placed biliary stent (*curved arrow*), passing through a mass (M) in the head of the pancreas. The pancreatic adenocarcinoma has almost obliterated the superior mesenteric vein (*arrowhead*) and abuts the superior mesenteric artery (*open arrow*). A retrocaval lymph node is noted (*thick arrow*).

less likely to show a difference in contrast between a mass and normal pancreatic tissue. Endoscopic retrograde cholangiopancreatography (ERCP) is useful for stent placement and to obtain brushings. MRCP is also useful in patients in whom ERCP is not technically feasible, and the technique continues to improve visualization of the ductal system (79). Recently, it has been shown that MRCP is as sensitive as ERCP for detecting pancreatic adenocarcinomas in patients with strong evidence of pancreatic tumors (80). For identification of an intraductal pancreatic mucinous neoplasm, communication with the ductal system is an important feature.

Postoperative patients with pancreatic cancer are difficult to image on all cross-sectional studies. Postoperative soft tissue infiltration cannot be discerned from recurrent tumor, and thus close follow-up is necessary. PET-CT combines the functional value of FDG and the anatomical detail of CT. Addition of PET-CT to routine staging has been shown in one study to change management in 16% of patients if used to stage preoperatively in patients deemed resectable (81).

Neuroendocrine tumors and cystic neoplasms of the pancreas are also well imaged on all cross-sectional imaging studies. Tumors of neuroendocrine origin have a different appearance from that of pancreatic adenocarcinoma. Neuroendocrine tumors are generally hypervascular and enhance intensely on postcontrast studies. On MRI, these lesions are usually hyperintense on T2-weighted images. Because most adenocarcinomas are not well seen on T2-weighted images, neuroendocrine tumors may be differentiated from the more common adenocarcinoma. Absence of FDG uptake 1 month following chemotherapy has been reported to be an indicator of improved overall survival in pancreatic cancer (82). This is particularly useful because the anatomy is distorted postoperatively, complicating cross-sectional imaging interpretation.

Cystic neoplasms of the pancreas have imaging features that allow them to be distinguished from one another. A classic microcystic cystadenoma is a mass with multiple small but discernible cysts. However, these masses may appear solid on CT if the cysts are too small to be distinguished individually, and a calcified scar may be present. The macrocystic subtype tends to be located in the body or tail portion of the pancreas. These lesions tend to be large (>10 cm) and multiloculated. The cystic component also tends to be >2 cm in size. The walls of the cyst may be thick and nodular, a finding not typically seen in the microcystic variety. Pancreatic cysts <1 cm are incidentally encountered in patients on CT and are too small to characterize. It is prudent to follow these lesions for at least 2 years at regular intervals to ensure stability because they may grow into a cystic neoplasm.

POSTOPERATIVE IMAGING

Postoperative imaging of oncologic patients may be problematic, depending on the type of surgical procedure performed. Early postoperative complications of esophageal resection, including leak from an anastomosis, are best evaluated with a barium swallow study using a water-soluble agent (Fig. 9.18). CT (Fig. 9.19) can also be used. In fact, due to its superior contrast resolution compared to plain film imaging, CT is an excellent method for evaluating the more subtle early postoperative complications.

After resection of colorectal carcinomas, patients may have residual soft tissue in the postoperative bed. These masses are difficult to characterize as benign or malignant on imaging. For example, presacral masses may represent postoperative fibrosis or recurrent disease (Fig. 9.20). PET-CT may be useful in selected patients in whom there is a rising carcinoembryonic antigen and in whom conventional imaging is negative or equivocal.

In many postoperative patients, the normal anatomy is distorted. In addition, recurrent disease in the liver may be difficult to identify due to chemotherapy-induced steatosis in the liver. Fatty infiltration of the liver is easily recognized on MRI, which is the preferred modality for evaluation of patients with fatty infiltration.

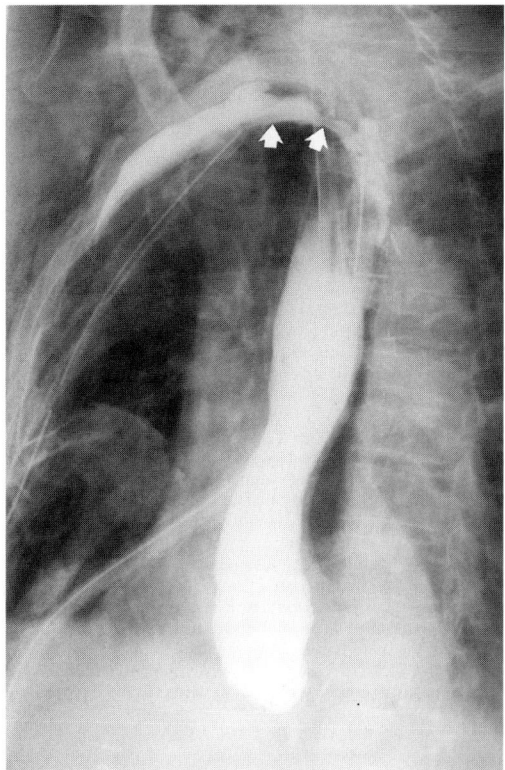

FIGURE 9.18. Postoperative leak from resection of esophageal carcinoma and gastric pull-through. Barium swallow study shows contrast extravasation (*arrows*) from the proximal anastomosis near the tip of the chest tube.

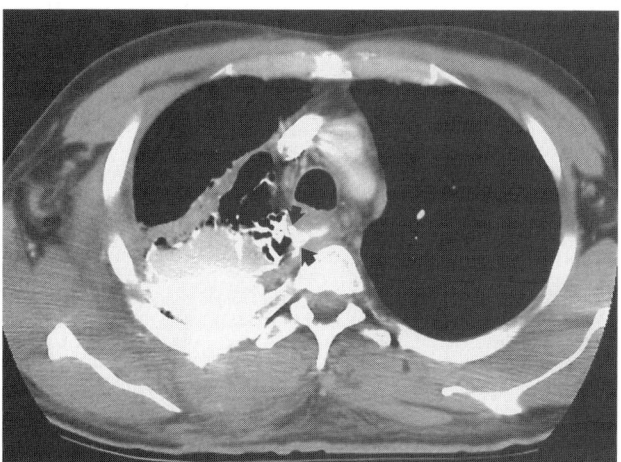

FIGURE 9.19. Postoperative leak from resection of esophageal carcinoma and gastric pull-through. Barium swallow study shows contrast extravasation (*arrows*) from the proximal anastomosis near the tip of the chest tube.

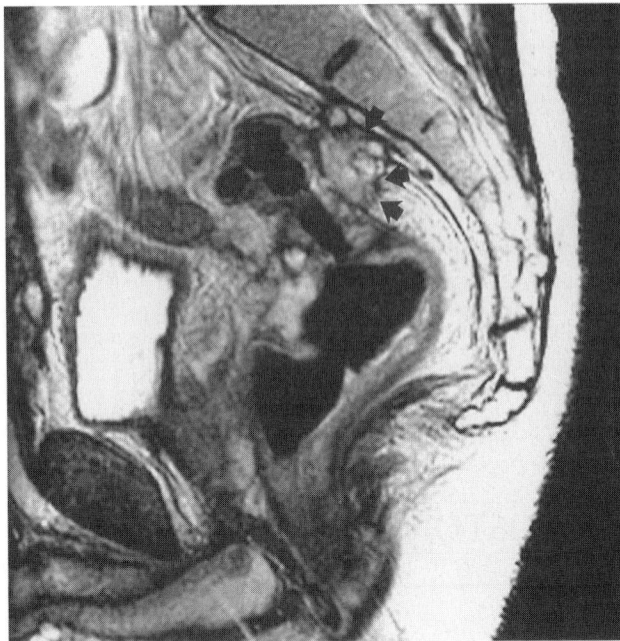

FIGURE 9.20. Recurrent colon carcinoma. Sagittal T2-weighted magnetic resonance image through the pelvis demonstrating a presacral mass (arrows). The patient had previously undergone resection of a colorectal carcinoma. This mass was proven to be a recurrence at exploration.

The afferent loop in patients who have undergone a Whipple procedure may also be mistaken for a mass on CT because it does not always fill with an orally administered contrast agent. In addition, postoperative scarring may be difficult to delineate from recurrent tumor and may warrant further investigation or short-term follow-up. PET scanning has been shown to be more accurate for the staging of patients with suspected recurrent CRC (83).

References

1. Collier BD. New radiographic techniques for colorectal cancer. *Cancer* 1993;71(12 suppl):4214–4216.
2. Stevenson GW. Radiology and endoscopy in the pretreatment diagnostic management of colorectal cancer. *Cancer* 1993;71(12 suppl):4198–4206.
3. Choi H, Charnsangavej C, de Castro Faria S, et al. CT evaluation of the response of gastrointestinal stromal tumors after imatinib mesylate treatment: a quantitative analysis correlated with FDG PET findings. *AJR Am J Roentgenol* 2004;183(6):1619–1628.
4. Kotanagi H, Fukuoka T, Shibata Y, et al. The size of regional lymph nodes does not correlate with the presence or absence of metastasis in lymph nodes in rectal cancer. *J Surg Oncol* 1993;54(4):252–254.
5. Maruyama M, Baba Y. Gastric carcinoma. *Radiol Clin North Am* 1994;32(6):1233–1252.
6. Akhurst T, Larson SM. Positron emission tomography imaging of colorectal cancer. *Semin Oncol* 1999;26(5):577–583.
7. Siegel BA, Dehdashti F. Oncologic PET/CT: current status and controversies. *Eur Radiol* 2005;15(suppl 4):D127–D132.
8. Williams SM, Harned RK. Double versus single contrast gastrointestinal radiology. *Curr Probl Diagn Radiol* 1983;12(2):1–41.
9. Gelfand DW, Ott DJ, Chen YM. Optimizing single- and double-contrast colon examinations. *Crit Rev Diagn Imaging* 1987;27(2):167–201.
10. Kelvin FM. Radiologic approach to the detection of colorectal neoplasia. *Radiol Clin North Am* 1982;20(4):743–759.
11. Strom E, Larsen JL. Colon cancer at barium enema examination and colonoscopy: a study from the county of Hordaland, Norway. *Radiology* 1999;211(1):211–214.
12. Bond JH. Screening guidelines for colorectal cancer. *Am J Med* 1999;106(1A):7S–10S.
13. Haseman JH, Lemmel GT, Rahmani EY, Rex DK. Failure of colonoscopy to detect colorectal cancer: evaluation of 47 cases in 20 hospitals. *Gastrointest Endosc* 1997;45(6):451–455.
14. Rex DK, Rahmani EY, Haseman JH, Lemmel GT, Kaster S, Buckley JS. Relative sensitivity of colonoscopy and barium enema for detection of colorectal cancer in clinical practice. *Gastroenterology* 1997;112(1):17–23.
15. Norfleet RG, Ryan ME, Wyman JB, et al. Barium enema versus colonoscopy for patients with polyps found during flexible sigmoidoscopy. *Gastrointest Endosc* 1991;37(5):531–534.
16. Dodd GD. Imaging techniques in the diagnosis of carcinoma of the colon. *Cancer* 1991;67(4 suppl):1150–1154.
17. Hull CC, Stellato TA, Ament AA, Gordon N, Galloway P. Endoscopic and radiographic evaluation of the murine colon. *Cancer* 1990;66(12):2528–2532.
18. Boudiaf M, Jaff A, Soyer P, Bouhnik Y, Hamzi L, Rymer R. Small-bowel diseases: prospective evaluation of multi-detector row helical CT enteroclysis in 107 consecutive patients. *Radiology* 2004;233(2):338–344.
19. Maglinte DD. Small bowel imaging—a rapidly changing field and a challenge to radiology. *Eur Radiol* 2006:1–5.
20. Noh HM, Fishman EK, Forastiere AA, Bliss DF, Calhoun PS. CT of the esophagus: spectrum of disease with emphasis on esophageal carcinoma. *Radiographics* 1995;15(5):1113–1134.
21. Levine MS, Chu P, Furth EE, Rubesin SE, Laufer I, Herlinger H. Carcinoma of the esophagus and esophagogastric junction: sensitivity of radiographic diagnosis. *AJR Am J Roentgenol* 1997;168(6):1423–1426.
22. Wolfman NT, Scharling ES, Chen MY. Esophageal squamous carcinoma. *Radiol Clin North Am* 1994;32(6):1183–1201
23. O'Brien MG, Fitzgerald EF, Lee G, Crowley M, Shanahan F, O'Sullivan GC. A prospective comparison of laparoscopy and imaging in the staging of esophagogastric cancer before surgery. *Am J Gastroenterol* 1995;90(12):2191–2194.
24. Holscher AH, Dittler HJ, Siewert JR. Staging of squamous esophageal cancer: accuracy and value. *World J Surg* 1994;18(3):312–320.
25. Lerut T, Flamen P, Ectors N, et al. Histopathologic validation of lymph node staging with FDG-PET scan in cancer of the esophagus and gastroesophageal junction: A prospective study based on primary surgery with extensive lymphadenectomy. *Ann Surg* 2000;232(6):743–752.
26. Himeno S, Yasuda S, Shimada H, Tajima T, Makuuchi H. Evaluation of esophageal cancer by positron emission tomography. *Jpn J Clin Oncol* 2002;32(9):340–346.
27. Yeung HW, Macapinlac HA, Mazumdar M, Bains M, Finn RD, Larson SM. FDG-PET in esophageal cancer. Incremental value over computed tomography. *Clin Positron Imaging* 1999;2(5):255–260.
28. Bar-Shalom R, Yefremov N, Guralnik L, et al. Clinical performance of PET/CT in evaluation of cancer: additional value for diagnostic imaging and patient management. *J Nucl Med* 2003;44(8):1200–1209.
29. Downey RJ, Akhurst T, Ilson D, et al. Whole body 18FDG-PET and the response of esophageal cancer to induction therapy: results of a prospective trial. *J Clin Oncol* 2003;21(3):428–432.
30. Kelly S, Harris KM, Berry E, et al. A systematic review of the staging performance of endoscopic ultrasound in gastro-oesophageal carcinoma. *Gut* 2001;49(4):534–539.
31. Hoppe H, Dinkel HP, Walder B, von Allmen G, Gugger M, Vock P. Grading airway stenosis down to the segmental level using virtual bronchoscopy. *Chest* 2004;125(2):704–711.
32. Gore RM, Levine MS, Ghahremani GG, Miller FH. Gastric cancer. *Radiologic diagnosis. Radiol Clin North Am* 1997;35(2):311–329.
33. Paramo JC, Gomez G. Dynamic CT in the preoperative evaluation of patients with gastric cancer: correlation with surgical findings and pathology. *Ann Surg Oncol* 1999;6(4):379–384.
34. Dux M, Richter GM, Hansmann J, Kuntz C, Kauffmann GW. Helical hydro-CT for diagnosis and staging of gastric carcinoma. *J Comput Assist Tomogr* 1999;23(6):913–922.
35. Rossi M, Broglia L, Maccioni F, et al. Hydro-CT in patients with gastric cancer: preoperative radiologic staging. *Eur Radiol* 1997;7(5):659–664.
36. Horton KM, Fishman EK. Current role of CT in imaging of the stomach. *Radiographics* 2003;23(1):75–87.
37. Kumano S, Murakami T, Kim T, et al. T staging of gastric cancer: role of multi-detector row CT. *Radiology* 2005;237(3):961–966.
38. Tsuburaya A, Noguchi Y, Matsumoto A, Kobayashi S, Masukawa K, Horiguchi K. A preoperative assessment of adjacent organ invasion by stomach carcinoma with high resolution computed tomography. *Surg Today* 1994;24(4):299–304.
39. Antoch G, Kanja J, Bauer S, et al. Comparison of PET, CT, and dual-modality PET/CT imaging for monitoring of imatinib (STI571) therapy in patients with gastrointestinal stromal tumors. *J Nucl Med* 2004;45(3):357–365.
40. Maglinte DD. Capsule imaging and the role of radiology in the investigation of diseases of the small bowel. *Radiology* 2005;236(3):763–767.
41. Macari M, Bini EJ, Jacobs SL, et al. Colorectal polyps and cancers in asymptomatic average-risk patients: evaluation with CT colonography. *Radiology* 2004;230(3):629–636.
42. Munikrishnan V, Gillams AR, Lees WR, Vaizey CJ, Boulos PB. Prospective study comparing multislice CT colonography with colonoscopy in the detection of colorectal cancer and polyps. *Dis Colon Rectum* 2003;46(10):1384–1390.
43. Kealey SM, Dodd JD, MacEneaney PM, Gibney RG, Malone DE. Minimal preparation computed tomography instead of barium enema/colonoscopy for suspected colon cancer in frail elderly patients: an outcome analysis study. *Clin Radiol* 2004;59(1):44–52.

44. Saar B, Beer A, Rosch T, Rummeny EJ. Magnetic resonance colonography: a promising new technique. *Curr Gastroenterol Rep* 2004;6(5):389–394.

45. Pickhardt PJ, Choi JR, Hwang I, et al. Computed tomographic virtual colonoscopy to screen for colorectal neoplasia in asymptomatic adults. *N Engl J Med* 2003;349(23):2191–2200.

46. Johnson CD, Harmsen WS, Wilson LA, et al. Prospective blinded evaluation of computed tomographic colonography for screen detection of colorectal polyps. *Gastroenterology* 2003;125(2):311–319.

47. Zalis ME, Barish MA, Choi JR, et al. CT colonography reporting and data system: a consensus proposal. *Radiology* 2005;236(1):3–9.

48. Hillman B. *American College of Radiology Imaging Network 2006*. Available at: http: //www.acrin.org. Accessed May 24, 2007.

49. Blomqvist L, Rubio C, Holm T, Machado M, Hindmarsh T. Rectal adenocarcinoma: assessment of tumour involvement of the lateral resection margin by MRI of resected specimen. *Br J Radiol* 1999;72(853):18–23.

50. Brown G, Richards CJ, Newcombe RG, et al. Rectal carcinoma: thin-section MR imaging for staging in 28 patients. *Radiology* 1999;211(1):215–222.

51. Massari M, De Simone M, Cioffi U, Rosso L, Chiarelli M, Gabrielli F. Value and limits of endorectal ultrasonography for preoperative staging of rectal carcinoma. *Surg Laparosc Endosc* 1998;8(6):438–444.

52. Zagoria RJ, Schlarb CA, Ott DJ, et al. Assessment of rectal tumor infiltration utilizing endorectal MR imaging and comparison with endoscopic rectal sonography. *J Surg Oncol* 1997;64(4):312–317.

53. Brown G, Richards CJ, Bourne MW, et al. Morphologic predictors of lymph node status in rectal cancer with use of high-spatial-resolution MR imaging with histopathologic comparison. *Radiology* 2003;227(2):371–377.

54. Beets-Tan RG, Beets GL, Vliegen RF, et al. Accuracy of magnetic resonance imaging in prediction of tumour-free resection margin in rectal cancer surgery. *Lancet* 2001;357(9255):497–504.

55. NCCN. NCCN *Clinical Practice Guidelines 2006*. Available at: http://www.nccn.org.

56. Lencioni R, Donati F, Cioni D, Paolicchi A, Cicorelli A, Bartolozzi C. Detection of colorectal liver metastases: prospective comparison of unenhanced and ferumoxides-enhanced magnetic resonance imaging at 1.5 T, dual-phase spiral CT, and spiral CT during arterial portography. *Magma* 1998;7(2):76–87.

57. Muller RD, Vogel K, Neumann K, et al. SPIO-MR imaging versus double-phase spiral CT in detecting malignant lesions of the liver. *Acta Radiol* 1999;40(6):628–635.

58. Semelka RC, Cance WG, Marcos HB, Mauro MA. Liver metastases: comparison of current MR techniques and spiral CT during arterial portography for detection in 20 surgically staged cases. *Radiology* 1999;213(1):86–91.

59. Semelka RC, Schlund JF, Molina PL, et al. Malignant liver lesions: comparison of spiral CT arterial portography and MR imaging for diagnostic accuracy, cost, and effect on patient management. *J Magn Reson Imaging* 1996;6(1):39–43.

60. Semelka RC, Worawattanakul S, Kelekis NL, et al. Liver lesion detection, characterization, and effect on patient management: comparison of single-phase spiral CT and current MR techniques. *J Magn Reson Imaging* 1997;7(6):1040–1047.

61. Ward J, Naik KS, Guthrie JA, Wilson D, Robinson PJ. Hepatic lesion detection: comparison of MR imaging after the administration of superparamagnetic iron oxide with dual-phase CT by using alternative-free response receiver operating characteristic analysis. *Radiology* 1999;210(2):459–466.

62. Outwater EK, Ito K, Siegelman E, Martin CE, Bhatia M, Mitchell DG. Rapidly enhancing hepatic hemangiomas at MRI: distinction from malignancies with T2-weighted images. *J Magn Reson Imaging* 1997;7(6):1033–1039.

63. Teefey SA, Hildeboldt CC, Dehdashti F, et al. Detection of primary hepatic malignancy in liver transplant candidates: prospective comparison of CT, MR imaging, US, and PET. *Radiology* 2003;226(2):533–542.

64. Ito K, Fujita T, Shimizu A, et al. Multiarterial phase dynamic MRI of small early enhancing hepatic lesions in cirrhosis or chronic hepatitis: differentiating between hypervascular hepatocellular carcinomas and pseudolesions. *AJR Am J Roentgenol* 2004;183(3):699–705.

65. Yamashita Y, Mitsuzaki K, Yi T, et al. Small hepatocellular carcinoma in patients with chronic liver damage: prospective comparison of detection with dynamic MR imaging and helical CT of the whole liver. *Radiology* 1996;200(1):79–84.

66. Murakami T, Kim T, Nakamura H. Hepatitis, cirrhosis, and hepatoma. *J Magn Reson Imaging* 1998;8(2):34–58.

67. Fraser C. Imaging of hepatocellular carcinoma. *J Gastroenterol Hepatol* 1999;14(8):750–756.

68. Earls JP, Theise ND, Weinreb JC, et al. Dysplastic nodules and hepatocellular carcinoma: thin-section MR imaging of explanted cirrhotic livers with pathologic correlation. *Radiology* 1996;201(1):207–214.

69. Kelekis NL, Semelka RC, Worawattanakul S, et al. Hepatocellular carcinoma in North America: a multiinstitutional study of appearance on T1-weighted, T2-weighted, and serial gadolinium-enhanced gradient-echo images. *AJR Am J Roentgenol* 1998;170(4):1005–1013.

70. Oliver JH, III, Baron RL, Federle MP, Rockette HE, Jr. Detecting hepatocellular carcinoma: value of unenhanced or arterial phase CT imaging or both used in conjunction with conventional portal venous phase contrast-enhanced CT imaging. *AJR Am J Roentgenol* 1996;167(1):71–77.

71. Trojan J, Schroeder O, Raedle J, et al. Fluorine-18 FDG positron emission tomography for imaging of hepatocellular carcinoma. *Am J Gastroenterol* 1999;94(11):3314–3319.

72. Becker CD. [Multidetector CT and MRI of biliary diseases]. *J Radiol* 2003;84(4 pt 2):473–479; discussion 480–483.

73. Loyer EM, Chin H, DuBrow RA, David CL, Eftekhari F, Charnsangavej C. Hepatocellular carcinoma and intrahepatic peripheral cholangiocarcinoma: enhancement patterns with quadruple phase helical CT—a comparative study. *Radiology* 1999;212(3):866–875.

74. O'Malley ME, Boland GW, Wood BJ, Fernandez-del Castillo C, Warshaw AL, Mueller PR. Adenocarcinoma of the head of the pancreas: determination of surgical unresectability with thin-section pancreatic-phase helical CT. *AJR Am J Roentgenol* 1999;173(6):1513–1538.

75. Lu DS, Vedantham S, Krasny RM, Kadell B, Berger WL, Reber HA. Two-phase helical CT for pancreatic tumors: pancreatic versus hepatic phase enhancement of tumor, pancreas, and vascular structures. *Radiology* 1996;199(3):697–701.

76. Megibow AJ, Zhou XH, Rotterdam H, et al. Pancreatic adenocarcinoma: CT versus MR imaging in the evaluation of resectability—report of the Radiology Diagnostic Oncology Group. *Radiology* 1995;195(2):327–332.

77. Catalano C, Pavone P, Laghi A, et al. Pancreatic adenocarcinoma: combination of MR imaging, MR angiography and MR cholangiopancreatography for the diagnosis and assessment of resectability. *Eur Radiol* 1998;8(3):428–434.

78. Neri E, Boraschi P, Braccini G, et al. MR virtual endoscopy of the pancreaticobiliary tract: a feasible technique? *Abdom Imaging* 1999;24(3):289–291.

79. Silva AC, Friese JL, Hara AK, Liu PT. MR cholangiopancreatography: improved ductal distention with intravenous morphine administration. *Radiographics* 2004;24(3):677–687.

80. Adamek HE, Albert J, Breer H, Weitz M, Schilling D, Riemann JF. Pancreatic cancer detection with magnetic resonance cholangiopancreatography and endoscopic retrograde cholangiopancreatography: a prospective controlled study. *Lancet* 2000;356(9225):190–193.

81. Heinrich S, Goerres GW, Schafer M, et al. Positron emission tomography/computed tomography influences on the management of resectable pancreatic cancer and its cost-effectiveness. *Ann Surg* 2005;242(2):235–243.

82. Maisey NR, Webb A, Flux GD, et al. FDG-PET in the prediction of survival of patients with cancer of the pancreas: a pilot study. *Br J Cancer* 2000;83(3):287–293.

83. Imbriaco M, Akhurst T, Hilton S, et al. Whole-body FDG-PET in patients with recurrent colorectal carcinoma. A comparative study with CT. *Clin Positron Imaging* 2000;3(3):107–114.

CHAPTER 10 ■ ENDOSCOPIC DIAGNOSIS, STAGING, AND MANAGEMENT OF GASTROINTESTINAL CANCERS

MARCIA IRENE CANTO

ENDOSCOPIC DIAGNOSIS AND TECHNIQUES

Gastrointestinal (GI) videoendoscopy has been a standard technique for visualizing and diagnosing GI cancers and their premalignant lesions. In addition, tissue samples in the form of brushings and mucosal biopsies are readily acquired for a pathological diagnosis (1). The most common clinical indications for performing videoendoscopy for suspected cancer are blood in the stool, chronic iron-deficiency anemia, change in bowel habits, anorexia, and dysphagia. Typically, GI cancers present as an ulcer, luminal narrowing (stricture), marked wall thickening (Fig. 10.1), and/or mass (Figs. 10.2 and 10.3).

In addition to standard videoendoscopy, endoscopic ultrasonography (EUS) was developed in the 1980s to improve visualization of the pancreas by allowing a transgastric or transduodenal placement of the ultrasound (US) probe unimpeded by bowel air. EUS combines videoendoscopy and high-frequency ultrasonography (Fig. 10.4). It allows visualization of the entire GI tract wall. Since the mid-1980s, it is still the best imaging modality of the GI tract wall. Importantly, it can also image adjacent organs such as pancreas, bile duct, adrenal gland, and liver (2). Hence, it has become an important diagnostic and staging modality for GI and pancreaticobiliary cancers. It is superior to dual-phase computed tomography (CT) for detection of pancreatic cancer (3,4) (particularly early cancers <2 cm [5,6]) and pancreatic neuroendocrine tumors (7). The negative predictive value of EUS for excluding a pancreatic tumor or mass in patients with a clinical suspicion of pancreatic cancer is very high (100%) (4), potentially obviating the need for further diagnostic testing when used as a first test (8).

In the 1990s, it became possible to obtain tissue samples from organs outside the GI tract via EUS guidance (EUS-guided fine-needle aspiration [EUS-FNA]) and a cytologic diagnosis of cancer in primary organs (pancreas, bile duct, gallbladder), lymph nodes, and distant organs, such as liver, adrenal gland, periportal area, and pancreas. The overall accuracy rate for EUS-FNA for diagnosing pancreatic cancer in suspicious lesions is 89% (compared to 74% for multidetector pancreatic protocol CT [4]) and 92% if there is no mass by CT (4). In another large prospective study, the sensitivity of EUS was 98% compared to 86% for multidetector CT detection of pancreatic cancer (9). EUS has a 22% negative predictive value in patients with obstructive jaundice, and 89% in those without obstructive jaundice (4). Hence, FNA does not seem to add much to the EUS alone in the diagnosis of pancreatic cancer in patients with obstructive jaundice. It can be argued that it is not neces-

sary prior to planned surgery except in two scenarios: (i) when the patient is unsure about surgery or has multiple medical comorbidities that increase risk for surgical complications, and (ii) if the patient will be treated in a neoadjuvant protocol before surgery and a histologic diagnosis is required.

ENDOSCOPIC SCREENING AND SURVEILLANCE

Patients at risk for the development of GI cancer can be identified by endoscopic screening and followed periodically using a variety of endoscopic techniques. Endoscopic screening with colonoscopy is commonly performed for average- and high-risk populations (13) (Tables 10.1 and 10.2). Both cancer and the premalignant adenomas can be accurately detected. Colonoscopy offers the advantages of complete visualization of the entire colon, detection and removal of polyps, and diagnostic sampling of cancers (14). Furthermore, colonoscopic polypectomy has been shown to significantly reduce the expected incidence of colorectal cancer by 76% to 90% in multiple cohort studies. In the National Polyp Study, patients who underwent colonoscopy with polypectomy had a 76% reduction in colorectal cancer incidence compared with a general population registry (15). Surveillance of patients with resected colonic adenomas for metachronous lesions is also recommended, depending on the type and number of adenomas detected at the index colonoscopy (16). People at increased risk have three or more adenomas, high-grade dysplasia, villous features, or an adenoma ≥1 cm in size. It is recommended that they have a 3-year follow-up colonoscopy. People at lower risk who have one or two small (<1 cm) tubular adenomas with no high-grade dysplasia can have a follow-up in 5 to 10 years, whereas people with hyperplastic polyps only should have a 10-year follow-up as average-risk people (16). Endoscopic screening of patients at risk for Barrett esophagus (BE)/esophageal adenocarcinoma and squamous dysplasia/carcinoma can also detect early neoplastic lesions (Table 10.1).

Screening of high-risk individuals with an inherited predisposition for familial esophageal gastric, colorectal, and pancreatic cancer is also performed (Table 10.2), with a view to potentially therapeutically intervene prior to the development of cancer. For example, endoscopic screening with chromoendoscopy performed on relatives from families with hereditary diffuse gastric cancer (E-cadherin mutation) is initiated at age 16 years after genetic testing (17,18). Screening with unsedated transnasal endoscopy can diagnose BE in asymptomatic

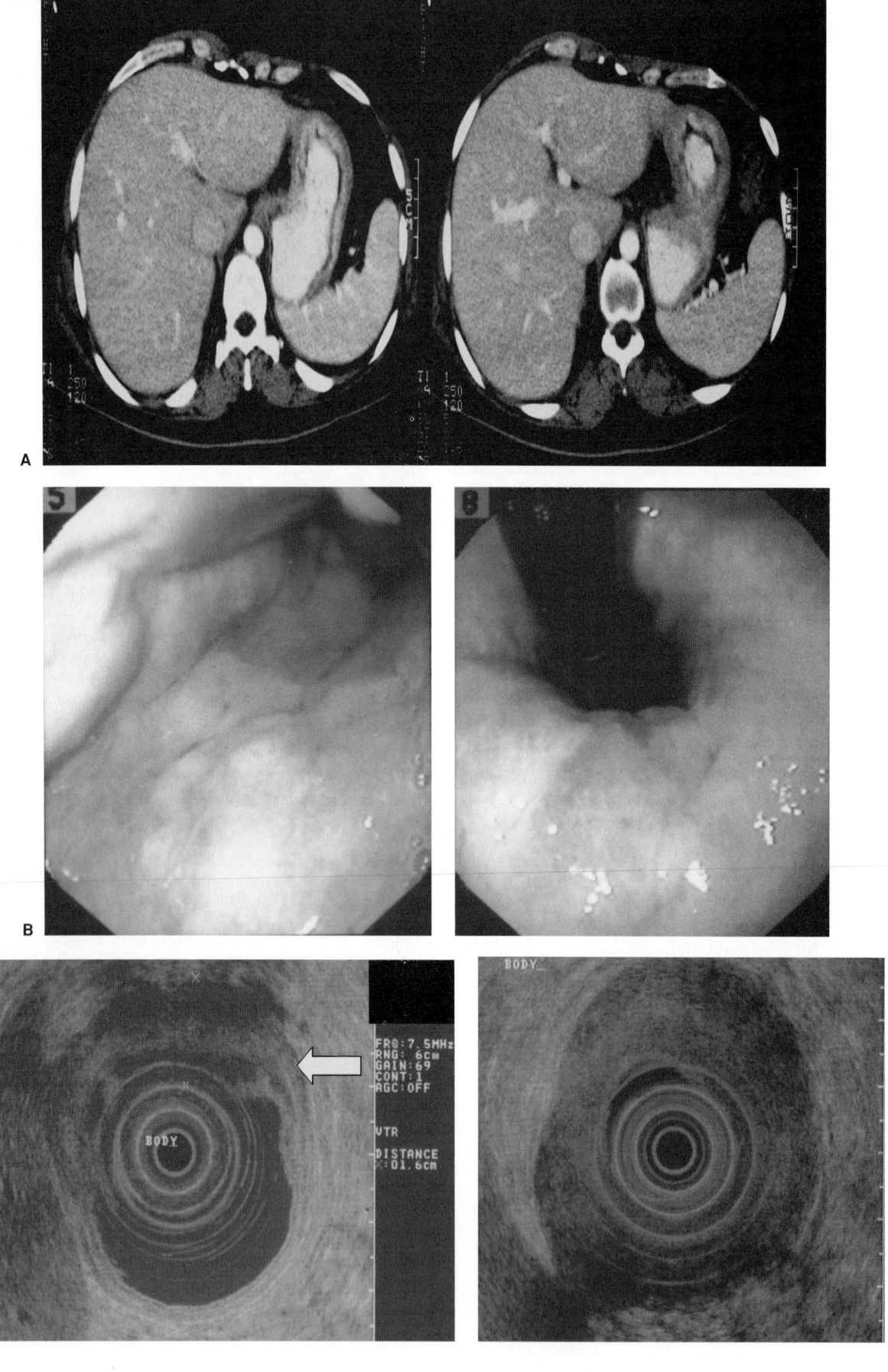

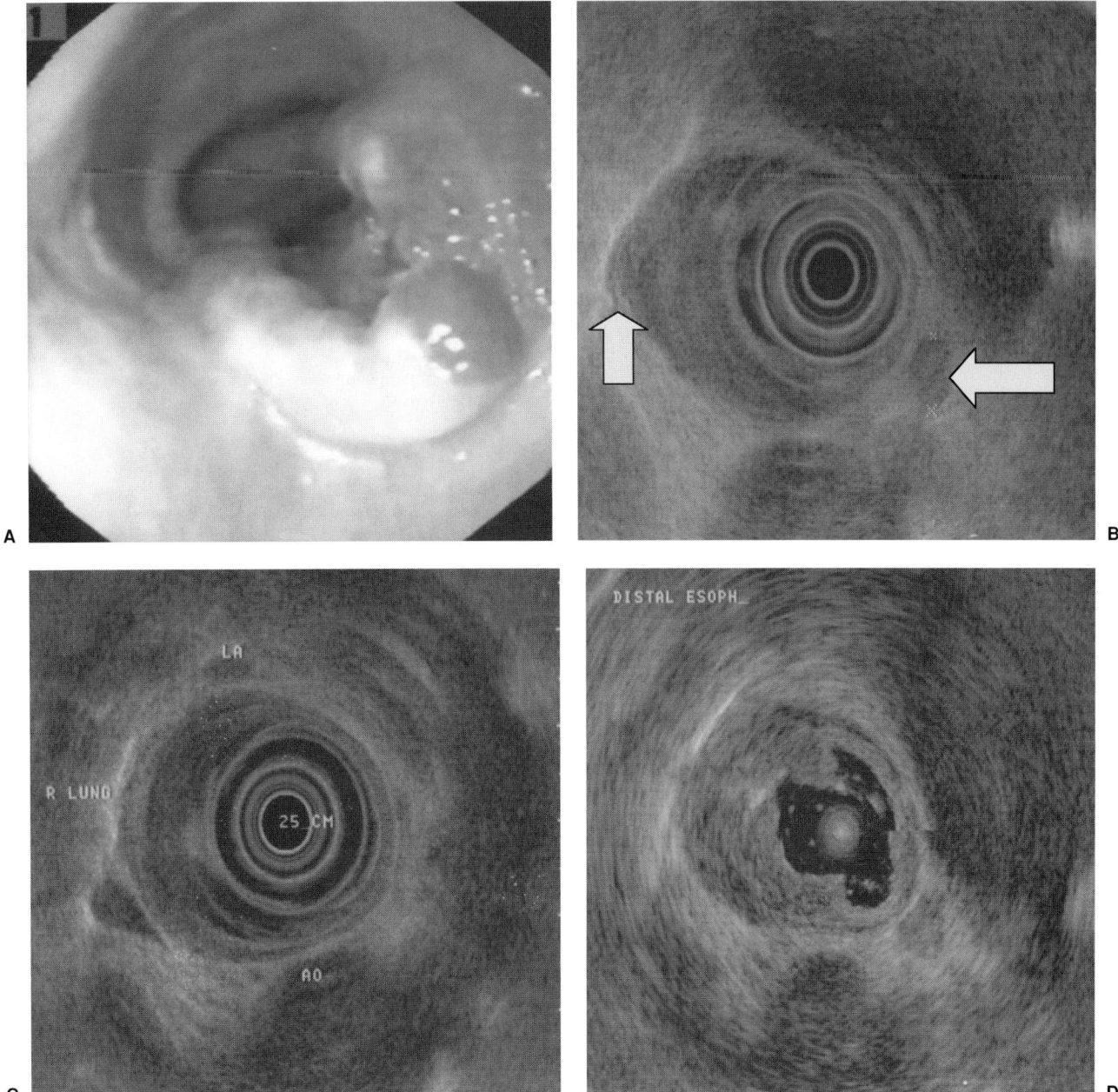

FIGURE 10.2. **A:** Endoscopic image of ulcerated esophageal adenocarcinoma arising in Barrett's esophagus. **B:** Endoscopic ultrasonography (EUS) image using 7.5-Mhz frequency demonstrates a cross-sectional view of the mass invading through the muscularis propria (*up arrow*) and abutting the pleura (*thin white line*), with an associated peritumor lymph node (*left arrow*), consistent with a T3 N1 cancer. **C** and **D:** Same tumor imaged with higher frequencies (**C:** 12 Mhz using the same radial echoendoscope; **D:** 20 Mhz using a catheter probe).

FIGURE 10.1. **(A)** CT scan images of the abdomen from a young woman with history of *Helicobacter pylori* infection who was found to have thick gastric folds by routine endoscopy and multiple nondiagnostic biopsies. The stomach (*arrow*) shows generalized thickening but no obvious mass. **(B)** Endoscopic images obtained at the time of the endoscopic ultrasonography (EUS) procedure showing markedly thickened gastric folds in the gastric body and antrum but no mass or ulcer. **(C)** EUS image from the proximal antrum showing marked expansion of all wall layers (*left arrow*) and normal five-layered wall structure on the opposite wall. **(D)** EUS image of the proximal body of the stomach showing complete effacement of normal wall layer structure and marked thickening. Targeted large capacity biopsies from these areas showed a poorly differentiated signet ring cell adenocarcinoma (linitis plastica).

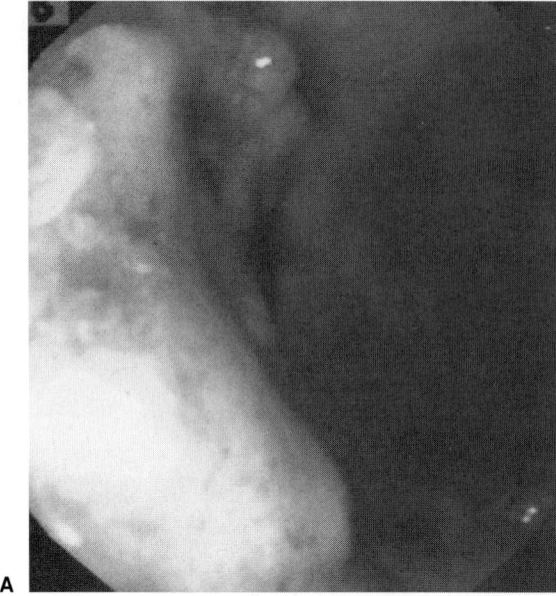
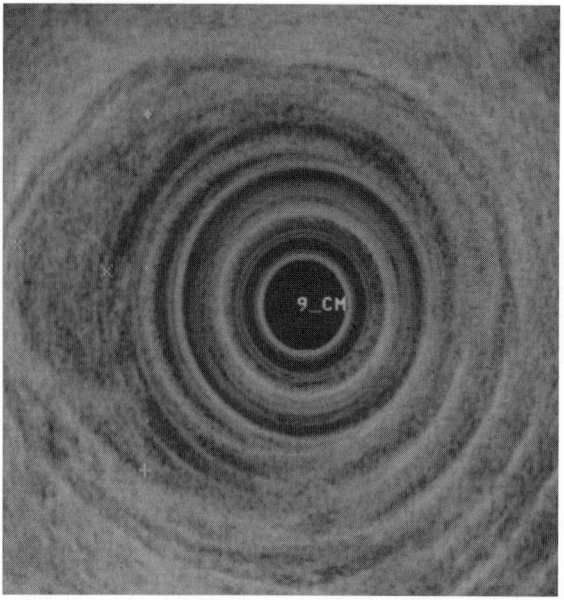

FIGURE 10.3. Endoscopic image (A) of a rectal mass biopsied to be adenocarcinoma. The endoscopic ultrasound staging procedure demonstrated this to be a T1 N0 lesion (B), and a transanal resection was performed instead of a more invasive abdominoperineal resection. The patient has been diseasefree for more than 5 years.

relatives from familial BE kindreds (19). Also, diagnosis of the precancerous lesion, such as the intraductal papillary mucinous neoplasm, can be made by EUS-FNA and surgical resection can be offered to asymptomatic relatives from familial pancreatic cancer kindreds (20) prior to the development invasive, incurable pancreatic adenocarcinoma.

ENDOSCOPIC STAGING OF LUMINAL CANCERS

The main endoscopic staging modality for GI cancers is EUS. It is superior to CT scan for staging the depth of invasion of esophageal (21,22) (Fig. 10.2), gastric (23) (Fig. 10.1), and rectal cancer (24) (Fig. 10.3). EUS is better than or comparable to CT and comparable to or better than positron emission to-

mography for regional lymph node metastasis from esophageal cancer (25). EUS is also better than standard pelvic magnetic resonance imaging (MRI), endorectal MRI (26), and CT for staging depth of tumor invasion, but equal to CT (24) and inferior to MRI for regional lymph node metastases for rectal cancer (27). Diagnosis of clinically suspected tumor regional esophageal (28), gastric (28), and rectal (26) cancer recurrence are better with EUS than CT or MRI. EUS is equal to multidetector, dual-phase pancreatic protocol CT for primary tumor assessment and locoregional staging of pancreatic cancer (3).

The accuracy of EUS for staging GI cancer is highest with advanced tumors that penetrate through the muscularis propria (T3) (Fig. 10.1) (accuracy rates usually ≥85%) and have regional lymph node involvement (N1) (accuracy rates typically 65%–75%). EUS staging results may impact patient management, particularly for esophageal (29) and rectal cancers (24) that are often treated with neoadjuvant chemoradiation therapy before surgery. EUS is generally least accurate with T2 lesions due to microscopic invasion into or through the muscularis propria that cannot be visualized. There has also been a need to improve the staging accuracy for T1 cancers because of the possibility of curative therapy of mucosal cancers with endoscopic mucosal resection (EMR) and/or photodynamic therapy. High-frequency (12-, 20-, and 30-Mhz) EUS probes (30) (Fig.10.2D) have been developed to improve the lateral resolution and help visualize the muscularis mucosae and submucosa. A few studies have shown improvement in staging accuracy of T1 mucosal and submucosal cancers in the esophagus (30) and stomach. Standard EUS with 5- and 7.5-Mhz frequencies (penetration depth of 6–10 cm) still needs to be performed with high-frequency EUS because the latter has limited depth of penetration (to 1–2 cm or less) and may miss regional lymph nodes. High-grade malignant esophageal strictures that do not allow passage of the echoendoscope can be staged with a 7 mm narrower instrument, the "blind" esophagoprobe (the standard echoendoscope minus the optics) that can be passed over a guidewire across the stricture (30) or a 2-mm catheter US probe (Fig. 10.2D).

When the accuracy rates for TNM (tumor, node, metastasis) staging for cancer at various sites are compared (Table 10.3), the highest reported accuracy rates are with esophageal and

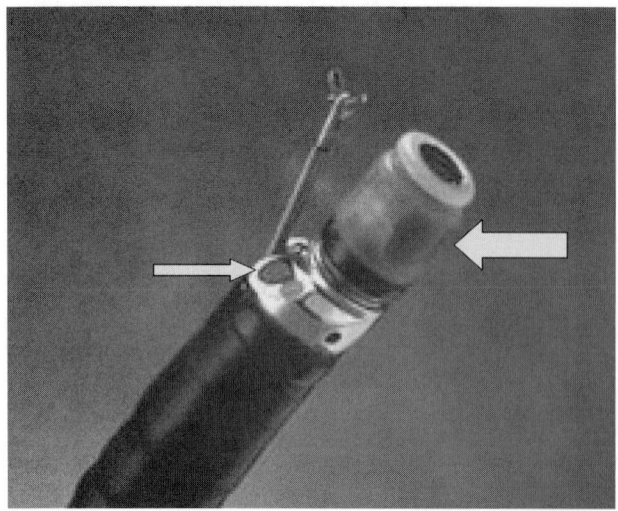

FIGURE 10.4. Radial scanning echoendoscope (Olympus America) used for endoscopic ultrasonography showing mechanical ultrasound transducer (*left arrow*) and oblique-viewing optics (*right arrow*).

AT-RISK GROUPS ELIGIBLE FOR ENDOSCOPIC SCREENING IN THE UNITED STATES

At-risk group	GI precursor lesion/GI cancer detected by endoscopy	Endoscopic methods used for screening
Chronic GERD	Barrett's esophagus/esophageal adenocarcinoma	Standard videoendoscopy (74), unsedated transnasal endoscopy, wireless capsule endoscopy (75,76)
Alcoholics, smokers, history of head and neck cancers	Esophageal squamous high grade dysplasia/squamous cell carcinoma	Standard videoendoscopy with Lugol's chromoendoscopy (77)
Adults 50 years of age or older	Colorectal adenoma/colorectal carcinoma	Colonoscopy (78)

GI, gastrointestinal; GERD, gastroesophageal reflux disease.

rectal cancer and lowest for gastric cancer, presumably due to peritumor inflammation and absence of the serosal layer in certain parts of the stomach (31).

EUS-FNA of regional and distant metastatic lymph nodes in the celiac, perigastric, and mediastinal regions increases the accuracy for N and M staging (32,33). Furthermore, detection and aspiration of small amounts of ascites not detected by CT or US can upstage cancer patients with occult peritoneal carcinomatosis (34).

ENDOSCOPIC STAGING FOR PANCREATIC AND BILIARY CANCER

EUS is highly accurate for staging primary pancreatic adenocarcinoma. Older studies had reported superior accuracy rates for T staging compared to CT (e.g., EUS 92% for T1, 85% for T2, and 93% for T3 lesions vs. 65%, 67%, and 38% for CT [35]), using surgical pathology as the reference standard. Furthermore, more recent studies using multidetector pancreatic protocol CT show variable results for the staging accuracy of EUS compared to CT, which may be due to interobserver variability for EUS and CT and technical differences in the

CT equipment and protocol. A large single-center study reported that EUS is superior to CT for T staging (67% vs. 41%, $p = 0.012$) and equivalent for nodal staging (44% vs. 47%) (9). However, these accuracy rates are lower than reported by other studies for both EUS and CT. EUS is also equivalent to CT for prediction of pancreatic cancer resectability based on vascular involvement (88% vs. 92%) (Fig. 10.5) (9). EUS is superior to angiography for detecting vascular invasion (36).

With regard to biliary cancers, EUS may be useful in the evaluation of cholangiocarcinoma. Intraductal US within the bile duct may help differentiate malignant from benign strictures. EUS-FNA can be helpful in the diagnosis of cholangiocarcinoma, especially in the region of the hilum (37).

ENDOSCOPIC DIAGNOSIS AND STAGING OF OTHER GASTROINTESTINAL-ASSOCIATED TUMORS

Low-grade gastric mucosa-associated lymphoid tumor (MALT) lymphoma can be staged and followed by EUS before and after treatment for *Helicobacter pylori* (38). Gastric

HIGH-RISK GROUPS ELIGIBLE FOR ENDOSCOPIC SURVEILLANCE

High-risk group	GI precursor lesion/GI cancer detected by endoscopy	Endoscopic methods used for surveillance
Barrett esophagus patients	Esophageal dysplasia/adenocarcinoma	Upper endoscopy and biopsy (79,80)
Familial Barrett esophagus/esophageal cancer relatives	Esophageal dysplasia/adenocarcinoma	Unsedated transnasal endoscopy (81)
Hereditary gastric cancer relative	Gastric dysplasia/diffuse gastric adenocarcinoma	Upper endoscopy and chromoendoscopy (82)
Hereditary colon cancer relative	Colorectal adenoma/carcinoma	Colonoscopy (83,84)
Chronic ulcerative colitis and Crohn disease (>8–10 years)	Colorectal adenoma/carcinoma	Colonoscopy with random biopsy or chromoendoscopy (85)
Family history of sporadic colorectal cancer	Colorectal adenoma/carcinoma	Colonoscopy (86)
Personal history of colon adenoma	Colorectal adenoma/carcinoma	Colonoscopy (87)
Peutz-Jeghers syndrome, familial adenomatous polyposis syndrome	Esophagus, gastric, small bowel, colon adenomas/adenocarcinoma	Upper endoscopy, colonoscopy, wireless capsule endoscopy (88,89)
Familial pancreatic cancer relatives, Peutz-Jeghers syndrome	Intraductal papillary mucinous neoplasm/pancreatic ductal adenocarcinoma	Endoscopic ultrasonography (90)

GI, gastrointestinal.

TABLE 10.3

COMPARISON OF ACCURACY RATES OF STAGING ENDOSCOPIC ULTRASOUND
±FNA FOR VARIOUS GASTROINTESTINAL CANCERS BY SITE

Organ site	Accuracy for T staging (depth of invasion)	Accuracy for N staging (regional lymph node metastases)
Esophagus	82%–89% (91)	70%–75% (91)
Stomach	68% (92)–83% (93)	63% (92)–78% (93)
Ampulla and duodenum	78% (94)–100% (95)	63%–66% (95)
Rectum	84% (96,97)–91% (98)	75% (96)–84% (99)
Pancreas	78% (100)–95% (101)	66% (102)–88% (101)

MALT can appear as ulcers, wall thickening by standard endoscopy, or obliteration or expansion of the normal wall-layered pattern by EUS (39). Normalization of the gastric wall layers highly correlates with complete response to antibiotic therapy for *H. pylori* (39).

EUS readily localizes neuroendocrine tumors in the duodenal wall and pancreas, even when these are not visible by US, CT (40,41), MRI, angiography (41), or somatostatin receptor scintigraphy (octreotide scan) (42). The detection rate of EUS for pancreatic neuroendocrine tumors is as high as 96.6%, compared to surgical pathology (43). EUS is superior to CT and somatostatin receptor scintigraphy for detection of insulinomas (sensitivity = 94% [7]) but comparable for diagnosis of gastrinomas (42). Hence, EUS may be the best test for localizing insulinomas, which are always in the pancreas. Octreotide scans are better than EUS, CT, or US for detecting liver metastases, with 92% accuracy (44). EUS screening of asymptomatic patients with multiple endocrine neoplasia type 1 can detect tumors prior to the development of biochemical test abnormalities (45). Furthermore, EUS-FNA can confirm the histologic type of the neuroendocrine tumor via immunohistochemical staining (43) and assist with intraoperative localization via EUS-guided fine-needle tattoo (46). The overall accuracy of EUS-FNA for preoperative diagnosis of neuroendocrine tumors is 83.3% (43). FNA specimens obtained by EUS guidance are more cellular and more likely to be adequate and diagnostic than those obtained by CT guidance (47). Overall, EUS is cost effective in the diagnosis of neuroendocrine tumors when used early in the diagnostic process due to reduced charges for preoperative localization studies ($2,620 vs. $4,846 per patient; $p < 0.05$), largely because of reductions in the number of diagnostic angiograms and venous sampling procedures performed (48). Surgical and total anesthesia times are also decreased (48).

LIMITATIONS OF ENDOSCOPY FOR DIAGNOSIS AND STAGING OF CANCER

Endoscopic diagnosis of luminal cancers is hampered by the inability to reliably distinguish between inflammation and tumor. For example, a nonhealing gastric ulcer may be benign or malignant, and a tissue diagnosis is required by sampling with multiple mucosal biopsies. Endoscopic assessment of mucosal

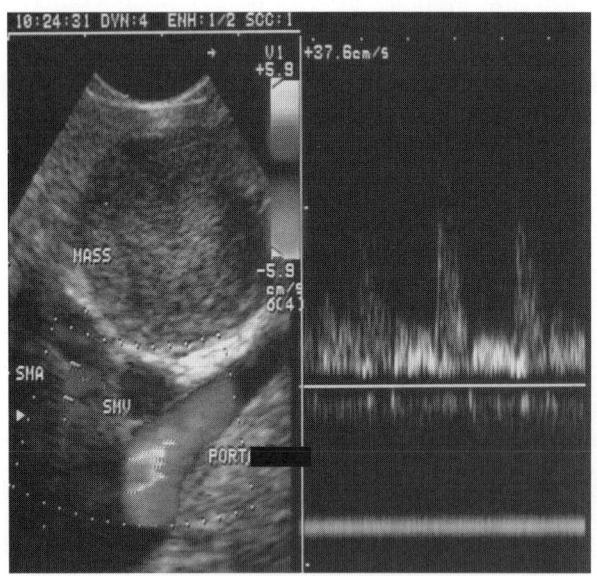
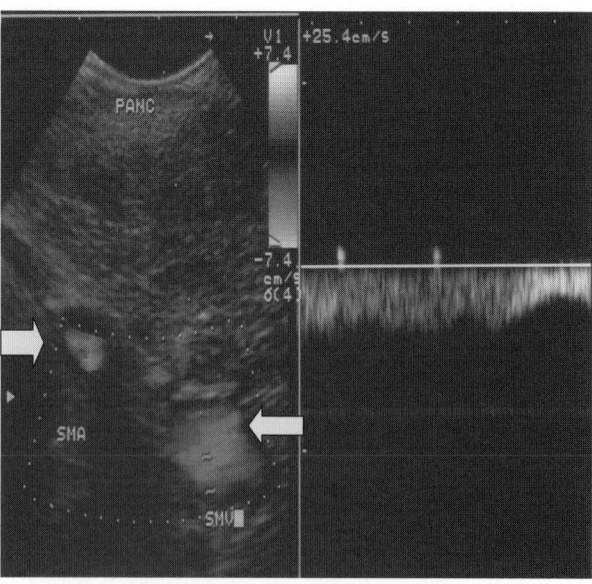

FIGURE 10.5. A: Endoscopic ultrasonography (EUS) image from a linear scanning ultrasound endoscope (Pentax Medical Systems, Montvale, New Jersey) showing a resectable pancreatic mass in the head. **B:** In contrast, this mass is clearly unresectable because of encasement of both the superior mesenteric artery and vein (*arrows*). At the same outpatient procedure, EUS-guided fine-needle aspiration obtained abundant cells consistent with adenocarcinoma, and celiac plexus neurolysis was performed to palliate cancer pain (See also color Figure 10.5a,b).

abnormalities is also operator dependent, and small tumors can be missed. For example, the miss rate between experienced academic endoscopists for colonic adenomas was 24%, particularly for small polyps (49). Furthermore, tissue samples obtained by standard and large capacity endoscopic biopsy samples typically contain only mucosa and little, if any, submucosa, which may misdiagnose cancers invading through the muscularis mucosae. Sampling of large areas of mucosa, such as in long BE or chronic ulcerative colitis, is currently not possible, except by obtaining multiple small random biopsies from the entire length of the involved esophageal or colonic mucosa. Hence, high-grade dysplasia or microscopic cancers in flat mucosa may be missed. A number of novel and advanced imaging techniques described here have been developed to enable scanning of large areas of mucosa in the upper and lower GI tract.

The main limitation of EUS is that it is highly operator dependent, and there is substantial interobserver variability (50,51). It is also less available in the United States compared to CT and MRI, primarily due to an insufficient number of trained endosonographers.

ENDOSCOPY AND MANAGEMENT OF GASTROINTESTINAL CANCERS

Curative and Preventive Therapies

If no invasive esophageal carcinoma is found in patients with a BE and high-grade dysplasia, there are several options. These are continued endoscopic surveillance, endoscopic mucosal ablation or resection, and surgery. Endoscopic surveillance consists of repeat endoscopy with intense mucosal sampling every 3 months until a cancer is detected (53). This option is attractive for patients who have only a limited focus of high-grade dysplasia (a few glands or small area). The incidence of adenocarcinoma in patients with confirmed high-grade dysplasia treated only with omeprazole was 39% in a prospective multicenter trial (54). Hence, "watchful waiting" may be appropriate, but only if endoscopic surveillance is intensified.

If the patient prefers to forestall esophagectomy or prevent cancer from developing, several choices are available for endoscopic therapy These include, but are not limited to, mucosal ablation with porfimer sodium-photodynamic therapy (PDT) (54) and argon plasma coagulation therapy (55,56). The techniques can be used in combination with EMR and can eliminate or delay the need for esophagectomy.

PDT involves administration of a photosensitizing agent. The typical agent is porfimer sodium (given intravenously), which is an inactive compound until it is exposed to light. The others in clinical use are 5-aminolevulinic acid (which is given orally and metabolized by the liver to protoporphyrin) and hematoporphyrin derivatives. Essentially these compounds function by inducing iatrogenic acquired porphyria in the patient. Porphyria is a disorder of heme synthesis that results in the accumulation of light-sensitive molecules in affected individuals. When exposed to the appropriate light wavelength, the agents produce cytotoxic oxygenfree radicals that kill nearby cells. Porfimer accumulates in normal cells but more so in neoplastic cells. When light is delivered by dye laser or diode laser, cancer cells are killed, and nearby vessels are damaged due to photochemical reaction. Patients treated with porfimer sodium need to avoid direct sunlight for about 4 to 6 weeks after receiving the compound. Active photobleaching by indirect exposure to sunlight decreases the period of photosensitivity. The main complication of PDT is esophageal strictures, which occur in 10% to 30% of treated patients, depending on the depth of tissue damage. In addition, a subset of patients has incomplete eradication of their neoplastic cells, so lesions may recur and, thus, continued surveillance is indicated after treatment.

PDT has been advocated by many due to the results of several prospective cohort studies and a large randomized controlled multicenter phase 3 study (54,57). But PDT is expensive, and the majority of patients have side effects such as photosensitivity, chest pain, anorexia, nausea, and dehydration. Only about three fourths of the patients in the multicenter study (57) had complete ablation of their high-grade dysplasia at some point in the study. However, more important, PDT is the only ablative technique that has been shown to decrease the incidence of cancer (57), compared to treatment with omeprazole alone, and 5-year follow-up data suggest the effects are long lasting and durable (57).

An argon plasma coagulator (APC) is a noncontact device that uses a high-frequency monopolar current conducted to a tissue via flow of ionized argon gas. The depth of tissue necrosis is a function of the power setting of the generator, the distance from the probe to the mucosa, the amount of gas flow, and the duration of the application such that tissue injury can involve a depth of 6 mm. APC and PDT may be equally effective for eradicating BE, but for ablation of high-grade dysplasia in BE, APC appears to be slightly less effective but less costly than PDT (56). Newer ablative therapies still under evaluation are radiofrequency ablation and cryotherapy (58). Both devices are approved for clinical use by the U.S. Food and Drug Administration, but there is little published evidence of their long-term safety and efficacy for treating BE and associated neoplasia.

EMR was developed in Japan as a minimally invasive technique for curative treatment of gastric cancer (59). It has been adopted in the United States and other parts of the world. EMR offers the opportunity for histopathological assessment of the maximum depth and lateral extent, as well as complete removal of the diseased area. This technique can be used in combination with other ablative techniques, achieving excellent results in terms of removing high-grade neoplastic lesions (60). Furthermore, EMR improves the diagnosis and staging of BE-associated neoplasia as compared with endoscopic biopsy and EUS (61). Moreover, the evaluation of lateral and deep margins of the EMR specimen can predict local recurrence and may potentially modify patient management (61). Finally, the morbidity and mortality of this EMR are favorable compared to the alternative of esophagectomy (62). There are few studies reporting long-term results, but gastroenterologists are optimistic that the approach of combined EMR and PDT may be curative in a high percentage of patients. Certainly, the patient presented here has had excellent results over a period of 32 months.

Patients with visible macroscopic lesions may undergo EUS to exclude periesophageal lymphadenopathy and a cancer infiltrating into and through the submucosa. The type of endoscopic therapy offered is influenced by the patient's age, preferences, medical status, comorbidities, endoscopic features of Barrett mucosa, and pathology results. If the patient has no invasive lesion in the BE segment and high-grade dysplasia is either multifocal or not localized, PDT is performed, particularly if he or she has long BE, which is not easily resected using current techniques (63). Porfimer sodium-PDT should include all dysplastic areas (63). Complete ablation of high-grade dysplasia and any synchronous undetected cancer is the primary goal.

If the patient has dysplastic lesion or a short length of BE with high-grade dysplasia, EMR is performed as the first and potentially only treatment. Multiple EMR can be performed to completely remove Barrett mucosa, but no more than half of the circumference is resected at one time to minimize stricture formation.

After EMR, the stage of any cancer, if present, and the lateral and deep margins of the EMR specimen are assessed by the pathologist. If the deep margin is positive for cancer and invasion of the submucosa is present, then surgery is recommended. If a lateral margin is positive, or there is multifocal dysplasia or dysplasia that cannot be localized in a long BE segment, then PDT can be performed 2 to 4 weeks after EMR to either remove or ablate the remaining BE (63). Alternatively, EMR of the remaining BE can be performed to resect the remaining neoplastic tissue. The long term outcomes of endoscopic treatments are now being reported. These complete responses to EMR (60,64) and/or PDT (57,63,65) with minimal to no major morbidity (63,66), no treatment-related mortality (60,63,65), and comparable long-term survival (57,62,63,65,66) provide patients with a safe, outpatient treatment as a favorable alternative to surgery.

Palliative Therapies

EUS-guided therapies are also highly promising alternatives to conventional treatments for cancer patients. Endoscopic therapies for palliation of pancreatic cancer include endoscopic biliary stenting for obstructive jaundice in patients with malignant bile duct strictures from cholangiocarcinoma and pancreatic cancer, and stenting for duodenal obstruction. Self-expanding metal stents can be placed on an outpatient basis by experienced endoscopists, thereby obviating the need for palliative surgical biliary and duodenal bypass procedure. The endoscopic approach may help avoid the complications and hospitalization resulting from surgery performed only for palliation.

Palliation of pancreatic cancer pain can also be successfully provided by celiac plexus neurolysis via an EUS-guided approach. This can be performed at the same outpatient visit as the diagnostic/staging EUS-FNA procedure (Fig. 10.5) in patients with obvious locally unresectable or metastatic disease and a pancreatic mass. Similar to operative and percutaneous celiac plexus neurolysis, alcohol is injected into the area of the celiac plexus. However, the EUS-guided approach is a potentially safer and better tolerated because of the proximity of the needle in the echoendoscope within the stomach to the celiac trunk and adjacent celiac ganglia immediately posterior to the gastric wall. Furthermore, the anterior approach and accurate real-time guidance of the injection during EUS minimizes complications associated with a posterior approach (e.g., trauma or inadvertent injection into the spinal arteries and nerves and traversal of the pleura and diaphragm). EUS-guided celiac plexus neurolysis results in pain relief in 80% to 90% of patients, similar to CT- and fluoroscopy-guided techniques.

FUTURE DIRECTIONS FOR ENDOSCOPIC DIAGNOSIS AND STAGING

Techniques to Improve the Miss Rate for Detection of Mucosal Lesions

Emerging endoscopic techniques offer an opportunity for better evaluation of patients with Barrett-associated neoplasia. A number of strategies have been introduced to improve detection of dysplastic foci in BE. Methylene blue chromoendoscopy has been used to improve identification of the most suspicious mucosal foci to biopsy (67); however, the technique is operator dependent, and variability in the results of various studies has limited its use for routine screening and surveillance (68). A new generation of endoscopes linked to modern imaging devices may improve diagnostic yield and limit the number of biopsies needed for detection of intraepithelial neoplasia, but there are few published studies. Some examples of these emerging endoscopic techniques are confocal laser endomicroscopy (69), optical coherence tomography (70), autofluorescence endoscopy (71), high-resolution and high-magnification endoscopy, and narrow band imaging (72).

Confocal laser endomicroscopy (CLE) is a novel method for examining mucosal morphology in real time during an endoscopic procedure (73). The confocal endomicroscope (EC3870K; Pentax, Tokyo, Japan, in cooperation with Optiscan, Victoria, Australia) is a standard videoendoscope with "close focus" optics, allowing imaging at a distance of 2 to 100 mm from the mucosal surface and optical magnification to approximately $30\times$ to $50\times$. The endomicroscope functions like a standard endoscope, but it also has a laser light and a miniaturized confocal microscope built into the tip. Using the device, high-resolution endomicroscopic images of mucosal cells, crypt architecture, and lamina propria are obtained up to a depth of 200 μm from the surface, equivalent to $1{,}000\times$ magnification and lateral resolution of <1 μm. Confocal microscopy itself is a fluorescent microscopy technique. A laser is used to provide the excitation light (to obtain very high intensities). The laser light reflects off a dichroic mirror. From there, the laser hits two mirrors mounted on motors; these mirrors serially scan the laser across the sample. Dye in the sample fluoresces, and the emitted light is descanned by the same mirrors that are used to scan the excitation light from the laser. The emitted light passes through the dichroic mirror and is focused onto a pinhole, which excludes out-of-focus light. The light that passes through the pinhole is measured by a detector. The detector is therefore attached to a computer that builds up the image, 1 pixel at a time. A single-center study suggests that confocal endomicroscopy may enable accurate in vivo imaging and targeted biopsy of BE and associated neoplasia (69).

Optical coherence tomography (OCT) relies on light scattering by tissues. The optical delay of back-scattered/reflected light is measured; the scatter is a function of the distance between the light source and the scattering object. Data from OCT are converted into gray scale images. This technique allows identification of distinctive features found in Barrett epithelium and reasonable sensitivity (83%) and specificity (75%) for diagnosis of high-grade dysplasia and intramucosal carcinoma using an OCT dysplasia index (70). The resolution is approximately 3 to 4 m (half the size of an erythrocyte). However, the volume of tissue in a single OCT image is quite small; therefore, imaging of a large surface area is cumbersome and time consuming. OCT must therefore be coupled with either high-resolution endoscopy or a technique that allows accurate but efficient scanning of the mucosa.

Autofluorescence imaging (AFI) involves stimulation of the tissue during endoscopy with laser light, detection of intrinsic (auto) fluorescence and reflected light, and computer-aided compositing of images to create a combined pseudocolor endoscopic image. This results in differential coloration of normal from nonnormal mucosa, which in turn can be readily detected during endoscopy. AFI has a potential to be an excellent method for scanning large areas of mucosa for neoplastic tissue. In a single-center prospective study (71), there was a small but significant 10% incremental benefit (23%−33% diagnostic rate of BE with endoscopically inapparent high-grade dysplasia or early adenocarcinoma) of AFI over standard white light endoscopy. Hence, the standard white light image and autofluorescence image can potentially allow the endoscopist to obtain targeted biopsies after examination of the mucosal surface for suspicious areas.

Narrow band imaging (NBI) is a method that uses special filters on the endoscope (Olympus America, Center Valley, PA) to narrow the band-pass ranges of red, green, and blue light and increase the relative intensity of blue light (72). Hence, when used in combination with high-magnification or high-resolution endoscopy, the mucosal and vascular pattern in BE can be readily visualized with the mere flick of a button and without having to spray dyes. The overall sensitivity for detection of high-grade dysplasia or early adenocarcinoma can be slightly increased beyond that for high-resolution endoscopy alone (i.e., 89% for high-resolution endoscopy, and 86% with the addition of NBI) (72). However, even more important is the incremental benefit of adding NBI to high-resolution endoscopy. In one small randomized single-center study, 3 more out of a total of 14 patients were diagnosed with high-grade dysplasia or early cancer using NBI. But like other novel imaging techniques, the true incremental benefit of NBI to standard or high-resolution endoscopy detecting BE-intraepithelial neoplasia outside centers with special interest in imaging and BE remains unknown, and studies are ongoing.

These novel techniques offer the potential to enhance real-time diagnosis of mucosal lesions. They may allow reduction in the number of biopsies required to manage such patients and eliminate the need for biopsies in others. The need for conventional histology may ultimately be subsumed by these techniques, but until they are validated and endoscopists are trained in interpreting images, conventional histologic evaluation, although imperfect, remains the foundation of assessment of surveillance biopsies. Furthermore, advances in endoscopic therapy, particularly techniques for endoscopic mucosal resection, may also eliminate the need for multiple surveillance biopsies, as complete resection of the Barrett mucosa becomes a more cost-effective approach to managing intraepithelial neoplasia.

References

1. Hendlisz A, Bleiberg H. Diagnosis and treatment of gastric cancer. *Drugs* 1995;49:711–20.
2. Takemoto T, Aibe T, Fuji T, Okita K. Endoscopic ultrasonography. *Clin Gastroenterol* 1986;15:305–319.
3. Dewitt J, Devereaux BM, Lehman GA, Sherman S, Imperiale TF. Comparison of endoscopic ultrasound and computed tomography for the preoperative evaluation of pancreatic cancer: a systematic review. *Clin Gastroenterol Hepatol* 2006;4:717–725; quiz 664.
4. Agarwal B, Abu-Hamda E, Molke KL, Correa AM, Ho L. Endoscopic ultrasound-guided fine needle aspiration and multidetector spiral CT in the diagnosis of pancreatic cancer. *Am J Gastroenterol* 2004;99:844–850.
5. Yasuda K, Mukai H, Nakajima M, Kawai K. Staging of pancreatic carcinoma by endoscopic ultrasonography. *Endoscopy* 1993;25:151–155.
6. Legmann P, Vignaux O, Dousset B, et al. Pancreatic tumors: comparison of dual-phase helical CT and endoscopic sonography. *AJR Am J Roentgenol* 1998;170:1315–1322.
7. McLean AM, Fairclough PD. Endoscopic ultrasound in the localisation of pancreatic islet cell tumours. *Best Pract Res Clin Endocrinol Metab* 2005;19:177–193.
8. Klapman JB, Chang KJ, Lee JG, Nguyen P. Negative predictive value of endoscopic ultrasound in a large series of patients with a clinical suspicion of pancreatic cancer. *Am J Gastroenterol* 2005;100:2658–2661.
9. DeWitt J, Devereaux B, Chriswell M, et al. Comparison of endoscopic ultrasonography and multidetector computed tomography for detecting and staging pancreatic cancer. *Ann Intern Med* 2004;141:753–763.
10. Levy MJ, Smyrk TC, Reddy RP, et al. Endoscopic ultrasound-guided Tru-Cut biopsy of the cyst wall for diagnosing cystic pancreatic tumors. *Clin Gastroenterol Hepatol* 2005;3:974–979.
11. Gines A, Wiersema MJ, Clain JE, Pochron NL, Rajan E, Levy MJ. Prospective study of a Tru-Cut needle for performing EUS-guided biopsy with EUS-guided FNA rescue. *Gastrointest Endosc* 2005;62:597–601.
12. Wittmann J, Kocjan G, Sgouros SN, Deheragoda M, Pereira SP. Endoscopic ultrasound-guided tissue sampling by combined fine needle aspiration and Tru-Cut needle biopsy: a prospective study. *Cytopathology* 2006;17:27–33.
13. Itzkowitz SH, Present DH. Consensus conference: colorectal cancer screening and surveillance in inflammatory bowel disease. *Inflamm Bowel Dis* 2005;11:314–321.
14. Davila RE, Rajan E, Baron TH, et al. ASGE guideline: colorectal cancer screening and surveillance. *Gastrointest Endosc* 2006;63:546–557.
15. Winawer SJ, Zauber AG, Ho MN, et al. Prevention of colorectal cancer by colonoscopic polypectomy. The National Polyp Study Workgroup. *N Engl J Med* 1993;329:1977–1981.
16. Winawer SJ, Zauber AG, Fletcher RH, et al. Guidelines for colonoscopy surveillance after polypectomy: a consensus update by the US Multi-Society Task Force on Colorectal Cancer and the American Cancer Society. *CA Cancer J Clin* 2006;56:143–159; quiz 184–185.
17. Blair V, Martin I, Shaw D, et al. Hereditary diffuse gastric cancer: diagnosis and management. *Clin Gastroenterol Hepatol* 2006;4:262–275.
18. Shaw D, Blair V, Framp A, et al. Chromoendoscopic surveillance in hereditary diffuse gastric cancer: an alternative to prophylactic gastrectomy? *Gut* 2005;54:461–468.
19. Chak A, Faulx A, Kinnard M, et al. Identification of Barrett's esophagus in relatives by endoscopic screening. *Am J Gastroenterol* 2004;99:2107–2114.
20. Canto M, Goggins M, RH H, et al. Screening for early pancreatic neoplasia in high-risk individuals: a prospective controlled study. *Clin Gastroenterol Hepatol* 2006;4:766–781.
21. Botet JF, Lightdale CJ, Zauber AG, Gerdes H, Urmacher C, Brennan MF. Preoperative staging of esophageal cancer: comparison of endoscopic US and dynamic CT [see comments]. *Radiology* 1991;181:419–425.
22. Kienle P, Buhl K, Kuntz C, et al. Prospective comparison of endoscopy, endosonography and computed tomography for staging of tumours of the oesophagus and gastric cardia. *Digestion* 2002;66:230–236.
23. Polkowski M, Palucki J, Wronska E, Szawlowski A, Nasierowska-Guttmejer A, Butruk E. Endosonography versus helical computed tomography for locoregional staging of gastric cancer. *Endoscopy* 2004;36:617–623.
24. Harewood GC, Wiersema MJ, Nelson H, et al. A prospective, blinded assessment of the impact of preoperative staging on the management of rectal cancer. *Gastroenterology* 2002;123:24–32.
25. Lowe VJ, Booya F, Fletcher JG, et al. Comparison of positron emission tomography, computed tomography, and endoscopic ultrasound in the initial staging of patients with esophageal cancer. *Mol Imaging Biol* 2005;7:422–430.
26. Meyenberger C, Huch Boni RA, Bertschinger P, Zala GF, Klotz HP, Krestin GP. Endoscopic ultrasound and endorectal magnetic resonance imaging: a prospective, comparative study for preoperative staging and follow-up of rectal cancer. *Endoscopy* 1995;27:469–479.
27. Bianchi P, Ceriani C, Palmisano A, et al. A prospective comparison of endorectal ultrasound and pelvic magnetic resonance in the preoperative staging of rectal cancer. *Ann Ital Chir* 2006;77:41–46.
28. Lightdale CJ, Botet JF, Kelsen DP, Turnbull AD, Brennan MF. Diagnosis of recurrent upper gastrointestinal cancer at the surgical anastomosis by endoscopic ultrasound. *Gastrointest Endosc* 1989;35:407–412.
29. Slater MS, Holland J, Faigel DO, Sheppard BC, Deveney CW. Does neoadjuvant chemoradiation downstage esophageal carcinoma? *Am J Surg* 2001;181:440–444.
30. Menzel J, Hoepffner N, Nottberg H, Schulz C, Senninger N, Domschke W. Preoperative staging of esophageal carcinoma: miniprobe sonography versus conventional endoscopic ultrasound in a prospective histopathologically verified study. *Endoscopy* 1999;31:291–297.
31. Tsendsuren T, Jun SM, Mian XH. Usefulness of endoscopic ultrasonography in preoperative TNM staging of gastric cancer. *World J Gastroenterol* 2006;12:43–47.
32. Vazquez-Sequeiros E, Norton ID, Clain JE, et al. Impact of EUS-guided fine-needle aspiration on lymph node staging in patients with esophageal carcinoma. *Gastrointest Endosc* 2001;53:751–757.
33. Eloubeidi MA, Wallace MB, Reed CE, et al. The utility of EUS and EUS-guided fine needle aspiration in detecting celiac lymph node metastasis in patients with esophageal cancer: a single-center experience. *Gastrointest Endosc* 2001;54:714–719.
34. Lee YT, Ng EK, Hung LC, et al. Accuracy of endoscopic ultrasonography in diagnosing ascites and predicting peritoneal metastases in gastric cancer patients. *Gut* 2005;54:1541–1545.
35. Gress FG, Hawes RH, Savides TJ, et al. Role of EUS in the preoperative staging of pancreatic cancer: a large single-center experience. *Gastrointest Endosc* 1999;50:786–791.
36. Ahmad NA, Kochman ML, Lewis JD, et al. Endosonography is superior to angiography in the preoperative assessment of vascular involvement among patients with pancreatic carcinoma. *J Clin Gastroenterol* 2001;32:54–58.
37. Moparty B, Bhutani MS. Endoscopic ultrasonography for choledocholithiasis and biliary malignancy. *Curr Treat Options Gastroenterol* 2005;8:135–142.
38. Yeh HZ, Chen GH, Chang WD, et al. Long-term follow up of gastric low-grade mucosa-associated lymphoid tissue lymphoma by endosonography emphasizing the application of a miniature ultrasound probe. *J Gastroenterol Hepatol* 2003;18:162–167.
39. Lugering N, Menzel J, Kucharzik T, et al. Impact of miniprobes compared to conventional endosonography in the staging of low-grade gastric malt lymphoma. *Endoscopy* 2001;33:832–837.
40. Gines A, Vazquez-Sequeiros E, Soria MT, Clain JE, Wiersema MJ. Usefulness of EUS-guided fine needle aspiration (EUS-FNA) in the diagnosis of functioning neuroendocrine tumors. *Gastrointest Endosc* 2002;56:291–296.

41. Anderson MA, Carpenter S, Thompson NW, Nostrant TT, Elta GH, Scheiman JM. Endoscopic ultrasound is highly accurate and directs management in patients with neuroendocrine tumors of the pancreas. *Am J Gastroenterol* 2000;95:2271–2277.

42. Zimmer T, Stolzel U, Bader M, et al. Endoscopic ultrasonography and somatostatin receptor scintigraphy in the preoperative localisation of insulinomas and gastrinomas. *Gut* 1996;39:562–568.

43. Ardengh JC, de Paulo GA, Ferrari AP. EUS-guided FNA in the diagnosis of pancreatic neuroendocrine tumors before surgery. *Gastrointest Endosc* 2004;60:378–384.

44. Gibril F, Jensen RT. Comparative analysis of diagnostic techniques for localization of gastrointestinal neuroendocrine tumors. *Yale J Biol Med* 1997;70:509–522.

45. Wamsteker EJ, Gauger PG, Thompson NW, Scheiman JM. EUS detection of pancreatic endocrine tumors in asymptomatic patients with type 1 multiple endocrine neoplasia. *Gastrointest Endosc* 2003;58:531–535.

46. Gress FG, Barawi M, Kim D, Grendell JH. Preoperative localization of a neuroendocrine tumor of the pancreas with EUS-guided fine needle tattooing. *Gastrointest Endosc* 2002;55:594–597.

47. Jhala D, Eloubeidi M, Chhieng DC, et al. Fine needle aspiration biopsy of the islet cell tumor of pancreas: a comparison between computerized axial tomography and endoscopic ultrasound-guided fine needle aspiration biopsy. *Ann Diagn Pathol* 2002;6:106–112.

48. Bansal R, Tierney W, Carpenter S, Thompson N, Scheiman JM. Cost effectiveness of EUS for preoperative localization of pancreatic endocrine tumors. *Gastrointest Endosc* 1999;49:19–25.

49. Rex DK, Cutler CS, Lemmel GT, et al. Colonoscopic miss rates of adenomas determined by back-to-back colonoscopies. *Gastroenterology* 1997;112:24–28.

50. Meining A, Rosch T, Wolf A, et al. High interobserver variability in endosonographic staging of upper gastrointestinal cancers. *Z Gastroenterol* 2003;41:391–394.

51. Fusaroli P, Buscarini E, Peyre S, et al. Interobserver agreement in staging gastric MALT lymphoma by EUS. *Gastrointest Endosc* 2002;55:662–668.

52. Ell C, May A, Gossner L, et al. Endoscopic mucosal resection of early cancer and high-grade dysplasia in Barrett's esophagus. *Gastroenterology* 2000;118:670–677.

53. Levine DS, Haggitt RC, Blount PL, Rabinovitch PS, Rusch VW, Reid BJ. An endoscopic biopsy protocol can differentiate high-grade dysplasia from early adenocarcinoma in Barrett's esophagus [see comments]. *Gastroenterology* 1993;105:40–50.

54. Overholt BF, Lightdale CJ, Wang KK, et al. Photodynamic therapy with porfimer sodium for ablation of high-grade dysplasia in Barrett's esophagus: international, partially blinded, randomized phase III trial. *Gastrointest Endosc* 2005;62:488–498.

55. Van Laethem JL, Jagodzinski R, Peny MO, Cremer M, Deviere J. Argon plasma coagulation in the treatment of Barrett's high-grade dysplasia and in situ adenocarcinoma. *Endoscopy* 2001;33:257–261.

56. Ragunath K, Krasner N, Raman VS, Haqqani MT, Phillips CJ, Cheung I. Endoscopic ablation of dysplastic Barrett's oesophagus comparing argon plasma coagulation and photodynamic therapy: a randomized prospective trial assessing efficacy and cost-effectiveness. *Scand J Gastroenterol* 2005;40:750–758.

57. Overholt B, Wang K, Burdick S, et al. A 5-year randomized phase III trial of efficacy and safety of photodynamic therapy using porfimer sodium in high grade dysplasia in Barrett's esophagus. *Gastrointest Endosc* 2006;63:AB82.

58. Johnston MH. Technology insight: ablative techniques for Barrett's esophagus—current and emerging trends. *Nat Clin Pract Gastroenterol Hepatol* 2005;2:323–330.

59. Inoue H, Takeshita K, Hori H, Muraoka Y, Yoneshima H, Endo M. Endoscopic mucosal resection with a cap-fitted panendoscope for esophagus, stomach, and colon mucosal lesions [see comments]. *Gastrointest Endosc* 1993;39:58–62.

60. Behrens A, May A, Gossner L, et al. Curative treatment for high-grade intraepithelial neoplasia in Barrett's esophagus. *Endoscopy* 2005;37:999–1005.

61. Mino-Kenudson M, Brugge WR, Puricelli WP, et al. Management of superficial Barrett's epithelium-related neoplasms by endoscopic mucosal resection: clinicopathologic analysis of 27 cases. *Am J Surg Pathol* 2005;29:680–6.

62. Pacifico RJ, Wang KK, Wongkeesong LM, Buttar NS, Lutzke LS. Combined endoscopic mucosal resection and photodynamic therapy versus esophagectomy for management of early adenocarcinoma in Barrett's esophagus. *Clin Gastroenterol Hepatol* 2003;1:252–257.

63. Canto M, Gress FG, Wolfsen HC. Long term outcomes of curative bare fiber porfimer sodium (Ps)-photodynamic therapy (PDT) for T1N0 cancers of the esophagus and esophagogastric junction: a multicenter prospective cohort study. *Gastrointest Endosc* 2005;61:AB128.

64. Peters FP, Kara MA, Rosmolen WD, et al. Endoscopic treatment of high-grade dysplasia and early stage cancer in Barrett's esophagus. *Gastrointest Endosc* 2005;61:506–514.

65. Pech O, Gossner L, May A, et al. Long-term results of photodynamic therapy with 5-aminolevulinic acid for superficial Barrett's cancer and high-grade intraepithelial neoplasia. *Gastrointest Endosc* 2005;62:24–30.

66. May A, Gossner L, Pech O, et al. Local endoscopic therapy for intraepithelial high-grade neoplasia and early adenocarcinoma in Barrett's oesophagus: acute-phase and intermediate results of a new treatment approach. *Eur J Gastroenterol Hepatol* 2002;14:1085–1091.

67. Canto MI, Setrakian S, Willis J, et al. Methylene blue-directed biopsies improve detection of intestinal metaplasia and dysplasia in Barrett's esophagus. *Gastrointest Endosc* 2000;51:560–568.

68. Canto MI. Methylene blue chromoendoscopy for Barrett's esophagus: coming soon to your GI unit? *Gastrointest Endosc* 2001;54:403–409.

69. Kiesslich R, Gossner L, Goetz M, et al. In vivo histology of Barrett's esophagus and associated neoplasias by confocal laser endomicroscopy. *Clin Gastroenterol Hepatol* 2006:in press.

70. Evans JA, Poneros JM, Bouma BE, et al. Optical coherence tomography to identify intramucosal carcinoma and high-grade dysplasia in Barrett's esophagus. *Clin Gastroenterol Hepatol* 2006;4:38–43.

71. Kara MA, Peters FP, Ten Kate FJ, Van Deventer SJ, Fockens P, Bergman JJ. Endoscopic video autofluorescence imaging may improve the detection of early neoplasia in patients with Barrett's esophagus. *Gastrointest Endosc* 2005;61:679–685.

72. Kara MA, Peters FP, Rosmolen WD, et al. High-resolution endoscopy plus chromoendoscopy or narrow-band imaging in Barrett's esophagus: a prospective randomized crossover study. *Endoscopy* 2005;37:929–936.

73. Kiesslich R, Neurath MF. Endoscopic confocal imaging. *Clin Gastroenterol Hepatol* 2005;3:S58–S60.

74. Rex DK, Cummings OW, Shaw M, et al. Screening for Barrett's esophagus in colonoscopy patients with and without heartburn. *Gastroenterology* 2003;125:1670–1677.

75. Eliakim R, Yassin K, Shlomi I, Suissa A, Eisen GM. A novel diagnostic tool for detecting oesophageal pathology: the Pill CAM oesophageal video capsule. *Aliment Pharmacol Ther* 2004;20:1083–1089.

76. Ramirez FC, Shaukat MS, Young MA, Johnson DA, Akins R. Feasibility and safety of string, wireless capsule endoscopy in the diagnosis of Barrett's esophagus. *Gastrointest Endosc* 2005;61:741–746.

77. Yokoyama A, Ohmori T, Makuuchi H, et al. Successful screening for early esophageal cancer in alcoholics using endoscopy and mucosa iodine staining. *Cancer* 1995;76:928–934.

78. Levin B, Barthel JS, Burt RW, et al. Colorectal cancer screening clinical practice guidelines. *J Natl Compr Canc Netw* 2006;4:384–420.

79. Sampliner RE. Updated guidelines for the diagnosis, surveillance, and therapy of Barrett's esophagus. *Am J Gastroenterol* 2002;97:1888–1895.

80. Sharma P, McQuaid K, Dent J, et al. A critical review of the diagnosis and management of Barrett's esophagus: the AGA Chicago Workshop. *Gastroenterology* 2004;127:310–30.

81. Chak A, Faulx A, Kinnard M, Brock W, et al. Identification of Barrett's esophagus in relatives by endoscopic screening. *Am J Gastroenterol* 2004;99:2107–2114.

82. Blair V, Martin I, Shaw D, et al. Hereditary diffuse gastric cancer: diagnosis and management. *Clin Gastroenterol Hepatol* 2006;4:262–275.

83. Green SE, Chapman PD, Burn J, Bishop DT, Varma JS. Clinical impact of colonoscopic screening in first-degree relatives of patients with hereditary non-polyposis colorectal cancer. *Br J Surg* 1995;82:1338–1340.

84. Cruz-Correa M, Giardiello FM. Diagnosis and management of hereditary colon cancer. *Gastroenterol Clin North Am* 2002;31:537–549.

85. Kiesslich R, Fritsch J, Holtmann M, et al. Methylene blue-aided chromoendoscopy for the detection of intraepithelial neoplasia and colon cancer in ulcerative colitis. *Gastroenterology* 2003;124:880–888.

86. Guillem JG, Forde KA, Treat MR, Neugut AI, O'Toole KM, Diamond BE. Colonoscopic screening for neoplasms in asymptomatic first-degree relatives of colon cancer patients. A controlled, prospective study. *Dis Colon Rectum* 1992;35:523–529.

87. Winawer SJ, Zauber AG, Fletcher RH, et al. Guidelines for colonoscopy surveillance after polypectomy: a consensus update by the US Multi-Society Task Force on Colorectal Cancer and the American Cancer Society. *CA Cancer J Clin* 2006;56:143–159; quiz 184–185.

88. Cobrin GM, Pittman RH, Lewis BS. Increased diagnostic yield of small bowel tumors with capsule endoscopy. *Cancer* 2006;107:22–27.

89. Mata A, Llach J, Castells A, et al. A prospective trial comparing wireless capsule endoscopy and barium contrast series for small-bowel surveillance in hereditary GI polyposis syndromes. *Gastrointest Endosc* 2005;61:721–725.

90. Canto MI, Goggins M, Hruban RH, et al. Screening for early pancreatic neoplasia in high-risk individuals: a prospective controlled study. *Clin Gastroenterol Hepatol* 2006;4:766–81; quiz 665.

91. Rasanen JV, Sihvo EIT, Knuuti MJ, et al. Prospective analysis of accuracy of positron emission tomography, computed tomography, and endoscopic ultrasonography in staging of adenocarcinoma of the esophagus and the esophagogastric junction. *Ann Surg Oncol* 2003;10:954–960.

92. Tsendsuren T, Jun SM, Mian XH. Usefulness of endoscopic ultrasonography in preoperative TNM staging of gastric cancer. *World J Gastroenterol* 2006;12:43–47.

93. Ganpathi IS, So JB, Ho KY. Endoscopic ultrasonography for gastric cancer: does it influence treatment? *Surg Endosc* 2006;20:559–562.

94. Mukai H, Nakajima M, Yasuda K, Mizuno S, Kawai K. Evaluation of endoscopic ultrasonography in the pre-operative staging of carcinoma of the ampulla of Vater and common bile duct. *Gastrointest Endosc* 1992;38:676–683.

95. Rosch T, Lorenz R, Zenker K, et al. Local staging and assessment of resectability in carcinoma of the esophagus, stomach, and duodenum by endoscopic ultrasonography. *Gastrointest Endosc* 1992;38:460–467.

96. Spinelli P, Schiavo M, Meroni E, et al. Results of EUS in detecting perirectal lymph node metastases of rectal cancer: the pathologist makes the difference. *Gastrointest Endosc* 1999;49:754–758.

97. Meyenberger C, Huch Boni RA, Bertschinger P, Zala GF, Klotz HP, Krestin GP. Endoscopic ultrasound and endorectal magnetic resonance imaging: a prospective, comparative study for preoperative staging and follow-up of rectal cancer. *Endoscopy* 1995;27:469–479.

98. Harewood GC, Wiersema MJ, Nelson H, et al. A prospective, blinded assessment of the impact of preoperative staging on the management of rectal cancer. *Gastroenterology* 2002;123:24–32.

99. Hünerbein M, Pegios W, Rau B, Vogl TJ, Felix R, Schlag PM. Prospective comparison of endorectal ultrasound, three-dimensional endorectal ultrasound, and endorectal MRI in the preoperative evaluation of rectal tumors. Preliminary results. *Surg Endosc* 2000;14(11):1005–1009.

100. Cannon ME, Carpenter SL, Elta GH, et al. EUS compared with CT, magnetic resonance imaging, and angiography and the influence of biliary stenting on staging accuracy of ampullary neoplasms. *Gastrointest Endosc* 1999;50:27–33.

101. Chang KJ, Nguyen P, Erickson RA, Durbin TE, Katz KD. The clinical utility of endoscopic ultrasound-guided fine-needle aspiration in the diagnosis and staging of pancreatic carcinoma. *Gastrointest Endosc* 1997;45:387–393.

102. Yasuda K, Mukai H, Nakajima M, Kawai K. Staging of pancreatic carcinoma by endoscopic ultrasonography. *Endoscopy* 1993;25:151–155.

CHAPTER 11 ■ AN OVERVIEW OF OUTCOMES RESEARCH IN GASTROINTESTINAL CANCER

HANNA K. SANOFF AND DEBORAH SCHRAG

INTRODUCTION TO OUTCOMES RESEARCH

Definition of Outcomes Research

Despite great progress in cancer therapeutics, cancer continues to place a tremendous burden on patients' physical, emotional, and financial health. Although better supportive care has made treatments more tolerable, the lives of patients and their families are still disrupted. In addition, many effective treatments never reach those in need. These aspects of cancer care lie outside the realm of most therapeutic clinical trials and thus have not been studied nearly as well as traditional clinical end points of efficacy. Outcomes research (OR) is a field of study that encompasses important aspects of cancer care that extend beyond traditional survival end points. Goals of OR are to fully characterize how cancer therapy impacts patients, assess the quality of care being delivered, determine why it is delivered in that manner, and include analyses of how health care is organized and delivered. Many OR investigations approach these questions from the patient's perspective, although OR also investigates cancer care from the perspective of other decision makers, including physicians, health care payers, and policy makers.

Types of Outcomes Research

Although some may argue about what technically falls under its rubric, OR typically uses patient-oriented end points, such as quality of life (QOL), long-term impact, patient preferences, or patient satisfaction as ways to evaluate delivered care. By comparison, cancer clinical trials classically use the more clear-cut measures of survival, diseasefree survival, and toxicity (Table 11.1) (1,2). Many studies can be defined as outcomes research, and therefore OR can be categorized along a number of dimensions. The four most common classifications are theme, end point, arena of application, and method (1,3). For example, clinical decision making and quality of care are two broad themes in OR. However, a single theme, such as quality of care, might be measured by the distinct end points of patient satisfaction, receipt of recommended care, or survival. Another classification scheme uses arenas of application to subdivide OR studies into the following: macrolevel analyses that examine population trends in end points such as QOL; mesolevel analyses that examine a diverse range of topics such as effec-tiveness, cancer impact, and care utilization; and microlevel analyses that focus on improving patient–physician decision making (3).

Finally, OR investigations may be categorized according to the method they employ. In some circumstances, OR is embedded alongside a traditional clinical trial; in this case, the methods are analogous to those used for trials designed with primary clinical end points. For example, a recent randomized clinical trial evaluating the efficacy of laparoscopic colectomy had patient survival as its primary outcome but included both QOL and cost effectiveness as secondary outcomes (4). Because OR is very concerned with understanding real world practice and how therapies delivered in the clinical trial setting translate into real world practice, outcomes researchers often rely on observational study designs. These studies are of most interest when they describe the experience of large segments of the population and when the experience of the studied segment is perceived to be relevant and generalizable to the population as a whole. The most notable example of this type of OR is secondary database analysis. These studies rely on resources such as the Surveillance, Epidemiology, and End Results (SEER) registries and administrative data from health insurance providers, including Medicare. These resources can be used to evaluate disparities of care and to characterize experience in real world settings. The drawback of these studies is that the lack of random assignment of therapies makes inferences about the effectiveness based on comparisons of treated and untreated persons extremely challenging. Another methodology, meta-analyses of clinical trials, which are predominantly used to answer therapeutic trial questions that are unanswerable by a smaller trial, are sometimes classified as OR. Health services research is a particular type of OR that typically focuses on health care delivery and organization outside the clinical trial setting.

Application of Outcomes Research

The concept of using patient-oriented outcomes to assess care dates back to the early 20th century when practitioners suggested that care should be measured not by the numbers of patients being treated, but by the impact of treatment on the health of patients (1). It was not until the 1990s, however, that OR gained traction and recognition as an important way to investigate cancer care. During this decade, the number of outcomes studies focused on cancer and cancer care has markedly increased, and systematic reviews show that this effort has

TABLE 11.1

OUTCOMES RESEARCH END POINTS AND DATA SOURCES

Traditional end points			Outcomes research end points	
Overall survival			Quality adjusted life-years	
Toxicity grade			Health-related quality of life	
Relapsefree survival			Preference	
Diseasefree survival			Satisfaction	

	Data source	Strength	Limitation	Example
SEER	Registry	■ 25% of U.S. cancer pts ■ Readily accessible	■ Minimal treatment info	Yancik et al. (12)
SEER- Medicare	Registry-claims	■ Treatment information available	■ Treatment defined by codes, may be missed ■ Does not reliably report drugs; no dose information ■ Only older than 65 years	Schrag et al. (10)
NCDB	Hospital reporting	■ 75% of new cancer cases	■ Minimal treatment info	Jessup et al. (34)
Clinical trials	Retrospective analysis of trials Prospective secondary end point	■ Randomized ■ Treatment well specified ■ Prospectively collected	■ May not be generalizable ■ Cannot assess care disparities ■ May be inadequately powered if not accounted for in study design	Meyerhardt et al. (14) Weeks et al. (4)

SEER, Surveillance, Epidemiology, and End Results; NCDB, National Cancer Data Base.

been largely led by investigators in the field of breast cancer (1). In gastrointestinal (GI) malignancy, the initial forays into OR methodology were undertaken by those studying colorectal cancer (CRC) screening, generally not practicing oncologists (5). These trends have begun to change, however, and outcomes methods—such as secondary analyses of large databases and the incorporation of QOL measures as secondary end points of clinical trials—are commonly used today. Mainstream oncology groups have begun to recognize the importance of this emerging field to the study of cancer. The American Cancer Society, the National Cancer Institute, and the American Society of Clinical Oncology, among others, have initiated OR teams or have integrated health services researchers into their organizations. Increasingly, there are dedicated research funds to support this type of research. Despite this gathering momentum, there are still large gaps in the application of outcomes methods to treatment of cancer, and specifically to GI malignancy.

This chapter provides an overview of OR by describing some representative typologies in CRC. It is not intended to be a comprehensive review, but rather this chapter is meant to convey why OR is valuable for a comprehensive understanding of cancer care. Because OR has been applied less frequently to noncolorectal GI cancers, CRC studies are highlighted for this purpose. However, this is unfortunate because gastroesophageal and pancreatic cancers are diseases for which treatments are both rigorous and inadequate. In such a setting, OR topics such as communication of patient preference, information exchange, and impact of treatment on QOL should all be integral components of the treatment process. Hopefully, subsequent editions of this text will comprise separate chapters describing the newer OR pertaining to each GI cancer.

OUTCOMES RESEARCH IN COLORECTAL CANCER

Patterns of Care/Access to Care: Database Analysis

Patterns of care and access to care studies both aim to assess what treatments cancer patients are actually receiving outside the realm of the clinical trial. In addition, they hope to uncover what factors predict the receipt of care. The primary methodology for this research question is secondary analysis of existing databases. These investigations allow for the identification of treatments or interventions that are not being used as recommended; in addition, because they are clinically annotated, they allow for the identification of groups—such as the elderly, the poor, and racial minorities—that are less likely to receive recommended care. However, although a study using a database may demonstrate an association between a clinical characteristic (e.g., black race) and an outcome (e.g., survival), such a study is unable to identify the cause of the outcome disparity. Thus, the associations that emerge from analyses of patient outcomes from large databases are generally used to generate hypotheses. These investigations identify target areas for further study and future interventions that might improve the quality of care for cancer patients.

Data Sources

Data sources that are available for study of the real world treatment and outcomes of cancer patients include the SEER program from the National Cancer Institute (NCI), the

SEER-Medicare database that includes the SEER program data linked to Medicare claims data, the National Cancer Data Base (NCDB) sponsored by the American College of Surgeons, and individual data sets from either large single or pooled clinical trials (Table 11.1).

SEER collects population-based information on cancer incidence and survival by identifying incident cancers through selected U.S. cancer registries. Currently, registries that participate in the SEER program represent 26% of the U.S. population (6). The SEER database includes patient demographics, cancer site, stage, histology, first course of treatment, and survival. The SEER program is particularly useful because it is updated frequently, contains a huge proportion of the U.S. population, and the demographics of the areas included in SEER are representative of the demographics of the entire United States (6). Use of the SEER database is limited, however, primarily because it only records information on the first treatment given at the time of cancer diagnosis. Therefore, for CRC patients, SEER captures radiotherapy that is given as part of the first course of treatment. Information regarding chemotherapy treatment in SEER is not considered reliable. This is because the SEER registries are largely hospital based and chemotherapy is typically administered in private office settings subsequent to hospital discharge.

The NCI and the Centers for Medicare and Medicaid Services have addressed this information deficit by linking the SEER registry with claims from Medicare. Through this effort, 93% of Medicare claims for persons older than 65 years have been matched to their SEER registry information (6,7). As the majority of Medicare recipients enroll in both Medicare part A (which covers hospitalizations) and Medicare part B (which covers outpatient departments and physicians' offices), this linkage offers investigators the opportunity to assess surgical, radiation, and chemotherapeutic treatments given for cancer, and markedly improves the utility of the SEER program for OR in cancer. In just a few years, hundreds of papers have been published relying on the SEER-Medicare linked data.

Maintained through a partnership with the American College of Surgeons and the American Cancer Society, the NCDB collects data on incident cancer cases from hospitals that voluntarily contribute to the database. The NCDB includes nearly 75% of all new cancer cases each year (8). Like SEER, the NCDB contains patient demographic information, primary tumor site, histology, and tumor stage, and only contains information about the first cancer treatment received.

Single or pooled clinical trial data can also be used to address questions about cancer care. Although these data do not accurately represent patterns of care or access to care in a routine clinical setting in the general population, trial data do allow differences in outcomes among patient subsets to be addressed because stratification by prognostic factor (e.g., tumor stage) and the randomization process should make prognostic factors, treatments, and other confounding factors equal.

Examples of Database Analyses: Age and Adjuvant Therapy for Stage III Colon Cancer

Adjuvant therapy for stage III colon cancer has been the standard of care since the release of the National Institutes of Health consensus statement in 1990 (9). However, because dissemination of new information often takes time, practice may not always conform to the recommended standard. In addition, other barriers to care—such as distance to travel for treatment, comorbid illness, and physician bias—may result in some groups being less likely to receive treatment that is concordant with consensus opinion.

In a 2001 report, Schrag et al. used the SEER-Medicare linkage to address whether the age at diagnosis of colon cancer is related to the use of adjuvant chemotherapy (10). Their investigation included 6,262 patients older than 65 years enrolled in Medicare parts A and B in the SEER database. All patients had stage III colon cancer and had been operated on for their cancer within 3 months of diagnosis. Patients were considered to have received adjuvant chemotherapy if they were treated with chemotherapy within 3 months of their surgery.

In this study, advanced age was significantly associated with decreased use of chemotherapy. Overall, 55% of the cohort received adjuvant treatment. When stratified by age, however, disparities in treatment use emerged clearly: 11% of 85- to 89-year-olds received adjuvant therapy, as opposed to 34% of 80- to 84-year-olds, 58% of 75- to 79-year-olds, 74% of 70- to 74-year-olds, and 78% of 65- to 69-year-olds (10). Although race, gender, income, and the number of positive lymph nodes were also associated with the use of adjuvant therapy, these factors did not predict the use of chemotherapy as strongly as age. Furthermore, the decline in therapy with increasing age persisted even in patients without comorbidity. Based on these results, the authors were able to conclude that chemotherapy use clearly declines with age and that there are likely nonmedical reasons for this decline. Although the reasons underlying this variation were unknown, Schrag et al. were able to identify an important area for future research. Subsequently, an indepth study has been launched by the NCI to help understand the cause for disparities or variations in cancer care. The Cancer Care Outcomes Research and Surveillance Consortium has undertaken an observational study that uses patient surveys, physician surveys, and medical record data to identify clinically important differences in treatment and outcomes in lung and CRC patients, and to uncover causes for these differences (11).

Examples of Data Set Analyses Using Existing Clinical Trial Data: Impact of Diabetes on Adjuvant Colon Cancer Therapy

Although the immediate health effects of diabetes mellitus have been widely documented, prior investigations have also shown that diabetes is associated with diminished survival in CRC patients (12,13). However, because these studies were limited in their ability to control for potentially significant prognostic information such as treatment, results were potentially confounded by treatment differences between diabetics and nondiabetics rather than the presence of comorbid disease. To overcome this limitation, Meyerhardt et al. used patient data from the GI Intergroup trial 0089, a four-arm trial of adjuvant therapy in stage II and III colon cancer that enrolled nearly 3,550 patients (14,15). Because study participants received uniform surgical care and adjuvant chemotherapy (all arms of this trial were equivalent), the investigators were able to assess stage- and treatment-independent predictors of outcome.

Eight percent of all patients enrolled on INT 0089 were diabetic (14). Consistent with prior investigations, study participants with diabetes were more likely to suffer relapse or death than those without diabetes. Five-year survival of nondiabetics was 66%, compared with 57% for diabetics, indicating an adjusted hazard of death of 1.42 for diabetics. Diseasefree survival was similarly decreased in diabetics, with only 48% of diabetics surviving without cancer recurrence compared to 59% of nondiabetics. Interestingly, although diabetics did not suffer an overall increase in the risk of severe or life-threatening toxicities, they did have a moderate increase in the risk of severe treatment-related diarrhea; 29% of diabetics experienced grade 3 or 4 diarrhea compared with 20% of nondiabetics. This side effect did not explain differences in survival.

Both studies augment the understanding of existing treatment patterns and important considerations in the care of colon cancer patients. Because healthy elders seem to benefit equally from adjuvant therapy as their younger counterparts (15–17), a better understanding of the discrepancy in chemotherapy use in elders should be sought, especially as the U.S. population ages. Because diabetes affects approximately 7% of the adult population (18), further inquiry into poor outcomes for diabetics with cancer is important for reasons of public health and perhaps the biology of CRC.

Quality of Care

In 1999, the Institute of Medicine's National Cancer Policy Board reported that some individuals were receiving substandard care for their cancer and thus charged cancer researchers with finding new ways to measure and monitor the quality of cancer care over time (19). Cancer investigators have responded by assessing quality in three main ways that address its various aspects. The first way is comparing actual care in the population to the standard of care documented by organizations such as the National Comprehensive Cancer Network and by medical journals. A second way is to look at patient determinants of quality, such as satisfaction. A third way is to compare patient outcomes, such as overall survival, across various settings.

Examples of Quality of Care Studies: Hospital Volume and Patient Outcomes

To assess the quality of care for colon cancer surgery, Schrag et al. used the SEER-Medicare linkage to determine whether hospital procedure volume (the number of colon cancer surgeries performed) predicts survival following initial surgery for colon cancer (20). The study examined differences in the outcomes of 30-day survival, overall survival, and colon cancer–specific survival between Medicare-enrolled patients in the SEER database operated on at high or low volume centers. Hospital volume was determined by the number of surgeries performed between 1991 and 1996, and then split into quartiles of low (1–57), medium (58–112), high (113–165), and very high (166–383). The investigators found that 30-day postoperative mortality increased with decreasing volume of operation; however, the

absolute difference in survival between the very high-volume and low-volume hospitals, 2%, was small. Overall mortality was also increased with decreasing center volume. There was a 4.4% absolute difference in mortality at 5 years between low-volume and very high-volume centers. The association between hospital volume and both short- and long-term mortality was most pronounced in those with stage III cancers, even when adjusted for adjuvant chemotherapy use, and translated into substantial difference (62.5% mortality in low-volume hospitals and 56% in high-volume centers) in mortality at 5 years. A number of patient characteristics predicted surgery at a low-volume center, including nonwhite race and low socioeconomic status.

Given the potential of regionalization to improve outcomes, the authors asked what effect rerouting patients from low-volume to very high-volume hospitals would have on mortality. Of approximately 70,000 cases of CRC diagnosed each year, they found that 770 deaths at 5 years could be avoided by diverting patients from low-volume to high-volume hospitals. However, this would require shifting a large number of patients to different hospitals—a feat that may or may not be feasible for patients or hospitals outside urban areas.

Examples of Quality of Care Studies: Proportion Receiving Recommended Care

Another way that investigators assess the quality of cancer care is by comparing the actual treatment received to the established standard of care. Such studies aim not only to define the proportion of patients receiving suboptimal care but also to identify patient subgroups or types of treatments associated with the most pronounced disparities in quality. In February 2006, Malin et al. reported the findings of the 1998 National Initiative for Cancer Care Quality study on quality of care (11), which included patients diagnosed with stages I to III breast cancer and stage II or III CRC approximately 4 years after their original diagnosis. Using existing guidelines, reviews, and expert opinion, the investigators identified 25 management items that they considered essential to high-quality care (Table 11.2). These items were all eligibility specific; for example, only stage II and III rectal cancer patients were assessed for referral to a radiation oncologist. Actual patient care, as determined by

---

TABLE 11.2

MEASURING QUALITY

Examples of required elements	Scoring domains	
	Care domains	Components of care
Referrals If a patient has stage II or III rectal cancer, *then* the patient should have a consultation with a radiation oncologist.	■ Diagnostic evaluation ■ Surgery ■ Adjuvant therapy ■ Management of toxicity ■ Posttreatment surveillance	■ Testing ■ Pathology ■ Documentation of key clinical factors ■ Referral ■ Receipt of treatment ■ Technical quality of treatment ■ Respect for patient preferences ■ Timing
Systemic adjuvant therapy If a patient is treated with chemotherapy, *then* the planned dose should fall within a range that is consistent with published regimens.		

Examples from ref. 11.

chart review, was compared to these 25 quality measures. The investigators calculated a mean percent adherence to quality measures in the following care domains: diagnostic evaluation, surgery, adjuvant therapy, management of treatment toxicity, and posttreatment surveillance. In addition, they determined the adherence to a number of components of care (Table 11.2).

The quality analysis was based on the records of 478 CRC patients identified through hospital databases in five metropolitan areas: Atlanta; Cleveland; Houston; Kansas City, KS; and Los Angeles. Based on thorough chart reviews, CRC patients received 78% of recommended care. Actual care best approximated recommended care for surgical therapies, with 93% of required items met. The least compliant with recommended care, with 64% and 50% of cases complying respectively, were adjuvant therapy and posttreatment surveillance. Additional breakdown into the specific components of care identified timing of care (57% compliance) and referral (59% compliance) as areas for which actual care most diverged from recommended care. Promisingly, these results indicate that the majority of patients do, in fact, receive care that is consistent with recommended guidelines. As noted by the authors, 27% of potentially eligible patients had died at the time of this study; these patients may have received lower quality care, and thus, their exclusion might have biased the results in favor of good quality care.

Both quality-of-care investigations suggest that the majority of patients appeared to be receiving good CRC care; however, they also highlight the fact that minorities and patients with lower socioeconomic status may be at elevated risk of inferior medical treatment. In addition, despite the good compliance with CRC treatments overall, low compliance in adjuvant therapies (64%) suggests that necessary improvements remain.

Quality of Life

QOL has become one of the most widely adopted themes of the OR movement in cancer (21). It is an end point that can be tangibly applied to the treatment of cancer patients. Because a good QOL scale combines efficacy (tumor symptoms) with measures of the effect of cancer treatment on the life of the patient (social, emotional, and physical function) into a gestalt measure of impact of both treatment and cancer on an individual (1), a QOL scale can be used as a means to select or reject a treatment.

QOL measures are most commonly used as secondary end points in therapeutic clinical trials. In some cases, however, QOL is used as a primary outcome measure. For example, QOL was the primary end point of a study of cancer survivors identified through the National Health Interview Survey, which showed that cancer survivors have a more impaired QOL and decreased productivity versus their cancerfree peers (22).

Example of Quality of Life Study: Laparoscopic versus Open Colectomy for Colon Cancer

The Clinical Outcomes of Surgical Therapy (COST) trial (4), a multigroup collaboration led by the North Central Cancer Treatment Group, was designed to test whether diseasefree survival and overall survival are equivalent in CRC patients randomly assigned to treatment with laparoscopic colectomy (LAC) or open colectomy. Because the benefit of LAC in the postoperative period must be weighed against the risk of a compromised oncologic outcome that might result from adopting LAC for colon cancer, the investigators designed COST so it could also measure whether patients treated with LAC had superior QOL.

The a priori QOL areas of interest included the composite score of the QOL Index, a global QOL score, and the pain

distress item from the Symptoms Distress Scale; differences in these outcomes were based on responses from 213 patients assigned to open colectomy and 215 patients assigned to LAC. Consistent with prior studies that suggest patients recover more quickly after laparoscopic surgery than open procedures (23), LAC patients used oral and parenteral analgesic therapy for 0.3 fewer days and left the hospital 0.8 days sooner. Although these clinical proxies suggest LAC is easier on patients, there was essentially no difference between the pain distress, QOL Index, or global QOL scores between study groups at any time during the 2 months of follow-up. The ostensible conflict between comparable patient-reported symptom or QOL scores and the clear benefits of LAC may be explained by the more rigorous methods used to assess symptoms and QOL. The authors concluded that until further results are available, LAC should only be performed in the setting of a clinical trial.

The COST trial is an example of how adding rigorous QOL end points to clinical trials can help select therapy. Based on these results that refute that LAC is easier on patients, open colectomy would have to prove an inferior cancer operation for LAC to be accepted as the standard of care.

Clinical Decision Making and Patient Preferences

Studies of decision making and patient preference aim to improve care by helping patients select therapies that are concordant with both their life goals and individual clinical situation. Studies of clinical decision making assess the adequacy of information exchange and patient–physician communication (24). Investigations of patient preferences ask patients what they want and to what degrees these wants are met in actual practice. Fulfilling decision-making needs and patient preferences requires good patient–physician communication, with the result that certain patient subgroups—particularly the elderly, minorities, or nonnative English speakers—may be at greater risk for receiving treatment that does not reflect their preferences. Because groups with compromised communication abilities are also less likely to receive aggressive therapies and more likely to die of their cancer (10,25,26), it is critical to understand what causes underlie these variations. Once the causes of discrepant care are understood, interventions can be directed to correct these factors and thereby all groups can be provided an equal chance for optimal treatment.

Example of Clinical Decision-Making Study: Decisions in Advanced Cancer Patients

To better understand the treatment decisions made by patients with incurable malignancies, investigators from Australia asked to what degree patients with advanced cancer were enabled by their physician to make an informed decision about their care (27). To answer this question, they enrolled 118 patients with advanced cancer who were eligible for palliative therapy and also being seen in consultation at an outpatient tertiary care oncology clinic. To analyze the decision-making process, the consultation was audiotaped, and transcripts were analyzed with attention to (a) information disclosure as measured by seven elements (Table 11.3) and (b) physician encouragement to participate in the decision as measured by five elements. Just prior to their doctor visit, participants were administered a questionnaire that included questions regarding their anxiety about the decision, preferences for emotional support, preferences for information exchange, and preferred level of involvement in decision making. Immediately after the visit, they were again asked about their anxiety. Seven days later, telephone interviews were used to assess patient recall. A follow-up interview was administered 14 days after the consultation.

TABLE 11.3

ASSESSING INFORMED DECISION MAKING

Information disclosure elements	Encouragement to participate elements
■ Effect of treatment on tumor ■ Aim of treatment ■ Disease is incurable ■ Drawbacks of treatment ■ Information about life expectancy ■ Treatment alternatives ■ Effect of treatment on quality of life	■ Acknowledges uncertainty that treatment will achieve aim ■ Elicits patient values ■ Acknowledges trade-offs ■ Offers treatment choice ■ Checks patient's understanding

Examples from ref. 27.

TABLE 11.4

MEASURING PATIENT PERCEPTIONS OF CARE

Domains of care	Examples of elements within domains
■ Coordination of care ■ Confidence in providers ■ Treatment information ■ Health information ■ Access to cancer care ■ Psychosocial care ■ Symptom control	**Coordination of care** How often were your providers aware of changes in your treatment that other providers recommended? **Treatment information** Were you given as much information as you wanted or needed about the treatment options for treating your cancer?

Examples from ref. 28.

In this interview, patients were queried with regard to their anxiety about their decision, satisfaction with the consultation, and perceived level of involvement in the decision-making process.

Based on review of the transcripts, most consultations provided patients with adequate information on important elements, including the fatal nature of their cancer, the goal of treatment, how treatment would act on the tumor, and the adverse effects or other drawbacks to therapy. Unfortunately, information exchange was not uniformly good. Only 44% of patients were presented with an alternative to anticancer treatment such as best supportive care, and only 36% were presented with information about the impact of treatment on QOL. The degree to which physicians encouraged the patients to participate in treatment decisions was also poor. Doctors presented alternatives to their patients just 30% of the time, and only confirmed that the patient understood the information 10% of the time.

Patients were more likely to be encouraged to participate in the decision-making process if they had metastatic disease at presentation (rather than recurrent disease), were younger, asked more questions, and consulted with a medical oncologist rather than a radiation oncologist. Neither information disclosure nor doctor encouragement to participate in the decision predicted a patient's perception of his or her involvement in the decision. Interestingly, encouragement to participate (not the degree of information provided) was predictive of a patient's 7-day information recall; however, patients who received greater encouragement to participate in the decision making also reported more anxiety. Although information disclosure did not predict recall, anxiety increased in patients who received less information. The results of this study clearly demonstrate that patient encouragement to participate and information exchange both impact cancer patients' understanding of their disease and their resulting anxiety.

Example of Patient Preferences Study: Patient Perceptions of Care

To study racial differences in care, Ayanian et al. examined racial and ethnic differences in the areas of cancer care that patients had identified as inadequate (28). They identified a racially and ethnically diverse cohort of CRC patients through the California Cancer Registry. The cohort of 1,067 patients, all within 4 months of a CRC diagnosis, were administered a survey that asked about their experiences with cancer care (Table 11.4), their health-related QOL, their comorbid illnesses, and their sociodemographic characteristics.

As demonstrated by the survey responses, access to information, psychosocial support, and coordination of care are the domains of care that cancer patients believe are most problematic. Compared with whites, minorities and non-English speakers reported greater difficulty in accessing all aspects of care. However, coordination of care and access to information were the most problematic domains for minorities compared to whites. In addition, African American respondents reported greater problems with access to psychosocial care. The proportion of respondents who rated their cancer care as excellent or very good was significantly influenced by race, with 82% of whites, 74% of African Americans, 61% of Asian/Pacific Islanders, and 67% of Hispanics reporting that they received excellent or very good care. Language had the most profound impact on patients' perception of their care, with 81% of all who spoke English at home reporting their care to be excellent or very good compared with only 52% who spoke a language other than English at home.

Patient perceptions of the quality of their cancer care clearly demonstrate that at least part of the racial discrepancy in the quality of cancer care may be related to communication, both between patient and physician and between physicians of different subspecialties. Communication interventions should focus on improving the discourse between the physician and non-white patient, in addition to addressing language barriers.

The results of these two very different studies of decision making and patient preferences support the notion that an area for quality improvement is patient–physician communication.

Cost-Effectiveness Analysis

Now that five effective drugs are available for CRC, the median survival of patients with metastatic CRC has nearly doubled from 10 to 12 months in the early 1990s with 5-FU and leucovorin, to approximately 21 months with irinotecan, oxaliplatin, and 5-FU (29); furthermore, the risk of cancer recurrence in the adjuvant setting has decreased by nearly 25% (30). Unfortunately, the financial cost of this progress is staggering: Two months of the common frontline palliative regimen of FOLFOX and bevacizumab costs 340 times more than 2 months of the Mayo Clinic bolus 5-FU/LV regimen (31).

One way to address the cost of emerging therapies is to measure the cost effectiveness of the new therapy compared to the standard to care. Cost-effectiveness analyses incorporate both clinical outcomes and cost into one measure so the overall value of a new treatment relative to an old one can be assessed (32). This can be done in a retrospective fashion by assigning costs to the known potential outcomes derived from clinical trials (e.g., cost of admission for neutropenic fever or cost of second-line chemotherapy at disease recurrence), and then creating a model that compares the cost of the new therapy, based on the chance of each clinical outcome, with the cost of the old therapy, based on the chance of each clinical outcome. Using these retrospective modeling techniques, Hillner et al. analyzed the cost of first-line FOLFOX compared with IFL for metastatic disease using data from the North Central Cancer Treatment Group trial N9741 (33). Based on their results, switching from first-line IFL to FOLFOX costs $111,000 per quality adjusted life-year.

Another approach to assessing the cost of new therapies is to prospectively incorporate cost end points into clinical trials. For example, the Cancer and Leukemia Group B 80405, which compares FOLFOX or FOLFIRI with bevacizumab, cetuximab, or both in untreated metastatic CRC, includes a prospective assessment of cost. Hopefully, this will become a more common practice as more effective drugs emerge, so that cost–benefit discussions can occur concurrently with risk–benefit discussions.

An additional cost that may be overlooked in the discussion of the cost of emerging therapies is the cost to the patient. Patients may suffer financially from direct treatment costs; however, the indirect effect from lost days of work for the patient and his or her family, as well as the loss of potential future employment, may also have a significant impact on the financial well-being of those treated for cancer. Patient costs have not been well studied, although they may often be a critical component of the effect of cancer treatment on many.

SUMMARY

OR encompasses a broad range of research topics. These topics are related largely through their mutual aim of improving the quality of patient care by documenting the care that patients actually receive and how this care impacts life from the patient's perspective. Breast cancer researchers have led the way in cancer OR, with more studies using outcomes end points devoted to breast cancer than any other malignancy (1). Although outcomes end points are increasingly incorporated into CRC treatment trials, outcomes studies of screening modalities still outpace treatment trials (5). When funding sources are limited, OR-related objectives are typically the first place that clinical trial budgets are trimmed. Increasing reliance on wireless and web-based tools for collecting information directly from patients may help ensure that the complement of information about the patient experience is obtained without sacrificing efficiency or the ability to perform important studies in a timely fashion. Many OR themes, including patient preferences, decision making, and cost effectiveness, have not been well explored in CRC. Furthermore, outcomes end points have rarely been applied to the study of end-of-life care and noncolorectal GI cancers.

Going forward, it is hoped that OR will become an integral part of the investigation of emerging therapies. Ideally, analyses of these questions will contribute to the patient experience and the overall quality of care. Although OR will not cure cancer, by shortening cancer's reach, it can nevertheless improve lives.

References

1. Lee SJ, Earle CC, Weeks JC. Outcomes research in oncology: history, conceptual framework, and trends in the literature. *J Natl Cancer Inst* 2000; 92(3):195–204.
2. Lipscomb J, Donaldson MS, Hiatt RA. Cancer outcomes research and the arenas of application. *J Natl Cancer Inst Monogr* 2004(33):1–7.
3. Lipscomb J, Donaldson MS, Arora NK, et al. Cancer outcomes research. *J Natl Cancer Inst Monogr* 2004(33):178–197.
4. Weeks JC, Nelson H, Gelber S, Sargent D, Schroeder G. Short-term quality-of-life outcomes following laparoscopic-assisted colectomy vs open colectomy for colon cancer: a randomized trial. *JAMA* 2002;287(3):321–328.
5. Provenzale D, Gray RN. Colorectal cancer screening and treatment: review of outcomes research. *J Natl Cancer Inst Monogr* 2004(33):45–55.
6. National Cancer Institute. Overview of the SEER program. Available at http://seer.cancer.gov/about/. Accessed March 6, 2007.
7. Potosky AL, Riley GF, Lubitz JD, Mentnech RM, Kessler LG. Potential for cancer related health services research using a linked Medicare-tumor registry database. *Med Care* 1993;31(8):732–748.
8. American College of Surgeons. National Cancer Database. Available at http://www.facs.org/cancer/ncdb/. Accessed March 6, 2007.
9. NIH consensus conference. Adjuvant therapy for patients with colon and rectal cancer. *JAMA* 1990;264(11):1444–1450.
10. Schrag D, Cramer LD, Bach PB, Begg CB. Age and adjuvant chemotherapy use after surgery for stage III colon cancer. *J Natl Cancer Inst* 2001;93(11): 850–857.
11. Malin JL, Schneider EC, Epstein AM, et al. Results of the National Initiative for Cancer Care Quality: how can we improve the quality of cancer care in the United States? *J Clin Oncol* 2006;24(4):626–634.
12. Yancik R, Wesley MN, Ries LA, et al. Comorbidity and age as predictors of risk for early mortality of male and female colon carcinoma patients: a population-based study. *Cancer* 1998;82(11):2123–2134.
13. Payne JE, Meyer HJ. The influence of other diseases upon the outcome of colorectal cancer patients. *Aust N Z J Surg* 1995;65(6):398–402.
14. Meyerhardt JA, Catalano PJ, Haller DG, et al. Impact of diabetes mellitus on outcomes in patients with colon cancer. *J Clin Oncol* 2003;21(3):433–440.
15. Sargent DJ, Goldberg RM, Jacobson SD, et al. A pooled analysis of adjuvant chemotherapy for resected colon cancer in elderly patients. *N Engl J Med* 2001;345(15):1091–1097.
16. Goldberg RM, Sargent DJ, Bleiberg H, et al. A pooled safety and efficacy analysis of the FOLFOX4 regimen (bi-monthly oxaliplatin plus fluorouracil/leucovorin) in elderly compared to younger patients with colorectal cancer. Abstract 228. *GI Cancers Symposium* 2006:199.
17. Folprecht G, Cunningham D, Ross P, et al. Efficacy of 5-fluorouracil-based chemotherapy in elderly patients with metastatic colorectal cancer: a pooled analysis of clinical trials. *Ann Oncol* 2004;15(9):1330–1338.
18. National Institute of Diabetes and Digestive and Kidney Diseases. National diabetes statistics. Available at http://diabetes.niddk.nih.gov/dm/pubs/statistics/. Accessed March 6, 2007.
19. Hewitt M, Simone J. *National Cancer Policy Board, Institute of Medicine: Ensuring Quality Cancer Care.* Washington, DC: National Academy Press; 1999.
20. Schrag D, Cramer LD, Bach PB, Cohen AM, Warren JL, Begg CB. Influence of hospital procedure volume on outcomes following surgery for colon cancer. *JAMA* 2000;284(23):3028–3035.
21. Gotay CC, Lipscomb J, Snyder CF. Reflections on findings of the Cancer Outcomes Measurement Working Group: moving to the next phase. *J Natl Cancer Inst* 2005;97(21):1568–1574.
22. Yabroff KR, Lawrence WF, Clauser S, Davis WW, Brown ML. Burden of illness in cancer survivors: findings from a population-based national sample. *J Natl Cancer Inst* 2004;96(17):1322–1330.
23. Schwenk W, Hasse O, Neudecker J, Muller J. Short term benefits for laparoscopic colorectal resection. *Cochran Database Syst Rev* 2005;2. Art No. CD003145.
24. Charles C, Gafni A, Whelan T. Shared decision-making in the medical encounter: what does it mean? (or it takes at least two to tango). *Soc Sci Med* 1997;44(5):681–692.
25. Shavers VL, Brown ML. Racial and ethnic disparities in the receipt of cancer treatment. *J Natl Cancer Inst* 2002;94(5):334–357.
26. Hodgson DC, Fuchs CS, Ayanian JZ. Impact of patient and provider characteristics on the treatment and outcomes of colorectal cancer. *J Natl Cancer Inst* 2001;93(7):501–515.
27. Gattellari M, Voigt KJ, Butow PN, Tattersall MH. When the treatment goal is not cure: are cancer patients equipped to make informed decisions? *J Clin Oncol* 2002;20(2):503–513.
28. Ayanian JZ, Zaslavsky AM, Guadagnoli E, et al. Patients' perceptions of quality of care for colorectal cancer by race, ethnicity, and language. *J Clin Oncol* 2005;23(27):6576–6586.
29. Grothey A, Sargent D, Goldberg RM, Schmoll HJ. Survival of patients with advanced colorectal cancer improves with the availability of fluorouracil-leucovorin, irinotecan, and oxaliplatin in the course of treatment. *J Clin Oncol* 2004;22(7):1209–1214.

30. Andre T, Boni C, Mounedji-Boudiaf L, et al. Oxaliplatin, fluorouracil, and leucovorin as adjuvant treatment for colon cancer. *N Engl J Med* 2004; 350(23):2343–2351.

31. Schrag D. The price tag on progress—chemotherapy for colorectal cancer. *N Engl J Med* 2004;351(4):317–319.

32. Russell LB, Gold MR, Siegel JE, Daniels N, Weinstein MC. The role of cost-effectiveness analysis in health and medicine. Panel on Cost-Effectiveness in Health and Medicine. *JAMA* 1996;276(14):1172–1177.

33. Hillner BE, Schrag D, Sargent DJ, Fuchs CS, Goldberg RM. Cost-effectiveness projections of oxaliplatin and infusional fluorouracil versus irinotecan and bolus fluorouracil in first-line therapy for metastatic colorectal carcinoma. *Cancer* 2005;104(9):1871–1884.

34. Jessup JM, Stewart A, Greene FL, Minsky BD. Adjuvant chemotherapy for stage III colon cancer: implications of race/ethnicity, age, and differentiation. *JAMA* 2005;294(21):2703–2711.

CHAPTER 12 ■ INTEGRATIVE ONCOLOGY: COMPLEMENTARY THERAPIES IN GASTROINTESTINAL CANCER CARE

BARRIE R. CASSILETH AND GARY DENG

INTRODUCTION

Until more recently, unconventional cancer therapies were typically underground or available outside the United States, their proponents claiming benefits beyond anything that mainstream medicine could offer. Such claims still accompany many contemporary methods, but today the field of unconventional cancer therapies, no longer underground, is crowded with openly promoted, widely available alternative products and regimens.

At the same time, harsh therapies cured increasing numbers of patients, while producing serious and often lasting side effects. The use of adjunctive complementary therapies expanded to meet cancer patients' needs for better symptom control during treatment and as survivors. Helpful interventions such as massage therapies, relaxation and other mind-body interventions, acupuncture, music therapy, yoga, fitness programs, and so on escalated.

Because both alternative and complementary therapies developed primarily outside mainstream cancer care, they were linguistically merged as *unconventional, alternative, complementary*, or *complementary and alternative medicine (CAM)*. This unfortunate linking created a confusing collection of unrelated remedies, all known by the same terms.

This chapter defines and describes the current status of complementary therapies in cancer care and distinguishes it from alternative practices. It also delineates mainstream acceptance, concerns, and regulatory issues, and discusses the implications of the health care trend represented by this growth industry. Recommended complementary therapies and potentially dangerous regimens also are listed.

TERMINOLOGY AND DEFINITIONS

The National Institutes of Health (NIH), National Center for Complementary and Alternative Medicine (NCCAM) and the National Cancer Institute (NCI) Office of Cancer Complementary and Alternative Medicine (OCCAM) support research in this area. *CAM* is defined by NCCAM as a group of diverse medical and health care systems, practices, and products that are not part of conventional medicine. An advantage of the phrase *complementary and alternative* is that it enables important distinctions between the two. *Alternative therapies* may be perceived literally as such; they are promoted as cancer treatments to be used instead of mainstream therapy. *Complemen-tary therapies*, in contrast, are used to manage symptoms and to enhance quality of life as adjuncts to mainstream care. Increasingly, the term "integrative oncology" is applied, especially in academic settings, thus emphasizing the adjunctive utility of complementary modalities.

Alternative regimens remain big business. These are unproved or disproved bogus therapies, typically promoted as independent treatments for use instead of surgery, chemotherapy, and radiation. They are usually invasive, biologically active, expensive, and potentially harmful. Alternative regimens may harm directly through biological activity or indirectly when patients postpone receipt of mainstream care. Examples of alternative therapies include the metabolic therapies available in Tijuana, Mexico, and elsewhere; shark cartilage; high-dose vitamins and other products sold over the counter and delivered intravenously in alternative clinics; electromagnetic cures; energy healing; "dietary cures"; and many other products and regimens.

Conversely, complementary therapies are used as part of supportive care to help reduce symptoms related to cancer or cancer treatment. They do not have clinically significant effects on cancer per se. Their evidence-based benefits lie in symptom control and enhancing quality of life with noninvasive, pleasant interventions desired and appreciated by patients. They are associated with few adverse events and have substantial appeal for many cancer patients.

IMPACT OF COMPLEMENTARY THERAPIES ON THE HEALTH CARE SYSTEM

The popularity of complementary therapies has affected every component of the health care system and all specialties of medicine, including oncology. It left its mark on the thinking and practice of physicians and other health professionals, and, importantly, broadened patients' involvement and influence in their own care.

We use the acronym "CAM" in the following review of related surveys because investigators have typically failed to distinguish between these two qualitatively different categories. A recent report presented the most comprehensive and reliable findings to date on Americans' use of CAM in general. The National Center for Health Statistics' 2002 National Health Interview Survey of 31,044 adults found that 75% used some form of CAM (1). When prayer specifically for health reasons was excluded, the percentage was 50%. As found in virtually all previous surveys, CAM use was most common among women, better educated people, those hospitalized in the previous year, and former smokers, indicating a more health-conscious segment of the population.

In cancer patients, CAM use is highly prevalent, according to scores of surveys from North America, going back to a systematic review in 1998 (2) and before then to 1984 (3), when different terminology applied. The prevalence of CAM use ranges from 15% to more than 70%. This wide range is explained by varying or absent definitions of "complementary therapies," "alternative medicine," or the "CAM" umbrella term. Recent large-scale surveys from Europe (4) and Japan (5) showed similar results. Another consistent finding in cancer patient surveys is that users are typically younger, more educated, and more affluent, a function of these patients' desires and ability to play an active role in their own care. Patients get most of their CAM information not from their physicians, but rather, for better or worse, from sources more knowledgeable about these therapies.

CAM today is very much an open and public issue, discussed widely in the media and readily found on the Internet. Magazines and television specials provide the general public with details about new therapies. The yellow pages of telephone books in most cities and towns list various types of CAM practitioners.

Information available to the public varies widely in accuracy. Many Web sites and publications that appear to be objective are actually sponsored by commercial enterprises that promote and sell the products they report. Misinformation about health issues is widespread. In 1999, the U.S. Federal Trade Commission announced that it had identified hundreds of Web sites promoting and selling phony cures for cancer and other serious ailments among the estimated 15,000 to 17,000 health-related Web sites. A Google search of "alternative cancer therapy" in February 2006 yielded 23 million Web pages, whereas the same search in 2004 produced only 8 million Web pages. It is likely that those selling bogus treatments have increased accordingly.

MAINSTREAM ACCEPTANCE OF COMPLEMENTARY AND ALTERNATIVE MEDICINE

A survey of 295 family physicians in the Maryland-Virginia region (6) revealed that up to 90% view complementary therapies such as diet and exercise, behavioral medicine, and hypnotherapy as legitimate medical practices. The majority refers patients to nonphysicians for these therapies or provides the services themselves. Homeopathy, Native American medicine, and traditional Oriental medicine were not seen as legitimate practices.

Two hundred Canadian general practitioners held similar views, noting their patients' particular interest in chiropractic medicine. These physicians perceive chiropractic care, hypnosis, and acupuncture for chronic pain as the most effective CAM therapies, and homeopathy and reflexology as less efficacious (7). A meta-analysis of 12 studies in Great Britain suggests that British physicians view complementary medicine as only moderately effective (8), a level of enthusiasm that contrasts with the fervent efforts of the British Royal Family to promote homeopathy and other complementary therapies, and to merge them with mainstream care.

In addition to increasing coverage of CAM services by health insurers, a final marker of mainstream interest noted here is the publication of CAM research articles in major mainstream medical journals. Articles in major journals shifted from commentaries through the 1970s expressing realistic concern about quackery, to surveys of patients' knowledge and use of unproven methods in the 1980s, and to reports of actual research results starting primarily in the mid-1990s.

The *Journal of the American Medical Association*, the *New England Journal of Medicine*, *The Lancet*, the *British Medical Journal*, and specialty journals such as *Cancer* and the *Journal of Clinical Oncology* have published reports of research on complementary therapies in recent years. In 1996 and 1997, the National Library of Medicine added many new CAM search terms to its medical subject headings and began to cover alternative medicine journals previously not reviewed for inclusion in Medline. In large part, mainstream science opposition is being replaced by emphasis on the importance of methodologically sound research, which now increasingly occurs in numerous respected institutions around the world. Integrative oncology has become an informal subspecialty of oncology and is increasingly the focus of good quality scientific research.

Activity of the National Institutes of Health

An Office of Alternative Medicine was established at the NIH by congressional mandate in 1992. In 1998, the U.S. Congress elevated the Office of Alternative Medicine to the NCCAM, appropriating $50 million for its support. Its budget steadily grew to $120 million in fiscal year 2006.

Although recognizing overlap, NCCAM groups CAM therapies into four domains: biologically based practices, mind-body medicine, manipulative and body-based practices, and energy medicine. In addition, whole medical systems cut across all domains. Traditional Chinese medicine, for example, includes biologically active botanicals, mind-body practices, manipulative techniques, and acupuncture.

Within the NCI, the OCCAM was established in 1998. Its role is to coordinate and enhance activities of the NCI in CAM research on prevention, diagnosis, and treatment of cancer, cancer-related symptoms, and side effects of conventional cancer treatment. Since OCCAM's creation, the NCI's expenditure in related research more than quadrupled from $28 million in 1998 to $129 million in 2004. The research portfolio includes more than 400 projects in the form of grants, cooperative agreements, supplements, or contracts.

Medical Schools and Medical Centers

Another marker of mainstream interest is the emergence of medical school courses in CAM. Elective courses in CAM and portions of required courses were taught in 75 medical schools in the United States in 1997 (9), and the number has increased since then (10). Numerous hospitals and medical centers have developed research and clinical service programs in CAM. Cancer programs, as well as many comprehensive cancer centers, have implemented or are creating complementary or integrative medicine programs.

Hospital programs differ by departmental base, types of clients served (inpatients, outpatients, community), access (physician or self-referral), administrative staff (physician, nurse, CAM expert), and services provided. Services range from mind-body sessions only, to massage and exercise, to the provision of herbs and food supplements, and to services even more removed from mainstream care, such as colonic irrigation and homeopathy. Some clinical CAM programs are repackaged support services, previously available to patients as spiritual care, group and individual counseling, art therapy, nutritional guidance, and so on.

Professional Societies

Concerted efforts are now made to raise awareness and encourage the use of evidence-based complementary therapies in oncology. An international organization, the Society for Integrative Oncology, was established to encourage appropriate clinical integration, scientific evaluation, and dissemination of evidence-based information. Members of the Society for Integrative Medicine are oncology professionals and researchers who study complementary therapies, including botanicals and other over-the-counter remedies, with scientific methodology. The organization's goal is to apply knowledge generated through research to clinical practice and to educate the public and professional colleagues in the proper use of complementary therapies in cancer care.

COSTS AND INSURANCE COVERAGE

Health insurance programs increasingly cover CAM services and providers. More than 30 major insurers, half of them Blue Cross plans, cover more than one method. Expanding insurance coverage of complementary and alternative therapies reflects consumer demand, but it also represents managed care efforts to control costs. Most alternative practitioners typically provide an opportunity for cost savings, and food supplements are less costly than prescription pharmaceuticals if used instead of the latter. Coverage varies according to the state. Naturopathic care is covered by approximately 100 insurance companies in the United States; most are concentrated in Alaska, Connecticut, and Washington State. Acupuncture, massage therapy, and other CAM services are variably covered by insurers, and most given a physician's prescription for that therapy. In the state of Washington, which requires the inclusion of nonmainstream practitioners in private, commercial insurance products, billings were less than 2% of overall costs for cancer patients (11).

COMMON "ALTERNATIVE" CANCER THERAPIES

These approaches are unproved methods promoted as literal alternatives to mainstream cancer care. Helpful complementary or adjunctive therapies are discussed separately at the end of this chapter.

Diet and Nutrition Regimens as Cancer Treatment

Advocates of dietary cancer treatments typically extend mainstream assumptions about the protective effects of fruits, vegetables, fiber, and avoidance of excessive dietary fat in reducing cancer risk, to the idea that food or vitamins can cure cancer. Proponents of this belief make their claims in books with titles such as *The Food Pharmacy: Dramatic New Evidence That Food Is Your Best Medicine*, *Prescription for Nutritional Healing*, and *New Choices in Natural Healing*.

The macrobiotic diet is a persistently popular example of such dietary approaches. As currently constructed, it is similar to recent U.S. Department of Agriculture dietary pyramid recommendations for healthful eating, except that the macrobiotic diet omits dairy products and meat. This diet derives 50% to 60% of its calories from whole grains; 25% to 30% from vegetables; and the remainder from beans, seaweed, and soups. All animal meat and certain vegetables and processed foods are to be avoided, and soybean consumption is promoted. Despite claims in publications and Web sites, there is no evidence that this or any other diet can cure cancer.

Another diet regimen promoted by some alternative medicine practitioners is the "alkaline diet." The theory goes like this—cancer tissue tends to be acidic; thus, acidity promotes cancer growth; by eating alkaline foods, one would create an environment hostile to cancer cells. This theory neglects the fact that it is the rapid growth of cancer cells that creates an acidic environment, not an acidic environment that creates cancer. In addition, the pH in the body is tightly regulated and not significantly changed by eating alkaline foods. Although "alkaline foods" include fruits and vegetables, the "acidic foods" list includes grains and animal proteins, important components of a healthy, balanced diet. Such extreme dietary plans do more harm than good for cancer patients.

Metabolic Therapies and Detoxification

Metabolic therapies continue to draw patients from North America to the many clinics in Tijuana, Mexico. They are also popular in parts of Europe and elsewhere. These therapies involve practitioner-specific combinations of diet plus vitamins, minerals, enzymes, and detoxification. One of the best known sites for metabolic therapy is the Gerson Clinic, where treatment is based on the belief that toxic products of cancer cells accumulate in the liver, leading to liver failure and death. The Gerson treatment aims to counteract liver damage with a low-salt, high-potassium diet; coffee enemas; and a gallon of fruit and vegetable juice daily (12). The clinic's use of liquefied raw calf liver injections was suspended in 1997, following sepsis in a number of patients.

Other clinics and practitioners provide their own versions of metabolic therapy, each applying an individualized dietary and detoxification regimen. Additional components of treatment are included according to practitioners' preferences. Metabolic regimens are based on belief in the importance of detoxification, which is believed necessary for the body to heal itself. Practitioners view cancer and other illnesses as symptoms of the accumulation of toxins. This is a nonphysiological but venerable concept that originated in ancient Egyptian, Ayurvedic, and other early efforts to understand illness and death, both of which were believed to be caused by the putrefaction of food in the colon. Decay and purging were major themes in early cultures' therapeutic regimens. Neither the existence of toxins nor the benefit of colonic cleansing has been documented.

Modern variations on the older approach to internal cleansing are drinkable cleansing formulas, said to detoxify and rejuvenate the body. Many variations are available in health food stores, in books, and on the Internet. A shake of liquid clay, psyllium seed husks, and fruit juice, for example, is said to remove harmful food chemicals and air pollutants. These products tend to function as major laxatives, potentially dangerous when taken over days or weeks, or on the regular basis recommended by promoters, and are of special concern for cancer patients.

Megavitamin and Orthomolecular Therapy

Some patients and alternative practitioners believe that large dosages of vitamins—typically hundreds of pills a day—or intravenous infusions of high-dose vitamin C can cure disease. In 1968, Nobel Laureate Linus Pauling coined the term "orthomolecular" to describe the treatment of disease with large quantities of nutrients. His claims that massive doses of vitamin C could cure cancer were disproved in clinical trials (13), but megavitamin and orthomolecular therapy—the latter adding minerals and other nutrients—remain popular among cancer patients. There is no evidence that megavitamin or orthomolecular therapy is effective in treating any disorder. Supplementation of beta-carotene was associated with higher risk of lung cancer in selected populations (14).

Mind-Body Techniques as Cancer Treatment

The potential for people to influence health with their minds is an extremely appealing concept in the United States. It affirms the power of the individual, a belief intrinsic to U.S. culture. Some mind-body interventions have moved from the category of alternative, unconventional therapies into mainstream complementary or supportive care. Good documentation exists, for example, for the effectiveness of meditation, biofeedback, and yoga in stress reduction and the control of some physiological reactions (15).

The argument that patients can use mental attributes or mind-body work to cure cancer is not tenable (16,17). Attending to the psychological health of cancer patients is a fundamental component of good cancer care. Support groups, good doctor–patient relationships, and the emotional and instrumental help of family and friends are vital. However, the idea that patients can influence the course of their disease through mental or emotional work is not substantiated and can evoke feelings of guilt and inadequacy when disease continues to advance despite patients' best spiritual or mental efforts (18).

Bioelectromagnetics

Bioelectromagnetics is the study of interactions between living organisms and their electromagnetic fields. According to proponents, magnetic fields penetrate the body and heal damaged tissues, including cancers. No peer-reviewed publications could be located for this work or for any clinical cancer-related claims regarding bioelectromagnetics. Despite the lack of data and the patent absurdity of these claims, proponents continue to sell electromagnetic therapy as a cure for cancer and other major illnesses.

Electromagnetic therapy and the related group of energy therapies, discussed in the Manual Healing Methods section, illustrate a striking difference between previous and currently popular alternative practices. Whereas many earlier alternatives reflected concepts important to scientific study of the time, many of today's popular alternatives are mystical and explicitly contrary to contemporary scientific and medical thought. It is as though the new millennium encouraged deeper adoption of explanatory notions applied in millennia past.

Alternative Medical Systems

This category includes ancient systems of healing typically based on concepts of human physiology that differ from those accepted by modern Western science. Two of the most popular healing systems are traditional Chinese medicine and India's Ayurvedic medicine, popularized by best-selling author Deepak Chopra, MD (19).

Ayurveda comes from the Sanskrit words "ayur" (life) and "veda" (knowledge). The ancient healing techniques of Ayurveda are based on the classification of people into one of three predominant body types. There are specific remedies for disease and regimens to promote health for each body type.

This medical system has a strong mind-body component, stressing the need to keep consciousness in balance. It uses techniques such as yoga and meditation to do so. Ayurveda also emphasizes regular detoxification and cleansing through all bodily orifices.

Traditional Chinese medicine explains the body in terms of its relationship to the environment and the cosmos. Concepts of human physiology and disease are interwoven with geographic features of ancient China and the forces of nature. Chi, the life force said to run through all of nature, flows in the human body through vertical energy channels known as meridians.

The 12 main meridians are believed to be dotted with acupoints. Each acupoint corresponds to a specific body organ or system, so that needling (acupuncture) or pressing an acupoint (acupressure) can redress the life force imbalance causing the problem in that particular organ.

Although the very existence of chi or a "vital energy force" remains unproved, acupuncture has been shown to induce measurable neurophysiological change. It also helps reduce certain symptoms experienced by cancer patients. Tai chi, a gentle exercise technique with a mind-body component to foster the smooth flow of chi, is useful in preventing falls among the frail or elderly (20). Traditional Chinese medicine also includes a full herbal pharmacopoeia with remedies for most ailments, including cancer (21). The potential anticancer and immunomodulatory benefits of many Chinese herbs and other botanicals are under investigation in the United States and elsewhere.

Pharmacologic and Biological Treatments

Because pharmacologic and biological alternative treatments are invasive and biologically active, they tend to be highly controversial. An example is *antineoplastons*, developed by Dr. Stanislaw Burzynski and available in his clinic in Houston, Texas. Laboratory analysis conducted by a respected scientist concluded that antineoplastons did not normalize tumor cells (22). Promising anecdotal reports encouraged a clinical trial for pediatric patients with brain tumors, but an NCI research effort failed to accrue patients. Further research at the Burzynski Institute was permitted under an investigational new drug, but preliminary data were criticized as uninterpretable, and the therapy as useless and toxic, by respected mainstream scientists. Burzynski and his patients continue the antineoplaston therapy and remain vocal advocates of its efficacy.

Immunoaugmentive therapy (IAT) was developed by the late Dr. Lawrence Burton and offered in his clinic in the Bahamas. Injected IAT is said to balance four protein components in the blood and to strengthen the patient's immune system. Burton claimed that IAT was particularly effective in treating mesothelioma. Documentation of the efficacy of IAT remains anecdotal. The clinic has continued to operate after Burton's death, but its popularity seems to have waned.

Interest in shark cartilage as a cancer therapy was activated by I. William Lane's 1992 book *Sharks Don't Get Cancer* and by a television special that displayed apparent remissions in patients treated with shark cartilage in Cuba. The televised outcome was strongly disputed by oncologists in the United States. Advocates base their therapy on its putative antiangiogenic properties. A recent randomized controlled trial found neither survival benefit nor improved quality of life in advanced cancer patients (23). The product was poorly tolerated due to its unpleasant taste.

Cancell is another biological remedy that appears to be especially popular in Florida and the midwestern United States. Proponents claim that it returns cancer cells to a "primitive state" from which they can be digested and rendered inert.

U.S. Food and Drug Administration (FDA) laboratory studies, which showed Cancell to be composed of common chemicals, including nitric acid, sodium sulfite, potassium hydroxide, sulfuric acid, and catechol, found no basis for proponent claims of Cancell's effectiveness against cancer (24).

Manual Healing Methods

Osteopathic and chiropractic doctors were among the earliest groups to use manual methods. Today, there are numerous approaches involving touch and manipulation technique, including hands-on massage. The benefit of chiropractic treatment of low back pain was supported by a NIH consensus conference (25), but its value is widely disputed by mainstream physicians. Its application in oncology is problematic because of potential neurologic and other injuries.

A manual healing method especially popular among nurses is therapeutic touch (TT), which, despite its name, involves no direct contact. In TT, healers move their hands a few inches above a patient's body and sweep away "blockages" to the patient's energy field. Although a study in the *Journal of the American Medical Association* showed that experienced TT practitioners were unable to detect the investigator's "energy field" (26) and despite mainstream scientists' unwillingness to accept its fundamental premises, TT is taught in North American nursing schools and practiced by nurses in the United States and other countries.

Similarly, Reiki, defined as spiritually guided life force, is the manipulation of energy surrounding the patient and involves no touch. This energy is called "ki" in Japanese lore or "qi or chi" in Chinese tradition. A small study reported better pain control in advanced cancer patients receiving Reiki when compared to usual care (27). Reduction of heart rate and diastolic blood pressure has been reported in a randomized controlled trial of 45 subjects (28). However, the existence of the bioenergy field and its subjection to a practitioner's manipulation has never been convincingly demonstrated.

Several other therapies also involve manipulation of a putative human energy field or use of an individual's special gift for energy healing. Healing of this type, which has remained popular over the centuries in less developed areas of the world (29), has gained increasing public interest and acceptance in the United States. Healers in many areas of the United States claim the ability to cure people of cancer. Although they may cause only minor difficulties when patients also receive mainstream care, many patients are firmly convinced of healers' abilities and decline even to have tumors removed surgically in favor of healers' ministrations.

Herbal Treatments for Cancer

Herbal remedies are typically part of traditional and folk healing methods with long histories of use. Herbal medicine is found in most areas of the world and across all cultures historically. Although many herbal remedies are claimed to have anticancer effects, only a few have gained substantial popularity as alternative cancer therapies.

For decades, Essiac has remained a popular herbal cancer alternative in North America. Developed initially by a native healer from southwestern Canada, it was popularized by a Canadian nurse, Rene Caisse (Essiac is Caisse spelled backward). Essiac is comprised of four herbs: burdock, turkey rhubarb, sorrel, and slippery elm. Researchers at the NCI and elsewhere found that it has no anticancer effect.

Iscador, a derivative of mistletoe, is a popular cancer remedy in Europe, where it is said to have been in continuous use as folk treatment since the Druids. It is used in many main-stream European cancer clinics, typically in conjunction with chemotherapy. Despite many studies, definitive data in support of the usefulness of Iscador have not emerged.

Because plants are the source of many highly successful chemotherapeutic agents, such as paclitaxel, irinotecan, and vinorelbine, it is not surprising that serious efforts have been devoted to the development of new cancer therapies from herbal medicine. Although laboratory data are usually promising, clinical data have been disappointing mainly due to bioavailability and pharmacokinetic issues. It is difficult to achieve an effective concentration of the active compounds in target tissues by oral administration of the herbs.

Despite such limitations, some Asian herbal remedies show promise in oncology. Several mushroom-derived compounds are approved for use as cancer treatments in Japan, and there is evidence of effectiveness in randomized Phase III trials. Polysaccharide kureha (PSK), an extract of the mushroom *Coriolus versicolor*, or schizophyllan has been subjected to a number of studies. PSK is extracted from the culture medium of *Schizophyllum commune Fries*. Trials typically compared chemotherapy or radiotherapy plus mushroom extract or conventional treatment alone, and found superior survival with PSK as compared to controls in esophageal and gastric cancer patients (30−32).

Two randomized trials of PSK extract given after curative resection for colorectal cancer have been conducted. In the first ($n =$120), median survival in the PSK group was approximately 5 years compared with slightly more than 4 years in controls (33). A subsequent trial randomized 462 colorectal cancer patients scheduled for curative resection to chemotherapy with or without PSK (34). Diseasefree and overall survival was significantly higher in the PSK group. In recent randomized trials, oral PSK with tegafur/uracil reduced recurrence and increased survival in stage III patients with colorectal cancer (35,36). Results are less encouraging in breast cancer (37,38) and leukemia (39).

PC-SPES (PC for prostate cancer, SPES is the Latin word for hope), a combination of eight herbs, all but one from traditional Chinese medicine, reduces prostate-specific antigen levels in men with advanced prostate cancer regardless of whether disease is androgen dependent (40−42). Improvements in quality of life also have been reported (41). PC-SPES was suspended from the market in early 2002, when undisclosed contamination with anxiolytic and antithrombotic agents was uncovered.

Sho-saiko-to (Xiao-Chai-Hu-Tang) is a traditional Asian medicine for liver disease comprised of seven botanicals. It has marked antiproliferative effects on various cancer lines, particularly hepatoma (43). In a Phase III randomized trial, 260 patients with cirrhosis were randomized to treatment with Sho-saiko-to or control (44). At 5 years, Sho-saiko-to led to a one-third reduction in the incidence of hepatocellular carcinoma (23% vs. 34%) and a 40% reduction in deaths (24% vs. 40%).

In a separate study, SV Soup, a formula of 19 vegetables from traditional Chinese medicine believed to have antitumor activity, was added to the diets of 12 patients with stages III and IV non–small-cell lung cancer. Thirteen clinically similar patients were selected as controls. All patients received conventional therapies. The median survival of control patients was 4 months (mean 4.8 months). The median survival of patients who received the vegetable remedy was 15.5 months (mean 15 months). This nontoxic vegetable brew was reported to improve quality of life (45).

These investigations suggest that historical herbal cancer remedies, pretested to ensure purity and consistency of product and studied carefully, may produce potentially useful, nontoxic cancer treatments. The difficulty with time-honored herbal remedies is that they are rarely tested for purity, examined for consistency, or studied carefully. They are, nonetheless, in common use.

Complementary Therapies

Complementary therapies are safe, nontoxic, noninvasive, easy to use, and inexpensive. Many may be self-managed, meaning that practitioners often are unnecessary, which gives patients the rare and important opportunity to maintain a measure of control over their well-being. Supportive or complementary modalities are also soothing, comforting, distracting, and backed by good efficacy data.

Some complementary therapies, such as relaxing in a warm bath or painting soothing mental pictures, are intuitively comforting and helpful. Major supportive therapies have been singled out here for more detailed review. These therapies—music therapy, therapeutic massage, acupuncture, and mind-body modalities—address some of the most pervasive and difficult problems faced by patients under palliative care. Although data do not always come from the patient population of concern, research shows that these minimally invasive, side effect–free therapies effectively reduce anxiety, depression, pain, dyspnea, nausea, and fatigue (46).

Music Therapy

Music therapy is provided by professional musicians who are also trained music therapists. They often hold professional degrees in music therapy, and are adept in dealing with the psychosocial and clinical issues faced by patients and family members. Music therapy is particularly effective in the palliative care setting. Formal music therapy programs in palliative medicine exist in many major institutions. Although music therapy extends back to folklore and Greek mythology (Apollo was the god of both music and medicine), it has been studied scientifically only in recent years.

Controlled trials indicate that music therapy produces emotional and physiological benefits, reducing anxiety, stress, depression, and pain. Music intervention significantly reduced heart rate, respiratory rate, and anxiety scores among inpatients after myocardial infarction, ventilatory assistance, and patients undergoing flexible sigmoidoscopy (47). Live versus recorded music more effectively reduced anxiety.

In the preoperative setting, randomized trials found that music reduced anxiety and its physiological correlates such as blood pressure and salivary cortisol, a biochemical marker of stress and anxiety. Music lowered blood pressure and anxiety scores during and after eye surgery (48) and among women undergoing hysterectomies in a randomized, controlled trial (49).

Music therapy was shown to be effective against laboratory-induced pain, among cancer patients (50) and among cancer patients with chronic pain (51). Music reduced intraoperative analgesic requirements compared to controls, and patients randomized to a music intervention reported significantly less pain and required less pain medication. In what was possibly the largest trial of its type, 500 surgical patients were randomized to control, recorded music, jaw relaxation, or a music/jaw relaxation combination. Music led to significant decreases in both pain intensity and related distress associated with pain (52). Music also can help reduce depression (53).

In a randomized controlled trial of cancer patients undergoing autologous stem cell transplantation, anxiety, depression, and total mood disturbance scores were significantly lower in music therapy group when compared with standard care controls (54).

Massage Therapy

The benefits of massage therapy are documented for end-of-life populations (55), and the pain-reducing effects of this intervention are well documented for cancer patients at various stages of illness (56). In the largest study to date, 87 hospitalized cancer patients were randomized to foot massage (also called "reflexology") or to control on a crossover basis. Pain and anxiety scores fell with massage, with differences between groups achieving substantial significance ($p = 0.001$) (50). Pain scores fell by two-thirds immediately after the first massage of patients with postburn itching and pain, and improvements appeared to be cumulative. No similar changes were seen in controls. Other studies found similar results for patients with postoperative pain. In an analysis of 1,290 patient reports of symptom severity pre and post massage therapy, 0 to 10 ratings of pain, fatigue, stress/anxiety, nausea, depression, and "other" were reduced by approximately 50%, even for patients reporting high baseline scores. Benefits persisted with no return toward baseline scores throughout 48-hour follow-up (57).

Acupuncture

Pain is the most common and the best studied indication for acupuncture. It relieves both acute (e.g., postoperative dental pain) and chronic (e.g., headache) pain (58,59). A recent randomized controlled trial of 570 patients with osteoarthritis of the knee found that a 26-week course of acupuncture significantly improved pain and dysfunction when compared to sham-acupuncture control. In this study, all patients received other usual care for osteoarthritis. At week 8, improvement in function but not in pain was observed, indicating that long-term treatment may be required to achieve full effect (60).

Acupuncture appears effective against cancer-related pain. A randomized placebo-controlled trial tested auricular acupuncture for patients with pain despite stable medication. A total of 90 patients were randomized to needles placed at correct acupuncture points (treatment group) versus acupuncture or pressure at nonacupuncture points. Pain intensity decreased by 36% at 2 months from baseline in the treatment group, a statistically significant difference compared with the two control groups, for whom little pain reduction was seen (61). Skin penetration per se showed no significant analgesic effect. The authors selected acupuncture points by measuring electrodermal signals. These results are especially important because most of the patients had neuropathic pain, which is often refractory to conventional treatment.

Acupuncture helps lessen chemotherapy-induced nausea and vomiting. In one study, 104 breast cancer patients receiving highly emetogenic chemotherapy were randomized to receive electroacupuncture at the PC6 acupuncture point, minimal needling at nonacupuncture points, or pharmacotherapy alone. Electroacupuncture significantly reduced the number of episodes of total emesis when compared with pharmacotherapy only. Most patients did not know the group to which they had been assigned (62). The effects of acupuncture do not appear entirely due to attention, clinician–patient interaction, or placebo.

Acupuncture has been reported to reduce xerostomia (severe dry mouth). Radiotherapy for head and neck cancer causes acute and chronic xerostomia, which may persist despite the use of pilocarpine (Salagen) and amifostine (Ethyol). Acupuncture improved Xerostomia Inventory scores in 18 patients with head and neck cancer and pilocarpine-resistant xerostomia in uncontrolled trials. Patients with breast or prostate cancer may experience vasomotor symptoms (hot flashes) during estrogen or androgen ablation therapy. A few uncontrolled studies investigated acupuncture to treat these symptoms. Self-stimulation of implanted miniature acupuncture needles attenuated tamoxifen-related hot flashes in 8 of 12 patients with breast cancer (63), and similar results were found in a case series of patients with breast (64) and prostate cancer (65). Controlled trials are under way at several centers.

Fatigue following chemotherapy or irradiation, another major and common problem, has few reliable treatments in patients without a correctable cause such as anemia. In an uncontrolled trial of fatigue after chemotherapy, acupuncture reduced fatigue 31% after 6 weeks of treatment. Among those with severe fatigue at baseline, 79% had nonsevere fatigue scores at follow-up (66), whereas fatigue was reduced only in 24% of patients receiving usual care in another center (67).

Mind-Body Therapies for Improvement of Quality of Life

The varied group of mind-body therapies is geared to decrease stress and promote relaxation in different ways. Hypnotherapy has been shown to reduce chemotherapy-related nausea and vomiting in children, and possibly to control anxiety and nausea. Hypnosis for pain is well supported (68). Other techniques, including visualization and progressive relaxation, also decrease pain and promote well-being (69).

Meditation can help stress reduction. In a randomized wait-list control study of 109 cancer patients, participation in a 7-week mindfulness-based stress reduction program was associated with significant improvement in mood disturbance and symptoms of stress (70). A single arm study of breast and prostate cancer patients showed significant improvement in overall quality of life, stress, and sleep quality, but symptom improvement was not significantly correlated with program attendance or minutes of home practice (71).

Yoga, which combines physical movement, breath control, and meditation, improved sleep quality in a controlled trial of 39 lymphoma patients. Practicing a form of yoga that incorporates controlled breathing and visualization significantly decreased sleep disturbance when compared to wait-list controls (72). Mindfulness-based stress reduction techniques must be practiced to produce beneficial effects (73).

Other Therapies

The use of pet animals (pet therapy) is believed to help reduce loneliness and improve quality of life, especially for those who are elderly, alone, or demented. Most pet therapy research has been conducted in psychiatric settings. A randomized clinical trial with pain and palliative care cancer patients, conducted at the NIH Clinical Center, began enrollment in 2005. This study will examine how animal-assisted therapy affects pain in cancer patients receiving pain and palliative care at the NIH Clinical Center.

Art therapy is a behavioral modality that uses creative expression to help develop coping skills. Many cancer centers provide access to artistic expression on a recreational basis or guided by professional art therapists. A few reports showed association of art therapy with better collaboration of children with leukemia undergoing painful procedures or reduced stress and lowered anxiety in family caregivers of patients with cancer. Although scientific study of art therapy is minimal, it is clear that many patients enjoy creative activity, and the enjoyment per se is an important end in and of itself.

Other complementary therapies, such as spiritual care, counseling, and group support, have been part of supportive and palliative care in cancer for decades. The complementary therapies discussed here represent an extension of those efforts to decrease symptoms and enhance patients' quality of life. Our challenge is to help patients avoid the pitfalls of useless unproved therapies, while ensuring their access to the safe, noninvasive, beneficial complementary modalities reviewed here (74).

REGULATORY AND SAFETY ISSUES OF DIETARY SUPPLEMENTS

Dietary supplements, which include vitamins and minerals, homeopathic remedies, herbal treatments, antioxidants, and other over-the-counter products, are probably the most popular unconventional remedies used today by cancer patients, as well as by the public in general. Legal standards for the processing and packaging of herbs, as well as quality control standards and oversight, are very much needed. Because they are not yet mandatory, few food supplement companies voluntarily self-impose quality evaluation and control. Consumer protection and enforcement agencies cannot provide protection against contaminated or falsely advertised products. Current federal regulations do not permit such oversight, and regulatory capability would prohibit full analysis and ongoing oversight of the estimated 20,000 food supplement items now sold over the counter.

Cancer patients use many over-the-counter herbal products in addition to or instead of those promoted specifically as cancer treatments. It is therefore important to recognize herbal remedies that are toxic or tend to interact with other medications as well as those that may help cancer patients. Because neither the FDA nor any other agency examines herbal remedies for safety and effectiveness, few products have been formally tested for side effects or quality control, but information is beginning to emerge on the basis of public experience with over-the-counter supplements.

Reports in the literature describe severe liver and kidney damage from some herbal remedies. These reports underscore the fact that "natural" products, contrary to apparent consumer belief, are not necessarily safe or harmless (24). Most members of the public are apparently unaware that herbs are essentially dilute natural drugs that contain scores of different chemicals, most of which have not been documented. Effects are not always predictable.

Moreover, the potential for herb–drug interaction is sufficiently problematic that patients on chemotherapy or other major medications should not use herbal remedies. Similar cautions are necessary for patients receiving radiation because some herbs photosensitize the skin and cause severe reactions. Some herbs interfere with coagulation and produce dangerous blood pressure swings and other unwanted interactions with anesthetics (24). Herbs such as feverfew, garlic, ginger, and ginkgo have anticoagulant effects and should be avoided by patients on warfarin sodium (Coumadin), heparin sodium, aspirin, and related agents. The risk of herb–drug interactions appears to be greatest for patients with kidney or liver problems. Herbs can alter metabolism of prescription medicine via the cytochrome P450 system, possibly worsening side effects or compromising efficacy (24).

The California Department of Health found unsafe levels of mercury and other toxic metals in more than one third of Asian patent medicines studied. Several instances of heart problems resulting from digitalis-contaminated supplements have been reported (75). PC-SPES, an herbal mixture popular in 2002 as a treatment for prostate cancer, was found to be contaminated

TABLE 12.1

REPUTABLE SOURCES OF ONLINE INFORMATION ON COMPLEMENTARY AND ALTERNATIVE MEDICINE

Organization/source	Web site
National Center for Complementary and Alternative Medicine	http://nccam.nih.gov/
National Cancer Institute, Office of Cancer Complementary and Alternative Medicine	http://www.cancer.gov/cam/index.html
American Cancer Society	http://www.cancer.org/docroot/ETO/ETO_5.asp?sitearea=ETO
U.S. Department of Agriculture, Food and Nutrition Information Center	http://www.nal.usda.gov/fnic
National Institutes of Health, Office of Dietary Supplements	http://dietary-supplements.info.nih.gov
U.S. Pharmacopeia (USP), USP Verified Dietary Supplements	http://www.usp.org/USPVerified/dietarySupplements/
Medline Plus, All Herbs and Supplements	http://www.nlm.nih.gov/medlineplus/druginfo/herb_All.html
Memorial Sloan-Kettering Cancer Center, About Herbs, Botanicals and Other Supplements	http://www.mskcc.org/aboutherbs
M.D. Anderson Cancer Center, Complementary/Integrative Medicine	http://www.mdanderson.org/departments/CIMER
Institute of Medicine of the National Academies, Food and Nutrition Board	http://www.iom.edu/board.asp?id=3788

with prescription medicine (76). Concerns have been raised even about dietary antioxidants, which may interact with radiation therapy and certain groups of chemotherapeutic agents (77).

The magnitude and seriousness of the problem hopefully will result in the establishment of government oversight programs of some kind, despite anticipated efforts on the part of the food supplement industry to block efforts that could lead to regulation. Information provided by manufacturers and marketeers are not without bias and conflict of interest. Reputable sources of information are listed in Table 12.1. Some of the herbal products or other dietary supplements associated with potentially serious adverse effects are listed in Table 12.2.

COMPLEMENTARY AND ALTERNATIVE MEDICINE PRACTITIONERS AND PRACTICES

Major categories of CAM practitioners outside mainstream medicine include chiropractors, naturopaths, and acupuncturists, who often practice a broader range of traditional Chinese medicine involving herbal therapeutics (78).

Chiropractic medicine requires 4 years of training and prepares students to provide primary clinical services, including wellness maintenance, diagnosis of illness, and primary care, in addition to musculoskeletal care. Fifteen percent of clinical

TABLE 12.2

HERBAL PRODUCTS AND OTHER DIETARY SUPPLEMENTS WITH POTENTIALLY SERIOUS ADVERSE EFFECTS

Product	Adverse effects
Products containing aristolochic acid (*Aristolochia, Bragantia,* or *Asarum* species)	Renal toxicity that can lead to renal failure
Comfrey products containing pyrrolizidine alkaloids (*Symphytum officinale* [common comfrey], *Symphytum asperum* [prickley comfrey], and *Symphytum x uplandicum* [Russian comfrey])	Hepatic toxicity, veno-occlusive disease
Products containing ephedrine alkaloids (various names such as ephedra, Ma huang, *Sida cordifolia* and *Pinellia,* usually used for weight loss and fatigue)	Sympathomimetic activity; hypertension; tachycardia; increased risks for stroke, heart attack, and heart failure
Products containing androstenedione, or "andro," used to build muscles and enhance athletic performance	Androgenic and estrogenic effects
Kava-containing products commonly used for anxiety and stress reduction	Hepatic toxicity
St. John's wort commonly used for depression	Potent cytochrome P450 3A4 inducer, altered metabolism of many drugs
Cesium therapy used to "make to body alkaline" as a cancer treatment	Hypokalemia, prolonged QT interval, cardiac arrhythmia

From U.S. Food and Drug Administration.
Adapted from USFDA website.

training is devoted to organ systems other than the musculoskeletal system. All 50 states and the District of Columbia have licensure programs for chiropractors. The accrediting agency for chiropractic medicine was established in 1971, and a standardized national examination was created in 1982 (78,79).

Naturopathic doctoral degrees are awarded after 4 years of training. Naturopathic education is designed to prepare primary care providers. Training emphasizes health promotion, disease prevention, and the use of natural remedies, such as botanicals. As of January 2005, all 13 states that license naturopaths permit the designation ND—Doctor of Naturopathic Medicine (80). The accrediting agency for naturopathy was established in 1978, and standardized tests were first offered in 1986.

Practitioners of acupuncture and herbal medicine are trained for 3 years. They learn to diagnose disease, using pulse diagnosis and other traditional Chinese medicine techniques, and to treat common problems with acupuncture and herbal remedies. Acupuncturists are recognized and licensed in 34 states, and three additional jurisdictions permit practice under MD supervision (81). Acupuncturists were accredited and their standardized national test was created in 1982 (82). In some states, physicians are authorized to practice acupuncture without additional training. Other states require a minimal of 200 to 300 hours of special training in acupuncture before a physician can use acupuncture in his or her medical practice.

SUMMARY

Alternative cancer therapies take advantage of patient desperation and fear. Fraudulent products and regimens abound; there are no viable alternatives to mainstream cancer care. Complementary therapies, conversely, are rational, evidence-based therapies used adjunctively to relieve symptoms and enhance quality of life. Massage therapy, acupuncture, music therapy, meditation, self-hypnosis, and other mind-body therapies are examples of complementary interventions that effectively reduce physical and emotional symptoms experienced by cancer patients. These should be made available by certified practitioners trained to treat patients with cancer. Herbs and other botanicals, many of which hold great promise and are currently under study, can be risky due to quality control, toxicity, and herb–drug interaction issues. Their use by patients under active treatment or on prescription medications should be discouraged. Oncologists should be able to discuss the pros and cons of usage of complementary and alternative therapies, or at least be able to direct patients to reliable information from reputable sources and professionals.

References

1. Barnes PM, Powell-Griner E, McFann K, Nahin RL. Complementary and alternative medicine use among adults: United States, 2002. *Adv Data* 2004; 343:1–19.
2. Ernst E, Cassileth BR. The prevalence of complementary/alternative medicine in cancer: a systematic review. *Cancer* 1998;83(4):777–782.
3. Cassileth BR, Lusk EJ, Strouse TB, Bodenheimer BJ. Contemporary unorthodox treatments in cancer medicine. A study of patients, treatments, and practitioners. *Ann Intern Med* 1984;101(1):105–112.
4. Molassiotis A, Fernadez-Ortega P, Pud D, et al. Use of complementary and alternative medicine in cancer patients: a European survey. *Ann Oncol* 2005;16(4):655–663.
5. Hyodo I, Amano N, Eguchi K, et al. Nationwide survey on complementary and alternative medicine in cancer patients in Japan. *J Clin Oncol* 2005; 23(12):2645–2654.
6. Berman BM, Singh BK, Lao L, Singh BB, Ferentz KS, Hartnoll SM. Physicians' attitudes toward complementary or alternative medicine: a regional survey. *J Am Board Fam Pract* 1995;8(5):361–366.

7. Verhoef MJ, Sutherland LR. General practitioners' assessment of and interest in alternative medicine in Canada. *Soc Sci Med* 1995;41(4):511–515.
8. Ernst E, Resch KL, White AR. Complementary medicine. What physicians think of it: a meta-analysis. *Arch Intern Med* 1995;155(22):2405–2408.
9. Wetzel MS, Eisenberg DM, Kaptchuk TJ. Courses involving complementary and alternative medicine at US medical schools. *JAMA* 1998;280(9):784–787.
10. Brokaw JJ, Tunnicliff G, Raess BU, Saxon DW. The teaching of complementary and alternative medicine in U.S. medical schools: a survey of course directors. *Acad Med* 2002;77(9):876–881.
11. Lafferty WE, Bellas A, Corage Baden A, Tyree PT, Standish LJ, Patterson R. The use of complementary and alternative medical providers by insured cancer patients in Washington State. *Cancer* 2004;100(7):1522–1530.
12. Green S. A critique of the rationale for cancer treatment with coffee enemas and diet. *JAMA* 1992;268(22):3224–3227.
13. Moertel CG, Fleming TR, Creagan ET, Rubin J, O'Connell MJ, Ames MM. High-dose vitamin C versus placebo in the treatment of patients with advanced cancer who have had no prior chemotherapy. A randomized double-blind comparison. *N Engl J Med* 1985;312(3):137–141.
14. The Alpha-Tocopherol, Beta Carotene Cancer Prevention Study Group. The effect of vitamin E and beta carotene on the incidence of lung cancer and other cancers in male smokers. *N Engl J Med* 1994;330(15):1029–1035.
15. NIH Technology Assessment Panel on Integration of Behavioral and Relaxation Approaches into the Treatment of Chronic Pain and Insomnia. Integration of behavioral and relaxation approaches into the treatment of chronic pain and insomnia. *JAMA* 1996;276(4):313–318.
16. Cunningham AJ, Edmonds CV, Jenkins GP, Pollack H, Lockwood GA, Warr D. A randomized controlled trial of the effects of group psychological therapy on survival in women with metastatic breast cancer. *Psychooncology* 1998; 7(6):508–517.
17. Gellert GA, Maxwell RM, Siegel BS. Survival of breast cancer patients receiving adjunctive psychosocial support therapy: a 10-year follow-up study. *J Clin Oncol* 1993;11(1):66–69.
18. Cassileth BR. The social implications of mind-body cancer research. *Cancer Invest* 1989;7(4):361–364.
19. Chopra D. *Ageless Body, Timeless Mind*. New York, NY: Harmony Books; 1993.
20. Henderson NK, White CP, Eisman JA. The roles of exercise and fall risk reduction in the prevention of osteoporosis. *Endocrinol Metab Clin North Am* 1998;27(2):369–387.
21. Cai Y, Luo Q, Sun M, Corke H. Antioxidant activity and phenolic compounds of 112 traditional Chinese medicinal plants associated with anticancer. *Life Sci* 2004;74(17):2157–2184.
22. Green S. 'Antineoplastons'. An unproved cancer therapy. *JAMA* 1992;267 (21):2924–8.
23. Loprinzi CL, Levitt R, Barton DL, et al. Evaluation of shark cartilage in patients with advanced cancer. *Cancer* 2005;104(1):176–182.
24. Memorial Sloan-Kettering Cancer Center. About herbs, botanicals and other products. Available at http://www.mskcc.org/mskcc/html/11570.cfm. Accessed March 6, 2007.
25. Lawrence DJ. Report from the Consensus Conference on the Validation of Chiropractic Methods. *J Manipulative Physiol Ther* 1990;13(6):295–296.
26. Rosa L, Rosa E, Sarner L, Barrett S. A close look at therapeutic touch. *JAMA* 1998;279(13):1005–1010.
27. Olson K, Hanson J, Michaud M. A phase II trial of Reiki for the management of pain in advanced cancer patients. *J Pain Symptom Manage* 2003; 26(5):990–997.
28. Mackay N, Hansen S, McFarlane O. Autonomic nervous system changes during Reiki treatment: a preliminary study. *J Altern Complement Med* 2004; 10(6):1077–1081.
29. Cassileth BR, Vlassov VV, Chapman CC. Health care, medical practice, and medical ethics in Russia today. *JAMA* 1995;273(20):1569–1573.
30. Niimoto M, Hattori T, Tamada R, Sugimachi K, Inokuchi K, Ogawa N. Postoperative adjuvant immunochemotherapy with mitomycin C, futraful and PSK for gastric cancer. An analysis of data on 579 patients followed for five years. *Jpn J Surg* 1988;18(6):681–686.
31. Nakazato H, Koike A, Saji S, Ogawa N, Sakamoto J. Efficacy of immunochemotherapy as adjuvant treatment after curative resection of gastric cancer. Study Group of Immunochemotherapy with PSK for Gastric Cancer. *Lancet* 1994;343(8906):1122–1126.
32. Ogoshi K, Satou H, Isono K, Mitomi T, Endoh M, Sugita M. Immunotherapy for esophageal cancer. A randomized trial in combination with radiotherapy and radiochemotherapy. Cooperative Study Group for Esophageal Cancer in Japan. *Am J Clin Oncol* 1995;18(3):216–222.
33. Torisu M, Hayashi Y, Ishimitsu T, et al. Significant prolongation of disease-free period gained by oral polysaccharide K (PSK) administration after curative surgical operation of colorectal cancer. *Cancer Immunol Immunother* 1990;31(5):261–268.
34. Mitomi T, Tsuchiya S, Iijima N, et al. Randomized, controlled study on adjuvant immunochemotherapy with PSK in curatively resected colorectal cancer. The Cooperative Study Group of Surgical Adjuvant Immunochemotherapy for Cancer of Colon and Rectum (Kanagawa). *Dis Colon Rectum* 1992;35 (2):123–130.
35. Ohwada S, Kawate S, Ikeya T, et al. Adjuvant therapy with protein-bound polysaccharide K and tegafur uracil in patients with stage II or III colorectal

cancer: randomized, controlled trial. *Dis Colon Rectum* 2003;46(8):1060–1068.

36. Ohwada S, Ikeya T, Yokomori T, et al. Adjuvant immunochemotherapy with oral tegafur/uracil plus PSK in patients with stage II or III colorectal cancer: a randomised controlled study. *Br J Cancer* 2004;90(5):1003–1010.

37. Toi M, Hattori T, Akagi M, et al. Randomized adjuvant trial to evaluate the addition of tamoxifen and PSK to chemotherapy in patients with primary breast cancer. 5-Year results from the Nishi-Nippon Group of the Adjuvant Chemoendocrine Therapy for Breast Cancer Organization. *Cancer* 1992;70(10):2475–2483.

38. Iino Y, Yokoe T, Maemura M, et al. Immunochemotherapies versus chemotherapy as adjuvant treatment after curative resection of operable breast cancer. *Anticancer Res* 1995;15(6B):2907–2911.

39. Ohno R, Yamada K, Masaoka T, et al. A randomized trial of chemoimmunotherapy of acute nonlymphocytic leukemia in adults using a protein-bound polysaccharide preparation. *Cancer Immunol Immunother* 1984;18(3):149–154.

40. Small EJ, Frohlich MW, Bok R, et al. Prospective trial of the herbal supplement PC-SPES in patients with progressive prostate cancer. *J Clin Oncol* 2000;18(21):3595–3603.

41. Pfeifer BL, Pirani JF, Hamann SR, Klippel KF. PC-SPES, a dietary supplement for the treatment of hormone-refractory prostate cancer. *BJU Int* 2000;85(4):481–485.

42. Oh WK, George DJ, Hackmann K, Manola J, Kantoff PW. Activity of the herbal combination, PC-SPES, in the treatment of androgen-independent prostate cancer. *Urology* 2001;57(1):122–126.

43. Yano H, Mizoguchi A, Fukuda K, et al. The herbal medicine Sho-saiko-to inhibits proliferation of cancer cell lines by inducing apoptosis and arrest at the G0/G1 phase. *Cancer Res* 1994;54(2):448–454.

44. Oka H, Yamamoto S, Kuroki T, et al. Prospective study of chemoprevention of hepatocellular carcinoma with Sho-saiko-to (TJ-9). *Cancer* 1995;76(5):743–749.

45. Sun AS, Ostadal O, Ryznar V, et al. Phase I/II study of stage III and IV non-small cell lung cancer patients taking a specific dietary supplement. *Nutr Cancer* 1999;34(1):62–69.

46. Deng G, Cassileth BR, Yeung KS. Complementary therapies for cancer-related symptoms. *J Support Oncol* 2004;2(5):419–426; discussion 27–29.

47. Chlan L, Evans D, Greenleaf M, Walker J. Effects of a single music therapy intervention on anxiety, discomfort, satisfaction, and compliance with screening guidelines in outpatients undergoing flexible sigmoidoscopy. *Gastroenterol Nurs* 2000;23(4):148–156.

48. Allen K, Golden LH, Izzo JL, Jr, et al. Normalization of hypertensive responses during ambulatory surgical stress by perioperative music. *Psychosom Med* 2001;63(3):487–492.

49. Mullooly VM, Levin RF, Feldman HR. Music for postoperative pain and anxiety. *J N Y State Nurses Assoc* 1988;19 (3):4–7.

50. Beck SL. The therapeutic use of music for cancer-related pain. *Oncol Nurs Forum* 1991;18(8):1327–1337.

51. Zimmerman L, Pozehl B, Duncan K, Schmitz R. Effects of music in patients who had chronic cancer pain. *West J Nurs Res* 1989;11(3):298–309.

52. Good M, Stanton-Hicks M, Grass JA, et al. Relaxation and music to reduce postsurgical pain. *J Adv Nurs* 2001;33(2):208–215.

53. Hanser SB, Thompson LW. Effects of a music therapy strategy on depressed older adults. *J Gerontol* 1994;49(6):P265–P269.

54. Cassileth BR, Vickers AJ, Magill LA. Music therapy for mood disturbance during hospitalization for autologous stem cell transplantation: a randomized controlled trial. *Cancer* 2003;98(12):2723–2729.

55. Wilkinson S, Aldridge J, Salmon I, Cain E, Wilson B. An evaluation of aromatherapy massage in palliative care. *Palliat Med* 1999;13(5):409–417.

56. Ferrell-Torry AT, Glick OJ. The use of therapeutic massage as a nursing intervention to modify anxiety and the perception of cancer pain. *Cancer Nurs* 1993;16(2):93–101.

57. Cassileth BR, Vickers AJ. Massage therapy for symptom control: outcome study at a major cancer center. *J Pain Symptom Manage* 2004;28(3):244–249.

58. NIH Consensus Conference. Acupuncture. *JAMA* 1998;280(17):1518–1524.

59. Melchart D, Linde K, Fischer P, et al. Acupuncture for recurrent headaches: a systematic review of randomized controlled trials. *Cephalalgia* 1999;19(9):779–786; discussion 65.

60. Berman BM, Lao L, Langenberg P, Lee WL, Gilpin AM, Hochberg MC. Effectiveness of acupuncture as adjunctive therapy in osteoarthritis of the knee: a randomized, controlled trial. *Ann Intern Med* 2004;141(12):901–910.

61. Alimi D, Rubino C, Pichard-Leandri E, Fermand-Brule S, Dubreuil-Lemaire ML, Hill C. Analgesic effect of auricular acupuncture for cancer pain: a randomized, blinded, controlled trial. *J Clin Oncol* 2003;21(22):4120–4126.

62. Shen J, Wenger N, Glaspy J, et al. Electroacupuncture for control of myeloablative chemotherapy-induced emesis: a randomized controlled trial. *JAMA* 2000;284(21):2755–2761.

63. Towlerton G, Filshie J, O'Brien M, Duncan A. Acupuncture in the control of vasomotor symptoms caused by tamoxifen. *Palliat Med* 1999;13(5):445.

64. Porzio G, Trapasso T, Martelli S, et al. Acupuncture in the treatment of menopause-related symptoms in women taking tamoxifen. *Tumori* 2002;88(2):128–130.

65. Hammar M, Frisk J, Grimas O, Hook M, Spetz AC, Wyon Y. Acupuncture treatment of vasomotor symptoms in men with prostatic carcinoma: a pilot study. *J Urol* 1999;161(3):853–856.

66. Vickers AJ, Straus DJ, Fearon B, Cassileth BR. Acupuncture for postchemotherapy fatigue: a phase II study. *J Clin Oncol* 2004;22(9):1731–1735.

67. Escalante CP, Grover T, Johnson BA, et al. A fatigue clinic in a comprehensive cancer center: design and experiences. *Cancer* 2001;92(suppl 6):1708–1713.

68. Sellick SM, Zaza C. Critical review of 5 nonpharmacologic strategies for managing cancer pain. *Cancer Prev Control* 1998;2(1):7–14.

69. Walker LG, Walker MB, Ogston K, et al. Psychological, clinical and pathological effects of relaxation training and guided imagery during primary chemotherapy. *Br J Cancer* 1999;80(1–2):262–268.

70. Speca M, Carlson LE, Goodey E, Angen M. A randomized, wait-list controlled clinical trial: the effect of a mindfulness meditation-based stress reduction program on mood and symptoms of stress in cancer outpatients. *Psychosom Med* 2000;62(5):613–622.

71. Carlson LE, Speca M, Patel KD, Goodey E. Mindfulness-based stress reduction in relation to quality of life, mood, symptoms of stress and levels of cortisol, dehydroepiandrosterone sulfate (DHEAS) and melatonin in breast and prostate cancer outpatients. *Psychoneuroendocrinology* 2004;29(4):448–474.

72. Cohen L, Warneke C, Fouladi RT, Rodriguez MA, Chaoul-Reich A. Psychological adjustment and sleep quality in a randomized trial of the effects of a Tibetan yoga intervention in patients with lymphoma. *Cancer* 2004;100(10):2253–2260.

73. Shapiro SL, Bootzin RR, Figueredo AJ, Lopez AM, Schwartz GE. The efficacy of mindfulness-based stress reduction in the treatment of sleep disturbance in women with breast cancer: an exploratory study. *J Psychosom Res* 2003;54(1):85–91.

74. Cassileth B. *The Alternative Medicine Handbook: The Complete Reference Guide to Alternative and Complementary Therapies*. New York, NY: WW Norton; 1998.

75. Slifman NR, Obermeyer WR, Aloi BK, et al. Contamination of botanical dietary supplements by *Digitalis lanata*. *N Engl J Med* 1998;339(12):806–811.

76. Walsh PC. Prospective, multicenter, randomized phase II trial of the herbal supplement, PC-SPES, and diethylstilbestrol in patients with androgen-independent prostate cancer. *J Urol* 2005;173(6):1966–1967.

77. Labriola D, Livingston R. Possible interactions between dietary antioxidants and chemotherapy. *Oncology (Huntingt)* 1999;13(7):1003–1008; discussion 8, 11, 12.

78. Cooper RA, Henderson T, Dietrich CL. Roles of nonphysician clinicians as autonomous providers of patient care. *JAMA* 1998;280:795–802.

79. American Chiropractic Association. *Chiropractic: State of the Art*. Arlington, Va.: American Chiropractic Association; 1994.

80. Lawton S. Naturopathy online Web site. Available at http://www.naturopathyonline.com/. Accessed March 6, 2007.

81. Ergil KV. *Acupuncture*. 1997;15:1–34.

82. Council of Colleges of Acupuncture and Oriental Medicine Web site. Available at http://www.ccaom.org/. Accessed March 6, 2007.

CHAPTER 13 ■ PAIN AND SYMPTOM CONTROL

RUSSELL K. PORTENOY AND CRAIG D. BLINDERMAN

INTRODUCTION

Approximately 30% to 50% of cancer patients undergoing antineoplastic therapy and 75% to 90% of patients with advanced disease have chronic pain severe enough to warrant opioid therapy (1–3). Symptoms other than pain are also highly prevalent in this population, particularly when the disease is advanced (4). Unfortunately, there are numerous obstacles to effective pain and symptom management, and symptom distress caused by inadequately treated pain and other problems is commonly encountered in practice. These obstacles relate to deficiencies in clinician knowledge and skills, health care systems that limit access to care, and the tendency to underreport pain on the part of patients. To improve patient outcomes, strategies are needed to address these obstacles. Clinician education must focus on both the assessment of pain and other symptoms, and the many approaches that now exist to manage it.

DEFINITIONS AND MODELS OF CARE

Pain, Nociception, and Suffering

According to the International Association for the Study of Pain, pain is "an unpleasant sensory and emotional experience associated with actual or potential tissue damage, or described in terms of such damage" (5). To clarify the approach to pain assessment, it is useful to distinguish pain from both nociception and suffering.

Nociception is the activity produced in the afferent nervous system by potentially tissue-damaging stimuli. Nociception is clinically inferred whenever tissue damage is identified. Pain is the *perception* of nociception and can be sustained in the absence of ongoing tissue injury by any of a variety of factors. Neuropathic pain syndromes are presumably sustained through plastic changes in the nervous system; so-called psychogenic pains are attributed to psychological disturbances.

Suffering has been described as any threat to the integrity of the person and may be due to unrelieved symptoms (including pain), psychological or psychosocial disturbances, or spiritual distress (6,7). Other factors, such as financial concerns, may also be prominent. Patients vary in psychosocial and spiritual strengths and weaknesses, and consequently suffer in different ways when dealing with symptoms or other experiences.

Supportive Care and Palliative Care

It is best to define supportive care as those interventions that are intended to manage the adverse effects of antineoplastic therapy. From this perspective, supportive care includes the use of blood products, growth factors, antibiotics, symptom management approaches, and interventions that address the psychosocial consequences of therapy.

The World Health Organization (WHO) has defined *palliative care* as "an approach that improves the quality of life of patients and their families facing ... life-threatening illness ... [palliative care relieves] suffering by means of early identification and impeccable assessment and treatment of pain and other problems, physical, psychosocial, and spiritual" (8). Palliative care is relevant throughout the course of the illness and must intensify as the end of life approaches. Its goals include symptom control; effective communication among patient, family, treatment team, and others; management of psychological distress and comorbid psychiatric disorders; and support for efforts to address social isolation and spiritual distress. Palliative care recognizes the need to provide practical support in the home and to manage caregiver distress and burden. For the patient with advanced illness, palliative care strives to remove the obstacles to a comfortable and dignified death, and to assist families in the process of effective grieving through support and formal bereavement services.

Palliative care should be considered an essential element in oncology practice. The routine efforts of the oncologist and other members of the oncology treatment team to address a broad array of patient concerns may be considered "generalist-level" palliative care. When distress continues despite this care, the oncologist typically refers the patient for specialist services. Specialist-level palliative care may be accessed through institution-based programs and, for eligible patients, hospice patients. In the United States, hospice and palliative medicine will soon be a formal subspecialty of medicine and other medical specialties, and will be largely provided by certified physicians who work in teams maintained through institutions or hospices. Recognition of the need for specialist-level palliative care and appropriate referral to a specialist team should be considered a necessary competency of oncologists and others who treat populations with progressive incurable disease.

ASSESSMENT AND MANAGEMENT OF CANCER PAIN

Pain is a prevalent and distressing symptom, and is often considered the model for guidelines that have been developed to assist in the management of other cancer-related symptoms. For most patients, multidimensional assessment, followed by simple management strategies, can yield satisfactory control of pain.

Pain Characteristics

The pain complaint should be characterized in terms of clinically relevant descriptors: temporal features, location and patterns of radiation, intensity, quality, and factors that provoke or alleviate the pain. This information, combined with the physical examination and imaging studies, may identify a specific pain syndrome and allow inferences regarding the underlying pathophysiology.

Acute pain usually has a well-defined onset and a readily identifiable cause (e.g., surgical incision). If it is associated with other features, these usually are anxiety, moaning or grimacing, and signs of sympathetic hyperactivity (including tachycardia, hypertension, and diaphoresis).

In contrast, chronic pain is characterized by an ill-defined onset and a prolonged, fluctuating course. Overt pain behaviors and sympathetic hyperactivity are typically absent, and vegetative signs, including lassitude, sleep disturbance, and anorexia, may be present. A clinical depression evolves in some patients.

Most patients with chronic cancer pain also experience periodic flares of pain, or "breakthrough pain" (9). An important subtype of breakthrough pain is "incident pain," which is precipitated by voluntary activity. The recognition of breakthrough pain as a significant problem has supported the use of so-called "rescue" doses—a short-acting opioid administered on an as-needed basis—during long-term opioid therapy.

Etiology and Inferred Pathophysiology

In most patients with cancer, pain can be related to an underlying nociceptive lesion, usually direct invasion of pain-sensitive structures by the neoplasm (10). Bone injury is most common, but pain can also occur as a result of damage to neural tissue, obstruction of hollow viscus, distention of organ capsules, distortion or occlusion of blood vessels, and infiltration of soft tissues. The etiology of pain relates to an antineoplastic treatment in about one fourth of patients, and fewer than 10% have pain unrelated to the neoplasm or its treatment (10). Identification of the etiology of the pain can provide an opportunity for a primary therapy, such as radiotherapy (11).

The history, findings on examination, and objective data may allow inferences about the pathophysiological processes that may be sustaining the pain. These processes are categorized as nociceptive, neuropathic, psychogenic, idiopathic, or mixed. Although these labels represent constructs, they are clinically relevant, in many cases suggesting the use of specific therapies.

Nociceptive pain refers to pain that is sustained predominantly by ongoing tissue injury and may involve either somatic or visceral structures. Somatic pain is often described as aching, stabbing, throbbing, or pressurelike. Visceral pain is usually gnawing or crampy when arising from obstruction of a hollow viscus and aching or stabbing when arising from other visceral structures.

Pain is labeled *neuropathic* if the evaluation suggests that it is sustained by abnormal somatosensory processing in the peripheral or central nervous system. Neuropathic mechanisms are involved in approximately 40% of cancer pain syndromes and can be caused by disease or treatment (12). Dysesthesia, or abnormal uncomfortable sensations that may be described using words such as "burning," "shocklike," and "electrical,"

are suggestive of neuropathic mechanisms. On physical examination, the presence of allodynia (pain induced by nonpainful stimuli) and hyperalgesia (increased perception of painful stimuli) also suggests this diagnosis. Patients may or may not develop motor or autonomic dysfunction in the distribution of the involved nerve.

TABLE 13.1

ACUTE PAIN SYNDROMES IN CANCER PATIENTS

Acute pain associated with diagnostic procedures
- Lumbar puncture headache
- Bone marrow biopsy
- Lumbar puncture
- Venipuncture
- Paracentesis
- Thoracentesis

Acute pain associated with analgesic techniques
- Spinal opioid hyperalgesia syndrome
- Acute pain after radiopharmaceutical therapy of metastatic bone pain

Acute postoperative pain
Acute pain associated with other therapeutic procedures
- Pleurodesis
- Tumor embolization
- Nephrostomy insertion
- Pain associated with bone marrow transplantation

Acute pain associated with chemotherapy
- Pain from intravenous or intra-arterial infusion
- Intraperitoneal chemotherapy
- Headache due to intrathecal chemotherapy
- Painful oropharyngeal mucositis
- Painful peripheral neuropathy
- Bone or muscle pain from colony-stimulating factors or chemotherapies
- 5-Fluorouracil-induced angina

Acute pain associated with hormonal therapy
- Painful gynecomastia
- Luteinizing hormone-releasing factor tumor flare in prostate cancer
- Hormone-induced acute pain flare in breast cancer

Acute pain associated with immunotherapy
- Arthralgia and myalgia from interferon and interleukin

Acute pain associated with radiation therapy
- Painful oropharyngeal mucositis
- Acute radiation enteritis or proctitis
- Early onset brachial plexopathy following radiation for breast cancer

Acute tumor-related pain
- Vertebral collapse and other pathological fractures
- Acute obstruction of hollow viscus (e.g., bowel, ureter, bladder outlet)
- Headache from intracranial hypertension
- Hemorrhage from tumor

Acute pain associated with infection
- Myalgia and arthralgia associated with sepsis
- Pain associated with superficial wounds or abscesses

Adapted from Portenoy RK. Pain syndromes in patients with cancer and HIV/AIDS. In: Portenoy RK, ed. *Contemporary Diagnosis and Management of Pain in Oncologic and AIDS Patients.* Newton, Pa.: Handbooks on Healthcare; 1998.

The term *psychogenic pain* refers to pain that is believed to be sustained predominantly by psychological factors and is a generic label applied to a number of syndromes described in the *Diagnostic and Statistical Manual of Mental Disorders* of the American Psychiatric Association. An assessment of these pains should reveal positive evidence for the psychopathology that is believed to be causally related to the pain. Although psychological factors commonly influence the presentation of the pain and the patient's adaptation, psychogenic pain appears to be rare in the cancer population.

In the absence of sufficient evidence to label the pain by a more definitive term, it can be considered *idiopathic*. In the cancer population, this label usually suggests the need to reassess etiology and pathophysiology at a later time.

Cancer Pain Syndromes

Efforts to improve the assessment of cancer pain have been greatly encouraged by the description of numerous pain syndromes, each of which is defined by a cluster of symptoms and signs (10,12). Syndrome identification can help direct the diagnostic evaluation, clarify the prognosis, and target therapeutic interventions.

Acute pain syndromes are commonly caused by diagnostic or therapeutic interventions, including surgery (Table 13.1). Chronic pain syndromes may be directly related to the neoplasm or to antineoplastic therapy (Tables 13.2 and 13.3).

TABLE 13.2

CHRONIC PAIN SYNDROMES IN PATIENTS WITH CANCER: TUMOR-RELATED PAIN SYNDROMES

NOCICEPTIVE PAIN SYNDROMES

Bone, joint, and soft tissue pain syndromes
- Multifocal or generalized pain (focal metastases or marrow expansion)
- Base of skull metastases
- Vertebral syndromes
- Pain syndromes of the bony pelvis and hip
- Tumor invasion of joint, soft tissue, or both

Paraneoplastic pain syndromes
- Hypertrophic osteoarthropathy
- Tumor-related gynecomastia

Neoplastic involvement of viscera
- Hepatic distension syndrome
- Rostral retroperitoneal syndrome
- Chronic intestinal obstruction and peritoneal carcinomatosis
- Malignant pelvic and perineal pain
- Chronic ureteral obstruction

NEUROPATHIC PAIN SYNDROMES

Painful peripheral mononeuropathies

Painful polyneuropathies

Plexopathy
- Cervical
- Brachial
- Lumbosacral
- Sacral

Radiculopathy

Epidural spinal cord compression

Adapted from Portenoy RK, Lesage P. Management of cancer pain. *Lancet* 1999;353:1696–1697.

TABLE 13.3

CHRONIC PAIN SYNDROMES IN PATIENTS WITH CANCER: TREATMENT-RELATED PAIN SYNDROMES

NOCICEPTIVE PAIN SYNDROMES

Painful osteonecrosis
- Radiation-induced or corticosteroid-induced necrosis of femoral or humeral head
- Osteoradionecrosis of other bones

Painful lymphedema

Painful gynecomastia

Chronic abdominal pain
- Due to intraperitoneal chemotherapy
- Due to radiation therapy

Radiation-induced chronic pelvic pain

NEUROPATHIC PAIN SYNDROMES

Postsurgical neuropathic pain syndromes
- Postmastectomy syndrome
- Postthoracotomy syndrome
- Postradical neck dissection syndrome
- Postnephrectomy syndrome
- Stump pain and phantom pain

Postradiotherapy pain syndrome
- Radiation fibrosis of cervical, brachial, or lumbosacral plexus
- Radiation-induced neoplasm
- Radiation myelopathy

Postchemotherapy pain syndromes
- Polyneuropathies

Adapted from Portenoy RK, Lesage P. Management of cancer pain. *Lancet* 1999;353:1696–1697.

MANAGEMENT OF CHRONIC CANCER PAIN

Role of Primary Therapy

Primary treatments for the pain include antineoplastic therapies and interventions directed at other pathologies. Although the palliative role of chemotherapy is widely accepted (13–15), the specifics have received limited study. Nonetheless, it is a common observation that patients who attain a partial or complete tumor response also experience symptom improvement. Two chemotherapies, mitoxantrone for prostate cancer and gemcitabine for pancreatic cancer, received regulatory approval largely on the basis of symptom palliation.

Radiation therapy has been reported to provide effective palliation of pain in up to 50% of patients treated for bone metastases (16,17), and pain control is the reason for treatment in the majority of patients who receive this intervention. Analgesia also commonly results when radiation is used to treat other disorders, including epidural disease, tumor ulceration, cerebral metastases, superior vena cava obstruction, and bronchial obstruction. Patients with limited prognosis (i.e., months) may benefit from single doses or a shortened fractionation schedule, thereby decreasing treatment burden (18).

Pharmacotherapy of Chronic Cancer Pain

Although primary therapies can be helpful in selected patients, most patients require symptomatic analgesic therapy.

Prospective trials indicate that 70% to 90% of patients can achieve adequate relief of cancer pain using a pharmacologic approach (3,19,20). Effective pain management requires expertise in the use of the nonsteroidal anti-inflammatory drugs (NSAIDs), opioid analgesics, and the so-called adjuvant analgesics.

A model approach to the selection of analgesic drugs for cancer pain, known as the "analgesic ladder," was developed in the 1980s by an expert panel for WHO (3). Although the analgesic ladder approach has evolved since it was created and rigid adherence to its guidelines is no longer justified, key elements are still accepted. Most important, the approach reinforces the consensus view that persistent moderate to severe cancer pain should be treated with an opioid-based drug regimen. From this perspective, the analgesic ladder has been useful as a tool to educate policy makers and others about the need for access to opioids.

Nonsteroidal Anti-inflammatory Drugs

NSAIDs have a well-established role in the treatment of cancer pain (21). A recent meta-analysis suggests that NSAIDs can be effective initial monotherapy for cancer pain and that NSAIDs combined with opioids may lead to a slight short-term improvement in pain compared with either agent alone (22). The long-term efficacy and safety of NSAIDs for cancer pain have not been established.

In practice, a NSAID may be used as the sole analgesic for patients with generally mild pain and should be considered for combination therapy when pain is moderate or severe. NSAIDs appear to be especially useful in patients with nociceptive pain, particularly bone pain and pain related to grossly inflammatory lesions, and relatively less useful in patients with neuropathic pain (23–25). Recent studies in the neurobiology of bone pain suggest that there may be an even greater role for NSAIDs in managing pain secondary to bony metastases (26–28).

The therapeutic limitations of NSAIDs are primarily due to their side effects. All NSAIDs have the potential for nephrotoxicity, with effects that range from peripheral edema to acute or chronic renal failure. Clinical effects and serum creatinine must be monitored periodically in the medically frail cancer patient who receives one of these drugs for ongoing treatment of pain. In addition, NSAIDs increase the risk of gastrointestinal ulcers and bleeding. The selective cyclo-oxygenase (COX)-2 inhibitors reduced the risk of the latter outcomes, and many clinicians recommend these drugs as first-line therapy for all patients at relatively high risk of ulcer, including the elderly, those concurrently receiving a corticosteroid, those with a prior history of peptic ulcer disease or NSAID-induced gastroduodenopathy, and patients who are medically frail and less able to tolerate a gastrointestinal hemorrhage. Recently, there has been recognition that that COX-2 inhibition can increase the risk of thrombotic disease, and the U.S. Food and Drug Administration has required a special warning about this risk on the labels of all NSAIDs, including the nonselective COX inhibitors and the COX-2 selective drugs. Although this risk appears to be relatively small, it may influence the decision to offer a NSAID to patients at relatively high risk of thrombotic complications for other reasons.

Adjuvant Analgesics

The adjuvant analgesics are a diverse group of drugs, most of which have primary indications other than pain but can be effective analgesics in specific circumstances (29) (Table 13.4). Treatment with one of these drugs is generally considered if an optimally administered opioid regimen fails to provide a satisfactory balance between pain relief and side effects. These drugs are particularly useful in the treatment of neuropathic pain, bone pain, and pain related to bowel obstruction.

Corticosteroids are multipurpose adjuvant analgesics. In addition to their use in neuropathic pain, these drugs may improve anorexia, nausea, and fatigue associated with advanced cancer. They are empirically used to treat the pain associated with lymphedema, liver metastases, bowel obstruction, metastatic bone pain, headache associated with intracranial mass lesions, and superior vena cava syndrome.

Corticosteroids, anticonvulsants, antidepressants, and other drugs have analgesic effects in neuropathic pain (29). The safety and efficacy of gabapentin has been established in both nonmalignant (30,31) and cancer-related neuropathic pain syndromes (32–34), and this drug, or a similar, recently approved drug, pregabalin, is therefore usually tried first. Of the newer anticonvulsants, the evidence of analgesic efficacy is strongest for pregabalin, and there is also some evidence for lamotrigine; other anticonvulsants are tried empirically in refractory cases, despite limited supporting data.

Although there is substantial evidence for the analgesic efficacy of the tricyclic antidepressants, particularly amitriptyline (35), the use of these drugs is often limited by the high likelihood of side effects. In the medically ill, the secondary amine tricyclics, desipramine and nortriptyline, are typically used because of their relatively better side effect profile. Newer antidepressants, such as duloxetine, venlafaxine, paroxetine, citalopram, and bupropion, are also analgesic and are better tolerated in the cancer population; of these, duloxetine is now approved for one type of neuropathic pain, and therefore, should be considered first.

There are relatively fewer data supporting a role for other drugs and drug classes as adjuvant analgesics. Sodium channel blockers, cannabinoids, alpha-2 adrenergic agonists, and n-methyl-D-aspartate inhibitors have all been used for neuropathic cancer pain.

Topical agents represent another adjuvant analgesic strategy. Lidoderm, a lidocaine transdermal patch, has been shown to be effective in postherpetic neuralgia (36,37). In a study in cancer patients with surgical neuropathic pain (e.g., postmastectomy syndrome), topical capsaicin, a peptide that depletes substance P in small primary afferent neurons, was found to significantly decrease pain (38).

Like neuropathic pain that has not responded adequately to an opioid, malignant bone pain may be an appropriate target for therapy with an adjuvant analgesic. The preferred drugs include bisphosphonates, radiopharmaceuticals, and calcitonin. The bisphosphonates, including pamidronate, zoledronate, ibandronate, and clodronate (not available in the United States), are usually considered first because of established efficacy in reducing the risk of adverse skeletal events (39).

Opioid Analgesics

Expertise in the administration of opioid analgesics is the foundation of cancer pain management. The clinician should have knowledge of opioid pharmacology and a clear grasp of practical guidelines for dosing.

Opioid Selection. The distinction between so-called "weak" and "strong" opioids, which was originally incorporated into the WHO analgesic ladder approach, is more operational than pharmacologic. The weak opioids are conventionally administered orally for moderate pain in those patients with limited prior opioid exposure. The strong opioids are conventionally used to treat severe pain and pain in those already receiving opioid therapy. In the United States, the former group includes codeine, hydrocodone (only with acetaminophen or ibuprofen), dihydrocodeine (only with aspirin), oxycodone (when combined with aspirin, acetaminophen, or ibuprofen), propoxyphene, and, occasionally, meperidine. Tramadol, a unique centrally acting analgesic with a mechanism that is partly opioid, is also generally included in this group.

TABLE 13.4

ADJUVANT ANALGESICS

Indication	Class	Examples
Neuropathic pain	Steroids	Dexamethasone
		Prednisone
	Antidepressants	Amitriptyline
	Tricyclics	Desipramine
		Nortriptyline
	SSRIs/SNRIs	Duloxetine
		Venlafaxine
		Citalopram
		Paroxetine
	Anticonvulsants	Pregabalin
		Gabapentin
		Lamotrigine
		Carbamazepine
		Clonazepam
		Valproate
	Sodium channel blockers	Mexiletine
		Tocainide
	Alpha-2 adrenergic agonists	Tizanidine
		Clonidine
	NMDA receptor antagonists	Ketamine
		Dextromethorphan
		Amantadine
		Memantine
	GABA agonists	Baclofen
	Topical agents	5% Lidocaine patch
		Local anesthetic creams
		Capsaicin
Bone pain	Bisphosphonates	Pamidronate
		Ibandronate
		Zoledronate
	Other osteoclast inhibitor	Calcitonin
	Radiopharmaceuticals	Strontium-89
		Samarium-153
Bowel obstruction	Steroid	Dexamethasone
	Anticholinergic drugs	Scopolamine
		Glycopyrrolate
	Somatostatin analogue	Octreotide

SSRI, selective serotonin reuptake inhibitor; SNRI, serotonin-norepinephrine reuptake inhibitor; NMDA, N-methyl-D-aspartate; GABA, gamma-aminobutyric acid.

Opioids used conventionally for severe pain include morphine, fentanyl, oxycodone, (without acetaminophen or aspirin), hydromorphone, oxymorphone, levorphanol, and methadone. There is no one preferred opioid, and the decision to choose one over another is usually based on the available formulation, cost, and prior experience. Therapeutic failure with one drug may be followed by remarkable success with another (40).

Routes of Administration. Long-term administration of an opioid is best accomplished by the oral or transdermal route. Numerous oral formulations are available, and the long-acting, modified-release drugs are usually preferred in an effort to improve therapeutic adherence and convenience. The modified-release drugs include oral morphine (with dosing intervals of 12 hours or 24 hours), oxycodone (12-hour dosing interval), and transdermal fentanyl (48- to 72-hour interval). The latter formulation is preferred by some patients and may be associated with less constipation (41). Modified-release oral hydromorphone and oxymorphone are in development.

Long-term parenteral dosing can be used for patients who are poor candidates for oral or transdermal formulations. Continuous intravenous infusion is most feasible for patients with an indwelling central venous port. In addition, ambulatory infusion via the subcutaneous route has been made possible with the development of small infusion pumps.

Opioids and other drugs may also be delivered into the epidural or intrathecal spaces. Neuraxial infusion can provide opioid analgesia at doses far lower than those required systemically and can therefore provide equivalent or better analgesia with fewer side effects. The strongest indication for neuraxial analgesia is the presence of intolerable somnolence or confusion in patients who experience some degree of analgesia from systemic therapy. In a recent controlled trial, continuous intrathecal infusion of morphine via an implanted drug delivery system yielded better pain control, less fatigue, and improved survival than comprehensive medical management alone (42).

The oral transmucosal form of fentanyl has been shown to be safe and efficacious when used to treat breakthrough pain in cancer patients receiving a fixed-dose opioid regimen for persistent pain (9,43). Absorption through the oral cavity is theoretically possible with any opioid, particularly those that are, like fentanyl, highly lipophilic (44). Other oral transmucosal formulations of fentanyl, including an effervescent tablet, a patch, and a sublingual tablet, are currently available. Although injectable formulations of any opioid therefore could be tried, practical considerations and the variable absorption of most drugs do not support wider use of this approach.

Rectal formulations of oxymorphone, hydromorphone, and morphine are available in the United States and have potencies that are believed to approximate oral dosing. This route is generally used in opioid-naive patients who are transiently unable to take oral drugs.

Dosing. Optimal opioid therapy requires individualization of the dose through a process of repeated dose titration. As the dose is titrated, most patients experience a favorable balance between analgesia and side effects, and this balance generally persists unless there is progression in the pain-producing pathology. The absolute dose of the opioid is immaterial as long as the balance between analgesia and side effects remains acceptable to the patient. Conventionally, the size of the increment at each dose escalation is between 30% and 100% of the total daily dose on the prior day. The lower end of this range is used if the pain is not severe or the patient is medically frail; the upper part of the range is appropriate for severe pain in the patient who is more robust.

TABLE 13.5

OPIOID ANALGESICS USED FOR THE TREATMENT OF PERSISTENT CANCER PAIN

Drug	Dose (mg) equianalgesic to morphine 10 mg IM[a]		Half-life (h)	Duration (h)	Comment
	PO	IM			
Morphine	20–30[b]	10	2–3	2–4	Standard for comparison
Morphine, modified release	20–30	10	2–3	8–12	Various formulations are not bioequivalent
Oxycodone	20	—	2–3	3–4	
Oxycodone, modified release	20	—	2–3	12	
Hydromorphone	7.5	1.5	2–3	2–4	Potency may be greater during prolonged use (i.e., hydromorphone:morphine = 3:1 rather than 6.7:1)
Methadone	20	10	12–190	4–12	Although 1:1 IM:IM potency ratio with morphine was found in single dose study, there is a change with chronic dosing, and large dose reduction (75%–90%) is needed when switching to methadone
Oxymorphone	10	1	2–3	2–4	Available in rectal and injectable formulations
Levorphanol	4	2	12–15	4–6	
Fentanyl	—	—	7–12	—	Can be administered as a continuous IV or SQ infusion; based on clinical experience, 100 μg/h is roughly equianalgesic to morphine IV 4 mg/h
Fentanyl TTS	—	—	16–24	48–72	Based on clinical experience, 100 μg is roughly equianalgesic to morphine 4 mg/h IV. A ratio of oral morphine:transdermal fentanyl of 70:1 may also be used clinically
Oral transmucosal fentanyl citrate	—	—	7–12	1–2	Recommended starting dose for breakthrough pain, 200–400 μg, even with high "baseline" opioid doses

PO, oral; IM, intramuscular; IV, intravenous; SQ, subcutaneous.
[a] Studies to determine equianalgesic doses of opioids have used morphine by the IM route. The IM and IV routes are considered to be equivalent, and IV is the most common route used in clinical practice.
[b] Although the PO:IM morphine was 6:1 in single dose study, other observations indicate a ratio of 2–3:1 with repeated administration.
Adapted from Derby S, Chin J, Portenoy RK. Systemic opioid therapy for chronic cancer pain: practical guidelines for converting drugs and routes of administration. *CNS Drugs* 1998;9:99–109.

TABLE 13.6

COMMONLY USED APPROACHES IN THE MANAGEMENT OF OPIOID SIDE EFFECTS

Side effect	Treatment
Constipation	**General approach** ■ Increase fluid intake and dietary fiber ■ Encourage mobility and ambulation if appropriate ■ Ensure comfort and convenience for defecation ■ Rule out and treat impaction if present **Pharmacologic approach** ■ Contact laxative plus stool softener (e.g., senna plus docusate) ■ Osmotic laxative (e.g., milk of magnesia) ■ Lavage agent (e.g., oral propylethylene glycol) ■ Prokinetic agent (e.g., metoclopramide) ■ Oral naloxone
Nausea	**General approach** ■ Hydrate as appropriate ■ Progressive alimentation ■ Good mouth care ■ Correct contributory factors ■ Adjust medication **Pharmacologic approach** ■ Vertigo → antihistamine (e.g., scopolamine, meclizine) ■ Early satiety → prokinetic (e.g., metoclopramide) ■ Dopamine antagonists (e.g., prochlorperazine, chlorpromazine, haloperidol, metoclopramide)
Somnolence or cognitive impairment	**General approach** ■ Reassurance ■ Education ■ Treatment of potential etiologies **Pharmacologic approach** ■ If analgesia is satisfactory, reduce opioid dose by 25%–50% ■ If analgesia is satisfactory and the toxicity is somnolence, consider a trial of psychostimulant (e.g., methylphenidate)

Administration of the opioid on a fixed schedule is preferred when pain is persistent or frequently recurring. Given the high prevalence of breakthrough pain, however, the coadministration of a short-acting drug along with a long-acting baseline regimen—a technique called "rescue" dosing—is common practice (9). An oral rescue dose can be prescribed every two hours "as needed," at a dose equal to 5% to 15% of the total daily opioid consumption.

Among the approaches that may be used to manage the patient with poor response to an opioid trial is a switch of the opioid, or so-called "opioid rotation." When patients are switched from one opioid to another, the dose of the new drug is calculated based on well-accepted equianalgesic doses (45) (Table 13.5). The calculated dose of the new drug is reduced to account for incomplete cross-tolerance and individual variation. With two exceptions, a reduction in dose by 25% to 50% is typical practice. A safety factor has already been built into the conversion to transdermal fentanyl, and the dose of this formulation is usually not reduced. When converting to methadone, the dose should be reduced by 75% to 90% because of the possibility of a greater-than-expected potency from this drug.

Management of Side Effects. The most common opioid side effects during long-term therapy are constipation and cognitive impairment. Effective side effect management is a fundamental aspect of opioid therapy (46) (Table 13.6), and may improve the quality of analgesia and the likelihood of treatment adherence.

Patients who experience poor responsiveness during titration of an opioid may also become more responsive if the treatment-limiting toxicity can be addressed.

MANAGEMENT OF OTHER SYMPTOMS AND DISORDERS RELATED TO CANCER

Fatigue

The pathophysiology of cancer-related fatigue, or asthenia, presumably varies with the etiology. Proposed mechanisms include abnormalities in energy metabolism related to increased requirements (e.g., due to tumor growth, infection, fever, or surgery); decreased availability of metabolic substrate (e.g., due to anemia, hypoxemia, or poor nutrition); or the abnormal production of substances that impair metabolism or normal functioning of muscles (e.g., cytokines or antibodies). Other proposed mechanisms link fatigue to the pathophysiology of sleep disorders and major depression. There is no clear evidence in support of any of these mechanisms, and further research is needed.

In some cases, evaluation of the cancer patient with fatigue reveals one or more potentially treatable etiologies (Table 13.7). The interventions to address these conditions are diverse,

TABLE 13.7

POTENTIAL ETIOLOGIES OF CANCER-RELATED FATIGUE

Directly related to the disease

Related to antineoplastic therapy
  Radiotherapy
  Chemotherapy
  Immunotherapy
  Surgery

Related to metabolic or other disorders
  Anemia
  Electrolyte disturbances
  Malnutrition
  Infection
  Cardiopulmonary disorders
  Renal disorders
  Hepatic disorders
  Neuromuscular disorders

Related to the use of centrally acting drugs

Related to mood disorder
  Depression
  Anxiety

Related to sleep disorder

Related to other symptoms
  Pain

Related to immobility and deconditioning

and the decision to pursue one or another must be based on a case-by-case analysis of the feasibility, risks and benefits, goals of care, and other factors. Some of these interventions may be relatively simple (e.g., eliminating nonessential centrally acting drugs or using a hypnotic to improve sleep), indicated for physiological reasons (e.g., correction of metabolic disturbances or anemia), or likely to independently benefit quality of life (e.g., treatment of depression or pain).

In addition to the treatment of potential etiologies, a variety of symptomatic therapies can be considered. Among the pharmacologic approaches, the corticosteroids and the psychostimulants (methylphenidate, modafinil, and dextroamphetamine) are usually tried first. Nonpharmacologic symptomatic therapies include education in sleep hygiene, stress reduction, and regular exercise.

Chronic Nausea

Persistent nausea may be a consequence of the tumor, various antineoplastic therapies, or any of a large number of comorbid conditions. It may be highly distressing in itself and contribute to anorexia and weight loss. In the absence of controlled trials comparing various therapies for the persistent nausea, treatment is empirical (46). The pathophysiology of nausea is presumably complex. It may be caused by direct stimulation of the chemoreceptor trigger zone located in the floor of the fourth ventricle, activation of afferent nerves emanating from the gastrointestinal tract, sensitization of the vestibular-labyrinthine system, cortical mechanisms (e.g., anxiety or learned responses), and other processes (47). Gastroparesis may be suspected if the patient complains of early satiety or postprandial nausea, and vestibular-related nausea is suspected if vertigo is present or nausea is worsened by movement.

Although the mechanisms responsible for the antiemetic efficacy of corticosteroids are unclear and may be multiple,

these drugs are clearly beneficial for some patients and are typically tried in the context of advanced illness. Most patients with opioid-induced nausea respond promptly to drugs that are active at the chemoreceptor trigger zone. A dopamine antagonist, such as prochlorperazine or haloperidol, is a reasonable initial therapy. Refractory nausea or nausea related to chemotherapy can be treated with a 5-HT$_3$ antagonist, such as ondansetron, granisetron, or dolasetron. Based on limited observations, olanzapine is sometimes tried in refractory cases, as is the commercially available cannabinoid, dronabinol.

Patients with postprandial nausea should be considered for a trial of a prokinetic drug, such as metoclopramide. A proton pump inhibitor is often added. Nausea that is associated with vertigo or movement may be alleviated by an anticholinergic (e.g., scopolamine), an antihistamine (e.g., meclizine or promethazine), or a benzodiazepine (e.g., lorazepam).

Dyspepsia

Dyspepsia is a syndrome that encompasses a range of upper gastrointestinal (GI) symptoms, with upper abdominal pain being the most common feature. Dyspepsia can be classified by etiology into three distinct types: acid-related disease of the upper GI tract, gastric/duodenal dysmotility, and esophageal dysmotility (48). Causes of dyspepsia in patients with advanced cancer may include the disease process itself (e.g., gastric carcinoma, gastrinoma, or paraneoplastic autonomic neuropathy resulting in gastroparesis), a medical or surgical treatment (e.g., radiotherapy-induced, partial gastrectomy, or use of anti-inflammatory agents), or comorbid conditions (e.g., mucosal damage from candidiasis, reflux disease, *Helicobacter pylori*, uremia, alcoholism). Rational treatment begins with an effort to reverse the likely etiology. Dyspepsia that may be related to reflux or to NSAID treatment might respond to a proton pump inhibitor (49,50). If dysmotility is suspected, a trial of a prokinetic agent (e.g., metoclopramide) should be considered (51).

Constipation

There are many causes of constipation in the patient with cancer. The tumor itself, consequences of therapy, comorbidities that may be related or unrelated to the cancer, any of numerous constipating drugs, and poor nutrition or hydration may be involved (52). If appropriate, reversible causes should be sought and treated.

Opioid treatment often contributes to constipation. Opioids act both centrally and on mu and delta receptors in the myenteric plexus, and are also involved in the modulation of acetylcholine and vasoactive intestinal peptide (52). As a result, peristalsis is slowed and luminal secretions are reduced.

The management of opioid-induced constipation begins with prevention. Nonessential constipating drugs should be eliminated, and if possible, fluid and fiber intake should be increased. Fiber should not be given to debilitated patients or those with partial bowel obstruction because of the potential for worsening obstruction. Laxative therapy should be administered prophylactically to patients who are starting opioid therapy and have other risk factors for constipation.

There are numerous types of laxatives, including bulk-forming agents, osmotic agents, lubricants, surfactants, contact cathartics, prokinetic drugs, agents for colonic lavage, and oral opioid antagonists (52). The conventional first-line approach is a combination of a stool softener, such as docusate, and a cathartic agent, such as senna or bisacodyl. Most patients respond to this therapy. For patients who do not, lactulose (an osmotic agent) or polyethylene glycol (a lavage agent) might be considered (53). In refractory cases, a prokinetic drug such as metoclopramide can be added. In addition, oral opioid antagonist therapy can reverse opioid-induced constipation without causing systemic opioid withdrawal through local action on opioid receptors in the gut (54,55). Oral naloxone is now used occasionally for this purpose, and other compounds, including alvimopan and methylnaltrexone, are in development.

Diarrhea

The most common causes of diarrhea in the population with advanced cancer are laxative therapy and other drugs, such as antibiotics and chemotherapy agents (especially 5-flourouracil), and NSAIDs (56). Malignant intestinal obstruction and fecal impaction may cause a partial obstruction and lead to diarrhea or an alternating picture of diarrhea and constipation. Radiotherapy to the abdomen or pelvis may also cause diarrhea, with a peak incidence in the second or third week of therapy. Other causes include malabsorption, infectious gastroenteritis, and hormone-secreting tumors (52).

The management of diarrhea should include rehydration and correction of electrolyte imbalances. Treatment may be available for specific etiologies (52). For example, cholestyramine, a bile acid−binding resin, has been used for both cholagenic diarrhea and radiation-induced diarrhea (57), and aspirin has been tried in radiation-induced diarrhea (58). Pancreatin, a combination of amylase, lipase and protease, is indicated for diarrhea secondary to fat malabsorption. Metronidazole is the recommended first-line treatment for *Clostridium difficile* colitis and can be tried in patients in which diarrhea is a result of bacterial overgrowth. Cyproheptadine, a serotonin antagonist, may be useful for diarrhea due to carcinoid syndrome (59).

Most patients benefit from nonspecific treatments. These include absorbent agents (e.g., methyl cellulose, pectin, kaolin), mucosal prostaglandin inhibitors (e.g., aspirin, mesalazine, bismuth subsalicylate), and opioid agents (e.g., codeine). The somatostatin analogue, octreotide, may be considered for patients with refractory diarrhea.

Dysphagia

Cancer-related dysphagia may be related to mechanical obstruction by tumor, fibrosis following surgery or radiotherapy, postoperative disruption of normal anatomy, mucosal inflammation, drugs that cause abnormal motility or dry mouth, or an intercurrent neurologic disorder (60). Simple bedside screening examinations can be carried out by any clinician. Further examination and investigations are performed with a speech therapist specializing in swallowing disorders.

Treatment of a defined etiology may be possible in some patients. Antibiotic treatment can address presumed candidiasis or herpetic infections, and endoscopic dilatation and stenting of a mechanical obstruction may be helpful, if feasible (61). Pain related to mucositis may be treated with topical and systemic analgesics, as well as oral coating agents, including sucralfate suspension (62,63).

Anticancer treatment may be indicated for tumor-related dysphagia. External beam or intraluminal radiotherapy or, in more recent reports, chemotherapy may reduce obstruction directly (64), and dysphagia related to peritumor edema may be diminished with a corticosteroid such as dexamethasone (65).

Adjuvant Analgesics for Bowel Obstruction

Patients with malignant bowel obstruction who are not candidates for surgical decompression require intensive palliative interventions to reduce pain and other obstructive symptoms, including distention, nausea, and vomiting (66,67). Surveys of patients with far advanced disease suggest that the use of opioids, a corticosteroid, anticholinergic drugs, and the somatostatin analog octreotide can provide good symptom control for most patients, and, on occasion, a drainage percutaneous endoscopic gastroscopy may be considered (68). Of the anticholinergic drugs, scopolamine is available in a transdermal system and is often tried first. Hyoscyamine is available in a sublingual formation, and glycopyrrolate has lesser penetration through the blood−brain barrier and, therefore, may be less likely to produce central nervous system toxicity. Octreotide inhibits the secretion of gastric, pancreatic, and intestinal secretions, and reduces gastrointestinal motility. Like the anticholinergic drugs, the use of this compound in the symptomatic treatment of bowel obstruction is supported by favorable anecdotal experience (69,70).

CONCLUSION

The goal of palliative care is to assist the patient and family in their effort to maintain a good quality of life throughout the course of the illness and, if necessary, prepare well for the end of life. Pain and symptom distress is a major concern for the oncology patient and expertise in the assessment and management of common systems is an essential element in oncology practice. Other factors contribute to quality of life and should also be assessed and managed by the oncologist. Referral to specialists in palliative care may be needed to provide more comprehensive services, particularly in the setting of advanced illness. Continuing education to acquire and maintain the competencies needed to provide optimal supportive care and palliative care deserves high priority in oncology practice.

References

1. Kanner RM. The scope of the problem. In: Portenoy RK, Kanner RM, eds. *Pain Management: Theory and Practice*. Philadelphia, Pa.: FA Davis; 1996:40.
2. Vainio A, Auvinen A. Prevalence of symptoms among patients with advanced cancer: an international collaborative study. *J Pain Symptom Manage* 1996;12:3–10.
3. World Health Organization (WHO). *Cancer Pain Relief with a Guide to Opioid Availability*. 2nd ed. Geneva: WHO; 1996.
4. Portenoy RK, Thaler HT, Kornblith AB, et al. Symptom prevalence, characteristics and distress in a cancer population. *Quality Life Res* 1994;3(3):183–189.
5. Merskey H, Bogduk N, eds. *Classification of Chronic Pain: Descriptions of Chronic Pain Syndromes and Definitions of Pain Terms*. 2nd ed. Seattle, Wash.: IASP Press; 1994.
6. Saunders C. A personal therapeutic journey. *BMJ* 1996;313:1599–1601.
7. Cassell EJ. The nature of suffering and the goals of medicine. *N Engl J Med* 1982;306(11):639–645.
8. Sepulveda C, Marlin A, Yoshida T, Ullrich A. Palliative care: the World Health Organization's global perspective. *J Pain Symptom Manage* 2002;24:91–96.
9. Fine PG. Breakthrough pain. In: Bruera E, Portenoy R, eds. *Cancer Pain*. New York, NY: Cambridge University Press; 2003:408–412.
10. Cherny NI, Portenoy RK. Cancer pain: principles of assessment and syndromes. In: Wall PD, Melzack R, eds. *Textbook of Pain*. 4th ed. Edinburgh: Churchill Livingstone; 1999:1017–1064.
11. Gonzales GR, Elliott KJ, Portenoy RK, et al. The impact of a comprehensive evaluation in the management of cancer pain. *Pain* 1991;47:141–144.
12. Caraceni A, Portenoy RK. A working group of the IASP task force on cancer pain: an international survey of cancer pain characteristics and syndromes. *Pain* 1999;82:263–274.
13. Ellison NM. Palliative chemotherapy. In: Berger A, Weissman D, Portenoy RK, eds. *Principles and Practice of Supportive Oncology*. Philadelphia, Pa.: Lippincott-Raven; 2002:667.
14. Hoy AM, Lucas CF. Radiotherapy, chemotherapy and hormone therapy: treatment for pain. In: Wall P, Melzack R, eds. *Textbook of Pain*. 3rd ed. New York, NY: Churchill Livingstone; 1994:1279.
15. McIllmurray M. Palliative medicine and the treatment of cancer. In: Doyle D, Hanks GWC, Cherny NI, Calman K, eds. *Oxford Textbook*

of Palliative Medicine. 3rd ed. Oxford, UK: Oxford University Press; 2004:229.

16. Hoskin PJ, Paice P, Easton D, et al. A prospective randomized trial of 4 Gy or 8 Gy single doses in the treatment of metastatic bone pain. *Radiother Oncol* 1992;23:74–78.

17. Pereira J. Management of bone pain. In: Portenoy RK, Bruera E, eds. *Topics in Palliative Care*. New York, NY: Oxford University Press; 1998:79.

18. Fine PG. Palliative radiation therapy in end-of-life care: evidence-based utilization. *Am J Hosp Palliat Care* 2002;19:166–170.

19. Zech DFJ, Grong S, Lynch J, et al. Validation of the World Health Organization guidelines for cancer pain relief: a 10-year prospective study. *Pain* 1995;63:5–76.

20. Schug SA, Zech D, Dorr U. Cancer pain management according to WHO analgesic guidelines. *J Pain Symptom Manage* 1990;5:27–32.

21. Eisenberg E, Berkey CS, Carr DB, et al. Efficacy and safety of nonsteroidal anti-inflammatory drugs for cancer pain: a meta-analysis. *J Clin Oncol* 1994; 12:2756–2765.

22. McNicol E, Strassels S, Goudas L, et al. Nonsteroidal anti-inflammatory drugs, alone or combined with opioids, for cancer pain: a systematic review. *J Clin Oncol* 2004;22:1975–1992.

23. Mercadante S, Cassucio A, Agnello A, et al. Analgesic effects of nonsteroidal anti-inflammatory drugs in cancer pain due to somatic or visceral mechanisms. *J Pain Symptom Manage* 1999;17:351–356.

24. Mercadante S, Sapio M, Caligara M, et al. Opioid-sparing effect of diclofenac in cancer pain. *J Pain Symptom Manage* 1997;14:15–20.

25. Mercadante S, Fulfaro F, Casuccio A. A randomized controlled study on the use of anti-inflammatory drugs in patients with cancer pain on morphine therapy: effects of dose-escalation and a pharmacoeconomic analysis. *Eur J Cancer* 2002;38:1358–1363.

26. Sabino MA, Mantyh PW. Pathophysiology of bone cancer pain. *J Support Oncol* 2005;3(1):15–24.

27. Sevcik MA, Ghilardi JR, Halvorson KG, Lindsay TH, Kubota K, Mantyh PW. Analgesic efficacy of bradykinin B1 antagonists in a murine bone cancer pain model. *J Pain* 2005;6(11):771–775.

28. Sabino MAC, Ghilardi JR, Jongen LM, et al. Simultaneous reduction of cancer pain, bone destruction, and tumor growth by selective inhibition of cyclooxygenase 2. *Cancer Res* 2002;62(24):7343–7349.

29. Lussier D, Portenoy RK. Adjuvant analgesics in pain management. In: Doyle D, Hanks GWC, Cherny NI, Calman K, eds. *Oxford Textbook of Palliative Medicine*. 3rd ed. Oxford, UK: Oxford University Press; 2004:349.

30. Backonja M, Beydoun A, Edwards KR, et al. Gabapentin for the symptomatic treatment of painful neuropathy in patients with diabetes mellitus: a randomized controlled trial. *JAMA* 1998;280:1831–1836.

31. Rice ASC, Maton S. Gabapentin in postherpetic neuralgia: a randomized, double blind, placebo controlled study. *Pain* 2001;94:215–224.

32. Caraceni A, Zecca E, Marini C, et al. Gabapentin as an adjuvant to opioid analgesia for neuropathic cancer pain. *J Pain Symptom Manage* 1999; 17:441–445.

33. Caraceni A, Zecca E, Bonezzi C, et al. Gabapentin for neuropathic cancer pain: a randomized controlled trial from the Gabapentin Cancer Pain Study Group. *J Clin Oncol* 2004;22:2909–2917.

34. Bosnjak S, Jelic S, Susnjar S, et al. Gabapentin for relief of neuropathic pain related to anticancer treatment: a preliminary study. *J Chemother* 2002; 14:214–219.

35. Kalso E, Tasmuth T, Neuronen PJ. Amitriptyline effectively relieves neuropathic pain following treatment of breast cancer. *Pain* 1995;64:293.

36. Galer BS, Rowbotham MC, Perander J, et al. Topical lidocaine patch relieves postherpetic neuralgia more effectively than a vehicle topical patch: results of an enriched enrollment study. *Pain* 1999;80:533–538.

37. Gammaitoni AR, Davis MW. Pharmacokinetics and tolerability of lidocaine patch 5% with extended dosing. *Ann Pharmacother* 2002;36:236–240.

38. Ellison N, Loprinzi CL, Kugler J, et al. Phase III placebo-controlled trial of capsaicin cream in the management of surgical neuropathic pain in cancer patients. *J Clin Oncol* 1997;15:2974–2980.

39. Bloomfield DJ. Should bisphosphonates be part of the standard therapy of patients with multiple myeloma or bone metastases from other cancers? An evidence-based review. *J Clin Oncol* 1998;16:1218–1225.

40. Galer BS, Coyle N, Pasternak GW, et al. Individual variability in the response to different opioids: report of five cases. *Pain* 1992;49:87–91.

41. Ahmedzai S, Brooks O. Transdermal fentanyl versus sustained-release oral morphine in cancer pain: preference, efficacy and quality of life. *J Pain Symptom Manage* 1997;13:254–261.

42. Smith TJ, Staats PS, Stearns LJ, et al. Randomized clinical trial of an implantable drug delivery system compared with comprehensive medical management for refractory cancer pain: impact on pain, drug-related toxicity, and survival. *J Clin Oncol* 2002;19:4040–4049.

43. Christie JM, Simmonds M, Patt R, et al. A dose-titration, multicenter study of oral transmucosal fentanyl citrate (OTFC) for the treatment of breakthrough pain in cancer patients using transdermal fentanyl for persistent pain. *J Clin Oncol* 1998;16:3238–3245.

44. Weinberg OS, Inturrisi CE, Reidenberg B, et al. Sublingual absorption of selected opioid analgesics. *Clin Pharmacol Ther* 1988;44:335–342.

45. Indelicato RA, Portenoy RK. Opioid rotation in the management of refractory cancer pain. *J Clin Oncol* 2002;20:348–352.

46. Cherny N, Ripamonti C, Pereira J, et al. Strategies to manage the adverse effects of oral morphine: an evidence-based report. *J Clin Oncol* 2001;19:2542–2554.

47. Mannix K. Palliation of nausea and vomiting. In: Doyle D, Hanks G, Cherny N, Calman K, eds. *Oxford Textbook of Palliative Medicine*. 3rd ed. Oxford, UK: Oxford University Press; 2004:459–468.

48. Regnard C. Dysphagia, dyspepsia, and hiccup. In: Doyle D, Hanks G, Cherny N, Calman K, eds. *Oxford Textbook of Palliative Medicine*. 3rd ed. Oxford, UK: Oxford University Press; 2004:468–483.

49. Delaney BC, Innes MA, Deeks J, et al. Initial management strategies for dyspepsia. *Cochrane Database Syst Rev* 2002;2:CD001961.

50. Hawkey CJ, Karrasch JC, Szepanski L, et al. Omeprazole compared with misoprostol for ulcers associated with non steroidal anti inflammatory drugs. *N Engl J Med* 1998;338:727–734.

51. Twycross RG. The use of prokinetic drugs in palliative care. *Eur J Palliat Care* 1995;4:141–145.

52. Sykes N. Constipation and diarrhoea. In: Doyle D, Hanks G, Cherny NI, Calman K, eds. *Oxford Textbook of Palliative Medicine*. 3rd ed. Oxford, UK: Oxford University Press; 2004:513–525.

53. Andorsky RI, Goldner F. Colonic lavage solution (polyethylene glycol electrolyte lavage solution) as a treatment for chronic constipation: a double-blind, placebo-controlled study. *Am J Gastroenterol* 1990;85:261–265.

54. Culpepper-Morgan JA, Inturrisi CE, Portenoy RK, et al. Treatment of opioid-induced constipation with oral naloxone: a pilot study. *Clin Pharm* 1992;52:90–95.

55. Sykes NP. An investigation of the ability of oral naloxone to correct opioid-related constipation in patients with advanced cancer. *Palliat Med* 1996;10:135–144.

56. Twycross RG, Lack SA. Diarrhea. In: *Control of Alimentary Symptoms in Far Advanced Cancer*. London: Churchill Livingstone; 1986:208–229.

57. Condon JR, South M, Wolveson RL, Brinkley D. Radiation diarrhea and cholestyramine. *Postgrad Med J* 1996;54:838–839.

58. Menni AT, Dalley VM, Dinneen LC, Collier HO. Treatment of radiation-induced gastrointestinal distress with acetylsalicylate. *Lancet* 1975;ii:942–943.

59. Norton JA, Doppman JL, Jensen RT. Cancer of the endocrine system. In: DeVita VT, Hellman S, Rosenberg SA, eds. *Cancer: Principles and Practice of Oncology*. 3rd ed. Philadelphia, Pa: Lippincott; 1989:1269–1344.

60. Regnard C. Dysphagia, dyspepsia, and hiccup. In: Doyle D, Hanks G, Cherny N, Calman K, eds. *Oxford Textbook of Palliative Medicine*. 3rd ed. Oxford, UK: Oxford University Press; 2004:468–483.

61. Aste H, Munizzi F, Martines H, Pugliese V. Esophageal dilatation in malignant dysphagia. *Cancer* 1985;11:2713–2715.

62. Solomon MA. Oral sucralfate suspension for mucositis. *N Engl J Med* 1986; 314:29–32.

63. Shaiova L, Lapin J, Manco LS, et al. Tolerability and effects of two formulations of oral transmucosal fentanyl citrate (OTFC; ACTIQ) in patients with radiation-induced oral mucositis. *Support Care Cancer* 2004;12(4):268–273.

64. Brewster AE, Davidson SE, Makin WP, Stout R, Burt PA. Intraluminal brachytherapy using the high dose rate microselection in the palliation of carcinoma of the esophagus. *Clin Oncol* 1995;7:102–105.

65. Carter R, Smith JS, Anderson JR. Laser canalization versus endoscopic intubation in the palliation of malignant dysphagia: a randomized prospective study. *Br J Surg* 1992;79:1167–1170.

66. Ripamonti C. Management of bowel obstruction in advanced cancer patients. *J Pain Symptom Manage* 1994;9:193–200.

67. Fainsinger RL, Spachynski K, Hanson J, et al. Symptom control in terminally ill patients with malignant bowel obstruction (MBO). *J Pain Symptom Manage* 1994;9:12–18.

68. Mercadante S. Tolerability of continuous subcutaneous octreotide used in combination with other drugs. *J Palliat Care* 1995;4:14–16.

69. Mercadante S, Spoldi E, Caraceni A, et al. Octreotide in relieving gastrointestinal symptoms due to bowel obstruction. *Palliat Med* 1993;7: 295–299.

70. Ripamonti C, Twycross R, Baines M, et al. Clinical-practice recommendations for the management of bowel obstruction in patients with end-stage cancer. *Support Care Cancer* 2001;9:223–233.

ESOPHAGEAL CANCER

CHAPTER 14 ■ ESOPHAGEAL CANCER: EPIDEMIOLOGY, SCREENING, AND PREVENTION

EVAN S. DELLON AND NICHOLAS J. SHAHEEN

Esophageal malignancies are relatively uncommon in the United States, and because they are often diagnosed at an advanced stage, prognosis is poor. These cancers have attracted attention due to changing epidemiology, ongoing attempts to identify risk factors, and the large percentage of the population purportedly at risk for disease. This chapter focuses on the two major forms of esophageal neoplasm: squamous cell carcinoma (SCC) and adenocarcinoma of the esophagus (ACE). The epidemiologies of these diseases are reviewed, issues pertaining to screening are discussed, and strategies for prevention are presented.

EPIDEMIOLOGY

Worldwide, esophageal cancer is the eighth most common malignancy, responsible for approximately 462,000 new cases in 2002, with SCC as the most common pathological subtype (1). Although SCC was the predominant histologic form of esophageal cancer in the United States until the 1960s, the incidence of ACE has risen steadily since then (2). Various studies place the rate of increase of incidence at approximately 4% to 10% per year, with a total increase of 300% to 500% in that time frame (3–7), a rate greater than seen in any other type of cancer (Fig. 14.1). The underlying cause of this shifting epidemiologic pattern is not known, but proposed contributing factors include the current epidemic of obesity, increasing use of endoscopy leading to better detection, changing demographics of the U.S. population, alteration in the prevalence of other risk factors, and perhaps even widespread treatment of *Helicobacter pylori* (5,6). Although a rapid change in epidemiology is not suggestive of an underlying genetic etiology, host factors are also likely of importance for these neoplasms (see Chapter 15). Several analyses have assessed possible factors that might explain this increase, including misclassification bias and increasing endoscopy utilization. After controlling for numerous factors, the increasing incidence of ACE does not appear to be explained by these biases (8,9).

Despite these impressive changes in histologic subtype, the overall number of esophageal malignancies has only increased slightly in the United States because as the incidence of ACE has increased, the incidence of SCC has decreased. Overall, there were estimated to be 14,520 new cases of esophageal cancers in 2005, and esophageal cancer was responsible for 13,570 deaths (2). Although esophageal cancer was only the 19th most common cause of cancer in the United States (the most common gastrointestinal cancer was colorectal cancer, with an estimated 145,290 new cases in 2005), it was the sixth leading cause of cancer deaths in men, and the 16th cause in women. The 5-year survival rate of 14% is worse than most other malignancies, with the exception of pancreatic and hepatobiliary cancers, and has improved only trivially since the 1970s and 1980s (2,10). Of new diagnoses of esophageal cancer in the United States in 2005, more than half were ACE (compared with approximately 5% prior to 1970); the majority of the remainder of cancers were SCC (3,4,6,11). Risk factors and other issues pertaining to these cancers are discussed in separate sections of this chapter. Other uncommon benign and malignant neoplasms of the esophagus comprise less than 7% of all esophageal tumors (12); several of these are discussed in Chapter 16.

Risk Factors for Squamous Cell Carcinoma of the Esophagus

Geographic

There are multiple well-established risk factors for esophageal SCC (Table 14.1). Worldwide, there is a marked discrepancy in incidence by geographic region (1,13). For example, in the United States and several Western European countries, rates are relatively low (1–5 cases per 100,000). In contrast, in parts of Asia, India, and Africa, the rates can be substantially higher (50–200 cases per 100,000). Although a particular geographic area may be a proxy for genetic or environmental factors, a person's country of origin may nonetheless be helpful in stratifying risk.

Demographic

Similar to other cancers of the digestive tract, the incidence of SCC of the esophagus increases with age, and the mean age of diagnosis is in the seventh and eighth decades of life (14). Males are two to four times more likely to be affected by SCC than females, and African Americans have four to five times the risk of Caucasians (3,15). The risk for other nonwhite ethnic minorities has not been well delineated. Poor socioeconomic status is also independently associated with increased risk of SCC of the esophagus (15).

Tobacco and Alcohol

Multiple studies have found that exposure to tobacco and alcohol is strongly associated with an increased risk of SCC in a dose-dependent manner, and when present together, the risk increases synergistically (16–23). For both substances, relative risk increases are in the 2- to 10-fold range, but some reports

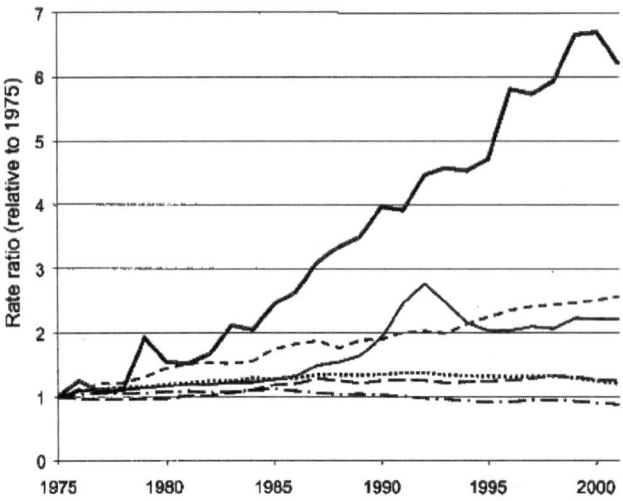

FIGURE 14.1. Comparison of relative rates of increase of esophageal adenocarcinoma (*solid black line*) and other malignancies in the United States. Short dashed line—melanoma, line—prostate cancer, dashed line—breast cancer, dotted line—lung cancer, dashes and dotted line—colorectal cancer. *Source:* From Pohl H, Welch HG. The role of over-diagnosis and reclassification in the marked increase of esophageal adenocarcinoma incidence. *J Natl Cancer Inst* 2005;97:142–146, with permission.

find increases in risk of up to 25-fold. In addition, although some studies suggest that the type of alcohol, such as hard liquor, may be more significant (16,19), others suggest that the total quantity of alcohol ingested is the most important factor (22). Interestingly, head and neck cancers, which are also associated with tobacco and alcohol use, demonstrate an association with esophageal SCC (24).

TABLE 14.1

RISK FACTORS FOR SQUAMOUS CELL CARCINOMA AND ADENOCARCINOMA OF THE ESOPHAGUS

Squamous cell carcinoma	Adenocarcinoma
Geographic location	Geographic location
Demographic	Demographic
■ Increasing age	■ Increasing age
■ Male	■ Male
■ African American	■ White
■ Low socioeconomic status	
Environmental	Environmental
■ Tobacco	■ Obesity
■ Alcohol	■ Tobacco
■ Few fruits and vegetables	■ Cholecystectomy
■ Low selenium	Increased acid exposure (GERD, medications)
■ Low zinc	
■ Vitamin deficiency (A, C, E, B₁₂, folate, riboflavin)	Barrett esophagus
Other	
■ Achalasia	
■ Caustic injury	
■ Radiation	
Plummer-Vinson syndrome	
Human papillomavirus	
Tylosis palmaris	

GERD, gastroesophageal reflux disease.

Diet and Nutrition

Dietary factors may explain some of the wide geographic variation in the incidence of esophageal SCC. Foods that contain N-nitrosamines are associated with increasing rates of SCC of the esophagus (25,26). These may not only cause direct toxicity to esophageal mucosa but may also injure DNA over time. Chronic chewing of the Betel nut, a practice in Asia, has been associated with increased SCC (27), as has the Iranian custom of drinking very hot beverages (28). General malnutrition; deficiencies of selenium and zinc; and deficiencies of vitamins A, C, E, folate, riboflavin, and B12 have also been associated with esophageal SCC (29–35).

Nonmalignant Esophageal Disease

Underlying disease processes of the esophagus can predispose to cancer. It has been well established that over time, patients with achalasia have between a 15- and 30-fold increased risk of developing SCC of the esophagus (36–38). The mechanism of this association is not understood. In addition, caustic ingestions (e.g., of lye) have been shown to increase the risk of esophageal SCC (39,40). Radiation exposure, either environmental or medical (41–43); Plummer-Vinson syndrome (44); and Zenker diverticula (45) have also been associated with SCC.

Infections

Human papillomavirus has been implicated as an oncogenic factor in SCC of the cervical and anal epithelium. Similarly, it may be associated with SCC of the esophagus (46,47).

Other

Tylosis palmaris is a rare autosomal dominant condition characterized by hyperkeratosis of the palms and soles. Patients with this disorder are at high risk for development of esophageal SCC (48,49). Because rates have been reported as high as 50% at the age of 45 and 95% at the age of 65, the American Society for Gastrointestinal Endoscopy recommends that patients with this condition be screened with upper endoscopy starting at age 30 (50,51).

Risk Factors for Adenocarcinoma of the Esophagus

Demographic

The risk factors for ACE are distinct from those for esophageal SCC (Table 14.1). Although increasing age, with a mean onset in the seventh and eighth decades of life, and a male predominance are similar to SCC of the esophagus, the demographic similarities end there (3–7,11). In general, ACE is approximately five times more common in Caucasians than in African Americans, and the association with socioeconomic status seen in SCC is not found in ACE. However, regional variation of ACE in the United States has been described (52). In addition, there does not appear to be a strong heritability, although host factors likely do play a role (53,54).

Obesity

Numerous studies have found that increasing obesity, as measured by body mass index, is a risk factor not only for acid reflux and Barrett esophagus but also for development of ACE (55–58). Further exploration of this relationship suggests that central or visceral obesity may modulate this effect.

Acid Exposure

As both a pathogenic mechanism and a risk factor, increased acid exposure is well recognized to play a role in ACE. Chronic gastroesophageal reflux disease (GERD) has been shown to increase the risk of ACE both in case-control studies and in a recent meta-analysis (59–62). Although this is an important risk factor, it has been shown that approximately 40% to 50% of patients diagnosed with ACE do not have pre-existing reflux symptoms (59,60). Similar to associations seen in GERD, data suggest that medications such as nitrates, aminophylline, anticholinergics, and benzodiazepines, which lower the tone of the lower esophageal sphincter, may be linked to ACE (63,64). Finally, *H. pylori* does not appear to be an independent risk factor; in fact, some data suggest that *H. pylori* infection may actually be protective against the development of ACE.

Barrett Esophagus

Barrett esophagus (BE) remains the most significant and widely studied risk factor for ACE. Initially described in the 1950s (65), BE is defined today by a combination of endoscopic and histologic findings. Suspected on endoscopy as tongues of salmon-colored mucosa in the distal esophagus that replace the normal squamous esophagus epithelium and displace the Z-line cephalad from the gastroesophageal junction, the diagnosis is confirmed by demonstrating specialized (or intestinalized) metaplasia with the presence of goblet cells on histologic examination (66,67). It is believed that the majority of adenocarcinomas arise in areas with Barrett mucosa, and that there is likely a pathway by which metaplasia progresses first to dysplasia, and then to carcinoma (68–71) (see Chapter 15). BE may be a response to chronic mucosal injury from GERD (72) and may also be associated with intra-abdominal obesity (73). GERD has also been linked to BE in numerous studies (74–77). However, new data demonstrate that many subjects do not have GERD symptoms but are found to have BE (78–81). Although environmental factors may interact with host factors to generate BE, specific genes have yet to be identified, and BE does not appear to have a strong heritable component (71).

The presence of BE independently increases the risk of developing ACE between 30 and 400 times (82–87), although a more accurate estimate is believed to be in the 30 to 60 range (11). The rate of progression from BE to ACE has been estimated in many investigations, and recent meta-analyses suggest that the rate of progression to cancer is approximately 0.5% per year (71,88). However, the risk is significantly higher in dysplastic BE. For example, in high-grade dysplasia (HGD) the rate can be 10% to 30% per year (69,71,89,90). In addition, surgical series show that in patients who undergo esophagectomy for HGD, there is a high rate of metachronous, previously undetected cancers in the resected specimen (70,91). But there is not an inexorable progression from BE to ACE. Several natural history and treatment trials show spontaneous regression from BE to normal squamous epithelium in some cases, as well as from HGD to low-grade dysplasia (LGD) and LGD to nondysplastic BE (72,92,93). Although this apparent regression may be partially explained by sampling error from diagnostic biopsy protocols (94), resolution of BE and/or dysplasia in some patients has been repeatedly demonstrated and is likely a true phenomenon. Finally, although BE is a strong risk factor for ACE, the presence of BE has not been definitively shown to increase mortality (95–98). Indeed, several studies have shown that patients with BE have the same life expectancy as those subjects without BE, and that, in many cases, even if BE progresses to esophageal AC, the eventual cause of death is not related to the cancer (97–99). Because ACE is a disease of the elderly, comorbidities can accumulate and compete with cancer as a cause of death in these subjects.

Other

In addition to BE, there are several other risk factors that might predispose to ACE. Smoking appears to elevate risk, although this increase is less impressive than seen with esophageal SCC, and some reports in the literature do not demonstrate an association (100–102). Alcohol has not consistently been shown to be a risk factor for either BE or ACE (102). Finally, one study reports an association with cholecystectomy and ACE (103), but this finding has yet to be replicated.

Clinical Presentation and Diagnosis

Unless incidentally identified early in its course on upper endoscopy performed for screening or for other gastrointestinal (GI)-related symptoms, both esophageal SCC and AC tend to present at an advanced stage (104). Symptoms are generally related to local growth and invasion. Patients can note dysphagia, odynophagia, food impaction or regurgitation of just-swallowed food, early satiety, weight loss, fatigue, malaise, poor appetite, chest pain, nausea, vomiting, or GI bleeding symptoms.

Diagnosis can be made by barium swallow, but in most cases it is now made during upper endoscopy. Endoscopic ultrasound can be used to effectively stage the tumor. These issues are discussed in more depth in Chapter 18.

SCREENING

Although esophageal malignancies are uncommon compared with many other tumors, their poor prognosis and disappointing response to treatment make the possibility of screening for the cancers attractive. For esophageal SCC in the United States, the incidence is too low and the population at risk too poorly defined to justify routine screening programs; however, in areas of the world with very high rates of SCC, population-based programs have been used (51). In the United States, two commonly used indications for screening for SCC are tylosis palmaris and caustic ingestion (50,51). In addition, screening might be justified in long-standing achalasia (38).

In contrast, screening for ACE is a widespread practice in the United States (105). The rising incidence of ACE, the large pool of identifiable at-risk individuals (patients with GERD), and the recognizable premalignant lesion (BE) have all raised enthusiasm for endoscopic screening and surveillance for ACE in this country. However, several logistical and theoretical issues suggest that endoscopic screening and surveillance as it is currently practiced in the United States is likely to be minimally effective (106,107). Most of the debate focuses around using esophagogastroduodenoscopy (EGD), an invasive test, to diagnosis BE; reliable serum biomarkers have yet to be developed for screening purposes. The two major U.S. GI societies have issued somewhat conflicting statements regarding screening upper endoscopy in the setting of heartburn symptoms. The American College of Gastroenterology notes that "patients with chronic GERD symptoms are those most likely to have Barrett's esophagus and should undergo upper endoscopy" (66). Those patients found to have BE would then be enrolled in endoscopic surveillance programs, in which periodic endoscopic examinations and biopsies are performed to allow early detection of HGD and/or cancer. The American Gastroenterological Association, however, convened an international panel of experts in the field to review the available evidence regarding endoscopic screening. This group concluded that current evidence did not support endoscopic screening for those with chronic heartburn symptoms (67).

Although endoscopic screening for BE and ACE is appealing, multiple difficulties plague the process. First, even though many risk factors are known for both BE and ACE, it remains difficult to isolate the population at high enough risk to warrant endoscopic screening. Also, if patients with GERD are to be the target screening group, then the 40% to 50% of cases of ACE that arise in patients with no history of GERD will be missed (59,60,107). There are also data to suggest that not all cancers may arise from Barrett mucosa (95) and that not all upper endoscopies identify BE, even when it is present (95,96), so the negative predictive value of EGD may be unacceptably low. Second, despite a clear definition of the criteria required for diagnosing BE, errors in interpretation of biopsy specimens are common (108,109). There can be endoscopic false positives due to improper techniques of either visualization or biopsy. If the GE junction is not appropriately identified, such as in a hiatal hernia, then biopsies of the gastric cardia may be inadvertently taken and labeled as esophagus. Furthermore, variability exists in pathological diagnosis of metaplasia. There is good interobserver reliability for distinguishing normal mucosa from either HGD or carcinoma, but relatively moderate correlation for separating normal mucosa from LDG, or even HDG from adenocarcinoma (89,110,111). Third, and probably most important, outcomes data for screening are lacking. There has never been a randomized controlled trial showing decreased mortality as a result of a screening program. Some data are suggestive of a benefit from endoscopic screening and surveillance (112–114), but these data are derived from retrospective trials where lead time and other biases can be introduced (71). Similarly, some data suggest that endoscopic screening programs may be cost effective, but these decision analyses are based on several poorly described assumptions, and sensitivity analysis suggests that the results may not be robust (115,116). Finally, although upper endoscopy is a safe test, when applied to an enormous screening population, serious complications due to its use may be greater than the number of incident ACEs identified (71,107,117). For these reasons, the current evidence does not support widespread endoscopic screening for BE and ACE. However, changes in potential screening techniques (e.g., with noninvasive testing or biomarkers, or better identification of at-risk individuals) may affect the calculus for screening in the future.

PREVENTION

Because endoscopic screening for esophageal cancer may not be currently practical, strategies for prevention of these malignancies have been considered. There are little data on risk factor modification for primary prevention. Once a premalignant lesion such as BE has developed, secondary strategies have been used to attempt to prevent progression to ACE. Possibilities include endoscopic surveillance, ablative techniques, and chemoprevention.

Risk Factor Modification

Risk factor modification can be used for both SCC and ACE. Several of the known risk factors outlined previously are amenable to intervention. Cessation of tobacco use and abstinence from alcohol can be recommended for all patients. Weight loss programs can be prescribed. Consumption of diets high in fruits, vegetables, and fiber can be encouraged. Although these measures make good sense in practice, in theory it is difficult for patients to make long-term lifestyle changes, particularly for a relatively uncommon and possibly asymptomatic condition. The data on efficacy of these strategies are limited (118–120). In patients with reflux symptoms, routine

testing and treatment of *H. pylori* is not warranted because some data suggest that this micro-organism may be protective against the development of dysplasia (121–123).

Endoscopic Surveillance

For patients who are diagnosed with BE, American College of Gastroenterology guidelines suggest intermittent endoscopic surveillance to monitor for development of ACE and to assess for progression from metaplasia to dysplasia (66,67). In this setting, biopsies are obtained according to a set protocol, usually using jumbo forceps every 2 cm and in four quadrants in the involved esophagus (Fig. 14.2) (124). For nondysplastic BE, a 3-year interval between studies is suggested. Patients with LGD are recommended to have annual endoscopic surveillance, whereas patients with HGD may require endoscopy as frequently as every 3 months. Some evidence does suggest that surveillance may decrease incidence of ACE (92,95,112–114). In these series, incident cancers are diagnosed at earlier stages than historical or matched controls not participating in surveillance programs. Despite concerns of lead time and length bias, many investigators cite these results as indirect evidence that surveillance is effective. As with endoscopic screening of subjects with GERD for BE, no prospective randomized data substantiate endoscopic surveillance practices in prevalent BE cases.

Ablative Techniques

Rather than intermittently surveying the esophagus, are there techniques to ablate Barrett epithelium? There are multiple strategies that have been studied for ablation, but no definitive comparative trials demonstrate the superiority of one modality over another. Because of the relatively low risk of progression to cancer from nondysplastic BE and LGD, ablative techniques are generally reserved for HGD or early ACE, or for patients who cannot, or do not want to, undergo esophagectomy.

Thermal therapies studied include electrocoagulation (both catheter and balloon guided), various lasers modalities, and argon beam plasma coagulation (125–130). However, there is building evidence, including a recent randomized control trial of photodynamic therapy (PDT) in patients with HGD (91), to support PDT as an effective thermal ablative technique (131–133). The principle is that when a photosensitizing chemical

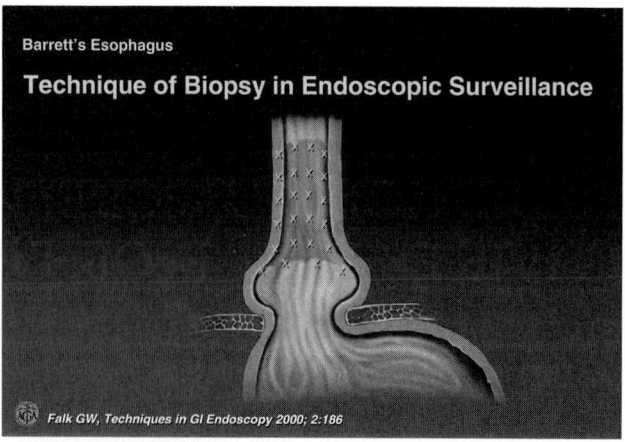

FIGURE 14.2. Surveillance biopsy protocol in Barrett esophagus (BE). Note that biopsies are obtained in each of the four quadrants at 2-cm intervals in the segment of esophagus with BE. Used with permission. Copyright American Gastroenterologic Association Institute, Bethesda, MD (See also color Figure 14.2).

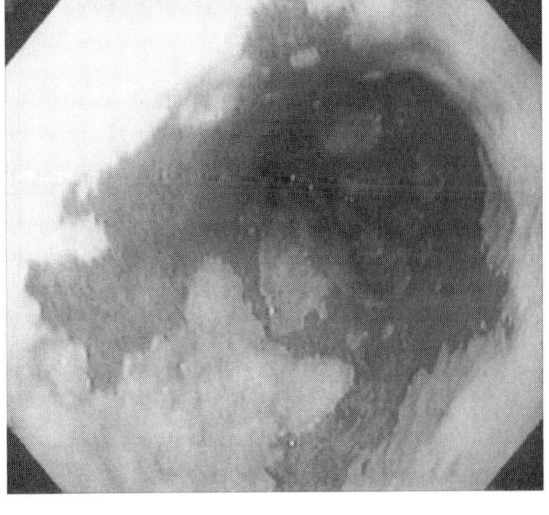

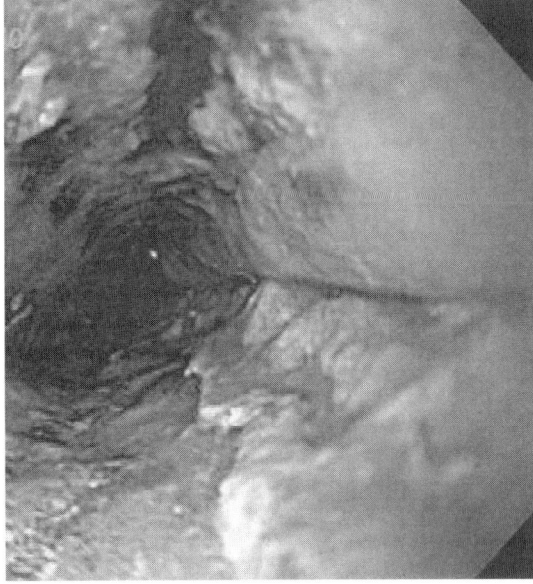

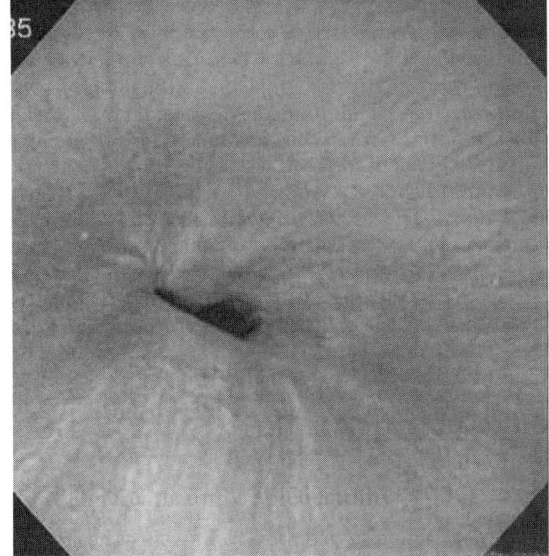

FIGURE 14.3. Photodynamic therapy for ablation of Barrett esophagus (BE). **A:** BE at baseline. **B:** The esophageal tissue injury 48 hours after the initial exposure to 630 nm light. **C:** The esophagus 4 weeks later with healing and a normal layer of esophageal squamous mucosa (See also color Figure 14.3a,b,c).

such as porfimer sodium is infused and the esophageal mucosa is exposed to light of a wavelength of 630 nm, the porfimer reacts to the light, and the resultant free oxygen radicals cause cell death and tissue injury (72). After this injury, the esophagus heals with a layer of normal squamous epithelium (Fig. 14.3). There are significant side effects to PDT, including chest pain, systemic photosensitization with a risk of severe sunburn, and stricture formation (93,131,132). Avoidance of significant sunlight exposure for the 4 to 6 weeks that the porfimer remains in the system is recommended. Esophageal strictures have been seen in 20% to 50% of patients undergoing PDT, depending on the number of treatment sessions required (134). In general, these strictures can be treated with endoscopic dilation using standard techniques. Although PDT has been approved by the U.S. Food and Drug Administration for treatment of patients with BE and HGD, its role in LGD and nondysplastic BE has not been defined, and research is ongoing.

Another approach to ablation of BE is endoscopic resection, and again there are multiple techniques available. Researchers have reported experience with endoscopic mucosal resection (EMR) using various devices (135–137). Here, saline is injected to separate the mucosa from the submucosa, and a snare is used to resect the abnormal area. This technique has been modified in several ways. In one version, a specialized EMR cap is placed on the tip of the endoscope, and an area of mucosa up to 2 cm in diameter can be removed at once (138). In another version, a device similar to that used for variceal band ligation is used to resect areas of the mucosa (139). With these techniques, Barrett mucosa may be removed, although problems with stricture formation have been reported if large areas of mucosa are resected at once (140).

Inherent in all ablative techniques is the assumption that the Barrett mucosa will be removed in a durable fashion with normal squamous epithelium regrowing in its place. However, this assumption may not always hold. Patients undergoing protocolized surveillance and biopsies after ablation did indeed show endoscopic healing, but in rare cases biopsies revealed either intact, but buried, subsquamous Barrett glands or, worse, incident ACEs under what appeared to be normal mucosa (141–143). This phenomenon, now referred to as buried glands or buried cancer, casts a cautionary light on ablative therapy, and indicates the continued need for close endoscopic follow-up with biopsies in patients who undergo ablation.

Chemoprevention

There is a developing body of literature addressing the issue of chemoprevention, the use of medications to attempt to alter the natural history of BE and ACE. Several studies and one

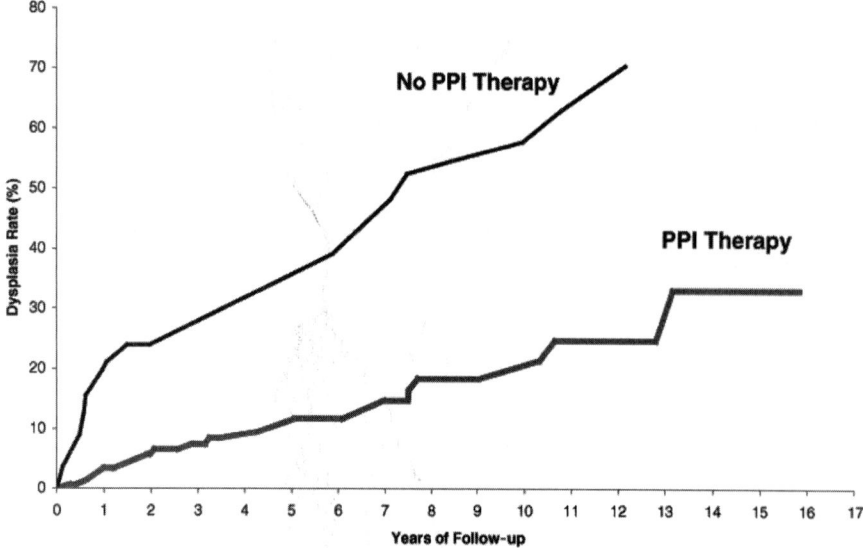

FIGURE 14.4. Decreased dysplasia in Barrett esophagus with use of proton pump inhibitors (PPIs). *Source:* From El Serag HB, Aguirre TV, Davis S, et al. Proton pump inhibitors are associated with reduced incidence of dysplasia in Barrett's esophagus. *Am J Gastroenterol* 2004;99:1877–1883.

recent meta-analysis have demonstrated that the use of non-steroidal anti-inflammatory medications (NSAIDs) can decrease the risk of BE and ACE (144–150), but none of these studies have yet proven causality. Some clinicians have proposed giving NSAIDs routinely as chemoprevention in the setting of BE. No randomized controlled trial of chemoprevention of ACE with NSAIDS has been published. In addition, it is unknown at what point in the pathogenesis of ACE that NSAIDs may exert their effect, and if their primary effect is to halt the metaplasia from squamous to columnar tissue (as opposed to retarding the development of dysplasia in already metaplastic tissue), such therapy would be useless in those subjects who already harbor BE. Finally, these medications can have serious adverse effects. For these reasons, routine use of NSAIDs in the setting of BE is currently not supported.

Similarly, recent prospective data have shown that the long-term proton pump inhibitor (PPI) use appears to lower the rate of dysplasia in BE (Fig. 14.4) (151–154). Although there are no direct data to suggest that PPIs prevent ACE, most experts would now recommend that given the favorable side effect and safety profiles of these medications, patients with BE should be treated with PPIs (72), although the degree of acid suppression needed for optimal result remains open to debate.

CONCLUSION

This chapter reviews the epidemiology and discusses screening and prevention strategies for the two major forms of esophageal neoplasm: SCC and adenocarcinoma. SCC is the most common esophageal malignancy worldwide. In the United States, the incidence of ACE has been increasing faster than any other cancer, and ACE is now more common than SCC. The reasons for this change in epidemiology are not fully understood, but proposed contributing factors include the current epidemic of obesity, increasing use of endoscopy leading to better detection, and changing demographics of the U.S. population. Despite these evolving trends, esophageal malignancies are still relatively uncommon compared with other GI neoplasms such as colon cancer. In the United States, the incidence of SCC is too low and the population at risk too poorly defined to justify screening programs. Screening for ACE and BE is a widespread practice in the United States, but this remains a controversial area. It is believed that the current available evidence does not support routine screening for ACE. Risk factor modification is the primary preventative strategy for SCC, and it can

also be applied to ACE. Endoscopic ablative techniques appear to have utility in preventing ACE, particularly when dysplasia is detected in areas of Barrett mucosa. Patients with BE are also placed in endoscopic surveillance programs. Although the role of PDT for thermal ablation continues to evolve, chemoprevention with NSAIDs is not routinely recommended. Most experts do use PPIs in patients with BE because these agents are well tolerated over the long term. Given the number of unanswered questions in this field, continuing research will likely provide new insight and alter clinical practice in the coming years.

References

1. Parkin DM, Bray F, Ferlay J, Pisani P. Global cancer statistics 2002. *CA Cancer J Clin* 2005;55:74–108.
2. Jemal A, Murray T, Ward E, et al. Cancer statistics, 2005. *CA Cancer J Clin* 2005;55:10–30.
3. Yang PC, Davis S. Incidence of cancer of the esophagus in the US by histologic type. *Cancer* 1988;61:612–617.
4. Blot WJ, Devesa SS, Kneller RW, et al. Rising incidence of adenocarcinoma of the esophagus and gastric cardia. *JAMA* 1991;265:1287–1289.
5. Daly JM, Karnell LH, Menck HR. National cancer database report on esophageal carcinoma. *Cancer* 1996;78:1820–1828.
6. Devesa SS, Blot WJ, Fraumeni JF. Changing patterns in the incidence of esophageal and gastric carcinoma in the United States. *Cancer* 1998;83:2049–2053.
7. Bytzer P, Christensen PB, Damiker P, et al. Adenocarcinoma of the esophagus and Barrett's esophagus: a population-based study. *Am J Gastroenterol* 1999;94:86–91.
8. Corley DA, Kubo A. Influence of site classification on cancer incidence rates: an analysis of gastric cardia carcinomas. *J Natl Cancer Inst* 2004;96:1383–1387.
9. Pohl H, Welch HG. The role of overdiagnosis and reclassification in the marked increase of esophageal adenocarcinoma incidence. *J Natl Cancer Inst* 2005;97:142–146.
10. Eloubeidi MA, Mason AC, Desmond RA, El-Serag HB. Temporal trends (1973–1997) in survival of patients with esophageal adenocarcinoma in the United States: a glimmer of hope? *Am J Gastroenterol* 2003;98:1627–1633.
11. Lagergren J. Adenocarcinoma of oesophagus: what exactly is the size of the problem and who is at risk? *Gut* 2005;54:1–5.
12. Daly JM, Fry WA, Little AG, et al. Esophageal cancer: results of an American College of Surgeons Patient Care Evaluation Study. *J Am Coll Surg* 2000;190:562–572.
13. Parkin DM, Laara E, Muir CS. Estimates of the world-wide frequency of sixteen major cancers in 1980. *Int J Cancer* 1988;41:184–197.
14. Engel LS, Chow WH, Vaughan TL, et al. Population attributable risks of esophageal and gastric cancers. *J Natl Cancer Inst* 2003;95:1404–1413.
15. Gammon MD, Schoenberg JB, Ahsan H, et al. Tobacco, alcohol, and socioeconomic status and adenocarcinomas of the esophagus and gastric cardia. *J Natl Cancer Inst* 1997;89:1277–1284.

16. Pottern LM, Morris LE, Blot WJ, et al. Esophageal cancer among black men in Washington, D.C. I. Alcohol, tobacco, and other risk factors. *J Natl Cancer Inst* 1981;67:777–783.

17. Burch PR. Esophageal cancer in relation to cigarette and alcohol consumption. *J Chronic Dis* 1984;37:793–814.

18. La Vecchia C, Liati P, Decarli A, et al. Tar yields of cigarettes and the risk of oesophageal cancer. *Int J Cancer* 1986;38:381–385.

19. Brown LM, Blot WJ, Schuman SH, et al. Environmental factors and high risk of esophageal cancer among men in coastal South Carolina. *J Natl Cancer Inst* 1988;80:1620–1625.

20. Yu MC, Garabrant DH, Peters JM, et al. Tobacco, alcohol, diet, occupation, and carcinoma of the esophagus. *Cancer Res* 1988;48:3843–3848.

21. Thun MJ, Peto R, Lopez AD, et al. Alcohol consumption and mortality among middle-aged and elderly U.S. adults. *N Engl J Med* 1997;337:1705–1714.

22. Brown LM, Hoover R, Gridely G, et al. Drinking practices and risk of squamous-cell esophageal cancer among black and white men in the United States. *Cancer Causes Control* 1997;8:605–609.

23. Hori H, Kawano T, Endo M, et al. Genetic polymorphisms of tobacco- and alcohol-related metabolizing enzymes and human esophageal squamous cell carcinoma susceptibility. *J Clin Gastroenterol* 1997;25:568–575.

24. Abemayor E, Moore DM, Hanson DG. Identification of synchronous esophageal tumors in patients with head and neck cancer. *J Surg Oncol* 1988;38:94–96.

25. Siddiqi M, Tricker AR, Preussmann R. The occurrence of preformed N-nitroso compounds in food samples from a high risk area of esophageal cancer in Kashmir, India. *Cancer Lett* 1988;39:37–43.

26. Pickwell SM, Schimelpfening S, Palinkas LA. "Betelmania." Betel quid chewing by Cambodian women in the United States and its potential health effects. *West J Med* 1994;160:326–331.

27. Lu SH, Montesano R, Zhang MS, et al. Relevance of N-nitrosamines to esophageal cancer in China. *J Cell Physiol* 1986;4(suppl):51–58.

28. Ghadirian P. Thermal irritation and esophageal cancer in northern Iran. *Cancer* 1987;60:1909–1914.

29. Ziegler RG, Morris LE, Blot WJ, Pottern LM, Hoover R, Fraumeni JF. Esophageal cancer among black men in Washington, D.C. II. Role of nutrition. *J Natl Cancer Inst* 1981;67:1199–1206.

30. Mark SD, Qiao YL, Dawsey SM, et al. Prospective study of serum selenium levels and incident esophageal and gastric cancers. *J Natl Cancer Inst* 2000;92:1753–1763.

31. Blot WJ, Li JY, Taylor PR, et al. Nutrition intervention trials in Linxian, China: supplementation with specific vitamin/mineral combinations, cancer incidence, and disease-specific mortality in the general population. *J Natl Cancer Inst* 1993;85:1483–1492.

32. Abnet CC, Lai B, Qiao YL, et al. Zinc concentration in esophageal biopsy specimens measured by x-ray fluorescence and esophageal cancer risk. *J Natl Cancer Inst* 2005;97:301–306.

33. Chen LH, Boissonneault GA, Glauert HP. Vitamin C, vitamin E, and cancer. *Anticancer Res* 1988;8:739–748.

34. Santhi Swaroop V, Damle SR, Advani SH, et al. Nutrition and esophageal cancer. *Semin Surg Oncol* 1989;5:370–373.

35. Thurnham D, Rathakette P, Hambridge K, et al. Riboflavin, vitamin A, and zinc status in Chinese subjects in a high-risk area of oesophageal cancer in China. *Hum Nutr Clin Nutr* 1982;36C:337–349.

36. Chuong JJ, Dubovik S, McCallum RW. Achalasia as a risk factor for esophageal carcinoma: a reappraisal. *Dig Dis Sci* 1984;29:1105–1108.

37. Meijssen MA, Tilanus HW, van Blankenstein M, et al. Achalasia complicated by oesophageal squamous cell carcinoma: a prospective study in 195 patients. *Gut* 1992;33:155–158.

38. Sandler RS, Nyren O, Ekbom A, et al. The risk of esophageal cancer in patients with achalasia: a population-based study. *JAMA* 1995;274:1359–1362.

39. Appelqvist P, Salmo M. Lye corrosion carcinoma of the esophagus: a review of 63 cases. *Cancer* 1980;45:2655–2658.

40. Isolauri J, Markkula H. Lye ingestion and carcinoma of the esophagus. *Acta Chir Scand* 1989;155:269–271.

41. Beebe GW, Kato H, Land CE. Studies of the mortality of A-bomb survivors. 6. Mortality and radiation dose, 1950–1974. *Radiat Res* 1978;75:138–201.

42. Gofman TE, McKeen EA, Curtis RE, et al. Esophageal carcinoma following irradiation for breast cancer. *Cancer* 1983;52:1808–1809.

43. Ogino T, Kato H, Tsukiyama I, et al. Radiation-induced carcinoma of the esophagus. *Acata Oncol* 1992;31:475–477.

44. Larsson LG, Sandstrom A, Westling P. Relationship of Plummer-Vinson disease to cancer of the upper alimentary tract in Sweden. *Cancer Res* 1975;35:3308–3316.

45. Huang BS, Unni KK, Payne WS. Long-term survival following diverticulectomy for cancer in pharyngoesophageal (Zenker's) diverticulum. *Ann Thorac Surg* 1984;38:207–210.

46. Chang F, Syrjanen S, Shen Q, et al. Human papillomavirus involvement in esophageal carcinogenesis in the high-incidence area of China: a study of 700 cases by screening and type-specific in situ hybridization. *Scand J Gastroenterol* 2000;35:123–130.

47. Togwa K, Jaskiewica K, Takahashi H, et al. Human papilloma virus DNA sequences in esophageal squamous cell carcinoma. *Gastroenterology* 1994;107:128–136.

48. Iwaya T, Maesawa C, Ogasawara S, et al. Tylosis esophageal cancer locus on chromosome 17q25.1 is commonly deleted in sporadic esophageal cancer. *Gastroenterology* 1998;114:1206–1210.

49. Harper PS, Harper RM, Howel-Evans AW. Carcinoma of the oesophagus with tylosis. *Q J Med* 1970;39:317–333.

50. American Society for Gastrointestinal Endoscopy. The role of endoscopy in the surveillance of premalignant conditions of the upper gastrointestinal tract. *Gastrointest Endosc* 1998;48:663–668.

51. Brown A, Shaheen N. Screening for upper gastrointestinal tract malignancies. *Semin Oncol* 2004;31:487–497.

52. Kubo A, Corley DA. Marked regional variation in adenocarcinomas of the esophagus and the gastric cardia in the United States. *Cancer* 2002;95:2096–2102.

53. Chak A, Lee T, Kinnard MF. Familial aggregation of Barrett's oesophagus, oesophageal carcinoma, and oesophageal junctional adenocarcinoma in Caucasian adults. *Gut* 2002;51:323–328.

54. Dhillon PK, Farrow DC, Vaughan TL, et al. Family history of cancer and risk of esophageal and gastric cancers in the United States. *Int J Cancer* 2001;93:148–152.

55. Lagergren J, Bergstrom R, Nyren O, et al. Association between body mass and adenocarcinoma of the esophagus and gastric cardia. *Ann Intern Med* 1999;130:883–890.

56. Brown LM, Swanson CA, Gridley G, et al. Adenocarcinoma of the esophagus: role of obesity and diet. *J Natl Cancer Inst* 1995;87:104–109.

57. Chow WH, Blot WJ, Vaughan TL, et al. Body mass index and the risk of adenocarcinoma of the esophagus and gastric cardia. *J Natl Cancer Inst* 1998;90:150–155.

58. Wu AH, Wan P, Bernstein L. A multiethnic population-based study of smoking, alcohol and body size and risk of adenocarcinomas of the stomach and esophagus (United States). *Cancer Causes Control* 2001;12:721–732.

59. Lagergren J, Bergstrom R, Lindren A, et al. Symptomatic gastroesophageal reflux as a risk factor for esophageal adenocarcinoma. *N Engl J Med* 1999;340:825–831.

60. Farrow DC, Vaughan TL, Sweeny C, et al. Gastroesophageal reflux disease, use of H2 receptor antagonists, and risk of esophageal and gastric cancer. *Cancer Causes Control* 2000;11:231–238.

61. Ye W, Chow WH, Lagergren J, et al. Risk of adenocarcinomas of the esophagus and gastric cardia in patients with gastroesophageal reflux diseases and after antireflux surgery. *Gastroenterology* 2001;121:1286–1293.

62. Hampel H, Abraham NS, El-Serag HB. Meta-analysis: obesity and the risk for gastroesophageal reflux disease and its complications. *Ann Intern Med* 2005;143:199–211.

63. Lagergren J, Bergstrom R, Adami HO, et al. Association between medications that relax the lower esophageal sphincter and risk for esophageal adenocarcinoma. *Ann Intern Med* 2000;133:165–175.

64. Vaughan TL, Farrow DC, Hansten PD, et al. Risk of esophageal and gastric adenocarcinomas in relation to use of calcium channel blockers, asthma drugs, and other medications that promote gastroesophageal reflux. *Cancer Epidemiol Biomarkers Prev* 1998;7:749–756.

65. Barrett NR. The oesophagus lined by columnar epithelium. *Gastroenterologia* 1956;86:183–186.

66. Sampliner RE, Practice Parameters Committee of the American College of Gastroenterology. Updated guidelines for the diagnosis, surveillance, and therapy of Barrett's esophagus. *Am J Gastroenterol* 2002;97:1888–1895.

67. Sharma P, McQuaid K, Dent J, et al. A critical review of the diagnosis and management of Barrett's esophagus: the AGA Chicago workshop. *Gastroenterology* 2004;127:310–330.

68. Hameeteman W, Tytgat GNJ, Houthoff HJ, et al. Barrett's esophagus: development of dysplasia and adenocarcinoma. *Gastroenterology* 1989;96:1249–1256.

69. Miros M, Kerlin P, Walker N. Only patients with dysplasia progress to adenocarcinoma in Barrett's oesophagus. *Gut* 1991;32:1441–1446.

70. Cameron AJ, Carpenter HA. Barrett's esophagus, high-grade dysplasia, and early adenocarcinoma: a pathological study. *Am J Gastroenterol* 1997;92:586–591.

71. Shaheen N, Ransohoff DF. Gastroesophageal reflux, Barrett esophagus, and esophageal cancer: scientific review. *JAMA* 2002;287:1972–1981.

72. Shaheen NJ. Advances in Barrett's esophagus and esophageal adenocarcinoma. *Gastroenterology* 2005;128:1544–1566.

73. El-Serag HB. Kvapil P, Hacken-Bitar J, Kramer JR. Abdominal obesity and the risk of Barrett's esophagus. *Am J Gastroenterol* 2005;100:2151–2156.

74. Romero, Y, Cameron AJ, Schnaid DJ, et al. Barrett's esophagus: prevalence in symptomatic relatives. *Am J Gastroenterol* 2002;97:1127–1132.

75. Lieberman DA, Oehlke M, Helfand M. Risk factors for Barrett's esophagus in community-based practice—GORGE consortium. *Am J Gastroenterol* 1997;92:1293–1297.

76. Eisen GM, Sandler RS, Murray S, et al. The relationship between gastroesophageal reflux disease and its complications with Barrett's esophagus. *Am J Gastroenterol* 1997;92:27–31.

77. Avidan B, Sonnenberg A, Schnell TG, et al. Hiatal hernia size, Barrett's length, and severity of acid reflux are all risk factors for esophageal adenocarcinoma. *Am J Gastroenterol* 2002;97:1930–1936.

78. Conio M, Filiberti R, Blanchi S, et al. Risk factors for Barrett's esophagus: a case-control study. *Int J Cancer* 2002;97:225–229.

79. Gerson LB, Shetler K, Triadafilopoulous G. Prevalence of Barrett's esophagus in asymptomatic individuals. *Gastroenterology* 2002;123:461–467.

80. Rex DK, Cummings OW, Shaw M, et al. Screening for Barrett's esophagus in colonoscopy patients with and without heartburn. *Gastroenterology* 2003;125:1670–1677.

81. DeVault KR, Ward EM, Wolfsen HC, et al. Barrett's esophagus is common in older patients undergoing screening colonoscopy regardless of gastroesophageal reflux symptoms [abstract]. *Gastroenterology* 2004;126(suppl 2):680A.

82. Cameron AJ, Ott BJ, Payne WS, et al. The incidence of adenocarcinoma in columnar-lined (Barrett's) esophagus. *N Engl J Med* 1985;313:857–858.

83. Rosenberg JC, Budev H, Edwards RC, et al. Analysis of adenocarcinoma in Barrett's esophagus utilizing a staging system. *Cancer* 1985;55:1353–1360.

84. Van Der Veen AH, Dees J, Blankenstein JD, et al. Adenocarcinoma in Barrett's oesophagus: an overstated risk. *Gut* 1989;30:14–18.

85. Drewitz DJ, Sampliner RE, Garewal HS. The incidence of adenocarcinoma in Barrett's esophagus: a prospective study of 170 patients followed 4.8 years. *Am J Gastroenterol* 1997;92:212–215.

86. O'Connor JB, Falk GW, Richter JE. The incidence of adenocarcinoma and dysplasia in Barrett's esophagus: report of the Cleveland Clinic Barrett's Esophagus Registry. *Am J Gastroenterol* 1999;94:2037–2042.

87. Conio M, Blanchi S, Lapertosa G, et al. Long-term endoscopic surveillance of patients with Barrett's esophagus: incidence of dysplasia and adenocarcinoma: a prospective study. *Am J Gastroenterol* 2003;98:1931–1939.

88. Shaheen NJ, Crosby MA, Bozymsky EM, Sandler RS. Is there publication bias in the reporting of cancer risk in Barrett's esophagus? *Gastroenterology* 2000;119:333–338.

89. Reid BJ, Haggitt RC, Rubin CE, et al. Observer variation in the diagnosis of dysplasia in Barrett's esophagus. *Hum Pathol* 1988;19:166–178.

90. Buttar NS, Wang KK, Sebo TJ, et al. Extent of high-grade dysplasia in Barrett's esophagus correlates with risk of adenocarcinoma. *Gastroenterology* 2001;120:1630–1639.

91. Heitmiller RF, Redmond M, Hamilton SR, et al. Barrett's esophagus with high-grade dysplasia: an indication for prophylactic esophagectomy. *Ann Surg* 1996;224:66–71.

92. Schnell TG, Sontag SJ, Chejfec G, et al. Long-term nonsurgical management of Barrett's esophagus with high-grade dysplasia. *Gastroenterology* 2001;120:1607–1619.

93. Overholt BF, Lightdale CJ, Wang KK, et al. Photodynamic therapy with porfimer sodium for ablation of high-grade dysplasia in Barrett's esophagus: international, partially blinded, randomized phase III trial. *Gastrointest Endosc* 2005;62:488–498.

94. Falk GW, Rice TW, Goldblum JR, Richter JE. Jumbo biopsy forceps protocol still misses unsuspected cancer in Barrett's esophagus with high-grade dysplasia. *Gastrointest Endosc* 1999;49:170–176.

95. Corley DA, Levin TR, Habel LA, et al. Surveillance and survival in Barrett's adenocarcinomas: a population-based study. *Gastroenterology* 2002;122:633–640.

96. Dulai GS, Guha S, Kahn KL, et al. Preoperative prevalence of Barrett's esophagus in esophageal adenocarcinoma: a systematic review. *Gastroenterology* 2002;122:26–33.

97. Eckardt VF, Kanzler G, Bernhard G. Life expectancy and cancer risk in patients with Barrett's esophagus: a prospective controlled investigation. *Am J Med* 2001;111:33–37.

98. Anderson LA, Murray LJ, Murphy SJ, et al. Mortality in Barrett's oesophagus: results from a population based study. *Gut* 2003;52:1081–1084.

99. van der Burgh A, Dees J, Hop WC, et al. Oesophageal cancer is an uncommon cause of death in patients with Barrett's oesophagus. *Gut* 1996;39:5–8.

100. Zhang ZF, Kurtz RC, Sun M, et al. Adenocarcinomas of the esophagus and gastric cardia: medical conditions, tobacco, alcohol, and socioeconomic factors. *Cancer Epidemiol Biomarkers Prev* 1996;5:761–768.

101. Gray MR, Donnelly RJ, Kingsnorth AN. The role of smoking and alcohol in metaplasia and cancer risk in Barrett's columnar line oesophagus. *Gut* 1993;34:727–731.

102. Brown LM, Silverman DT, Pottern LM, et al. Adenocarcinoma of the esophagus and esophagogastric junction in white men in the United States: alcohol, tobacco, and socioeconomic factors. *Cancer Causes Control* 1994;5:333–340.

103. Freedman J, Ye W, Naslund E, et al. Association between cholecystectomy and adenocarcinoma of the esophagus. *Gastroenterology* 2001;121:548–553.

104. Enzinger PC, Mayer RJ. Esophageal cancer. *N Engl J Med* 2003;349:2241–2252.

105. Falk GW, Ours TM, Richter JE. Practice patterns for surveillance of Barrett's esophagus in the United States. *Gastrointest Endosc* 2000;52:197–203.

106. Shaheen NJ, Provenzale D, Sandler RS. Upper endoscopy as a screening and surveillance tool in esophageal adenocarcinoma: a review of the evidence. *Am J Gastroenterol* 2002;97:1319–1327.

107. Dellon ES, Shaheen NJ. Does Screening for Barrett's esophagus and adenocarcinoma of the esophagus prolong survival? *J Clin Oncol* 2005;23:4478–4482.

108. Sharma P. Prevalence of Barrett's oesophagus and metaplasia at the gastro-oesophageal junction. *Aliment Pharmacol Ther* 2004;20(suppl 5):48–54.

109. Armstrong D. Towards consistency in the endoscopic diagnosis of Barrett's oesophagus and columnar metaplasia. *Aliment Pharmacol Ther* 2004;20(suppl 5):40–47.

110. Ormsby AH, Petras RE, Henricks WH, et al. Observer variation in the diagnosis of superficial oesophageal adenocarcinoma. *Gut* 2002;51:671–676.

111. Montgomery E, Goldblum JR, Greenson JK, et al. Dysplasia as a predictive marker for invasive carcinoma in Barrett esophagus: a follow-up study based on 138 cases from a diagnostic variability study. *Hum Pathol* 2001;32:379–388.

112. Peters JH, Clark GW, Ireland AP, et al. Outcome of adenocarcinoma arising in Barrett's esophagus in endoscopically surveyed and nonsurveyed patients. *J Thorac Cardiovasc Surg* 1994;108:813–821.

113. van Sandick JW, van Lanschot JJ, Kuiken BW, et al. Impact of endoscopic biopsy surveillance of Barrett's oesophagus on pathological stage and clinical outcome of Barrett's carcinoma. *Gut* 1998;43:216–222.

114. Eloubeidi MA, Mason AC, Desmond RA, et al. Temporal trends (1973–1997) in survival of patients with esophageal adenocarcinoma in the United States: a glimmer of hope? *Am J Gastroenterol* 2003;98:1627–1633.

115. Soni A, Sampliner RE, Sonnenberg A. Screening for high-grade dysplasia in gastroesophageal reflux disease: is it cost effective? *Am J Gastroenterol* 2000;95:2086–2093.

116. Inadomi JM, Sampliner R, Lagergren J, et al. Screening and surveillance for Barrett Esophagus in high-risk groups: a cost-utility analysis. *Ann Intern Med* 2003;138:176–186.

117. Eisen GM, Baron TH, Dominitz JA, et al. Complications of upper GI endoscopy. *Gastrointest Endosc* 2002;55:784–793.

118. Mayne ST, Risch HA, Dubrow R, et al. Nutrient intake and risk of subtypes of esophageal and gastric cancer. *Cancer Epidemiol Biomarkers Prev* 2001;10:1055–1062.

119. Terry P, Lagergren J, Hansen H, et al. Inverse association between intake of cereal fiber and risk of gastric cardia cancer. *Gastroenterology* 2001;120:387–391.

120. Terry P, Lagergren J, Ye W, et al. Fruit and vegetable consumption in the prevention of esophageal and cardia cancers. *Eur J Cancer Prev* 2001;10:365–369.

121. Chow WH, Blaser MJ, Blot WJ, et al. An inverse relation between cagA+ strains of *Helicobacter pylori* infection and risk of esophageal and gastric cardia adenocarcinoma. *Cancer Res* 1998;58:588–590.

122. Weston AP, Badr AS, Topalovski M, et al. Prospective evaluation of the prevalence of gastric *Helicobacter pylori* infection in patients with GERD, Barrett's esophagus, Barrett's dysplasia, and Barrett's adenocarcinoma. *Am J Gastroenterol* 2000;95:387–394.

123. Ye W, Held M, Lagergren J, et al. *Helicobacter pylori* infection and gastric atrophy: risk of adenocarcinoma and squamous cell carcinoma of the esophagus and gastric cardiac adenocarcinoma. *J Natl Cancer Inst* 2004;96:388–396.

124. Reid BJ, Blount PL, Feng Z, Levine DS. Optimizing endoscopic biopsy detection of early cancers in Barrett's high-grade dysplasia. *Am J Gastroenterol* 2000;95:3089–3096.

125. Barham CP, Jones RL, Biddlestone LR, et al. Photothermal laser ablation of Barrett's oesophagus: endoscopic and histological evidence of squamous re-epithelialisation. *Gut* 1997;41:281–284.

126. McCarthy M, Wilkinson ML. Treatment of Barrett's esophagus by endoscopic laser ablation and antireflux surgery. *Gastrointest Endosc* 1999;49:129–130.

127. Dumoulin FL, Terjung B, Neubrand M, et al. Treatment of Barrett's epithelium by endoscopic argon plasma coagulation. *Endoscopy* 1997;29:751–753.

128. Attwood SE, Lewis CJ, Caplin S, et al. Argon beam plasma coagulation as therapy for high-grade dysplasia in Barrett's esophagus. *Clin Gastroenterol Hepatol* 2003;1:258–263.

129. Weston AP, Sharma P. Neodymium:yttrium-aluminum garnet contact laser ablation of Barrett's high grade dysplasia and early adenocarcinoma. *Am J Gastroenterol* 2002;97:2998–3006.

130. Ganz RA, Utley DS, Stern RA, et al. Complete ablation of esophageal epithelium with a balloon-based bipolar electrode: a phased evaluation in the porcine and in the human esophagus. *Gastrointest Endosc* 2004;60:1002–1010.

131. Panjehpour M, Overhold BF, Haydek JM, et al. Results of photodynamic therapy for ablation of dysplasia and early cancer in Barrett's esophagus and effect of oral steroids on stricture formation. *Am J Gastroenterol* 2000;95:2177–2184.

132. Overholt BF, Panjehpour M, Haydek JM, et al. Results of photodynamic therapy for Barrett's esophagus: follow-up in 100 patients. *Gastrointest Endosc* 1999;49:1–7.

133. Shaheen NJ, Inadomi JM, Overholt BF, Sharma P. What is the best management strategy for high grade dysplasia in Barrett's oesophagus? A cost effectiveness analysis. *Gut* 2004;53:1736–1744.

134. Panjehpour M, Overholt BF, Phan MN, Haydek JM. Optimization of light dosimetry for photodynamic therapy of Barrett's esophagus: efficacy vs.incidence of stricture after treatment. *Gastrointest Endosc* 2005;61:13–18.

135. Van Laethem JL, Peny MO, Salmon I, et al. Intramucosal adenocarcinoma arising under squamous re-epithelialisation of Barrett's oesophagus. *Gut* 2000;46:574–577.

136. Macey N, Le Dreau G, Volant A, et al. Adenocarcinoma of the esophagogastric junction arising after endoscopic laser photocoagulation ablation of the short segment of Barrett's esophagus. *Gastroenterol Clin Biol* 2001;25:204–206.

137. Shand A, Dallal H, Palmer K, et al. Adenocarcinoma arising in columnar lined oesophagus following treatment with argon plasma coagulation. *Gut* 2001;48:580–581.

138. Nijhawan PK, Wang KK. Endoscopic mucosal resection for lesions with endoscopic features suggestive of malignancy and high-grade dysplasia within Barrett's esophagus. *Gastrointest Endosc* 2000;52:328–332.

139. Ell C, May A, Gossner L, et al. Endoscopic mucosal resection of early cancer and high-grade dysplasia in Barrett's esophagus. *Gastroenterology* 2000;118:670–677.

140. Seewald S, Akaraviputh T, Seitz U, et al. Circumferential EMR and complete removal of Barrett's epithelium: a new approach to management of Barrett's esophagus containing high-grade intraepithelial neoplasia and intramucosal carcinoma. *Gastrointest Endosc* 2003;57:854–859.

141. Harada M, Nagashima R, Takeda H, Takahashi T. Endoscopic resection of adenocarcinoma arising in a tongue of Barrett's esophagus. *Gastrointest Endosc* 2000;52:427–429.

142. Nwakakwa V, Fleischer D. Endoscopic mucosal resection of the esophagus: band ligation technique. *Gastrointest Endosc Clin N Am* 2001;11:479–488.

143. Seewald S, Akaraviputh T, Seitz U. Circumferential EMR and complete removal of Barrett's epithelium: a new approach to management of Barrett's esophagus containing high-grade intraepithelial neoplasia and intramucosal carcinoma. *Gastrointest Endosc* 2003;57:854–859.

144. Thun MJ, Namboodiri MM, Calle EE, et al. Aspirin and risk of fatal cancer. *Cancer Res* 1993;53:1322–1327.

145. Funkhouser EM, Sharp GB. Aspirin and reduced risk of esophageal carcinoma. *Cancer* 1995;76:1116–1119.

146. Farrow DC, Vaughan TL, Hansten PD, et al. Use of aspirin and other nonsteroidal anti-inflammatory drugs and risk of esophageal and gastric cancer. *Cancer Epidemiol Biomarkers Prev* 1998;7:97–102.

147. Corely DA, Kerlikowske K, Verma R, et al. Protective association of aspirin/NSAIDs and esophageal cancer: a systematic review and meta-analysis. *Gastroenterology* 2003;124:47–56.

148. Sonnenberg A, Fennerty MB. Medical decision analysis of chemoprevention against esophageal adenocarcinoma. *Gastroenterology* 2003;124:1758–1766,

149. Gammon MD, Terry MB, Arber N, et al. Nonsteroidal anti-inflammatory drug use associated with reduced incidence of adenocarcinomas of the esophagus and gastric cardia that overexpress cyclin D1: a population-based study. *Cancer Epidemiol Biomarkers Prev* 2004;13:34–39.

150. Hur C, Nishioka NS, Gazelle GS. Cost-effectiveness of aspirin chemoprevention for Barrett's esophagus. *J Natl Cancer Inst* 2004;96:316–325.

151. Sharma P, Sampliner RE, Camargo E. Normalization of esophageal pH with high-dose proton pump inhibitor therapy does note results in regression of Barrett's esophagus. *Am J Gastroenterol* 1997;92:582–585.

152. Peters FT, Ganesh S, Kuipers EJ, et al. Endoscopic regression of Barrett's oesophagus during omeprazole treatment: a randomized double blind study. *Gut* 1999;45:489–494.

153. Hillman LC, Chiragakis L, Shadbolt B, et al. Proton-pump inhibitor therapy and the development of dysplasia in patients with Barrett's esophagus. *Med J Aust* 2004;180:387–391.

154. El Serag HB, Aguirre TV, Davis S, et al. Proton pump inhibitors are associated with reduced incidence of dysplasia in Barrett's esophagus. *Am J Gastroenterol* 2004;99:1877–1883.

CHAPTER 15 ■ THE MOLECULAR GENETICS OF ESOPHAGEAL CANCER

JAMES P. HAMILTON AND STEPHEN J. MELTZER

INTRODUCTION

Esophageal cancer (EC) is the eighth most common malignancy and the sixth most common cause of cancer death in the world (1). Worldwide, esophageal squamous cell cancer (ESCC) remains the most common histologic type of EC (1). However, since the 1960s, the incidence of esophageal adenocarcinoma (EAC) in the United States has risen from 300% to 500% (2). Therefore, intensive efforts have been underway since the 1990s to improve the molecular understanding of this deadly disease, with the hope that this knowledge will translate into earlier detection and more effective treatments.

Many studies of EC biology have included ESCC and EAC together. In some respects, these two histologic subtypes share biological features; however, in many other ways, they are distinct entities. A large body of information has accumulated regarding the molecular genetic pathophysiology of both EAC and ESCC. Increasingly, attention has focused on a transition from purely descriptive to translational research so that molecular genetic findings may be applied clinically. The molecular genetic events in EC in general follow the classic colon cancer paradigm. That is, the development of cancer is accompanied by cumulative alterations in proto-oncogenes, tumor suppressor genes, and, to a much lesser extent, DNA mismatch repair genes. In addition, recent discoveries implicate tumor suppressor gene inactivation by promoter region hypermethylation in esophageal tumorigenesis. This chapter describes molecular biology germane to both histologic subtypes of EC and also addresses the current potential of translational research in this area.

FAMILIAL ESOPHAGEAL CARCINOMA

Genetic Predisposition of Esophageal Squamous Cell Carcinoma

Although there is a genetic basis for pathogenesis of the sporadic form of ESCC, genetic predisposition appears to be rare (3). Tylosis is a rare autosomal dominant disease characterized by diffuse hyperkeratosis of the squamous epithelium of the esophagus, palms of the hands, and soles of the feet, and is associated with a high incidence of SCC (4). Also known as *keratosis palmaris et plantaris*, this syndrome may also present with oral leukokeratosis and follicular hyperkeratosis (5). The early dermatologic manifestations usually begin between 7 and 8 years of age, and Howel-Evans et al. are credited with the ini-

tial observation that these patients develop EC at an early age (average age 45 years) (6). The disease locus, termed the *tylosis oesophageal cancer (TOC)* locus, has been mapped to chromosome band 17q25 by linkage analyses (7). Thus, a target gene locus of potential importance in sporadic ESCC has been unearthed, in keeping with the principle that genes mutated in familial syndromes are also implicated in sporadic forms of the same cancer (8). Iwaya et al. reported frequent loss of heterozygosity (LOH) on chromosome arm 17q using 20 microsatellite markers from the *TOC* locus in ESCC. They observed LOH within the region of the TOC locus in 33 of 52 informative cases (63%) (8). However, despite these findings, research until recently was unable to identify the culpable gene (9). At the time of this writing, however, a group from the University of Liverpool, led by John K. Field and Janet M. Risk, appears to have identified a promising candidate gene at 17q25, cytoglobin, which is downregulated and transallelically repressed in TOC (10).

The Shanxi Province in north-central China has among the highest rates of ESCC in the world (11). Studies have shown a strong tendency toward familial aggregation in this high-risk area, suggesting a potential genetic mechanism of carcinogenesis (12). Researchers have identified a high degree of genetic instability in the early precursor lesions of ESCC in patients from this region (13). In particular, germline mutations of BRCA2 in patients from this high-risk area of China are more frequent in ESCC patients who have a positive family history of ESCC (9 of 78, 12%) than in those without a family history of ESCC (0 of 48, 0%; $p = 0.013$) (14). In addition, GSTM1 (glutathione S-transferase) deletions were found to be a predisposing risk factor (OR 1.91, 95% CI 1.03–3.81) for ESCC development in Chinese patients who smoked tobacco, drank alcohol, and had a positive family history of EC (15). It should be noted that these GSTM1 deletions represent constitutive (i.e., germline) polymorphisms, rather than acquired (i.e., somatic) events that occur during tumorigenesis. The GSTM1 gene product is a metabolic enzyme that can detoxify a number of reactive electrophilic compounds, including carcinogenic polyaromatic hydrocarbons, and polymorphisms of this gene have been implicated in the pathogenesis of multiple human cancers (16). GSTM1 deletions have also been described in Indian, French, and Brazilian patients who smoked tobacco and had ESCC (17–19).

Genetic Predisposition of Adenocarcinoma of the Esophagus

A familial form of EAC has been described in the setting of families with increased gastroesophageal reflux. There are case reports of families in which multiple members are affected by gastroesophageal reflux disease (GERD), Barrett esophagus (BE), and EAC (20–22). Pedigree analysis suggests an autosomal dominant inheritance, with variable degrees of penetrance (23). Thus far, the only report of a susceptibility locus (at chromosome 13q14) was identified in a kindred of patients with pediatric esophageal reflux, and the incidence of BE or EAC in these patients was not known (24).

SPORADIC ESOPHAGEAL CARCINOMA

Etiologic Factors of Esophageal Squamous Cell Carcinoma

ESCC is one of the leading causes of cancer mortality in men, particularly among African Americans (3). Tobacco smoking and excessive alcohol intake constitute the largest risk factors for the development of ESCC in North America and Western Europe (25,26). In certain high-risk regions, such as the Henan Province of China, northern Iran, southern Turkey, and northern Africa, dietary factors may represent additional major determinants of carcinoma risk (3).

The pathogenesis of sporadic ESCC is driven largely by these environmental factors; this topic has been reviewed in depth elsewhere (27). Underscoring the importance of environmental factors is the fact that seven of eight ESCCs in an American pedigree with tylosis occurred in smokers, which suggests that even in the presence of familial genetic predisposition, environmental triggers are necessary for tumorigenesis (28).

Additional risk factors for ESCC are achalasia, Plummer-Vinson syndrome (dysphagia, iron deficiency, and esophageal webs), caustic injury to the esophagus, a history of head and neck cancer, a history of breast cancer treated with radiotherapy, and poverty (27).

Etiologic Factors of Adenocarcinoma

BE is the most important precursor condition to sporadic EAC (29–31). BE results from long-standing GERD. Patients with weekly reflux symptoms are at greatest risk for developing both BE and EAC (27,32). Risk factors for GERD (and therefore BE and EAC) are obesity, decreased lower esophageal sphincter pressure, and the presence of a hiatal hernia (27,33). In addition, scleroderma is a condition characterized by diminished lower esophageal pressure and complicated by BE and an increased likelihood of EAC (34). Patients with BE have a 2% to 5% lifetime risk of developing EAC (35).

In addition to reflux of gastric acid per se, there is some evidence suggesting that reflux of alkaline small bowel contents may contribute to metaplastic transformation of the esophagus (36). The controversy surrounding the relative clinical importance of alkaline reflux has not been resolved. Some authors suggest that alkaline reflux is a minor contributor, whereas others believe that the mixture of gastric and duodenal contents may cause synergistic damage to the esophageal epithelium (37). In one study of patients who received gastric surgery for benign peptic ulcers, no increased incidence of BE was found, suggesting that bile reflux alone is not sufficient to produce a metaplastic change in the distal esophagus (38).

GENETICS AND EPIGENETICS OF ESOPHAGEAL CANCER

Gene Promoter Hypermethylation in Esophageal Cancer

In recent years, promoter hypermethylation–associated inactivation of gene expression has been demonstrated for a number of tumor suppressor genes in neoplasia, and has created a paradigm shift in the understanding of the molecular pathogenesis of EC and cancer in general. Genes frequently methylated in cancer include, but are not limited to, adenomatous polyposis coli (APC), tissue inhibitor of metalloproteinase 3 (TIMP3), p16 (CDKN2A), p15 (CDKNB), retinoblastoma (RB1), E-cadherin (CDH1), GSTP1, and O^6-methylguanine-DNA methyltransferase (MGMT) (39–43). A host of genes found to be abnormally methylated in EC are shown in Table 15.1. The mutL homolog 1 (MLH1) mismatch repair gene promoter is often hypermethylated in cancers with high frequencies of mismatch repair deficiency, such as colorectal, endometrial, and gastric cancers (42,44–46). In fact, some of the best evidence for promoter hypermethylation as a direct cause of diminished gene expression derives from the study of MLH1 in repair-proficient and -deficient colorectal cancer cells (47). Colorectal cancer cells defective in DNA mismatch repair and known to be hypermethylated at MLH1 were demethylated with 5-azacytidine. Not only did this demethylation restore expression of MLH1, but the return of effective DNA repair was also documented (47). The precise mechanism whereby promoter hypermethylation inhibits gene expression is not well understood. One theory asserts that promoter methylation facilitates histone deacetylation, thereby altering the DNA ultrastructure so that transcription factor binding is inhibited (48).

This additional putative mechanism of gene inactivation in cancer has resulted in a dramatic shift in the understanding of molecular alterations. Now, in addition to mutation and deletion, a third epigenetic mechanism is understood to account for the silencing of genes in cancer. Loci harboring tumor suppressor genes in any cancer need not undergo accompanying mutations, but rather become hypermethylated at one or both alleles to explain diminished or silenced expression. Previous studies suggesting the role of a known gene contained within a particular locus frequently deleted in a given cancer can now be extended to investigate hypermethylation of its target gene promoter within the specific locus.

This approach has already been successfully applied to the study of CDKN2A in EC. As previously stated, the CDKN2A locus at 9p21 is frequently deleted but is infrequently mutated in EC. Reports of frequent CDKN2A hypermethylation in EC have been forthcoming (49,50). In addition, it appears that hypermethylation of multiple genes is an early, easily detectable abnormality that predicts which patients progress from Barrett metaplasia to develop high-grade dysplasia or adenocarcinoma (51,52). However, future research is needed to fully validate methylation biomarkers before they are clinically applicable.

Aneuploidy in Esophageal Squamous Cell Cancer

The first genetic abnormalities to be described in EC were aneuploidy and abnormal chromosome complement. Aneuploidy refers to abnormal DNA content and encompasses both structural and numerical DNA abnormalities. Aneuploidy does not correlate with any single mutation but reflects widespread

TABLE 15.1

HYPERMETHYLATED GENES IN ESOPHAGEAL CANCER[a]

Gene	NE	D	ESCC	BE	BE-D	EAC	References
APC	6.3	—	50	80	89	70	(40,51,182,183,220)
CDH1	17	—	70	10	0	70	(40,183,184,201,221,222)
DAPK	5.6	—	—	—	—	20	(183,184)
GSTP1	0	—	—	0	0	5	(40,184)
MLH1	0	—	—	0	0	12	(40,184,223)
HPP1	3	—	—	44	—	68	(51,178,223)
MGMT	21	—	39	43	89	59	(40,51,183,224)
CDK2AP2	0	—	18	4	0	0	(40,51,220,225–227)
CDKN2B	3	—	13	12	0	4.5	(40,225,227)
CDKN2A	1.3	71	56	20	43	45	(40,51,183,184,220,221,225,228–231)
RARβ	25	58	63	—	—	—	(232,233)
RASSF1A	3.7	—	51	—	—	—	(184,234,235)
RUNX3	0.8	—	—	25	—	48	(51,178,184)
TIMP3	4.8	—	—	60	78	56	(40,51,178,183)
RPRM	0	—	13	36	64	63	(236)

NE, normal esophagus; D, dysplasia; ESCC, esophageal squamous cell carcinoma; BE, Barrett esophagus; BE-D, Barrett esophagus with dysplasia; EAC, esophageal adenocarcinoma.
[a]Numbers represent the median value of reported prevalence and are expressed as a percentage.
Adapted from Sato F, Meltzer SJ. CpG island hypermethylation in progression of esophageal and gastric cancer. *Cancer* 2006;106:484.

DNA changes due to genomic instability (53). Abnormal DNA content has been detected in ESCC and its precursor lesion, squamous dysplasia (54,55). Aneuploidy occurs in 84% to 94% of ESCCs (54–57). The prevalence of aneuploidy in squamous dysplasia and carcinoma in situ has been reported at 22% to 28% (55). Aneuploidy also occurs in histologically normal mucosa adjacent to aneuploid tumors and is believed to represent increased potential for malignant transformation in response to environmental stimuli, such as cigarette smoke and alcohol (56). However, the reported prevalence of aneuploidy in normal mucosa varies widely, and brings into question the histologic classification of mucosa in some studies (55,56). One of these studies demonstrated that the percentage of S-phase fraction tends to increase with degree of dysplasia and correlates with progression from premalignant tissue to invasive carcinoma (55). A relationship between poorly differentiated tumors and aneuploidy has also been shown (54). Knowledge of specific genetic alterations implicated in esophageal tumorigenesis has expanded in recent years, allowing the study of associations between molecular findings and aneuploidy. One study established that ESCCs with aneuploidy are more likely to have genetic alterations, including amplification of the genes v-myc myelocytomatosis viral oncogene homolog (MYC), cyclin D1 (CCND1), and epidermal growth factor receptor (EGFR); LOH of multiple tumor suppressor loci including RB1; and APC (58). This latter study suggested that aneuploidy not only may constitute a marker for large-scale genomic alterations but also may be associated with specific genetic abnormalities important in esophageal tumorigenesis.

There is a preponderance of published data associating aneuploidy with advanced stages of disease and a poor prognosis (57–59). However, a role for the testing of DNA ploidy in the clinical management of patients with ESCC remains to be established.

Aneuploidy in Esophageal Adenocarcinoma

Cellular subpopulations with aneuploidy or increased tetraploid (4N) DNA content occur within more than 90% to 95%

of EAC, arise in premalignant epithelium, and appear to predict progression (60–63). One early study suggested that alterations in ploidy correlated with dysplasia in BE, although the histologic classification of dysplasia in this report was controversial (60). In another series of patients, the presence of aneuploid cells as detected by flow cytometric analyses of histologically equivocal biopsy specimens allowed for the identification of mildly dysplastic areas. Furthermore, aneuploidy was always associated with some morphologic abnormality, varying from mild dysplasia to frank carcinoma (64). Others have found that aneuploidy and dysplasia can be discordant (31,65). In a seminal study involving DNA ploidy analysis of mapped Barrett epithelium, clonal growth similar to that seen in fully developed cancer was present in metaplastic Barrett mucosa (66). Finally, in a prospective evaluation of patients with BE who were enrolled in a rigorous endoscopic biopsy protocol, patients with neither aneuploidy nor increased 4N fractions had a 0% 5-year cumulative cancer incidence. In comparison, patients with increased 4N fractions had a 56% 5-year cancer incidence, and patients with aneuploidy had a 43% 5-year cancer incidence (67).

In summary, although the results of certain studies indicate that flow cytometry appears to be useful in detecting a subset of patients who do not have high-grade dysplasia and yet show an increased risk of progression to EAC that cannot be identified by dysplasia grade (68), no precisely defined role for the determination of tetraploidy or aneuploidy in clinical practice has yet been proven for either EAC or ESCC.

Specific Chromosomal Alterations

Karyotypic Abnormalities in Esophageal Adenocarcinoma and Esophageal Squamous Cell Cancer

Multiple studies have detected specific chromosomal alterations in BE and EAC. Diverse karyotypic abnormalities have been documented, including Y chromosome loss, trisomies, translocations of chromosomes 7 and 11, overrepresentation of chromosome 8, and loss of chromosome 17 (69–71). Similar chromosomal abnormalities were detected in ESCC (72,73). In addition, there are data indicating that DNA copy number changes on 2q, 3q, 7p, 17q, and 22q may be involved in the metastatic process of EAC (74). Furthermore, gain of chromosome 12p is indicative of a poor prognosis after esophagectomy in patients with ESCC (75). Despite these scientific advances, analysis of karyotypic abnormalities does not yet have a role in the clinical arena. For the most part, changes in the number of copies of a chromosome or a segment of a chromosome have served as a target or screening tool that researchers use to identify specific genes that may be abnormally expressed or inactivated in EC.

Proto-oncogenes in Esophageal Adenocarcinoma and Esophageal Squamous Cell Cancer

Early studies of EC focused on abnormalities in proto-oncogenes. Amplification of the genes encoding the EGFR (76,77), MYC (76,78), fibroblast growth factor 4 (FGF4) (79), fibroblast growth factor 3 (FGF3) (80), and CCND1 (81) have all been reported in esophageal tumors.

The significance of many molecular alterations in gastrointestinal cancers to some extent revolves around the cell cycle (82). For example, transitions between cell cycle phases are partially controlled by cyclins and cyclin-dependent kinases (CDKs). In EC, G_1 is perhaps the most important cell cycle phase in which molecular abnormalities have been described. Proteins implicated in EC that affect CDK-cyclin complex–mediated acceleration through G_1 include the products of the RB1 tumor suppressor gene, the CDK inhibitor CDKN2A, the TP53-inducible proapoptotic gene p21 (CDKN1A), and TP53 itself. In addition, other growth factor receptor–initiated and signaling pathways are important in esophageal tumorigenesis. These include the APC/β-catenin and EGFR/RAS/MAP (mitogen-activated protein) kinase pathways. Evidence implicating specific proto-oncogenes in esophageal carcinogenesis is discussed later in this chapter.

CCND1 in Esophageal Squamous Cell Cancer

In ESCC, perhaps the most critical proto-oncogene is CCND1 or cyclin D1. CCDN1 is the catalytic subunit of a complex containing the CDK inhibitor CDKN2A and CDK4 and CDK6, which phosphorylate RB1 and block the inhibitory effect of RB1 on progression beyond the G_1 phase of the cell cycle. In vitro studies revealed that overexpression of antisense cyclin decreases CCND1 expression and diminishes cellular proliferation in ESCC-derived cells containing amplified CCDN1 (83). Moreover, amplification or overexpression of CCND1 has been documented in up to 65% of EC cell lines and is associated with morphologic neoplastic transformation (84,85). Finally, targeting of the CCND1 oncogene by an Epstein-Barr virus promoter in transgenic mice has been shown to lead to esophageal dysplasia (86). This transgenic model may ultimately prove useful in demonstrating a tumor-initiating effect for CCND1 overexpression in upper aerodigestive epithelial tissues (86).

In the clinical arena, CCND1 was shown to be overexpressed in 22% to 71% of ESCCs (81,87,88). Moreover, an overwhelming preponderance of evidence suggests a correlation between CCND1 dysregulation, tumor recurrence, and poor prognosis (89–92). Additional studies correlated CCND1 amplification, messenger RNA, and protein overexpression with distal organ (i.e., hematogenous) rather than lymph node spread (93,94). This point is relevant because prognosis is worse in patients with distal organ spread than in those with lymph node spread (95). In addition, increased CCND1 expression, both independently and in conjunction with *p53* protein

overexpression, has been associated with multiple primary malignant neoplasms of the hypopharynx and esophagus (96). Of note, however, one study of 53 ESCCs did not find CCND1 expression to be an independent predictor of poor survival; moreover, another study of 64 patients found that patients with CCND1-negative disease had a worse prognosis (97,98). Finally, overexpression of CCND1 protein has also been associated with a poorer response to chemotherapy in patients receiving multimodality therapy (89).

Other Cyclins Implicated in Esophageal Carcinogenesis. Other cyclins have also been implicated in ESCC. High levels of cyclin A expression were documented by immunohistochemistry in 39.5% of 124 tumors; furthermore, these levels correlated with advanced stage and a poor prognosis (99). Increased expression of cyclins A, D1, D3, and E were found in 23.1%, 65.4%, 15.4%, and 57.7% of 26 human EC cell lines, respectively (85). High levels of cyclin B1, which activates CDC2 and upregulates progression through the G_2 and M phases of the cell cycle, were detected in 72.4% of 87 ESCCs by immunohistochemical analysis. This overexpression was associated with tumor invasion beneath the muscularis propria and with a worse prognosis (100). Finally, the fact that the tumor suppressor genes RB1 and CDKN2A have been shown to be involved in EC is noteworthy. These genes also interact with cyclins and exert effects on the cell cycle.

Epidermal Growth Factor Receptor in Esophageal Squamous Cell Cancer. EGFR is one of a family of four closely related transmembrane receptors that include ERBB2, ERBB3, and ERBB4. Up to 71% of ESCCs show EGFR overexpression (76,77,101). The EGFR activates the tyrosine kinase activity of its own intracellular domain. Binding of EGF ligand to EGFR triggers activation of guanosine diphosphate–bound ras to guanosine triphosphate–bound ras and permits subsequent steps in intracellular signaling (102). When EGFR is altered, for example, by point mutations, it can become constitutively activated and result in impaired growth control (103–106). Evidence exists that EGFR may be stimulated by autocrine secretion of EGF and transforming growth factor-α in squamous carcinoma cells (107). A role for EGFR expression as a prognostic marker has been suggested. An early study dividing 32 patients with ESCC into two groups according to EGF binding levels demonstrated decreased survival in the group with higher EGF-binding capacity (108).

More recent studies have suggested prognostic value for EGFR either alone or in conjunction with a panel of other molecular markers, including CCND1 and CDH1 (91,109). However, one study of 39 patients with ESCC undergoing esophagectomy documented increased expression of EGFR, ERBB2, and ERBB3, but no prognostic significance of overexpression of any of these genes (110).

Biological agents that target EGFR are at the forefront of novel anticancer therapies (111). Several monoclonal antibodies directed against EGFR have been designed and are in early phase clinical trials for the treatment of EC, and results are encouraging (112,113).

ERBB2 in Esophageal Adenocarcinoma and Esophageal Squamous Cell Cancer

In EC cells, evidence suggests that ERBB2 (HER-2/neu) plays an important role in immortalization or maintenance of the transformed phenotype (114). For ESCC, little information exists as to the prognostic significance of ERBB2 expression. One report demonstrated that 30% of ESCC (n = 66) tumors were positive for ERBB2 and that increased expression was associated with a poor prognosis (115). In adenocarcinoma associated with BE, there are contradictory data. However, most of the information available indicates that this marker has significant prognostic value (101). Expression of the ERBB2 proto-oncogene has been evaluated in cases of BE. Jankowski et al. found immunodetectable ERBB2 in 9 of 15 patients with Barrett metaplasia as well as in 11 of 15 additional patients with EAC (116). Another study showed ERBB2 overexpression in 64% of ECs, but expression and prognosis did not correlate with one another (110). In yet another study, ERBB2 oncoprotein overexpression was seen in 7 of 66 (11%) EACs but not in surrounding dysplastic tissue and nondysplastic epithelium. In addition, in this latter report, expression of ERBB2 was associated with poor survival (117). Finally, ERBB2 amplification in serum using quantitative real-time polymerase chain reaction has been detected in EC patients (118). This finding, along with observations of other serum DNA abnormalities, encourages analyses of therapeutic response in patients with advanced EC.

MYC in Esophageal Adenocarcinoma and Esophageal Squamous Cell Cancer

MYC encodes a transcription factor implicated in many cellular processes such as proliferation, differentiation, transformation, and apoptosis (119). The MYC gene has been shown to render cells' growth factor independent and to accelerate their passage through G1 (120). In addition, in tumor cells that exhibit MYC deregulation, activation of survival pathways that convey resistance to oxidative stress appears to depend on MYC phosphorylation (121). As with most proto-oncogenes, the precise role of MYC amplification in cancer is complex and continues to be defined. The MYC gene is located on chromosome band 8q24; this locus is amplified in 14% to 25% of ECs (76,122). Jankowski et al. detected upregulated MYC expression in 50% of BE cases and in 90% of EAC samples. In addition, the proliferation of MYC was demonstrated in vitro by the administration of acidified bile (123). Another group from Germany found that normal esophageal tissues and low-grade dysplastic lesions had no amplification of MYC, but amplification of MYC was found in 6 of 24 BE specimens with high-grade dysplasia and in 17 of 39 cases (44%) of EAC (124). It appears that MYC amplification is also important in sporadic ESCC. In one study, MYC amplification was detected in 8 of 77 surgically treated ESCCs and in 13 of 43 cases (30%) of ESCC that required multimodality therapy, suggesting that MYC amplification is found more frequently in advanced stages of cancer (78). Furthermore, a novel gene, *mimitin*, was recently found to be directly stimulated by MYC and highly expressed in 80% (28 of 35 cases) of ESCC (125). Thus, there are significant data that suggest increased expression of MYC is an important and late event in the pathogenesis of both EAC and ESCC.

FGF3 and FGF4 in Esophageal Squamous Cell Carcinoma. The FGF3 and FGF4 genes, located 35 kilobases apart on chromosome band 11q13, encode members of the fibroblast growth factor family. Amplification of FGF4, as well as coamplification of FGF3 and FGF4, has been noted in ESCC (79,126). Coamplification of FGF3 and FGF4 or amplification of either gene alone has been correlated with a poor prognosis and increased likelihood of distant metastases (127,128). Moreover, sevenfold or greater amplification of the FGF4 gene has been associated with hematogenous recurrence of EC after resection (129). However, the precise relationship between 11q13 amplification and overexpression of FGF3 and FGF4 in EC is unclear. A review by Yoshida et al. noted minimal expression of FGF3 and FGF4 even though they are coamplified (130). This finding is particularly relevant, considering that the CCND1 gene lies within the 11q13 amplicon containing *FGF3* and *FGF4*, and that CCND1 is overexpressed in EC (81). One study of ESCC noted no prognostic significance for FGF4 amplification (131).

KRAS. A notable feature of both ESCC and EAC that distinguishes them from other cancers, such as colorectal cancer, lung adenocarcinoma, and pancreatic carcinoma, is the striking rarity or absence of KRAS proto-oncogene mutations. Mutations of KRAS were completely absent in most published studies of EC (132,133).

Tumor Suppressor Genes

The following list of known and putative tumor suppressor genes in esophageal carcinogenesis is intended not to be exhaustive but to point out several important genes that may be involved in esophageal tumorigenesis. A discussion of tumor suppressor gene inactivation is difficult to separate from a consideration of chromosomal deletions, LOH, and promoter hypermethylation. During the process of cancer evolution, molecular events that lead to a growth or survival advantage result in clonal expansion. Moreover, normal DNA repair mechanisms check replication fidelity before permitting progression through subsequent stages of the cell cycle. Deletions and other DNA alterations may permit unhampered progress through the cell cycle, which leads to proliferation and expansion of abnormal or mutated clones of cells. These deletions and mutations form the basis for Nicholl's two-hit hypothesis (cited and popularized by Knudson) describing the inactivation of both alleles of a tumor suppressor gene (134,135). For example, the APC gene on chromosome arm 5q is frequently mutated, and its locus frequently undergoes allelic deletion in sporadic colorectal cancers (136). Based on this principle, chromosomal areas showing frequent LOH in a given type of sporadic tumor might predict the presence of a tumor suppressor gene at the deleted locus. This approach proved successful in early work that suggested that the RB1 and TP53 genes, localized to regions of frequent LOH on chromosome bands 13q14 and 17p13, respectively, were potential tumor suppressor genes (137,138).

Studies report varying frequencies of LOH involving multiple chromosomes in EC. These chromosomal loci, in many instances, are associated with genes important in tumorigenesis, and these candidate tumor suppressor genes are indicated. Since the 1990s, a large body of evidence has accumulated in support of promoter hypermethylation as an additional mechanism by which tumor suppressor genes are inactivated (43). Promoter methylation is discussed in detail later in this chapter, as well as within the section for individual genes.

p53 (TP53). The first tumor suppressor gene shown to undergo frequent point mutation in primary ECs and cell lines was TP53 on chromosome band 17p13.1 (139). Similar findings were soon reported in noncancerous Barrett metaplasia, BE with high-grade dysplasia, and metaplastic or dysplastic tissues adjacent to adenocarcinomas (140–142). Mutations are also commonly detected in precancerous squamous tissues as well as ESCC itself (143–145). Thus, perhaps the key tumor suppressor gene in both ESCC and EAC is TP53. It has many functions, including cell cycle arrest, induction of apoptosis, and transcriptional regulation (146). Up to 70% of ECs carry TP53 mutation, TP53 deletion, or both (139,147). The prevalence of TP53 alteration in nondysplastic Barrett mucosa, however, is relatively low when compared to adenocarcinoma (148).

The TP53 phosphoprotein possesses sequence-specific DNA binding properties. In normal cells, TP53 does not accumulate to high levels because of its rapid turnover (half-life of 2–15 minutes) (149). In the setting of DNA damage or cellular stress, however, TP53 becomes stabilized and transactivates several important genes, including (a) CDKN1A, which arrests cells in G_1; and (b) genes affecting apoptosis. Thus, TP53 is able to prevent DNA replication after DNA damage, either by arresting cells in G_1 or by inducing the apoptotic death of cells containing damaged DNA. Mutations of TP53 are believed to prevent transactivation of these growth-controlling physiological gene targets. Furthermore, mutant TP53 may possess an oncogenic gain of function (dominant-negative mutation). Precise mechanisms whereby mutated TP53 exerts tumor-promoting effects are still being elucidated. Many mutants of TP53 are expressed at high levels in cancer tissue (150), which suggests clonal expansion of cancer cells bearing mutant TP53. High levels of expression of mutant TP53 permit its detection by immunohistochemical and Western blotting assays.

Due to its frequent mutation and allelic deletion frequencies, TP53 is regarded as the most important known tumor suppressor gene in esophageal carcinomas of both major types. The high prevalence of TP53 mutations in ESCC and EAC has been confirmed in several studies (122,143,144,146). Most studies assessed mutation of TP53 based on evaluation of exons 5 to 8. These exons encode the entire DNA binding domain and flanking splice sites. Mutations of *p53* in the remaining exons 1 to 4 and 9 to 11 have rarely been evaluated in EC (151). The localization of mutations is different in ESCC and EAC. In EAC, mutational hot spots occur at codons 175 (exon 5), 248 (exon 8), and 273 (exon 8). These three codons are also the most frequently mutated in all cancer types documented in a TP53 gene mutational database (152). Another hot spot for mutation in cancer is at codon 249; however, there are no documented mutations at this codon in EAC (149). Another distinguishing feature of EAC is that TP53 mutations show transitions at CpG dinucleotides in up to 69% of cases, and this represents the highest frequency of such transitions in any cancer (153–155). In ESCC, mutations at codons 248 or 273 account for only 3% of all point mutations detected, whereas relatively high frequencies of mutation at codon 270 (4%, compared with 0% in adenocarcinoma and 0.4% in other cancers) have been documented. Furthermore, a relatively high frequency of mutation at codons 193, 194, and 195 contributes to a unique mutational profile distinguishing esophageal SCC from other cancers (149,153). In addition, 30% of mutations in esophageal SCC occur at sites encoding the hydrophobic core, whereas most mutations in adenocarcinoma are limited to sites encoding the DNA binding domain (149). Current efforts are directed at the correlation of specific mutational events with particular carcinogens in EC (156). Mutation of TP53 is considered an early event in EC because it is found in noninvasive and early malignant tissues of both ESCC and EAC (145,146). Hypermethylation of TP53 does not result in functional silencing because the promoter region of this gene lacks a CpG island.

TP53 and Barrett esophagus. Frequent LOH of the TP53 locus on 17p13.1 is seen not only in EAC but also in Barrett metaplasia and dysplasia (63). In most patients with high-grade dysplasia, Barrett mucosa contains a mosaic of clones and subclones with differing patterns of LOH (157). In BE, frequency of TP53 overexpression correlates with degree of dysplasia (158). Furthermore, early dysplastic lesions with TP53 expression have been associated with a higher likelihood of progression to high-grade dysplasia, which suggests that determining TP53 status in BE patients with low-grade dysplasia may have value (159). Mutational analysis of TP53 has recently been shown to identify patients with BE that are at greater risk for progression to EAC (160). In a large prospective series, patients with loss of TP53 over an area of >5 cm of Barrett increases the cancer risk by threefold (161). However, low frequencies of elevated *p53* expression in BE without dysplasia seem to preclude widespread use as a screening tool (162).

TP53 and prognosis in esophageal cancer. Although TP53 is mutated frequently in EC, the prognostic value of TP53 has not been substantiated in several studies (163–165). One of these studies failed to demonstrate prognostic significance for the combination of TP53 expression and diminished expression of retinoblastoma when evaluated by multivariate analysis (163). Furthermore, TP53 expression did not correlate with diminished apoptosis index in ESCC (166). However,

TP53 expression has been correlated with occurrence of distal metastases in patients treated with radiotherapy alone for ESCC (167). One report suggested poor response to preoperative chemotherapy or radiation therapy in patients with TP53-expressing tumors who subsequently underwent surgical resection (168). Finally, determining TP53 status may be of some value in predicting response to trimodal therapy for EC (169).

Although not directly related to prognosis per se, in as many as 15% of cases of upper aerodigestive tract cancers, at least two primaries are present (96). Expression of TP53 (and CCND1), which reflects underlying gene mutation, is seen more frequently in cancers presenting with multiple primaries (96,170). Furthermore, the presence of TP53 mutations in EC correlates positively with cigarette smoking (153).

P16 (CDKN2A). The tumor suppressor gene CDKN2A, located on chromosome band 9p21, is an inhibitor of CDK4. A principle emerging from studies of ESCC is that either CCND1 overexpression or CDKN2A inactivation seems to be required to accelerate the cell through G_1 (171,172). The CDKN2A locus undergoes frequent LOH in EC, however, relatively low frequencies of CDKN2A-inactivating mutations have been documented in EC (173–175). Promoter hypermethylation of CDKN2A has been reported in numerous studies involving esophageal carcinomas of both histologic subtypes (49,50,172,175,176), which strongly suggests that this epigenetic phenomenon is the dominant mode of inactivation for this gene. Methylation of this tumor suppressor gene has been associated with neoplastic progression of BE to EAC (51,176). Finally, although the prognostic value of diminished CDKN2A expression has been disputed (91,177), methylation of a panel of genes that includes CDKN2A is associated with a poor response to chemotherapy and radiation in EC (178).

Adenomatous Polyposis Coli. APC is regarded as the gatekeeper gene for colorectal cancer, in which it is the most frequently mutated and allelically deleted (179). The APC locus on 5q21 is allelically deleted in up to 80% of ECs, but inactivating mutations of APC are seen in only 2% (180,181). Several studies suggested that the APC gene promoter region is frequently hypermethylated in EAC and slightly less so in ESCC (182,183). Therefore, APC inactivation by mechanisms other than mutation is likely to be important in esophageal carcinogenesis. In addition, these data suggest that additional gene targets located on 5q21 are less likely to be involved in esophageal tumorigenesis. In addition, a recently published study proposed that methylation of a panel of genes that includes APC is indicative of progression from Barrett metaplasia to EAC (52). However, there is evidence from autopsy studies to suggest methylation of APC is common in normal esophageal tissue and is associated with aging rather than tumorigenesis (184); thus, more studies are needed to confirm the importance of methylation of APC in EC.

Retinoblastoma (RB1). Loss or inactivation of both alleles of the RB1 gene is the primary mechanism underlying retinoblastoma (134). Moreover, a high incidence of second primary tumors among patients inheriting one inactive RB1 allele suggested that this cancer gene plays a key role in the etiology of several other primary malignancies (185). EC cells show decreased expression of RB1 protein by both Western blotting and immunohistochemical analyses (186,187). Most important, LOH or abnormal messenger RNA transcripts involving RB1 or both have been demonstrated in 36% to 67% of esophageal tumors, and in one study were associated with unfavorable survival (180,188). Additional research has determined that loss of RB1 is one of the main genetic alterations accompanying the progression through dysplasia to adenocarcinoma of the esophagus (189). The transcription factor E2F-1, a downstream regulator of the RB pathway, is required for cell cycle progression and has been found to be overexpressed and related to poor prognosis in ESCC (190).

E-Cadherin (CDH1). CDH1 is a calcium-dependent adhesion molecule that plays a major role in mediating homophilic cell–cell interactions (191), establishing cell polarity (192), and maintaining intercellular junctions in normal epithelial cells in most organs (193). In EC, downregulation of CDH1 and the cytoplasmic protein β-catenin is associated with tumor dedifferentiation, infiltrative growth, and lymph node metastasis (194). Diminished CDH1 expression has also been demonstrated in BE (195), and this reduction in expression appears to grow as the metaplasia-dysplasia-carcinoma sequence progresses (196). Reports have associated diminished expression of CDH1 with hematogenous spread and poor prognosis of ESCC (91,197). One study, however, found that aberrant CDH1 expression conferred a better, rather than worse, prognosis in Dutch patients undergoing high-dose radiation therapy (198). Mutations of CDH1 are rare in EAC, even in the setting of frequent (36%–65%) LOH involving its chromosomal locus, 16q22.1 (199,200). Hypermethylation of the CDH1 promoter is common in EAC and appears to correlate inversely with survival and tumor recurrence (183,201). In addition, methylation and the subsequent reduced expression CDH1 has been reported in 61% of ESCC cases (202). There was also a significant correlation between CDH1 methylation and tumor invasion and vascular invasion (202).

P21 (CDKN1A). The CDK inhibitor CDKN1A arrests the cell cycle after DNA damage at the G_1-S checkpoint. The literature has also demonstrated a role for CDKN1A in G_2 arrest. Studies with ESCC cell lines have shown that radiation-induced CDKN1A protein induction is associated with G_2 arrest (203). Reports on the prognostic significance of CDKN1A expression in ESCC are conflicting. Although increased CDKN1A expression was associated with worse prognosis in one study (204), diminished CDKN1A protein expression in surgically resected ESCC specimens was associated with a poor prognosis in another (205). The results from another study suggested that CDKN1A expression is potentially useful for predicting the response to chemoradiotherapy and survival of patients with advanced ESCC (206). A gradual reduction in CDKN1A expression has been observed in the multistep process of esophageal adenocarcinogenesis (207).

TCF-2 Locus. LOH with a frequency of up to 66% of the locus containing TCF-2 on 17q has been documented in EAC (208). However, a specific gene within this locus has not yet been studied.

BRCA1. Among 94 ESCCs, allelic deletion of the area around loci 17q21.1–3 containing the BRCA1 gene was observed in up to 62% of cases (209). A significant role for BRCA1 in esophageal carcinogenesis is not established.

ESOPHAGEAL CANCER AND APOPTOSIS

Apoptosis is defined as programmed cell death. Dysregulation of apoptosis, specifically downregulation, is a finding germane to most neoplastic or tumorigenic processes. The machinery of apoptosis includes the cell death receptors DR4 and DR5 as well as their ligand TRAIL. In addition to regulating DR5, TP53 appears to exert a regulating effect on an antagonist decoy receptor, TRID, which is overexpressed in gastrointestinal malignancies, including ECs (210). This overexpressed decoy receptor may assist neoplastic cells in escaping apoptotic suicide. In addition, high levels of BCL2 (an antiapoptotic factor) correlated inversely with apoptotic index by terminal deoxynucleotidyl transferase–mediated deoxyuridine triphosphate nick end labeling in ESCC (166).

LIMITATIONS OF SURVEILLANCE IN BARRETT ESOPHAGUS

Despite the paucity of data supporting its use, screening upper endoscopy for patients with chronic GERD symptoms to assess for BE and EAC has become a widely accepted practice and an issue of significant debate (23,211,212). A limitation of screening for dysplasia and cancer in BE is the danger of type II error (i.e., high false-negative rate) associated with mucosal biopsies. To sample the entire mucosa altered by the Barrett process is impossible. The fear of the endoscopist is that areas of dysplasia will go undetected. For this reason, some gastroenterologists recommend performing two endoscopies 2 to 3 months apart in any patient who is newly diagnosed with BE. Some studies have validated a "mucosal mapping" approach, showing predictable molecular and pathological findings in Barrett tissue sampled at different times in the same individuals (213). These studies require modified endoscopes, however, and may be too tedious to use in routine or nontertiary care centers. Further complicating the detection of dysplasia is significant interobserver variation in the histopathological diagnosis of dysplasia (214). Surveillance of patients with BE has not been shown to prolong survival (211).

OTHER TYPES OF ESOPHAGEAL CANCER

It has been suggested that basaloid-squamous carcinoma of the esophagus should be regarded as a discrete but rare entity with distinctive molecular genetic features, including increased DNA ploidy and altered TP53 protein levels by immunohistochemistry. In one study, 371 cases of esophageal malignancies were reviewed, and 7 cases of basaloid-squamous carcinoma (1.9%) were documented. Histologically, these tumors displayed a biphasic pattern of basaloid and squamous components. The former component predominated in three cases, the latter in four cases. All tumors contained solid growth of basaloid cells with microcystic patterns and stromal hyalinosis as well as palisading of cells (215). The molecular genetic basis of basaloid-squamous esophageal carcinomas has not been extensively studied.

TRANSLATIONAL POTENTIAL OF MOLECULAR ALTERATIONS IN ESOPHAGEAL CANCER

Although serologic markers such as cancer antigen 72.4 in gastric cancer, cancer antigen 19-9 in pancreatic cancer, carcinoembryonic antigen in colorectal cancer, and α-fetoprotein in hepatocellular carcinoma may sometimes be useful in diagnosis and in monitoring for the possibility of recurrent disease, no such marker has proven to be of high sensitivity or specificity in ESCC or EAC. In fact, few known biological markers have correlated consistently with stage and overall survival in either SCC or adenocarcinoma.

Therefore, development of a panel of biological markers to identify the propensity of EC of a given stage to progress will help in the future selection of appropriate therapeutic modalities (51,178,183,216,217). Moreover, future improvements in prognosis will require a panel of biomarkers to diagnose early cancer.

Future attempts to improve traditionally dismal outcomes in EC must rely on advances in molecular medicine. Researchers now have an extensive understanding of the molecular alterations accompanying EC of both major histologic types.

Accordingly, huge strides have been made during recent years (218). These therapeutic strategies include EGFR inhibitors, antiangiogenic agents, cell cycle inhibitors, and apoptosis promoters. The emerging data from the clinical development of these compounds have provided novel opportunities in the treatment of EC that will likely translate into successes for the treatment of EC (113).

In summary, accurate prognostication of ECs is often problematic. Markers of individuals at high risk of cancer development or rapid cancer progression are needed. One such potential marker is serum DNA. DNA from tumors may escape into the bloodstream and can be extracted for analysis of methylation, mutation, or other abnormalities (219). This approach holds significant promise for the future management of these patients. Moreover, functional genomics approaches, such as those using microarray technology, also appear to offer significant potential in discovering biomarkers for earlier detection and more accurate prognostication of EC.

References

1. Parkin DM, Bray F, Ferlay J, Pisani P. Global cancer statistics, 2002. *CA Cancer J Clin* 2005;55:74–108.
2. Shaheen NJ. Advances in Barrett's esophagus and esophageal adenocarcinoma. *Gastroenterology* 2005;128:1554–1566.
3. Ginsberg GG, Fleischer DE. Esophageal tumors. In: Feldman M, Friedman LS, Sleisenger MH, eds. *Sleisenger & Fordtran's Gastrointestinal and Liver Disease: Pathophysiology, Diagnosis, Management*. Philadelphia, Pa.: WB Saunders; 2002:647–671.
4. Harper PS, Harper RM, Howel-Evans AW. Carcinoma of the oesophagus with tylosis. *Q J Med* 1970;39:317–333.
5. Kelsell DP, Risk JM, Leigh IM, et al. Close mapping of the focal nonepidermolytic palmoplantar keratoderma (PPK) locus associated with oesophageal cancer (TOC). *Hum Mol Genet* 1996;5:857–860.
6. Howel-Evans W, Clarke CA, Sheppard PM. Carcinoma of the oesophagus with keratosis palmaris et plantaris (tylosis): a study of two families. *Q J Med* 1958;27:413–429.
7. Risk JM, Evans KE, Jones J, et al. Characterization of a 500 kb region on 17q25 and the exclusion of candidate genes as the familial tylosis oesophageal cancer (TOC) locus. *Oncogene* 2002;21:6395–6402.
8. Iwaya T, Maesawa C, Ogasawara S, Tamura G. Tylosis esophageal cancer locus on chromosome 17q25.1 is commonly deleted in sporadic human esophageal cancer. *Gastroenterology* 1998;114:1206–1210.
9. Langan JE, Cole CG, Huckle EJ, et al. Novel microsatellite markers and single nucleotide polymorphisms refine the tylosis with oesophageal cancer (TOC) minimal region on 17q25 to 42.5 kb: sequencing does not identify the causative gene. *Hum Genet* 2004;114:534–540.
10. McRonald FE, Liloglou T, Xinarianos G, et al. Down-regulation of the cytoglobin gene, located on 17q25, in tylosis with oesophageal cancer (TOC): evidence for trans-allele repression. *Hum Mol Genet* 2006;15:1271–1277.
11. Li JY. Epidemiology of esophageal cancer in China. *Natl Cancer Inst Monogr* 1982;62:113–120.
12. Li GH, He LJ. A survey of the familial aggregation of esophageal cancer in Yangcheng County, Shanxi Province. In: Wu M, Neberg DW, eds. *Genes and Disease*. Beijing: Science Press; 1986:43–47.
13. Roth MJ, Hu N, Emmert-Buck MR, et al. Genetic progression and heterogeneity associated with the development of esophageal squamous cell carcinoma. *Cancer Res* 2001;61:4098–4104.
14. Hu N, Wang C, Han XY, et al. Evaluation of BRCA2 in the genetic susceptibility of familial esophageal cancer. *Oncogene* 2004;23:852–858.
15. Wang AH, Sun CS, Li LS, Huang JY, Chen QS, Xu DZ. Genetic susceptibility and environmental factors of esophageal cancer in Xi'an. *World J Gastroenterol* 2004;10:940–944.
16. Parl FF. Glutathione S-transferase genotypes and cancer risk. *Cancer Lett* 2005;221:123–129.
17. Jain M, Kumar S, Rastogi N, et al. GSTT1, GSTM1 and GSTP1 genetic polymorphisms and interaction with tobacco, alcohol and occupational exposure in esophageal cancer patients from north India. *Cancer Lett* 2005;242:60–67.
18. Abbas A, Delvinquiere K, Lechevrel M, et al. GSTM1, GSTT1, GSTP1 and CYP1A1 genetic polymorphisms and susceptibility to esophageal cancer in a French population: different pattern of squamous cell carcinoma and adenocarcinoma. *World J Gastroenterol* 2004;10:3389–3393.
19. Ribeiro Pinto LF, Teixeira Rossini AM, Albano RM, et al. Mechanisms of esophageal cancer development in Brazilians. *Mutat Res* 2003;544:365–373.
20. Drovdlic CM, Goddard KA, Chak A, et al. Demographic and phenotypic features of 70 families segregating Barrett's oesophagus and oesophageal adenocarcinoma. *J Med Genet* 2003;40:651–656.
21. Jochem VJ, Fuerst PA, Fromkes JJ. Familial Barrett's esophagus associated with adenocarcinoma. *Gastroenterology* 1992;102:1400–1402.
22. Romero Y, Cameron AJ, Locke GR III, et al. Familial aggregation of gastroesophageal reflux in patients with Barrett's esophagus and esophageal adenocarcinoma. *Gastroenterology* 1997;113:1449–1456.
23. Fitzgerald RC. Complex diseases in gastroenterology and hepatology: GERD, Barrett's, and esophageal adenocarcinoma. *Clin Gastroenterol Hepatol* 2005;3:529–537.
24. Hu FZ, Preston RA, Post JC, et al. Mapping of a gene for severe pediatric gastroesophageal reflux to chromosome 13q14. *JAMA* 2000;284:325–334.
25. Burch P. Esophageal cancer in relation to cigarette and alcohol consumption. *J Chronic Dis* 1984;37:793–814.
26. Yu MC, Garabrant DH, Peters JM, Mack TM. Tobacco, alcohol, diet, occupation, and carcinoma of the esophagus. *Cancer Res* 1988;48:3843–3848.
27. Enzinger PC, Mayer RJ. Esophageal cancer. *N Engl J Med* 2003;349:2241–2252.
28. Stevens HP, Kelsell DP, Bryant SP, et al. Linkage of an American pedigree with palmoplantar keratoderma and malignancy (palmoplantar ectodermal dysplasia type III) to 17q24. Literature survey and proposed updated classification of the keratodermas. *Arch Dermatol* 1996;132:640–651.
29. Pera M, Trastek VF, Pairolero PC, Cardesa A, Allen MS, Deschamps C. Barrett's disease: pathophysiology of metaplasia and adenocarcinoma. *Ann Thorac Surg* 1993;56:1191–1197.
30. Haggitt RC. Barrett's esophagus, dysplasia, and adenocarcinoma. *Hum Pathol* 1994;25:982–993.
31. Fennerty MB, Sampliner RE, Way D, Riddell R, Steinbronn K, Garewal HS. Discordance between flow cytometric abnormalities and dysplasia in Barrett's esophagus. *Gastroenterology* 1989;97:815–820.
32. Lagergren J, Bergstrom R, Lindgren A, Nyren O. Symptomatic gastroesophageal reflux as a risk factor for esophageal adenocarcinoma. *N Engl J Med* 1999;340:825–831.
33. Pandolfino JE, Shi G, Trueworthy B, Kahrilas PJ. Esophagogastric junction opening during relaxation distinguishes nonhernia reflux patients, hernia patients, and normal subjects. *Gastroenterology* 2003;125:1018–1024.
34. Katzka DA, Reynolds JC, Saul SH, et al. Barrett's metaplasia and adenocarcinoma of the esophagus in scleroderma. *Am J Med* 1987;82:46–52.
35. Prach AT, MacDonald TA, Hopwood DA, et al. Increasing incidence of Barrett's oesophagus: education, enthusiasm, or epidemiology? *Lancet* 1997;350:933.
36. Champion G, Richter JE, Vaezi MF, et al. Duodenogastroesophageal reflux: relationship to pH and importance in Barrett's esophagus. *Gastroenterology* 1994;107:747–754.
37. D'Onofrio V, Bovero E, Iaquinto G. Characterization of acid and alkaline reflux in patients with Barrett's esophagus. G.O.S.P.E. Operative Group for the Study of Esophageal Precancer. *Dis Esophagus* 1997;10:16–22; discussion 22–23.
38. Avidan B, Sonnenberg A, Schnell TG, et al. Gastric surgery is not a risk for Barrett's esophagus or esophageal adenocarcinoma. *Gastroenterology* 2001;121:1281–1285.
39. Tamura G, Yin J, Wang S, et al. E-Cadherin gene promoter hypermethylation in primary human gastric carcinomas. *J Natl Cancer Inst* 2000;92:569–573.
40. Eads CA, Lord RV, Wickramasinghe K, et al. Epigenetic patterns in the progression of esophageal adenocarcinoma. *Cancer Res* 2001;61:3410–3418.
41. Esteller M, Corn PG, Baylin SB, Herman JG. A gene hypermethylation profile of human cancer. *Cancer Res* 2001;61:3225–3229.
42. Fleisher AS, Esteller M, Tamura G, et al. Hypermethylation of the hMLH1 gene promoter is associated with microsatellite instability in early human gastric neoplasia. *Oncogene* 2001;20:329–335.
43. Herman JG, Baylin SB. Gene silencing in cancer in association with promoter hypermethylation. *N Engl J Med* 2003;349:2042–2054.
44. Leung SY, Yuen ST, Chung LP, Chu KM, Chan AS, Ho JC. hMLH1 promoter methylation and lack of hMLH1 expression in sporadic gastric carcinomas with high-frequency microsatellite instability. *Cancer Res* 1999;59:159–164.
45. Kane MF, Loda M, Gaida GM, et al. Methylation of the hMLH1 promoter correlates with lack of expression of hMLH1 in sporadic colon tumors and mismatch repair-defective human tumor cell lines. *Cancer Res* 1997;57:808–811.
46. Esteller M, Catasus L, Matias-Guiu X, et al. hMLH1 promoter hypermethylation is an early event in human endometrial tumorigenesis. *Am J Pathol* 1999;155:1767–1772.
47. Herman JG, Umar A, Polyak K, et al. Incidence and functional consequences of hMLH1 promoter hypermethylation in colorectal carcinoma. *Proc Natl Acad Sci U S A* 1998;95:6870–6875.
48. Jones PA, Laird PW. Cancer epigenetics comes of age. *Nat Genet* 1999;21:163–167.
49. Maesawa C, Tamura G, Nishizuka S, et al. Inactivation of the CDKN2 gene by homozygous deletion and de novo methylation is associated with advanced stage esophageal squamous cell carcinoma. *Cancer Res* 1996;56:3875–3878.
50. Wong DJ, Barrett MT, Stoger R, Emond MJ, Reid BJ. p16INK4a promoter is hypermethylated at a high frequency in esophageal adenocarcinomas. *Cancer Res* 1997;57:2619–2622.

51. Schulmann K, Sterian A, Berki A, et al. Inactivation of p16, RUNX3, and HPP1 occurs early in Barrett's-associated neoplastic progression and predicts progression risk. *Oncogene* 2005;24:4138–4148.

52. Clement G, Braunschweig R, Pasquier N, Bosman FT, Benhattar J. Methylation of APC, TIMP3, and TERT: a new predictive marker to distinguish Barrett's oesophagus patients at risk for malignant transformation. *J Pathol* 2006;208:100–107.

53. Morales CP, Souza RF, Spechler SJ. Hallmarks of cancer progression in Barrett's oesophagus. *Lancet* 2002;360:1587–1589.

54. Robaszkiewicz M, Reid BJ, Volant A, Cauvin JM, Rabinovitch PS, Gouerou H. Flow-cytometric DNA content analysis of esophageal squamous cell carcinomas. *Gastroenterology* 1991;101:1588–1593.

55. Chanvitan A, Puttawibul P, Casson AG. Flow cytometry in squamous cell esophageal cancer and precancerous lesions. *Dis Esophagus* 1997;10:206–210.

56. Wang LS, Wu LH, Chang CJ, et al. Flow-cytometric DNA content analysis of oesophageal carcinoma: comparison between tumour and sequential non-tumour mucosae. *Scand Cardiovasc J* 1998;32:205–212.

57. Yuan Z, Jiang H, Xu C. (Study of heterogeneity in DNA ploidy and its clinical-pathological significance in esophageal squamous cell carcinoma). *Zhonghua Bing Li Xue Za Zhi* 1996;25:159–161.

58. Watanabe M, Kuwano H, Tanaka S, Toh Y, Sadanaga N, Sugimachi K. Flow cytometric DNA analysis is useful in detecting multiple genetic alterations in squamous cell carcinoma of the esophagus. *Cancer* 1999;85:2322–2328.

59. Chanvitan A, Nekarda H, Casson AG. Prognostic value of DNA index, S-phase fraction and p53 protein accumulation after surgical resection of esophageal squamous-cell carcinoma in Thailand. *Int J Cancer* 1995;63:381–386.

60. Reid BJ, Haggitt RC, Rubin CE, Rabinovitch PS. Barrett's esophagus. Correlation between flow cytometry and histology in detection of patients at risk for adenocarcinoma. *Gastroenterology* 1987;93:1–11.

61. Reid BJ, Blount PL, Rubin CE, Levine DS, Haggitt RC, Rabinovitch PS. Flow-cytometric and histological progression to malignancy in Barrett's esophagus: prospective endoscopic surveillance of a cohort. *Gastroenterology* 1992;102:1212–1219.

62. Galipeau PC, Cowan DS, Sanchez CA, et al. 17p (p53) Allelic losses, 4N (G2/tetraploid) populations, and progression to aneuploidy in Barrett's esophagus. *Proc Natl Acad Sci U S A* 1996;93:7081–7084.

63. Barrett MT, Sanchez CA, Prevo LJ, et al. Evolution of neoplastic cell lineages in Barrett oesophagus. *Nat Genet* 1999;22:106–109.

64. James PD, Atkinson M. Value of DNA image cytometry in the prediction of malignant change in Barrett's oesophagus. *Gut* 1989;30:899–905.

65. Garewal HS, Sampliner RE, Fennerty MB. Chemopreventive studies in Barrett's esophagus: a model premalignant lesion for esophageal adenocarcinoma. *J Natl Cancer Inst Monogr* 1992:51–54.

66. Raskind WH, Norwood T, Levine DS, Haggitt RC, Rabinovitch PS, Reid BJ. Persistent clonal areas and clonal expansion in Barrett's esophagus. *Cancer Res* 1992;52:2946–2950.

67. Reid BJ, Levine DS, Longton G, Blount PL, Rabinovitch PS. Predictors of progression to cancer in Barrett's esophagus: baseline histology and flow cytometry identify low- and high-risk patient subsets. *Am J Gastroenterol* 2000;95:1669–1676.

68. Reid BJ, Blount PL, Rabinovitch PS. Biomarkers in Barrett's esophagus. *Gastrointest Endosc Clin N Am* 2003;13:369–397.

69. Garewal H, Meltzer P, Trent J, Prabhala R, Sampliner R, Korc M. Epidermal growth factor receptor overexpression and trisomy 7 in a case of Barrett's esophagus. *Dig Dis Sci* 1990;35:1115–1120.

70. Garewal HS, Sampliner R, Liu Y, Trent JM. Chromosomal rearrangements in Barrett's esophagus: a premalignant lesion of esophageal adenocarcinoma. *Cancer Genet Cytogenet* 1989;42:281–286.

71. Menke-Pluymers MB, van Drunen E, Vissers KJ, Mulder AH, Tilanus HW, Hagemeijer A. Cytogenetic analysis of Barrett's mucosa and adenocarcinoma of the distal esophagus and cardia. *Cancer Genet Cytogenet* 1996;90:109–117.

72. Rosenblum-Vos LS, Meltzer SJ, Leana-Cox J, Schwartz S. Cytogenetic studies of primary cultures of esophageal squamous cell carcinoma. *Cancer Genet Cytogenet* 1993;70:127–131.

73. Yamaki H, Sasano H, Ohashi Y, et al. Alteration of X and Y chromosomes in human esophageal squamous cell carcinoma. *Anticancer Res* 2001;21:985–990.

74. Walch AK, Zitzelsberger HF, Bink K, et al. Molecular genetic changes in metastatic primary Barrett's adenocarcinoma and related lymph node metastases: comparison with nonmetastatic Barrett's adenocarcinoma. *Mod Pathol* 2000;13:814–824.

75. Kwong D, Lam A, Guan X, et al. Chromosomal aberrations in esophageal squamous cell carcinoma among Chinese: gain of 12p predicts poor prognosis after surgery. *Hum Pathol* 2004;35:309–316.

76. Lu SH, Hsieh LL, Luo FC, Weinstein IB. Amplification of the EGF receptor and c-myc genes in human esophageal cancers. *Int J Cancer* 1988;42:502–505.

77. Hollstein MC, Smits AM, Galiana C, et al. Amplification of epidermal growth factor receptor gene but no evidence of ras mutations in primary human esophageal cancers. *Cancer Res* 1988;48:5119–5123.

78. Bitzer M, Stahl M, Arjumand J, et al. C-myc gene amplification in different stages of oesophageal squamous cell carcinoma: prognostic value in relation to treatment modality. *Anticancer Res* 2003;23:1489–1493.

79. Tsuda T, Nakatani H, Matsumura T, et al. Amplification of the hst-1 gene in human esophageal carcinomas. *Jpn J Cancer Res* 1988;79:584–588.

80. Wagata T, Ishizaki K, Imamura M, Shimada Y, Ikenaga M, Tobe T. Deletion of 17p and amplification of the int-2 gene in esophageal carcinomas. *Cancer Res* 1991;51:2113–2117.

81. Jiang W, Kahn SM, Tomita N, Zhang YJ, Lu SH, Weinstein IB. Amplification and expression of the human cyclin D gene in esophageal cancer. *Cancer Res* 1992;52:2980–2983.

82. Jankowski JA, Wright NA, Meltzer SJ, et al. Molecular evolution of the metaplasia-dysplasia-adenocarcinoma sequence in the esophagus. *Am J Pathol* 1999;154:965–973.

83. Zhou P, Jiang W, Zhang YJ, et al. Antisense to cyclin D1 inhibits growth and reverses the transformed phenotype of human esophageal cancer cells. *Oncogene* 1995;11:571–580.

84. Watanabe M, Kuwano H, Tanaka S, Toh Y, Masuda H, Sugimachi K. A significant morphological transformation is recognized in human esophageal cancer cells with an amplification/overexpression of the cyclin D1 gene. *Int J Oncol* 1999;15:1103–1108.

85. Fujii S, Tominaga O, Nagawa H, et al. Quantitative analysis of the cyclin expression in human esophageal cancer cell lines. *J Exp Clin Cancer Res* 1998;17:491–496.

86. Nakagawa H, Wang TC, Zukerberg L, et al. The targeting of the cyclin D1 oncogene by an Epstein-Barr virus promoter in transgenic mice causes dysplasia in the tongue, esophagus and forestomach. *Oncogene* 1997;14:1185–1190.

87. Sunpaweravong P, Sunpaweravong S, Puttawibul P, et al. Epidermal growth factor receptor and cyclin D1 are independently amplified and overexpressed in esophageal squamous cell carcinoma. *J Cancer Res Clin Oncol* 2005;131:111–119.

88. Arber N, Gammon MD, Hibshoosh H, et al. Overexpression of cyclin D1 occurs in both squamous carcinomas and adenocarcinomas of the esophagus and in adenocarcinomas of the stomach. *Hum Pathol* 1999;30:1087–1092.

89. Sarbia M, Stahl M, Fink U, et al. Prognostic significance of cyclin D1 in esophageal squamous cell carcinoma patients treated with surgery alone or combined therapy modalities. *Int J Cancer* 1999;84:86–91.

90. Matsumoto M, Furihata M, Ishikawa T, Ohtsuki Y, Ogoshi S. Comparison of deregulated expression of cyclin D1 and cyclin E with that of cyclin-dependent kinase 4 (CDK4) and CDK2 in human oesophageal squamous cell carcinoma. *Br J Cancer* 1999;80:256–261.

91. Shimada Y, Imamura M, Watanabe G, et al. Prognostic factors of oesophageal squamous cell carcinoma from the perspective of molecular biology. *Br J Cancer* 1999;80:1281–1288.

92. Itami A, Shimada Y, Watanabe G, Imamura M. Prognostic value of p27(Kip1) and CyclinD1 expression in esophageal cancer. *Oncology* 1999;57:311–317.

93. Inomata M, Uchino S, Tanimura H, Shiraishi N, Adachi Y, Kitano S. Amplification and overexpression of cyclin D1 in aggressive human esophageal cancer. *Oncol Rep* 1998;5:171–176.

94. Shinozaki H, Ozawa S, Ando N, et al. Cyclin D1 amplification as a new predictive classification for squamous cell carcinoma of the esophagus, adding gene information. *Clin Cancer Res* 1996;2:1155–1161.

95. Ishikawa T, Furihata M, Ohtsuki Y, Murakami H, Inoue A, Ogoshi S. Cyclin D1 overexpression related to retinoblastoma protein expression as a prognostic marker in human oesophageal squamous cell carcinoma. *Br J Cancer* 1998;77:92–97.

96. Kohmura T, Hasegawa Y, Ogawa T, et al. Cyclin D1 and p53 overexpression predicts multiple primary malignant neoplasms of the hypopharynx and esophagus. *Arch Otolaryngol Head Neck Surg* 1999;125:1351–1354.

97. Ikeda G, Isaji S, Chandra B, Watanabe M, Kawarada Y. Prognostic significance of biologic factors in squamous cell carcinoma of the esophagus. *Cancer* 1999;86:1396–1405.

98. Kuwahara M, Hirai T, Yoshida K, et al. p53, p21(Waf1/Cip1) and cyclin D1 protein expression and prognosis in esophageal cancer. *Dis Esophagus* 1999;12:116–119.

99. Furihata M, Ishikawa T, Inoue A, et al. Determination of the prognostic significance of unscheduled cyclin A overexpression in patients with esophageal squamous cell carcinoma. *Clin Cancer Res* 1996;2:1781–1785.

100. Murakami H, Furihata M, Ohtsuki Y, Ogoshi S. Determination of the prognostic significance of cyclin B1 overexpression in patients with esophageal squamous cell carcinoma. *Virchows Arch* 1999;434:153–158.

101. Ross JS, McKenna BJ. The HER-2/neu oncogene in tumors of the gastrointestinal tract. *Cancer Invest* 2001;19:554–568.

102. Barnard JA, Beauchamp RD, Russell WE, Dubois RN, Coffey RJ. Epidermal growth factor-related peptides and their relevance to gastrointestinal pathophysiology. *Gastroenterology* 1995;108:564–580.

103. Khazaie K, Schirrmacher V, Lichtner RB. EGF receptor in neoplasia and metastasis. *Cancer Metastasis Rev* 1993;12:255–274.

104. Dou Y, Hoffman P, Hoffman BL, Carlin C. Ligand-induced protein tyrosine kinase activity in living cells coexpressing intact EGF receptors and receptors with an extensive cytosolic deletion. *J Cell Physiol* 1992;153:402–407.

105. Walton GM, Chen WS, Rosenfeld MG, Gill GN. Analysis of deletions of the carboxyl terminus of the epidermal growth factor receptor reveals

self-phosphorylation at tyrosine 992 and enhanced in vivo tyrosine phosphorylation of cell substrates. *J Biol Chem* 1990;265:1750–1754.

106. Wells A, Welsh JB, Lazar CS, Wiley HS, Gill GN, Rosenfeld MG. Ligand-induced transformation by a noninternalizing epidermal growth factor receptor. *Science* 1990;247:962–964.

107. Yoshida K, Kyo E, Tsuda T, et al. EGF and TGF-alpha, the ligands of hyperproduced EGFR in human esophageal carcinoma cells, act as autocrine growth factors. *Int J Cancer* 1990;45:131–135.

108. Ozawa S, Ueda M, Ando N, Shimizu N, Abe O. Prognostic significance of epidermal growth factor receptor in esophageal squamous cell carcinomas. *Cancer* 1989;63:2169–2173.

109. Inada S, Koto T, Futami K, Arima S, Iwashita A. Evaluation of malignancy and the prognosis of esophageal cancer based on an immunohistochemical study (p53, E-cadherin, epidermal growth factor receptor). *Surg Today* 1999;29:493–503.

110. Friess H, Fukuda A, Tang WH, et al. Concomitant analysis of the epidermal growth factor receptor family in esophageal cancer: overexpression of epidermal growth factor receptor mRNA but not of c-erbB-2 and c-erbB-3. *World J Surg* 1999;23:1010–1018.

111. Mendelsohn J. Targeting the epidermal growth factor receptor for cancer therapy. *J Clin Oncol* 2002;20:1S–13S.

112. Vanhoefer U, Tewes M, Rojo F, et al. Phase I study of the humanized antiepidermal growth factor receptor monoclonal antibody EMD72000 in patients with advanced solid tumors that express the epidermal growth factor receptor. *J Clin Oncol* 2004;22:175–184.

113. Tabernero J, Macarulla T, Ramos FJ, Baselga J. Novel targeted therapies in the treatment of gastric and esophageal cancer. *Ann Oncol* 2005;16:1740–1748.

114. Shiga K, Shiga C, Sasano H, et al. Expression of c-erbB-2 in human esophageal carcinoma cells: overexpression correlated with gene amplification or with GATA-3 transcription factor expression. *Anticancer Res* 1993;13:1293–1301.

115. Mimura K, Kono K, Hanawa M, et al. Frequencies of HER-2/neu expression and gene amplification in patients with oesophageal squamous cell carcinoma. *Br J Cancer* 2005;92:1253–1260.

116. Jankowski J, Coghill G, Hopwood D, Wormsley KG. Oncogenes and onco-suppressor gene in adenocarcinoma of the oesophagus. *Gut* 1992;33:1033–1038.

117. Flejou JF, Paraf F, Muzeau F, et al. Expression of c-erbB-2 oncogene product in Barrett's adenocarcinoma: pathological and prognostic correlations. *J Clin Pathol* 1994;47:23–26.

118. Chiang PW, Beer DG, Wei WL, Orringer MB, Kurnit DM. Detection of erbB-2 amplifications in tumors and sera from esophageal carcinoma patients. *Clin Cancer Res* 1999;5:1381–1386.

119. Nilsson JA, Cleveland JL. Myc pathways provoking cell suicide and cancer. *Oncogene* 2003;22:9007–9021.

120. Baudino TA, McKay C, Pendeville-Samain H, et al. c-Myc is essential for vasculogenesis and angiogenesis during development and tumor progression. *Genes Dev* 2002;16:2530–2543.

121. Benassi B, Fanciulli M, Fiorentino F, et al. c-Myc phosphorylation is required for cellular response to oxidative stress. *Mol Cell* 2006;21:509–519.

122. Esteve A, Lehman T, Jiang W, et al. Correlation of p53 mutations with epidermal growth factor receptor overexpression and absence of mdm2 amplification in human esophageal carcinomas. *Mol Carcinog* 1993;8:306–311.

123. Tselepis C, Morris CD, Wakelin D, et al. Upregulation of the oncogene c-myc in Barrett's adenocarcinoma: induction of c-myc by acidified bile acid in vitro. *Gut* 2003;52:174–180.

124. Sarbia M, Arjumand J, Wolter M, Reifenberger G, Heep H, Gabbert HE. Frequent c-myc amplification in high-grade dysplasia and adenocarcinoma in Barrett esophagus. *Am J Clin Pathol* 2001;115:835–840.

125. Tsuneoka M, Teye K, Arima N, et al. A novel Myc-target gene, mimitin, that is involved in cell proliferation of esophageal squamous cell carcinoma. *J Biol Chem* 2005;280:19977–19985.

126. Tsuda T, Nakatani H, Tahara E, Sakamoto H, Terada M, Sugimura T. HST1 and INT2 gene coamplification in a squamous cell carcinoma of the gallbladder. *Jpn J Clin Oncol* 1989;19:26–29.

127. Kitagawa Y, Ueda M, Ando N, Shinozawa Y, Shimizu N, Abe O. Significance of int-2/hst-1 coamplification as a prognostic factor in patients with esophageal squamous carcinoma. *Cancer Res* 1991;51:1504–1508.

128. Ikeda Y, Ozawa S, Ando N, Kitagawa Y, Ueda M, Kitajima M. Meanings of c-erbB and int-2 amplification in superficial esophageal squamous cell carcinomas. *Ann Thorac Surg* 1996;62:835–838.

129. Chikuba K, Saito T, Uchino S, et al. High amplification of the hst-1 gene correlates with haematogenous recurrence after curative resection of oesophageal carcinoma. *Br J Surg* 1995;82:364–367.

130. Yoshida T, Sakamoto H, Terada M. Amplified genes in cancer in upper digestive tract. *Semin Cancer Biol* 1993;4:33–40.

131. Shiga C, Shiga K, Hirayama H, Katayama M, Nishihira T, Mori S. Prognostic significance of hst-1 gene amplification in primary esophageal carcinomas and its relationship to other prognostic factors. *Anticancer Res* 1994;14:651–656.

132. Victor T, Du Toit R, Jordaan AM, Bester AJ, van Helden PD. No evidence for point mutations in codons 12, 13, and 61 of the ras gene in a high-incidence area for esophageal and gastric cancers. *Cancer Res* 1990;50:4911–4914.

133. Jiang W, Kahn SM, Guillem JG, Lu SH, Weinstein IB. Rapid detection of ras oncogenes in human tumors: applications to colon, esophageal, and gastric cancer. *Oncogene* 1989;4:923–928.

134. Knudson AG, Jr. Mutation and cancer: statistical study of retinoblastoma. *Proc Natl Acad Sci U S A* 1971;68:820–823.

135. Nicholls EM. Somatic variation and multiple neurofibromatosis. *Hum Hered* 1969;19:473–479.

136. Vogelstein B, Fearon ER, Hamilton SR, et al. Genetic alterations during colorectal-tumor development. *N Engl J Med* 1988;319:525–532.

137. Baker SJ, Markowitz S, Fearon ER, Willson JK, Vogelstein B. Suppression of human colorectal carcinoma cell growth by wild-type p53. *Science* 1990;249:912–915.

138. Harbour JW, Lai SL, Whang-Peng J, Gazdar AF, Minna JD, Kaye FJ. Abnormalities in structure and expression of the human retinoblastoma gene in SCLC. *Science* 1988;241:353–357.

139. Hollstein MC, Metcalf RA, Welsh JA, Montesano R, Harris CC. Frequent mutation of the p53 gene in human esophageal cancer. *Proc Natl Acad Sci U S A* 1990;87:9958–9961.

140. Casson AG, Mukhopadhyay T, Cleary KR, Ro JY, Levin B, Roth JA. p53 gene mutations in Barrett's epithelium and esophageal cancer. *Cancer Res* 1991;51:4495–4499.

141. Schneider PM, Casson AG, Levin B, et al. Mutations of p53 in Barrett's esophagus and Barrett's cancer: a prospective study of ninety-eight cases. *J Thorac Cardiovasc Surg* 1996;111:323–331; discussion 331–333.

142. Greenwald B, Huang Y, Baum R, et al. Barrett's carcinoma in a 25-year-old man with point mutation of the p53 tumor suppressor gene. *Intl J Oncol* 1992;1:271–275.

143. Hollstein MC, Peri L, Mandard AM, et al. Genetic analysis of human esophageal tumors from two high incidence geographic areas: frequent p53 base substitutions and absence of ras mutations. *Cancer Res* 1991;51:4102–4106.

144. Gao H, Wang LD, Zhou Q, Hong JY, Huang TY, Yang CS. p53 Tumor suppressor gene mutation in early esophageal precancerous lesions and carcinoma among high-risk populations in Henan, China. *Cancer Res* 1994;54:4342–4346.

145. Mandard AM, Hainaut P, Hollstein M. Genetic steps in the development of squamous cell carcinoma of the esophagus. *Mutat Res* 2000;462:335–342.

146. Wang LD, Hong JY, Qiu SL, Gao H, Yang CS. Accumulation of p53 protein in human esophageal precancerous lesions: a possible early biomarker for carcinogenesis. *Cancer Res* 1993;53:1783–1787.

147. Meltzer SJ, Yin J, Huang Y, et al. Reduction to homozygosity involving p53 in esophageal cancers demonstrated by the polymerase chain reaction. *Proc Natl Acad Sci U S A* 1991;88:4976–4980.

148. Gonzalez MV, Artimez ML, Rodrigo L, et al. Mutation analysis of the p53, APC, and p16 genes in the Barrett's oesophagus, dysplasia, and adenocarcinoma. *J Clin Pathol* 1997;50:212–217.

149. Montesano R, Hollstein M, Hainaut P. Genetic alterations in esophageal cancer and their relevance to etiology and pathogenesis: a review. *Int J Cancer* 1996;69:225–235.

150. Hainaut P. The tumor suppressor protein p53: a receptor to genotoxic stress that controls cell growth and survival. *Curr Opin Oncol* 1995;7:76–82.

151. Wagata T, Shibagaki I, Imamura M, et al. Loss of 17p, mutation of the p53 gene, and overexpression of p53 protein in esophageal squamous cell carcinomas. *Cancer Res* 1993;53:846–850.

152. Hainaut P, Soussi T, Shomer B, et al. Database of p53 gene somatic mutations in human tumors and cell lines: updated compilation and future prospects. *Nucleic Acids Res* 1997;25:151–157.

153. Hollstein M, Shomer B, Greenblatt M, et al. Somatic point mutations in the p53 gene of human tumors and cell lines: updated compilation. *Nucleic Acids Res* 1996;24:141–146.

154. Gleeson CM, Sloan JM, McGuigan JA, Ritchie AJ, Russell SE. Base transitions at CpG dinucleotides in the p53 gene are common in esophageal adenocarcinoma. *Cancer Res* 1995;55:3406–3411.

155. Hamelin R, Flejou JF, Muzeau F, et al. TP53 gene mutations and p53 protein immunoreactivity in malignant and premalignant Barrett's esophagus. *Gastroenterology* 1994;107:1012–1018.

156. Hollstein M, Hergenhahn M, Yang Q, Bartsch H, Wang ZQ, Hainaut P. New approaches to understanding p53 gene tumor mutation spectra. *Mutat Res* 1999;431:199–209.

157. Prevo LJ, Sanchez CA, Galipeau PC, Reid BJ. p53-Mutant clones and field effects in Barrett's esophagus. *Cancer Res* 1999;59:4784–4787.

158. Blount PL, Ramel S, Raskind WH, et al. 17p Allelic deletions and p53 protein overexpression in Barrett's adenocarcinoma. *Cancer Res* 1991;51:5482–5486.

159. Gimenez A, de Haro LM, Parrilla P, Bermejo J, Perez-Guillermo M, Ortiz MA. Immunohistochemical detection of p53 protein could improve the management of some patients with Barrett esophagus and mild histologic alterations. *Arch Pathol Lab Med* 1999;123:1260–1263.

160. Dolan K, Walker SJ, Gosney J, Field JK, Sutton R. TP53 mutations in malignant and premalignant Barrett's esophagus. *Dis Esophagus* 2003;16:83–89.

161. Maley CC, Galipeau PC, Li X, et al. The combination of genetic instability and clonal expansion predicts progression to esophageal adenocarcinoma. *Cancer Res* 2004;64:7629–7633.

162. Klump B, Hsieh CJ, Holzmann K, et al. Diagnostic significance of nuclear p53 expression in the surveillance of Barrett's esophagus—a longitudinal study. *Z Gastroenterol* 1999;37:1005–1011.

163. Hashimoto N, Tachibana M, Dhar DK, Yoshimura H, Nagasue N. Expression of p53 and RB proteins in squamous cell carcinoma of the esophagus: their relationship with clinicopathologic characteristics. *Ann Surg Oncol* 1999;6:489–494.

164. Kanamoto A, Kato H, Tachimori Y, et al. No prognostic significance of p53 expression in esophageal squamous cell carcinoma. *J Surg Oncol* 1999;72:94–98.

165. Soontrapornchai P, Elsaleh H, Joseph D, Hamdorf JM, House A, Klacopetta B, TP53 gene mutation status in pretreatment biopsies of oesophageal adenocarcinoma has no prognostic value. *Eur J Cancer* 1999;35:1683–1687.

166. Azmi S, Dinda AK, Chopra P, Chattopadhyay TK, Singh N. Bcl-2 expression is correlated with low apoptotic index and associated with histopathological grading in esophageal squamous cell carcinomas. *Tumour Biol* 2000;21:3–10.

167. Pomp J, Blom J, Zwinderman AH, Van Krimpen C. P53 and radiotherapy for oesophageal carcinoma: a comparison between 4 different antibodies. *Oncol Rep* 2000;7:1075–1078.

168. Nasierowska-Guttmejer A, Szawlowski A, Jastrzebska M, Jeziorski K, Radziszewski J. p53 Protein accumulation as a prognostic marker of preoperative radiotherapy and/or chemotherapy in advanced squamous cell esophageal carcinoma—preliminary report. *Dis Esophagus* 1999;12:128–131.

169. Krasna MJ, Mao YS, Sonett JR, et al. P53 gene protein overexpression predicts results of trimodality therapy in esophageal cancer patients. *Ann Thorac Surg* 1999;68:2021–2024; discussion 2024–2025.

170. Fukuzawa K, Noguchi Y, Yoshikawa T, et al. High incidence of synchronous cancer of the oral cavity and the upper gastrointestinal tract. *Cancer Lett* 1999;144:145–151.

171. Liu Q, Yan YX, McClure M, Nakagawa H, Fujimura F, Rustgi AK. MTS-1 (CDKN2) tumor suppressor gene deletions are a frequent event in esophagus squamous cancer and pancreatic adenocarcinoma cell lines. *Oncogene* 1995;10:619–622.

172. Klump B, Hsieh CJ, Holzmann K, Gregor M, Porschen R. Hypermethylation of the CDKN2/p16 promoter during neoplastic progression in Barrett's esophagus. *Gastroenterology* 1998;115:1381–1386.

173. Suzuki H, Zhou X, Yin J, et al. Intragenic mutations of CDKN2B and CDKN2A in primary human esophageal cancers. *Hum Mol Genet* 1995;4:1883–1887.

174. Igaki H, Sasaki H, Tachimori Y, et al. Mutation frequency of the p16/CDKN2 gene in primary cancers in the upper digestive tract. *Cancer Res* 1995;55:3421–3423.

175. Esteve A, Martel-Planche G, Sylla BS, Hollstein M, Hainaut P, Montesano R. Low frequency of p16/CDKN2 gene mutations in esophageal carcinomas. *Int J Cancer* 1996;66:301–304.

176. Sato F, Meltzer SJ. CpG island hypermethylation in progression of esophageal and gastric cancer. *Cancer* 2006;106:483–493.

177. Takeuchi H, Ozawa S, Ando N, et al. Altered p16/MTS1/CDKN2 and cyclin D1/PRAD-1 gene expression is associated with the prognosis of squamous cell carcinoma of the esophagus. *Clin Cancer Res* 1997;3:2229–2236.

178. Hamilton JP, Sato F, Greenwald BD, et al. Promoter methylation and response to chemotherapy and radiation in esophageal cancer. *Clin Gastroenterol Hepatol* 2006;4(6):701–708.

179. Kinzler KW, Vogelstein B. Lessons from hereditary colorectal cancer. *Cell* 1996;87:159–170.

180. Dolan K, Garde J, Gosney J, et al. Allelotype analysis of oesophageal adenocarcinoma: loss of heterozygosity occurs at multiple sites. *Br J Cancer* 1998;78:950–957.

181. Powell SM, Papadopoulos N, Kinzler KW, Smolinski KN, Meltzer SJ. APC gene mutations in the mutation cluster region are rare in esophageal cancers. *Gastroenterology* 1994;107:1759–1763.

182. Kawakami K, Brabender J, Lord RV, et al. Hypermethylated APC DNA in plasma and prognosis of patients with esophageal adenocarcinoma. *J Natl Cancer Inst* 2000;92:1805–1811.

183. Brock MV, Gou M, Akiyama Y, et al. Prognostic importance of promoter hypermethylation of multiple genes in esophageal adenocarcinoma. *Clin Cancer Res* 2003;9:2912–2919.

184. Waki T, Tamura G, Sato M, Motoyama T. Age-related methylation of tumor suppressor and tumor-related genes: an analysis of autopsy samples. *Oncogene* 2003;22:4128–4133.

185. Murphree AL, Benedict WF. Retinoblastoma: clues to human oncogenesis. *Science* 1984;223:1028–1033.

186. Jiang W, Zhang YJ, Kahn SM, et al. Altered expression of the cyclin D1 and retinoblastoma genes in human esophageal cancer. *Proc Natl Acad Sci U S A* 1993;90:9026–9030.

187. Coppola D, Schreiber RH, Mora L, Dalton W, Karl RC. Significance of Fas and retinoblastoma protein expression during the progression of Barrett's metaplasia to adenocarcinoma. *Ann Surg Oncol* 1999;6:298–304.

188. Huang Y, Meltzer SJ, Yin J, et al. Altered messenger RNA and unique mutational profiles of p53 and Rb in human esophageal carcinomas. *Cancer Res* 1993;53:1889–1894.

189. Jenkins GJ, Doak SH, Parry JM, D'Souza FR, Griffiths AP, Baxter JN. Genetic pathways involved in the progression of Barrett's metaplasia to adenocarcinoma. *Br J Surg* 2002;89:824–837.

190. Ebihara Y, Miyamoto M, Shichinohe T, et al. Over-expression of E2F-1 in esophageal squamous cell carcinoma correlates with tumor progression. *Dis Esophagus* 2004;17:150–154.

191. Guilford P, Hopkins J, Harraway J, et al. E-cadherin germline mutations in familial gastric cancer. *Nature* 1998;392:402–405.

192. Richards FM, McKee SA, Rajpar MH, et al. Germline E-cadherin gene (CDH1) mutations predispose to familial gastric cancer and colorectal cancer. *Hum Mol Genet* 1999;8:607–610.

193. Shiozaki H, Tahara H, Oka H, et al. Expression of immunoreactive E-cadherin adhesion molecules in human cancers. *Am J Pathol* 1991;139:17–23.

194. Streit M, Schmidt R, Hilgenfeld RU, Thiel E, Kreuser ED. Adhesion receptors in malignant transformation and dissemination of gastrointestinal tumors. *J Mol Med* 1996;74:253–268.

195. Swami S, Kumble S, Triadafilopoulos G. E-cadherin expression in gastroesophageal reflux disease, Barrett's esophagus, and esophageal adenocarcinoma: an immunohistochemical and immunoblot study. *Am J Gastroenterol* 1995;90:1808–1813.

196. Bailey T, Biddlestone L, Shepherd N, Barr H, Warner P, Jankowski J. Altered cadherin and catenin complexes in the Barrett's esophagus-dysplasia-adenocarcinoma sequence: correlation with disease progression and dedifferentiation. *Am J Pathol* 1998;152:135–144.

197. Tamura S, Shiozaki H, Miyata M, et al. Decreased E-cadherin expression is associated with haematogenous recurrence and poor prognosis in patients with squamous cell carcinoma of the oesophagus. *Br J Surg* 1996;83:1608–1614.

198. Pomp J, Blom J, van Krimpen C, et al. E-cadherin expression in oesophageal carcinoma treated with high-dose radiotherapy; correlation with pretreatment parameters and treatment outcome. *J Cancer Res Clin Oncol* 1999;125:641–645.

199. Wijnhoven BP, de Both NJ, van Dekken H, Tilanus HW, Dinjens WN. E-cadherin gene mutations are rare in adenocarcinomas of the oesophagus. *Br J Cancer* 1999;80:1652–1657.

200. van Dekken H, Geelen E, Dinjens WN, et al. Comparative genomic hybridization of cancer of the gastroesophageal junction: deletion of 14Q31-32.1 discriminates between esophageal (Barrett's) and gastric cardia adenocarcinomas. *Cancer Res* 1999;59:748–752.

201. Corn PG, Heath EI, Heitmiller R, et al. Frequent hypermethylation of the 5′ CpG island of E-cadherin in esophageal adenocarcinoma. *Clin Cancer Res* 2001;7:2765–2769.

202. Takeno S, Noguchi T, Fumoto S, Kimura Y, Shibata T, Kawahara K. E-cadherin expression in patients with esophageal squamous cell carcinoma: promoter hypermethylation, snail overexpression, and clinicopathologic implications. *Am J Clin Pathol* 2004;122:78–84.

203. Rigberg DA, Blinman TA, Kim FS, Cole MA, McFadden DW. Antisense blockade of p21/WAF1 decreases radiation-induced G2 arrest in esophageal squamous cell carcinoma. *J Surg Res* 1999;81:6–10.

204. Lam KY, Law S, Tin L, Tung PH, Wong J. The clinicopathological significance of p21 and p53 expression in esophageal squamous cell carcinoma: an analysis of 153 patients. *Am J Gastroenterol* 1999;94:2060–2068.

205. Nita ME, Nagawa H, Tominaga O, et al. p21Waf1/Cip1 expression is a prognostic marker in curatively resected esophageal squamous cell carcinoma, but not p27Kip1, p53, or Rb. *Ann Surg Oncol* 1999;6:481–488.

206. Nakamura T, Hayashi K, Ota M, et al. Salvage esophagectomy after definitive chemotherapy and radiotherapy for advanced esophageal cancer. *Am J Surg* 2004;188:261–266.

207. Riegman PH, Vissers KJ, Alers JC, et al. Genomic alterations in malignant transformation of Barrett's esophagus. *Cancer Res* 2001;61:3164–3170.

208. Swift A, Risk JM, Kingsnorth AN, Wright TA, Myskow M, Field JK. Frequent loss of heterozygosity on chromosome 17 at 17q11.2–q12 in Barrett's adenocarcinoma. *Br J Cancer* 1995;71:995–998.

209. Dunn J, Garde J, Dolan K, et al. Multiple target sites of allelic imbalance on chromosome 17 in Barrett's oesophageal cancer. *Oncogene* 1999;18:987–993.

210. Sheikh MS, Huang Y, Fernandez-Salas EA, et al. The antiapoptotic decoy receptor TRID/TRAIL-R3 is a p53-regulated DNA damage-inducible gene that is overexpressed in primary tumors of the gastrointestinal tract. *Oncogene* 1999;18:4153–4159.

211. Dellon ES, Shaheen NJ. Does screening for Barrett's esophagus and adenocarcinoma of the esophagus prolong survival? *J Clin Oncol* 2005;23:4478–4482.

212. Spechler SJ. Dysplasia in Barrett's esophagus: limitations of current management strategies. *Am J Gastroenterol* 2005;100:927–935.

213. Eisen GM, Montgomery EA, Azumi N, et al. Qualitative mapping of Barrett's metaplasia: a prerequisite for intervention trials. *Gastrointest Endosc* 1999;50:814–818.

214. Reid BJ, Haggitt RC, Rubin CE, et al. Observer variation in the diagnosis of dysplasia in Barrett's esophagus. *Hum Pathol* 1988;19:166–178.

215. Abe K, Sasano H, Itakura Y, Nishihira T, Mori S, Nagura H. Basaloid-squamous carcinoma of the esophagus: a clinicopathologic, DNA ploidy, and immunohistochemical study of seven cases. *Am J Surg Pathol* 1996;20:453–461.

216. Meltzer SJ. The molecular biology of esophageal carcinoma. *Recent Results Cancer Res* 1996;142:1–8.

217. Koppert LB, Wijnhoven BP, van Dekken H, Tilanus HW, Dinjens WN. The molecular biology of esophageal adenocarcinoma. *J Surg Oncol* 2005;92:169–190.
218. Schrump DS, Nguyen DM. Novel molecular targeted therapy for esophageal cancer. *J Surg Oncol* 2005;92:257–261.
219. Esteller M, Sanchez-Cespedes M, Rosell R, Sidransky D, Baylin SB, Herman JG. Detection of aberrant promoter hypermethylation of tumor suppressor genes in serum DNA from non-small cell lung cancer patients. *Cancer Res* 1999;59:67–70.
220. Sarbia M, Geddert H, Klump B, Kiel S, Iskender E, Gabbert HE. Hypermethylation of tumor suppressor genes (p16INK4A, p14ARF and APC) in adenocarcinomas of the upper gastrointestinal tract. *Int J Cancer* 2004;111:224–228.
221. Hibi K, Taguchi M, Nakayama H, et al. Molecular detection of p16 promoter methylation in the serum of patients with esophageal squamous cell carcinoma. *Clin Cancer Res* 2001;7:3135–3138.
222. Si HX, Tsao SW, Lam KY, et al. E-cadherin expression is commonly downregulated by CpG island hypermethylation in esophageal carcinoma cells. *Cancer Lett* 2001;173:71–78.
223. Geddert H, Kiel S, Iskender E, et al. Correlation of hMLH1 and HPP1 hypermethylation in gastric, but not in esophageal and cardiac adenocarcinoma. *Int J Cancer* 2004;110:208–211.
224. Zhang L, Lu W, Miao X, Xing D, Tan W, Lin D. Inactivation of DNA repair gene O6-methylguanine-DNA methyltransferase by promoter hypermethylation and its relation to p53 mutations in esophageal squamous cell carcinoma. *Carcinogenesis* 2003;24:1039–1044.
225. Wong DJ, Paulson TG, Prevo LJ, et al. p16(INK4a) lesions are common, early abnormalities that undergo clonal expansion in Barrett's metaplastic epithelium. *Cancer Res* 2001;61:8284–8289.
226. Esteller M, Cordon-Cardo C, Corn PG, et al. p14ARF silencing by promoter hypermethylation mediates abnormal intracellular localization of MDM2. *Cancer Res* 2001;61:2816–2821.
227. Xing EP, Nie Y, Song Y, et al. Mechanisms of inactivation of p14ARF, p15INK4b, and p16INK4a genes in human esophageal squamous cell carcinoma. *Clin Cancer Res* 1999;5:2704–2713.
228. Tokugawa T, Sugihara H, Tani T, Hattori T. Modes of silencing of p16 in development of esophageal squamous cell carcinoma. *Cancer Res* 2002;62:4938–4944.
229. Xing EP, Nie Y, Wang LD, Yang GY, Yang CS. Aberrant methylation of p16INK4a and deletion of p15INK4b are frequent events in human esophageal cancer in Linxian, China. *Carcinogenesis* 1999;20:77–84.
230. Hibi K, Koike M, Nakayama H, et al. A cancer-prone case with a background of methylation of p16 tumor suppressor gene. *Clin Cancer Res* 2003;9:1053–1056.
231. Bian YS, Osterheld MC, Fontolliet C, Bosman FT, Benhattar J. p16 Inactivation by methylation of the CDKN2A promoter occurs early during neoplastic progression in Barrett's esophagus. *Gastroenterology* 2002;122:1113–1121.
232. Kuroki T, Trapasso F, Yendamuri S, et al. Allele loss and promoter hypermethylation of VHL, RAR-beta, RASSF1A, and FHIT tumor suppressor genes on chromosome 3p in esophageal squamous cell carcinoma. *Cancer Res* 2003;63:3724–3728.
233. Wang Y, Fang MZ, Liao J, et al. Hypermethylation-associated inactivation of retinoic acid receptor beta in human esophageal squamous cell carcinoma. *Clin Cancer Res* 2003;9:5257–5263.
234. Kuroki T, Trapasso F, Yendamuri S, et al. Promoter hypermethylation of RASSF1A in esophageal squamous cell carcinoma. *Clin Cancer Res* 2003;9:1441–1445.
235. Wong ML, Tao Q, Fu L, et al. Aberrant promoter hypermethylation and silencing of the critical 3p21 tumour suppressor gene, RASSF1A, in Chinese oesophageal squamous cell carcinoma. *Int J Oncol* 2006;28:767–773.
236. Hamilton JP, Sato F, Jin Z, et al. Reprimo methylation is a potential biomarker of Barrett's-Associated esophageal neoplastic progression. *Clin Cancer Res* 2006;12(22):6637–6642.

CHAPTER 16 ■ ESOPHAGEAL CANCER: PATHOLOGY

SUSAN C. ABRAHAM AND TSUNG-TEH WU

Esophageal cancer is an aggressive disease with a poor prognosis. In 2005, it is estimated that there will be approximately 14,000 new esophageal cancers, and an equal number of cancer deaths are expected (1). The dismal prognosis of esophageal carcinoma is mainly due to late diagnosis with presentation at an advanced stage. The 5-year survival is approximately 14% for all stages of esophageal carcinoma (1). Histologically, esophageal cancer can be subclassified into epithelial and nonepithelial tumors. Similar to other regions of the gastrointestinal tract, carcinomas are the most common esophageal cancer with more than 90% of cancers representing either squamous cell carcinoma (SCC) or adenocarcinoma. SCC is the most common malignant esophageal cancer worldwide, especially in Asian populations and in parts of Africa and Europe. In the United States, SCC accounted for more than 90% of all esophageal cancers in 1960, but the pattern of esophageal cancers has changed since then (2). The incidence of esophageal adenocarcinomas, including those of the gastroesophageal junction (GEJ), has increased markedly in Western countries and in the United States, now constituting almost 50% of all esophageal cancers (3,4).

Esophagectomy has been the mainstay of therapy for localized esophageal carcinomas. Their prognosis is influenced by pathological features, including depth of tumor invasion, lymph node status, and completeness of resection as determined on the resected esophagus (5–7). Multimodality strategies using preoperative chemoradiation followed by esophagectomy are frequently used to treat locoregional esophageal carcinomas (8), based on the assumption of early therapy of micrometastasis, reduced local relapse, and a higher rate of curative surgery after chemoradiation despite equivocal benefits in randomized trials (9–13). The prognosis appears to be predicted by pathological stage determined on the resected esophagus after preoperative chemoradiation (14). In patients with high-grade precursor lesions (squamous or columnar epithelial dysplasia) or superficial esophageal carcinomas, noninvasive therapeutic modalities such as endoscopic mucosal resection have become attractive alternatives to esophagectomy. Pathological evaluation, including diagnosis of esophageal carcinoma by endoscopic biopsy or evaluation of detailed pathological features in esophagectomy or endoscopic mucosal resections, is essential for treatment planning and communication with patients regarding prognosis.

SQUAMOUS CELL CARCINOMA

Pathogenesis

SCC of the esophagus affects males more commonly than females. The pathogenesis of SCC is multifactorial and may vary among different regions of the world (15). The most significant contributing factors include tobacco and alcohol use, food and water contamination with nitrates and nitrosamines, and various vitamin deficiencies. Human papillomavirus (HPV) infection has been found in esophageal SCC by identification of HPV DNA either by in situ hybridization or polymerase chain reactions with a variable rate between 0% and 66% (16–18). It is more consistently detected in China but generally absent in SCC arising in Western countries. There are also several predisposing conditions for the development of SCC, including achalasia, Plummer-Vinson syndrome, esophageal strictures secondary to lye or acid ingestion, and the autosomal dominant disease tylosis palmaris et plantaris. Esophageal SCC also develops in up to 60% of patients surviving a previous head and neck carcinoma associated with smoking (19). In addition, distal esophageal SCC can also occur in regions of Barrett esophagus, a condition more predisposed to develop adenocarcinoma (20).

Pathological Features

Gross Pathology

SCCs are located predominantly in the middle (50%–60%) and lower (30%) esophagus, and only infrequently in the upper (10%–15%) esophagus (21). The gross appearance of esophageal SCC varies according to the stage of disease at the time of diagnosis. Superficial SCC—defined as tumor invading only the mucosa or submucosa irrespective of the presence of lymph node metastasis (22)—accounts for 10% to 20% of resected SCC in Japan but is much less frequently reported in Western countries. The gross appearance of superficial SCC can be polypoid, plaquelike, depressed, or grossly inconspicuous (23). Superficial SCC can also present with multiple tumors in up to 14% to 31% of cases (24–26).

Most esophageal SCCs are diagnosed at an advanced stage, and these tumors can be classified into three major gross patterns: fungating, ulcerating, or infiltrative (Fig. 16.1A, B) (21). The fungating pattern is characterized by exophytic or polypoid growth and is the most common type (60% of cases). In contrast, tumors with the ulcerating pattern (25% of cases) typically have intramural growth with a central ulceration. The infiltrative pattern is the least common type (15% of cases), containing intramural tumor growth but only a small mucosal defect. The gross appearance of advanced SCC, however, is not a significant prognostic factor. The gross appearance can also change substantially after preoperative adjuvant therapy depending on individual tumor response to treatment.

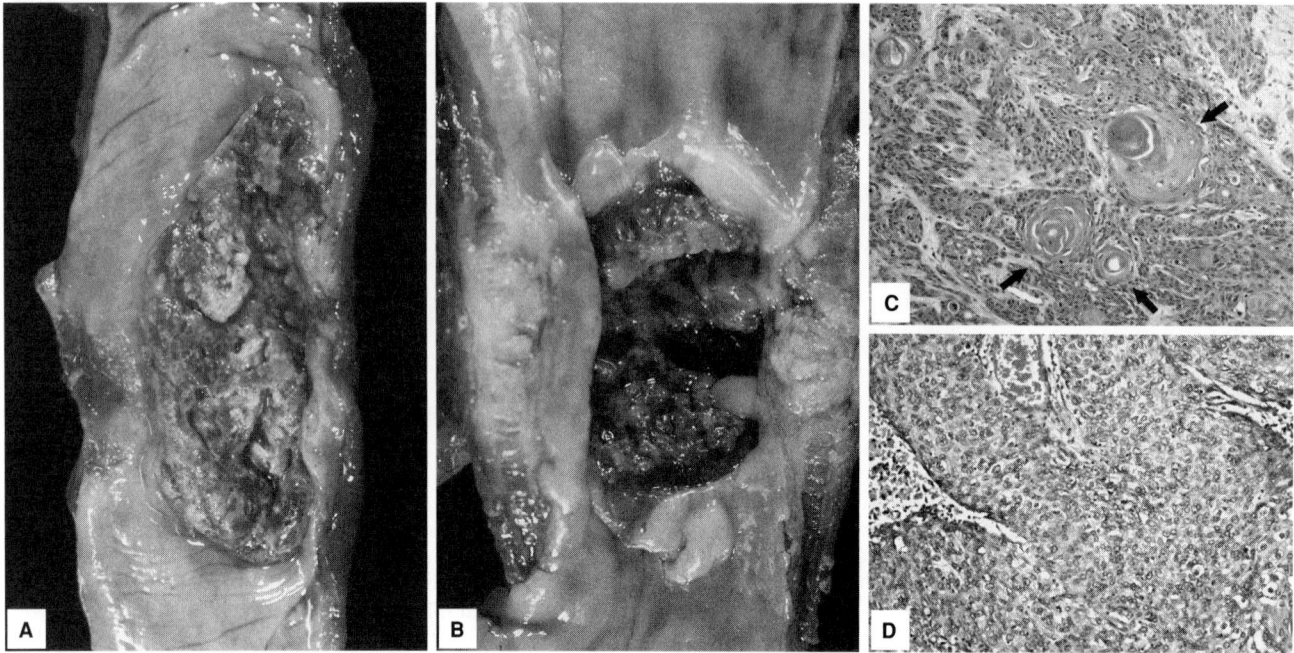

FIGURE 16.1. Gross appearance and histologic features of esophageal squamous cell carcinoma (SCC). **A:** A large fungating and exophytic SCC. **B:** Ulcerating SCC with heaped-up borders. **C:** Well-differentiated SCC characterized by sheets of neoplastic squamous cells with individual cell keratinization and prominent squamous pearl formation (*arrows*). **D:** Poorly differentiated SCC with a solid growth pattern and marked nuclear pleomorphism. No obvious keratinization is present.

Microscopic Pathology

Tumor Differentiation. Esophageal SCC has a range of differentiation and can be classified into well, moderately, and poorly differentiated based on the degree of squamous differentiation. In well-differentiated tumors, the epithelial tumor nests have mild nuclear atypia and cellular pleomorphism, distinct intercellular bridges, prominent eosinophilic cytoplasm representing individual cell keratinization, and squamous pearl formation (Fig. 16.1C). Moderately differentiated tumors typically have higher degrees of cellular atypia and nuclear pleomorphism and a lesser degree of keratinization as compared to well-differentiated tumors; moderately differentiated SCC accounts for a majority (two-thirds) of esophageal SCC. Poorly differentiated SCCs tend to grow in solid sheets or single cells, cytologic atypia and nuclear pleomorphism are more pronounced, and keratinization is less appreciable (Fig. 16.1D).

The distinction between poorly differentiated SCC and adenocarcinoma can occasionally be subtle. Immunohistochemical labeling for cytokeratin (CK) 5/6 and p63—markers for squamous differentiation positive in up to 75% to 93% of SCC (27)—can be used to support the diagnosis of poorly differentiated SCC. The presence of poor tumor differentiation may be a prognostic factor, but its significance remains controversial (28,29). Focal neuroendocrine or glandular differentiation, tumors with mixed SCC and adenocarcinoma (adenosquamous carcinoma), or mixed SCC and neuroendocrine carcinoma can also occur (30,31).

Tumor Spread and Metastasis. The depth of tumor invasion (T stage) correlates well with the presence of lymphovascular invasion and regional lymph node metastasis (N stage) (6). Positive lymph nodes are present in 50% to 60% of esophagectomies for locally advanced SCC (32). The carcinoma, in fact, can invade into intramural lymphatic vessels at an early stage of disease. In superficial (T1) esophageal SCCs, the risk of lymph node metastasis is lower than in advanced SCCs and has been shown to depend on the depth of invasion. Tumors invading only into lamina propria (intramucosal carcinomas) have lymph node metastasis in only 5% of cases, whereas tumors invading submucosa have a 35% risk of lymph node involvement (21,33).

Occurrence of intramural metastasis, manifested by intramural or submucosal lymphatic spread with the establishment of secondary tumor deposits, has been found in 11% to 16% of resected esophageal SCCs and is associated with advanced stage and poorer survival (24,34). Frozen section evaluation of the proximal esophageal resection margin for the presence of submucosal lymphatic spread is justified to ensure curative resection. The most frequent sites of distant metastases are lung and liver, present in up to 50% of autopsied cases (35). Other organs such as bones, adrenal glands, and brain are less frequently involved. Disseminated tumor cells identified by cytokeratin immunolabeling in bone marrow have been detected in 40% of resected esophageal SCC (36), and may account for poor survival and high recurrence rate despite curative surgery.

Variants of Squamous Cell Carcinoma

Basaloid Squamous Cell Carcinoma

Basaloid SCC is an uncommon but distinct variant of esophageal SCC that affects predominantly older men (37). Basaloid SCCs typically present as bulky fungating tumors with ulceration and stricture. Histologically, these tumors are composed of large solid or compact tumor nests with hyperchromatic nuclei, scant basophilic cytoplasm, peripheral palisading, and central comedo-type necrosis (Fig. 16.2A, B). Foci of myxoid matrix and hyalinized stroma surrounding tumor nests and occasional small glandlike structures are also seen (Fig. 16.2 C). Basaloid SCCs are often associated with squamous dysplasia, invasive SCC, or islands of squamous differentiation.

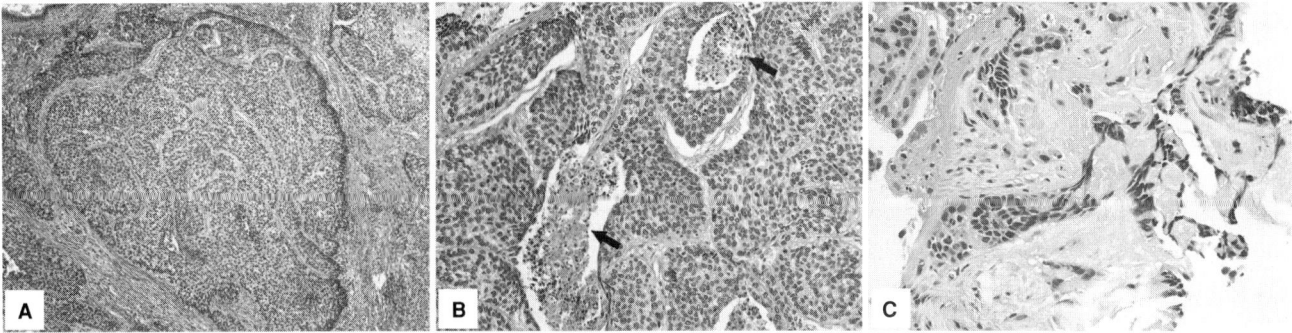

FIGURE 16.2. Basaloid squamous cell carcinoma (SCC). **A:** Low-power image of typical basaloid SCC with large round nests of basaloid cells and peripheral palisading. **B:** Central comedo-type necrosis (*arrows*) in basaloid SCC. **C:** Hyalinized stroma surrounding compressed tumor nests with occasional small glandlike structures.

Proliferation activity and apoptosis rate are higher than in classical SCC.

Basaloid SCC needs to be differentiated from true adenoid cystic carcinoma of the esophagus—a rare and less aggressive subtype than basaloid SCC—and from high-grade neuroendocrine (small cell) carcinoma. Immunohistochemical labeling for S-100 and actin can be used to highlight the basal cells of adenoid cystic carcinoma. Basaloid SCC is positive for CK 5/6 but negative for neuroendocrine markers such as chromogranin and synaptophysin, which are positive in neuroendocrine carcinoma.

Verrucous Squamous Cell Carcinoma

Verrucous carcinoma is a rare variant of SCC, histologically similar to verrucous carcinomas arising in other organ sites (38). An association with chronic esophagitis has been reported in one study (39). Grossly, these tumors have an exophytic, papillary, and cauliflowerlike appearance, and tend to grow large and involve the entire circumference of the esophageal wall before symptoms occur and a diagnosis can be made. Microscopically, the tumors are composed of large fronds of well-differentiated squamous epithelium with parakeratosis, hyperkeratosis, and minimal cytologic atypia mimicking benign squamous epithelium. They grow with an expansile or pushing border rather than the infiltrative pattern seen in classical SCC.

These deceptively benign histologic features make definitive diagnosis of verrucous carcinoma (usually >3 cm) versus large squamous papilloma (usually <3 cm) challenging for pathologists in endoscopic mucosal biopsy specimens. Careful endoscopic-pathological correlation is required. Esophageal verrucous carcinoma is a low-grade malignant neoplasm, which grows slowly and invades locally with only infrequent lymph node metastasis.

Sarcomatoid Carcinoma

This is a rare variant of SCC also known as carcinosarcoma, polypoid carcinoma, and spindle cell carcinoma (40,41). This tumor has a polypoid gross appearance and may grow to a large size averaging 6 cm in diameter. Histologically, sarcomatoid carcinoma is characterized by the presence of a biphasic pattern with both carcinomatous and spindle cell (sarcomatoid) components. The carcinomatous component is typically well to moderately differentiated SCC; infrequently, adenocarcinoma or undifferentiated carcinoma has been described. The sarcomatous component is more variable, ranging from rather innocuous spindle cells to high-grade sarcoma with pleomorphic, bizarre giant cell cells and numerous mitoses. Maturation

and differentiation into bone, cartilage, or skeletal muscle can also be present in the sarcomatoid component.

The sarcomatous component appears to arise from the carcinomatous component by metaplasia, judging from immunohistochemical and electron microscopic analyses (42). However, carcinosarcoma arising from two distinct malignant clones has been suggested by a recent molecular analysis that sarcomatous and carcinomatous components contain different genetic alteration profiles in 13 cases (41). The prognosis of sarcomatoid carcinoma appears to be more favorable than classical SCC due to the fact that sarcomatoid carcinoma has a luminal polypoid exophytic growth pattern. However, lymph node metastasis is present in 40% to 50% of the cases at the time of diagnosis, and in a stage-by-stage comparison, the prognosis is similar to SCC (40,41).

Precursor Lesion: Squamous Dysplasia (Intraepithelial Neoplasia)

Esophageal SCC is believed to arise from a multistage process through progression of a premalignant precursor lesion (squamous dysplasia or squamous intraepithelial neoplasia) into invasive SCC (43). Squamous dysplasia was present adjacent to invasive SCC in 14% to 20% of resected SCC in one study (44) and 60% to 90% in another study (25). Squamous dysplasia is commonly present in patients at high risk for developing SCC (44). Dysplasia is defined by the presence of cytologically and architecturally neoplastic epithelial cells confined within the mucosa. Squamous dysplasia can be further classified using a two-tiered system as either low-grade or high-grade dysplasia (25).

Grossly, squamous dysplasia appears erythematous, friable, and irregular in shape. In some cases, erosions, plaquelike lesions, nodules, or even a normal appearance can also be seen by endoscopic examination (44). Mucosal spread of Lugol's iodine can be used to highlight the dysplastic lesions to increase the yield of biopsies in surveillance of high-risk patients (45).

Histologically, low-grade squamous dysplasia is characterized by neoplastic squamous epithelial cells with irregular and hyperchromatic nuclei and increased nuclear:cytoplasmic ratio that are confined to the lower half of the epithelium (Fig. 16.3A). In high-grade squamous dysplasia, a greater degree of cytologic atypia is present with involvement of the upper half of the epithelium (Fig. 16.3B). Dysplasia involving esophageal submucosal gland ducts can occasionally occur and needs to be distinguished from invasive SCC (46). In this two-tiered grading system, carcinoma in situ is included in the high-grade dysplasia category and carries the same clinical implication (21).

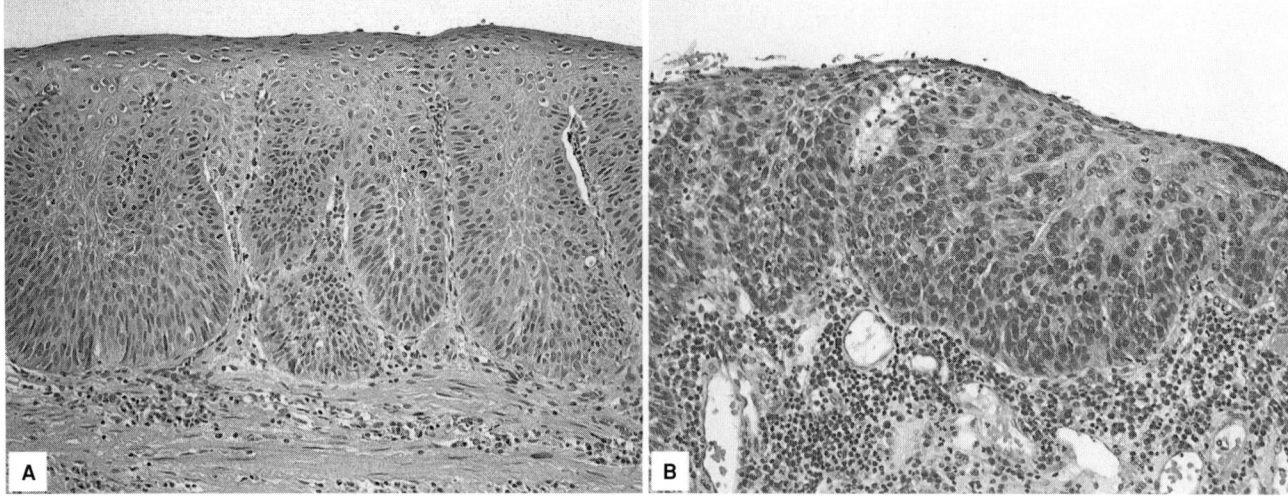

FIGURE 16.3. Squamous dysplasia (intraepithelial neoplasia) of the esophagus. **A:** Low-grade squamous dysplasia is characterized by neoplastic squamous epithelial proliferation confined to the lower half of the epithelium. **B:** High-grade squamous dysplasia is manifested by involvement of the entire thickness of epithelium by neoplastic squamous cells with a greater degree of architectural disarray and cytologic atypia.

Patients with squamous dysplasia have an increased risk of developing invasive SCC. Regression of low-grade squamous dysplasia can occur (and is more frequent than regression of high-grade dysplasia), but progression to high-grade dysplasia occurs in 15% of patients (47). In prospective follow-up studies conducted in China, invasive SCC arose in 9% of patients with squamous dysplasia over a 15-year period (48) and in 30% of patients with high-grade dysplasia over an 8-year period (47). The high incidence of SCC arising in patients with high-grade squamous dysplasia warrants close endoscopic surveillance for early diagnosis of invasive SCC or, alternatively, removal of visible lesions by endoscopic mucosal resection.

NEUROENDOCRINE CARCINOMA

Carcinoid Tumor

Carcinoid tumors (well-differentiated neuroendocrine neoplasms) of the esophagus are rare. They can present as isolated tumor nodules or be associated with adenocarcinoma (49). The histologic features are the same as in carcinoid tumors of the gastrointestinal tract in general. Carcinoid tumor is composed of solid nests of relatively monotonous tumor cells with "salt and pepper" nuclear chromatin that express neuroendocrine differentiation by immunohistochemical labeling for chromogranin or synaptophysin.

Small Cell Carcinoma (Poorly Differentiated Neuroendocrine Carcinoma)

Poorly differentiated neuroendocrine carcinomas constitute only 1% to 2% of all esophageal cancer (50). They are frequently located in the lower esophagus and tend to form large exophytic masses. Small cell carcinomas of the esophagus are histologically similar to small cell carcinomas of the lung. Microscopically, the tumor is composed of sheets or nests of small round to oval tumor cells with scant cytoplasm and hyperchromatic nuclei with molding. Foci of squamous differentiation or glandular differentiation have been reported in as many as 50% of esophageal small cell carcinomas (51).

Esophageal small cell carcinomas are aggressive malignancies, and their prognosis is poor, with a median survival of only 6 to 12 months (50). As previously mentioned, distinction between small cell carcinoma and basaloid SCC is important for choosing appropriate preoperative neoadjuvant therapy.

ADENOCARCINOMA

Pathogenesis

Adenocarcinoma has become the predominant histologic type of esophageal carcinoma in Western countries due to a marked increased rate of adenocarcinoma in the distal esophagus and esophagogastric junction (EGJ) since the 1970s (3,4). A majority (>95%) of esophageal adenocarcinomas arise in association with Barrett esophagus, a precursor of adenocarcinoma. Barrett esophagus is characterized by the presence of intestinal metaplasia (goblet cells) in the tubular esophagus and develops in approximately 10% of patients with chronic gastroesophageal reflux disease (52). Patients with Barrett esophagus have a 125-fold increased risk of developing adenocarcinoma as compared to the general population (53); however, this risk may be overestimated as shown in more recent studies (54–57).

A small subset (<5%) of esophageal adenocarcinomas arise from submucosal glands or ducts, or from gastric heterotopia in the upper esophagus. Adenocarcinoma at the EGJ can arise either from the gastric cardia or from short segment Barrett esophagus (58,59). The disposition of adenocarcinomas arising near the EGJ remains problematic, but clinically they should be treated as distal esophageal adenocarcinomas if significant involvement of the proximal gastric wall (>2 cm from EGJ) can be excluded.

Pathological Features

Gross Pathology

Most esophageal adenocarcinomas arise in the distal esophagus within a segment of Barrett metaplasia. Gross appearance

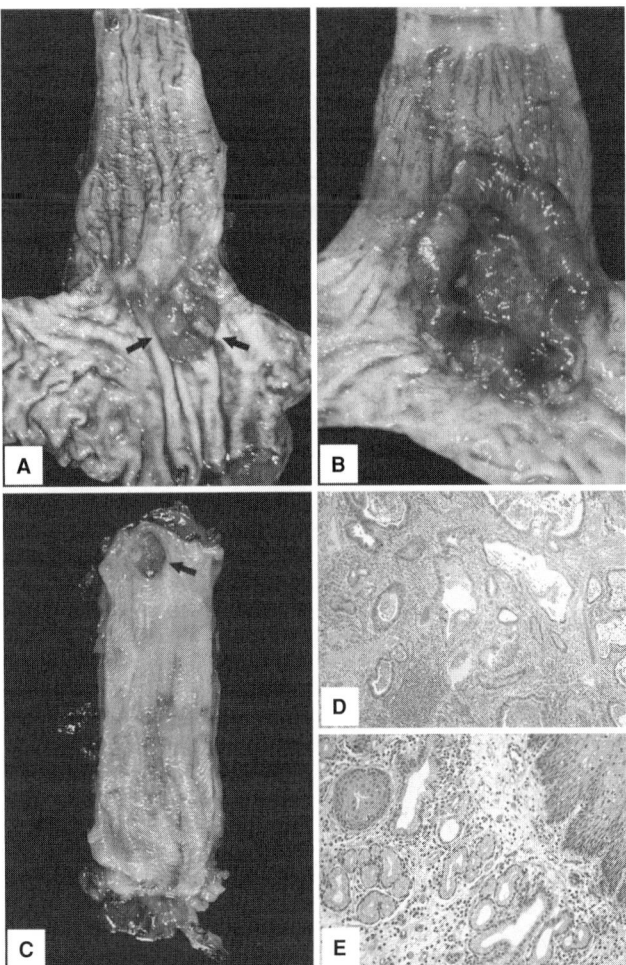

FIGURE 16.4. Gross appearance of esophageal adenocarcinoma. **A:** A polypoid superficially invasive adenocarcinoma (*arrows*) of the distal esophagus, arising in Barrett mucosa. **B:** A large ulcerated fungating mass of the distal esophagus with extension into gastric cardia. The background of Barrett esophagus has the classical salmon-pink appearance. **C:** Adenocarcinoma with polypoid growth (*arrow*) in the upper esophagus, arising from gastric heterotopia (inlet patch). Microscopically, there is well- to moderately differentiated adenocarcinoma (**D**) adjacent to a focus of heterotopic gastric cardia-type epithelium (**E**).

varies according to tumor stage at the time of diagnosis. In superficially invasive (early stage) adenocarcinomas, the appearance can be subtle with small nodules, plaques, or irregular mucosal bumps in a background of typical salmon-pink Barrett mucosa (Fig 16.4A). Extensive sectioning of the Barrett segment for histologic examination, especially in areas of mucosa irregularity, is necessary to identify microscopic foci of intramucosal adenocarcinoma that invade into lamina propria or muscularis mucosae.

The gross pathology of more advanced esophageal adenocarcinoma is similar to that of SCC, with the infiltrative type being most common (40%–50%), followed by fungating or polypoid type (25%–35%) and flat type (10%–15%) (60). Secondary involvement of the EGJ and gastric cardia by direct tumor extension from the distal esophagus is also frequently observed (Fig. 16.4B). The presence of Barrett mucosa can be masked in some cases of advanced adenocarcinoma due to overgrowth of Barrett epithelium by large tumor masses.

Multifocal tumors can occur occasionally, and these are more common in early stage tumors arising in long segment

Barrett esophagus (21,61). Adenocarcinomas of the upper or cervical esophagus typically arise from heterotopic gastric mucosa (inlet patch). In these cases, normal-appearing esophageal squamous mucosa is present between the tumor and EGJ (Fig. 16.4C–E). The gross appearance of adenocarcinoma following preoperative adjuvant therapy is similar to SCC and depends on the degree of tumor response to treatment.

Microscopic Pathology

Tumor Differentiation. Adenocarcinomas are graded as well-, moderately, or poorly differentiated based on the degree of glandular differentiation. Most esophageal adenocarcinomas are either well- or moderately differentiated (60). Well-differentiated adenocarcinomas are defined as tumors containing more than 95% cystic or tubular glands lined by cuboidal or columnar epithelium. In some cases, the cytologic atypia can be quite minimal, posing a diagnostic challenge in superficial mucosal biopsy specimens; in such cases, invasion into submucosa or the muscular wall may be needed to make a correct diagnosis. Moderately differentiated adenocarcinomas are composed of glands (50%–95% of tumor) and solid tumor nests with a higher degree of cellular atypia and nuclear pleomorphism (Fig 16.5A). Tumors growing in solid sheets or as single cells with only occasional (<5%) gland formation are classified as poorly differentiated (Fig. 16.5B); these typically also have pronounced cytologic atypia and nuclear pleomorphism. Specific subtypes of esophageal adenocarcinoma include mucinous adenocarcinoma (characterized by abundant mucin pools with floating tumor clusters), which accounts for 5% to 10% of cases (Fig 16.5C), and signet ring cell adenocarcinoma, which accounts for approximately 5% of cases (Fig 16.5D) (60).

Neuroendocrine differentiation is present in a significant minority (20%–30%) of esophageal adenocarcinomas (62,63). Tumor cells with neuroendocrine differentiation identified by immunohistochemistry for chromogranin and synaptophysin tend to be focal in distribution and mostly located at the periphery of tumor glands, but occasional esophageal adenocarcinomas contain a significant component of neuroendocrine differentiation. The presence of neuroendocrine differentiation appears to have no effect on patients' prognosis, however (63). Primary esophageal choriocarcinoma is extremely rare (64), but occasional aberrant expression of human chorionic gonadotropin can be seen in poorly differentiated adenocarcinoma.

Most esophageal adenocarcinomas have cytokeratin 7 (CK7) positivity and are negative for cytokeratin 20 (CK20) (65,66). This CK7/CK20 profile distinguishes esophageal adenocarcinoma from colorectal adenocarcinoma but does not help in distinguishing primary esophageal carcinoma from metastatic adenocarcinoma originating in the lung, breast, or stomach. The presence of Barrett esophagus can support the diagnosis of primary esophageal adenocarcinoma. Immunolabeling for TTF-1 and estrogen and progesterone receptors can be used to support lung or breast primaries, respectively.

Tumor Spread and Metastasis. Esophageal adenocarcinomas initially spread locally and infiltrate the esophageal wall. Direct extension of tumor into the proximal gastric wall is commonly seen in tumors with involvement of the EGJ. Tumors can also invade through the esophageal wall into periesophageal adventitia and adjacent organs such as lung, trachea, or pericardium. Similar to SCC, depth of tumor invasion (T stage) correlates well with the presence of lymphovascular invasion and regional lymph node metastasis (N stage) (67,68). Lymph nodes with metastases are present in 50% to 60% of resected specimens and are correlated with depth of tumor invasion (67–69). Tumor invasion into intramural lymphatic vessels can occur at early stages of disease (70). The most frequent sites of distant metastases are lung and liver.

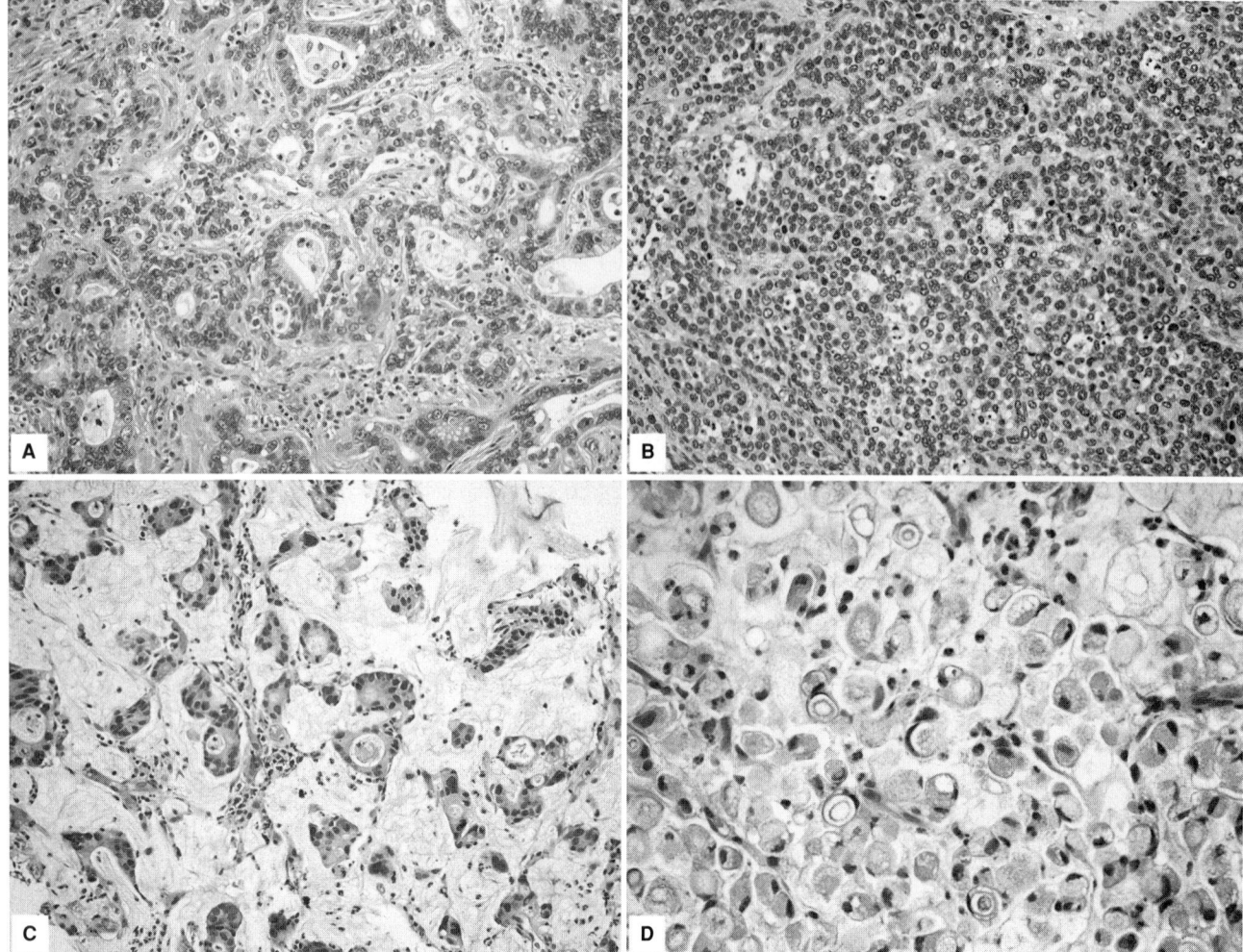

FIGURE 16.5. Histologic features of adenocarcinoma. **A:** Moderately differentiated adenocarcinoma with gland formation. **B:** Poorly differentiated adenocarcinoma with solid or sheetlike growth pattern and no obvious gland formation. **C:** Mucinous adenocarcinoma characterized by clusters of adenocarcinoma cells floating in extracellular mucin pools. **D:** Signet ring cell carcinoma containing classic individual neoplastic tumor cells with a signet ring appearance.

Superficially invasive (T1) adenocarcinomas account for 16% to 38% of esophageal adenocarcinomas (29,60,67,71). Within this group, depth of tumor invasion also affects outcome because adenocarcinomas confined to the mucosa (T1a) have significantly better overall survival and recurrencefree survival than adenocarcinomas that invade submucosa (T1b) (70). Lymphovascular invasion is present in only 6% of adenocarcinomas confined to the mucosa but in up to 41% of carcinomas invading submucosa (70,72). Similarly, lymph node metastases are only rarely associated with intramucosal carcinomas, but occur in up to 33% of submucosal tumors (70,71).

Precursor Lesion: Barrett Dysplasia (Intraepithelial Neoplasia)

Barrett esophagus is the precursor of most esophageal adenocarcinoma. The accumulated morphologic and molecular evidence indicates that esophageal adenocarcinomas arise through a Barrett metaplasia-dysplasia-adenocarcinoma sequence (53,73). Barrett dysplasia, a premalignant precursor lesion for esophageal adenocarcinoma, is present adjacent to inva-

sive adenocarcinoma in more than 90% of cases (60,70,71). Barrett dysplasia is defined by presence of cytologically and architecturally neoplastic columnar epithelial cells confined in the mucosa. Barrett dysplasia generally has no distinctive gross appearance and is detected by systematic sampling of the salmon-pink, flat Barrett mucosa. In some cases, dysplastic lesions can appear as erosions, nodules, or polyps (74).

Barrett dysplasia can be further subclassified in a two-tiered system as either low-grade or high-grade dysplasia, using a similar scheme for grading of dysplasia in idiopathic inflammatory bowel disease (75). A diagnosis of "indefinite for dysplasia" is made when the histologic distinction between dysplasia and regenerative atypia is not clear.

Indefinite for Dysplasia

Barrett esophagus is a metaplastic process due to chronic gastroesophageal reflux, and most patients have ongoing reflux with active inflammation, erosion, and even ulceration. Biopsies of Barrett epithelium in the presence of active inflammation can have marked cytologic atypia, architectural distortion, and nuclear crowding or stratification; however, in contrast to definite dysplasia, there is typically maturation to the surface

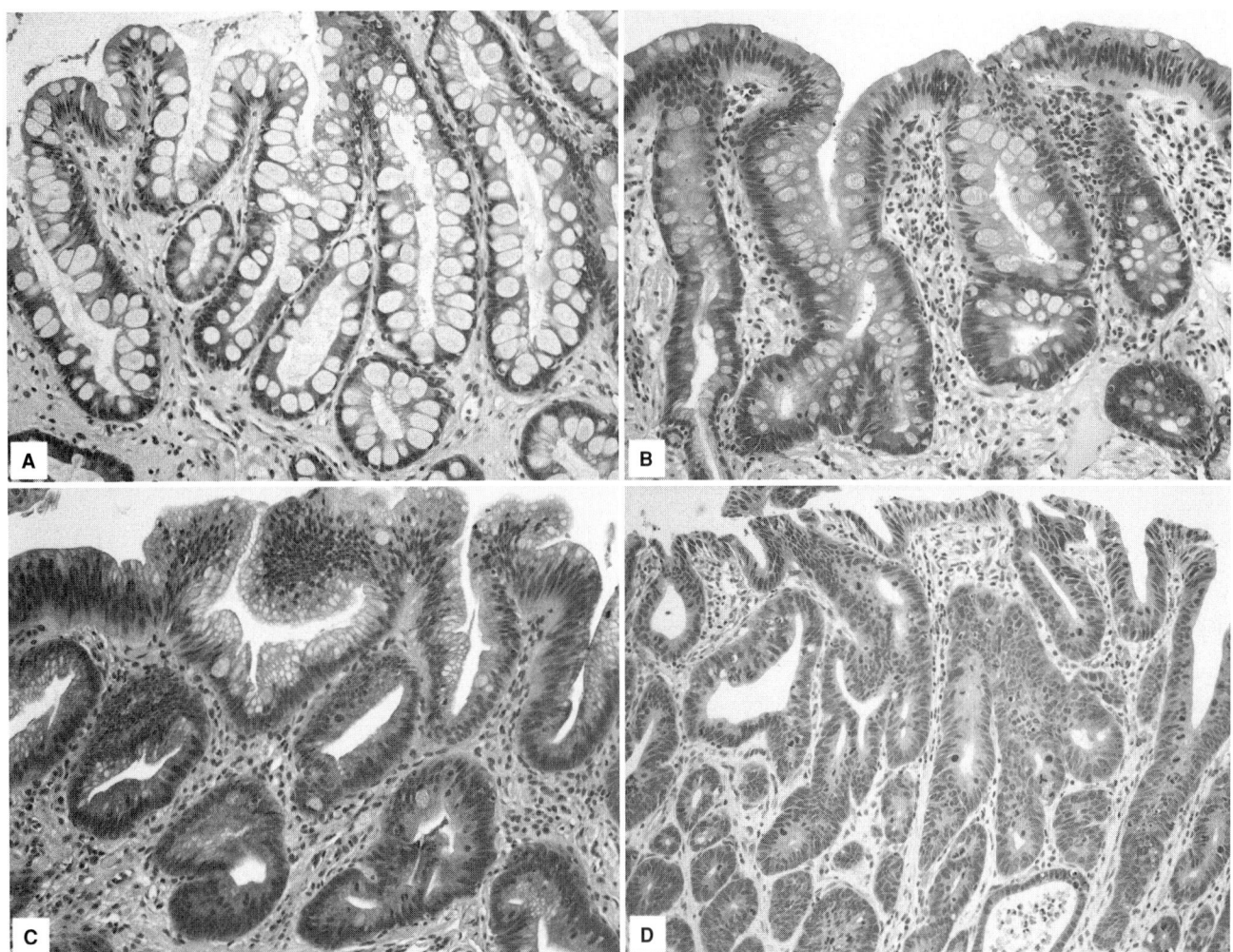

FIGURE 16.6. Histologic grading of dysplasia in Barrett esophagus. **A:** Negative for dysplasia. The columnar epithelium contains goblet cells with small basally located nuclei. **B:** Indefinite for dysplasia. The columnar epithelium has a mild degree of nuclear pseudostratification and crypt architectural disarray, but there is maturation at the surface epithelium. **C:** Low-grade dysplasia. Neoplastic columnar epithelial proliferation with a mild to moderate degree of nuclear hyperchromatism and pseudostratification limited to the lower half of the epithelium. **D:** High-grade dysplasia characterized by loss of cytoplasmic mucin, marked nuclear hyperchromatism, increased nuclear:cytoplasmic ratio, and marked crypt architectural disarray.

epithelium (Fig. 16.6A, B). In this situation, a definitive distinction between dysplasia and regenerative atypia is impossible, and such biopsies should be classified as indefinite for dysplasia. It is important to note that there are no uniform and reproducible diagnostic criteria for this category, and it is subject to significant interobserver variation (76,77). For practical clinical management purposes, patients with a diagnosis of indefinite for dysplasia should be followed as low-grade dysplasia. A repeat biopsy after adequate control of reflux disease is normally indicated.

Low-Grade Dysplasia

The dysplastic columnar epithelium has mild to moderate crypt distortion, decreased cytoplasmic mucin, mild nuclear pleomorphism, and nuclear pseudostratification or crowding. In contrast to high-grade dysplasia, nuclear pseudostratification is limited to the lower half of the epithelial layer (Fig. 16.6C). These histologic features typically present from the basal crypts and extend onto the surface epithelium. Similar to the indef-

inite category, a substantial degree of interobserver variation also exists in grading low-grade dysplasia (76,77).

High-Grade Dysplasia

The cytologic atypia and architectural distortion are more pronounced in high-grade dysplasia. High-grade dysplasia is characterized by marked nuclear hyperchromatism, increased nuclear/cytoplasmic ratio, full-thickness nuclear pseudostratification, marked decrease in cytoplasmic mucin, and marked crypt architectural disarray (Fig. 16.6D). A cribriform glandular pattern without disruption of the basement membrane is also a feature of high-grade dysplasia, but in these cases the distinction from adenocarcinoma invading into lamina propria (intramucosal adenocarcinoma) can be difficult when only small biopsy fragments are examined. In contrast to low-grade/indefinite for dysplasia, there is an excellent agreement in grading high-grade dysplasia among gastrointestinal pathologists (76,77).

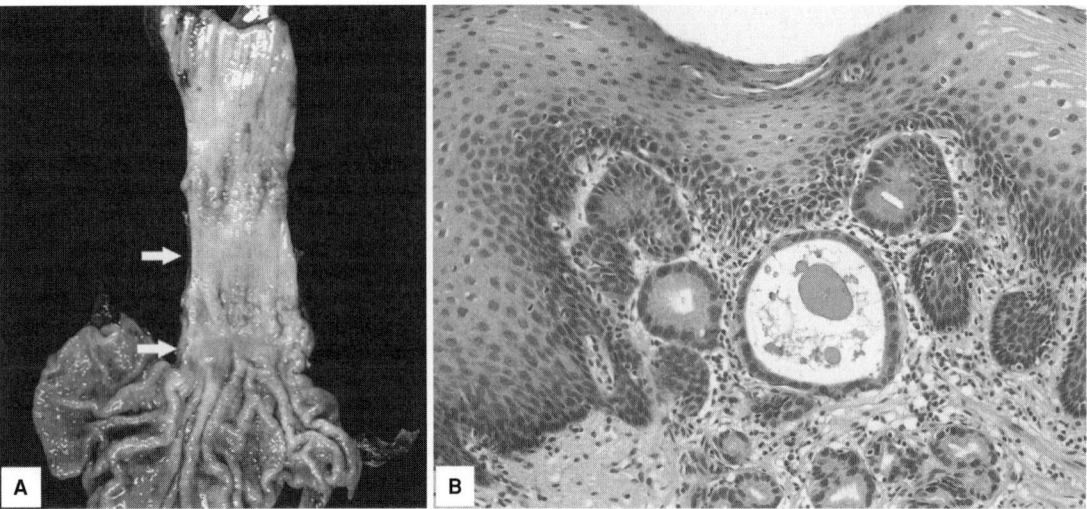

FIGURE 16.7. Barrett esophagus after photodynamic therapy (PDT). **A:** Gross image of Barrett esophagus with high-grade dysplasia after PDT. Residual Barrett mucosa is interposed with normal-appearing squamous esophageal mucosa (*arrows*). **B:** Microscopically, the areas of grossly normal squamous mucosa contain residual dysplastic Barrett mucosa that is covered by squamous epithelium ("pseudoregression").

Occult invasive adenocarcinoma can be detected in up to 43% of patients who undergo esophagectomy for high-grade dysplasia in Barrett esophagus (78,79). For this reason, a diagnosis of high-grade dysplasia should be confirmed by an experienced gastrointestinal pathologist, and extensive sampling of Barrett esophagus should be undertaken to identify any coexisting adenocarcinoma.

The natural history of low-grade dysplasia in Barrett esophagus is difficult to predict, mainly due to significant interobserver variation in the diagnosis of low-grade dysplasia. An increased risk of progression to high-grade dysplasia or invasive adenocarcinoma has been shown in cases with a consistent diagnosis of low-grade dysplasia (80). High-grade dysplasia, however, has been widely accepted as a precursor of invasive adenocarcinoma. Published progression rates from high-grade dysplasia into invasive adenocarcinoma vary significantly among different studies, ranging from 16% to 53% in patients with long-term follow-up (55,81). The extent of high-grade dysplasia in Barrett esophagus correlates with risk of developing invasive adenocarcinoma; patients with diffuse high-grade dysplasia have a 3.7-fold increased risk of esophageal adenocarcinoma as compared to patients with only focal high-grade dysplasia (82). Close endoscopic surveillance with intensive sampling of Barrett esophagus for early diagnosis of occult invasive adenocarcinoma, photodynamic therapy (PDT), or removal of visible lesions by endoscopic mucosal resection (EMR) are alternatives to esophagectomy for treatment of high-grade dysplasia.

Treated Barrett Dysplasia

A variety of noninvasive techniques such as argon plasma coagulation, laser ablation, and PDT have been used to treat Barrett esophagus with dysplasia (83). The aim of these types of treatment is to destroy Barrett mucosa and dysplastic lesions with subsequent re-epithelialization by normal squamous epithelium. Residual Barrett epithelium typically presents with isolated islands, and squamous epithelium overlying Barrett glands is commonly seen—in up to 52% of cases—after therapy (84,85). High-grade dysplasia or intramucosal adenocarcinomas arising in Barrett esophagus have persisted in

approximately 50% of cases after PDT (85). The endoscopic appearance of the esophagus following PDT can be deceptively normal because re-epithelialization by squamous mucosa can cover residual Barrett glands (Fig. 16.7A). One alarming histologic finding that warrants specific attention is the presence of squamous re-epithelialization over dysplastic Barrett epithelium or even adenocarcinoma, which has been documented in 27% of cases after PDT (Fig. 16.7B) (85). Similarly, genetic abnormalities such as p53 mutations or p16 hypermethylation can persist after PDT despite histologic improvement (86).

Endoscopic Mucosal Resection

Endoscopic mucosal resection (EMR) has been recently used in the treatment of early esophageal carcinoma or high-grade dysplastic lesions as an alternative for esophagectomy (87). The therapeutic utility has been limited due to the high rate of positive lateral and/or deep resection margins based on series from Europe and North America (88). Complete resection of dysplastic lesions or adenocarcinomas as judged by histologic examination can only be achieved in 4% of cases, and 86% of cases with positive margins have residual disease on follow-up biopsies (88). However, EMR can be used as a diagnostic and staging tool, and offers more information than endoscopic biopsy for further management decisions (89). The study by Mino-Kenudson et al. showed that EMR can improve the diagnosis and staging of Barrett dysplasia and adenocarcinoma as compared to biopsy; three of their ten cases with a biopsy diagnosis of high-grade dysplasia had intramucosal adenocarcinoma in subsequent EMR specimens (88).

EMR specimens need to be handled carefully by endoscopists and pathologists. Orientation of the EMR specimens is critical for pathological examination. The peripheral and deep resection margins need to be inked, and the specimen needs to be sectioned according to the location of the gross lesion (Fig. 16.8A, B). The two ends away from the lesion should be submitted as en face margins, and perpendicular sections should be taken in-between. Microscopic examination should include the histologic grade of dysplasia and/or adenocarcinoma as

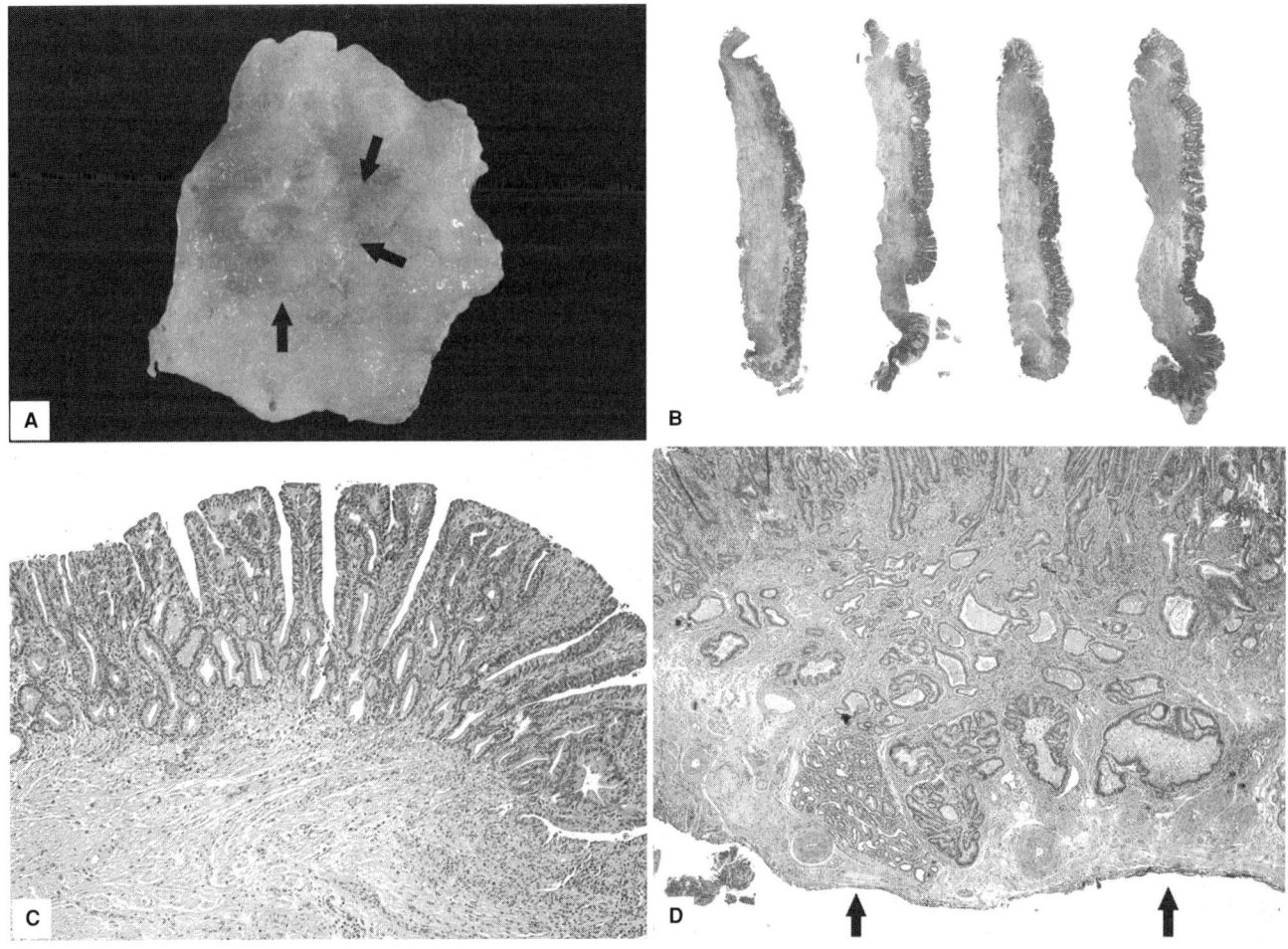

FIGURE 16.8. Pathological evaluation of Barrett dysplasia and adenocarcinoma after endoscopic mucosal resection. **A:** Gross image of Barrett mucosa containing a slightly elevated lesion (*arrows*) after endoscopic mucosal resection. **B:** Low-power image of a hematoxylin-and-eosin–stained cross section through the lesion (shown in **A**), containing Barrett mucosa with high-grade dysplasia (**C**). **D:** In another case, adenocarcinoma invades into submucosa and extends close to the inked deep endoscopic mucosal resection margin (*arrows*).

well as resection margin status (Fig. 16.8C, D). In cases with adenocarcinoma, the depth of tumor invasion and presence or absence of lymphovascular invasion should also be recorded (Fig. 16.8D).

PATHOLOGY AFTER PREOPERATIVE CHEMORADIATION

Positron emission tomography scan is a promising technique for assessing response to preoperative therapy (90), but at present there are no reliable clinical diagnostic tools that accurately predict pathological response after preoperative chemoradiation. Pathological evaluation of the resected esophagus after preoperative chemoradiation remains the gold standard for assessing response until specific molecular markers can be identified. In a retrospective study, posttherapy pathological stage was the best predictor of outcome for patients with locoregional esophageal carcinoma treated with preoperative chemoradiation followed by surgery, irrespective of different chemotherapy regimens used (14). Patient outcome after preoperative chemoradiation is significantly better when no residual carcinoma (complete patho-

logical response) is found in the resected esophagus specimen (91–95).

Gross Pathology

The gross appearance of the chemoradiated esophagus will vary depending on the extent of tumor response to treatment. In approximately 25% of cases, there is minimal response to preoperative chemoradiation, and these specimens present with grossly identifiable tumor similar to untreated carcinoma, although the surrounding esophageal mucosa typically has therapy-related erosions or ulcerations (Fig. 16.9A). The presence of gross residual disease is associated with poor outcome (14). In the remaining 75% of treated cases, there is no grossly identifiable residual tumor, but the esophageal wall may be thickened secondary to fibrosis and there may be extensive mucosal ulceration (Fig 16.9B). In specimens without gross residual tumor, it is necessary to completely embed the treatment field for histologic evaluation in order to separate patients with complete pathological response from patients with microscopic residual disease. Patients with microscopic residual disease have a prognosis that is intermediate between complete response and gross residual disease (14).

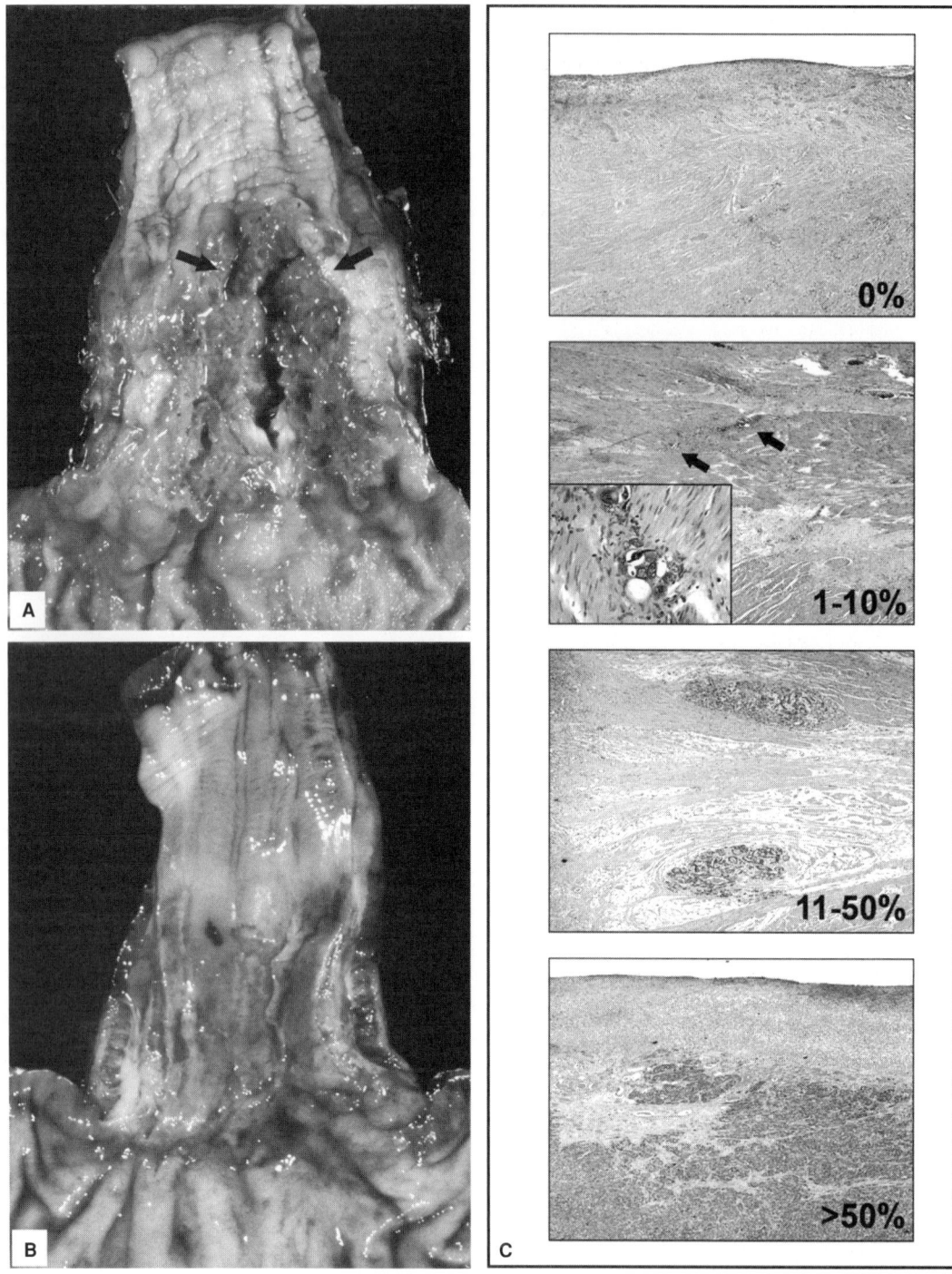

FIGURE 16.9. Esophageal carcinoma after preoperative chemoradiation. **A:** Gross residual carcinoma with a fungating and ulcerating tumor mass (*arrows*) indicates minimal or no treatment response. **B:** Diffuse ulceration, fibrotic esophageal wall and no grossly identifiable tumor are more frequently present after preoperative chemoradiation. **C:** Histologic assessment of residual esophageal carcinoma after preoperative chemoradiation. The extent of residual carcinoma is semiquantitatively classified into 0% (no residual carcinoma), 1% to 10% residual carcinoma, 11% to 50% residual carcinoma, and >50% residual carcinoma.

Microscopic Pathology

Therapy-related histologic changes can include mucosal ulceration with granulation tissue, stromal cell atypia, transmural fibrosis, and radiation-induced perivascular fibrosis. Degree of response to preoperative chemoradiation can be evaluated by estimation of the ratio of residual carcinoma to the original carcinoma area. In a large retrospective histologic evaluation of esophageal specimens after preoperative chemoradiation, the degree of residual carcinoma was assigned semiquantitatively into four categories: no residual carcinoma, 1% to 10% residual carcinoma, 11% to 50% residual carcinoma, and >50% residual carcinoma (Fig. 16.9C) (14). In this scheme, the original carcinoma area was considered to represent the area of radiotherapy-induced tissue injury on histologic examination (14,96). Patient outcome was shown to be correlated with the percent of residual carcinoma as divided into three categories— no residual carcinoma, 1% to 50% residual carcinoma, and >50% residual carcinoma (14). A subsequent study showed this to be a relatively simple and reproducible method for grading the extent of residual carcinoma and for assessing pathological response after preoperative chemoradiation (97).

Extracellular mucin pools are present in 17% of esophagectomy specimens after preoperative chemoradiation, usually in patients who had pretreatment tumor biopsies that contained mucinous or signet ring cell carcinoma. In 40% of cases with extracellular mucin pools, the mucin pools are acellular (containing no residual adenocarcinoma cells), and these acellular mucin pools can present in the submucosa, muscularis propria, or even periesophageal adventitia (98). The presence of acellular mucin pools should be considered as a complete pathological response and does not represent residual disease. In particular, acellular mucin pools present at the radial resection margin are not associated with increased risk for developing recurrent tumor (98). In a recent study, all 13 patients with only acellular mucin pools in their esophagectomy specimens following preoperative chemoradiation were alive after an average of 3-years follow-up (98).

Neuroendocrine differentiation is present in 20% to 30% of esophageal adenocarcinomas and can persist after preoperative chemoradiation (62,63). Some residual carcinomas are composed predominantly of tumor cells with abundant eosinophilic cytoplasm that suggests neuroendocrine differentiation, an impression that can be supported by positive immunohistochemistry for chromogranin or synaptophysin. The proportion of tumor cells with neuroendocrine differentiation appears to increase after chemoradiation as compared to pretreatment biopsy material. The clinical significance of neuroendocrine differentiation in residual adenocarcinoma, however, remains to be clarified.

Endoscopic biopsies of the esophagus after chemoradiation have sometimes been used to evaluate treatment response, but their clinical utility is limited. This is due to the fact that residual carcinoma is not often present in a superficial location that would be amenable to endoscopic biopsy. One study demonstrated that as many as 77% of patients had residual carcinoma in their esophagectomy specimens, yet the preoperative mucosal biopsies had been negative in 80% of these cases (99). Another potential pitfall in evaluation of mucosal biopsies after chemoradiation is overdiagnosis due to the reactive atypia that typically accompanies chemoradiation. In evaluating these biopsies, pathologists need to be aware of the patient's history and cognizant of treatment-related epithelial atypia to avoid overdiagnosis of dysplasia or residual carcinoma (100).

References

1. Jemal A, Tiwari RC, Murray T, et al. Cancer statistics, 2004. *CA Cancer J Clin* 2004;54:8–29.
2. Hesketh PJ, Clapp RW, Doos WG, et al. The increasing frequency of adenocarcinoma of the esophagus. *Cancer* 1989;64:526–530.
3. Devesa SS, Blot WJ, Fraumeni JF, Jr. Changing patterns in the incidence of esophageal and gastric carcinoma in the United States. *Cancer* 1998;83: 2049–2053.
4. Pickens A, Orringer MB. Geographical distribution and racial disparity in esophageal cancer. *Ann Thorac Surg* 2003;76:S1367—S1369.
5. Ando N, Ozawa S, Kitagawa Y, Shinozawa Y, et al. Improvement in the results of surgical treatment of advanced squamous esophageal carcinoma during 15 consecutive years. *Ann Surg* 2000;232:225–232.
6. Holscher AH, Bollschweiler E, Bumm R, et al. Prognostic factors of resected adenocarcinoma of the esophagus. *Surgery* 1995;118:845–855.
7. Steup WH, De Leyn P, Deneffe G, Van Raemdonck D, Coosemans W, Lerut T. Tumors of the esophagogastric junction: long-term survival in relation to the pattern of lymph node metastasis and a critical analysis of the accuracy or inaccuracy of pTNM classification. *J Thorac Cardiovasc Surg* 1996;111:85–94.
8. Coia LR, Minsky BD, Berkey BA, et al. Outcome of patients receiving radiation for cancer of the esophagus: results of the 1992–1994 Patterns of Care Study. *J Clin Oncol* 2000;18:455–462.
9. Walsh TN, Noonan N, Hollywood D, et al. A comparison of multimodal therapy and surgery for esophageal adenocarcinoma. *N Engl J Med* 1996; 335:462–467.
10. Kelsen DP, Ginsberg R, Pajak TF, et al. Chemotherapy followed by surgery compared with surgery alone for localized esophageal cancer. *N Engl J Med* 1998;339:1979–1984.
11. Herskovic A, Martz K, al-Sarraf M, et al. Combined chemotherapy and radiotherapy compared with radiotherapy alone in patients with cancer of the esophagus. *N Engl J Med* 1992;326:1593–1598.
12. Urba SG, Orringer MB, Turrisi A, et al. Randomized trial of preoperative chemoradiation versus surgery alone in patients with locoregional esophageal carcinoma. *J Clin Oncol* 2001;19:305–313.
13. Bosset JF, Gignoux M, Triboulet JP, et al. Chemoradiotherapy followed by surgery compared with surgery alone in squamous cell cancer of the esophagus. *N Engl J Med* 1997;337:161–167.
14. Chirieac LR, Swisher SG, Ajani JA, et al. Posttherapy pathologic stage predicts survival in patients with esophageal carcinoma receiving preoperative chemoradiation. *Cancer* 2005;103:1347–1355.
15. Ribiero U, Posner MC, Safatle-Ribiero AV, et al. Risk factors for squamous cell carcinoma of the oesophagus. *Br J Surg* 1996;83:1174–1183.
16. Turner JR, Shen LH, Crum CP, et al. Low prevalence of human papillomavirus infection in esophageal squamous cell carcinomas from North America: analysis by a highly sensitive and specific polymerase chain reaction–based approach. *Hum Pathol* 1997;28:174–178.
17. Poljak M, Cerar A, Seme K. Human papillomavirus infection in esophageal carcinomas: study of 121 lesions using multiple broad spectrum polymerase chain reactions and literature review. *Hum Pathol* 1998;29: 266–271.
18. Chang F, Syrjanen S, Shen Q, et al. Human papillomavirus involvement in esophageal carcinogenesis in the high-incidence area of China: a study of 700 cases by screening and type-specific in situ hybridization. *Scand J Gastroenterol* 2000;35:123–130.
19. Norton GA, Postlethwait RW, Thompson WM. Esophageal carcinoma: a survey of populations at risk. *South Med J* 1980;73:25–27.
20. Rosengard AM, Hamilton SR. Squamous carcinoma of the esophagus in patients with Barrett esophagus. *Mod Pathol* 1989;2:2–7.
21. Lewin KJ, Appelman HD. *Tumors of the Esophagus and Stomach. Atlas of Tumor Pathology, 3rd Series, Vol. 18.* Washington, DC: Armed Forces Institute of Pathology; 1996.
22. Schmidt LW, Dean PJ, Wilson RT. Superficially invasive squamous cell carcinoma of the esophagus: a study of seven cases in Memphis, Tennessee. *Gastroenterology* 1986;91:1456–1461.
23. Bogomoletz WV, Molas G, Gayet B, et al. Superficial squamous cell carcinoma of the esophagus: a report of 76 cases and review of the literature. *Am J Surg Pathol* 1989;13:535–546.
24. Kuwano H, Ohno S, Matsuda H, Mori M, Sugimachi K. Serial histologic evaluation of multiple primary squamous cell carcinomas of the esophagus. *Cancer* 1988;61:1635–1638.
25. Mandard AM, Marnay J, Gignoux M, et al. Cancer of the esophagus and associated lesions: detailed pathologic study of 100 esophagectomy specimens. *Hum Pathol* 1984;15:660–669.
26. Pesko P, Rakic S, Milicevic M, et al. Prevalence and clinicopathologic features of multiple squamous cell carcinoma of the esophagus. *Cancer* 1994;73:2687–2690.
27. Kaufman O, Fietze E, Mengs J, Dietel M. Value of p63 and cytokeratin 5/6 as immunohistochemical markers for the differential diagnosis of poorly differentiated and undifferentiated carcinomas. *Am J Clin Pathol* 2001;116:823–830.
28. Tajima Y, Nakanishi Y, Ochai A, et al. Histopathologic findings predicting lymph node metastasis and prognosis of patients with superficial esophageal carcinoma: analysis of 240 surgically resected tumors. *Cancer* 2000;88:1285–1293.
29. Torres C, Turner JR, Wang HH, et al. Pathologic prognostic factors in Barrett's associated adenocarcinoma: a follow-up study of 96 patients. *Cancer* 1999;85:520–528.
30. Kuwano H, Nagamatsu M, Ohno S, et al. Coexistence of intraepithelial carcinoma and glandular differentiation in esophageal squamous cell carcinoma. *Cancer* 1988;62:1568–1572.
31. Fujiwara Y, Nakagawa K, Tanaka T, et al. Small cell carcinoma of the esophagus combined with superficial esophageal cancer. *Hepatogastroenterology* 1996;43:1360–1369.
32. Ide H, Nakamura T, Hayashi K, et al. Esophageal squamous cell carcinoma: pathology and prognosis. *World J Surg* 1994;18:321–330.
33. Soga J, Tanaka O, Sasaki K, Kawaguchi M, Muto T. Superficial spreading carcinoma of the esophagus. *Cancer* 1982;50:1641–1645.
34. Takubo K, Sasajima K, Yamashita K, et al. Prognostic significance of intramural metastasis in patients with esophageal carcinoma. *Cancer* 1990;65: 1816–1819.
35. Mandard AM, Chasle J, Marnay J, et al. Autopsy findings in 111 cases of esophageal cancer. *Cancer* 1981;48:329–335.

36. Thorban S, Roder JD, Nekarda H, et al. Immunocytochemical detection of disseminated tumor cells in the bone marrow of patients with esophageal carcinoma. *J Natl Cancer Inst* 1996;88:1222–1227.

37. Abe K, Sasano H, Itakura Y, et al. Basaloid-squamous carcinoma of the esophagus: a clinicopathologic, DNA ploidy, and immunohistochemical study of seven cases. *Am J Surg Pathol* 1996;20:453–461.

38. Agha FP, Weatherbee L, Sams JS. Verrucous carcinoma of the esophagus. *Am J Gastroenterol* 1984;79:844–849.

39. Kavin H, Yaremko L, Valatis J, Chowdhury L. Chronic esophagitis evolving to verrucous squamous cell carcinoma: possible role of exogenous chemical carcinogens. *Gastroenterology* 1996;110:904–914.

40. Iasone C, Barreca M. Carcinosarcoma and pseudosarcoma of the esophagus: two names, one disease—comprehensive review of the literature. *World J Surg* 1999;23:153–157.

41. Lauwers GY, Grant Ld, Scott GV, et al. Spindle cell squamous carcinoma of the esophagus: analysis of ploidy and tumor proliferative activity in a series of 13 cases. *Hum Pathol* 1998;29:863–868.

42. Balercia G, Bhan AK, Dickersin GR. Sarcomatoid carcinoma: an ultrastructural study with light microscopic and immunohistochemical correlation of 10 cases from various anatomic sites. *Ultrastruct Pathol* 1995;19:249–263.

43. Dawsey SM, Lewin KJ. Histologic precursors of squamous esophageal cancer. *Pathol Annu* 1995;30:209–226.

44. Dawsey SM, Wang GQ, Weinstein WM, et al. Squamous dysplasia and early esophageal cancer in the Linxian region of China: distinctive endoscopic lesions. *Gastroenterology* 1993;105:1333–1340.

45. Dawsey SM, Fleischer DE, Wang GQ, et al. Mucosal iodine staining improves endoscopic visualization of squamous dysplasia and squamous cell carcinoma of the esophagus in Linxian, China. *Cancer* 1998;83:220–231.

46. Tajima Y, Nakanishi Y, Tachimori Y, et al. Significance of involvement by squamous cell carcinoma of the ducts of esophageal submucosal glands: analysis of 201 surgically resected superficial squamous cell carcinomas. *Cancer* 2000;89:248–254.

47. Qui S, Yang G. Precursor lesions of esophageal cancer in high-risk populations in Henan Province, China. *Cancer* 1998;62:551–557.

48. Dawsey SM, Lewin KJ, Liu FS, et al. Esophageal morphology from Linxian, China: squamous histologic findings in 754 patients. *Cancer* 1994;73:2027–2037.

49. Hoang MP, Hobbs CM, Sobin LH, Albores-Saavedra J. Carcinoid tumor of the esophagus: a clinicopathologic study of four cases. *Am J Surg Pathol* 2002;26:517–522.

50. Casas F, Ferrer F, Farrus B, et al. Primary small cell carcinoma of the esophagus: a review of the literature with emphasis on therapy and prognosis. *Cancer* 1997;80:1366–1372.

51. Takubo K, Nakamura K, Sawabe M, et al. Primary undifferentiated small cell carcinoma of the esophagus. *Hum Pathol* 1999;30:216–221.

52. Spechler SJ. Barrett's esophagus. *N Engl J Med* 2002;346:836–842.

53. Hameeteman W, Tytgat GN, Houthoff HJ, van den Tweel JG. Barrett's esophagus: development of dysplasia and adenocarcinoma. *Gastroenterology* 1989;96:1249–1256.

54. Shaheen NJ, Crosby MA, Bozymski EM, Sandler RS. Is there publication bias in the reporting of cancer risk in Barrett's esophagus? *Gastroenterology* 2000;119:333–338.

55. Weston AP, Sharma P, Topalovski M, et al. Long-term follow-up of Barrett's high-grade dysplasia. *Am J Gastroenterol* 2000;95:1888–1893.

56. Avidan B, Sonnenberg A, Schnell TG, et al. Hiatal hernia size, Barrett's length, and severity of acid reflux are all risk factors for esophageal adenocarcinoma. *Am J Gastroenterol* 2002;97:1930–1936.

57. Conio M, Cameron AJ, Romero Y, et al. Secular trends in the epidemiology and outcome of Barrett's oesophagus in Olmsted County, Minnesota. *Gut* 2001;48:304–309.

58. Hamilton SR, Smith RL, Cameron JL. Prevalence and characteristics of Barrett's esophagus in patients with adenocarcinoma of the esophagus or esophagogastric junction. *Hum Pathol* 1988;19:942–948.

59. Cameron AJ, Lomboy CT, Pera M, Carpenter HA. Adenocarcinoma of the esophagogastric junction and Barrett's esophagus. *Gastroenterology* 1995;109:1541–1546.

60. Paraf F, Flejou JF, Pignon JP, et al. Surgical pathology of adenocarcinoma arising in Barrett's esophagus: analysis of 67 cases. *Am J Surg Pathol* 1995;19:183–191.

61. Smith RR, Hamilton SR, Boinott JK, Rogers EL. The spectrum of carcinoma arising in Barrett's esophagus: a clinicopathologic study of 26 patients. *Am J Surg Pathol* 1984;8:563–573.

62. Griffin M, Sweeney EC. The relationship of endocrine cells, dysplasia and carcinoembryonic antigen in Barrett's mucosa to adenocarcinoma of the oesophagus. *Histopathology* 1987;11:53–62.

63. Hamilton K, Chiappori A, Olson S, et al. Prevalence and prognostic significance of neuroendocrine cells in esophageal adenocarcinoma. *Mod Pathol* 2000;13:475–481.

64. Kikuchi Y, Tsuneta Y, Kawai T, Aizawa M. Choriocarcinoma of the esophagus producing chorionic gonadotropin. *Acta Pathol Jpn* 1988;38:489–499.

65. Ormsby AH, Goldblum JR, Rice TW, et al. The utility of cytokeratin subsets in distinguishing Barrett's-related esophageal adenocarcinoma from gastric adenocarcinoma. *Histopathology* 2001;38:307–311.

66. Taniere P, Scoazec GB, Saurin JC, et al. Cytokeratin expression in adenocarcinomas of the esophagogastric junction. *Am J Surg Pathol* 2002;26:1213–1221.

67. Rice TW, Zuccaro GJ, Adelstein DJ, et al. Esophageal carcinoma: depth of tumor invasion is predictive of regional lymph node status. *Ann Thorac Surg* 1998;65:787–792.

68. Hagen JA, DeMeester SR, Peters JH, Chandrasoma P, DeMeester TR. Curative resection for esophageal adenocarcinoma: analysis of 100 en bloc esophagectomies. *Ann Surg* 2001;234:520–531.

69. Siewert JR, Stein HJ, Feith M, et al. Histologic tumor type is an independent prognostic parameter in esophageal cancer: lessons from more than 1,000 consecutive resections at single center in the Western world. *Ann Surg* 2001;234:360–367.

70. Liu L, Hofstetter WL, Rashid A, et al. Significance of the depth of tumor invasion and lymph node metastasis in superficially invasive (T1) esophageal adenocarcinoma. *Am J Pathol* 2005;29:1079–1085.

71. van Sandick JW, van Lanschot JJ, ten Kate FJ, et al. Pathology of early invasive adenocarcinoma of the esophagus or esophagogastric junction: implications for therapeutic decision making. *Cancer* 2000;88:2429–2437.

72. Hosch SB, Stoecklein NH, Pichlmeier U, et al. Esophageal cancer: the mode of lymphatic tumor cell spread and its prognostic significance. *J Clin Oncol* 2001;19:1970–1975.

73. Reid BJ, Blount PL, Rubin CE, et al. Predictors of progression to malignancy in Barrett's esophagus: endoscopic, histologic and flow cytometric follow-up of a cohort. *Gastroenterology* 1992;102:1212–1219.

74. Lee RG. Adenomas arising in Barrett's esophagus. *Am J Clin Pathol* 1986;85:629–632.

75. Haggitt RC. Barrett's esophagus, dysplasia and adenocarcinoma. *Hum Pathol* 1994;25:982–993.

76. Reid BJ, Haggitt RC, Rubin CE, et al. Observer variation in the diagnosis of dysplasia in Barrett's esophagus. *Hum Pathol* 1988;19:166–178.

77. Montgomery E, Bronner M, Goldblum JR, et al. Reproducibility of the diagnosis of dysplasia in Barrett esophagus (BE): a reaffirmation. *Hum Pathol* 2001;32:368–378.

78. Hamilton SR, Smith RRL. The relationship between columnar epithelial dysplasia and invasive adenocarcinoma arising in Barrett's esophagus. *Am J Clin Pathol* 1987;87:301–312.

79. Heitmiller RF, Redmond M, Hamilton SR. Barrett's esophagus with high-grade dysplasia: an indication for prophylactic esophagectomy. *Ann Surg* 1996;224:66–71.

80. Skacel M, Petras RE, Gramlich TL, et al. The diagnosis of low-grade dysplasia in Barrett's esophagus and its implications for disease progression. *Am J Gastroenterol* 2000;95:3383–3387.

81. Schnell TG, Sontag SJ, Chejfec G, et al. Long-term-non-surgical management of Barrett's esophagus with high-grade dysplasia. *Gastroenterology* 2001;120:1607–1619.

82. Buttar NS, Wang KK, Sebo TJ, et al. Extent of high-grade dysplasia in Barrett's esophagus correlates with risk of adenocarcinoma. *Gastroenterology* 2001;120:1630–1639.

83. Gossner L, Stolte M, Sroka R, et al. Photodynamic ablation of high-grade dysplasia and early cancer in Barrett's esophagus by means of 5-aminolevulinic acid. *Gastroenterology* 1998;114:448–455.

84. Biddlestone LR, Barham CP, Wilkinson SP, et al. The histopathology of treated Barrett's esophagus. *Am J Surg Pathol* 1998;22:239–245.

85. Ban S, Mino M, Nishioka NS, et al. Histopathologic aspects of photodynamic therapy for dysplasia and early adenocarcinoma arising in Barrett's esophagus. *Am J Surg Pathol* 2004;28:1466–1473.

86. Krishnadath KK, Wang KK, Taniguchi K, et al. Persistent genetic abnormalities in Barrett's esophagus after photodynamic therapy. *Gastroenterology* 2000;119:624–630.

87. Ell C, May A, Gossner L, Pech O, et al. Endoscopic mucosal resection of early cancer and high-grade dysplasia in Barrett's esophagus. *Gastroenterology* 2000;118:670–677.

88. Mino-Kenudson M, Brugge WR, Puricelli WP, et al. Management of superficial Barrett's epithelium-related neoplasms by endoscopic mucosal resection: clinicopathologic analysis of 27 cases. *Am J Surg Pathol* 2005;29:680–686.

89. Maish MS, DeMeester SR. Endoscopic mucosal resection as a staging technique to determine depth of invasion of esophageal adenocarcinoma. *Ann Thorac Surg* 2004;78:1777–1782.

90. Swisher SG, Erasmus J, Maish M, et al. 2-Fluoro-2-deoxy-D-glucose positron emission tomography imaging is predictive of pathologic response and survival after preoperative chemoradiation in patients with esophageal carcinoma. *Cancer* 2004;101:1776–1785.

91. Heath EI, Burtness BA, Heitmiller RF, et al. Phase II evaluation of preoperative chemoradiation and postoperative adjuvant chemotherapy for squamous cell and adenocarcinoma of the esophagus. *J Clin Oncol* 2000;18:868–876.

92. Darnton SJ, Archer VR, Stocken DD, et al. Preoperative mitomycin, ifosfamide, and cisplatin followed by esophagectomy in squamous cell carcinoma of the esophagus: pathologic complete response induced by chemotherapy leads to long-term survival. *J Clin Oncol* 2003;21:4009–4015.

93. Meluch AA, Greco FA, Gray JR, et al. Preoperative therapy with concurrent paclitaxel/carboplatin/infusional 5-FU and radiation therapy in

locoregional esophageal cancer: final results of a Minnie Pearl Cancer Research Network phase II trial. *Cancer J* 2003;9:251–260.

94. Leichman L, Steiger Z, Seydel HG, et al. Preoperative chemotherapy and radiation therapy for patients with cancer of the esophagus: a potentially curative approach. *J Clin Oncol* 1984;2:75–79.

95. Poplin E, Fleming T, Leichman L, et al. Combined therapies for squamous cell carcinoma of the esophagus: a Southwest Oncology Group Study (SWOG-8037). *J Clin Oncol* 1987;5:622–628.

96. Mandard AM, Dalibard F, Mandard JC, et al. Pathologic assessment of tumor regression after preoperative chemoradiotherapy of esophageal carcinoma: clinicopathologic correlations. *Cancer* 1994;73:2680–2686.

97. Wu T-T, Chirieac LR, Abraham SC, et al. Excellent interobserver agreement on grading the extent of residual carcinoma following preoperative chemoradiation in esophageal carcinoma: a reliable predictor for patient outcome. *Mod Pathol* 2006;19:124A.

98. Chirieac LR, Swisher SG, Correa AM, et al. Signet-ring cell or mucinous histology after preoperative chemoradiation and survival in patients with esophageal or esophagogastric junction adenocarcinoma. *Clin Cancer Res* 2005;11:2229–2236.

99. Yang Q, Cleary KR, Yao JC, et al. Significance of post-chemoradiation biopsy in predicting residual esophageal carcinoma in the surgical specimen. *Dis Esophagus* 2004;17:3843.

100. Brien TP, Farraye FA, Odze RD. Gastric dysplasia-like epithelial atypia associated with chemoradiotherapy for esophageal cancer: a clinicopathologic and immunohistochemical study of 15 cases. *Mod Pathol* 2001;14:389–396.

CHAPTER 17 ■ ESOPHAGEAL CANCER: ANATOMY AND STAGING

RICHARD P.M. KOEHLER, FRANK C. DETTERBECK, AND DAVID A. DEAN

The surgical treatment of esophageal cancer requires today's surgeons to not only have a thorough knowledge of anatomy and surgical techniques, but also to understand and interpret the medical literature in order to efficiently work up and appropriately stage patients. Accurate staging is essential to defining prognosis, selecting appropriate treatment, and describing patient populations so studies can be compared. As is the case with most malignancies, staging of esophageal cancer uses the TNM (Tumor invasion, Nodal involvement, Metastatic disease) classification as defined by the American Joint Commission on Cancer (AJCC) (1).

ANATOMY

Although it plays no role in digestive, absorptive, or endocrine functions, the esophagus is an important part of the gastrointestinal system. It serves as a conduit for solids and liquids from the oropharynx to the stomach as it traverses the posterior mediastinum from the lower neck into the upper abdomen. Despite having distinct layers (mucosa, submucosa, and muscularis propria), the esophagus lacks both mesentery and serosal layers. The mucosal layer is comprised of nonkeratinized squamous epithelium, basement membrane, lamina propria, and muscularis mucosa. The submucosal (or strength) layer of the esophagus contains connective tissue, blood vessels, lymphatics, and submucosal glands. The muscularis propria allows for the propulsive abilities of the esophagus, and is comprised of an inner circular muscle layer and an outer longitudinal oriented muscle layer.

The blood supply to the cervical esophagus arises from branches of the superior and inferior thyroid arteries in the neck, while the upper and middle thoracic esophagus receives blood from bronchial branches. The blood supply to the lower thoracic esophagus comes directly from the aorta, which are the only "true" dedicated esophageal arterial branches. The lower thoracic and abdominal esophagus receives blood supply from branches of the left gastric and splenic arteries. Venous drainage is accomplished by an extensive submucosal venous plexus, which ultimately drains into inferior thyroid, brachiocephalic, azygous, hemiazygous, and left gastric and splenic veins. Mucosal lymphatics drain directly into a rich submucosal plexus that spans the entire length of the esophagus, accounting for the often rapid and early dissemination seen in many esophageal cancers. Innervation of esophagus arises from both sympathetic and parasympathetic fibers. Vagal parasympathetics supply motor input to the muscularis propria, whereas secretomotor provides input to the submucosal glands. Sympathetic innervation, which arises from both the sympathetic chain and the celiac plexus, causes constriction of the esophageal sphincters and blood vessels and increases parastatic and glandular activity.

DEFINITION OF STAGING

The stage of esophageal cancer can be defined in the context of several distinct clinical situations. The pathological stage, which is generally accepted as the gold standard, is the stage as evaluated by the pathologist after examining all tissue sampled during the course of surgical resection. At the time patients are evaluated and decisions regarding the treatment approach are made, only clinical staging is possible. Clinical staging is the stage determined from all available information, including invasive techniques, *before any treatment* (e.g., surgery). Finally, in the context of induction chemotherapy or radiotherapy, consideration of the stage *after completion of the induction treatment*, often referred to as restaging, is useful. Pathological stage, clinical stage, and restaging after initial treatment are denoted by the prefixes p, c, or y (e.g., pI or cT3N1M0). Clarity about which type of staging is being referred to is important because the implication of a particular stage can be different in each situation.

The pathological stage is usually accepted as the most accurate representation of the true stage of esophageal cancer, at least as far as intrathoracic or intraabdominal disease is concerned. The issue with regard to clinical staging or restaging after treatment is how reliably this stage correlates with the ultimate pathological stage. That is the focus of this chapter. The questions of particular interest to clinicians working with patients with esophageal cancer are regarding accurate determination of T0 to T2 versus T3 versus T4 tumors, identification of nodal involvement, and the presence of metastatic disease.

STATISTICS

The reliability of tests used in staging is usually measured with indices such as sensitivity, specificity, false-positive (FP) rate, false-negative (FN) rate, and accuracy. Appropriate interpretation of these indices requires a thorough understanding of these parameters, how they are calculated, their inherent limitations, and how factors such as prevalence affect them. These indices are often misunderstood, as evidenced by the frequency with which people use the wrong parameter when interpreting or presenting clinical data (e.g., using the sensitivity rather than the FN rate in interpreting a negative result in a patient). To avoid confusion, the definitions of these parameters are provided in Figure 17.1.

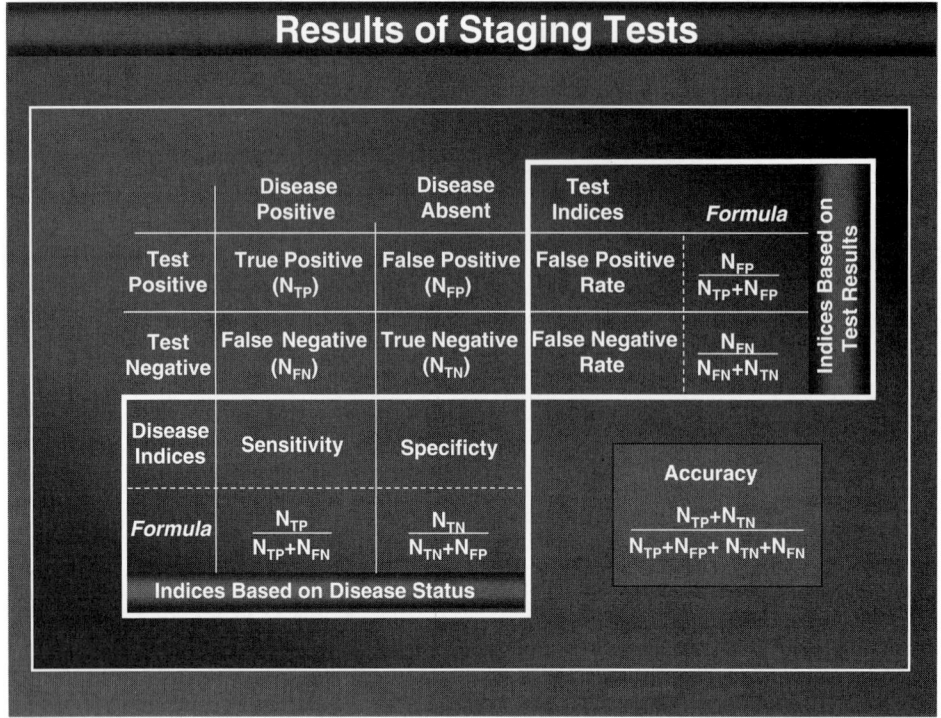

FIGURE 17.1. Results of Staging Tests.

Sensitivity and *specificity* are useful in selecting a test to be performed in a population of patients, but these parameters are limited because they pertain to *theoretical* populations, *all members of which* either have or do not have the condition in question. In contrast, FP and FN rates allow interpretation of the test result in individual patients, which permits a more refined estimate of the true disease status. These latter parameters are generally of more practical use to the clinician. The FP and FN rates are often expressed a bit less concretely as the positive and negative predictive values. *Accuracy* represents the fraction of "correct results" and is strongly affected by disease prevalence. It represents a combination of these other measures, but with such a loss of detail that interpretation of the results is rendered nearly impossible. For example, a test may be highly "accurate" but have a sensitivity of zero if the specificity is high and the prevalence is low. Therefore, although accuracy may satisfy a desire to express the reliability as a single parameter, it has virtually no practical application and is of limited value.

FP and FN rates are affected by the overall prevalence of the condition in the entire population. This probably makes these parameters less appealing to statisticians and may explain why more emphasis has been placed on sensitivity and specificity in the medical literature. The prevalence has little effect on FP and FN rates, however, unless extremes of prevalence are encountered (i.e., <10% or >90% prevalence), at least in the case of tests that have a reasonable sensitivity and specificity (i.e., >80%). Therefore, this chapter focuses on FP and FN rates but attempts to exclude data from studies that had a prevalence of <10% or >90%.

TNM DEFINITIONS

Esophageal cancer is usually classified according to the TNM system. Definitions of these TNM classes are based on pathological findings and are shown in Table 17.1. Tis and T1 (in-

vasion into the submucosa but not muscle) tumors represent minimal invasion of the esophageal wall. T2 tumors invade into, but not through, the muscle into the periesophageal tissue; the latter type of invasion is the definition of T3 tumors. T4 tumors invade adjacent structures such as the aorta, trachea, or pericardium (Fig. 17.2). Nodal status (N) is based solely on the presence (N1) or absence (N0) of involvement of periesophageal lymph nodes by standard histologic evaluation. M1 disease represents distant metastases. The latest revision of the TNM system defines positive lymph nodes in cervical and celiac nodal regions as distant metastatic disease (M1a) and solid organ metastatic disease as M1b. Table 17.2 shows the TNM categories that comprise the stage groups in esophageal carcinoma (2).

Although the pathological definition of esophageal cancer has been clearly defined by the AJCC, the definitions used in clinical staging are slightly different, at least in the case of computed tomography (CT) definition of the T status. The criteria commonly used for CT and endoscopic ultrasound (EUS) are shown in Table 17.1. The clinically important issues in clinical staging are the differentiation between T1 and T2, T3, and T4 tumors; identification of N1 involvement; and recognition of the presence of M1 disease.

DIAGNOSTIC MODALITIES

Computed Tomography

A staging CT for esophageal carcinoma includes the supraclavicular area; the lungs and mediastinum; the liver, adrenal glands, and gastrohepatic ligament; and the celiac nodal areas. CT is often used as an initial study for the assessment of T status and M status, but it is quite unreliable in determining N status. The normal thoracic esophagus varies in the degree of

TABLE 17.1

DEFINITION OF TNM FOR CARCINOMA OF THE ESOPHAGUS

T	Pathological	CT/MRI	EUS
PRIMARY TUMOR (T)			
Tis	Carcinoma in situ		
T1	Invades submucosa	Wall thickness 5–10 mm[a]	Invasion into first three layers
T2	Invades muscularis propria		Invasion into fourth layer
T3	Invades adventitia	Wall thickness >10 mm	Invasion into fifth layer
T4	Invades adjacent structures	Extraesophageal invasion	Invasion into adjacent organs
REGIONAL LYMPH NODES (N)			
N0	No lymph nodes involved		
N1	Regional lymph nodes involved	Lymph nodes >10 mm	Lymph nodes >10 mm, rounded, hypoechoic, sharp borders
DISTANT METASTASIS (M)			
M0	None present		
M1a	Nonregional lymph nodes[b]		Celiac lymph nodes >5 mm
M1b	Other distant metastasis		

TNM, tumor, node, metastasis; CT, computed tomography; MRI, magnetic resonance imaging; EUS, endoscopic ultrasound.
[a]T1/T2 CT/MRI unable to differentiate individual layers.
[b]Cervical or celiac.

wall thickness, depending on distention with oral contrast, but measurements of >5 mm are routinely considered abnormal (3). Small primary tumors of the esophagus may be difficult to see by CT. Furthermore, CT cannot discriminate between the histologic layers of the wall of the esophagus, making it difficult to differentiate between T stages. Tumor invasion is suggested when normal fat planes are lost between tumor and adjacent structures or when a mass effect is present (4–6). CT also occasionally plays a role in guiding a fine-needle aspiration (FNA) biopsy.

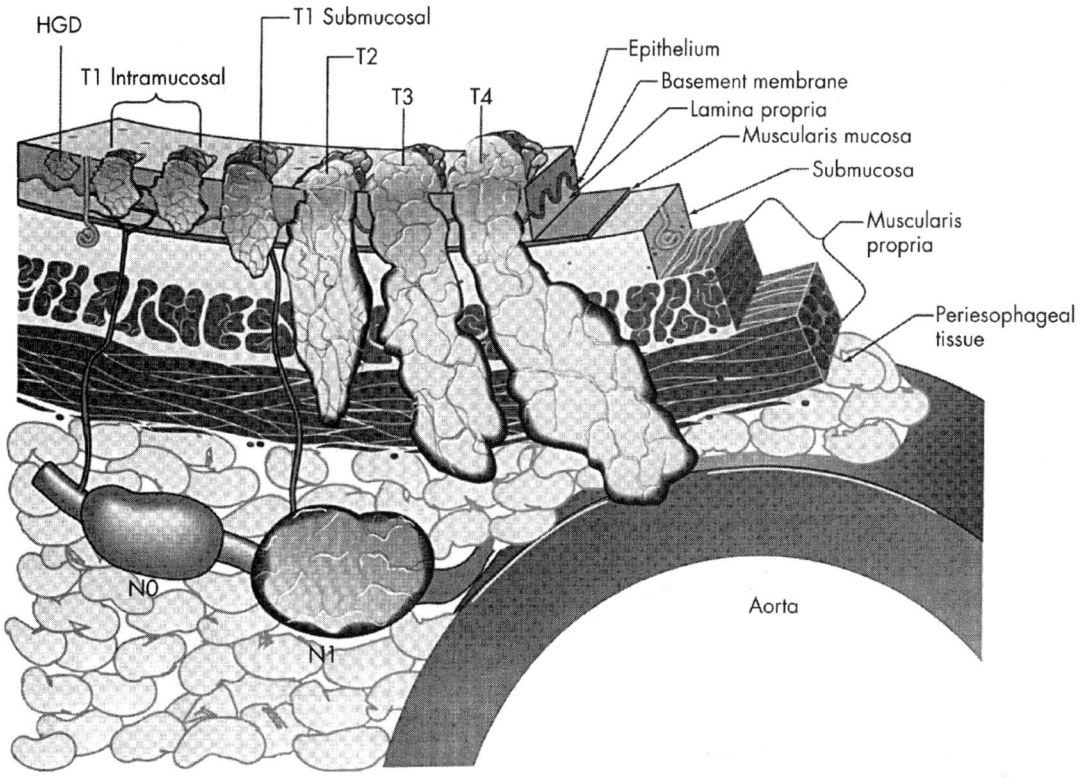

FIGURE 17.2. Schematic of tumor (T) staging. *Source:* Reprinted from Rice TW. Clinical staging of esophageal carcinoma. *Chest Surg Clin N Am* 2000;10:473, with permission of Elsevier.

TABLE 17.2

STAGE GROUPINGS FOR CARCINOMA OF THE ESOPHAGUS

Stage	T	N	M
0	Tis	N0	M0
I	T1	N0	M0
IIa	T2,3	N0	M0
IIb	T1,2	N1	M0
III	T3	N1	M0
	T4	N_{any}	M0
IVa	T_{any}	N_{any}	M1a
IVb	T_{any}	N_{any}	M1b

T, tumor; N, node; M, metastasis; Tis, carcinoma in situ.
From ref. 2.

Magnetic Resonance Imaging

Magnetic resonance imaging (MRI) uses nonionizing magnetic radiation to obtain data that can be used to reconstruct anatomy in many different planes. Results have been comparable to CT (4,7–9), and CT is used in most institutions.

Endoscopic Ultrasound

EUS uses high-frequency (5- to 20-MHz) transducers incorporated into the tip of a flexible endoscope or in a separate fiber-optic instrument passed through a normal scope to create ultrasonic images. A 7.5-MHz transducer provides reasonable resolution to a depth of 5 to 7 cm, whereas a 12-MHz transducer provides resolution to a depth 2 to 3 cm with spatial resolution of 2 mm. Ultrasound of a normal esophagus produces an image consisting of five layers (Fig. 17.3). The innermost first layer is hyperechoic (white) and represents the mucosal interface. The second layer is hypoechoic (black) and corresponds to the muscularis mucosa. The third layer is hyperechoic and

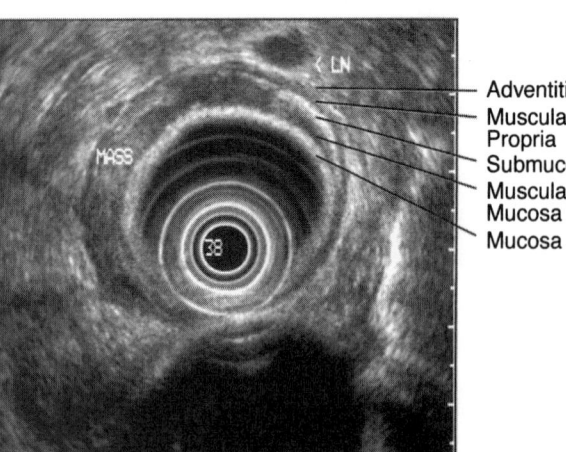

FIGURE 17.3. Endoscopic ultrasound demonstrating a T3 lesion (mass), with penetration through the adventitia and a positive lymph node (LN) that is hypoechoic and rounded with distinct borders.

corresponds to the submucosa. The fourth layer (hypoechoic) corresponds to the muscularis propria and the fifth layer (hyperechoic) to the adventitial interface (Table 17.1). EUS provides not only reliable T staging but can also be used to assess regional lymph nodes. Criteria for abnormal pathology include lymph node shape, border characteristics, and central echogenicity (10). EUS-directed FNA is a useful modality for obtaining tissue samples of suspicious periesophageal lymph nodes during ultrasound staging procedures.

Positron Emission Tomography

Positron emission tomography (PET) is an imaging modality that provides an assessment based on differences in the cellular metabolism as opposed to the anatomical abnormalities that serve as the basis for CT, MRI, and EUS. Most commonly, this involves administration of 2-deoxyglucose labeled with fluorine 18 (FDG), a radionucleotide that decays by positron emission. FDG is taken up into cells in proportion to glucose utilization, and as such, tumor cells, which have high energy requirements, take up large amounts of FDG. In these tumor cells, FDG is phosphorylated but then cannot be rapidly metabolized because many types of tumor cells have very low levels of glucose-6-phosphatase. Normal cells, in contrast, with higher levels of glucose-6-phosphatase can more rapidly dephosphorylate and thereby metabolize FDG-6-phosphate; this provides the physiological basis of the PET scan. Simply put, this means that FDG is in essence trapped within tumor cells, and thus, tumor cells can be detected because of higher rates of positron emission as the FDG decays (11). A limitation of PET scanning is the poor anatomical definition, particularly of the early generation scanners, so that separation of the primary tumor from adjacent lymph nodes can be difficult. In an attempt to improve on the lack of precise anatomical detail, many modern PET scanners have incorporated CT imaging capabilities, creating fusion PET/CT images. This allows for the simultaneous acquisition of both PET and CT data, and with real-time comparison and integration of the images, it is now possible to interpret PET data with more anatomical precision.

Other Noninvasive Tests

Few other imaging studies or laboratory tests are warranted in the staging of patients with esophageal cancer. A chest radiograph is usually obtained but is of limited value because it is normal in >70% of patients with esophageal cancer (16). CT imaging and PET scans both provide a better overall assessment for metastatic disease, and unlike chest radiographs, are not limited to the chest. Screening blood tests are neither sensitive nor specific for determining possible liver metastases unless liver involvement is massive. Although a barium swallow is routinely performed in the initial workup of a patient with dysphagia, it provides only a limited amount of information regarding the degree of luminal narrowing and the location and length of the lesion and provides no staging information. With the availability of endoscopy and CT, a barium study has become less important, and most clinical staging issues are better addressed by CT or EUS, once the diagnosis of esophageal cancer has been made.

Invasive Modalities

Invasive staging consists of surgical evaluation of the primary tumor and the lymph nodes, as well as surveying the liver for possible metastases. Invasive staging can be justified by the fact that several groups have demonstrated nodal involvement in remote areas at the time of resection that was not appreciated by conventional preoperative noninvasive staging studies. Akiyama et al. found that 32% of patients with upper esophageal tumors had disease in abdominal lymph nodes (17). Two additional studies evaluating the three-field lymphadenectomy demonstrated positive cervical lymph nodes in 20% to 30% of patients with thoracic and abdominal esophageal carcinoma (18,19). Furthermore, current techniques in molecular biology and immunohistochemistry allow a more sensitive evaluation of nodes for malignant involvement than was previously possible by routine histologic assessment (20–22).

In 1977, Murray et al. described preoperative surgical staging of esophageal cancer with mediastinoscopy and a minilaparotomy in a prospective study involving 30 patients (23). Celiac nodal involvement was found in 53% and mediastinal involvement in 23%, although these authors believed that this staging technique did not optimally stage the chest. Krasna et al. examined the utility of combined preoperative thoracoscopy and laparoscopy in a prospective multiinstitutional phase II trial (CALGB 9380) (24). This study established that thoracoscopy and laparoscopy for staging of esophageal cancer was safe and feasible. Later, Krasna et al. compared thoracoscopic and laparoscopic staging with conventional staging; they found that invasive staging provided more accurate information about local tumor invasion, regional lymph node involvement, and distant metastases (25). Clements et al. confirmed the utility of laparoscopy as part of a preoperative staging algorithm for distal esophageal and proximal gastric cancers. By using this invasive staging technique, they were able to prevent unnecessary laparotomy in 18% of patients who had been deemed "resectable" by conventional imaging modalities (26). However, a substantial learning curve exists with laparoscopy and thoracoscopy. In addition, invasive staging usually requires 3 to 4 hours of general anesthesia and 2 to 3 days of hospitalization.

ESOPHAGEAL CARCINOMA STAGING: TNM

Tumor

The T stage of esophageal carcinoma has marked prognostic implications (5-year survival is approximately 80% for patients with Tis or T1 disease, approximately 65% for those with T2 tumors, 25% for those with T3 disease, and nonexistent with T4 tumors) (27). Furthermore, the T stage correlates with the chance of nodal involvement (0% with Tis, 10% with T1, 33%–50% with T2, 70%–80% with T3, and 85%–90% with T4 tumors) (28–32). Although the optimal treatment of different stages of esophageal cancer lacks consensus, most institutions base treatment protocols on the clinical T and N staging. Therefore, determining the ability of a clinical staging test to correctly predict the pathological T status is important, particularly with regard to the differentiation between Tis through T2, T3, and T4 tumors.

Historically, accurate T staging of esophageal cancer occurred in only 25% to 30% of cases using barium studies, endoscopy, and early generation CT scans (33). Current generation helical CT scanners have much better resolution, and various indices of reliability for these tests are shown in Table 17.3. In the studies shown in Table 17.3, the gold standard was pathological staging at the time of surgical exploration. The criteria for tumor wall invasion by CT and EUS as defined in Table 17.1 are well accepted and used consistently in these studies. Table 17.3 and subsequent tables display data from relevant studies involving 25 or more patients and report data

from which FN and FP rates could be calculated. Although the FN rates from studies with high prevalence rates (>90%) and the FP rates from studies with low prevalence rates (<10%) are shown, they are excluded from calculated averages because of questionable validity.

The FP rates for CT in predicting T3 and T4 involvement are consistently low (7%), whereas the FN rate is high (57%). Thus, a CT suggesting T3 or T4 disease is reliable, but a CT suggesting tumor confined to the muscularis propria is *not* reliable. One-half to two-thirds of advanced tumors in these studies involved T3 and not T4 tumors. Although the presence of a T3 tumor may alter some physicians' recommendations for therapy, in the opinion of most physicians, the presence of a T4 tumor is a much clearer contraindication to surgical resection. Tumors with T4 involvement have not been consistently addressed as a group, but both aortic and tracheal invasion (the major categories of T4 involvement) have been addressed individually. The results in Table 17.3 indicate that the FN rate of CT is low in these instances, but the FP rate is high. This means that one should be very cautious in excluding patients from surgery on the basis of a CT scan that suggests aortic or tracheal involvement. Conclusions drawn from the reported data are fairly convincing in general, even though there is a fair amount of unexplained variability in the FP rates among individual studies. MRI has demonstrated similar sensitivity, specificity, and FP and FN rates for the determination of T status (4,7).

EUS is largely accepted as the gold standard, nonsurgical, staging modality for accurately determining T status in esophageal cancers (Table 17.3). The ability to predict T3 or T4 tumors from earlier stage T1 and T2 tumors is quite good, with low FP and FP rates (average, 5% and 7%, respectively). In 20% to 30% of cases, the probe cannot be passed through the tumor, given that EUS probes are typically >12 mm in size (30,31,34,35). Hordijk et al. showed that the traversability of lesions also impacts T staging, finding that accuracy decreased from 92% to 46% if lesions were difficult to pass as compared to easily traversable lesions (36). Attempts at dilating nontraversable lesions are fraught with unacceptably high perforation rates, nearly one-fourth of patients in one early series (37). Attempts at staging tumors proximal to the stricture have shown very high FN rates (35), whereas attempts at dilation have had equally poor results (38). Despite these potential drawbacks, EUS is currently the single best staging modality for determining T stage in patients with esophageal cancer.

Nodes

The presence of tumor in lymph nodes is associated with a poor prognosis (5-year patient survival of approximately 50% for N0, approximately 20% for N1, and <10% for distant nodal involvement) (27,28,31,39,40). The prediction of nodal involvement by CT or MRI relies on node size, with almost all studies using a threshold of 1 cm, above which is worrisome for lymph node involvement. EUS also uses a size threshold of 1 cm but can further evaluate characteristics of the echo signal and the borders (Fig. 17.3). In one study that examined various categories of node size, the chance of malignant involvement was 3% (3 of 99 cases) for nodes <5 mm, 8% (4 of 49 cases) for nodes 5 to 10 mm, and 21% (3 of 14 cases) for nodes >10 mm (41). Reactive inflammation and granulomatous disease can lead to FP results, whereas microscopic disease can lead to FN results (5,20,22,40).

Table 17.4 summarizes the results of studies examining nodal status using CT or MRI, EUS, PET, and invasive approaches. As one would expect based on size criteria alone, CT and MRI have relatively poor reliability in predicting nodal status, with both FN and FP rates being quite high. Both EUS

TABLE 17.3

EFFICACY OF STAGING TUMOR INFILTRATION

Study	Test	n	Prevalence (%)	Sensitivity (%)	Specificity (%)	FP rate (%)	FN rate (%)
T3/T4 VS. T1/T2							
Nishimaki et al. (56)	CT	138	89	94	13	10	80
Tio et al. (3)	CT	66	83	85	82	4	47
Botet et al. (57)	CT	42	86	94	50	8	40
Average for CT				91	48	7	56
Dittler and Siewert (31)	EUS	167	65	94	93	4	11
Nishimaki et al. (56)	EUS	160	52	94	92	7	7
Tio et al. (30)	EUS	103	75	97	88	4	8
Grimm et al. (58)	EUS	63	60	97	92	5	4
Botet et al. (57)	EUS	50	86	100	71	4	0
Ziegler et al. (59)	EUS	37	76	96	89	4	11
Siewert et al. (60)	EUS	37	59	91	87	9	13
Sugimachi et al. (41)	EUS	33	52	100	100	0	0
Average for EUS				96	89	5	7
AORTIC INFILTRATION							
Lehr et al. (4)	CT	55	13	14	71	93	15
Quint et al. (7)	CT	33	6	100	87	(67)[a]	0
Picus et al. (5)	CT	30	20	67	96	20	8
Average for CT				60	85	57	8
Lehr et al. (4)	MRI	55	11	67	67	80	6
TRACHEAL INFILTRATION							
Lehr et al. (4)	CT	57	17	40	81	69	14
Quint et al. (7)	CT	33	6	100	97	(33)[a]	0
Picus et al. (5)	CT	30	20	100	100	0	0
Average for CT				80	93	35	5
Lehr et al. (4)	MRI	53	21	45	79	64	15

FP, false positive; FN, false negative; CT, computed tomography; EUS, endoscopic ultrasound; MRI, magnetic resonance imaging.
[a]Value should be interpreted with caution because of low prevalence.

and PET scanning appear to be much more reliable if a positive node is found. Both tests, however, have fairly high FN rates. FN results with PET may be due to the inability to detect small nodes using the current technology, and FN results with EUS may be due to difficulties in reliably visualizing periesophageal lymph nodes. The best results are seen with invasive staging—with sensitivity, specificity, PPV, and NPV of approximately 50%, 100%, 100%, and 90%, respectively, for N1 disease in the thorax, and 87%, 100%, 100%, and 94%, respectively, for N1 disease in the abdomen (25,42).

Metastasis

Disease with metastasis to the liver, lung, adrenal glands, or bone (M1b) has a very poor prognosis, with a mean survival of several months. Identification of patients with metastatic disease is of particular importance because it is a contraindication to aggressive surgical therapy. The prognosis of patients with nonregional nodal metastases (M1a indicates metastasis to cervical or celiac nodes) is also poor, although the most appropriate therapy remains controversial. The most common sites of distant metastases from esophageal cancer are the celiac lymph nodes and the liver, both of which are adequately visualized by typical staging studies such as CT or EUS. The reliability of these tests for assessing each site is discussed in Table 17.5.

The identification of metastases to the brain, bone, lung, and adrenal glands from esophageal cancer is the same as that of metastases from any cancer and is not discussed.

The reliability of CT, EUS, PET, and minimally invasive staging in assessing celiac lymph nodes has been reported, and tends to show similar results when compared to the gold standard of surgical exploration. The sensitivity is rather poor, the FP rates are quite high at almost 25%, and the FN rates are lower at approximately 15%. Thus, a negative scan justifies proceeding with treatment appropriate for M0 disease, whereas a positive scan warrants further confirmation to determine the true status of the suspicious celiac nodes by either needle aspiration or minimally invasive staging. In a limited study (17 patients), laparoscopy, like thoracoscopy, had a 0% FP rate and an 8% FN rate (43).

The assessment of hepatic metastases by CT or EUS has a relatively low sensitivity, with FP and FN rates of 20% and 15%, respectively. The reliability of CT greatly depends on the appropriate timing of intravenous contrast injection; many metastatic deposits can be missed on a noncontrasted scan, or on one in which the equilibrium phase has been reached (similar density of contrast in the aorta and the inferior vena cava) (44,45). The suggestion is often made that MRI is theoretically better for evaluation of the liver (46). However, this notion is based primarily on the data showing that MRI is better at identifying hepatic hemangiomas, rather than on consistent data showing

TABLE 17.4

RELIABILITY OF STAGING TESTS IN PREDICTING N0 AND N1 STATUS

Study	Test	n	Prevalence (%)	Sensitivity (%)	Specificity (%)	FP rate (%)	FN rate (%)
Nishimaki et al. (56)	CT	210	66	60	75	18	54
Tio et al. (3)	CT	74	68	34	88	15	61
Botet et al. (57)	CT	42	69	79	62	18	43
Ziegler et al. (59)	CT	37	65	42	69	29	61
Block et al. (14)	CT	35	60	29	79	33	58
Quint et al. (7)	CT	33	54	61	60	35	44
Sihvo et al. (49)	CT	43	60	42	82	21	52
Cerfolio et al. (52)	CT	41	20	78	78	22	22
Average for CT				53	74	24	49
Krasna et al. (61)	MRI	33	15	100	61	69	0
Dittler and Siewert (31)	EUS	167	68	75	70	16	44
Nishimaki et al. (56)	EUS	166	66	80	59	21	40
Tio et al. (30)	EUS	111	69	95	50	19	19
Grimm et al. (58)	EUS	63	67	88	81	10	23
Botet et al. (57)	EUS	50	72	97	64	13	10
Lightdale and Botet (62)	EUS	37	73	85	60	15	40
Siewert et al. (60)	EUS	37	73	85	60	15	40
Ziegler et al. (59)	EUS	37	68	64	75	16	50
Luketich et al. (63)	EUS	21	86	67	67	8	75
Rice et al. (34)	EUS	20	50	70	70	30	30
Vazquez-Sequeiros et al. (65)	EUS	33	67	64	82	13	47
Cerfolio et al. (52)	EUS-FNA	41	20	78	78	22	22
Average for EUS				79	68	17	37
Luketich et al. (12)	PET	21	95	45	100	0	(92)[a]
Block et al. (14)	PET	35	60	52	79	21	48
Cerfolio et al. (52)	PET	41	20	92	92	7	7
Sihvo et al. (49)	PET	43	60	26	100	0	50
Average for PET				54	93	7	49
Krasna et al. (43)	Surgery	30	13	50	100	0	7
Krasna et al. (61)	Surgery	33	15	40	100	0	10
Krasna and Xiaolong (42)	Surgery	47	17	63	100	0	7
Average for surgery				53	100	0	8

FP, false positive; FN, false negative; CT, computed tomography; MRI, magnetic resonance imaging; EUS, endoscopic ultrasound; FNA, fine-needle aspiration; PET, positron emission tomography.
[a] Value should be interpreted with caution because of high prevalence.

that metastases are detected in more patients (47). EUS plays only a minor role in the detection of hepatic metastasis, given its limited depth of penetration of the ultrasound waves (up to 5–10 cm). The patients included in most of these studies have been considered as potential surgical candidates, and all underwent confirmation of suspected hepatic metastases. As a result, the population may be skewed toward patients in whom the positive test results are suspected of being FP. It is likely that the reliability of CT and EUS in demonstrating liver metastases is probably higher when patients with multiple typical metastases are included.

PET scanning has been evaluated more recently for detecting distant metastases from esophageal cancer. The sensitivity and specificity are acceptable, and the FP and FN rates are low at approximately 15%. The patients in some of the initial studies were referred to centers as potential resection candidates because they met all other requirements by standard staging modalities. They then underwent PET as an additional staging tool. These studies used a reasonable gold standard, with positive findings being confirmed by surgical biopsy or clinical correlation with another noninvasive modality with clinical follow-up. Negative findings were confirmed

by a follow-up of longer than 6 months (13). PET picked up unsuspected metastatic disease in 16% of cases in one large study (negative clinical evaluation and standard radiographic studies) and had an FN rate of 20% (all lesions reported as >10 mm) (13). Although multiple studies have been unable to show that PET scanning by itself increases the accuracy of preoperative staging, several authors have shown that when PET is added to CT and EUS, it does, however, improve detection of stage IV disease (48,49). PET has also been shown to pick up unexpected synchronous primary neoplasms in approximately 5.5% (20/366) of patients with esophageal cancer (50). As with nodal disease, the best results are seen with invasive staging, although the available data are limited.

NEOADJUVANT THERAPY AND STAGING

Although still somewhat controversial, most esophageal surgeons are using neoadjuvant chemoradiotherapy in the treatment of esophageal cancer. This so-called trimodality therapy

TABLE 17.5

EFFICACY OF STAGING METASTATIC DISEASE (M1A AND M1B)

Study	Test	n	Prevalence (%)	Sensitivity (%)	Specificity (%)	FP rate (%)	FN rate (%)
M1a (CLN)							
Tio et al. (3)	CT	65	28	50	96	18	17
Quint et al. (7)	CT	33	9	67	87	(67)	4
Picus et al. (5)	CT	28	32	56	89	39	19
Cerfolio et al. (52)	CT	41	13	0	100	0	13
Average for CT				43	93	31	14
Tio et al. (30)	EUS	80	30	58	96	12	15
Reed et al. (64)	EUS	57	46	73	97	5	19
Cerfolio et al. (52)	EUS-FNA	48	13	33	100	0	9
Average for EUS				55	98	6	14
Krasna et al. (43)	Laparoscopy	17	35	83	100	0	8
M1b							
Luketich et al. (13)	CT	91	43	46	73	44	36
Tio et al. (3)	CT	50	6	67	96	(50)[a]	2
Botet et al. (57)	CT	42	38	75	100	0	13
Average for CT				63	90	22	17
Tio et al. (30)	EUS	62	10	67	96	33	4
Botet et al. (57)	EUS	46	43	25	100	0	37
Average for EUS				46	98	17	21
Luketich et al. (13)	PET	91	43	69	94	10	20

FP, false positive; FN, false negative; CLN, celiac lymph node; CT, computed tomography; EUS, endoscopic ultrasound; FNA, fine-needle aspiration; PET, positron emission tomography.
[a]Value should be interpreted with caution because of low prevalence.

has been reported to have pathological complete responses ranging from 20% to 40% of patients. Follow-up of those patients who are found to be stage 0 on restaging at the time of resection have demonstrated excellent 5-year survivals of around 50% (39). Restaging has posed a problem, with many authors reporting overstaging by both EUS and CT. In one study of 31 consecutively examined patients, EUS had an FP rate of 53% and an FN rate of 67% following neoadjuvant treatment (51). Cerfolio et al. presented data from a prospec-tive trial of 48 patients who had undergone neoadjuvant ther-apy with restaging CT, EUS-FNA, and CT/PET (integrated), and showed FP rates of 89%, 91%, and 93%, respectively, and FN rates of 20%, 19%, and 7%, respectively (52). Dittler et al. examined 25 patients with T3 tumors, all of whom had received neoadjuvant therapy and underwent EUS (53). The FP rate of EUS for predicting tumor invasion was 60%. CT scan is also unable to differentiate between posttherapy inflamma-tion and scar and residual tumor. Jones et al. showed that in

TABLE 17.6

EFFICACY OF RESTAGING FOLLOWING NEOADJUVANT THERAPY

Study	Test	n	Prevalence (%)	Sensitivity (%)	Specificity (%)	FP rate (%)	FN rate (%)
T3/T4 VS. T1/T2							
Jones et al. (54)	CT	50	28	29	92	43	23
Dittler et al. (53)	EUS	25	40	100	0	60	–
Isenberg et al. (51)	EUS	23	52	67	18	53	67
Average for EUS				84	9	57	67
REGIONAL LYMPH NODES							
Dittler et al. (53)	EUS	41	39	100	12	58	0
Isenberg et al. (51)	EUS	23	52	67	45	43	44
Average for EUS				84	29	51	22

FP, false positive; FN, false negative; CT, computed tomography; EUS, endoscopic ultrasound.

50 patients receiving adjuvant therapy who were restaged with CT, the FN rate was 23% and the FP rate was 43% (54). Swisher et al. evaluated the utility of using standardized uptake values (SUVs); in their series of 100 consecutive patients, they found that FDG-PET SUVs were more accurate than both CT and EUS in predicting long-term survival following neoadjuvant chemoradiation (55). Despite some limited success of "restaging" patients' responses to neoadjuvant chemoradiotherapy, CT, PET, EUS-FNA, and PET-CT are all of limited value in predicting pathological response to chemoradiotherapy (Table 17.6).

CONCLUSION

Accurate staging is essential to defining prognosis and selecting appropriate treatment for patients with esophageal cancer. Currently, no test is 100% reliable in determining clinical stage with respect to pathological stage. Therefore, no strict guidelines can be proposed with the current modalities of staging.

One way of approaching this problem is to base the choice of the staging test on the specific clinical question being asked, which is often affected by the policy toward treatment. For most institutions, the determination of resectability is based on the absence of distant metastatic disease. In most instances, distant metastatic disease can be ruled out with a standard CT in addition to clinical findings. Positive results should be confirmed with biopsy because of the 22% FP rate.

If distant metastases are excluded, the next issue is the presence or absence of nodal disease, but the best test depends on the question being asked. For example, if the major question is to *rule out* nodal involvement because this would lead to treatment with surgery alone, invasive staging with laparoscopy and thoracoscopy may be the best approach because of the low FN rate. In contrast, for clinicians wanting to identify patients with positive N1 nodes in the belief that positive nodal involvement rules out an aggressive or curative approach, a test such as EUS or PET may be best because of the low FP rate. Of course, some patients with nodal involvement will be missed altogether despite these tests. At any rate, treatment decisions should probably not be based on the results of CT because this test is not very reliable for assessing nodal involvement. Resectability evaluation based on tumor size and local infiltration is best answered with EUS. CT can rule out infiltration of adjacent structures fairly well (low FN rate), but by itself it is unreliable in identifying patients who are not resectable.

In patients who have been treated with induction chemotherapy and radiation, the ability to restage the tumor may be an issue. For example, if patients can be identified as having no residual disease, theoretically these patients would not need to undergo surgical resection. However, given the high FP and FN rates of EUS, CT, and even PET, no adequate method of restaging exists at this time.

In summary, optimal use of staging tests should be based on the clinical question being asked and on the approach that will be taken with either a positive or a negative result. The best approach may be to combine a test with a low FN rate with one with a low FP rate with respect to a specific clinical question. Because the clinical questions asked vary according to the policy of treatment of esophageal cancer in different institutions, a universally acceptable algorithm cannot be devised at this time.

References

1. American Joint Committee on Cancer (AJCC). *AJCC Cancer Staging Manual.* 5th ed. Chicago, Ill.: AJCC; 1997.

2. American Joint Commission on Cancer. *Manual for Staging Cancer.* Philadelphia, Pa.: JB Lippincott; 1988.

3. Tio TL, Cohen P, Coene PP, et al. Endosonography and computed tomography of esophageal carcinoma: preoperative classification compared to the new (1987) TNM system. *Gastroenterology* 1989;96:1478–1486.

4. Lehr L, Rupp N, Siewert JR. Assessment of resectability of esophageal cancer by computed tomography and magnetic resonance imaging. *Surgery* 1988;103:344–350.

5. Picus D, Balfe DM, Koehler RE, et al. Computed tomography in the staging of esophageal carcinoma. *Radiology* 1983;146:433–438.

6. Halvorsen RA, Jr., Thompson WM. Computed tomographic staging of gastrointestinal tract malignancies. Part I. Esophagus and stomach. *Invest Radiol* 1987;22:2–16.

7. Quint LE, Glazer GM, Orringer MB, et al. Esophageal carcinoma: CT findings. *Radiology* 1985;155:171–175.

8. Takashima S, Takeuchi N, Shiozaki H, et al. Carcinoma of the esophagus: CT vs MR imaging in determining resectability. *AJR Am J Roentgenol* 1991;156:297–302.

9. Koch J, Halvorsen RA, Jr. Staging of esophageal cancer: computed tomography, magnetic resonance imaging, and endoscopic ultrasound. *Semin Roentgenol* 1994;29:364–372.

10. Grimm H, Hamper K, Binmoeller KF, et al. Enlarged lymph nodes: malignant or not? *Endoscopy* 1992;24(suppl 1):320–323.

11. Rigo P, Paulus P, Kaschten BJ, et al. Oncological applications of positron emission tomography with fluorine-18 fluorodeoxyglucose. *Eur J Nucl Med* 1996;23:1641–1674.

12. Luketich JD, Schauer PR, Meltzer CC, et al. Role of positron emission tomography in staging esophageal cancer. *Ann Thorac Surg* 1997;64:765–769.

13. Luketich JD, Friedman DM, Weigel TL, et al. Evaluation of distant metastases in esophageal cancer: 100 consecutive positron emission tomography scans. *Ann Thorac Surg* 1999;68:1133–1137.

14. Block MI, Patterson GA, Sundaresan RS, et al. Improvement in staging of esophageal cancer with the addition of positron emission tomography. *Ann Thorac Surg* 1997;64:770–777.

15. Rankin SC, Taylor H, Cook GJ, et al. Computed tomography and positron emission tomography in the pre-operative staging of oesophageal carcinoma. *Clin Radiol* 1998;53:659–665.

16. Lindell MM, Jr., Hill CA, Libshitz HI. Esophageal cancer: radiographic chest findings and their prognostic significance. *AJR Am J Roentgenol* 1979;133:461–465.

17. Akiyama H, Tsurumaru M, Kawamura T, et al. Principles of surgical treatment for carcinoma of the esophagus: analysis of lymph node involvement. *Ann Surg* 1981;194:438–446.

18. Altorki NK, Girardi L, Skinner DB. En bloc esophagectomy improves survival for stage III esophageal cancer. *J Thorac Cardiovasc Surg* 1997;114:948–956.

19. Akiyama H, Tsurumaru M, Udagawa H, et al. Radical lymph node dissection for cancer of the thoracic esophagus. *Ann Surg* 1994;220:364–373.

20. Luketich JD, Kassis ES, Shriver SP, et al. Detection of micrometastases in histologically negative lymph nodes in esophageal cancer. *Ann Thorac Surg* 1998;66:1715–1718.

21. Porte H, Triboulet JP, Kotelevets L, et al. Overexpression of stromelysin-3, BM-40/SPARC, and MET genes in human esophageal carcinoma: implications for prognosis. *Clin Cancer Res* 1998;4:1375–1382.

22. Izbicki JR, Hosch SB, Pichlmeier U, et al. Prognostic value of immunohistochemically identifiable tumor cells in lymph nodes of patients with completely resected esophageal cancer. *N Engl J Med* 1997;337:1188–1194.

23. Murray GF, Wilcox BR, Starek PJK. The assessment of operability of esophageal carcinoma. *Ann Thorac Surg* 1977;23:393–399.

24. Krasna MJ, Reed CE, Nedzwiecki D, et al. CALGB 9380: a prospective trial of the feasibility of thoracoscopy/laparoscopy in the staging of esophageal cancer. *Ann Thorac Surg* 2001;71(4):1073–1079.

25. Krasna M, Xiaolong J, You SM, et al. Thoracoscopy/laparoscopy in the staging of esophageal cancer: Maryland experience. *Surg Laparosc Endosc Percutan Tech* 2002;12:213–218.

26. Clements DM, Bowrey DJ, Havard TJ. The role of staging investigations for oesophago-gastric carcinoma. *Eur J Surg Oncol* 2004;30:309–312.

27. Korst RJ, Rusch VW, Venkatraman E, et al. Proposed revision of the staging classification for esophageal cancer. *J Thorac Cardiovasc Surg* 1998;115:660–670.

28. Ellis FH, Jr., Heatley GJ, Krasna MJ, et al. Esophagogastrectomy for carcinoma of the esophagus and cardia: a comparison of findings and results after standard resection in three consecutive eight-year intervals with improved staging criteria. *J Thorac Cardiovasc Surg* 1997;113:836–848.

29. Catalano MF, Sivak MV, Jr., Rice TW, et al. Depth of tumor invasion of esophageal carcinoma (ECA) is predictive of lymph node metastasis: role of endoscopic ultrasonography (EUS) [abstract]. *Am J Gastroenterol* 1992;87:1245A.

30. Tio TL, Coene PPLO, den Hartog Jager FCA, et al. Preoperative TNM classification of esophageal carcinoma by endosonography. *Hepatogastroenterology* 1990;37:376–381.

31. Dittler HJ, Siewert JR. Role of endoscopic ultrasonography in esophageal carcinoma. *Endoscopy* 1993;25:156–161.

32. Van Dam J. Endosonographic evaluation of the patient with esophageal cancer. *Chest* 1997;112:184S–190S.

33. Fein R, Kelsen DP, Geller N, et al. Adenocarcinoma of the esophagus and gastroesophageal junction: prognostic factors and results of therapy. *Cancer* 1985;56:2512–2518.

34. Rice TW, Boyce GA, Sivak MV. Esophageal ultrasound and the preoperative staging of carcinoma of the esophagus. *J Thorac Cardiovasc Surg* 1991; 101:536–544.

35. Catalano MF, Van Dam J, Sivak MV, Jr. Malignant esophageal strictures: staging accuracy of endoscopic ultrasonography. *Gastrointest Endosc* 1995;41:535–539.

36. Hordijk ML, Zander H, van Blankenstin M, et al. Influence on tumor stenosis on the accuracy of endosonography in preoperative T staging of esophageal cancer. *Endoscopy* 1993;25:171–175.

37. Lightdale C, Kulkarni K. Role of endoscopic ultrasonography in the staging and follow-up of esophageal cancer. *J Clin Oncol* 2005;20:4483–4489.

38. Kallimanis GE, Gupta PK, al-Kawas FH, et al. Endoscopic ultrasound for staging esophageal cancer, with or without dilation, is clinically important and safe. *Gastrointest Endosc* 1995;41:540–546.

39. Orringer MB, Marshall B, Iannettoni MD. Transhiatal esophagectomy: clinical experience and refinements. *Ann Surg* 1999;230:392–403.

40. Skinner DB, Little AG, Ferguson MK, et al. Selection of operation for esophageal cancer based on staging. *Ann Surg* 1986;204:391–401.

41. Sugimachi K, Ohno S, Fujishima H, et al. Endoscopic ultrasonographic detection of carcinomatous invasion and of lymph nodes in the thoracic esophagus. *Surgery* 1990;107:366–371.

42. Krasna MJ, Xiaolong J. Thoracoscopic and laparoscopic staging for esophageal cancer. *Semin Thorac Cardiovasc Surg* 2000;3:186–194.

43. Krasna MJ, Flowers JL, Attar S, et al. Combined thoracoscopic/laparoscopic staging of esophageal cancer. *J Thorac Cardiovasc Surg* 1996;111:800–807.

44. Burgener FA, Hamlin DJ. Contrast enhancement of hepatic tumors in CT: comparison between bolus and infusion techniques. *AJR Am J Roentgenol* 1983;140:291–295.

45. Wernecke K, Rummeny E, Bongartz G, et al. Detection of hepatic masses in patients with carcinoma: comparative sensitivities of sonography, CT, and MR imaging. *AJR Am J Roentgenol* 1991;157:731–739.

46. Reinig JW, Dwyer AJ, Miller DL, et al. Liver metastasis detection: comparative sensitivities of MR imaging and CT scanning. *Radiology* 1987;162:43–47.

47. Birnbaum BA, Weinreb JC, Megibow AJ, et al. Definitive diagnosis of hepatic hemangiomas: MR imaging versus Tc-99m-labeled red blood cell SPECT. *Radiology* 1990;176:95–101.

48. Kneist W, Schreckenberger M, Bartenstein P, et al. Prospective evaluation of PET in the preoperative staging of esophageal carcinoma. *Arch Surg* 2004;139:1043–1049.

49. Sihvo E, Rasanen J, Knuuti J, et al. Adenocarcinoma of the esophagus and the esophagogastric junction: PET improves staging and prediction of survival in distant but not in locoregional disease. *J Gastrointest Surg* 2004;8:988–996.

50. van Westreenen H, Westerterp M, Jager P, et al. Synchronous primary neoplasms detected on ^{18}F-FDG PET in staging of patients with esophageal cancer. *J Nucl Med* 2005;8:1321–1325.

51. Isenberg G, Chak A, Canto MI, et al. Endoscopic ultrasound in restaging of esophageal cancer after neoadjuvant chemoradiation. *Gastrointest Endosc* 1998;48:158–163.

52. Cerfolio R, Bryant A, Buddhiwardhan O, et al. The accuracy of endoscopic ultrasonography with fine-needle aspiration, integrated positron emission tomography with computed tomography, and computed tomography in restaging patients with esophageal cancer after neoadjuvant chemoradiotherapy. *J Thorac Cardiovasc Surg* 2005;6:1232–1241.

53. Dittler HJ, Rosch U, Fink JR, et al. Endoscopic restaging of esophagus and cardia following radio- and chemotherapy [abstract]. *Gastrointest Endosc* 1992;38:241.

54. Jones DR, Parker LA, Jr., Detterbeck FC, et al. Inadequacy of computed tomography in assessing patients with esophageal carcinoma after induction chemoradiotherapy. *Cancer* 1999;85:1026–1032.

55. Swisher S, Maish M, Erasmus J, et al. Utility of PET, CT and EUS to identify pathologic responders in esophageal cancer. *Ann Thor Surg* 2004;78:1152–1160.

56. Nishimaki T, Tanaka O, Ando N, et al. Evaluation of the accuracy of preoperative staging in thoracic esophageal cancer. *Ann Thorac Surg* 1999;68:2059–2064.

57. Botet JF, Lightdale CJ, Zauber AG, et al. Preoperative staging of esophageal cancer: comparison of endoscopic US and dynamic CT. *Radiology* 1991;181:419–425.

58. Grimm H, Binmoeller KF, Hamper K, et al. Endosonography for preoperative locoregional staging of esophageal and gastric cancer. *Endoscopy* 1993;25:224–230.

59. Ziegler K, Sanft C, Zeitz M, et al. Evaluation of endosonography in TN staging of oesophageal cancer. *Gut* 1991;32:16–20.

60. Siewert JR, Hölscher AH, Dittler HJ. Preoperative staging and risk analysis in esophageal carcinoma. *Hepatogastroenterology* 1990;37:382–387.

61. Krasna MJ, Reed CE, Jaklitsch MT, Cushing D, Sugarbaker DJ and the Cancer and Leukemia Group B Thoracic Surgeons. Thoracoscopic staging of esophageal cancer: a prospective, multiinstitutional trial. *Ann Thorac Surg* 1995;60:1337–1340.

62. Lightdale CJ, Botet JF. Staging of esophageal cancer. *Endoscopy* 1993;25:655–659.

63. Luketich JD, Schauer P, Landreneau R, et al. Minimally invasive surgical staging is superior to endoscopic ultrasound in detecting lymph node metastases in esophageal cancer. *J Thorac Cardiovasc Surg* 1997;114:817–823.

64. Reed CE, Mishra G, Sahai AV, et al. Esophageal cancer staging: improved accuracy by endoscopic ultrasound of celiac lymph nodes. *Ann Thorac Surg* 1999;67:319–322.

65. Vazquez-Sequeiros E, Norton I, Clain J, et al. Impact of EUS-guided fine-needle aspiration on lymph node staging in patients with esophageal carcinoma. *Gastrointest Endosc* 2001;7:751–757.

CHAPTER 18 ■ ESOPHAGEAL CANCER: CLINICAL MANAGEMENT

J. RÜDIGER SIEWERT, MICHAEL MOLLS, FRANK ZIMMERMANN, AND FLORIAN LORDICK

In contrast to gastric cancer incidence, which is decreasing worldwide, the incidence and prevalence of esophageal carcinoma are rising at an alarming rate in the Western world. This rise is due primarily to an increase in the rate of adenocarcinoma of the distal esophagus (1). At many institutions in the Western world, adenocarcinomas of the esophagus now outnumber squamous cell esophageal cancers. Because of marked differences in the pathogenesis, tumor location, tumor biology, and characteristics of the affected patients (Table 18.1), squamous cell carcinoma and adenocarcinoma of the esophagus should be treated as separate entities to a certain extent (2). This differentiation is frequently not made when treatment results for esophageal cancer are reported.

Despite marked advances in the surgical treatment of squamous cell carcinoma and adenocarcinoma of the esophagus, the overall prognosis for affected patients has not improved much over the past decades. This is because these tumors continue to be diagnosed at an advanced stage in the majority of the affected patients. An improvement of early diagnosis in the Western Hemisphere is only visible in Barrett Ca. Furthermore, systemic and local recurrences are still common even after a complete tumor resection, extensive lymphadenectomy, or multidisciplinary approaches (2). In the future, a valuable improvement in the overall survival of patients with esophageal cancer most likely can be achieved by the development of tailored therapeutic strategies based on the individual histologic tumor type, tumor location, tumor stage at time of presentation, response to induction radiochemotherapy (RCT), and consideration of other established prognostic factors (2). A clear classification of the underlying tumor entity, a profound knowledge of the prognostic factors applicable, and a thorough preoperative staging are therefore essential for the selection of the optimal therapeutic modality in a given situation.

TOPOGRAPHIC CLASSIFICATION

The classification of squamous cell esophageal cancer according to its location in the proximal, middle, and distal third of the esophagus should be abandoned. Rather, these tumors should be classified into tumors of the cervical esophagus ("cervical esophageal cancer"); tumors arising above the level of the tracheal bifurcation ("suprabifurcal esophageal cancer"), which means with contact to the tracheal-bronchial tree; and tumors arising below the level of the tracheal bifurcation ("infrabifurcal esophageal cancer") (3), which means without contact to the tracheal-bronchial tree. The selection of treatment strategy is guided by this topographic classification. Whereas tumors located below the level of the tracheal bifurcation can frequently be resected with adequate margins, an extensive resection of

transmural suprabifurcal or cervical tumors is usually prohibited by the proximity to the tracheoesophageal tree. The pattern of lymphatic spread also depends on the location of the primary tumor. The direction of lymphatic flow is primarily directed to the upper mediastinum and cervical region in patients with suprabifurcal tumors, and to the lower posterior mediastinum and celiac axis in patients with infrabifurcal tumors. Tumors located at the level of the tracheal bifurcation tend to metastasize in both directions (3,4).

An even better classification is based on a direct assessment of the relationship between the primary tumor and the tracheobronchial tree, that is, a differentiation of tumors with and without contact to the trachea or mainstem bronchi. These two classification systems are not identical because a tumor arising below the level of the tracheal bifurcation may still have contact with the tracheobronchial tree. In this situation, the area of contact is usually in the region of the left mainstem bronchus.

Adenocarcinoma of the esophagus, which is usually located in the distal esophagus, should be differentiated from other tumor entities arising in the vicinity of the esophagogastric junction. Due to the borderline location and the ambiguous use of the term *cardia carcinoma*, many discrepancies exist in the current literature regarding the classification of these tumors. Although some classify all such tumors as esophageal carcinomas, others classify them as gastric carcinomas or regard them as an entity separate from esophageal and gastric cancer. To clarify these issues, adenocarcinomas of the esophagogastric junction (AEG) are defined here as tumors that have their center within 5 cm proximal and distal of the anatomical cardia and have differentiated three distinct tumor entities within this area (5,6):

- AEG type I—adenocarcinoma of the distal esophagus that usually arises from an area with specialized intestinal metaplasia of the esophagus (i.e., Barrett esophagus) and may infiltrate the esophagogastric junction from above
- AEG type II—true carcinoma of the cardia arising from the cardiac epithelium or short segments with intestinal metaplasia at the esophagogastric junction
- AEG type III—subcardial gastric carcinoma that infiltrates the esophagogastric junction and distal esophagus from below

The assignment to each type is purely morphologic and is based on the anatomical location of the tumor center or, in patients with advanced tumor, the location of the tumor mass.

This differentiation of esophagogastric junction tumors is supported by several observations. Patients with AEG type I tumors are more likely to have a hiatal hernia and a long history of gastroesophageal reflux disease than are patients with AEG type II or type III tumors. Specialized intestinal epithelial

TABLE 18.1

COMPARISON OF PATIENT CHARACTERISTICS FOR THOSE WITH SQUAMOUS CELL ESOPHAGEAL CANCER AND ADENOCARCINOMA OF THE DISTAL ESOPHAGUS

	Squamous cell esophageal carcinoma	Adenocarcinoma of the distal esophagus	p Value
Median age	53.4 y	62.6 y	<0.001
Male-to-female ratio	7:1	8:1	NS
Profession (prevalence)			
Academic	20.8%	52.9%	
White collar	27.2%	27.7%	<0.001
Blue collar	52.2%	20.2%	
Alcohol abuse (prevalence)	69.7%	42.3%	<0.001
Smoking (prevalence)	69.3%	51.9%	<0.05
Malnutrition (prevalence)	24.1%	1.9%	<0.001
Pulmonary function (mean FEV$_1$,% of normal)	82.5%	93.7%	<0.05
Cardiovascular risk factors (prevalence)	19.5%	34.8%	<0.01
Impaired liver function (prevalence)	35.3%	24.9%	<0.05

FEV$_1$, forced expiratory volume in 1 s; NS, not significant.
Data are for patients treated at the Department of Surgery, Klinikum rechts der Isar, Technische Universität München, 1982–2000.

metaplasia in the distal esophagus (Barrett esophagus) with subsequent development of progressively severe dysplastic changes has been clearly identified as the main precursor lesion for adenocarcinoma in the distal esophagus (AEG type I) (7,8). Although an association with short segments of intestinal metaplasia at or below the gastric cardia has also been reported for AEG type II and III tumors, this is rather uncommon (6). In addition, there appears to be a strong association between *Helicobacter pylori* infection and intestinal metaplasia at or below the gastric cardia; this is not the case for specialized intestinal metaplasia in the distal esophagus, which is clearly reflux related (8). Furthermore, the prevalence of undifferentiated tumors and tumors with a "nonintestinal" growth pattern is rather low in AEG type I tumors and increases significantly from AEG type II to AEG type III tumors (6). Accordingly, the expression of cytokeratins and cell adhesion molecules, as well as the prevalence and pattern of genetic abnormalities detected by comparative genomic hybridization, show marked differences among the three AEG tumor types (5). Finally, lymphographic studies indicate that the main lymphatic pathways originating from the lower esophagus advance both upward into the mediastinum and downward along the celiac axis, whereas those from the gastric cardia and subcardial region preferentially make their way to the celiac axis, the splenic hilus, and the para-aortic lymph nodes (9). This is reflected in the different patterns of lymphatic spread of the three tumor entities at the esophagogastric junction (6). The most important aspect (with therapeutical consequences) is the differentiation of Barrett Ca from gastric Ca. Some imaging is helpful for this differentiation. Based on these observations, which support a possible heterogeneity in the pathogenesis and biological behavior of the different tumor types, all experts at a consensus conference and the International Society for Diseases of the Esophagus agreed that this classification should form the basis for defining, assessing, and reporting treatment of adenocarcinoma arising in the vicinity of the esophagogastric junction (6) and differentiating adenocarcinoma of the distal esophagus from

the other tumor entities. This classification is now accepted worldwide, and an increasing number of publications on this topic are based on it.

PROGNOSTIC FACTORS

The presence of distant hematogenous metastases constitutes the single most important prognostic factor in patients with squamous cell carcinoma and adenocarcinoma of the esophagus. The median survival of such patients is in the order of 6 to 12 months irrespective of the location and histologic subtype of the primary tumor, and can not usually be prolonged significantly by any of the available therapeutic modalities.

In patients without systemic metastases, a complete macroscopic and microscopic tumor resection (i.e., a R0 resection according to the guidelines of the International Union Against Cancer and the American Joint Committee on Cancer [10]) constitutes the most powerful independent prognostic factor (Fig. 18.1A, B) (11). The chance for achieving a complete tumor resection in these patients with primary surgery clearly depends on the tumor location and the pathological T (pT) category (Table 18.2).

In the subgroup of patients who undergo a complete tumor resection, the lymph node status and the number of positive lymph nodes represent the major independent prognostic factors (11) (Fig. 18.2A, B). The prevalence of lymph node metastases depends on the tumor location and the pT category (Table 18.3). An independent prognostic effect of "microinvolvement" of lymph nodes that were negative by routine histologic examination has also been demonstrated for patients with squamous cell esophageal carcinoma (12,13). In primarily resected adenocarcinoma of the esophagus, the invasion of lymphatic vessels has also been shown to be an independent prognostic factor (14).

The clinical relevance of immunohistochemical detection of epithelial tumor cells in the bone marrow of patients with

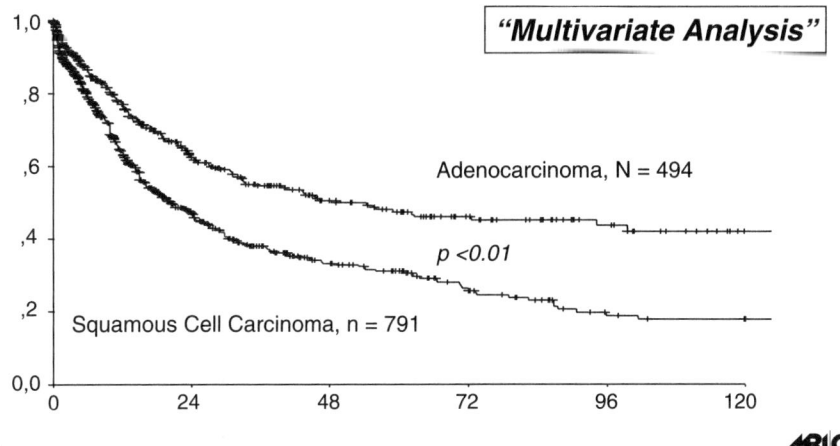

A

Esophageal Ca	Independent prognostic factors (stepwise Cox regression analysis)		
Parameter	**p-value**	**Relative Risk Exp (B)**	**95% Confidence Interval Exp (B)**
All resected patients (*n* = 1,059)			
R Category	<0.0001	1.550	1.304–1.842
N Category	<0.0001	1.806	1.500–2.175
T Category	<0.0001	1.421	1.260–1.603
Histologic Tumor Type	<0.0001	1.673	1.348–2.077
Patients with primary resection only (*n* = 722)			
R Category	<0.0001	1.557	1.279–1.941
N Category	<0.0001	1.917	1.547–2.375
T Category	<0.0001	1.420	1.235–1.633
Histologic Tumor Type	=0.001	1.528	1.193–1.958
Patients with primary resection and R0 category only (*n* = 578)			
N Category	<0.0001	1.986	1.533–2.572
T Category	<0.0001	1.359	1.162–1.590
Histologic Tumor Type	=0.001	1.626	1.224–2.161

B

FIGURE 18.1. Ten-year survival rates for patients with resected squamous cell carcinoma (**A**) and adenocarcinoma (**B**) of the esophagus. Data are shown for patients with complete macroscopic and microscopic tumor resection (R0 resection) and for patients with residual disease after resection (R1/R2 resection). *Source:* Data from the Chirurgische Klinik und Poliklinik, Klinikum rechts der Isar der Technische Universität München, 1982–1999.

esophageal cancer is still debated. At least in some of the published reports, this observation was identified as a strong predictor of early relapse and overall poor prognosis.

Of the treatment-related factors, the experience of the treatment center and the surgeon performing the resection have been clearly identified as independent prognostic factors for long-term survival in patients with esophageal cancer (15–18). The amount of perioperative blood transfusion required and the postoperative morbidity appear to constitute further independent prognostic factors for duration of survival (11,19).

A clear overall survival benefit has not yet been demonstrated for extended lymphadenectomy in patients with squamous cell carcinoma and adenocarcinoma of the esophagus. Nevertheless, several studies indicate that extended lymphadenectomy may improve survival in the subgroup of patients with a limited number of positive lymph nodes or early stages of lymphatic spread, that is, lymph node microinvolvement (20). The lymph node ratio—the ratio of positive nodes to total nodes removed—is a parameter for estimating the extent of lymph node dissection in relation to lymphatic tumor spread. A lymph node ratio of <0.2 constitutes an independent favorable prognostic factor for patients with squa-

mous cell carcinoma and adenocarcinoma of the esophagus (21,22). The potential benefit of extended lymphadenectomy may be nullified, however, if an associated increase in postoperative morbidity occurs. A new aspect brings the so-called induction chemotherapy. In patients with complete resection, the response to induction chemotherapy is a decisive prognostic factor. Discussion regarding the therapeutic consequences of induction chemotherapy is ongoing. So far, patient-related factors (i.e., age, gender, general status) have not convincingly been shown to have an independent effect on long-term survival after complete tumor resection in patients with esophageal cancer (11).

STAGING AS A PREREQUISITE FOR TAILORED THERAPY

A tailored therapeutic approach requires exact pretherapeutic staging for selection of an adequate treatment modality. After histologic confirmation, classification, and exact topographic localization of the tumor, determination of the depth of tumor

TABLE 18.2

RATE OF COMPLETE MACROSCOPIC AND MICROSCOPIC TUMOR RESECTION (R0 RESECTION BY UICC/AJCC DEFINITION) IN SQUAMOUS CELL CARCINOMA AND ADENOCARCINOMA OF THE ESOPHAGUS ACCORDING TO PATHOLOGICAL T (pT) CATEGORY (UICC/AJCC classification)

	Squamous cell carcinoma of the esophagus (%)	Adenocarcinoma of the distal esophagus (%)
pT1		
Mucosa	100	100
Submucosa	91	100
pT2	84	84
pT3	70	68
pT4	48	59

UICC, International Union Against Cancer; AJCC, American Joint Committee on Cancer.
Data from the Chirurgische Klinik und Poliklinik, Klinikum rechts der Isar, Technische Universität München 1982–2000.

TABLE 18.3

PREVALENCE OF LYMPH NODE METASTASES IN SQUAMOUS CELL CARCINOMA AND ADENOCARCINOMA OF THE ESOPHAGUS BY PATHOLOGICAL T (pT) CATEGORY (UICC/AJCC classification)

	Squamous cell carcinoma of the esophagus (%)	Adenocarcinoma of the distal esophagus (%)
pT1	30,8	11,5
Mucosa	7,7	0
Submucosa	36,4	20,7
pT2	50	67
pT3	74	85
pT4	79	89

UICC, International Union Against Cancer; AJCC, American Joint Committee on Cancer. Data from the Chirurgische Klinik und Poliklinik, Klinikum rechts der Isar, Technische Universität München, 1982–2000.

infiltration into the organ wall (T category), the lymph node status (N category), and the presence or absence of distant metastases (M category) thus becomes essential.

Today, the pT category of an esophageal, esophagogastric junction, or gastric carcinoma can be predicted by endoscopic

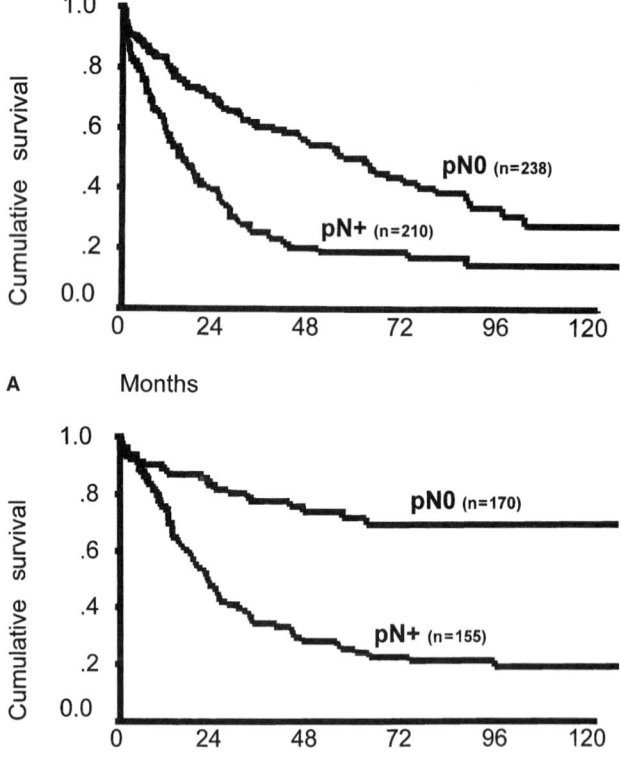

A   Months

B   Months

FIGURE 18.2. Ten-year survival rates for patients with resected squamous cell carcinoma (**A**) and adenocarcinoma (**B**) of the esophagus. Data are shown for patient pN0 and pN+ cancers. *Source:* Data from the Chirurgische Klinik und Poliklinik, Klinikum rechts der Isar der Technische Universität München, 1982–1999.

sonography with a diagnostic accuracy of approximately 85% in experienced hands. Problems still arise in the differentiation of a T2 from a T3 tumor and a T1a from a T1b tumor. The presence and extent of infiltration into neighboring organs in patients with esophageal cancer can best be assessed by computed tomography (CT) and bronchoscopy. The multislice contrast-enhanced CT scan can answer nearly all important topographic questions and is now the most decisive diagnostic procedure. Unfortunately, it has only a low accuracy to separate T1a from T1b and T2 from T3 cancer (<80%). Magnetic resonance imaging (MRI) does not add any useful information in principle but may be done if rare aortal infiltration is suspected.

None of the available imaging techniques (CT, MRI, endoscopic ultrasonography) can reliably predict the presence of lymph node metastases. The problem with all imaging techniques is that lymphatic spread can only be inferred by the documentation of enlarged nodes, which gives an accuracy of <70%.

Percutaneous ultrasonography of the upper abdomen, plain chest radiography, CT scanning, positron emission tomography (PET), and diagnostic laparoscopy are used to assess for distant metastases. (These staging techniques are described in other chapters.) PET/CT can give complete diagnostic information such as follows:

- Topographic information that is essential for radiation and surgical treatment concepts (CT and PET)
- Distant lymph nodes (LN) and distant visceral metastases (CT and PET)
- Information about the tumor metabolism

By doing this, PET/CT offers a new approach to response evaluation of neoadjuvant treatment.

If neoadjuvant therapy is considered, the patient should also be evaluated for adequate liver, renal, and bone marrow function. Because preoperative radiation or combined RCT appears to increase postoperative morbidity after an esophagectomy (23), a thorough evaluation of the physiological reserve and general status is essential in these patients to make sure that they can withstand a potentially prolonged and complicated postoperative course. In the authors' experience, a detailed risk analysis using a dedicated organ function scoring system has proved helpful in patient selection (24).

THERAPEUTIC OPTIONS

Surgical Resection

General Principles

Most surgeons agree that complete resection (R0 resection) of the tumor and its entire lymphatic drainage offers the best chance for long-term survival in patients with esophageal cancer. In patients in whom tumor resection is incomplete (R1 or R2 resection), the procedure must be considered palliative. These patients gain no survival benefit from resection. Today, palliation of dysphagia in patients with nonresectable esophageal cancer can be achieved better and more safely by endoscopic intervention, intraluminal irradiation, external beam RT, or combined RCT. A complete macro- and microscopic tumor resection must consequently be the aim of any surgical approach to squamous cell carcinoma and adenocarcinoma of the esophagus. Palliative resections have been abandoned at most institutions.

With standardized resection and reconstruction techniques, advances in complication management, and careful patient selection, a transthoracic or transmediastinal esophagectomy with en bloc two-field lymphadenectomy can be performed with a postoperative mortality of <5%. In the authors' experience, postoperative mortality can be decreased to <2% by application of a procedure-specific risk scoring system and exclusion of high-risk patients from surgery (24). Such results, however, can be achieved only in experienced centers with a high patient load (high-volume centers). Concentration of esophageal cancer surgery in centers with high experience and a documented history of excellence are therefore recommended.

The role and optimal extent of lymphadenectomy for esophageal cancer remains controversial. In the Western world, the benefits of lymphadenectomy for esophageal cancer so far have not been proven in large and well-designed prospective randomized trials, except in the Dutch trial for Barrett Ca. A comparison of the results from phase III trials from various centers using different strategies for lymphadenectomy, however, indicates that extended lymphadenectomy can improve the prognosis for patients with an early stage of lymphatic spread (15). In the authors' experience, an en bloc esophagectomy with two-field lymphadenectomy (abdominal lymph node dissection and extended mediastinal lymphadenectomy) resulted in an overall 10-year survival rate of approximately 20% for patients with squamous cell carcinoma, and the survival for patients with adenocarcinoma of the esophagus was slightly better (~35%) (21,22). The lymph node ratio constituted one of the major independent predictors of long-term survival in this analysis. The prognosis was dismal if >20% of the removed lymph nodes contained metastatic tumor on routine histologic assessment. The gain that can be achieved with lymph node dissection is thus highest for tumors at the early stage of lymphatic spread, that is, with only a limited number of positive lymph nodes. Consequently, the Dutch trial (25) was able to demonstrate a strong trend in favor of the transthoracic resection (vs. transhiatal resection). In the authors' experience, the transthoracic resection is therefore the standard procedure for Barrett Ca.

Even more extended forms of lymphadenectomy have been reported by some centers, particularly for patients with squamous cell esophageal cancer (19–22). Although a number of retrospective series showed evidence of improved survival and a reduction of local recurrence rates after extended three-field lymphadenectomy (abdominal lymph node dissection, extended mediastinal lymphadenectomy, and cervical lymphadenectomy), more recent prospective studies indicate that this may only be the case for patients with tumors located in the proximal esophagus and for patients with less than five positive lymph nodes (26–29). Of importance is that, in most of the more recent series, extended three-field lymph node dissection was associated with a marked increase in pulmonary complications and recurrent laryngeal nerve injuries requiring tracheotomy. This limits the potential benefits of three-field lymphadenectomy. In the authors' practice, a two-field lymphadenectomy is therefore considered standard in any potentially curative surgical approach to esophageal cancer (20).

Surgical Approach to Squamous Cell Esophageal Cancer

In patients with squamous cell esophageal cancer, a subtotal esophagectomy is usually indicated due to the frequent longitudinal submucosal lymphangiosis. The subtotal esophagectomy and reconstruction can be best performed via a right transthoracic and abdominal approach. A right transthoracic and abdominal approach is also required for adequate mediastinal and upper abdominal lymphadenectomy (two-field lymphadenectomy). At most institutions, a two-field lymphadenectomy constitutes an essential part of the procedure and comprises the following (30):

- Periesophageal lymph nodes above the diaphragm and along the vena cava superior
- Lymph nodes at the tracheal bifurcation
- Paratracheal lymph nodes together with the nodes along the left recurrent nerve
- Abdominal suprapancreatic lymphatic compartment along the celiac axis

Because of the early lymphatic spread with a risk of about 20% even in T1 tumors, lymphadenectomy is also performed in patients with T1 tumors. In the authors' opinion, limited resection has no place in early tumor stages. Limited procedures, as proposed by some Japanese centers, are indicated only for patients with high-grade dysplasia and mucosal carcinoma. This situation is rare in Western countries.

Reconstruction after transthoracic en bloc esophagectomy is usually performed with a gastric tube and cervical anastomosis (31). A high intrathoracic anastomosis may be justified in patients who have had previous surgical procedures or radiation in the neck area, in those for whom recurrent nerve injury must definitively be avoided (i.e., singers and public speakers), or in those with a tumor located below the tracheal bifurcation.

After RCT, differentiating scars from residual tumor is frequently difficult, even during the surgical procedure. The extent of resection after neoadjuvant therapy therefore matches that of the primary surgical resection. The postoperative course after combined RCT is more severe than after neoadjuvant chemotherapy without radiation or after a primary resection. A radiation-induced compromise in immune function appears to account for this observation (32). This has prompted us to perform the reconstruction after a delay of 1 to 2 weeks following esophagectomy in patients who had neoadjuvant RCT to increase the safety of the procedure. This safety concept has resulted in a marked decrease of postoperative mortality to <5% after neoadjuvant combined RCT.

In contrast to treatment of intrathoracic squamous cell esophageal cancer, neoadjuvant treatment of squamous cell cancer of the cervical esophagus allows a limitation of the subsequent surgical resection in those who respond to preoperative therapy. The simultaneous laryngectomy that is usually required can frequently be omitted after neoadjuvant therapy, and a limited resection of the cervical esophagus with reconstruction by a free jejunal graft becomes possible. This limited procedure is associated with a markedly better quality of life than is radical esophagolaryngectomy, without compromising the long-term prognosis.

Surgical Approach to Adenocarcinoma of the Distal Esophagus

The standard procedure today for the resection of adenocarcinoma of the distal esophagus is the transhiatal esophagectomy ending with an intrathoracic anastomosis. This procedure is well proven in a prospective controlled randomized trial (25). In comparison to the transhiatal esophagectomy, the transthoracic esophagectomy allows for an adequate lymphadenectomy in the mediastinum and an en bloc resection of the tumor. The reconstruction is performed by a gastric tube with a high located intrathoracic anastomosis. In the authors' experience, this intrathoracic anastomosis has many advantages: better swallowing function, better healing of the anastomosis, fewer paresis of the recurrent laryngeal nerve, and simplified management of complications. In case of insufficiency, this type of anastomosis can be covered easily and effectively by an endoscopically inserted stent. As a consequence of this effective complication management, the mortality is now <3% and the morbidity around 20%.

The reported surgical approaches to adenocarcinoma of the distal esophagus include abdominothoracic en bloc esophagogastrectomy, subtotal esophagectomy with resection of the proximal stomach, total gastrectomy with transhiatal resection of the distal esophagus, and limited resection of the esophagogastric junction. Since the late 1980s, the authors have performed resections in more than 1,500 patients with adenocarcinoma of the esophagogastric junction and have assessed a variety of surgical approaches (6). In patients with adenocarcinoma of the distal esophagus (i.e., AEG type I tumors), the Dutch trial could demonstrate a significant difference in long-term survival in favor of patients undergoing transthoracic resection, if the tumor was removed completely. As a consequence, the transhiatal esophagectomy is now accepted as the authors' standard procedure.

The experience with systematic lymph node dissection in patients with adenocarcinoma of the distal esophagus shows that lymph node metastases are virtually never present in patients with tumors limited to the mucosa (pT1a about 0%) and are uncommon in patients with tumors limited to the submucosa (pT1b <20%) (Table 18.3). Data indicate that this is also true when immunohistochemical techniques are used to search for micrometastases in the lymph nodes of such patients (33). In patients with more advanced tumors, lymph node metastases occur in decreasing order of prevalence in the paracardial region, the posterior lower mediastinum, the lesser and greater curve of the stomach, along the left gastric artery toward the celiac axis, at the superior border of the pancreas along the splenic artery toward the splenic hilum, and in the area of the left adrenal gland and the left renal vein (34). Lymph node metastases in the upper mediastinum or cervical region occur only in patients with locally advanced adenocarcinoma who also have numerous positive locoregional nodes.

Given this pattern of lymphatic spread, an extended lymph node dissection in patients with adenocarcinoma of the distal esophagus should include the removal of lymph nodes along the splenic artery, at the splenic hilus, and along the left renal vein behind the pancreas. To perform this retroperitoneal lymph node dissection, a left-sided pancreatic resection with splenectomy should be avoided because this procedure is associated with a substantial number of septic complications due to pancreatic fistula and abscess formation. Although pancreas-preserving splenectomy allows a similar clearance of lymph nodes in this area without the risk of pancreatic fistula, splenectomy itself may result in significant morbidity. Because postoperative complications independently influence long-term survival, safe resection and reconstruction techniques are essential. Consequently, the potential benefits of a more extensive lymph node dissection achieved with splenectomy may be nullified by the associated morbidity. Splenectomy is therefore only justified in patients with frank lymph node metastases or infiltration of the splenic hilum.

The morbidity associated with extended total gastrectomy or esophagectomy and the compromised quality of life after these procedures have in recent years stimulated efforts to assess more limited forms of resection for adenocarcinoma of the distal esophagus. Based on the virtual absence of lymph node metastases and micrometastases in patients with tumors limited to the mucosa and the low prevalence and number of lymph node metastases found in patients with tumors extending to the submucosa, a limited resection of the distal esophagus, cardia, and proximal stomach has been evaluated in such patients (33). To avoid postoperative reflux, reconstruction is performed by interposition of a pedicled jejunal segment. In the authors' experience of performing more than 100 such procedures for tumors staged as uT1 on endoscopic ultrasonography, a complete resection (R0) could be achieved in all instances. No evidence of lymph node metastases or micrometastases was found in a mean of 20 removed nodes per patient. So far, in a 2-year follow-up, no recurrences or deaths have occurred. Quality-of-life assessment showed no evidence of gastroesophageal reflux and good to excellent swallowing function in >90% of the patients (33). Similar encouraging data with limited resection in patients with early tumors at the esophagogastric junction, particularly those in which the vagus nerve can be preserved during the resection, are also reported by several Japanese authors.

Endoscopic Mucosa Resection

The new technology of endoscopic mucosa resection offers an even more limited approach to early tumors of the distal esophagus (35). Because a lymphadenectomy is not possible with this technique, endoscopic mucosa resection can only be recommended for patients with pT1a tumors. The frequent multicentric tumor growth; the inaccuracy of current preoperative staging modalities, including high-frequency endoscopic ultrasonography, in differentiating mucosal from submucosal tumors; and the persistence of precancerous lesions (i.e., Barrett esophagus) currently restrict the clinical application of trial protocols.

Combined Modality Treatment

Despite the remarkable progress that has been documented over the past decades in the surgical treatment of esophageal cancer, prospects for long-term survival of these patients, even after complete resection, are still dismal. This is because more than two-thirds of patients present with tumors that have grown beyond the esophageal wall, such as tumors invading the adventitia (T3) or adjacent structures (T4). A complete resection can be achieved in only a minority of these patients (Table 18.2). Furthermore, esophageal carcinoma metastasizes early during the course of the disease. Autopsy studies demonstrate that a large percentage of patients already have systemic disease at the time of presentation (36). Lymphatic spread is common in tumors that extend beyond the mucosal layers (Table 18.3). Finally, the close anatomical relationship of the proximal esophagus to the tracheobronchial tree prohibits extensive resection in patients with esophageal tumors located at or above the level of the tracheal bifurcation. Thus, primary surgical resection is reasonable only in those patients for whom preoperative staging indicates that a R0 resection can be achieved with a high degree of certainty.

Consequently, multidisciplinary approaches using adjuvant, neoadjuvant, or additive therapeutic methods have received increasing attention. Targets for the additional treatment are the local extraesophageal tumor growth in T3 and T4 tumors (tumor bed) and occult locoregional and distant micrometastases. Modalities include radiotherapy, chemotherapy, or combined chemoradiation.

Despite numerous phase II and phase III trials, the role of multimodal therapy in the treatment of esophageal cancer is still under discussion. This is because most studies are not comparable. Some studies show remarkable shortcomings in study design, others lack adequate pretherapeutic staging, and yet others use confusing terminology. The major limitations of most available studies are (2,37) as follows:

- Inaccurate staging and patient stratification according to prognostic factors
- Major differences in the staging systems (American Joint Committee on Cancer/International Union Against Cancer) applied before 1997
- Different definition of locoregional and locally advanced disease
- Imprecise information concerning the quality and extent of surgical resection and lymphadenectomy
- Variations in the definition of "curative resection": curative according to the surgeon (who misses microscopic residual disease in up to 20% of the patients) versus macroscopic and microscopic complete resection (R0) according to the surgeon and pathologist
- Differences in the quality of the pathological-histologic workup of the resected specimen and pathological reporting
- Failure to discriminate squamous cell carcinoma and adenocarcinoma of the esophagus
- A broad spectrum of variably defined radiation schedules

Each factor listed here can influence the prognosis of a patient to a greater extent than the potentially beneficial multimodal therapy. This must be kept in mind when analyzing the published reports.

Postoperative Adjuvant Treatment

By definition, *adjuvant* therapy is postoperative treatment after macroscopic and microscopic complete resection (R0), as far as surgeon and pathologist can exclude micrometastases beyond the resection margins. The aim is to eradicate left tumor cells beyond resection margin and occult regional and distant micrometastases to prevent or delay locoregional and distant recurrence. An advantage of adjuvant treatment is that pathological evaluation of the resected specimen and intraoperative staging provide definitive pretreatment information. The surgeon can define areas of risk and thus focus postoperative therapy. However, one major shortcoming of adjuvant therapy in contrast to neoadjuvant therapy is that it cannot lead to tumor shrinkage, and therefore, it will not contribute to a higher potentially curative R0 resection rate. In the light of the limited chances for R0 resection in locally advanced esophageal cancer (Table 18.2), this consideration constitutes a strict hypothesis against the adjuvant approach in this setting.

Even after a complete resection, patients with pT3 and pT4 or pN-positive tumors are at a high risk for recurrence. For example, patients with disease classified as pT3 N0 have a risk of at least 60% of dying from local or distant tumor recurrence within 5 years after the operation. Such patients are therefore potential candidates for postoperative adjuvant treatment. Only a minority of eligible patients, however, tolerate an intensive postoperative treatment protocol. This is due to a generally reduced performance status after esophagectomy, which is accompanied by a potentially increased toxicity of the treatment with subsequent poor compliance. Furthermore, adjuvant therapy is often initiated after a long delay due to postoperative complications. From an anatomical and physiological point of view, postoperative therapy is also hindered by tumor cell entrapment, hypo-oxygenation, and altered blood supply in the areas of interest.

Postoperative Radiotherapy. Postoperative changes in the anatomy may result in the presence of larger areas of uninvolved tissue (e.g., the organ used for reconstruction) in the irradiated volume. This leads to an increase in morbidity. The assumed decreased oxygenation of residual tumor cells results in decreased radiosensitivity and possibly in the selection of tumor clones resistant to cytotoxic therapy (38).

The rationale for using adjuvant radiation is based on the pattern of failure after a complete resection; only a few surgical series have reported such data. The rates of local failure in the surgical control arms of two randomized trials of preoperative radiation therapy were 12% and 67%, respectively (39,40). Local failure rates in the surgical control arm of the randomized postoperative radiation therapy trial of Teniere et al. were 35% for patients with negative locoregional lymph nodes and 38% for those with positive nodes (41). Although the majority of patients with esophageal cancer die of distant metastasis, the incidence of local failure after surgery alone is high enough to examine the use of adjuvant radiation therapy.

Nonrandomized trials have reported encouraging results with postoperative radiation therapy. In a study by Kasai et al., patients with lymph node–negative disease had a 5-year survival rate of 88% (42). Yamamoto et al. reported a 2-year local control rate of 94% in node-negative patients (43).

Data on five randomized trials comparing postoperative radiotherapy and resection with resection alone are reported. Only three trials suggested that postoperative radiation may actually decrease the local failure rate (43–45), but at the expense of significant morbidity in two trials, with one single trial even demonstrating an adverse but nonsignificant effect of additional radiotherapy on overall survival, perhaps due to hypofractionated schedule (single dose of 3.5 Gy) (44). None of these trials observed an overall survival benefit for patients receiving adjuvant radiation; this was also confirmed by a negative meta-analysis (46).

Teniere et al. reported on 221 patients with squamous cell esophageal cancer randomly assigned to receive surgery alone or surgery plus postoperative radiation therapy (45–55 Gy at 1.8 Gy per fraction). After a minimum follow-up of 3 years, adjuvant radiation was not found to prolong survival (41) (Table 18.4). These data were confirmed by further clinical trials with no significant difference in 2-, 3-, or 5-year overall survival even with large total doses of up to 60 Gy (45,47), although the latter was conducted in nearly 500 patients. A second trial by Fok et al. included patients with squamous cell carcinoma and adenocarcinoma of the esophagus (44). Patients with a complete or palliative resection were included in this trial. Even in this study with an extraordinary risk of postoperative local tumor progression after incomplete tumor resection, the addition of postoperative radiation therapy did not significantly decrease local (31%–15%) or distant failure, or improve median survival.

Adjuvant radiation therapy is sometimes recommended for patients with positive locoregional lymph nodes. Although the data from Teniere et al. suggest that postoperative radiation therapy may reduce local failures, the benefit was limited to node-negative patients. In this subset, adjuvant radiation therapy decreased the local failure rate from 35% to 10%.

That means there is no indication for postoperative radiation after complete or incomplete resection. Side effects are increased by postoperative radiotherapy, which may be due to high total doses in some trials (45,47) and lack of modern conformal radiotherapy with optimal sparing of critical organs as lung in all studies published in the 1990s from trials started in the 1980s. Therefore, postoperative

TABLE 18.4

POSTOPERATIVE RADIOTHERAPY AND SURVIVAL FOR ESOPHAGEAL CARCINOMA AFTER COMPLETE RESECTION: RANDOMIZED PHASE III TRIALS

Study	Protocol	No. patients	Histology	Stage	Survival (mo)	Survival rate (%)				p Value
						1 y	2 y	3 y	5 y	
Teniere et al. (41)	Surgery	119	SCC	I–III	18	75	NS	24	19	NS
	Surg. + 45–55 Gy	102			18	67		26	19	
Fok et al. (44)	Surgery	30	SCC	I–II	21	—	NS	—	—	NS
	Surg. + 49 Gy	30			15	—		—	—	
Zieren et al. (167)	Surgery	35	SCC	I–III	NA	53	NS	20	—	NS
	Surg. + 56 Gy	33				57		22	—	
JEOG (168)	Surg. + CDDP/VDS	130	SCC	I–IV	NA	90	NS	52	—	NS
	Surg. + 49 Gy	128				80		50	—	

SCC, squamous cell carcinoma; NS, not significant; NA, not available; JEOG, Japanese Esophageal Oncology Group; CDDP, cisplatin; VDS, vindesine.

radiotherapy might be offered if the risk of distant metastases is estimated comparatively low, and the patient has recovered rapidly and completely after resection. It is an individual decision that should be based on multidisciplinary discussion and the decision of an informed patient. The use of conformal radiotherapy is a prerequisite then.

Intraoperative radiotherapy (IORT) constitutes a special form of adjuvant radiotherapy. Different IORT techniques and doses have been examined in patients with esophageal carcinoma. Single IORT doses of 25 Gy caused tracheal damage in almost 30% of patients (48). Because patients receiving IORT were not compared with untreated controls, the effect on local recurrence rates and long-term survival in esophageal cancer remains unknown.

In summary, although the limited data available suggest that the use of adjuvant radiation therapy in esophageal cancer may decrease local failure in node-negative patients, it has no proven impact on overall survival (46). The only established role for postoperative radiation therapy might be in patients who have positive tumor margins after resection. Based on the positive survival results from combined modality therapy trials, postoperative radiation should be combined with systemic chemotherapy, if used at all.

Postoperative Chemotherapy. The use of postoperative chemotherapy has been assessed in four randomized trials, with three trials comparing it with surgery alone. A French multicentric study investigated the effect of cisplatin-based combination therapy (cisplatin and 5-fluorouracil [5-FU]) after complete resection versus surgery alone. No difference in survival was seen between the two groups (49). Significantly more patients in the treated group had hematologic, neurologic, or renal complications. In a randomized trial, the Japanese Esophageal Oncology Group compared postoperative chemotherapy with cisplatin and vindesine to surgery alone in 205 patients with squamous cell esophageal cancer (50). They reported no significant differences in survival between groups, even after stratification for lymph node status. A newer Japanese trial randomized 402 patients to surgery alone or surgery and chemotherapy (two courses of cisplatin and 5-FU). Again, this trial revealed no statistical significant difference in survival and diseasefree survival between the two groups, but the risk reduction by postoperative chemotherapy was remarkable for patients with lymph node metastases, with an absolute improvement in 5-year overall survival of 14% (51) (Table 18.5). However, there was stratification only based on resection margin and not on nodal status, which means that this study does

TABLE 18.5

POSTOPERATIVE CHEMOTHERAPY FOR ESOPHAGEAL CARCINOMA: PROSPECTIVE, RANDOMIZED TRIALS

Study	Protocol	No. patients	Stage	Survival rate (%)			p Value
				2 y	3 y	5 y	
Pouliquen et al.[a] (49)	Surgery	38	IIb–III	30	17	NA	NS
	Surg. + CDDP/5-FU	24		30	10	—	
Ando et al.[a] (50)	Surgery	100	I–IV	65	NA	45	NS
	Surg + CDDP/VDS	105		65	—	48	
Ando et al. (51)	Surgery	122	IIa–IV (M1lymph)	NA	NA	52	NS
	Surg + CDDP/5-FU	120		NA	NA	61	
JEOG (168)	Surg. + 50 Gy	128	I–IV	61	50	NA	NS
	Surg. + CDDP/VDS	128		59	52	—	

NA, not available; NS, not significant; CDDP, cisplatin; 5-FU, 5-fluorouracil; VDS, vindesine; JEOG, Japanese Esophageal Oncology Group.
[a]The subgroup that underwent complete resection was analyzed separately.

not sufficiently justify postoperative chemotherapy in clinical routine.

All studies that investigated chemotherapy using a "sandwich method" (i.e., preoperative and postoperative chemotherapy) reported failure. The projected postoperative chemotherapy could not be administered due to unacceptable toxicity after the operation. In a study by Heath et al., the combination of cisplatin and paclitaxel to be given postoperatively could be administered to <50% of the patients due to unacceptable myelosuppression and fatigue (52).

Postoperative Radiochemotherapy. Postoperative chemoradiation has so far been studied in only one phase II trial (53), which does not allow any conclusions.

Based on these data, postoperative adjuvant chemotherapy after complete resection of esophageal cancer has so far shown no efficacy in prolonging diseasefree and overall survival, and consequently, has no established role outside clinical trials. The potential reduction of local recurrences after postoperative radiation therapy did not result in a prolonged overall survival. Neither is there evidence that supports the idea of postoperative radio-, chemo- or RCT even in R1–2 resection. However, in a single situation with informed consent of the patient, it might be justifiable to offer an additional treatment to patients after incomplete tumor resection, to avoid an early local tumor progression. The high toxicity after previous esophagectomy (hematotoxicity CTC°III–IV >20%, gastrointestinal toxicity CTC°III–IV >30%) should be taken into account, and the patient should be offered an optimal supportive care program.

Preoperative Treatment

Three major approaches to preoperative combined modality therapy have been explored in patients with locoregional or advanced esophageal cancer since the 1970s: preoperative radiotherapy, chemotherapy, and chemoradiation. After phase II trials demonstrated the safety of these techniques, random assignment studies were performed in an effort to improve the chances for a complete tumor resection and to prolong overall survival.

Several theoretical and clinical factors favor the use of preoperative therapy over postoperative therapy (2,54):

- Blood and lymph vessels are undamaged, which provides an effective drug concentration in the problem areas around the tumor, and tumor oxygenation and radiosensitivity are preserved.
- The performance status of the patient is better than it is postoperatively, which allows the administration of a more aggressive cisplatin-based combination chemotherapy.
- The performance status of responding patients is improved preoperatively.
- The tumor is "downsized" (or, better, "downshrunk"); thus, the possibility for a complete resection is improved.
- Systemic micrometastases are eliminated early.
- Preoperative therapy may devitalize tumor cells and minimize the risk of intraoperative spillage and seeding of viable tumor cells.
- The efficacy of preoperative radiation, chemotherapy, or both can be studied histopathologically in the resected specimen.
- Patients who may not tolerate aggressive combined preoperative treatment and resection can be detected before resection to avoid high perioperative mortality.
- Patients with minor tumor response and severe toxicity of preoperative treatment may be omitted for resection to avoid high mortality.

Prerequisite for neoadjuvant treatment is an exact pretherapeutic staging. This is lacking in most reported trials. More than 90% of studies published so far use only on endoscopic or radiographic staging criteria. Endoscopic ultrasonography is used in <20% of hospitals dealing with esophageal cancer patients, and the overall availability of endoscopic ultrasonography in all hospitals in the United States does not exceed 5% (55).

Preoperative Radiotherapy. Preoperative radiotherapy (20–55 Gy) was studied in seven randomized trials, starting as early as 1968 (Table 18.6), with five trials against surgery alone, one trial within a four-arm setting against surgery alone and against postoperative radiotherapy, and one trial against postoperative radiotherapy (46). Some studies observed that resectability was slightly higher in patients treated with preoperative radiotherapy than in untreated patients (56–59), whereas others reported the opposite. In two studies, the treatment-related mortality rate of patients receiving preoperative radiotherapy was higher than that of patients treated by esophageal resection alone (40,44), but both trials used high single doses (2.4–3.3 Gy) known to disproportionately

TABLE 18.6

PREOPERATIVE RADIOTHERAPY FOR PATIENTS WITH ESOPHAGEAL CANCER: RANDOMIZED PHASE III TRIALS

Study	Protocol	Histology	No. patients	Resection rate (%)	Mortality (%)	Median Survival (mo)	Survival rate (%) 2 y	Survival rate (%) 5 y	p Value
Launois et al. (56)	Surgery	SCC	47	70	23	12	35	12	NS
	40 Gy		62	76	23	10	22	10	
Gignoux et al. (40)	Surgery	SCC	106	82	18	45	28	9	NS
	35 Gy		102	74	24	48	26	10	
Wang et al. (57)	Surgery	SCC	102	85	6	NA	NA	30	NS
	40 Gy		104	93	5	—	—	35	
Arnott et al. (58)	Surgery	SCC	86	72	13	8	30	17	NS
	20 Gy		90	74	15	8	25	9	
Fok et al. (59)	Surgery	SCC	39	NA	8	22	40	16	NS
	35–53 Gy		40		37	11	35	10	

SCC, squamous cell carcinoma; NS, not significant; NA, not available.

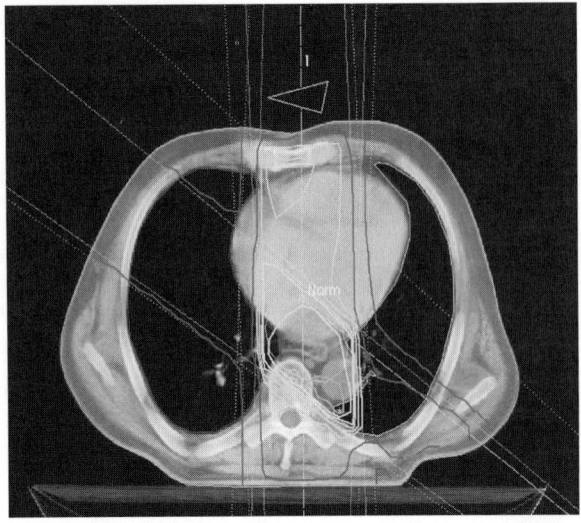

FIGURE 18.3. Example of three-dimensional conformational planning of radiotherapy for esophageal cancer. The isodose distribution is shown.

increase side effects (59). No survival benefit compared to primary resection has been reported from any single randomized trial; some studies even recorded a slight reduction in overall survival after preoperative radiotherapy. However, an analysis by the Cochrane Collaboration found an overall reduction of 11% in the risk of death, making an absolute survival benefit of 3% at 2 years and 4% at 5 years, respectively, with a borderline significance ($p = 0.062$) in pooled data of five properly designed randomized trials including 1,147 patients with a median follow-up of 9 years. The studies used for the meta-analysis mostly included patients with squamous cell cancer, making it impossible to give any advice on treatment of adenocarcinoma of the lower esophagus (AEG I). However, due to the borderline significance, preoperative radiotherapy is not recommended as standard procedure even in squamous cell carcinoma of the oesophagus (60). According to a meta-analysis by Arnott et al., inclusion of more than 3,000 patients would be necessary to perform a valid study to prove the benefits of preoperative radiotherapy (61).

Controversy still exists regarding fractionation (conventional fractionation vs. hyperfractionation or hyperfractionation and acceleration), dosage, target volume of radiotherapy, and timing of surgery after radiation. Because of recent advances in delivery of radiation, additional studies are required to define the role of preoperative radiation as a single modality or combined with chemotherapy. Innovative radiation approaches are under study in an attempt to maximize tumor cell damage while sparing normal tissue.

The use of three-dimensional conformational radiation planning is essential, which may allow higher doses to be delivered with less morbidity (Fig. 18.3). The use of hyperfractionated schedules allows a better repair of sublethal damage in critical organs between two smaller fractions, and the combination of accelerated fractionation with reduction of overall treatment time may overcome relative radioresistance of tumor cells.

Preoperative Chemotherapy. The impact of neoadjuvant chemotherapy on the prognosis for patients with esophageal cancer can be assessed only if patients with resectable tumors and those with locally advanced and irresectable tumors are evaluated separately. Resectable tumors include T1 and T2 categories, whereas T3 and T4 and N+ categories are considered locally advanced tumors. At least 30% of this latter group is not completely resectable (R0). Unfortunately, due to inadequate staging procedures, a lack of multidisciplinary assessment, and

inconsistent definitions in clinical trials, the majority of studies does not clearly separate these two distinct clinical situations.

Phase II studies involving patients with potentially resectable tumors. By far, the majority of studies of preoperative chemotherapy in patients with potentially resectable tumors have been uncontrolled phase II trials. The first cisplatin-based combination therapy study was initiated by Kelsen's group more than 25 years ago (62). In subsequent trials, higher response rates were observed with a combination of cisplatin, bleomycin sulfate, and vindesine (DBV, a "first-generation" chemotherapy regimen) (63–66). The rate of pathological complete responses, however, was disappointingly low (approximately 5%). Because of a significant number of postoperative deaths, which might be attributed to the potential pulmonary toxicity of bleomycin, this substance was omitted in later trials and replaced by drugs that have shown some single-agent activity against esophageal cancer. The overall results were not changed significantly.

The combination of cisplatin and 5-FU given by continuous infusion ("second-generation" combination chemotherapy) has been studied extensively in preoperative chemotherapy trials in squamous cell and adenocarcinoma of the esophagus (67–77). Major responses have been observed in 42% to 66% of patients, with pathologically determined complete response rates of 7% to 11%. Resectability after a preoperative regimen of cisplatin and 5-FU has ranged from 38% to 94%. Toxicity has been tolerable. Chemotherapy-related deaths were rare, and operative mortality did not seem to be increased in these studies. Next, the biomodulation of 5-FU–containing combinations by addition of leucovorin calcium (68) or interferon-α (77) or both was investigated in the "third-generation" chemotherapy protocols. The response and resectability rates, postoperative mortality, and survival reported in these trials were comparable to those with cisplatin and 5-FU alone. The toxicity, however, appeared to be higher.

Recently, the taxanes (paclitaxel and docetaxel) and irinotecan hydrochloride in combination with cisplatin ("fourth-generation" chemotherapy regimen) were introduced for the preoperative treatment of esophageal cancer. As yet, the experience is limited but promising (78–80).

Overall, the use of preoperative chemotherapy in patients with localized esophageal cancer is feasible and does not appear to increase postoperative morbidity and mortality. Major responses were achieved with cisplatin-based combinations in 41% to 69% of patients. Pathologically determined complete responses were reported in less than 10% of patients. Although the percentage of distant treatment failures appeared to decrease, locoregional failures remained constant with local recurrences of 30% to 40%, even after complete resection. Median overall survival times have been reported to be between 12 and 24 months, and survival rates are 40% at 2 years after resection. The phase II studies indicated that the administration of preoperative chemotherapy is tolerable and without demonstrable adverse effects on survival outcome.

Phase III studies involving patients with potentially resectable tumors. Final results of nine randomized trials have thus far been reported (66,81–89) (Table 18.7). Seven trials included only patients with squamous cell esophageal cancer, whereas in the trials with the largest number of enrolled patients (INT 0113, MRC), 54% and 67%, respectively, had adenocarcinoma (85,88). No postoperative treatment after potential curative resection was allowed in six studies, whereas in two studies postoperative chemotherapy was administered to responding patients (66,85). Additional postoperative radiation was given to patients with T3 tumors and to those with positive lymph nodes in one of the trials (66).

Seven of these nine trials failed to demonstrate a significant prolongation of overall survival, whereas two trials found a significant benefit from preoperative treatment. In the trial with positive results reported by Kok et al. (86,88), 163 patients

TABLE 18.7

PREOPERATIVE CHEMOTHERAPY FOR POTENTIALLY RESECTABLE ESOPHAGEAL CARCINOMA: RANDOMIZED PHASE III TRIALS

Study	Protocol	Histology	No. patients	Resection rate (%)	R0[a] (%)	Postoperative mortality (%)	Major resp./pCR (%)	Madian survival (mo) All	Madian survival (mo) Resected	p Value
Roth et al. (66)	Surgery	SCC	19	NA	21	0	—	9	NA	NS
	CDDP/BLM/VDS		17	NA	35	12	47/6	9	NA	
Nygaard et al. (81)	Surgery	SCC	41	68	37	13	—	8	NA	NS
	CDDP/BLM		50	58	44	15	NA	8	NA	
Schlag (82)	Surgery	SCC	24	79	42	10	—	10	NA	NS
	CDDP/5-FU ci		22	50	32	21	38	10	NA	
Maipang et al. (83)	Surgery	SCC	22	NA	NA	NA	—	17	NA	NS
	CDDP/BLM/VBL		24	NA	NA	NA	NA	17	NA	
Law (169)	Surgery	SCC	73	95	33	9	—	13	NA	NS
	CDDP/5-FU ci		74	89	54	8	58/7	16.8	NA	
Ancona et al. (170)	Surgery	SCC	47	87	75	4	—	22	NA	NS
	CDDP/5-FU ci		47	85	79	4	40/15	27	—	
Kelsen et al. (85)	Surgery	SCC + AC	227	89	59	6	—	16.1	25	NS
	CDDP/5-FU ci		213	76	62	6	19/2.5	14.9	27.4	
Kok et al. (86)	Surgery	SCC	82	85	45	4	—	12	15	0.01
	CDDP/Etop		81	83	72	3	38/3	19	26	
MRC (88)	Surgery	SCC+AC	400	91	71	10	—	13	15	0.01
	CDDP/5-FU		402	91	84	9	NA	17	26	

R0, complete resection; pCR, pathohistologic response after surgery; SCC, squamous cell carcinoma; NA, not available; NS, not significant; CDDP, cisplatin; BLM, bleomycin sulfate; VDS, vindesine; 5-FU, 5-fluorouracil; ci, continuous infusion; VBL, vinblastine sulfate; AC, adenocarcinoma; Etop, etoposide.
[a]Calculation based on all patients enrolled for preoperative chemotherapy.

with squamous cell cancer of the esophagus were randomly assigned to undergo surgery alone or to receive preoperative cisplatin plus etoposide (two cycles, with two additional cycles for patients showing a major response). Patients receiving preoperative chemotherapy had a median survival of 19 months and an actuarial 3-year survival rate of 41% compared with a median survival of 12 months and a 21% 3-year survival rate in the surgery-only arm. Compared to the other trials, this trial differed with respect to the chemotherapy regimen applied, the use of a flexible number of cycles according to the response achieved after two cycles, and the type of surgical resection (transmediastinal approach). Questions arise as to whether the choice of a different chemotherapy regimen and a more intense scheduling for responding patients led to superior survival rates. Another possible explanation is that the results of limited lymphadenectomy can be improved with the help of preoperative chemotherapy.

In Intergroup Trial 0113, 440 patients with both squamous cell carcinoma and adenocarcinoma of the esophagus were enrolled (85). The study randomly assigned patients to receive surgery alone or up to three cycles of cisplatin plus 5-FU chemotherapy followed by resection. Patients in the neoadjuvant group who underwent a potentially curative resection were to receive two additional chemotherapy cycles postoperatively. In the intention-to-treat analysis, no significant increase in overall survival was seen: median survival was 14.5 months in patients treated with the multimodal approach and 16.1 months in those undergoing surgery alone. In addition, the 2-year survival rates (35% vs. 37%) and 3-year survival rates (26% for both groups) were nearly identical. No significant

difference in survival was seen for either histologic subgroup. No differences were noted in diseasefree survival. After complete resection, locoregional failures were equally common in patients who received preoperative chemotherapy (31%) and those who did not (32%). A slightly higher frequency of first failures at distant sites was observed in patients who underwent surgery alone. Preoperative chemotherapy was tolerated fairly well and did not increase postoperative morbidity and mortality. Twenty percent of patients with potentially resectable esophageal cancer were not referred to surgery, however. This might have had a negative effect in the intention-to-treat analysis. Overall, the resection rates were consistently lower in patients who received preoperative chemotherapy; nevertheless, complete resections could be achieved in a higher percentage (78%). The response rate of 19% to cisplatin plus 5-FU was disappointingly low in comparison to the response rate of 38% to 53% reported in other trials. This may reflect the true antitumor activity of this combination regimen.

In contrast to the studies mentioned previously, a Medical Research Council trial of chemotherapy before surgery versus surgery alone shows a significant improvement in survival after combined therapy (88). Between 1992 and 1998, 802 patients with resectable esophageal cancer of any cell type were randomly assigned to receive either two 4-day cycles, 3 weeks apart, of cisplatin 80 mg/m^2 by 4-hour infusion plus 5-FU 1 g/m^2/day by infusion for 4 days followed by resection, or surgery alone. Two-thirds of the patients in each group had adenocarcinoma. The resection rate was 91%, with 84% complete resections after chemotherapy and 71% after surgery alone. Postoperative morbidity was 48% and 41% for the combined therapy group and surgery-only group, respectively; 30-day mortality was 9% and 10%, respectively. In the intent-to-treat analysis, median survival (17.4 months vs. 13.4 months) and 2-year survival (45% vs. 35%) ($p = 0.002$) were significantly better after combined treatment. No evidence was seen of a different treatment effect according to histology. This trial might underline the fact that, even when conventional agents are used in a large trial, significant improvements after neoadjuvant chemotherapy can be reached. The Medical Research Council study stresses that trials of neoadjuvant therapy in esophageal cancer must be adequately powered so clinically meaningful improvements in outcome will not be missed.

Generally, most trials of preoperative chemotherapy show that patients who have a major response to preoperative therapy live significantly longer than patients who do not respond and patients who are treated with surgery alone. However, non-responding patients appear to have a significantly worse prognosis than those who are treated with surgery alone, even after a potentially curative resection. In other words, responders to chemotherapy live significantly longer but at the expense of causing treatment toxicity in nonresponders without improvement in tumor control. Whether this is the result of chemotherapy or whether sensitivity to chemotherapy merely identifies a subgroup of patients with good prognosis remains unclear. The identification of responders to chemotherapy is clearly of high clinical importance. Molecular profiling and early metabolic response evaluation by means of PET may gain importance in this field in the near future.

In conclusion, in patients with potentially resectable squamous cell carcinoma or adenocarcinoma, the clinical benefit by preoperative chemotherapy compared with surgery alone remains unclear. Further investigation not only should be based on sophisticated pretherapeutic staging but also should explore the possibilities of "molecular staging" and early metabolic response evaluation to predict which patients will respond and to exclude nonresponding patients, who might be harmed by a prolonged, ineffective, and toxic therapy that could lead to a delay of surgery.

Neoadjuvant chemotherapy for patients with locally advanced tumors. The experience with the use of neoadjuvant therapy to treat locally advanced esophageal cancer is still limited. Patients who respond to the therapy may be offered a second chance for local treatment, which might be chemoradiation, surgery, or both. In the largest study, neoadjuvant therapy with cisplatin plus 5-FU allowed subsequent resection in 52% of the 163 enrolled patients with locally advanced (presumable stage T4) esophageal carcinoma (90). Complete resection could be achieved in 32% of the patients (87). The authors report an impressive 23-month median survival and a 5-year survival rate of 29% for patients who had an R0 resection. However, the rate of locoregional failure, even after R0 resection, was disappointingly high (85%). This finding again reflects the inefficacy of chemotherapy in achieving local control in locally advanced primary tumors and underlines the need for additional radiotherapy.

Preoperative Chemoradiation Therapy. In the majority of patients with esophageal cancer, immediate resection or resection after preoperative chemotherapy has failed to eradicate disease left at the circumferential margins of resection (tumor bed). Preoperative radiotherapy improves locoregional control. A combination of all three modalities—preoperative chemotherapy and radiotherapy followed by surgery (trimodality therapy)—may offer the greatest potential for increasing cure rates. The primary objectives of combined modality therapy in a preoperative setting are both to increase local control by intensifying radiotherapy with concurrent chemotherapy used as a radiosensitizer and to eradicate clinical occult micrometastases by means of systemic chemotherapy.

Phase II studies involving patients with potentially resectable tumors. In the initial pilot study, Leichmann et al.

treated 21 patients with squamous cell esophageal cancer with 30 Gy of radiation plus two cycles of cisplatin plus infusional 5-FU (91). In 5 of 15 resected specimens, no tumor could be detected in the esophagus or the lymph nodes. To confirm the initial work, studies were conducted by the Southwest Oncology Group and the Radiation Therapy Oncology Group (92). The results of the Southwest Oncology Group trial reflect the problems encountered in performing preoperative chemoradiation in a larger multicentric trial (93). Of 113 eligible patients with potentially resectable tumors, 27% of patients were not referred to surgery after treatment. A complete resection could be performed in only 37% of all patients.

To increase the rate of complete remissions, the total radiation dose was increased from 30 to 45 Gy in the following studies (73–75). The chemotherapy protocol was changed (a) to increase the time of exposure during concurrent radiation with the aim of maximizing radiosensitizing by applying all chemotherapy during radiation or delivering 5-FU by means of protracted infusion over the total period of radiation (94–97), and (b) to reduce the risk of distant metastasis by increasing the total dose and thus antitumor activity of the chemotherapy applied. Despite the numerous changes in the application of chemoradiation, no major breakthrough was achieved in identifying the most effective chemoradiation strategy. In the initial reports, complete response rates of approximately 25% were cited; median overall survival was 18 months, and some patients survived for 3 years. Some of the more intense regimens achieved higher histopathological complete response and superior survival rates. This was usually achieved, however, at the expense of increased acute toxicity, postoperative mortality, or both. Preliminary reports of studies using paclitaxel combinations with radiotherapy did not show this regimen to be either less toxic or more effective than cisplatin plus 5-FU and radiation treatment (98–100). Recently, active and tolerable chemoradiation regimens have been implemented in the clinical routine, omitting the continuous infusion of 5-FU (101,102) or replacing cisplatin by its analogue oxaliplatin (103), but data on overall survival data are either not yet convincing or missing.

The following lessons have been learned from these trials on preoperative RCT:

- Patients with a histopathologically determined complete response have a longer diseasefree survival, but the majority of patients develops recurrent disease and dies from distant metastases.
- Postoperative morbidity and mortality are significantly greater than with preoperative chemotherapy or radiotherapy alone.
- A considerable number of patients with initially potentially resectable disease are not referred to surgery, mainly due to tumor progression, deterioration of performance status, or the presence of pre-existing medical conditions, as well as refusal of surgery after improvement of dysphagia.
- Locoregional disease control is increased, but elimination of distant metastases remains a difficult problem that requires novel therapeutic strategies.

Randomized phase III studies involving patients with potentially resectable tumors. Final results of nine randomized trials have been reported (81,104–111) (Table 18.8). Six trials included only patients with squamous cell esophageal cancer; one trial enrolled patients with adenocarcinoma; in two other trials, 75% and 69% of the patients, respectively, had adenocarcinoma. The chemotherapy regimens used in these trials differed considerably: single-drug cisplatin, cisplatin plus bleomycin, and cisplatin plus 5-FU, given either as a continuous infusion for 5 to 7 days or as a protracted infusion over 21 days together with vinblastine sulfate.

TABLE 18.8

PREOPERATIVE CHEMORADIATION FOR POTENTIALLY RESECTABLE ESOPHAGEAL CANCER: PHASE III TRIALS

Study	RTx/CTx protocol	Histology	No. patients	Resection rate (%)	R0 (%)	Mortality (%)	pCR (%)	Median survival (mo)	Survival (%)	p Value
Nygaard et al. (81)	Surgery	SCC	41	68	37	13	—	7.5	3 y: 9	NS
	CDDP/BLM + 35 Gy		47	66	55	24	NA	7.5	17	
LePrise et al. (105)	Surgery	SCC	45	84	84	7	—	10	3 y: 13.8	NS
	CDDP/5-FU + 20 Gy		41	85	85	8.5	11.4	10	19.2	
Apinop et al. (104)	Surgery	SCC	34	100	NA	15	—	7.4	5 y: 10	NS
	CDDP/5-FU + 40 Gy		35	74	NA	14	27	9.7	24	
Walsh et al. (107)	Surgery	AC	55	100	NA	4	—	11	3 y: 6	0.01
	CDDP/5-FU + 40 Gy		58	88	NA	8	25	16	32	
Bossett et al. (106)	Surgery	SCC	139	NA	68	4	—	18.6	5 y: 25	NS
	CDDP + 37 Gy		143	NA	78	12.3	21	18.9	25	
Law et al. (110)	Surgery	SCC	60 (total)	90	42	0	—	26	NA	NS
	CDDP/5-FU + 40 Gy			95	80	0	25	27	NA	
Walsh et al. (109)	Surgery	SCC	52	NA	NA	17.3	—	8	5 y: 11	0.017
	CDDP/5-FU + 40 Gy		46	NA	NA	19.5	30	12	36	
Urba et al. (108)	Surgery	SCC (25%), AC (75%)	50	90	90	2	—	17.5	3 y: 16	NS
	CDDP/VBL/5-FU + 45 Gy		50	90	90	7	28	17	30	
Burmeister et al. (111)	Surgery	SCC (36%), AC (61%), Other (3%)	128	86	59	5	—	19	NA	
	CDDP/5-FU + 35 Gy		128	82	80	5	15	22	NA	

RTx/CTx, chemoradiation; R0, complete resection; pCR, pathohistologic response after surgery; SCC, squamous cell carcinoma; CDDP, cisplatin; BLM, bleomycin sulfate; NA, not available; NS, not significant; 5-FU, 5-fluorouracil; AC, adenocarcinoma; VBL, vinblastine.

Major differences also exist in the mode of radiation therapy and in the sequencing of chemotherapy and radiation. Concurrent radiation with single daily fractionation was performed in four studies, whereas in one study hyperfractionated radiotherapy was applied with two times 1.2 Gy/day. In the early trials, chemotherapy preceded radiation or was applied alternately with low total dose radiation (20 Gy) administered between two cycles of chemotherapy. In the largest study reported by Bossett et al. (106), radiation was administered as a split course with large fraction size (3.7 Gy/day over 5 days in weeks 1 and 4), resulting in a broad variation of total radiation doses (20−45.6 Gy).

A trend was seen toward an increase in the number of curative resections after preoperative chemoradiation, which reached the level of statistical significance in three trials. Postoperative mortality was increased after preoperative therapy. The rate of pathologically determined complete responses (11%−30%) was comparable to that in the majority of phase II trials. Five of these nine trials, however, failed to demonstrate a significant prolongation in the overall survival. The overall modest results can be explained at least in part by the small number of patients in six trials with <58 patients per arm each, and unusual biological treatment concepts in two trials using sequential RCT or a very pure dose of radiation (81,105).

In a large study of the European Organization for Research and Treatment of Cancer (EORTC), Bossett et al. compared the combination of cisplatin and radiation therapy followed by surgery with surgery alone in 282 patients with squamous cell esophageal cancer (106). The rate of curative resection was significantly higher in patients receiving combined radi-

ation and chemotherapy; however, this increase was obtained at the expense of a significant increase in postoperative mortality (13% vs. 4%). The diseasefree 3-year survival was significantly higher in the combined treatment group (40% vs. 28%), but median overall survival (18.6 months) and 5-year-overall survival (33% vs. 32%) was similar for both groups. Cancer-related deaths were more common in the group receiving surgery alone. The authors concluded that the potential benefits of combined modality treatment followed by surgery were annihilated by the high postoperative mortality, mostly due to pulmonary complications. One must emphasize that this combined modality treatment protocol was unconventional in design. Not only was the radiation administered as a split course with unusually high doses per fraction (3.7 Gy ∞ 5), increasing the risk of lung sequelae, but also the dosages of chemotherapy (cisplatin as a single drug) were inadequate for systemic therapy.

The preliminary findings of a trial yielding positive results in patients with squamous cell esophageal cancer have been published (109). Forty-six patients were randomly assigned to receive combined therapy (cisplatin plus 5-FU and 45 Gy of radiation), and 52 were assigned to receive surgery alone. The complete response rate after RCT was 30%. Hospital mortality was high in both treatment arms (19.5% in the combined treatment group vs. 17.3% for the group receiving surgery alone). Based on intention-to-treat analysis, the median survival was 12 months after combined therapy versus 8 months after surgery alone ($p = 0.017$). These preliminary results are compromised by the small size of the population investigated and the unusually high postoperative mortality in both treatment groups.

At the University of Michigan, Urba et al. (108) randomly assigned 100 patients (75% with adenocarcinoma) to either preoperative chemoradiation plus surgery or surgery alone. The primary objective was to increase median survival from 12 months (surgery alone) to 24 months (combined therapy); however, median overall survival was not improved after preoperative chemoradiation (17.5 months vs. 17 months), although 5-year survival was increased from 10% to 20%. A major problem of the study is the small sample size, with only 50 patients assigned to each arm.

Another trial involved both patients with adenocarcinoma (69%) and squamous cell carcinoma (31%) of the esophagus (111). This trial was designed to show a significant improvement in progressionfree survival. Neither progressionfree survival nor overall survival differed between groups [hazard ratio (HR) 0.82 (95% confidence interval [CI] 0.61−1.10) and 0.89 (95% CI 0.67−1.19), respectively]. The chemoradiotherapy and surgery group had more complete resections with clear margins than did the surgery-alone group [103 of 128 (80%) vs. 76 of 128 (59%), $p = 0.0002$] and had fewer positive lymph nodes [44 of 103 (43%) vs. 69 of 103 (67%), $p = 0.003$]. Subgroup analysis showed that patients with squamous cell tumors had better progressionfree survival with chemoradiotherapy than did those with nonsquamous tumors [HR 0.47 (0.25−0.86) vs. 1.02 (0.72−1.44)]. However, the trial was underpowered to determine the real magnitude of benefit in this subgroup.

Walsh et al. (107) reported a significant survival benefit after preoperative combined modality therapy in 113 patients with adenocarcinoma of the esophagus and the esophagogastric junction, including cardia and proximal stomach cancers. A histopathologically determined complete remission rate of 25% was observed. Operative mortality was 9% in the pretreated patient group versus 4% for those receiving surgery alone. After a median follow-up of 18 months for the surviving patients, the group receiving preoperative chemoradiation showed a significant improvement in both median survival (16 months vs. 11 months) and 3-year survival rate (32% vs. 6%) compared to patients receiving surgery alone. The major criticisms of this trial are the inclusion of entities of different natural histories; the lack of accurate pretherapeutic staging procedures with using no CT scan, which might have led to imbalances with respect to tumor stages; the high postoperative mortality rate of 9% in the combined modality arm; the low 3-year survival rate of 6% in the surgical control arm; and premature closure, having accrued only 113 patients at the end.

As reported in preoperative chemotherapy, responders also did better after preoperative RCT. One study described superior outcome for patients with tumor response on preoperative treatment, with significantly improved overall survival in this subgroup (104), and an improvement of 5-year overall survival for the trimodality group (24% vs. 10%).

Although two of these randomized trials revealed a survival advantage for combined modality therapy and two recently published meta-analyses showing a borderline significant statistical advantage in favor of the trimodality approach (23,112), this advantage did not become obvious prior to 3 years postoperation for all histologies, despite the small number of patients with adenocarcinoma (inclusion criteria only in two trials) (107,108). At 3 years, the improvement was 11%, with a relative risk for multimodal treatment of 0.53 ($p = 0.03$) even more pronounced for concurrent RCT (relative risk 0.45, $p = 0.005$) (23,46). However, the most recent randomized trials have not been included in any of these meta-analyses (112,113), and these trials were not in favor of neoadjuvant treatment, at least in part due to a high local recurrence rate probably based on the extraordinarily high dropout rate of esophagectomy in the combined treatment arm, mainly caused by patients' refusal to participate (113). This latter study demonstrates the difficulties in neoadjuvant protocols, providing a hint that preoperative RCT should be offered in a guarded manner and only under optimal supportive care. Toxicity can be severe, with each having >50% CTC°II−IV hematologic and gastrointestinal sequelae. Therefore, and based on studies comparing combined neoadjuvant RCT with definite RCT (114,115), neoadjuvant RCT cannot be recommended as standard of care outside clinical trials. To help clarify this controversy, further randomized trials enrolling a larger number of patients and including a stratification of both histologic subtypes and a longer follow-up are necessary. Despite the widespread use of preoperative chemoradiation therapy, as reported in the 1992 to 1994 Patterns of Care study, trimodal treatment of patients with resectable esophageal cancer is still an investigational approach (55).

Neoadjuvant chemoradiation in patients with locally advanced tumors. Phase II trials of the use of neoadjuvant chemoradiation to treat patients with locally advanced esophageal cancer are shown in Table 18.9. Only studies that included classifications of the primary tumor based on CT scans (presumably T4), endoscopic ultrasonography (T3 and T4 primaries), or both were selected. In the majority of studies, concurrent chemotherapy with cisplatin plus 5-FU and radiation with conventional fractionation were used.

After chemoradiation, improvement of swallowing was reported in up to 58% of patients. The resection rates ranged between 50% and 100% (mean, 77%); a complete resection was accomplished in approximately two-thirds of patients (range, 44%−93%). Pathologically determined complete remission was observed in approximately 25% of the resected specimens (range, 14%−44%). In studies that used endoscopic ultrasonography for T staging, a downstaging of the primary based on the pathological findings was reported in 60% of cases (116−118). Increased postoperative mortality rates of more than 10% were reported in four studies. Therapy-related deaths ranged from 0% to 18%, mainly due to pulmonary complications. Median survival for all patients was 15 months (11.5−18 months), with an actuarial 3-year survival of approximately 35% (20%−43%). For those showing a pathologically determined complete response, the projected 3-year survival was 65% to 100% (117). One-third of the patients who had gross or microscopic residual tumor in the resection specimen after complete resection were long-term survivors (117,118). In the survival analysis, no significant differences were reported for patients with squamous cell carcinoma and those with adenocarcinoma. Unrelated causes of death or death due to treatment toxicity appeared to be more likely, however, in patients with squamous cell cancer (119).

Preoperative chemoradiation remarkably improved the locoregional control. Rates of local failure <10% were reported for patients who underwent complete resection. This applied not only to patients with a complete pathologically demonstrated remission but also to patients in whom residual tumor could be completely resected (117). Control of distant disease remains a major problem, however. Even patients for whom no viable tumor remains in the resected specimen may die from systemic disease 3 years or longer after surgical resection.

More recently, it has been intensively discussed whether nonoperative treatment with chemotherapy combined with radiation alone can replace a multimodality approach, including resection in locally advanced cancer of the esophagus. A randomized phase III trial of the German Esophageal Cancer Study Group compared chemoradiation (60 Gy) alone with chemoradiation (40 Gy) followed by surgery in patients with esophageal squamous cell cancer staged T3−4, N0−1, M0 (114). One hundred and seventy-seven randomized patients were assigned to either chemoradiotherapy and surgery (arm A) or chemoradiotherapy without surgery (arm B). Overall survival at 2 years was equivalent between both treatment groups

TABLE 18.9

PREOPERATIVE CHEMORADIATION FOR LOCALLY ADVANCED ESOPHAGEAL CANCER: PHASE II TRIALS

Study	RTx/CTx protocol	Histology	No. patients	Resection rate (%)	R0 (%)	pCR (%)	Postoperative mortality (%)	Median survival (mo)	Survival (%)
Bidoli et al. (171)	CDDP/5-FU + 30 Gy	SCC	34	74	62	24	20	18	2 y: 38
Sielezneff et al. (172)	CDDP/5-FU + 30 Gy	SCC, 4 AC	25	100	84	28	8	18	2 y: 22
Van Raemdonck et al. (173)	CDDP/5-FU + 36 Gy	SCC	18	83	78	17	0	18	3 y: 43 R0: 55 pCR: 100
Adelstein et al. (174)	CDDP/5-FU + 45 Gy	24 SCC, 48 AC	72	90	90	27	18	18	3 y: 38 pCR: 67
Yano et al. (175)	CDDP/5-FU + 40 Gy	SCC	45	62	44	23	0	11.5 res.: 32	NA
Laterza et al. (118)	CDDP/5-FU + 30 Gy	SCC	111	72	44	14	10.3	14	5 y: 17.5
Alexander et al. (176)	5-FU + 60 Gy	SCC, 3 AC	34	50	47	23.5	6	14	3 y: 20
Adelstein et al. (177)	CDDP/PAC/5-FU + 45 Gy	12 SCC, 25 AC, 3 UD	40	93	93	16	15	15	3 y: 30

RTx/CTx, chemoradiation; R0, complete resection; pCR, pathohistologic response after surgery; CDDP, cisplatin; 5-FU, 5-fluorouracil; SCC, squamous cell carcinoma; AC, adenocarcinoma; NA, not available; PAC, paclitaxel; res., resected patients only; UD, undifferentiated.

(arm A: 39.9%; 95% CI, 29.4%–50.4%; arm B: 35.4%; log-rank test for equivalence with $\delta = -0.15$, $P = 0.007$). However, at 3 years, survival already differed by 7%, and freedom from local progression was better in the surgery group (2-year freedom from progression, 64.3%) than in the chemoradiotherapy group (2-year freedom from progression, 40.7%; HR for arm B vs. arm A, 2.1; 95% CI, 1.3–3.5; $P = 0.003$). This has been confirmed by Liao et al. (120) in a retrospective study with stage II and III esophageal cancer, where local tumor control was significantly improved by esophagectomy after previous RCT, but radiation dose was poor in that trial.

Moreover, in the randomized trial of Stahl et al. (114), postoperative morbidity was high, with 70% of the patients developing at least one severe complication, and the postoperative mortality rate was 11.3%. Five of 11 centers included less than ten patients within 8 years. Therefore, the question remains open as to whether this trial was too small to detect a significant but clinically meaningful survival difference in favor of resection. Furthermore, survival results of the trimodality arm may have been much better if only highly specialized centers had implemented this study. However, definite RCT was not optimally scheduled, starting with chemotherapy alone first.

The results of the German group have been confirmed in part by a study of the French Gastrointestinal Study Group that started with 455 patients and randomized 259 patients with locally advanced esophageal squamous cancer who responded to induction chemoradiation to either definitive chemoradiation or surgery (115). Although the final results of this study are not yet fully published, difference in survival between the two study groups was only marginal and in favor of conservative treatment (2-year survival 40% vs. 34%, not significant), and quality of life at first follow-up was worse after surgical treatment but did not differ after a longer follow-up (121). However, interpretation of this trial is again hampered by the poor treatment compliance in the surgery arm, by a high postoperative mortality rate approximating 10% and by the fact that overall survival (median, 17.7 months) was surprisingly poor in a patient subpopulation that was deemed to respond to preoperative treatment. As in the trial of Stahl et al. (114), RCT was also suboptimal, with a break for response evaluation allowing tumor regrowth in-between.

In summary, suitable patients, especially those who are medically fit for aggressive preoperative combined modality therapy and subsequent surgery, can be offered preoperative therapy with the chance of subsequent resection. The main candidates are patients with locally advanced tumors adjacent to the tracheobronchial tree for which primary complete resection is anatomically impossible. Due to the marginal activity of chemotherapy in reducing locoregional failure, radiotherapy is essential for these patients. Use of this kind of high-risk surgery should be restricted to highly specialized centers in the context of innovative trials.

Patients who benefit from neoadjuvant therapy. All available studies show that a prognostic benefit from multimodal therapy can only be expected in patients who respond to preoperative therapy and subsequently have a complete tumor resection. Treatment-related morbidity and mortality are high, and the prognosis is dismal for those who do not respond to neoadjuvant therapy (122,123). Prognosis for patients who do not respond is poor in comparison to that for patients receiving surgery alone or chemoradiation alone. Consequently, correct evaluation—and, even more important, the prediction of response before treatment—are important areas of research. Nevertheless, it is under discussion whether patients with tumors responding to RCT really need a resection or whether they might have good results with conservative treatment alone.

Problems still exist in evaluating response because primary tumors are not measurable bidimensionally. A relief of symptoms or normalization of the barium esophagography does not necessarily indicate a change of tumor stage. With a CT scan of the chest, only changes in tumor length and wall infiltration can be visualized. In a systematic review, CT revealed inaccuracy in assessing response to preoperative treatment (124). Endoscopic ultrasonography cannot differentiate between fibrotic tissue and vital tumor residuals. Clinical response correlates with pathological-histologic assessment in <30% of cases. Furthermore, biopsies are not helpful. Despite negative biopsy results, vital tumor cells were found in 30% of resected specimens. Therefore, to predict complete pathological-histologic response with currently available clinical methods is impossible. PET with 2-(fluorine-18)fluoro-2-deoxy-D-glucose is a promising approach for assessment of response. In particular, the early metabolic response assessment, as shown in several single-institutional studies (125–128), may offer new avenues for response-based tailored treatment algorithms, but this approach is still being investigated.

The results of preoperative chemosensitivity testing are inconclusive so far. The most promising approach is to investigate molecular markers in pretherapeutic biopsy specimens. Because cytotoxic response seems to be mediated mainly through mechanisms leading to apoptosis, genes involved in this programmed cell death are potential candidates for preoperative testing (e.g., p53 family, genes of the bax family). Expression of thymidylate synthase seems to be the best candidate for response prediction in adenocarcinoma when chemotherapy containing 5-FU is used. Complex genetic analysis by means of gene profiling may also be helpful in discerning chemotherapy or radiotherapy responders from nonresponders (129).

In summary, preoperative neoadjuvant treatment for esophageal cancer is safe, postoperative mortality after chemotherapy is comparable to that in surgery-only series, and overall survival remains dismal (median survival, 10–20 months). In several trials, however, a trend toward improved survival has been reported in patients with complete (or major) response to preoperative treatment. Even patients with no viable tumor cells in the resected specimen may die from systemic recurrence 3 years or more after surgical resection. The present data indicate that currently available neoadjuvant treatments should be considered investigational for patients with potentially re-sectable esophageal cancer but may become standard treatment for patients with locally advanced tumors. Meticulous preoperative staging is mandatory for all patients, but the overall staging sensitivity of 80% is still unsatisfactory.

Nonoperative Therapy

Chemotherapy

Chemotherapy for esophageal cancer was first used in the treatment of recurrent or metastatic disease. For both histologic subtypes of esophageal carcinoma, >50% of patients are age 60 years or older. Hence, a large number of patients present with not only tumor-related but also tumor-unrelated medical problems, which makes them poor candidates for clinical chemotherapy trials. Furthermore, 70% to 80% of all patients exhibit advanced disease, which is often associated with reduced performance status, malnourishment, or complications such as liver cirrhosis or liver metastasis, all of which severely limit patients' tolerance for toxic chemotherapy regimens.

The activity of chemotherapy clearly is stage dependent, with significantly higher response rates of 40% to 60% in patients with locoregional disease compared with rates of approximately 30% in unselected patients with metastatic disease. Response rates for selected single agents for treatment of esophageal cancer are summarized in Table 18.10. Generally, the clinical responses associated with single-agent therapy have been brief, lasting 2 to 4 months, and are associated with little palliative and no survival benefit. In clinical practice, cisplatin, 5-FU, vinorelbine, irinotecan, and the taxanes are the drugs used for purely palliative care. In contrast, carboplatin has shown a disappointing low response rate of 0% to 9% in treating both squamous cell carcinoma and adenocarcinoma (130–134). No data on single agent activity of oxaliplatin in esophageal cancer have been published so far.

The first generation of combination protocols was based on regimens containing cisplatin plus bleomycin or cisplatin plus methotrexate in a two-, three-, or four-drug schedule. The regimen of cisplatin, bleomycin, and vindesine was introduced by Kelsen and Ilson. In patients with unresectable or metastatic

---

TABLE 18.10

SINGLE-AGENT CHEMOTHERAPY FOR ESOPHAGEAL CANCER

Agent	Histology	No. patients	Response rate (%)[b]	95% CI (%)	References
Cisplatin[a]	SCC	152	42 (28)	20–35	178–181
	AC	12	1 (8)	0–26	182
Bleomycin sulfate[a]	SCC	80	12 (15)	7–23	183–186
Mitomycin C[a]	SCC	58	15 (26)	15–37	187–189
5-Fluorouracil	SCC	26	4 (15)	1–29	190
Etoposide	SCC	26	5 (19)	7–41	191
Vindesine[a]	SCC	86	19 (22)	13–32	192–195
Vinorelbine	SCC	30	6 (20)	8–39	196
Paclitaxel	SCC	18	5 (28)	8–48	197
	AC	32	11 (34)	15–51	
Docetaxel	SCC	27	8 (30)	NA	198
Irinotecan	AC	21	3 (14)	3–36	199

CI, confidence interval; SCC, squamous cell carcinoma; AC, adenocarcinoma; NA, not available.
[a]Pooled response.
[b]Patients (%).
Adapted from Enzinger PC, Ilson DH, Kelsen DP. Chemotherapy in esophageal cancer. *Semin Oncol* 1999;26:12–20.

TABLE 18.11

CISPLATIN/5-FLUOROURACIL–BASED COMBINATION CHEMOTHERAPY FOR LOCALLY ADVANCED AND METASTATIC ESOPHAGEAL CANCER

Treatment	Dose (mg/m^2) and schedule	Histology	Tumor extension	No. evaluable patients	Response: CR or PR (%)	Median survival (mo)	References
CDDP/5-FU	100, day 1 1,000 ci, days 1–5	SCC	M1	37	43	NA	201
CDDP/5-FU	100, day 1 1,000 ci, days 1–5	SCC	LAD + M1	34	35	8	136
CDDP/5-FU	70, day 1 700 ci, days 1–5	SCC	LAD + M1	36	36	NA	202
CDDP/5-FU/FA	100, day 1 370, days 1–5 200, days 1–5	SCC	LAD + M1	17	23	6+	203
CDDP/5-FU/FA	20, days 1–5 600, days 1–5 200, days 1–5	SCC	LAD + M1	31	58	11[a]	68
CDDP/5-FU/IFN	100, day 1 750, days 1–5 3 million IU daily	SCC + AC	LAD + M1	27	50	8	204
CDDP/5-FU/IFN	100, day 1, then 25 weekly[b] 750 ci, days 1–5 weekly[b] 10 million IU 3 × week	SCC + AC	LAD + M1	23	65	8.6[a]	205

CR, complete response; PR, partial response; CDDP, cisplatin; 5-FU, 5-fluorouracil; ci, continuous infusion; SCC, squamous cell carcinoma; M1, metastatic disease; NA, not available; LAD, locally advanced disease; FA, folinic acid; AC, adenocarcinoma; IFN, interferon-α.
[a]Partly local radiotherapy after chemotherapy.
[b]Starting on day 15.
Adapted from Stahl M. Chemotherapy of esophageal carcinoma. *Onkologie* 1999;22:98–104.

squamous cell esophageal cancer, remission rates of 30% to 35% were achieved with response duration of 5 to 6 months and a median survival of 6 to 8 months (135). Despite increased toxicity, the first protocols did not show higher efficacy than with single-agent treatment. In the late 1980s, cisplatin- and 5-FU–based regimens were introduced (Table 18.11). Cisplatin was administered either in a single dose of 100 mg/m^2 or at a dosage of 20 mg/m^2/day on 5 consecutive days. 5-FU was given as a continuous infusion over 5 days at a dosage of 1,000 mg/m^2/day. In patients with locoregional and locally advanced tumors, response rates between 47% and 64% were reported (206).

The efficacy of cisplatin plus 5-FU in patients with unresectable or metastatic squamous cell esophageal cancer was assessed in one randomized phase II trial of the EORTC comparing cisplatin plus 5-FU with cisplatin given as a single agent (136). Because the combination of cisplatin and 5-FU is widely regarded as standard therapy for patients with esophageal cancer, the results of the EORTC trial are of special interest. In this multicenter trial, administration of cisplatin plus 5-FU yielded a higher response rate (35%) than single-agent cisplatin (19%); however, this did not translate into a significant survival benefit (median survival of 8 months for cisplatin plus 5-FU vs. 7 months for cisplatin only; 1-year survival, 34% vs. 27%; 2-year survival, 18% vs. 9%). This might be due to the higher toxicity and treatment-related deaths (16% vs. 0%) observed in the cisplatin plus 5-FU arm. Of note is the low response rate of 19% in patients with resectable squamous cell carcinoma and adenocarcinoma in Intergroup Trial 0113 (85). This also raises questions concerning the role of cisplatin plus 5-FU as standard therapy for patients with advanced esophageal cancer. The platin-analogue oxaliplatin was studied in combination with 5-fluorouracil and leucovorin in 35 patients with advanced irresectable esophageal cancer who had undergone a maximum of one prior session of chemotherapy (137). The overall response rate was 40%, the median response duration was 4.6 months, and the median survival was 7.1 months. These results indicate that oxaliplatin may replace cisplatin in combination with 5-FU and leucovorin, at least when there are contraindications against treatment with cisplatin.

The taxane paclitaxel, which has been identified as a promising single agent, was added either alone or together with 5-FU to cisplatin (Table 18.12). In a phase II multicenter study, paclitaxel (175 mg/m^2 over 3 hours, day 1), cisplatin (20 mg/m^2, days 1–5), and a continuous infusion of 5-FU (750 mg/m^2, days 1–5) were given to patients with metastatic or recurrent esophageal cancer. Of 60 patients available for response, major responses were observed in 48%, which included complete responses in seven patients. The median duration of response was 5.7 months; median survival was 10.8 months. Toxicity was severe but manageable. Of special interest was the development of cumulative irreversible sensory neuropathy in 18% of the patients, which usually occurred after four cycles (138). In a phase II study organized by the EORTC therapy, vinorelbine 25 mg/m^2 on days 1 and 8 plus cisplatin 80 mg/m^2 on day 1, every 3 weeks, was assessed in first-line metastatic squamous cell cancer of the esophagus. Seventy-one eligible patients were entered. Twenty-four achieved a confirmed partial response (33.8%; 95% CI 23–46); the median duration of response was 6.8 months, progressionfree survival was 3.6 months, and median survival was 6.8 months. Toxicity was mainly related to neutropenia (grade 3/4 in 41% of patients) (139). In a phase II

TABLE 18.12

PACLITAXEL/CISPLATIN-BASED COMBINATION CHEMOTHERAPY FOR ADVANCED ESOPHAGEAL CANCER

Treatment	Dose (mg/m^2) and schedule	Histology	Tumor extension	No. evaluable patients	Response (%)	Median survival (mo)	References
Pac/CDDP/5-FU	175 (3 h), day 1 20, days 1–5 750 ci, days 1–5	SCC + AC	LAD, M1	60	48 (35–61)	10.8	138
Pac/CDDP	200 (24 h), day 1 75, day 2	SCC + AC	LAD, M1	37	49	NA	207
Pac/CDDP	90 (3 h), day 1 50, day 1, q14d	SCC + AC	LAD, M1	20	40	7	208
Pac/CDDP	180 (3 h), day 1 60, day 1; q14d	SCC + AC + UD	LAD, M1	51	41	NA	209

Pac, paclitaxel; CDDP, cisplatin; 5-FU, 5-fluorouracil; SCC, squamous cell carcinoma; AC,adenocarcinoma; LAD, locally advanced disease; M1, metastatic disease; ci, continuous infusion; UD, undifferentiated; NA, not available.

study, Ilson et al. evaluated the combination of weekly cisplatin plus irinotecan given to 35 patients with metastatic esophageal cancer in an outpatient setting (140). Major objective responses were observed in 57% of patients, including 6% complete responses. Similar response rates were observed for adenocarcinoma and squamous cell carcinoma. The median duration of response was 4.2 months. In patients with excellent response to protocol therapy, definitive local therapy was attempted in five such patients; this treatment resulted in a median actuarial survival of 14.6 months. These promising results indicate the need for further evaluation of the combination of weekly irinotecan and cisplatin, including the addition of other agents to this regimen.

Platinfree combination regimens have also been investigated recently. Although the combination of irinotecan plus docetaxel yielded disappointing results (141), the combination of docetaxel and capecitabine showed promising activity in metastatic esophageal cancer. The latter study included 24 patients with advanced disease (17 squamous cell carcinoma and 7 adenocarcinoma) who received oral capecitabine (1,000 mg/m^2 twice daily on days 1–14) plus intravenous docetaxel (75 mg/m^2 on day 1) every 3 weeks as first-line ($n = 16$) or second-line ($n = 8$) therapy. Intent-to-treat efficacy analysis showed an overall response rate of 46%. Of the 11 responders (1 complete and 10 partial responses), 9 of 16 (56%) received first-line and 2 of 8 (25%) received second-line therapy. The median time to progression was 6.1 months (95% CI, 4.5–7.7 months). The median survival was 15.8 months (95% CI, 7.8–23.9 months) (142). These results indicate that platinfree therapy merits further investigation in larger studies. Docetaxel and capecitabine is an alternative schedule in case of cisplatin contraindications, and it is an option for patients who are fit for second-line treatment after failure from platin-based first-line chemotherapy.

Clinical experience with biologically targeted therapies is limited at this stage. One study enrolled 36 chemotherapy refractory patients with advanced disease who were treated with the endothelial growth factor receptor (EGFR) tyrosine kinase inhibitor gefitinib 500 mg/day. Clinical activity was reported to be moderate but somehow more promising in patients with squamous cell histology and high EGFR gene copy numbers (143). Additional laboratory experiments demonstrate that novel compounds that inhibit survival signaling markedly enhance the efficacy of conventional therapeutic regimens for esophageal cancer. These data clearly support evaluation of combination treatment regimens in well-designed clinical protocols (144). Among the most promising poten-

tial targets in esophageal cancer are proteins of growth regulation (EGFR, Her-2, ki 67), angiogenesis (vascular endothelial growth factor), inflammation (cyclooxygenase-2), cell cycle control (p16, p21, cyclin D1), apoptosis (p53, bax, bcl-2), and adhesion/invasion molecules (E-cadherin, matrix metalloproteinases) (145).

In summary, the use of combination chemotherapy to treat advanced esophageal carcinoma appears to yield higher response rates than single-agent treatment. This increase, however, does not translate into prolonged survival for patients with metastatic disease. Therefore, combination chemotherapy may be recommended only for patients with good performance status (Karnofsky index >70). In this situation, cisplatin plus 5-FU has been regarded as standard treatment. In view of the results of the randomized trial of the EORTC, this regimen must be questioned. The preliminary experiences with paclitaxel-based combinations, the regimen of weekly irinotecan and cisplatin, and the results from platinfree combination chemotherapy with docetaxel and capecitabine clearly indicate that eligible patients should be treated within clinical trials.

Radiotherapy

External beam radiation therapy is usually given to total doses of 40 to 70 Gy through ports that typically encompass the primary tumor with a 5-cm margin proximally and distally and with at least 40 to 45 Gy to all locoregional lymph node areas. Radiation therapy techniques must meet the requirement that, with conventional fractionation (single dose of 1.8 or 2.0 Gy), the total dose to the spinal cord is limited to 50 Gy. Irradiation is now performed as conformal radiotherapy with multiple individual-shaped beams based on three-dimensional treatment planning. The treatment techniques are influenced by tumor localization (neck and thoracic inlet vs. middle and lower chest). Modern brachytherapy uses remote afterloading following esophageal intubation. The use of radiation therapy with curative intent for esophageal cancer up to a total dose of about 70 also requires careful patient selection. Patients with stage I or II disease are especially amenable to radiotherapy alone.

Many series have reported the results of the use of external beam radiation therapy alone. Most of these trials included patients with unfavorable features, such as clinical T4 disease and positive lymph nodes. For example, in the series reported by De-Ren (146), 184 of the 678 patients had stage IV disease. Overall, the 5-year survival rates for patients treated with radiation therapy alone are 0% to 10% (146). One report of the use of radiation therapy alone to treat patients with clinically early stage disease has been published. The trial by Sykes et al. was limited to 101 patients (90% of whom had squamous cell carcinoma) with tumors of <5 cm. Patients received 45 to 52 Gy in 15 to 16 fractions. The 5-year survival rate was 20% (147). In general, however, radiation therapy has been used to treat patients who were not surgical candidates due to either tumor extent or poor medical condition. Despite this inherent selection bias, trials of radiation therapy as primary therapy show results comparable to those of surgery, with a median survival of 6 to 12 months and 5-year survival rates of 6% to 17%. To overcome this tumor resistance and to attain long-lasting local tumor control, radiation doses might be increased by endoluminal brachytherapy—which is not yet proven effective in curative treatments—or by shortening the overall treatment time, usually done by hyperfractionated accelerated schedules (i.e., 2×1.5 Gy/day from the third week onward to a total dose of 68.4 Gy). The latter has been tested advantageous in two randomized trials (148,149). The authors have found an improvement in mean survival of up to 3 years, which is also in the range of resection and optimized RCT. These schedules should be used if resection and/or combined RCT is not feasible, but the patient is compliant and in good condition. Randomized trials comparing external beam radiation therapy to surgery in the primary treatment of resectable disease have not been performed.

Symptomatically, external beam radiation therapy is effective in palliating dysphagia in 60% to 80% of patients for up to 10 months. Complications include mucositis, esophageal strictures, and generation of tracheoesophageal fistulas. If tumors infiltrate the tracheobronchial tree with impending fistula or if the adventitia of the aorta appears to be involved with impending rupture, the daily dose should be reduced from the conventional 1.8 or 2.0 Gy to 1.5 Gy per fraction (150) if indication for radiotherapy still exists.

Brachytherapy

Intraluminal brachytherapy allows the escalation of the dose to the primary tumor while protecting the surrounding dose-limiting structures, such as the lung, heart, and spinal cord. Brachytherapy has been used both as a primary therapy and as a boost after external beam radiation therapy. It can be delivered at high- or low-dose rates. Although technical and radiobiological differences exist between the two dose rates, neither has shown a clear therapeutic advantage. A major limitation of brachytherapy is the effective treatment distance. The isotope is iridium 192, which is usually prescribed to treat to a distance of 1 cm from the source. Therefore, any portion of the tumor that is more than 1 cm from the source will receive a suboptimal radiation dose (i.e., the locoregional lymph nodes).

As primary therapy, brachytherapy results in a local control rate of 25% to 35%. A randomized trial conducted by Sur et al. found no significant difference in local control or survival with high-dose rate brachytherapy and with external beam radiation (151). In the Radiation Therapy Oncology Group (RTOG) 92-07 trial, 75 patients with squamous cell carcinoma (92%) or adenocarcinoma (8%) of the thoracic esophagus received the RTOG 85-01 combined modality regimen, followed during cycle 3 of chemotherapy by a boost with either low-dose rate (19 patients) or high-dose rate intraluminal brachytherapy (56 patients). The choice of dose rate was made at the discretion of the investigator. Due to low patient accrual, the low-dose rate option was discontinued and the analysis was limited to patients who received the high-dose rate treatment, which was delivered in weekly fractions of 5 Gy during weeks 8, 9, and 10. Because of the development of fistulas, delivery of an additional fraction at week 10 was discontinued (152). Although the complete response rate was 73%, with a median follow-up of only 11 months, the rate of local failure was 27%. Acute toxicities included a 58% incidence of grade 3 events, 26% in-

cidence of grade 4 toxicity, and 8% incidence of grade 5 events (treatment-related death). The cumulative incidence of fistulas was 18% per year, and the crude incidence was 14%. Of the six treatment-related fistulas, three were fatal. Given the significant toxicity, this treatment approach should be used with caution.

Randomized trials comparing stent insertion with brachytherapy in palliative intent could demonstrate a slow but significant improvement of dysphagia with better long-term relief after brachytherapy than following stent placement. Because brachytherapy produced better long-lasting health-related quality of life in both trials, it should be the treatment of choice if no rapid improvement of dysphagia within less than 1 month is necessary (153,154).

The American Brachytherapy Society has developed guidelines for esophageal cancer brachytherapy (155). For patients treated in the curative setting, brachytherapy should be limited to tumors of ≤10 cm with no evidence of distant metastasis. Contraindications to brachytherapy include tracheal or bronchial involvement, tumor location in the cervical esophagus, and stenosis that cannot be passed. The applicator should have an external diameter of 6 to 10 mm. Finally, brachytherapy should be delivered either alone as palliation or after the completion of external beam radiation therapy, and not concurrently with chemotherapy.

In summary, radiation therapy should be used if resection and/or combined RCT is not feasible, but the patient is compliant and in good condition, or as palliative treatment with a high chance of improving cancer-related symptoms.

Radiochemotherapy

In the mid-1980s, nonoperative pilot trials of concurrent chemotherapy and radiotherapy were initiated (156). The local failure rate was 25%, with 50% of patients alive at 3 years and 30% alive at 5 years (156). Coia et al. treated patients with early disease with mitomycin and 5-FU administered concurrently with 60 Gy of radiation. The local failure rate again was 25%, and the 5-year survival rate was 30% (157). Based on these promising results, the Eastern Cooperative Oncology Group initiated a randomized trial comparing combined chemoradiation with radiotherapy alone for early stage squamous cell esophageal cancer. Patients who received combined modality therapy had a significantly longer median survival than those receiving radiation alone (14.8 months vs. 9.2 months; $p = 0.04$); the 5-year survival rate was similar for both groups (9% vs. 7%). This was not a pure nonsurgical trial because 39% of all patients (approximately half in each arm) underwent surgery after receiving 40 Gy of radiation. Surgical therapy did not have an impact on survival in this trial (158).

Meanwhile, almost 20 randomized trials on definite RCT have been conducted, comparing either primary RCT with primary radiotherapy alone (159,160), definite RCT with preoperative RCT (114,115), or definite RCT with primary resection—the latter with preliminary data from China (161).

There is a tremendous heterogeneity across all studies, with the sequence of chemotherapy (simultaneous > sequential RCT) appearing the most apparent prognostic factor. Unfortunately, the results of the studies on sequential RCT were heterogeneous so they could not be pooled by the Cochrane Collaboration (159). So far, the outcome of all randomized trials does not support a recommendation of sequential RCT. In contrast, it became evident that concomitant RCT provided significant improvement in overall survival (7% improvement at 1 and 2 years follow-up), disease-specific survival, and local tumor control (12% improvement, up to about 45%) compared to radiotherapy alone (Table 18.13).

Unfortunately, even in simultaneous combined RCT, most trials used suboptimal doses of radiation and/or inadequate doses of systemic chemotherapy.

TABLE 18.13

CHEMORADIATION VERSUS RADIATION ALONE FOR ESOPHAGEAL CARCINOMA: RANDOMIZED PHASE III TRIALS

Study	Protocol	Histology	No. patients	Local failure rate (%)	Median survival (mo)	Overall survival rate (%) 2 y	Overall survival rate (%) 5 y	p Value
Araujo et al. (210)	50 Gy	SCC	31	84	12		6	NS
	+ 5-FU/MMC/BLM		28	61	NA		16	
Roussel et al. (211)	40 Gy	SCC	110	NA	8	16	NA	NS
	+ CDDP		111		10	20		
al-Sarraf et al. (162)	64 Gy	SCC	62	68	9		0	0.001
	50 Gy + CDDP/5-FU		61	45[a]	14		27	
Smith et al.[b] (158)	50–60 Gy	SCC	60	NA	9	12	7	NS
	+ 5-FU, MMC		59		15[a]	27	9	
Slabber et al. (212)	50–60 Gy	SCC	60	NA	5	NA		NS
	+ CDDP/5-FU		59		6			

SCC, squamous cell carcinoma; NS, not significant; NA, not available; 5-FU, 5-fluorouracil; MMC, mitomycin C; BLM, bleomycin sulfate; CDDP, cisplatin.
[a]Statistically significant.
[b]Approximately 50% of patients in each arm underwent surgery.

So far, two sequential clinical trials yielded the idea to define the optimal concept of RCT (162–165). The first trial designated to deliver adequate doses of systemic chemotherapy with concurrent radiation therapy was the RTOG 85-01 trial. Patients randomly assigned to be given radiation alone received 64 Gy. The chemoradiation group received four cycles of 5-FU (1,000 mg/m^2/24 hours for 4 days) and cisplatin (75 mg/m^2 on day 1); radiation therapy (50 Gy) was given concurrently on day 1 of chemotherapy (162). The group who received combined modality therapy had a significantly longer median survival time (14.1 months vs. 9.3 months) and higher 5-year survival rate (27% vs. 0%; $p < 0.001$) than the group receiving radiation alone (163). The incidence of local failure as first site of failure was also significantly decreased in the combined modality group (45% vs. 68%). The protocol was closed early due to these positive results. After this early closure, an additional 69 patients were treated with the same combined modality regimen, and similar results were seen (median survival, 17.2 months; 3-year survival, 30%) (163). Overall, treatment with radiation alone or combined modality therapy was reasonably well tolerated. However, the combined treatment arm showed higher levels of severe and life-threatening acute side effects (grade 4 toxicity of 10% vs. 2% in the radiation-alone group). No significant differences were seen between groups in the incidence of severe late toxic effects. Chemother-

apy could be administered as planned in only 68 of 130 patients.

In the final report after a minimum follow-up of 5 years, the 8-year survival for the group randomized to receive chemoradiation was 22% (projected 10-year survival, 20%). No patient alive at 5 years has died of recurrence of the disease, which indicates that these patients are cured of their disease. No statistical difference in survival related to histologic type was seen in those patients treated with combined modality therapy; however, 88% of the randomly assigned patients had squamous cell esophageal cancer (164). Based on the findings of this trial, chemoradiation does not merely delay the time to failure (local, regional, or distant) but cures more patients than radiation alone. Therefore, the conventional nonsurgical treatment for esophageal carcinoma is combined modality therapy. In this RTOG 85-01 trial, the local failure rate in the chemoradiation group was still 45%, demanding further improvement of therapy.

In the second sequential trial, concomitant RCT was given in both arms at two different dose levels (50.4 Gy vs. 64.8 Gy total dose, 5 × 1.8 Gy/week), while chemotherapy was the same as in the former study (four cycles of cisplatin and 5-FU) (randomized phase III Intergroup Trial 0123). The trial was discontinued prematurely after an interim analysis that showed no survival benefit or increase in local control when

TABLE 18.14

COMBINED DATA ON PATTERNS OF FAILURE OF CHEMORADIATION THERAPY (CTx/RTx) for esophageal carcinoma with and without resection

	No. patients	Recurrences (%) Total	Recurrences (%) Local	Recurrences (%) Distant	Recurrences (%) Local + distant
CTx/RTx without surgical resection	273	175	34	15	16
CTx/RTx with surgical resection	218	122	13	27	16

Adapted from Fink U, Stein HJ, Wilke H, et al. Multimodal treatment for squamous cell esophageal cancer. World J Surg 1995;19:198–204.

high-dose chemoradiation was administered (165), probably due to a higher mortality rate in the high-dose arm. It is difficult to explain the results because the majority of the adverse events happened before the 50 Gy were exceeded, but it confirms that a combined RCT can cause severe side effects, and the increase of radiation dose has do be done cautiously. Optimal supportive care is a prerequisite that means to secure nutrition and carry out blood tests in regular and close intervals in order to direct the application of chemotherapy. Using conventional fractionation schedules (5 × 1.8–2.0 Gy/week) and a concomitant chemotherapy, total dose between 50 and 60 Gy might be optimal for locally advanced, nonresectable esophageal carcinoma. About four cycles of cisplatin- and 5-FU–based chemotherapy are also recommended.

Based on the convincing data of pure radiotherapy given in an accelerated and hyperfractionated manner (148), the idea to combine an altered fractionation schedule with concomitant chemotherapy is interesting and was followed by Zhao et al. in a randomized trial (160). A total dose of 68.4 Gy was applied in 41 fractions within 44 days—either alone or combined with cisplatin and 5-FU. There was a nonsignificant difference in survival data (5-year survival, 40% vs. 28%; median survival, 30.8 vs. 23.9 months) in favor of RCT ($p = 0.31$). It can be speculated as to whether significance was not reached due to an increase in severe acute toxicity (CTC°III/IV: 46% vs. 25%; death: 6% vs. 0%), with poor nutrition and inadequate supportive care being major reasons, and/or due to the low number of patients in the trial. Therefore, altered fractionation schedules in RCT cannot be recommended without further evaluation.

The conclusion was that the results obtained with conventional chemoradiation supported a new standard of care for patients with potentially curable esophageal cancer, supported already by the 1992 to 1994 Pattern of Care study (55). In this study, 20% of patients received radiation alone, and 54% received concurrent chemoradiation. A significant survival advantage (39% vs. 21% at 2 years) and a significantly lower locoregional failure rate (30% vs. 58%) were seen for those who had combined chemoradiation.

These results indicate that radiation alone should not be used in the definitive management of esophageal cancer and that the results obtained with chemoradiation in a clinical trial can also be achieved in a nationwide practice setting. Therefore, in particular, if R0 resection is really questionable, a definite simultaneous RCT will be the treatment of choice, presupposed that supportive care is optimal and the patient is under close supervision. Chemoradiation administered outside a study protocol should use standard radiation dosing. Future directions should include the use of new radiosensitizing chemotherapy combinations (e.g., paclitaxel, docetaxel, irinotecan).

These rather impressive results, together with the low treatment-related mortality rate obtained with definitive chemoradiation, led several investigators to question the role of surgical resection in the context of a combined modality approach. A review of the literature shows that the use of combined chemoradiation alone in patients with resectable tumors results in a median survival time of 10 to 19 months and a 2-year survival rate of 20% to 44% (166). However, survival data for chemoradiation alone from nonrandomized trials compare unfavorably with the survival data for surgery alone in patients with potentially resectable tumors and with the survival data for combined preoperative chemoradiation followed by surgical resection in patients with locally advanced tumors. In the Pattern of Care study, patients who received preoperative chemoradiation had a higher survival rate than those who received definitive chemoradiation (63% vs. 39% survival at 2 years). This difference, however, was not statistically significant (55).

An analysis of the patterns of failure of chemoradiation with and without subsequent surgical resection underlines the integral role of surgery in the combined modality approach to esophageal cancer (Table 18.14). The rate of local tumor recurrence is much higher in patients with potentially resectable esophageal cancer who undergo chemoradiation alone than in patients who undergo surgical resection after preoperative chemoradiation. At present, surgical resection is essential for improved local tumor control after chemoradiation, which might have a subsequent impact on overall survival after longer follow-up (114). However, the rather high rate of distant failures after chemoradiation, with or without resection, shows that current neoadjuvant protocols are so far insufficient to control systemic disease.

TAILORED THERAPEUTIC APPROACH

Diagnostic and therapeutic algorithms for patients with squamous cell carcinoma and adenocarcinoma of the esophagus at Klinikum rechts der Isar are shown in Figs. 18.4 and 18.5. The selection of the therapeutic modality is based on resectability of the primary tumor and the general status of the patient. In both squamous cell carcinoma and adenocarcinoma, a primary surgical resection is considered the therapy of choice if a complete tumor resection can be anticipated with a high likelihood based on pretherapeutic staging and if the risk analysis indicates that the patient will tolerate an extensive surgical procedure. In cases in which, based on pretherapeutic staging, a complete tumor resection appears uncertain, a neoadjuvant protocol with subsequent resection if the patient responds to preoperative therapy is considered, provided the patient's general status permits an extensive treatment protocol. The presence of enlarged lymph nodes at the lesser curvature of the stomach or along the celiac axis does not constitute a contraindication to a surgical or multimodal approach with curative intent. Primary nonsurgical treatment modalities with curative intent are used for patients with poor general status. Purely palliative treatment modalities (chemotherapy alone, brachytherapy, stents, laser ablation, feeding tubes) are considered only if staging shows distant metastases or an esophagorespiratory fistula.

In patients with potentially resectable squamous cell esophageal cancer—that is, T1 to T4 tumors located below the

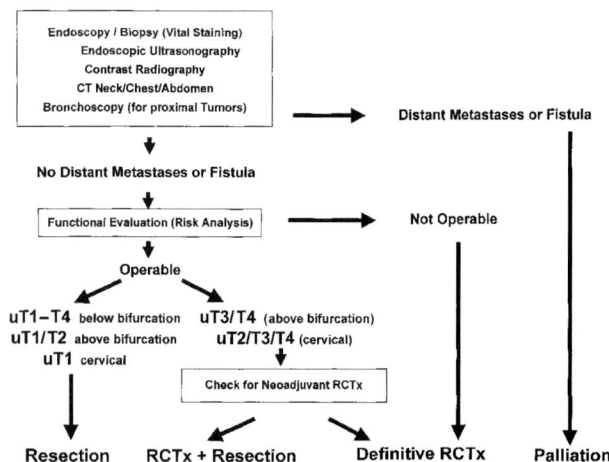

FIGURE 18.4. Algorithm outlining the diagnostic and individualized therapeutic approach for patients with squamous cell esophageal cancer followed at the Chirurgische Klinik und Poliklinik, Klinikum rechts der Isar der TU München. CT, computed tomography; RCTx, radiochemotherapy.

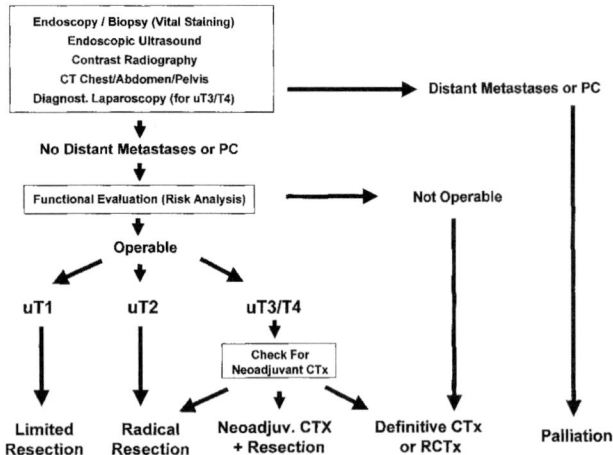

FIGURE 18.5. Algorithm outlining the diagnostic and individualized therapeutic approach for patients with adenocarcinoma of the distal esophagus followed at the Chirurgische Klinik und Poliklinik, Klinikum rechts der Isar der TU München. CT, computed tomography; PC, peritoneal carcinosis; RCTx, radiochemotherapy.

level of the tracheal bifurcation and T1 or T2 tumors located at or above the level of the tracheal bifurcation—multimodal treatment protocols have so far not been tested in well-designed randomized trials. Therefore, a transthoracic en bloc esophagectomy with two-field lymphadenectomy (mediastinum and upper abdominal compartment) constitutes the treatment of choice in these patients at Klinikum rechts der Isar. Primary chemoradiation is used if the risk analysis indicates that the patient will not tolerate this extensive surgical procedure. Because of the close anatomical relationship between the proximal esophagus and the tracheobronchial tree, a complete tumor resection is unlikely in patients with locally advanced squamous cell esophageal cancer (i.e., uT3 or T4 tumors) located at or above the level of the tracheal bifurcation. Multimodal therapeutic approaches with preoperative combined chemoradiation are used in these patients within clinical trials. In patients who respond to preoperative treatment, a subsequent transthoracic en bloc esophagectomy with two-field lymphadenectomy is performed if the tumor is located below the thoracic inlet, and a limited resection of the cervical esophagus with interposition of a free jejunal graft is performed if the tumor is located above the thoracic inlet.

In patients with adenocarcinoma of the distal esophagus, a complete tumor resection is possible with a high degree of likelihood even if the tumor has grown through the esophageal wall. A transmediastinal or transthoracic esophagectomy with en bloc removal of the lymph nodes in the lower posterior mediastinum and the upper abdominal compartment is the treatment of choice in these patients. Data indicate that early adenocarcinoma of the distal esophagus—that is, a category T1 tumor on preoperative staging—can also be treated adequately by a limited transabdominal resection of the distal esophagus and esophagogastric junction, locoregional lymphadenectomy, and interposition of a pedicled jejunal loop. This procedure is associated with less morbidity than esophagectomy and provides a good quality of life. Due to increasing evidence for the potential benefit of neoadjuvant chemotherapy in responders, patients are offered to be enrolled in clinical trials assessing new preoperative treatment strategies, including early metabolic response assessment and individualization of the therapeutic algorithm according to the tumor's sensitivity to chemotherapy.

The authors' experience with this tailored therapeutic strategy based on the histologic tumor type, topographic location, and preoperatively determined tumor stage in more than 1,500

patients shows survival rates superior to those reported with more indiscriminate approaches.

References

1. Devesa SS, Blot WJ, Fraumeni JF, Jr. Changing patterns in the incidence of esophageal and gastric carcinoma in the United States. *Cancer* 1998;83: 2049–2053.
2. Lordick F, Stein HJ, Peschel C, Siewert JR. Neoadjuvant therapy in oesophago-gastric cancer. *Br J Surg* 2004;91:540–551.
3. Liebermann-Meffert D, Stein HJ, Duranceau A. Anatomy and embryology of the esophagus. In: Zuidema GD, Yeo CJ, eds. *Surgery of the Alimentary Tract*. Vol 1. 5th ed. Philadelphia, Pa: WB Saunders; 2001:3–39.
4. Nishimaki T, Tanaka O, Suzuki T, et al. Patterns of lymphatic spread in thoracic esophageal carcinoma. *Cancer* 1994;74:4–11.
5. Siewert JR, Stein HJ. Classification of carcinoma of the esophagogastric junction. *Br J Surg* 1998;85:1457–1459.
6. Siewert JR, Feith M, Werner M, et al. Adenocarcinoma of the esophagogastric junction: results of surgical therapy based on anatomical/topographic classification in 1,002 consecutive patients. *Ann Surg* 2000;232:353–361.
7. Spechler SJ, Goyal RK. The columnar-lined esophagus, intestinal metaplasia, and Norman Barrett. *Gastroenterology* 1996;110:614–621.
8. Stein HJ, Feith M, Siewert JR. Malignant degeneration of Barrett's esophagus: clinical point of view. *Recent Results Cancer Res* 2000;155:119–122.
9. Aikou T, Shimazu H. Difference in main lymphatic pathways from the lower esophagus and gastric cardia. *Jpn J Surg* 1989;19:290–295.
10. International Union Against Cancer. *TNM Classification of Malignant Tumors*. 6th ed. Berlin: Springer; 2002.
11. Stein HJ. Prognostic factors in cancer of the esophagus. In: Gospodarowicz M, Wittekind U, eds. *Prognostic Factors in Cancer*. 2nd ed. New York, NY: Wiley-Liss; 2001:137–249.
12. Natsugoe S, Mueller J, Stein HJ, et al. Micrometastasis and tumor cell microinvolvement of lymph nodes in esophageal squamous cell cancer: frequency, associated tumor characteristics and impact on prognosis. *Cancer* 1998;83:858–866.
13. Izbicki JR, Hosch SB, Pichlmeier U, et al. Prognostic value of immunohistochemically identifiable tumor cells in lymph nodes of patients with completely resected esophageal cancer. *N Engl J Med* 1997;337:1188–1194.
14. von Rahden BH, Stein HJ, Feith M, et al. Lymphatic vessel invasion as a prognostic factor in patients with primary resected adenocarcinomas of the esophagogastric junction. *J Clin Oncol* 2005;23:874–879.
15. Miller JD, Jain MK, de Gara CJ, et al. Effect of surgical experience on results of esophagectomy for esophageal carcinoma. *J Surg Oncol* 1997;65:20–21.
16. Birkmeyer JD, Siewers AE, Finlayson EV, et al. Hospital volume and surgical mortality in the United States. *N Engl J Med* 2002;346:1128–1137.
17. Birkmeyer JD, Stukel TA, Siewers AE, et al. Surgeon volume and operative mortality in the United States. *N Engl J Med* 2003;349:2117–2127.
18. Birkmeyer JD, Dimick JB, Staiger DO. Operative mortality and procedure volume as predictors of subsequent hospital performance. *Ann Surg* 2006;243:411–417.
19. Langley SM, Alexiou C, Bailey DH, Weeden DF. The influence of perioperative blood transfusion on survival after esophageal resection for carcinoma. *Ann Thorac Surg* 2002;73:1704–1709.
20. Siewert JR, Stein HJ. Lymphadenectomy for esophageal cancer. *Langenbecks Arch Surg* 1999;384:141–148.
21. Roder JD, Busch R, Stein HJ, et al. Ratio of invaded to removed lymph nodes as a predictor of survival in squamous cell carcinoma of the esophagus. *Br J Surg* 1994;81:410–413.
22. Hölscher AH, Bollschweiler E, Bumm R, et al. Prognostic factors of resected adenocarcinoma of the esophagus. *Surgery* 1995;118:845–855.
23. Fiorica F, Di Bona D, Schepis F, et al. Preoperative chemoradiotherapy for oesophageal cancer: a systematic review and meta-analysis. *Gut* 2004;53:925–930.
24. Bartels H, Stein HJ, Siewert JR. Preoperative risk-analysis and postoperative mortality of oesophagectomy for resectable oesophageal cancer. *Br J Surg* 1998;85:840–844.
25. Hulscher JB, van Sandick JW, de Boer AG, et al. Extended transthoracic resection compared with limited transhiatal resection for adenocarcinoma of the esophagus. *N Engl J Med* 2002;347:1662–1669.
26. Akiyama H, Tsurumaru M, Udagawa H, et al. Radical lymph node dissection for cancer of the thoracic esophagus. *Ann Surg* 1994;220:364–372.
27. Baba M, Aikou T, Yoshinak H, et al. Long-term results of subtotal esophagectomy with three-field lymphadenectomy for carcinoma of the thoracic esophagus. *Ann Surg* 1994;219:310–316.
28. Fujita H, Kakegawa T, Yamana H, et al. Mortality and morbidity rates, postoperative course, quality of life, and prognosis after extended radical lymphadenectomy for esophageal cancer. *Ann Surg* 1995;222:654–662.
29. Nishihira T, Hirayama K, Mori S. A prospective randomized trial of extended cervical and superior mediastinal lymphadenectomy for carcinoma of the thoracic esophagus. *Am J Surg* 1998;175:47–51.
30. Fumagalli U, Panel of Experts. Resective surgery for cancer of the thoracic esophagus: results of a consensus conference. *Dis Esophagus* 1996;9:3–19.

31. Siewert JR, Stein HJ, Liebermann D, et al. The gastric tube as esophageal substitute. *Dis Esophagus* 1995;8:11–19.
32. Heidecke CD, Weighardt H, Feith M, et al. Neoadjuvant treatment of esophageal cancer: immunosuppression following combined radiochemotherapy. *Surgery* 2002;132:495–501.
33. Stein HJ, Feith M, Müller J, et al. Limited resection for early Barrett's cancer. *Ann Surg* 2000;232:733–742.
34. Siewert JR, Stein HJ. Barrett's cancer: indications, extent and results of surgical resection. *Semin Surg Oncol* 1997;13:245–252.
35. Ell C, May A, Gossner L, et al. Endoscopic mucosal resection of early cancer and high grade dysplasia in Barrett's esophagus. *Gastroenterology* 2000;118:670–677.
36. Bosch A, Frias Z, Caldwell WL, et al. Autopsy findings in carcinoma of the esophagus. *Acta Radiol Oncol Radiat Phys Biol* 1979;18:103–112.
37. Fink U, Stein HJ, Wilke H, et al. Multimodal treatment for squamous cell esophageal cancer. *World J Surg* 1995;19:198–204.
38. Molls M, Vaupel P, eds. *Blood Perfusion and Microenvironment of Human Tumors. Implications for Clinical Radiooncology.* Heidelberg: Springer-Verlag; 1998.
39. Mei W, Xian-Zhi G, Weibo Y. Randomized clinical trial on the combination of preoperative irradiation and surgery in the treatment of esophageal carcinoma: report on 206 patients. *Int J Radiat Oncol Biol Phys* 1989;16:325–327.
40. Gignoux M, Roussel A, Paillot B, et al. The value of preoperative radiotherapy in esophageal cancer: results of a study of the E.O.R.T.C. *World J Surg* 1987;11:426–432.
41. Teniere P, Hay JM, Fingerhut A, et al. Postoperative radiation therapy does not increase survival after curative resection for squamous cell carcinoma of the middle and lower esophagus as shown by a multicenter controlled trial. French University Association for Surgical Research. *Surg Gynecol Obstet* 1991;173:123–130.
42. Kasai M, Mori S, Watanabe T. Follow-up results after resection of thoracic esophageal carcinoma. *World J Surg* 1978;2:543–551.
43. Yamamoto M, Yamashita T, Matsubara T, et al. Reevaluation of postoperative radiotherapy for thoracic esophageal carcinoma. *Int J Radiat Oncol Biol Phys* 1997;37:75–78.
44. Fok M, Sham JS, Choy D, et al. Postoperative radiotherapy for carcinoma of the esophagus: a prospective, randomized controlled study. *Surgery* 1993;113:138–147.
45. Zieren HU, Müller JM, Jacobi CA, et al. Adjuvant postoperative radiation therapy after curative resection of squamous cell carcinoma of the thoracic esophagus: a prospective randomized study. *World J Surg* 1995;19:444–449.
46. Malthaner RA, Wong RK, Rumble RB, Zuraw L, Members of the Gastrointestinal Cancer Disease Site Group of Cancer Care Ontario's Program in Evidence-based Care. Neoadjuvant or adjuvant therapy for resectable esophageal cancer: a systematic review and meta-analysis. *BMC Med* 2004;2:35–52.
47. Xiao ZF, Yang ZY, Liang J, et al. Value of radiotherapy after radical surgery for eophageal carcinoma: a report of 495 patients. *Ann Thorac Surg* 2003;75:331–336.
48. Arimoto T, Takamura A, Tomita M, et al. Intraoperative radiotherapy for esophageal carcinoma—significance of IORT dose for the incidence of fatal tracheal complication. *Int J Radiat Oncol Biol Phys* 1993;27:1063–1067.
49. Pouliquen X, Levard H, Hay JM, et al. 5-Fluorouracil and cisplatin therapy after palliative surgical resection of squamous cell carcinoma of the esophagus: a multicenter randomized trial. French Associations for Surgical Research. *Ann Surg* 1996;223:127–133.
50. Ando N, Iizuka T, Kakegawa T, et al. A randomized trial of surgery with and without chemotherapy for localized squamous carcinoma of the thoracic esophagus: the Japan Clinical Oncology Group Study. *J Thorac Cardiovasc Surg* 1997;114:205–209.
51. Ando N, Iizuka T, Ide H, et al. Surgery plus chemotherapy compared with surgery alone for localized squamous cell carcinoma of the thoracic esophagus: a Japan Clinical Oncology Group Study—JCOG9204. *J Clin Oncol* 2003;21:4592–4596.
52. Heath EI, Burtness BA, Heitmiller RF, et al. Phase II evaluation of preoperative chemoradiation and postoperative adjuvant chemotherapy for squamous cell and adenocarcinoma of the esophagus. *J Clin Oncol* 2000;18:868–871.
53. Hoffman PC, Haraf DJ, Ferguson MK, et al. Induction chemotherapy, surgery, and concomitant chemoradiotherapy for carcinoma of the esophagus: a long-term analysis. *Ann Oncol* 1998;9:647–651.
54. Fink U, Stein HJ, Bochtler H, et al. Neoadjuvant therapy for squamous cell esophageal cancer. *Ann Oncol* 1994;5:17–26.
55. Coia LR, Minsky BD, Berkey BA, et al. Outcome of patients receiving radiation for cancer of the esophagus: results of the 1992–1994 Patterns of Care study. *J Clin Oncol* 2000;18:455–462.
56. Launois B, Delarue D, Campion JP, et al. Preoperative radiotherapy for carcinoma of the esophagus. *Surg Gynecol Obstet* 1981;153:690–692.
57. Wang M, Gu XZ, Yin WB, et al. Randomized clinical trial on the combination of preoperative irradiation and surgery in the treatment of esophageal carcinoma: report on 206 patients. *Int J Radiat Oncol Biol Phys* 1989;16:325–327.
58. Arnott SJ, Duncan W, Kerr GR, et al. Low dose preoperative radiotherapy for carcinoma of the oesophagus: results of a randomized clinical trial. *Radiother Oncol* 1992;24:108–113.
59. Fok M, McShane J, Law S, et al. Prospective randomized study of radiotherapy and surgery in the treatment of oesophageal carcinoma. *Asian J Surg* 1994;17:223–229.
60. Arnott SJ, Duncan W, Gignoux M, et al. Preoperative radiotherapy for esophageal carcinoma. Oeosphageal Cancer Collaborative Group. *Cochrane Database Syst Rev* 2005;(4):CD001799.
61. Arnott SJ, Duncan W, Gignoux M, et al. Preoperative radiotherapy in esophageal carcinoma: a meta-analysis using individual patient data. Oesophageal Cancer Collaborative Group. *Int J Radiat Oncol Biol Phys* 1998;41:579–583.
62. Coonley CJ, Bains M, Hilaris B, et al. Cisplatin and bleomycin in the treatment of esophageal carcinoma: a final report. *Cancer* 1984;54:2351–2355.
63. Kelsen D, Hilaris B, Coonley C, et al. Cisplatin, vindesine, and bleomycin chemotherapy of local-regional and advanced esophageal carcinoma. *Am J Med* 1983;75:645–652.
64. Schlag P, Herrmann R, Raeth V, et al. Preoperative chemotherapy in esophageal cancer: a phase II study. *Acta Oncol* 1988;27(6b):811–814.
65. Kelsen DP, Minsky B, Smith M, et al. Preoperative therapy for esophageal cancer: a randomized comparison of chemotherapy versus radiation therapy. *J Clin Oncol* 1990;8:1352–1361.
66. Roth JA, Pass HI, Flanagan MM, et al. Randomized clinical trial of preoperative and postoperative adjuvant chemotherapy with cisplatin, vindesine, and bleomycin for carcinoma of the esophagus. *J Thorac Cardiovasc Surg* 1988;96:242–248.
67. Kies MS, Rosen ST, Tsang TK, et al. Cisplatin and 5-fluorouracil in the primary management of squamous esophageal cancer. *Cancer* 1987;60:2156–2160.
68. Feliu J, Gonzalez BM, Garcia GC, et al. Phase II study of cisplatin, 5-fluorouracil, and leucovorin in inoperable squamous cell carcinoma of the esophagus. ONCOPAZ Cooperative Group, Spain. *Am J Clin Oncol* 1996;19:577–580.
69. Carey RW, Hilgenberg AD, Wilkins EW, Jr, et al. Long-term follow-up of neoadjuvant chemotherapy with 5-fluorouracil and cisplatin with surgical resection and possible postoperative radiotherapy and/or chemotherapy in squamous cell carcinoma of the esophagus. *Cancer Invest* 1993;11:99–105.
70. Temeck BK, Liebmann JE, Theodossiou C, et al. Phase II trial of 5-fluorouracil, leucovorin, interferon-alpha-2a, and cisplatin as neoadjuvant chemotherapy for locally advanced esophageal carcinoma. *Cancer* 1996;77:2432–2439.
71. Vignoud J, Visset J, Paineau J, et al. Pre-operative chemotherapy in 60 cases of squamous cell carcinoma of the esophagus. Proceedings of the Third International Congress on Neo-Adjuvant Chemotherapy; February 6–9, 1991; Paris.
72. Ajani JA, Roth JA, Ryan B, et al. Evaluation of pre- and postoperative chemotherapy for resectable adenocarcinoma of the esophagus or gastroesophageal junction. *J Clin Oncol* 1990;8:1231–1238.
73. Carey RW, Hilgenberg AD, Choi NC, et al. A pilot study of neoadjuvant chemotherapy with 5-fluorouracil and cisplatin with surgical resection and postoperative radiation therapy and/or chemotherapy in adenocarcinoma of the esophagus. *Cancer* 1991;68:489–492.
74. Ajani JA, Roth JA, Ryan MB, et al. Intensive preoperative chemotherapy with colony-stimulating factor for resectable adenocarcinoma of the esophagus or gastroesophageal junction. *J Clin Oncol* 1993;11:22–28.
75. Ajani JA, Ryan B, Rich TA, et al. Prolonged chemotherapy for localised squamous carcinoma of the oesophagus. *Eur J Cancer* 1992;28A:880–884.
76. Wright CD, Mathisen DJ, Wain JC, et al. Evolution of treatment strategies for adenocarcinoma of the esophagus and gastroesophageal junction. *Ann Thorac Surg* 1994;58:1574–1578.
77. Ajani JA, Roth JA, Putnam JB, et al. Feasibility of five courses of preoperative chemotherapy in patients with resectable adenocarcinoma of the oesophagus or gastrooesophageal junction. *Eur J Cancer* 1995;31A:665–670.
78. Ilson DH, Forastiere A, Arquette M, et al. A phase II trial of paclitaxel and cisplatin in patients with advanced carcinoma of the esophagus. *Cancer J* 2000;6:316–323.
79. Ilson DH. Phase II trial of weekly irinotecan/cisplatin in advanced esophageal cancer. *Oncology (Huntingt)* 2004;18(suppl 14):22–25.
80. Rigas JR, Dragnev KH, Bubis JA. Docetaxel in the treatment of esophageal cancer. *Semin Oncol* 2005;32(suppl 4):S39—S51.
81. Nygaard K, Hagen S, Hansen HS, et al. Pre-operative radiotherapy prolongs survival in operable esophageal carcinoma: a randomized, multicenter study of pre-operative radiotherapy and chemotherapy: the second Scandinavian trial in esophageal cancer. *World J Surg* 1992;16:1104–1109.
82. Schlag PM. Randomized trial of preoperative chemotherapy for squamous cell cancer of the esophagus. Chirurgische Arbeitsgemeinschaft für Onkologie der Deutschen Gesellschaft für Chirurgie Study Group. *Arch Surg* 1992;127:1446–1450.
83. Maipang T, Vasinanukorn P, Petpichetchian C, et al. Induction chemotherapy in the treatment of patients with carcinoma of the esophagus. *Surg Oncol* 1994;56:191–197.
84. Law S, Fok M, Chow S, et al. Preoperative chemotherapy versus surgical therapy alone for squamous cell carcinoma of the esophagus: a prospective randomized trial. *J Thorac Cardiovasc Surg* 1997;114:210–217.

85. Kelsen DP, Ginsberg R, Pajak TF, et al. Chemotherapy followed by surgery compared with surgery alone for localized esophageal cancer. *N Engl J Med* 1998;339:1979–1984.

86. Kok TC, van Lanschot J, Siersema PD, et al. Neoadjuvant chemotherapy in operable squamous cell cancer: final report of a phase III multicenter randomized trial [abstract]. *Proc Am Soc Clin Oncol* 1997;17:A984.

87. Ancona E, Merigliano S, Petrin G, et al. First-line chemo-radiotherapy neoadjuvant treatment in locally advanced (T4) epidermoid carcinoma of the esophagus. *Chir Ital* 1999;51:91–97.

88. Medical Research Council Oesophageal Cancer Working Party. Surgical resection with or without preoperative chemotherapy in oesophageal cancer: a randomized controlled trial. *Lancet* 2002;359:1727–1733.

89. Seydel HG, Leichman L, Byhardt R, et al. Preoperative radiation and chemotherapy for localized squamous cell carcinoma of the esophagus: a RTOG study. *Int J Radiat Oncol Biol Phys* 1988;14:33–35.

90. Ancona E, Ruol A, Castoro C, et al. First-line chemotherapy improves the resection rate and long-term survival of locally advanced (T4, any N, M0) squamous cell carcinoma of the thoracic esophagus: final report on 163 consecutive patients with 5-year follow-up. *Ann Surg* 1997;226:714–723.

91. Leichman L, Steiger Z, Seydel HG, et al. Combined preoperative chemotherapy and radiation therapy for cancer of the esophagus: the Wayne State University, Southwest Oncology Group and Radiation Therapy Oncology Group experience. *Semin Oncol* 1984;11:178–185.

92. Seydel HG, Leichman L, Byhardt R, et al. Preoperative radiation and chemotherapy for localized squamous cell carcinoma of the esophagus: a RTOG study. *Int J Radiat Oncol Biol Phys* 1988;14:33–35.

93. Poplin E, Fleming T, Leichman L, et al. Combined therapies for squamous-cell carcinoma of the esophagus, a Southwest Oncology Group study (SWOG-8037). *J Clin Oncol* 1987;5:622–628.

94. Naunheim KS, Petruska P, Roy TS, et al. Preoperative chemotherapy and radiotherapy for esophageal carcinoma. *J Thorac Cardiovasc Surg* 1992;103:887–893.

95. Forastiere AA, Orringer MB, Perez-Tamayo C, et al. Concurrent chemotherapy and radiation therapy followed by transhiatal esophagectomy for local-regional cancer of the esophagus. *J Clin Oncol* 1990;8:119–127.

96. Jones DR, Detterbeck FC, Egan TM, et al. Induction chemoradiotherapy followed by esophagectomy in patients with carcinoma of the esophagus. *Ann Thorac Surg* 1997;64:185–191.

97. Forastiere AA, Heitmiller RF, Lee DJ, et al. Intensive chemoradiation followed by esophagectomy for squamous cell and adenocarcinoma of the esophagus. *Cancer J Sci Am* 1997;3:144–152.

98. Weiner LM, Colarusso P, Goldberg M, et al. Combined-modality therapy for esophageal cancer: phase I trial of escalating doses of paclitaxel in combination with cisplatin, 5-fluorouracil, and high-dose radiation before esophagectomy. *Semin Oncol* 1997;24:S19.

99. Blanke CD, Choy H, Teng M, et al. Concurrent paclitaxel and thoracic irradiation for locally advanced esophageal cancer. *Semin Radiat Oncol* 1999;9:43–52.

100. Safran H, Gaissert H, Akerman P, et al. Neoadjuvant paclitaxel, cisplatin and radiation for esophageal cancer [abstract]. *Proc Am Soc Clin Oncol* 1998;17:A994.

101. Brenner B, Ilson DH, Minsky BD, et al. Phase I trial of combined-modality therapy for localized esophageal cancer: escalating doses of continuous-infusion paclitaxel with cisplatin and concurrent radiation therapy. *J Clin Oncol* 2004;22:45–52.

102. Ilson DH, Bains M, Kelsen DP, et al. Phase I trial of escalating-dose irinotecan given weekly with cisplatin and concurrent radiotherapy in locally advanced esophageal cancer. *J Clin Oncol* 2003;21:2926–2932.

103. Khushalani NI, Leichman CG, Proulx G, et al. Oxaliplatin in combination with protracted-infusion fluorouracil and radiation: report of a clinical trial for patients with esophageal cancer. *J Clin Oncol* 2002;20:2844–2850.

104. Apinop C, Puttisak P, Preecha N. A prospective study of combined therapy in esophageal cancer. *Hepatogastroenterology* 1994;41:391–393.

105. Le Prise E, Etienne PL, Meunier B, et al. A randomized study of chemotherapy, radiation therapy, and surgery versus surgery for localized squamous cell carcinoma of the esophagus. *Cancer* 1994;73:1779–1784.

106. Bosset JF, Gignoux M, Triboulet JP, et al. Chemoradiotherapy followed by surgery compared with surgery alone in squamous-cell cancer of the esophagus. *N Engl J Med* 1997;337:161–167.

107. Walsh TN, Noonan N, Hollywood D, et al. A comparison of multimodal therapy and surgery for esophageal adenocarcinoma. *N Engl J Med* 1996;335:462–467.

108. Urba SG, Orringer MB, Turrisi A, et al. Randomized trial of preoperative chemoradiation versus surgery alone in patients with locoregional esophageal carcinoma. *J Clin Oncol* 2001;19:305–313.

109. Walsh TN, McDonell CO, Mulligan ED, et al. Multimodal therapy versus surgery alone for squamous cell carcinoma of the esophagus: a prospective randomized trial [abstract]. *Gastroenterology* 2000;118:A1008.

110. Law S, Kwong DLW, Tung HM, et al. Preoperative chemoradiation for squamous cell esophageal cancer: a prospective randomized trial [abstract]. *Can J Gastroenterol* 1998;12(suppl B):A161.

111. Burmeister BH, Smithers BM, Gebski V, et al. Surgery alone versus chemoradiation followed by surgery for resectable cancer of the oesophagus: a randomised controlled phase III trial. *Lancet Oncol* 2005;6:659–668.

112. Urschel JD, Vasan H. A meta-analysis of randomised controlled trials that compared neoadjuvant chemoradiation and surgery alone for resectable esophageal cancer. *Am J Surg* 2003;185:538–543.

113. Lee J-L, Park SI, Kim S-B, et al. A single institutional phase III trial of preoperative chemotherapy with hyperfractionation radiotherapy plus surgery versus surgery alone for resectable esophageal squamous cell carcinoma. *Ann Oncol* 2004;15:947–954.

114. Stahl M, Stuschke M, Lehmann N, et al. Chemoradiation with and without surgery in patients with locally advanced squamous cell carcinoma of the esophagus. *J Clin Oncol* 2005;23:2310–2317.

115. Bedenne L, Michel P, Bouche O, et al. Final results of a randomised multicentric phase III trial in locally advanced esophageal cancer: radiochemotherapy followed by surgery versus radiochemotherapy alone (FFCD 9102) [abstract]. *Proc Am Soc Clin Oncol* 2002;21:A130.

116. Wright CD, Wain JC, Lynch TJ, et al. Induction therapy for esophageal cancer with paclitaxel and hyperfractionated radiotherapy: a phase I and II study. *J Thorac Cardiovasc Surg* 1997;114:811–815.

117. Adelstein DJ, Rice TW, Becker M, et al. Use of concurrent chemotherapy, accelerated fractionation radiation, and surgery for patients with esophageal carcinoma. *Cancer* 1997;80:1011–1020.

118. Laterza E, deManzoni G, Tedesco P, et al. Induction chemo-radiotherapy for squamous cell carcinoma of the thoracic esophagus: long-term results of a phase II study. *Ann Surg Oncol* 1999;6:777–784.

119. Rice T, Adelstein D, Saxton J, et al. A phase II trial of post-operative adjuvant chemoradiotherapy for patients (pts) with high-risk cancer of the esophagus and gastroesophageal junction (GEJ) [abstract]. *Proc Am Soc Clin Oncol* 2000;19:A1057.

120. Liao Z, Zhang Z, Jin J, et al. Esophagectomy after concurrent chemoradiotherapy improves locoregional control in clinical stage II or III esophageal cancer patients. *Int J Radiat Oncol Biol Phys* 2004;60:1484–1493.

121. Bonnetain F, Bouche O, Michel P, et al. A comparative longitudinal quality of life study using the Spitzer quality of life index in a randomized multicenter phase III trial (FFCD 9102): chemoradiation followed by surgery compared with chemoradiation alone in locally advanced squamous resectable thoracic esophageal cancer. *Ann Oncol* 2006;17:827–834.

122. Rohatgi P, Swisher SG, Correa AM, et al. Characterization of pathologic complete response after preoperative chemoradiotherapy in carcinoma of the esophagus and outcome after pathologic complete response. *Cancer* 2005;104:2365–2372.

123. Brucher BL, Becker K, Lordick F, et al. The clinical impact of histopathologic response assessment by residual tumor cell quantification in esophageal squamous cell carcinomas. *Cancer* 2006;106:2119–2127.

124. Westerterp M, van Westreenen HL, Reitsma JB, et al. Esophageal cancer: CT, endoscopic US, and FDG PET for assessment of response to neoadjuvant therapy—systematic review. *Radiology* 2005;236:841–851.

125. Weber WA, Ott K, Becker K, et al. Prediction of response to preoperative chemotherapy in adenocarcinomas of the esophagogastric junction by metabolic imaging. *J Clin Oncol* 2001;19:3058–3065.

126. Wieder HA, Brucher BL, Zimmermann F, et al. Time course of tumor metabolic activity during chemoradiotherapy of esophageal squamous cell carcinoma and response to treatment. *J Clin Oncol* 2004;22:900–908.

127. Wieder HA, Beer AJ, Lordick F, et al. Comparison of changes in tumor metabolic activity and tumor size during chemotherapy of adenocarcinomas of the esophagogastric junction. *J Nucl Med* 2005;46:2029–2034.

128. Beer AJ, Wieder HA, Lordick F, et al. Adenocarcinomas of esophagogastric junction: multi-detector row CT to evaluate early response to neoadjuvant chemotherapy. *Radiology* 2006;239:472–480.

129. Luthra R, Wu TT, Luthra MG, et al. Gene expression profiling of localized esophageal carcinomas: association with pathologic response to preoperative chemoradiation. *J Clin Oncol* 2006;24:259–267.

130. Albertsson M, Fagerberg J, Jacobsen A, et al. Preliminary results of a phase II study with Taxotere (docetaxel) in patients with primary untreated or recurrent oesophagus cancer [abstract]. *Proc Am Soc Clin Oncol* 2000;19:A1218.

131. Mannell A, Winters Z. Carboplatin in the treatment of oesophageal cancer. *S Afr Med J* 1989;76:213–214.

132. Queisser W, Preusser P, Mross KB, et al. Phase II evaluation of carboplatin in advanced esophageal carcinoma: a trial of the Phase I/II Study Group of the Association for Medical Oncology of the German Cancer Society. *Onkologie* 1990;13:190–193.

133. Sternberg C, Kelsen D, Dukeman M, et al. Carboplatin: a new platinum analog in the treatment of epidermoid carcinoma of the esophagus. *Cancer Treat Rep* 1985;69:1305–1307.

134. Einzig A, Kelsen DP, Cheng E, et al. Phase II trial of carboplatin in patients with adenocarcinomas of the upper gastrointestinal tract. *Cancer Treat Rep* 1985;69:1453–1454.

135. Ilson DH, Kelsen DP. Chemotherapy in esophageal cancer. *Anticancer Drugs* 1993;4:287–299.

136. Bleiberg H, Conroy T, Paillot B, et al. Randomised phase II study of cisplatin and 5-fluorouracil (5-FU) versus cisplatin alone in advanced squamous cell oesophageal cancer. *Eur J Cancer* 1997;33:1216–1220.

137. Mauer AM, Kraut EH, Krauss SA, et al. Phase II trial of oxaliplatin, leucovorin and fluorouracil in patients with advanced carcinoma of the esophagus. *Ann Oncol* 2005;16:1320–1325.

138. Ilson DH, Ajani J, Bhalla K, et al. Phase II trial of paclitaxel, fluorouracil,

and cisplatin in patients with advanced carcinoma of the esophagus. *J Clin Oncol* 1998;16:1826–1834.

139. Conroy T, Etienne PL, Adenis A, et al. Vinorelbine and cisplatin in metastatic squamous cell carcinoma of the oesophagus: response, toxicity, quality of life and survival. *Ann Oncol* 2002;13:721–729.

140. Ilson DH, Saltz L, Enzinger P, et al. Phase II trial of weekly irinotecan plus cisplatin in advanced esophageal cancer. *J Clin Oncol* 1999;17:3270–3275.

141. Lordick F, von Schilling C, Bernhard H, et al. Phase II trial of irinotecan plus docetaxel in cisplatin-pretreated relapsed or refractory oesophageal cancer. *Br J Cancer* 2003;89:630–633.

142. Lorenzen S, Duyster J, Lersch C, et al. Capecitabine plus docetaxel every 3 weeks in first- and second-line metastatic oesophageal cancer: final results of a phase II trial. *Br J Cancer* 2005;92:2129–2133.

143. Janmaat ML, Gallegos-Ruiz MI, Rodriguez JA, et al. Predictive factors for outcome in a phase II study of gefitinib in second-line treatment of advanced esophageal cancer patients. *J Clin Oncol* 2006;24:1612–1619.

144. Schrump DS, Nguyen DM. Novel molecular targeted therapy for esophageal cancer. *J Surg Oncol* 2005;92:257–261.

145. Tew WP, Kelsen DP, Ilson DH. Targeted therapies for esophageal cancer. *Oncologist* 2005;10:590–601.

146. De-Ren S. Ten-year follow-up of esophageal cancer treated by radical radiation therapy: analysis of 869 patients. *Int J Radiat Oncol Biol Phys* 1989;16:329–334.

147. Sykes AJ, Burt PA, Slevin NJ, et al. Radical radiotherapy for carcinoma of the oesophagus: an effective alternative to surgery. *Radiother Oncol* 1998;48:15–21.

148. Shi XH, Yao W, Liu T. Late course accelerated fractionation in radiotherapy of esophageal carcinoma. *Radiother Oncol* 1999;51:21–26.

149. Wang Y, Shi XH, He SQ, et al. Comparison between continuous accelerated hyperfractionated and late-course accelerated hyperfractionated radiotherapy for esophageal carcinoma. *Int J Radiat Oncol Biol Phys* 2002;54(1):131–136.

150. Perez CA, Brady LW. *Principles and Practice of Radiation Oncology.* 2nd ed. Philadelphia, Pa.: JB Lippincott; 1992.

151. Sur RK, Singh DP, Sharma SC, et al. Radiation therapy of esophageal cancer: role of high dose rate brachytherapy. *Int J Radiat Oncol Biol Phys* 1992;22:1043–1046.

152. Gaspar LE, Winter K, Kocha WI, et al. A phase I/II study of external beam radiation, brachytherapy, and concurrent chemotherapy for patients with localized carcinoma of the esophagus (Radiation Therapy Oncology Group Study 9207): final report. *Cancer* 2000;88:988–995.

153. Bergquist H, Wenger U, Johnsson E, et al. Stent insertion or endoluminal brachytherapy as palliation of patients with advanced cancer of the esophagus and gastroesophageal junction: results of a randomized controlled clinical trial. *Dis Esophagus* 2005;18:131–139.

154. Homs MYV, Steyerberg EW, Eijkenboom WMH, et al. Single dose brachytherapy versus metal stent placement for the palliation of dysphagia from oesophageal cancer: multicentre randomised trial. *Lancet* 2004;364:1497–1504.

155. Gaspar LE, Nag S, Herskovic A, et al. American Brachytherapy Society (ABS) consensus guidelines for brachytherapy of esophageal cancer. Clinical Research Committee, American Brachytherapy Society, Philadelphia, PA. *Int J Radiat Oncol Biol Phys* 1997;38:127–132.

156. Leichman L, Herskovic A, Leichman CG, et al. Nonoperative therapy for squamous-cell cancer of the esophagus. *J Clin Oncol* 1987;5:365–370.

157. Coia LR, Engstrom PF, Paul AR, et al. Long-term results of infusional 5-FU, mitomycin-C and radiation as primary management of esophageal carcinoma. *Int J Radiat Oncol Biol Phys* 1991;20:29–36.

158. Smith TJ, Ryan LM, Douglass HO, et al. Combined chemoradiotherapy vs. radiotherapy alone for early stage squamous cell carcinoma of the esophagus: a study of the Eastern Cooperative Oncology Group. *Int J Radiat Oncol Biol Phys* 1998;42:269–276.

159. Wong R, Malthaner R. Combined chemotherapy and radiotherapy (without surgery) compared with radiotherapy alone in localized carcinoma of the esophagus. *Cochrane Database Syst Rev* 2006;(1):CD002092.

160. Zhao KL, Shi XH, Jiang GL, et al. Late course accelerated hyperfractionated radiotherapy plus concurrent chemotherapy for squamous cell carcinoma of the esophagus: a phase III randomized study. *Int J Radiat Oncol Biol Phys* 2005;62:1014–1420.

161. Chiu PWY, Chan ACW, Leung SF, et al. Multicenter prospective randomized trial comparing standard esophagectomy with chemoradiotherapy for treatment of squamous esophageal cancer: early results from the Chinese university research group for esophageal cancer (CURE). *J Gastrointest Surg* 2005;9:794–802.

162. Herskovic A, Martz K, al-Sarraf M, et al. Combined chemotherapy and radiotherapy compared with radiotherapy alone in patients with cancer of the esophagus. *N Engl J Med* 1992;326:1593–1598.

163. al-Sarraf M, Martz K, Herskovic A, et al. Progress report of combined chemoradiotherapy versus radiotherapy alone in patients with esophageal cancer: an intergroup study. *J Clin Oncol* 1997;15:277–284. [erratum appears in *J Clin Oncol* 1997;15(2):866].

164. Cooper JS, Guo MD, Herskovic A, et al. Chemoradiotherapy of locally advanced esophageal cancer: long-term follow-up of a prospective randomized trial (RTOG 85-01). Radiation Therapy Oncology Group. *JAMA* 1999;281:1623–1627.

165. Minsky BD, Pajak TF, Ginsberg RJ, et al. INT 0123 (Radiation Therapy Oncology Group 94-05) phase III trial of combined-modality therapy for esophageal cancer: high-dose versus standard-dose radiation therapy. *J Clin Oncol* 2002;20:1167–1174.

166. Kavanagh B, Anscher M, Leopold K, et al. Patterns of failure following combined modality therapy for esophageal cancer, 1984–1990. *Int J Radiat Oncol Biol Phys* 1992;24:633–642.

167. Zieren HU, Müller JM, Jacobi CA, et al. Adjuvant postoperative radiation therapy after curative resection of squamous cell carcinoma of the thoracic esophagus: a prospective randomized study. *World J Surg* 1995;19:444–449.

168. Japanese Esophageal Oncology Group. A comparison of chemotherapy and radiotherapy as adjuvant treatment to surgery for esophageal carcinoma. *Chest* 1993;104:203–207.

169. Law S, Wong J. The roles of multimodality treatment and lymphadenectomy in the management of esophageal cancer. *Chin Med J* 1997;110:819–825.

170. Ancona E, Ruol A, Santi S, et al. Only pathologic complete response to neoadjuvant chemotherapy improves significantly long-term survival in resectable esophageal squamous cell carcinoma: final report of a randomized controlled trial of preoperative chemotherapy versus surgery alone. *Cancer* 2001;91:2165–2174.

171. Bidoli P, Spinazze S, Valente M, et al. Combined chemotherapy (CT)-radiotherapy (RT) ± esophagectomy (E) in squamous cell cancer of the esophagus (SCCE) [abstract]. *Proc Am Soc Clin Oncol* 1990;9:A424.

172. Sieleznelf I, Thomas P, Giovannini M, et al. Esophageal carcinoma with doubtful extirpability: value of preoperative chemotherapy plus radiotherapy. *Eur J Cardiothorac Surg* 1993;7:606–611.

173. Van Raemdonck D, Van Cutsem E, Menten J, et al. Induction therapy for clinical T4 oesophageal carcinoma: a plea for continued surgical exploration. *Eur J Cardiothorac Surg* 1997;11:828–837.

174. Adelstein DJ, Rice TW, Rybicki LA, et al. Concurrent chemoradiotherapy and surgery for esophageal cancer: updated results [abstract]. *Can J Gastroenterol* 1998;12(suppl B):A26.

175. Yano M, Tsujinaka T, Shiozaki H, et al. Concurrent chemotherapy (5-fluorouracil and cisplatin) and radiation therapy followed by surgery for T4 squamous cell carcinoma of the esophagus. *J Surg Oncol* 1999;70:25–32.

176. Alexander EP, Lipman T, Harmon J, et al. Aggressive multimodality therapy for stage III esophageal cancer: a phase I/II study. *Ann Thorac Surg* 2000;69:363–368.

177. Adelstein DJ, Rice TW, Rybicki LA, et al. Does paclitaxel improve the chemoradiotherapy of locoregionally advanced esophageal cancer? A nonrandomized comparison with fluorouracil-based therapy. *J Clin Oncol* 2000;18:2032–2039.

178. Panettiere FJ, Leichman L, O'Bryan R, et al. Cis-diamminedichloride platinum(II), an effective agent in the treatment of epidermoid carcinoma of the esophagus: a preliminary report of an ongoing Southwest Oncology Group study. *Cancer Clin Trials* 1981;4:29–31.

179. Ravry MJ, Moore MR, Omura GA, et al. Phase II evaluation of cisplatin in squamous carcinoma of the esophagus: a Southeastern Cancer Study Group trial. *Cancer Treat Rep* 1985;69:1457–1458.

180. Davis S, Shanmugathasa M, Kessler W. cis-Dichlorodiammineplatinum(II) in the treatment of esophageal carcinoma. *Cancer Treat Rep* 1980;69:709–711.

181. Murthy SK, Prabhakaran PS, Chandrashekar M, et al. Neoadjuvant Cis-DDP in esophageal cancers: an experience at a regional cancer centre, India. *J Surg Oncol* 1990;45:173–176.

182. Ajani J, Kantarjian H, Kanojia M, et al. Phase II trial of cisplatinum in advanced upper gastrointestinal cancer [abstract]. *Proc Am Soc Clin Oncol* 1984;2:C-573.

183. Stephens FO. Bleomycin—a new approach in cancer chemotherapy. *Med J Aust* 1973;1:1277–1283.

184. Bonadonna G, De Lena M, Monfardini S, et al. Clinical trials with bleomycin in lymphomas and in solid tumors. *Eur J Cancer* 1972;8:205–215.

185. Tancini G, Bajetta E, Bonadonna G. Bleomycin alone and in combination with methotrexate in the treatment of carcinoma of the esophagus. *Tumori* 1974;60:65–71.

186. Ravry M, Moertel CG, Schutt AJ, et al. Treatment of advanced squamous cell carcinoma of the gastrointestinal tract with bleomycin (NSC-125066). *Cancer Chemother Rep* 1973;57:493–495.

187. Engstrom PF, Lavin PT, Klaassen DJ. Phase II evaluation of mitomycin and cisplatin in advanced esophageal carcinoma. *Cancer Treat Rep* 1983;67:713–715.

188. Desai PB, Borges EJ, Vohra VG, et al. Carcinoma of the esophagus in India. *Cancer* 1969;23:979–989.

189. Whittington RM, Close HP. Clinical experience with mitomycin C (NSC-26980). *Cancer Chemother Rep* 1970;54:195–198.

190. Ezdinli EZ, Gelber R, Desai DV, et al. Chemotherapy of advanced esophageal carcinoma: Eastern Cooperative Oncology Group experience. *Cancer* 1980;46:2149–2153.

191. Harstrick A, Bokemeyer C, Preusser P, et al. Phase II study of single-agent etoposide in patients with metastatic squamous-cell carcinoma of the esophagus. *Cancer Chemother Pharmacol* 1992;29:321–322.

192. Bezwoda WR, Derman DP, Weaving A, et al. Treatment of esophageal cancer with vindesine: an open trial. *Cancer Treat Rep* 1984;68:783–785.
193. Kelsen DP, Bains M, Cvitkovic E, et al. Vindesine in the treatment of esophageal carcinoma: a phase II study. *Cancer Treat Rep* 1979;63:2019–2021.
194. Popkin J, Bromer R, Byrne R, et al. Continuous 48-hour infusion of vindesine in squamous cell carcinoma of the upper aero-digestive tract. Proceedings of the 13th International Cancer Congress; September 8–12, 1982; Seattle, Wash.
195. Bedikian AY, Valdivieso M, Bodey GP, et al. Phase II evaluation of vindesine in the treatment of colorectal and esophageal tumors. *Cancer Chemother Pharmacol* 1979;2:263–266.
196. Conroy T, Etienne PL, Adenis A, et al. Phase II trial of vinorelbine in metastatic squamous cell esophageal carcinoma. European Organization for Research and Treatment of Cancer Gastrointestinal Treat Cancer Cooperative Group. *J Clin Oncol* 1996;14:164–170.
197. Ajani JA, Ilson DH, Daugherty K, et al. Activity of taxol in patients with squamous cell carcinoma and adenocarcinoma of the esophagus. *J Natl Cancer Inst* 1994;86:1086–1091.
198. Slabber CF, Falkson CI, Musi NNM, et al. A phase II study of docetaxel in advanced, inoperable squamous carcinoma of the esophagus [abstract]. *Proc Am Soc Clin Oncol* 1999;18:A1151.
199. Lin L, Hecht J. A phase II trial of irinotecan in patients with advanced adenocarcinoma of the gastroesophageal (GE) junction [abstract]. *Proc Am Soc Clin Oncol* 2000;19:1130.
200. Enzinger PC, Ilson DH, Kelsen DP. Chemotherapy in esophageal cancer. *Semin Oncol* 1999;26:12–20.
201. De Besi P, Sileni VC, Salvagno L, et al. Phase II study of cisplatin, 5-FU, and allopurinol in advanced esophageal cancer. *Cancer Treat Rep* 1986;70:909–910.
202. Iizuka T, Kakegawa T, Ide H, et al. Phase II evaluation of cisplatin and 5-fluorouracil in advanced squamous cell carcinoma of the esophagus: a Japanese Esophageal Oncology Group trial. *Jpn J Clin Oncol* 1992;22:172–176.
203. Zaniboni A, Simoncini E, Tonini G, et al. Cisplatin, high dose folinic acid and 5-fluorouracil in squamous cell carcinoma of the esophagus: a pilot study. *Chemioterapia* 1987;6:387–389.
204. Ilson DH, Sirott M, Saltz L, et al. A phase II trial of interferon alpha-2A, 5-fluorouracil, and cisplatin in patients with advanced esophageal carcinoma. *Cancer* 1995;75:2197–2202.
205. Wadler S, Haynes H, Beitler JJ, et al. Phase II clinical trial with 5-fluorouracil, recombinant interferon-alpha-2b, and cisplatin for patients with metastatic or regionally advanced carcinoma of the esophagus. *Cancer* 1996;78:30–34.
206. Stahl M. Chemotherapy of esophageal carcinoma. *Onkologie* 1999;22:98–104.
207. Kelsen D, Ginsberg R, Bains M, et al. A phase II trial of paclitaxel and cisplatin in patients with locally advanced metastatic esophageal cancer: a preliminary report. *Semin Oncol* 1997;24:S19-77–S1981.
208. Petrasch S, Welt A, Reinacher A, et al. Chemotherapy with cisplatin and paclitaxel in patients with locally advanced, recurrent or metastatic oesophageal cancer. *Br J Cancer* 1998;78:511–514.
209. Polee M, Eskens F, van der Burg T, et al. Phase II study of a bi-weekly treatment with cisplatin and paclitaxel in patients with advanced esophageal cancer [abstract]. *Proc Am Soc Clin Oncol* 2000;19:A1117.
210. Araujo CM, Souhami L, Gil RA, et al. A randomized trial comparing radiation therapy versus concomitant radiation therapy and chemotherapy in carcinoma of the thoracic esophagus. *Cancer* 1991;67:2258–2261.
211. Roussel A, Haegele P, Paillot B, et al. Results of the EORTC-GTCCG phase III trial of irradiation vs irradiation and CDDP in inoperable esophageal cancer [abstract]. *Proc Am Soc Clin Oncol* 1994;13:A583.
212. Slabber CF, Nel JS, Schoeman L, et al. A randomized study of radiotherapy alone versus radiotherapy plus 5-fluorouracil and platinum in patients with inoperable, locally advanced squamous cancer of the esophagus. *Am J Clin Oncol* 1998;21:462–465.

GASTRIC CANCER

CHAPTER 19 ■ GASTRIC CANCER: EPIDEMIOLOGY, SCREENING, SURVEILLANCE, AND PREVENTION

RENE LAMBERT AND DONALD M. PARKIN

INCIDENCE SURVIVAL AND MORTALITY FROM GASTRIC CANCER

Despite a declining incidence, stomach cancer is still one of the most common causes of cancer, and the second most common cause of death from cancer worldwide (1). The areas of highest incidence and mortality are in eastern Asia (Japan, Korea, China), in the Andes in South America, and in eastern Europe (2), as shown in Table 19.1 and Fig. 19.1. Incidence in men is about twice that of women in both high- and low-risk countries, although close inspection of age-specific incidence data (3) shows that rates in women exceed those of men in the youngest age groups (younger than age 40).

In Japan, stomach cancer is still the most common type of cancer overall (4–6). In an estimate based on data from 11 population-based registries, stomach cancer accounted for 23% of cancer cases in males in 1999 and 15% in females (6). Although the lifetime risk of developing gastric cancer has been decreasing in Japan, the increasing proportion of elderly persons means that the actual toll, in terms of new cases per year, is still increasing despite a declining age-specific and age-standardized incidence.

In the Western world, the declining incidence of cancer in the distal stomach contrasts with an increase of cancer at the esophagogastric junction (including the cardia) (7). Although there is some inaccuracy in attributing the site of origin of cancers at the esophagogastric junction to stomach or oesophagus (8), such misclassification cannot account for the large changes observed.

In its early stage, stomach cancer is either asymptomatic or presents with nonspecific symptoms that suggest dyspepsia. In the Western world, most cases are detected at an advanced stage, with invasion of the muscularis propria or the serosa, and with a correspondingly poor prognosis. In the United States and Europe, the 5-year relative survival rate is around the 20% level (9,10), as shown in Table 19.2, despite a weak trend to improvement (Fig. 19.2). In the United States, an analysis of 57,407 cases in the National Cancer Data Base (11) showed that most cases in the 1987–1988 cohort were still detected at an advanced stage, with as many as 39.9% in stage IV. In the 1992–1993 cohort, at each stage of the disease, the number of cases that received no treatment is surprisingly high (28.7% on average), and there were many nontreated patients even with early stage disease (38.5% in stage IA, 26.1% in stage IB).

Survival in developing countries is still lower (<15%) than in developed countries (12)

In Japan, survival is considerably better (>40%) than in the Western world, even in population-based series (13,14), as shown in Fig. 19.2. The trend to increased survival during the last 25 years also concerns the cases detected outside the official screening programs (Table 19.3). This difference suggests that the national policy of prevention is beneficial. Survival is influenced by the distribution of cases by stage and by survival within stage:

- The *localized* (curable) stage is much more frequent in Japan than in the West.
- The regional stage has better survival in Japan than in the West. The respective 5-year survival rates (both genders) in the first half of the 1980s were 32.0% in the Osaka Cancer Registry (5) and only 15.0% in the Surveillance, Epidemiology, and End Results (SEER) registries (white) of the United States (9).
- The *distant* stage (metastases) has the same poor prognosis in the East as in the West.

The declining incidence in Japan shows that the "unplanned prevention" (15) observed in other countries is also occurring in Japan, presumably as a result of changing lifestyle. Nevertheless, secondary prevention has been a priority in Japan since 1963; it aims at early diagnosis of gastric cancer in asymptomatic persons. Time trends in incidence and mortality may help assess the role of screening. The sustained decrease of the mortality-to-incidence ratio after 1970 in Japan strongly supports a beneficial effect. The trend is shown in Table 19.4 with data from the Osaka Cancer Registry (16). However, favorable survival and mortality to incidence ratios may also be due to other factors:

- Incidence may be somewhat inflated by the detection of cancers (by screening) that would not otherwise have been diagnosed within the life span of some individuals (overdiagnosis).
- A different classification of intramucosal neoplasia without invasion increases the numbers of favorable cases, including as "cancer" many of the so-called high-grade dysplasia lesions in the Western world.
- Stage migration (17) is linked to lymphadenectomy D2 in the classification of cancer at the regional stage, so tumors previously classified N1 are classified N2.

TABLE 19.1

ASR INCIDENCE (FOR 100,000) OF STOMACH
CANCER (1993–1997) IN SOME REGIONS WITH A
HIGH RISK AS COMPARED TO THE LOW INCIDENCE
RATE IN THE UNITED STATES

	Men	Women
China, Changle	145.0	34.5
China, Cixian	78.1	31.9
Japan, Hiroshima	85.5	33.9
Japan, Yamagata	91.6	38.9
Korea, Seoul	68.0	28.5
Belarus	40.5	17.4
Portugal, Vila nova de gaia	33.3	19.9
Italy, Romagna	32.3	17.8
Estonia	31.9	14.8
Costa Rica	40.1	20.8
Colombia, Cali	30.5	18.8
United States, SEER, white	6.6	2.6
United States, SEER, black	13.4	5.3

From ref. 2.

TABLE 19.2

RELATIVE 5-YR SURVIVAL RATE (BOTH GENDERS)
FOR STOMACH CANCER IN JAPAN, AMERICA,
AND EUROPE

Country	Period	Relative 5-yr survival rate	
		Male	Female
Japan (Osaka)[a]	1997	49.0%	47.9%
Europe[b]	1990–1994	20.0%	25.4%
United States, white (SEER)[c]	1995–2001	19.9%	23.9%
United States, black (SEER)[c]	1995–2001	21.5%	24.2%

[a]Data from ref. 13.
[b]Data from ref. 10.
[c]Data from ref. 9.

1992). In urban areas, the rate decreased by 23.8%, whereas in rural areas it increased by 25.8%.

Role of Genetic Susceptibility

Family relatives of gastric cancer patients have a higher risk of cancer, with a high prevalence of *Helicobacter pylori* infection and intestinal metaplasia in the stomach (19). However, only a small proportion of gastric cancers are due to genetic predisposition, as characterized by familial clustering and a dominant inheritance pattern. The rare syndrome of hereditary diffuse gastric cancer has been described in New Zealand and is attributed to a germline mutation in a gene encoding the cell adhesion protein E-cadherin (20,21). This cancer is a diffuse, poorly differentiated infiltrative adenocarcinoma. In contrast, gastric cancer of the intestinal differentiated type may occur in hereditary nonpolyposis colon cancer (22) or in patients with gastrointestinal polyposis, including familial

ETIOLOGY IN RELATION TO PREVENTION

Most gastric cancers occur sporadically and are related to environmental factors, linked to diet and infection. Atrophic gastritis may be an important intermediary because it results in the increased intraluminal pH, which may promote the genesis of carcinogens in the gastric lumen. A study in cancer registries of China (18) illustrates the role of lifestyle: Mortality from gastric cancer (ASR/100,000) has been compared in the urban and rural populations in two periods (1973–1975 and 1990–

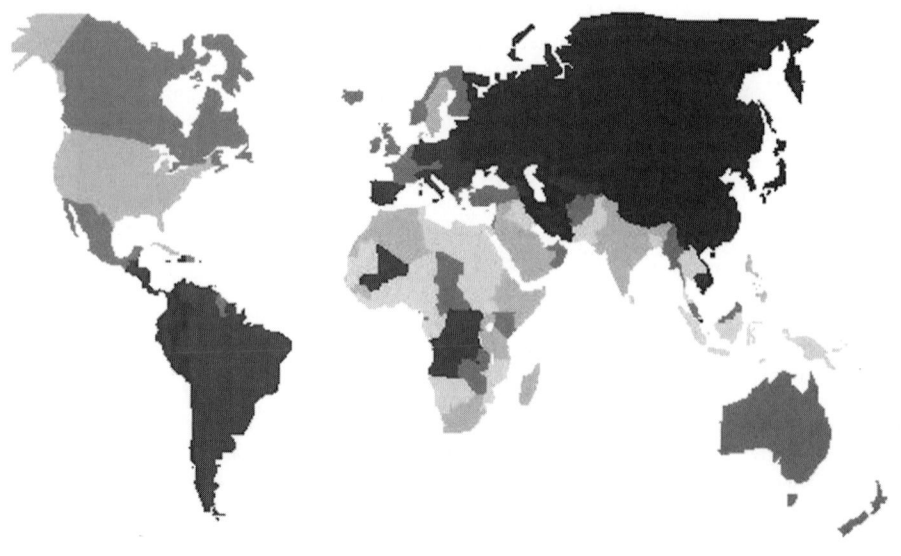

■ < 5.5   ■ < 8.9   ■ < 13.9   ■ < 21.7   ■ < 69.6

GLOBOCAN 2002

FIGURE 19.1. Incidence of stomach cancer in the world in men in 2002. *Source*: From ref. 148.

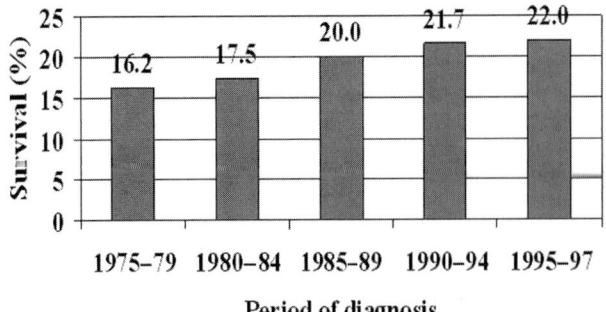

FIGURE 19.2. Five-year relative survival of stomach cancer in the United States. *Source:* From ref. 9.

TABLE 19.3

TIME TRENDS IN DETECTION AND RELATIVE 5-YR SURVIVAL RATE OF STOMACH CANCER IN JAPAN: THE OSAKA CANCER REGISTRY, 1975–1989, IN MEN

Period	Screen detected (relative 5-yr survival rate [%])	Others (relative 5-yr survival rate [%])
1975–1977	5.1% (73.4)	81.5% (26.0)
1981–1983	6.0% (70.8)	83.2% (38.7)
1987–1989	11.6% (85.0)	81.5% (44.8)

Comparison between screen detected and other conditions of detection. The difference up to 100% when adding the two groups is for unknown.
From ref. 13.

adenomatous polyposis and Peutz-Jeghers syndrome. With respect to the infectious factor, genetic polymorphisms may play a role, both for *H. pylori* and for the human host. A small increase in the risk of gastric cancer (23) is linked to the blood group A phenotype and explained by the higher risk of atrophic gastritis with the adhesion of *H. pylori* to the Lewis[b] blood group antigen.

Role of Dietary Factors

A high intake of mucosal irritants such as salt and nitrates causes chronic inflammation and superficial gastritis, which can develop into atrophic gastritis (24,25). The fact that dietary salt also influences the more advanced pathological changes of the gastric mucosa was demonstrated in a cohort study in Japan (26), where during a 6-year follow-up of 5,373 persons, 69 developed gastric cancer. The risk of gastric cancer increased 2.2-fold in subjects with atrophic gastritis at enrollment; in the presence of atrophic gastritis, the risk was 1.8-fold by the consumption of spicy food and decreased 0.6-fold by a reduction in intake of salty food.

Reduced acid secretion in the presence of atrophy increases gastric pH, thus favoring the growth of anaerobic bacteria, which reduces nitrate to nitrite and can eventually form N-nitroso mutagens. In contrast, a high intake of fruit and vegetables is associated with a reduced risk of gastric cancer (27). Antioxidants such as beta-carotene, alpha-tocopherol (vitamin E), and ascorbic acid (vitamin C) prevent the formation of mutagens and carcinogens in the stomach. The exact role of these vitamins in the etiology of gastric cancer is not known, and it may be that low ascorbic acid in gastric juice is simply a marker of the extension of inflammation and infection.

Role of Tobacco and Alcohol

In its recent review, the International Agency for Research on Cancer (IARC) (28) concluded that there was a consistent and causal association of cancer of the stomach with cigarette smoking in both men and women. Confounding by other factors (alcohol, *H. pylori* infection, and dietary factors) could be reasonably ruled out. Risk increases with duration of smoking and number of cigarettes smoked, and decreases with increasing duration of successful quitting.

With respect to alcohol, the 1988 review by IARC (29) concluded that "there is little . . . to suggest a causal role for drinking alcoholic beverages in stomach cancer." Despite a host of studies in the last 18 years, this remains a fair summary of the evidence today (30).

Role of *Helicobacter pylori*

In 1994, *H. pylori* was classified by IARC (31) as being carcinogenic for humans, with sufficient evidence for a causal association with both carcinomas of the stomach and gastric lymphoma. At that time, much of the evidence came from retrospective case-control studies. However, these studies are limited in that the presence of *H. pylori* infection is evaluated after the development of cancer. *H. pylori* tends to disappear as intestinal metaplasia and atrophy develop, so prevalence of infection may be seriously underestimated in cases, even if anti–*H. pylori* antibody is used as an indicator of infection. Prospective studies

TABLE 19.4

TIME TREND OF AGE-STANDARDIZED (WORLD STANDARD) INCIDENCE AND MORTALITY PER 100,000 FOR STOMACH CANCER IN JAPAN

Period	Males			Females		
	Incidence	Mortality	Ratio M/I	Incidence	Mortality	Ratio M/I
1963–1965	108.13	83.82	0.77	51.98	41.18	0.80
1975–1977	79.01	58.78	0.74	38.85	29.17	0.75
1987–1989	68.28	41.21	0.60	29.68	18.31	0.61

M/I, mortality to incidence.
Figures per 100,000 in the Osaka Cancer Registry between 1963 and 1989, in males and females (5).

give a more accurate assessment. Several case-control studies nested within cohorts have now been published in which infection is evaluated in cases and controls before the onset of disease. The results of these studies have been the subject of several meta-analyses (32–35). In the review by the Helicobacter and Cancer Collaborative Group (35), 12 prospective studies were included, with a total of 1,228 gastric cancer cases and 3,406 controls. Overall, the odds ratio (OR) for the association between *H. pylori* infection and the subsequent development of gastric cancer was 2.36 (95% confidence interval [CI], 1.98–2.81). Analyzing cancers of the gastric cardia and noncardia separately, the authors found no increase in risk for cardia cancers (OR = 0.99), while the overall risk for noncardia cancers was 2.97 (95% CI, 2.34–3.77). The risk varied with the interval between sample collection and cancer diagnosis (as might be expected, if infection is progressively lost as gastric atrophy develops). The increase in risk was 5.9-fold (95% CI, 3.4–10.3) for *H. pylori* positivity 10 years or more prior to diagnosis. The associations were not related to histologic type of gastric cancer (intestinal vs. diffuse) or gender.

In the human host, *H. pylori* infection can be detected by anti–*H. pylori* antibodies. It is an exceedingly common infection with an estimated overall prevalence of infection in middle-age adults of 74% in developing countries and 58% in developed countries (36). The prevalence of infection increases rapidly with age, is associated with childhood living conditions (37), and may persist during a long period. In adults undergoing a periodic health check, the rate of seroconversion to positive and of seroreversion to negative over 9 years was estimated as 6.3% and 7.1%, respectively (38).

Prevalence of infection correlates reasonably well with the risk of gastric cancer in the same population (31) but is not perfect. The "African enigma" (39) refers to the supposed low incidence of gastric cancer in Africa, where there is high prevalence of *H. pylori* infection. However, the incidence of gastric cancer in Africa (particularly central Africa) is not especially low (40), and even if it were, there is no reason to suppose that the risk related to *H. pylori* could not be modified by other (protective) factors. An evidence-based review (41) of 40 prospective endoscopic studies from 17 African countries (20,531 persons) did not suggest dissociation between the prevalence of *H. pylori* infection and *H. pylori*–related diseases: *H. pylori*–related clinical outcomes included duodenal ulcers in 21.1%, gastric ulcers in 3.4%, and gastric cancers in 2.4%.

Studies using serum banks suggest that there has been a decline in prevalence of infection with *H. pylori* between successive generations (42–45). Banatvala et al. (44), for example, using 631 sera collected in 1969, 1979, and 1989, observed that the odds of being *H. pylori* seropositive decrease by 26% per decade. An early age of infection favors the development of atrophic gastritis and increases the risk of stomach cancer. From 1973 to 1994 in Finland (45), the proportion of subjects infected by *H. pylori* strains has declined. However, the prevalence of cag-A (+) strains among those younger than 45 years declined more than for cag-A (–) strains. In Japan (46), middle-age persons have a pattern of infection similar to that in developing countries, whereas young generations have a much lower rate of infection. Time trends in the incidence of gastric cancer in Japan were analyzed from 1976 to 1996 and compared to changes in the prevalence of *H. pylori* infection (47), which declined in both genders between 1989 and 1998, with young age groups experiencing more change. In addition, a marked decline in gastric cancer incidence occurred in the young population ages 20 to 39 years. An estimation of the numbers of stomach cancer attributable to *H. pylori* infection in the world for 2002 (29) is shown in Table 19.5.

The recent determination of the complete DNA sequence of the *H. pylori* genome (48) has shown specific islands common to various strains, but all strains of *H. pylori* may not play the same role in the development of gastric cancer. In humans, subjects infected with cag-A–positive strains have a higher prevalence of atrophic gastritis and higher levels of IgG anti–*H. pylori* antibodies than those with cag-A–negative infections (49–51). *H. pylori* can also produce a vacuolating cytotoxin named vac-A. In Colombia, the relative frequency of cag-A and vac-A s1 and m1 phenotypes was higher in gastric biopsies from high-risk areas for gastric cancer (49) than in low-risk areas.

The etiologic role of *H. pylori* in gastric carcinogenesis is supported by animal experiments showing that inoculation of cag-A– and vac-A–positive strains was able to induce intestinal metaplasia and gastric carcinoma in Mongolian gerbils (52). Research is ongoing to determine whether strain-specific genes could be associated with gastric carcinogenesis (53).

The carcinogenic effect of *H. pylori* is indirect and linked to the increased proliferation of the gastric epithelium occurring in the *H. Pylori*–infected stomach. This effect depends on the ability of *H. pylori* to produce ammonia via its potent urease action on intragastric urea. Cell replication potentiates the action of carcinogens targeting DNA (54–58). The bacterial organisms are hosted in the mucus layer overlying the normal gastric epithelium but not in areas overlying intestinal metaplasia where neoplasia originates; this suggests that soluble carcinogens present in the gastric lumen play a role. *H. pylori* infection causes oxidative stress in the gastric mucosa; inducible nitric oxide synthetase (iNOS) is expressed in inflammatory cells and located in the lamina propria at the early stage of gastritis (58). Nitric oxide (NO) is active on the renewal sector of epithelial

---

TABLE 19.5

ESTIMATED NUMBERS OF GASTRIC CANCER CASES (BOTH GENDERS) IN 2002 CAUSED BY *H. PYLORI*, IN DEVELOPED AND DEVELOPING COUNTRIES

	All cases stomach cancer	Noncardia stomach cancer	Cases attributable to *H. pylori*
Developed countries	312,400	259,000	192,000 (61.4%)
Developing countries	621,500	571,000	400,000 (64.4%)
World	933,900	770,000	592,000 (63.4%)

The estimate is based on the following assumptions: (a) *H. pylori* infection plays no role in cancer of the cardia (approximately 18% of cases overall), (b) the prevalence of *H. pylori* infection is lower in developed (58%) than in developing countries (74%), and (c) the relative risk of noncardia gastric cancer associated with *H. pylori* infection is 5.9 (36).

cells in the deep foveolar epithelium and in lymphoid follicles. In the precancerous mucosa, iNOS migrates in the superficial foveolar epithelium, where protein and DNA damage can be produced. At this stage, bacterial eradication diminishes the markers without preventing new DNA damage. The higher intragastric pH following atrophic gastritis provoked by *H. pylori* may rather modify external or endogenous carcinogens. Nitrosated compounds are recognized as gastric carcinogens in the experimental setting. Transformation of nitrite (NO_2) to NO produces the reactive dinitrogen trioxide (N_2O_3) that forms nitrosothiols and nitrosamines. This chain reaction toward nitrosation is inhibited in the presence of antioxidants, explaining the preventive action of ascorbic acid; however *H. pylori* also interferes with antioxidant functions by decreasing intragastric ascorbic acid concentrations.

PROGRESSION OF THE DISEASE

The pathological changes that precede cancer are chronic atrophic gastritis, metaplasia of the intestinal type, and dysplasia. Dysplasia is intraepithelial neoplasia without invasion of the stroma; it arises in either the normal gastric epithelium or in intestinal metaplasia. In gastric oncogenesis, dysplasia lies between atrophic metaplastic lesions and invasive cancer. Progression of the disease was studied in a follow-up study of 1,400 asymptomatic subjects in an area of high gastric cancer risk in Colombia (59,60); endoscopy and biopsy were performed twice, at an average interval of 5 years, and showed an overall progression to more advanced lesions. Atrophic gastritis preceded gastric cancer in a Japanese prospective study (26), which reported a relative risk of 2.3 of developing cancer for those affected by severe atrophy. The less severe types of lesions—both nonatrophic and mild atrophic gastritis—have also been shown to occur more often in cases of gastric cancer than in control subjects. A case-control study (61) in Finland, including 243 cases with gastric cancer and 1,408 controls for which gastric histology was available found a relative risk of gastric cancer in patients with nonatrophic antral gastritis of 1, 8, and 2.5 in patients with nonatrophic pangastritis. The same group (62) observed a declining prevalence of gastritis in Finland from 1977 to 1992 in young age groups (similar to the decrease in incidence of gastric cancer). The diagnosis of gastric epithelial dysplasia includes (a) the distinction between true dysplasia and the reactive changes associated with inflammation, and (b) the distinction between dysplasia and truly invasive cancer.

In a meta-analysis of the literature (63), 80% of cases of high-grade dysplasia will progress to cancer after 6 months, whereas the rate of transformation of low-grade dysplasia is 10% in 1.5 years. The speed of progression from early to advanced cancer is not constant, and it is possible that some of the tumors detected might not have manifested themselves later. The potential role of this bias has been examined in Japan (64) in a series of 43 early gastric cancer cases who received no treatment for at least 6 months and had some follow-up (diagnostic tests, late operation). Advanced gastric cancer occurred in 27 subjects (63%); the median duration of early gastric cancer after diagnosis was 37 months. This suggests that most such early cancers diagnosed through screening will progress to more advanced symptomatic disease.

In Western countries, the term "adenoma" is applied when the mucosal proliferation produces a macroscopic protruding lesion. Gastric adenomas are less common than hyperplastic polyps; they account for approximately 10% of gastric polyps. Malignant transformation of adenomas is rare in lesions measuring <2 cm but frequent (40%) in lesions >2 cm. Flat adenomas may have a greater tendency to develop into carcinomas, even when small.

In Japan, intraepithelial neoplasia with severe dysplastic changes and no invasion of the lamina propria is also called *intramucosal carcinoma*. In Western countries, a diagnosis of intramucosal carcinoma is made only if there is demonstration of malignant cells in the lamina propria. The East/West divergence, confirmed by multidisciplinary teams (65), disappears when there is tumor invasion across the muscularis mucosae. The inclusion of these noninvasive "intramucosal" carcinomas in Japanese series of gastric cancers accounts, at least in part, for the markedly better prognosis of gastric cancer in Japan.

A significant distinction in the morphology of gastric cancer is between the differentiated intestinal and the poorly differentiated diffuse types (66). The first is linked to chronic atrophic gastritis and intestinal metaplasia, and is responsible for most geographic variations in risk (67). In Japan, the decline in incidence of gastric cancer is largely attributed to decline in the intestinal type of gastric carcinoma (68). Similar, although less clear, changes have been seen in U.S. data (69). Molecular genetics is becoming increasingly important, and several loci have been identified, indicating possible tumor-suppressor genes. As yet, none of these tests is currently used in the screening of the early stages of gastric cancer.

DIRECT DIAGNOSIS OF CANCER

Gastroscopy

Gastroscopy has not been used as the primary test in mass screening. Leaving aside issues of cost, it does not satisfy several other criteria for a screening test, one of which relates to complete safety. There is a very small (but not nil) risk of severe complications, either respiratory or digestive (hemorrhage or perforation). In a retrospective study of 211,410 procedures (70), complications and mortality occurred in 0.13% and 0.04%, respectively, and in a prospective study from a single institution; the rate of complications was as high as 1.9% (70). Although not used as a screening test, gastroscopy is considered as a "gold standard" against which to evaluate sensitivity of other procedures in the detection of gastric malignancy and permit biopsies. Gastroscopy also proved efficacy in the morphologic distribution of superficial cancer in the subtypes of a type 0 occurring in superficial cancer (Table 19.6) (71).

When gastroscopy is used to diagnose the nature of suspicious lesions detected by other screening procedures, a substantial number of persons will undergo diagnostic gastroscopy, without malignancy being confirmed. There is no doubt that the extensive practice of endoscopy in Japan has improved the yield of early cases, and in consequence, the survival of gastric cancer, as compared to other countries (the proportion of early cases is currently around 40% in Japan). Recent figures from population registries (13,14) show that the 5-year survival increased from around 20% in 1965 to almost 50% by 1997. In contrast, in population registries from Western countries, the 5-year survival rate from gastric cancer has been stable, in the 20% range during the same period (9,10).

Although considered to constitute a gold standard, the validity of gastroscopic diagnosis may be low if the procedure is performed incorrectly. The miss rates of gastroscopy in the detection of gastric cancer in Japan have been shown in a study comparing negative endoscopies of the Prefectural Hospital, with cases recorded in the population-based cancer Fukui Registry after a 3-year interval (72). The sensitivity of gastroscopy for gastric cancer was only 81%.

In the Western world (73–75), population-based questionnaires have shown that approximately 25% of persons have symptoms of dyspepsia (annual prevalence). When endoscopy

TABLE 19.6

PROPORTION OF MAJOR MACROSCOPIC SUBTYPES
WITHIN TYPE 0 OF SUPERFICIAL GASTRIC CANCER
(m + sm)

Subtype 0	% of all type 0	% sm
0-Ip/s, polypoid pedunculated/ sessile	3%	57%
0-IIa, nonpolypoid elevated	17%	29%
0-IIb, nonpolypoid flat	<1%	20%
0-IIc, nonpolypoid depressed	71%	37%
0-IIc+IIa, nonpolypoid depressed + elevated	1%	47%
0-IIa+IIc, nonpolypoid elevated + depressed	6.2%	65%
0-III, ulcerated	1.3%	40%

In a surgical series (2,098 lesions from 1990 to 1999), with pathology
control from National Cancer Center Hospital in Tokyo (71). Type I
lesions are polypoid, pedunculated, or sessile. Type II lesions are
nonpolypoid, slightly elevated, flat, or slightly depressed. Type III
lesions are ulcerated.

is performed, structural disease is usually detected in only
30% to 35% of cases, and gastric malignancy is rare (1% or
2%) and quite exceptional in persons younger than 40 years.
This is why in a patient younger than 45 years and com-
plaining of dyspepsia, the American College of Physicians has,
since 1985, recommended avoiding prompt endoscopy and giving empirical treatment instead. This policy has been complemented more recently by testing for *H. pylori* and treating patients found to be infected. Cost effectiveness has been a major argument against the prompt endoscopy strategy, although
the excessive cost observed in the short term has not been
proved in long-term analyses (74–75). The small proportion
of stomach cancers detected at the early stage in the Western
world justifies more attention to the quality control of gastroscopy.

Radiography and Photofluorography

When used in the detection of stomach cancer, radiology uses
either full-size films with double-contrast or miniature films
in photofluorography. Since 1963 in Japan (76–84), full-size
x-ray testing has been used less often for screening than miniature seven-exposure photofluorography. There is a tendency to
adopt full-size x-rays in large cities and miniature photos in
rural areas. The target of the Japanese program is to examine 30% of the population age 40 years and older each year
(77). Any suspicious result is followed by gastroscopy, which
is necessary in 13% to 23% of subjects (79,80). Radiology is
less sensitive than endoscopy in the detection of early cancer;
however, the aim of radiology in a mass screening program
is to detect silent cancer in the preclinical stage, rather than
early cancer (78,82). In a study (81) linked to the Osaka Cancer Registry, the sensitivity of plain x-rays films was estimated
at 90.8% and that of miniature photofluorography at 88.5%.
Another study (83) compared the diagnostic validity of miniature photofluorography with that of endoscopy: In a group of
17,976 randomly selected screened individuals submitted to
both explorations, 93% of 80 advanced cancer cases detected
by endoscopy were also detected by radiology. The percentage
was lower (39%) for 207 early cancers detected by endoscopy,
and only 22% for lesions <2 cm in diameter. Radiology has the
potential hazard of exposure to radiation, although modern
equipment and image intensification have lowered exposure
doses dramatically. A population-based case-control study of
leukemia (84) found no excess risk among persons screened at
least once within the preceding 10 years.

DIAGNOSIS OF AN INCREASED RISK OF STOMACH CANCER

Tumor Antigens

Studies (85) have been conducted in Scandinavia on the discriminative value of various tumor antigens, either in the sera
(CEA, CA19-9, CA 50) or in the gastric juice (fetal sulfoglyco-
protein antigen). Such studies aim to detect a specific tumoral
signature. Although they do not yet contribute to a screening
policy, this could change in the future with the explosive progression of cancer genetics.

Pepsinogen

In the gastric mucosa, the progression from chronic superficial to atrophic gastritis, intestinal metaplasia, and cancer is
associated with changes in serum levels of pepsinogens (Pg),
which are proenzymes of pepsin (86). There are four pepsinogens, precursors of four proteolytic enzymes (pepsin A, B, C,
D). The level of Pg C has proved discriminant for the risk of
cancer in persons positive for *H. pylori* infection: The level of
Pg-C is high in superficial gastritis in *H. pylori*–positive persons and decreases in atrophic gastritis and gastric cancer (87).
Most assays are based on the distinction between Pg I, which is
produced in the gastric fundus (chief cells of gastric glands and
mucous neck cells), and Pg II, which is also produced in the
antrum. Atrophic gastritis of the fundic mucosa is associated
with a specific decrease in Pg I and a reduction in the ratio of Pg
I/II (88–91). Nomura et al. (90), in a follow-up study of 7,498
Japanese Americans in Hawaii, found that a Pg I/II ratio <2
had better sensitivity for predicting later gastric cancer than Pg
I levels alone. Prospective studies have demonstrated that low
Pg I levels are associated with an increased risk of gastric cancer, and nested case-control studies suggest that changes in Pg
levels are most marked close to the time of diagnosis of stomach cancer. Thus, in a follow-up of 39,268 individuals age 15
or older in Finland (92), a Pg I level <50 ng/mL was associated with diagnosis of gastric cancer in the next 8 to 14 years
(OR = 2.7), with a stronger association (OR = 6.3) for cases
diagnosed within 2 years. The current trend is to use the two
serologic tests, with cut-off levels adequately selected for the Pg
I and Pg I/II ratios. The interaction between *H. pylori* infection
and pepsinogen status on gastric cancer risk was analyzed in
a prospective cohort study in Japan (93), with a follow-up of
4.7 years. The risk of incident gastric relative to that in persons
who are *H. pylori* negative with a normal pepsinogen was 1.1
for those who are *H. pylori* positive with a normal pepsinogen, 6.0 for those *H. pylori* positive with a low pepsinogen,
and 8.2 for those *H. pylori* negative with a low pepsinogen
(this group had the most complete degree of gastric atrophy).
In Japan, the efficacy of the pepsinogen test was analyzed in 878
subjects (94) who underwent a gastroscopy with a urea test a
H. pylori serology and a measure of the pepsinogen I/II ratio. The prevalence of intestinal metaplasia in the stomach

was higher in persons with a cut-off value of the PG-I/PG-2 ratio <3.

Serology to *Helicobacter pylori*

The association between infection with *H. pylori*, as shown by the presence of antibodies in serum, and the development of atrophic gastritis gastric cancer has been described previously. Although *H. pylori* infection is quite a sensitive predictor of subsequent gastric cancer (95), (some authors [96] going so far as to claim that it is a "necessary cause"), it is very nonspecific, which is unsurprising when half or more of the population is infected. Nomura et al. (97), testing for serum IgG antibody to cag-A toxin, obtained a sensitivity of 94.5% and a specificity of 92.5%. Several prospective studies have shown that the combination of *H. pylori* infection and atrophic gastritis (as evaluated by the PG test) provides a high level of prediction of development of gastric cancer, with fewer false positives than either test alone (93,97,98).

SCREENING

Screening entails the examination of asymptomatic individuals so they can be separated into those who probably do, and those who probably do not, have the disease of interest. A second diagnostic examination is needed for those selected by the positive test. Mass screening for stomach cancer has been encouraged in Japan since 1963 and has been covered by the Health Services Law for the Aged since 1983. Widespread use of the method has had a positive impact on the prognosis of the disease. Outside Japan, mass screening has proved too costly and opportunistic screening, or no screening at all, is the usual situation.

Screening Based on Photofluorography

Since the introduction of mass screening in Japan, a progressively greater proportion of cases of gastric cancers have been diagnosed at an early stage of disease, and mortality rates from stomach cancer have declined (13,14,77–79). However, the change toward a westernized lifestyle that helps prevent gastric cancer complicates interpretation of time trends. The screening programs in Japan reach a large proportion of the population. In 1985, a national survey of the Ministry of Health and Welfare estimated the percentage of ever-screened subjects in Japan at 59.8%; however, only 15.1% had had tests regularly (79).

The decline in mortality from gastric cancer in different areas of Japan is associated with the intensity of screening (79,80,99). Time trends of incidence and mortality for stomach cancer were analyzed from 1960 to 1985 in Miyagi Prefecture (80): Both indexes follow the general trend toward decline, and after 1970, the rate of decline was greater for mortality. This implies improved survival, also observed in the Osaka Cancer Registry (13), and is compatible with a beneficial effect of the mass screening policy. The *Japanese Journal of Gastroenterological Mass Survey* published a report on the results of mass screening for stomach cancer throughout Japan in 1995 (100). This report concerns the mass survey program based on photofluorography followed by endoscopy, applied either in "Japanese communities" or by private companies. In 1995, 6,765,268 persons were examined, with 841,795 workup tests proposed and 576,545 performed. Screening detected a gastric cancer in 6,718 persons (0.1% of those screened). The characteristics of the screen-detected cancers are presented in Table 19.7: Small lesions (up to 2 cm in diameter) occur in 40%, the endoscopic pattern is predominantly depressed, and the cancer is confirmed T1 in 66.7%. Surgical treatment is performed in most cases (88%). The proportion of cases detected by screening has tended to increase in recent times, but it is still a minority, as shown in Table 19.3, with data from the Osaka Cancer Registry from 1975 to 1987. During the same period in the same registry, the proportion of cancers with distant extension was stable, while localized cases increased and cases with regional extension decreased, as shown in Table 19.8. In the SEER registries in the United States (9), the proportion of localized cases is about half of that observed in Japan (Table 19.9).

Randomized Controlled Trials

Randomized studies are difficult to conduct in Japan, in the presence of an ongoing screening program. One study was begun in 1985 in the Miyagi Prefecture (80), where inhabitants of 39 municipalities were randomized to receive an invitation to attend gastric cancer screening, whereas those in the control municipalities received no invitation letter. However, after the first year, the difference in the proportion of subjects attending screening in the intervention areas versus the control areas

---

TABLE 19.7

NATIONAL RESULTS OF MASS SCREENING OF STOMACH CANCER IN JAPAN IN 1995

A – Diameter of stomach cancer (n = 5,066)

<1 cm	1.1–2.0 cm	2.1–5.0 cm	5.1 and over
15.5%	24.9%	42.3%	17.3%

B – Cancer depth of penetration in the gastric wall (n = 5,267)

Mucosa	Submucosa	Muscularis	Subserosa	Serosa
39.3%	27.4%	10.4%	12.0%	10.9%

C – Treatment of screen-detected stomach cancer (n = 5,574)

Surgical Treatment	Endoscopic Treatment	Laparoscopic Treatment	Other Treatment	No Treatment
88%	8%	0.5%	1.1%	1.4%

Data from ref. 100.

TABLE 19.8

TIME TREND IN STAGE DISTRIBUTION OF STOMACH CANCER AT DETECTION IN JAPAN: THE OSAKA CANCER REGISTRY, 1975–1989, IN MALES

Period	Localized (relative 5-yr survival rate [%])	Regional (relative 5-yr survival rate [%])	Distant (relative 5-yr survival rate [%])
1975–1977	26.4% (65.9)	54.8% (24.0)	18.8% (1.5)
1981–1983	32.1% (86.0)	47.2% (31.4)	20.7% (1.3)
1987–1989	42.8% (88.1)	37.0% (33.4)	20.2% (2.7)

The difference up to 100% when adding the three groups is for unstaged.
From ref. 5.

was so small that there was no possibility of observing any difference in the mortality rates due to screening.

Cohort Studies

In the Osaka Prefecture, a follow-up study conducted from 1967 to 1970 and using the Osaka Cancer Registry (101) was organized in 33,000 individuals, screened at least once, and then followed for an average 6.1 years. The number of gastric cancer cases diagnosed in the cohort was 1.37 times higher than expected, based on the general population rates, while there was a very slight reduction in the number of deaths. Some of the excess incidence may be due to overdiagnosis of gastric cancer. A survey in Miyagi Prefecture (102) has shown that those taking part in the gastric cancer screening program had a lower prevalence of smoking and higher intakes of dietary items such as milk and fruit, which are usually associated with a reduced risk of gastric cancer. Another Japanese study concerned a cohort of 24,134 persons followed for a period of 40 months (103) after self-report of being screened or not screened. The risk of death from gastric cancer in males who reported having been screened was 0.72 (CI, 0.31–1.66), and in females the figure was 1.46 (CI, 0.43–4.90); it was concluded that the screening program did not contribute greatly to decreasing cancer mortality. In an 18-year follow-up study of 7,008 residents of Miyagi Prefecture (104), incidence from gastric cancer did not differ between screened and unscreened subjects, but mortality decreased significantly in screened subjects compared with unscreened subjects for both men (61.9 vs. 137.2 per 100,000 person-years, $p < 0.005$) and women (28.1 vs. 53.8 per 100,00 person-years, $p < 0.01$). In a population-based cohort of 42,150 persons (105), the persons who had undergone a screening photofluorography during the preceding 12 months at the beginning of the study (36%) were considered as the screened group. The others were the control group. After a 13-year follow-up, there was a twofold decrease in gastric mortality in the screened group (RR = 0.52), although the overall incidence rate was not influenced.

Case-Control Studies

Several case-control studies have been reported from Japan. The first study (77) was conducted in an area covered by the population-based cancer registry of Osaka, which allowed the identification of all residents who died from stomach cancer from 1969 to 1981. A total of 87 deaths from gastric cancer (cases) and three times as many controls were included in the analysis. The odds ratio for screened versus unscreened subjects was 0.59 in men and 0.38 in women. The protective effect was greater for those who had more than one examination. A second study adopted the same sampling design, which compared screening histories of 367 cases of advanced stomach cancer with the same number of controls matched for gender, age, and residence (106). Significant protective effect was detected up to 3 years since the last negative test, with an odds ratio for those screened at 0.34. A third study (107) compared 198 dead cases and 577 live controls matched by gender, age, and residence (district) with respect to their screening histories in the 5 years preceding the diagnosis of the case. Recent examinations were associated with an odds ratio of 0.41 (0.28–0.61) forever versus never screened within 5 years

Screening for Gastric Cancer Outside Japan

There has been little screening for gastric cancer outside Japan. However, a program using the same methodology was introduced in Venezuela in 1980 (108). The 241 cases that died from stomach cancer from 1985 to 1989 were compared to 2,410 controls from the same population. An excess risk of dying from stomach cancer was observed for those who had tests occurring within the 6 months preceding the diagnosis of the case, and no benefit from screening was detected when such recent examinations were excluded from the screening histories of both cases and controls. This result suggested that the screening program was being used primarily by symptomatic individuals at high risk of death from gastric cancer (selection bias). To try to control for this, an analysis was confined to subjects who had tests taking place just before diagnosis of the case. The odds ratio at 0.47 was then consistent with a protective effect.

TABLE 19.9

STAGE DISTRIBUTION OF STOMACH CANCER AT DETECTION IN THE UNITED STATES: THE SEER REGISTRY, MALE AND FEMALES, 1989–1995

Race	Localized	Regional	Distant
White	20%	30%	35%
Black	19%	29%	38%

The difference up to 100% when adding the three groups is for unstaged.
From ref. 9

Screening Based on Serum Pepsinogen

Using the Pepsinogen (Pg) test requires determination of cutoff levels adapted to screening studies. Various thresholds have been proposed for the two parameters (Pg I and Pg I/Pg II ratio) that are usually analyzed simultaneously (109–111). For levels of Pg I, various thresholds have been proposed: <30, 50, or 70 ng. The sensitivity for concurrent gastric cancer increases, and the specificity decreases with the higher levels. The other one is the Pg I/II ratio, where the usual thresholds are <3 or <2. The sensitivity varies with the morphologic pattern of early cancer and is higher for elevated or depressed nonulcerated lesions (112). The Pg test has been proposed to increase compliance in mass screening official survey protocols. It has been shown (113) that 82% of persons who agree to give a blood sample would attend the stomach examination when told that they had an increased risk of stomach cancer. The Pg test has also been combined to the presence of Ig-G against *H. pylori* infection (114).

Of more importance is whether the Pg test could be used as a relatively low-cost primary screening test (with follow-up of positive screening tests by gastroscopy) in place of photofluorography. The performance of Pg as a screening test has been evaluated in Japan. Miki et al. (115) screened 4,647 company employees (mean age 49 years) by measuring serum Pg levels and submitting those with Pg I levels <50 ng/mL, together with a PgI/II ratio of <3.0, to follow-up endoscopy. Overall, 18.8% of subjects were positive (29% older than 50 years), and four gastric cancers were detected. Although there was no proper evaluation of sensitivity, the authors imply that it could have been equal to that of x-rays screening because the detection rate (0.86/1,000) was somewhat better than mass screening in the same company using x-rays (0.66/1,000). However, the comparability of the screened groups, even in terms of age, was unclear, and the Pg test represented a prevalent screen, rather than a mixture of new and repeat tests, as for x-rays. In later studies, using the same methods and criteria for positive cases, about 20% of the subjects who were screened were positive, representing a predictive value of 1.3% to 1.4% (113–116). With this limited definition, sensitivity was estimated at 66.7% and specificity as 81.5% (116). Another Japanese group (112) adopted the following indicators of a high risk of cancer: Pg I <30 ng/mL and Pg I/II ratio <2. Using these parameters, screening was conducted in 5,620 persons in 1991 and 1992. The prevalence of gastric cancer in subjects with a positive Pg test was 0.12%, a figure just comparable to that obtained with photofluorography (0.11%). Another group (109), using the cut-off points for identifying risk for gastric cancer (<70 ng/mL for Pg I, and <3 for the Pg I/II ratio) in 5,113 subjects also screened by endoscopy (13 gastric cancers detected), obtained a sensitivity for gastric cancer at 84.6%, with a specificity at 73.5%. Eleven of the 13 cancers were detected by the Pg test. The Pg test missed 2 out of 4 cancers with mild atrophic gastritis and 1 of those with atrophic gastritis. In summary, it can be concluded that the Pg test is just as effective and that it could replace photofluorography.

In another study (117), 17,647 persons were screened with two procedures: barium digital radiography, which is better than photofluorography, and the pepsinogen test. Pepsinogen was more adapted to the detection of asymptomatic early cancer with intestinal type, while radiology was more adapted to the detection of ulcerated forms with a diffuse type. The study called Hisayama (118) showed that the test combining PG-I and the PG-I/PG-2 ratio was effective in the screening for gastric cancer. The incidence of gastric cancer was higher in strongly positive tests (RR = 4.5 in men and 5.8 in women). Pepsinogen as a screening tool has been compared to photofluorography: The positive predictive value of the test for gastric cancer was 0.8% in the x-ray method and 1.4% with a pepsinogen test (119).

Screening Based on the Serology of *Helicobacter pylori*

Although theoretically possible to screen for gastric cancer using anti–*H. pylori* antibody testing, the high prevalence of infection would mean that many individuals would test positive and require follow-up. Testing for anti–*H. pylori* antibody has been primarily advocated to select groups of the population as candidates for *H. pylori* eradication.

SURVEILLANCE

Endoscopy is the main procedure used worldwide for surveillance of persons at high risk; for example, in genetic syndromes, gastroscopy is used for examination of members of probands in families with E-cadherin mutations, and with the familial adenomatous colorectal polyposis, where lesions in the upper digestive tract must be sought. However, at present, the most frequent reason for surveillance is the presence of chronic acquired atrophic gastritis in the following circumstances:

- In the postoperative stomach following partial gastrectomy for a benign lesion, an increased risk of cancer in the gastric stump has been shown in the long term (15–20 years), and the literature, until recently (120), has recommended endoscopic surveillance. Annual endoscopic screening is proposed only for the late period after gastrectomy, but its benefit is unclear because most cases are detected at the advanced noncurable stage even during surveillance. However, fewer cases need such surveillance because of the considerable decrease in the indications of gastrectomy for peptic ulcer.
- In pernicious anemia and the genetically linked autoimmune gastritis type A, the risk of gastric cancer has been found to be increased some two- to fivefold in studies in the Nordic countries (121–123).
- In focal lesions with low- or high-grade dysplasia occurring in a mucosa altered by atrophic gastritis with intestinal metaplasia, the risk of confirmed malignancy is very high in all lesions >2 cm (54). Thus, the recent trend is for endoscopic treatment (endoscopic mucosal resection) rather than surveillance.

PRIMARY PREVENTION

The decline in incidence and mortality of stomach cancer in many, if not most, populations might be considered to be "unplanned" primary prevention (15). Quite probably, it is the result of changes in lifestyle, particularly for diet and hygiene, occurring in younger generations. The effect of a changing lifestyle and diet on gastric cancer risk is clearly illustrated by studies of migrants. Migrant populations from high-risk parts of the world show a marked diminution in risk when they move to a lower-risk area. The change is quite gradual and seems to depend on age at migration. In Japanese migrants to the United States, there is quite a substantial fall in the risk between the migrant generation and U.S.-born Japanese (124). These data fit with observations concerning the importance of childhood environment in determining risk (125). The dietary changes in Japan to which the decline in gastric cancer risk have been attributed include a decrease in consumption of salted and pickled foods, and an increase in consumption of fruits and vegetables; these have been accompanied by the widespread use of refrigerators for food storage (126). Despite a wealth of observational data, as well as recommendations in most dietary guidelines to increase consumption of green and yellow vegetables and to decrease salt intake, there is little objective evidence that change does actually result in a decrease in cancer risk. However, in a well-known cohort study in Japan, Hirayama not only observed that there was a lower risk of stomach cancer in persons consuming green or yellow vegetables, but also that high-risk subjects, who changed their diet, could benefit from the protective effects (127).

Chemoprevention

Chemoprevention of stomach cancer has been proposed through dietary supplementation with beta-carotene, retinol, alpha-tocopherol, and vitamin C (128–131). In most studies, the design is a double-blind placebo control. The end point is the occurrence of precancerous lesions but not the occurrence of cancer. Some protocols require a preliminary testing for *H. pylori* and eradication of infection in patients with a positive test. In the Linxian Trial, 30,000 adults were randomized to receive eight mineral/vitamin combinations. Significantly lower total mortality occurred among those receiving supplementation with carotene, vitamin E, and selenium (RR = 0.91, $P < 0.03$). The reduction was mainly due to lower cancer rates (RR = 0.87), especially gastric cancer (132).

Two studies have been conducted in Europe: one in various countries in 1,200 persons with vitamin C (128) and the other in Finland (130), with daily supplementation over a period of 5 to 8 years with 50 mg alpha-tocopherol and 20 mg beta-carotene, or a placebo, in a cohort of 29,133 male smokers. All persons were followed for gastric cancer in addition to other end points. In this cohort, 2,132 persons had a low Pg and were invited for gastroscopy. Gastric neoplasia (cancer or dysplasia) was detected in 63 of the 1,344 persons who accepted gastroscopy after 5.1 years of supplementation. Neither alpha-tocopherol nor beta-carotene had any impact on the occurrence of neoplasia. Two prevention trials occurred in South America. A study in Venezuela on 2,200 persons (129) with vitamin C, beta-carotene, and vitamin E has been ongoing since 1996 in 2,200 patients of ages 35 to 69 after the initial eradication of *H. pylori* gave disappointing results. A study in the high-risk area of Colombia involved 852 subjects with confirmed histologic diagnoses of multifocal nonmetaplastic atrophy and/or intestinal metaplasia. Both beta-carotene and ascorbic acid supplementation resulted in significant regression of these preneoplastic lesions after 3 years of follow-up (131). The overall disappointing results of chemoprevention trials suggest that a more complex intervention with multiple factors, including eradication of infection by *H. pylori*, may be required for prevention.

Eradication of *Helicobacter pylori*

H. pylori, the most frequent cause of chronic gastritis, is acknowledged as a factor causing inflammation and atrophy, which are fundamental steps in the carcinogenic process. *H. pylori* infection is curable with relatively simple courses of antibiotics, and this has suggested that eradication of *H. pylori* may be a valuable prevention strategy (133), although the benefit would extend only to distal stomach cancer because proximal stomach cancer, at the cardia, is not related to this infectious factor.

There have been several studies of the effectiveness of treating *H. pylori* in promoting regression or nonprogression of preneoplastic lesions. In a study in Colombia (131), 387 subjects randomized to treatment of *H. pylori* (96% were infected)

showed significantly higher regression of both multifocal non-metaplastic atrophy and intestinal metaplasia compared to the 386 controls, although progression rates were similar. In a longer-term follow-up, a cohort of 795 persons in Colombia (134) with altered gastric mucosa on biopsy (nonatrophic or atrophic gastritis), of whom 97% were infected by *H. pylori*, was randomized for anti–*H. pylori* treatment and/or antioxidants (beta-carotene). Gastric biopsies were obtained at 3, 6, or 12 years. The annual rate of reinfection was 5.4%. In patients who were *H. pylori* negative, the chronic lesions of the gastric mucosa showed less progression and more regression than in patients who were *H. pylori* positive. A smaller study in Mexico (248 subjects randomized to anti–*H. pylori* therapy or control) found that more than three-fourths of treated patients were free of infection at 1 year and had a more favorable histology (index score) than controls (135). In a randomized trial in Japan, the group in whom eradication of *H. pylori* had been performed (1 week combined antibiotic treatment) showed histopathological evidence of regression of inflammation, atrophy, and metaplasia, although there was little apparent change on gastroscopy, compared to the controls (136). In a randomized trial of eradication in China (137), the incidence of gastric cancer development at the population level was similar between participants receiving *H. pylori* eradication treatment and those receiving placebo during a period of 7.5 years follow-up; however, in the subgroup of *H. pylori* carriers without precancerous lesions, eradication of *H. pylori* significantly decreased the development of gastric cancer (0 vs. 6 cases). Other trials are currently underway.

A potential drawback of *H. pylori* eradication lies in the promotion of gastroesophageal reflux (GERD) by preserving the parietal cell mass in the fundic mucosa, and GERD is considered as an etiologic factor in adenocarcinoma at the esophagogastric junction (138).

In practice, eradication strategies would be confined to individuals found to be infected with *H. pylori* through a preliminary screening for anti–*H. pylori* antibody. It has been suggested that this could be a cost-effective strategy for prevention of gastric cancer and other *H. pylori*–related disease (139–141). A simulated cost-effectiveness Markov analysis of a cohort conducted in the United States estimated that population-based *H. pylori* screening and treatment of patients with a positive test could yield some benefit (142). Another U.S. study estimated that the cost would be around $23,900 per life-year gained with the cag-A serology or $25,100 using standard serology, in contrast with much lower values in Japan: $5,100 (143). An Australian simulation analysis (144) concluded that such a program (screening and treatment) would achieve no more of a reduction in incidence of gastric cancer than is likely to occur naturally in a 15-year period.

It must be concluded that further studies of the effectiveness of different strategies of eradication, particularly in preventing cancer in different subgroups, and cost-effectiveness studies are needed before decisions about the desirability of embarking on screening programs that will require rather large-scale medication of the population becomes clearer (145).

An alternative to eradication of *H. pylori* with antibiotic therapy is vaccination. This is a potentially promising approach, especially in developing countries where there is a high prevalence of infection (146). To be effective, vaccination would have to occur during childhood. Various bacterial proteins are being assessed as vaccine candidates; some, such as urease, are involved in bacterial colonization, whereas others, such as the vacuolating cytotoxin vac-A, are involved in the induction of the disease. Two vaccine candidates are being tested: one with the recombinant urease, produced in genetically engineered *Escherichia coli*, and the other with the vac-A toxin. The vaccines have prophylactic effects in animal models and a recent trial in infected humans suggested that the vaccine was immunogenic and well tolerated (147). There is not yet proof that a large-scale vaccination program would be cost effective.

STRATEGIES FOR THE PREVENTION OF STOMACH CANCER

Unplanned prevention is occurring worldwide with a strong impact on incidence and mortality; however, there is still a large number of stomach cancers occurring in the older generations, and absolute numbers of cases are increasing. The two elements for primary prevention depend on a westernized lifestyle during childhood: more fruit and less salt in the diet, and more hygiene to delay and slow down the rate of contamination by *H. pylori*.

An active program of prevention, supported by health authorities, is justified only if the risk for stomach cancer is very high, such as in many countries of East Asia, in the Andean sector of South America, and in some countries in North Europe. Secondary prevention aims at the early detection of cancer through screening, but there is a general belief that concentration on primary prevention is more appropriate, even though there may be debate about whether the most appropriate approach is through dietary change or eradication of *H. pylori*. Trials with vitamin supplementation have not yet proved any efficacy, and vaccination is still in the experimental phase.

In developing countries, priority should be given to education about hygiene and healthy diet. In developed countries with a low risk of stomach cancer, intervention is not a priority, and spontaneous regression is enough. The consensus view is that screening for gastric cancer does not deserve a public health policy in countries other than Japan. The persisting and nonnegligible mortality toll from gastric cancer in the Western world is linked to the poor quality of endoscopic detection outside Japan. The test (*H. pylori*) and treat (eradication) strategy proposed as an alternative to prompt endoscopy in the Western world has a negative impact on the quality standard of the procedure. More emphasis should be given to quality assurance in gastroscopy and to the role of endoscopic exploration in patients with nonalarming digestive symptoms. It should be recalled that a major advantage of screening programs is to draw attention to the early detection and prevention of cancer in other situations. In contrast, to neglect the detection may have a negative impact on daily practices.

In Japan, where the incidence of stomach cancer has been very high, screening is likely to be continued. Cost-effectiveness analyses of x-ray screening has been conducted in Miyagi (80) and present marginal costs (screening program vs. none) per "lives saved" for the Japanese program, the assumptions were 85% sensitivity and 90% specificity of the examination, and 70% survival of screen-detected cancer versus 25% survival in those diagnosed with symptoms. As compared to colorectal cancer screening in the same country, the cost per life saved was considered to be five times less for men and two to three times less for women. However, most of this difference can be accounted for by the incidence of gastric cancer being, at the time of the analysis, considerably higher than that of colon cancer in Japan. This situation has dramatically changed, and the incidence of large bowel cancer in Japan is now among the highest in the world (148). Other indicators point to a decrease in cost effectiveness in Japan, and the photofluorography-endoscopy sequence could be replaced by a less costly and probably as effective Pg test-endoscopy sequence. The age groups proposed for screening should also be revised—it has been suggested that interventions are not cost effective for the age classes younger than 50 years (149). Finally, the direct effects of the screening program for stomach cancer in Japan are limited to the 10%

of all incident cases detected by screening. In contrast, the program had an indirect advertising impact in Japan, resulting in a general improvement of all other situations of detection. This is an important consideration not taken into account in the evaluation of cost effectiveness in Japan and other countries.

References

1. Parkin DM, Bray F, Ferlay J, Pisani P. Global cancer statistics, 2002. *CA Cancer J Clin* 2005;55:74–108.
2. Parkin DM, Whelan SL, Ferlay J, Teppo L, Thomas DB, eds. *Cancer Incidence in Five Continents Vol VIII*. IARC Scientific Publication No. 155. Lyon, France: IARC Press; 2003.
3. Parkin DM, Bray F, Devesa S. Cancer burden in the year 2000: the global picture. *Eur J Cancer* 2001;37:S4–S66.
4. The Research Group for Population Based Cancer Registration in Japan. Cancer incidence in Japan, 1985–89: re-estimation based on data from eight population based cancer register. *Jpn J Clin Oncol* 1998;28:54–67.
5. Fujimoto I, Hanai A, Oshima A, et al. *Cancer Incidence and Mortality in Osaka, 1963–1989*. Tokyo: Shinohara; 1993.
6. Ajiki W, Tsukuma H, Oshima A. Cancer incidence rates in Japan in 1999: estimates based on data from 11 population-based cancer registries. *Jpn J Clin Oncol* 2004;34:352–356.
7. Devesa SS, Blot WJ, Fraumeni JF. Changing patterns in the incidence of esophageal and gastric carcinoma in the United States. *Cancer* 1998;83:2049–2053.
8. Ekstrom AM, Signorello LB, Hansson LE, Bergstrom R, Lindgren A, Nyren O. Evaluating gastric cancer misclassification: a potential explication for the rise in cardia cancer incidence. *J Natl Cancer Inst* 1999;91:786–789.
9. Ries LAG, Eisner MP, Kosary CL, et al., eds. *SEER Cancer Statistics Review, 1975–2002*. Bethesda, Md.: National Cancer Institute; 2005.
10. Sant M, Aareleid T, Berrino F, et al. EUROCARE-3: survival of cancer patients diagnosed 1990–94—results and commentary. *Ann Oncol* 2003;14(suppl 5):v61–v118.
11. Hundahl SA, Menck HR, Mansour EG, Winchester DP. The National Cancer Data Base report on gastric carcinoma. *Cancer* 1997;80:2333–2341.
12. Sankaranarayanan R, Black RJ, Parkin DM, eds. *Cancer Survival in Developing Countries*. IARC Scientific Publication No. 145. Lyon, France: IARC; 1998.
13. Osaka Cancer Registry. *Survival of Cancer Patients in Osaka (1975–89)*. Tokyo: Shinohara; 1998.
14. Hanai A, Tsukuma H, Hiyama T, Fujimoto I. Survival of patients with stomach cancer: results from population based cancer registries. In: Sugimura T, Sasako M, eds. *Gastric Cancer*. Oxford: Oxford University Press; 1997:1–30.
15. Howson CP, Hiyama T, Wynder EL. The decline in gastric cancer: epidemiology of an unplanned triumph. *Epidemiol Rev* 1986;8:1–27.
16. Lambert R, Guilloux A, Oshima A, et al. Incidence and mortality from stomach cancer in Japan, Slovenia and USA. *Int J Cancer* 2002;97:811–818.
17. Bunt AM, Hermans S, Smit VT, van de Velde CJ, Fleuren GJ, Bruijn JA. Surgical pathologic stage migration confounds comparison of gastric cancer survival rates between Japan and Western countries. *J Clin Oncol* 1995;13:19–25.
18. Yang L. Incidence and mortality of gastric cancer in China. *World J Gastroenterol* 2006;12:17–20.
19. Leung WK, Ng EK, Chan WY, et al. Risk factors associated with the development of intestinal metaplasia in first-degree relatives of gastric cancer patients. *Cancer Epidemiol Biomarkers Prev* 2005;14:2982–2886.
20. Guilford P, Hopkins J, Grady W, et al. E-cadherin germline mutations define an inherited cancer syndrome dominated by diffuse gastric cancer. *Hum Mutat* 1999;14:249–255.
21. Gayther SA, Gorringe KL, Ramus SJ, et al. Identification of germ-line E-cadherin mutations in gastric cancer families of European origin. *Cancer Res* 1998;58:4086–4089.
22. Aarnio M, Salovaara R, Aaltonen LA, Mecklin JP, Jarvinen HJ. Features of gastric cancer in hereditary non-polyposis colorectal cancer syndrome. *Int J Cancer* 1997;74:551–555.
23. Carneiro F, Amado M, Lago P, et al. *Helicobacter pylori* infection and blood groups. *Am J Gastroenterol* 1996;91:2646–2647.
24. Hill MJ. Diet and cancer: a review of scientific evidence. *Eur J Cancer Prev* 1995;4(suppl 2):3–42.
25. Hirohata T, Kono S. Diet/nutrition and stomach cancer in Japan. *Int J Cancer* 1997;(suppl 10):34–36.
26. Inoue M, Tajima K, Kobayashi S, et al. Protective factor against progression from atrophic gastritis to gastric cancer—data from a cohort study in Japan. *Int J Cancer* 1996;66:309–314.
27. Vainio H, Bianchini F, eds. *IARC Handbooks of Cancer Prevention, Vol 8: Fruit and Vegetables*. Lyon, France: IARC Press; 2003.
28. International Agency for Research on Cancer (IARC). *IARC Monographs on the Evaluation of Carcinogenic Risks to Humans, Vol 83: Tobacco Smoke and Involuntary Smoking*. Lyon, France: IARC Press; 2004.

29. International Agency for Research on Cancer (IARC). *IARC Monographs on the Evaluation of Carcinogenic Risks to Humans, Vol 44: Alcohol Drinking.* Lyon, France: IARC; 1988.

30. Terry MB, Gaudet MM, Gammon MD. The epidemiology of gastric cancer. *Semin Radiat Oncol* 2002;12:111–127.

31. International Agency for Research on Cancer (IARC). *IARC Monographs on the Evaluation of Carcinogenic Risks to Humans, Vol 61: Schistosomes, Liver Flukes and Helicobacter pylori.* Lyon, France: IARC Press; 1994:177–240.

32. Huang J-Q, Sridhar S, Chen Y, Hunt RH. Meta-analysis of the relationship between *Helicobacter pylori* seropositivity and gastric cancer. *Gastroenterology* 1998;114:1169–1179.

33. Eslick GD, Lim LL, Byles JE, Xia HH, Talley NJ. Association of *Helicobacter pylori* infection with gastric carcinoma: a meta-analysis. *Am J Gastroenterol* 1999;94:2373–2379.

34. Danesh, J. *Helicobacter pylori* infection and gastric cancer: systematic review of the epidemiological studies. *Aliment Pharmacol Ther* 1999;13:851–856.

35. Helicobacter and Cancer Collaborative Group. Gastric cancer and *Helicobacter pylori*: a combined analysis of 12 case-control studies nested within prospective cohorts. *Gut* 2001;49:347–353.

36. Parkin DM. The global health burden of infection-associated cancers in the year 2002. *Int J Cancer* 2006;118:3030–3044.

37. Webb PM, Knight T, Greaves S, et al. Relation between infection with *Helicobacter pylori* and living conditions in childhood: evidence for person to person transmission in early life. *BMJ* 1994;308:750–753.

38. Kikuchi S, Ohgihara A, Hasegawa A, Miki K, Kaneko E, Mizukochi H. Seroconversion and seroreversion of *Helicobacter pylori* antibodies over a 9-year period and related factors in Japanese adults. *Helicobacter* 2004;9:335–341.

39. Holcombe C. *Helicobacter pylori*: the African enigma. *Gut* 1992;33:429–431.

40. Parkin DM, Ferlay J, Hamdi-Chérif M, et al, eds. *Cancer in Africa: Epidemiology and Prevention.* IARC Scientific Publication No. 153. Lyon, France: IARC Press; 2003.

41. Agha A, Graham DY. Evidence-based examination of the African enigma in relation to *Helicobacter pylori* infection. *Scand J Gastroenterol* 2005;40:523–529.

42. Kosunen TU, Aromaa A, Knekt P, et al. *Helicobacter* antibodies in 1973 and 1994 in the adult population of Vammala, Finland. *Epidemiol Infect* 1997;119:29–34.

43. Roosendaal R, Kuipers EJ, Buitenwerf J, et al. *Helicobacter pylori* and the birth cohort effect: evidence of a continuous decrease of infection rates in childhood. *Am J Gastroenterol* 1997;92:1480–1482.

44. Banatvala N, Mayo K, Megraud F, Jennings R, Deeks JJ, Feldman RA. The cohort effect and *Helicobacter pylori*. *J Infect Dis* 1993;168:219–221.

45. Perez-Perez GI, Salomaa A, Kosunen TU, et al. Evidence that cagA(+) *Helicobacter pylori* strains are disappearing more rapidly than cagA(–) strains. *Gut* 2002;50:295–298.

46. Shimoyama T, Tominaga Y, Sagakami T, Fukuda Y. Epidemiological study for infection with *H. pylori* in Japan compared with that in the USA, Europe and Asian Pacific area. *Nippon Rinsho* 1999;57:11–16.

47. Kobayashi T, Kikushi S, Lin Y, et al. Trends in the incidence of gastric cancer in Japan and their associations with *Helicobacter pylori* infection and gastric mucosal atrophy. *Gastric Cancer* 2004;7:233–239.

48. Tomb JF, White O, Kerlavage AR, et al. The complete genome sequence of the gastric pathogen *Helicobacter pylori*. *Nature* 1997;388:539–547.

49. Bravo LE, van Doom LJ, Realpe JL, Correa P. Virulence-associated genotypes of *Helicobacter pylori*: do they explain the African enigma? *Am J Gastroenterol* 2002;97:2839–2842.

50. Kuipers EJ, Perez-Perez GI, Meuwissen SGM, Blaser MJ. *Helicobacter pylori* and atrophic gastritis: importance of the CagA status. *J Natl Cancer Inst* 1995;87:1777–1780.

51. Blaser MJ, Perez-Perez GI, Kleanthous H, et al. Infection with *Helicobacter pylori* strains possessing cagA is associated with an increased risk of developing adenocarcinoma of the stomach. *Cancer Res* 1995;55:2111–2115.

52. Watanabe T, Tada M, Nagai H, Sasaki S, Nakao M. *Helicobacter pylori* infection induces gastric cancer in mongolian gerbils. *Gastroenterology* 1998;115:642–648.

53. Kato S, Onda M, Matsukura N, et al. *Helicobacter pylori* infection and genetic polymorphisms for cancer related genes in gastric carcinogenesis. *Biomed Pharmacother* 1997;51:145–149.

54. Correa P, Miller MJ. Carcinogenesis, apoptosis and cell proliferation. *Br Med Bull* 1998;54:151–162.

55. Grisham MB, Ware K, Gilleland HEJ, Gilleland LB, Abell CL, Yamada T. Neutrophil-mediated nitrosamine formation: role of nitric oxide in rats. *Gastroenterology* 1992;103:1260–1266.

56. Mannick EE, Bravo LE, Zarama G, et al. Inducible nitric oxide synthase, nitrotyrosine, and apoptosis in *Helicobacter pylori* gastritis: effect of antibiotics and antioxidants. *Cancer Res* 1996;56:3238–3243.

57. Felley CP, Pignatelli B, Van Melle GD, et al. Oxidative stress in gastric mucosa of asymptomatic humans infected with *Helicobacter pylori*: effect of bacterial eradication. *Helicobacter* 2002;7:342–348.

58. Pignatelli B, Bancel B, Plummer M, Toyokuni S, Patricot LM, Ohshima H. *Helicobacter pylori* eradication attenuates oxidative stress in human gastric mucosa. *Am J Gastroenterol* 2001;96:1758–1766.

59. Correa P, Haenszel W, Cuello C, et al. Gastric precancerous process in a high risk population: cohort follow-up. *Cancer Res* 1990;50:4737–4740.

60. Correa P. Human gastric carcinogenesis: a multistep and multifactorial process-first American Cancer Society Award lecture on cancer epidemiology and prevention. *Cancer Res* 1992;52:6735–6740.

61. Sipponen P, Riihela M, Hyvarinen H, Seppala K. Chronic nonatrophic ('superficial') gastritis increases the risk of gastric carcinoma: a case control study. *Scand J Gastroenterol* 1994;29:336–340.

62. Sipponen P, Kimura K. Intestinal metaplasia, atrophic gastritis and stomach cancer: trends over time. *Eur J Gastroenterol Hepatol* 1994;6(suppl 1):S79–S83.

63. Hamilton SR, Aaltonen LA, eds. *Pathology & Genetics: Tumours of the Digestive System.* Lyon, France: IARC Press; 2000.

64. Tsukaemia H, Mishima T, Oshima A. Prospective study of 'early' gastric cancer. *Int J Cancer* 1983;31:421–426.

65. Schlemper RJ, Itabashi M, Kato Y, et al. Differences in diagnostic criteria for gastric carcinoma between Japanese and Western pathologists. *Lancet* 1997;349:1725–1729.

66. Lauren P. The two histological main types of gastric carcinoma: diffuse and so-called intestinal-type carcinoma. *Acta Pathol Microbiol Scand* 1965;64:31–49.

67. Muñoz N, Correa P, Cuello C, Duque E. Histologic types of gastric carcinoma in high- and low-risk areas. *Int J Cancer* 1968;3(6):809–818.

68. Hanai A, Fujimoto I, Taniguchi H. Trends on stomach cancer incidence and histological types in Osaka. In: Magnus K, ed. *Trends in Cancer Incidence.* New York, NY: McGraw-Hill; 1982:143–154.

69. Correa P, Chen VW. Gastric cancer. *Cancer Surv* 1994;19–20:55–76.

70. Chan MF. Complications of upper gastrointestinal endoscopy. *Gastrointest Endosc Clin N Am* 1996;6:287–303.

71. Endoscopic Classification Review Group. Update on the Paris classification of superficial neoplastic lesions in the digestive tract. *Endoscopy* 2005;37(6):570–578.

72. Hosokova O, Tsuda S, Kidani E, et al. Diagnosis of gastric cancer up to three years after negative upper GI endoscopy. *Endoscopy* 1998;30:669–674.

73. Lambert R. The role of endoscopy in the prevention of esophagogastric cancer. *Endoscopy* 1999;31:180–199.

74. Lambert R. Digestive endoscopy: relevance of negative findings. *Ital J Gastroenterol Hepatol* 1999;31:761–772.

75. Axon ATR. Chronic dyspepsia: who needs endoscopy? *Gastroenterology* 1998;112:1376–1380.

76. Oshima A, Hirata N, Ubukata T, Umeda K, Fujimoto L. Evaluation of a mass screening program for stomach cancer with a case-control study design. *Int J Cancer* 1986;38:829–833.

77. Oshima A. Screening for stomach cancer: the Japanese program. In: Chamberlain J, Miller AB, eds. *Screening for Gastrointestinal Cancer.* Toronto, Ontario, Canada: Hans Huber; 1988:65–70.

78. Oshima A. Secondary prevention: screening methods in high incidence areas. In: Sugimura T, Sasaki M, eds. *Gastric Cancer.* Oxford: Oxford University Press; 1997:199–212.

79. Yamagata S, Sugawara N, Hisamichi S. Mass screening for cancer in Japan—present and future. In: Yamagata S, Hirayama T, Hisamichi S, eds. *Recent Advances in Cancer Control: Proceedings of 6th Asia Pacific Cancer Conference, Sendai, Japan, September 23–30, 1983.* Amsterdam: Excepta Medica; 1983.

80. Hisamichi S, Fukao A, Sugawara N, et al. Evaluation of mass screening programme for stomach cancer in Japan. In: Miller AB, Chamberlain J, Day NE, Hakama M, Prorok PC, eds. *Cancer Screening.* Cambridge: Cambridge University Press; 1991:357–370.

81. Murakami R, Tsukuma H, Ubukata T, et al. Estimation of validity of mass screening program for gastric cancer in Osaka, Japan. *Cancer* 1990;65:1255–1260.

82. Kawai K, Watanabe Y. The impact of mass screening on gastric cancer mortality in Japan. *Gastrointest Endosc* 1998;47:320–322.

83. Shiga T, Nishizawa M, Hosoi K, et al. Evaluation of gastric mass survey from the point of view of the prevalence of gastric cancer among seemingly healthy individuals. *Stom Intest* 1991;26:1371–1387.

84. Fukao A, Hisamichi S, Kamatsu S, Sugawara N, Takano A. Risk of leukaemia among participants of gastric mass screening survey in Japan: a population-based case control study. *Cancer Detect Prev* 1992;16:283–286.

85. Hakama M, Stenman UH, Knekt P, et al. Tumour markers and screening for gastrointestinal cancer: a follow up study in Finland. *J Med Screen* 1994;I:60–64.

86. Samloff IM, Varis K, Ibamaki T, Sicerala M, Rotter JI. Relationships among serum pepsinogen I, serum pepsinogen II and gastric mucosal histology: a study in relatives of patients with pernicious anemia. *Gastroenterology* 1982;83:204–209.

87. Ning PF, Liu HJ, Yuan Y. Dynamic expression of pepsinogen C in gastric cancer, precancerous lesions and *Helicobacter pylori* associated gastric diseases. *World J Gastroenterol* 2005;11:2545–2548.

88. Westerveld BD, Pals G, Lamers CBHW, et al. Clinical significance of pepsinogen A isozymogens, serum pepsinogen A and C levels, and serum gastrin levels. *Cancer* 1987;59:952–958.

89. Miki K, Ichinose M, Shimizu A, et al. Serum pepsinogens as a screening test of extensive chronic gastritis. *Gastroenterol Jpn* 1987;22:133–141.

90. Nomura AM, Stemmermann GN, Samloff IM. Serum pepsinogen I as a predictor of stomach cancer. *Ann Intern Med* 1980;93:537–540.

91. Stemmermann GN, Samloff LM, Normura AMY, Heilbrun LK. Serum pepsinogens I and II and stomach cancer. *Clin Chim Acta* 1987;163:191–198.

92. Aromaa A, Kosunen TU, Knekt P, et al. Circulating anti-*Helicobacter pylori* immunoglobulin A antibodies and low serum pepsinogen I level are associated with increased risk of gastric cancer. *Am J Epidemiol* 1996;144:142–149.

93. Watabe H, Mitsushima T, Yamaji Y, et al. Predicting the development of gastric cancer from combining *Helicobacter pylori* antibodies and serum pepsinogen status: a prospective endoscopic cohort study. *Gut* 2005;54:764–768.

94. Urita Y, Hike K, Torri N, et al. Serum pepsinogens as a predicator of the topography of intestinal metaplasia in patients with atrophic gastritis. *Dig Dis Sci* 2004;49:795–801.

95. Parsonnet J, Friedman GD, Vandersteen DP, et al. *Helicobacter pylori* infection and the risk of gastric carcinoma. *N Engl J Med* 1991;325:1127–1131.

96. Brenner H, Arndt V, Stegmaier C, Ziegler H, Rothenbacher D. Is *Helicobacter pylori* infection a necessary condition for noncardia gastric cancer? *Am J Epidemiol* 2004;159:252–258.

97. Nomura AM, Kolonel LN, Miki K, et al. *Helicobacter pylori*, pepsinogen, and gastric adenocarcinoma in Hawaii. *J Infect Dis* 2005;191:2075–2081.

98. Ohata H, Kitauchi S, Yoshimura N, et al. Progression of chronic atrophic gastritis associated with *Helicobacter pylori* infection increases risk of gastric cancer. *Int J Cancer* 2004;109:138–143.

99. Kuroishi T, Hirose K, Nakagawa N, Tominaga S. Comparison of time trends of stomach cancer death rates between the model area of the screening program and the control area. *J Gastroenterol* 1983;58:45–52.

100. National Report of the Group Medical Examinations for Digestive Cancer in 1995. *J Gastroenterol Mass Survey* 1998;36:251–269.

101. Oshima A, Hanai A, Fujimoto L. Evaluation of a mass screening program for stomach cancer. *NCI Monogr* 1979;53:181–186.

102. Fukao A, Hisamichi S, Komatsu S, et al. Comparison of characteristics between frequent participants and non–participants in screening program for stomach cancer. *Tohoku J Exp Med* 1992;166:459–469.

103. Inaba S, Hirayama H, Nagata C, et al. Evaluation of a screening program on reduction of gastric cancer mortality in Japan: preliminary results from a cohort study. *Prev Med* 1999;29:102–106.

104. Tsubono Y, Nishino Y, Tsuji I, Hisamichi S. Screening for gastric cancer in Miyagi, Japan: evaluation with a population-based cancer registry. *Asian Pac J Cancer Prev* 2000;1:57–60.

105. Lee KJ, Inoue M, Otani T, Iwasaki M, Sasakusi S, Tsugana S. Gastric cancer screening and subsequent risk of gastric cancer: a large-scale population-based cohort study, with a 13-year follow-up in Japan. *Int J Cancer* 2006;118:2315–2321.

106. Fukao A, Hisamichi S, Sugawara N. A case-control study on evaluating the effect of mass screening on decreasing advanced stomach cancer. *J Gastroenterol* 1987;75:112–116.

107. Fukao A, Tsubono Y, Tsuji L, Hisamichi S, Sugahara N, Takano A. The evaluation of screening for gastric cancer in Miyagi Prefecture, Japan: a population-based case-control study. *Int J Cancer* 1995;60:45–48.

108. Pisani P, Oliver WE, Parkin DM, Alvarez N, Vivas J. Case-control study of gastric cancer screening in Venezuela. *Br J Cancer* 1994;69:1102–1105.

109. Kitahara F, Kobayashi H, Sato T, Kojima Y, Araki T, Fujino MA. Accuracy of screening for gastric cancer using serum pepsinogen concentrations. *Gut* 1999;44:693–697.

110. Yoshihara M, Sumii K, Haruma K, et al. The usefulness of gastric mass screening using serum pepsinogen levels compared with photofluorography. *Hiroshima J Med Sci* 1997;46:81–86.

111. Aoki K, Misumi J, Kimura T, Zhao W, Xie T. Evaluation of cut off levels for screening of gastric cancer using serum pepsinogens and distributions of levels of serum pepsinogen I, II and of PGI/PGII ratios in a gastric cancer case control study. *J Epidemiol* 1997;7:143–151.

112. Kodoi A, Yoshihara M, Sumii K, Haruma K, Kajuyama G. Serum pepsinogen in screening for gastric cancer. *J Gastroenterol* 1995;30:452–560.

113. Kurosawa M, Kikuchi S, Arisue T, Fukao A. Effectiveness and feasibility of a strategy for increasing participation in the Japanese Stomach Cancer Examination programs by incorporating serum pepsinogen tests. *Nippon Koshu Eisei Zasshi* 1998;45:352–360.

114. Parsonnet J, Samloff IM, Nelson LM, Orentreich N, Vogelman JH, Friedman GD. *Helicobacter pylori*, pepsinogen, and risk for gastric adenocarcinoma. *Cancer Epidemiol Biomarkers Prev* 1993;2:461–466.

115. Miki K, Ichinose M, Ishikawa KB, et al. Clinical application of serum pepsinogen I and II levels for mass screening to detect gastric cancer. *Jpn J Cancer Res* 1993;84:1086–1090.

116. Hattori Y, Tashiro H, Kawamoto T, Kodama Y. Sensitivity and specificity of mass screening for gastric cancer using the measurement of serum pepsinogens. *Jpn J Cancer Res* 1995;86:1210–1215.

117. Ohata H, Oka M, Yanaoka K, et al. Gastric cancer screening of a high-risk population in Japan using serum pepsinogen and barium digital radiography. *Cancer Sci* 2005;96:713–720.

118. Oishi Y, Kiyohara Y, Kubo M, et al. The serum pepsinogen test as a predictor of gastric cancer. *Am J Epidemiol* 2006;163:629–637.

119. Miki K, Morita M, Sasajima M, Hoshina R, Kanda E, Urita Y. Usefulness of gastric cancer screening using the serum pepsinogen test method. *Am J Gastroenterol* 2003;98:735–739.

120. Greene FL. Management of gastric remnant carcinoma based on the results of a 15 year endoscopic screening program. *Ann Surg* 1996;223:701–706.

121. Mellemkjoer L, Gridley G, Moller H, et al. Pernicious anemia and cancer risk in Denmark. *Br J Cancer* 1996;73:998–1000.

122. Kokkola A, Sjoblom SM, Haapiainen R, Sipponen P, Puolakkainen P, Jarvinen H. The risk of gastric carcinoma and carcinoid tumours in patients with pernicious anaemia: a prospective follow up study. *Scand J Gastroenterol* 1998;33:88–92.

123. Hsing AW, Hansson LE, McLaughin JK, et al. Pernicious anemia and subsequent cancer: a population based cohort study. *Cancer* 1993;71:745–750.

124. Kolonel LN, Nomura AM, Hirohata T, Hankin JH, Hinds MW. Association of diet and place of birth with stomach cancer incidence in Hawaii Japanese and Caucasians. *Am J Clin Nutr* 1981;34:2478–2485.

125. Coggon D, Osmond C, Barker DJ. Stomach cancer and migration within England and Wales. *Br J Cancer* 1990;61:573–574.

126. Tominaga S. Decreasing trend of stomach cancer in Japan. *Jpn J Cancer Res* 1987;78:1–10.

127. Hirayama T. Does daily intake of green-yellow vegetables reduce the risk of cancer in man? An example of the application of epidemiological methods to the identification of individuals at low risk. In: Bartsch H, Armstrong B, eds. *Host Factors in Human Carcinogenesis*. IARC Scientific Publication No. 39. Lyon, France: IARC Press; 1982:531–540.

128. Buiatti E, Munoz N. Chemoprevention of stomach cancer. In: Hakama M, et al., eds. *Chemoprevention in Cancer Control*. IARC Publication No. 136. Lyon, France: IARC Press; 1996:35–39.

129. Munoz N, Vivas J, Buaitti E, Kato I, Oliver W. *Chemoprevention Trial on Precancerous Lesions of the Stomach in Venezuela: Summary of Study Design and Baseline Data*. IARC Scientific Publication No. 139. Lyon, France: IARC; 1996:125–133.

130. Varis K, Taylor PR, Sipponen P, et al. Gastric cancer and premalignant lesions in atrophic gastritis: a controlled trial on the effect of supplementation with alpha tocopherol and beta-carotene. The Helsinki Gastritis Study Group. *Scand J Gastroenterol* 1998;33:294–300.

131. Correa P, Fontham ET, Bravo JC, et al. Chemoprevention of gastric dysplasia: randomized trial of antioxidant supplements and anti-*Helicobacter pylori* therapy. *J Natl Cancer Inst* 2000;92:1881–1888.

132. Blot WJ, Li J-Y, Taylor PR, et al. Nutrition intervention trials in Linxian, China: supplementation with specific vitamin/mineral combinations, cancer incidence and disease-specific mortality in the general population. *J Natl Cancer Inst* 1993;85:1483–1492.

133. Graham DY, Shiotani A. The time to eradicate gastric cancer is now. *Gut* 2005;54:735–738.

134. Mera R, Fontham ET, Bravo LE, et al. Long term follow up of patients treated for *Helicobacter pylori* infection. *Gut* 2005;54:1536–1540.

135. Ley C, Mohar A, Guarner J, et al. *Helicobacter pylori* eradication and gastric preneoplastic conditions: a randomized, double-blind, placebo-controlled trial. *Cancer Epidemiol Biomarkers Prev* 2004;13:4–10.

136. Saito D. [*H. pylori* infection and gastric cancer: Japanese intervention trial.] *Nippon Rinsho* 2005;63(suppl 11):35–40.

137. Wong BC, Lam SK, Wong WM, et al. *Helicobacter pylori* eradication to prevent gastric cancer in a high-risk region of China: a randomized controlled trial. *JAMA* 2004;291:187–194.

138. Spechler SJ. The role of gastric carditis in metaplasia and neoplasia at the gastroesophageal junction. *Gastroenterology* 1999;117:21888–218228.

139. Parsonnet J, Harris RA, Hack HM, Owens DK. Modelling cost-effectiveness of *Helicobacter pylori* screening to prevent gastric cancer: a mandate for clinical trials. *Lancet* 1996;348:150–154.

140. Mason J, Axon AT, Forman D, et al. The cost-effectiveness of population *Helicobacter pylori* screening and treatment: a Markov model using economic data from a randomized controlled trial. Leeds HELP Study Group. *Aliment Pharmacol Ther* 2002;16:559–568.

141. Wang Q, Jin PH, Lin GW, Xu SR, Chen J. Cost-effectiveness of *Helicobacter pylori* screening to prevent gastric cancer: Markov decision analysis (in Chinese). *Zhonghua Liu Xing Bing Xue Za Zhi* 2003;24:135–139.

142. Fendrick AM, Chernew ME, Hirth RA, Bloom BS, Bandekar RR, Scheiman JM. Clinical and economic effects of population based *Helicobacter pylori* screening to prevent gastric cancer. *Arch Intern Med* 1999;159:142–148.

143. Harris RA, Owens DK, Wittherell H, Parsonnet J. *Helicobacter pylori* and gastric cancer: what are the benefits of screening only for the CagA phenotype of *H. pylori*? *Helicobacter* 1999;4:69–76.

144. Forbes GM, Threlfall TJ. Treatment of *Helicobacter pylori* infection to reduce gastric cancer incidence: uncertain benefits of a community based programme in Australia. *J Gastroenterol Hematol* 1998;13:1091–1095.

145. Parsonnet J, Forman D. *Helicobacter pylori* infection and gastric cancer—for want of more outcomes. *JAMA* 2004;291:244–245.

146. Chui SY, Clay TM, Lyerly HK, Morse MA. The development of therapeutic and preventive vaccines for gastric cancer and *Helicobacter pylori*. *Cancer Epidemiol Biomarkers Prev* 2005;14:1883–1889.

147. Michetti P. Oral immunization with urease and *Escherichia coli* heat labile enterotoxin is safe and immunogenic in *Helicobacter pylori*-infected adults. *Gastroenterology* 1999;116:804–812.

148. Ferlay J, Bray F, Pisani P, Parkin DM. *GLOBOCAN 2002: Cancer Incidence, Mortality and Prevalence*. Worldwide IARC Cancer Base No. 5, Version 2.0. Lyon, France: IARC Press; 2004.

149. Babazono A, Hillman AL. Declining cost effectiveness of screening for disease: the case of gastric cancer in Japan. *Int J Technol Assess Health Care* 1995;11:354–364.

CHAPTER 20 ■ GASTRIC CANCER: MOLECULAR BIOLOGY AND GENETICS

RAJNISH MISHRA AND STEVEN M. POWELL

INTRODUCTION

General Epidemiology

Gastric carcinoma remains one of the world's most common cancers and a leading cause of cancer death worldwide (1). Global estimates suggest that 933,937 new cases of gastric carcinoma will be diagnosed and 700,349 will die from this disease each year (2). The American Cancer Society projects that 21,760 new cases of gastric cancer will be diagnosed in the United States this year (2). Neoplasia of the stomach is largely composed of adenocarcinomas, accounting for more than 95% of cases. Primary lymphoma, stromal tumors (i.e., leiomyosarcoma, liposarcoma), and carcinoid tumors can also arise in the stomach, but malignant tumors of these types do not occur as often.

Interestingly, a sharp increase in incidence of gastroesophageal junction adenocarcinomas was recently noted in the white male population of the United States as well as in other populations (3,4). Significant geographic variability in incidence both intra- and internationally is observed (5). Epidemiologic studies that include migration and temporal analyses indicate that environmental factors, especially in the first decades of life, are important in the etiology of gastric cancers (6,7). Notably, a consistent predominance (2:1 ratio) of gastric cancers in males is seen worldwide. With such a temporal and regional variation in gastric cancer incidence rates, a better understanding of these phenomena through molecular studies of gastric tumorigenesis will provide important insights into cancer development in general, and it is anticipated to lead to earlier diagnosis and better management options in combating this devastating cancer. In addition, multiple gastric tumor pathological classification systems have been formulated in efforts to identify various subgroups with different biological behavior and prognostic indicators. Molecular markers should help facilitate the classification of the various subgroups of gastric carcinomas.

Helicobacter pylori infection appears to lead to a five- to sixfold increase in risk of gastric malignancy, both adenocarcinoma and primary non-Hodgkin lymphoma (8,9). Yet, most of those infected with this micro-organism do not develop gastric cancer. Evidence of Epstein-Barr virus infection has been noted in a small proportion of gastric carcinomas, especially those that exhibit lymphoepithelial histopathology. The relative importance of bacterial virulence factors, environmental factors, and host factors (i.e., age of acquisition, immune responses, acid secretion changes) involved in the clinical outcome of these infections and other environmental exposures are currently pressing issues, and molecular studies may help discern the true influential factors. Indeed, Park et al. noted that gene–environment interactions between CYP2E1 gene polymorphism and smoking may alter the susceptibility for cancer development in the stomach (10).

Host Observations

A population association study recently demonstrated the more frequent occurrence (54%) of the human leukocyte antigen (HLA) DQB1*0301 allele in Caucasian patients with gastric cancer than in a control noncancerous group (27%) (11). If confirmed not to represent ethnic heterogeneity, this association may imply that this locus itself directly influences susceptibility to gastric cancer development or is a marker in linkage disequilibrium with a nearby cancer-predisposing locus. In another study, the frequency of allele DQB1*0401 was significantly higher in those infected with *H. pylori* who developed atrophic gastritis than in those who were infected and did not develop atrophic gastritis or those not infected (12). The potential role of the HLA locus in gastric tumorigenesis has implications for the importance of a potential escape mechanism from immune surveillance as a causative factor for this disease. The fact that most people with these alleles do not develop gastric cancer illustrates the complexity of this multifactorial disease.

Of note, the blood group A phenotype was reported to be associated with gastric cancers in the 1950s (13,14). Interestingly, *H. pylori* was shown to adhere to the Lewis blood group antigen, indicating a potentially important host factor that might facilitate this chronic infection and subsequent risk of gastric cancer (15). In addition, small variant alleles of a mucin gene, *Muc1*, were found to be associated with gastric cancer patients compared to a blood donor control population (16). Confirmation or studies demonstrating the relevance of these findings are still awaited. In fact, a recent study found no correlation between blood group phenotype including A and Lewis and the occurrence of gastric cancer (17).

Several precursor lesions have been identified in the development of intestinal-type gastric carcinomas (18). Dysplasia is generally regarded as a true precancerous lesion; however, the magnitude of atrophic gastritis and intestinal metaplastic (incomplete type) lesions as precancerous lesion remains to be defined. Although an association of chronic atrophic gastritis and gastric intestinal metaplasia has been observed in patients with gastric carcinoma, most individuals harboring these lesions do not develop gastric cancers (19). Furthermore, a low serum pepsinogen 1-to-pepsinogen 2 ratio has been used to identify patients harboring gastric atrophy (20).

Familial Epidemiology

Most cases of gastric cancer appear to occur sporadically without an obvious inherited component. It is estimated that as many as 8% to 10% of gastric cancer cases are related to an inherited familial component (21). Familial clustering has been observed in 12% to 25% of gastric carcinoma cases and dominant inheritance patterns observed (22,23). Notably, Napoleon Bonaparte was apparently afflicted with gastric cancer involving most of his stomach and may have also had other family members (e.g., father, sister) afflicted with this cancer (24,25). In the Swedish Family Cancer Database, which is the largest study of familial gastric cancer published to date, the standardized incident rates were 1.31 (95% confidence interval [CI], 0.97–1.70) and 1.7 (95% CI, 1.08–1.92) when a patient presented with gastric carcinoma. Risk was 1.59 (95% CI, 1.10–2.16) in offspring whose diagnosis was at an age younger than 50 years (26).

Case-control studies have observed consistent, up to three-fold increases in risk for gastric cancer among relatives of gastric cancer patients (23,27). A population-based control study found increased risk for gastric cancer when first-degree relatives were affected (OR = 1.7 with a parent, OR = 2.6 with a sibling), with the risk increasing (OR up to 8.5) if more than one first-degree relative was affected (28). Interestingly, a higher risk was noted in individuals with an affected mother versus an affected father. Studies of monozygotic twins have even shown a slight trend toward increased concordance of gastric cancers compared to dizygotic twins (29,30).

Several genetic susceptibility traits with an inherited predisposition to gastric cancer development are described in this chapter. A few are well-characterized inherited predisposition syndromes potentially involving gastric cancer development, such as hereditary nonpolyposis colorectal cancer (HNPCC). Other clinical entities with a predisposition to gastric tumorigenesis are just being unveiled, such as kindreds manifesting diffuse, poorly differentiated gastric cancers and cosegregating germline E-cadherin alterations.

INHERITED GENETIC SUSCEPTABILITY

E-cadherin in Diffuse Gastric Cancers

Large families with an obvious autosomal dominant, highly penetrant inherited predisposition for the development of gastric cancer, having the potential power to link disease markers, are rare. A large Maroi kindred manifesting early onset diffuse gastric cancers was investigated for linkage analysis, and disease was found to be linked to the E-cadherin/CDH1 locus on 16q and associated with significant mutations in this gene (31). Since then, more than 14 truncating germline E-cadherin mutations have been reported scattered across 8 of the 16 exons this gene encompasses (31–36). The age of onset and diagnosis of diffuse gastric cancer in those who harbored germline mutations of E-cadherin ranged from 14 to 69 years of age. The incomplete penetrance of germline E-cadherin mutation was seen with obligatory carriers who remained unaffected in their eighth and ninth decades of life. One of the larger studies of ten kindreds manifesting diffuse gastric cancers identified three families with germline E-cadherin mutations (32). No germline mutations of this gene were detected in apparent "sporadic" diffuse gastric cancer cases in Britain with a mean age of 62 years (35).

Based on the results of E-cadherin mutation, screening of the probands from 42 new families with diffuse gastric can-

cers, Brooke-Wilson et al. determined that 40% of families with multiple gastric cancers and at least one diffuse gastric cancer diagnosed in an individual younger than 50 years had a pathological germline E-cadherin mutation and thus recommended it as a screening criteria (37). Therefore, genetic counseling for those kindreds manifesting a strong predisposition for the development of diffuse gastric cancer is imperative in their medical management (Fig. 20.1). The diffuse familial gastric cancer families are one of the subgroup of kindreds for which genetic testing can now be offered. It is noteworthy though that two-thirds of hereditary diffuse gastric cancer families reported to date have proved negative for E-cadherin gene mutation (37).

Hereditary Nonpolyposis Colorectal Cancer

A now well-characterized inherited predisposition syndrome that can involve gastric cancer development is HNPCC (38). Germline genetic abnormalities of mismatch repair (MMR) genes underlying this disease entity have been unveiled and include potential tumor development in a variety of tissue types (39). Gastric carcinomas that occur in this setting were predominantly diagnosed at the mean age of 56 years, of the intestinal type, without H. pylori infection detected, and most exhibited microsatellite instability (MSI) in a Finnish HNPCC registry study (40). Renkonen-Sinisalo et al. studied gastric histopathology comparing 73 mutation-positive and 32 mutation-negative families for difference in occurrence of H. pylori, atrophy, inflammation, intestinal metaplasia (IM), and dysplasia. They identified only a single case of duodenal cancer among the mutation-positive individuals, but there was no evidence of gastric neoplastic lesions in either group. Thus, abnormalities of MMR genes rarely cause gastric cancer (41).

Interestingly, the occurrence of gastric cancers associated with HNPCC has decreased, similar to the recent general decline in incidence of gastric cancer in developed countries (42). The isolation and characterization of these predisposing gene alterations should allow better definition of the fraction of gastric cancers that result from this trait. Testing for MSH2 and MLH1 gene alterations is currently readily available and can be used to identify those gastric cancer cases that are part of this specific cancer predisposing trait.

Other Inherited Traits

There has even been a report of gastric carcinoma in an extended Li-Fraumeni kindred with an underlying p53 germline alteration (43). Gastric cancers have also been noted to occur in patients with gastrointestinal polyposis disease entities such as familial adenomatous polyposis (FAP) and Peutz-Jeghers syndrome (PJS) (44,45). Interestingly, an increased risk of gastric cancer associated with FAP (patients with germline APC mutations) has been reported in high-risk regions such as Asia (46), whereas no increased risk was exhibited in other populations (47). Overall, gastric carcinoma is rare in these settings, and the exact contribution of the polyposis and underlying germline alterations of APC (FAP) and LKB1/STK11 (PJS) to gastric cancer development in these cases is unclear.

Rare kindreds exhibiting site-specific gastric cancer predilection have been reported, occasionally associated with other inherited abnormalities (48,49). A constitutional deletion of 18p inherited from her mother with subsequent loss of 18q and the whole chromosome was observed in the gastric carcinoma of a 14-year-old patient with associated mental and cardiac abnormalities, suggesting a predisposing condition (50). A kindred manifesting the autosomal dominant inheritance of familial gastric polyposis and gastric cancer development was demonstrated not to have a germline E-cadherin mutation,

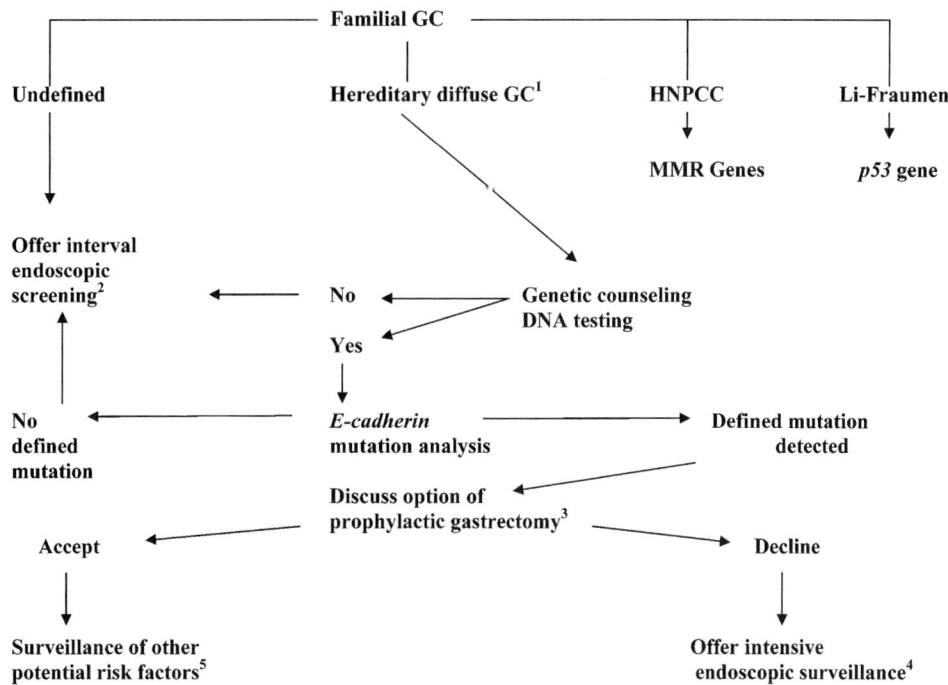

FIGURE 20.1. Algorithm for guidance in managing familial gastric cancer (GC) kindreds. Those identified to meet clinical criteria for hereditary nonpolyposis colon cancer syndrome (HNPCC) and the Li-Fraumeni syndrome are counseled for consideration of genetic testing. MMR, mismatch repair. Microsatellite instability testing can aid in diagnosing HNPCC. [1]This algorithm was initially formulated at the consensus symposia where clinical criteria were generated to define hereditary diffuse gastric cancer: two or more cases in first/second-degree relatives, at least one diagnosed before the age of 50 years, or three or more cases of documented diffuse gastric cancer in first/second-degree relatives (33). [2]Consider individual age-dependent familial expression to determine the initiation, interval, and intensity of screening exams. Prophylactic gastrectomies have been performed in kindreds expressing highly penetrant phenotypes without prior knowledge of causative mutations. [3]Consider age-dependent familial expression in determining management. [4]Endoscopic ultrasound and chromographic (methylene blue or indigo carmine staining) endoscopy can be applied in attempts to increase the sensitivity of detecting early lesions in the stomach. [5]One should have a high index of suspicion for the potential development of other cancers such as that of the breast, colon, and endometrium.

and on linkage analysis, was not linked to 16q, the locus of E-cadherin (32,51). Thus, other loci appear to exist that when altered may predispose an individual to gastric cancer development.

SOMATIC MOLECULAR GENETICS

General

Most molecular analyses of this cancer have involved studies of sporadic tumors for critical, acquired alterations. A detailed, clear working model of gastric tumorigenesis has yet to be formulated. Multiple somatic alterations have been described, but the significance of these changes in gastric tumorigenesis remains to be established in most instances. Molecular studies may provide new avenues for lowering the dismal gastric cancer mortality rate.

Cytogenetic studies of gastric adenocarcinomas are few in number, with a variable number of numerical or structural aberrations, and have failed to identify any consistent or noteworthy chromosomal abnormalities (52,53). Comparative genomic hybridization analyses of xenografted and primary gastric and gastroesophageal junctional adenocarcinomas have revealed several regions of consensus change in DNA copy number that may indicate the location of candidate oncogenes

and tumor suppressor genes involved in gastric tumorigenesis (54,55). Chromosomal arms 4q, 5q, 9p, 17p, and 18q showed frequent decreases in DNA copy number. However, chromosomes 7, 8, and 20q showed frequent increases in DNA copy number of cases analyzed in this fashion. Loss of heterozygosity (LOH) analyses have identified several arms and regions of chromosomes that contain or potentially harbor tumor suppressor genes important in gastric tumorigenesis, including 17p (>60% at *p53*'s locus) (56), 18q (>60% at *SMAD4* and *DCC*'s loci) (57), and 5q (30%–40% at or near *APC*'s locus) (56,58). Comprehensive LOH analysis in xenografted adenocarcinomas identified 3p, 4p, 4q, 5p, 8q, 13p, 17p, and 18q to be frequently lost well above background (59). In LOH analysis of more than 100 archived stomach cancers, allelic loss was most frequently noted on chromosome 3p (60). Moreover, three distinct regions of chromosome 4q were found to be frequently lost in gastroesophageal junctional adenocarcinomas, indicating the potential of multiple tumor suppressor genes on this chromosomal arm (61).

Notable allelic loss of both 17p and 18q in proximal or gastroesophageal junctional tumors was associated with a poorer survival than those cases without allelic loss or just one allelic loss at their loci (62). Knowledge of these critical alterations is important because gastric cancers of different histopathological features have been shown to be associated with distinct patterns of genetic alterations, supporting the notion that they evolve through distinct genetic pathways. As described later in this section, both known and candidate tumor suppressor genes have been isolated in some of these frequently lost regions, but the actual targets of genetic loss that provide gastric neoplastic cells with additional survival or growth advantages for clonal expansion remain to be clarified for many of these loci.

Instability: Chromosomal and Microsatellite

The majority of gastric cancers exhibit significant gross chromosomal aneuploidy. One study found that 72% of differentiated tumors and 43% of undifferentiated gastric tumors were aneuploid (63). However, MSI has been found in a subset of sporadic gastric carcinomas ranging from 13% to 44% of tumors (64). Variability in classification of instability or histopathological subtype and number of loci examined in studies account for some variation of this phenotype's frequency, with a trend toward more frequent occurrence in intestinal-type cancers at more advanced stages observed. The degree of genomewide instability also varies with more significant instability (e.g., microsatellite instability-high [MSI-H] exhibiting >33% unstable loci of those tested) occurring in only 10% to16% of gastric cancers (65).

Alterations responsible for producing the MSI-H phenotype in a subset of sporadic gastric cancers have been elucidated. Abnormal loss of protein expression of either MLH1 or MSH2 was demonstrated in all cases exhibiting MSI-H (66). Altered expression of MLH1 was associated with increased methylation of the promoter region of MLH1 in MSI-H cases, suggesting a silencing role of hypermethylation (67,68). Distinct methylation of the promoter of hMLH1 was noted in five of eight MSI-H cases, whereas none of 43 microsatellite instability-low (MSI-L) or microsatellite stable (MSS) cases exhibited this methylation (69).

MSI-H gastric tumors exhibit distinct clinicopathological characteristics. Consistent associations of the MSI-H phenotype with intestinal subtype, distal location (e.g., antral), and more favorable prognosis have been observed (65,70–74). In addition, some but not all studies have noted associations between the MSI-H phenotype and less frequent lymph node metastasis (65,71,72), greater depth of invasion (72), near-diploid DNA content (65), and tumoral lymphoid infiltration (65,71,72). A possible explanation for the unique clinicopathological phenotype observed in MSI-H gastric tumors may be the occurrence of mutations in a distinct set of cancer-related genes differing from those in tumors with no or low-level MSI. Because MSI-H gastric carcinomas appear to be clinicopathologically distinct, it may ultimately prove valuable to have markers that identify this subgroup of gastric cancers, such as BAT-26 (66). Several tumor suppressor genes have been shown to be critical targets of defective MMR in MSI-H tumors. Moreover, a proapoptotic gene and additional MMR genes have been demonstrated to be altered in MSI gastric cancer cases. These same genes are observed to be infrequently mutated or altered in MSI-L or MSS tumors (71,75,76).

At least one important target of MSI appears to be the transforming growth factor (TGF)-β type II receptor ($TGF\beta R2$) at a polyadenine tract within its gene (77). Altered $TGF\beta R2$ could also be found in gastric cancers not displaying MSI. Several gastric cancer cell lines resistant to the growth inhibitory and apoptotic effects of TGF-β were shown to have abnormal $TGF\beta R2$ genes and/or transcripts (78). Moreover, some gastric cancer cell lines and 5 of 40 primary gastric cancers (12.5%) exhibited hypermethylation of the promoter region of TGF-β type 1 receptor gene and decreased mRNA expression (79). Another gene involved in this signaling pathway, ACVR2, was found to be similarly mutated, even in a biallelic fashion, in gastric tumors exhibiting MSI (80). Thus, alteration of TGF-β receptors and other members of this signaling path appears to be

a critical event in the development of at least a subset of gastric cancers, allowing escape from the growth control signal of TGF-β.

Additional genes with simple tandem repeat sequences within their coding regions found to be altered in gastric cancers displaying MSI include BAX, $IGFRII$, and $E2F-4$, which are known to be involved in regulation of cell cycle progression and apoptotic signaling (81–84). Furthermore, somatic non-frameshift mutations have been reported in BAX (81). Moreover, the relatively frequent missense mutations at codon 169 of BAX were shown to impair its proapoptotic activity (85).

Specific Alterations

The $p53$ gene has consistently been demonstrated to be significantly altered in gastric adenocarcinomas. Allelic loss occurs in more than 60% of cases, and mutations are identified in approximately 30% to 50% of cases, depending on the mutational screening method employed and variable sample sizes (86). Some mutations of $p53$ have even been identified in early dysplastic and apparent intestinal metaplasia gastric lesions; however, most alterations occurred in the advanced stages of neoplasia. The spectrum of mutations in this gene within gastric tumors is not unusual with a predominance of base transitions, especially at CpG dinucleotides. Many studies have used immunohistochemical analysis of tumors in an effort to detect excessive expression of p53 as an indirect means to identify mutations of this gene, but this assay does not appear to have consistent prognostic value in patients with gastric cancers (87,88).

Several sporadic gastric cancers have displayed altered E-cadherin, mainly diffuse types. E-cadherin is a transmembrane, calcium ion-dependent adhesion molecule important in epithelial cell homotypic interactions that, when decreased in expression, is associated with invasive properties (89). Reduced E-cadherin expression determined by immunohistochemical analysis was noted in the majority (92% of 60 cases) of gastric carcinomas when compared to the adjacent normal tissue (90). Furthermore, absent expression of E-cadherin was observed to be significantly associated with undifferentiated, diffuse-type cancers ($n = 30$) compared to intestinal-type cancers ($n = 30$). Genetic abnormalities of the E-$cadherin$ gene (located on chromosome 16q22.1) and transcripts were demonstrated in 13 of 26 diffuse gastric cancers on reverse transcriptase polymerase chain reaction (RT-PCR) analysis (91). Moreover, a study of ten gastric cancer cell lines displaying loose intracellular adhesion found absent E-cadherin transcripts in four lines, and insertions or deletions in two other lines (92). E-$cadherin$ splice site alterations producing exon deletion and skipping, large deletions including allelic loss and point mutations, mostly of the missense nature, have been demonstrated in diffuse-type cancers, some even exhibiting alterations in both alleles (93). Seven of ten diffuse-type gastric carcinomas were found to contain somatic E-$cadherin$ alterations, including the diffuse component in five of six mixed-type tumors (94). Methylation of the promoter region of E-$cadherin$ was found in 16 (26%) of 61 gastric cancers studied (69). In addition, α-catenin, which binds to the intracellular domain of E-cadherin and links it to actin-based cytoskeletal elements, was noted to have reduced immunohistochemical expression in 70% of 60 gastric carcinomas and correlated with infiltrated growth and poor differentiation (95).

Evidence of tumor suppressor loci on chromosome 3p has accumulated from a variety of studies, including allelic loss in primary gastric tumors (46%) and homozygous deletion in a gastric cancer cell line (KATO III) as well as xenografted tumors (96). The $FHIT$ gene was recently isolated from the common fragile site FRA3B region at 3p14.2 and found to have abnormal transcripts with deleted exons in five of nine gastric cancers (97). Furthermore, loss of FHIT protein expression was demonstrated immunohistochemically in the majority of gastric carcinomas (98). One somatic missense mutation was identified in exon 6 of the *FHIT* gene during a coding region analysis of 40 gastric carcinomas (99). Additional studies are needed to identify the critically altered targets on this chromosome, clarify the role *FHIT* plays in gastric tumorigenesis, and determine the role breakpoints in this region of 3p have in gastric cancer development.

Loss of the trefoil peptide TFF1(pS2), a stable three-loop molecule synthesized in mucus-secreting cells, has been described in approximately 50% of gastric carcinomas (100–103). The biological significance of this loss was reported in a knockout mouse model of gastric antral neoplasia (104). In addition, expression of TFF1 was observed to be lower in some gastric intestinal metaplasia and gastric adenomatous lesions compared to adjacent normal or hyperplastic mucosa (105,106). *TFF1* resides on chromosome 21q22, a region noted to be deleted in some gastric cancers in LOH studies (107,108). Overexpression of TFF1 in the gastric cancer cell line, AGS, inhibited its growth (109). Furthermore, the overwhelming majority of gastric cancers studied had absent to minimal transcript levels compared to normal gastric mucosa (110). Moreover, C/EBP-*β* was found to be overexpressed in the majority of gastric cancers in a corresponding manner and to bind to the promoter of TFF1, suggesting a regulatory factor role (111,112).

Several members of the Wnt signaling pathway, *APC* and *β-catenin*, have had several somatic alterations noted in a few cases of gastric cancer. *β*-Catenin participates with the Tcf-Lef family of transcription factors in the transfer of cellular proliferation signals to the nucleolus. Thus, inactivating mutations of APC or mutations in specific serine and threonine residues in the NH$_2$ terminus of *β*-catenin would be expected to lead to the stabilization of *β*-catenin and the loss of cellular growth control as demonstrated in colon cancers (113).

Somatic *APC* mutations, mostly missense in nature and of relatively low frequency, have been reported in Japanese patients' gastric adenocarcinomas and adenomas on partial screening (114). However, several other reports including Japanese patients have not identified significant *APC* mutations in gastric carcinomas on similar partial screening analysis of the commonly mutated region, including direct nucleotide sequencing (115–117). Significant allelic loss at the loci of *APC* suggests the nearby existence of a tumor suppressor gene important in gastric tumorigenesis. Indeed, the interferon regulatory factor-1 gene has been mapped to this commonly deleted region in gastric cancers (118). Thus, defining the critical alteration(s) on chromosome 5q with frequent loss remains to be delineated.

Missense somatic mutations in *β-catenin*, which also has connections with the cell adhesion complex involving E-cadherin, were identified in a few cases of intestinal-type gastric cancer (119). However, the functional consequences of these changes remain to be determined because the four commonly mutated serines or threonines that are known to be involved in regulatory phosphorylation of this signaling pathway were not affected. No *β-catenin* mutations were observed in diffuse-type gastric cancers (120). The gastric cancer cell line, HSC-39, established from a patient with a signet ring cell carcinoma, contains a 321 base pair (bp) in-frame deletion in the NH$_2$ terminal region, including the GSK3-*β* phosphorylation and *α*-catenin–binding site (121). Decreased normal membranous expression of *β*-catenin was found to be associated with poor differentiation and shorter patient survival (122).

No inactivating somatic mutations of *p16^{INK4}* were detected in more than 70 cases of gastric carcinoma screened by polymerase chain reaction-single strand polymorphism (PCR-SSCP) analysis (123). However, *p16^{INK4}* somatic mutations were noted in several esophageal adenocarcinomas with LOH, and others with loss of p16 expression were found to have abnormal hypermethylation of the *p16^{INK4}* promoter, suggesting that this epigenetic gene expression silencing may play a role in esophageal tumorigenesis (124–126). A significant number (41%) of gastric cancers exhibited CpG island methylation in a study of the promoter region of p16 (69). Many of these cases with hypermethylation of promoter regions displayed the MSI-H phenotype and multiple sites of methylation, including the *MLH1* promoter region (127). Only 1 of 35 gastric cancers contained an intragenic mutation of *SMAD4* along with allelic loss, suggesting that this gene is infrequently altered in gastric tumorigenesis (128,129). In addition, only one missense change of uncertain functional significance in the *LKB1* (STK11) gene was noted in a study of 28 sporadic gastric carcinomas (130).

Other Molecular Biological Alterations

Overexpression of DARP32 and a novel truncated isoform were found in the majority of gastric cancers (131). Moreover, an antiapoptotic effect of this overexpression of DARP32 and t-DARP was observed in vitro (132). Overexpression of ERBB2 (HER-2/neu), a transmembrane tyrosine kinase receptor proto-oncogene, has been implicated as a potential marker of poor prognosis (133–135). ERBB2 has even been detected immuno-histochemically in the serum of gastric cancer patients (136). Other studies, however, have not found any prognostic value of ERBB expression in these cancers (137,138).

Overexpression of the *MET* gene, which encodes a tyrosine kinase receptor for the hepatocyte growth factor, has been reported to have prognostic value to indicate poorer survival in multivariate analysis (139). There have been numerous reports in the literature indicating that the *MET* gene is amplified in approximately 15%, and its expression elevated in as many as 50%, of gastric tumors (140–144). Interestingly, *MET* amplification in colon carcinomas rarely occurs. This evidence, along with the infrequent mutations in the *ras* proto-oncogene found in gastric cancer (145,146), provides good indication that the mechanisms involved in the development of colon and gastric cancers are distinct.

Overexpression of *MET* gene by itself may not be sufficient for cancer progression because interaction of the precancerous cells with stromal fibroblast-derived growth factors, including hepatocyte growth factor (HGF), may promote the progression of disease. Tahara proposed that stromal fibroblasts stimulated by IL-1 or TGF-*β* secrete HGF that can then bind to the MET protein on cancer cells and promote the morphogenesis and progression of the cancer (147). In the absence of (or at low levels of) E-cadherin and catenins, HGF may cause the scattering of cancer cells and the development of the poorly differentiated phenotype. Thus, interactions between the stromal and epithelial layers of the stomach may have profound effects on the development of disease. This notion has been borne out in several studies. Inoue et al. demonstrated that TGF-*β* and HGF produced by a culture of gastric fibroblasts could stimulate the invasiveness of a human scirrhous-type gastric cancer cell line in vitro (148). In addition, several reports in the literature have indicated that prostaglandins can induce the expression of HGF from gastric and colonic fibroblasts, implying the potential for a paracrine loop between epithelial-derived PGE$_2$ and stromal-derived HGF (149–151). It is tempting to speculate that this may be one of the mechanisms through which *H. pylori* could act to promote the development of gastric cancers. Infection with *H. pylori* has in fact been shown to result in an increase in gastric mucosal HGF levels and an increase in HGF gene expression (152–154).

Tumor and stromal cell interaction have been suggested for several other growth factor signaling systems. Approximately

15% of gastric cancers have been observed to express both epidermal growth factor (EGF) and epidermal growth factor receptor (EGFR), suggesting the presence of an autocrine mechanism of growth stimulation in these cases. Some studies suggest a worse prognosis for tumors with positive expression of EGF, EGFR, or both. Involvement of several other growth factor signaling paths have been implicated in gastric tumorigenesis, including TGF-alpha, interleukin-1, criptor, amphiregulin, platelet-derived growth factor, and K-sam (155). Expression of basic fibroblast growth factor and fibroblast growth factor receptor have been found in 70% and 60% of gastric cancers, respectively, and noted to be frequently undifferentiated and in a more advanced invasive stage (156). Rare amplification of MYC and KSAM has also been reported in gastric cancers (144).

A role for cyclo-oxygenase (COX)-2 in the development and progression of gastric cancer has also been suggested. In normal gastric mucosa, cox-1, but not cox-2, is expressed and is found almost exclusively in epithelium. As one explanation for high levels of PGE$_2$ in cancerous tissue, Ristimaki et al. reported increased cox-2 expression in tumor-bearing mucosa at both the mRNA and protein levels. Evidence that cox-2 participates in the proliferation of gastric cancer cells (MKN45) was suggested by Tsuji et al., who also later showed that a role for cox-2 in cancer progression is clearly not limited to tumors of the gastric epithelium (157). Furthermore, dysregulated expression of cox-2 was shown to be an important factor in the progression and growth of gastrointestinal tumors (158).

RUNX3, a tumor suppressor gene, apparently suppresses gastric epithelial cell growth by inducing p21 (WAF1/Cip1) expression in cooperation with TGF-β–activated SMAD (128). RUNX3 was found to be altered in 82% of gastric cancers through either gene silencing or protein mislocalization to the cytoplasm (159). Significant downregulation of RUNX3 through methylation on the promoter region was observed in primary tumors (75%) as well as in all clinical peritoneal metastasis of gastric cancers (100%) compared with normal gastric mucosa. Silencing of RUNX3 affects expression of important genes such as p21 and others involved in aspects of metastasis, including cell adhesion, proliferation, and apoptosis. They potentially promote the peritoneal metastasis of gastric cancer (160).

In vitro studies suggest that hedgehog signaling contributes to gastric cancer cell growth. Elevated expressions of hedgehog target genes human patched gene 1 (PTCH1) or Glil occurs in 63 of 99 primary gastric cancers. Activation of the hedgehog pathway is associated with poorly differentiated and more aggressive tumors. Treatment of gastric cancer cells with KAAD-cyclonamine, a hedgehog signaling inhibitor, decreases expressions of Glil and PTCH1, resulting in cell growth inhibition and apoptosis (161).

A number of other alterations have been reported in gastric carcinomas that remain to be fully characterized in gastric tumorigenesis. Several splice variants of a transmembrane glycoprotein that participates in cell–substrate and cell–cell interactions, CD44, seem to be preferentially expressed in gastric tumors cells (162). Membrane-type matrix metalloproteinase (MMP) was preferentially expressed in some gastric cancer cells with colocalization and activation of the zymogen, proMMP-2 (163). In addition, increased plasminogen activation has been reported in several gastric tumors (164). A somatic mitochondrial deletion of 50 bp was even demonstrated in four gastric adenocarcinomas (165). Telomerase activity, which appears necessary for cell immortality, has been detected by a PCR-based assay frequently in the late stages of gastric tumors and observed to be associated with a poor prognosis (166). Furthermore, Tahara et al. identified telomerase activity in the vast majority of primary gastric tumor tissues, whereas no activity was observed in the corresponding normal gastric mucosa (147). Specific alterations and the true prevalence of significant changes in these genes, gene products, or phenotypes in human gastric tumors remain to be characterized. Table 20.1 lists alterations that appear consistently in human gastric carcinomas; others will undoubtedly be added as studies accumulate.

Animal Model Observations

Animal models have greatly enhanced the understanding of gastric carcinogenesis. Loss of TFF1 expression in homozygous knockout mice invariably led to neoplastic growth in the antropyloric mucosa at 5 months of age (104). Moreover, decreased TFF1 expression was found in mice genetically engineered to have an altered gp130 gene, and these mice also developed hyperplasia and adenoma formation in their gastric mucosa (167). Zavros et al. showed that in the hypochlorhydric mouse stomach, the chronic gastritis, atrophy, metaplasia, and dysplasia paradigm can be recapitulated in mice (168).

Cdx2, a transcription factor whose expression is limited to the intestine, has been detected in gastric intestinal metaplasia. Cdx2 expression in the gastric mucosa was achieved in mice through the derivation of transgenic mice in which the mouse having Cdx2 cDNA was under the control of the cis-regulatory elements of the winged helix transcription factor Foxa3 in yeast artificial chromosome (YAC). Histologic examination of the gastric mucosa of the Foxa3/Cdx2 mice revealed the presence of Alcian blue positive intestinal-type goblet cells, a hallmark of intestinal metaplasia. Gastric expression of Cdx2 alone was sufficient to induce intestinal metaplasia in mice. The phenotype generated suggests involvement of Cdx2 in the early initiation of the metaplastic process potentially facilitating the

TABLE 20.1

SOMATIC ALTERATIONS IN HUMAN GASTRIC ADENOCARCINOMAS

Frequent	Specifically in MSI-H cases	Infrequent
p53 inactivation	Loss of hMLH1 or hMSH2 protein	APC
TFF1 loss and C/EBP-ß increase	TGF-βIIR	Smad4
FHIT loss	Bax	LKB1
DARP32/t-DARP/c-MET increase	IGFIIR	
HER-2/neu increase	E2F-4	
EGFR /K-sam increase	hMSH3	
E-cadherin loss (diffuse type)	hMSH6	
P16/p27/ PAI-1 loss		
VEGF/MMP-9/Cox-2 increase		

eventual development of gastric neoplasia because gastric cancer in humans is often preceded by intestinal metaplasia (169).

Findings by Houghton et al. suggest that epithelial cancers can originate from bone marrow–derived sources and thus have broad implications on the multistep model progression of cancer (170). Chronic infection of C57BL/6 mice with *Helicobacter*, a known carcinogen, induces repopulation of the stomach with bone marrow–derived cells (BMDCs). Subsequently, these cells progress through metaplasia and dysplasia to intraepithelial cancer. Using two independent markers (GFP and Y chromosome), it was confirmed that BMDCs may give rise to gastric epithelial cancer in *Helicobacter*-infected mice. Because this study was not designed to evaluate for reductive division, further work in this field will elucidate if the epithelial cells that differentiate from BMDCs after irradiation of the recipient are not the result of cell fusion (170).

Phenotypic consequences of the Car9 null mutation show the important role of CAIX in morphogenesis and homeostasis of the glandular gastric epithelium via the control of cell proliferation and differentiation. Mice homozygous for null mutation of the Car9 gene deficient in carbonic anhydrase developed gastric hyperplasia of the glandular epithelium with numerous cysts (171). In humans, SMAD4, a signal transducer, has been believed to play different roles in human gastric carcinogenesis, especially between intestinal type and diffuse type of gastric adenocarcinoma. A study in SMAD4 mice suggested that haploinsufficiency of SMAD4 facilitates gastric tumor initiation and may provide a valuable model for screening factors that promote or prevent gastric tumorigenesis (172).

The only wild-type rodent species to develop gastric cancer following *H. pylori* infection is the Mongolian gerbil. Animal studies have suggested that development of a Th1 immune response following *Helicobacter* infection increased levels of the hormone gastrin; expression of other growth factors, such as TGF-α; and alteration of other growth factors, such an SMAD4 and RUNX3, which may all be important in rendering the host-susceptible gastric carcinogenesis. Finally, animal models have shown that carcinogenesis may also be modulated by environmental factors, such as the amount of salt, carcinogens, and antioxidants in the diet (173).

POTENTIAL BIOMARKERS

Elevated tissue levels of certain proteins have been shown to be associated with increased invasiveness of tumor cells, and some even associated with poorer survival including: urokinase-type plasminogen activator, vascular endothelial growth factor, MET , MYC, tie-1 protein tyrosine kinase, CD44v6, PDGF-A, TGF-ß1, and cyclin D2 (164,174–180). However, decreased levels of other proteins have been noted to be associated with more invasiveness and poorer survival, including loss of p27 (Kip1), p21 (CIP1), plasminogen activator inhibitor type 1, and tissue-type plasminogen activator (164,181–184). In a study by Zafirellis et al., the expression of p53 and bcl-2 proteins had no significant impact on the outcome of patients with gastric cancer (185). The combined analysis of p53 and p27 (kip1) was of added prognostic value, but these findings alone are not compelling for a specific role in gastric tumorigenesis and may represent only nonspecific changes accompanying tumor development (186). Nishigaki et al. identified nine proteins with increased expression and 13 proteins with decreased expression in gastric carcinomas, notably including proteins that function at mitotic checkpoints (MAD1L1 and EB1) and mitochondrial functions (CLPP, COX5A, and ECH1) (187). Thus, some of these molecules could potentially provide diagnostic and/or prognostic markers that can be evaluated in gastric cancer tissues for clinical utilities. Thymidine phosphorylase has been noted to correlate with angiogenesis in gastric cancers (188).

The KLK6 gene is markedly overexpressed in gastric cancer tissue, and its expression status may be an important prognostic indicator for patients with gastric cancer. KLK6 gene silencing with KLK6 small interfering RNA effectively suppressed the cell proliferation rate ($P = 0.002$), cell population in the S phase ($p < 0.01$), and invasiveness ($p < 0.01$) in comparison to mock-transfected cells. Furthermore, patients with a high KLK6 expression had a significantly poorer survival rate than those with a low KLK6 expression ($P = 0.03$) (189).

Additional diagnostic and prognostic markers for gastric cancer patients have been sought in bone marrow and peripheral blood samples. Concentrations of MMP-9 were higher in the plasma of gastric cancer patients compared to normal controls (190). High concentrations of tissue inhibitor of metalloproteinase (TIMP)-1, interleukin-10, HGF, soluble receptor for interleukin-2, and soluble fragment of E-cadherin in the serum or plasma of gastric carcinoma patients have been observed to be associated with more invasiveness and poorer survival (191–195). Furthermore, detection of cytokeratin 20, CD44 variants, CA-125, CEA, CA 19-9, CA 72-4, and anti-p53 antibodies in the peripheral blood of gastric cancer patients tend to indicate disseminated disease (196–200).

Tumor progression in gastric cancer patients has been attributed to the persistence of disseminated tumor cells (DTCs) in various body compartments as a sign of minimal disease. In a study of 70 cancer patients whose venous blood was sampled intraoperatively before surgical manipulation, the expression of cytokeratin 20 (CK20) by RT-PCR as a marker of DTC was an independent prognostic marker, especially in early stages (T1 and T2) (N0; $p < 0.0032$) (201).

Multiple tumor suppressor genes and candidates, including CDKN2A, GSTP1, APC, MGMT, MLH1, DAKP, THBS-1, RUNX1, and CDH1, have been shown to be methylated in gastric cancers and provide potential candidate molecular markers for these cancers. In addition, the methylation of some of these genes may occur early in gastric carcinogenesis, potentially providing optimal diagnostic markers (202).

GASTRIC STROMAL TUMORS

The most common mesenchymal tumor of the gastrointestinal tract is a gastrointestinal stromal tumor (GIST). Most GISTs are solitary, and activating gain-of-function mutations of the *KIT* proto-oncogene have been demonstrated in these tumors (203). A germline mutation of *KIT* between the transmembrane and tyrosine kinase domains similar to the somatic changes previously noted in sporadic cases was also demonstrated in a family manifesting multiple GISTs that cosegregated with disease (204). Interestingly, affected members of this family also displayed hyperpigmentation and mast cell hyperplasia, which is consistent with the known function of KIT to be important in melanocyte and mast cell development. Alterations of KIT in GIST tumor development provides evidence that interstitial cells of Cajal may give rise to these tumors because these cells also depend on this signal for development and express this protein as well as CD34.

IMPLICATIONS

Because gastric cancer appears to be a rather heterogeneous disease biologically and genetically, characterization of the various pathways and events along the way should afford multiple opportunities to design more specific and therefore more effective therapies in the treatment of this tumor. Critical molecular alterations in these cancers once fully characterized may ultimately provide new avenues to combat this lethal disease. These concepts provide a deeper understanding of cancer initiation and progression, and have broad implications for the development of anticancer therapies. For example, antibodies to the oncogene ERBB2 and EGF receptor have shown promise in inhibiting growth of gastric cancer cell lines and xenografts (205,206). The potential of gene therapy to help replace altered tumor suppressor gene function has been demonstrated in the administration of wild-type p53 in an engineered adenovirus to promote growth arrest and apoptosis in a gastric cell line (207). The ability to specifically seek out and destroy tumor cells has been demonstrated in experiments on gastric cancer cell lines infected with adenoviral vectors expressing the herpes simplex virus thymidine kinase or cytosine deaminase, specifically in CEA-producing tumor cells to enhance treatments (208,209). Demonstration of malignant progression of a marrow-derived progenitor cell in the setting of chronic inflammation offers the basis for a new model of epithelial cancer. Many features of cancer cells become much clearer when viewed within the context of this model: their undifferentiated nature, ability for self-renewal, relative resistance to apoptosis, and propensity for metastasis and early spread.

Transfection of a gastric cell line with TIMP-1 to generate exogenous expression demonstrated potential to decrease metastatic spread to the liver when transplanted into nude mice (210). Moreover, infection of three gastric cancer cell lines with an adenovirus vector that expressed antisense RNA for EGFR decreased this protein's cell surface expression and inhibited growth of these cells both in vivo and in vitro (211). Improved prognostic markers are also eagerly awaited to help guide more aggressive surgical or systemic therapies (i.e., chemotherapy and/or radiotherapy) and may ultimately be derived from molecular alterations indicated above or from as yet unidentified critical change in gastric cancer cells. Relatively noninvasive tests, such as detection of DTCs in venous blood of gastric patients, may serve as an independent predictive marker of poor prognosis and could help define patients for adjuvant therapy with this tumor entity (201).

ACKNOWLEDGMENTS

This work was supported in part by National Institutes of Health grant CA67900-01.

References

1. Parkin DM, Pisani P, Ferlay J. Estimates of the worldwide incidence of eighteen major cancers in 1985. *Int J Cancer* 1993;54(4):594–606.
2. Parkin DM, Bray F, Ferlay J, Pisani P. Global cancer statistics. *CA Cancer J Clin* 2005;55(2):74–108.
3. Blot WJ, Devesa SS, Kneller RW. Rising incidence of adenocarcinoma of the esophagus and gastric cardia. *JAMA* 1991;265:1287–1289.
4. Locke GR, Talley NJ, Carpenter HA, Harmsen WS, Zinsmeister AR, Melton L, Jr. Changes in the site- and histology-specific incidence of gastric cancer during a 50-year period. *Gastroenterology* 1995;109(6):1750–1756.
5. Parker SL, Tong T, Bolden S, Wingo PA. Cancer statistics, 1996. *CA Cancer J Clin* 1996;46(1):5–28.
6. Correa P, Chen V, eds. *Trends in Cancer Incidence and Mortality: Gastric Cancer.* New York, NY: Cold Spring Harbor Laboratory Press; 1994.
7. Haenszel W, Kurihara M, Segi M, Lee R. Stomach cancer among Japanese in Hawaii. *J Natl Cancer Inst* 1972;49:969–988.
8. Parsonnet J, Friedman G, Vandersteen D. *Helicobacter pylori* infection and the risk of gastric carcinoma. *N Engl J Med* 1991;325:1127–1131.
9. Parsonnet J, Hansen S, Rodriguez L, et al. *Helicobacter pylori* infection and gastric lymphoma. *N Engl J Med* 1994;330:1267–1271.
10. Park GT, Lee OY, Kwon SJ, et al. Analysis of CYP2E1 polymorphism for the determination of genetic susceptibility to gastric cancer in Koreans. *J Gastroenterol Hepatol* 2003;18(11):1257–1263.
11. Lee J, Lowry A, Thompson W, et al. Association of gastric adenocarcinoma with the HLA class II gene DQB1*0301. *Gastroenterology* 1996;111:426–432.
12. Sakai t, Aoyama N, Satonaka K, et al. HLA-DQB1 locus and the development of atrophic gastritis with *Helicobacter pylori* infection. *J Gastroenterol* 1999;34:24–27.
13. Aird I, Bentall H. A relationship between cancer of stomach and ABO groups. *Br J Med* 1953;1:799–780.
14. Buckwalter JA, Wholwend CB, Colter DC. The association of the ABO blood groups to gastric carcinoma. *Surg Gynecol Obstet* 1957;104:176–179.
15. Boren T, Per F, Roth KA, Larson G, Normark S. Attachment of *Helicobacter pylori* to human gastric epithelium mediated by blood group antigens. *Science* 1993;262:1892–1895.
16. Carvalho F, Seruca R, David L, et al. Muc1 gene polymorphism and gastric cancer—an epidemiological study. *Glycoconj J* 1997;14:107–111.
17. Umlauft F, Keeffe EB, Offner F, et al. *Helicobacter pylori* infection and blood group antigens: lack of clinical association. *Am J Gastroenterol* 1996;91(10):2135–2138.
18. Correa P, Shiao YH. Phenotypic and genotypic events in gastric carcinogenesis. *Cancer Res* 1994;54:1941–1943.
19. Stemmerman GN. Intestinal metaplasia of the stomach. *Cancer* 1994;74(2):556–564.
20. Yoshihara M, Sumii K, Haruma K, et al. Correlation of ratio of serum pepsinogen 1 and 2 with prevalence of gastric cancer and adenoma in Japanese subjects. *Am J Gastroenterol* 1998;93:1090–1096.
21. La Vecchia C, Negri E, Franceschi S, Gentile A. Family history and the risk of stomach and colorectal cancer. *Cancer* 1992;70:50–55.
22. Goldgar DE, Easton DF, Cannon-Albright LA, Skolnock MH. Systematic population-based assessment of cancer risk in the first-degree relatives of cancer probands. *J Natl Cancer Inst* 1994;86:1600–1608.
23. Videbaek A, Mosbech J. The etiology of gastric carcinoma elucidated by a study of 302 pedigrees. *Acta Med Scand* 1954;149:173–159.
24. Antommarchi F. *Les derniers moments de Napoleon, en compement du memorial de Sainte-Helene.* Brussels, Belgium: H Tarlier; 1825.
25. Kubba A, Young M. The Napoleonic cancer gene? *J Med Biogr* 1977;7:175–181.
26. Hemminki K, Jiang Y. Familial and second gastric carcinomas: a nationwide epidemiologic study from Sweden. *Cancer* 2002;94(4):1157–1165.
27. Zangheiri G, Di Gregorio C, Sacchetti C, et al. Familial occurrence of gastric cancer in the 2-year experience of a population-based registry. *Cancer* 1990;66:2047–2051.
28. Palli D, Galli M, Caporaso NE, et al. Family history and risk of stomach cancer in Italy. *Cancer Epidemiol Biomarkers Prev* 1994;3:15–18.
29. Gorer PA. Genetic interpretation of studies on cancer in twins. *Ann Eugenics* 1938;8:219–232.
30. Lee FI. Carcinoma of the gastric antrum in identical twins. *Postgrad Med J* 1971;47:622–624.
31. Guilford P, Hopkins J, Harraway J, et al. E-cadherin germline mutations in familial gastric cancer. *Nature* 1998;392(6674):402–405.
32. Gayther SA, Gorringe KL, Ramus SJ, et al. Identification of germ-line E-cadherin mutations in gastric cancer families of European origin. *Cancer Res* 1998;58(18):4086–4089.
33. Caldas C, Carneiro F, Lynch HT, et al. Familial gastric cancer: overview and guidelines for management. *J Med Genet* 1999;36:873–880.
34. Yoon KA, Ku JL, Yang HK, Kim WH, Park SY, Park JG. Germline mutations of E-cadherin gene in Korean familial gastric cancer patients. *J Hum Genet* 1999;44(3):177–180.
35. Stone J, Bevan S, Cunningham D, et al. Low frequency of germline E-cadherin mutations in familial and nonfamilial gastric cancer. *Br J Cancer* 1999;79(11–12):1935–1937.
36. Shinmura K, Kohno T, Takahashi M. Familial gastric cancer: clinicopathological characteristics, RER phenotype, and germline p53 and E-cadherin mutations. *Carcinogenesis* 1999;20:1127–1131.
37. Lynch HT, Grady W, Suriano G, Huntsman D. Gastric cancer: new genetic developments. *J Surg Oncol* 2005;90(3):114–133; discussion 133.
38. Lynch HT, Smyrk TC, Watson P, et al. Genetics, natural history, tumor spectrum, and pathology of hereditary nonpolyposis colorectal cancer. *Gastroenterology* 1993;104:1535–1549.
39. Kinzler KW, Vogelstein B. Lessons from hereditary colorectal cancer. *Cell* 1996;87:159–170.
40. Aarnio M, Salovaara R, Aaltonen LA, Mecklin JP, Jarvinen HJ. Features of gastric cancer in hereditary non-polyposis colorectal cancer syndrome. *Int J Cancer* 1997;74(5):551–555.
41. Renkonen-Sinisalo L, Sipponen P, Aarnio M, et al. No support for endoscopic surveillance for gastric cancer in hereditary non-polyposis colorectal cancer. *Scand J Gastroenterol* 2002;37(5):574–577.
42. Lynch HT, Krush AJ. Cancer family "G" revisited: 1895–1970. *Cancer* 1971;27:1505–1511.
43. Varley JM, McGown G, Thorncroft M, et al. An extended Li-Fraumeni kindred with gastric carcinoma and a codon 175 mutation of TP53. *J Med Genet* 1995;32:942–945.
44. Lindor NM, Greene MH. The concise handbook of family cancer syndromes: Mayo Familial Cancer Program. *J Natl Cancer Inst* 1998;90:1039–1071.
45. Hofgartner WT, Thorp M, Ramus MW, et al. Gastric adenocarcinoma associated with fundic gland polyps in a patient with attenuated familial adenomatous polyposis. *Am J Gastroenterol* 1999;94:2275–2281.

46. Utsunomiya J. The concept of hereditary colorectal cancer and the implications of its study. *Hereditary Colorectal Cancer* 1990;3–16.
47. Offerhaus G, Giardiello G, Krush A, et al. The risk of upper gastrointestinal cancer in familial adenomatous polyposis. *Gastroenterology* 1992;102:1980–1982.
48. Maimon S, Zinninger M. Familial gastric cancer. *Gastroenterology* 1953;25:139–152.
49. Wolf C, Isaacson E. An analysis of 5 stomach cancer families in the state of Utah. *Cancer* 1961;14:1005–1016.
50. Dellavecchia C, Guala A, Olivieri C, et al. Early onset of gastric carcinoma and constitutional deletion of 18p. *Cancer Genet Cytogenet* 1999;113:96–99.
51. Seruca R, Carneiro F, Castedo S, David L, Lopes C, Sobrinho-Simones M. Familial gastric polyposis revisited: autosomal dominant inheritance confirmed. *Cancer Genet Cytogent* 1991;53:97–100.
52. Seruca R, Castedo S, Correia C, et al. Cytogenetic findings in eleven gastric carcinomas. *Cancer Genet Cytogenet* 1993;68:42–48.
53. Panani AD, Ferti A, Malliaros S, Raptis S. Cytogenetic study of 11 gastric adenocarcinomas. *Cancer Genet Cytogenet* 1995;81:169–172.
54. Moskaluk CA, Hu J, Perlman EJ. Comparative genomic hybridization of esophageal and gastroesophageal adenocarcinomas shows consensus areas of DNA gain and loss. *Genes Chromosomes Cancer* 1998;22:305–311.
55. El-Rifai W, Harper JC, Cummings OW, et al. Consistent genetic alterations in xenografts of proximal stomach and gastro-esophageal junction adenocarcinomas. *Cancer Res* 1998;58(1):34–37.
56. Sano T, Tsujino T, Yoshida K, et al. Frequent loss of heterozygosity on chromosomes 1q, 5q, and 17p in human gastric carcinomas. *Cancer Res* 1991;51(11):2926–2931.
57. Uchino S, Tsuda H, Noguchi M, et al. Frequent loss of heterozygosity at the DCC locus in gastric cancer. *Cancer Res* 1992;52:3099–3102.
58. Rhyu MG, Park WS, Jung YJ, Choi SW, Meltzer SJ. Allelic deletions of MCC/APC and p53 are frequent late events in human gastric carcinogenesis. *Gastroenterology* 1994;106(6):1584–1588.
59. Yustein AS, Harper JC, Petroni GR, Cummings OW, Moskaluk CA, Powell SM. Allelotype of gastric adenocarcinoma. *Cancer Res* 1999;59(7):1437–1341.
60. Schneider BG, Pulitzer DR, Brown RD, et al. Allelic imbalance in gastric cancer: an affected site on chromosome arm 3p. *Genes Chromosomes Cancer* 1995;13(4):263–271.
61. Rumpel CA, Powell SM, Moskaluk CA. Mapping of genetic deletions on the long arm of chromosome 4 in human esophageal adenocarcinomas. *Am J Pathol* 1999;154:1329–1334.
62. Wu T-T, Watanabe T, Heitmiller R, Zahurak M, Forastiere AA, Hamilton SR. Genetic alterations in Barrett esophagus and adenocarcinomas of the esophagus and esophagogastric junction region. *Am J Pathol* 1998;153:287–294.
63. Sasaki O, Soejima K, Korenage D, Haraguchi Y. Comparison of the intratumor DNA ploidy distribution pattern between differentiated and undifferentiated gastric carcinoma. *Anal Quant Cytol Histol* 1999;21:161–165.
64. Iacopetta BJ, Soong R, house AK, Hamelin R. Gastric carcinomas with microsatellite instability: clinical features and mutations to the TGF-beta type II receptor, IGFII receptor, and BAX genes. *J Pathol* 1999;187:428–432.
65. dos Santos NR, Seruca R, Constancia M, Seixas M, Sobrinho-Simoes M. Microsatellite instability at multiple loci in gastric carcinoma: clinicopathologic implications and prognosis. *Gastroenterology* 1996;110(1):38–44.
66. Halling KC, Harper J, Moskaluk CA, et al. Origin of microsatellite instability in gastric cancer. *Am J Pathol* 1999;155(1):205–211.
67. Leung SY, Yuen ST, Chung LP, Chu KM, Chan ASY, Ho JCI. hMLH1 promoter methylation and lack of hMLH1 expression in sporadic gastric carcinomas with high-frequency microsatellite instability. *Cancer Res* 1999;59:159–164.
68. Fleisher AS, Esteller M, Wang S, et al. Hypermethylation of the hMLH1 gene promoter in human gastric cancers with microsatellite instability. *Cancer Res* 1999;59(5):1090–1095.
69. Suzuki H, Itoh F, Toyota M, et al. Distinct methylation pattern and microsatellite instability in sporadic gastric cancer. *Int J Cancer* 1999;83:309–313.
70. Yamamoto H, Perez-Piteira J, Yoshida T, et al. Gastric cancers of the microsatellite mutator phenotype display characteristic genetic and clinical features. *Gastroenterology* 1999;116:1348–1357.
71. Olivera C, Seruca R, Seixas M, Sobrinho-Simons M. The clinicopathological features of gastric carcinomas with microsatellite instability may be mediated by mutations of different "target genes": a study of the TGF–betaRII, IGFRII, and BAX genes. *Am J Pathol* 1998;153:1211–1219.
72. Wu MS, Lee CW, Shun CT, et al. Clinicopathological significance of altered loci of replication error and microsatellite instability-associated mutations in gastric cancer. *Cancer Res* 1998;58:1494–1497.
73. Ottini L, Palli D, Falchetti M, et al. Microsatellite instability in gastric cancer is associated with tumor location and family history in a high-risk population from Tuscany. *Cancer Res* 1997;57(20):4523–4529.
74. Strickler JG, Zheng J, Shu Q, Burgart LJ, Alberts SR, Shibata D. p53 mutations and microsatellite instability in sporadic gastric cancer: when guardians fail. *Cancer Res* 1994;54(17):4750–4755.

75. Ottini L, Falchetti M, D'Amico C, et al. Mutations at coding mononucleotide repeats in gastric cancer with the microsatellite mutator phenotype. *Oncogene* 1998;16(21):2767–2772.
76. Yamamoto H, Itoh F, Fukushima H, et al. Frequent Bax frameshift mutations in gastric cancer with high but not low microsatellite instability. *J Exp Clin Cancer Res* 1999;18:103–106.
77. Myeroff LL, Parsons R, Kim SJ, et al. A transforming growth factor beta receptor type II gene mutation common in colon and gastric but rare in endometrial cancers with microsatellite instability. *Cancer Res* 1995;55(23):5545–5547.
78. Park K, Kim S-J, Bang Y-J, et al. Genetic changes in the transforming growth factor beta (TGF-b) type II receptor gene in human gastric cancer cells: correlation with sensitivity to growth inhibition by TGF-b. *Proc Natl Acad Sci U S A* 1994;91:8772–8776.
79. Kang SH, Bang YJ, Im YH, et al. Transcriptional repression of the transforming growth factor-beta type 1 receptor gene by DNA methylation results in the development of TGF-beta resistance in human gastric cancer. *Oncogene* 1999;18:7280–7286.
80. Mori Y, Sato F, Selaru FM, et al. Instabilotyping reveals unique mutational spectra in microsatellite-unstable gastric cancers. *Cancer Res* 2002;62(13):3641–3645.
81. Yamamoto H, Sawai H, Perucho M. Frameshift somatic mutations in gastrointestinal cancer of the microsatellite mutator phenotype. *Cancer Res* 1997;57(19):4420–4426.
82. Yin J, Kong D, Wang S, et al. Mutation of hMSH3 and hMSH6 mismatch repair genes in genetically unstable human colorectal and gastric carcinomas. *Hum Mutat* 1997;10(6):474–478.
83. Souza RF, Appel R, Yin J, et al. Microsatellite instability in the insulin-like growth factor II receptor gene in gastrointestinal tumours [letter]. *Nat Genet* 1996;14(3):255–257. [Erratum appears in *Nat Genet* 1996;14(4):488].
84. Souza RF, Yin J, Smolinski KN, et al. Frequent mutations of the E2F-4 cell cycle gene in primary human gastrointestinal tumors. *Cancer Res* 1997;57:2350–2353.
85. Gil J, Yamamoto H, Zapata JM, Reed JC, Perucho M. Impairment of the proapoptotic activity of BAX by missense mutations found in gastrointestinal cancers. *Cancer Res* 1999;59:2034–2037.
86. Hollstein M, Shomer B, Greenblatt M, et al. Somatic point mutations in the p53 gene of human tumors and cell lines: updated compilation. *Nucleic Acids Res* 1996;24(1):141–146.
87. Gabber HE, Muller W, Scnheiders A, Meier S, Hommel G. The relationship of p53 expression to the prognosis of 418 patients with gastric carcinoma. *Cancer* 1997;76(5):720–726.
88. Hurlimann J, Saraga EP. Expression of p53 protein in gastric carcinomas. *Am J Surg Pathol* 1994;18(12):1247–1253.
89. Birchmeier W, Behrens J. Cadherin expression in carcinomas: role in the formation of cell junctions and the prevention of invasiveness. *Biochem Biophys Acta* 1994;1198:11–26.
90. Mayer B, Johnson JP, Leitl F, et al. E-cadherin expression in primary and metastatic gastric cancer: down-regulation correlates with cellular dedifferentiation and glandular disintegration. *Cancer Res* 1993;53(7):1690–1695.
91. Becker KF, Atkinson MJ, Reich U, et al. E-cadherin gene mutations provide clues to diffuse type gastric carcinomas. *Cancer Res* 1994;54:3845–3852.
92. Oda T, Kanai Y, Oyama T, et al. E-cadherin gene mutations in human gastric carcinoma cell lines. *Proc Natl Acad Sci U S A* 1994;91:1858–1862.
93. Berx G, Becker KF, Hofler H, van Roy F. Mutations of the human E-cadherin (CDH1) gene. *Hum Mutat* 1998;12(4):226–237.
94. Machado JC, Soares P, Carneiro F, et al. E-cadherin gene mutations provide a genetic basis for the phenotypic divergence of mixed gastric carcinomas. *Lab Invest* 1999;79(4):459–465.
95. Matsui S, Shiozaki H, Masatoshi I, et al. Immunohistochemical evaluation of alpha-catenin expression in human gastric cancer. *Virchows Archiv* 1997;424:375–381.
96. Kastury K, Baffa R, Druck T, et al. Potential gastrointestinal tumor suppressor locus at the 3p14.2 FRA3b site identified by homozygous deletions in tumor cell lines. *Cancer Res* 1996;56:978–983.
97. Ohta M, Hiroshi I, Citticelli MG, Kastury K. The *FHIT* gene, spanning the chromosome 3p14.2 fragile site and renal carcinoma (associated t(3;8) breakpoint, is abnormal in digestive tract cancers. *Cell* 1996;84:587–597.
98. Baffa R, Veronese ML, Santoro R, et al. Loss of FHIT expression in gastric carcinoma. *Cancer Res* 1998;58(20):4708–4714.
99. Gemma A, Hagiwara K, Ke Y, et al. FHIT mutations in human primary gastric cancer. *Cancer Res* 1997;57(8):1435–1437.
100. Luqmani Y, Bennett C, Paterson I, et al. Expression of the pS2 gene in normal, benign, and neoplastic human stomach. *Int J Cancer* 1989;44:806–812.
101. Wu M-S, Shun C-T, Wang H-P, Lee W-J, Wang T-H, Lin J-T.Loss of pS2 protein expression is an early event of intestinal-type gastric cancer. *Jpn J Cancer Res* 1998;89:278–282.
102. Henry JA, Bennett MK, Piggott NH, Levett DL, May FE, Westley BR. Expression of the pNR-2/pS2 protein in diverse human epithelial tumours. *Br J Cancer* 1991;64:677–682.
103. Muller W, Borchard F. pS2 protein in gastric carcinoma and normal mucosa: association with clinicopathological study. *Eur J Cancer* 1996;32:1585–1590.

104. Lefebvre O, Chenard MP, Masson R, et al. Gastric mucosa abnormalities and tumorigenesis in mice lacking the pS2 trefoil protein. *Science* 1996;274(5285):259–262.

105. Machado JC, Carneiro F, Blin N, Sobrinho-Simoes M. Pattern of pS2 protein expression in premalignant and malignant lesions of gastric mucosa. *Eur J Cancer Prev* 1996;5:169–179.

106. Nogueira AMMF, Machado JC, Carneiro F, Celso AR, Gott P, Sobrinho-Simoes M. Pattern of expression of trefoil peptides and mucins in gastric polyps with and without malignant transformation. *J Pathol* 1999;187:541–548.

107. Sakata K, Tamura G, Nishizuka S, et al. Commonly deleted regions on the long arm of chromosome 21 in differentiated adenocarcinoma of the stomach. *Genes Chromosomes Cancer* 1997;18:318–321.

108. Nishizuka S, Tamura G, Terashima M, Satodate R. Loss of heterozygosity during the development and progression of differentiated adenocarcinoma of the stomach. *J Pathol* 1998;185:38–43.

109. Calnan DP, Westley BR, May FEB, Floyd DN, Marchbank T, Playford RJ. The trefoil peptide TFF1 inhibits the growth of the human gastric adenocarcinoma cell line AGS. *J Pathol* 1999;188:312–317.

110. Beckler AD, Roche JK, Harper JC, et al. Decreased abundance of trefoil factor 1 transcript in the majority of gastric carcinomas. *Cancer* 2003;98(10):2184–2191.

111. Sankpal NV, Mayo MW, Powell SM. Transcriptional repression of TFF1 in gastric epithelial cells by CCAAT/enhancer binding protein-beta. *Biochim Biophys Acta* 2005;1728(1–2):1–10.

112. Sankpal NV, Moskaluk CA, Hampton GM, Powell SM. Overexpression of CEBPbeta correlates with decreased TFF1 in gastric cancer. *Oncogene* 2006;25(4):643–649.

113. Morin PJ. Beta-catenin signaling and cancer. *Bioassays* 1999;21:1021–1030.

114. Nagase H, Nakamura Y. Mutation of the APC (adenomatous polyposis coli) gene. *Hum Mutat* 1993;2:425–434.

115. Ogaswara S, Maesawa C, Tamura G, Satodate R. Lack of mutations of the adenomatous polyposis coli gene in oesophageal and gastric carcinomas. *Virchows Archiv* 1994;424(6):607–611.

116. Maesawa C, Tamura G, Suzuki Y, et al. The sequential accumulation of genetic alterations characteristic of the colorectal adenoma-carcinoma sequence does not occur between gastric adenoma and adenocarcinoma. *J Pathol* 1997;176:249–258.

117. Powell SM, Cummings OW, Mullen JA, et al. Characterization of the APC gene in sporadic gastric adenocarcinomas. *Oncogene* 1996;12(9):1953–1959.

118. Tamura G, Ogasawara S, Nishizuka S, et al. Two distinct regions of deletion on the long arm of chromosome 5 in differentiated adenocarcinomas of the stomach. *Cancer Res* 1996;56(3):612–615.

119. Park WS, Oh RR, Park JY, et al. Frequent somatic mutations of the beta-catenin gene in intestinal-type gastric cancer. *Cancer Res* 1999;59:4257–4260.

120. Candidus S, Bischoff P, Becker KF, Hofler H. No evidence for mutations in the alpha- and beta-catenin genes in human gastric and breast carcinomas. *Cancer Res* 1996;56(1):49–52.

121. Kawanishi J, Kato J, Sasaki K, Jujii S, Watanabe N, Niitsu Y. Loss of E-cadherin—dependent cell–cell adhesion due to mutation of the beta-catenin gene in a human cancer cell line, HSC-39. *Mol Cell Biol* 1995;15:1175–1181.

122. Ramesh S, Nash J, McCulloch PG. Reduction in membranous expression of beta-catenin and increased cytoplasmic E-cadherin expression predict poor survival in gastric cancer. *Br J Cancer* 1999;81(8):1392–1397.

123. Igaki H, Sasaki H, Tachimori Y, et al. Mutation frequency of the p16/CDKN2 gene in primary cancers in the upper digestive tract. *Cancer Res* 1995;55(15):3421–3423.

124. Wong DJ, Barrett MT, Stoger R, Emond MJ, Reid BJ. p16INK4a promoter is hypermethylated at a high frequency in esophageal adenocarcinomas. *Cancer Res* 1997;57(13):2619–2622.

125. Klump B, Hsieh CJ, Holzmann K, Gregor M, Porschen R. Hypermethylation of the CDKN2/p16 promoter during neoplastic progression in Barrett's esophagus. *Gastroenterology* 1998;115(6):1381–1386.

126. Barrett MT, Sanchez CA, Galipeau PC, Neshat K, Emond M, Reid BJ. Allelic loss of 9p21 and mutation of the CDKN2/p16 gene develop as early lesions during neoplastic progression in Barrett's esophagus. *Oncogene* 1996;13(9):1867–1873.

127. Toyota M, Nita A, Suzuki H, et al. Aberrant methylation in gastric cancer associated with the CpG island methylator phenotype. *Cancer Res* 1999;59:5438–5442.

128. Chi XZ, Yang JO, Lee KY, et al. RUNX3 suppresses gastric epithelial cell growth by inducing p21(WAF1/Cip1) expression in cooperation with transforming growth factor {beta}-activated SMAD. *Mol Cell Biol* 2005;25(18):8097–8107.

129. Powell SM, Harper JC, Hamilton SR, Robinson CR, Cummings OW. Inactivation of Smad4 in gastric carcinomas. *Cancer Res* 1997;57(19):4221–4224.

130. Park WS, Moon YW, Yang YM, et al. Mutations of the STK11 gene in sporadic gastric carcinoma. *Int J Oncol* 1998;13(3):601–604.

131. El-Rifai W, Smith MF, Jr, Li G, et al. Gastric cancers overexpress DARPP-32 and a novel isoform, t-DARPP. *Cancer Res* 2002;62(14):4061–4064.

132. Belkhiri A, Zaika A, Pidkovka N, Knuutila S, Moskaluk C, El-Rifai W. Darpp-32: a novel antiapoptotic gene in upper gastrointestinal carcinomas. *Cancer Res* 2005;65(15):6583–6592.

133. Uchino S, Tsuda H, Maruyama K, et al. Overexpression of c-erbB-2 protein in gastric cancer. *Cancer* 1993;72:3179–3184.

134. Yonemura Y, Ninomiya I, Yamaguchi A, Fushida S, Kimura H, Ohoyama S. Evaluation of immunoreactivity for erbB-2 protein as a marker of poor short term prognosis in gastric cancer. *Cancer Res* 1991;51:1034–1038.

135. Mizutani T, Onda M, Tokunaga A, Yamanaka N, Sugisaka Y. Relationship of c-erb B-2 protein expression and gene amplification to invasion and metastasis in human gastric cancer. *Cancer* 1993;72:2083–2088.

136. Chariyalertsak S, Sugano K, Ohkura H, Mori Y. Comparison of c-erbB-2 oncoprotein expression in tissue and serum of patients with stomach cancer. *Tumor Biol* 1994;15:294–303.

137. Freiss H, Fukuda A, Tang WH, et al. Concomitant analysis of the epidermal growth factor receptor family in esophageal cancer: overexpression of epidermal growth factor receptor mRNA but not of c-erbB-2 and c-erbB-3. *World J Surg* 1999;23:1010–1018.

138. Tateishi M, Toda T, Minamisono Y, Nagasaki S. Clinicopathological significance of c-erbB-2 protein expression in human gastric carcinoma. *J Surg Oncol* 1992;49:209–212.

139. Matsuda M, Sakaguchi T, Hirao T, Nakano H. The prognostic significance of amplification and overexpression of c-met and c-erbB2 in human gastric carcinomas. *Cancer* 1999;85:1894–1902.

140. Kuniyasu H, Yasui W, Kitadai Y, Yokozaki H, Ito H, Tahara E. Frequent amplification of the c-met gene in scirrhous type stomach cancer. *Biochem Biophys Res Commun* 1992;189(1):227–232.

141. Kuniyasu H, Yasui W, Yokozaki H, Kitadai Y, Tahara E. Aberrant expression of c-met mRNA in human gastric carcinomas. *Int J Cancer* 1993;55(1):72–75.

142. Taniguchi K, Yonemura Y, Nojima N, et al. The relation between the growth patterns of gastric carcinoma and the expression of hepatocyte growth factor receptor (c-met), autocrine motility factor receptor, and urokinase-type plasminogen activator receptor. *Cancer* 1998;82(11):2112–2122.

143. Tsugawa K, Yonemura Y, Hirono Y, et al. Amplification of the c-met, c-erbB-2 and epidermal growth factor receptor gene in human gastric cancers: correlation to clinical features. *Oncology* 1998;55(5):475–481.

144. Hara T, Ooi A, Kobayashi M, Mai M, Yanagihara K, Nakanishi I. Amplification of c-myc, K-sam, and c-met in gastric cancers: detection by fluorescence in situ hybridization. *Lab Invest* 1998;78(9):1143–1153.

145. Koshiba M, Ogawa O, Habuchi T, et al. Infrequent K-ras mutation in human stomach cancers. *Jpn J Cancer Res* 1993;84:163–167.

146. Lee K-H, Lee J-S, Suh C, et al. Clinicopathologic significance of the K-ras gene codon 12 point mutation in stomach cancer. *Cancer* 1995;75:2794–2801.

147. Tahara E. Molecular biology of gastric cancer. *World J Surg* 1995;19(4):484–488.

148. Inoue T, Chung YS, Yashiro M, et al. Transforming growth factor-beta and hepatocyte growth factor produced by gastric fibroblasts stimulate the invasiveness of scirrhous gastric cancer cells. *Jpn J Cancer Res* 1997;88(2):152–159.

149. Bamba H, Ota S, Kato A, Matsuzaki F. Nonsteroidal anti-inflammatory drugs may delay the repair of gastric mucosa by suppressing prostaglandin-mediated increase of hepatocyte growth factor production. *Biochem Biophys Res Commun* 1998;245(2):567–571.

150. Ota S, Tanaka Y, Bamba H, Kato A, Matsuzaki F. Nonsteroidal anti-inflammatory drugs may prevent colon cancer through suppression of hepatocyte growth factor expression. *Eur J Pharmacol* 1999;367(1):131–138.

151. Takahashi M, Ota S, Hata Y, et al. Hepatocyte growth factor as a key to modulate anti-ulcer action of prostaglandins in stomach. *J Clin Invest* 1996;98(11):2604–2611.

152. Yasunaga Y, Shinomura Y, Kanayama S, et al. Increased production of interleukin 1 beta and hepatocyte growth factor may contribute to foveolar hyperplasia in enlarged fold gastritis [see comments]. *Gut* 1996;39(96):787–794.

153. Taha AS, Curry GW, Morton R, Park RH, Beattie AD. Gastric mucosal hepatocyte growth factor in Helicobacter pylori gastritis and peptic ulcer disease. *Am J Gastroenterol* 1996;91(7):1407–1409.

154. Kondo S, Shinomura Y, Kanayama S, et al. Helicobacter pylori increases gene expression of hepatocyte growth factor in human gastric mucosa. *Biochem Biophys Res Commun* 1995;210(3):960–965.

155. Tahara E, Semba S, Tahara H. Molecular biological observations in gastric cancer. *Semin Oncol* 1996;23(3):307–315.

156. Ueki T, Koji T, Tamiya S, Nakane PK, Tsuneyoshi M. Expression of basic fibroblast growth factor and fibroblast growth factor receptor in advanced gastric carcinoma. *J Pathol* 1995;177:353–361.

157. Tsuji S, Kawano S, Sawaoka H, et al. Evidences for involvement of cyclooxygenase-2 in proliferation of two gastrointestinal cancer cell lines. *Prostaglandins Leukot Essent Fatty Acids* 1996;55(3):179–183.

158. Oshima M, Dinchuk JE, Kargman SL, et al. Suppression of intestinal polyposis in APC delta-716 knockout mice by inhibition of cyclooxygenase 2 (COX-2). *Cell* 1996;87:803–809.

159. Ito K, Liu Q, Salto-Tellez M, et al. RUNX3, a novel tumor suppressor, is frequently inactivated in gastric cancer by protein mislocalization. *Cancer Res* 2005;65(17):7743–7750.

160. Sakakura C, Hasegawa K, Miyagawa K, et al. Possible involvement of RUNX3 silencing in the peritoneal metastases of gastric cancers. *Clin Cancer Res* 2005;11(18):6479–6488.

161. Ma X, Chen K, Huang S, et al. Frequent activation of the hedgehog pathway in advanced gastric adenocarcinomas. *Carcinogenesis* 2005;26(10):1698–1705.

162. Dammrich J, Vollmers HP, Heider K-H, Muller-Hermelink H-K. Importance of different CD44v6 expression in human gastric intestinal and diffuse type cancers for metastatic lymphogenic spreading. *J Mol Med* 1995;73:395–401.

163. Nomura H, Hiroshi S, Motoharu S, Masyoshi M, Yasunori O. Expression of membrane-type matrix metalloproteinase in human gastric carcinomas. *Cancer Res* 1995;55:3263–3266.

164. Ito H, Yonemura Y, Fujita H, et al. Prognostic relevance of urokinase-type plasminogen activator (uPA) and plasminogen activator inhibitors PAI-1 and PAI-2 in gastric cancer. *Virchows Arch* 1996;427:487–496.

165. Burgart LJ, Zheng J, Shu Q, Strickler JG, Shibata D. A somatic mitochondrial mutation in gastric cancer. *Am J Pathol* 1995;147(4):1105–1111.

166. Hiyama E, Yokoyama T, Tatsumato N, et al. Telomerase activity in gastric cancer. *Cancer Res* 1995;55:3258–3262.

167. Tebbutt NC, Giraud AS, Inglese M, et al. Reciprocal regulation of gastrointestinal homeostasis by SHP2 and STAT-mediated trefoil gene activation in gp130 mutant mice. *Nat Med* 2002;8(10):1089–1097.

168. Zavros Y, Eaton KA, Kang W, et al. Chronic gastritis in the hypochlorhydric gastrin-deficient mouse progresses to adenocarcinoma. *Oncogene* 2005;24(14):2354–2366.

169. Silberg DG, Sullivan J, Kang E, et al. Cdx2 ectopic expression induces gastric intestinal metaplasia in transgenic mice. *Gastroenterology* 2002;122(3):689–696.

170. Houghton J, Stoicov C, Nomura S, et al. Gastric cancer originating from bone marrow-derived cells. *Science* 2004;306(5701):1568–1571.

171. Gut MO, Parkkila S, Vernerova Z, et al. Gastric hyperplasia in mice with targeted disruption of the carbonic anhydrase gene Car9. *Gastroenterology* 2002;123(6):1889–1903.

172. Xu X, Brodie SG, Yang X, et al. Haploid loss of the tumor suppressor Smad4/Dpc4 initiates gastric polyposis and cancer in mice. *Oncogene* 2000;19(15):1868–1874.

173. Pritchard DM, Przemeck SM. Review article: how useful are the rodent animal models of gastric adenocarcinoma? *Aliment Pharmacol Ther* 2004;19(8):841–859.

174. Duffy MJ, Maguire TM, McDermott EW, O'Higgins N. Urokinase plasminogen activator: a prognostic marker in multiple types of cancer. *J Surg Oncol* 1999;71:130–135.

175. Maeda K, Kang SM, Onaoda N, et al. Vascular endothelial growth factor expression in the preoperative biopsy specimens correlates with disease recurrence in patients with early gastric carcinoma. *Cancer* 1999;86:566–571.

176. Han S, Kim HT, Park K, et al. c-myc Expression is related with cell proliferation and associated with poor clinical outcome in human gastric cancer. *J Korean Med Sci* 1999;14:526–530.

177. Lin WC, Li AFY, Chi CW, et al. tie-1 Protein tyrosine kinase: a novel independent prognostic marker for gastric cancer. *Clin Cancer Res* 1999;5:1745–1751.

178. Yamamichi K, Uehara Y, Kitamura N, Nakane Y, Hioki K. Increased expression of CD44v6 mRNA significantly correlates with distant metastasis and poor prognosis in gastric cancer. *Int J Cancer* 1998;79:256–262.

179. Kuwahara A, Katano M, Nakamura M, et al. New therapeutic strategy for gastric carcinoma: a two-step evaluation of malignant potential from its molecular biologic and pathologic characteristics. *J Surg Oncol* 1999;72:142–149.

180. Takano Y, Kato Y, Masuda M, Ohshima Y, Okayasu I. Cyclin D2 but not cyclin D1, overexpression closely correlates with gastric cancer progression and prognosis. *J Pathol* 1999;189:194–200.

181. Kwon OJ, Kang HS, Suh JS, Chang MS, Jang JJ, Chung JK. The loss of p27 protein has an independent prognostic significance in gastric cancer. *Anticancer Res* 1999;19:4215–4220.

182. Jang SJ, Park YW, Park MH, et al. Expression of cell-cycle regulators, cyclin E and p21 (WAF1/CIP1) potential prognostic markers for gastric cancer. *Eur J Surg Oncol* 1999;25:157–163.

183. Che XM, Hokita S, Natsugoe S, et al. C0-ocurrence of reduced expression of alpha-catenin and overexpression of p53 is a predictor of lymph node metastasis in early gastric cancer. *Oncology* 1999;57:131–137.

184. Ganesh S, Sier CFM, Heerding MM, et al. Prognostic value of the plasminogen activation system in patients with gastric carcinoma. *Cancer* 1996;77:1035–1043.

185. Zafirellis K, Karameris A, Milingos N, Androulakis G. Molecular markers in gastric cancer: can p53 and bcl-2 protein expressions be used as prognostic factors? *Anticancer Res* 2005;25(5):3629–3636.

186. Liu XP, Kawauchi S, Oga A, et al. Combined examination of p27(Kip1), p21(Waf1/Cip1) and p53 expression allows precise estimation of prognosis in patients with gastric carcinoma. *Histopathology* 2001;39(6):603–610.

187. Nishigaki R, Osaki M, Hiratsuka M, et al. Proteomic identification of differentially-expressed genes in human gastric carcinomas. *Proteomics* 2005;5(12):3205–3213.

188. Saito H, Tsujitani S, Oka S, et al. The expression of thymidine phosphorylase correlates with angiogenesis and the efficacy of chemotherapy using fluorouracil derivatives in advanced gastric carcinoma. *Br J Cancer* 1999;81:484–489.

189. Nagahara H, Mimori K, Utsunomiya T, et al. Clinicopathologic and biological significance of kallikrein 6 overexpression in human gastric cancer. *Clin Cancer Res* 2005;11(19 pt 1):6800–6806.

190. Torii A, Kodera Y, Uesaka K, et al. Plasma concentration of matrix metalloproteinase 9 in gastric cancer. *Br J Surg* 1997;84:133–136.

191. Yoshikawa T, Saitoh M, Tsuburaya A, et al. Tissue inhibitor of matrix metalloproteinase-1 in the plasma of patients with gastric carcinoma-a possible marker for serosal invasion and metastasis. *Cancer* 1999;86:1929–1935.

192. De Vita F, Orditura M, Galizia G, et al. Serum interleukin-10 levels in patients with advanced gastrointestinal malignancies. *Cancer* 1999;86:1936–1943.

193. Han SU, Lee JH, Kim WH, Cho YK, Kim MW. Significant correlation between serum level of hepatocyte growth factor and progression of gastric carcinoma. *World J Surg* 1999;23:1176–1180.

194. Saito H, Tsujitani S, Ikeguchi M, Maeta M, Kaibara N. Serum level of a soluble receptor for interleukin-2 as a prognostic factor in patients with gastric cancer. *Oncology* 1999;56:253–258.

195. Gofuku J, Shiozaki H, Doki Y, et al. Characterization of soluble E-cadherin as a disease marker in gastric cancer patients. *Br J Cancer* 1998;78:1095–1101.

196. Chausovsky G, Luchansky M, Figer A, et al. Expression of cytokeratin 20 in the blood of patients with disseminated carcinoma of the pancreas, colon, stomach, and lung. *Cancer* 1999;86:2398–2405.

197. Pituch-Noworolska A, Wieckiewicz J, Krzeszowiak A, et al. Evaluation of circulating tumour cells expressing CD44 variants in the blood of gastric cancer patients by flow cytometry. *Anticancer Res* 1998;18:3747–3752.

198. Nakata B, Chung KH-Y, Kato Y, et al. Serum CA 125 level as a predictor of peritoneal dissemination in patients with gastric carcinoma. *Cancer* 1998;83:2488–2492.

199. Marrelli D, Roviello F, de Stefano A, et al. Prognostic significance of CEA, CA 19-9, and CA 72-4 preoperative serum levels in gastric carcinoma. *Oncology* 1999;57:55–62.

200. Wu CW, Lin YY, Chen GD, Chi CW, Carbone DP, Chen JY. Serum anti-p53 antibodies in gastric adenocarcinoma patients are associated with poor prognosis, lymph node metastasis and poorly differentiated nuclear grade. *Br J Cancer* 1999;80:483–488.

201. Illert B, Fein M, Otto C, et al. Disseminated tumor cells in the blood of patients with gastric cancer are an independent predictive marker of poor prognosis. *Scand J Gastroenterol* 2005;40(7):843–849.

202. Tamura G. Promoter methylation status of tumor suppressor and tumor-related genes in neoplastic and non-neoplastic gastric epithelia. *Histol Histopathol* 2004;19(1):221–228.

203. Hirota S, Isoazki K, Moriyama Y, et al. Gain-of-function mutations of c-kit in human gastrointestinal stromal tumors. *Science* 1998;279:577–580.

204. Nishida T, Hirota S, Taniguchi M, et al. Familial gastrointestinal stromal tumours with germline mutation of the KIT gene. *Nature Genetics* 1998; 19:323–324.

205. Tokunaga A, Onda M, Okuda T, et al. Clinical significance of epidermal growth factor (EGF), EGF receptor, and c-erbB-2 in human gastric cancer. *Cancer* 1995;75:1418–1425.

206. Kasprzyk PG, Song SU, Di Fiore PP, King CR. Therapy of an animal model of human gastric cancer using a combination of anti-*erb*B-2 monoclonal antibodies. *Cancer Res* 1992;52:2771–2776.

207. Tatebe S, Matsuura T, Endo K, et al. Adenovirus-mediated transfer of wild-type p53 gene results in apoptosis or growth arrest in human cultured gastric carcinoma cells. *Int J Oncol* 1999;15(2):229–235.

208. Kijima H, Osaki T, Nishino K, et al. Application of the Cre recombinase/loxP system further enhances antitumor effects in cell type-specific gene therapy against carcinoembryonic antigen-producing cancer. *Cancer Res* 1999;59:4906–4911.

209. Lan K-H, Kanai F, Shiratori Y, et al. In vivo selective gene expression and therapy mediated by adenoviral vectors for human carcinoembryonic antigen-producing gastric carcinoma. *Cancer Res* 1997;57:4279–4284.

210. Watanabe M, Takahashi Y, Ohta T, Mai M, Sasake T, Motoharu S. Inhibition of metastasis in human gastric cancer cells transfected with tissue inhibitor of metalloproteinase 1 gene in nude mice. *Cancer* 1996;77(8):1676–1680.

211. Hirao T, Sawada H, Koyama F, et al. Antisense epidermal growth factor receptor delivered by adenoviral vector blocks tumor growth in human gastric cancer. *Cancer Gene Therapy* 1999;6:423–427.

CHAPTER 21 ■ GASTRIC CANCER: PATHOLOGY

GRANT N. STEMMERMANN AND CECILIA M. FENOGLIO-PREISER

Gastric cancers represent a heterogeneous group of tumors, most lesions being adenocarcinomas. The less common gastric cancers, such as lymphomas, neuroendocrine tumors, and stromal tumors, are discussed elsewhere in this volume.

Gastric adenocarcinoma shows striking temporal, geographic, and subsite variations in frequency, with more than 10-fold differences in incidence existing between countries with high and low rates of the disease (1). High rates are observed in Japan, Korea, and northeast China; in the Andean areas of Latin America; and in Eastern Europe. Once the most common cancer in the United States, gastric cancer distal to the cardia has shown a dramatic decrease in frequency since the 1940s, while the frequency of cancer of the cardia among white American men has more than doubled since 1975 (2). Studies of migrants from high-risk countries, such as Japan, to lower-risk countries, such as the United States, indicate that first-generation migrants continue to experience the high noncardia gastric cancer rates of Japan, whereas their children and grandchildren show rates approaching that of the host country (3). These data support the concept that environmental factors in early life generate precursors to cancer distal to the cardia. These persist into adulthood and are not reversed by living in a more favorable environment.

Gastric adenocarcinoma behaves not as one but as several distinct diseases, depending on the location of the tumor and its histologic type. Gastric cancers may be classified by site of origin into cardiac (gastroesophageal), body, or antral types. Tumors arising in each location differ in their epidemiology, their histology, and their molecular biology. Differences in gastric cancer growth patterns were first recognized by Lauren, who divided gastric cancers into "intestinal" and "diffuse" types based on their histologic characteristics (4). Intestinal cancers have a glandular appearance and expand through the gastric wall, whereas diffuse cancers infiltrate as single discohesive cells and demonstrate an infiltrating growth pattern. The intestinal-type of tumor predominates in populations at high risk of cancer in the distal stomach. This tumor most commonly arises in the antrum in the setting of a multifocal gastritis that is initiated by *Helicobacter pylori* infection and characterized by extensive atrophy and intestinal metaplasia (5–7). Cancers arising in the cardia are also usually of the intestinal type but are not associated with the extensive corpus atrophy that precedes more distal cancers. Diffuse gastric cancers are less common and frequently arise in a nonatrophic corpus that shows *H. pylori*–induced superficial gastritis. Intestinal-type cancers are more frequent in males and the elderly, and are associated with better survival. Diffuse cancers, in contrast, occur more frequently in women and individuals younger than age 50 (8). They generally have a poor prognosis, and have been associated with blood type A (8) and mutations that inactivate the E-cadherin gene (9,10).

GASTRIC CANCER PRECURSORS

Gastritis resulting from exposure to environmental hazards in early life precedes the development of cancer distal to the cardia. These include *H. pylori* infection, a high intake of salt and nitrates, and a diet deficient in fresh fruits and vegetables (11). Middle age, obesity, gastrointestinal reflux disease, and smoking precede the development of cardia cancer (12–14).

Gastric carcinomas do not arise de novo from normal gastric epithelium. Like other cancers, gastric carcinomas arise from epithelium that has been altered in some way. The precursor lesions associated with the intestinal-type of antral gastric cancer are well characterized, and include chronic gastritis and intestinal metaplasia. The metaplastic glands resemble those of the small gut, but there are subsite variations in the glycocalyceal enzymes and mucins produced by them. Some metaplastic glands reproduce the cell types of the small bowel. This histologic pattern is termed "complete" metaplasia. Other glands may lack Paneth cells, lose the ability to make some glycocalyceal enzymes, and produce mucosubstances similar to those in the colon, the so-called "incomplete" metaplasia (15). Hybrid goblet cells, sharing both gastric and intestinal phenotypes have also been identified in the metaplastic mucosa (16), as well as gastric and intestinal types of neuroendocrine cells (17). It has been proposed that, in the presence of inflammation, circulating bone marrow–derived stem cells with the potential of differentiating into gastric or intestinal type may take part in gastric cell replication (18). This could account for the observed heterogeneity of intestinal metaplasia. The immunohistochemical labeling indices for cell replication progressively increase with increasing severity of gastritis and are highest in and near areas of intestinal metaplasia. Intestinal metaplasia first appears as discrete foci at the antrocorpus junction (Fig. 21.1). As the process expands, metaplastic glands replace the gastric glands throughout the antrum and extend proximally to replace the acid-producing oxyntic glands of the corpus. The risk of gastric cancer peaks when acid production is at its nadir (Fig. 21.2). Incomplete metaplasia appears in the later stages of this process and is a feature of the extensive metaplasia that results in achlorhydria (7). Serum pepsinogen assays give indirect evidence of the extent of metaplastic replacement of gastric mucosa. Pepsinogen group I (PGI) production is limited to the oxyntic mucosa of the corpus of the stomach, although pepsinogen group II (PGII) is made in all gastric glands. The replacement of oxyntic mucosa by intestinalized mucosa results in decreasing levels of circulating PGI (19). A PGI level <30 ng/mL or a PGI:PGII ratio <2 serve as useful cut points for the identification of extensive intestinal metaplasia, and have been used to identify persons who should be screened because they are at high risk of stomach cancer distal to the cardia (20).

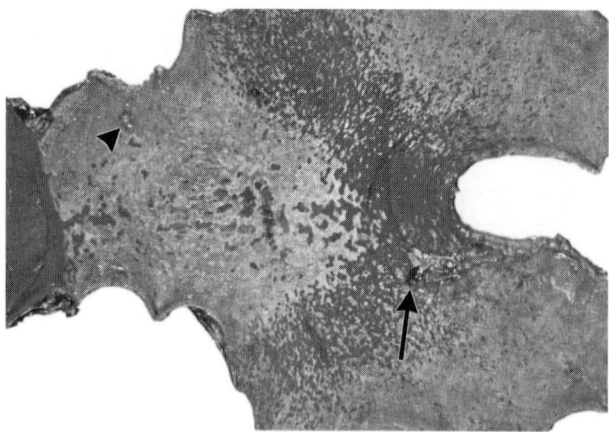

FIGURE 21.1. A gastric resection specimen containing early phase, multifocal gastritis. Foci of intestinal metaplasia are demonstrated by staining for alkaline phosphatase and are limited to the antrocorpus junction and antral lesser curvature. An ulcer (*arrow*) is present on the posterior wall of the junction zone, and a hyperplastic polyp (*arrowhead*) is present on the anterior wall of the antrum.

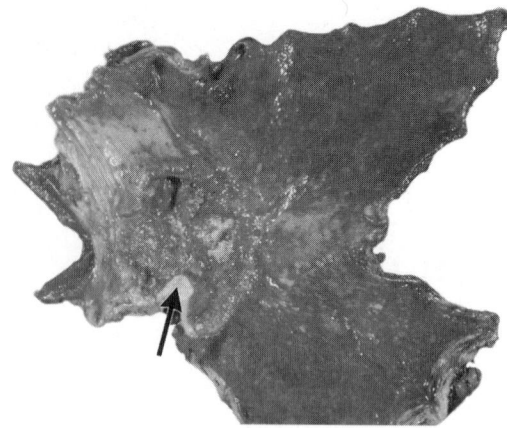

FIGURE 21.2. A resected stomach in which all but a small portion of the greater curvature of the antrum has been converted to alkaline phosphatase—positive intestinalized mucosa. The achlorhydria associated with this change incurs a high risk of carcinoma that, as in this case, characteristically develops at or near the proximal antrum (*arrow*).

This is especially useful when the PGI level is combined with measurements of the serum *H. pylori* antibody levels, as shown in Table 21.1, adapted from a recent case-control study (21). Similar trends are observed with PGI:PGII ratios.

The mechanisms that underlie in the development of intestinal metaplasia of the gastric mucosa are complex. The maintenance of specific organ structures and functions in the gastrointestinal tract has been attributed to CDX, a homologue of the *Drosophila caudal* homeobox gene during intestinal development (22). CDX1 and CDX2 are not expressed in the normal stomach, but their mRNAs are expressed in metaplastic glands. CDX2 expression precedes CDX1 expression and appears to be the trigger that initiates the metaplastic process. Mutoh et al. (23) generated transgenic mice that express CDX2 in the gastric parietal cells. By day 37, all gastric mucosal cells are replaced by a full array of intestinal cells, including goblet cells and absorption cells that express alkaline phosphatase. A mechanism for the insertion of this gene into the gastric mucosa is suggested by the recent studies of Houghton and Wang (18). They found that, in the presence of *Helicobacter*-generated gastritis, circulating bone marrow—derived stem cells may be recruited and engrafted into the replicating zone of the gastric mucosa. This mechanism could account for the observation of hybrid metaplastic epithelium with both gastric and intestinal features in association with *H. pylori* gastritis (24).

H. pylori infection is closely associated with increased cancer risk, but it does not act alone and not all strains of the organism are equally pathogenic. Strains that possess the cagA gene (25) and those that produce a vacuolating toxin (26) induce a more intense inflammatory reaction, incur greater cell damage, and are associated with greater risk of stomach cancer than other strains. *H. pylori* infection increases the risk of cancer induction in several ways:

- Its metabolic products may function as direct carcinogens.
- More rapid replication of gastric stem cells in response to mucosal injury increases the number of cells vulnerable to ingested carcinogens (Fig. 21.3A, B).
- Endogenous byproducts of inflammation, such as superoxide and hydroxyl radicals, may initiate mutations through oxidative damage.
- The appearance of a bacterial flora with the capacity of generating carcinogenic nitroso compounds from ingested amines is a feature of the achlorhydria, whether associated with end-stage *H. pylori* infection or pernicious anemia (27).

Fifty percent of patients with gastric juice pH >4 have nitrate-reducing bacteria in their stomachs (28).

H. pylori attach to the surface epithelium (Fig. 21.4) but produce cell damage in the area of the mucus neck region, which contains actively replicating cells (Fig. 21.5). The inflammatory cells generate free radicals and reactive nitrogen

TABLE 21.1

AGE, GENDER, AND ETHNICITY ADJUSTED ODDS RATIOS FOR COMBINATIONS OF SERUM PGI LEVELS AND *HELICOBACTER PYLORI* ANTIBODY STATUS, ACCORDING TO HISTOLOGIC TYPES OF GASTRIC CANCER

	All cancer distal to cardia	Intestinal type	Diffuse type
H pyl/CagA negative, PGI normal	1.00	1.00	1.00
Hpyl/CagA negative, PGI low	5.40 (2.61–11.2)[a]	5.06 (2.43–10.97)	8.92 (1.48–53.65)
Hpyl/CagA positive, PGI normal	4.86 (2.90–8.13)	3.64 (2.05–6.45)	14.84 (4.04–54.4)
Hpyl/CagA positive, PGI low	9.21 (4.95–17.13)	6.91 (3.53–13.53)	40.74 (9.51–174.6)

PGI, Pepsinogen group I.
[a] 95% Confidence level.

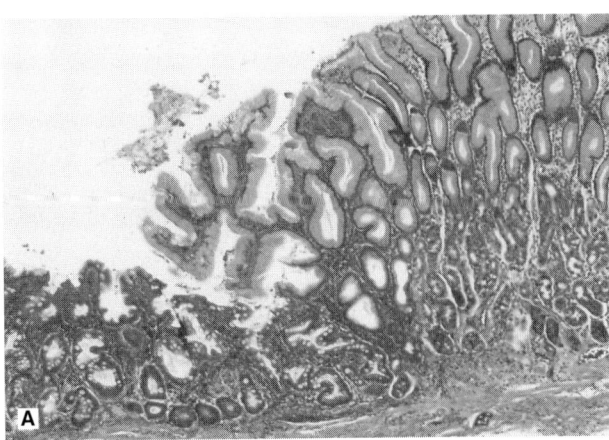
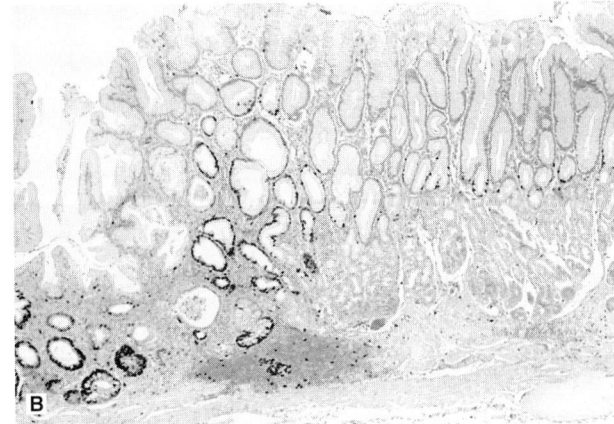

FIGURE 21.3. **A:** A hematoxylin-and-eosin—stained section has a focus of intestinal metaplasia (*left*). The adjacent gastric mucosa is hyperplastic. **B:** Ki-67 immunohistochemistry reflects the increased cell replication in the metaplastic mucosa and the gastric mucosa adjacent to it.

molecules that are capable of damaging cellular DNA and presumably increase gastric cancer risk through induction of mutations in genes critical to cell division and repair.

H. pylori gastritis evolves from an acute to a chronic gastritis that is characterized by a polymorphic infiltrate in the upper lamina propria, consisting of neutrophils, eosinophils, basophils, monocytes, and plasma cells (Fig. 21.6). Foci of atrophy associated with lymphocytic follicles and isolated metaplastic glands follow (Fig. 21.7).

Mucosal inflammation also precedes other types of gastric cancer. As noted previously, diffuse carcinomas arise in patients whose stomachs show intense, *H. pylori*—induced superficial gastritis. The risk of acquiring diffuse cancer is especially high when CagA is the infecting strain (21). The onset of diffuse cancers in the nonatrophic corpus of young patients suggests an increased vulnerability to cancer induction, either from an intense immunologic response to infection, from infection by toxic strains of *H. pylori*, or from greater exposure to exogenous carcinogens. Inherited mutations or polymorphisms may also contribute to this increase in risk.

Gastric Ulcer

In the early stages of the expansion of *H. pylori*—induced multifocal gastritis, the intestinalized mucosa at the antrocorpus junction is exposed to acid and pepsin produced by the still intact oxyntic mucosa. The intestinalized mucosa lacks the protective mucus barrier of the normal stomach and is therefore vulnerable to peptic ulceration. Patients with chronic gastric ulcers are at greatly increased risk of gastric cancer. Re-epithelialization of the ulcerated surface associates with expansion of the replication zones in the intact glands adjacent to the ulcer (29). This exposes a larger number of replicating cells to genotoxic damage and accounts for the observation that dysplasia and early cancers arise in the gastric mucosa bordering ulcers, rather than in the ulcer itself (30). An example of this phenomenon is shown in Fig. 21.8A and B.

Autoimmune Gastritis

Autoimmune gastritis, like environmental gastritis, increases the risk of gastric cancer. Patients with autoimmune gastritis produce autoantibodies to parietal cell membranes (31–33), intrinsic factor, and the gastrin receptor (34). Patients show progressive destruction of the acid-secreting mucosa, ultimately leading to hypochlorhydria or achlorhydria. Inflammation centering on the fundic glands is characterized by the accumulation of lymphocytes and plasma cells in the lamina propria. Depending on the stage of the disease, variable degrees of parietal and chief cell loss are present. The sustained inflammatory process

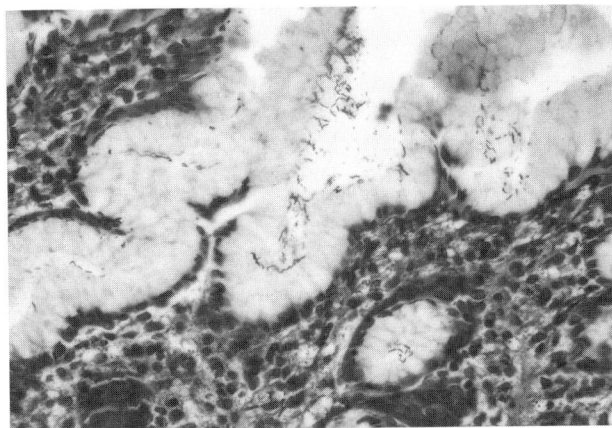

FIGURE 21.4. A Steiner stain shows the characteristic superficial location of *Helicobacter pylori* organisms in the infected stomach.

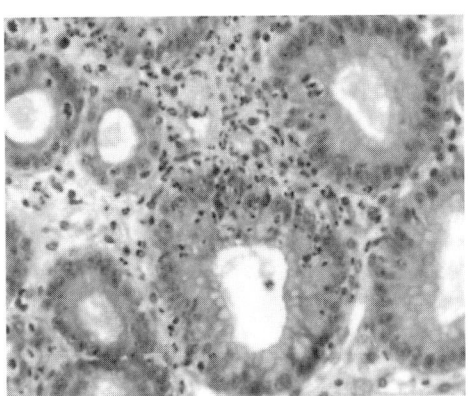

FIGURE 21.5. A hematoxylin-and-eosin stain showing a characteristic tissue reaction to *Helicobacter pylori* infection—mononuclear infiltration of the replication zones of the gastric glands.

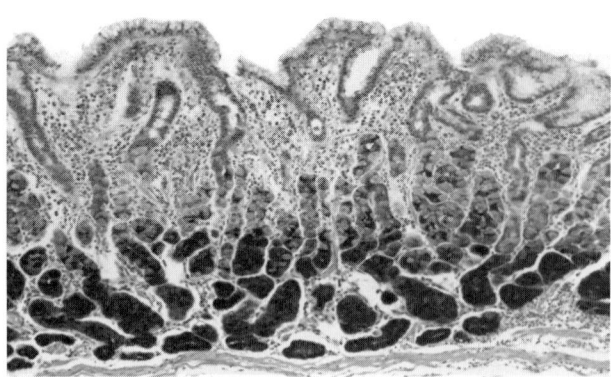

FIGURE 21.6. An immunohistochemical study of an antrum containing the superficial gastritis that characterizes the early phases of *Helicobacter pylori* gastritis. The pepsinogen group II–expressing antral glands are not yet atrophic.

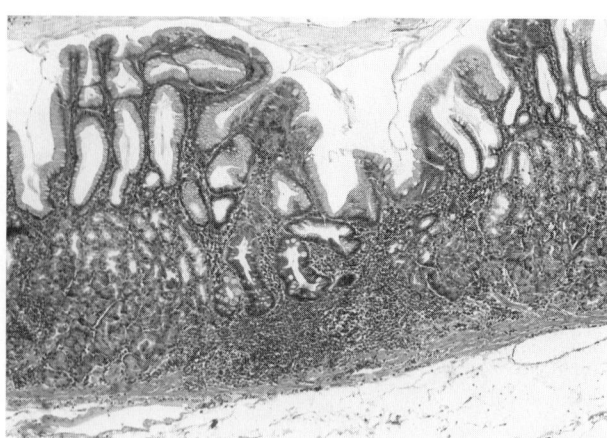

FIGURE 21.7. A hematoxylin-and-eosin–stained section of stomach contains an early focus of atrophy and intestinal metaplasia in the oxyntic mucosa of the corpus. These foci typically consist of one or two intestinalized glands and are associated with a lymphocytic follicle.

and the gastrin-induced growth promotion that accompanies achlorhydria results in increased cell replication. The foveolar epithelium is unaffected by this process and may even be hyperplastic (Fig. 21.9), sometimes to the point of forming hyperplastic polyps (Fig. 21.10A, B). Eventually, the fundic mucosa is completely replaced by pyloric and, later, by intestinalized glands. As in end-stage environmental gastritis, the achlorhydric stomach favors the generation of a bacterial flora that may generate carcinogenic nitroso compounds. The areas of intestinal metaplasia may undergo dysplastic alterations that can progress to invasive cancer.

Reflux Gastritis

Long-term exposure to refluxed bile salts and pancreatic juice in the gastric remnant after subtotal gastrectomy elicits mucosal inflammation. This associates with increased risk of cancer in the gastric remnant starting at 17 years after the resection (35). Reflux of bile and pancreatic juice may also occur in patients with an intact stomach, and this has been associated with an increased risk of gastric and gastroesophageal cancer (36).

Dysplasia

Dysplasia represents intraepithelial neoplasia and is the immediate precursor to invasive cancer. The dysplastic cells may be either gastric or intestinal in type, or may be hybrid forms from each lineage. Dysplastic gastric cells may be encountered at the margins of chronic gastric ulcers, while the intestinal forms predominate in stomachs showing confluent intestinal metaplasia. Both forms associate with immunohistochemical overexpression of p53 (Figs. 21.8B and 21.11). The dysplastic mucosa may be polypoid or flat, whether intestinal or gastric in type. The dysplastic cells show increased nuclear size, hyperchromasia, and irregularity in shape. These cytologic changes may be superimposed on a disorganized mucosal architecture.

The World Health Organization (WHO) classification for gastric dysplasia divides it into mild, moderate, and severe

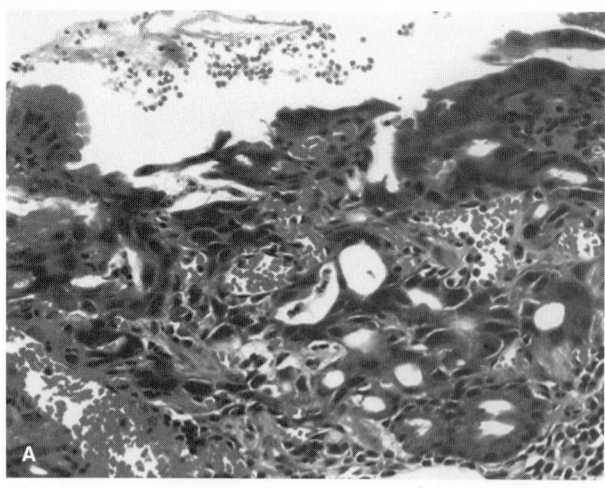

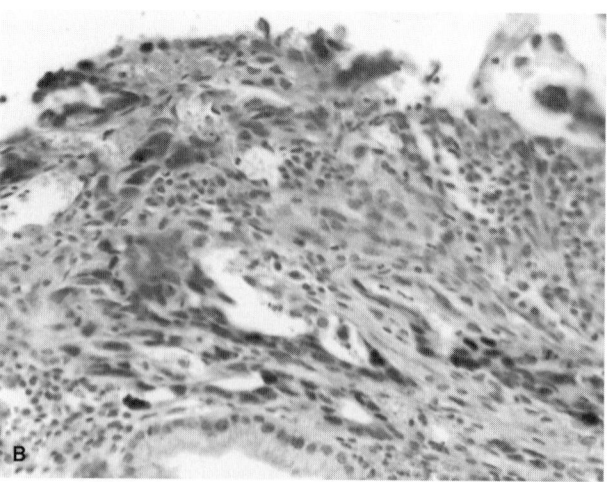

FIGURE 21.8. A: Hematoxylin-and-eosin–stained ulcer margin has a small area of dysplastic mucosa bordering a healing ulcer. **B:** This dysplastic mucosa has p53 overexpression shown by immunohistochemistry (See also color Figure 21.8a,b).

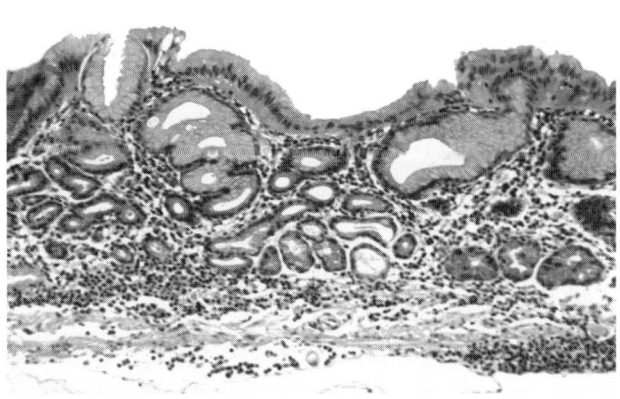

FIGURE 21.9. Severe mucosal atrophy of the corpus in a patient with autoimmune gastritis. Neither parietal cells nor corpus chief cells remain. The stomach lining consists of a somewhat hyperplastic foveolar epithelium and actively replicating neck zones. A uniform lymphocytic infiltrate occupies the lamina propria.

categories (37,38), but we believe that it is sufficient to classify dysplasia as either high or low grade. Dysplasia may be limited to the upper third of the mucosa, as shown in Fig. 21.11, or may involve the full thickness of the mucosa (Fig. 21.12). Correa described the now widely accepted sequence of steps that begins with gastritis, leading to intestinal metaplasia, then dysplasia, and ultimately to invasive gastric cancer (39), as shown in Fig. 21.13. Both genetic (40,41) and epigenetic (42,43) alterations increase in frequency with each step from the normal mucosa to gastritis, to metaplasia, to dysplasia, and to invasive cancer.

Progression of Dysplasia to Invasive Cancer

The risk of progression of dysplasia to cancer is highest in individuals with moderate to severe dysplasia (44). One study of 93 cases of gastric dysplasia showed progression to a more severe grade of dysplasia or evolution to invasive cancer in 21% of low-grade dysplasias, 33% of moderate dysplasias, and 57% of severe dysplasias (45). Dysplasia progresses slowly, usually over a period of months to years (44). However, it may also remain stable or even regress (46,47). A high percentage of closely followed cases of severe dysplasia ultimately develop into invasive carcinoma (47).

Gastric Adenomas

Some forms of gastric dysplasia present as sessile or pedunculated adenomas closely resembling colorectal tubular adenomas (Fig. 21.14). Gastric adenomas and carcinomas have similar epidemiologic backgrounds, are more commonly identified in the antrum or the midstomach than in the corpus, and arise in association with intestinal metaplasia (48). Only a minority of early gastric cancers arises in adenomas, but adenomas are clearly precancerous and their treatment must be aimed at total removal (49).

Hyperplastic Polyps

Hyperplastic polyps represent the most commonly encountered polyps in the stomach (49). These lesions often develop adjacent to gastric remnants, ulcers, or gastroenterostomy stomas. They also commonly arise in stomachs with chronic gastritis. Hyperplastic polyps are exuberant regenerative responses of the gastric foveolar cells rather than true neoplasms, but hyperplasia may coexist with either adenoma or carcinoma in the same polyp (49). The synchronous appearance of hyperplastic polyps and gastric cancers may merely reflect the propensity of both lesions to arise in a setting of chronic gastritis or atrophy.

Fundic Gland Polyps

Fundic gland polyps were initially described in patients with familial adenomatous polyposis (FAP) (48). Fundic gland polyps also develop in the absence of familial polyposis and usually affect individuals in middle age. Most fundic gland polyps do not have malignant potential, but those found in FAP may be dysplastic.

HISTOGENESIS OF GASTRIC CANCERS

Little is known about the exact cell of origin of gastric carcinomas. Many tumors arise on a background of chronic atrophic gastritis with intestinal metaplasia. Metaplastic changes in the mucosa adjacent to intestinal-type carcinomas are quite common but are less frequent in diffuse-type cancers (50,51). As discussed previously, analysis of early intestinal-type carcinomas demonstrates that areas of intestinal metaplasia commonly

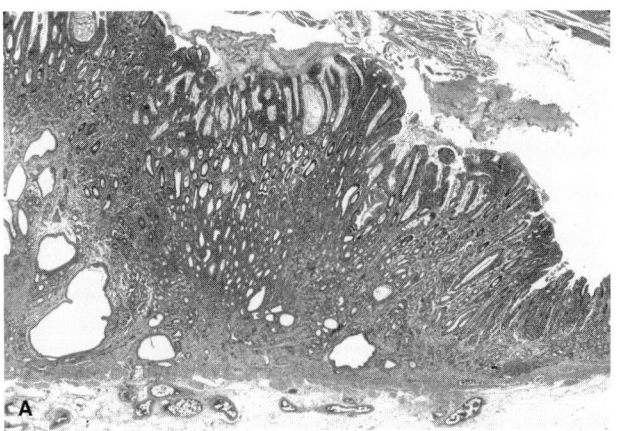

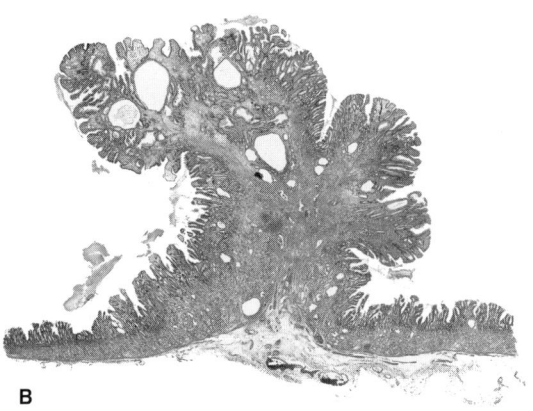

FIGURE 21.10. A: A hyperplastic polyp in the corpus in a patient with autoimmune gastritis. B: An antral hyperplastic polyp in this patient.

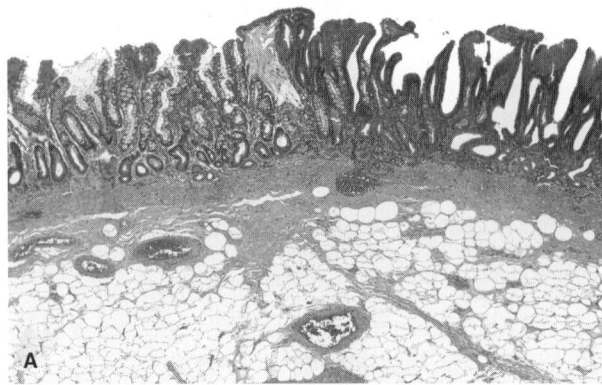
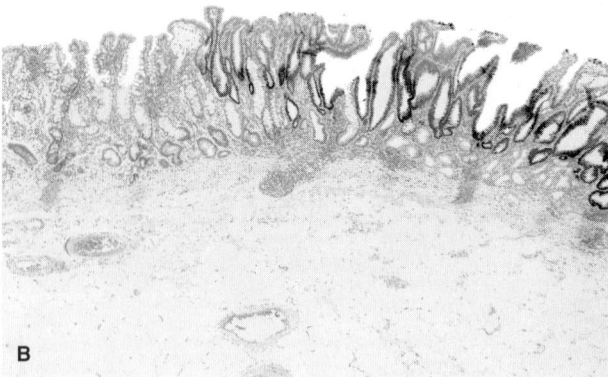

FIGURE 21.11. A: A hematoxylin-and-eosin–stained section of stomach containing confluent intestinal-ization. A well-defined area of flat dysplasia is characterized by cells with large dark nuclei and loss of mucus production. **B:** p53 Overexpression, shown by immunohistochemistry, highlights the dysplastic mucosa.

occur adjacent to the tumors. In contrast, in small diffuse-type cancers, the neoplastic cells form an intimate association with the replication zone in the neck of the gland, suggesting that they originate from the undifferentiated cells residing in this region (52).

Identification of a single cell of origin is often difficult in gastric cancers. Gastric carcinomas are heterogeneous lesions that may contain numerous cell types, including those with features of intestinal columnar cells (53–55), intestinal goblet cells, pyloric mucous cells (54–56), foveolar cells (53,54), Paneth cells (56), parietal cells (57,58), squamous cells (54), and endocrine cells (59,60). In addition, numerous hybrid cell forms occur (53). The identification of multiple cell types in gastric cancers probably reflects the fact that most of the gastric epithelial cells originate from a single multipotential progenitor cell.

TOPOGRAPHY OF GASTRIC CANCER

Gastric carcinomas in high-risk populations most commonly arise on the lesser curvature of the antrum and are especially common at mucosal junctional areas, such as the prepyloric region and incisura on the lesser curvature at the antrocorpus junction (7). Less common sites of origin include the cardia (2,61) and the greater curvature of the corpus (7). Identification of the point of origin of an esophageal adenocarcinoma

or cancer of the cardia is not always possible (62). Some observers favor the designation of "gastroesophageal junction tumors" to these cancers because the two tumors share similar epidemiologic backgrounds, recent increases in frequency among middle-age white males, an association with intestinal metaplasia of the distal esophagus, and similar molecular features (62,63). Neither cancer associates with *H. pylori* gastritis nor the multifocal gastritis that the infection produces. It has even been suggested that *H. pylori* could be protective against these tumors (64,65).

EARLY GASTRIC CANCER

Gastric carcinomas are divided into early and advanced stages, depending on the depth of invasion into the gastric wall. *Early gastric carcinoma* is defined as a cancer that remains limited to the mucosa or the submucosa, regardless of the presence or absence of nodal metastases. The subtypes of early cancer, first defined in Japan, are now generally accepted worldwide (Fig. 21.15) (66).

In countries with a high incidence of gastric cancer, improvements in gastric radiology, and refined fiber-optic endoscopy, combined with adequate cytologic and histologic sampling, have allowed large-scale screening programs to be implemented and have resulted in the identification of a high percentage of early carcinomas. The proportion of early gastric cancer in Japanese resections ranges from 30% to 50% (67–69).

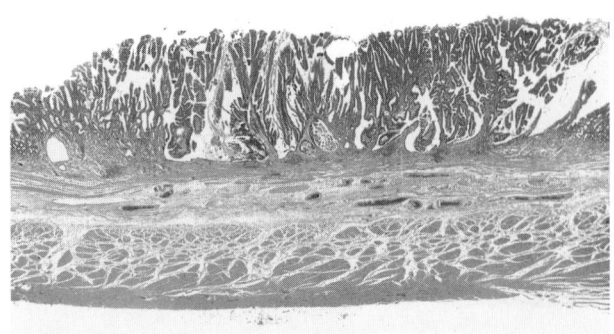

FIGURE 21.12. A hematoxylin-and-eosin–stained section of full-thickness dysplastic intestinalized mucosa. The lesion resembles a colonic villous adenoma.

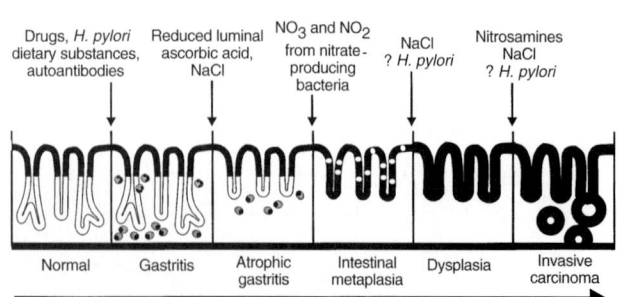

FIGURE 21.13. A diagram of the sequence of well-defined steps leading to invasive sporadic gastric cancer, including gastritis, atrophic gastritis, intestinal metaplasia, dysplasia, intramucosal cancer, and invasive cancer. Various factors influencing each step in the progression are indicated.

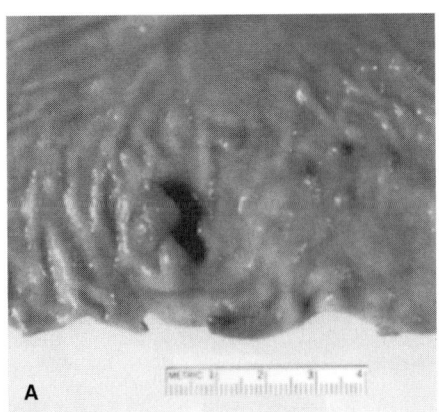 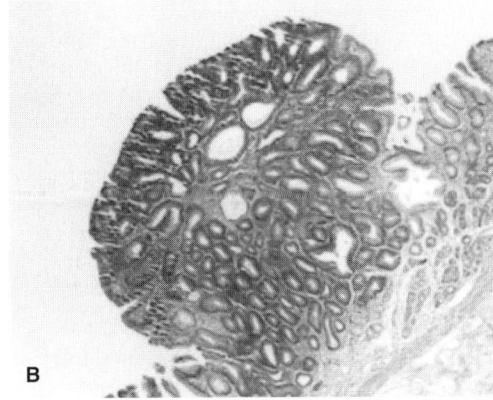

FIGURE 21.14. A: A gross specimen of an adenomatous polyp arising in the gastric mucosa. **B:** A hematoxylin-and-eosin—stained section of this polyp, which resembles a tubular adenoma of the large bowel.

Between 1962 and 1991, a broad application of community screening in Japan resulted in a marked reduction in the size of early gastric cancers (68). In Western countries, where screening programs are less common, early gastric cancers are identified less frequently (70–72).

The ability to diagnose early gastric cancer has allowed surgeons to devise function-preserving, minimally invasive, methods of treatment that give the patient a better quality of life than conventional gastric resections. These include endoscopic mucosal resection (EMR) (73) and wedge resection, with or without adjacent lymphadenectomy (74). Selection of either approach depends on the probability that a tumor will recur. The risk factors that favor lymph node involvement and subsequent recurrence are large tumor size (>30 mm), submucosal penetration, undifferentiated or diffuse histology, ulceration,

and lymphatic invasion (68,75). The incidence of node involvement in cases from multiple Japanese institutions in mucosal lesions was 4% and 19% for submucosal tumors, but the presence of ulceration increased the frequency to 23% (68). The currently accepted indications for EMR include well- or moderately well-differentiated mucosal adenocarcinoma without ulceration measuring <2 cm if elevated (type IIa), or <1 cm if flat (types IIb and IIc). An EMR may be considered potentially curable if the cancer has been completely removed with histologically tumorfree margins and minimal or no risk of lymph node metastases.

ADVANCED GASTRIC CANCER

The gross appearance of gastric cancer formed the basis for the first classification system for stomach cancers, the Borrmann classification (76). Four gross growth patterns are recognized: polypoid, fungating, ulcerated, and infiltrative (Fig. 21.16). Any of the four types may coexist. Polypoid cancers

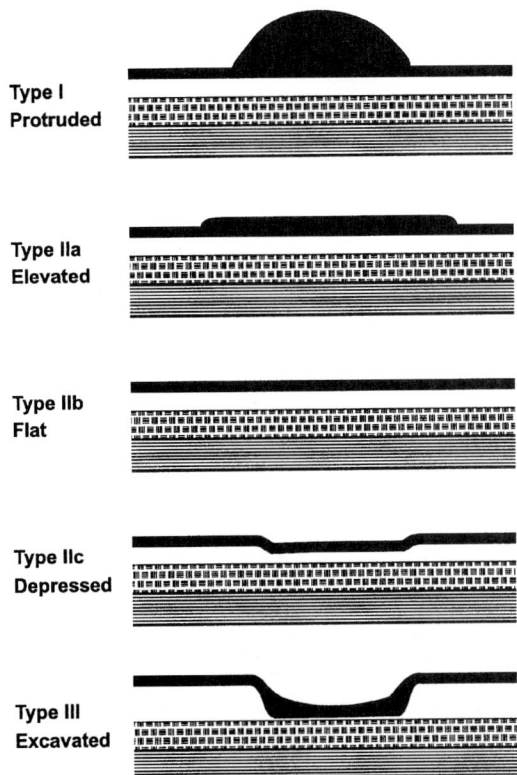

FIGURE 21.15. A diagram of the classification of early gastric cancer, developed by the Japan Gastroenterological Endoscopic Society.

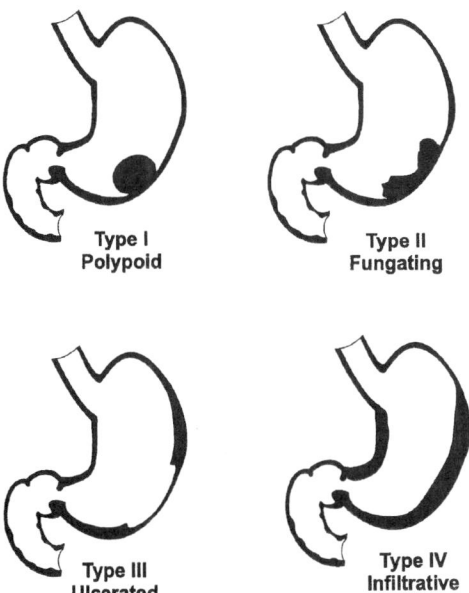

FIGURE 21.16. A diagram of the gross configuration of gastric cancer, based on the Borrmann classification.

protrude into the gastric lumen without major areas of ulceration. In contrast, fungating tumors are irregularly shaped and variably sized exophytic growths with areas of ulceration. The ulcerated type of gastric cancer consists of an irregular, variably sized ulcer with raised edges. The frequently overhanging margins appear hard and stiff. The ulcer base appears irregular with areas of necrosis. The mucosal folds surrounding the ulcer have a more irregular shape and distribution than is seen in benign ulcers. Infiltrative tumors spread superficially in the mucosa and submucosa, producing flat, plaquelike lesions, with or without shallow areas of ulceration. Massive neoplastic infiltration combined with a marked desmoplastic reaction produces gastric rigidity.

Gastric cancers exhibit considerable heterogeneity, not only from tumor to tumor, but also within a tumor. This heterogeneity results from the complex cellular composition of the gastric mucosa and the multiple types of cells in metaplastic mucosa. Because of the common association of intestinal metaplasia gastric carcinoma, a gastric cancer may contain cells reminiscent of intestinal and gastric epithelium (54,78). Finally, some cancers contain diverging clones of cell types that arise from postinduction mutations. The intestinal characteristics may be evident in hematoxylin and eosin (H&E)–stained sections, or may become apparent when the cells are examined for their secretory products, biological markers (77), or ultrastructural features (54,78). In some cases, however, the cell structure and functions of the neoplastic cells remain gastric in nature or may revert to a gastric phenotype from an intestinal form (79). Thus, although numerous histologic classifications have been proposed, none satisfactorily account for the cellular variability that may be seen within an individual neoplasm.

GASTRIC CANCER CLASSIFICATION

Lauren Classification

The approach to the classification of gastric cancers elaborated by Lauren (4) is simple and well accepted by epidemiologists. In this scheme, gastric cancers are divided into two major types, intestinal and diffuse, based on their histologic features (Fig. 21.17). A third type of carcinoma with mixed features is called *unclassified*. The intestinal-type carcinoma is usually sufficiently differentiated to contain recognizable glands lined by goblet cells containing acid mucin and absorptive cells with a brush border. When present, secretion is mostly extracellular. The cells of diffuse-type carcinomas usually appear round and rather small, and are either arranged as single cells or structured in abortive glandlike formations. Characteristically, these cells do not cause gross distortion of the gastric architecture but are scattered in the lamina propria, widening the distances between the pits and the glands. Intercellular cohesion is minimal. Signet ring cells with nuclei compressed against the cell membrane are most commonly encountered in the superficial aspects of diffuse cancers. In contrast to the discohesive diffuse cancer cells that infiltrate the stomach wall, cell cycle markers such as ^{3}H-tdr and Ki-67 may fail to label the most superficial signet ring cells that are so characteristic of these cancers (80). An intense desmoplastic reaction is the hallmark of the diffuse cancer and may be more conspicuous than the neoplastic cells that elicited it. A recently discovered hereditary type of gastric cancer resulting from mutation in the E-cadherin gene has been associated with familial gastric cancer (81–83) and is usually a diffuse cancer. Prophylactic gastrectomies in asymptomatic members of at-risk families have found very early mucosal and submucosal diffuse cancers (83). These familial cancers lack the

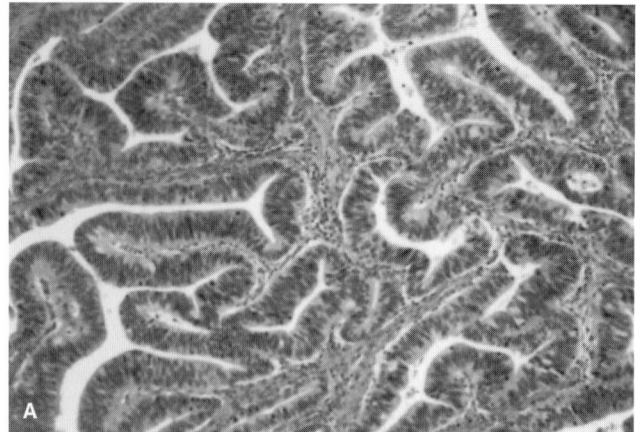
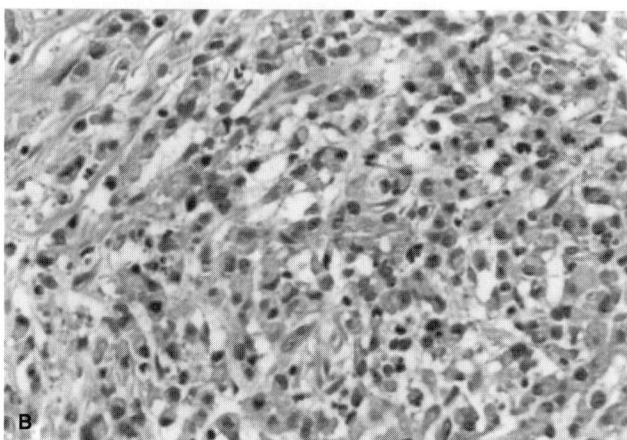

FIGURE 21.17. Typical examples of intestinal and diffuse cancer according to the Lauren classification. **A:** Intestinal type with cohesive epithelial cells forming tubules and glands. **B:** Diffuse type with discohesive cells that invade individually.

intense *H. pylori*–induced superficial gastritis that associates with sporadic diffuse cancer (Fig. 21.18). Paneth cells and neuroendocrine cells may be present in either diffuse or intestinal types of cancer.

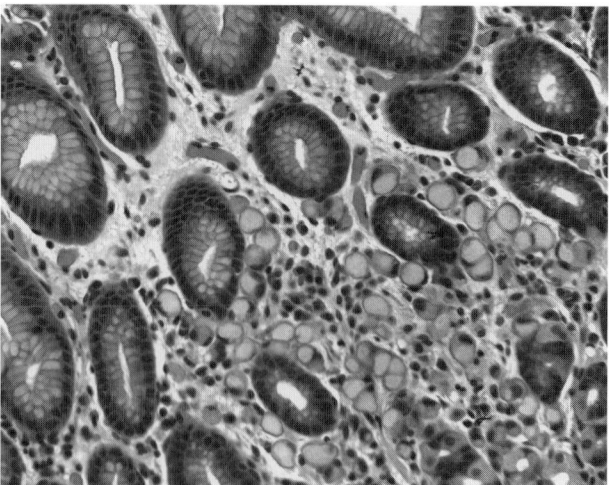

FIGURE 21.18. An extremely early signet ring cancer arising in the gastric corpus of an asymptomatic young man with an inherited E-cadherin mutation. Note the absence of inflammation that usually accompanies sporadic cancers.

World Health Organization Classification

The WHO International Reference Center for the Histologic Classification of Gastric Tumors recognizes the epithelial tumors listed in Table 21.2 (84). In this classification scheme, adenocarcinomas are graded into well-, moderately, and poorly differentiated subtypes. Well-differentiated carcinomas produce well-formed glandular structures that often resemble the metaplastic intestinal epithelium from which they are believed to arise. Poorly differentiated tumors, in contrast, are composed of irregular, poorly formed glands, or infiltrate as single cells or small cell clusters. Moderately differentiated cells demonstrate characteristics that are intermediate between well- and poorly differentiated lesions.

In addition to the degree of differentiation, subtyping may also take into account traditional histopathological features, such as intestinal or diffuse growth patterns. According to the WHO classification system, most gastric cancers represent one of four major types: papillary, tubular, mucinous, or signet ring cell cancers.

Tubular carcinomas (Fig. 21.19A) form glands with prominent lumina that may be accompanied by papillary structures. Dilated and branching tubules with acinar structures may be present. This histologic subtype shows wide variation in the degree of differentiation between individual tumors. Poorly differentiated adenocarcinomas of the tubular type are

TABLE 21.2
WORLD HEALTH ORGANIZATION HISTOLOGIC CLASSIFICATION OF GASTRIC TUMORS—EPITHELIAL TUMORS
Intraepithelial neoplasia—adenoma
Carcinoma
Adenocarcinoma
Intestinal type
Diffuse type
Papillary adenocarcinoma
Tubular adenocarcinoma
Mucinous adenocarcinoma
Signet ring carcinoma
Adenosquamous carcinoma
Squamous carcinoma
Undifferentiated carcinoma
Others

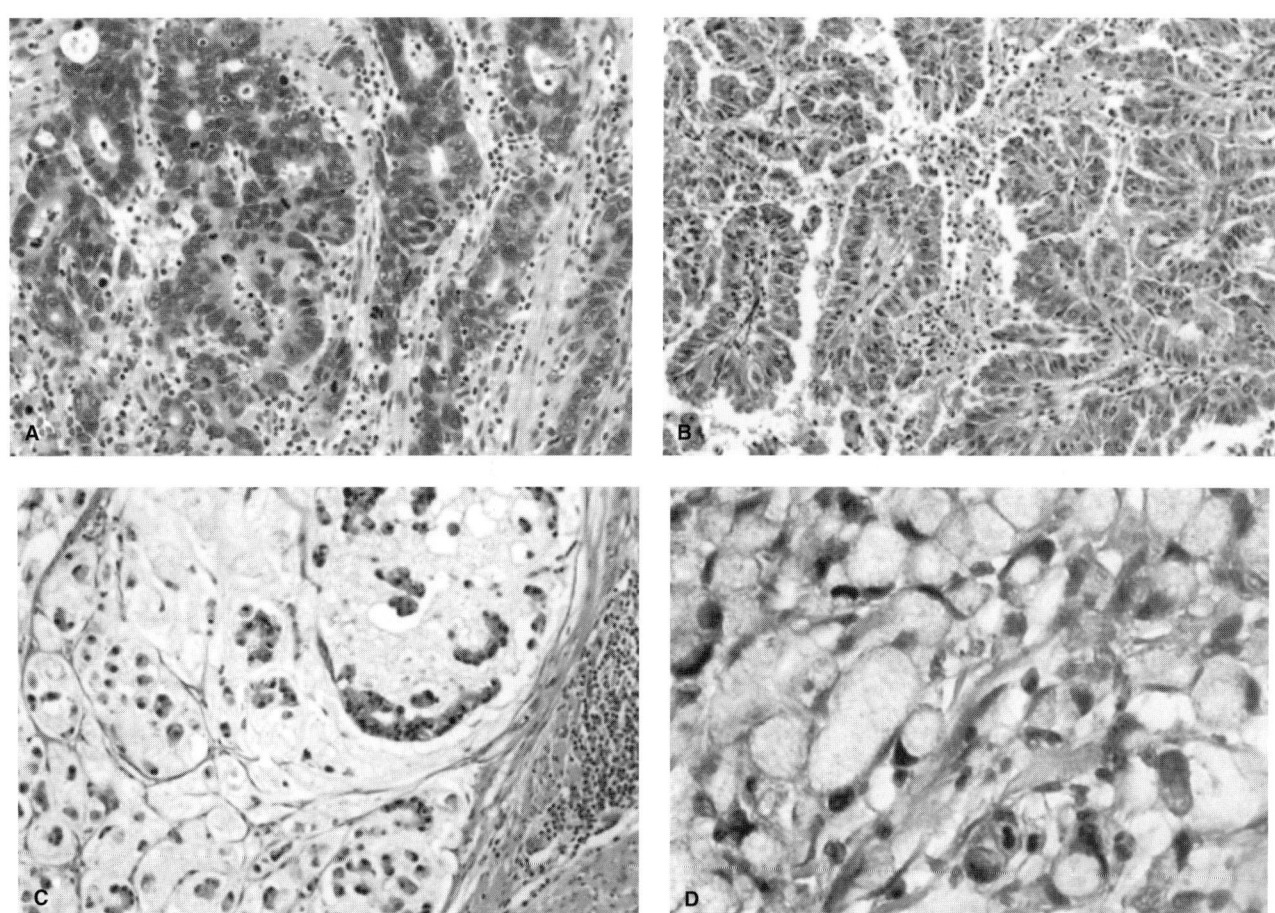

FIGURE 21.19. World Health Organization classification of gastric cancer. **A:** Intestinal type with well-formed glandular structures. **B:** Papillary type with the papillae composed of fronds of columnar cell supported by a delicate fibrovascular core. **C:** Mucinous type, consisting of individual and aggregates of tumor cells in mucus lakes. **D:** Signet ring carcinoma composed of large amounts of intracytoplasmic mucus that compresses the nuclei to the periphery of the cells.

sometimes referred to as solid carcinomas. The degree of desmoplasia varies and may be conspicuous.

Papillary carcinomas (Fig. 21.19B) are usually well-differentiated, exophytic lesions with elongated slender or plump fingerlike processes lined by cylindrical or cuboidal cells. The neoplastic cells are supported by fibrovascular cores and connective tissue. The degree of cellular atypia and the mitotic index varies and does not necessarily indicate low-grade malignancy despite an orderly appearance.

Mucinous carcinomas (Fig. 21.19C) are sometimes also referred to as colloid carcinomas. The glands are lined by mucus-producing cells whose secretions are retained in the lumina. Subsequently, the mucin compresses the lining epithelium, which detaches and is found as small cellular clusters floating free in mucinous lakes. There may also be mucus accumulation in the stroma between glands. Scattered signet ring cells are present, but they do not dominate the histologic picture.

Signet ring cell carcinomas consist of cells containing prominent intracytoplasmic mucin. Classic signet ring cells are characterized by the presence of an eccentric nucleus and abundant, optically clear cytoplasm containing acid mucin (Fig. 21.19D). Other tumors have cells with more central nuclei and cytoplasm containing neutral periodic acid Schiff (PAS)–positive diastase-resistant mucin. Signet ring cell carcinomas often demonstrate an infiltrative growth pattern. Desmoplasia may be prominent; the number of malignant cells in the lesion may be relatively small. Single, widely dispersed, neoplastic cells may be hard to detect on routine H&E-stained preparations (Fig. 21.20A, B). As a result, special stains are often used to document their presence. The most commonly used stains are mucin stains (PAS, mucicarmine, or Alcian blue) or immuno-histochemical staining with antibodies to cytokeratin (Fig. 21.20C, D). We prefer the latter because nonneoplastic muci-phages stain with mucin stains and because a greater percentage of the neoplastic cells are detectable with the anticytokeratin antibodies.

LESS COMMON TYPES OF GASTRIC CARCINOMA

Epstein-Barr Virus—Associated Carcinoma

It is now widely recognized that from 5% to 15% of gastric cancers are infected with Epstein-Barr virus (EBV) (85–88) (Fig. 21.21A–C). These cancers have distinct histologic features. They may arise in any part of the stomach, but they are most frequent in the proximal corpus. Gastric cancers that are heavily infiltrated with lymphocytes (so-called medullary cancers) are frequently EBV infected. Most of the infiltrating lymphocytes are T cells, while follicular aggregates containing B cells may be found at the periphery of the cancer. The infiltrating lymphocytes may be so numerous that the carcinoma cells may be difficult to identify on standard H&E-stained sections. Another common growth pattern seen in EBV-infected cancers consists of slender interlacing glands supported by a loose stroma—the so-called lacelike pattern. Both growth patterns may occur in different parts of the same cancer, the lacelike pattern predominating in the superficial portions of the cancer. A specific tumor phenotype may be vulnerable to infection with EBV because synchronous multicentric cancers have been observed in which only one cancer was infected (85,86,88).

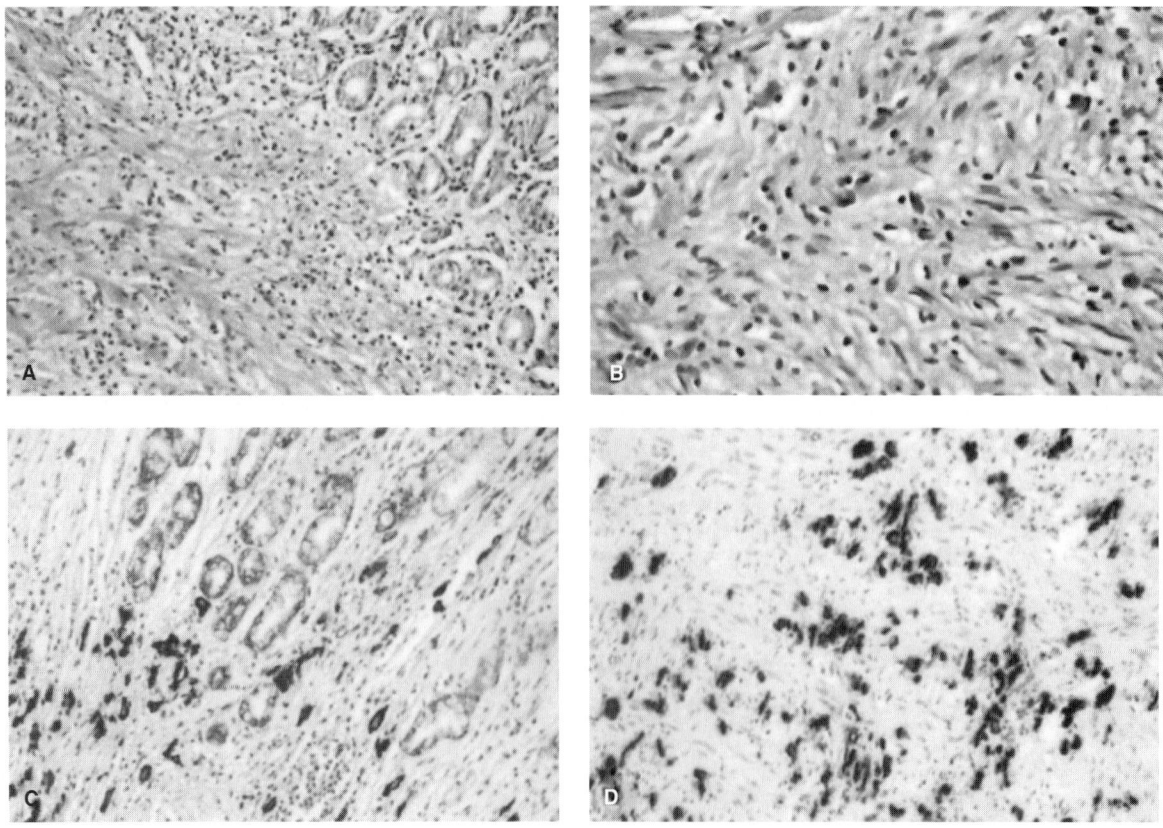

FIGURE 21.20. Diffuse cancer. The cancer cells may be very difficult to identify on hematoxylin-and-eosin stains (**A,B**), but immunohistochemistry for cytokeratin (**C,D**) clearly indicates their infiltrative nature.

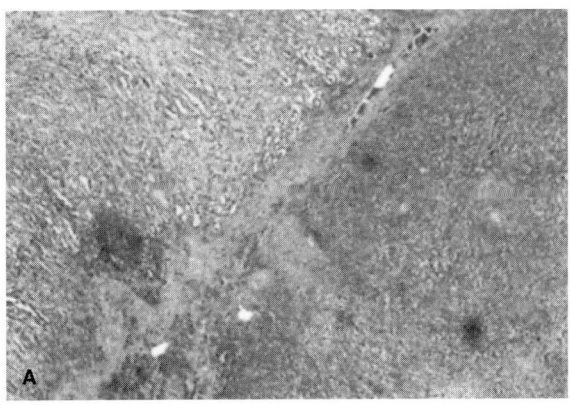

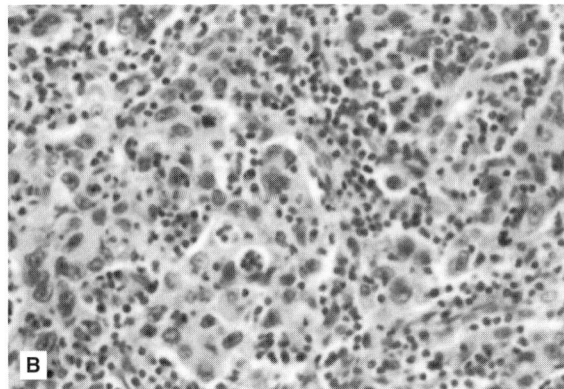

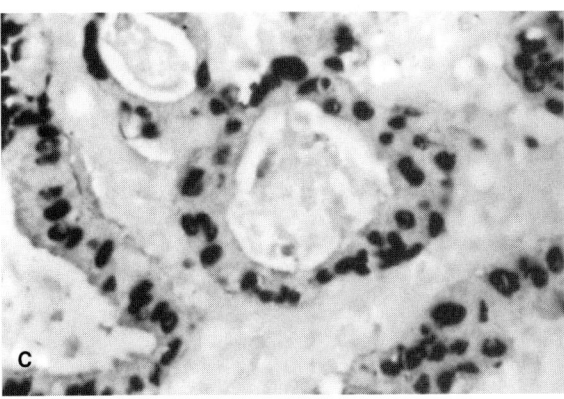

FIGURE 21.21. Epstein-Barr virus (EBV)–associated gastric cancer. Gastric cancers that are heavily infiltrated with lymphocytes (**A,B**), are usually EBV infected. This should be confirmed by in situ hybridization (**C**).

The survival of patients with EBV-infected cancers is similar to that of uninfected gastric cancers when assessed by stage, but these cancers are more likely to be diagnosed at low stage than uninfected cancers (89). Indeed, it is not unusual for EBV-infected cancers to exceed 10 cm in diameter without acquiring lymph node metastases.

Paneth Cell Cancer

Gastric cancers composed of Paneth cells are very uncommon, but they do occur (56,90). They arise in areas of complete intestinal metaplasia. H&E stains of these cancers reveal conspicuous red cytoplasmic granules that label with markers for lysozyme (91) (Fig. 21.22A–C).

Gastric Parietal Cell Carcinoma and Parietal Cell-like Carcinoma (Oncocytic Adenocarcinoma)

Gastric parietal cell carcinoma is rare. Histologically, the tumor has a solid or medullary appearance, with occasional tubular differentiation. The round cells contain abundant eosinophilic granular cytoplasm lacking mucin or neuroendocrine granules. The tumor cells demonstrate light microscopic staining characteristics and ultrastructural features similar to those of normal parietal cells (57). A well-differentiated adenocarcinoma has been observed in elderly patients that is rich in mitochondria and mimics parietal cell cancer by light and ultrastructural microscopy. These cancers have been termed oncocytic adenocarcinomas and have been distinguished from parietal cell cancers by the absence of staining with any of four antiparietal antibodies (58).

Adenosquamous Carcinoma

Adenosquamous carcinomas contain coexisting areas of adenocarcinoma and squamous cell carcinoma (Fig. 21.23A–C). The glandular part of adenosquamous carcinoma may be more or less differentiated and bears some influence on survival. The overall prognosis of adenosquamous carcinoma is less favorable than that of adenocarcinoma, probably because the tumors are advanced and frequently demonstrate vascular invasion (92).

Squamous Cell Carcinoma

Pure squamous carcinomas are rare in the stomach. They are believed to arise from areas of squamous metaplasia, in ectopic squamous epithelium, or possibly from an undifferentiated mucosal stem cell (93). Histologically, they resemble squamous cell carcinomas arising at other sites in the body.

Choriocarcinoma

The association between adenocarcinoma and choriocarcinoma in the stomach has been known since the turn of the 21st century (94–97). Most tumors contain combinations of variably differentiated gastric cancer and choriocarcinoma. Pure choriocarcinomas, otherwise indistinguishable from gestational and gonadal tumors, also occur (96). Metastases involve the lymph nodes, lungs, liver, pancreas, and intraabdominal organs due to direct or transperitoneal spread. The metastases may show both mixed and pure patterns, although a pure choriocarcinomatous overgrowth is more common.

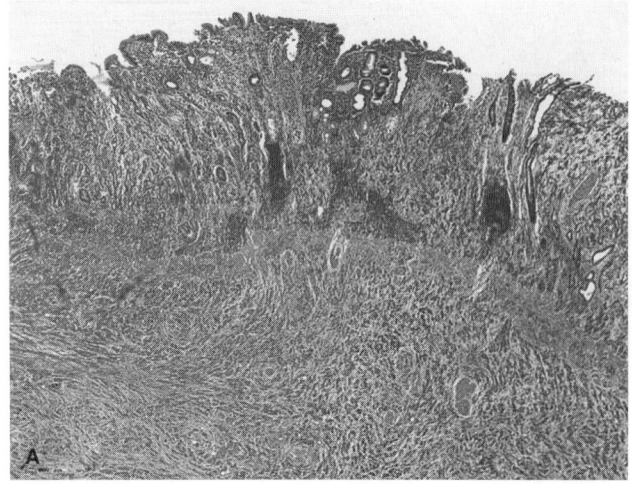

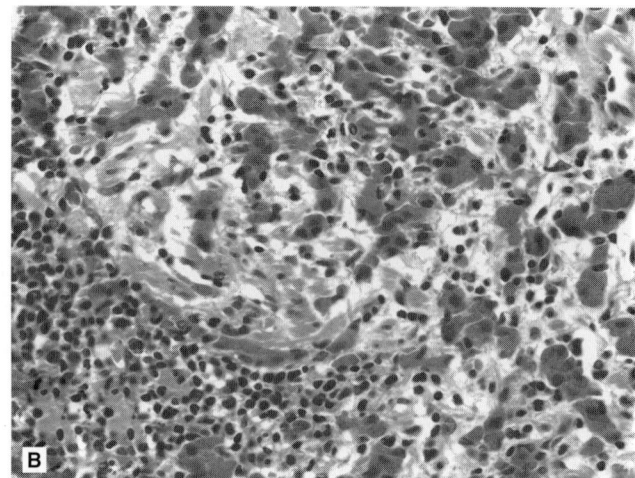

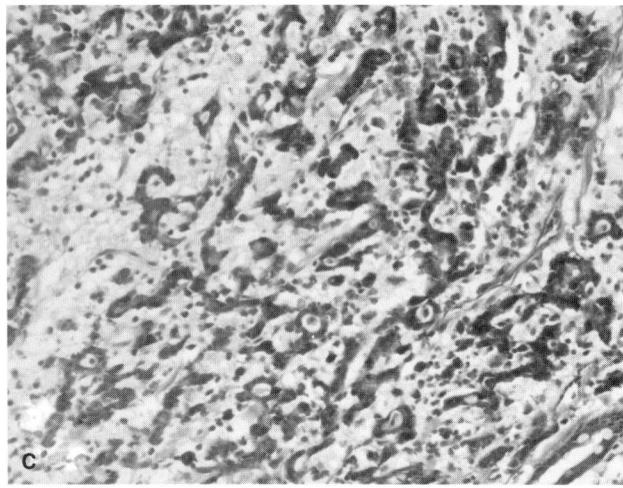

FIGURE 21.22. Paneth cell cancer arising in the setting of complete intestinal metaplasia. This flat, stage 1, infiltrating cancer (**A**) is composed of cells with bright red cytoplasmic granules (**B**). Immunohistochemistry for lysozomes (**C**) confirms the nature of these granules. This patient developed a peritoneal recurrence 7 years after subtotal resection (See also color Figure 21.22a,b,c).

Hepatoid Adenocarcinoma

A small number of gastric carcinomas show focal hepatocellular differentiation (98–100). Most cases are advanced tumors, and death occurs mostly because of massive intravenous spread to the liver. The hepatoid component may appear trabecular, medullary, or pseudoglandular, sometimes with obvious bile secretion. Transitions between adenocarcinomatous and hepatoid areas occur.

Carcinosarcomas and Spindle Cell Carcinomas

Carcinosarcomas rarely arise in the stomach but usually do so in elderly men (101). The lesions usually present grossly as large polypoid or fungating masses containing areas of adenocarcinoma and sarcoma. The sarcomatous component usually has spindle cell morphology, and when differentiated, most often shows smooth muscle differentiation. Chondrosarcoma has also been reported on several occasions. The sarcomatous components sometimes stain with markers usually associated with epithelial cells (102), supporting the concept that the mesenchymal component represents a mesenchymal metaplasia of epithelial cells, or that the carcinoma has a spindle cell component.

SPREAD OF GASTRIC CARCINOMA

In countries with a low incidence of gastric cancer and where screening does not take place, most patients are diagnosed and undergo surgery when their cancer is already advanced. There may be direct extension to adjacent organs, such as the pancreas, splenic hilum, transverse colon, hepatic hilum, omentum, diaphragm, abdominal wall, or esophagus (103). Lymphatic and vascular invasion carries a poor prognosis (104,105) and is often seen in advanced cases (106). In many cases, lymphatic spread occurs early, even in patients who appear to be surgically curable. In addition to the nodes nearest the lesion, other commonly involved nodes include those of the lesser curvature and in the left gastropancreatic, juxtacardiac, gastroduodenal, gastropyloric, suprapyloric, pancreaticoduodenal, splenic, and hepatic lymph nodes. Carcinomas arising in the cardia may metastasize to the pancreaticolienal, pericardial, and superior gastric nodes. Second-station lymph nodes include the paraaortic nodes and those of the celiac axis. Supradiaphragmatic and mediastinal nodes may also become involved by metastatic tumor. Gastric cancers rarely metastasize to the left supraclavicular nodes via the thoracic duct.

Distant bloodborne metastases occur, even in the absence of lymphatic involvement, and can occur in the liver, lungs, bones, and skin. Bilateral massive ovarian involvement (Krukenberg tumor) results from transperitoneal spread, together with

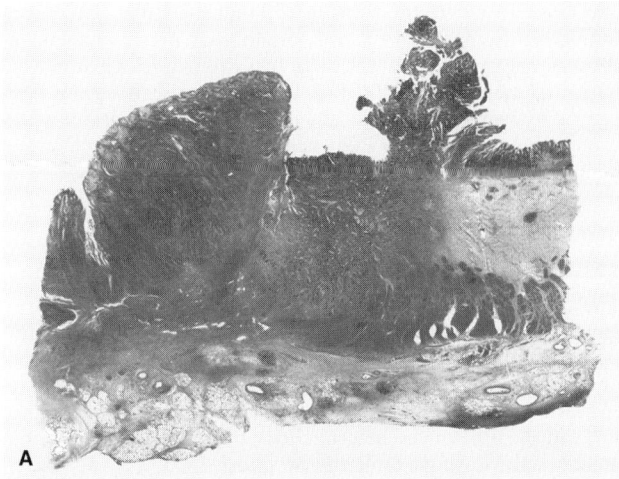

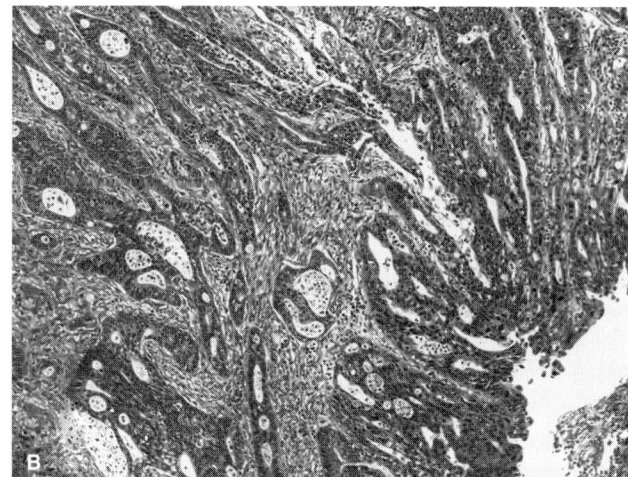

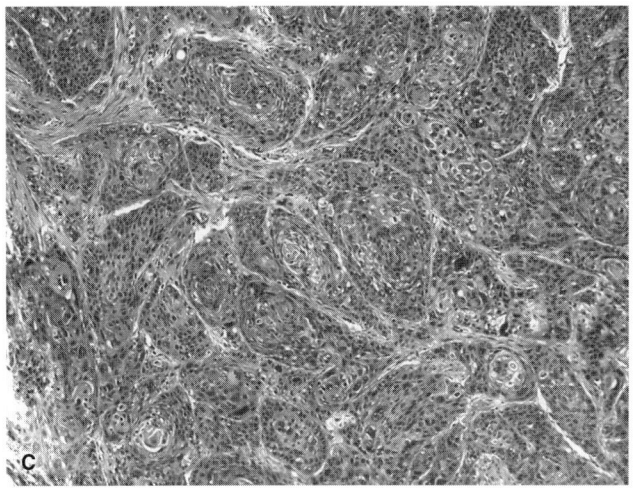

FIGURE 21.23. Adenosquamous carcinoma. A low-power view (**A**) of this large, stage 3 antral cancer reveals two distinct, clearly defined growth patterns, one composed of well-defined glands (*) (**B**), the other composed of sheets of keratinizing squamous cells (**) (**C**). The patient died of recurrent disease 19 months after resection.

other neoplastic seeding within the peritoneum, mesentery, and omentum. Similar transperitoneal spread may involve the uterus and present with endometrial bleeding (107). Pelvic metastases of this type are most frequent in premenopausal women. Intestinal cancers preferentially metastasize to the liver (108), whereas diffuse cancers preferentially involve lymph nodes and peritoneal surfaces.

PROGNOSIS

The 5-year survival of advanced gastric cancer when a potentially curative operation has been carried out is approximately 10% to 20% (109–111). Early gastric cancer has a much more favorable prognosis. The most important determinant of prognosis of gastric cancer is the depth of invasion into the stomach wall (112). Patients with stage T1 cancers limited to the mucosa and submucosa have a 5-year survival of approximately 95%. Tumors that invade the muscularis propria (T2) have a 60% to 80% 5-year survival, whereas tumors invading the subserosa (T3) have a 50% 5-year survival (113,114). The presence or absence of duodenal invasion is next in importance in determining prognosis (115). Factors such as growth pattern, tumor size, and degree of differentiation also have prognostic value. As a result, accurate staging and grading of gastric cancers is vital in determining subsequent strategies for patient management (111,116,117). Nodal involvement is a strong prognostic factor. The 45% 5-year survival for patients with three or fewer

lymph nodes containing metastatic carcinoma compares with 25% in patients with larger numbers of involved lymph nodes (118–120). Unfortunately, in the United States, most patients with advanced gastric cancer already have lymph node metastases at the time of diagnosis.

IMMUNOHISTOCHEMICAL BIOMARKERS

It is now common practice to use immunohistochemical (IHC) studies to assess the prognosis of gastric cancers; to characterize their phenotype; and to identify tumor characteristics that might make them more, or less, responsive to chemotherapeutic agents. The literature on this subject is vast and expanding. A short, and necessarily incomplete, review of the subject follows.

Markers for Phenotype

Antibodies are now available to identify the different gastric and intestinal cells from which cancers may arise. These antibodies have been used to characterize cancer phenotypes, but loss of specific traits through dedifferentiation and the accumulation of other traits through postinduction metaplasia complicate attempts to identify the progenitor cells of specific cancers.

Analysis of large numbers of cancers, however, provides levels of probability that a tumor in the proximal stomach derives from the cardia, the distal esophagus, or the corpus, or that a cancer in the distal stomach is derived from metaplastic intestinal cells or residual antral glands. Thus, cytokeratin 20 (CK20) is a marker for antral epithelium, while CK7 marks the columnar epithelium of the cardia (121). Tumors from these sites are less consistent in the expression of these markers, but adenocarcinomas in the distal esophagus are more likely to express CK7, and those in the antrum are more likely to express CK20 (122). The mucin peptide cores (MUC) vary from site to site in the gastrointestinal tract. Two of these, MUC1 and MUC5AC, are more frequent in tumors distal to the cardia than in cardia cancers (123).

Sucrase is a disaccharidase normally present in the small intestine. IHC uniformly labels sucrase in the glycocalyx of intestinalized gastric mucosa. Its expression in gastric cancer is less consistent. As might be expected, sucrase expression is more frequent in well-differentiated cancers than in poorly differentiated tumors, suggesting that these cancers derive from intestinalized mucosa. Sucrase expression increases in frequency with the depth of invasion for both well- and poorly differentiated tumors, but this trend is unexpectedly stronger for the less well-differentiated tumors (124). This suggests that sucrase expression in some late stage cancers is the result of postinduction intestinal metaplasia of cancers that had originated from gastric stem cells.

PGII is normally produced in all gastric glands. Approximately 40% of gastric cancers express this product (125), suggesting a gastric rather than metaplastic intestinal origin of some of these cancers. This may be misleading, however, because PGII expression is most frequent in patients with poorly differentiated, high-stage tumors that arise from a totally intestinalized gastric mucosa (Fig. 21.24) (79,126). This suggests the possibility that, as with sucrase, postinduction metaplasia may change a cancer phenotype, in this case, by reversion from an intestinal to a gastric form.

IHC has a practical, but limited, use in the identification of the primary site of a metastatic cancer. Thus, PGII expression is a fairly specific marker for gastric origin but lacks sensitivity. It is well recognized that lobular carcinoma of the breast may metastasize to the stomach and that these metastases may mimic diffuse gastric cancer. Most lobular breast cancers express estrogen receptor (ER), whereas this is infrequent (<5%) in gastric cancers (127,128). A PGII-positive cancer in a perigastric tissue sample is almost certainly of gastric origin whatever its ER status, but a PGII-negative cancer is most likely to be of mammary origin if it is ER positive.

Markers of Prognosis

The cell division cycle is controlled by the coordinated expression of many regulatory proteins. Biomarkers are labeled antibodies that identify the expression of these proteins in normal and neoplastic cells. Amplification of a growth factor, or inactivation of a tumor suppressor, associates with a poor prognosis, and the greater the heterogeneity of tumor markers within a cancer, the less favorable the prognosis (79).

The overexpression of growth factors, such as epithelial growth factor and epithelial growth factor receptor (EGFR), associates with higher indices of cell turnover, and this relationship is enhanced when they are coexpressed with other growth factors (TGFα, p185$^{c-erB-2}$) (129). As might be expected, EGFR overexpression also associates with more frequent metastases and less favorable 5-year survival (130,131). The influence of growth factors on tumor progression is augmented when associated with abnormalities in cell cycling. Thus, adenocarcinomas that are dependent on the TGFα-EGFR autocrine loop exhibit increased aggressiveness in the presence of aberrant p53 (132). Clonal heterogeneity of EGFR and other tumor markers within an advanced cancer is especially ominous, with the overexpressing components of the tumor showing a selective advantage in vascular invasion (Fig. 21.25).

Cyclin D1 is a protooncogene that regulates the progression from G1 to S in the cell cycle (133). The role of cyclin D1 has been studied in the normal, hyperplastic, and neoplastic gastric mucosa (134). Cyclin D1 was not identified in the normal or hyperplastic mucosa but was found in 40.5% of gastric cancers. Although there was no correlation between amplification of cyclin D1 and lymph node metastases, age, or histologic grade, patients with cancers showing cyclin D1 amplification had a less favorable 5-year survival than those who did not.

Loss of a tumor-suppression factor, such as p53 (135), spurs abnormal cell growth. Normal or wild-type p53 has a very short half-life, and IHC identifies p53 missense mutations that increase the protein half-life (136). Because it does not detect deletions of the p53 gene or nonsense mutations and because rapidly replicating cancers may express wild-type p53, IHC expression does not exactly correlate with molecular analysis (136). Observed differences respecting the influence of p53 immunohistochemical expression on prognosis (137–139) suggest that it is less consistent in this respect than are growth factors. A higher cancer stage is more likely, however, when p53 expression is associated with an overexpressed growth factor than with growth factor expression alone (79,134).

A cancer must degrade the extracellular matrix, acquire motility, and be able to penetrate vascular channels in order to migrate to a new location. Matrix metalloproteases (MMPs) are proteolytic enzymes that target extracellular matrix. Among these, MMP7 has the highest activity, has been shown to associate with penetration of lymphatic channels, and may be detected by IHC in cancer cell membranes at the invasion boundaries of aggressive intestinal and diffuse gastric cancers (140). As may be expected, MMP7 expression has also been associated with poor survival with this cancer (141). Activated urokinase plasminogen activator also induces destruction

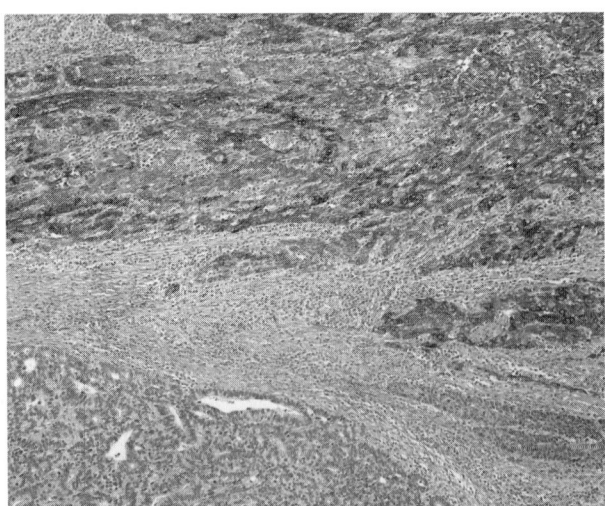

FIGURE 21.24. Heterogeneity of pepsinogen group II (PGII) expression. Immunohistochemistry for PGII labels a poorly differentiated portion of a stage 3, intestinal-type antral cancer. An adjacent, well-differentiated component of the cancer does not label for this product. This patient died 5 months after a palliative resection (See also color Figure 21.24).

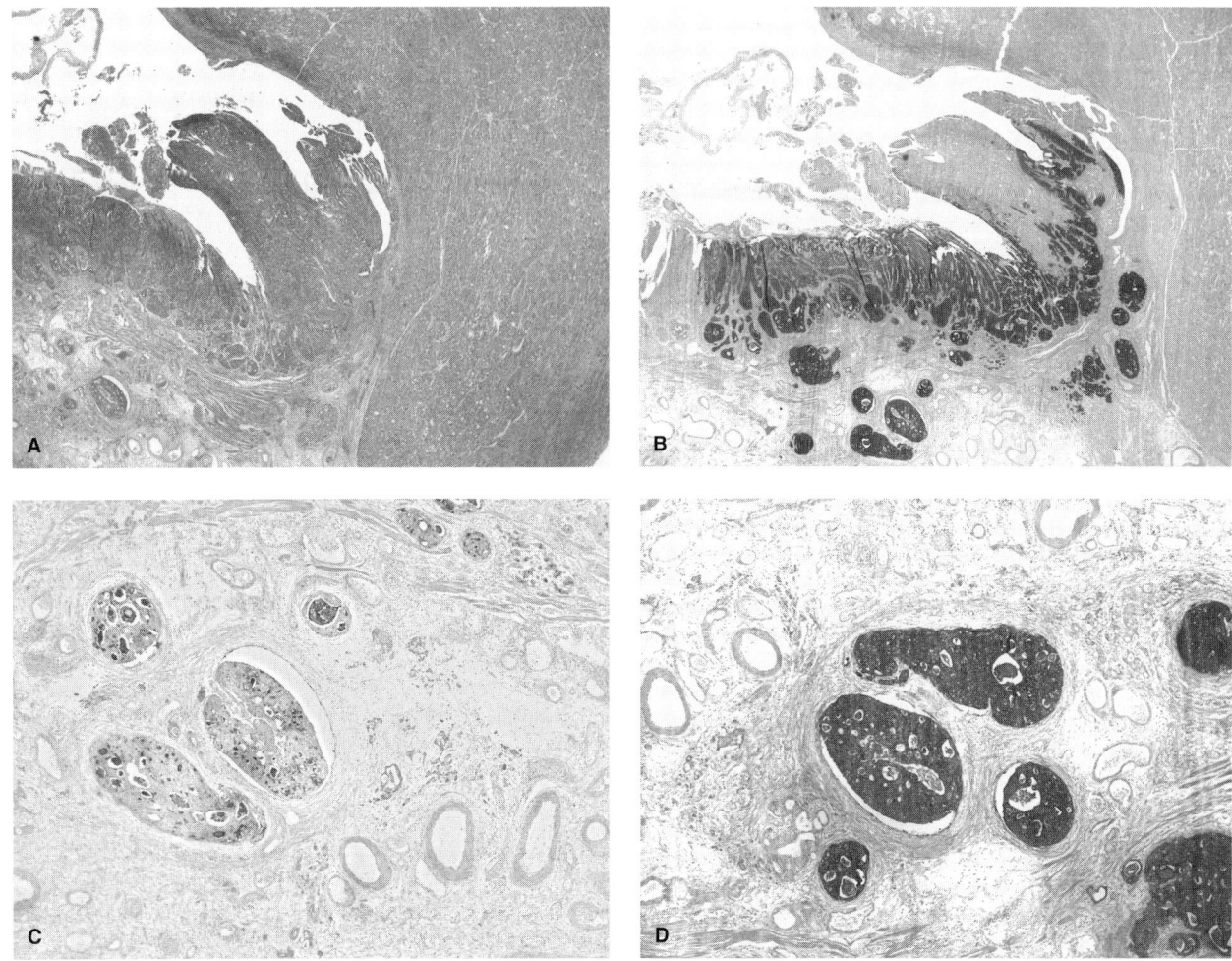

FIGURE 21.25. Epithelial growth factor receptor (EGFR) heterogeneity in gastric cancer. A low-power hematoxylin-and-eosin stain (**A**) shows a large, stage 4 gastric cancer. An immunohistochemical study (**B**) indicates overexpression of EGFR in a clone of this tumor. High-power pictures indicate the EGFR-positive component of the cancer has a selective advantage for vascular invasion, as compared to the EGFR-negative tumor (**C**). The intravascular tumor is also MET positive (**D**). This patient died 7 months after a palliative resection.

of extracellular matrix. Expression of its receptor (uPAR) promotes cancer cell invasion and has been independently associated with gastric cancer progression (142).

Two motility factors have been identified in gastric cancer. Fascin, an actin-bundling protein, increases cell motility in various transformed cells. Fascin-positive gastric cancers are frequently high-stage tumors and have a poorer prognosis than fascin-negative cancers (143,144). Autocrine motility factor is a cytokine that also regulates the motility of cancer cells. Expression of autocrine motility factor receptor (AMFR) is closely associated with progression and poor prognosis of gastric cancer (142).

A cancer may enhance its chances of dissemination by expressing vascular endothelial growth factors (VEGFs) that stimulate angiogenesis. Two members of the VEGF family, VEGF-C and VEGF-D, activate a tyrosine kinase that is expressed in lymphatic channels and the blood vessels of malignant tumors VEGF-3 (145). Expression of VEGF-C and VEGF-D in gastric cancer and VEGF-3 receptor in the endothelial cells of vascular channels of gastric cancers is associated with lymphatic channel invasion and lymph node metastases (145,146), as well as increased mortality (145).

A large number of other gastric cancer IHC biomarkers have been associated with tumor aggression and/or poor prognosis.

The mechanism of action of some these has not been determined, while others may function in more than one way. These include thioredoxin, a putative oncogene product that associates with increased gastric cancer cell proliferation (147). MET, the receptor of hepatocyte growth factor, is an oncogene that has been independently associated with gastric cancer progression, an association that is strengthened when coexpressed with AMFR and uPAR (142). It has been suggested, on the basis of cell culture studies, that the cag-A strain of *H. pylori* targets MET, leading to a forceful motility response in gastric cancer cell lines (148). This could account for the association of MET expression with tumor progression.

Androgen receptor (AR) activation enhances VEGF gene transcription and may have antiapoptotic activity as well. A more recent report indicates that approximately 17% of gastric cancers express AR, with no gender difference in frequency (128). AR-expressing gastric cancers are more likely to have lymph node metastases ($p = 0.03$) and have a less favorable prognosis than tumors that do not.

Overexpression of cyclooxygenase-2 (Cox2) associates with deep invasion and lymph node metastases, but the mechanisms of its upregulation are not well understood (149). Cox2 is frequently overexpressed in tumors with increased expression of Her2 or in tumors with reduced expression of Smad4 (an intracellular signal transducer), suggesting that signal transduction through the Her2 and Smad system may regulate COX-2 expression.

Biomarkers as Guides to Chemotherapy

At first sight, the almost limitless heterogeneity of most advanced gastric cancers creates an impassible barrier to the development of customized chemotherapeutic approaches. Surgery therefor remains the mainstay of the treatment of this cancer, even when it is associated with locoregional or distant recurrence. Palliation, rather than cure, is the primary goal of adjuvant therapy (150). Most patients who have had a resection for gastric cancers with extensive lymph node metastases will have a disease relapse. No randomized clinical trial has shown a benefit for this subset of patients, and no single regimen has proven to be effective for postoperative adjuvant chemotherapy (150). This is not unexpected because a successful response to treatment with drugs that may target specific oncogenes could also allow other subsets of neoplastic cells to survive and serve as the seed beds for recurrent tumors.

Handling of Gastric Resection Specimens

Gastrectomy specimens should be sent to surgical pathology as soon as possible after removal from the patient. The stomach should be opened along the greater curvature, pinned to a corkboard, and floated upside down in 10% neutral buffered formalin for at least 12 hours. The gross limits of the tumor are more easily assessed if the specimen is well fixed, and small unsuspected multicentric tumors may more easily be identified.

The gross description of the fixed specimen should include the type of resection (proximal subtotal, distal subtotal, or total), the lengths of the greater and lesser curvatures, the length of attached esophagus, duodenum, or both, the axial and transverse diameters of the tumor, and the location of the tumor within the stomach. The gross configuration and size of the tumor should be noted (e.g., fungating, ulcerated, diffuse). All lesions should be described and sampled, including areas of ulceration and polypoid or elevated lesions. The location of such lesions should be accurately described in relation to the main tumor mass. In many cases, an explanatory diagram or photograph is useful for documenting the distance of the tumor from resection margins and its relationship to other lesions present in the stomach.

Circumferential sections should be obtained from the margins of resection to rule out grossly inapparent intramural spread to the surgical margin. Two to four sections should be taken from the tumor, depending on its size. The sections should include the full thickness of the gastric wall so the maximum depth of penetration of the tumor can be determined. A generous sample of the intact nonneoplastic mucosa on the proximal and distal sides of the tumor should be included with the neoplasm to identify precursor lesions, including intestinal metaplasia, atrophic gastritis, or areas of dysplasia. The pathologist should harvest as many lymph nodes as possible from the lesser curvature and the distal and proximal greater curvature, separately identifying those <3 cm or >3 cm from the tumor.

All of the following should be determined at the time of histologic examination:

- Tumor, node, metastasis (TNM) status of the tumor
- Histologic type of the cancer using the Lauren or WHO classification, and its degree of differentiation
- Presence and extent of vascular and perineural invasion
- Histologic findings in the nonneoplastic gastric mucosa
- Presence or absence of lymph node metastasis

Each report should contain, at a minimum, the information needed to assign an accurate TNM stage, the gastric subsite location of the tumor, a histologic classification of the tumor, and an estimate of its degree of differentiation.

References

1. Parkin DM, Whelan SL, Ferlay J, Teppo L, Thomas DB, eds. *Cancer Incidence in Five Continents*. Vol VIII. Lyon, France: IARC Scientific Publications No 155. 2002:546–548.
2. Devesa SS, Blot WJ, Fraumeni JF, Jr. Changing patterns in the incidence of esophageal and gastric cancer in the United States. *Cancer* 1998;83:2049–2053.
3. Kolonel LN, Hanken J, Nomura AMY. Multiethnic studies of diet, nutrition and cancer in Hawaii. In: Hayashi Y, Nagao M, Sugimura T, eds. *Diet, Nutrition and Cancer*. Tokyo: Japan Scientific Societies Press; 1986:29–40.
4. Lauren T. The two histologic main types of gastric carcinoma. *Acta Pathol Microbiol Scand* 1965;49:969–988.
5. Parsonnet J, Friedman GD, Vandersteen, et al. Helicobacter pylori infection and the risk of gastric cancer. *N Engl J Med* 1991;325:1127–1131.
6. Nomura AMY, Stemmermann GN, Chyou H, et al. Helicobacter pylori infection and gastric cancer among Japanese Americans in Hawaii. *N Engl J Med* 1991;325:1132–1136.
7. Stemmermann GN, Fenoglio-Preiser CM. Gastric carcinoma distal to the cardia: a review of the epidemiological pathology of the precursors to a preventable cancer. *Pathology* 2002;34:494–503.
8. Correa P, Sasano N, Stemmermann GN, Haenszel W. Pathology of gastric cancer in Japanese populations: comparisons between Miyagi prefecture, Japan and Hawaii. *J Natl Cancer Inst* 1973;51:1449–1459.
9. Caldas C, Carneiro F, Lynch HT, et al. Familial gastric cancer: overview and guidelines for management. *J Med Genet* 1999;36:873–880.
10. Cheng XX, Wang ZC, Chen XY, et al. Frequent loss of membranous E-cadherin in gastric cancers: a cross-talk with Wnt in determining the fate of β-catenin. *Clin Exp Metastasis* 2005;22:85–93.
11. Nomura AMY, Hankin JH, Kolonel L, et al. Case-control study of diet and other risk factors for gastric cancer in Hawaii. *Cancer Causes Control* 2003;14:547–558.
12. Wu A, Wan P, Bernstain LA. A multiethnic population-based study of smoking, alcohol and body size and risk of adenocarcinoma of the stomach and esophagus. *Cancer Causes Control* 2001;12:721–732.
13. Chow WH, Blot WJ, Vaughn TL, et al. Body mass index and risk of adenocarcinomas of the esophagus and gastric cardia. *J Natl Cancer Inst* 1998;90:150–5.
14. Lindblat M, Garcia-Rodriguez LA, Lagergren J. Body mass, tobacco, and alcohol and risk of esophageal, gastric cardia, and gastric non-cardia adenocarcinoma among men and women in a nested case-control study. *Cancer Causes Control* 2005;16:285–94.
15. Matsukura N, Suzuki K, Kawachi T, et al. Distribution of marker enzymes and mucin in intestinal metaplasia of the stomach in relation to complete and incomplete types of metaplasia to minute gastric cancer. *J Natl Cancer Inst* 1980;65:231–6.
16. Aihara I, Ajioka Y, Watanabe H, et al. Incidence and distribution of hybrid goblet cells in complete type intestinal metaplasia of the stomach. *Pathol Res Pract* 2005;201:11–19.
17. Otsuka T, Tsukamoto T, Mizoshita T, et al. Coexistence of gastric- and intestinal-type endocrine cells in gastric and intestinal mixed intestinal metaplasia of the human stomach. *Pathol Int* 2005;55:17–19.
18. Houghton J, Wang TG. Helicobacter pylori and gastric cancer: a new paradigm for inflammation-associated epithelial cancers. *Gastroenterology* 2005;128:1567–78.
19. Stemmermann GN, Samloff IM, Nomura AMY, et al. Serum pepsinogen I and gastrin in relation to extent and location of intestinal metaplasia in the surgically resected stomach. *Dig Dis Sci* 1980;25:680–687.
20. Miki K, Ichinose M, Shimizu A, et al. Serum pepsinogen as a screening test for chronic gastritis. *Gastroenterol Jpn* 1987;22:133–141.
21. Nomura AMY, Kolonel L, Miki K, et al. Helicobacter pylori, pepsinogen and gastric carcinoma Hawaii. *J Infect Dis* 2005;191:2075–2081.
22. Chiba T. Key molecules in metaplastic gastritis: sequential analysis of CSX1/2 homeobox gene expression. *J Gastroenterol* 2002;37:147–148.
23. Mutoh H, Hakamata Y, Sato K, et al. Conversion of gastric mucosa to intestinal metaplasia in Cdx2-expressing transgenic mice. *Biochem Biophys Res Commun* 2002;294:470–479.
24. Ota H, Katsuyama T, Nakajima S, et al. Intestinal metaplasia with adherent Helicobacter pylori: a hybrid epithelium with both gastric and intestinal features. *Hum Pathol* 1998;29:846–850.
25. Peek RM, Miller GG, Tham KT, et al. Heightened inflammatory response and cytokine expression in vivo to cagA+ Helicobacter strains. *Lab Invest* 1995;71:760–770.
26. Shimoyama T, Yoshimura T, Mikami T, et al. Evaluation of Helicobacter pylori vacA genotype in Japanese patients with gastric cancer. *J Clin Pathol* 1998;51:299–301.
27. Mirvish SS. The etiology of gastric cancer: intragastric nitrosamide formation and other theories. *J Natl Cancer Inst* 1983;71:631–647.

28. Pignatelli B, Melaveille C, Rogatko A, et al. Mutagens, N-nitroso compounds and their precursors in gastric juice from patients with and without precancerous lesions of the stomach. *Eur J Cancer* 1993;29A:2031–2039.

29. Hayashi T, Papla B, Stemmermann GN. Gastric organ culture: a model for re-epithelialization. *Am J Pathol* 1975;78:23–32.

30. Nagayo T. Microscopical cancer of the stomach. *Int J Cancer* 1975;16:52–57.

31. Carmel R. Reassessment of the relative prevalence of antibodies to gastric parietal cell and intrinsic factor in patients with pernicious anemia: influence of patient age and race. *Clin Exp Immunol* 1992;89:74–77.

32. Burman P, Mardh S, Norberg L, et al. Parietal cell antibodies in pernicious anemia inhibit H+, K+-adenosine triphosphatase, the proton pump of the stomach. *Gastroenterology* 1989;96:1434–1438.

33. Kaye MD. Immunologic aspects of pernicious anemia. *Clin Gastroenterol* 1987;1:487–506.

34. DeAizpuria HJ, Ungar B, Toh BH. Antibody to the gastrin receptor in pernicious anemia. *N Engl J Med* 1985;311:479–483.

35. Fisher S, Davis S, Nelson R, et al. A cohort study of cancer after gastric surgery for benign disease. *J Natl Cancer Inst* 1993;85:1303–1310.

36. Miwa K, Hattori T, Miyazaki I. Duodenogastric reflux and foregut carcinogenesis. *Cancer* 1995;75:1426–1432.

37. Morson BC, Sobin LH, Grundmann E, et al. Precancerous conditions and epithelial dysplasia in the stomach. *J Clin Pathol* 1980;33:711–721.

38. Nagayo T. Dysplasia of the gastric mucosa and its relation to the precancerous state. *Jpn J Cancer Res* 1981;72:813–823.

39. Correa P. A human model of gastric carcinogenesis. *Cancer Res* 1988;48:3554–3560.

40. Nakatsuru S, Yanagisawa A, Furukawa Y, et al. Somatic mutations of the APC gene in precancerous lesions of the stomach. *Hum Mol Genet* 1993;2:1463–1465.

41. Wu LB, Kushima R, Borchard F, et al. Intramucosal carcinomas of the stomach: phenotypic expression and loss of heterozygosity at microsatellites linked to the APC gene. *Pathol Res Pract* 1998;194:405–412.

42. Kang GH, Shim YH, Jung HY, et al. CpG island methylation in premalignant stages of gastric carcinoma. *Cancer Res* 2001;61:2847–2851.

43. Sato F, Meltzer SJ. CpG island methylation in progression of esophageal and gastric cancer. *Cancer* 2006;106:483–493.

44. Coma del Corral MJ, Pardo-Mindan FJ, Razquin S, et al. Risk of cancer in patients with gastric dysplasia. *Cancer* 1990;65:2078–2085.

45. Rugge M, Farinati F, Baffa R, et al. Gastric epithelial dysplasia in the natural history of gastric cancer: a multicenter follow-up study. *Gastroenterology* 1994;107:1288–1296.

46. Oehlert W, Keller P, Henke M, et al. Gastric mucosal dysplasia: what is its clinical significance? *Front Gastrointest Res* 1979;4:173–182.

47. Saraga E-P, Gardiol D, Costa J. Gastric dysplasia: a histological follow-up study. *Ann Surg Pathol* 1987;11:788–796.

48. Hirota T, Okada T, Itabashi M, et al. Histogenesis of human gastric cancer: with special reference to the significance of adenoma as a precancerous lesion. In: Ming SC, ed. *Precursors to Gastric Cancer*. New York, NY: Praeger; 1984:233–252.

49. Ming SC. Malignant potential of epithelial polyps of the stomach. In: Ming SC, ed. *Precursors to Gastric Cancer*. New York, NY: Praeger; 1984:219–231.

50. Correa P, Cuello C, Duque E, et al. Gastric cancer in Colombia. III. Natural history of precursor lesions. *J Natl Cancer Inst* 1976;57:1027–1035.

51. Munoz N, Matko I. Histological types of gastric cancer and its relationship with intestinal metaplasia. *Recent Results Cancer Res* 1972;39:99–105.

52. Yamashina M. A variant of early gastric carcinoma: histologic and histochemical studies of earl signet ring cell carcinomas discovered beneath preserved surface epithelium. *Cancer* 1986;58:1333–1339.

53. Fiocca R, Villani L, Tenti P, et al. Characterization of four main cell types in gastric cancer: foveolar, mononleptic, intestinal columnar and goblet cells. An histopathologic, histochemical, and ultrastructural study of "early" and "advanced" tumours. *Pathol Res Pract* 1987;182:308–325.

54. Sasano N, Nakamura K, Arai M, et al. Ultrastructural cell patterns in human gastric carcinoma compared with non-neoplastic gastric mucosa: histiogenic analysis of carcinoma by mucin histochemistry. *J Natl Cancer Inst* 1969;43:783–802.

55. Nevalainen T, Jarvi OH. Ultrastructure of intestinal and diffuse type of gastric carcinoma. *J Pathol* 1977;122:129–136.

56. Capella C, Cornaggia M, Usellini L, et al. Neoplastic cells containing lysozyme in gastric carcinomas. *Pathology* 1984;16:87–92.

57. Capella C, Frigerio B, Cornaggia M, et al. Gastric parietal cell carcinoma—a newly recognized entity. *Histopathology* 1984;8:813–824.

58. Takubo K, Honma N, Sawabe M, et al. Oncocytic adenocarcinoma of the stomach. *Am J Surg Pathol* 2002;26:458–463.

59. Prade M, Bara J, Gardenne C, et al. Gastric carcinomas with argyrophilic cells: light microscopic and immunochemical study. *Hum Pathol* 1982;13:588–592.

60. Tahara E, Ito H, Nakagami K, et al. Scirrhous argyrophil cell carcinoma of the stomach with multiple production of polypeptide hormones, amine, CEA, lysozyme and hCG. *Cancer* 1982;49:1904–1915.

61. Antonioli DA, Goldman H. Changes in the location and type of gastric adenocarcinoma. *Cancer* 1982;50:775–781.

62. Dolan K, Morris AI, Gosney JR, et al. Three different subsite classification systems for carcinomas of the GEJ, but is it all one disease? *J Gastroenterol Hepatol* 2004;19:24–30.

63. Ruol A, Parenti A, Zaninotto G, et al. Intestinal metaplasia is the probable common precursor of adenocarcinoma in Barrett esophagus and adenocarcinoma of the gastric cardia. *Cancer* 2000;88:2520–2528.

64. Blaser MJ. Not all *Helicobacter pylori* strains are created equal: should all be eliminated? *Lancet* 1997;349:1020–1022.

65. Yamaji Y, Mitsushima T, Ikuma H, et al. Inverse background of *Helicobacter pylori* antibody and pepsinogen in reflux oesophagitis compared to gastric cancer: analysis of 5732 Japanese subjects. *Gut* 2001;49:335–340.

66. Murakami T. Pathomorphological diagnosis: definition and gross classification of early gastric cancer. In: Nishi T, ed. *Early Gastric Cancer*. Gann Monograph on CancerResearch No 11. Tokyo: University of Tokyo Press; 1972:53–55.

67. Ohta H, Noguchi Y, Takagi K, et al. Early gastric carcinoma with special reference to macroscopic classification. *Cancer* 1987;60:1099–1106.

68. Hirota T, Ming SC, Itabashi M. Pathology of early gastric cancer. In: Nishi M, Ichikawa H, Nakajima T, et al., eds. *Gastric Cancer*. Tokyo: Springer-Verlag; 1993:66–85.

69. Hisamachi S, Sugawara N. Mass screening for gastric cancer by x-ray examination. *Jpn J Clin Oncol* 1984;14:211–212.

70. Green PHR, O'Toole KM, Weinberg LM, et al. Early gastric cancer. *Gastroenterology* 1981;81:247–256.

71. Carter KJ, Schaffer HA, Ritchie WP, Jr. Early gastric cancer. *Ann Surg* 1984;199:604–609.

72. Biasco G, Paganelli GM, Azzaroni D, et al. Early gastric cancer in Italy: clinical and pathological observations on 80 cases. *Dig Dis Sci* 1987;32:113–120.

73. Otsuka K, Murakami M, Aoki T, et al. Minimally invasive treatment of stomach cancer. *Cancer J* 2005;11:18–25.

74. Shimoyama S, Seto Y, Yasuda H, et al. Concepts, rationale, and current outcomes of less invasive surgical strategies for early gastric cancer: data from a quarter-century of experience in a single institution. *World J Surg* 2005;29:58–65.

75. Noh SH, Hyung WJ, Cheong JH. Minimally invasive treatment for gastric cancer: approaches and selection process. *J Surg Oncol* 2005;90:188–194.

76. Bormann R. Makroskopishen Formen des vorgeschritteten Magenkrebses. In: Henke E, Lubarsch O, eds. *Handbuch der Speziellen Pathologischen Anatomie und Histologie*. Vol 4/1. Berlin: Springer; 1926:236–242.

77. Stemmermann GN. Comparative study of histochemical patterns in non-neoplastic and neoplastic gastric epithelium: a study of Japanese in Hawaii. *J Natl Cancer Inst* 1967;39:375–383.

78. Nevalainen TJ. Electron microscopy of malignant and premalignant gastric epithelium. In: Filipe MI, Jass JR, eds. *Gastric Carcinoma*. Edinburgh: Churchill Livingstone; 1986:236.

79. Stemmermann GN, Nomura AMY. The relation of pepsinogen group II (PGII) expression to intestinal metaplasia and gastric cancer. *Histopathology* 2006;49:45–51.

80. Sugihara H, Hattori T, Fujita S, et al. Cell proliferation and differentiation in intramucosal and advanced signet ring cell carcinomas of the stomach. *Virchows Arch* 1989;411:117–127.

81. Guilford P, Hopkins J, Harraway J, et al. E-cadherin germline mutations in familial gastric cancer. *Nature* 1998;392:402–405.

82. Gayther SA, Gorringe KL, Ramus SJ, et al. Identification of germ-line E-cadherin mutations in gastric cancer patients of European origin. *Cancer Res* 1998;58:4086–4089.

83. Chun YS, Lindor NM, Smyrk TC. Germline E-cadherin gene mutations. Is prophylactic total gastrectomy indicated? *Cancer* 2001;92:181–187.

84. Fenoglio-Preiser CM, Carneiro F, Correa P, et al. Gastric cancer. In: Hamilton SR, Aaltonen LA, eds. *World Health Organization Classification of Tumours. Pathology & Genetics*. Lyon, France: IARC Press; 2000:39–52.

85. Shibata D, Tokunaga M, Uemura Y, et al. Association of Epstein-Barr virus with undifferentiated gastric carcinomas with intense lymphoid infiltration. *Am J Pathol* 1991;139:10–16.

86. Tokunaga M, Land CE, Uemura Y, et al. Epstein-Barr virus in gastric carcinoma. *Am J Pathol* 1993;143:1250–1254.

87. Shibata D, Hawes D, Stemmermann GN, Weiss LM. Epstein-Barr associated gastric adenocarcinoma among Japanese in Hawaii. *Cancer Epidemiol Biomarkers Prev* 1993;2:213–217.

88. Uemura Y, Tokunaga M, Arikawa J, et al. A unique morphology of Epstein-Barr virus-related early gastric cancer. *Cancer Epidemiol Biomarkers Prev* 1994;3:607–611.

89. Matsunou H, Konishi F, Hori H, et al. Characteristics of Epstein-Barr virus-associated gastric cancer with lymphoid stroma in Japan. *Cancer* 1996;77:1998–2004.

90. Tokunaga M, Land CE. Epstein-Barr virus involvement in gastric cancer: biomarker for lymph node metastases. *Cancer Epidemiol Biomarkers Prev* 1998;7:449–450.

91. Lev R, DeNucci TD. Neoplastic Paneth cells in the stomach. *Arch Pathol* 1989;113:129–133.

92. Heitz PU, Wegmann W. Identification of neoplastic Paneth cells in an adenocarcinoma of the stomach using lysozyme as a marker, and electron microscopy. *Virchows Arch A Pathol Anat Histol* 1980;386:107–116.

93. Mori M, Iwashita A, Enjoji M. Adenosquamous carcinoma of the stomach. *Cancer* 1986;57:333–339.

94. Ruck P, Wehrmann M, Campbell M, et al. Squamous carcinoma of the gastric stump: a case report and review of the literature. *Am J Surg Pathol* 1989;13:317–324.

95. Jindrak K, Bochetto JF, Alpert LL. Primary gastric choriocarcinoma: case report with review of world literature. *Human Pathol* 1986;7: 595–604.

96. Mori H, Soeda O, Kamano T, et al. Choriocarcinomatous change with immunocytochemically hCG-positive cells in gastric carcinoma in the male. *Virchows Arch* 1982;396:141–153.

97. Wurzel J, Brooks JJ. Primary gastric choriocarcinoma: immunohistochemistry, and postmortem documentation, and hormonal effects in a postmenopausal female. *Cancer* 1981;48:2756–2761.

98. Maher JC, Donohoe JF, Fennelly JJ, et al. Extragenital choriocarcinoma in a female presenting as a gastric tumour. *Br J Surg* 1970;57:73–75.

99. Kodama T, Kameya T, Hirota T, et al. Production of alpha-fetoprotein, normal serum proteins and human chorionic gonadotropin in stomach cancer: histologic and immunohistochemical analyses of 35 cases. *Cancer* 1981;48:1647–1655.

100. Ishikura H, Fukusawa Y, Ogasawara K, et al. An AFP-producing gastric carcinoma with features of hepatic differentiation: a case report. *Cancer* 1985;56:840–848.

101. Cho KJ, Myong MH, Choi DW, et al. Carcinosarcoma of the stomach: a case report with light microscopic, immunohistochemical, and electron microscopic study. *APMIS* 1990;98:991–995.

102. Sotelo-Avila C, Gooch WMN. Neoplasms associated with Beck-Wiedemann syndrome. *Perspect Pediatr Pathol* 1976;3:255–272.

103. Lundh G, Burn JI, Kolig G, et al. A cooperative international: study of gastric cancer. *Ann R Coll Surg Engl* 1974;54:214–228.

104. Okada M, Kojima S, Murakami M, et al. Human gastric carcinoma: prognosis in relation to macroscopic and microscopic features of primary tumor. *J Natl Cancer Inst* 1983;71:275–279.

105. Serlin O, Keehn RJ, Higgins GA, et al. Factors related to survival following resection for gastric cancer: analysis of 903 cases. *Cancer* 1977;40:1318–1329.

106. Noguchi Y. Blood vessel invasion in gastric carcinoma. *Surgery* 1990;107:140–148.

107. Stemmermann GN. Extrapelvic carcinoma metastatic to the uterus. *Am J Obstet Gynecol* 1961;82:1261–1266.

108. Esaki Y, Hirayama R, Hirokawa K. A comparison of patterns of metastasis in gastric cancer by histologic age and type. *Cancer* 1990;65:2086–2090.

109. Bizer S. Adenocarcinoma of the stomach: current results of treatment. *Cancer* 1983;51:743–745.

110. Tuech JJ, Cervi C, Pessaux P, et al. Early gastric cancer: univariate and multivariate analysis for survival. *Hepatogastroenterology* 1999;46:3276–3280.

111. Wanebo HJ, Kennedy BJ, Chmiel J, et al. Cancer of the stomach: a patient care study by the American College of Surgeons. *Ann Surg* 1993;218:3276–3280.

112. Adashek K, Sanger J, Longmire WP. Cancer of the stomach: review of consecutive ten year intervals. *Ann Surg* 1979;189:6–10.

113. Harrison JC, Dean PJ, Vander Zwaag R, et al. Adenocarcinoma of the stomach with invasion limited to the muscularis propria. *Hum Pathol* 1991;22:111–117.

114. Yoshikawa K, Maruyama K. Characteristics of gastric cancer invading to the propria muscle layer with special reference to mortality and cause of death. *Jpn J Clin Oncol* 1985;15:499–503.

115. Paramanandhan TL. The duodenal spread of gastric carcinoma. *Br J Surg* 1967;54:169–174.

116. Maruyama K. The most important prognostic factors for gastric cancer patients: a study using univariate and multivariate analyses. *Scand J Gastroenterol* 1987;22(suppl):63–68.

117. Siewert JR, Boucher K, Roder JD, et al. Prognostic relevance of systematic lymph node dissection in gastric carcinoma. *Br J Surg* 1993;80:1015–1018.

118. Ichikura T, Tomimatsu, Okusa Y, et al. Comparison of the prognostic significance between the number of metastatic lymph nodes and nodal stage base on their location in patients with gastric cancer. *J Clin Oncol* 1993;11:1894–1900.

119. Kim JP, Jung SE. Patients with gastric cancer and their prognosis in accordance with number of lymph node metastases. *Scand J Gastroenterol* 1987;22:33–37.

120. Pagnini CA, Rugge M. Advanced gastric carcinoma and prognosis. *Virchows Arch* 1985;406:213–221.

121. Ectors N, Driessen A, De Hertog G, et al. Is adenocarcinoma of the esophagogastric junction or cardia different from Barrett adenocarcinoma? *Arch Pathol Lab Med* 2005;128:183–185.

122. Taniere P, Borghi-Scoazec G, Saurin J-C, et al. Cytokeratin expression in adenocarcinomas of the esophagogastric junction: a comparative study of adenocarcinomas of the distal esophagus and of the proximal stomach. *Am J Surg Pathol* 2002;26:1213–1221.

123. Kim Ma, Lee SH, Yang H-K, Kim WH. Clinicopathologic and protein expression differences between cardia carcinoma and noncardia carcinoma of the stomach. *Cancer* 2005;103:1439–1446.

124. Nakamura W, Inada K, Hirano K, et al. Increased expression of sucrase and intestinal-type phosphatase in human gastric carcinomas with progression. *Jpn J Cancer Res* 19;89:186–191.

125. Stemmermann GN, Samloff IM, Hayashi T. Pepsinogens I and II in carcinoma of the stomach: an immunohistochemical study. *Appl Pathol* 1985;3:375–383.

126. Fiocca R, Cornaggia M, Villani L, et al. Expression of pepsinogen II in gastric cancer: its relation to local invasion and lymph node metastases. *Cancer* 1988;61:956–962.

127. Matsuyama S, Ohkura Y, Eguchi H, et al. Estrogen receptor beta is expressed in human stomach adenocarcinoma. *J Cancer Res Clin Oncol* 2002;128:319–324.

128. Kominea A, Konstantinopoulos PA, Kapranos N, et al. Androgen receptor (AR) expression is an independent unfavorable prognostic factor in gastric cancer. *J Cancer Res Clin Oncol* 2004;130:253–260.

129. Suzuki T, Tsuda T, Haruma K, et al. Growth of gastric carcinomas and expression of epidermal growth factor, transforming growth factor-a, epidermal growth factor receptor and p185 c-erbB-2. *Oncology* 1995;52:3856–3891.

130. Tokunaga A, Onda M, Okuda T, et al. Clinical significance of epidermal growth factor (EGF), EGF receptor and c-erB-2 in human gastric cancer. *Cancer* 1995;75:1418–1425.

131. Hirono Y, Tsugawa K, Fushida S, et al. Amplification of epidermal growth factor receptor gene and its relationship to survival in human gastric cancer. *Oncology* 1995;52:182–188.

132. Espinoza LA, Tone LG, Neto JB, et al. Enhanced TGFa-EGFR expression and p53 alterations contributes to gastric tumors aggressiveness. *Cancer Lett* 2004;212:33–41.

133. Tam SW, Theodoras AM, Shay JW, et al. Differential expression and regulation of cyclin D1 protein in normal and tumor human cells: association with Cdk4 is required for cyclin D1 function in G1 progression. *Oncogene* 1994;9:2663–2674.

134. Gao P, Zhou G-Y, Liu Y, et al. Alteration of cyclin D1 in gastric carcinoma and its clinicopathologic significance. *World J Gastroenterol* 2004;10:2936–2939.

135. Yamada Y, Yoshida T, Hayashi K, et al. p53 Gene mutations in gastric cancer metastases and in gastric cancer cell lines derived from metastases. *Cancer Res* 1991;51:5800–5803.

136. Stemmermann GN, Heffelfinger SC, Noffsinger A, et al. The molecular biology of esophageal and gastric cancer and their precursors: oncogenes, tumor suppressor genes, and growth factors. *Hum Pathol* 1994;25:968–981.

137. Motojima K, Furui J, Kohara N, et al. Expression of p53 protein in gastric cancer is not independently prognostic. *Surgery* 1994;116:890–895.

138. Martin H, Filipe MI, Morris RW, et al. p53 Expression and prognosis in gastric carcinoma. *Int J Cancer* 1992;50:859–862.

139. Pinto-de-Sousa J, Siva F, David L, et al. Clinicopathological significance and survival influence of p53 protein expression in gastric cancer expression. *Histopathology* 2004;44:323–331.

140. Kitoh T, Yanai H, Saitoh Y, et al. Increased expression of matrix metalloproteinase-7 in invasive early cancer. *J Gastroenterol* 2004;39:434–440.

141. Liu XP, Kawauchi S, Oga A, et al. Prognostic significance of matrix metalloproteinase-7 (MMP-7) expression at the invasive front in gastric cancer. *Jpn J Cancer Res* 2002;93:291–295.

142. Taniguchi K, Yonemura Y, Nojima N, et al. The relation between the growth patterns of gastric carcinoma and the expression of hepatocyte growth factor (c-met), autocrine motility factor receptor, and urokinase-type plasminogen activator receptor. *Cancer* 1997;82:2112–2122.

143. Hashimoto Y, Skacel M, Adams JC. Roles of fascin in human carcinoma motility and signaling: prospects for a novel biomarker? *Int J Biochem Cell Biol* 2005;37:1787–1804.

144. Hashimoto Y, Shimada Y, Kawamura J, et al. The prognostic relevance of fascin expression in human gastric carcinoma. *Oncology* 2004;67:262–270.

145. Juttner S, Wissmann C, Jöns T, et al. Vascular endothelial growth factor-D and its receptor VEGFR-3: two novel independent prognostic markers in gastric adenocarcinoma. *J Clin Oncol* 2006;24:228–240.

146. Kitidai Y, Kodama M, Cho S, et al. Quantitative analysis of lymphangiogenic markers for predicting metastases of human gastric carcinoma to lymph nodes. *Int J Cancer* 2005;115:388–392.

147. Grogan TM, Fenoglio-Preiser CM, Zeheb R, et al. Thioredoxin, a putative oncogene product, is overexpressed in gastric cancer and associated with increased cell proliferation and increased cell survival. *Hum Pathol* 2000;31:475–481.

148. Churin Y, Al-Ghoul L, Kepp O, et al. *Helicobacter pylori* CagA protein targets c-Met receptor and enhances motogenic response. *J Cell Biol* 2003;161:249–255.

149. Okano H, Shinohara H, Miyamotao A, et al. Concomitant overexpression of cyclooxygenase-2 in Her-2-positive on Smad4-reduced human gastric carcinomas is associated with a poor outcome. *Clin Cancer Res* 2004;10:6938–6945.

150. Catalano V, La Bianca R, Beretta GD, et al. Gastric cancer. *Oncol Hematol* 2005;54:209–241.

CHAPTER 22 ■ GASTRIC CANCER: STAGING SYSTEMS AND TECHNIQUES

MARK GREAVES, ARNOLD MARKOWITZ, AND HANS GERDES

In the early 1900s, it was observed that survival rates for cancer were higher for patients in whom the tumor had not yet spread beyond the organ of origin (1). These observations led to the beginnings of cancer staging, classifying cancers according to anatomical location, tumor size, and extent of spread. The Lockhart-Mummery system of rectal cancer was one such example (2). First reported in 1927, and later modified by Dukes (3) and others, it helped form the foundation for an international standard in colorectal cancer staging.

The rationale for cancer staging systems is to develop a reproducible method of categorizing neoplasms to permit the accurate description of tumors, to facilitate communication between clinicians caring for patients, to guide therapy, to predict prognosis, and to help standardize enrollment criteria and evaluate results in investigative research (4). Staging systems have evolved from institution-based schemes or national-based schemes into international systems that are now widely applied. Advances in radiology, endoscopy, and histopathology have allowed for improved staging capabilities, while advances in surgery, chemotherapy, and radiation oncology have increased the demand for accurate staging.

Historically, long-term survival has been poor for patients with gastric carcinoma, with 5-year survival rates ranging from 5% to 15% (5). Recurrent disease has traditionally been noted in up to 80% of patients after "curative" resection (5). The presence of distant metastases at the time of diagnosis has meant an even poorer prognosis because of the failure of surgical attempts to completely resect the disease and the lack of effective systemic therapy in patients with such advanced disease.

For many years, surgery was the standard of care for locoregional spread of disease. However, 5-year survival for stage III disease remained poor, with rates of 13% to 18% in most American series (6,7). These findings demonstrated that surgery alone is not always adequate therapy, and since the 1980s, there has been a focus on combined modality protocols. Neoadjuvant therapy has now become the standard of care at the authors' institution for stage III disease.

The American and Japanese literature, however, have consistently shown that earlier stage gastric cancer has a better prognosis than more advanced disease (8,9). This fact, coupled with the high cost and poor outcome of attempted surgical intervention in advanced disease, highlights the importance of preoperative staging. The evolution of computed tomography (CT) has played an important role in this area, significantly reducing the number of unnecessary laparotomies by identifying patients with intraabdominal, hepatic, or intrathoracic metastases before surgical exploration. CT, however, has been less accurate when it comes to locoregional staging. The depth of primary tumor invasion and the presence of lymph node involvement (i.e., locoregional disease) have emerged as the two most important prognostic markers in such patients and are now influencing the choice of treatment.

The emphasis on extent of tumor invasion (T) and the presence of lymph node involvement (N) has led to the increased utilization of endoscopic ultrasonography (EUS). This modality is described and compared with more traditional staging modalities such as radiography, standard endoscopy, and staging laparoscopy. In addition, advances in immunohistochemistry and molecular genetics have also been shown to further aid in predicting prognosis, although these are not yet widely used. Applying this technology to the analysis of various tissues such as lymph nodes, for example, may increase the sensitivity for identifying malignant cells not seen on routine staining and thereby help refine current staging modalities (10,11).

TUMOR, NODE, METASTASIS SYSTEM

The American Joint Committee on Cancer (AJCC) Staging and End Results Reporting was organized in 1959 with the support of medical, surgical, radiologic, and pathological societies; the American Cancer Society; and the National Cancer Institute. The AJCC published the first comprehensive manual on cancer staging in 1977 (12). The emphasis was on simplicity, practicality, and credibility, and the staging system was based on published data.

These guidelines were originally created in parallel to those published by the International Union Against Cancer (UICC), which is a consortium of multiple national tumor, node, metastasis (TNM) committees, including American, British, Canadian, French, German, Italian, and Japanese. The AJCC manual, together with the UICC guidelines, have since been revised several times and together have become an internationally recognized system of cancer staging. The sixth revision of the joint manual was published in 2002 (13), and efforts continue to encourage the universal application of this system.

The approach of these international classifications has been to standardize cancer staging according to groups for each anatomical site based on the extent of the primary tumor (T), the presence and extent of lymph node disease (N), and the presence or absence of distant organ metastases (M) (Table 22.1). This system is based largely on the premise that an untreated cancer initially increases in size, invades locally, and then spreads to local and regional lymph nodes before finally metastasizing to distant sites. Clinical trials have shown that tumors of larger size and with more sites of metastases carry a poorer prognosis than smaller localized tumors and should be treated differently.

TABLE 22.1

GASTRIC ADENOCARCINOMA TUMOR, NODE, METASTASIS (TNM) STAGING CLASSIFICATION OF THE AMERICAN JOINT COMMITTEE ON CANCER

Primary tumor stage (T)	Definition
Tx	Primary tumor cannot be assessed
T0	No evidence of primary tumor
Tis	Carcinoma in situ: intraepithelial tumor without invasion of the lamina propria
T1	Tumor invades lamina propria or submucosa
T2a	Tumor invades muscularis propria
T2b	Tumor invades subserosa
T3	Tumor penetrates serosa without invasion of adjacent structures
T4	Tumor invades adjacent structures
Regional lymph nodes (N)	
Nx	Regional lymph nodes cannot be assessed
N0	No regional lymph node metastases
N1	Metastases in 1 to 6 lymph nodes
N2	Metastases in 7 to 15 lymph nodes
N3	Metastases in >15 lymph nodes
Distant metastasis (M)	
Mx	Distant metastases cannot be assessed
M0	No distant metastases
M1	Distant metastases

TABLE 22.2

STAGE GROUPING FOR GASTRIC ADENOCARCINOMA ACCORDING TO AMERICAN JOINT COMMITTEE ON CANCER CLASSIFICATION

Stage grouping			
0	Tis	N0	M0
IA	T1	N0	M0
IB	T1	N1	M0
	T2a,b	N0	M0
II	T1	N2	M0
	T2a,b	N1	M0
	T3	N0	M0
IIIA	T2a,b	N2	M0
	T3	N1	M0
	T4	N0	M0
IIIB	T3	N2	M0
IV	T4	N1	M0
	T1	N3	M0
	T2a,b	N3	M0
	T3	N3	M0
	T4	N2	M0
	T4	N3	M0
	Any T	Any N	M1

fication were the most significant prognostic factors (16). More recently, a study compared survival rates for 1,244 gastric cancer patients using the Japanese Classification system versus the AJCC/UICC system, and found that the AJCC/UICC system was more rational and homogenous than the Japanese system (17).

Japanese Classification of Gastric Carcinoma

For many years, the staging of gastric carcinoma in Japan has followed the TNM model, similar to the AJCC system. The Japanese system, though, has several differences. In addition to the level of invasion of the primary tumor, it looks at the gross morphologic characteristics of the tumor. The Japanese system also puts greater emphasis on the location and groups of lymph nodes involved and separates the location of distant metastases into peritoneal, hepatic, and distant sites. These classifications were published for the first time in English in 1995 (18). The Japanese classification criteria are presented in Table 22.3, and the stage groupings are shown in Table 22.4.

METHODS OF STAGING

Barium Radiography and Endoscopy

Barium radiography and upper gastrointestinal endoscopy are both useful modalities in the diagnosis and assessment of gastric adenocarcinoma, but neither modality has been shown to accurately predict the stage of cancer so they both remain strictly diagnostic tools. Although barium radiography has an excellent record as an effective screening tool for high-risk mass population screening in Japan, endoscopy has become the procedure of choice in the United States and Japan for the

Gastric Carcinoma Staging

The AJCC approach to staging of gastric adenocarcinoma is based on the TNM classification. Using the TNM classification, cancers are grouped from a stage of best prognosis (stage 0: Tis N0 M0) to poorest prognosis (stage IV: T4 N1 M1) (Table 22.2). The disease stage is stated according to actual information for each TNM factor. Both clinical TNM (cTNM) and pathological TNM (pTNM) staging schemes exist for tumors because histopathological confirmation of stage may not always be available when treatment decisions are being made, and the two types of staging may each predict outcome differently.

In the fifth revision of the AJCC classification of gastric adenocarcinoma, the classification of nodal metastases (N staging) was restructured to reflect the number of involved lymph nodes as opposed to their anatomical stations. The sixth revision did not bring about any major changes to the staging of gastric cancer. The current classification is reflected in Table 22.1, and the stage groupings are shown in Table 22.2.

Several groups, including the Japanese, have retrospectively evaluated their respective cohorts of gastric adenocarcinoma patients in the context of the nodal staging classifications brought about in the fifth edition (14,15). A multivariate analysis of various factors in gastric adenocarcinoma demonstrated that the depth of tumor invasion and the new nodal stage classi-

TABLE 22.3

GASTRIC ADENOCARCINOMA JAPANESE CLASSIFICATION SYSTEM

1. Location of tumor in proximal, mid, or distal third of the stomach

2. Depth of tumor invasion:
   T1: invasion of mucosa or submucosa
   T2: invasion of muscularis propria or subserosa
   T3: penetration of serosa
   T4: invasion of adjacent structures

3. Macroscopic type of tumor according to gross endoscopic or radiographic appearance:
   Type 0: superficial, flat tumor with or without minimal elevation or depression
   Type 1: polypoid tumor, sharply demarcated from the surrounding mucosa, usually attached on a wide base
   Type 2: ulcerated tumor with sharply demarcated and raised margins
   Type 3: ulcerated tumor without definite limits, infiltrating into the surrounding wall
   Type 4: diffusely infiltrating tumor in which ulceration is usually not a marked feature
   Type 5: nonclassifiable tumor that cannot be categorized into any of the above types

4. Regional lymph node metastases classified according to the numbered lymph node stations and placed in groups:
   N0: no evidence of lymph node metastases
   N1: metastases to group 1 lymph nodes but not groups 2, 3, and 4
   N2: metastases to group 2 lymph nodes but not groups 3 and 4
   N3: metastases to group 3 lymph nodes but not group 4
   N4: metastases to group 4 lymph nodes

5. Peritoneal metastases:
   P0: no peritoneal metastases
   P1: metastases to adjacent peritoneum but not to the distant peritoneum
   P2: a few metastases to the distant peritoneum
   P3: numerous metastases to the distant peritoneum

6. Liver metastases:
   H0: no liver metastases
   H1: (dext/sin): metastases limited to either the right or the left lobe
   H2: a few metastases to both lobes
   H3: numerous metastases to both lobes

7. Distant metastases:
   M0: no distant metastases other than peritoneal or liver metastases
   M1: distant metastases other than peritoneal or liver metastases

TABLE 22.4

STAGE GROUPING FOR GASTRIC ADENOCARCINOMA ACCORDING TO JAPANESE CLASSIFICATION

Stage grouping					
IA	T1	N0	P0	H0	M0
IB	T1	N1	P0	H0	M0
	T2	N0	P0	H0	M0
II	T1	N2	P0	H0	M0
	T2	N1	P0	H0	M0
	T3	N0	P0	H0	M0
IIIA	T1	N3	P0	H0	M0
	T2	N2	P0	H0	M0
	T3	N1	P0	H0	M0
	T4	N0	P0	H0	M0
IIIB	T2	N3	P0	H0	M0
	T3	N2	P0	H0	M0
	T4	N1	P0	H0	M0
IVA	T1-3	N0-3	P0	H1	M0
	T4	N2	P0	H0	M0
	T1-3	N0-2	P1	H0	M0
IVB	All other tumors including T4 tumors involving two organs or more and M1 tumors				

Computed Tomography

Traditionally, the major usefulness of CT scan imaging in staging gastric cancer is related to its ability to identify metastatic disease to the liver, peritoneum, intraabdominal or retroperitoneal lymph nodes, or other more distant locations. However, in prospective studies comparing the results of CT with intraoperative findings, the sensitivity of CT for staging gastric cancer has been called into question (19). In the staging of hepatic and peritoneal metastases, preoperative staging by CT has been suggested in one study to have an accuracy of 79% for hepatic disease and 81% for peritoneal disease; however, the sensitivity for each in the same study was quite low, 52% and 8%, respectively (20). In another prospective study of a series of 111 patients undergoing laparoscopic staging for gastric cancer, preoperative CT was shown to have missed as many as 37% of small metastatic lesions that were detected by laparoscopy or laparotomy (21). The majority of these lesions were small peritoneal implants, with only 3 of 38 representing liver metastases. This suggests that although CT provides important information regarding liver metastases in gastric carcinoma, it misses a substantial proportion of peritoneal disease. In the staging of the primary tumor and locoregional lymph node metastases, CT has performed even more poorly, with accuracy rates ranging from 25% to 43% for T staging and 33% to 51% for N staging (22,23).

Newer studies have focused on the role of spiral or thin-section CT in gastric cancer staging. Early investigations using this technology were disappointing, demonstrating results similar to traditional CT, with a sensitivity of 71% for peritoneal metastases and 57% for hepatic metastases in one study (24). The sensitivity for lymph node staging in that same study was 24% for N1 disease and 43% for N2 disease. Subsequent studies have shown more promise, with locoregional staging capabilities comparable to EUS (25,26). In one study of 51 patients, helical CT achieved correct T staging in 76% and correct

diagnostic evaluation of symptomatic patients. Endoscopy offers the advantage of biopsy at the time of the procedure, thus providing a definitive diagnosis. The location, extent, and gross morphologic characteristics of a tumor are readily identified by either method, but the depth of tumor invasion and the assessment of lymph nodes cannot be achieved by either technique. Therefore, neither procedure alone provides enough information to allow for complete staging of gastric carcinoma.

N staging in 70% of cases (26). As with EUS, the greatest difficulty in T staging with helical CT relates to differentiating between T2 and T3 lesions. Another study demonstrated that the ability to accurately predict T and N staging has improved with progressive CT technology and with physician experience in using that technology (27).

Finally, some of the most recent studies have looked at the use of contrast-enhanced helical hydro-CT scanning in staging gastric cancer. For this exam, patients must first ingest 1 to 1.5 L of water to help distend the stomach, and then undergo a helical CT with contrast. One trial using this new technology showed a detection rate of lymph node metastases of 60%, with an overall accuracy in staging gastric cancer of 86% (28).

Despite the concerns over the limitations of CT scan imaging, our institution continues to rely on spiral CT early in the evaluation to identify those patients with metastatic disease. The detection of metastatic disease at presentation permits immediate triage of these patients to systemic therapy and avoidance of the unnecessary risks and morbidity of laparotomy, except in those cases in which surgical palliation of obstruction or bleeding may be indicated. Patients in whom initial CT does not reveal metastatic disease then undergo more advanced staging evaluation with EUS and laparoscopy, and are more appropriately offered curative surgical treatment or multimodality treatment protocols with curative intent.

Endoscopic Ultrasonography

EUS involves the introduction of an endoscope-mounted ultrasonic transducer directly into the gastrointestinal lumen, bringing the instrument into close proximity to the tumor. This eliminates the artifacts usually created by intraluminal air and food that is seen with traditional transcutaneous ultrasonography and CT scan imaging. Although it does require conscious sedation, EUS is performed with the same ease and comfort as routine upper gastrointestinal endoscopy, with minimal risk, and is well tolerated by most patients.

The 5-, 7.5-, and 12-MHz probes fitted on these echoendoscopes permits assessment of the microscopic tissue planes of the gastrointestinal tract, including the mucosa, submucosa, muscularis propria, and serosa (Fig. 22.1). The lower frequen-

cies permit the evaluation of nearby extramural disease, including local and regional lymphadenopathy and adjacent organs such as the liver, spleen, and pancreas in addition to the identification of perigastric ascites. Thus, EUS allows for both accurate assessment of the depth of tumor invasion into and through the wall of the stomach (Fig. 22.2A–H), as well as the identification of local lymph node metastases (Fig. 22.3), making it an ideal modality for determining a tumor's T and N stages.

Early studies helped establish the role of endoscopic ultrasonography in gastric cancer staging. In one study, preoperative EUS was found to be concordant with pathological staging for depth of tumor invasion in 92% of patients, compared with only 42% concordance for CT scanning (29). In that same study, EUS findings were concordant with pathological findings for lymph node staging in 78% of patients, compared with 48% for CT. In another early study, EUS accuracy for T staging was 67% to 92% and for N staging was 50% to 87% (30). Finally, in one study, preoperative EUS was shown to be more accurate than either preoperative CT or intraoperative manual assessment by the surgeon for T stage (86% vs. 43% and 56%, respectively) and for N stage (74% vs. 51% and 54%, respectively) (23).

The past several years have seen similar positive results concerning EUS in gastric cancer staging published from other countries around the world because they, too, have adopted EUS as part of the preoperative staging evaluation (31,32). One study in Singapore, for example, looked at 126 patients with gastric cancer and found an overall accuracy for EUS of 80.4% for T stage and an overall accuracy of 77.7% for N stage (33). In another study from Japan, the role of EUS in staging adenocarcinoma of the gastric cardia was demonstrated (34). This study is important because most previous studies evaluating EUS staging of gastric cancer have focused on tumors located in the body and antrum of the stomach, and there were concerns that lesions in the cardia might be harder to assess due to the difficulties in positioning the tip of the echoendoscope into that part of the stomach.

One of the main strengths of EUS has been the demonstration that the depth of tumor invasion as assessed by preoperative EUS is highly predictive of disease recurrence and overall prognosis in patients undergoing curative surgery (35). In this series, with a median follow-up of 25 months, only 15% of patients found to have T1 or T2 tumors on preoperative EUS developed recurrent cancer after curative resection. In contrast, 77% of patients with T3 or T4 disease by preoperative EUS developed recurrent disease after curative resection, and 73% died of recurrent disease after a median follow-up of 23 months. A more recent report from the author's institution that is awaiting publication showed that although the accuracy of EUS for T and N staging was less than what has been reported in previous studies, EUS was still highly sensitive in identifying patients with transmural tumors, which have a poorer prognosis when managed by surgery alone (36).

Attempts to accurately characterize the depth of tumor invasion according to histologic layers have demonstrated that distinguishing between T2 and T3 disease in gastric carcinoma may at times be difficult. Histologically, T3 disease is defined as penetration by infiltrating cancer through the serosa. The serosal layer is only a few cells thick and is represented by a very thin, bright signal on EUS imaging (Fig. 22.1). The classification of T2 tumors by EUS is made when the tumor invades the muscularis propria, but the outer surface of this layer appears smooth and intact as demonstrated by the preservation of the bright signal caused by the serosa. In contrast, T3 tumors on EUS have an irregular outer surface to the muscularis propria with the disruption or loss of the bright serosal signal (37). Tumors that have penetrated through the muscularis propria and into the subserosal fat but not through the serosal layer are

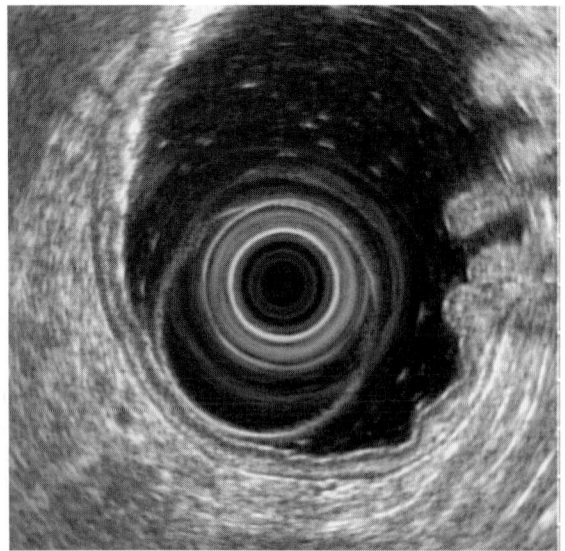

FIGURE 22.1. Normal gastric wall on endoscopic ultrasonography. Mucosa, submucosa, muscularis propria, and serosa layers visible.

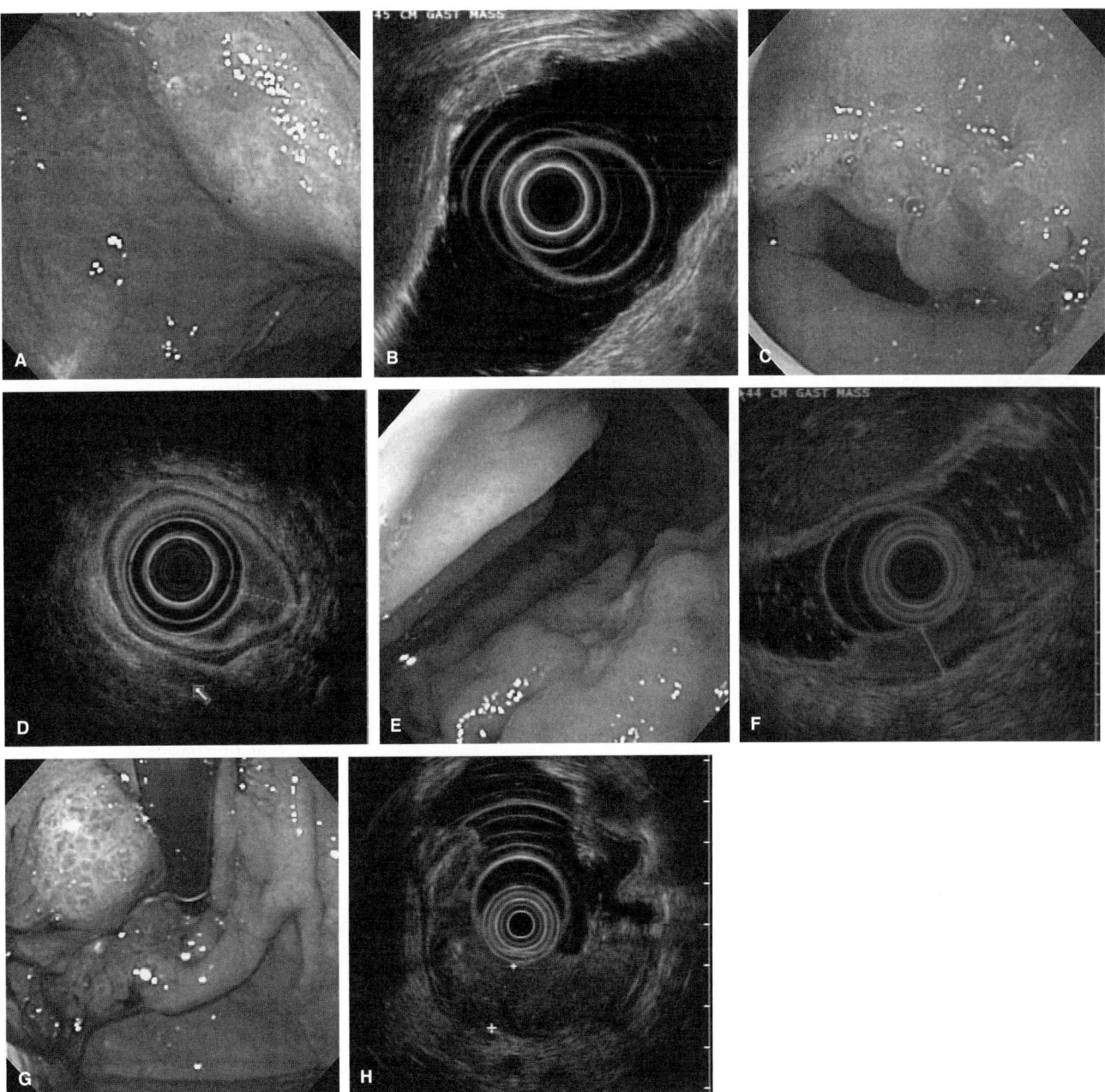

FIGURE 22.2. The endoscopic and corresponding endoscopic ultrasonography (EUS) images of different T-staged gastric cancers. **A, B:** T1 lesion. The tumor involves both the mucosal and submucosal layers, but the muscularis propria layer remains intact in the EUS image (**B**). **C, D:** Another T1 lesion. Note how, despite being a larger tumor, this is still a T1 lesion because the muscularis propria layer again remains intact (**D**). **E, F:** T2 lesion. The tumor penetrates the muscularis propria in the EUS image (**F**). **G, H:** T3 lesion. Note how the entire thickness of the gastric wall appears involved by the tumor in the EUS image (**H**) (See also color Figure 22.2a,c,e,g).

classified histologically as T2, but may be misclassified as T3 by EUS because of the irregular outer surface of the muscularis propria on imaging (Fig. 22.4). Furthermore, tumors invading into the gastrohepatic or gastrocolic ligaments may have deep extension beyond the muscularis propria without penetrating the serosa and thus may also be misinterpreted as T3 by EUS. The importance of this misclassification needs further study because experience demonstrates that tumors such as these that invade beyond the muscularis propria but do not penetrate the serosa behave more like pathological T3 tumors than T2 tumors (8,36). In other words, the overstaging of such tumors by EUS may more accurately predict the prognosis than the actual histologic stage. Such tumors would perhaps be more appropriately treated with combined modality therapy than solely by surgical resection.

The evaluation of deeply ulcerating tumors by EUS can also lead to misclassification. The intense adjacent inflammation caused by the ulcer can lead to an overestimation of the depth of tumor invasion (38). The inflammatory response can also lead to the development of enlarged reactive nearby lymph nodes that may be misinterpreted as being malignant.

As mentioned previously, reactive lymph nodes can pose a challenge to the endoscopist when attempting to assess the N stage of a tumor because reactive (inflammatory) nodes may

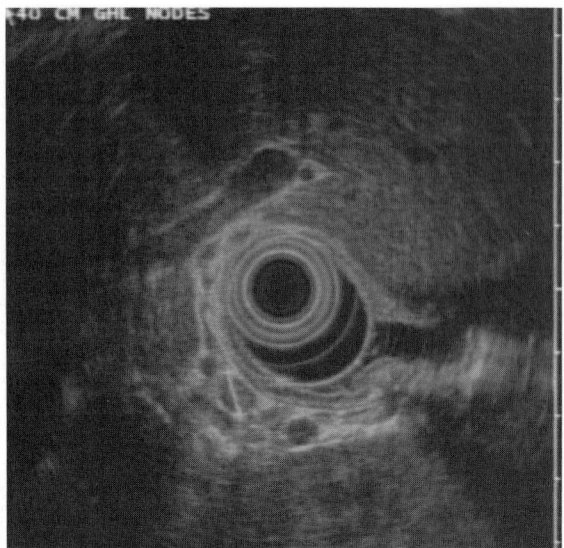

FIGURE 22.3. Malignant lymph nodes. There are two malignant lymph nodes seen in the lower half of the picture. The larger node (*left*) has a line across the center of it to mark it and to assess its size. Note the round shape, clear margin, and hypoechoic pattern of each node.

have some of the same features as malignant nodes. Lightdale and Mierop showed that those lymph nodes of "round shape, clear margin, and hypoecho pattern" similar to that of the primary tumor were more likely to be malignant (39). Heintz et al. reported that the sensitivity and specificity of lymph node staging would be 85% and 45% to 85%, respectively, if the following diagnostic criteria are used to characterize malignant lymph nodes: size larger than 10 mm in diameter, heterogeneous echo pattern, and a sharp border (40). Although not currently used for routine staging of gastric adenocarcinoma, EUS-guided fine-needle aspiration has been shown to be of value in distinguishing the nature (benign vs. malignant) of enlarged nodes (41,42). This technique, however, may be limited in gastric cancer because traversing the tumor with a

needle to aspirate a nearby perigastric lymph node may falsely result in the finding of cancer cells in the lymph node specimen.

EUS lacks the ability to accurately identify distant metastases such as liver, lung, and peritoneal disease. Although EUS may identify the presence of liver metastases in nearby adjacent liver segments close to the wall of the stomach, most of the right lobe of the liver is not seen well. Similarly, although EUS has the potential to detect the occasional small pocket of perigastric ascites missed on CT (43), EUS overall has performed poorly in identifying peritoneal disease. This is why, in most published studies, the sensitivity of EUS for M1 disease has been low (44) or has not been reported. EUS alone, therefore, has not generally been used to rule out distant metastases, but has been used instead to complement CT.

Finally, patients with locally advanced disease (T3 and/or N1) may be offered neoadjuvant therapy followed by surgery. Many oncologists attempt to restage patients after the neoadjuvant therapy and before surgery to identify those patients that have progressed (and are therefore no longer surgical candidates). Endoscopy, CT, positron emission tomography (PET), and EUS have all been used to restage gastric cancer. Recently though, studies have shown that the accuracy of EUS post chemotherapy is much lower (60% in one study) than the initial staging accuracy (45). This is largely due to the inflammation and edema that is associated with the response of tumors to the chemotherapy, and this may lead to errors in restaging, similar to that seen with deeply ulcerated tumors.

Despite its utility, EUS is not largely applied in the locoregional staging of gastric cancer. At our institution, EUS is not performed routinely on all newly diagnosed gastric carcinoma patients. It is, however, used to better stage a small proportion of patients who have equivocal findings at laparoscopy or those in whom the CT scan results suggest a posterior gastric tumor or an early tumor.

Laparoscopy

In the evaluation of gastric cancer by laparoscopy, the surgeon is able to fully assess external gastric anatomy, the serosal surface of the stomach, and perigastric lymph node stations. Accurate staging of gastric cancer requires the careful evaluation of both the anterior and the posterior gastric areas because tumors that penetrate into the lesser sac may not be visible unless the surgeon manipulates the stomach and exposes this area. However, the staging of depth of invasion varies, depending on whether the surgeon makes the determination based on visual inspection, brush cytology of the serosal surface, or through the application of laparoscopic ultrasonography. Similarly, abnormal lymph nodes that harbor metastatic disease may not be readily apparent without a systemic search by the operator. Celiac lymph nodes may require a great deal of manipulation or dissection for full assessment, and the determination of lymph node metastases depends on the surgeon's assessment of appearance, firmness, and mobility of these lymph nodes. The presence of large, matted lymph nodes is an obvious demonstration of metastases, but limited infiltration of lymph nodes by tumor may present a challenge for the surgeon. Excision or fine-needle aspiration at laparoscopy can sample lymph nodes, but this introduces the potential risk of seeding the peritoneum with tumor cells during a diagnostic staging examination and is subject to the inherent limitations of fine-needle aspiration itself.

Initial studies of laparoscopy of upper gastrointestinal malignancies indicate that laparoscopy is sensitive for detecting metastatic disease, particularly in identifying small tumor implants that are not identified by conventional imaging modalities (21,46). Prevalence rates of 30% to 40% for M1 disease in patients with gastric malignancies have been reported in cases

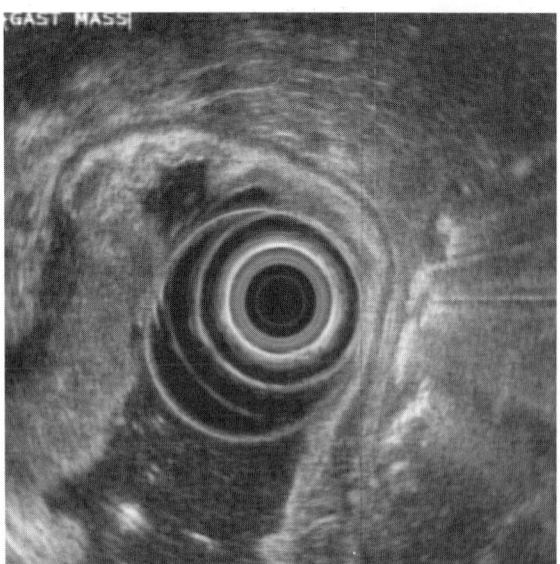

FIGURE 22.4. Example of overstaging. The lesion shown was staged as a T3 lesion based on the endoscopic ultrasonography image shown. On pathology, it was determined to be a T2 lesion.

in which current state-of-the-art imaging modalities have failed to reveal the metastatic disease (46). The most common sites of metastatic disease detected are the peritoneal surface and the liver. Such results have improved the selection of patients for surgery and have increased the curative resection rates at some hospitals while reducing the number of unnecessary laparotomies (21,47).

A recent retrospective review looked at 657 patients in whom laparoscopy detected M1 disease that had been previously missed with other imaging modalities (48). M1 disease was significantly more prevalent with tumors located at the gastroesophageal (GE) junction or whole stomach, poorly differentiated tumors, or patients diagnosed at younger than age 70. On preoperative spiral CT, lymphadenopathy >1 cm or T3/T4 tumors were associated with significantly higher prevalence of M1. On multivariate analyses, only tumor location (GE junction or whole stomach) and lymphadenopathy were independently significant, and M1 was not detected in any patient with neither risk factor. Based on these results, the authors concluded that laparoscopy may be avoided if the primary tumor was not at the GE junction or whole stomach, and there is no lymphadenopathy (48).

Positron Emission Tomography

PET scanning is a unique imaging modality in cancer care that allows visualization of tumors by virtue of differences in metabolic activity between tumor and normal tissue. Tumor tissue is generally more metabolically active than normal nonneoplastic tissue and has increased glycolytic activity. The administration of 2-[^{18}F]-fluoro-2-deoxy-D-glucose (FDG) to an individual with cancer results in a greater uptake of FDG by tumor tissue than by most normal tissues. Once FDG enters cancer cells, it is phosphorylated and trapped within the cells, rendering the cells radioactive. Tumors of sufficient size and uptake of FDG are therefore readily detected using a gamma camera. PET images can then be superimposed on conventional CT scans to correlate the areas of increased radioisotope activity with anatomical sites of disease.

Currently, the role of PET scan in the evaluation of cancer is being defined because the full capabilities of this technology are still being explored. The utility of PET has been studied in both cancer staging and in assessing treatment response, with mixed results. Although PET has been demonstrated to have a high sensitivity in detecting the primary tumor location in gastrointestinal malignancies (49), it has not been shown to be helpful in defining the depth of primary tumor invasion, and therefore is not of value in determining T stage. Thus, the usefulness of PET presently relies on its ability to detect lymph node disease (N stage) and distant metastases (M stage).

In one study that looked at PET in staging gastric cancer, the sensitivity for detecting the primary lesion was 93%, with a specificity of 100%, and an accuracy of 95% (50). PET has also proven effective in gastric cancer for detecting distant metastases (51). The controversy with PET in gastric cancer staging has pertained to its ability to detect regional lymph node disease. Earlier studies showed that PET scanning had difficulties in distinguishing involved local lymph nodes from the primary tumor (49,52). A more recent study found that PET had a similar accuracy to spiral CT for diagnosing local and distant lymph node metastases and peritoneal disease. In addition, PET had a higher specificity than CT (92% vs. 62%) in assessing the local lymph node status (53). Of note, in the same study, PET combined with CT was more accurate for preoperative staging than either modality alone (66% vs. 51% and 66% vs. 47%, respectively). A second recent trial also compared preoperative PET to spiral CT in patients with gastric cancer. Using the Japanese system for classification of lymph node status, this study reported a sensitivity, specificity, positive predictive value, and negative predictive value of PET for lymph node metastases of 40%, 95%, 91%, and 56%, respectively (54). In this study, CT was superior to PET in terms of sensitivity, but PET was superior to CT in terms of specificity and positive predictive value.

It is important to note that in approximately 20% of patients with gastric cancer, the primary tumor cannot be visualized by PET. These patients are said to have a "noninformative PET" because one cannot determine the presence or absence of metastatic disease in a patient whose primary tumor does not show up on PET. The physiological accumulation of FDG in the stomach may prevent the detection of small malignancies (55). This was highlighted in a study that showed that larger (size >30 mm), more advanced gastric cancers had a higher detection rate by PET than smaller, early gastric cancers (56). It has also been shown that there are lower levels of expression of glucose transporter-1 (glut-1) in signet cells and mucinous gastric carcinoma (57). This low expression seems to affect diffuse-type gastric cancer more so than intestinal type, explaining why Stahl et al. found that the detection rate for diffuse type (41%) was significantly lower than for intestinal type (83%) (58).

Although PET has not become a standard of care, there is increasing interest in using PET in the staging of gastric cancer. Specifically, PET could prove to be a useful adjunct to EUS staging of gastric cancer, offering an attractive alternative to fine-needle aspiration in improving the accuracy of lymph node staging by EUS.

Potential Future Staging Approaches

Immunohistochemistry is an investigational tool that may allow for the detection of micrometastases in lymph nodes, microinvasion of the muscularis propria, and microdissemination in the peritoneal cavity by studying the tissues or fluid in the peritoneal cavity at the time of surgery (11,59). Using antibodies directed at cytokeratins, this technology has been applied to gastric carcinoma. In one series of patients with early-stage gastric carcinoma, 1,945 lymph nodes and 79 gastric tumors were studied using the anticytokeratin antibody CAM 5.2 (60). Micrometastases were found in 25% of lymph nodes believed to be negative for malignancy by routine histology and in all histologically positive nodes. Microinvasion of the muscularis propria was also found in 11 of 68 patients (16%) believed to have invasion limited to the submucosa. Importantly, those patients with micrometastases or microinvasion had poorer survival than those with less invasive disease.

Molecular genetics has been shown to aid in predicting prognosis in gastric cancer patients. In one study that looked at 259 cases of gastric cancer, expression of CDX2 (an intestinal transcription factor) by gastric cancer cells was shown to be associated with less invasive tumors, meaning that CDX2 was associated with a more favorable prognosis (61). In a second study, gastric cancer patients that had overexpression of EZH2 (enhancer of zeste homolog 2, a known repressor of gene transcription) had a poorer prognosis than those patients with no or low levels of EZH2. This was due to the fact that EZH2 levels were directly correlated with tumor size, depth of invasion, and lymph node metastases (62). Studies such as these may ultimately lead to the development of biomarkers that can be routinely applied to all gastric cancer patients at the time of diagnosis, for the purpose of predicting the prognosis of gastric cancers, thereby redefining the way in which we currently stage the disease and impacting the current treatment algorithm.

SUMMARY

The management of gastric adenocarcinoma continues to evolve as technologic advances improve the ability to diagnose, stage, and treat this disease. International experiences have clearly shown the effect of early detection on the ability to cure this cancer, as early-stage disease is associated with a much better rate of survival. Current understanding of the causative agents and premalignant states has not yet provided clues to effective prevention. Clinical strategies for treating the majority of affected patients therefore focus on radical surgical resection for patients with earlier stages of disease, combined modality protocols for patients with locoregional spread of disease, and palliative chemotherapy for patients with advanced metastatic disease.

These approaches depend on accurate preoperative clinical staging for all patients with newly diagnosed adenocarcinoma of the stomach. The international staging system, which emphasizes the TNM scheme of staging in gastric adenocarcinoma, predicts the clinical course and outcome with reasonable accuracy. It is a simple system that is reproducible, and allows for staging to be readily ascertained by existing noninvasive and minimally invasive imaging modalities.

The approach to staging and management of gastric carcinoma varies, depending on the availability of new instruments, technical expertise, and effective therapeutic modalities. As demonstrated in this chapter, spiral CT, EUS, laparoscopy, and PET represent state-of-the-art methods for accurate preoperative staging of gastric cancer. Although each modality has its limitations, taken together they represent a relatively safe and accurate way to stage the majority of patients.

It is our opinion that, for the majority of patients, a good-quality spiral CT scan with oral and intravenous contrast can effectively identify distant metastases. Patients identified with metastatic disease can then be immediately triaged to palliative care and spared the risk, morbidity, and cost of unnecessary surgery. For patients in whom CT scan imaging does not demonstrate distant metastases, additional staging should then be performed with either EUS or laparoscopy (based on institutional expertise) to determine the TNM stage so patients with early stage disease (T1, T2, N0, M0) can then be scheduled for immediate surgery. Neoadjuvant therapy is then available for those patients with T3 or N+ disease, in the absence of distant metastases. Patients found to have metastatic disease via these methods that were not originally detected by CT can then also be offered palliative treatment. Finally, although PET imaging may prove to be an important complement to CT and even EUS in improving the accuracy of preoperative staging, more refinements in this field need to occur before it is adopted as a routine tool in gastric cancer staging.

References

1. Rubin P. Concepts of cancer staging. In: Calabresi P, Schein P, Roseberg S, eds. *Medical Oncology, Basic Principles and Clinical Management of Cancer.* New York, NY: Macmillan; 1986:157–177.
2. Lockhart-Mummery JP. Two hundred cases of cancer of the rectum treated by perineal excision. *Br J Surg* 1927;14:110–124.
3. Dukes C. The classification of cancer of the rectum. *J Pathol* 1932;35:323–332.
4. Grunberg SM, Groshen S. Concepts of cancer staging. In: Calabresi P, Schein PS, eds. *Medical Oncology.* 2nd ed. New York, NY: McGraw-Hill; 1993:229–236.
5. Alexander HR, Kelsen DP, Tepper JE. Cancer of the stomach. In: DeVita VT, Hellman S, Rosenberg SA, eds. *Cancer: Principles and Practice of Oncology.* 4th ed. Philadelphia, Pa.: JB Lippincott; 1993:818–848.
6. Hundahl SA, Menck HR, Mansour EG, et al. The national cancer data base report on gastric carcinoma. *Cancer* 1997;80:2333–2341.
7. Brennan MF, Karpeh MS. Surgery for gastric cancer: the American view. *Semin Oncol* 1996;23:352–359.
8. Wanebo HJ, Kennedy BJ, Chmiel J, et al. Cancer of the stomach: a patient care study by the American College of Surgeons. *Ann Surg* 1993;218:583–592.
9. Maruyama K, Okabayashi K, Kinoshita T. Progress in gastric cancer surgery in Japan and its limits of radicality. *World J Surg* 1987;11:418–425.
10. Heiss MM, Allgayer H, Gruetzner KU, et al. Clinical value of extended biologic staging by bone marrow micrometastases and tumor-associated proteases in gastric cancer. *Ann Surg* 1997;226:736–744.
11. Harrison LE, Choe JK, Goldstein M, et al. Prognostic significance of immunohistochemical micrometastases in node negative gastric cancer patients. *J Surg Oncol* 2000;73:153–157.
12. Bears OH, Carr DJ, Rubin P, eds. *American Joint Committee on Cancer Manual for Staging of Cancer.* Philadelphia, Pa.: JB Lippincott; 1978.
13. Greene FL, Page DL, Fleming ID, eds. *American Joint Committee on Cancer Manual for Staging of Cancer.* 6th ed. New York, NY: Springer-Verlag; 2002.
14. Ichikura T, Tomimatsu S, Uefuji K, et al. Evaluation of the new American Joint Committee on Cancer/International Union Against Cancer classification of lymph node metastasis from gastric carcinoma in comparison with the Japanese classification. *Cancer* 1999;86:553–558.
15. De Manzoni G, Verlato G, Guglielmi A, et al. Classification of lymph node metastases from carcinoma of the stomach: comparison of the old (1987) and the new (1997) TNM systems. *World J Surg* 1999;23:664–669.
16. Yoo CH, Noh SH, Kim YI, et al. Comparison of prognostic significance of nodal staging between old (4th edition) and new (5th edition) UICC TNM classification for gastric carcinoma. *World J Surg* 1999;23:492–498.
17. Kunisaki C, Shimada H, Nomura M, et al. Comparative evaluation of gastric carcinoma staging: Japanese classification versus new American Joint Committee on Cancer/International Union Against Cancer Classification. *Ann Surg Oncol* 2004;11:203–206.
18. Mitsumasa N, Omori Y, Miwa K, eds. *Japanese Classification of Gastric Carcinoma.* Japanese Research Society for Gastric Cancer. Tokyo: Kanehara & Co.; 1995.
19. Sussman SK, Halvorsen RA, Illescas FF, et al. Gastric adenocarcinoma: CT versus surgical staging. *Radiology* 1988;167:335–340.
20. Stell DA, Carter CR, Stewart I, et al. Prospective comparison of laparoscopy, ultrasonography and computed tomography in the staging of gastric cancer. *Br J Surg* 1996;83:1260–1262.
21. Burke EC, Karpeh MS, Conlon KC, et al. Laparoscopy in the management of gastric adenocarcinoma. *Ann Surg* 1997;225:262–267.
22. Botet JF, Lightdale CJ, Zauber AG, et al. Preoperative staging of gastric cancer: comparison of endoscopic US and dynamic CT. *Radiology* 1991;181:426–432.
23. Ziegler K, Sanft C, Zimmer T, et al. Comparison of computed tomography, endosonography, and intraoperative assessment in TN staging of gastric carcinoma. *Gut* 1993;34:604–610.
24. Davies J, Chalmers AG, Sue-Ling HM, et al. Spiral computed tomography and operative staging of gastric adenocarcinoma: a comparison with histopathological staging. *Gut* 1997;41:314–319.
25. Polkowski M, Palucki J, Wronska E, et al. Endosonography versus helical computed tomography for locoregional staging of gastric cancer. *Endoscopy* 2004;36:617–623.
26. Habermann CR, Weiss F, Riecken R, et al. Preoperative staging of gastric adenocarcinoma: comparison of helical CT and endoscopic US. *Radiology* 2004;230:465–471.
27. Blackshaw GR, Stephens MR, Lewis WG, et al. Progressive CT system technology and experience improve the perceived preoperative stage of gastric cancer. *Gastric Cancer* 2005;8:29–34.
28. Wei WZ, Yu JP, Li J, et al. Evaluation of contrast-enhanced helical hydro-CT in staging gastric cancer. *World J Gastroenterol* 2005;11:4592–4595.
29. Botet JF, Lightdale CJ, Zauber AG, et al. Endoscopic ultrasound in the preoperative staging of gastric cancer: a comparative study with dynamic CT. *Radiology* 1991;181:426–432.
30. Pollack BJ, Chak A, Sivak M. Endoscopic ultrasonography. *Semin Oncol* 1996;23:336–346.
31. Mesihovic R, Vanis N, Husic-Selimovic A, et al. Evaluation of the diagnostic accuracy of the endoscopic ultrasonography results in the patients examined in a period of three years. *Med Arh* 2005;59:299–302.
32. Tsendsuren T, Jun S, Mian X. Usefulness of endoscopic ultrasonography in preoperative TNM staging of gastric cancer. *World J Gastroenterol* 2006;12:43–47.
33. Ganpathi IS, So JB, Ho K. Endoscopic ultrasonography for gastric cancer. Does it influence treatment? *Surg Endosc* 2006;20:559–562.
34. Shimoyama S, Yasuda H, Hashimoto M, et al. Accuracy of linear-array EUS for preoperative staging of gastric cardia cancer. *Gastrointest Endosc* 2004;60:50–55.
35. Smith JW, Brennan MF, Botet JF, et al. Preoperative endoscopic ultrasound can predict the risk of recurrence after operation for gastric carcinoma. *J Clin Oncol* 1993;11:2380–2385.
36. Bentrem D, Gerdes H, Tang L, et al. Clinical correlation of endoscopic ultrasound with pathologic stage and outcome in patients undergoing curative resection for gastric cancer. *Annals Surg Oncol* 2007;14(6):1853–1859.
37. Kimmey MB, Martin RW, Haggitt RC, et al. Histologic correlates of gastrointestinal ultrasound images. *Gastroenterology* 1989;96:433–441.
38. Fein J, Gerdes H, Karpeh M, et al. Overstaging of ulcerated gastric cancers by endoscopic ultrasonography. *Gastrointest Endosc* 1993;39:274.

39. Lightdale CJ, Mierop FV. Staging gastric cancer: the New York experience. In: Dam JV, Sivak VM, eds. *Gastrointestinal Endosonography*. Philadelphia: WB Saunders; 1999:185–192.

40. Heintz A, Mildenberger P, Georg H, et al. Endoscopic ultrasonography in the diagnosis of regional lymph nodes in esophageal and gastric cancer. *Endoscopy* 1993;25:231–235.

41. Wiersema MJ, Kochman ML, Cramer HM, et al. Endosonography-guided real-time fine-needle aspiration biopsy. *Gastrointest Endosc* 1994;40:700–707.

42. Vilmann P, Hancke S, Henriksen FW, et al. Endoscopic ultrasonography-guided fine-needle aspiration biopsy of lesions in the gastrointestinal tract. *Gastrointest Endosc* 1995;41:230–235.

43. Lee YT, Ng EKW, Hung LCT, et al. Accuracy of endoscopic ultrasonography in diagnosing ascites and predicting peritoneal metastases in gastric cancer patients. *Gut* 2005;54:1541–1545.

44. Tio TL, Schouwink MH, Cikot RJLM, et al. Preoperative TNM classification of gastric carcinoma by endosonography in comparison with the pathological TNM system: a prospective study of 72 cases. *Hepatogastroenterology* 1989;36:51–56.

45. Ribeiro A, Franceschi D, Parra J, et al. Endoscopic ultrasound restaging after neoadjuvant chemotherapy in esophageal cancer. *Am J Gastroenterol* 2006;101:1216–1221.

46. Conlon KC, Karpeh MS. Laparoscopy and laparoscopic ultrasound in the staging of gastric cancer. *Semin Oncol* 1996;23:347–351.

47. Sotiropoulos GC, Kaiser GM, Lang H, et al. Staging laparoscopy in gastric cancer. *Eur J Med Res* 2005;10:88–91.

48. Sarela AI, Lefkowitz R, Brennan MF, et al. Selection of patients with gastric adenocarcinoma for laparoscopic staging. *Am J Surg* 2006;191:134–138.

49. Kole AC, Plukker JT, Nieweg OE, et al. Positron emission tomography for staging oesophageal and gastroesophageal malignancy. *Br J Cancer* 1998;78:521–527.

50. Yeung HW, Macapinlac H, Karpeh M, et al. Accuracy of FDG-PET in gastric cancer. Preliminary experience. *Clin Positron Imaging* 1998;1:213–221.

51. Couper GW, McAteer D, Wallis F, et al. Detection of response to chemotherapy using positron emission tomography in patients with oesophageal and gastric cancer. *Br J Surg* 1998;85:1403–1406.

52. Lerut T, Flamen P, Ectors N, et al. Histopathologic validation of lymph node staging with FDG-PET scan in cancer of the esophagus and gastroesophageal junction: a prospective study based on primary surgery with extensive lymphadenectomy. *Ann Surg* 2000;232:743–752.

53. Chen J, Cheong JH, Yun MJ, et al. Improvement in preoperative staging of gastric adenocarcinoma with positron emission tomography. *Cancer* 2005; 103:2383–2390.

54. Kim SK, Kang KW, Lee JS, et al. Assessment of lymph node metastases using 18F-FDG PET in patients with advanced gastric cancer. *Eur J Nucl Med Mol Imaging* 2006;33:148–155.

55. Koga H, Sasaki M, Kuwabara Y, et al. An analysis of the physiological FDG uptake pattern in the stomach. *Ann Nucl Med* 2003;17: 733.

56. Mukai K, Ishida Y, Okajima K, et al. Usefulness of pre-operative FDG-PET for detection of gastric cancer. *Gastric Cancer* 2006;9:192.

57. Kawamura T, Kusakabe T, Sugino T, et al. Expression of glucose transporter-1 in human gastric carcinoma. *Cancer* 2001;92:634.

58. Stahl A, Ott K, Weber WA, et al. FDG PET imaging of locally advanced gastric carcinomas: correlation with endoscopic and histopathological findings. *Eur J Nucl Med* 2003;30:288.

59. Tsutsumi S, Asao T, Shimura T, et al. A novel rapid colorimetric assay of carcinoembryonic antigen level in the abdominal cavity to detect peritoneal micrometastasis during gastric cancer surgery. *Cancer Lett* 2000;149: 1–5.

60. Cai J, Ideguchi M, Mateo M, et al. Micrometastasis in lymph nodes and microinvasion of the muscularis propria in primary lesions of submucosal gastric cancer. *Surgery* 2000;127:32–39.

61. Kim H, Song A, Park Y, et al. CDX2 expression is increased in gastric cancers with less invasiveness and intestinal mucin phenotype. *Scand J Gastroenterol* 2006;41:880–886.

62. Matsukawa Y, Semba S, Kato H, et al. Expression of the enhancer of zeste homolog 2 is correlated with poor prognosis in human gastric cancer. *Cancer Sci* 2006;97:484–491.

CHAPTER 23 ■ GASTRIC CANCER: CLINICAL MANAGEMENT

DAVID P. KELSEN, CORNELIS J. H. VAN DE VELDE, AND BRUCE D. MINSKY

CLINICAL PRESENTATION: SIGNS AND SYMPTOMS

In the West, the majority of patients with gastric cancer present with symptoms that lead to the diagnosis of malignancy. This means that, for these patients, the disease is almost always at a more advanced stage. The symptoms usually associated with gastric cancer can be relatively nonspecific. They may include anorexia with associated weight loss, fatigue, and mild to moderate epigastric distress. Hematemesis is an uncommon presenting symptom of gastric cancer and occurs in only 10% to 15% of patients (1). The association of abdominal pain with relief by meals that may be caused by an ulcerated lesion is frequently confused with benign peptic ulcer disease. More proximal gastric tumors may cause dysphagia, and more distal tumors may cause gastric outlet obstruction.

Signs on physical examination include ascites, if peritoneal metastases have occurred, or a palpable left upper quadrant mass. Both mean that locally advanced or metastatic cancer is present. Jaundice may occur if obstruction of the biliary tree occurs from portal lymph node metastasis or from extensive hepatic replacement. Occasionally, the first sign of gastric cancer is a metastasis to the ovary (Krukenberg's tumor) or a mass in the pelvis felt on rectal examination (Blumer's shelf). As is the case with other abdominal malignancies, gastric cancer may metastasize to the left supraclavicular lymph node area or occasionally to the left axilla. Metastasis to the periumbilical area (Sister Joseph's nodule) may represent the first sign of gastric cancer at either presentation or recurrence. As is the case with supraclavicular lymph node involvement, tissue diagnosis by needle biopsy can be easily performed in this situation. In summary, the symptoms of gastric cancer are usually vague and nonspecific. Positive signs and findings on physical examination frequently mean that the patient has advanced incurable disease. Unfortunately, in the absence of effective prevention and screening programs, the majority of patients present with more advanced cancer.

Approaches to diagnosis and staging have been described in earlier chapters of this section. In summary, upper endoscopy with biopsy is the preferred technique for establishing tissue diagnosis in patients newly diagnosed with gastric adenocarcinoma limited to the stomach. Evaluation of the extent of the disease should include computed tomography (CT) scans of the abdomen. Pelvic CT scans may reveal ascites or ovarian metastases. CT scans of the chest are appropriate in patients with tumors of the cardia or gastroesophageal junction (GEJ). Endoscopic ultrasonography (EUS) has proven useful in determining depth of invasion (T) but is only modestly accurate in determining nodal metastasis. For patients who do not have clear evidence of metastatic, unresectable disease by physical examination or CT scan, laparoscopy (which can be performed immediately before laparotomy or, in investigational programs, before neoadjuvant therapy) is an accurate test and helps identify patients who have unsuspected intraabdominal metastasis, usually to the peritoneum or liver. The use of positron emission tomography (PET) as part of staging is becoming more widespread (see Chapter 22 and later in this chapter).

SURGICAL MANAGEMENT

In the 19th century, gastric cancer was the most important form of cancer, and many patients died of upper gastrointestinal obstruction. In 1881, Billroth was the first to perform a successful gastric resection. In fact, as he removed several enlarged lymph nodes, he also performed a lymph node dissection (2). The patient died 14 months later of recurrent disease. In 1889, Mikulicz advocated lymph node dissection in addition to gastrectomy, with removal of the pancreas tail if necessary (3). Basic research on lymph drainage was performed in 1900 by Cunéo and in 1907 by Jamieson, who injected coloring agents. Jamieson divided locoregional lymph node groups into 10 stations that show an amazing resemblance to the current Japanese classification (4). Unfortunately, the importance of the work of Cunéo and Jamieson was not recognized at the time.

After reviewing reports on 298 total gastrectomies performed in the early 1900s, Pack and McNeer found a postoperative mortality rate of 37.6% and therefore rejected the use of total gastrectomy (5). From then on, discussion was ongoing about what type of resection should be performed to achieve the best survival with the least morbidity and postoperative mortality. In a review of articles published in English since 1970, the proportion of surgical patients undergoing resection, or the resectability rate, was found to increase from 37% in the series ending before 1970 to 48% in those ending before 1990 (Table 23.1) (6,7). The 5-year survival rate after all resections increased significantly from 21% in the series ending before 1970 to 28% in those ending before 1990, and the 5-year survival rate after curative resection rose from 38% to 55% during the same period (6). Reports from Japanese institutions have shown an even better prognosis; moreover, they have demonstrated that the improvement in 5-year survival has exceeded the decline in incidence, which has resulted in an improved overall cure rate (8). The most important current surgical controversy is the extent of lymphadenectomy, which the Japanese believe to be the most important explanation for the improved outlook for patients with gastric cancer.

TABLE 23.1

HISTORY OF RESECTABILITY, HOSPITAL MORTALITY, AND 5-YEAR SURVIVAL

Period	Resectability (%)	Mortality (%)	5-yr survival (%)
Before 1960	—	25	19.4
Before 1970	37.1	15	38
Before 1980	52.7	13	52
Before 1990	47.7	4.6	55

Data from Macintyre IMC, Akoh JA. Improving survival in gastric cancer. *Br J Surg* 1991;78:771–776; Akoh JA, Macintyre IM. Improving survival in gastric cancer: review of 5-year survival rates in English language publications from 1970. *Br J Surg* 1992;79:293–299.

Surgical Methods

The Japanese Research Society for the Study of Gastric Cancer (JRSGC) has provided guidelines for the standardization of surgical treatment and pathological evaluation of gastric cancer (8). These guidelines are also recommended by the American Joint Committee on Cancer (AJCC) and the International Union Against Cancer (UICC) in their fourth manual for the staging of cancer (9,10). In these guidelines, 16 different lymph node compartments (stations) are identified surrounding the stomach (Fig. 23.1). In general, the perigastric lymph node stations along the lesser (stations 1, 3, and 5) and greater (stations 2, 4, and 6) curvature are grouped N1, whereas the nodes along the left gastric (station 7), common hepatic (station 8), celiac (station 9), and splenic (stations 10 and 11) arteries are grouped N2. Minor modifications to this schedule are made, depending on the location of the tumor. Further lymph node dissections of stations 13 to 16 (N3 and N4) are also described. Lymph node dissection is classified accordingly as D1 to D4. A D1 dissection entails removal of the involved part of the stomach (distal or total), including greater and lesser omentum. The spleen and pancreas tail are resected only when necessitated by tumor invasion. For a D2 dissection, the omental bursa is removed with the front leaf of the transverse mesocolon, and the mentioned vascular pedicles of the stomach are cleared completely. Resection of the spleen and pancreatic tail was initially regarded as necessary to achieve adequate removal of D2 lymph node stations 10 and 11 in proximal tumors, but spleen- and pancreas-preserving lymphadenectomies are becoming more popular.

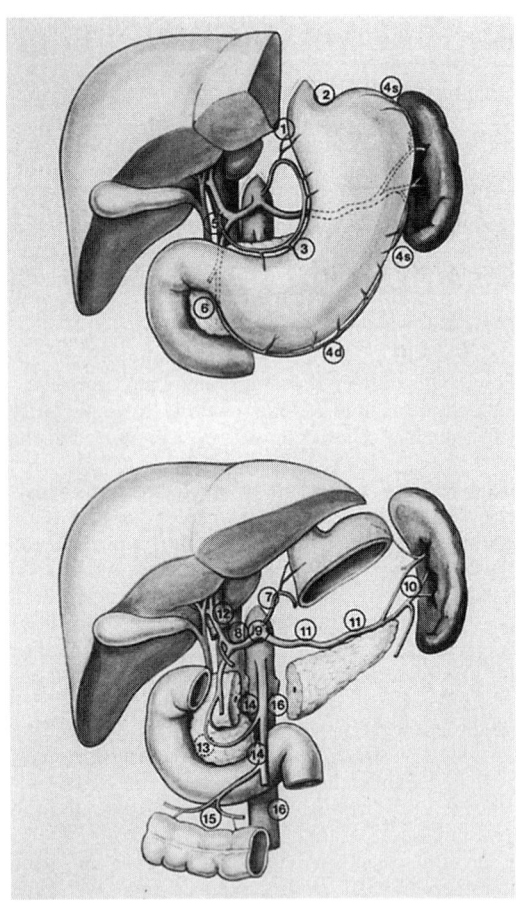

Grouping and location of lymph node stations according to the Japanese Research Society for the Study of Gastric Cancer

Lymph node level	A, AM	M, MA, MC	C, CM	CMA
N1		1	1	1
			2	2
	3	3	3	3
	4	4	4	4
	5	5		5
	6	6		6
	1	2[a]	5	
			6	
	7	7	7	7
N2	8	8	8	8
	9	9	9	9
		10[a]	10	10
		11	11	11
	2			
	10			
N3	11			
	12	12	12	12
	13	13	13	13
	14	14	14	14
N4	15	15	15	15
	16	16	16	16

Anatomical location of lymph node stations:

1. Right paracardial	7. Left gastric artery	13. Retropancreatic
2. Left paracardial	8. Hepatic artery	14. Root of mesentery
3. Lesser curvature	9. Celiac axis	15. Transverse mesocolon
4. Greater curvature	10. Splenic hilus	16. Paraaortic
5. Suprapyloric	11. Splenic artery	
6. Infrapyloric	12. Hepatoduodenal ligament	

FIGURE 23.1. Lymph node locations and grouping. A, distal one-third; C, upper one-third; CMA, entire stomach; M, middle one-third.
[a]Dissection only indicated in case of total gastrectomy.

Furthermore, the stomach can be divided into a proximal, middle, and distal one-third zone. For tumors in the lower two-thirds of the stomach, a subtotal gastrectomy can be performed.

The standard treatment of gastric cancer in the Western world for many years was a total or subtotal gastrectomy, with more or less complete removal of omentum and perigastric lymph nodes (D1 dissection). Hospital mortality, most often defined as death within 30 days postoperatively, has decreased over the years. Before the 1970s, a median mortality rate of 15% was reported, but in the 1980s this rate was decreased to 4.6% (Table 23.1) (7). The 5-year survival in curative resections also improved in these years from 38% before 1970 to 55% in the 1980s (6). A survey by the American College of Surgeons showed a 77.1% resection rate in 18,365 patients, with a postoperative mortality of 7.2% and 5-year survival of 19%. Only 4.7% of these were D2 dissections. Stage-related 5-year survival was 50% for stage I, 29% for stage II, 13% for stage III, and 3% for stage IV (11). Japanese centers report 5-year overall survival rates higher than 50%, as well as higher than 70% for curative resections, whereas hospital mortality is approximately 2% (6,12,13). Japanese national stage-related 5-year survival is reported at 96.6% for stage I disease, 72% for stage II, 44.8% for stage III, and 7.7% for stage IV (12). Differences in surgical techniques may be responsible in part for these better outcomes. In Japan, a total gastrectomy in combination with en bloc resection of adjacent organs, as well as a standard extended lymph node dissection, is performed more often than in Western countries. This aggressive approach is believed by the Japanese to be the main explanation for the difference in stage-specific survival (14–16). Other factors may

contribute, however, such as the lower age of Japanese patients, the lower rates of systemic (e.g., cardiovascular) disease and obesity among gastric cancer patients, earlier diagnosis due to screening programs, stage migration, and the more aggressive chemotherapy policy in Japan. Since the 1990s, D2 dissections have become more popular in Western countries as well. Nonrandomized gastric cancer studies from Germany, England, Norway, and the United States have reported postoperative mortality between 4% and 5%, morbidity between 22% and 30.6%, and 5-year survival between 26.3% and 55% for patients undergoing D2 dissections (Table 23.2) (17–20). The variability in outcomes is substantial, likely because of the different definitions of D2 dissections in most series. Comparison of outcomes with those of patients who had a limited (D1) lymph node dissection (usually in historical comparison) showed better results for D2 dissection, although morbidity rates seemed to be higher. D2 dissection thus appears to improve survival even in Western countries, but results are still not near those reported by the Japanese.

Based on these retrospective data, four randomized studies comparing D1 and D2 dissections have been conducted (Table 23.2). The first was by Dent et al., who described a selected group of only 43 patients (21). In 21 D2 dissections, no hospital mortality was seen, but morbidity, hospital stay, and blood transfusion requirements were significantly higher than for those in the D1 dissection group. No difference in survival was noted between the two groups. A randomized study by McKenzie and Robertson encompassing 55 patients was set up to determine the difference in outcomes between a D1 subtotal gastrectomy with omentectomy (n = 25) and a D3 total

TABLE 23.2

D1 AND D2 GASTRECTOMIES: NONRANDOMIZED AND RANDOMIZED STUDIES

| Study | Period | Setup | D1 | | | | D2 | | |
			No.	Morbidity (%)	Mortality (%)	5-yr survival rate (%)	No.	Morbidity (%)	Mortality (%)
Siewert et al. (17), Germany	1986–1989	MC, Pros	558	29	5.2	51.2	1,096	30.6	5.0
Sue-Ling et al. (18), England	1970–1989	SI, Pros					207	22	5.0
Viste (29), Norway	1980–1990	SI, Retr	78	37	13	30	105	30	4
Wanebo et al. (20), United States	1982–1987	MC, Pros	1,529			30	695		
Dent et al. (21), South Africa	1982–1985	SS, Rand	22	22	0	69	21	43	0
Robertson (22), Hong Kong	1987–1991	SI, Rand	25	0	0	45	30 (D3)	58.6	3.3
Cuschieri et al. (24), Great Britain	1987–1994	MC, Rand	200	28	6.5	35	200	46	13.0
Hartgrink et al. (23), The Netherlands	1989–1993	MC, Rand	380	25	4.0	45	331	43	10.0

MC, multicenter; Pros, prospective study; SI, single institution; Retr, retrospective study; SS, single surgeon; Rand, randomized study.

gastric resection, including pancreatic-splenectomy ($n = 30$) in patients with adenocarcinoma of the gastric antrum (22). Postoperative death occurred in only one patient in the D3 group due to abdominal sepsis. Morbidity was significantly increased for those undergoing extended resections because half of the patients who had D3 dissections developed a subphrenic abscess. Survival was significantly better among patients undergoing a D1 dissection than among those who had a D3 resection. In both studies, no benefit was seen from more extended resections.

Two large randomized multicenter studies comparing D1 and D2 dissections have been published: the Dutch Gastric Cancer Trial (DGCT) (14,23) and the British Medical Research Council Gastric Cancer Surgical Trial (MRC) (24).

Dutch Gastric Cancer Trial

In the Netherlands, 80 hospitals participated in a randomized trial to compare morbidity, hospital mortality, survival, and cumulative relapse risk after D1 or D2 lymph node dissection for gastric cancer. Between 1989 and 1993, 996 patients were centrally randomly assigned to different treatment groups; 711 patients (380 assigned to D1 dissection and 331 to D2 dissection) underwent the allocated treatment with curative intent, and 285 patients required palliative treatment. For definition of D1 and D2 dissection, the guidelines of the JRSGC were used. Because these guidelines were not regularly used in the Netherlands, a Japanese surgeon experienced in the treatment of gastric cancer was invited to instruct the participating Dutch surgeons. Continuous quality control was believed to be necessary to maintain the appropriate level of lymph node dissection. This quality control was substantiated by relating the number and location of lymph nodes detected at pathological examination to the guidelines of the protocol (25). If lymph nodes were harvested from stations that were not supposed to be present according to protocol, this was called contamination. If lymph nodes were not harvested from stations that should have been harvested, this was termed noncompliance. These differences from the study protocol could occur in patients undergoing both D1 and D2 dissection. Contamination in the D1 group and noncompliance in the D2 group, in particular, could lead to decreased distinction between the trial arms.

After curative resection, patients in the D2 arm had higher postoperative mortality (10% vs. 4% for the D1 arm; $P = 0.004$). They also had significantly more complications (43% vs. 25% for the D1 arm; $P <0.001$), which led to significant prolonged hospital stay for patients with a D2 dissection. Hemorrhage (5% for D2 vs. 2% for D1), anastomotic leakage (9% for D2 vs. 4% for D1), and intraabdominal infection (17% for D2 vs. 8% for D1) were the most frequent complications. After curative resection, D2 patients had higher postoperative mortality (10% vs. 4% for D1; $P = 0.004$). They also showed significantly more complications (43% vs. 25% for D1; $P \leq 0.001$) that led to significant prolonged hospitalization for patients after D2 dissection. Hemorrhage (5% vs. 2% for D1), anastomotic leakage (9% vs. 4% for D1), and intraabdominal infection (17% vs. 8% for D1) were the most frequent complications. In the most recent evaluation, the median follow-up for all eligible patients is 11 years (range, 6.8–13.1 years). At 11 years, survival rates are 30% for D1 and 35% for D2 ($P = 0.53$). The risk of relapse is 70% for D1 and 65% for D2 ($P = 0.43$). If hospital deaths are excluded, survival rates are 32% for D1 ($n = 365$) and 39% for D2 ($n = 299$, $P = 0.10$). The relapse risk of these patients ($n = 664$) is in favor of the D2 dissection group ($P = 0.07$).

In a univariate analysis of all 711 patients, no significant impact on survival rates was found for any of the subgroups based on the selected prognostic variables between D1 and D2 dissection. Analysis of interaction between covariate and extent of lymph node dissection shows no significance either. The only subgroup with a trend to benefit is the N2 disease group. If patients with hospital mortality are excluded, there is a significant survival and relapse advantage for patients with N2 disease who had a D2 dissection ($P = 0.01$). Other stages show no significant difference (N0 $P = 0.42$; N1 $P = 0.31$; N3 $P = 0.24$) in this subset analysis. Furthermore, there is no difference in survival after 11 years whether <15 lymph nodes, between 15 and 25 lymph nodes, or >25 lymph nodes are harvested.

British Medical Research Council: Gastric Cancer Surgical Trial

In a prospective randomized trial conducted by the British Medical Research Council, D1 dissection was compared with D2 dissection. Central random assignment of patients to treatment groups followed a staging laparotomy. Of 737 patients with histologically proven gastric adenocarcinoma registered, 337 patients were judged ineligible by staging laparotomy because of advanced disease, and 400 were randomly assigned to treatment (200 to D1 dissection and 200 to D2 dissection). Postoperative mortality was significantly higher in the D2 group (13% vs. 6.5% for D1 dissection; $P = 0.04$). Postoperative complications were also significantly higher in the D2 group (46% vs. 28% for the D1 group; $P <0.001$). In this study, anastomotic leakage (26% for D2 vs. 11% for D1), cardiac complications (8% for D2 vs. 2% for D1), and respiratory complications (8% for D2 vs. 5% for D1) were most frequent. The 5-year survival rates were 35% for patients undergoing D1 dissection and 33% for those having D2 dissection (24).

These major randomized studies, the MRC and the DGCT, obviously show the same tendency. Although the timing of randomization was different in the two trials and no quality control was carried out in the British trial, the postoperative mortality and morbidity rates in both trials were significantly higher in the group undergoing D2 dissection. Furthermore, no 5-year survival advantage was found for extended (D2) dissections in either study. The conclusion from these randomized studies was that generally no support exists for the standard use of extended (D2) lymph node dissections in patients with gastric cancer in the West (14,24).

Is the Debate on Nodal Dissection Solved?

More recently, a randomized trial from Taipei on 221 patients indicated a survival benefit at 5 years from 53.6% to 59.5% as a result of extended lymph node dissection (26). Critical is low mortality rate, which is usually shown in high-volume centers and was also confirmed in a randomized trial on extended lymph node dissection from Japan. The first presentation, however, in 2006 (ASCO abstract LBA 4015) (27) indicated no survival benefit with a mortality of 0.8% in both arms. The Italian Gastric Cancer Study Group showed similar results on postoperative mortality but has not produced long-term survival results (28). Results suggest that D2 gastrectomy with pancreas preservation is safe and acceptable when performed on high-volume centers and that an extensive lymphadenectomy in selected cases may confer a survival benefit.

Surgical Prognostic Factors

Besides the issue of D1 versus D2 dissections, other aspects of gastric surgery have generated controversies. These include type of gastrectomy (subtotal vs. total), pancreatectomy-splenectomy, stage and stage migration, patient selection, and the experience of the surgeon as a prognostic factor.

Total versus Subtotal Gastrectomy

Surgical complications are influenced by the extent of the operation, and a number of studies have addressed this topic. In a Norwegian study, morbidity was significantly lower after subtotal resection (28%) than after total gastrectomy (38%), although in this study proximal gastrectomy had the highest morbidity (52%) (29). In a German study, these differences in morbidity were also found (23% for subtotal resection vs. 48% for total gastrectomy) (30). Gennari et al. found a decreased morbidity for subtotal resections without any significant influence on survival (31). Comparison of their results with those of 15 previous studies led to the conclusion that subtotal gastrectomy should be standard provided that a safe proximal margin is guaranteed. In the DGCT and the MRC, hospital mortality in the groups undergoing D1 dissection and D2 dissection was significantly lower for subtotal gastrectomy (3% and 7%, respectively) than for total gastrectomy (5% and 14%, respectively) (23,32,33). In both trials, the complication rate was also lower after subtotal resections. In the DGCT, this difference was statistically significant. The prognostic value of microscopic resection line involvement in the DGCT was studied by Songun et al. (34). Tumor-positive resection lines were seen in 5.9% of evaluable patients. Resection line involvement was significantly associated with T stage, N stage, tumor location, and tumor differentiation. Presence of resection line involvement was also associated with significantly worse survival. The conclusion from this study was that preoperative frozen-section examination is mandatory in patients undergoing a curative resection for gastric cancer, especially in those with poorly differentiated, signet ring cell, or anaplastic tumors. In this context, arguments can be made for performing a total gastrectomy in all patients with poor tumor differentiation.

Pancreatectomy-Splenectomy

Resection of spleen, pancreas, or both plays an important role in surgical complications. Although one study failed to find significant differences (35), most studies find a significant increase of morbidity and hospital mortality if a pancreaticosplenectomy is performed (19,36,37). Two studies in Japan did not show any beneficial effect on survival if pancreaticosplenectomy was combined with total gastrectomy, whereas morbidity was increased in these patients (35,39). In the DGCT, pancreatectomy and type of gastrectomy were the only factors significantly influencing the occurrence of major surgical complications (37). Although the number of dissected lymph nodes increases, septic complications occur more often due to anastomotic leakage, intraabdominal infections, and pancreatic fistula (39).

Preferably, the spleen should also be spared because this might reduce concomitant morbidity (33,40). An increase of anastomotic leakage was seen, particularly in subtotal D2 gastrectomies. The most likely explanation for this finding is that in D2 dissections, the left gastric artery is divided at its origin and the rest of the stomach is dependent on the blood supply of its short gastric arteries. In D1 dissections, in which the left gastric artery is divided more peripherally, the vascularization of the rest of the stomach is probably less compromised. Immunologic factors may play a role in this as well, associated first with resection of the spleen itself (41,42) and second with the immunosuppression induced by blood transfusions, which may be needed for increased hemorrhage (43–45). A recent randomized trial on splenectomy indicated no advantages in survival as reported by Yu et al. (46).

Cancer Stage

Tumor stage is an important prognostic factor for survival in gastric cancer. Although not all studies find size of the tumor to be an independent prognostic factor for survival (47,48), a clear relation is seen between increasing depth of invasion and survival (15). With increasing depth of invasion, a steady increase is seen in the number of cases with positive lymph nodes, from 45.7% when the tumor invades the muscularis propria to 79.6% when adjacent organs are directly invaded. Also, the frequency with which the more distant tiers of nodes (second, third, and fourth) is involved rises steadily with depth of invasion (49).

The incidence of metastasis and 5-year survival rate shows a strong correlation. Moreover, with increasing distance between involved node and the primary tumor, the proportion of 5-year survivors decreases. Involvement of node station 13 is associated with a zero 5-year survival rate (49). In the DGCT, surgery with an involved N4 node was regarded as a noncurative operation. Benefit from extended dissections (stations 7–12 and 16) in Japanese studies is estimated to be between 0% and 10.5% (49), although as discussed previously, this benefit was not found in randomized studies in the West (14,32). In Japan, dissections even beyond the D2 level are now being studied in two randomized studies, results are not expected before 2008 (50).

Lymph Node Staging Systems and Stage Migration

Recommendations for stage grouping from the JRSGC and from the fourth edition of the AJCC/UICC manual are more or less comparable (8–10). Most studies until now have used these classifications. The fifth edition of the UICC manual, however, classifies N stage by the number of affected regional lymph node metastases and not by the location of the lymph node metastases (51,52). Details of the sixth edition AJCC staging system can be found in Chapter 22. This new staging method has three advantages:

1. The pathologist can stage the cases directly on the resection specimens and is not dependent on the preparation by surgeons or the surgical information on the location of the separately submitted nodes.
2. The problematic assessment of the distance of involved nodes to the edge of the primary tumors is eliminated.
3. The histopathological method can be simplified because the nodes need not be embedded separately for the different node positions.

Hermanek et al. compared this staging system with the previously used systems and found an improvement in estimation of outcome with the new staging system (53). Other studies comparing these staging systems are now underway. Also, the data of the DGCT are being used for evaluation of this new system.

With more accurate staging, a stage migration phenomenon may arise (54). As a result of extended lymphadenectomy, a proportion of patients will be assigned to a more advanced stage than would otherwise be the case, although their prognosis is the same. If this occurs, the overall results for each stage improve, and the proportion of patients in more advanced stages increases. This stage migration is often held responsible for the differences in survival between Japanese and Western patients (52).

In the DGCT, 5-year survival for tumor, node, metastasis (TNM) stage II was 38% after D1 dissection and 43% after D2 dissection. For TNM stage IIIA, 5-year survival was 10% after D1 dissection and 29% after D2 dissection (14). Stage migration occurred in 30% of the patients undergoing D2 dissection. Given the observed 5-year survival rates, we calculated that stage migration leads to a drop in TNM stage-specific survival of 3% for UICC stage I, 8% for stage II, 6% for stage IIIA, and 12% for stage IIIB (55). In a large German study, the disease stages of patients that benefited most in 5-year survival from D2 dissections were stages II and IIIA (stage II: standard dissection 27% and radical dissection 55%; stage IIIA: standard dissection 25.3% and radical dissection 38.4%) (17). The significant or marginally significant differences in survival for patients undergoing D1 and D2 dissections for disease of TNM stages II and IIIA have now shown to be largely attributable to stage migration.

Patient Selection

With the aging of Western society, gastric cancer will be diagnosed in more elderly patients. Population-based data from the Netherlands from 1982 to 1992 show that 27% of newly diagnosed patients were older than 80 (56). A study of gastric cancer in the elderly by Kranenbarg et al. (57) found no difference in resectability and curability rates between different age groups (Table 23.3), but hospital mortality increases with age, especially in those older than 75. Performance of extended (D2) dissections in elderly patients was associated with significantly higher hospital mortality. Multivariate analysis of these data showed that the older than 65 age group had a relative risk of 4.35 for hospital death, compared to patients younger than 65 (33). Also, 5-year survival was found to be significantly better for patients younger than 65. Some investigators do not consider age to be an important prognostic factor (58); however, the present authors believe that, although gastrectomies should not be withheld from elderly patients, extended dissections should be avoided in Western patients older than 70.

Maruyama et al. compiled a computer-based database containing pathological data from 3,040 patients (59). With the knowledge of tumor size, position, and depth of invasion (judged preoperatively by endoscopy and double-contrast barium meal or by endosonography), the likelihood of lymph node metastasis in each of the 16 lymph node stations can be predicted accurately. This enables the correct level of lymph node dissection to be determined. Applicability of this program to Western patients is shown by Peeters et al. (60). A blinded, retrospective analysis of Dutch (D1 vs. D2) trial data suggests that low Maruyama Index (MI) surgery is associated with significantly increased survival. A dose–response effect with respect to the MI and survival is also apparent. We advocate using the Maruyama program, a computerized tool based on patient experience, to identify nodal stations at risk, either preoperatively or intraoperatively, to customize surgical lymphadenectomy and routinely generate a low-MI operation.

Experience and Learning Curves

Gastric resections are performed less frequently, especially because H$_2$ antagonists have reduced the need for them and because the incidence of malignant gastric disease throughout the world has declined. Nevertheless, resection remains the only possible cure for gastric cancer. With the improvement of surgical techniques, postoperative mortality and morbidity have decreased in the past decades, and anesthesia, metabolic care, and nutrition still play important roles. Because extended resections are recommended to increase survival, the question arises as to whether the influence of surgical skill on outcomes has grown (61).

McCulloch et al. retrospectively studied the results of 206 gastrectomies performed by 17 consultant surgeons and showed a considerable variation among surgeons with respect to judgments of resectability, adequacy of resection, anastomotic leakage, and patient mortality (62). Although in this study the number of resections performed by a surgeon had no significant influence, the conclusion was that having fewer surgeons perform all resections might improve outcomes. In the German Gastric Cancer Study, the experience of surgeons was also studied (30). A significantly higher rate of anastomotic leakage occurred when patients were operated on by surgical trainees under supervision than when they were operated on by experienced surgeons (19% vs. 6%, respectively). In the DGCT, all D2 dissections were supervised by referent surgeons, whereas nearly all D1 dissections were attended by the study coordinator. All referent surgeons had at least some experience with D2 dissections before the trial. To standardize the procedure, all referent surgeons were trained by a single Japanese surgeon experienced in this surgery (23). Referent surgeons performed, on average, 41 D2 dissections (range, 23–61) during the trial (Table 23.4) (63). No serious heterogeneity in morbidity and postoperative mortality rates was seen among referent operators, nor between referent surgeons and the Japanese

---

TABLE 23.3

AGE AS A PROGNOSTIC FACTOR IN THE DUTCH GASTRIC CANCER TRIAL OF D1 AND D2 DISSECTIONS

Age (yr)	<65	65–69	70–74	75–79	>80
No. of patients	444	192	166	143	51
Resectability (%)	88	86	84	88	90
Curability (%)	82	80	85	82	78
Dissection (mortality %)					
D1%	50 (0.6)	56 (4.1)	59 (5.7)	49 (8.0)	69 (12.0)
D2%	50 (5.0)	44 (8.6)	41 (12.5)	51 (20.8)	31 (18.2)
Gastrectomy (mortality %)					
Total (%)	35 (3.6)	39 (7.7)	35 (10.4)	34 (30.2)	27 (27.3)
Subtotal (%)	65 (3.5)	61 (8.0)	65 (6.6)	66 (9.6)	76 (11.4)
Overall mortality (%)	3.6	7.9	7.9	16.7	15.2
5-yr Survival (%)[a]	62	44	44	42	22

[a]After curative resection.

TABLE 23.4

COMPLICATIONS AND MORTALITY IN 331 PATIENTS UNDERGOING D2 DISSECTION, GROUPED BY REFERENT SURGEON

Reference No. of surgeon[a]	No. of D2 dissections	Complications	Hospital mortality
1	61	23 (38%)	7 (12%)
2	49	22 (45%)	4 (8%)
3	38	18 (47%)	4 (11%)
4	36	11 (31%)	5 (14%)
5	31	13 (42%)	3 (10%)
6	30	12 (40%)	1 (3%)
7	29	17 (59%)	4 (14%)
8	23	19 (39%)	2 (9%)
M.S.	34	17 (50%)	2 (6%)

M.S., Japanese instructor surgeon.
[a]Surgeons ordered by number of D2 dissections performed.

instructing surgeon in operations on Dutch patients (64). Neither univariate nor multivariate analysis showed a learning curve for the referent surgeons throughout the study (33). In his own experience, McCulloch found that he had to perform at least 30 dissections independently before reaching a plateau (65). In a 3-year prospective study of his own learning curve for D2 gastrectomy, a significant decrease in morbidity and postoperative mortality was shown to occur in the third year, which suggests a learning curve lasting 18 to 24 months, or 15 to 25 procedures, before a plateau is reached. Explanations given for this improvement in outcome, besides operative skill, include better patient selection and performance of less extensive dissections (66). As McCulloch gradually moved away from pancreaticosplenectomy, the idea that only the change of tactics, and not the operative skill, improved outcome during these years is not unthinkable. A plateau may have been reached before or may not yet have been reached. Furthermore, the learning period differs for every surgeon—some are quick learners and some are slow learners. Thus, the number of operations or time needed to reach a plateau for a certain procedure differs for each surgeon. Finally, some surgeons are just better surgeons. In addition, the means of learning may be of influence. Supervision and training very likely lead to quicker and better learning of a certain procedure than "self-tuition."

The experience of the hospital might also influence outcomes for gastric resection. Comparison of results for resections at Japanese ($n = 845$), German ($n = 564$), and Dutch ($n = 50$) hospitals showed a significantly better outcome for Japanese patients. The reasons for these differences between Japanese and Western results have often been discussed (15,18,59). No difference in outcomes was noted between the German hospital and the smaller Dutch hospital. The impact of hospital volume on postoperative mortality was also studied by Begg et al. (67). In this retrospective cohort study of 5,013 patients older than 65, a low hospital volume was shown to be strongly associated with excess mortality. In the German Gastric Cancer Study, 19 hospitals participated and together performed 1,654 resections (range, 12–243). In a multivariate analysis in this study, the experience of the hospitals had a significant influence on morbidity and postoperative mortality (30). These findings are in line with those of McCulloch (62,66).

Surgical Therapy: Summary

Since the first successful gastric resection by Billroth in 1881, substantial research has been performed to evaluate results and improve outcomes of gastrectomy. Fortunately, results have indeed improved. Still, the risk–benefit ratio should be calculated for each patient so the procedure is known to represent optimal treatment. The extent of disease, the operative procedure, and the selection of the patient all play a crucial role in optimizing outcome.

The JRSGC has provided guidelines for the standardization of surgical treatment and pathological evaluation (8). As a result of these guidelines, physicians now speak the same language concerning gastric cancer, and the possibility has been created to compare different studies on this subject. Nevertheless, considerable variation is still seen in results of gastric cancer treatment. Several surgical-, patient-, tumor-, and treatment-related factors may play a role in this variation.

Resectability of gastric cancer has increased in the past decades, not only because of earlier detection but also due to the technical ability to perform extended operations. Pessimism about outcomes may prevail, however, and lead to negative attitudes that may become self-fulfilling. If the surgeon performs palliative procedures because of a belief that gastric cancer is nearly always incurable at presentation, this low expectation will be fulfilled (62). Conversely, inappropriately aggressive surgery in unfit patients may lead to increased postoperative morbidity and postoperative mortality without improving long-term outcome (68).

Tumor stage is an important prognostic factor in gastric cancer. A strong relationship is found between depth of invasion and the occurrence of lymph node metastasis. The occurrence of lymph node metastasis is in itself strongly related to 5-year survival. Because the incidence of lymph node metastasis is known to be greater in the node stations near the tumor than in more distant ones (69), and the distance between tumor and lymph node shows a direct relationship with survival (49), the question remains as to which patients can benefit from an extended lymph node dissection.

In Japan, where extended (D2) dissections are standardized, results from gastric cancer treatment are encouraging. In

Western countries, nonrandomized trials seemed to indicate that survival may be better for patients undergoing a D2 dissection, although the Japanese results could not be matched. As noted previously, two large randomized Western studies, the DGCT and the MRC, have compared D1 and D2 dissections (23,32), and final results are now available (14,24). These studies show that the group undergoing D2 dissection experienced higher morbidity and hospital mortality without showing a significantly longer survival. The conclusion is that these studies do not generally support the standard use of extended (D2) lymph node dissection in Western patients with gastric cancer.

With a mean survival of 45% at 5 years, the results of the Dutch D1 and D2 trials for both treatment arms are far better than the previous experience in Western countries. This indicates the benefit of trial participation with optimal selection, use of surgical techniques, compliance in dissecting the appropriate lymph nodes, and postoperative care throughout the study.

The use of subtotal versus total gastrectomy for tumors in the distal part of the stomach has often been a point of discussion. From previous studies, subtotal gastrectomy appears to carry less morbidity and achieve the same survival rates, provided that an adequate tumorfree margin can be obtained. Resection line involvement should be evaluated perioperatively by frozen-section examination. In all studies, resection of spleen and pancreas led to increased hospital mortality and increased morbidity, which eventually resulted in a decreased survival. Therefore, in Western countries, resection of the pancreas and spleen are recommended only if tumor ingrowth prohibits a possible curative resection.

Age is found to be an important prognostic factor among Western patients. Although the resectability and curability rates do not differ across age groups, both a significant increase in morbidity and mortality and a markedly worse survival rate are seen with increasing age.

The presence of disease in lymph node station 16 (N4) or a positive result on cytologic examination of abdominal fluid is associated with poor prognosis. Consequently, extended resections should be avoided in these situations.

The technical skills of the surgeon may also influence outcomes in gastric surgery. Only in the German Gastric Cancer Study was a significant difference in outcomes found between surgeons with more or less experience, especially with regard to the occurrence of anastomotic leakage. Other trials failed to show a significant difference. Although morbidity in Western countries exceeds that in Japan, no significant difference in morbidity and hospital mortality is found for Japanese surgeons operating on Western patients and for Western surgeons (63). Thus, the difference in results between Japanese and Western studies does not seem to be caused by the skills of the surgeons. Nevertheless, a learning curve for performance of extended resections has been shown by McCulloch (62,66). This may be one of the reasons that more experienced hospitals show a lower morbidity and hospital mortality (70). Other reasons for better results may be better patient selection, a better pathological analysis (stage migration phenomenon), better preoperative staging, and the possibility of (neo)adjuvant chemotherapy. In view of the much lower postoperative mortality rates reported by specialized centers, the treatment of gastric cancer should be the territory of a multidisciplinary team of committed specialists in all areas to achieve optimal results. Preoperative assessment of the lesion and the patient, as well as perioperative management, are as important as the operation itself (33). Promising results from genomic profiling and from nomograms that predict disease-specific survival may, in the near future, help discriminate between patients with a high risk of relapse and select those patients who will most likely benefit from tailored multimodality treatment.

PATTERNS OF SPREAD AND RECURRENCE

Understanding the patterns of spread of gastric cancer can help direct therapeutic approaches, particularly those using systemic or regional (intraperitoneal) chemotherapy and radiation. For malignancies in which locoregional disease alone is the major clinical problem, the use of aggressive surgical resection and radiation (with or without chemotherapeutic sensitization) is a rational approach. However, for tumors such as gastric cancer, especially in the more advanced stages in which the propensity for systemic metastasis is high, surgery alone (or any local modality alone) is unlikely to offer long-term benefit.

The pattern of spread of gastric cancer has been evaluated both in patients with newly diagnosed cancer and in patients undergoing potentially curative surgical resection. Some studies, especially those performed in Japan, have evaluated the lymph node drainage from various portions of the stomach to direct the extent of resection for tumors in relatively early stages. As noted previously, Maruyama et al. extensively studied the incidence of metastasis to different lymph node groups (69). In their study, lymph node metastases were seen in 49% of patients. The likelihood of metastasis was analyzed based on the location of the primary tumor within the stomach (proximal, middle, or distal third) and its location on the lesser or greater curvature and anterior or posterior wall. Not surprisingly, metastases were considerably more likely in lymph node groups closest to the primary tumor and in the nodal chain immediately adjacent. The risk of metastasis to more distant lymph node sites could be predicted using this database. This type of data might direct the extent of resection. Sunderland et al. evaluated lymph node metastasis for proximal versus distal lesions (71). Proximal tumors were much more likely to have lymph node involvement than were distal lesions. The extent of spread within the stomach also varies widely. Tumor invasion of intramural lymphatics may extend into the distal esophagus or the proximal duodenum. As mentioned previously, inadequate resection margins resulting in an R1 resection (with a concomitant high likelihood of local failure) may occur because of lymphatic vessel invasion. Deep penetration of primary lesions may increase the risk of intraperitoneal contamination. Positive findings on cytologic examination of abdominal lavage fluid in gastric cancer are associated with a poor prognosis (72). In the DGCT, cytologic examination was performed for 535 patients, 457 (85%) after curative resection and 78 (15%) after palliative resection. A clear association was seen between positive cytologic findings and serosal invasion (12.4% positive cytologic results) and lymph node invasion (7.5% positive cytologic findings). Survival was significantly lower for those for whom cytologic findings were positive than for those for whom they were negative, irrespective of the procedure used (curative or palliative).

Kodera et al. (73) studied peritoneal fluid obtained during laparotomy in 90 patients with gastric cancer. Carcinoembryonic antigen (CEA) mRNA levels were quantified using real-time reverse transcriptase polymerase chain reaction (RT-PCR). With a median follow-up of approximately 2 years, 13 patients had clinical evidence of peritoneal metastasis. Conventional cytology was relatively insensitive (31%) for detection of peritoneal disease at the time of laparotomy. CEA mRNA accuracy was better (77% sensitive and 94% specific). They concluded that quantitative RT-PCR peritoneal washes for CEA were useful tools to predict intraperitoneal recurrence. Hayes et al. performed a similar study involving 85 patients undergoing operation (74). Peritoneal cytology samples were collected first by laparoscopy, and then again before resection by intraperitoneal lavage and serosal brushings. Preoperative lavage demonstrated malignant cells in 19% of patients, with an additional small group of patients also having positive cytologic findings at laparotomy, found by examination of serosal brushings or imprint cytology. All patients had 13 tumors. As was the case for the previous study, the risk of recurrence was significantly higher in patients in whom free intraperitoneal malignant cells were present. Because peritoneal recurrence is common, these data might influence the design of clinical trials by, for example, supporting the use of intraperitoneal chemotherapy in selected patients.

The type of adjuvant therapy that might be proposed (systemic vs. locoregional) also depends, as noted previously, on recurrence sites after potentially curative (R0) resection. Treatment failure patterns in patients who have undergone resection for primary gastric cancer have been evaluated by autopsy series, second-look laparotomy, and clinical evaluation. In one early study, McNeer et al. reviewed the autopsy results of 92 patients who had undergone potentially curative resections (75). In 50% of patients, local failure was noted, either in the gastric remnant or at the gastroenterostomy. An additional 21% of patients had recurrence in the gastric bed. Thirteen percent of patients had distant failure only without any local component. Wisbeck et al. reviewed the autopsy data for 85 patients with primary gastric cancer (76). Only 16 of these patients had undergone potentially curative resections. For the group as a whole, peritoneal involvement was seen in 47% of patients. Hepatic metastases were also common, occurring in 39% of patients. Lung metastases occurred in 34% of patients.

Of more relevance to patients treated with potentially curative resection, Gunderson and Sosin reviewed failure patterns in patients undergoing second-look laparotomies (77). Not all patients in this group were asymptomatic, however, and other patients with extraabdominal metastatic disease (e.g., to supraclavicular lymph nodes) were probably not explored because distant disease could be proven by other techniques. Nonetheless, this analysis is valuable in that it might demonstrate the earliest sites of failure. Sixty-nine percent of patients had locoregional disease, and, in keeping with other studies, 42% had peritoneal recurrence. A similar high rate of local failure was reported by the British Stomach Cancer Group in patients undergoing operation alone (54%) (78). Landry et al. reviewed failure patterns among a group of 130 patients who had curative resections at the Massachusetts General Hospital from 1969 to 1979 (79). Treatment failure was clinically documented in approximately one-third of patients and pathologically documented in the remainder. Forty-six percent of patients experienced failure in the locoregional area, although distant metastasis was frequently found as well. Only locoregional failure was found in 38% of patients. Slightly more than half of all patients had distant metastasis, either alone or in association with locoregional recurrence. Recurrence was mostly within the abdominal cavity; 30% of patients had liver involvement and 23% peritoneal metastasis. As part of the random assignment DGCT study comparing D1 dissection with D2 dissection, Bonenkamp et al. commented on failure patterns among patients whose disease had recurred. In this large study involving 1,078 patients, death from recurrent disease was noted in a total of 289 patients. Thirty percent of patients had locogional recurrence only, and 51% had locoregional and distant disease (14). In summary, both older and more recent studies indicate that patients with gastric cancer frequently have intraabdominal metastasis, even at the time of diagnosis. The most common sites of intraabdominal distant metastases are hepatic and peritoneal.

ADJUVANT THERAPY

Rationale

As discussed previously, patients with early (AJCC stage 0 or 1A) tumors have a good to excellent prognosis, with cure rates exceeding 70% to 80% after surgery alone, and those with disease of more advanced stage have a far worse outcome. The risk of recurrence after potentially curative resection increases steadily as stage increases, and for patients with locally advanced disease (T3 or T4), performing an R0 resection can be difficult. The pattern of spread and the failure pattern for patients with gastric cancer have been discussed. The high rate of intraabdominal metastasis, especially to the peritoneum, liver, and distant lymph node sites, as well as the lower but still substantial risk of extraabdominal recurrence, makes the use of combined modality therapy an important investigational approach.

Adjuvant therapy is the use of an additional treatment to increase the cure rate in patients who have already undergone a potentially curative resection. In the case of gastric cancer, such therapy follows an R0 surgical procedure in which all gross disease has been removed and no distant metastases are present. Additional treatment for patients undergoing R1 or R2 resections should not be considered adjuvant therapy, but rather treatment of known residual cancer. Neoadjuvant therapy usually means treatment given before the definitive (curative) therapy; in gastric cancer, the term implies preoperative treatment.

In general, postoperative adjuvant therapy should be started as soon after surgery as practical. Several theoretical reasons can be cited for not delaying treatment. Preclinical studies have shown a rapid increase in labeling index of metastasis after resection of the primary tumor. Newer data suggest that this observation may be due to the removal of primary tumor–related factors that in themselves block angiogenesis. Earlier research studies using systemic therapy commonly allowed delays of up to 8 to 12 weeks after surgery before starting treatment. A long delay may allow metastatic disease to grow to the point at which its eradication is much more difficult, if not impossible.

The rationale for neoadjuvant therapy, as opposed to postoperative adjuvant chemotherapy or chemoradiation, is based on the low rate of R0 resections in patients with more advanced tumors and the high likelihood that micrometastatic disease is already present. Preoperative (or primary) chemotherapy is an attractive concept in gastric cancer as a means of decreasing the size of the primary tumor, which results in a higher rate of R0 resections. It also allows a simultaneous and early treatment of micrometastatic disease before surgical intervention.

Adjuvant Postoperative Systemic Therapy

Table 23.5 summarizes the results of selected random assignment trials in which postoperative adjuvant chemotherapy was compared to surgery alone in patients with gastric cancer. The data shown focus on more recent trials with larger numbers of patients. Older data have been extensively discussed in the previous edition this textbook, in other textbooks, and in reviews. As can be seen, the majority of these studies also involved small numbers of patients, and so are seriously underpowered. Even larger trials have only approximately 130 to 160 patients per arm. With rare exceptions, these studies did not show a significant advantage to systemic chemotherapy following surgery versus surgery alone.

The following discussion renews regimens grouped by agent. Almost all studies include fluorouracil.

TABLE 23.5

INTRAVENOUS POSTOPERATIVE ADJUVANT THERAPY FOR GASTRIC CANCER: SELECTED PHASE III TRIALS

Study	Regimen	No. of patients	Median survival (mo)	5-yr survival rate (%)	P value
MacDonald et al. (81)	Control	93	28	NS	
	FAM	83	32	NS	0.52
Tsavaris et al. (84)	Control	42	NS	81	
	FU-epirubicin-mitomycin	42	NS	64	NS
Lise et al. (82)	Control	159	NS	≈43	
	FAM	155	NS	≈43	0.3
Hallissey et al. (83)	Control	145	14.7	20	
	RT 4,500 cGy	153	12.9	12	
	FAM	138	17.3	19	0.14
Coombes et al. (80)	Control	133	36	46	
	FAM	148	36	35	0.17
Krook et al. (85)	Control	61	36	32	
	FA	64	34	33	0.88
Neri et al. (87)	Control	68	18	13	
	FU-leucovorin-epirubicin	69	31	30	0.01
DeVita (88)	Control	116	NS	43	
	ELFE	112	NS	48	0.6
Bajetta et al. (90)	Control	136	NS	48	
	EAP-FU-LV	135	NS	52	0.8

Control, surgery followed by observation; FAM, fluorouracil-doxorubicin-mitomycin; NS, not stated; FU, fluorouracil; RT, radiotherapy; FA, fluorouracil-doxorubicin-hydrochloride; ELFE, epirubicin-leucovorin-fluorouracil-etoposide; EAP, etoposide-doxorubicin-cisplatin; LV, leucovorin.

Regimens Containing Anthracyclines

Both doxorubicin and epirubicin have been used in the adjuvant setting. Several of the combinations also included mitomycin C.

Several trials have used the fluorouracil-doxorubicin-mitomycin (FAM) regimen or a variant. Coombes et al. reported the results of a trial in which patients undergoing curative resection received either FAM or observation only (80). A total of 281 patients were evaluable. Entrance into the trial was allowed as late as 6 weeks postoperation. After a median follow-up of 68 months, 61% of patients in the control arm experienced recurrence versus 56% in the treated arm. No significant difference was seen in either diseasefree or overall survival (overall survival was 45.7% in the FAM arm vs. 35.4% in the observation arm). A trend toward improved outcome was noted for patients with T3 or T4 tumors who had positive lymph nodes ($P = 0.07$ in favor of the FAM group). In a similar study, investigators from the Southwest Oncology Group examined the use of FAM therapy versus expectant observation. Of 193 eligible patients, 100 were randomly assigned to observation and 93 to receive FAM chemotherapy (81). After an overall median follow-up of 9.5 years, no significant differences were found in diseasefree or overall survival (overall survival at 5 years was 37% for the FAM group vs. 32% for the observation group; $P = 0.59$). As was the case in the study by Coombes et al., an unplanned subgroup analysis indicated a trend toward benefit for patients with stage III disease. In a third FAM study, Lise et al. randomly assigned 159 patients to receive surgery only and 155 to receive a modification of the FAM regimen (82). After a median follow-up of 80 months, no significant differences in survival were seen, with approximately 43% of patients in each arm surviving for 5 years.

An improvement was found in diseasefree survival ($P = 0.02$). Hallissey et al. reported the results of a three-arm study in which patients undergoing resection were followed with observation only, received radiation therapy to 45 Gy, or received the FAM regimen. One hundred and forty-five patients were observed; 153 received radiation, and 138 received chemotherapy (83). The FAM regimen was modified from that in the original treatment report. No significant differences in outcome were seen; 5-year survival rates were 20% for the control group, 12% for the group receiving radiation, and 19% for the group receiving FAM chemotherapy.

Tsavaris et al. (84) examined the use of FAM chemotherapy versus observation in a group of 84 patients. Sixty-four percent of patients receiving chemotherapy experienced recurrence or death versus 81% of patients in the control group. For this small group of patients, however, this difference was not statistically significant.

Krook et al. studied 120 evaluable patients who were randomly assigned either to observation or to three cycles of fluorouracil and doxorubicin (85). The median survival was 31 months for patients undergoing observation versus 36 months for patients receiving therapy, and 5-year survival was almost identical for the two groups (33% vs. 32%, respectively). These differences were not statistically significant. Two treatment-related deaths occurred.

Dutch investigators performed a small random assignment trial using the fluorouracil-Adriamycin-methotrexate (FAMTX) regimen (86). Fifty-six patients were entered into this trial, which was closed early because of poor accrual. Four cycles of chemotherapy were given prior to surgery with the control arm undergoing operation alone. The study was initially powered for a total of 225 patients in each arm, with an interim analysis after 100 patients had been studied. The objectives included an improvement in curable resectability rate and disease-free survival. Fifty-six percent of patients in the FAMTX arm had R0 resections versus 62% in the surgery-only arm. There was no significant difference in "downstaging." Toxicity in the FAMTX arm included neutropenia. There was no significant difference in median survival.

Epirubicin has also been used in the adjuvant setting. In a small trial, Neri et al. compared an epirubicin-fluorouracil-leucovorin regimen to expectant observation in a group of 137 patients (87). Chemotherapy was delivered over a 7-month period. The median survival for patients receiving this therapy was 31 months and was superior to survival of those undergoing observation only (18 months) ($P = 0.01$). At 5 years, 30% of patients receiving adjuvant therapy remained alive versus 13% of patients randomly assigned to observation. The results are different from those of the study by Krook et al. (85), who treated a similar number of patients with a similar anthracycline regimen. A confirmatory trial is not yet available.

Recently, the final results of a phase III trial performed by Italian investigators have been reported in abstract form. This study used systemic chemotherapy, including epirubicin, leucovorin, fluorouracil, and etoposide, after operation versus operation alone in patients having at least a D1 lymph node dissection. Two hundred twenty-eight patients were randomized to surgery only or surgery followed by chemotherapy. With a median follow-up of 60 months, 5-year overall survival was 48% for those receiving postoperative chemotherapy and 45% for those undergoing surgery only ($P = 0.6$). There also was no difference in disease-free survival. They concluded that adjuvant therapy using this regimen had a 4% to 5% difference in overall disease-free survival, which was not statistically different between the two arms. Of note, this is the same magnitude of difference reported from meta-analyses (88).

Nitti et al. recently reported the combined experience of two trials using either FAMTX or FEMTX after surgery compared to surgery alone in patients with locally advanced gastric cancer (89). One trial had been performed by EORTC Gastrointestinal Group, and the second was a study by the International Collaborative Cancer Group. In both studies, patients who were undergoing potentially curative operation were randomly assigned to operation alone or to receive either FAMTX or FEMTX. The primary end point was overall survival with secondary end points of toxicity and disease-free survival. A total of 397 patients were randomized; 191 in the ICCG trial and 206 in the EORTC study. With a median follow-up of 6.4 to 6.6 years, there was no difference in overall survival between patients receiving postoperative chemotherapy and those who did not (hazard ratio for overall survival 0.89 in the EORTC trial and 1.05 in the ICCG trial). The 5-year overall survival was 52% in the FAMTX arm and 51% in the surgery only arm. Similarly, in the ICCG trial, the overall survival was 33% in the FEMTX arm and 36% in the surgery-only arm. A pooled analysis also failed to see a significant difference. They concluded that the use of these agents in the postoperative period was not effective in preventing recurrence.

In summary, one trial using an anthracycline has demonstrated benefit, but results of this study have not yet been confirmed. These regimens remain an investigational treatment for patients undergoing curative gastric resections.

Regimens Containing Cisplatin

Cisplatin has become an important agent in the treatment of patients with advanced metastatic gastric cancer. Trials using many regimens combining cisplatin with an anthracycline, a fluorinated pyrimidine, taxanes, or irinotecan to treat patients with recurrent or inoperable stomach cancer have been reported. However, although response rates and, in some studies, survival appear to be improved for patients receiving cisplatin/fluorouracil-containing regimens, only one random assignment postoperative adjuvant trial is currently available in which patients who have undergone a curative resection are randomly assigned to receive cisplatin-containing treatment versus expectant observation. Bajetta et al. reported the results of a random assignment trial using the etoposide-doxorubicin-cisplatin (EAP) regimen, which was followed by fluorouracil and leucovorin (90). Two hundred seventy-four patients were entered into this trial, all of whom had undergone potentially curative resection. One hundred and thirty-five evaluable patients received postoperative chemotherapy, and 136 were followed expectantly. The 5-year overall survival for patients receiving treatment was 52%, while for those in the surgery-only group, 5-year survival was 48% ($P = 0.869$). There were two treatment-related deaths due to sepsis in patients receiving postoperative chemotherapy. Neoadjuvant studies using Cisplatin have been performed; these are discussed later in this chapter.

Meta-analysis of Adjuvant Chemotherapy Trials

Several meta-analyses of adjuvant therapy for gastric cancer have been performed. Hermans et al. reviewed 11 trials that had been reported since 1980 (91). These studies were random assignment trials in which patients who had had resections were randomly assigned to observation alone or one of a variety of chemotherapeutic regimens. Data were available on a total of 2,096 patients. However, these studies did not involve a pooled analysis of individual patient data, but rather reviewed each trial result. The odds ratio was 0.88 (95% confidence limits, 0.78–1.08). Although this trend was in favor of treatment, adjuvant therapy was not significantly superior to observation alone. In a letter to the editor updating their initial report, the authors added two additional trials to their database, which then indicated a slight benefit overall for postoperative adjuvant therapy. Earle and Maroun performed a meta-analysis of 13 trials involving postoperative systemic chemotherapy versus observation (92). As is the case for the review by Hermans et al., individual studies were reviewed, but individual data within those studies were not analyzed. The 13 trials involved a total of 1,990 patients. All studies involved Western (non-Asian) patients. They found an odds ratio of 0.8 (95% confidence limits, 0.66–0.97), which had a borderline statistical significance of 0.02. They noted that the analysis became significant only with the addition of the trial by Neri et al., discussed previously. The relative risk was 0.94 (95% confidence limits, 0.89–1.0) in favor of adjuvant chemotherapy suggesting an absolute risk reduction of approximately 4%.

As is the case for the earlier analysis by Hermans et al., they concluded that using older chemotherapeutic regimens in patients undergoing curative resection yielded a small survival benefit. Hu et al. performed a meta-analysis of postoperative studies using intravenous chemotherapy (93). Both Asian and Western trials were included. Fourteen studies involving a total of 4,543 patients were identified and included in the analysis. As is the case for the two earlier studies, individual patient data were not included in the analysis. Fourteen trials were identified, including the meta-analysis by Hermans et al. Although a benefit to postoperative therapy was suggested, if low-quality trials were excluded (not small number of studies), the odds ratio is almost identical to that found by Hermans and Earle and Maroun (odds ratio, 0.81, 95% confidence interval [CI], 0.70–0.94). They also concluded that the low quality of many of these studies made it impossible to make a definitive conclusion regarding the value of postoperative adjuvant therapy.

Panzini et al. evaluated 17 studies in which chemotherapy was compared to no treatment after radical surgery. Information on 3,118 patients was collected (94). Again, whether individual patient information was included in this analysis is unclear. In their review, chemotherapy was found to reduce the risk of death by 17% (hazard ratio, 0.83; 95% CI, 0.76–0.90). However, they also recommend that adequately powered prospective trials were needed. Their conclusion matches those of the earlier trials.

Mari et al. reviewed randomized trials with a surgery-only controlled arm, which had been published before 2000 (95). Twenty studies were considered for analysis. Three used single-agent chemotherapy, 7 used fluorouracil-anthracycline, and 10 used fluorouracil without anthracycline. A total of 3,658 patients were in the study. Chemotherapy reduced the risk of death by 18% (hazard ratio, 0.82, 95% CI, 0.75–0.89, P <0.001). They concluded that chemotherapy had a small survival benefit when given after surgery. However, this was not an individual patient data analysis; therefore, the authors further concluded that postoperative adjuvant chemotherapy could not routinely be recommended. Overall, the meta-analyses suggest modest benefit, at most, for systemic postoperative adjuvant therapy using these regimens.

Summary of Postoperative Systemic Adjuvant Chemotherapy

The rationale for the use of systemic treatment in patients with resected but high-risk gastric cancers is similar to that used in treating other tumors such as colorectal or breast cancer. In the latter diseases, clear evidence of benefit has been reported in many trials, and the standard of care is the use of postoperative chemotherapy. Compared to the number of patients included in meta-analyses involving other diseases such as breast cancer or colon cancer, the number of patients studied in the gastric cancer review is relatively small. In gastric cancer, however, confirmed random assignment trials using chemotherapy only in which treatment has a significant advantage over observation are not yet available. The meta-analyses have not yet shown convincing evidence of benefit. The individual studies reported to date are seriously handicapped by the small number of patients studied in each trial. A statistically significant benefit could have been demonstrated only if very large differences in outcome were seen. Newer, more effective chemotherapeutic regimens have been developed, and data (discussed later) indicate that postoperative chemoradiation therapy offers an improvement in outcome. The MAGIC study of perioperative (pre- and post-) chemotherapy also demonstrated a significantly improved outcome. As more effective regimens are identified, a high priority should be placed on designing studies with adequate numbers of patients (similar to colorectal and breast cancer trials), which allow appropriate power to assess benefit.

Adjuvant Radiation Therapy

Rationale

As discussed earlier, the incidence of local regional failure increases with deeper penetration of the tumor through the muscle wall and the presence of lymph node metastases. The failure sites documented in the reoperation series of the University of Minnesota, as well as idealized radiation fields covering these failure sites, are shown in Fig. 23.2. The patterns-of-failure data presented suggest that, even in patients in whom a complete resection is performed, local regional failure remains a significant problem.

Results of Treatment

Adjuvant Postoperative Radiation Therapy With or Without Chemotherapy. Three randomized trials of postoperative radiation therapy with or without chemotherapy after a "curative" resection have been performed (Table 23.6). Two of these are small trials. The most recent, the Intergroup 0116 trial, is a large definitive study.

In 1984, Moertel et al. reported the results of a randomized trial at the Mayo Clinic of postoperative radiation (37.5 Gy) plus fluorouracil versus surgery alone (96). Although the report does not state that the margins of resection were negative because the therapy was described as "adjuvant," the assumption will be that patients underwent curative surgery. Although a significant improvement in survival was seen among patients who were in the arm receiving postoperative radiation plus chemotherapy compared with those in the surgery-alone arm (23% vs. 4%), this improvement may have been due to the fact that 10 patients who were randomly assigned to receive the postoperative therapy refused it. The 5-year survival of the 10 patients who refused the treatment was higher than that of the remaining 29 who were randomly assigned to the treatment arm and accepted the treatment (30% vs. 20%). Local regional failure was lower in the patients who received postoperative therapy, however, than in those who were assigned to surgery alone or who refused the postoperative therapy (39% vs. 54%). These data illustrate the problems both with interpretation of studies that allow prerandomization and with small trials with low power.

The second trial involves a subset analysis of a randomized trial by Dent et al. (97). When the analysis is limited to

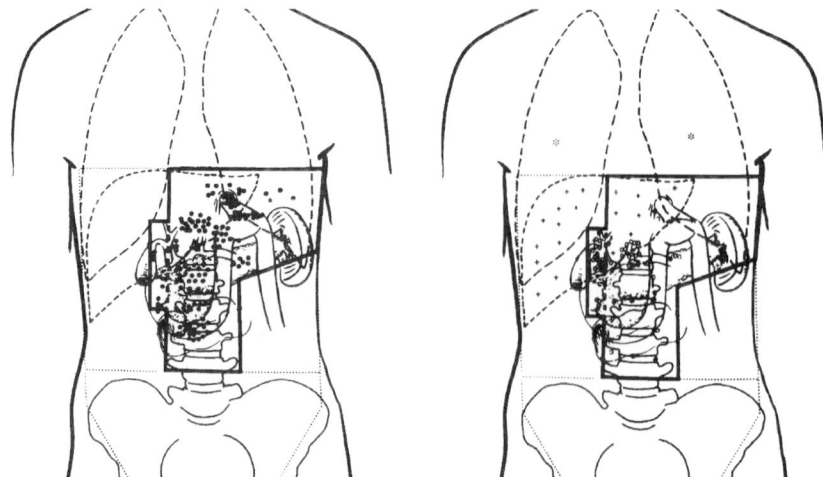

FIGURE 23.2. Patterns of failure observed in 82 evaluable patients in the University of Minnesota reoperation series for gastric cancer. The superimposed radiation fields cover the areas of lymph node drainage, gastric remnant, anastomosis, duodenal stump, and gastric bed structures. (Adapted from Gunderson LL, Sosin H. Adenocarcinoma of the stomach: areas of failure in a re-operation series (second or symptomatic look): clinicopathologic correlation and implications for adjuvant therapy. *Int J Radiat Oncol Biol Phys* 1992;8:1–11.)

TABLE 23.6

EXTERNAL RADIATION THERAPY WITH OR WITHOUT CHEMOTHERAPY FOR GASTRIC CANCER: SELECTED RANDOMIZED TRIALS

Series	Curative resections (%)	No. of patients	Treatment	Survival rate	Local failure (%)
PREOPERATIVE					
Zhang et al. (105)	83	171	Preop 40 Gy	30% 5-yr[a]	33%[a]
		199	Surgery	20% 5-yr[a]	47%
POSTOPERATIVE					
Allum et al. (78);	15	138	Chemo	19% 5-yr	12
Hallissey et al. (83)		153	45–50 Gy	12% 5-yr	8
		245	Surgery	20% 5-yr	22[b]
Dent et al. (97)	43	35	20 Gy+chemo	30% 2-yr	
	48	31	Surgery	40% 2-yr	
			Subset analysis		
	100	15	20 Gy+chemo	38% 2-yr	
	100	15	Surgery	60% 2-yr	
Schein et al. (GITSG	0	45	Chemo	6% 4-yr	
8274) (109)	0	45	50 Gy+chemo	18% 4-yr[b]	
Gastrointestinal Tumor	0	50	Chemo	11% 3-yr	
Study Group (GITSG10932) (110)	0	45	43.2 Gy+chemo	7% 3-yr	
Moertel et al. (96)	0	25	35–40 Gy+chemo	13 mo (mean)[b]	
			Surgery	6 mo (mean)	
	100	23			
	100	39			
			37.5 Gy+chemo	4% 5-yr	
				23% 5-yr	
		29			39
		10	*Subset analysis*		
		33	(Accepted Rx)	20% 5-yr	54
			(Refused Rx)	30% 5-yr	
			Either surgery or refused Rx		
MacDonald et al. (81)	100		45 Gy-FU-LV	36 mo	50% 3-yr
	100		Surgery	27 mo	41% 3-yr

GITSG, Gastrointestinal Tumor Study Group; NA, information not available from report; Rx, treatment consisting of combined chemotherapy + radiation.
[a] "Division I" only (T1 3N1 2M0).
[b] Statistically significant difference.

the 30 patients with local regional disease who underwent a potentially curative resection (division I), postoperative radiation plus chemotherapy is found to have a negative impact on 2-year survival compared with surgery alone. Virtually all other randomized and nonrandomized trials of postoperative radiation therapy alone or in combination with chemotherapy have included patients with residual disease.

MacDonald et al. reported results of the phase III intergroup INT 0116 trial comparing postoperative chemotherapy plus radiation (combined modality therapy) with observation (Fig. 23.3). In this study, 603 patients with stages IB to IIIB disease were registered, 557 of which were eligible (98). Pretreatment characteristics were similar in both arms, and most patients had locally advanced disease (69% had T_{3-4} tumors and 85% had positive local/regional nodes). All patients had undergone an R0 resection. Patients were randomly assigned to observation or to receive chemotherapy followed by combined modality therapy and then additional chemotherapy. Patients receiving postoperative treatment began with fluorouracil 425 mg/m^2 and leucovorin 20 mg/m^2 given daily for 5 days in a row.

One month later, radiation and additional chemotherapy were started. A dose of 45 Gy given in fractions of 180 cGy/day was delivered with fluorouracil 400 mg/m^2 and leucovorin 20 mg/m^2 on days 1 to 4, and then the same doses of 5-FU were given on the last 3 days of radiation. One month after completion of radiation, two additional cycles of fluorouracil

T3 and/or N+ Adenocarcinoma of the Stomach or GE Junction

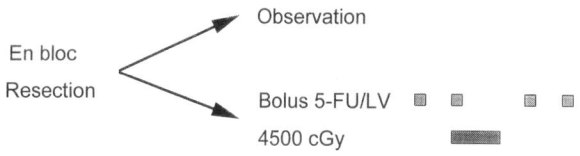

FIGURE 23.3. Treatment structure for Intergroup Gastric Adjuvant Trial 0116. 5-FU, 5-fluorouracil; GE, gastroesophageal; LV, leucovorin calcium.

425 mg/m^2 and leucovorin 20 mg/m^2 were given at once-monthly intervals. Patients were stratified on the basis of T stage and the number of lymph nodes involved. Overall, 65% of patients randomized to combined modality therapy completed treatment.

The most common acute toxicities were hematologic and gastrointestinal, and the incidence of grade 4 toxicity was higher with combined modality therapy (41% vs. 32%). Although 17% could not complete all therapy as planned, there was only one treatment-related death. Importantly, although all patients had an R0 resection, 54% of patients had less than a D1 resection. Only 10% of patients had a D2 resection, and 36% had a D1 resection. Radiation therapy treatment planning was centralized. The investigators noted that 35% of cases required a change in the radiation therapy planning after a pretreatment central review. Furthermore, 7% still had minor or major deviations at final review. This illustrates the difficulty in designing gastric adjuvant radiation fields. As part of an educational effort, Smalley et al. reviewed the gastric anatomy, patterns of failure following surgery, and offer detailed radiation treatment planning recommendations (99).

Patients who received postoperative therapy had a significant improvement in median survival (36 months vs. 27 months, $P = 0.005$) and 3-year overall survival (50% vs. 41%, $P = 0.005$). A subset analysis revealed that the benefit in survival was seen in all stages of disease. Patterns of failure defined as the first site of failure in the treated group versus the observation group revealed a decrease in local failure (19% vs. 29%) and regional failure (65% vs. 72%), but a higher incidence of distant failure (33% vs. 18%).

The results of the INT 0116 trial indicate that, at least among this group of patients in whom surgery was less than optimal, postoperative combined modality therapy had a clinically significant survival benefit. Therefore, it has become a standard option for postoperative adjuvant treatment for patients with stage II, IIIA, and IIIB gastric cancer undergoing resection. However, the number of patients with stage IB disease (36 patients in total, 18 in each arm) was too small to draw firm conclusions regarding the role of postoperative therapy in that subset.

A major criticism of the trial is that because the majority of patients underwent less than a D1 resection, the impact of postoperative combined modality therapy after a D1 or D2 resection is unclear. Although there are no randomized data, a recent large retrospective analysis by Kim et al. from South Korea examines the impact of postoperative adjuvant combined modality therapy after a D2 resection (100). They reviewed 990 patients with stages IIA to IV (non-M1) gastric cancer of whom 544 received postoperative combined modality therapy using the INT 0116 regimen and compared the results to 446 who underwent surgery alone. Patients who received postoperative therapy had a significant improvement in median survival (95 vs. 63 months, $P = 0.02$), 5-year relapsefree survival (55% vs. 48%, $P = 0.0161$), 5-year survival (57% vs. 51%, $P = 0.005$), and a decrease in local recurrence (15% vs. 22%, $P = 0.005$), but no difference in distant recurrence (38%). Grade 3+ toxicity was 30% hematologic and 15% gastrointestinal, and there was only one treatment-related death. Although retrospective, these data suggest that postoperative adjuvant combined modality is appropriate even for patients who undergo a D2 resection. However, randomized data are clearly needed.

New Postoperative Combined Modality Therapy Regimens

The chemotherapy regimen used in the INT 0116 regimen was designed in the 1980s, and advances in systemic chemotherapy have been incorporated in more contemporary chemoradiation regimens. Paclitaxel is both an active agent and a radiosensitizer. Phase II trials from Kollmannsberger et al. combining 45 Gy with continuous infusion 5-FU, leucovorin, and paclitaxel, with or without cisplatin, reveal 2-year progressionfree survival of 61% to 64% with acceptable acute toxicity (101). The RTOG 0114 phase II randomized trial compared 45 Gy plus paclitaxel and cisplatin, with or without 5-FU (102). A total of 78 patients were entered, and the 5-FU—containing arm closed early due to unacceptable grade 3+ acute toxicity. In the 45 patients treated on the non—5-FU—containing arm, the total grade 3+ acute toxicity rate was 71%, the median diseasefree survival was 35 months, and 2-year diseasefree survival was 57%.

The epirubicin-cisplatin-5-FU (ECF) regimen has been successfully combined with postoperative radiation (103,104). A postoperative pilot trial of ECF, followed by 45 Gy plus 5-FU and additional ECF by Fuchs et al. in 21 patients, revealed acceptable (<30%) acute grade 3+ toxicity, which has led to the cancer and leukemia group B (CALGB) 80101 postoperative adjuvant trial. This phase III randomized trial compares combined modality regimens using the ECF regimen with the 5-FU/LV arm from INT 0116 and is actively accruing. Of note, the dose of radiation in this trial is 50.4 Gy compared with 45 Gy in INT 0116.

Adjuvant Preoperative Radiation Therapy With or Without Chemotherapy. In contrast to the experience with postoperative therapy, a randomized trial of preoperative radiation therapy by Zhang et al. revealed a significant improvement in survival (105). A total of 370 patients younger than age 65 with adenocarcinoma of the gastric cardia who had clinically resectable disease based on endoscopy and CT criteria were randomly assigned to preoperative radiation (40 Gy in 20 fractions) followed by surgery 2 to 4 weeks later or to surgery alone. After a median follow-up of 123 to 128 months for the total patient group, a significant improvement in survival was found among those receiving preoperative radiation (30% vs. 20%; $P = 0.0094$). The subset of 311 patients who underwent surgery also had a survival benefit with preoperative radiation, although it did not reach statistical significance (33% vs. 25%, $P = 0.15$). Use of preoperative radiation increased the R0 resection rate (80% vs. 62%; $P < 0.001$) without increasing the postoperative morbidity or mortality. The cumulative incidence of local failure and regional lymph node failure was lower in patients who received preoperative radiation than in those who received surgery alone (33% vs. 47% for local failure and 31% vs. 55% for regional failure). No difference in distant failure was noted (24% for the radiation group vs. 25% for the surgery-only group). These data suggest that preoperative radiation improves local control and survival. However, randomized trials are needed to confirm the results in Western patients.

Given the positive results of combined modality therapy in INT 0116, there is increasing interest in preoperative regimens. The potential advantages include more accurate identification of the tumor volume at the time of radiation simulation, and, in contrast with postoperative treatment where the gastric pull-up is in the radiation field, the radiated stomach is removed. Allal et al. reported a phase I trial of preoperative hyperfractionated radiation plus 5-FU, leucovorin, and cisplatin (106). A total of 19 patients with cT3-4 or N+ gastric cancers were treated and 5-year survival was 35%. There was no increase in the operative risk compared with their prior experience of surgery alone. The RTOG 99-04 trial included 43 patients with cT2-3, many of whom were M0 by laparoscopy and received induction 5-FU, leucovorin, and cisplatin, followed by 45 Gy plus 5-FU and paclitaxel preoperatively (107). The pathological CR rate was 27%, and 77% underwent a R0 resection.

Radiation Therapy After "Noncurative" Surgery

The use of postoperative combined modality therapy in gastric cancer was reported in 1969 by Moertel et al. (108). After laparotomy, patients with advanced gastric cancers were randomly assigned to receive 40 Gy of radiation or 40 Gy of radiation plus fluorouracil as a radiation sensitizer. As seen in Table 23.6, a significant improvement in survival was seen in patients receiving the combination of radiation plus fluorouracil.

The remaining randomized trials listed in Table 23.6 also included patients with unresectable or residual disease. None of the trials has delivered adequate doses of radiation to control residual disease. In general, after a complete resection with negative margins, a dose of 45 to 50 Gy is recommended. Patients with residual disease require at least 55 to 65 Gy, a dose that exceeds the tolerance of the stomach and small intestines.

In a study by Allum et al. of the British Stomach Cancer Group, the interim report revealed a significantly lower rate of local recurrence in patients who received postoperative radiation therapy than in those who received surgery alone (8% vs. 22%) (78). In the final report with a 5-year minimum follow-up, however, no improvement in survival was seen (83). In this trial, the chemotherapy was not delivered concurrently with the radiation therapy.

The Gastrointestinal Tumor Study Group (GITSG) conducted two consecutive trials comparing radiation therapy plus chemotherapy with radiation therapy alone in patients with locally unresectable gastric cancer. In the first GITSG study, reported by Schein et al., almost 25% of patients who received radiation plus chemotherapy either died or deteriorated clinically within the first 10 weeks of treatment (109). With further follow-up, however, a significant improvement was seen in 4-year survival for those receiving combined therapy (18%) compared with those receiving chemotherapy alone (6%).

Due to the high incidence of early morbidity and mortality in this trial, the GITSG designed a replacement trial in which the combined modality treatment was modified. Modifications included delivery of chemotherapy before administration of combined modality therapy, the addition of doxorubicin, a rigorous review of surgical entry criteria, and delivery of radiation therapy in a continuous rather than a split course (110). Patients were randomly assigned to receive postoperative chemotherapy alone (fluorouracil, methyl CCNU, and doxorubicin) or combined radiation plus chemotherapy. The incidence of grade 3+ toxicity varied from 52% to 59%. In contrast with the results of the initial GITSG trial, combined modality therapy in this modified GITSG trial did not improve survival.

In summary, randomized trials comparing postoperative combined modality therapy with surgery alone or with postoperative chemotherapy in patients with locally unresectable disease have generated conflicting data. The conflicting results may be explained, in part, by the use of suboptimal doses of chemotherapy and radiation as well as the selection of patients with unresectable disease for whom the prognosis is poor.

Intraoperative Radiation Therapy

An alternative method of delivering radiation therapy is intraoperative radiation therapy (IORT). The theoretical advantage of this approach is the ability to deliver a more intensive dose of radiation to the tumor bed while excluding the surrounding normal tissues from the high-dose field. The results of selected trials of electron beam IORT (with or without external beam radiotherapy) are given in Table 23.7. The trials by Sindelar and Kinsella (111), Takahashi and Abe (112), and Abe et al. (113)

are randomized phase III trials. The limited data suggest that IORT may be beneficial in selected patients with gastric cancer. The optimal method by which to combine it with surgery and external beam radiation has yet to be determined. The use of IORT in gastric cancer, although encouraging, remains investigational.

Palliative Radiation Therapy

In the palliative setting, radiation therapy provides relief of symptoms such as bleeding, obstruction, and pain in the majority of patients (114). Patients who have favorable prognostic factors such as high performance status and microscopic rather than gross residual disease, as well as those who received fluorouracil-based chemotherapy, tend to have a higher response rate. Overall, the median duration of palliation is 4 to 18 months (114–116). Rhomberg et al. treated 28 patients with gross unresectable disease (23 patients) or with positive margins after an R1 resection (5 patients) with a median of 50 Gy of radiation plus the radiosensitizer razoxane (117). The partial response rate was 89%, local control was achieved in 64%, and rapid pain relief was achieved in 96%.

Recommendations

In summary, the INT 0116 trial revealed that postoperative combined modality therapy is an appropriate option in patients with stage II, IIIA, and IIIB disease, especially those undergoing less than a D1 lymph node dissection. Almost all the other series examining the role of postoperative radiation therapy in gastric cancer included patients who had microscopic or gross residual disease, which makes the data difficult to interpret.

One trial of preoperative radiation conducted in China revealed a significant improvement in local control and survival; however, its results need to be confirmed in Western patients. Preoperative combined modality therapy regimens are promising and need to be examined in phase III trials.

In the setting of locally unresectable or residual disease, postoperative combined modality therapy may decrease local failure and improve survival. Although it is a reasonable approach, it is still not the standard of care at this time. In those patients who are selected to receive radiation therapy, it should be combined with adequate doses of chemotherapy. IORT, although promising, remains investigational. In the palliative setting, radiation therapy offers symptomatic relief to the majority of patients.

Technical Aspects of Radiation Simulation and Treatment. The design and delivery of radiation therapy for gastric cancer requires knowledge of the natural history of the disease, patterns of failure, anatomy, and radiobiological principles. The dose-limiting organs primarily include the kidneys and liver with other sensitive organs, such as the small bowel, spinal cord, bone marrow, and gastric stump (118).

For most abdominal and pelvic malignancies, a multiple-field technique allows a larger volume of small bowel to be excluded from the radiation field than an anteroposterior/posteroanterior (AP/PA) technique. For gastric cancer, however, due to the location of the target volume and the proximity of adjacent organs (especially the kidneys and liver), a multiple-field technique may not always be advantageous. Leong et al. compared dose to the kidneys and liver using three-dimensional (3-D) conformal plans with AP/PA techniques (119). There was no comparison to a four-field technique. In the 15 patients, the mean doses to one-third of the kidney with 3-D conformal versus AP/PA was left (18 Gy vs. 40 Gy) and right (18 Gy vs. 35 Gy). There was little difference

TABLE 23.7

INTRAOPERATIVE RADIATION THERAPY WITH OR WITHOUT POSTOPERATIVE EXTERNAL BEAM RADIATION THERAPY FOR GASTRIC CANCER: SELECTED SERIES

Series	No. of patients	Intraoperative radiation (Gy)	External beam (Gy)	Chemotherapy	Severe complications	Survival rate (%)				Local failure
						Stage	No.	IORT	5-yr	
Takahashi and Abe (112); Abe et al. (113)	110	28–35	None	No	NA	I	24	Yes	87	
							43	No	93	
						II	20	Yes	84	
							11	No	62	
						III	30	Yes	62	
							38	No	37	
						IV	27	Yes	15	
							18	No	0	
Ogata (200)	58	28–30	None	No	NA	II	11	Yes	100	
							38	No	63	
						III	13	Yes	80	
							34	No	60	
						IV	34	Yes	12	
							48	No	13	
Sindelar and Kinsella (111)	10	20	None	No	40%	Median: 21 mo				Mean 21 mo[a] to local failure
Coquard et al. (201)	63	12–23 (median, 15)	44–46	Yes	5% postop death	I	17	Yes	82	0
						II	11	Yes	55	30
						IIIA	9	Yes	78	22
						IIIB	20	Yes	20	35
						IV	6	Yes	0	60
						Total	63	Yes	47	25
Calvo et al. (202)	48	15	40–46	Yes	13% GI 13% Bone 19% Bowel	39% with maxim follow-up of 71 mo				None for primary cancers without residual disease
Avizonis et al. (203)	27	12.5–16.5	45 (in 23 patients)	No	15% postoperative 14% long term	Median: 19 mo 2-y disease free: 27% 2-y overall: 47%				15% as the only site 37% as a component

IORT, intraoperative radiation therapy; NA, not available; GI, gastrointestinal.
[a]Versus 8 mo with 50 Gy external beam radiation ($p = 0.02$).

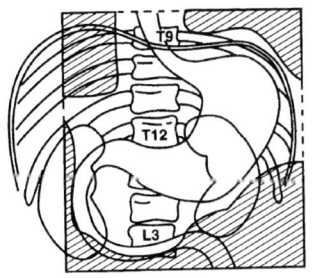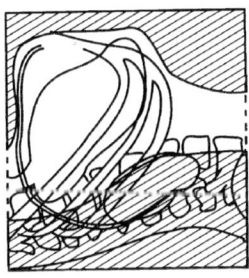

FIGURE 23.4. Idealized treatment fields for gastric cancer. In this example, a four-field technique is used.

in doses to two-thirds of the kidneys. However, the 3-D conformal techniques increased rather than decreased the dose to the liver.

If the dose delivered is 45 Gy, use of the AP/PA technique with high-energy photons may offer the best compromise between decreasing the small bowel volume in the radiation field and limiting the dose to the adjacent organs. However, if 50.4 Gy becomes the new standard based on the CALGB trial, multiple field techniques will be mandatory.

CT-based treatment planning using dose volume histograms are essential to determine if an AP/PA or a multiple field technique should be used. In general, if the dose to a given volume of an organ exceeds its functional tolerance, then a slightly higher dose to that volume is recommended to limit the dose to the remaining portion of the organ. For example, if 20% of the kidney receives 30 Gy, that 20% will not function. Therefore, delivering 45 Gy to that 20% will not further decrease function, whereas it may allow the delivery of a tolerable dose (<20 Gy) to the remaining 80% of the kidney. With this approach, the largest volume of the organ receives the smallest dose and thereby maintains function. The exception to this approach is the spinal cord, for which the dose should be <50 Gy. An example of the use of a four-field technique is shown in Fig. 23.4.

Verheij et al. compared the dose received by the kidneys from intensity modulated radiation therapy (IMRT) versus AP/PA (120). A total of 58 patients received 45 Gy AP/PA, and for comparison, the dose was recalculated using an IMRT plan. Although IMRT reduced the left kidney dose at least 50%, it did not change the right kidney dose. They also examined renal function by renography, and at 6 months, there was a 20% decrease in left renal function.

Adjuvant Postoperative Intraperitoneal Chemotherapy. The use of postoperative intraperitoneal chemotherapy, either alone or with systemic chemotherapy, is based on the high risk of peritoneal recurrence as a component for first failure in patients undergoing R0 resections. As discussed previously, a large percentage of patients develop clinically evident peritoneal carcinomatosis, either alone or with other sites of metastasis. A strong pharmacokinetic rationale exists for the use of intraperitoneal treatment. Drug concentrations obtained within the peritoneal cavity after intraperitoneal administration are from severalfold to up to 2 log units higher than drug concentrations achievable using the oral or intravenous route. Clinical trials involving other diseases in which peritoneal failure is a frequent component of recurrence, such as ovarian cancer, have demonstrated a small but statistical and clinically significant advantage to women receiving a portion of their treatment intraperitoneally. Several models have demonstrated the effectiveness of intraperitoneal treatment, both in destroying peritoneal metastasis and in decreasing the frequency of liver metastasis. Archer and Grey, using a rat model, demonstrated that intraperitoneal chemotherapy decreased the incidence of peritoneal and liver metastasis (121). Murthy et al. used a

mouse model to show that the frequency of metastatic disease in the peritoneal cavity was dependent on surgical trauma and on the type of incision made (122). Other studies confirmed the high rate of peritoneal implantation in animals undergoing laparotomy (123). Thus, preclinical models, pharmacokinetic analysis, and clinical evidence from random assignment trials in ovarian cancer support the use in gastric cancer of an approach maximizing the effectiveness of currently available antineoplastic agents by using intraperitoneal treatment as part of adjuvant therapy.

Although increasing numbers of reports have been published in which immediate postoperative intraperitoneal therapy was given to patients with gastric cancer, the applicability of these data in a noninvestigational setting is hampered by flaws in the design of these studies. Some are retrospective. Many prospective trials are pilot, phase II trials in which small numbers of patients were treated to test feasibility and safety. Although several phase III trials have been reported, these generally involve only small numbers of patients and are thus severely underpowered. At this point, no definitive conclusions can be drawn regarding the effectiveness of intraperitoneal chemotherapy in gastric cancer patients.

With these caveats, selected reports are described in which intraperitoneal chemotherapy was given as adjuvant therapy in the postoperative period. Several themes have begun to emerge. First, most studies administer intraperitoneal treatment, using either heated chemotherapy solutions (continuous hyperthermic peritoneal perfusion [CHPP]) or nonhyperthermic therapy, after resection of all gross disease. Thus, initial intraperitoneal chemotherapy is given either in the operating or recovery room, or within several days after resection. Particularly for therapy given postoperatively, after closure of the abdomen, an intraperitoneal catheter may be placed to allow delivery of repeated courses of treatment. Currently, no random assignment studies have been performed to compare the use of single doses given in the operating or recovery room, and multiple doses delivered over several weeks via catheter. The theoretical advantage of the former is better drug distribution, whereas the advantage of the latter is the ability to deliver repeated courses. Note that in ovarian cancer, the phase III studies demonstrating benefit used intraperitoneal catheters with therapy started up to weeks after surgery; CHPP was not used. Because both techniques have also been used in patients who have established peritoneal carcinomatosis (in which the primary tumor has been removed, but the patient had stage IV disease at presentation), drawing definitive conclusions is even more difficult. Most studies have used either a fluorinated pyrimidine such as fluorouracil or floxuridine with or without mitomycin C. Several trials have included cisplatin.

Regimens Containing Mitomycin C

The use of mitomycin C (Table 23.8), alone or in combination with other agents, for the adjuvant treatment of resected gastric cancer has been fairly extensively studied. Most of these trials, however, have included relatively small groups of patients. Hagiwara et al. reported a marked improvement in survival for patients with locally advanced gastric cancer who received mitomycin absorbed to a carbon-containing solution given immediately at the end of the operative procedure (124). In their study, 49 patients were randomly assigned either to receive mitomycin C (24 patients) or to undergo observation alone (25 patients). Both 2- and 3-year survival rates were highly significantly improved in patients receiving intraperitoneal therapy (2-year survival 68.6% vs. 26.9% for patients not receiving intraperitoneal therapy). This study with positive results was followed by several subsequent trials. Retrospective reviews and phase II studies using mitomycin C in

TABLE 23.8

INTRAPERITONEAL THERAPY FOR GASTRIC CANCER: SELECTED PHASE III TRIALS

Study	Regimen	No. of patients	Median survival	2-Year survival rate (%)	p Value
Hagiwara et al. (124)	Mitomycin C	24	>3 yr	69	.01
	Control	25	1.2 yr	27	
Rosen et al. (127)	Mitomycin C	46	738 days	NS	.44
	Control	45	515 days	NS	
Schiessel et al. (131)	Cisplatin	31	15 mo	38	NS
	Control	33	12 mo	36	
Sautner et al. (132)	Cisplatin	33	17	33	.6
	Control	34	16	30	
Yu (130)	Mitomycin-FU	125	NS	38.7[a]	.2
	Control	123	NS	29.3[a]	

NS, not stated.
[a] 5-year survival
Adapted from Karpeh M, Kelsen D, Tepper J. Gastric cancer. In: Devita VT Jr, Hellman S, Rosenberg SA, eds. *Principles and practice of oncology.* Philadelphia: Lippincott Williams & Wilkins, 2001, with permission.

similar doses (with or without absorption to charcoal) noted an increase in toxicity with an associated increase in operative mortality (125,126). As a result, Rosen et al. conducted a confirmatory random assignment trial in which patients either received carbon-absorbed mitomycin C 50 mg postoperatively or were followed with observation only (127). Ninety-one patients were entered into this study. The trial was closed early when an interim analysis revealed a marked increase in postoperative complications in the group receiving mitomycin (25% vs. 16%) and, more important, a marked increase in perioperative mortality for this group: 11% of the patients receiving intraperitoneal therapy died in the immediate postoperative period versus 2% of patients in the control group. Furthermore, no survival advantage was seen for patients receiving mitomycin. More recently, Hall et al. (128) reported a single institution review using operation, postoperative CHPP plus mitomycin C. Thirty-four patients received intraperitoneal therapy, and 40 patients treated during the same period (but not in a random assignment trial) underwent operation alone. There was no difference in median survival for patients undergoing operation alone versus those receiving intraperitoneal therapy. It should be noted that many of the patients receiving intraperitoneal therapy had gross residual disease.

Regimens Containing Fluorinated Pyrimidines

Several phase II trials have used fluorouracil or floxuridine, usually in combination with leucovorin and other agents such as cisplatin. Some of these trials also include low-dose mitomycin in addition to fluorouracil.

In single-institution studies, cisplatin and fluorouracil or cisplatin and floxuridine were used. In one trial reported by Atiq et al., 35 patients received intraperitoneal cisplatin and intraperitoneal fluorouracil. Concurrent systemic intravenous fluorouracil was given (129). At a median follow-up of 2 years, 51% of patients were alive without evidence of recurrence. Although toxicity was in general acceptable, sclerosing encapsulating peritonitis was noted in 15% of patients. This was believed to be due to the high pH of fluorouracil-containing solutions and the fact that fluorouracil and cisplatin were combined

in the same solution before administration. When the drugs were given sequentially from separate containers, no further episodes of sclerosing encapsulating peritonitis were noted. In a trial reported by Crookes et al., postoperative intraperitoneal therapy followed neoadjuvant chemotherapy. Again, no significant toxicities were noted, and no increase was seen in operative morbidity or mortality (85). The preliminary survival data were encouraging (see Neoadjuvant Chemotherapy section).

Yu reported the results of a phase III trial comparing intraperitoneal fluorouracil and mitomycin with expectant observation (130). This study enrolled patients with both early and advanced gastric cancers, including patients with stage IV disease. As is the case with other trials involving mitomycin, morbidity and mortality were higher among the group of patients receiving postoperative intraperitoneal chemotherapy (5.6% vs. 0.8%). No difference was seen in overall survival (38.7% vs. 29.3%; P = 0.219), although a subset analysis did show benefit for patients with stage II or III disease.

The use of cisplatin with or without systemic thiosulfate has been studied in patients with both resected and residual disease. Schiessel et al. administered intraperitoneal cisplatin 90 mg/m² with systemic thiosulfate, starting treatment within 4 weeks of surgery (131). Although toxicity was acceptable, no survival advantage was found for those receiving intraperitoneal therapy compared with those followed with observation only. In a similar trial, Sautner et al. administered cisplatin 90 mg/m² once a month intraperitoneally (132). Thiosulfate was not used. This study also included patients with stage IV residual disease. Again, no significant difference in outcome was seen between patients receiving intraperitoneal therapy and those followed expectantly.

Hyperthermic intraperitoneal therapy (CHPP) involves the use of heated solutions of chemotherapeutic agents. As is the case for studies using chemotherapy without hyperthermia, the pharmacokinetic advantages have been well described. Hyperthermia is used because of the possible synergistic cytotoxicity with heated chemotherapeutic solutions. Many of these studies have been reported by investigators in Asia, particularly Japan. In most earlier trials, patients had visible peritoneal involvement, and such therapy could not be considered adjuvant. Mitomycin C, fluorinated pyrimidines, and cisplatin were the most common agents used. In a random assignment phase III trial, Koga et al. studied 47 patients with serosal invasion (133). They found a substantial but not significant improvement in 3-year survival for patients receiving hyperthermic intraperitoneal therapy compared with those followed expectantly. Toxicity, primarily anastomotic leak or postoperative ileus, was increased in patients receiving CHPP. Fujimura et al. compared CHPP to unheated intraperitoneal chemotherapy and to surgery alone in patients with locally advanced gastric cancers (134). Chemotherapeutic agents were cisplatin and mitomycin. Although survival with chemotherapy using either intraperitoneal approach was better than survival with observation only, the number of patients in each group was very small. Hamazoe et al. compared CHPP with expectant observation in a group of 82 patients (135). No significant differences in outcome were found.

Yu reviewed the results of postoperative adjuvant therapy, in general, as well as intraperitoneal chemotherapy (130). He updated the results of the study in which patients were randomly assigned to receive 5 days of intraperitoneal mitomycin C and fluorouracil via catheter placed at the time of operation or operation alone. At 5 years, 40% of patients undergoing operation alone were alive versus 67% of those receiving postoperative intraperitoneal chemotherapy ($P = 0.008$). Xu et al. performed a meta-analysis of intraperitoneal therapy for gastric cancer (136). They included 11 trials involving 1,161 patients. Independent patient data were not included in this analysis. The studies involved trials in which patients were randomly assigned to receive intraperitoneal therapy after operation or undergo operation alone. The majority of the studies used mitomycin C; most trials were performed in Asia, and most were quite small (<100 patients per arm). A total of 552 patients underwent operation alone, and 609 patients operation followed by chemotherapy (odds ratio, 0.51; 95% CI, 0.4–0.65). They concluded that the meta-analysis suggested benefit to postoperative intraperitoneal chemotherapy, but only a few of the studies were believed to be high-quality trials. They suggested that larger, more rigorously designed trials would be necessary before definitive conclusions could be reached.

In summary, intraperitoneal chemotherapy with or without hyperthermia is a rational experimental strategy to pursue until more highly effective systemic agents can be developed. In addition to offering an improvement in survival, intraperitoneal chemotherapy serves the important palliative goal of preventing abdominal carcinomatosis and recurrent bowel obstruction. The data available now demonstrate fairly clearly that certain agents, particularly high-dose mitomycin C, do increase the risks of operative morbidity and mortality. Fluorinated pyrimidines and cisplatin-containing treatments appear to be better tolerated. Newer, more active systemic agents such as the taxanes are only now beginning intraperitoneal trials. As is the case for all postoperative adjuvant studies, large-scale adequately powered trials are needed to definitively test the hypothesis that intraperitoneal therapy offers an improvement in outcome.

IMMUNOCHEMOTHERAPY

Asian investigators have studied the use of immunostimulants and systemic treatment as preventative therapy after resection of primary gastric cancer. These studies used either a protein-bound polysaccharide (PSK) or a *Streptococcus pyogenes* preparation, OK432. PSK is extracted from *Coriolus versicolor*. Phase III trials have been performed using both agents; however, in a number of studies, the control arm received chemotherapy. Only a few studies included an observation-only arm.

Nakazato et al. studied 262 patients receiving mitomycin C intravenously and oral fluorouracil or an identical chemotherapy regimen plus PSK (137). Patients who were eligible for this study were immunocompetent as indicated by positive results on a purified protein derivative (tuberculin) test. Ten cycles of chemotherapy were given. The experimental group received 36 months of PSK treatment. After a minimum follow-up of 5 years, a significant advantage was seen for patients receiving immunochemotherapy: 70.7% for those receiving PSK plus chemotherapy versus 59.4% for those receiving chemotherapy alone. In a similar study, Ochiai compared chemotherapy using mitomycin, fluorouracil, and Ara-C with the same treatment plus an immunostimulant of *Nocardia* Rubra cell wall skeleton extract (138). Treatment was begun on the day of surgery. Ninety patients received chemotherapy, and 97 patients received immunochemotherapy. No survival advantage was found for patients receiving immunochemotherapy who had undergone curative resection. In an unplanned subgroup analysis involving 71 patients who had had noncurative resections, a survival advantage was seen for those receiving immunochemotherapy.

Mitomycin, fluorouracil, and Ara-C chemotherapy plus OK432 were given to 74 patients in a Korean study; a control group of 64 patients underwent operation and observation (139). At 5-year follow-up, a survival advantage was seen for patients receiving immunochemotherapy (44.6% vs. 23.4% for those not receiving immunochemotherapy). In a second trial, some patients were randomly assigned to receive immunotherapy with OK432 plus mitomycin and fluorouracil, a second group received mitomycin and fluorouracil alone, and control patients were followed expectantly after operation (140). Again, a survival advantage was seen for immunochemotherapy compared with either chemotherapy alone or observation (45.3% of those receiving immunochemotherapy, 29.8% of those given chemotherapy, and 24.4% of patients receiving surgery alone were alive at 5 years). Kim et al. used the FAM chemotherapy regimen with or without OK432 (141). In this trial, 50 patients received chemotherapy alone, and 49 were given immunochemotherapy. The immunochemotherapy group had superior survival (62% vs. 52%; $P = 0.04$). Sakamoto et al. (142) performed a meta-analysis involving six trials in which patients received chemotherapy alone or chemotherapy plus OK-432. The analysis was of the overall study data rather than individual patient data. In these six trials, 765 patients received chemotherapy alone and 757 patients had received chemotherapy plus OK-432. The 3-year overall survival curves, based on the published data from trials, showed a 3-year survival of 67.5% for patients receiving OK-432 and 62.6% for those in the controlled group. The authors noted that in three of the six trials, published results were used for their calculations. In three unpublished studies, individual patient data were used. In a comment on this trial, Panzini et al. (94) noted the nephrologic difficulties in interpreting these data and concluded that larger-scale prospective trials would be needed (142). In summary, data from Asian investigators suggest that immunochemotherapy is superior to chemotherapy alone and perhaps to observation alone in patients undergoing potentially curative resection. As is the case in Western trials, however, the number of patients in any given study was quite small and the power of the trials relatively weak. Before accepting immunotherapy as a standard part of adjuvant therapy, larger-scale confirmatory trials are necessary.

THERAPY WITH OTHER AGENTS

H₂ Blockers

Anecdotal evidence suggested that the use of ranitidine or cimetidine may decrease the risk of recurrence in patients undergoing resection of primary gastric cancer. Therefore, Primrose et al. performed a random assignment, double-blind, placebo-controlled trial of ranitidine 150 mg twice daily versus placebo (143). Therapy was given for up to 5 years. No chemotherapy was used. Patients with all stages of disease, including stage IV, were allowed entrance into this study. In this trial, which included only 87 patients total (41 patients receiving treatment vs. 46 receiving placebo), no difference was seen in survival. A trend was noted toward benefit in patients with stage IV disease. A second study with a similar design used cimetidine (144). Again, no evidence of benefit was noted. Thus, to date, therapy using H$_2$ blockers has not shown benefit in preventing recurrence.

Tamoxifen

On the basis of data showing that estrogen receptor protein was expressed in a variety of tumors, Harrison et al. studied 100 patients who were given tamoxifen as postoperative therapy (145). This study included patients who had residual gross disease and is thus not truly a test of adjuvant therapy. Fifty-five percent of patients had estrogen receptor–positive tumors; however, no survival benefit was seen for the patients receiving tamoxifen. The control group had a slightly better outcome than did those receiving hormonal therapy.

NEOADJUVANT CHEMOTHERAPY

The rationale for giving systemic treatment prior to operation is based on several factors. The first is that many Western patients with newly diagnosed gastric cancer are found to have locally advanced tumors (T3 or T4 or lymph node–positive tumors); patients with such deeply penetrating primary tumors are frequently found to have extensive disease, making performance of an R0 resection difficult. In addition, particularly for patients with lymph node involvement, the risk of distant disease is high. Adopting a strategy of systemic therapy prior to operation thus has two goals: downstage the primary tumor to increase the likelihood that R0 resection can be performed, and begin an early assault on micrometastatic disease. Last, many patients have long postoperative recovery periods or may never receive postoperative systemic therapy. Preoperative therapy is given when the patient is most likely to tolerate it. The ultimate aim is to increase the cure rate.

Many pilot phase II trials using preoperative (neoadjuvant) had been reported. In general, these phase II studies have been designed to assess the efficacy of preoperative chemotherapy when measured as potential downstaging, as well as to demonstrate tolerance to such therapy in the patient population being studied. This includes an increase in anticipated surgical morbidity or mortality. Evaluating efficacy when measured as objective tumor regression for patients with primary gastric cancer is difficult. Endoscopy, barium contrast studies, CT, and EUS have all been employed. None have been demonstrated to be validated surrogates. Kelsen et al. and others have compared EUS to pathological stage in assessing TNM stage in patients receiving preoperative chemotherapy (146). After preoperative chemotherapy, EUS performed immediately prior to operation was found to be relatively inaccurate, particularly in separating T2 from T3 tumors and in measuring overall lymph node status. The conclusion of the studies was that EUS, although accurate in assessing the T stage in patients who have not received prior therapy, is not reliable in patients who have received systemic treatment. Most recently, serial PET scans have been studied to evaluate response to therapy. Ott et al. studied 44 patients with locally advanced gastric cancer (147). This study suggested that PET scanning could differentiate between patients who would receive benefit from preoperative therapy and those who would not. Several other trials have now been reported in complete or abstract form for patients with esophageal and gastric tumor, suggesting that PET scan performed soon after initiation of chemotherapy might be able to distinguish between those who are obtaining benefit and those who are not, including an improvement in survival for those receiving chemotherapy followed by operation who were "PET responders" versus "PET nonresponders" (148). Of issue in gastric cancer is that approximately one-fifth to one-fourth of patients will not have an informative PET scan, presumably because tumor cells lack or have an inefficient glucose transport. One of the rationales in looking for a predictive marker to guide therapy is the development of systemic regimens that may lack cross-resistance. In theory, an early assessment by PET scanning will allow patients who are nonresponders to go directly to surgery, while chemotherapy would be continued in patients who are obtaining benefit. Alternatively, patients not responding to initial chemotherapy might cross over to receive a non–cross-resistant regimen. Such studies are in the design stage but have not yet been reported.

Kang et al. performed a small random assignment trial using cisplatin, etoposide, and fluorouracil, or operation alone. There was no difference in 5-year survival (149).

Recently, the final results of a large, adequately powered prospective random assignment control trial of perioperative chemotherapy versus operation alone have been reported (Table 23.9). Cunningham et al. studied the ECF regimen in patients (see combination chemotherapy on page 307) with operable adenocarcinoma of the stomach, GEJ, or lower esophagus, compared with patients undergoing operation alone (150). Five

TABLE 23.9

NEOADJUVANT THERAPY FOR LOCALLY ADVANCED GASTRIC CANCER: PHASE III TRIALS

Study	Regimen	No. of patients	Operable	Resectable	Median survival (mo)	2-yr survival rate (%)	5-yr survival rate (%)
Kang et al. (182)	Cisplatin-etoposide-FU	53	89%	71%	33	55	
		54	100%	61%	32	55	
	Surgery alone						
Cunningham et al. (150) (MAGIC Trial)	ECF	250	88%	69%	NS	50	36
	Surgery alone	253	95%	66%	NS	41	23

FU, fluorouracil; ECF, epirubicin-cisplatin-fluorouracil; NS, not stated.

hundred and three patients were randomized to pre- and post-operative ECF chemotherapy or to surgery alone; 74% had gastric cancers, 11% GEJ tumors, and 15% lower esophageal adenocarcinomas. With a median follow-up of 4 years, the group receiving pre- and postoperative ECF had a hazard ratio for survival of 0.75 (95% CI, 0.6–0.9, $P = 0.009$) when compared with those undergoing surgery alone. The 5-year survival rates for patients receiving chemotherapy was 36%, while for surgery it was 23%. Progressionfree survival was also significantly prolonged. Toxicity was tolerable, with no apparent increase in operative morbidity and mortality. They concluded that preoperative ECF chemotherapy significantly improved resectability rate, as well as progressionfree and overall survival in patients with operable gastric and lower esophageal junction tumors. This important trial is the first study to demonstrate an advantage to systemic therapy plus operation over operation alone.

Summary for Neoadjuvant Chemotherapy

In summary, the promising results of the MAGIC trial have demonstrated that systemic chemotherapy using moderately effective regimens when given before surgery, as well as when possible postoperatively, improves survival when compared to surgery alone. Newer chemotherapy regimens, which may be more effective than ECF, are now undergoing their initial trials. The combination of the results of the MAGIC trial and the postoperative intragroup 116 trial strongly suggest the role of multimodality therapy in the treatment of patients with gastric cancer. Whether all therapies should be given prior to operation or whether there is a role for chemotherapy first followed by surgery and postoperative radiation remains to be demonstrated.

TREATMENT OF ADVANCED GASTRIC CANCER

Noncurative Treatment

Palliative Surgery

Due to better preoperative staging, the proportion of all patients with gastric cancer who undergo surgery decreased from 92% before 1970 to 71% in 1990. Resectability of gastric cancer has increased in the past years, from 37% before 1970 to 48% in 1990. This is due mainly to earlier diagnosis of gastric cancer but is also a result of the performance of extended operations and improved patient selection. Nevertheless, only 31% of all patients undergo a curative resection (6). Whether patients benefit from a palliative resection remains a point of discussion. In most studies of palliative treatment, resection is associated with prolongation of survival and alleviates complaints such as pain, anemia, and intolerance of food intake (151–154). Although D2 and D3 dissections are sometimes performed for palliation in Japan, this is very uncommon in the West (155). In the DGCT, 29% of the randomly assigned patients were found have noncurable disease at laparotomy. A wide variation of tumor load was found in these patients, ranging from extensive local growth to lymph node metastasis beyond the D2 level, hepatic metastasis, peritoneal metastasis, and combinations of these. Extensive local growth was found in 150 patients, 103 patients had metastases at two sites, and 32 had metastases at more than two sites. Median survival was 253 days after palliative resection compared to 169 days after a nonresective procedure ($P = 0.002$). This survival advantage for patients undergoing resection disappeared when

two or more signs of noncurability were found. Morbidity was significantly higher and hospital stay significantly longer in the resection group (55).

Studies of palliative surgical treatment are always limited by the inability to confirm the results in randomized trials; therefore, conclusions must be regarded cautiously. For the group of patients requiring palliation in general, the data mentioned earlier confirm that a resection can on occasion be beneficial, especially for those patients with limited tumor load restricted to one metastatic site. Palliative surgery may be beneficial in patients with persistent signs of gastric obstruction or bleeding, particularly when palliative chemotherapy cannot be used due to poor nutritional intake.

Palliative Systemic Chemotherapy

Chemotherapy for Gastric Cancer. Because many patients with gastric cancer present with locally advanced primary tumors or with clinically evident metastatic disease, there is a pressing need to develop more effective systemic treatments. In addition, agents that are effective in palliation may improve outcome in patients with potentially curable disease. Many different chemotherapy agents have been tested in patients with advanced gastric cancer; to date, all of these have only modest activity, at most, when used as single agents. Since the early 21st century, new classes of agents have been studied. Several have been identified as having activity, and newer targeted therapies have entered clinical trial. This section summarizes the data for the use of systemic chemotherapy in palliation. The first edition of this textbook, as well as several other textbooks and reviews, have an extensive discussion of older agents. This section focuses on newer agents, standard of care recommendations, and some major research initiatives.

Chemotherapy versus Best Supportive Care. Wagner et al. reported the results of a review of random assignment trials in gastric cancer for the Cochrane Collaboration (156). They performed a meta-analysis for chemotherapy versus best supportive care, single-agent chemotherapy versus combination chemotherapy, and a variety of combination chemotherapy studies.

For chemotherapy versus best supportive care, a total of 184 patients from three random assignment trials were evaluated (Table 23.10). Overall survival was superior for patients receiving chemotherapy compared to best supportive care as initial treatment with an overall hazard ratio of 0.39 (95% CI, 0.28–0.52). The overall improvement in median survival was 4.3 months for best supportive care to 11 months for chemotherapy. They concluded that there was convincing evidence for chemotherapy as an initial approach compared to best supportive care. Time to progression (TTP) to chemotherapy was approximately 7 months for patients receiving chemotherapy and approximately 2.5 months for patients receiving best supportive care. Quality of life was not formally analyzed in any of the three studies included in the Cochrane evaluation. Among studies evaluating the potential advantage of immediate initiation of systemic chemotherapy versus best supportive care, Glimelius et al. allowed a crossover to chemotherapy when requested by patients assigned to the best supportive care arm (157). This study was excluded from the Cochrane analysis because of this factor. However, of interest, quality of life was assessed in this trial. The average quality-adjusted survival for patients receiving chemotherapy was superior to that of patients initially assigned to best supportive care (median of 6 months vs. 2 months). In all chemotherapy versus best supportive care trials, the only patients who had longer-term survival (≤ 24 months) were patients receiving chemotherapy. A 2-year survival rate of 5% to 14% for patients receiving combination chemotherapy has been confirmed by other authors.

TABLE 23.10

CHEMOTHERAPY FOR ADVANCED GASTRIC CANCER: TREATMENT VERSUS BEST SUPPORTIVE CARE

| Regimen | No. of patients | Median survival (mo) | Survival rate (%) | |
			1-yr	2-yr
FAMTX	30	10	40	6
BSC	10	3	10	0
FEMTX	17	12	NS	NS
BSC	19	3	NS	NS
ELF	10	10	NS	NS
BSC	8	4	NS	NS

FAMTX, fluorouracil-doxorubicin-methotrexate sodium; BSC, best supportive care; FEMTX, fluorouracil-epirubicin-methotrexate sodium; ELF, epirubicin-leucovorin-fluorouracil; NS, not specified.
Adapted from Wils J. The treatment of advance gastric cancer. *Semin Oncol* 1996;23:397–406.

Single-Agent Chemotherapy

For the large majority of single agents, a variety of doses and schedules have been employed. Because these are not comparative trials, there is no clear evidence that one schedule is markedly superior to another.

A substantial number of single agents has been studied in gastric cancer from all or most of the major classes of cytotoxic drugs. Shown in Table 23.11 is a summary of important agents that are currently considered for use in the treatment of patients with gastric cancer. Agents that had been studied in the period before the year 2000 and that have little activity are not included Table 23.11. These data may be found in the first edition of this textbook, in other textbooks, and in reviews. For some of the agents shown, some data come from trials performed in the 1960s, 1970s, and early 1980s. These early studies used criteria for response that were much more liberal than those currently employed. As a result, the reported response rates for a number of drugs are almost certainly substantially overestimated.

Among the antimetabolites, fluorinated pyrimidines have been the most extensively studied. 5-FU has been used in a variety of different schedules and doses. Earlier studies used rapid bolus injections given either weekly or daily for 5 days in a row. Cycles were repeated every 3 to 4 weeks. More recently, fluorouracil has been given as a prolonged intravenous infusion. Data from the 1990s involve fluorouracil as a single agent, when used as one of the arms of random assignment trials. This aggregate data indicate an overall response rate of 10% to 20%, with a median duration of response or TTP of 2 to 4 months (158–161). The major toxicities of fluorouracil include mucositis, diarrhea, and myelosuppression. Several oral fluorinated pyrimidines have also been studied. These included UFT, S1, and capecitabine. These agents have attracted considerable attention in the treatment of gastrointestinal malignancies in general. Capecitabine, for example, has undergone extensive study in colorectal cancer, and in that disease is a standard of care palliative option. It is also used in the adjuvant setting for colon cancer for those patients who might be treated with fluorouracil leucovorin therapy alone. Data for gastric cancer are also shown in Table 23.10. Capecitabine has now been extensively studied in combination regimens. S1 is an oral fluoropyrimidine. When used as a single agent, response rates range from 26% to 45% in patients with advanced gastric cancer (162,163). In one study in European patients, a dose of 40 mg/m^2 twice daily was found to be too toxic. Among 22 evaluable patients, 6 responded for an overall response rate of 26.1%. The median TTP was 140 days, and the median duration survival was not reported. In several studies reported in Japan, a higher response rate of 44% to 54% was reported. S1 has been combined with other agents, including cisplatin.

UFT is a combination of ftorafur and uracil. This oral fluorinated pyrimidine has been extensively used in Japan for a variety of malignancies, including gastric cancer. When used as a single agent, responses of 27.7% have been seen among gastric cancer patients in Japanese reports (164). More recently, on behalf the EORTC, Ravaud et al. reported the results of a phase II trial using UFT and leucovorin in previously untreated patients with gastric cancer (165). UFT was given at 300 mg/m^2

TABLE 23.11

ACTIVITY OF SELECTED SINGLE AGENTS IN ADVANCED GASTRIC CANCER

Drug	Response rate (%)
FLUORINATED PYRIMIDINES	
5-Fluorouracil	21
UFT	28
S1	49
Capecitabine	26
ANTIBIOTICS	
Doxorubicin hydrochloride	17
Epirubicin hydrochloride	19
HEAVY METALS	
Cisplatin	19
TAXANES	
Paclitaxel	17
Docetaxel	19
CAMPTOTHECINS	
Irinotecan hydrochloride	23

for 28 days on and 7 days off. Twenty-three patients were considered evaluable for response. A 16% response rate was seen among 23 evaluable patients.

Cisplatin remains an important part of combination chemotherapy. Single-agent data dates primarily from the 1980s. The major objective response rate is approximately 15%, including previously treated patients. The major toxicities of cisplatin include nephrotoxicity, ototoxicity, and peripheral neuropathy. Nausea and vomiting has been considerably ameliorated with the use of newer antiemetics. Carboplatin has been less well studied but appears to have less activity than cisplatin.

More recently, oxaliplatin, a diamino cyclohexane, which is a standard agent in the treatment of colorectal cancer, has been studied as part of combination chemotherapy in gastric cancer. As is the case for colon cancer, it is most frequently combined with fluorouracil. Data for the FOLFOX regimen are reviewed later in this chapter.

The taxanes, paclitaxel and docetaxel, have also been studied as single agents in gastric cancer. Docetaxel is probably the most extensively studied taxane in gastric cancer. Cosimo et al. reviewed phase II trials in which docetaxel was given as a single agent to previously treated or previously untreated patients (166). They identified 262 patients who were evaluable for response. The average response rate was 19.1%. In most of the trials, docetaxel was given at 100 mg/m^2 on an every 3-week basis. Toxicity was that expected from docetaxel as seen in other diseases, primary neutropenia, alopecia, and fluid retention. Allergic reactions were seen in approximately one-fourth of patients. When reported, the median TTP was 6 months.

Docetaxel has been recently approved by the U.S. Food and Drug Administration (FDA) for treatment of patients with advanced gastric cancer when given in combination with fluorouracil and cisplatin (see combination chemotherapy). Paclitaxel has also been studied and has similar activity.

The camptothecin irinotecan has been fairly extensively studied in gastric cancer in the late 1990s (167). A response rate of 15% to 25% was seen in both previously treated and untreated patients. The major toxicities were myelosuppression and diarrhea. The anthracyclines also have activity in gastric cancers. Again, as is the case for earlier studies with fluorouracil, much of these data date from the 1960s and 1970s. Doxorubicin has a major objective response rate of 17%, and epirubicin, while widely used in combination therapy, has been studied in smaller groups of patients. An aggregate response rate of 19% has been noted.

Wagner et al. also evaluated the difference in overall survival for patients receiving single-agent therapy versus those receiving combination chemotherapy (156). Here, the hazard ratio of 0.85 (0.75–0.96) favored combination chemotherapy in providing a statistically significant survival benefit when compared to an initial treatment with single agents. The average survival for patients receiving combination chemotherapy was 7 months versus slightly less than 6 months for patients receiving single agents. They included secondary analyses to evaluate the effect of second-line therapy and to explore possible differences between Asian and non-Asian patients as possible causes of heterogeneity. Again, combination chemotherapy was favored with an overall hazard ratio of 0.79 (range, 0.69–0.91). TTP favored combination versus single-agent chemotherapy (hazard ratio, 0.62). Toxicity was higher in the combination chemotherapy arms but not usually statistically significant. Treatment-related mortality was 2.1% for patients receiving combination chemotherapy versus 0.9% for patients receiving single-agent therapy with fluorouracil.

Of interest from the point of view of the ECF regimen, they also evaluated the role of anthracycline chemotherapy as a portion of combination chemotherapy versus nonanthracycline-containing combinations. Three studies were included in their analysis with a total of 501 patients. The analysis indicated an advantage in overall survival for fluorouracil-cisplatin-anthracycline combinations when compared to fluorouracil-cisplatin alone (hazard ratio, 0.77–0.62–0.95). Similarly, studies including cisplatin-fluorouracil-anthracycline (vs. fluorouracil-anthracycline alone) also demonstrated a modest improvement in outcome (hazard ratio for overall survival, 0.83–0.76–0.91).

It is important to note that this recent Cochrane review did not evaluate newer agents including taxanes or irinotecan.

In summary, several single agents have modest activity in gastric cancer. Response rates range from 10% to 25%, with relatively short durations of response. Fluorouracil, cisplatin, docetaxel and paclitaxel, doxorubicin and epirubicin, and irinotecan are the major components of conventional regimens. Oxaliplatin and capecitabine are also now being used in combination therapy.

Combination Chemotherapy

Multidrug regimens combining agents that have demonstrated single-agent activity have been extensively studied in gastric cancer over the past several decades. As is the case for other malignancies, the assumption is that combinations of single agents that have different mechanisms of action and different toxicity spectrums will increase efficacy. This section concentrates on data from random assignment phase III trials. For more recent combinations, only phase II data are available. This is indicated where appropriate.

Cisplatin-Fluorouracil. Shown in Table 23.12 are data from recent random assignment trials in which the combination of cisplatin and fluorouracil (CF) was the control arm of one of the control arms. These studies have been reported since the year 2000; several have been reported to date in abstract form only. As can be seen, the doses of cisplatin delivered in all four trials are 100 mg/m^2/course; three studies gave cisplatin on day 1 only. The dose of fluorouracil is 1,000 mg/m^2/day as a continuous 24-hour infusion from days 1 to 5 in three of the four studies, with a slightly lower dose in a Japanese trial. Cycles are repeated on an every 28-day basis. The trials are moderately sized with between 100 and 224 patients per arm.

Response rates, progressionfree survival, and overall survival are consistent across the four trials. Responses were seen in-between one-fifth and one-third of patients, with the two most recent trials reporting approximately one-fourth of patients having major objective regression. Complete remissions are rare.

Van Hoefer et al. reported the final results of an EORTC study in patients with advanced gastric cancer (168). CF was compared to methotrexate, fluorouracil, and doxorubicin (FAMTX), with a third arm of etoposide, leucovorin, and fluorouracil. One hundred and thirty-four patients received CF with a dosing schedule as shown in Table 23.13. Efficacy was assessed as objective regression, progressionfree, and overall survival. In this study, no significant differences in outcome were seen in any of the three arms.

A Japan Clinical Oncology Group study (JCO 9205) compared fluorouracil alone versus CF versus ftorafur/tegafur plus mitomycin. CF was not superior to fluorouracil alone in their study (169). The TAX325 trial compared docetaxel plus CF alone and is described in more detail later (170). In this study, an advantage was seen to the TCF arm.

Last, irinotecan-fluorouracil was compared to CF by Dank et al. (171). The CF arm data are shown in Table 23.13. This trial is also discussed in more detail later in this section. In summary, CF is still widely used in the treatment of advanced metastatic or locally unresected gastric cancer. The recent random assignment studies described previously used almost identical doses and schedules. The aggregate of these trials indicates

TABLE 23.12

COMBINATION CHEMOTHERAPY IN ADVANCED GASTRIC CANCER:
CISPLATIN-FLUOROURACIL—CONTAINING REGIMENS USED AS THE CONTROL
ARM IN RANDOM ASSIGNMENT TRIALS

Study	Drug	Dose (mg/MI)	Schedule (d)	No. of Patients	RR (%)	Median TTP/PFS (mo)	Median survival (mo)	2-yr survival
EORTC (204)	C	100	1	127	20%	4.1	7.2	~10%
	F	1,000	1–5					
JCOG (158)	C	20	1–5	105	36%	3.9	7.3	7%
	F	800	1–5					
DANK (171)	C	100	1	163	26%	4.2	8.7	~10%
	F	1,000	1–5					
TAX325 (170)	C	100	1	224	25%	3.7	8.6	9%
	F	1,000	1–5					
REAL-2 (180)	E	50	1	289	41%	6.2	9.9	~15%
	C	60	1					
	F	200	Daily					

MI, Maruyama Index; TTP, time to progression; PFS, progression free survival; C, cisplatin; F, fluorouracil; E, epirubicin.

that the response rate for CF is approximately 25%, median progressionfree survival is about 4 months, and median overall survival is approximately 8.5 months. Two-year survival is 8% to 10%. Two-year survival in the TAX325 and irinotecan-fluorouracil-leucovorin (IF) versus CF study was 15% to 20% for the TCF and IF arms and 15% to 20% for ECF. Thus, at least some patients with advanced gastric cancer may have longer survival using multidrug chemotherapeutic regimens, including docetaxel or irinotecan. In the TCF study, the 2-year survival for CF was 9%.

Toxicity with CF, although tolerable in most patients, can be severe. In the EORTC trial reported by Vanhoefer et al., grade 3 to 4 neutropenia was seen in 35% of patients, and approximately one-fourth of patients had grade 3 to 4 nausea or vomiting. In the more recent TAX325 trial, grade 3 to 4 treatment-related adverse events occurred in 75% of patients receiving CF. The development of better antiemetic therapy, such as aprepitant, should decrease the incidence of severe nausea and vomiting; the use of cytokine supports may decrease the incidence of neutropenic fever. Nonetheless, the CF regimen is associated with substantial toxicity.

Docetaxel, Cisplatin, and Fluorouracil. Ajani et al. reported the results of a random assignment trial comparing the three-drug combination of docetaxel-cisplatin-fluorouracil (DCF) to a regimen of CF alone (TAX325) (170). In this trial, previously untreated patients with metastatic gastric cancer were randomly assigned to receive DCF using the regimen shown in Table 23.13 or CF. The study, reported in abstract

TABLE 23.13

DOSAGE SCHEDULES OF SELECTED TREATMENT REGIMENS FOR
GASTRIC CANCER

Drug	Dose (mg/m^2)	Day(s)	Week(s)
Cisplatin-FU			
Cisplatin	100	1	Every 4 wk
5-Fluorouracil	1,000	1–5 CI	
DCF			
Docetaxel	75	1	Every 3 wk
Cisplatin	75	1	
Fluorouracil	750	1–5 CI	
IF			
Irinotecan	80	1	Weekly for 6 wk
Fluorouracil	2,000	1 CI	
Leucovorin	500	1	
mFOLFOX-6			
Fluorouracil	2,600	1–2 CI	Every 2 wk
Leucovorin	200	1	
Oxaliplatin	85	1	

FU, fluorouracil; CI, continuous infusion; DCF, docetaxel-cisplatin-fluorouracil; IF, irinotecan-fluorouracil-leucovorin FOLFOX, fluorouracil-leucovorin-oxaliplatin.

form at the time of the preparation of this chapter, included 221 analyzable patients who were assigned to receive DCF, and 224 CF. The primary end point was TTP. The study was powered to detect an increase in median TTP from 4 months for the control arm to 6 months for the experimental arm. The two arms appeared well balanced for prognostic factors, including weight loss >10%, performance status, and extent of disease when measured as the number of organs involved. Patients assigned to DCF received a median of six cycles versus four cycles for those receiving CF. This difference was not surprising because the TTP was significantly better for patients receiving DCF. The median TTP was 3.7 months for patients receiving CF and 5.6 months for those receiving DCF (hazard ratio 1.47, $P = 0.0004$). Overall survival was also improved, with a median survival of 8.6 months for patients receiving CF and 9.2 months for those receiving DCF. Perhaps more impressively, the 2-year survival rate was 8.8% for those receiving CF and 18.4% for those receiving DCF. A response rate difference also favored the DCF arm, with a 25% response rate for patients receiving CF and 37% for those receiving DCF. In contrast, toxicity with the DCF regimen was substantial. Eighty-one percent of patients receiving DCF had at least one grade 3-4 nonhematologic toxicity. The toxicity on the CF arm was also substantial, with 75% of patients having grade 3-4 toxicity. Hematologic toxicity, however, was substantially greater for the DCF arm. Grade 3-4 neutropenia was seen in 82% of patients receiving DCF versus 57% for those receiving CF. More striking, febrile neutropenia was seen in 13.5% of CF patients and 30% of those receiving DCF. There was, however, no difference in a total toxic death rate between the two arms. On the basis of this trial, the FDA recently approved docetaxel for use in patients with metastatic gastric cancer.

Effort is under way at a variety of centers to develop a more tolerable DCF regimen. Several phase II trials have already been reported using modifications of DCF. In general, these used somewhat lower doses of docetaxel or a different fluorouracil infusion schedule.

Irinotecan, Fluorouracil, and Leucovorin. The combination of irinotecan, fluorouracil, and leucovorin has undergone extensive study in patients with colorectal cancer. A FOLFIRI-type regimen is a standard care option in that disease. In advanced gastric cancer, irinotecan as a single agent, as described previously, has modest activity with response rates in the 14% to 25% range. After a random assignment phase II study of irinotecan, fluorouracil, and leucovorin showed an advantage over irinotecan cisplatin, a phase III definitive trial was performed comparing FOLFIRI to CF (171,172). Three hundred and thirty-seven patients were randomly assigned to receive either IF or CF. One hundred and seventy patients received IF, and 163 received CF. The primary end point of the study was TTP; if a nonsignificant trend toward superiority for TTP was observed a noninferiority comparison was to be performed. The doses of the IF arm are shown in Table 23.13. The two arms were reasonably well balanced. Approximately one-fifth of patients had GEJ tumors. The major objective response rate (CR+PR) was 31.8% for IF and 25.8% for CF. The median time to tumor progression was 5 months for IF and 4.2 months for CF, with a noninferiority margin of 0.93. There was no significant difference between the two arms ($P = 0.08$). There was also no difference in median survival (9 months for IF and 8.7 months for CF). Toxicity was less for the IF arm, particularly for neutropenic fever and stomatitis. It was greater for diarrhea. The investigators concluded that IF was less toxic than CF with similar efficacy. They proposed this regimen as an alternative for previously untreated patients in whom a noncisplatin-containing regimen is considered.

ECF. Cisplatin, as noted previously, has been widely used in combination with a variety of agents, particularly fluorouracil. A three-drug combination of ECF has been extensively studied by English investigators. After phase II data demonstrated toler-

ance and encouraging activity, Waters et al., updating the initial report of Webb et al., reported the results of a random assignment trial comparing ECF to an older noncisplatin-containing combination, FAMTX (fluorouracil modulated by methotrexate and doxorubicin) (173,174). One hundred and twenty-six patients received ECF, and 130 received FAMTX. ECF was significantly more effective than FAMTX in terms of overall response rate (46% vs. 21%) and median survival (8.7 months vs. 6.1 months). It was also superior in terms of long-term survival: at 2 years, 14% of patients receiving ECF were alive versus 5% of those receiving FAMTX. The long-term survival rate reported is in concert with data from other regimens, noted previously.

In a follow-up study, Ross et al. compared ECF to mitomycin-cisplatin-fluorouracil (MCF) (175). Essentially, mitomycin replaced epirubicin. A total of 574 patients were randomly assigned to receive either ECF (289 patients) or MCF (285 patients). This study included patients with gastric and GEJ tumors. The primary end point was 1-year survival.

The objective response rates for the two arms were similar (ECF 49.6%, MCF 55.4%). Approximately 10 patients randomized to ECF underwent resection after chemotherapy, as did 14 patients receiving MCF. Toxicity was tolerable with more myelosuppression for patients receiving MCF. The median duration of survival was 9.4 months for ECF and 8.7 months for MCF. One-year survival was slightly better with ECF (40% vs. 32% for MCF). At 2 years, 15.8% of ECF and 14.2% of MCF patients were alive, again consistent with results from several other trials. The authors concluded that there was no advantage for MCF over ECF, and that ECF could be considered a reference regimen for patients with GEJ and gastric cancers.

The data for ECF from the REAL-2 trial are shown in Table 23.12.

Cisplatin and Irinotecan. As noted previously in the discussion for irinotecan-fluorouracil-leucovorin, irinotecan has single-agent activity in patients with previously treated and untreated gastric cancer. Irinotecan was combined with cisplatin in several phase II studies. Toxicity was tolerable, with encouraging response rates.

These preliminary trials led to a larger-scale random assignment phase II trial in which IF was compared to irinotecan-cisplatin. Pozzo et al. reported the results of this study (172). The irinotecan-cisplatin arm used a dosing schedule of irinotecan 200 mg/m^2, followed by cisplatin 60 mg/m^2 once every 3 weeks. Note that this relatively high-dose regimen is somewhat different from other irinotecan-cisplatin regimens tested previously.

Sixty-five eligible patients were entered into each arm; 62 receiving the IF regimen were evaluable compared to 61 on the irinotecan-cisplatin arm. The trial was designed to choose the better of the two regimens based on the complete response rate. Secondary end points included safety, TTP, and survival. The overall response rate was 42.4% in the IF arm and 32.1% in the IC arm. Complete responses were seen in 5% of patients in the IF and 1.8% of patients in the IC arm. The time to disease progression also favored the IF arm (6.5 months vs. 4.2 months). The IF arm was chosen for further study compared with CF as the standard arm, with results as described previously.

Although irinotecan-cisplatin as used in this random assignment phase II trial was less encouraging than the IF arm, there is still substantial interest in this regimen using different schedules. IC has been studied in both esophageal and GEJ and gastric cancers (176–178). Discussed previously, in the section on targeted therapy, are data for a phase II trial using this regimen when combined with Bevacizumab.

Fluorouracil-Leucovorin-Oxaliplatin. The fluorouracil-leucovorin-oxaliplatin (FOLFOX) regimen is a standard care option in patients with advanced colorectal cancer. When given as adjuvant therapy for patients with stage III colon cancer, it has been demonstrated to be superior to fluorouracil and leucovorin alone. In gastric cancer, several phase II trials have been performed investigating the use of a FOLFOX-type regimen (179). In general, toxicity was acceptable and similar to that seen in patients with colorectal cancers. The dose-limiting toxicity for oxaliplatin is a peripheral neuropathy. Myelosuppression, mucositis, and diarrhea toxicity rates were similar to those reported in bowel tumors. Efficacy measured as overall response rate ranges from 50% to 60%. The median TTP is 5 to 6 months, with overall median survival of 10 to 12 months. Phase III studies comparing this regimen to cisplatin-containing combinations have now been reported. Cunningham et al. reported the results of the REAL2 trial in abstract form (180). In this study, fluorouracil-epirubicin-oxaliplatin was compared to ECF; a second comparison was between capecitabine-epirubicin-cisplatin and capecitabine-oxaliplatin-epirubicin. Stratification for performance status and extent of disease was followed by randomization to receive ECF, EOF (epirubicin-oxaliplatin-fluorouracil), ECX (epirubicin-cisplatin-capecitabine), or epirubicin oxaliplatin capecitabine (EOX). The doses of the different chemotherapy regimens are shown in Table 23.14. The primary end point was overall survival. The goal was to demonstrate noninferiority of capecitabine compared with fluorouracil and oxaliplatin compared with cisplatin. One thousand and two patients were randomized with approximately 250 patients per arm; 2×2 comparisons were performed. Forty percent of the patients had gastric primaries, and the rest GEJ or esophageal tumors (approximately 10% had squamous cell cancers of the esophagus). With a median follow-up of 17 months, median overall survival did not differ significantly among the groups (ECF 9.9 months, EOF 9.3 months, ECX 9.9 months, EOX 11.2 months). One-year overall survival was also similar, ranging from 37.7% to 46.8%, with the highest value seen with EOX and the lowest for ECF. The oxaliplatin

and capecitabine combinations were not inferior to ECF, thus meeting the primary goal of the study. They concluded that EOF was an acceptable substitute for ECF, and similarly, that ECX could replace ECF.

In a second study, al-Batran et al. reported the preliminary results of a random assignment phase III trial comparing FOL (fluorouracil-oxaliplatin-leucovorin) with FLP (fluorouracil-leucovorin-cisplatin) (181). The oxaliplatin regimen was an mFOLFOX 6 schedule involving fluorouracil 2,600 mg/m^2 over 24 hours, leucovorin 200 mg/m^2, and oxaliplatin 85 mg/m^2 given every 2 weeks. The FLP regimen was similar, delivering 2,000 mg/m^2 of fluorouracil every week, leucovorin 200 mg/m^2 every week, and cisplatin 50 mg/m^2 every 2 weeks. The study was designed to assess an improvement in median TTP from 3.5 to 5 months. A total of 220 patients were randomized, 112 for FLO and 108 to FLP. There was no significant difference in TTP between the two arms ($P = 0.08$). Although superiority was not demonstrated, the results support the REAL-2 data indicating noninferiority for oxaliplatin-FU–containing regimens. FLO was somewhat less toxic than FLP with a higher objective response rate (34% vs. 27%).

Last, Kang et al. also reported, in abstract form, the results of a random assignment phase III trial testing for noninferiority of a capecitabine platinum regimen versus CF (182). The dosing schedule involved cisplatin 80 mg/m^2 on day 1 and a continuous infusion of fluorouracil 800 mg/m^2/day for 5 days in a row, given on an every 3-week schedule, somewhat more frequently than described for standard CF. The CAPP (cisplatin-capecitabine) regimen used the same dose of cisplatin with capecitabine given at 1,000 mg/m^2 twice daily for 14 days every 3 weeks. One hundred and sixty patients received CAPP, and 156 patients received FP. The study demonstrated noninferiority for the CAPP arm, with a median progression free oraviral of 5.6 months for CAPP versus 5 months for FP. There was also no difference in overall survival. They concluded that CAPP was not inferior to FP.

TABLE 23.14

REAL-2 REGIMENS

Drug	Dose	Day(s)	Week(s)
ECF			
Epirubicin	50 mg/m^2 IV	1	Every 3 wk
Cisplatin	60 mg/m^2 IV	1	
PVI 5-FU	200 mg/m^2/d^a	1	
EOF			
Epirubicin	50 mg/m^2 IV	1	Every 3 wk
Oxaliplatin	130 mg/m^2 IV	1	
PVI 5-FU	200 mg/m^2/d^a	1	
ECX			
Epirubicin	50 mg/m^2 IV	1	Every 3 wk
Cisplatin	60 mg/m^2 IV	1	
Capecitabine	625 mg/m^2/bd	1	
EOX			
Epirubicin	50 mg/m^2 IV	1	Every 3 wk
Oxaliplatin	130 mg/m^2 IV	1	
Capecitabine	625 mg^2 bd	1	

ECF, epirubicin-cisplatin-5-FU; IV, intravenous; PVI 5-FU, protracted venous-infusion fluorouracil; EOF, epirubicin-oxaliplatin-fluorouracil; ECX, epirubicin-cisplatin-capecitabine; EOX, epirubicin oxaliplatin capecitabine.
Planned treatment duration: 24 wk (eight cycles).
^{a}PVI 5-FU delivered by central venous access catheter.

It is of interest that these regimens (FOLFOX, FOLFIRI, capecitabine-containing, and other oxaliplatin-containing regimens) are widely used in colon cancer. In that disease, median TTP for patients with advanced cancer is 7 to 8 months, and median survivals are now 20 to 21 months, even without the use of Bevacizumab. With these regimes, 1-year survival for patients with metastatic colon cancer is approximately 70%, and 2-year survival is approximately 40%. The results in gastric and GEJ tumors are substantially inferior. This may be because of biological differences between the two tumors, with gastroesophageal tumors being inherently more resistant to the same regimens. However, it is also of interest that there are more classes of active drugs in gastroesophageal tumors than there are in colon tumors. It addition to oxaliplatin, cisplatin, fluorouracil, irinotecan, and capecitabine, the taxanes and anthracyclines are active in gastric and gastroesophageal tumors and not in colon cancer. Better preclinical models and tissue correlates would be helpful in exploring biological differences between the two diseases. It is also possible that we are not as effective in sequencing these agents in gastroesophageal tumors. In the REAL-2 trial, for example, only 15% of patients received additional therapy at the TTP of disease.

TARGETED THERAPY

Bevacizumab

Bevacizumab, a humanized monoclonal antibody directed against the VEGF ligand, has undergone extensive study in patients with solid tumors over the past several years. In patients with advanced colorectal cancer, Bevacizumab plus cytotoxic chemotherapy is superior to cytotoxic chemotherapy alone, and the agent is approved for this indication in the United States. Similar increase in efficacy has been seen in pivotal phase III trials in patients with non–small cell lung cancer and in women with breast cancer. In gastric cancer, Shah et al. reported in abstract form the results of a phase II trial studying use of Bevacizumab-cisplatin-irinotecan (183). Bevacizumab was given at a dose of 15 mg/kg on day 1 and repeated every 3 weeks. The irinotecan-cisplatin regimen studied used a dose schedule of irinotecan 65 mg/m^2 and cisplatin 30 mg/m^2 given once a week 2 weeks in a row with a 1-week break. Forty-seven previously untreated patients with gastric or GEJ tumors were studied. Median TTP was 9.9 months, which met the primary end point of the study for a 50% improvement in TTP over historical controls. Among 35 patients whose primary tumor was still in place, two gastric perforations were seen. There was only 1 patient with significant bleeding, and there were no toxicity-related deaths. Thromboembolic events were seen in 25% of patients, including 4 patients with asymptomatic pulmonary embolism (184). It was unclear, however, whether this was due to Bevacizumab. In a companion study, patients with local regional disease receiving neoadjuvant cisplatin-irinotecan alone had a similar rate of thromboembolic events. The authors concluded that Bevacizumab can safely be combined with cytotoxic chemotherapy in patients with advanced gastric and GEJ adenocarcinomas, including patients in whom the primary tumor was still in place. Phase III trials comparing chemotherapy with and without Bevacizumab are planned.

Epidermal Growth Factor Receptor Tyrosine Kinase Inhibitors

Both erlotinib and gefitinib have been studied in phase II trials in patients with gastric and GEJ cancers. Most of these data are available in abstract form only at this point. Five studies have evaluated the use of EGFR-TK inhibitors in esophagus, gastroesophageal, or gastric cancers. These studies indicate modest single-agent activity for gefitinib and erlotinib. In the largest study from Dragovich et al., 26 patients with gastric and 44 with GEJ tumors received single-agent erlotinib (185). There were no responses among patients with gastric cancers; 4/44 (12%) of GEJ tumor responded. Toxicity was as expected for these agents.

To date, the data indicate the same modest level of activity for single-agent EGFR-TK inhibitors as has been reported in other tumors including non–small cell lung cancers.

Cetuximab, an antibody to the EGFR receptor, is now undergoing a clinical trial as a single agent, as well as when combined with irinotecan-cisplatin–containing regimens, in patients with advanced esophageal and GEJ tumors.

Molecular Markers and Prediction of Response

For many years, techniques that would allow medical oncologists to customize treatment for the individual patient have been recognized to be a high priority. This strategy assumes that outcome will be better if patients are treated with agents chosen because pretreatment tests have indicated a high likelihood of response so they will be spared the toxicity of ineffective therapy, and the chance for regression will be maximized using agents that are active in that individual. This is particularly important because most currently available cytotoxic agents for gastric cancer have only modest to moderate activity. Toxicities, as noted previously, can be substantial. Initial predictive assays used live tumor cell samples for in vitro assays. With fresh tumor cell assays, however, formidable logistic problems and the poor positive predictive value in choosing an individual agent have not yet been overcome. An alternative approach measures, on a qualitative or semiquantitative basis, levels of individual target molecules or molecules associated with the mechanism action of an individual agent that could predict the likelihood of response. Several studies suggest that such molecular analysis of tumor tissue may be a more accurate and reliable method of predicting outcome.

Several techniques are being studied. Both immunohistochemistry and reverse transcriptase polymerase chain reaction (RT-PCR) technology have been used to measure markers of interest. Immunohistochemical techniques allow a visual assessment of the level of expression of the marker of interest, usually indicated as none, intermediate, or high. With RT-PCR, relative gene expression is measured on a semiquantitative or quantitative basis. The general hypothesis is that levels of gene expression correlate with relative resistance or sensitivity to individual chemotherapeutic agents. With regard to gastric cancer, at this point, most of the data to evaluate this hypothesis are available for patients with locoregional disease; little information exists regarding patients with advanced measurable metastatic disease. Because of the difficulty of assessing response in the primary tumor, interpretation of the predictive value of measurement of molecular markers depends to a large extent on survival data.

Several studies in gastric cancer, similar to those performed for colorectal tumors, evaluated individual molecular markers, such as thymidine phosphorylase (TS) as a marker for fluorouracil sensitivity or resistance or excision repair cross-complementary gene (ERCC-1) as a marker of cisplatin sensitivity or resistance. Additional markers for predicting efficacy of fluorouracil included thymidine phosphorylase and dipyrimidine dehydrogenase. These studies suggested a correlation between a level of gene expression of TS, TP, DPD, or ERCC-1 and improved outcome. These data have yet to be confirmed in prospective trials. As is the case for several other tumors, mutations of a variety of genes, particularly p53 oncogene, have also been studied (186–191). Again, prospective trials indicating a relationship between outcome and mutational status of p53 have not yet been reported in gastric cancer.

A high priority is to conduct a definitive prospective study in which adequate numbers of patients with advanced measurable gastric cancer (for whom response is the measure of outcome) or patients with locoregional disease (in whom survival is the outcome) receive the same chemotherapy irrespective of their molecular marker profile and are then followed. Clearly, the identification of molecular markers measured by immunohistochemistry, RT-PCR, or other techniques that could predict outcome would be of substantial aid in directing individualized therapy for patients with gastric cancer.

Predictive markers that accurately indicate which agents will be effective in gastric cancer and/or which will be particularly toxic in the individual patient have yet to be identified, but there is more progress in other solid tumors. In breast cancer, for example, predictive markers have long been identified and accepted to guide therapeutic intervention. This includes not only the measurement of estrogen and progesterone receptor status from primary or metastatic tumor, but also analysis HER-2 to determine whether trastuzumab should be used. Women whose tumors do not have overamplification of HER-2 will not respond to trastuzumab (192). Preliminary data from other common tumors, such as lung cancer, suggest that future use of epidermal growth factor receptor tyrosine kinase inhibitors may be based on the presence or absence of a mutation in the molecular target (193). Studies in less common tumors, such as GIST (see Chapter 50) and glioblastoma multiforme, indicate that analysis of a limited set of molecular markers or genetic abnormalities may predict outcome. Extensive studies are under way in gastric and GEJ tumors to identify a similar set of predictive markers (194,195).

Functional imaging has already undergone initial study in predicting outcome in patients with gastric cancer. As briefly described previously, Ott et al. studied 44 consecutive patients with locally advanced gastric cancer using FDG-PET (196). A FDG-PET scan was performed before and after cisplatin-fluorouracil-leucovorin chemotherapy (FLP). Surgery was planned 3 to 4 weeks after completing a course of neoadjuvant chemotherapy. In this study, measurement of effectiveness was a decrease in subtraction uptake value (SUV). Changes in PET were compared to tumor response assessed pathologically. A grading system that ranged from near complete tumor regression (<10% residual tumor) to minimal or no tumor regression (>50% residual tumor) was used. Responding patients were classified as having <10% viable tumor. Thirteen patients were considered pathological responders.

The decrease in SUV was markedly higher among responding patients (median of −49% in responders and −17% in nonresponders). Survival was also better for patients who had a PET/CT response compared with those who did not. More recently, Wieder et al. (197) evaluated 20 patients with GEJ adenocarcinomas using FDG-PET/CT. FDG-PET was again performed prior to and 14 days after initiation of chemotherapy. They concluded that changes in PET scan were more sensitive in assessing the effects of chemotherapy than measurements of tumor size by CT scan. Weber (198) reviewed the use of PET scanning to identify active systemic agents. PET/CT is now able to measure targets such as HER-2 expression of tumors. Thus, preliminary data indicate that PET scanning may allow the early identification of patients responding to systemic therapy, at a time considerably earlier than that by traditional measures. A decision could then be made for nonresponding patients to either proceed directly to definitive local therapy (surgical intervention) or for patients with locally advanced disease to change to an alternative form of systemic therapy. Investigationally, PET may be used to assess whether a targeted agent is "hitting the target."

Expression profiling has been performed among a variety of solid tumors in an attempt to identify molecular signatures that were prognostic. More recently, Luthra et al. (199) studied patients with esophageal and GEJ tumors who were to receive preoperative chemoradiation therapy. Endoscopic biopsies were obtained prior to treatment. Sixteen patients had adenocarcinoma, two squamous cell, and one adenosquamous cell carcinoma. RNA was isolated from each biopsy and oligonucleotide microarray performed. A hierarchical clustering algorithm was used to group genes. The analysis segregated the specimens into two major categories: subtype I and subtype II. They found that five of six patients who had pathological complete response to chemoradiation therapy had clustering in what they described as subtype I of their analysis. They noted a differential expression among 400 genes between two subtypes. Only preliminary clinical data were available. This indicated a slightly shorter diseasefree survival of 22 months for patients in subtype II versus 28 months for patients in subtype I. They concluded that these preliminary data were encouraging and that further studies in larger groups of patients were appropriate. Three marker genes, PERP, S1082, and SPRR3, were able to discriminate between patients who would eventually have complete pathological remissions and those who would not.

In summary, although studies are underway to identify predictive markers to individualize therapy in gastric cancer, they are still an experimental approach.

References

1. Moertel CG. The stomach. In: Holland JF, Frei EI, eds. *Cancer Medicine.* Philadelphia, Pa.: Lea & Febiger; 1982:1760.
2. Wolfler A. *Uber die Herrn Professor Billroth Ausgefuerten Resectionen des Ccarcinomatosen Pylorus.* (Braumuller W, ed.) Wien; 1881.
3. Mikulicz J. Beitrage zur technik der operation des magencarcinoms. *Arch Clin Chir Berl* 1898;1(vii):524–532.
4. Jamieson JK, Dobson JF. The lymphatic system of the stomach. *Lancet* 1907:1061–1066.
5. Pack GT, McNeer GP. Total gastrectomy for cancer: a collective review of the literature and an original report on 20 cases. *Int Abstr Surg* 1943;77:265–299.
6. Akoh JA, Macintyre IM. Improving survival in gastric cancer: review of 5-year survival rates in English language publications from 1970. *Br J Surg* 1992;79(4):293–299.
7. Macintyre IM, Akoh JA. Improving survival in gastric cancer: review of operative mortality in English language publications from 1970. *Br J Surg* 1991;78:771–776.
8. Kajitani T. The general rules for the gastric cancer study in surgery and pathology. Part I. Clinical classification. *Jpn J Surg* 1981;11(2):127–139.
9. Beahrs OH, Henson DE, Hutter RVP, Kennedy BJ. *Manual for Staging of Cancer.* 4th ed. American Joint Committee on Cancer. Philadelphia, Pa.: JB Lippincott; 1992.
10. Hermanek P, Sobin LH. *International Union Against Cancer: TNM Classification of Malignant Tumors.* 4th ed. Berlin: Springer; 1992.
11. Wanebo HJ, Kennedy BJ, Chmiel J, Steele G, Winchester D, Osteen R. Cancer of the stomach. A patient care study by the American College of Surgeons. *Ann Surg* 1993(218):583–592.
12. Kinoshita T, Maruyama K, Sasako M, et al. Treatment results of gastric cancer patients: Japanese experience. In: Nishi M, Ichakawa H, Nakajima T, et al, eds. *Gastric Cancer.* Tokyo: Springer-Verlag; 1993:319–330.
13. Soga J, Kobayashi K, Saito J, Fujimaki M, Muto T. The role of lymphadenectomy in curative surgery for gastric cancer. *World J Surg* 1979; 3(6):701–708.
14. Bonenkamp JJ, Hermans J, Sasako M, van de Velde CJ. Extended lymphnode dissection for gastric cancer. Dutch Gastric Cancer Group. *N Engl J Med* 1999;340(12):908–914.
15. Bonenkamp JJ, van de Velde CJ, Kampschoer GH, et al. Comparison of factors influencing the prognosis of Japanese, German, and Dutch gastric cancer patients. *World J Surg* 1993;17(3):410–414; discussion 5.
16. Cuschieri A. Recent advances in gastrointestinal malignancy. *Ann Chir Gynaecol* 1989;78(3):228–237.
17. Siewert JR, Bottcher K, Roder JD, et al. Prognostic relevance of systemic lymph node dissection in gastric carcinoma. *Br J Surg* 1993;80:1015–1018.

18. Sue-Ling HM, Johnston D, Martin IG, et al. Gastric cancer: a curable disease in Britain [see comments]. *BMJ* 1993;307(6904):591–596.

19. Arak A, Kull K. Factors influencing survival of patients after radical surgery for gastric cancer. A regional study of 406 patients over a 10-year period. *Acta Oncol* 1994;33(8):913–920.

20. Wanebo HJ, Kennedy BJ, Winchester DP, et al. Gastric carcinoma: does lymph node dissection alter survival? *J Am Coll Surg* 1996;183:616.

21. Dent DM, Madden MV, Price SK. Randomized comparison of R1 and R2 gastrectomy for gastric carcinoma. *Br J Surg* 1988;75:110–112.

22. McKenzie AD, Robertson HR. Gastro-ileostomy. *Ann Surg* 1953;138(6):911–914.

23. Hartgrink HH, van de Velde CJ, Putter H, et al. Extended lymph node dissection for gastric cancer: who may benefit? Final results of the randomized Dutch gastric cancer group trial. *J Clin Oncol* 2004;22(11):2069–2077.

24. Cuschieri A, Weeden S, Fielding J, et al. Patient survival after D1 and D2 resections for gastric cancer: long-term results of the MRC randomized surgical trial. Surgical Cooperative Group. *Br J Cancer* 1999;79(9–10):1522–1530.

25. Bunt AM, Hermans J, Boon MC, et al. Evaluation of the extent of lymphadenectomy in a randomized trial of Western- versus Japanese-type surgery in gastric cancer. *J Clin Oncol* 1994;12(2):417–422.

26. Wu CW, Hsjung CA, Lo SS, et al. Nodal dissection for patients with gastric cancer: a randomised controlled trial. *Eur J Surg Oncol* 2006;30:303–308.

27. Sasako M, Sano T, Yamamoto S, et al. Randomized phase III trial of standard D2 versus D2 + para-aortic lymph node (PAN) dissection (D) for clinically M0 advanced gastric cancer: JCOG9501. *J Clin Oncol* 2006;24(part I):18S.

28. Degiuli M, Sasako M, Calgaro M, et al. Morbidity and mortality after D1 and D2 gastrectomy for cancer: interim analysis of the Italian Gastric Cancer Study Group (IGCSG) randomised surgical trial. *Eur J Surg Oncol* 2004;30(3):303–308.

29. Viste A, Haùgstvedt T, Eide GE, Sreide O. Postoperative complications and mortality after surgery for gastric cancer. *Ann Surg* 1988;207:7–13.

30. Bottcher K, Siewert JR, Roder JD, Busch R, Hermanek P, Meyer HJ. Risk of surgical therapy of stomach cancer in Germany. Results of the German 1992 Stomach Cancer Study. *Chirurg* 1994;65(4):298–306.

31. Gennari L, Bozzetti F, Bonfanti G, et al. Subtotal versus total gastrectomy for cancer of the lower two-thirds of the stomach: a new approach to an old problem. *Br J Surg* 1986;73:534–538.

32. Cuschieri A, Fayers P, Fielding J, et al. Postoperative morbidity and mortality after D1 and D2 resection for gastric cancer: preliminary results of the MRC randomized controlled surgical trial. *Lancet* 1996;347:995–999.

33. Sasako M. Risk factors for surgical treatment in the Dutch Gastric Cancer Trial. *Br J Surg* 1997;84(11):1567–1571.

34. Songun I, Bonenkamp JJ, Hermans J, van Krieken JH, van de Velde CJ. Prognostic value of resection-line involvement in patients undergoing curative resections for gastric cancer. *Eur J Cancer* 1996;32A(3):433–437.

35. Kodera Y, Yamamura Y, Shimizu Y, et al. Lack of benefit of combined pancreaticosplenectomy in D2 resection for proximal-third gastric carcinoma. *World J Surg* 1997;21(6):622–627; discussion 7–8.

36. Degliulie M, Sasako M, Ponzetti A, et al. Extended lymph node dissection for gastric cancer: results of a prospective, multi-centre analysis of morbidity and mortality in 118 consecutive cases. *Eur J Surg Oncol* 1997;23:310–314.

37. Griffith J, Sue-Ling HM, Dixon MF, McMahon MJ, Axon AT, Johnston D. Preservation of the spleen improves survival after radical surgery for gastric cancer. *Gut* 1995;36:684.

38. Kitamura K, Nishida S, Ichikawa D, et al. No survival benefit from combined pancreaticosplenectomy and total gastrectomy for gastric cancer. *Br J Surg* 1999;86(1):119–122.

39. Siewert JR, Bottcher K, Stein HJ, Roder JD, Busch R. Problem of proximal third gastric carcinoma. *World J Surg* 1995;19(4):523–531.

40. Brady MS, Rogatko A, Dent LL, Shiu MH. Effect of splenectomy on morbidity and survival following curative gastrectomy for carcinoma. *Arch Surg* 1991;126:359–364.

41. Aldridge MC, Williamson RC. Distal pancreatectomy with and without splenectomy. *Br J Surg* 1991;78(8):976–979.

42. Meyers WC, Damiano RJ, Jr, Rotolo FS, Postlethwait RW. Adenocarcinoma of the stomach: changing patterns over the last 4 decades. *Ann Surg* 1987;205:1–8.

43. Kampschoer GH, Maruyama K, Sasako M, Kinoshita T, van de Velde CJ. The effects of blood transfusion on the prognosis of patients with gastric cancer. *World J Surg* 1989;13:637–643.

44. Kaneda M, Horimi T, Ninomiya M, et al. Adverse affect of blood transfusions on survival of patients with gastric cancer. *Transfusion* 1987;27:375–377.

45. Sugezawa A, Kaibara N, Sumi K, et al. Blood transfusion and the prognosis of patients with gastric cancer. *J Surg Oncol* 1989;42:113–116.

46. Yu W, Choi GS, Chung HY. Randomized clinical trial of splenectomy versus splenic preservation in patients with proximal gastric cancer. *Br J Surg* 2006;93(5):559–563.

47. Sanchez-Bueno F, Garcia-Marcilla JA, Perez-Flores D, et al. Prognostic factors in a series of 297 patients with gastric adenocarcinoma undergoing surgical resection. *Br J Surg* 1998;85(2):255–260.

48. Shiu MH, Perrotti M, Brennan MF. Adenocarcinoma of the stomach: a multivariate analysis of clinical, pathologic and treatment factors. *Hepatogastroenterology* 1989;36:7–12.

49. Sasako M, McCulloch P, Kinoshita T, Maruyama K. New method to evaluate the therapeutic value of lymph node dissection for gastric cancer. *Br J Surg* 1995;82(3):346–351.

50. Sano T, Sasako M, Yamamoto S, et al. gastric cancer surgery: morbidity and mortality results from a prospective randomized controlled trial comparing D2 and extended para-aortic lymphadenectomy—Japan Clinical Oncology Group Study 9501. *J Clin Oncol* 2004;22(14):2767–2773.

51. Fleming I, Cooper J, Henson D, et al. *American Joint Committee on Cancer Staging Manual*. Philadelphia, Pa.: Lippincott-Raven; 1997.

52. Sobin LH, Wittekind C. *International Union Against Cancer: TNM Classification of Malignant Tumors*. New York, NY: Wiley-Liss; 1997.

53. Hermanek P, Altendorf-Hofmann A, Mansmann U, et al. Improvements in staging of gastric carcinoma using the new edition of TNM classification. *Eur J Surg Oncol* 1998;24:536–541.

54. Feinstein AR, Sosin DM, Wells CK. The Will Rogers phenomenon. Stage migration and new diagnostic techniques as a source of misleading statistics for survival in cancer. *N Engl J Med* 1985;312(25):1604–1608.

55. Robertson CS, Chung SCS, Woods SDS et al. A prospective trial comparing R1 subtotal gastrectomy with R3 gastrectomy for antral cancer. *Ann Surg* 1994;220(2):176–182.

56. Damhuis RA, Tilanus HW. The influence of age on resection rates and postoperative mortality in 2773 patients with gastric cancer. *Eur J Cancer* 1995;31A(6):928–931.

57. Kranenbarg EK, van de Velde CJ. Gastric cancer in the elderly. *Eur J Surg Oncol* 1998;24(5):384–390.

58. Maruyama K. The most important prognostic factors for gastric cancer patients: a study using univariate and multivariate analysis. *J Gastroenterol* 1987;22(suppl 133):63.

59. Maruyama K, Okabayashi K, Kinoshita T. Progress in gastric cancer surgery in Japan and its limits of radicality. *World J Surg* 1987;11:418–425.

60. Peeters KC, Kattan MW, Hartgrink HH, et al. Validation of a nomogram for predicting disease-specific survival after an R0 resection for gastric carcinoma. *Cancer* 2005;103(4):702–707.

61. Kodama Y, Sugimachi K, Soejima K, Matsusaka T, Inokuchi K. Evaluation of extensive lymph node dissection for carcinoma of the stomach. *World J Surg* 1981;5:241.

62. McCulloch P, Niita ME, Kazi H, Gama-Rodrigues JJ. Gastrectomy with extended lymphadenectomy for primary treatment of gastric cancer. *Br J Surg* 2005;92(1):5–13.

63. Bonenkamp JJ, for the Dutch Gastric Cancer Group. D1 versus D2 dissection for gastric cancer [comment on letters]. *Lancet* 1995;345:1517–1518.

64. Bonenkamp JJ, van de Velde CJ, Sasako M, Hermans J. R2 compared with R1 resection for gastric cancer morbidity and mortality in a prospective, randomised trial. *Eur J Surg Oncol* 1992;158(8):413–418.

65. McCulloch P. D1 versus D2 dissection for gastric cancer [letter]. *Lancet* 1995;158:413–418.

66. Parikh D, Johnson M, Chagla L, Lowe D, McCulloch P. D2 gastrectomy: lessons from a prospective audit of the learning curve. *Br J Surg* 1996; 83(11):1595–1539.

67. Begg CB, Cramer LD, Hoskins WJ, Brennan MF. Impact of hospital volume on operative mortality for major cancer surgery. *JAMA* 1998; 280(20):1747–1751.

68. Gilbertsen VA. Results of treatment of stomach cancer. An appraisal of efforts for more extensive surgery and a report of 1,983 cases. *Cancer* 1969; 23(6):1305–1308.

69. Maruyama K, Gunven P, Okabayashi K, Sasako M, Kinoshita T. Lymph node metastases of gastric cancer. General pattern in 1931 patients. *Ann Surg* 1989;210:596–602.

70. Meyer HJ. The influence of case load and the extent of resection on the quality of treatment outcome in gastric cancer. *Eur J Surg Oncol* 2005;31(6):595–604.

71. Sunderland D. The lymphatic spread of gastric cancer. In: McNeer G, Pack G, eds. *Neoplasms of the Stomach*. Philadelphia, Pa.: Lippincott; 1967:408.

72. Nakajima T, Harashima A, Hirata M, Kajitani T. Prognostic and therapeutic values of peritoneal cytology in gastric cancer. *Acta Cytol* 1978;22(4):225–229.

73. Kodera Y, Nakanishi H, Ito S, et al. Quantitative detection of disseminated cancer cells in the greater omentum of gastric carcinoma patients with real-time RT-PCR: a comparison with peritoneal lavage cytology. *Gastric Cancer* 2002;5(2):69–76.

74. Hayes N, Wayman J, Wadehra V, Scott D, Raimes SA, Griffin SM. Peritoneal cytology in the surgical evaluation of gastric carcinoma. *Br J Cancer* 1999;79(3/4):520–524.

75. Mc Neer G, Vandenberg H, Jr, Donn FY, Bowden L. A critical evaluation of subtotal gastrectomy for the cure of cancer of the stomach. *Ann Surg* 1951; 134(1):2–7.

76. Wisbeck W, Becher E, Russel A. Adenocarcinoma of the stomach: autopsy observations with therapeutic implications for the radiation oncologist. *Radiother Oncol* 1986;7:13.

77. Gunderson LL, Sosin H. Adenocarcinoma of the stomach: areas of failure in a re-operation series (second or symptomatic look) clinicopathologic correlation and implications for adjuvant therapy. *Int J Radiat Oncol Biol Phys* 1992;8:1–11.

78. Allum WH, Hallissey MT, Ward LC, Hockey MS. A controlled, prospective, randomised trial of adjuvant chemotherapy or radiotherapy in resectable gastric cancer: interim report. British Stomach Cancer Group. *Br J Cancer* 1989;60:739–744.

79. Landry J, Tepper JE, Wood WC, Moulton EO, Koerner F, Sullinger J. Patterns of failure following curative resection of gastric carcinoma. *Int J Radiat Oncol Biol Phys* 1990;19:1357–1362.

80. Coombes RC, Schein PS, Chilvers CE, et al. A randomized trial comparing adjuvant fluorouracil, doxorubicin, and mitomycin with no treatment in operable gastric cancer. *J Clin Oncol* 1990;8(8):1362–1369.

81. MacDonald JS, Fleming TR, Peterson RF, et al. Adjuvant chemotherapy with 5-FU, Adriamycin, and mitomycin-C (FAM) versus surgery alone for patients with locally advanced gastric adenocarcinoma: a Southwest Oncology Group study. *Ann Surg Oncol* 1995;2(6):488–494.

82. Lise M, Nitti D, Buyse M, et al. Phase-III clinical trial of adjuvant FAM2 (5-FU, Adriamycin and mitomycin C) vs control in resectable gastric cancer: a study of the EORTC Gastrointestinal Tract Cancer Cooperative Group. *Recent Results Cancer Res* 1988;110:36–43.

83. Hallissey MT, Dunn JA, Ward LC, Allum WH. The second British Stomach Cancer Group trial of adjuvant radiotherapy or chemotherapy in resectable gastric cancer: five- year follow-up. *Lancet* 1994;343(8909):1309–1312.

84. Tsavaris N, Tentas K, Kosmidis P, et al. A randomized trial comparing adjuvant fluorouracil, epirubicin, and mitomycin with no treatment in operable gastric cancer. *Chemotherapy* 1996;42:220.

85. Krook JE, O'Connell MJ, Wieand HS, et al. A prospective, randomized evaluation of intensive course 5-fluorouracil plus doxorubicin as a surgical adjuvant chemotherapy for resected gastric cancer. *Cancer* 1991;67(10):2454–2458.

86. Songun I, Keizer HJ, Hermans J, et al. Chemotherapy for operable gastric cancer: results of the Dutch randomised FAMTX trial. The Dutch Gastric Cancer Group (DGCG). *Eur J Cancer* 1999;35(4):558–562.

87. Neri B, De Leonardis V, Romano S, et al. Adjuvant chemotherapy after gastric resection in node-positive cancer patients: a multicentre randomised study. *Br J Cancer* 1996;73(4):549–552.

88. DeVita F, Giuliani F, Gebbia V, et al. Surgery plus ELFE (epirubicin-leucovorin-fluorouracil-etoposide) versus surgery alone in radically resected gastric cancer. *J Clin Oncol* 2006;24(18S):182.

89. Nitti D, Wils J, Dos Santos JG, et al. Randomized phase III trials of adjuvant FAMTX or FEMTX compared with surgery alone in resected gastric cancer. A combined analysis of the EORTC GI Group and the ICCG. *Ann Oncol* 2006;17(2):262–269.

90. Bajetta E, Buzzoni R, Mariani L, et al. Adjuvant chemotherapy in gastric cancer: 5-year results of a randomised study by the Italian Trials in Medical Oncology (ITMO) Group. *Ann Oncol* 2002;13(2):299–307.

91. Hermans J, Bonenkamp JJ, Boon MC, et al. Adjuvant therapy after curative resection for gastric cancer: meta-analysis of randomized trials [see comments]. *J Clin Oncol* 1993;11(8):1441–1447.

92. Earle CC, Maroun JA. Adjuvant chemotherapy after curative resection for gastric cancer in non-Asian patients: revisiting a meta-analysis of randomised trials. *Eur J Cancer* 1999;35(7):1059–1064.

93. Hu JK, Chen ZX, Zhou ZG, et al. Intravenous chemotherapy for resected gastric cancer: meta-analysis of randomized controlled trials. *World J Gastroenterol* 2002;8(6):1023–1028.

94. Panzini I, Gianni L, Fattori PP, et al. Adjuvant chemotherapy in gastric cancer: a meta-analysis of randomized trials and a comparison with previous meta-analyses. *Tumori* 2002;88(1):21–27.

95. Mari E, Floriani I, Tinazzi A, et al. Efficacy of adjuvant chemotherapy after curative resection for gastric cancer: a meta-analysis of published randomised trials. A study of the GISCAD (Gruppo Italiano per lo Studio dei Carcinome dell'Apparato Digerente). *Ann Oncol* 2000;11:837–843.

96. Moertel CG, Childs DS, O'Fallon JR, Holbrook MA, Schutt AJ, Reitemeier RJ. Combined 5-fluorouracil and radiation therapy as a surgical adjuvant for poor prognosis gastric carcinoma. *J Clin Oncol* 1984;2(2):1249–1254.

97. Dent D, Werner I, Novis B, et al. Prospective randomized trial of combined oncological therapy for gastric carcinoma. *Cancer* 1979(44):385–391.

98. MacDonald J, Smalley S, Benedetti J, et al. Chemoradiotherapy after surgery compared with surgery alone for adenocarcinoma of the stomach or gastroesophageal junction. *N Engl J Med* 2001;345(10):725–730.

99. Smalley S, Gunderson L, Tepper J, et al. Gastric surgical adjuvant radiotherapy consensus report: rationale and treatment implementation. *Int J Radiat Oncol Biol Phys* 2002;52(2):283–293.

100. Kim SH, Lim DH, Lee J, et al. An observational study suggesting clinical benefit for adjuvant postoperative chemoradiation in a population of over 500 cases after gastric resection with D2 nodal dissection for adenocarcinoma of the stomach. *Int J Radiat Oncol Biol Phys* 2005;63:1279–1285.

101. Kollmannsberger C, Budach W, Stahl M, et al. Adjuvant chemoradiation using 5-fluorouracil/folinic acid/cisplatin with or without paclitaxel and radiation in patients with completely resected high-risk gastric cancer: two cooperative phase II studies of the AIO/ARO/ACO. *Ann Oncol* 2005;16(8):1326–1333.

102. Schwartz GK, Winter K, Minstky B, et al. A randomized phase II trial comparing two paclitaxel (P)-cisplatin (C) containing chemoradiation (CRT) regimens as adjuvant therapy in resected gastric cancer (RTOG 0114). *Int J Radiat Oncol Biol Phys* In press.

103. Fuchs C, Fitzgerald T, Mammon H, et al. Postoperative adjuvant chemoradiation for gastric or gastroesophageal adenocarcinoma using epirubicin, cisplatin, and infusional (CI) 5-FU (ECF) before and after CI 5-FU and radiotherapy (RT): a multicenter study. *Am Soc Clin Oncol* 2003;22:257.

104. Leong T, Michael M, Foo K, et al. Adjuvant and neoadjuvant therapy for gastric cancer using epirubicin/cisplatin/5-fluorouracil (ECF) and alternative regimens before and after chemoradiation. *Br J Cancer* 2003;89(8):1433–1438.

105. Zhang ZX, Gu XZ, Yin WB, Huang GJ, Zhang DW, Zhang RG. Randomized clinical trial on the combination of preoperative irradiation and surgery in the treatment of adenocarcinoma of gastric cardia (AGC)—report on 370 patients. *Int J Radiat Oncol Biol Phys* 1998;42(5):929–934.

106. Allal AS, Zwahlen D, Brundler MA, et al. Neoadjuvant radiochemotherapy for locally advanced gastric cancer: long-term results of a phase I trial. *Int J Radiat Oncol Biol Phys* 2005;63:1286–1289.

107. Okawara GS, Winter K, Donohue JH, et al. A phase II trial of preoperative chemotherapy and chemoradiotherapy for potentially resectable adenocarcinoma of the stomach (RTOG 99-04). *Proc Am Soc Clin Oncol* 2005;22:312s.

108. Moertel CG, Childs DS, Jr, Reitemeier RJ, Colby MY, Jr, Holbrook MA. Combined 5-fluorouracil and supervoltage radiation therapy of locally unresectable gastrointestinal cancer. *Lancet* 1969;2(7626):865–867.

109. Schein PS, Smith FP, Woolley PV, Ahlgren JD. Current management of advanced and locally unresectable gastric carcinoma. *Cancer* 1982;50(11 suppl):2590–2596.

110. Gastrointestinal Tumor Study Group. A comparison of combination chemotherapy and combined modality therapy for locally advanced gastric carcinoma. *Cancer* 1982;49:1771–1777.

111. Sindelar WF, Kinsella TJ. Randomized trial of resection and intraoperative radiotherapy in locally advanced gastric cancer. *Proc Am Soc Clin Oncol* 1987;6:91.

112. Takahashi M, Abe M. Intra-operative radiotherapy for carcinoma of the stomach. *Eur J Surg Oncol* 1986;12:247–250.

113. Abe M, Shibamoto Y, Ono K, Takahashi M. Intraoperative radiation therapy for carcinoma of the stomach and pancreas. *Front Radiat Ther Oncol* 1991;25:258–269.

114. Falkson G, van Eden E, Sandison A. A controlled clinical trial of fluorouracil plus imidazole carboxamide dimethyl triazeno plus vincristine plus bis-chloroethyl plus radiotherapy in stomach cancer. *Med Pediatr Oncol* 1976;1976(2):111–120.

115. Klaassen DJ, MacIntyre JM, Catton GE. Treatment of locally unresectable cancer of the stomach and pancreas: A randomized comparison of 5-fluorouracil alone with radiation plus concurrent and maintenance 5-fluorouracil. *J Clin Oncol* 2000;3(1985):373–81.

116. Mantell BS. Radiotherapy for dysphagia due to gastric carcinoma. *Br J Surg* 2000;69(1982):69–75.

117. Rhomberg W, Bohler F, Eiter H. Radiotherapy and razoxane in the palliative treatment of gastric cancer. *Radiat Oncol Invest* 1996;4(1996):27–32.

118. Minsky BD, Wagman RT. Cancer of the stomach. In: Leibel SA, Phillips TL, eds. *Textbook of Radiation Oncology.* 2nd ed. Philadelphia, Pa.: WB Saunders; 2004:825–836.

119. Leong T, Willis D, Joon DL, Condron S, Hui A, Ngan SY. 3D conformal radiotherapy for gastric cancer—results of a comparative planning study. *Radiother Oncol* 2005;74(3):301–306.

120. Verheij M, Oppedijk V, Boot H, et al. Late renal toxicity following postoperative chemoradiotherapy in gastric cancer. Proceedings of the ASCO/AGA/ASTRO/SSO GI Symposium; 2005.

121. Archer S, Grey B. Intraperitoneal 5-fluorouracil infusion for treatment of both peritoneal and liver micro-metastasis. *Surgery* 1990;108:502.

122. Murthy S, Goldschmidt RA, Rao LN. The influence of surgical trauma on experimental metastasis. *Cancer* 1989;64:2035.

123. Gunduz N, Fisher B, Saffer E. Effect of surgical removal on the growth and kinetics of residual tumor. *Cancer Res* 1979(39):1361–1365.

124. Hagiwara A, Takahashi T, Kojima O, et al. Prophylaxis with carbon-adsorbed mitomycin against peritoneal recurrence of gastric cancer. *Lancet* 1992(339):629–631.

125. Ubhi SS, McCulloch P, Veitch PS. Preliminary results of the use of intraperitoneal carbon-adsorbed mitomycin C in intra-abdominal malignancy. *Br J Cancer* 1997;76(12):1667–1669.

126. Francois Y, Grandclement E, Sayag AC, et al. Intraperitoneal chemohyperthermia with mitomycin in cancer of the stomach with peritoneal carcinosis. *J Chir (Paris)* 1997;134(5–6):237–242.

127. Rosen HR, Jatzko G, Repse S, et al. Adjuvant intraperitoneal chemotherapy with carbon-adsorbed mitomycin in patients with gastric cancer: results of a randomized multicenter trial of the Austrian Working Group for Surgical Oncology. *J Clin Oncol* 1998;16(8):2733–2738.

128. Hall JJ, Loggie BW, Shen P, et al. Cytoreductive surgery with intraperitoneal hyperthermic chemotherapy for advanced gastric cancer. *J Gastrointest Surg* 2004;8(4):454.

129. Atig OT, Kelsen DP, Shiu MH, et al. Phase II trial of postoperative adjuvant intraperitoneal cisplatin and fluorouracil and systemic fluorouracil chemotherapy in patients with resected gastric cancer. *J Clin Oncol* 1993;11(3):425–433.

130. Yu W. A review of adjuvant therapy for resected primary gastric cancer with an update on Taegu's phase III trial with intraperitoneal chemotherapy. *Eur J Surg Oncol* 2006;32(6):655–660.

131. Schiessel R, Funovics J, Schick B, et al. Adjuvant intraperitoneal cisplatin therapy in patients with operated gastric carcinoma: results of a randomized trial. *Acta Med Austriaca* 1989;16:68–69.

132. Sautner T, Hofbauer F, Depisch D, Schiessel R, Jakesz R. Adjuvant intraperitoneal cisplatin chemotherapy does not improve long-term survival after surgery for advanced gastric cancer. *J Clin Oncol* 1994;12(5):970–974.

133. Koga S, Hamazoe R, Maeta M, Shimizu N, Murakami A, Wakatsuki T. Prophylactic therapy for peritoneal recurrence of gastric cancer by continuous hyperthermic peritoneal perfusion with mitomycin C. *Cancer* 1988;61: 232–237.

134. Fujimura T, Yonemura Y, Muraoka K, et al. Continuous hyperthermic peritoneal perfusion for the prevention of peritoneal recurrence of gastric cancer: randomized controlled study. *World J Surg* 1994;18(1):150–155.

135. Hamazoe R, Maeta M, Kaibara N. Intraperitoneal thermochemotherapy for prevention of peritoneal recurrence of gastric cancer. *Cancer* 1994;73: 2048.

136. Xu DZ, Zhan YQ, Sun XW, et al. Meta-analysis of intraperitoneal chemotherapy for gastric cancer. *World J Gastroenterol* 2004;10(18): 2727–2730.

137. Nakazato H, Koike A, Saji S, Ogawa N, Sakamoto J. Efficacy of immunochemotherapy as adjuvant treatment after curative resection of gastric cancer. *Lancet* 1994;(343):1122–1126.

138. Ochiai T, Sato H, Hayashi R, et al. Randomly controlled study of chemotherapy versus chemoimmunotherapy in postoperative gastric cancer patients. *Cancer Res* 1983;(43):3001–3007.

139. Kim JP, Kwon OJ, Oh ST, Yang HK. Results of surgery on 6589 gastric cancer patients and immunochemosurgery as the best treatment of advanced gastric cancer. *Ann Surg* 1992;(216):269–279.

140. Kim JP. Immunochemosurgery as a new approach to reasonable treatment of advanced cancer. *Ann Acad Med Singapore* 1988;17:48–54.

141. Kim SY, Park HC, Yoon C, Yoon HJ, Choi YM, Cho KS. OK-432 and 5-fluorouracil, doxorubicin, and mitomycin C (FAM-P) versus FAM chemotherapy in patients with curatively resected gastric carcinoma. *Cancer* 1998;83(10):2054–2059.

142. Sakamoto J, Teramukai S, Nakazato H, et al. Efficacy of adjuvant immunochemotherapy with OK-432 for patients with curatively resected gastric cancer: a meta-analysis of centrally randomized controlled clinical trials. *J Immunother* 2002;25(5):405–412.

143. Primrose JN, Miller GV, Preston SR, et al. A prospective randomised controlled study of the use of ranitidine in patients with gastric cancer. Yorkshire GI Tumour Group [see comments]. *Gut* 1998;42(1):17–19.

144. Langman MJ, Dunn JA, Whiting JL, et al. Prospective, double-blind, placebo-controlled randomized trial of cimetidine in gastric cancer. British Stomach Cancer Group. *Br J Cancer* 1999;81(8):1356–1362.

145. Harrison JD, Morris DL, Ellis IO, Jones JA, Jackson I. The effect of tamoxifen and estrogen receptor status on survival in gastric carcinoma. *Cancer* 1989;64:1007–1010.

146. Kelsen D, Karpeh M, Schwartz G, et al. Neoadjuvant therapy of high-risk gastric cancer: a phase II trial of preoperative FAMTX and postoperative intraperitoneal fluorouracil-cisplatin plus intravenous fluorouracil. *J Clin Oncol* 1996;(14):1818.

147. Ott K, Fink U, Becker K, et al. Prediction of response to preoperative chemotherapy in gastric carcinoma by metabolic imaging: results of a prospective trial. *J Clin Oncol* 2003;21(24):4604–4610.

148. Weber WA. Use of PET for monitoring cancer therapy and for predicting outcome. *J Nucl Med* 2005;46(6):983–995.

149. Kang YK, Choi DW, Im YH, et al. Phase III randomized comparison of neoadjuvant chemotherapy followed by surgery versus surgery for locally advanced stomach cancer. *Proc Am Soc Clin Oncol* 1996;14(503).

150. Cunningham D, Allum WH, Stenning SP, et al. Perioperative chemotherapy versus surgery alone for resectable gastroesophageal cancer. *N Engl J Med* 2006;355(1):11–20.

151. Bozzetti F, Bonfanti G, Audisio RA, et al. Prognosis of patients after palliative surgical procedures for carcinoma of the stomach. *Sug Gynecol Obstet* 1987;164:151–154.

152. Haugstvedt T, Viste A, Eide GE, Soreide O. The survival benefit of resection in patients with advanced stomach cancer: the Norwegian multicenter experience. Norwegian Stomach Cancer Trial. *World J Surg* 1989;13:617–621; discussion.

153. Meijer S, De Bakker OJGB, Hoitsma HFW. Palliative resection in gastric cancer. *J Surg Oncol* 1983;23:77.

154. Monson JR, Donohue JH, McIlrath DC, Farnell MB, Ilstrup DM. Total gastrectomy for advanced cancer. A worthwhile palliative procedure. *Cancer* 1991;68:1863–1868.

155. Baba JM, Haehara Y, Inutsuka S, et al. Effectiveness of extended lymphadenectomy in non-curative gastrectomy. *Am J Surg* 1995;169:261–264.

156. Wagner AD, Grothe W, Behl S, et al. The Cochrane Collaboration. The Cochrane Library 2006(1).

157. Glimelius B, Hoffman K, Haglund U. Initial or delayed chemotherapy with best supportive care in advanced gastric cancer. *Ann Oncol* 1994;5:189.

158. Ohtsu A, Shimada Y, Shirao K, et al. Randomized phase III trial of fluorouracil alone versus fluorouracil plus cisplatin versus uracil and tegafur plus mitomycin in patients with unresectable, advanced gastric cancer: the Japan Clinical Oncology Group study (JCOG9205). *J Clin Oncol* 2003;21(1):54–59.

159. Lutz M, Wilke H, Wagener D, et al. Weekly infusional high-dose fluorouracil (HO-FU), HD-FU plus folinic acid (HD-FU/FA) or HD-FU/FA plus biweekly cisplatin in advanced gastric cancer. *J Clin Oncol* 2007;25(18):2580–2585.

160. Berenberg JL, Tangen C, MacDonald JS, et al. Phase II study of 5-fluorouracil and folinic acid in the treatment of patients with advanced gastric cancer. A Southwest Oncology Group study. *Cancer* 1995;76(5):715–719.

161. Cullinan SA, Moertel CG, Wieand HS, et al. Controlled evaluation of three drug combination regimens versus fluorouracil alone for the therapy of advanced gastric cancer. North Central Cancer Treatment Group. *J Clin Oncol* 1994;12(2):412–416.

162. Chollet P, Schoffski P, Weigang-Kohler K, et al. Phase II trial with S-1 in chemotherapy-naive patients with gastric cancer. A trial performed by the EORTC Early Clinical Studies Group (ECSG). *Eur J Cancer* 2003;39(9):1264–1270.

163. Koizumi W, Kurihara M, Nakano S, Hasegawa K. Phase II study of S-1, a novel oral derivative of 5-fluorouracil, in advanced gastric cancer. For the S-1 Cooperative Gastric Cancer Study Group. *Oncology* 2000;58(3):191–197.

164. Otak Taguchit T, Kimura K. Report of a nationwide poll data and cohorted investigation in UFT phase II trials. *Cancer Chemother Pharmacol* 1998;22:333–338.

165. Ravaud A, Borner M, Schellens JH, et al. UFT and leucovorin in first-line chemotherapy for patients with metastatic gastric cancer. An Early Clinical Studies Group (ECSG)/European Organization for Research Treatment of Cancer (EORTC) phase II trial. *Eur J Cancer* 2001;37(13):1642–1647.

166. Cosimo D. Docetaxel in advanced gastric cancer. *Acta ancologica* 2003;42: 693–700.

167. Bugat R. Irinotecan in the treatment of gastric cancer. *Ann Oncol* 2003; 14(suppl 2):ii37–ii40.

168. Vanhoefer U, Rougier P, Hansjochen W, et al. Final results of a randomized phase III trial of sequential high-dose methotrexate, fluorouracil, and doxorubicin versus etoposide, leucovorin, and fluorouracil versus infusional fluorouracil and cisplatin in advanced gastric cancer: a trial of the European Organization for Research and Treatment of Cancer Gastrointestinal Tract Cancer Cooperative Group. *J Clin Oncol* 2000;18(14): 2648–2657.

169. Ohtsu A, Shimada T, Shirao K, et al. Randomized phase III trial of fluorouracil alone versus fluorouracil plus cisplatin versus uracil and tegafur plus mitomycin in patients with unresectable, advanced gastric cancer: The Japan Clinical Oncology Group Study (JCOG9205). *J Clin Oncol* 2003;21(1):54–59.

170. Moiseyenko VM, Ajani JA, Tjulandin SA, et al. Final results of a randomized controlled phase III trial (TAX 325) comparing docetaxel (T) combined with cisplatin (C) and 5-fluorouracil (F) to CF in patients (pts) with metastatic gastric adenocarcinoma (MGC). *ASCO; June 1*, 2005; Orlando, Fla.

171. Dank M, Zaluski J, Barone C, et al. Randomized phase III trial of irinotecan (CPT-11) + 5FU/folinic acid (FA) vs CDDP + 5Fu in 1st line advanced gastric cancer patients. ASCO; June 1, 2005; Orlando, Fla.

172. Pozzo C, Barone C, Szanto J, et al. Irinotecan in combination with 5-fluorouracil and folinic acid or with cisplatin in patients with advanced gastric or esophageal-gastric junction adenocarcinoma: results of a randomized phase II study. *Ann Oncol* 2004;15(12):1773–1781.

173. Waters JS, Norman A, Cunningham D, et al. Long-term survival after epirubicin, cisplatin and fluorouracil for gastric cancer: results of a randomized trial. *Br J Cancer* 1999;80(1–2):269–272.

174. Webb A, Cunningham D, Scarffe JH, et al. Randomized trial comparing epirubicin, cisplatin, and fluorouracil versus fluorouracil, doxorubicin, and methotrexate in advanced esophagogastric cancer. *J Clin Oncol* 1997;15(1):261–267.

175. Ross P, Nicolson M, Cunningham D, et al. Prospective randomized trial comparing mitomycin, cisplatin and protracted venous-infusion fluorouracil (PVI 5-FU) with epirubicin, cisplatin and PVI 5-FU in advanced esophagogastric cancer. *J Clin Oncol* 2002;20(8):1996–2004.

176. Ajani JA, Baker J, Pisters PW, et al. CPT-11 plus cisplatin in patients with advanced, untreated gastric or gastroesophageal junction carcinoma: results of a phase II study. *Cancer* 2002;94(3):641–646.

177. Yoshida M, Boku N, Ohtsu A, Muto M, Nagashima F, Yoshida S. Combination chemotherapy of irinotecan plus cisplatin for advanced gastric cancer: efficacy and feasibility in clinical practice. *Gastric Cancer* 2001;4(3):144–149.

178. Boku N, Ohtsu A, Shimada Y, et al. Phase II study of combination of irinotecan and cisplatin against metastatic gastric cancer. *J Clin Oncol* 1999;17(1):319–323.

179. Zaniboni A, Meriggi F. The emerging role of oxaliplatin in the treatment of gastric cancer. *J Chemother* 2005;17(6):656–662.

180. Cunningham D, Rao S, Starling N, et al. Randomised multicentre phase III study comparing capecitabine with fluorouracil and oxaliplatin with cisplatin in patients with advanced oesophagogastric cancer: the REAL 2 trial. *Proc Am Soc Clin Oncol* 2006;25:182S.

181. Al-Batran SE, Atmaca A, Hegewisch-Becker S, et al. Phase II trial of biweekly infusional fluorouracil, folinic acid, and oxaliplatin in patients with advanced gastric cancer. *J Clin Oncol* 2004;22(4):658–663.

182. Kang Y, Kang WK, Shin DB, et al. Randomized phase III trial of capecitabine/cisplatin (XP) vs. continuous infusion of 5-FU/cisplatin (FP)

as first-line therapy in patients (pts) with advanced gastric cancer (AGC): efficacy and safety results. *J Clin Oncol* 2006;24(18S) supplement.

183. Shah MA, Ilson D, Ramanathan RK, et al. A multicenter phase ii study of irinotecan (CPT), cisplatin (CIS), and bevacizumab gastroesophageal junction (GEJ) adenocarcinoma. *J Clin Oncol* 2006;24(18S):183.

184. Shah MA, Ilson D, Kelsen DP. Thromboembolic events in gastric cancer: high incidence in patients receiving irinotecan- and bevacizumab-based therapy. *J Clin Oncol* 2005;23(11):2574–2576.

185. Dragovich T, McCoy S, Urba SG, et al. Phase II trial of erlotinib in GEJ and gastric adenocarcinomas, SWOG 0127. *Proc Am Soc Clin Oncol* 2005; 25(49).

186. Lenz HJ, Leichman CG, Danenberg K, et al. Thymidylate synthase mRNA level in adenocarcinoma of the stomach: a predictor for primary tumor response and overall survival. *J Clin Oncol* 1995;14(1):176–182.

187. Metzger R, Leichman CG, Danenberg KD, et al. ERCC1 mRNA levels complement thymidylate synthase mRNA levels in predicting response and survival for gastric cancer patients receiving combination cisplatin and fluorouracil chemotherapy. *J Clin Oncol* 1998;16(1):309–316.

188. Fata F, Baylor L, Karpeh M, et al. Thymidylate synthase (TS) is not an independent predictor of outcome in patients with operable gastric cancer. *Proc ASCO* 1998;17:280a.

189. Boku N, Chin K, Hosokawa K, et al. Biological markers as a predictor for response and prognosis of unresectable gastric cancer patients treated with 5-fluorouracil and cis-platinum. *Clin Cancer Res* 1998;4(6):1469–1474.

190. Cascinu S, Graziano F, Del Ferro E, et al. Expression of p53 protein and resistance to preoperative chemotherapy in locally advanced gastric carcinoma. *Cancer* 1998;83(9):1917–1922.

191. Yeh KH, Shun CT, Chen CL, et al. Overexpression of p53 is not associated with drug resistance of gastric cancers to 5-fluorouracil-based systemic chemotherapy. *Hepatogastroenterology* 1999;46:610–615.

192. Baselga J. Herceptin alone or in combination with chemotherapy in the treatment of HER2-positive metastatic breast cancer: pivotal trials. *Oncology* 2001;61(suppl 2):14–21.

193. Lynch TJ, Bell DW, Sordella R, et al. Activating mutations in the epidermal growth factor receptor underlying responsiveness of non–small–cell lung cancer to gefitinib. *N Engl J Med* 2004;350(21):2129–2139.

194. Heinrich MC, Corless CL, Demetri GD, et al. Kinase mutations and imatinib response in patients with metastatic gastrointestinal stromal tumor. *J Clin Oncol* 2003;21(23):4342–4349.

195. Mellinghoff IK, Wang MY, Vivanco I, et al. Molecular determinants of the response of glioblastomas to EGFR kinase inhibitors. *N Engl J Med* 2005;353(19):2012–2024.

196. Ott K, Fink U, Becker K, et al. Prediction of response to preoperative chemotherapy in gastric carcinoma by metabolic imaging: results of a prospective trial. *J Clin Oncol* 2003;21(24):4604–4610.

197. Wieder HA, Beer AJ, Lordick F, et al. Comparison of changes in tumor metabolic activity and tumor size during chemotherapy of adenocarcinomas of the esophagogastric junction. *J Nucl Med* 2005;46(12):2029–2034.

198. Weber WA. Chaperoning drug development with PET. *J Nucl Med* 2006;47(5):735–737.

199. Luthra R, Wu T-T, Luthra MG, et al. Gene expression profiling of localized esophageal carcinomas: association with pathologic response to preoperative chemoradiation. *J Clin Oncol* 2006;24(2):259–267.

200. Ogata T. A 10-year experience of intraoperative radiotherapy for gastric carcinoma and a new surgical method of creating a wider irradiation field for cases of total gastrectomy patients. *Int J Radiat Oncol Biol Phys* 1995;32:341.

201. Coquard R, Ayzac L, Gilly FN. Intraoperative radiation therapy combined with limited lymph node resection in gastric cancer: an alternative to extended resection? *Int J Radiat Oncol Biol Phys* 1997;39(1997):1093–1098.

202. Calvo FA, Aristu JJ, Azinovic I, et al. Intraoperative and external radiotherapy in resected gastric cancer: updated report of a phase II trial. *Int J Radiat Oncol Biol Phys* 1992;24(4):729–736.

203. Avizonis VN, Buzydlowski J, Lanciano R. Treatment of adenocarcinoma of the stomach with resection, intraoperative radiotherapy, and adjuvant external beam radiation. A phase two study from Radiation Therapy Oncology Group. *J Surg Oncol* 1995;2:295–302.

204. Vanhoefer U, Rougier P, Wilke H, et al. Final results of a randomized phase III trial of sequential high-dose methotrexate, fluorouracil, and doxorubicin versus etoposide, leucovorin, and fluorouracil versus infusional fluorouracil and cisplatin in advanced gastric cancer: a trial of the European organization for research and treatment of Cancer Gastrointestinal Tract Cancer Cooperative Group. *J Clin Oncol* 2000;18(14):2648–2657.

PANCREATIC CANCER

CHAPTER 24 ■ PANCREAS CANCER: EPIDEMIOLOGY AND RISK FACTORS

ALBERT B. LOWENFELS AND PATRICK MAISONNEUVE

INTRODUCTION

Compared to other digestive tract tumors, pancreatic cancer is infrequent, with an estimated world yearly total of about 230,000 new patients. Approximately 60% of patients live in developed countries, compared to 40% in developing countries. In the United States, there are about 31,000 new cases per year.

Although the tumor is comparatively rare, the survival rate is lower than for other digestive tract tumors and accounts for this tumor being ranked fourth or fifth as a cause of cancer mortality in Western countries. Even with early diagnosis and prompt intervention, nearly all patients who are diagnosed with pancreatic cancer tumor will eventually die from their cancer. A recent review of long-term survivors from the Finnish cancer registry discovered that the original diagnosis of pancreas cancer was often incorrect (1).

An additional difficulty with respect to pancreatic cancer is that it is located in the retroperitoneal space, where direct access for diagnostic purposes is much more difficult than in the tubular parts of the digestive tract. Although there has been substantial progress in visualizing the pancreas with new methodology such as helical computed tomography (CT) scans and endoscopic ultrasound, detecting pancreatic lesions is still not as simple as direct endoscopy, which can easily detect tumors in the upper and lower gastrointestinal tract—the most common sites for digestive cancer.

DESCRIPTIVE EPIDEMIOLOGY

Globally, pancreatic cancer is a rare tumor; it is much less common than breast, stomach, liver, large bowel, and prostate cancers, which comprise the bulk of world cancer. However, its high mortality makes pancreatic cancer the eighth most common international cause of cancer. Predictably, as lifespan in developing countries increases, this tumor will become even more frequent.

Age-Specific Rates

Similar to other digestive tract cancers, pancreatic cancer rates increase exponentially with age. Indeed, increasing age is the strongest known risk factor for pancreatic cancer; unfortunately, this risk factor is irreversible. The mean age at onset of pancreatic cancer is in the mid-60s, with only 10% of patients developing the tumor at or younger than age 50. In developed countries, cumulative risks (i.e., the probability of developing pancreatic cancer up to a given age, such as 65 or 70 years) is generally <1% for males and slightly less for females. Globally, the cumulative risk is 0.2% for males and 0.1% for females.

At present, surgery offers the best hope for increased survival from pancreatic cancer. However, the bulk of pancreatic cancer unfortunately occurs in elderly patients who often suffer from additional comorbidities, making them unsuitable for surgery. As an example, in New York State for the year 2001, only 15% of all patients with a diagnosis of pancreatic cancer underwent pancreatectomy—the best procedure for increasing survival.

Gender-Specific Differences

There are observable gender-specific differences in the overall frequency of pancreatic cancer (Table 24.1). A small fraction of these differences may be related to hormonal variations between males and females, but because smoking is the best known risk factor for pancreatic cancer, the main cause for the difference has to do with an excess of smoking in males as compared with females.

Racial Differences

Rates for pancreatic cancer are different in different racial groups. Black/white differences are particularly striking. For example, in a study from California, Chang et al. found that pancreatic cancer rates were about 50% higher in African Americans than in Caucasians (Table 24.2). Asian populations had the lowest rates (2). The explanation is not clear but could be due to racial differences in frequency of previously recognized risk factors (3).

Global Differences

Internationally, there are rather marked differences in mortality rates of pancreatic cancer (Table 24.3, Fig. 24.1). Low rates are found in Africa and parts of Asia; high rates are found in Australia/New Zealand, Europe, and North America. The average world age-standardized mortality rate is about 4.5/100,000/year.

TIME TRENDS

Even in the absence of any treatment-related factors, we can anticipate that there will be changes in the incidence and subsequent mortality of pancreatic cancer. With increasing longevity of population of several non-Western countries such as India

TABLE 24.1

SELECTED AGE-STANDARDIZED PANCREATIC CANCER INCIDENCE RATES PER 100,000 BY GENDER AND REGION, 1993–1997

Cancer registry	Men	Women
AMERICA		
Colombia, Cali	4.6	4.4
Costa Rica	4.0	3.5
Ecuador, Quito	3.9	3.7
Canada	7.3	5.6
United States, SEER: white	7.4	5.6
United States, SEER: black	12.8	9.2
ASIA		
China, Shanghai	5.6	4.8
India, Bombay	2.5	1.9
Israel: Jews	7.2	5.0
Japan, Osaka Prefecture	9.4	5.5
Philippines, Manila	3.9	3.8
Singapore: Chinese	5.4	3.3
Thailand, Chiang Mai	1.7	2.0
EUROPE		
Belarus	8.1	3.7
Czech Republic	11.3	7.0
Denmark	7.3	5.9
Estonia	11.5	5.3
Finland	8.9	6.3
France, Isere	7.5	4.8
Germany, Saarland	6.4	5.3
Iceland	7.3	6.1
Italy, Florence	7.7	5.4
Latvia	12.1	5.5
The Netherlands, Eindhoven	5.7	3.8
Norway	7.5	5.8
Poland, Lower Silesia	9.7	5.9
Slovakia	9.9	5.3
Slovenia	7.4	4.8
Spain, Navarra	8.2	4.4
Sweden	6.3	5.4
Switzerland, Zurich	7.1	4.4
UK, England, South Thames	7.5	5.2
OCEANIA		
Australia, New South Wales	6.4	5.0
New Zealand	6.4	5.0

SEER, Surveillance, Epidemiology, and End Results.
Data from ref. 48.

TABLE 24.2

RACE-SPECIFIC, AGE-ADJUSTED INCIDENCE RATES FOR PANCREATIC CANCER (MALES AND FEMALES COMBINED) IN CALIFORNIA, 1988–1998

Characteristics	No.	Incidence/100,000 (95% CI)
Race/ethnicity		
All races/ethnicities	16,679	5.8 (5.7–5.9)
Non-Hispanic whites	12,243	5.9 (5.8–6.0)
Hispanics	1,942	5.1 (4.9–5.3)
Asian/Pacific Islanders	1,069	4.8 (4.5–5.0)
African Americans	1,361	8.8 (8.3–9.3)

CI, confidence interval.
From ref. 2

ios (4). Unlike aging, where the effect of age on incidence will occur rapidly, the beneficial effects of smoking cessation will be more gradual because there is a time lag of 10 years after smoking cessation before the excess risk diminishes (5).

RISK FACTORS

Smoking

Of the several risk factors that are known to be linked with pancreatic cancer, smoking has been the most extensively studied. Research on smoking and lung cancer published in the 1960s led to an early publication on smoking as a risk factor for pancreatic cancer. Based on a case-control study of 100 patients with biopsy-proven pancreatic tumors and 194 control subjects, Wynder et al. detected a twofold increase in the risk of pancreatic cancer (6). This finding has been confirmed in nearly all subsequent publications that examined the relationship between smoking and lung cancer. The main findings are as follows:

- Smokers have a twofold increased risk of pancreatic cancer compared to nonsmokers.
- About 25% to 30% of all pancreatic cancer is caused by this single factor.
- There is a measurable dose response.
- Cigarettes are more harmful than other types of smoking exposure, but other tobacco delivery agents such as smokeless tobacco can cause pancreatic cancer (7,8).
- The lag period of approximately 40 years from onset of smoking to onset of pancreatic cancer is somewhat longer than the lag period from smoking to the onset of lung cancer.

Drinking

Heavy consumption of alcohol is the most common known risk factor for chronic pancreatitis, so it is reasonable to assume that alcohol might be a risk factor for pancreatic cancer. However, numerous studies of moderate drinkers have failed to find any link between consuming alcohol and pancreatic cancer. The best explanation is that the pancreas must be less sensitive to the toxic effects of alcohol than, say, the liver, where an occasional moderate drinker develops alcohol-induced cirrhosis eventually leading to liver cancer.

and China added to the already aging populations of Western countries, there will be a global increase in the number of elderly persons where the risk of pancreatic cancer is high. Therefore, based just on demographics, the number of patients diagnosed with pancreatic cancer will increase.

Smoking prevalence is the second important factor that will alter the incidence of pancreatic cancer. In the United States, the incidence of pancreatic cancer has already declined as a result of a decrease in smoking prevalence; this trend is more prominent in males than in females (Fig. 24.2). Several European countries have instituted partial restrictions on smoking that could eventually result in an overall reduction in smoking prevalence. Mulder et al. estimated the absolute reduction in pancreatic cancer deaths in relation to several different smoking scenar-

TABLE 24.3

ESTIMATED WORLD STANDARDIZED PANCREATIC CANCER MORTALITY RATES
PER 100,000 BY GENDER IN DIFFERENT GEOGRAPHIC AREAS, 2002

Country/region	Males		Females	
	Deaths	Rate	Deaths	Rate
World	119,544	4.4	107,479	3.3
More developed regions	71,119	8.0	67,549	5.4
Less developed regions	48,186	2.6	39,757	2.0
Eastern Africa	1,143	2.0	1,082	1.6
Middle Africa	324	1.3	1,069	3.7
Northern Africa	810	1.5	603	1.0
Southern Africa	240	1.8	220	1.2
Western Africa	698	1.2	704	1.1
Caribbean	706	4.1	668	3.3
Central America	1,931	4.4	2,244	4.4
South America	6,631	5.0	6,839	4.2
Northern America	16,598	7.7	17,022	6.0
Eastern Asia	34,512	4.4	26,818	3.1
South-Eastern Asia	3,424	1.8	2,929	1.4
South-Central Asia	7,048	1.3	4,451	0.8
Western Asia	1,902	2.9	1,347	1.9
Central and Eastern Europe	15,555	8.5	13,511	4.5
Northern Europe	5,603	7.2	6,132	5.8
Southern Europe	8,708	7.2	7,891	4.7
Western Europe	12,597	8.3	12,864	5.9
Australia/New Zealand	1,087	6.5	1,057	5.2
Australia	922	6.6	885	5.2
New Zealand	165	6.4	171	5.4

Data from ref. 49.

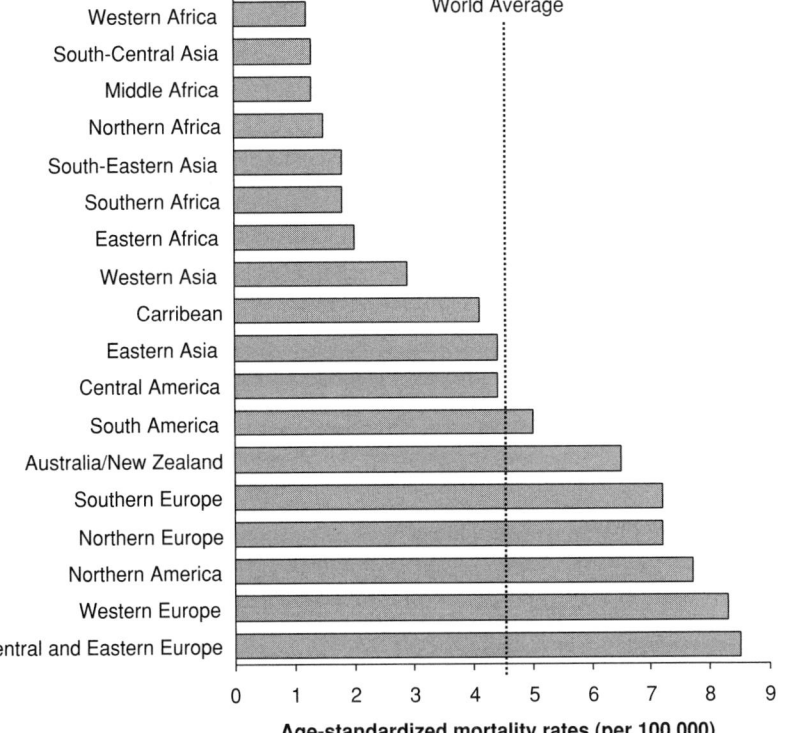

FIGURE 24.1. Estimated world standardized pancreatic cancer mortality rates per 100,000 in different geographic areas, 2002 (males). *Source:* Data from ref. 49.

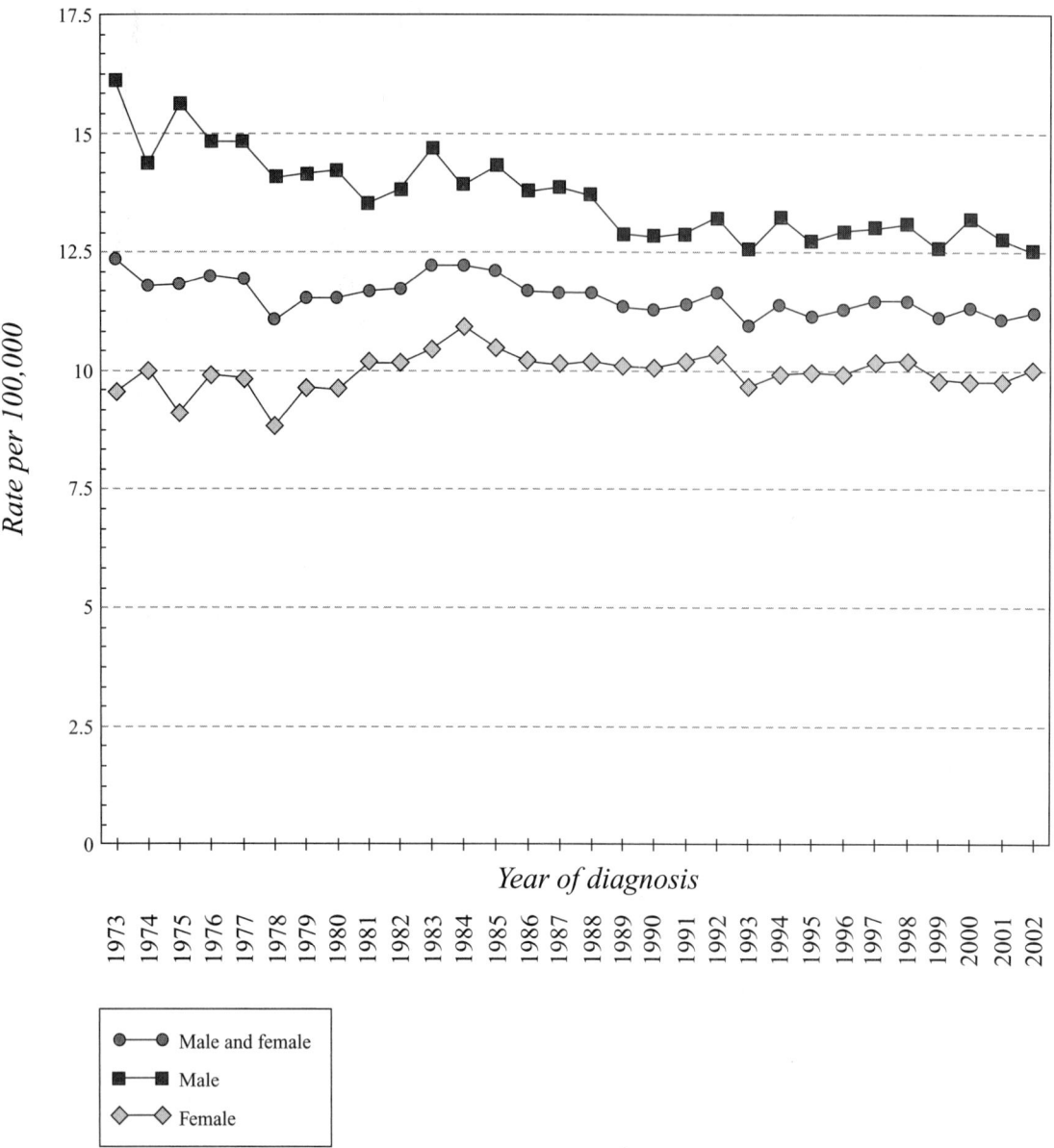

FIGURE 24.2. Age-standardized incidence rates per 100,000 for pancreatic cancer in the United States, 1973–2002. *Source:* From ref. 66.

Because heavy drinkers are nearly always heavy smokers, it is likely that any putative association between heavy drinking and pancreatic cancer can be explained by tobacco exposure, rather than by alcohol.

Diet

For many reasons, finding reliable evidence linking diet with pancreatic cancer has been difficult. Because the disease is so aggressive, recruitment of patients for case-control studies has been difficult and is certain to introduce unavoidable biases favoring patients with less aggressive disease. In any event, case-control studies are likely to be less informative than prospective studies, but only a few prospective studies have been performed because they are costly, time consuming, and require extremely accurate follow-up over prolonged time periods. For cancer to develop after any putative risk factor, there must be a prolonged exposure period. This causes a final difficulty—it is difficult to measure early dietary exposure, which is likely to be at least if not more important than recent dietary intake.

In one large prospective study performed in male smokers, a high intake of saturated fat increased the risk of pancreatic cancer by 40%. However, a strange finding in this study was that high intake of energy and carbohydrates lowered the risk (9). In another large prospective study of more than 124,000 persons, Michaud et al. failed to find any relationship between dietary patterns and the risk of pancreatic cancer (10). In contrast, a case-control study performed by Nkondjock et al. found that consumption of fruits and vegetables reduced the risk of pancreatic cancer (11). Omega-3 fatty acids have been suspected to be a beneficial dietary component, but a recent meta-analysis failed to find any reduction in the risk of pancreatic cancer (12).

Do dietary supplements reduce the risk of pancreatic cancer? This important area has been inadequately studied; one report suggests that neither beta-carotene nor alpha-tocopherol have any impact on the risk of pancreatic cancer (13).

TABLE 24.4

RISK OF PANCREATIC CANCER MORTALITY ACCORDING TO BODY MASS INDEX (BMI) AMONG MALES AND FEMALES IN THE CANCER PREVENTION STUDY II, 1982–1998

Gender	<25	25+	30+	35+	40+	p for Trend
			BMI			
Males	1	1.13 (1.0–1.2)	1.4 (1.2–1.7)	1.5 (0.99–2.2)		<0.001
Females	1	1.11 (1.0–1.2)	1.3 (1.1–1.5)	1.4 (1.0–2.0)	2.8 (1.7–4.4)	<0.001

Data from ref. 14.

As for many other types of cancer, the link between diet and pancreatic cancer remains elusive. However, rather than looking for a link between any individual dietary component and cancer, obesity resulting from either excessive caloric intake or reduced caloric expenditure may be the key factor. In a prospective study of 900,000 persons conducted by the American Cancer Society, obesity was strongly related to pancreatic cancer for both males and females (14) (Table 24.4).

In summary, we know less about diet as a risk factor for pancreatic cancer than we should, but available evidence is sufficient to recommend maintaining a normal body weight. Consuming healthy amounts of fruits and vegetables, although not of proven benefit, may also be helpful.

Diabetes

Diabetes afflicts at least 5% of adults in the United States, and because of the strong link between obesity and diabetes, the frequency of diabetes is increasing over time. Even though diabetes can be an early symptom in some patients with pancreatic cancer, nearly all published reports have found a link between diabetes and the subsequent development of pancreatic cancer. A meta-analysis based on 35 case-control and prospective studies detected a gender- and sex-adjusted odds ratio of 1.82 (95% CI, 1.66–1.89) (15). Results were stronger for studies with follow-up of less than 5 years, where pancreatic cancer may have already been present in some of the diabetic patients. However, in prospective studies, the excess risk persisted even after a follow-up period of more than 10 years (Fig. 24.3).

If diabetes is a risk factor for pancreatic cancer, is there a relationship between fasting blood sugar and pancreatic cancer? A large 10-year prospective study based on 1,298,385 Korean subjects found that the incidence of pancreatic cancer increased with increasing levels of fasting blood sugar (16). The authors concluded that elevated blood sugar levels and diabetes are

independent risk factors for this tumor (Table 24.5). The explanation for the association between diabetes and pancreatic cancer may be exposure to higher insulin levels and/or insulin resistance (17).

Pancreatitis

In all other parts of the digestive tract, prior inflammatory disease is a strong risk factor for pancreatic cancer. Is this true for the pancreas? Anecdotal evidence from individual case reports or case series provides weak evidence to support this concept. Stronger evidence comes from case-control studies, prospective studies, and record linkage studies. Nearly all reports confirm a link between chronic pancreatitis and pancreatic cancer. Fig. 24.4 describes a proposed pathway linking acute pancreatitis, chronic pancreatitis, and pancreatic cancer (18). Only a few patients with acute pancreatitis ever develop chronic pancreatitis, and similarly, pancreatic cancer is a rare complication of pancreatitis. The cumulative 20-year incidence of pancreatic cancer in patients with chronic pancreatitis is only about 5% (19).

In most studies, alcohol has not been a suspected risk factor of pancreatic cancer, but heavy drinking is a common cause for chronic pancreatitis. Thus, it is possible that alcohol, especially when consumed in large amounts, can lead first to chronic pancreatitis, and then in a small fraction of patients, to pancreatic cancer. The mechanism might be related to production of acetaldehyde, a degradation product of alcohol metabolism and a known carcinogen (20). Smoking is an important cofactor; most heavy drinkers are smokers, and smoking is a risk factor for both pancreatitis (21) and pancreatic cancer.

Mutations in K-ras are found in approximately 80% of patients with pancreatic cancer. They can sometimes be detected in patients with chronic pancreatitis; as the duration of pancreatitis increases, the proportion of patients with K-ras

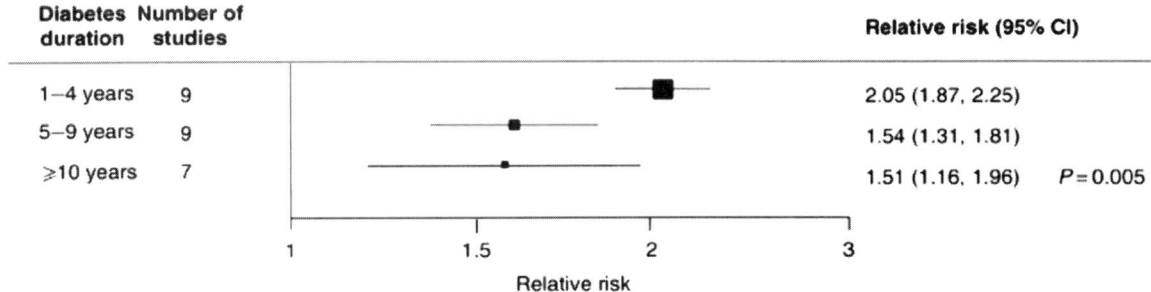

FIGURE 24.3. Association between preexisting diabetes and pancreas cancer stratified by duration of diabetes. *Source:* From ref. 15, with permission.

TABLE 24.5

RISK (HAZARD RATIO) OF PANCREATIC CANCER IN RELATION TO FASTING
GLUCOSE LEVEL AND PRESENCE OF DIABETES

Gender	<90	Fasting serum glucose (mg/dL) 90–109	110–125	126–139	140+	Diabetes
Male	1	1.1 (0.95–1.2)	1.3 (1.1–1.6)	1.4 (0.94–2.0)	2.1 (1.7–2.6)[a]	1.8 (1.5–2.1)
Female	1	1.3 (1.0–1.6)	1.4 (0.96–2.0)	2.0 (1.1–3.5)	1.7 (1.1–2.6)[b]	1.6 (1.1–2.1)

[a]p Value for trend = 0.03.
[b]p Value for trend = 0.04.
Data from ref. 16.

mutations increases (22). In a follow-up study of patients with chronic pancreatitis, pancreatic ductal adenocarcinoma developed in 4 of 44 patients with a K-ras mutations, compared to no cases in 68 K-ras–negative patients (23). When combined with other markers, the presence of K-ras mutations in patients with chronic pancreatitis may be useful as a screening tool for detecting early pancreatic cancer. Loss of p16 expression has also been observed in chronic pancreatitis and may be an additional factor in the development of pancreatic cancer (24).

Although alcoholic pancreatitis is the most common cause of pancreatitis, there are other causes. Hereditary pancreatitis is a rare genetic cause of chronic pancreatitis with an onset in childhood or early adulthood. The risk of pancreatic cancer is 40 to 50 times greater than in the background population. Similarly, tropical pancreatitis, which is common in southern India and parts of Africa, also has a high risk of pancreatic cancer (25).

Even though there seems to be a firm link between chronic pancreatitis and pancreatic cancer, the exact causal mechanism needs further investigation. Increased pancreatic cell turnover in patients with chronic pancreatitis could lead to defective DNA repair—a suspected cause of many human tumors.

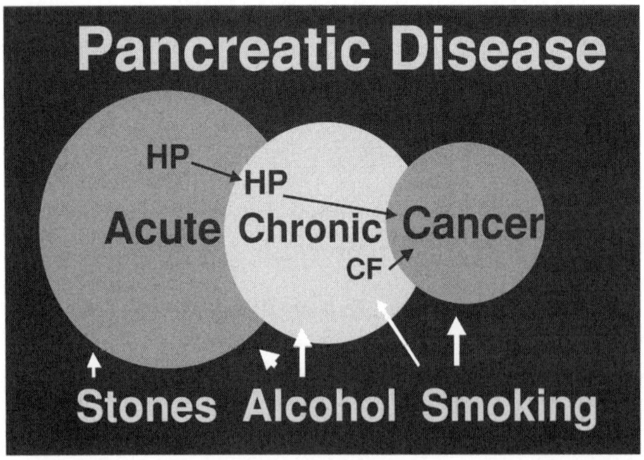

FIGURE 24.4. Possible relationship among acute pancreatitis, chronic pancreatitis, and pancreatic cancer. Shaded areas show extent of overlap between acute and chronic pancreatitis and between chronic pancreatitis and pancreatic cancer. Major risk factors are shown at the bottom of the diagram. Circle size approximates relative incidence of the three diseases. CF, cystic fibrosis; HP, hereditary pancreatitis. *Source:* From ref. 18 (See also color Figure 24.4).

Allergy

Some studies have found that allergic individuals have a decreased cancer risk, suggesting that allergy might be protective against pancreatic cancer. This hypothesis was investigated in a meta-analysis of 13 population-based studies, yielding evidence that allergic individuals do have a reduced risk of pancreatic cancer (RR = 0.7; 95% CI, 0.6–0.8) (26).

Occupation

Occupational exposure has not been proven to be a strong risk factor for pancreatic cancer; considerably <5% of all pancreatic cancers are believed to be due to work-related chemical exposure. A few studies have suggested a weak association between pesticide exposure of various types and pancreatic cancer; however, as in many occupational studies, it is difficult to adjust for other risk factors such as smoking, diabetes, or obesity (27,28). In a more recent case-control study where it was possible to adjust for smoking, diet, and family history, a few occupations, such as working with chemicals and transportation, had an increased risk of pancreatic cancer (29).

Aspirin and Nonsteroidal Antiinflammatory Drugs

Aspirin or other antiinflammatory drugs reduce the risk of colon cancer; do these agents also have a beneficial effect on pancreatic cancer? Aspirin has been the most widely studied drug, but unlike heart disease, where aspirin is clearly an effective preventive drug, the results are inconclusive (30–34). In two studies, aspirin use was associated with an increased risk of pancreatic cancer (35,36). It seems unlikely that aspirin will become an effective preventive agent against pancreatic cancer.

Infectious Agents

Is there evidence to support the hypothesis that an infectious agent could cause pancreatic cancer? Infectious agents are known to cause cancers of the liver, stomach, and cervix—three of the most common tumors throughout the world. Also, viral and other infectious agents are known to cause pancreatic disease (37). The mumps virus is pancreaticotrophic and can even lead to calcific pancreatitis (38). So, it is conceivable that a viral or bacterial agent might cause pancreatic cancer either directly or indirectly by first causing pancreatitis.

TABLE 24.6

RELATION BETWEEN *HELICOBACTER PYLORI* INFECTION AND PANCREATIC CANCER

Reference	Study type	No. pancreas cancers	Main finding
Borgström et al. (50)	Cohort	75	No increase over controls; patients were young
Nilsson et al. (51)	Case-control	6	5/6 Ductal pancreas cancer specimens were positive for *Helicobacter* by PCR with genus-specific primers compared with 0/3 controls
Stolzenberg-Solomon et al. (52)	Nested case-control within a prospective study	121	Odds ratio was 1.87 (95% CI, 1.05–3.34) for pancreas cancer patients seropositive for *H. pylori* CagA+
Raderer et al. (53)	Case-control	92	Odds ratio 2.1 (95% CI, 1.1–4.1) for pancreas cancer patients seropositive for *H. pylori* compared with controls without gastric cancer

PCR, polymerase chain reaction; CI, confidence interval.

TABLE 24.7

GERMLINE DISEASES ASSOCIATED WITH PANCREAS CANCER

Disease	Affected chromosome	Remarks
Familial pancreas cancer (U.S. National Familial Pancreatic Tumor Registry)	?	5- to 10-fold risk for first-degree relatives (54).
Familial pancreas cancer (Seattle cohort)	4q 32–34 (Unconfirmed)	High risk of pancreas cancer, pancreatitis, and diabetes. Smokers develop early onset pancreas cancer (44).
Hereditary nonpolyposis colon cancer	2,3	Some persons may develop pancreas cancer (55).
von Hippel-Lindau syndrome	3p25	Neuroendocrine tumors of pancreas are frequent (56).
Familial adenomatous polyposis	5q12–21	Mutation found in pancreas and in ampullary cancers (57).
Hereditary pancreatitis	7q35	Cumulative risk pancreas cancer at least 30% (58).
Familial atypical malignant melanoma syndrome	9p21	Patients carrying the p16 Leiden mutation have a 17% cumulative risk of pancreas cancer (59).
BRCA2	13	Most common inherited mutation leading to pancreas cancer (60).
Peutz-Jeghers syndrome	19p	Mutation may contribute to both sporadic and inherited disease (61).
Cystic fibrosis	7q31	Increased risk of digestive cancer, including pancreas tumors (62,63).
Ataxia-telangiectasia	11q	Breast cancer is most common tumor; a few patients with pancreas cancer (64).
Li-Fraumeni syndrome	17p13.1	Defect in *p53*. Moderate increased risk of pancreas cancer.
Fanconi anemia	Multiple chromosomes, including 3p22–26, 9p13, 9q22.3, 16q24.3	A few patients younger than 50 years with pancreas cancer carry FANCC or FANCG genes (65).

Helicobacter pylori is known to increase the risk of gastric cancer. Could it also cause pancreatic cancer? Three of the four studies that have examined this problem have noted an increased risk of pancreatic cancer following *Helicobacter pylori* infection. Patients in the single negative study were somewhat younger than patients in the other studies. The results are suggestive but not conclusive (Table 24.6).

INHERITED DISEASES AND PANCREATIC CANCER

Inherited germline disorders are suspected to cause no more than 5% to 10% of all pancreatic cancer, although the frequency was considerably lower in one carefully studied European population (39). The mode of inheritance is currently unproven, although the evidence from families with multiple afflicted members favors autosomal dominant inheritance of a rare allele with incomplete penetrance (40). There is some evidence for anticipation in that the disease appears to occur earlier in recent compared to older generations (41).

BRCA2, one of the two inherited genes known to cause breast cancer, has also been associated with pancreatic cancer. In a study of European families with at least two first-degree members afflicted with pancreatic cancer, BRCA2 mutations were the most common detected germline mutations, afflicting 19% of the families. Many of the families with this mutation had early onset pancreatic cancer. Table 24.7 lists several inherited germline disorders known to increase the risk of pancreatic cancer.

What is the impact on pancreatic cancer risk if a person with a known or suspected germline disorder is exposed to another risk factor, such as tobacco smoke? Several studies have looked at the interaction between smoking and genetics. Schenk et al. found an approximately eightfold increased risk of pancreatic cancer in persons who smoked and had a family member with early onset of pancreatic cancer (42). In patients with hereditary pancreatitis, smoking lowers the age of onset of pancreatic cancer by about 20 years (43). In a high-risk group of patients with familial pancreatic cancer, smoking was an independent risk factor and lowered the age of onset by about a decade (44).

In patients with sporadic rather than familial pancreatic cancer, heavy smokers with a deletion of the carcinogen-metabolizing GSTT-1 polymorphic gene have an increased risk of pancreatic cancer (45). Polymorphic genes that detoxify carcinogens may also be important for familial pancreatic cancer but have not been intensively investigated.

PREVENTION OF PANCREATIC CANCER

With an anticipated age-related increase in the frequency of pancreatic cancer, are there any preventive measures that will reduce the burden of this lethal tumor? The current most effective measure on the individual and population level is to reduce exposure to tobacco because smoking causes about one-fourth of all pancreatic cancer. Other measures, such as dietary intervention, are likely to be less effective, but maintaining normal body weight either by diet or exercise may be beneficial.

Screening for pancreatic cancer is currently not recommended, except for in very high-risk individuals, such as in those rare persons with hereditary pancreatitis or in selected individuals with a strong history of familial pancreatic cancer (46). The early results of screening family members who have three or more close relatives with pancreatic cancer appear promising (47).

References

1. Carpelan-Holmstrom M, Nordling S, Pukkala E, et al. Does anyone survive pancreatic ductal adenocarcinoma? A nationwide study re-evaluating the data of the Finnish Cancer Registry. *Gut* 2005;54(3):385–387.
2. Chang KJ, Parasher G, Christie C, Largent J, Anton-Culver H. Risk of pancreatic adenocarcinoma: disparity between African Americans and other race/ethnic groups. *Cancer* 2005;103(2):349–357.
3. Silverman DT, Hoover RN, Brown LM, et al. Why do black Americans have a higher risk of pancreatic cancer than white Americans? *Epidemiology* 2003;14(1):45–54.
4. Mulder I, Hoogenveen RT, van Genugten ML, et al. Smoking cessation would substantially reduce the future incidence of pancreatic cancer in the European Union. *Eur J Gastroenterol Hepatol* 2002;14(12):1343–1353.
5. Silverman DT, Dunn JA, Hoover RN, et al. Cigarette smoking and pancreas cancer: a case-control study based on direct interviews. *J Natl Cancer Inst* 1994;86(20):1510–1516.
6. Wynder EL, Mabuchi K, Maruchi N, Fortner JG. Epidemiology of cancer of the pancreas. *J Natl Cancer Inst* 1973;50:645–667.
7. Boffetta P, Aagnes B, Weiderpass E, Andersen A. Smokeless tobacco use and risk of cancer of the pancreas and other organs. *Int J Cancer* 2005;114(6):992–995.
8. Alguacil J, Silverman DT. Smokeless and other noncigarette tobacco use and pancreatic cancer: a case-control study based on direct interviews. *Cancer Epidemiol Biomarkers Prev* 2004;13(1):55–58.
9. Stolzenberg-Solomon RZ, Pietinen P, Taylor PR, Virtamo J, Albanes D. Prospective study of diet and pancreatic cancer in male smokers. *Am J Epidemiol* 2002;155(9):783–792.
10. Michaud DS, Skinner HG, Wu K, et al. Dietary patterns and pancreatic cancer risk in men and women. *J Natl Cancer Inst* 2005;97(7):518–524.
11. Nkondjock A, Krewski D, Johnson KC, Ghadirian P. Dietary patterns and risk of pancreatic cancer. *Int J Cancer* 2005;114(5):817–823.
12. MacLean CH, Newberry SJ, Mojica WA, et al. Effects of omega-3 fatty acids on cancer risk: a systematic review. *JAMA* 2006;295(4):403–415.
13. Rautalahti MT, Virtamo JR, Taylor PR, et al. The effects of supplementation with alpha-tocopherol and beta-carotene on the incidence and mortality of carcinoma of the pancreas in a randomized, controlled trial. *Cancer* 1999;86(1):37–42.
14. Calle EE, Rodriguez C, Walker-Thurmond K, Thun MJ. Overweight, obesity, and mortality from cancer in a prospectively studied cohort of U.S. adults. *N Engl J Med* 2003;348(17):1625–1638.
15. Huxley R, Ansary-Moghaddam A, Berrington DG, Barzi F, Woodward M. Type-II diabetes and pancreatic cancer: a meta-analysis of 36 studies. *Br J Cancer* 2005;92(11):2076–2083.
16. Jee SH, Ohrr H, Sull JW, Yun JE, Ji M, Samet JM. Fasting serum glucose level and cancer risk in Korean men and women. *JAMA* 2005;293(2):194–202.
17. Stolzenberg-Solomon RZ, Graubard BI, Chari S, et al. Insulin, glucose, insulin resistance, and pancreatic cancer in male smokers. *JAMA* 2005; 294(22):2872–2878.
18. Lowenfels AB, Maisonneuve P. Pancreas cancer: epidemiology and risk factors. In: Kelsen DP, Daly JM, Kern SE, Levin B, Tepper JE, eds. *Gastrointestinal Oncology: Principles and Practice*. Philadelphia, Pa.: Lippincott Williams & Wilkins; 2002:425–433.
19. Lowenfels AB, Maisonneuve P, Cavallini G, et al. Pancreatitis and the risk of pancreatic cancer. International Pancreatitis Study Group. *N Engl J Med* 1993;328:1433–1437.
20. Go VL, Gukovskaya A, Pandol SJ. Alcohol and pancreatic cancer. *Alcohol* 2005;35(3):205–211.
21. Maisonneuve P, Lowenfels AB, Mullhaupt B, et al. Cigarette smoking accelerates progression of alcoholic chronic pancreatitis. *Gut* 2005;54(4):510–514.
22. Lohr M, Kloppel G, Maisonneuve P, Lowenfels AB, Luttges J. Frequency of K-ras mutations in pancreatic intraductal neoplasias associated with pancreatic ductal adenocarcinoma and chronic pancreatitis: a meta-analysis. *Neoplasia* 2005;7(1):17–23.
23. Arvanitakis M, Van Laethem JL, Parma J, De Maertelaer V, Delhaye M, Deviere J. Predictive factors for pancreatic cancer in patients with chronic pancreatitis in association with K-ras gene mutation. *Endoscopy* 2004;36(6):535–542.
24. Rosty C, Geradts J, Sato N, et al. p16 Inactivation in pancreatic intraepithelial neoplasias (PanINs) arising in patients with chronic pancreatitis. *Am J Surg Pathol* 2003;27(12):1495–1501.
25. Tandon RK, Garg PK. Tropical pancreatitis. *Dig Dis* 2004;22(3):258–266.
26. Gandini S, Lowenfels AB, Jaffee EM, Armstrong TD, Maisonneuve P. Allergies and the risk of pancreatic cancer: a meta-analysis with review of epidemiology and biological mechanisms. *Cancer Epidemiol Biomarkers Prev* 2005;14(8):1908–1916.
27. Ji BT, Silverman DT, Stewart PA, et al. Occupational exposure to pesticides and pancreatic cancer. *Am J Ind Med* 2001;39(1):92–99.
28. Alguacil J, Kauppinen T, Porta M, et al. Risk of pancreatic cancer and occupational exposures in Spain. PANKRAS II Study Group. *Ann Occup Hyg* 2000;44(5):391–403.
29. Zhang Y, Cantor KP, Lynch CF, Zhu Y, Zheng T. Occupation and risk of pancreatic cancer: a population-based case-control study in Iowa. *J Occup Environ Med* 2005;47(4):392–398.

30. Schreinemachers DM, Everson RB. Aspirin use and lung, colon, and breast cancer incidence in a prospective study. *Epidemiology* 1994;5(2):138–146.
31. Coogan PF, Rosenberg L, Palmer JR, et al. Nonsteroidal anti-inflammatory drugs and risk of digestive cancers at sites other than the large bowel. *Cancer Epidemiol Biomarkers Prev* 2000;9(1):119–123.
32. Menezes RJ, Huber KR, Mahoney MC, Moysich KB. Regular use of aspirin and pancreatic cancer risk. *BMC Public Health* 2002;2(1):18.
33. Anderson KE, Johnson TW, Lazovich D, Folsom AR. Association between nonsteroidal anti-inflammatory drug use and the incidence of pancreatic cancer. *J Natl Cancer Inst* 2002;94(15):1168–1171.
34. Jacobs EJ, Connell CJ, Rodriguez C, Patel AV, Calle EE, Thun MJ. Aspirin use and pancreatic cancer mortality in a large United States cohort. *J Natl Cancer Inst* 2004;96(7):524–528.
35. Langman MJ, Cheng KK, Gilman EA, Lancashire RJ. Effect of anti-inflammatory drugs on overall risk of common cancer: case-control study in general practice research database. *BMJ* 2000;320(7250):1642–1646.
36. Schernhammer ES, Kang JH, Chan AT, et al. A prospective study of aspirin use and the risk of pancreatic cancer in women. *J Natl Cancer Inst* 2004;96(1):22–28.
37. Parenti DM, Steinberg W, Kang P. Infectious causes of acute pancreatitis. *Pancreas* 1996;13(4):356–371.
38. Graham JR. Mumps causing chronic calcific pancreatitis. *Med J Aust* 1980;2(8):454.
39. Bartsch DK, Kress R, Sina-Frey M, et al. Prevalence of familial pancreatic cancer in Germany. *Int J Cancer* 2004;110(6):902–906.
40. Klein AP, Beaty TH, Bailey-Wilson JE, Brune KA, Hruban RH, Petersen GM. Evidence for a major gene influencing risk of pancreatic cancer. *Genet Epidemiol* 2002;23(2):133–149.
41. McFaul CD, Greenhalf W, Earl J, et al. Anticipation in familial pancreatic cancer. *Gut* 2006;55(2):252–258.
42. Schenk M, Schwartz AG, O'Neal E, et al. Familial risk of pancreatic cancer. *J Natl Cancer Inst* 2001;93:640–644.
43. Lowenfels AB, Maisonneuve P, Whitcomb DC, Lerch MM, DiMagno EP. Cigarette smoking as a risk factor for pancreatic cancer in patients with hereditary pancreatitis. *JAMA* 2001;286(2):169–170.
44. Rulyak SJ, Lowenfels AB, Maisonneuve P, Brentnall TA. Risk factors for the development of pancreatic cancer in familial pancreatic cancer kindreds. *Gastroenterology* 2003;124(5):1292–1299.
45. Duell EJ, Holly EA, Bracci PM, et al. A population-based case-control study of polymorphisms in carcinogen-metabolizing genes, smoking and pancreatic adenocarcinoma risk. *J Natl Cancer Inst* 2002;94:297–306.
46. *Genetic Disorders of the Exocrine Pancreas: An Overview and Update.* Basel, Switzerland: Karger; 2002.
47. Canto MI, Goggins M, Yeo CJ, et al. Screening for pancreatic neoplasia in high-risk individuals: an EUS-based approach. *Clin Gastroenterol Hepatol* 2004;2(7):606–621.
48. Parkin DM, Whelan SL, Ferlay J, Storm HH. *Cancer Incidence in Five Continents (CI5) Volumes I to VIII.* Cancerbase No. 7. Lyon, France: International Agency for Research on Cancer; 2005.
49. Ferlay J, Bray F, Pisani P, Parkin DM. *GLOBOCAN 2002: Cancer Incidence, Mortality and Prevalence Worldwide.* 2nd ed. Lyon, France: International Agency for Research on Cancer Press; 2004.
50. Borgström A, Johansen D, Manjer J. Chronic *Helicobacter pylori* infection does not increase the risk to develop pancreatic cancer. *Pancreas* 2004;29: 330–331.
51. Nilsson HO, Stenram U, Ihse I, Wadstrom T. Re: *Helicobacter pylori* seropositivity as a risk factor for pancreatic cancer. *J Natl Cancer Inst* 2002;94(8): 632 633.
52. Stolzenberg-Solomon RZ, Blaser MJ, Limburg PJ, et al. *Helicobacter pylori* seropositivity as a risk factor for pancreatic cancer. *J Natl Cancer Inst* 2001;93(12):937–941.
53. Raderer M, Wrba F, Kornek G, et al. Association between *Helicobacter pylori* infection and pancreatic cancer. *Oncology* 1998;55(1):16–19.
54. Klein AP, Brune KA, Petersen GM, et al. Prospective risk of pancreatic cancer in familial pancreatic cancer kindreds. *Cancer Res* 2004;64(7):2634–2638.
55. Watson P, Lynch HT. Extracolonic cancer in hereditary nonpolyposis colorectal cancer. *Cancer* 1993;71:677–685.
56. Hammel PR, Vilgrain V, Terris B, et al. Pancreatic involvement in von Hippel-Lindau disease. The Groupe Francophone d'Étude de la Maladie de von Hippel-Lindau. *Gastroenterology* 2000;119(4):1087–1095.
57. Efthimiou E, Crnogorac-Jurcevic T, Lemoine NR, Brentnall TA. Inherited predisposition to pancreatic cancer. *Gut* 2001;48(2):143–147.
58. Lowenfels AB, Maisonneuve P, DiMagno EP, et al. Hereditary pancreatitis and the risk of pancreatic cancer. International Hereditary Pancreatitis Study Group. *J Natl Cancer Inst* 1997;89(6):442–446.
59. Vasen HF, Gruis NA, Frants RR, Der Velden PA, Hille ET, Bergman W. Risk of developing pancreatic cancer in families with familial atypical multiple mole melanoma associated with a specific 19 deletion of p16 (p16-Leiden). *Int J Cancer* 2000;87(6):809–811.
60. Hahn SA, Greenhalf B, Ellis I, et al. BRCA2 germline mutations in familial pancreatic carcinoma. *J Natl Cancer Inst* 2003;95(3):214–221.
61. Su GH, Hruban RH, Bansal RK, et al. Germline and somatic mutations of the STK11/LKB1 Peutz-Jeghers gene in pancreatic and biliary cancers. *Am J Pathol* 1999;154(6):1835–1840.
62. Maisonneuve P, FitzSimmons SC, Neglia JP, Campbell PW, III, Lowenfels AB. Cancer risk in nontransplanted and transplanted cystic fibrosis patients: a 10-year study. *J Natl Cancer Inst* 2003;95(5):381–387.
63. Neglia JP, FitzSimmons SC, Maisonneuve P, et al. The risk of cancer among patients with cystic fibrosis. *N Engl J Med* 1995;332:494–499.
64. Ghadirian P, Lynch HT, Krewski D. Epidemiology of pancreatic cancer: an overview. *Cancer Detect Prev* 2003;27(2):87–93.
65. van der Heijden MS, Yeo CJ, Hruban RH, Kern SE. Fanconi anemia gene mutations in young-onset pancreatic cancer. *Cancer Res* 2003;63(10):2585–2588.
66. U.S. National Institutes of Health, National Cancer Institute, Surveillance, Epidemiology, and End Results Web site. Available at: www.seer.cancer.gov. Accessed April 20, 2007.

CHAPTER 25 ■ PANCREATIC CANCER: MOLECULAR BIOLOGY AND GENETICS

SCOTT E. KERN, EIKE GALLMEIER, MICHAEL GOGGINS, AND RALPH H. HRUBAN

Pancreatic neoplasia is a genetic disease. In all of its manifestations, pancreatic cancer is inextricably molded by a microevolutionary process involving the serial steps of genetic mutation and the consequent emergence of subclones having selective growth advantages.

The utility of this perspective has been borne out. Molecular genetic analyses of pancreatic neoplasms have led to the recognition of new histopathological variants of pancreatic cancer and to a better understanding of the cellular basis for differences in the clinical behavior of distinct types of neoplasms of the pancreas. For example, although most common ductal adenocarcinomas are relatively uniform clinically, pathologically, and genetically, there are less common variant forms that have differing histologic and genetic characteristics and that carry clinical distinctions of importance. Genetic assays can enable conspicuous groupings among the tumors (because a given neoplasm either has a mutation or it does not); therefore, this mode of analysis has spurred the recognition of these variant forms.

DUCTAL NEOPLASIA OF THE PANCREAS

A variety of clinically and pathologically distinct neoplasms can involve the pancreas, and readers are encouraged to refer to the related chapters that review the histopathology (Chapter 27) and the epidemiology of pancreatic cancer (Chapter 24). Primary neoplasms of the pancreas are broadly divided into those having exocrine differentiation and those with endocrine differentiation. The infiltrating ductal adenocarcinoma is the most common malignant neoplasm having exocrine differentiation. The term *ductal adenocarcinoma* refers to a clinically aggressive neoplasm characterized by ductal differentiation, shown by its mucin production and the expression of certain cytokeratins. Ductal adenocarcinomas encompass the entire spectrum of histologic grades, from poorly differentiated to well differentiated, although the vast majority are moderately differentiated; the grades of differentiation per se have minimal clinical importance or demonstrable molecular associations. Among the ductal adenocarcinomas, however, there are some distinct molecular and histopathological variants (Fig. 25.1). In addition, there are a number of other exocrine neoplasms such as the intraductal papillary mucinous neoplasm (IPMN), which are clinically and pathologically distinct, although these variants are less well characterized at the molecular level.

Infiltrating ductal adenocarcinoma must also be distinguished from its precursor lesions, IPMNs, and pancreatic intraepithelial neoplasia (PanIN) (Fig. 25.2). PanINs are histologically distinct lesions in the pancreas, and molecular analyses of these distinct lesions provided hard evidence of the origins of and precursor lesions associated with infiltrating ductal adenocarcinoma (Fig. 25.2). IPMNs are usually larger than PanINs, although a unified classification independent of the size of the lesion may emerge on further work. IPMNs share some of the early genetic abnormalities of PanIN but lack some of the late stage genetic alterations, a difference that may help explain their more favorable tumorigenic course.

A "gatekeeper gene" analogous to the genes that prevent multiple adenomas in familial adenomatous polyposis in the colorectum (the *APC* gene) or endocrine hyperplasias in multiple endocrine neoplasia syndromes (e.g., the *MEN1* gene) (1,2) has not been identified in the pancreas. Nonetheless, recent studies of pancreata surgically resected from individuals with a strong family history of pancreatic cancer reveal multiple foci of PanIN (3), suggesting that one day a gatekeeper gene may be discovered in the pancreas as well. Finally, it is important to note that, in molecular terms even more so than in histologic terms, ductal carcinomas of the pancreas are distinct from other intestinal neoplasias, such as the neighboring entity, the duodenal carcinoma. It is, however, more difficult to distinguish pancreatic ductal adenocarcinoma from the carcinomas arising at the duodenal papilla and from the distal common bile duct. Pancreatic adenocarcinoma can also be contrasted to another ductal neoplasm, breast carcinoma. There is a relatively homogeneous genetic profile for conventional ductal adenocarcinomas of the pancreas that largely mirrors the homogeneity in the histopathological appearance and in the aggressive clinical course. In breast carcinoma, this is not the case because a remarkable heterogeneity of molecular genetic patterns parallels its clinical and histologic heterogeneity.

CYTOGENETICS AND PLOIDY

In the analysis of global patterns of chromosome number and structure by classical cytogenetics, the karyotypes of short-term and established cultures of pancreatic adenocarcinoma reveal a very complex set of abnormalities, as is typical for most other carcinomas of adulthood. Translocations, whole chromosome and partial deletions, gains of chromosomes and segments thereof, and occasional minute chromosomal fragments are present (4,5). Despite a considerable heterogeneity in karyotypic patterns among the cells of individual pancreatic cancers (6), dominant patterns exist. Some of the recurrent patterns include deletions of chromosomal arms 9p, 17p, and 18q, sites of known major tumor-suppressor gene abnormalities. The *CDKN2A/p16* tumor-suppressor gene resides on 9p, the *TP53/p53* gene on 17p, and the *SMAD4/DPC4* gene on 18q. The results of allelotyping, a molecular method of surveying the entire genome for chromosomal deletions (allelic losses), mirror these findings. The average allelotype indicates

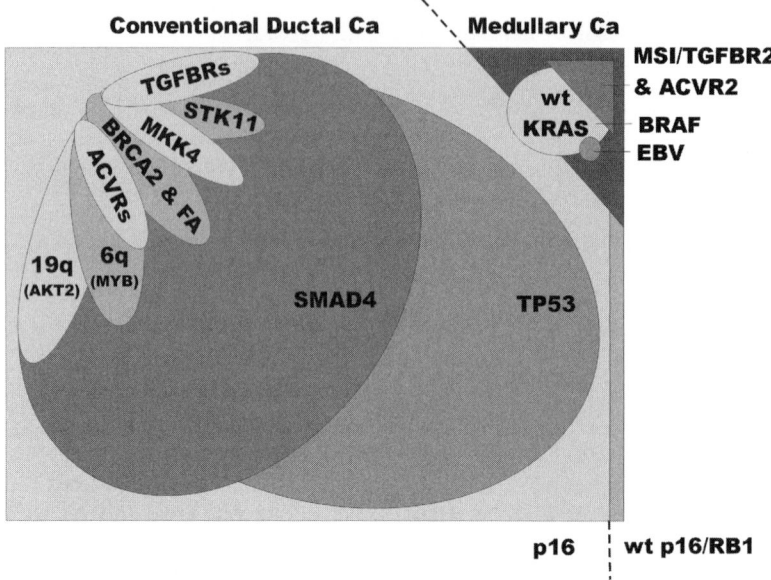

FIGURE 25.1. Venn diagram of the frequencies and relations of the gene mutations in pancreatic ductal adenocarcinoma. Each subset is labeled according to the histologic pattern or gene/chromosome abnormality and corresponds in area to the proportion of tumors having the genetic alteration (single alterations in the case of the *KRAS* oncogene, complex multiple alterations in the case of the amplifications of 19q and 6q, biallelic inactivation in the case of the tumor-suppressor genes). Medullary carcinomas encompass most cases having a wild-type *KRAS* gene and all cases having microsatellite instability (MSI). Most cases with MSI have a wild-type *KRAS* gene and a mutant *BRAF* gene, and all have had biallelic mutations of the polyadenine tract of the *TGFBR2* and *ACVR2* genes. Rare cases are reported to have mutation of the *RB1* gene and might overlap with the small subset having an unmethylated wild-type *p16* gene, reflecting a pattern of mutually exclusive gene mutation that is clearly defined in other tumor types. A single case harboring the Epstein-Barr virus episome is reported among the medullary cancers. The clustering of infrequently mutated genes in the upper left is meant to indicate the independent occurrence of these mutations that does not exclude their being present in the same tumors regardless of whether the tumors have alterations in *TP53* or *SMAD4*; the particular subset that adjoins another and the degree of overlap has no intended meaning here. FA refers to the genes of the Fanconi anemia core complex. The constellation of tumor-suppressor mutations present in the medullary cancers and in those having the unmethylated wild-type *p16* gene are currently poorly defined, and the diagram does not convey the relation of these tumors to this gene category.

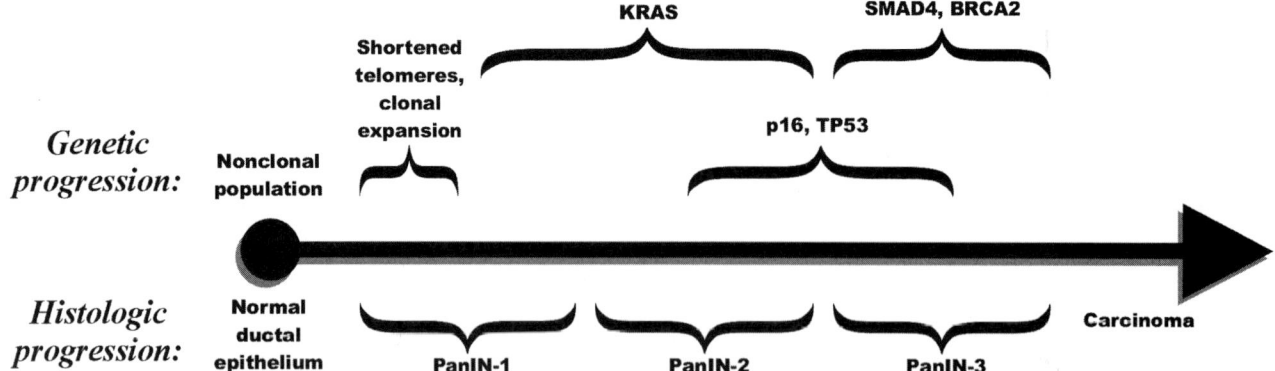

FIGURE 25.2. Genetic changes in the evolution of pancreatic ductal intraepithelial neoplasia (PanIN). PanIN is the new internationally defined system for classification of dysplasia (noninvasive epithelial neoplasia) of the pancreatic ducts. In brief, PanIN-1 comprises a flat mucosa of tall mucinous cells, PanIN-2 includes papillary architecture and some cytologic atypia, and PanIN-3 has a complex architecture with cytologic features resembling those of the invasive lesions, previously termed "carcinoma in situ." *KRAS* mutations are not observed in the majority of PanIN-1 lesions, suggesting that there might be another, perhaps more universal alteration that initiates this neoplastic process. p53 Overexpression is best studied in PanIN-3 but occurs in at least some instances of PanIN-2. To date, PanIN-3 lesions are the only precursor stage in which the inactivation of both alleles of *BRCA2* and *SMAD4* been observed; thus, these genes appear to play a "late" role as mutational targets.

that up to one-third of the chromosomal regions in ductal adenocarcinomas have suffered a loss of an allele and that the most common sites of loss involve chromosomal arms 9p, 17p, and 18q (7). Furthermore, there is a good correlation between the findings obtained with these two techniques, as a detailed comparison of cytogenetic abnormalities to allelotype data in a series of ductal adenocarcinomas demonstrated that most allelic losses are reflected in cytogenetic abnormalities (8).

The simple quantitation of total cellular DNA content by flow cytometry or static image cytometry can be used to compare the abnormal DNA content (termed *aneuploidy*) of cancer cells to normal cells, a ratio termed the *DNA index* (9). Measurements of DNA index have the advantage over classical cytogenetics in being applicable to the direct study of the primary tumor. However, these cytometric techniques can miss changes in individual chromosomes, and most tumors measured to have a normal DNA index do not in reality harbor a diploid chromosomal pattern (i.e., containing two copies of all 22 non–sex chromosomes).

There are many open questions regarding the cytogenetics of this pancreatic adenocarcinoma. For example, pancreatic cancer is similar to most carcinomas of adulthood in that a specific recurrent translocation has not been identified, although sensitive techniques to characterize the complex translocations of the carcinomas (in contrast to the simpler patterns seen in the hematopoietic malignancies) now exist. Spectral karyotyping is similar to karyotype analysis but is based on fluorescence in situ hybridization; it uses multiple fluorochromes, digital imaging, and computer analysis to represent a different color for each chromosome, allowing the recognition of constituent chromosomal parts involved in complex translocations in pancreatic cancers (10). Comparative genomic hybridization and related techniques such as the hybridization of tumor DNA to arrays of oligonucleotides, genes, and chromosomal segments have also been applied to pancreatic cancer (10,11); such techniques can be used to determine the relative copy number for each segment of chromosomal material and have proven useful for the identification of deletions and chromosome amplification (12). The most common sites of deletion and some notable sites of amplification are discussed later in this chapter. The findings of these techniques imply that pancreatic adenocarcinomas have considerable chromosomal instability, probably on the order of that seen in colorectal carcinoma.

MOLECULAR GENETICS

A simple molecular definition of a neoplasm is that it is a clone of cells distinguished from other tissues by autonomous growth and somatic mutations (13). These mutations lie within growth-controlling genes. Physiologically, neoplastic cells grow under what would otherwise be limiting conditions. Supporting and reactive tissues accompany the neoplastic cells in the formation of tumors. This definition clearly describes the infiltrating ductal adenocarcinomas of the pancreas and can be used to extend the concept of neoplasia to the precursor lesions (PanINs and IPMNs), where clonal genetic abnormalities in oncogenes and tumor-suppressor genes are readily demonstrable.

The molecular genetic alterations identified to date in infiltrating ductal adenocarcinomas of the pancreas now include instances of all five basic types of tumor mutation: translocation, amplification, deletion, subtle (intragenic) mutations, and the addition of exogenous (viral) sequences. As noted previously, only the translocations are not yet shown to form recurrent patterns that would indicate a specific selectable advantage, and the translocations observed might only represent the expected consequence of the general process that produces aneuploidy.

When a gene in a cancer is affected by mutation at a rate higher than would be expected by chance, we say that the gene is targeted by mutation. The mechanism increasing the prevalence of a mutation in a cancer is, of course, random, with selective pressures acting on the cellular population to favor the subclones harboring the mutated gene. The genes targeted by mutation can be grouped into three major classes. *Oncogenes* are genes whose function is *activated* by mutation (the normal gene is sometimes called a protooncogene). Oncogenes are said to be dominant because their appearance in a cell confers the subsequent cellular changes. *Tumor-suppressor genes* and *genome-maintenance genes* are inactivated by mutation. These are recessive gene classes in that the functional loss of both normal copies is needed to result in cellular changes, and the experimental transfer of a mutant version cannot be expected to confer a cellular change (an exception exists but represents yet another form of inactivated recessive gene: the dominant-negative mutation).

It is important to distinguish somatic mutations (those that occur during the life of the patient) from inherited (germline) mutations. Inherited mutations are transmitted from parent to child and will be present in all cells of the body. Inherited mutations usually, but not always, require a second (somatic) genetic event to manifest a cellular alteration. This second event, in the case of recessive genes such as the tumor-suppressor genes and genome-maintenance genes, is often the deletion of the remaining wild-type (normal) gene copy. In a line of analysis introduced by Nicholls and developed by Knudson, the neoplastic effects of an inherited mutation can be delayed because they are dependent on the chance occurrence of further somatic mutations (14,15).

Before considering a formal outline of molecular genetic events in pancreatic adenocarcinoma, it is appropriate to note a caveat of DNA methodology. Pancreatic carcinomas usually have a very characteristic and exuberant nonneoplastic host reaction, comprising dense scarring and chronic inflammatory reactions. For this reason, most cells in the mass formed by an invasive pancreatic ductal adenocarcinoma are genetically normal, reactive host cells such as fibroblasts and endothelial cells. Most genetic studies therefore use cell populations that are passaged in culture or in immunodeficient mice to enrich for neoplastic cells.

The following discussion presents the relationship of individual genetic changes to the major genetic and histologic classifications (Fig. 25.1), the means by which the genes were first discovered (Fig. 25.3), the frequencies of genetic changes, and major theories regarding their cancer-related functions (Fig. 25.4).

Oncogenes

The *KRAS* gene was first identified as the transforming gene of the Kirsten virus. Later, when DNA of human tumors was used to artificially transform mouse cells (i.e., conferring some of the properties associated with neoplastic cells), a mutated form of the ras genes was repeatedly isolated from multiple human tumor types (16). More than 90% of human pancreatic ductal adenocarcinomas have an activating point mutation in the *KRAS* gene (17). The occasional cases with wild-type *KRAS* genes tend to be the carcinomas with the medullary phenotype and *BRAF* gene mutations and include carcinomas with abnormalities in DNA mismatch repair (Fig. 25.1) (18–20). Most of the mutations in the *KRAS* gene result in codon 12 changing from glycine to aspartate or valine (although any possible mutation can be seen). In contrast, a broad spectrum of mutations is reported in colorectal carcinoma (21,22). The codon 12 *KRAS* gene mutations observed in most pancreatic cancers impair the GTPase function of the

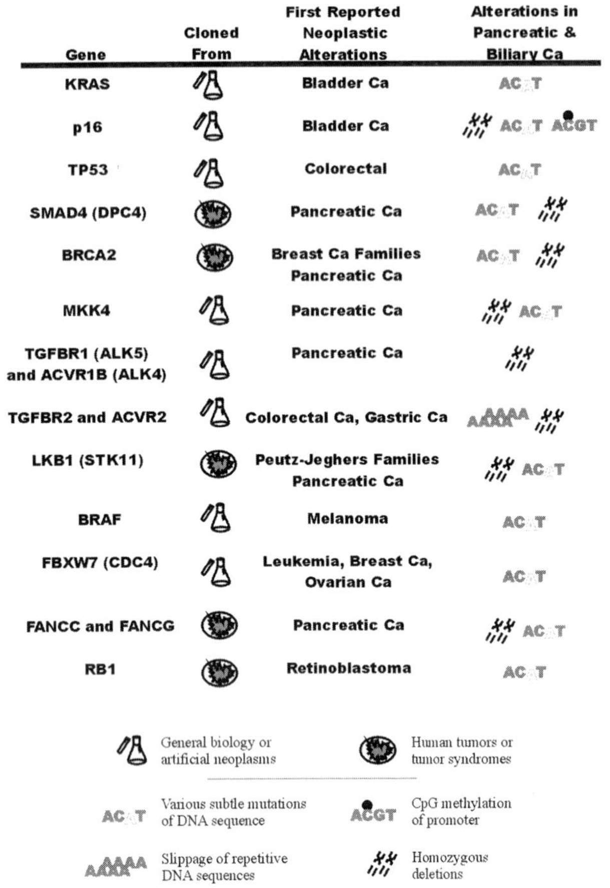

Gene	Cloned From	First Reported Neoplastic Alterations	Alterations in Pancreatic & Biliary Ca
KRAS	[flask]	Bladder Ca	AC..T
p16	[flask]	Bladder Ca	//// AC..T ACGT●
TP53	[flask]	Colorectal	AC..T
SMAD4 (DPC4)	[cell]	Pancreatic Ca	AC..T ////
BRCA2	[cell]	Breast Ca Families, Pancreatic Ca	AC..T ////
MKK4	[flask]	Pancreatic Ca	//// AC..T
TGFBR1 (ALK5) and ACVR1B (ALK4)	[flask]	Pancreatic Ca	////
TGFBR2 and ACVR2	[flask]	Colorectal Ca, Gastric Ca	AAAAA ////
LKB1 (STK11)	[cell]	Peutz-Jeghers Families, Pancreatic Ca	//// AC..T
BRAF	[flask]	Melanoma	AC..T
FBXW7 (CDC4)	[flask]	Leukemia, Breast Ca, Ovarian Ca	AC..T
FANCC and FANCG	[cell]	Pancreatic Ca	//// AC..T
RB1	[cell]	Retinoblastoma	AC..T

Legend:

[flask] General biology or artificial neoplasms

[cell] Human tumors or tumor syndromes

AC..T Various subtle mutations of DNA sequence

●ACGT CpG methylation of promoter

AAAA Slippage of repetitive DNA sequences

//// Homozygous deletions

FIGURE 25.3. The history of discovery of genes targeted for mutation in pancreatic ductal adenocarcinoma. Most genes were first described from studies of general biology (e.g., kinase signal pathways or cell cycle mechanisms) or from artificial tumor systems (e.g., virally induced tumors in animals and in culture), and were only later shown to be mutationally involved in human tumors. Others were first identified by positional genomic approaches in human families and tumors. Most tumor-suppressor genes can be inactivated by a variety of genetic mechanisms. Slippage of simple repetitive DNA sequences is most characteristic of tumors with microsatellite instability at sites of extended repeats such as the polyadenine tract of the *TGFBR2* and *ACVR2* genes. Methylation of gene promoter sequences can affect various genes but is distinctly associated with complete transcript silencing for the *p16* gene. There is a notable paucity of homozygous deletions among the mutational spectrum of the *TP53* gene, an unusual finding among the tumor-suppressor genes. The restricted mutational spectrum shown here for the *TGFBR1* and *RB1* genes is likely only a manifestation of the low numbers of affected tumors reported to date. Mutational profiles are similar among the cancers of the pancreatic ducts and those of the intrapancreatic distal common bile duct. Ca, cancer.

ras protein; because the GTP-bound form of ras is the active form, this is believed to cause overactivity in various intracellular signals (23). Ras genes mediate the signals arising from the binding of growth factors, and major mitogen-activated protein kinase (MAPK) pathways are activated by K-ras activity (24).

The *BRAF* gene is mutated in some medullary carcinomas of the pancreas (20). These same tumors have microsatellite instability and a wild-type *KRAS* gene. The *BRAF* gene stimulates the MAP kinase pathway, being positioned just downstream of ras genes.

Cyclin E is distinctly overexpressed in about 5% of pancreatic cancers, and, in one tumor subject to genetic analysis, this overexpression was attributed to a mutation of the *FBXW7*

(*CDC4*, a tumor suppressor) gene (20). Fbxw7 is an ubiquitin ligase responsible for the downregulation of the cyclin E protein. When mutated, cyclin E, an oncogene normally subject to cyclic expression during the cell division cycle, remains inappropriately expressed (25,26).

Gene amplification is seen in infiltrating ductal adenocarcinomas at a few chromosomal loci. These include the *AKT2* gene and its neighboring genes on chromosomal arm 19q (10%–20% of cases), *MYB* and its neighbors on 6q (10% of cases), cyclin E, and others (10,20,27–30). It is assumed that the maintenance and expansion of these arrays of repetitive DNA is the result of selective pressures conferred by overexpression of the oncogenes contained within their boundaries. Unfortunately, the DNA segments involved (termed *amplicons*) are so large as to impair the clear identification of the true target gene(s) of the amplification process.

Tumor-Suppressor Genes

The tumor-suppressor genes are recessive genes and have a close association with inherited syndromes. The presence of one mutated copy in the germline is well tolerated during early development. The human gene pool thus includes mutated tumor-suppressor genes in at least 1% of some populations. Some inherited mutations are associated with the subsequent development of multiple early neoplasms as part of an obviously recognizable clinical syndrome, such as familial adenomatous polyposis or multiple endocrine neoplasia syndromes. The gene involved is termed a *gatekeeper*, in that its full inactivation of both copies is sufficient to initiate a lesion (2,13). As discussed previously, it has been suggested that the pancreas uses a gatekeeper form of proliferative control; however, this still remains to be proven. The evidence indicates that some inherited mutations of tumor-suppressor genes do not play an early role in neoplastic development for some defects appear to become biologically significant only later in tumorigenesis (31).

The tumor-suppressor genes targeted by mutation in pancreatic ductal carcinoma include the *p16*, *TP53*, *SMAD4*, TGFβ and activin receptors I and II, *MKK4*, *STK11*, and *BRCA2* genes. These are discussed as follows. For these genes, intragenic sequence mutations act to inactivate the protein function and accompany loss of the wild-type gene copy. The intragenic mutations are of somatic origin, except where otherwise noted. All homozygous deletions noted are of somatic origin.

The *p16* gene (*CDKN2A*, chr. 9p) was first identified from studies of inhibitors of the cell division cycle mechanism (32). It was later identified to lie at a known common site of homozygous deletions affecting chromosomal arm 9p in multiple tumor types and is the mutant gene that causes familial melanoma (33,34). The *p16* gene may be the most commonly inactivated of the tumor-suppressor genes in humans. The p16 protein binds to the cyclin-dependent kinases Cdk4 and Cdk6 to inhibit their action. In the absence of p16, Cdk4 and Cdk6 phosphorylate and inactivate the cell cycle inhibitory protein Rb1 in late G1 phase, thereby initiating DNA replication. Because they lie within a single pathway, the *p16* and *RB1* genes have an inverse mutational relationship: when one is mutated in a particular tumor, the other is not (i.e., once *p16* is mutated in a particular neoplasm, there should be no selective advantage to the further inactivation of *RB1*). The *p16* gene is inactivated in virtually all pancreatic adenocarcinomas. Homozygous deletions or intragenic mutation are most common, although promoter methylation associated with the silencing of gene transcription occurs in the remainder (35,36). Rare mutations of *RB1* are reported in pancreatic cancer (37).

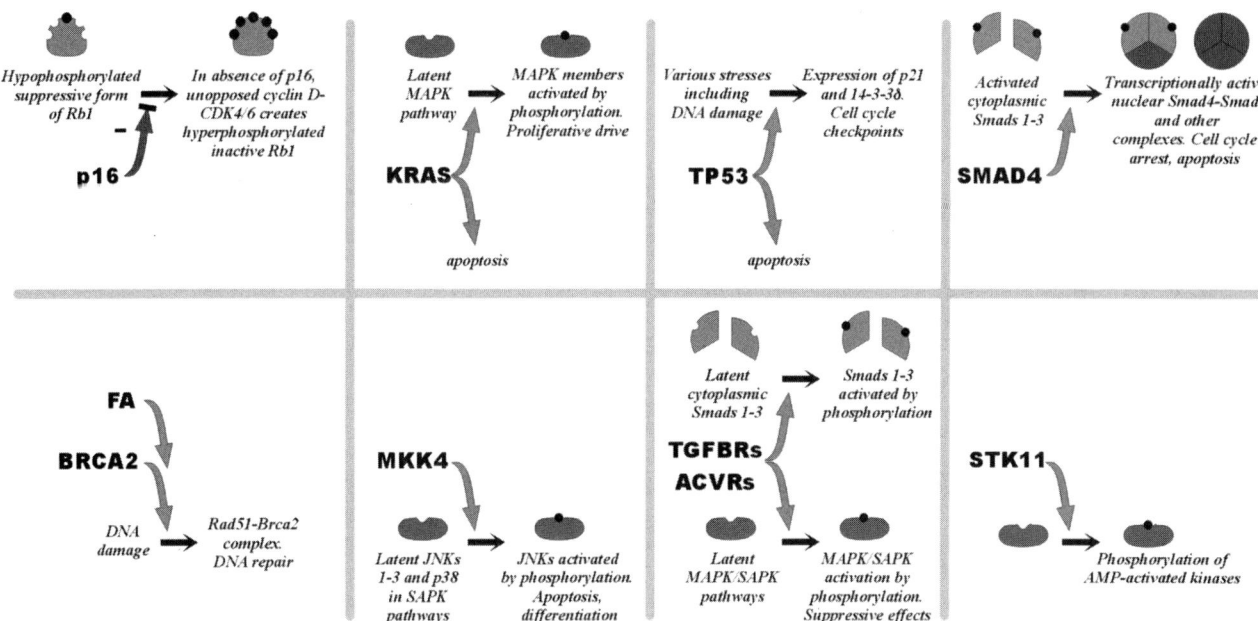

FIGURE 25.4. Pathways affected by mutation in pancreatic ductal adenocarcinoma. Major roles of each tumor-suppressor gene and the *KRAS* oncogene are indicated. Where the specific mechanism is known with some certainty, a straight arrow indicates the step mediated or facilitated, or in the case of *p16*, the step inhibited, by the wild-type gene. Mutations activate the function of the *KRAS* gene, whereas the other genes depicted are inactivated by mutation. Multiple additional properties are known for most of these genes; the discrimination of those functions with the highest relevance for tumorigenesis is an evolving subject of research and personal preference. Phosphorylation is depicted by occupation of a specific surface location of a protein by a filled circle. Apoptosis refers to the number of cells that commit to undergo cell death, and not to an augmentation of the basic cellular machinery by which this is accomplished. Checkpoints refer to highly patterned forms of cell cycle arrest in response to specific injurious agents. FA, genes of the Fanconi anemia core complex. TGFBRs and ACVRs, TGFß and activin receptors, types I and II.

The *TP53* gene (*p53*, chr. 17p) was identified as a protein bound by the major tumor antigen of the SV40 virus. Intragenic mutations were first found in colorectal cancer, and then in most types of malignancy (38,39). Next to *p16*, it is one of the most commonly mutated genes in human cancer. The mutations destroy the ability of the p53 protein to bind specific sequences of DNA (40), impairing its ability to stimulate the transcription of specific genes (41). These genes include the cell cycle inhibitor p21, which controls cell cycle checkpoints at the border of G1 and S (DNA synthesis) phases and in late G2 prior to M (mitosis) phase (42–45), and the 14–3-3σ protein, which maintains the late G2 checkpoint (46). These checkpoints involve the arrest of the cell division cycle in response to injurious exposures such as those resulting in DNA damage (47). p53 is also a powerful initiator of apoptotic mechanisms; the specific mechanism by which this is accomplished is not convincingly defined, but p53 is known to activate expression of the proapoptotic gene BAX (48). Fifty to 75% of pancreatic adenocarcinomas have intragenic mutations in *TP53* (49,50).

The *SMAD4* gene (*DPC4/MADH4*, chr. 18q), was identified in the search for the target gene of a hotspot of homozygous deletions affecting chromosomal arm 18q in pancreatic and biliary carcinomas (51). *SMAD4* encodes a member of a family of Smad genes that are important in development and that transmit signals initiated by the binding of TGFβ-like proteins to cell surface receptors (52,53). Signal transduction may require the formation of complexes of Smad proteins, and both homooligomers and heterooligomers of Smad4 are described (54,55). Smad4 binds to specific sequences of DNA to stimulate the transcription of neighboring genes (56–58). It remains unclear which of these downstream genes serve as the effectors of *SMAD4*'s tumor-suppressive effects; however, it is clear

that the nuclear localization of Smad4 causes growth suppression and increased apoptosis (59). Missense mutations in the N-terminal half of the protein inactivate the ability to bind DNA, while those of the C-terminal half impair nuclear localization, activation of gene transcription, and probably the ability to form oligomers (54). Homozygous deletions and intragenic mutations of the *SMAD4* gene occur in about half of pancreatic adenocarcinomas (51,60). Immunohistochemical analysis of Smad4 expression in tissues is an accurate means of identifying the tumors having genetic inactivation (Fig. 25.5) (61), in part because its missense mutations usually create an unstable protein (62,63).

The TGFβ and activin receptor genes encode a heterodimeric receptor pair comprising a type I receptor (for TGFβ, it is encoded by the *TGFBR1/ALK5* gene; for activin, the *ACVR1* and the *ACVR1B/ALK4* genes) and a type II receptor (for TGFβ, the *TGFBR2* gene; for activin, the *ACVR2* and *ACVR2B* genes). TGFβ and activin are secreted proteins that serve as extracellular "growth factors"—ligands that bind to cell surface receptors. These receptors were first identified as TGFβ- and activin-binding proteins. Subsequently, mutations of the *TGFBR2* gene, located at a polyadenine simple repeat within the gene, are nearly ubiquitous in cancers having microsatellite instability (MSI) and abnormalities of DNA-mismatch repair (64), and also, albeit at much lower frequencies, in non-MSI tumors of various organ sites (65). The ACVR2 gene accumulates similar mutations of a repeated sequence in MSI tumors (66,67). Genetic inactivation of the *TGFBR1* gene was first shown in non-MSI pancreatic and biliary carcinomas (68). The binding of TGFβ and activin ligands to their receptors usually results in growth arrest or even apoptosis of cells; to accomplish this, both TGFβ and activin

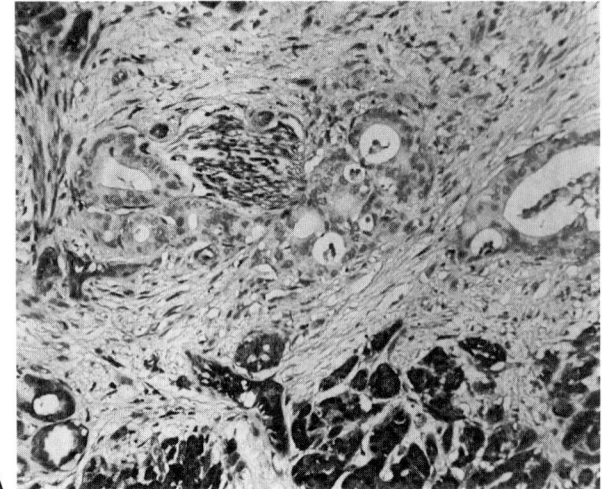

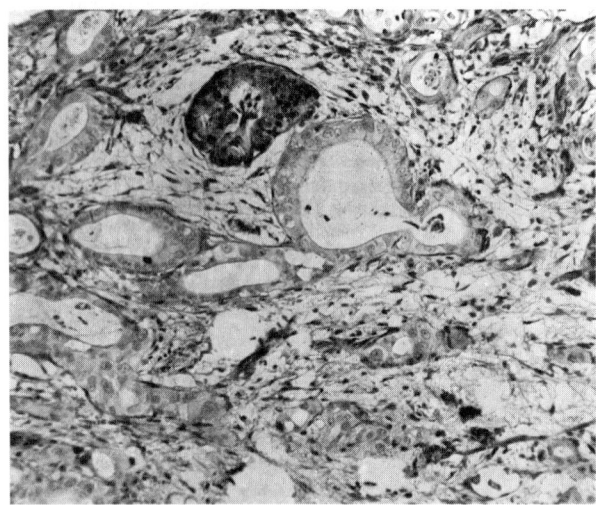

FIGURE 25.5. Immunohistochemistry accurately detects the genetic inactivation of the SMAD4 gene. This tumor had a homozygous deletion of the SMAD4 gene. **A:** Smad4 protein is immunolocalized within the epithelium of the remaining areas of pancreatic parenchyma (*bottom*), stromal fibroblasts (*scattered*), and within a nerve (*upper center*). Surrounding the nerve are the abortive duct structures of a moderately well-differentiated conventional type of pancreatic adenocarcinoma that lacks Smad4 immunoreactivity. A characteristic desmoplastic (scarring) reaction invests the area involved by carcinoma. **B:** A single pancreatic islet (*upper center*), expressing Smad4 protein, remains within a field of carcinoma lacking Smad4 expression. Monoclonal antibody B-8 (Santa Cruz) used with peroxidase detection, counterstained with hematoxylin.

receptors elicit the induction of expression of essentially similar sets of specific genes (69). These pathways can thus be considered as tumor suppressive. It is believed that to escape these effects, many cancers lose their responsiveness to TGFβ and activin. The type I receptors are kinases that phosphorylate Smad proteins 1–3. This event initiates the formation of Smad-Smad4 complexes, the nuclear localization of Smad4, and the induction of expression of downstream genes (70). The true relationship of TGFβ and *SMAD4* tumor suppression is, however, still not precisely defined. In some cells, *SMAD4* is necessary to convey the TGFβ-initiated growth arrest and transcriptional effects (71,72). In other cells, however, these actions of TGFβ persist even in the absence of *SMAD4* (73,74). The coexistent genetic inactivation of both *SMAD4* and a TGFβ receptor gene within individual tumors has also been described, suggesting

that the products of these genes are not as closely linked in the same pathway as, for example, are p16 and Rb1 (68,75). Pancreatic adenocarcinomas with MSI usually have mutations of the polyadenine tract of both copies of the *TGFBR2* gene and of the *ACVR2* gene (19,67,68). Occasional non-MSI pancreatic and biliary carcinomas harbor homozygous deletions involving the *TGFBR1* and *TGFBR2* genes (68).

The *MKK4* gene (*MAP2K4, SEK1*) was first identified as a member of the stress-activated protein kinase pathways that result in activation of Jun kinases and, although less well established, the p38 kinase (76,77). Activation of these pathways by exposure to ultraviolet light, hypoxia, certain cytokines and chemotherapeutic agents, etc., can result in apoptosis or differentiation. It was later found that a site of homozygous deletion, identified first in a pancreatic cancer, encompassed the *MKK4* gene (78). Homozygous deletions or intragenic mutations of the *MKK4* gene occur in about 4% of pancreatic cancers and in a similar fraction of other tumor types (78–80).

The *STK11* gene (*LKB1*) was identified from a search for the mutated gene that causes Peutz-Jeghers syndrome (81,82). It encodes a serine-threonine kinase that activates AMP-activated protein kinase–related kinases and their downstream effects, including inhibition of the proproliferative mTOR pathway (83,84). Peutz-Jeghers syndrome has been shown to be associated with nearly a 24-fold elevated risk of pancreatic cancer (85). Homozygous deletions or intragenic mutations involving *STK11* occur in about 4% of sporadic pancreatic and biliary carcinomas (86). In addition, loss of the wild-type allele was observed in a pancreatic cancer that arose in a patient with Peutz-Jeghers syndrome (86).

There are indications that other tumor-suppressor genes exist that are currently unknown (87). For examples, some chromosomal arms have rather high rates of deletion, sites of homozygous deletion are known that lie outside the known gene targets, and some familial patterns of pancreatic carcinoma remain unexplained by the known genetic syndromes.

The *DCC* (88,89), *FHIT* (90–92), and *DMBT1* (93) genes are occasionally affected by homozygous deletions in various human malignancies, including pancreatic adenocarcinoma, but sequence analysis of these genes has not yet strongly supported them to be mutational targets that would convey selective advantages during tumorigenesis. These genes may indeed be tumor suppressors or may only represent the innocent bystander genes at a genetic hotspot of structural alterations. The *FHIT* gene, for example, is located at a known chromosomal fragile site (94). It is also difficult to implicate a gene as a true tumor-suppressor gene based on the evidence of low expression levels in tumors because determination of the "normal" level of a gene's expression in a tumor is obscure at best.

Genome-Maintenance Genes

Two forms of genome-maintenance genes are implicated in pancreatic adenocarcinoma, affecting chromosomal maintenance and DNA-mismatch repair. The inactivation of genes involved in chromosome maintenance is implied by the number and complexity of the genomic deletions and rearrangements observed in cytogenetic analyses of pancreatic cancer, as discussed previously, and also by functional studies that show a defect in the mitotic spindle checkpoint in the non-MSI pancreatic cancers (95). Studies in colorectal cancer (see Chapter 40) indicate the existence of a quantitative abnormality termed chromosomal instability (CIN) to explain the emergence of the aneuploid carcinoma (96). Mutations in the mitotic checkpoint genes may account for this phenotype in colorectal cancer, and CIN is also associated with distinct patterns of whole genome methylation (96).

The *BRCA2* gene was identified from the convergence of two simultaneous searches: for the mutated gene that caused familial breast cancer, and for the target gene of a homozygous deletion identified in a pancreatic carcinoma (97–99). Brca2 protein binds the Rad51 protein, and Rad51 is involved in the repair of DNA double-strand breaks by the process of homologous recombination (100). However, cancers in which *BRCA2* has been inactivated do not typically develop a distinctive mutational profile such as might be expected for a faulty DNA-repair system (50). Only a single somatic homozygous deletion of *BRCA2* has been reported in pancreatic cancer (97,101). Instead, the vast majority of *BRCA2* mutations are of germline origin. Quite remarkably, these germline *BRCA2* mutations are seen in 5% to 7% of what appear to be clinically sporadic pancreatic cancers (97,101,102), and at even higher rates in familial pancreatic cancer (103,104), as well as in breast cancer families (105,106). Nonetheless, *BRCA2* mutations do not convey a high penetrance for malignant disease in most families having pancreatic cancer, and indeed most pancreas cancer patients with a germline *BRCA2* mutation do not have first-degree relatives with pancreatic or breast cancer (101,102).

Pancreatic cancers also can harbor occasional somatic and germline mutations in other genes related to DNA repair, especially repair of double-strand breaks and interstrand cross-links. Pancreatic cancers can have inactivation of the Fanconi anemia genes *FANCC* and *FANCG* (107–109). In noncancer systems in which Fanconi anemia genes are deficient, the prevalence of spontaneous chromosomal aberrations is elevated, and in otherwise near-diploid cancer cells engineered to lack specific Fanconi anemia genes, the actual rate of spontaneous chromosomal changes is increased (110). These data indicate that Fanconi and *BRCA2* mutations contribute to CIN in human neoplasms. Pancreatic cancer cells with inactivation of the Fanconi anemia genes or of *BRCA2* have a pronounced hypersensitivity to the toxicity of DNA interstrand cross-linking agents, such as melphalan, mitomycin C, and cisplatin (108, 110,111).

Another set of genes, the DNA-mismatch repair genes, maintains the integrity of the DNA sequence itself. MSI, indicative of alterations in genes of the DNA-mismatch repair system, is seen in about 3% of pancreatic adenocarcinomas. Pancreatic cancers with MSI tend to have a medullary histology, with wild-type *KRAS* genes (18,19), mutations of the *BRAF* gene (20), and biallelic mutation of the polyadenine tract of the *TGFBR2* and *ACVR2* genes (67,68). MSI is also reported in one of eight colloid (mucinous noncystic) carcinomas (112). The recognition of MSI pancreatic tumors is important because they can be associated with inherited mutations of the mismatch repair genes and can therefore be a manifestation of hereditary nonpolyposis colorectal cancer syndrome (113–119). Loss of expression of the *MLH1* gene was observed in some of the tumors and could offer a practical diagnostic aid.

Oncogenic Viruses

Epstein-Barr virus (EBV) is a DNA virus of the herpesvirus family. A role in neoplasia was originally postulated from its high prevalence among patients with Burkitt's lymphoma, and later supported by the presence of viral sequences in this lymphoma, in Hodgkin's lymphoma and posttransplant lymphoproliferative disease, in nasopharyngeal carcinomas, and in other tumor types, including occasional carcinomas of stomach (120,121). The infective virus has a linear DNA, which then circularizes and is propagated as an extrachromosomal circular DNA, termed an *episome*. Experimental studies indicate that in the absence of selective pressures, the episome is rapidly lost from proliferating cellular populations. Neoplasms containing EBV have cells sharing a single clonal ancestral circularization event.

The epidemiologic and experimental arguments thus show that EBV must confer survival advantages on the subclone of cells that acquires and maintains the episome, one or more of whose protein products may act as a dominant oncogene. A single pancreatic adenocarcinoma of medullary phenotype has been reported to contain EBV (18), but the epidemiologic patterns relative to EBV have not yet been studied in this disease.

MOLECULAR BIOLOGY

Patterns of global gene expression were evaluated in pancreatic cancer by serial analysis of gene expression, nucleic acid subtraction, and hybridization of tumor gene transcripts to arrays of cDNA or oligonucleotides (122–124). By these methods, a hierarchy of tens of thousands of expressed genes can be placed in order by quantitation of their relative numbers of mRNA transcripts. Genes that are overexpressed in the vast majority of pancreatic adenocarcinomas include mesothelin, prostate stem cell antigen (PSCA), Muc4, Koc1 (Igf2bp3), Claudin4, Mic1, and others (125–130). This technology has enormous potential for the development of new screening tests for pancreatic cancer. Some, such as mesothelin and PSCA, are rather specific for carcinoma and can be used in immunohistochemistry to aid the evaluation of difficult biopsies (131). To date, the sensitivity, specificity, and ease of blood-based assays based on the new markers are inadequate to serve as routine markers for clinical management, but exploration of the new markers is in an early phase.

Abnormalities of gene methylation accompany human cancers. Of special interest, the methylation of islands containing high numbers of the dinucleotide CpG occurs in the promoters of some genes during tumorigenesis. This methylation often accompanies the epigenetic silencing of gene expression, such as frequently occurs with the cell cycle regulatory genes *p16* and *CDKN1C/p57/KIP2* in pancreatic cancer (36,132). Methylation of the *PENK* (proenkephalin A) gene occurs in virtually all invasive pancreatic neoplasms and is associated with the more advanced PanIN lesions but is not present in normal ducts (133). Gene methylation of this and other genes might serve as a diagnostic marker in biopsies and pancreatic secretions (134). There is great interest in therapeutically reversing the abnormal methylation by use of drugs such as inhibitors of the DNA methyltransferase and histone deacetylase enzymes that otherwise help maintain the methylation patterns, in order to enable reexpression of the silenced genes.

Telomeres become shortened very early and universally in pancreatic neoplasia (135). Telomerase is expressed at low levels in many normal tissues and at significantly higher levels in many cancer types, including pancreatic ductal adenocarcinoma (136–138). It is unclear whether telomerase expression is "turned on" during tumorigenesis or whether there is a simple selection for those neoplastic clones best able to maintain enough telomerase activity to stabilize the chromosomal integrity of the genome. Early reports suggested that telomerase levels in pancreatic secretions might serve as a diagnostic aid (139).

Most human cells demonstrate a dependence on extracellular growth factors, opening the possibility of therapeutic approaches to block these stimulatory pathways. A number of growth factor receptors (e.g., Her2/Neu and epidermal growth factor receptors) are overexpressed, and tumor cells can be dependent on such signals (140,141). Pancreatic cancer cell lines often have a constitutive activation of NF-κB activity (142); this pathway is best studied in lymphoid tissues but is also known to have critical antiapoptotic effects in epithelial tissues (143). The hedgehog pathway, which is activated by mutations in basal cell carcinoma and medulloblastoma (144,145), is constitutively active for unknown reasons in pancreatic cancer (146).

The Stat3 DNA-binding transcription factor is also constitutively active, and would have a direct influence on gene expression (147,148). The overactivity of these growth-promoting or antiapoptotic pathways suggests potential targets for rational therapeutic approaches. For example, anti-EGFR therapeutics are being evaluated in clinical trials, drugs targeting the hedgehog and Jak-Stat pathways are being developed, and blockade of the hedgehog pathway causes regression of these cells in culture or when growing as xenografts in mice (146).

Patients with pancreatic cancer are especially susceptible to cachexia, a combination of loss of appetite, decreased anabolism, and increased catabolism of lipids and proteins. Studies of blood levels of various proteins released from the tumor site, including inflammatory cytokines, hint at a bewildering variety of potential effectors of the catabolic state. Nonetheless, biological studies of fractionated body fluids from animals and human patients with cancer cachexia have identified elevated levels of certain biochemically definable catabolic agents (149). One is a lipid-mobilizing factor and is synonymous with Zn $\alpha 2$ glycoprotein (150). Another mobilizes cellular protein and is associated with increased weight loss in patients with pancreatic carcinoma (151). The effects of the latter are antagonized by eicosapentaenoic acid (fish oil) (152), and fish oil therefore has been evaluated in clinical trials.

Given the extraordinary clinical aggressiveness of pancreatic ductal adenocarcinoma and the known genetic and biological features, it might be surprising to learn that slow growth is seen for many of the cell lines in tissue culture and that most primary tumors do not have high mitotic rates. Thus, it appears that the appropriateness, not simply the speed, of cell proliferation is abnormal. Pancreatic ductal cells located within stroma should not only be dividing slower, they should not be dividing at all. This perspective is poignant when considering the lack of responsiveness to conventional chemotherapeutic agents.

INHERITED MUTATIONS AND FAMILIAL SYNDROMES

Familial pancreatic cancer has an autosomal pattern and, by using segregation analysis of affected families, can be attributed to the action of rare mutant genes (153). Readers interested in the genetic epidemiology of pancreatic cancer are referred to Chapter 24 and to recent reviews (154,155).

In most kindred, unfortunately, the germline genetic alteration responsible for the aggregate of pancreatic cancer has not been identified. Even where the responsible gene has been identified, it should be noted that some of the carriers of these germline mutations in the relevant tumor-suppressor genes do not develop cancer. That is, the disease penetrance is relatively low. A number of reasons could be offered for this pattern. First, many superimposed somatic genetic events are required to produce the most advanced, invasive form of ductal neoplasia; because these events occur by chance and because the numeric population of duct cells is rather limited, not every susceptible individual would be expected to form a carcinoma. Second, the inherited gene abnormality would not produce a biological phenotype until the second (wild-type) allele is lost, which may be a late event in tumorigenesis as indicated in some cases for the BRCA2 gene (31).

The case for hereditary pancreatitis is entirely different. In some families with germline mutations of the PRSS1 (cationic trypsinogen) gene, the penetrance of cancer is >50% in gene carriers (156). This high rate for inherited cancer susceptibility is all the more remarkable in that the PRSS1 gene is neither an oncogene, tumor-suppressor gene, nor a genome maintenance gene. This may be an example where mitogenesis drives mutagenesis (i.e., the tissue requirements for continued cell division

as part of the reparative processes associated with chronic pancreatitis will create an increased incidence of mutations simply due to an increased number of DNA replicative cycles). Measured in cell division cycles, time moves faster in the pancreatic ducts of these patients. Interestingly, there are also suggestions that in cystic fibrosis patients and in heterozygous carriers of CFTR mutations, there is a slight increase in risk of pancreatic cancer (157). The mechanism may be similar.

PANCREATIC INTRAEPITHELIAL NEOPLASIA

Until recently, the nomenclature used to describe neoplastic lesions in the pancreas did not reflect ductal tumorigenesis as a continuum. It is now clear that there is a histologic and genetic progression series in the pancreatic ducts. Analogous to adenomas as the most common form of intestinal dysplasia and cervical intraepithelial neoplasia (CIN) as the form of uterine cervical dysplasia (among many other examples), the nomenclature for pancreatic intraepithelial neoplasia (PanIN) can be used to grade the noninvasive earlier manifestations of pancreatic ductal neoplasia. The current nomenclature has a surprising similarity to a long-overlooked grading system of Hulst published in 1905 (158–160).

From PanIN-1, which refers to the proliferation of columnar epithelial cells without significant architectural or cytologic atypia in the ducts, through to PanIN-3, which is architecturally and cytologically quite advanced, there is an associated progression of accumulated genetic abnormalities (Fig. 25.2). Telomere shortening and KRAS gene mutations frequently occur in relatively early (PanIN-1) lesions and are present in the vast majority of more advanced PanIN (135,161). Changes in the expression and genetic integrity of the p16 gene appear with significant frequency in intermediate lesions (PanIN-2) (162,163). Overexpression of p53 (which often accompanies mutations of that gene) (164), loss of expression of Smad4 protein (which is associated with SMAD4 genetic inactivation), and loss of the wild-type BRCA2 allele in carriers of germline BRCA2 mutations appears to occur late in the neoplastic progression of PanINs (PanIN-3) (31,165).

IMPLICATIONS FOR CLINICAL MANAGEMENT

Histologic, clinical, and genetic means now exist by which the primary care physicians can recognize inherited pancreatic cancer syndromes. The proximate clinical management then would most often be to recommend genetic counseling. This approach, however, may still not be appropriate for many of the families that could be recognized. In the absence of a clear clinical utility (would a real change in the clinical management of the patient be instituted based on the knowledge?), clinicians and/or families still often choose not to fully investigate the possibility of inherited susceptibility.

In families having two or more close relatives with pancreatic cancer, the risk of new incidents of the disease is increased many fold (166). Within these patients, multiple foci of centrilobular atrophy accompany the precursor lesions of the ducts (3). In a number of patients at very high inherited risk, IPMNs, PanINs, and even asymptomatic incipient carcinomas were identified by endoscopic ultrasound due to changes in the ducts and the accompanying atrophy (167), although such screening is only now being explored in larger populations of at-risk persons. The possibility of a mutation-based screening tool was supported when KRAS mutations were identified in the stool and in the pancreatic secretions of persons with pancreatic cancer (161,168).

An improved understanding of the molecular biology and genetics of pancreatic cancer also opens the door for the development of a potential "rational therapy" for pancreatic adenocarcinoma, by which one would target a specific molecular abnormality of the cancer. Cancers cells deficient in *BRCA2* and Fanconi anemia genes are hypersensitive to DNA interstrand cross-linking agents (108,110,111). This property has suggested that patients with such mutations in their cancers might be placed on protocols specifically incorporating this class of anticancer drugs (159,169).

Drugs to block the action of the ras oncogene have also been proposed. The localization of the H-ras, K-ras, and N-ras proteins at the cell membrane is required for their activity in signal transmission. Attachment of a farnesyl group to the end of the ras amino acid chain allows this association and is accomplished with the enzymatic catalysis of the ras farnesyl transferase protein. Compounds were developed that effectively inhibit this enzyme, and block the action of the H-ras and v-ras oncogenes in mammalian cells (170–172). However, the *KRAS* oncogene (the one mutated in pancreatic cancers) is unlike the H-ras protein in that it can bind to the cell membrane by additional means. Also, the membrane-dissociated ras produced by these agents would be expected to have a dominant-negative effect, a suppressive mechanism that would be more exaggerated under the conditions of artificial ras expression used in experimental models. There are multiple means of resistance to these agents, both ras independent and ras dependent (173). The antiproliferative actions of the compounds are not restricted to cells having mutant ras and may affect other ras-related genes. In taking advantage of these useful properties, the more optimistic expectations for rational therapy are not fully met (173–177).

Other intriguing but less developed approaches include the possibility of compounds that directly augment the action of tumor-suppressive pathways; in the case of mutated pathways members, effector mechanisms positioned further downstream in the pathway would serve as the appropriate target of therapeutic effect. It might be possible to stimulate immune responses against individual antigens, including the genes normally having highly tissue-restricted expression but that are specifically overexpressed in the cancer (178). Applying novel therapies to intraductal disease (PanIN), perhaps as part of the management of inherited susceptibility, is likely to attract more serious consideration. The use of gene therapy and infectious vectors for pancreatic carcinoma is difficult to envision due to the presence of disseminated disease.

Intraductal Papillary Mucinous Neoplasms

Activating point mutations in codon 12 of the *KRAS* gene occur in up to 50% of intraductal papillary mucinous neoplasms (IPMNs) (179,180). Nearly 11% have mutations in the *PIK3CA* kinase gene (F Schonleben et al.). In contrast to the high prevalence of loss of Smad4 in ductal adenocarcinomas, however, IPMNs almost always express Smad4 (181). Most IPMNs, particularly those with an "intestinal" pattern of differentiation, express the mucin antigen MUC2 rather than MUC1. In contrast, most PanIN lesions express MUC1, and almost all PanIN lesions are MUC2 negative (182).

Mucinous Cystic Neoplasms

Activating point mutations of the *KRAS* gene are reported in mucinous cystic neoplasms of the pancreas, especially those with an associated invasive cancer (183). The immunolabeling pattern retains a normal beta-catenin membranous localization. The Smad4 protein is present in almost all noninvasive mucinous cystic neoplasms but is lost in half of the invasive carcinomas that on occasion arise from genetic progression of these tumors (184,185).

Acinar Carcinoma of the Pancreas

Acinar carcinoma represents about 1% of the pancreatic exocrine carcinomas in adults. Genetic and biological studies of these tumors are limited to sparse reports, although in contrast to ductal adenocarcinomas, they usually do not harbor *KRAS* gene mutations (186). A subset of acinar cell carcinomas harbor mutations in the *Beta-Catenin* or *APC* gene, and these tumors have allelic losses indicative of the process of chromosomal instability (187). They thus have molecular genetic features similar to the histologically similar entity of pancreatoblastoma.

Pancreatoblastoma

Pancreatoblastomas are tumors that usually occur in the pediatric ages but can occur in adults. Most have mutations in the *Beta-Catenin* gene and nuclear accumulation of beta-catenin protein, but the tumor has also been reported as an extraintestinal manifestation of adenomatous polyposis coli caused by a germline *APC* gene mutation (188). The documentation of allelic losses confirmed the process of chromosomal instability (188).

Solid Pseudopapillary Neoplasms

Solid pseudopapillary neoplasms usually occur in adult females. A mutation in the *Beta-Catenin* gene and nuclear localization of beta-catenin protein are nearly always present, while the *KRAS* gene is wild type (189).

Neuroendocrine Neoplasms of the Pancreas

Functionally and histologically, the pancreas comprises two organs. Classification of the neuroendocrine tumors is complicated by the underappreciated fact that either system can give rise to carcinomas with features of neuroendocrine differentiation. Careful histologic examination can usually disentangle the two groups. Molecular discoveries may also provide distinguishing markers. For example, ductal carcinomas with features of neuroendocrine differentiation can harbor *SMAD4* abnormalities (60,190), while the tumors of more clear-cut endocrine origin lack such mutations in *SMAD4* (191,192).

The tumors of endocrine origin, whether benign or malignant, derive from the pancreatic endocrine system (i.e., the islets). Many tumors retain the capability to produce a particular hormone, and the overproduction of insulin, glucagon, gastrin, or VIP is often adequate to cause clinical manifestations. As discussed in Chapter 27, the clinical aggressiveness of the tumors is not closely tied to the histologic appearance of the primary tumor, and well-differentiated neuroendocrine tumors can metastasize. The tumors can occur sporadically, as part of multiple endocrine neoplasia type I (MEN I) syndrome, or occasionally in von Hippel-Lindau syndrome (193). Endocrine tumors often appear to involve the *MEN1* gene, but not the *KRAS* or *p53* genes, and have considerably fewer genetic deletions than the ductal carcinomas (194).

The *MEN1* gene was originally localized by genetic linkage studies in families with the MEN I syndrome (195). The precise localization was provided by the fine mapping of LOH patterns observed in the endocrine neoplasms of such patients (196). In patients with MEN I, the pancreatic endocrine tumors would be expected to harbor the inherited mutation and have somatic inactivation of the remaining wild-type allele, usually by a large deletion. Of the sporadic endocrine tumors, not associated with MEN I syndrome, nearly one-third contain *MEN1* inactivation (197). The gene is classified as a tumor suppressor and encodes a nuclear protein (198). It represses expression of telomerase, as one of a number of proposed functions (199).

Adenocarcinoma of the Distal Common Bile Duct

It is only with difficulty that the carcinomas of the distal (intrapancreatic) common bile duct can be distinguished from those of the pancreatic ducts. The distinction is anatomical and relies on careful histologic examination. There are as yet no clear-cut genetic distinctions. The biliary carcinomas, however, appear to be genetically somewhat less homogeneous than those of the pancreas, and the frequencies of mutation, when assessed for individual genes, are somewhat lower. Tumors of the proximal biliary tract, especially the intrahepatic tumors, are genetically dissimilar from those located at the pancreas. Thus, in clinical and in genetic studies, the best available characterization of a tumor should be determined according to experienced gross anatomical and histologic examination. The unqualified use of the term *biliary carcinoma* or *cholangiocarcinoma* to characterize the tumors in such studies is insufficient.

Adenocarcinoma of the Duodenum

Adenocarcinoma of the duodenum is an intestinal neoplasm. Neoplasia of the intestinal epithelium is in genetic terms quite distinct from the neoplasms of pancreatic epithelium. Intestinal neoplasia, including that of the duodenum, is characterized by mutations of the *APC/Beta-catenin* pathway and is not believed to include genetic alterations of the *p16* gene.

Adenocarcinoma at the Duodenal Papilla ("Ampullary Carcinoma")

Anatomically, the duodenal papilla is a raised mucosal orifice that forms the junction of the pancreatic duct with the duodenal lumen. The junction of the pancreatic and common bile duct to form a significant (>3 mm) straight or bulbous common intramucosal channel is the anatomical "ampulla," which in detailed histopathological and radiologic studies of the ducts and the papilla, is an inconstant feature found in nearly half of persons (200). If the anatomical variance of the population were not confusing enough, the invasive nature of carcinoma serves to obliterate the site of origin and the defining anatomical landmarks. Thus, it should be no surprise that the term *ampullary cancer* involves similar vagaries. In genetic terms, neoplasms at the duodenal papilla would be expected to represent an assortment of tumors having either ductal or intestinal origin, with features of the respective tumor type. Adjacent to some carcinomas, precursor neoplasia (dysplasia) of the duodenal mucosa or of the ductal system can aid in assigning the histogenesis.

Miscellaneous Tumors of the Pancreas

Mesenchymal tumors are, in terms of patterns of the somatic genetic alterations, unrelated to the carcinomas. Gastrointestinal stromal tumors are the most common form of mesenchymal tumors in the digestive tract. They can occur in the duodenal wall and often contain somatic mutations that activate the function of the *KIT* gene, a receptor for a ligand termed *stem cell factor* (201). These tumors respond to the tyrosine kinase inhibitor drug imatinib (202).

Lymphomas can appear as primary tumors within the pancreas. Their genetic profiles would mirror those of other lymphomas of the body.

Cysts of the pancreas occur in patients who have polycystic kidney disease caused by inherited inactivating mutations of the *PKD1* gene. The cysts develop from foci where there is loss of the remaining wild-type *PKD1* allele (203).

Among the nonneoplastic lumps and bumps of the pancreas, such as pseudocysts, scars, and simple strictures, no clonal genetic changes would be expected, except in the case of the coincidental presence and unintentional sampling of adjacent PanIN. This latter possibility must be taken into account if genetic assays are to be considered for use as a diagnostic aid.

References

1. Kinzler KW, Vogelstein B. Lessons from hereditary colorectal cancer. *Cell* 1996;87:159–170.
2. Kern SE. Clonality: more than just a tumor-progression model. *J Natl Cancer Inst* 1993;85:1020–1021.
3. Brune K, Abe T, Canto M, et al. Multifocal neoplastic precursor lesions associated with lobular atrophy of the pancreas in patients having a strong family history of pancreatic cancer. *Am J Surg Pathol* 2006;30:1067–1076.
4. Johansson B, Bardi G, Heim S, et al. Nonrandom chromosomal rearrangements in pancreatic carcinomas. *Cancer* 1992;69:1–8.
5. Griffin CA, Hruban RH, Long PP, Morsberger LA, Douna-Issa F, Yeo CJ. Chromosome abnormalities in pancreatic adenocarcinoma. *Genes Chrom Cancer* 1994;9:93–100.
6. Gorunova L, Hoglund M, Andren-Sandberg A, et al. Cytogenetic analysis of pancreatic carcinomas: intratumor heterogeneity and nonrandom pattern of chromosome aberrations. *Genes Chrom Cancer* 1998;23:81–99.
7. Iacobuzio-Donahue CA, van der Heijden MS, Baumgartner MR, et al. Large-scale allelotype of pancreaticobiliary carcinoma provides quantitative estimates of genome-wide allelic loss. *Cancer Res* 2004;64:871–875.
8. Brat DJ, Hahn SA, Griffin CA, Yeo CJ, Kern SE, Hruban RH. The structural basis of molecular genetic deletions: an integration of classical cytogenetic and molecular analyses in pancreatic adenocarcinoma. *Am J Pathol* 1997;150:383–391.
9. Allison DC, Bose KK, Hruban RH, et al. Pancreatic cancer cell DNA content correlates with long-term survival after pancreatoduodenectomy. *Ann Surg* 1991;214:648–655.
10. Ghadimi BM, Schröck E, Walker RL, et al. Specific chromosomal aberrations and amplification of the AIB1 nuclear receptor coactivator gene in pancreatic carcinomas. *Am J Pathol* 1999;154:525–536.
11. Solinas-Toldo S, Wallrapp C, Muller-Pillasch F, Bentz M, Gress T, Lichter P. Mapping of chromosomal imbalances in pancreatic carcinoma by comparative genomic hybridization. *Cancer Res* 1996;56:3803–3807.
12. Kallioniemi A, Kallioniemi O-P, Sudar D, et al. Comparative genomic hybridization for molecular cytogenetic analysis of solid tumors. *Science* 1992;258:818–821.
13. Kern SE. Progressive genetic abnormalities in human cancer. In: Mendelsohn MIJ, Liotta L, Howley PM, eds. *Molecular Basis of Cancer*. 2nd ed. Philadelphia WB Saunders; 2000:41–69.
14. Kern SE. Whose hypothesis? Ciphering, sectorials, D lesions, freckles and the operation of Stigler's law. *Cancer Biol Ther* 2002;1:571–581.
15. Nicholls EM. Somatic variation and multiple neurofibromatosis. *Hum Hered* 1969;19:473–479.
16. Bos JL. Ras oncogenes in human cancer: a review. *Cancer Res* 1989;49:4682–4689.
17. Almoguera C, Shibata D, Forrester K, Martin J, Arnheim N, Perucho M. Most human carcinomas of the exocrine pancreas contain mutant c-K-ras genes. *Cell* 1988;53:549–554.
18. Wilentz RE, Goggins M, Redston M, et al. Genetic, immunohistochemical, and clinical features of medullary carcinomas of the pancreas: a newly described and characterized entity. *Am J Pathol* 2000;156:1641–1651.

19. Goggins M, Offerhaus GJA, Hilgers W, et al. Adenocarcinomas of the pancreas with DNA replication errors (RER+) are associated with wild-type K-ras and characteristic histopathology: poor differentiation, a syncytial growth pattern, and pushing borders suggest RER+. *Am J Pathol* 1998;152:1501–1507.

20. Calhoun ES, Jones JB, Ashfaq R, et al. BRAF and FBXW7 (CDC4, FBW7, AGO, SEL10) mutations in distinct subsets of pancreatic cancer: potential therapeutic targets. *Am J Pathol* 2003;163:1255–1260.

21. Forrester K, Almoguera C, Han K, Grizzle WE, Perucho M. Detection of high incidence of K-ras oncogenes during human colon tumorigenesis. *Nature* 1987;327:298–303.

22. Bos JL, Fearon ER, Hamilton SR, et al. Prevalence of ras gene mutations in human colorectal cancers. *Nature* 1987;327:293–297.

23. Der CJ, Finkel T, Cooper GM. Biological and biochemical properties of human rasH genes mutated at codon 61. *Cell* 1986;44:167–176.

24. Elion EA. Routing MAP kinase cascades. *Science* 1998;281:1625–1626.

25. Moberg KH, Bell DW, Wahrer DC, Haber DA, Hariharan IK. Archipelago regulates cyclin E levels in *Drosophila* and is mutated in human cancer cell lines. *Nature* 2001;413:311–316.

26. Strohmaier H, Spruck CH, Kaiser P, Won KA, Sangfelt O, Reed SI. Human F-box protein hCdc4 targets cyclin E for proteolysis and is mutated in a breast cancer cell line. *Nature* 2001;413:316–222.

27. Batra SK, Metzgar RS, Hollingsworth MA. Isolation and characterization of a complementary DNA (PD-1) differentially expressed by human pancreatic ductal cell tumors. *Cell Growth Differ* 1991;2:385–390.

28. Miwa W, Yasuda J, Murakami Y, et al. Isolation of DNA sequences amplified at chromosome 19q13.1–q13.2 including the AKT2 locus in human pancreatic cancer. *Biochem Biophys Res Commun* 1996;225:968–974.

29. Cheng JQ, Ruggeri B, Klein WM, et al. Amplification of AKT2 in human pancreatic cancer cells and inhibition of AKT2 expression and tumorigenecity by antisense RNA. *Proc Natl Acad Sci U S A* 1996;93:3636–3641.

30. Wallrapp C, Muller-Pillasch F, Solinas-Toldo S, et al. Characterization of a high copy number amplification at 6q24 in pancreatic cancer identifies c-MYB as a candidate oncogene. *Cancer Res* 1997;57:3135–3139.

31. Goggins M, Hruban RH, Kern SE. BRCA2 is inactivated late in the development of pancreatic intraepithelial neoplasia: evidence and implications. *Am J Pathol* 2000;156:1767–1771.

32. Serrano M, Hannon GJ, Beach D. A new regulatory motif in cell-cycle control causing specific inhibition of cyclin D/CDK4. *Nature* 1993;366:704–707.

33. Kamb A, Gruis NA, Weaver-Feldhaus J, et al. A cell cycle regulator potentially involved in genesis of many tumor types. *Science* 1994;264:436–440.

34. Hussussian CJ, Struewing JP, Goldstein AM, et al. Germline p16 mutations in familial melanoma. *Nat Genet* 1994;8:15–21.

35. Caldas C, Hahn SA, da Costa LT, et al. Frequent somatic mutations and homozygous deletions of the p16 (MTS1) gene in pancreatic adenocarcinoma. *Nat Genet* 1994;8:27–31.

36. Schutte M, Hruban RH, Geradts J, et al. Abrogation of the Rb/p16 tumor-suppressive pathway in virtually all pancreatic carcinomas. *Cancer Res* 1997;57:3126–3130.

37. Huang L, Lang D, Geradts J, et al. Molecular and immunochemical analyses of RB1 and cyclin D1 in human ductal pancreatic carcinomas and cell lines. *Mol Carcinog* 1996;15:85–95.

38. Baker SJ, Fearon ER, Nigro JM, et al. Chromosome 17 deletions and p53 gene mutations in colorectal carcinomas. *Science* 1989;244:217–221.

39. Nigro JM, Baker SJ, Preisinger AC, et al. p53 Gene mutations occur in diverse human tumour types. *Nature* 1989;342:705–708.

40. Kern SE, Kinzler KW, Baker SJ, et al. Mutant p53 proteins bind DNA abnormally in vitro. *Oncogene* 1991;6:131–136.

41. Kern SE, Pietenpol JA, Thiagalingam S, Seymour A, Kinzler KW, Vogelstein B. Oncogenic forms of p53 inhibit p53-regulated gene expression. *Science* 1992;256:827–830.

42. El-Deiry WS, Tokino T, Velculescu VE, et al. WAF1, a potential mediator of p53 tumor suppression. *Cell* 1993;75:817–825.

43. Waldman T, Kinzler KW, Vogelstein B. p21 is necessary for the p53-mediated G1 arrest in human cancer cells. *Cancer Res* 1995;55:5187–5190.

44. Waldman T, Lengauer C, Kinzler KW, Vogelstein B. Uncoupling of S phase and mitosis induced by anticancer agents in cells lacking p21. *Nature* 1996;381:713–716.

45. Bunz F, Dutriaux A, Lengauer C, et al. Requirement for p53 and p21 to sustain G2 arrest after DNA damage. *Science* 1998;282:1497–1501.

46. Chan TA, Hermeking H, Lengauer C, Kinzler KW, Vogelstein B. 14-3-3Sigma is required to prevent mitotic catastrophe after DNA damage. *Nature* 1999;401:616–620.

47. Kastan MB, Onyekwere O, Sidransky D, Vogelstein B, Craig RW. Participation of p53 protein in the cellular response to DNA damage. *Cancer Res* 1991;51:6304–6311.

48. Zhan Q, Fan S, Bae I, et al. Induction of bax by genotoxic stress in human cells correlates with normal p53 status and apoptosis. *Oncogene* 1994;9:3743–3751.

49. Pellegata S, Sessa F, Renault B, et al. K-ras and p53 gene mutations in pancreatic cancer: ductal and nonductal tumors progress through different genetic lesions. *Cancer Res* 1994;54:1556–1560.

50. Rozenblum E, Schutte M, Goggins M, et al. Tumor-suppressive pathways in pancreatic carcinoma. *Cancer Res* 1997;57:1731–1734.

51. Hahn SA, Schutte M, Hoque ATMS, et al. DPC4, a candidate tumor-suppressor gene at 18q21.1. *Science* 1996;271:350–353.

52. Sekelsky JJ, Newfeld SJ, Raftery LA, Chartoff EH, Gelbart WM. Genetic characterization and cloning of Mothers against dpp, a gene required for decapentaplegic function in *Drosophila melanogaster*. *Genetics* 1995;139:1347–1358.

53. Savage C, Das P, Finelli AL, et al. Caenorhabditis elegans genes sma-2, sma-3, and sma-4 define a conserved family of transforming growth factor beta pathway components. *Proc Natl Acad Sci U S A* 1996;93:790–794.

54. Shi Y, Hata A, Lo RS, Massague J, Pavletich NP. A structural basis for mutational inactivation of the tumour suppressor Smad4. *Nature* 1997;388:87–93.

55. Zhang Y, Feng X, We R, Derynck R. Receptor-associated Mad homologues synergize as effectors of the TGF-beta response. *Nature* 1996;383:168–172.

56. Zawel L, Dai JL, Buckhaults P, et al. Human Smad3 and Smad4 are sequence-specific transcription activators. *Mol Cell* 1998;1:611–617.

57. Dai JL, Turnacioglu K, Schutte M, Sugar AY, Kern SE. Dpc4 transcriptional activation and dysfunction in cancer cells. *Cancer Res* 1998;58:4592–4597.

58. Dennler S, Itoh S, Vivien D, ten Dijke P, Huet S, Gauthier J-M. Direct binding of Smad3 and Smad4 to critical TGF-beta-inducible elements in the promoter of human plasminogen activator inhibitor-type I gene. *EMBO J* 1998;17:3091–3100.

59. Dai JL, Bansal RK, Kern SE. G1 cell cycle arrest and apoptosis induction by nuclear Smad4/Dpc4—phenotypes reversed by a tumorigenic mutation. *Proc Natl Acad Sci U S A* 1999;96:1427–1432.

60. Schutte M, Hruban RH, Hedrick L, et al. *DPC4* gene in various tumor types. *Cancer Res* 1996;56:2527–2530.

61. Wilentz RE, Su GH, Dai JL, et al. Immunohistochemical labeling for Dpc4 mirrors genetic status in pancreatic adenocarcinomas: a new marker of DPC4 inactivation. *Am J Pathol* 2000;156:37–43.

62. Iacobuzio-Donahue CA, Song J, Parmiagiani G, Yeo CJ, Hruban RH, Kern SE. Missense mutations of MADH4: characterization of the mutational hot spot and functional consequences in human tumors. *Clin Cancer Res* 2004;10:1597–1604.

63. Maurice D, Pierreux CE, Howell M, Wilentz RE, Owen MJ, Hill CS. Loss of Smad4 function in pancreatic tumors: C-terminal truncation leads to decreased stability. *J Biol Chem* 2001;276:43175–43181.

64. Markowitz S, Wang J, Myeroff L, et al. Inactivation of the type II TGF-beta receptor in colon cancer cells with microsatellite instability. *Science* 1995;268:1336–1338.

65. Garrigue-Antar L, Munoz-Antonia T, Antonia SJ, Gesmonde J, Vellucci VF, Reiss M. Missense mutations of the transforming growth factor beta type II receptor in human head and neck squamous carcinoma cells. *Cancer Res* 1995;55:3982–3987.

66. Mori Y, Yin J, Rashid A, et al. Instabilotyping: comprehensive identification of frameshift mutations caused by coding region microsatellite instability. *Cancer Res* 2001;61:6046–6049.

67. Hempen PM, Zhang L, Bansal RK, et al. Evidence of selection for clones having genetic inactivation of the activin A type II receptor (ACVR2) gene in gastrointestinal cancers. *Cancer Res* 2003;63:994–999.

68. Goggins M, Shekher M, Turnacioglu K, Yeo CJ, Hruban RH, Kern SE. Genetic alterations of the TGF beta receptor genes in pancreatic and biliary adenocarcinomas. *Cancer Res* 1998;58:5329–5332.

69. Ryu B, Kern SE. The essential similarity of TGFbeta and activin receptor transcriptional responses in cancer cells. *Cancer Biol Ther* 2003;2:164–170.

70. Macias-Silva M, Abdollah S, Hoodless PA, Pirone R, Attisano L, Wrana JL. MADR2 is a substrate of the TGFbeta receptor and its phosphorylation is required for nuclear accumulation and signaling. *Cell* 1996;87:1215–1224.

71. Zhou S, Buckhaults P, Zawel L, et al. Targeted deletion of Smad4 shows it is required for transforming growth factor-beta and activin signaling in colorectal cancer cells. *Proc Natl Acad Sci U S A* 1998;95:2412–2416.

72. de Winter JP, Roelen BA, ten Dijke P, van der Burg B, van den Eijnden-van Raaij AJ. DPC4 (SMAD4) mediates transforming growth factor-beta1 (TGF-beta1) induced growth inhibition and transcriptional response in breast tumour cells. *Oncogene* 1997;14:1891–1899.

73. Dai JL, Schutte M, Sugar A, Kern SE. TGF beta responsiveness in DPC4-null cancer cells. *Mol Carcinog* 1999;26:37–43.

74. Hocevar BA, Brown TL, Howe PH. TGF-beta induces fibronectin synthesis through a c-Jun N-terminal kinase-dependent, Smad4-independent pathway. *EMBO J* 1999;18:1345–1356.

75. Grady WM, Myeroff LL, Swinler SE, et al. Mutational inactivation of transforming growth factor receptor beta type II in microsatellite stable colon cancers. *Cancer Res* 1999;59:320–324.

76. Sanchez I, Hughes RT, Mayer BJ, et al. Role of SAPK/ERK kinase-1 in the stress-activated pathway regulating transcription factor c-Jun. *Nature* 1994;372:794–798.

77. Yan M, Dai T, Deak JC, et al. Activation of stress-activated protein kinase by MEKK1 phosphorylation of its activator SEK1. *Nature* 1994;372:798–800.

78. Teng DH-F, Perry WL, III, Hogan JK, et al. Human mitogen-activated protein kinase kinase 4 as a candidate tumor suppressor. *Cancer Res* 1997;57:4177–4182.

79. Su GH, Hilgers W, Shekher M, et al. Alterations in pancreatic, biliary, and breast carcinomas support MKK4 as a genetically targeted tumor-suppressor gene. *Cancer Res* 1998;58:2339–2342.

80. Parsons DW, Wang TL, Samuels Y, et al. Colorectal cancer: mutations in a signalling pathway. *Nature* 2005;436:792.
81. Hemminki A, Markie D, Tomlinson I, et al. A serine/threonine kinase gene defective in Peutz-Jeghers syndrome. *Nature* 1998;391:184–187.
82. Jenne DE, Reimann H, Nezu J, et al. Peutz-Jeghers syndrome is caused by mutations in a novel serine threonine kinase. *Nat Genet* 1998;18:38–43.
83. Hawley SA, Boudeau J, Reid JL, et al. Complexes between the LKB1 tumor suppressor, STRAD alpha/beta and MO25 alpha/beta are upstream kinases in the AMP-activated protein kinase cascade. *J Biol* 2003;2:28.
84. Shaw RJ, Bardeesy N, Manning BD, et al. The LKB1 tumor suppressor negatively regulates mTOR signaling. *Cancer Cell* 2004;6:91–99.
85. Giardiello FM, Welsh SB, Hamilton SR, et al. Increased risk of cancer in the Peutz-Jeghers syndrome. *N Engl J Med* 1987;316:1511–1514.
86. Su GH, Hruban RH, Bova GS, et al. Germline and somatic mutations of the STK11/LKB1 Peutz-Jeghers gene in pancreatic and biliary cancers. *Am J Pathol* 1999;154:1835–1840.
87. Hilgers W, Kern SE. The molecular genetic basis of pancreatic cancer. *Genes Chrom Cancer* 1999;26:1–12.
88. Fearon ER, Cho KR, Nigro JM, et al. Identification of a chromosome 18q gene that is altered in colorectal cancers. *Science* 1990;247:49–56.
89. Hilgers W, Song JJ, Hayes M, Hruban RR, Kern SE, Fearon ER. Homozygous deletions inactivate DCC, but not DPC4, in a subset of pancreatic and biliary cancers. *Genes Chrom Cancer* 2000;27:353–357.
90. Sorio C, Baron A, Orlandini S, et al. The *FHIT* gene is expressed in pancreatic ductular cells and is altered in pancreatic cancers. *Cancer Res* 1999;59:1308–1314.
91. Simon B, Bartsch D, Barth P, et al. Frequent abnormalities of the putative tumor suppressor gene *FHIT* at 3p14.2 in pancreatic carcinoma cell lines. *Cancer Res* 1998;58:1583–1587.
92. Hilgers W, Koerkamp BG, Geradts J, et al. Genomic *FHIT* alterations in RER+ and RER– adenocarcinomas of the pancreas. *Genes Chrom Cancer* 2000;27:239–243.
93. Mollenhauer J, Wiemann S, Scheurlen W, et al. DMBT1, a new member of the SRCR superfamily, on chromosome 10q25.3-26.1 is deleted in malignant brain tumours. *Nat Genet* 1997;17:32–39.
94. Le Beau MM, Drabkin H, Glover TW, et al. An *FHIT* tumor suppressor gene? *Genes Chrom Cancer* 1998;21:281–289.
95. Hempen PM, Kurpad H, Calhoun ES, Abraham S, Kern SE. A double missense variation of the BUB1 gene and a defective mitotic spindle checkpoint in the pancreatic cancer cell line Hs766T. *Hum Mutat* 2005;26:592.
96. Lengauer C, Kinzler KW, Vogelstein B. Genetic instability in colorectal cancers. *Nature* 1997;386:623–627.
97. Schutte M, da Costa LT, Hahn SA, et al. Identification by representational difference analysis of a homozygous deletion in pancreatic carcinoma that lies within the BRCA2 region. *Proc Natl Acad Sci U S A* 1995;92:5950–5954.
98. Wooster R, Neuhausen SL, Mangion J, et al. Localization of a breast cancer susceptibility gene, BRCA2, to chromosome 13q12–13. *Science* 1994;265:2088–2090.
99. Wooster R, Bignell G, Lancaster J, et al. Identification of the breast cancer susceptibility gene BRCA2. *Nature* 1995;378:789–792.
100. Mizuta R, LaSalle JM, Cheng HL, et al. RAB22 and RAB163/mouse BRCA2: proteins that specifically interact with the RAD51 protein. *Proc Natl Acad Sci U S A* 1997;94:6927–6932.
101. Goggins M, Schutte M, Lu J, et al. Germline *BRCA2* gene mutations in patients with apparently sporadic pancreatic carcinomas. *Cancer Res* 1996;56:5360–5364.
102. Ozcelik H, Schmocker B, Di Nicola N, et al. Germline BRCA2 6174delT mutations in Ashkenazi Jewish pancreatic cancer patients. *Nat Genet* 1997;16:17–18.
103. Murphy KM, Brune KA, Griffin C, et al. Evaluation of candidate genes MAP2K4, MADH4, ACVR1B, and BRCA2 in familial pancreatic cancer: deleterious BRCA2 mutations in 17%. *Cancer Res* 2002;62:3789–3793.
104. Hahn SA, Greenhalf B, Ellis I, et al. BRCA2 germline mutations in familial pancreatic carcinoma. *J Natl Cancer Inst* 2003;95:214–221.
105. Thorlacius S, Olafsdottir G, Tryggvadottir L, et al. A single *BRCA2* mutation in male and female breast carcinoma families from Iceland with varied cancer phenotypes. *Nat Genet* 1996;13:117–119.
106. Struewing JP, Hartge P, Wacholder S, et al. The risk of cancer associated with specific mutations of BRCA1 and BRCA2 among Ashkenazi Jews. *N Engl J Med* 1997;336:1401–1408.
107. van der Heijden MS, Yeo CJ, Hruban RH, Kern SE. Fanconi anemia gene mutations in young-onset pancreatic cancer. *Cancer Res* 2003;63:2585–2588.
108. van der Heijden MS, Brody JR, Gallmeier E, et al. Functional defects in the Fanconi anemia pathway in pancreatic cancer cells. *Am J Pathol* 2004;165:651–657.
109. Couch FJ, Johnson MR, Rabe K, et al. Germ line Fanconi anemia complementation group C mutations and pancreatic cancer. *Cancer Res* 2005;65:383–386.
110. Gallmeier E, Calhoun ES, Rago C, et al. Targeted disruption of FANCC and FANCG in human cancer provides a preclinical model of specific therapeutic options. *Gastroenterology* 2006;130:2145–2154.
111. van der Heijden MS, Brody JR, Dezentje DA, et al. In vivo therapeutic responses contingent on Fanconi anemia/BRCA2 status of the tumor. *Clin Cancer Res* 2005;11:7508–7515.
112. Luttges J, Beyser K, Pust S, Paulus A, Ruschoff J, Kloppel G. Pancreatic mucinous noncystic (colloid) carcinomas and intraductal papillary mucinous carcinomas are usually microsatellite stable. *Mod Pathol* 2003;16:537–542.
113. Aaltonen LA, Peltomäki P, Leach FS, et al. Clues to the pathogenesis of familial colorectal cancer. *Science* 1993;260:812–816.
114. Thibodeau SN, Bren G, Schaid D. Microsatellite instability in cancer of the proximal colon. *Science* 1993;260:816–819.
115. Ionov Y, Peinado MA, Malkhosyan S, Shibata D, Perucho M. Ubiquitous somatic mutations in simple repeated sequences reveal a new mechanism for colonic carcinogenesis. *Nature* 1993;363:558–561.
116. Bronner CE, Baker SM, Morrison PT, et al. Mutation in the DNA mismatch repair gene homologue hMLH1 is associated with hereditary non-polyposis colon cancer. *Nature* 1994;368:258–261.
117. Fishel R, Lescoe MK, Rao MRS, et al. The human mutator gene homolog MSH2 and its association with hereditary nonpolyposis colon cancer. *Cell* 1993;75:1027–1038.
118. Papadopoulos N, Nicolaides NC, Wei Y-F, et al. Mutation of a mutL homolog in hereditary colon cancer. *Science* 1994;263:1625–1629.
119. Leach FS, Nicolaides NC, Papadopoulos N, et al. Mutations of a mutS homolog in hereditary nonpolyposis colorectal cancer. *Cell* 1993;75:1215–1225.
120. Liebowitz D. Epstein-Barr virus—an old dog with new tricks. *N Engl J Med* 1995;332:55–57.
121. Shibata D, Weiss LM. Epstein-Barr virus-associated gastric adenocarcinoma. *Am J Pathol* 1992;140:769–774.
122. Zhang L, Zhou W, Velculescu VE, et al. Gene expression profiles in normal and cancer cells. *Science* 1997;276:1268–1272.
123. Gress TM, Wallrapp C, Frohme M, et al. Identification of genes with specific expression in pancreatic cancer by cDNA representational difference analysis. *Genes Chrom Cancer* 1997;19:97–103.
124. Iacobuzio-Donahue CA, Ashfaq R, Maitra A, et al. Highly expressed genes in pancreatic ductal adenocarcinomas: a comprehensive characterization and comparison of the transcription profiles obtained from three major technologies. *Cancer Res* 2003;63:8614–8622.
125. Mueller-Pillasch F, Lacher U, Wallrapp C, et al. Cloning of a gene highly overexpressed in cancer coding for a novel KH-domain containing protein. *Oncogene* 1997;14:2729–2733.
126. Argani P, Rosty C, Reiter RE, et al. Discovery of new markers of cancer through serial analysis of gene expression (SAGE): prostate stem cell antigen (PSCA) is overexpressed in pancreatic adenocarcinoma. *Cancer Res* 2001;61:4320–4324.
127. Argani P, Iacobuzio-Donahue CA, Ryu R, et al. Mesothelin is expressed in the vast majority of adenocarcinomas of the pancreas: identification of a new cancer marker by serial analysis of gene expression (SAGE). *Clin Cancer Res* 2001;7:3862–3868.
128. Michl P, Buchholz M, Rolke M, et al. Claudin-4: a new target for pancreatic cancer treatment using *Clostridium perfringens* enterotoxin. *Gastroenterology* 2001;121:678–684.
129. Hustinx SR, Cao D, Maitra A, et al. Differentially expressed genes in pancreatic ductal adenocarcinomas identified through serial analysis of gene expression. *Cancer Biol Ther* 2004;3:1254–1261.
130. Andrianifahanana M, Moniaux N, Schmied BM, et al. Mucin (MUC) gene expression in human pancreatic adenocarcinoma and chronic pancreatitis: a potential role of MUC4 as a tumor marker of diagnostic significance. *Clin Cancer Res* 2001;7:4033–4040.
131. McCarthy DM, Maitra A, Argani P, et al. Novel markers of pancreatic adenocarcinoma in fine-needle aspiration: mesothelin and prostate stem cell antigen labeling increases accuracy in cytologically borderline cases. *Appl Immunohistochem Mol Morphol* 2003;11:238–243.
132. Sato N, Matsubayashi H, Abe T, Fukushima N, Goggins M. Epigenetic down-regulation of CDKN1C/p57KIP2 in pancreatic ductal neoplasms identified by gene expression profiling. *Clin Cancer Res* 2005;11:4681–4688.
133. Fukushima N, Sato N, Ueki T, et al. Aberrant methylation of preproenkephalin and p16 genes in pancreatic intraepithelial neoplasia and pancreatic ductal adenocarcinoma. *Am J Pathol* 2002;160:1573–1581.
134. Matsubayashi H, Canto M, Sato N, et al. DNA methylation alterations in the pancreatic juice of patients with suspected pancreatic disease. *Cancer Res* 2006;66:1208–1217.
135. van Heek NT, Meeker AK, Kern SE, et al. Telomere shortening is nearly universal in pancreatic intraepithelial neoplasia. *Am J Pathol* 2002;161:1541–1547.
136. Hiyama E, Kodama T, Shinbara K, et al. Telomerase activity is detected in pancreatic cancer but not in benign tumors. *Cancer Res* 1997;57:326–331.
137. Kim NW, Piatyszek MA, Prowse KR, et al. Specific association of human telomerase activity with immortal cells and cancer. *Science* 1994;266:2011–2015.
138. Kyo S, Takakura M, Kohama T, Inoue M. Telomerase activity in human endometrium. *Cancer Res* 1997;57:610–613.
139. Iwao T, Hiyama E, Yokoyama T, et al. Telomerase activity for the preoperative diagnosis of pancreatic cancer. *J Natl Cancer Inst* 1997;89:1621–1623.

140. Korc M. Role of growth factors in pancreatic cancer. *Surg Oncol Clin N Am* 1998;7:25–41.

141. Day JD, DiGiuseppe JA, Yeo CJ, et al. Immunohistochemical evaluation of Her-2/neu oncogene expression in pancreatic adenocarcinoma and pancreatic intraepithelial neoplasms. *Human Pathol* 1996;27:119–124.

142. Wang W, Abbruzzese JL, Evans DB, Larry L, Cleary KR, Chiao PJ. The nuclear factor-kappa B RelA transcription factor is constitutively activated in human pancreatic adenocarcinoma cells. *Clin Cancer Res* 1999;5:119–127.

143. Baeuerle PA, Baltimore D. NF-kappa B: ten years after. *Cell* 1996;87:13–20.

144. Unden AB, Holmberg E, Lundh-Rozell B, et al. Mutations in the human homologue of *Drosophila* patched (PTCH) in basal cell carcinomas and the Gorlin syndrome: different in vivo mechanisms of PTCH inactivation. *Cancer Res* 1996;56:4562–4565.

145. Raffel C, Jenkins RB, Frederick L, et al. Sporadic medulloblastomas contain PTCH mutations. *Cancer Res* 1997;57:842–845.

146. Berman DM, Karhadkar SS, Maitra A, et al. Widespread requirement for Hedgehog ligand stimulation in growth of digestive tract tumours. *Nature* 2003;425:846–851.

147. Wei D, Le X, Zheng L, et al. Stat3 activation regulates the expression of vascular endothelial growth factor and human pancreatic cancer angiogenesis and metastasis. *Oncogene* 2003;22:319–329.

148. Scholz A, Heinze S, Detjen KM, et al. Activated signal transducer and activator of transcription 3 (STAT3) supports the malignant phenotype of human pancreatic cancer. *Gastroenterology* 2003;125:891–905.

149. Todorov P, Cariuk P, McDevitt T, Coles B, Fearon K, Tisdale M. Characterization of a cancer cachectic factor. *Nature* 1996;379:739–742.

150. Todorov PT, Deacon M, Tisdale MJ. Structural analysis of a tumor-produced sulfated glycoprotein capable of initiating muscle protein degradation. *J Biol Chem* 1997;272:12279–12288.

151. Wigmore SJ, Todorov PT, Barber MD, Ross JA, Tisdale MJ, Fearon KC. Characteristics of patients with pancreatic cancer expressing a novel cancer cachectic factor. *Br J Surg* 2000;87:53–58.

152. Smith HJ, Lorite MJ, Tisdale MJ. Effect of a cancer cachectic factor on protein synthesis/degradation in murine C2C12 myoblasts: modulation by eicosapentaenoic acid. *Cancer Res* 1999;59:5507–5513.

153. Klein AP, Beaty TH, Bailey-Wilson JE, Brune KA, Hruban RH, Petersen GM. Evidence for a major gene influencing risk of pancreatic cancer. *Genet Epidemiol* 2002;23:133–149.

154. Hruban RH, Canto MI, Griffin C, et al. Treatment of familial pancreatic cancer and its precursors. *Curr Treat Options Gastroenterol* 2005;8:365–375.

155. Lowenfels AB, Maisonneuve P. Risk factors for pancreatic cancer. *J Cell Biochem* 2005;95:649–656.

156. Lowenfels AB, Maisonneuve P, DiMagno EP, et al. Hereditary pancreatitis and the risk of pancreatic cancer. International Hereditary Pancreatitis Study Group. *J Natl Cancer Inst* 1997;89:442–446.

157. McWilliams R, Highsmith WE, Rabe KG, et al. Cystic fibrosis transmembrane conductance regulator gene carrier status is a risk factor for young onset pancreatic adenocarcinoma. *Gut* 2005;54:1661–1662.

158. Hulst SPL. Zur kenntnis der genese des adenokarzinoms und karzinoms des pankreas (Trans. T. van Heek and V. Koopman). *Virchows Arch B* 1905;180:288–316.

159. Kern SE, Hruban RH, Hidalgo M, Yeo CJ. An introduction to pancreatic carcinoma genetics, pathology, and therapy. *Cancer Biol Ther* 2002;1:607–613.

160. Hruban RH, Adsay NV, Albores-Saavedra J, et al. Pancreatic intraepithelial neoplasia: a new nomenclature and classification system for pancreatic duct lesions. *Am J Surg Pathol* 2001;25:579–586.

161. Caldas C, Hahn SA, Hruban RH, Redston MS, Yeo CJ, Kern SE. Detection of K-ras mutations in the stool of patients with pancreatic adenocarcinoma and pancreatic ductal hyperplasia. *Cancer Res* 1994;54:3568–3573.

162. Moskaluk CA, Hruban RH, Kern SE. p16 and K-ras mutations in the intraductal precursors of human pancreatic adenocarcinoma. *Cancer Res* 1997;57:2140–2143.

163. Wilentz RE, Geradts J, Offerhaus GHA, et al. Inactivation of the p16 (INK4A) tumor-suppressor gene early in pancreatic neoplasia: loss of intranuclear expression. *Cancer Res* 1998;58:4740–4744.

164. van Es JM, Polak MM, van den Berg FM, et al. Molecular markers for diagnostic cytology of neoplasms in the head region of the pancreas: mutation of K-ras and overexpression of the p53 protein product. *J Clin Pathol* 1995;48:218–222.

165. Wilentz RE, Iacobuzio-Donahue CA, Argani P, et al. Loss of expression of Dpc4 in pancreatic intraepithelial neoplasia: evidence that DPC4 inactivation occurs late in neoplastic progression. *Cancer Res* 2000;60:2002–2005.

166. Klein AP, Brune KA, Petersen GM, et al. Prospective risk of pancreatic cancer in familial pancreatic cancer kindreds. *Cancer Res* 2004;64:2634–2638.

167. Canto MI, Goggins M, Yeo CJ, et al. Screening for pancreatic neoplasia in high-risk individuals: an EUS-based approach. *Clin Gastroenterol Hepatol* 2004;2:606–621.

168. Shi C, Eshleman SH, Jones D, et al. LigAmp for sensitive detection of single-nucleotide differences. *Nat Methods* 2004;1:141–147.

169. Moynahan ME, Cui TY, Jasin M. Homology-directed DNA repair, mitomycin-c resistance, and chromosome stability is restored with correction of a Brca1 mutation. *Cancer Res* 2001;61:4842–4850.

170. Kohl NE, Mosser SD, deSolms SJ, et al. Selective inhibition of ras-dependent transformation by a farnesyltransferase inhibitor. *Science* 1993;260:1934–1937.

171. Kohl NE, Wilson FR, Mosser SD, et al. Protein farnesyltransferase inhibitors block the growth of ras-dependent tumors in nude mice. *Proc Natl Acad Sci U S A* 1994;91:9141–9145.

172. James GL, Goldstein JL, Brown MS, et al. Benzodiazepine peptidomimetics: potent inhibitors of ras farnesylation in animal cells. *Science* 1993;260:1937–1942.

173. Cox AD, Der CJ. Ras family signaling: therapeutic targeting. *Cancer Biol Ther* 2002;1:599–606.

174. Lerner EC, Qian Y, Blaskovich MA, et al. Ras CAAX peptidomimetic FTI-277 selectively blocks oncogenic Ras signaling by inducing cytoplasmic accumulation of inactive Ras-Raf complexes. *J Biol Chem* 1995;270:26802–26806.

175. James GL, Goldstein JL, Brown MS. Polylysine and CVIM sequences of K-RasB dictate specificity of prenylation and confer resistance to benzodiazepine peptidomimetic in vitro. *J Biol Chem* 1995;270:6221–6226.

176. Lebowitz PF, Prendergast GC. Non-Ras targets of farnesyltransferase inhibitors: focus on Rho. *Oncogene* 1998;17:1439–1445.

177. Du W, Prendergast GC. Geranylgeranylated RhoB mediates suppression of human tumor cell growth by farnesyltransferase inhibitors. *Cancer Res* 1999;59:5492–5496.

178. Thomas AM, Santarsiero LM, Lutz ER, et al. Mesothelin-specific CD8(+) T cell responses provide evidence of in vivo cross-priming by antigen-presenting cells in vaccinated pancreatic cancer patients. *J Exp Med* 2004;200:297–306.

179. Tada M, Omata M, Ohto M. Ras gene mutations in intraductal papillary neoplasms of the pancreas: analysis in five cases. *Cancer* 1991;67:634–637.

180. Sessa F, Solcia E, Capella C, et al. Intraductal papillary-mucinous tumours represent a distinct group of pancreatic neoplasms: an investigation of tumour cell differentiation and K-ras, p53 and c-erbB-2 abnormalities in 26 patients. *Virchows Arch* 1994;425:357–367.

181. Schonleben F, Qiu W, Ciau NT, et al. PIK3CA mutations in intraductal papillary neoplasm/carcinoma of the pancreas. *Clin Cancer Res* 2006;12:3851–3855.

182. Adsay NV, Merati K, Basturk O, et al. Pathologically and biologically distinct types of epithelium in intraductal papillary mucinous neoplasms: delineation of an "intestinal" pathway of carcinogenesis in the pancreas. *Am J Surg Pathol* 2004;28:839–848.

183. Bartsch D, Bastian D, Barth P, et al. K-ras oncogene mutations indicate malignancy in cystic tumors of the pancreas. *Ann Surg* 1998;228:79–86.

184. Iacobuzio-Donahue CA, Wilentz RE, Argani P, Yeo CJ, Kern SE, Hruban RH. Dpc4 protein in mucinous cystic neoplasms of the pancreas: frequent loss of expression in invasive carcinomas suggests a role in genetic progression. *Am J Surg Pathol* 2000;157:755–761.

185. Luttges J, Feyerabend B, Buchelt T, Pacena M, Kloppel G. The mucin profile of noninvasive and invasive mucinous cystic neoplasms of the pancreas. *Am J Surg Pathol* 2002;26:466–471.

186. Terhune PG, Heffess CS, Longnecker DS. Only wild-type c-Ki-ras codons 12, 13, and 61 in human pancreatic acinar cell carcinomas. *Mol Carcinog* 1994;10:110–114.

187. Abraham SC, Wu TT, Hruban RH, et al. Genetic and immunohistochemical analysis of pancreatic acinar cell carcinoma: frequent allelic loss on chromosome 11p and alterations in the APC/beta-catenin pathway. *Am J Pathol* 2002;160:953–962.

188. Abraham SC, Wu TT, Klimstra DS, et al. Distinctive molecular genetic alterations in sporadic and familial adenomatous polyposis-associated pancreatoblastomas: frequent alterations in the APC/beta-catenin pathway and chromosome 11p. *Am J Pathol* 2001;159:1619–1627.

189. Abraham SC, Klimstra DS, Wilentz RE, et al. Solid-pseudopapillary tumors of the pancreas are genetically distinct from pancreatic ductal adenocarcinomas and almost always harbor beta-catenin mutations. *Am J Pathol* 2002;160:1361–1369.

190. Bartsch D, Hahn SA, Danichevski KD, et al. Mutations of the DPC4/Smad4 gene in neuroendocrine pancreatic tumors. *Oncogene* 1999;18:2367–2371.

191. Allen E, Wilentz RE, Yeo CJ, Argani P, Kern SE, Hruban RH. Dpc4 expression is intact in neuroendocrine tumors of the pancreas. *NOGO* 2001;5:8.

192. Hessman O, Lindberg D, Einarsson A, et al. Genetic alterations on 3p, 11q13, and 18q in nonfamilial and MEN 1-associated pancreatic endocrine tumors. *Genes Chrom Cancer* 1999;26:258–264.

193. Lubensky IA, Pack S, Ault D, et al. Multiple neuroendocrine tumors of the pancreas in von Hippel-Lindau disease patients: histopathological and molecular genetic analysis. *Am J Pathol* 1998;153:223–231.

194. Chung DC, Brown SB, Graeme-Cook F, et al. Localization of putative tumor suppressor loci by genome-wide allelotyping in human pancreatic endocrine tumors. *Cancer Res* 1998;58:3706–3711.

195. Chandrasekharappa SC, Guru SC, Manickam P, et al. Positional cloning of the gene for multiple endocrine neoplasia-type 1. *Science* 1997;276:404–407.

196. Emmert-Buck MR, Lubensky IA, Dong Q, et al. Localization of the multiple endocrine neoplasia type I (MEN1) gene based on tumor loss of heterozygosity analysis. *Cancer Res* 1997;57:1855–1858.

197. Zhuang Z, Vortmeyer AO, Pack S, et al. Somatic mutations of the MEN1 tumor suppressor gene in sporadic gastrinomas and insulinomas. *Cancer Res* 1997;57:4682–4686.

198. Marx SJ, Agarwal SK, Heppner C, et al. The gene for multiple endocrine neoplasia type 1: recent findings. *Bone* 1999;25:119–122.

199. Lin SY, Elledge SJ. Multiple tumor suppressor pathways negatively regulate telomerase. *Cell* 2003;113:881–889.

200. DiMagno EP, Shorter RG, Taylor WF, Go VLW. Relationships between pancreaticobiliary ductal anatomy and pancreatic ductal and parenchymal histology. *Cancer* 1982;49:361–368.

201. Hirota S, Isozaki K, Moriyama Y, et al. Gain-of-function mutations of c-kit in human gastrointestinal stromal tumors. *Science* 1998;279:577–580.

202. Joensuu H, Roberts PJ, Sarlomo-Rikala M, et al. Effect of the tyrosine kinase inhibitor STI571 in a patient with a metastatic gastrointestinal stromal tumor. *N Engl J Med* 2001;344:1052–1056.

203. Qian F, Watnick TJ, Onuchic LF, Germino GG. The molecular basis of focal cyst formation in human autosomal dominant polycystic kidney disease type I. *Cell* 1996;87:979–987.

CHAPTER 26 ■ PANCREAS CANCER: ANATOMY, STAGING SYSTEMS, AND TECHNIQUES

KEVIN CONLON AND M. A. AREMU

INTRODUCTION

In clinical practice, pancreatic cancer is often used synonymously with pancreatic ductal adenocarcinoma, which constitutes more than 90% of all primary malignant tumors arising from the exocrine portion of the gland. Pancreatic cancer remains a highly lethal disease; on a worldwide basis, it affects as many as 545,000 patients per year (1) with a death–incidence ratio of 0.99% (2). In the United States, it ranks fourth in males and fifth in females as a leading cause of death behind lung, breast, prostate, colorectal, and ovarian cancer, and the disease now accounts for 10% of all cancers of the digestive tract, second behind colorectal cancer (3). Surgical resection remains the only potentially curative intervention for those patients with localized disease, yet only one in five patients will be resectable at presentation; the remainder will have locally advanced or metastatic disease (4).

Hence, precise staging of this disease is important to enable accurate patient stratification and assessment of response to therapy, as well as to avoid unnecessary morbidity and mortality and diminished quality of life in this population of patients with very poor prognosis (5). Staging should accurately define the extent of disease, direct appropriate therapy, and avoid unnecessary intervention in a safe and cost-efficient fashion.

ANATOMY OF THE PANCREAS

The pancreas is a retroperitoneal, lobulated, yellow organ that lies within the "C" curve of the first, second, and third parts of the duodenum and extends transversely in front of the inferior vena cava and aorta and behind the stomach to the hilum of the spleen. In adults, it measures between 12 and 15 cm in length and weighs about 100 g in men and 85 g in women (6).

Based on anatomical relations, the pancreas is divided into head, neck, body, and tail. The uncinate process is an accessory lobe that extends from the head of the gland lying posterior to the superior mesenteric vessels. The head is the broadest and thickest part and fits into the "C" curve of the duodenum, lying over the inferior vena cava. The neck joins the head and the body, and it is marked anteriorly by the gastroduodenal artery groove and posteriorly by the commencement of the portal vein. The body, which is the longest part of the gland, runs from the neck to the left toward the tail of the pancreas. The tail is the narrowest portion of the gland, and it extends to the hilum of the spleen (Fig. 26.1) (7).

Embryologically, the pancreas develops from two buds—the ventral and dorsal buds—which are outgrowths of the endoderm at the junction of foregut and midgut. The dorsal bud develops into the tail, body, neck, and part of the head, while the ventral bud gives rise to the rest of the head and the uncinate process. The normal rotation of the gut leads to the ventral bud rotating dorsally to fuse with the dorsal bud to form a single adult gland. Fusion of the ventral bud to the dorsal bud both posteriorly and anteriorly gives rise to annular pancreas in which a ring of pancreatic tissue encircles the second part of the duodenum, causing duodenal obstruction.

The pancreas is both an exocrine and an endocrine organ. Acini cells and ducts develop from endodermal tubules within both pancreatic buds, and secrete various digestive enzymes and bicarbonate (exocrine function). The endocrine function is by the islets cells, which are isolated clumps of endodermal cells derived from the tubules and comprises of alpha cells (produce glucagon), beta cells (produce insulin), delta cells (produce somatostatin), and PP cells (produce pancreatic polypeptides).

The exocrine secretions of the gland is drained by the main pancreatic duct (duct of Wirsung), which runs from the tail toward the head of pancreas and drains into the second part of the duodenum at the major papillae by joining with the common bile duct to form the ampulla of Vater. The main duct is formed by the fusion of the distal two-thirds of the dorsal duct and the ventral pancreatic duct. Persistence of the proximal one-third of the dorsal pancreatic duct gives rise to the accessory pancreatic duct (duct of Santorini), which drains the inferior part of the head and the uncinate process. The accessory duct empties into the duodenum via the minor papilla, which is located about 2 cm anterosuperior to the major papilla, or it may end blindly with some connecting channels to the main duct.

Pancreatic divisum is a congenital abnormality found in roughly 10% of the population in which the dorsal and ventral pancreatic ducts do not fuse. This results in the dorsal pancreatic duct, which drains the head, neck, body, and tail of the gland emptying into the duodenum via the minor papilla (predisposing to recurrent pancreatitis), and the ventral pancreatic duct, which drains the inferior portion of the head of pancreas and the uncinate process, emptying via the major papilla.

The pancreas receives the following main blood supply: the anterior and posterior superior pancreaticoduodenal arteries (from the gastroduodenal artery) supply the head, uncinate process, and the duodenum, together with anterior and posterior inferior pancreaticoduodenal arteries (from the superior mesenteric artery or its first jejunal branch). Many small branches from the splenic artery supply the neck, body, and tail of the pancreas, including arterial pancreatica magna (to the

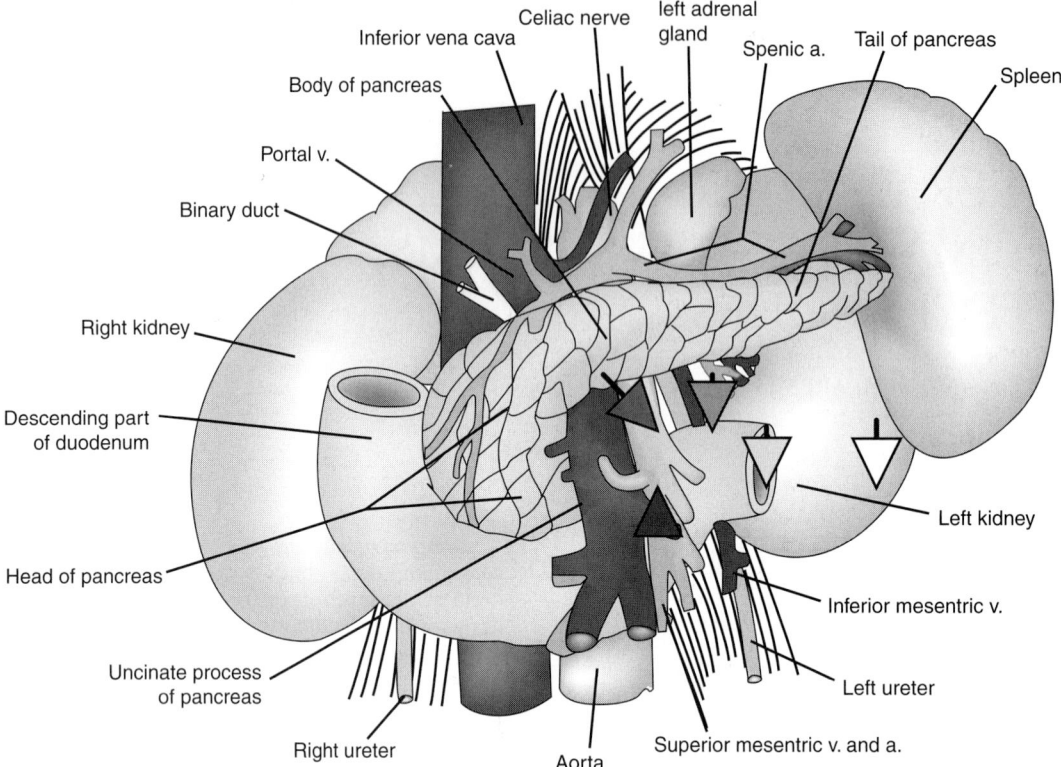

FIGURE 26.1. Anatomy of the pancreas and related structures. *Source:* Adapted from ref. 7 (See also color Figure 26.1).

body) and arteria cauda pancreatica (to the tail). Considerable variations in the blood supply to the pancreas have been described (8,9). The venous drainage of the head and neck is via the superior and inferior pancreaticoduodenal veins, and the body and tail drain by numerous small veins into the splenic vein; hence, the venous return is primarily into the portal system.

Lymphatic vessels from the pancreas follow the course of the arteries. The body and tail drain into the pancreaticosplenic nodes along the splenic artery, and the neck and head drain into pancreaticoduodenal, superior mesenteric, hepatic, and celiac lymph nodes. There is some direct drainage from the pancreas to the periaortic lymph nodes (10).

The innervation of the pancreas is by both sympathetic and parasympathetic systems. The sympathetic nerve supply, which regulates pancreatic blood flow by vasoconstriction, comes from T_6 to T_{10} segments of the spinal cord via splanchnic nerves and the celiac plexus. Parasympathetic innervation stimulates exocrine secretions and is derived from the posterior vagus nerve and the celiac plexus. Sensory fibers, including pain fibers, are carried by both the sympathetic and parasympathetic fibers.

STAGING SYSTEMS

In the United States, the most widely used staging system for pancreatic cancer is that developed by the American Joint Committee on Cancer in cooperation with the TMN Committee of the International Union Against Cancer. This classification represents an expression of the anatomical extent of the disease, taking into account the size and invasiveness of the primary tumor (T), the presence or absence of regional nodal metastases (N), and the existence or nonexistence of distant metastatic disease (M). Table 26.1 illustrates the components of this system

as it relates to pancreatic cancer. Histologic grade, although shown to have prognostic significance in some studies (11), is not included in the current classification. For pancreatic cancer, in particular, local extension of the tumor may lead to unresectability. This is reflected in the staging system because T3 tumors are those that do not involve unresectable structures and T4 tumors do (Table 26.1).

DIAGNOSIS AND STAGING

Clinical Presentation

Sener et al., reviewing the National Cancer Database, identified more than 100,000 patients diagnosed with pancreatic cancer between 1985 and 1995 (12). The head of the gland was the predominant site of disease (78%), while the body was the site in 11% and the tail in 11% of patients. Others have confirmed this distribution of disease (13–15). Sener et al. also noted that the ratio of limited (stage I) to advanced disease (stage IV) was 0.70 for lesions in the head of the gland, 0.24 for body tumors, and 0.10 for tail tumors (12).

Delayed presentation has been proposed as the reason for this apparent stage imbalance rather than inherent biological differences. Unlike tumors situated in the head of the gland in which obstructive jaundice may produce symptoms and signs, lesions of the pancreatic body and tail usually present with prolonged, nonspecific symptoms. Gastrointestinal symptoms such as nausea, anorexia, early satiety, and alteration in bowel function are common. These often prompt unsuccessful, empiric therapies that contribute to the delayed presentation.

The classic triad of abdominal pain, weight loss, and jaundice has generally been associated with pancreatic cancer. Modolell et al. (16) found abdominal pain to be the most

TABLE 26.1

AMERICAN JOINT COMMITTEE ON CANCER STAGING CLASSIFICATION FOR EXOCRINE PANCREATIC CANCER

DEFINITIONS

Primary Tumor (T)

Tx	Primary tumor cannot be assessed
T0	No evidence of primary tumor
Tis	Carcinoma in situ[a]
T1	Tumor limited to the pancreas ≤2 cm in greatest diameter
T2	Tumor limited to the pancreas >2 cm in greatest diameter
T3	Tumor extends beyond the pancreas but without involvement of the celiac axis or superior mesenteric artery
T4	Tumor involves the celiac axis or the superior mesenteric artery (unresectable primary tumor)

Regional Lymph Nodes (N)

NX	Regional lymph nodes cannot be assessed
N0	No regional node metastasis
N1	Regional lymph node metastasis

Distant Metastasis (M)

MX	Distant metastasis cannot be assessed
M0	No distant metastasis
M1	Distant metastasis

STAGE GROUPING

Stage 0	Tis	N0	M0
Stage IA	T1	N0	M0
Stage IB	T2	N0	M0
Stage IIA	T3	N0	M0
Stage IIB	T1	N1	M0
	T2	N1	M0
	T3	N1	M0
Stage III	T4	Any N	M0
Stage IV	Any T	Any N	M1

[a]This also includes the "PanIn III" classification.

common presenting complaint, whereas Maringhini et al. (17) reported weight loss and elevated bilirubin and alkaline phosphatase to have a negative predictive value of 95%. Nix et al. analyzing 123 patients with a carcinoma at the head of the pancreas found the frequencies of the classic triad and other symptoms to be abdominal pain (70.7%), weight loss (80.5%), jaundice (88.6%), tiredness and malaise (42.3%), change in bowel habits (41.5%), sudden onset of diabetes mellitus (33.3%), and upper abdominal discomfort (22.0%). However, they noted that jaundice and abdominal pain are late symptoms (18).

Dalton et al., reviewing the Mayo Clinic's experience, noted that the majority of their patients (92%) were symptomatic at presentation with the median duration of symptoms being 6 months (19). Generally, the symptoms were vague and nonspecific, with abdominal or back pain and weight loss predominating. Others have reported similar results (20). Physical signs are often lacking with <25% presenting with a palpable mass or ascites and less than one-third of patients have palpable gallbladder (21) (Courvoisier sign).

Laboratory investigations such as serum amylase or liver function tests are usually normal, except in obstructive jaundice or in association with liver metastases. Serum tumor markers such as CA 19-9 may be elevated but are not sensitive or specific enough to differentiate adenocarcinoma of the pancreas from benign pancreatic pathology or other gastrointestinal cancers. However, studies (22,23) have shown that >300 U/mL is associated with advanced pancreatic cancer and that

a threshold level of 150 U/mL has a specificity, sensitivity, and positive predictive value of 90%, 59%, and 88%, respectively, for predicting unresectability (24).

The goal of clinical staging for patients with pancreatic cancer is the identification of the subset of patients who would be candidates for curative surgical resection. Historically, surgical exploration has been the gold standard for determination of resectability. However, our current algorithm (Fig. 26.2) suggests that exploration be reserved for those patients considered to be resectable following laparoscopic staging or those patients in whom operative palliation is required. In the following discussion, we present the clinical staging modalities currently available, as well as their strengths and weaknesses, and relate our approach to the staging of patients with a pancreatic mass.

Before the advent of cross-sectional imaging, percutaneous cholangiography (PTC), and endoscopy, the workup of patients with painless jaundice, abdominal pain, or an abdominal mass was straightforward. An exploratory laparotomy would be performed for identification of the primary pathology and assessment of resectability.

Resection of the primary tumor with negative margins (R0 resection) remains the aim of the operating surgeon. In general, at exploration, the surgeon proceeds with visualization of the peritoneal surfaces, palpation of the liver, palpation of the retroperitoneal nodes, and dissection of the blood vessels. The primary tumor is also assessed. Tumors are considered unresectable by virtue of distant disease (peritoneal, nodal, or liver metastases) or local invasion involving the superior

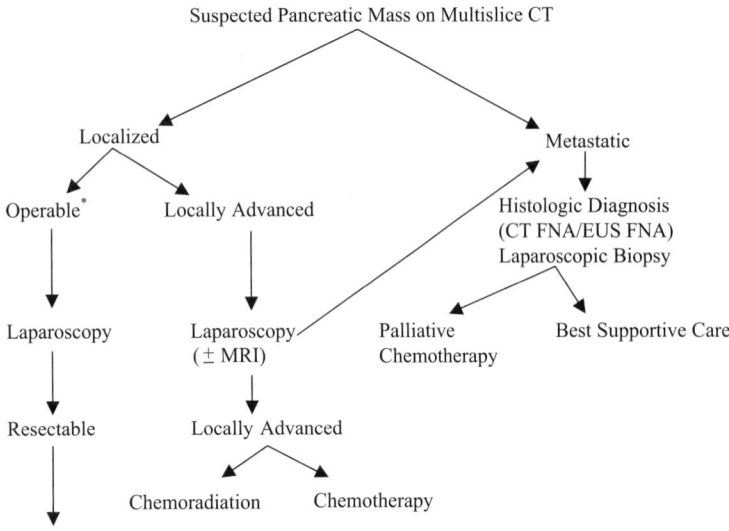

FIGURE 26.2. Staging algorithm. *, Clear fat plane around the splenic, mesenteric artery (and superior mesenteric vein and jejunal branches), the celiac and hepatic arteries. Less than 50% portal vein involvement, <1 cm portal, paraaortic, or superior mesenteric lymphadenopathy.

mesenteric artery, hepatic artery, or celiac trunk. Long segment involvement of the portal vein or its tributaries is also considered by most to be a barrier to resection. Invasion of the tumor into the stomach, colon, or duodenum is not in itself a contraindication to resection because these organs can be taken en bloc with the primary tumor if the vessels are free. However, in many cases, contiguous organ involvement also indicates vascular encasement. Lymphadenopathy located in the porta hepatis, the root of the transverse mesocolon, or the celiac region is considered metastatic, and although resectable, the patient is considered to have stage IV disease.

Although operation is considered the "gold standard" in regard to staging, the goal of staging is to select patients who have disease that is potentially curable by resection. However, as mentioned, 80% of patients presenting with pancreatic cancer have advanced disease. Contemporary studies of patients with unresectable disease have suggested that median survival is limited, and an exploratory operation may be associated with significant perioperative morbidity, potential mortality, and diminished quality of life (25). In addition, the development of improved nonoperative techniques for relieving both biliary and gastric obstruction has reduced the need for operation. Thus, simply put, the goal of clinical staging is to accurately identify patients who would benefit from a curative resection while directing others toward more appropriate therapy.

Diagnostic Procedures: Cholangiography—Endoscopic Retrograde Cholangiography and Percutaneous Cholangiography

Cholangiography has long been an important component of the initial evaluation of the patient with painless jaundice. The earliest reports of endoscopic retrograde cholangiography (ERCP) claimed a sensitivity and specificity ranging from 46% to 94% and 94% to 100% for the diagnosis of pancreatic cancer (25–27). ERCP allows for imaging of the biliary and pancreatic ductal systems, and in 90% to 100% of patients with pancreatic cancer, it shows morphologic changes in the bile and/or pancreatic ducts such as irregularities, strictures, stenoses, and the dilatation of both ducts ("double duct" sign) (28–31) (Fig. 26.3). However, these changes can also be seen

in chronic pancreatitis (32–35). The endoscopic and transhepatic approaches also allow for the collection of samples for cytologic confirmation of the cancer diagnosis. In addition, both approaches allow for the placement of temporary plastic stents to relieve biliary obstruction, and in unresectable patients, expanding metallic stents may be placed for long-term palliation. As a diagnostic modality, ERCP meets the criteria of high sensitivity and specificity with a minimally invasive risk profile (complication rates of 1%–2% after diagnostic ERCP and 5%–10% following therapeutic ERCP) (36–39). PTC is slightly more invasive (40); its role is less as a diagnostic tool and more for palliative therapy.

Since its introduction, computed tomography (CT) has replaced ERCP as the initial procedure of choice for diagnosis of pancreatic cancer (25–27), and the current primary role of ERCP is relieving malignant obstructive jaundice by placing plastic or expandable metallic stents (41,42). However, diagnostic ERCP could still be indicated in cases where the CT is normal but pancreatic cancer is suspected (43,44).

As staging modalities, ERCP and PTC do not address one of the main goals of staging, which is the determination of resectability.

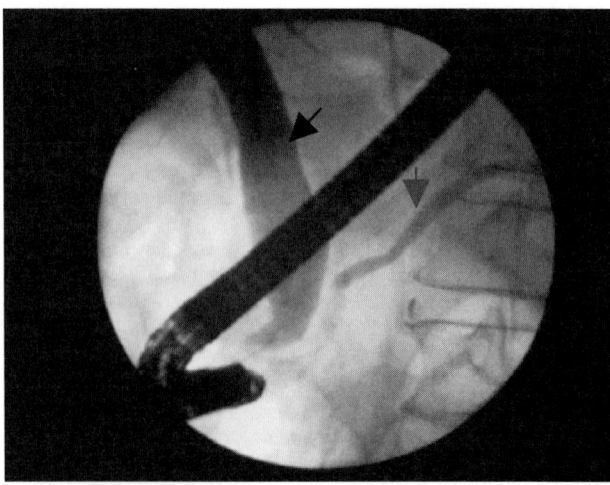

FIGURE 26.3. ERCP showing double duct sign—dilated pancreatic duct (*red arrow*) and dilated common bile duct (*black arrow*) (See also color Figure 26.3).

Endoscopic Ultrasound

Conventional transabdominal ultrasound (US) has limited value in pancreatic cancer (45). Although transabdominal US is a noninvasive, safe, and relatively inexpensive imaging modality that visualizes liver lesions and biliary dilatation well, it is operator dependent, and its signal is attenuated by gas in the intestine precluding adequate imaging of the pancreatic parenchyma and the retroperitoneum. Recently, however, the positive and negative predictive values for resection of US are reported to be 89% and 79%, respectively, when lesions are visualized (46).

In 1980, the concept of endoscopic ultrasound (EUS) was introduced. It uses an echoendoscope, which incorporates a small high-frequency US transducer at its tip, permitting a high-resolution, real-time, B-mode scanning of the pancreas and surrounding structures when passed into the lumen of the gut. It allows the endoscopist to see within and beyond the wall of the luminal gastrointestinal tract. Three types of echoendoscopes are available: radial endoscope, which has a rotating US probe integrated into its tip with no possibility for needle aspiration; linear array endoscope, which obtain images along a plane parallel to the endoscope axis and with the capability of diagnostic (fine-needle aspiration cytology) and therapeutic interventions; and endoscopic probe, which is passed through the channel of a regular endoscope and provides high-resolution images parallel to the endoscope axis. In their randomized study, Gress et al. (47) showed that the radial and linear array echoendoscopes are equally accurate in staging pancreatic cancer. In 1984, Yasuda et al. (48) reported on their initial experience with the early prototype endoscopic transducers. They reported 10 patients who had CT scan, EUS, ERCP, and angiogram. EUS identified one lesion seen only on angiogram, one lesion seen by ERCP and CT only, and one final lesion not seen by the other modalities. This study defined the role of EUS in identifying small pancreatic lesions that are identified by symptoms in the periampullary region and not well visualized by other cross-sectional imaging.

In a prospective study, Rosch et al. (49) compared EUS, transabdominal US, CT, and ERCP in the diagnosis of 132 patients with suspected pancreatic cancer. Sensitivity and specificity were significantly higher for EUS (99% and 100%) than for US (67%/40%) and CT (77%/53%) and equal to ERCP (sensitivity 90%). They found that this difference was even more significant in small pancreatic cancers of ≤3 cm, and they concluded that in the evaluation of patients with suspected pancreatic tumors, EUS should be considered early in the staging process.

A comparative study of Legmann et al. (80) of 32 patients with suspected pancreatic tumor comparing dual-phase helical CT and EUS for the diagnosis and staging of pancreatic tumors showed overall diagnostic sensitivity of 92% for dual-phase helical CT and 100% for EUS. Both dual-phase helical CT and EUS had overall accuracy for staging of pancreatic tumors of 93% and overall accuracy for predicting resectability of 90%; the accuracy of predicting unresectability was 100% and 86% for dual-phase helical CT and EUS, respectively (*p* >0.80). Other studies (50,51,66) have also shown that EUS is inaccurate in assessing superior mesenteric artery tumor involvement. This is because of the distance of superior mesenteric artery from the endoscopic probe in the lumen of the duodenum, and this obviously affects the prediction for unresectability. In the assessment of major venous invasion, spiral CT and gadolinium-enhanced MRI showed similar results as EUS (79). In a study of 62 patients with pancreatic cancer comparing EUS, helical CT, MRI, and angiography in the preoperative staging and tumor resectability assessment of pancreatic cancer, Soriano et al. (75) showed by using univariate logistic

regression analysis that helical CT had the highest accuracy in assessing extent of primary tumor locoregional extension, vascular invasion, distant metastases, tumor TNM stage, and tumor resectability, but in assessing tumor size and lymph node involvement, EUS had the highest accuracy. Very small lymph nodes <5 mm can be detected by EUS; however, nodal tumor involvement staging accuracy by EUS, although better than CT or MRI, has been shown to range from 64% to 82% (52). This is because of its inability to distinguish malignant infiltration from benign inflammation of the lymph nodes. Nodal staging of pancreatic tumors by EUS, however, has been enhanced by the addition of EUS-guided fine-needle aspiration, which allows for a tissue diagnosis of the primary tumor as well as lymph nodes, liver metastasis, and peritoneal/pleural fluid, useful in the context of unresectable disease or neoadjuvant therapy (53). Studies have shown it to have sensitivity and specificity rates of 75% to 90% and 94% to 100%, and a complication rate of 1% (54−56). These studies underscore the value of EUS in identifying small lesions and determining the status of peripancreatic vessels in patients with complex pancreatic pathology.

Another important role of EUS is its therapeutic capabilities, and as Fazel and Draganov (57) pointed out, EUS is evolving rapidly from a primarily diagnostic role to one of therapeutic intervention. Therapeutic interventions of EUS include celiac neurolysis and nerve block, fine-needle tumor injection with antitumor agents such as activated lymphocytes and viral gene vectors, delivery of photodynamic therapy, and transmural pseudocyst drainage (57,58).

Computed Tomography

CT was introduced into clinical practice in 1975 and subsequent refinements in CT technology have radically changed the staging of pancreatic cancer. It has become the standard staging modality for pancreatic tumors (59). CT can identify patients with significant metastatic disease without exploratory laparotomy. CT-guided needle biopsy allowed tissue confirmation in these advanced patients. The routine use of CT scanning in the staging of patients with pancreatic tumors has led to improved patient selection. CT yielded sensitivities in the range 66% to 97% and specificities of 53% to 69% in the studies of conventional dynamic CT in the diagnosis of pancreatic malignancy conducted in the 1980s and early 1990s (60−68). CT scanning allows accurate identification of hepatic metastases over 1 cm in diameter (69).

Although any lesion visualized outside the pancreas makes staging simple, the difficulty arises in the absence of visible metastatic disease. The determination of resectability by CT is based on a clear fat plane around the splenic, mesenteric artery and the celiac and hepatic arteries (Fig. 26.4).

Selections of recent studies (68,69,72−77,80−82,84) evaluating the utility of CT scanning in the determination of resectability by these criteria are displayed in Table 26.2. Studies by Freeny et al. (68) and McCarthy et al. (77) evaluated axial CT scanning coordinated with intravenous contrast injection (dynamic), and found adequate identification of the primary tumor and hepatic parenchymal lesions. However, there was reduced accuracy in assessment of portal nodes, portal vein involvement, extension into the root of the mesentery, and posterior extension of tumor. The introduction of spiral (helical) CT scanning with multiple detectors and dual-phase contrast enhancement have improved our ability to image the portal vein and the visceral arteries in relation to the primary tumor (82), a critical component of the determination of resectability. Spiral CT images a volume of tissue while the patient moves through the scanner tube, usually during a single breathhold (65). Dual-phase CT scanning takes advantage of the short

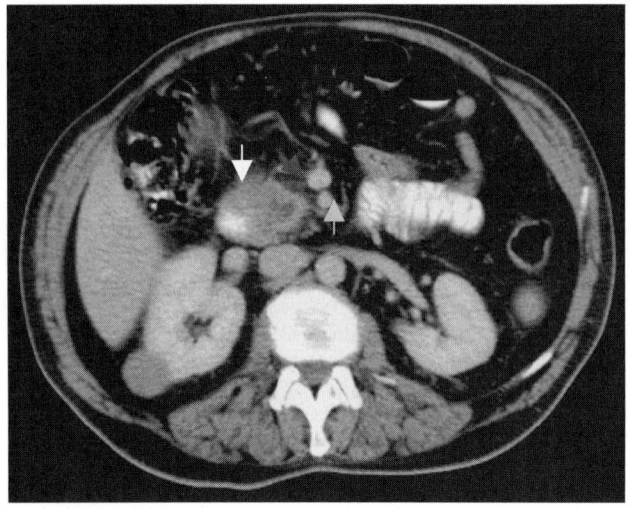

FIGURE 26.4. CT showing clear fat pad between head of pancreas tumor (*white arrow*) and the superior mesenteric vessels (*blue arrow*, superior mesenteric vein; *red arrow*, superior mesenteric artery) (See also color Figure 26.4).

acquisition time of the spiral CT scanner and images the pancreas first during its maximum enhancement and then rescans through the liver during the portal phase to obtain maximum enhancement of liver lesions. Subsequent reports with this technique have improved visualization of local tumor extension as well (69,80–83). In these studies, as in practice, prediction of resectability remains somewhat subjective, resulting in a number of reports with low positive predictive value of CT scanning for the identification of resectability. Saldinger et al. (84) defined unresectable to include only definitive evidence of metastasis or vascular invasion. Using these criteria when interpreting spiral CT angiography, they were able to increase the sensitivity and negative predictive value for resection to 100%. However, the specificity and positive predictive value remained disappointingly low at 39% to 86% and 50% to 89%, respectively, as also reported by other authors (60,66). Spiral CT angiogram uses a three-dimensional data set from spiral scan

to reconstruct the peripancreatic vessels. In addition, this data set can be displayed as an angiogram, allowing the surgeon to evaluate the important vessels without a conventional angiogram (79). These studies evaluated all patients with pancreatic tumors; the stage distribution was weighted toward advanced disease. This makes detection of metastatic disease or obvious signs of locally advanced disease more likely. However, spiral CT has been shown to miss small liver lesions and borderline lymphadenopathy identified at laparotomy or laparoscopy with studies reporting sensitivities of approximately 75% in the detection of small liver and/or peritoneal metastases (82), (83,85,86). Although approximately 25% to 30% of patients with radiologically resectable disease will ultimately be unresectable at surgery (61,68,87), CT scanning has nonetheless become the standard method for diagnosing and staging pancreatic cancer (54).

Magnetic Resonance Imaging

Magnetic resonance imaging (MRI) has been evaluated as a staging modality in pancreatic cancer (88), and since the 1980s, has developed into an effective and useful imaging tool for evaluation of pancreatic disorders. Conventional MRI was slow and cost prohibitive but more recently improved technology has reduced the acquisition time and improved the quality of the images. Most primary pancreatic tumors are found to be hypointense on the T1-weighted images; fat suppression on these images improves the delineation of anatomical structures in the retroperitoneum (Fig. 26.5). T1-weighted images also demonstrate abnormalities such as fatty infiltration of the pancreas, hemorrhage, and adenopathy very well. The T2-weighted images are useful for evaluating pancreatic or peripancreatic fluid collections, pancreatic neoplasms, calculi, and hepatic parenchyma (83) (Fig. 26.6). When gadolinium is used for intravenous contrast, smaller pancreatic tumors are more often identified as hypointense in the early phase post injection. Later acquisition of the images shows larger tumors as hyperintense relative to the surrounding parenchyma. These images allow for detection of dilated ducts and cystic lesions of the pancreas.

TABLE 26.2

MEASURES OF ACCURACY OF COMPUTED TOMOGRAPHY SCANNING FOR THE PREDICTION OF RESECTABILITY

Author	Year	N	Spiral	Sensitivity	Specificity	PPV	NPV
Freeny et al. (68)	1993	78	No	65	87	61	89
McCarthy et al. (77)	1998	67	No	72	80	77	76
Legmann et al. (80)	1998	30	Yes	100	78	90	100
Nishiharu et al. (81)	1999	31	Yes	74–89	87–90	NA	NA
Tabuchi et al. (69)	1999	25	Yes	55–88	50–100	50–100	55–82
Phoa et al. (82)	1999	56	Yes	76	78	79	75
Saldinger et al. (84)	2000	68	Yes angio	100	67	76	100
Valls et al. (72)	2001	39	Yes	75	35.7	73.5	100
Calculli et al. (73)	2002	95	Yes	98	79	87.5	96
Zhang and Zhao (74)	2002	31	Yes	60	91	92	91
Soriano et al. (75)	2004	62	Yes	55–79	93–100	89–100	66–88
Grenacher et al. (76)	2004	50	Yes	100	61	NA	NA

PPV, positive predictive value; NPV, negative predictive value; NA, not available.

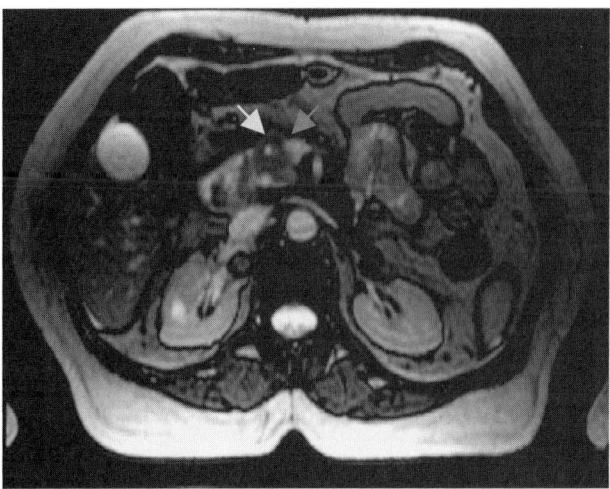

FIGURE 26.5. MRI–T_1-weighted image showing encroachment of the superior mesenteric vein (*blue arrow*) by pancreatic tumor (*yellow arrow*) (See also color Figure 26.5).

A benefit of the T2-weighted images is the visualization of stationary fluid; on these images, the gallbladder, bile ducts, and pancreatic duct are bright. A three-dimensional reconstruction of these structures is called magnetic resonance cholangiopancreatography (MRCP) (Fig. 26.7) and is displayed like an ERCP or PTC film. The added benefit of this technique, besides being minimally invasive, is the ability to visualize the surrounding parenchyma in order to identify lesions associated with the abnormal cholangiogram. MR angiography (MRA), which is a further enhancement of MRI, uses three-dimensional rendering to display the vessels in this area. In one study, Mueller et al. (89) compared MRI and CT in the evaluation of 49 patients with pancreatic adenocarcinoma. The sensitivity and overall specificity of MRI and CT were reported as 83% and 69% and 100% and 64%, respectively, showing the superiority of MRI in detecting pancreatic cancer.

Spencer et al. (90) prospectively evaluated 35 patients who were presumed resectable by CT or US examination using dynamic contrast-enhanced MRI. They found that >60% of patients were unresectable, 8 of these with metastatic disease and

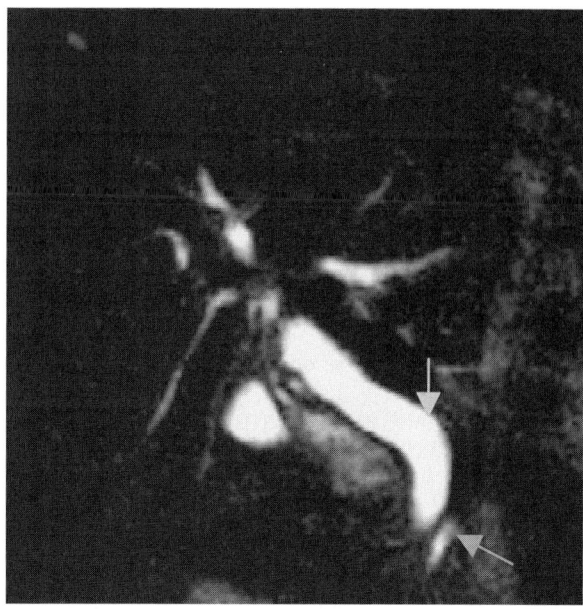

FIGURE 26.7. MRCP showing dilated common bile duct (*green arrow*) and obstructed pancreatic duct (*orange arrow*) (See also color Figure 26.7).

14 with vessel involvement. In patients deemed resectable, 2 of 11 had pancreatitis precluding resection not predicted by the MR scan. These authors concluded that MR should not be used for staging in all patients, only those deemed resectable on CT scan. The authors used spiral CT angiography to check their MRI interpretations with a 100% concordance. This suggested that either test is suitable for staging potentially resectable pancreatic tumors.

Other studies showed that MRI was more accurate than spiral CT in identifying extrapancreatic extension and vascular involvement (81,91). Vahldiek et al. (92) used both MRCP and MRA to determine resectability in their patients; however, they do not comment on their sensitivity or specificity. In a prospective comparison in 65 patients, Trede et al. found that ultrafast MRI was more accurate in determining extrapancreatic spread, lymph node involvement, and vascular invasion compared to CT, ERCP, angiography, or transabdominal ultrasonography (93). However, as in other studies that have assessed radiologic modalities, not all patients had adenocarcinoma of the pancreas, and for those that did, the stage of disease was advanced, making interpretation of the data difficult. Birchard et al. (94) most recently reported the use of three-dimensional gradient-echo (GRE) MRI in detecting pancreatic neoplasms with a mean size of 2.5 cm in 27 patients. The sensitivity of MRI was 86%, and the specificity was 89%. When high confidence ratings were also included, the sensitivity reached 98% without significantly compromising specificity (85%).

All in all, MRI, although accurate in imaging the pancreas, adds little to improve multidetector row helical CT scanning. We use MRI selectively when multidetector row helical CT scanning is normal or equivocal regarding resectability.

In summary, although not the first imaging study to be used for selecting indications, MRI scan may improve the decision regarding resection.

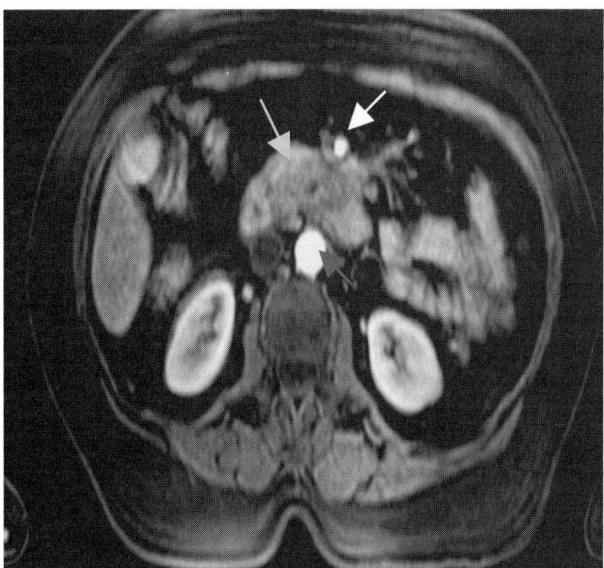

FIGURE 26.6. MRI–T_2-weighted image (*yellow arrow*, pancreatic tumor; *red arrow*, aorta; *black arrow*, superior mesenteric artery) (See also color Figure 26.6).

Positive Emission Tomography

Positron emission tomography (PET) is a functional, noninvasive study used extensively in oncologic medicine for tumor detection (95,96), staging (97,98), and grading (99). See Chapter 9 for further description of PET. Because of differential glucose metabolism in malignant and nonmalignant cells, PET has been proposed to functionally differentiate between pancreatic cancer and benign disease, including chronic pancreatitis (100–103).

Sperti et al. (104) assessed the reliability of 18-fluorodeoxyglucose (18-FDG) PET in distinguishing benign from malignant cystic lesions of the pancreas in 56 patients with suspected pancreatic cancer. They found that the sensitivity, specificity, and positive and negative predictive values for 18-FDG PET and CT scanning in detecting malignant tumors were 94%, 97%, 94%, and 97% and 65%, 87%, 69%, and 85%, respectively. Their conclusion was that in the preoperative evaluation of patients with pancreatic cystic lesions, FDG-PET should be used in combination with CT and tumor markers assay.

However, in more recent studies, PET seems not to have any advantage over helical CT in diagnostic value (105,106). Lytras et al. (107), in their recently published study of 112 patients with suspected cancer, reported a diagnostic sensitivity and specificity of 73% and 60% for PET and 89% and 65% for CT, and for detecting small-volume metastatic disease, 22% and 91% for PET and 20% and 94% for CT. CT was equivocal in 30 patients (14 malignant, 16 benign disease); 13 (6 malignant, 7 benign disease) of these were correctly diagnosed by PET, 4 (3 malignant, 1 benign disease) were interpreted as equivocal, and 13 (5 malignant, 8 benign disease) were wrongly diagnosed. They concluded that PET had a similar accuracy to that of CT for imaging pancreatic cancer, provided no additional information where CT findings were equivocal and in staging of pancreatic cancer would seem of little benefit.

Frohlich et al. (108) evaluated its use prospectively in patients selected for exploration for presumed pancreatic cancer. Of 168 patients studied with benign or malignant pancreatic disease, 22 were diagnosed with liver metastases from pancreatic cancer. Overall sensitivity was 68% for liver lesion detection, although it was 97% for lesions >1 cm in diameter. There were 8 false-positive and 7 false-negatives studies; cholestasis was responsible for the majority of the false-positive studies, whereas small size was the reason for negative results. The authors concluded that PET is helpful for the characterization of indeterminate lesions on CT or MRI, but it is not a helpful staging tool.

The ability of FDG-PET to identify the primary tumor as a carcinoma was evaluated by Delbeke et al. (109). They found that PET was more sensitive and specific than CT for identification of the primary tumor. For the staging of these patients, CT was able to identify vascular invasion, while PET could add no information about local resectability. PET did identify seven patients with metastatic disease that was missed by CT; in five of these patients CT, called the primary tumor resectable. Their conclusion was that PET cannot stage the primary tumor or determine resectability; however, it may increase the yield for detection of metastatic disease. Earlier studies established the superiority of PET over CT in the diagnosis of pancreatic cancer (109–111), although in the presence of hyperglycemia due to the competitive uptake of glucose, PET sensitivity is much lower (112,113).

In light of the previous studies, the determination of the clinical role of FDG-PET in the diagnosis and staging of pancreatic cancer is still ongoing. However, it has been shown to be useful in prediction of tumor response to chemotherapy, (114) and in identifying localized and distant tumor recurrence (115).

Laparoscopy and Laparoscopic Ultrasonography

The role of laparoscopy in the staging algorithm for patients with pancreatic malignancy has remained controversial since

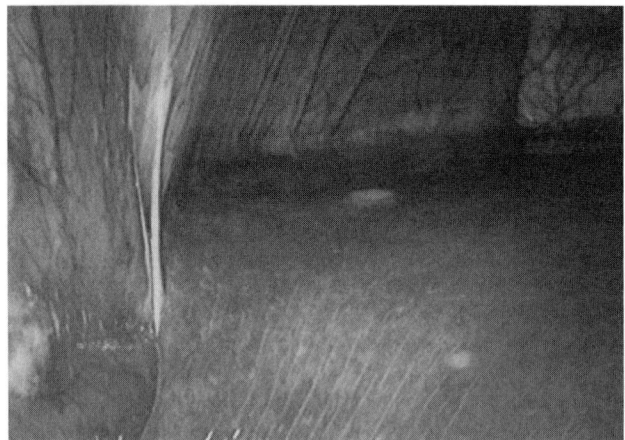

FIGURE 26.8. Laparoscopy showing liver metastases.

its introduction in the 1980s, despite the previous experience of Bernheim (116) in the early 1900s and, more recently, of Cuschieri in the United Kingdom (117) and Warshaw in the United States (118).

Laparoscopy is a sensitive technique in the detection of small-volume liver surface (Fig. 26.8) and peritoneal metastases (Fig. 26.9) being aided by the rapid technological improvements in light sources systems of modern cameras. Proponents of laparoscopic staging argue that if any group of patients should benefit from improved staging and a more rationale approach to therapy, it is those with pancreatic adenocarcinoma. It has been suggested that laparoscopy can prevent unnecessary open operations by identifying these small-volume liver surface and peritoneal metastases, thereby accurately defining resectability. Studies have shown up to 20% to 40% of unsuspected metastases revealed on laparoscopy in conjunction with peritoneal cytology in patients who were deemed resectable on preoperative high-quality CT scan (119–122).

Conlon and Minnard (4) demonstrated that multiport laparoscopic staging in conjunction with dynamic, contrast-enhanced, helical CT scanning had an overall accuracy of 94% in determining resectability (Fig. 26.10). Experience from Memorial Sloan-Kettering Cancer Center reported an improvement in resectability rate from 53% on the basis of CT alone to 91% when staging laparoscopy was introduced (122).

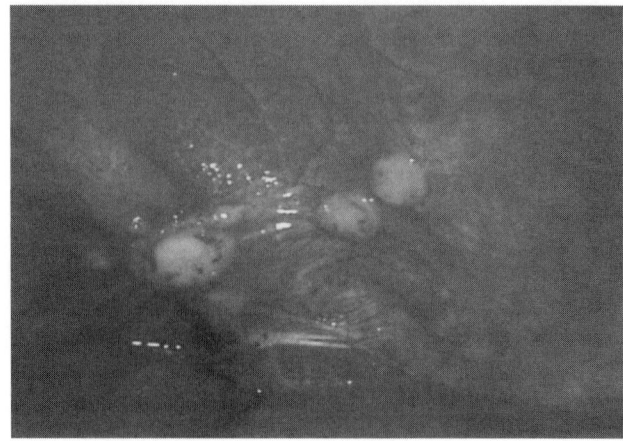

FIGURE 26.9. Laparoscopy showing peritoneal metastases.

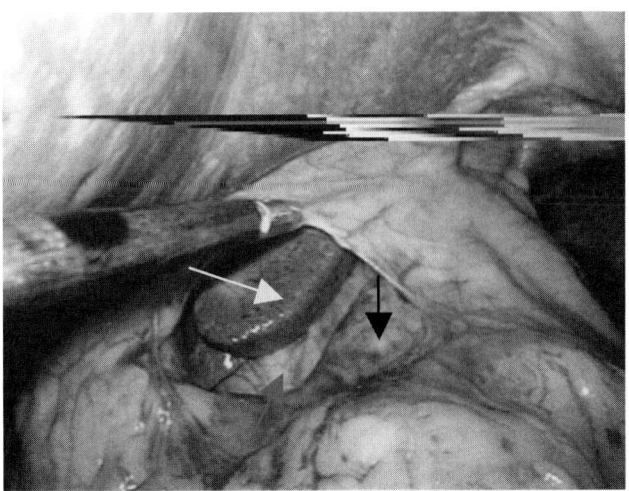

FIGURE 26.10. Laparoscopy showing the lesser sac via the lesser omentum (*yellow arrow*, caudate lobe; *blue arrow*, inferior vena cava; *black arrow*, celiac axis) (See also color Figure 26.10).

Despite advances in radiologic imaging, recent studies have demonstrated an incremental benefit for laparoscopy in conjunction with laparoscopic ultrasound (LUS) over conventional preoperative staging modalities in determining resectability of approximately 15% to 40% (117–120,123–130,147,165) (Table 26.3).

In contrast, the role of laparoscopic staging has been questioned. Some critics have argued that inoperable disease secondary to local extension and vascular encasement can best (and only) be determined at open exploration (131). Others have noted that because there are few patients who do not require an operation either for resection or surgical palliation,

the impact of laparoscopy in avoiding an operation is limited (126,132). More recently, some investigators argued that the incremental yield of laparoscopic staging over existing radiology is limited and, thus, not a cost-effective utilization of available resources (133,134).

The Memorial Sloan-Kettering Cancer Center experience has shown that the introduction of laparoscopic staging significantly altered both the requirements for open surgery and the type of procedure performed for pancreatic cancer. Prior to the introduction of laparoscopic staging in the early 1990s, only 35% of patients with "radiologically" resectable tumors were resected at the time of open exploration (135). In the most recent analysis, 91% of patients who had open operation were resected (122). This is mainly due to the avoidance of nonresective laparotomy.

More recently, Connor et al. (136) assessed the value of CA19.9 in improving patients' selection for staging laparoscopy. They analyzed 159 patients with resectable disease on CT that had laparoscopic staging. Sixty of 63 patients (95%) who had level of CA19.9 ≤150 U/mL were found resectable on laparoscopic staging. Also, patients undergoing laparoscopic staging alone for unresectable disease had a significantly reduced median hospital stay compared to those undergoing open exploration or gastric and biliary bypass (137).

The need for subsequent surgical palliation following laparoscopic staging was studied by Espat et al. (137). They reported on the prospective, nonrandom experience with 155 patients with pancreatic adenocarcinoma who had a laparoscopic staging procedure alone. The majority of patients had stage IV disease (115/155). On follow-up, only 4 patients (3%) required an operation for palliative purposes. This result is similar to reported "failure" rates after prophylactic open biliary or gastric bypass surgery (138).

In contrast, Van Dijkum et al. (139) studied 111 patients with pancreatic or periampullary cancer. Using staging laparoscopy, laparotomy was avoided in 17 patients (15%), but on follow-up, 5 of the 17 patients (29%) needed subsequent

TABLE 26.3

INCREMENTAL BENEFIT OF LAPAROSCOPIC STAGING FOLLOWING COMPUTED TOMOGRAPHY (CT) EXAMINATION

Author	Prospective study	Year	N	Spiral CT	Laparoscopic US	Deemed resectable by CT (%)	Resectable after laparoscopy (%)	Laparoscopy Yield (%)	Overall resectability rate (%)
Nieveen van Dijkum et al. (164)	Yes	2003	286	Yes	Yes	100	72.7	35	74
Menack et al. (123)	No	2001	27	Yes	Yes	100	74	26	90
Jimenez et al. (119)	No	2000	125	Yes	No	56	25	31	74.2
Schachter et al. (124)	Yes	2000	67	Yes	Yes	82	55	27	89
Reddy et al. (120)	No	1999	109	No	No	91	64	27	57
Pietrabissa et al. (125)	Yes	1999	50	Yes	Yes	84	64	20	90.6
Catheline et al. (121)	Yes	1999	26	Yes	Yes	50	19.2	30.8	100
Minnard et al. (146)	Yes	1998	90	Yes	Yes	72	45.5	26.5	97.5
Andren-Sandberg et al. (126)	Yes	1998	60	Yes	No	40	25	15	53.3
Conlon et al. (122)	Yes	1996	108	Yes	No	100	62	37.9	91

US, ultrasound.

surgical bypass for duodenal obstruction. Lillemoe et al. (156) from John Hopkins randomized 87 patients with unresectable periampullary cancer into two groups; 44 patients had prophylactic retrocolic gastrojejunostomy, whereas 43 did not undergo a gastric bypass. The mean survival duration was 8.3 months in both groups, and they reported that during this interval, none of the prophylactic gastric bypass group developed gastric outlet obstruction, whereas 8 of the 43 patients (19%) in the group that had no gastric bypass developed late gastric outlet obstruction that required therapeutic intervention.

Some studies have questioned the usefulness of routine staging laparoscopy in periampullary cancers, especially in subsets of ampullary and duodenal cancers. Vollmer et al. (140) studied 140 patients with periampullary and pancreatic cancers (72 with pancreatic head/uncinate, 12 with pancreatic body/tail, 11 with gallbladder, 23 with extrahepatic bile duct, 22 with ampulla of Vater/duodenum) who were considered to be resectable on preoperative conventional imaging. Laparoscopic yield of metastasis was 22%, 17%, 55%, 9%, and 0%, respectively. They concluded that routine laparoscopy in ampullary/duodenal cancers is of little or no value, and it should only be used in these cases selectively. Barreiro et al. (141), in their retrospective review of 188 patients who had preoperative CT and laparotomy for a potentially resectable periampullary and pancreatic cancers, determined the potential benefit of staging laparoscopy by identifying the number of patients with metastatic disease at laparotomy. They found that the potential yield of laparoscopy was 19.3%, 12%, 15.4%, 0%, and 52.9% for cancers in the pancreatic head, distal bile duct, duodenum, ampulla, and pancreatic body and tail, respectively. Their conclusion was that there is no need for routine use of laparoscopy in periampullary cancer but that it was useful in pancreatic body and tail tumors.

In a more recent study from Amsterdam, Tilleman et al. (142) compared the results of 186 patients with CT resectable periampullary cancers who had no diagnostic laparoscopy as part of their preoperative workup protocol with the results of another study of 198 patients with potentially resectable periampullary cancer who had staging laparoscopy (143). The resectability rate—32% and 34%, respectively—was similar in the two groups.

Laparoscopy has also been shown to have a role in staging patients with radiologically assessed locally advanced disease. Shoup et al. (144) studied 100 patients with locally advanced unresectable disease on preoperative CT or MRI. Metastatic disease (in the form of peritoneal metastasis, liver metastasis, or both) was found in 37 patients (37%) during laparoscopy. They found similar incidence of metastasis for pancreatic body/tail and head cancers (35% vs. 38%, respectively) and suggested that the biology of locally advanced cancers is more important in determining proneness to metastasis than the site of occurrence. In another more recent study, Liu and Traverso (145) carried out laparoscopy and peritoneal lavage cytology in a group of 74 patients with locally advanced nonmetastatic pancreatic cancer. All patients had high-quality CT; on laparoscopy, evidence of metastasis was found in 25 patients (34%) either as liver or peritoneal deposits or positive peritoneal cytology. The incidence of metastasis was 53% in body/tail cancers and 28% in the head tumors. They suggested that pancreatic body/tail tumors are more likely to give rise to unsuspected metastasis compared to pancreatic head tumors, although statistical significance was not reached.

The high incidence of unsuspected metastasis in locally advanced tumors in both studies suggested that laparoscopy should be part of the staging algorithm in these subsets of patients with locally advanced disease because positive findings will have major impact in their management. Laparoscopy is thus useful in the management of patients with pancreatic cancer in the accurate stratification of patients with unresectable

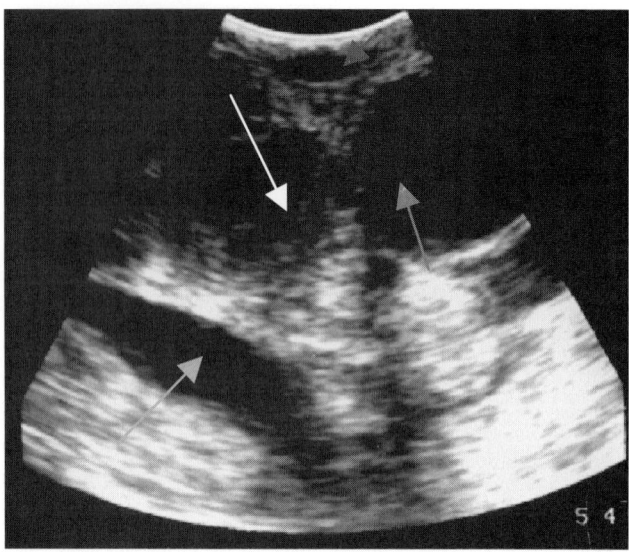

FIGURE 26.11. Laparoscopic ultrasound picture showing hepatic artery (*red arrow*), tumor inside the portal vein (*purple arrow*), common bile duct (*green arrow*), and inferior vena cava (*blue arrow*) (See also color Figure 26.11).

disease as either locally advanced or metastatic. For example, Jimenez et al. (119) used laparoscopy to stratify 125 patients with radiographic stage II to III pancreatic ductal adenocarcinoma into three groups: group 1, 39 patients with unsuspected metastases on laparoscopy (31.2%) who received palliation without further surgery; group 2, 55 patients with localized but unresectable carcinoma (44%) who received chemoradiation; and group 3, 31 patients with potentially resectable tumors with resection performed in 23 (resectability rate of 74.2%). The median survival was 7.5 months, 10.5 months, and 14.5 months in groups 1, 2, and 3, respectively. They concluded that staging laparoscopy in combination with spiral CT is useful in stratifying patients into treatment groups, and this stratification correlated with subsequent survival.

In patients who received neoadjuvant treatment before resection (see Chapter 28), laparoscopy could be used to assess tumor response. In patients with advanced disease undergoing novel chemotherapeutic treatments as part of experimental protocols, it could play a role in the accurate assessment of response.

LUS has been suggested to improve the diagnostic accuracy of laparoscopy alone in predicting hepatobiliary and pancreatic cancers resectability (Fig. 26.11). Callery et al. (128) performed staging laparoscopy with LUS in 50 patients with hepatobiliary and pancreatic malignancies that were considered resectable by traditional preoperative staging modalities. Twenty-two patients (44%) were found to be unresectable on staging laparoscopy with LUS. Unrecognized occult metastases in 11 patients (22%) were demonstrated by staging laparoscopy alone, while LUS established in 11 other patients (22%) who have been negative on staging laparoscopy alone, unresectability from vascular invasion (*n* = 5), lymph node metastases (*n* = 5), or intraparenchymal hepatic tumor (*n* = 1). Minnard et al. (146) in their prospective evaluation of 90 patients with pancreatic tumors undergoing laparoscopy and LUS reported a change in surgical treatment with the use of LUS for 13 patients (14%) in whom standard laparoscopic examination was equivocal and concluded that supplementing laparoscopy with LUS offers improved assessment and preoperative staging of pancreatic cancer. Other studies have shown that LUS improves diagnostic accuracy of staging laparoscopy, giving "additional value" in 14% to 25% of cases (147–149).

Laparoscopic Palliation

Only 20% of pancreatic cancers are resectable at presentation (150,151). The focus of management therefore in the majority of patients with nonresectable tumor will be palliation of symptoms such as jaundice, pain, and gastric outlet obstruction for quality of life maximization. Biliary obstruction causing jaundice occurs in about 70% to 80% of patients (151–153), whereas abdominal/back pain secondary to invasion of the celiac and mesenteric plexus by the tumor occurs in up to 80% of patients (154). For duodenal obstruction requiring bypass, an incidence of 2% to 19% have been reported (137,155–159).

The various methods of achieving palliation in these cases include endoscopic, radiologic, open surgical, and laparoscopic approaches. Endoscopic approach consists of biliary and/or duodenal stenting with plastic or metallic stents. It is less invasive when compared with open surgical approach and associated with shorter hospital stay but more late complications (160). Radiologic approach in the form of percutaneous transhepatic stent placement is associated with higher morbidity and mortality rates and lower success rate of drainage when compared with endoscopic drainage (161). Open surgical approach consists of biliary bypass (cholecystojejunostomy, choledochojejunostomy, or hepaticojejunostomy) and gastroenterostomy, and it is associated with morbidity rates of up to 35% (162) and a mortality rate of 0% to 2% (162,163). Laparoscopic bypass combined the advantages of minimal invasiveness with low morbidity rates (7%–25%) and shorter hospital stay (165–168). Laparoscopic biliary and/or gastric bypass can be done at the time of staging laparoscopy in patients with unresectable pancreatic disease.

In a retrospective review study (169), nine patients with unresectable pancreatic cancer had laparoscopic gastrojejunostomy for gastric outlet obstruction, eight of whom had previous failed duodenal stenting. Eight of the nine (88.8%) had successful palliation with no morbidity and mortality. Rothlin et al. (167), in a case-control study from Zurich, compared 14 patients who had laparoscopic palliation (3 had gastro- and biliary bypass, 7 had gastroenterostomy, and 4 had staging laparoscopy only) with 14 patients who had open palliative procedures. The results showed a morbidity of 7% versus 43% (p <0.05), mortality of 0% versus 29% (p <0.05), and mean hospital stay of 9 versus 21 days (p <0.06) for laparoscopic versus open palliation, respectively. Postoperative analgesic requirement was also significantly reduced for the laparoscopic group (p <0.03).

In a recent review article from the Manchester Royal Infirmary, Ravindra et al. (170) noted laparoscopic cholecystoenterostomy as the most common laparoscopic biliary bypass procedure done for palliation of periampullary cancers, accounting for 40 of the 52 reported cases in the literature (covering the period from January 1966 to December 2004) since the first report of laparoscopic biliary bypass in 1992. Others were 6 cases of laparoscopic choledochoduodenostomy and 6 cases of hepaticojejunostomy. They concluded that there is insufficient evidence at the present time for incorporating laparoscopic biliary bypass into the management algorithms of nonresectable periampullary cancer.

The initial treatment of pain from pancreatic cancer is by use of analgesic drugs such as paracetamol, nonsteroidal antiinflammatory drugs, and oral and transdermal opiates following World Health Organization guidelines (171). However, in intractable pain, relief could be obtained by chemical celiac block using alcohol, which can be performed under radiologic imaging, EUS guidance (172), or intraoperatively (173). Splanchnic nerves in which the pain fibers from the pancreas run after synapse in the celiac ganglion could also be disrupted in the thorax by video-assisted thoracoscopy (174,175).

Peritoneal Cytology

At Massachusetts General Hospital, Jimenez et al. (176) showed that by using staging laparoscopy and peritoneal cytology, approximately 30% of patients without metastases by CT harbor occult metastatic disease at laparoscopy. In their Sloan-Kettering Memorial Hospital study of 228 patients with radiographically resectable pancreatic adenocarcinoma who had laparoscopic staging and peritoneal cytology, Merchant et al. (177) indicated that positive peritoneal cytology (on the basis of cytomorphologic features using standard stains) had a positive predictive value of 94.1%, specificity of 98.1%, and sensitivity of 25.6% for determining unresectability of pancreatic adenocarcinoma. They concluded that positive peritoneal cytology is associated with advanced disease and is highly specific in predicting unresectability of pancreatic adenocarcinoma, resulting in decreased survival. Peritoneal cytology, in addition to laparoscopy, has been shown to disclose an additional 8% of patients with micrometastases who have an equally poor prognosis as those with visible metastases (178).

In a retrospective study by Konishi et al. (179) of 151 patients with radiologic resectable pancreatic cancer, the incidence of positive peritoneal cytology was 23.8%, and it increased significantly with disease progression. They also found that in patients with positive cytologic findings without visible metastases, survival and peritoneal metastasesfree survival were significantly better in the locally advanced group undergoing chemoradiotherapy than in the resectable group and suggested that chemoradiotherapy may be beneficial in this group of patients.

Positive peritoneal cytology (Fig. 26.12) has been shown to have implications for pancreatic cancer management. Makary et al. (180), in a retrospective cohort study of 32 consecutive pancreatic cancer patients with positive results from peritoneal washings during a 4-year period, showed median survival among patients with and without visible metastasis was 7.8 months and 8.6 months, respectively (p = 0.95). Their conclusion was that pancreatic cancer patients with peritoneal micrometastases have a poor prognosis and that the finding of a positive result from peritoneal fluid cytologic testing contraindicates further irradiation or surgery.

In contrast, Yachida et al. (181) performed peritoneal washings cytology using both standard cytologic technique and

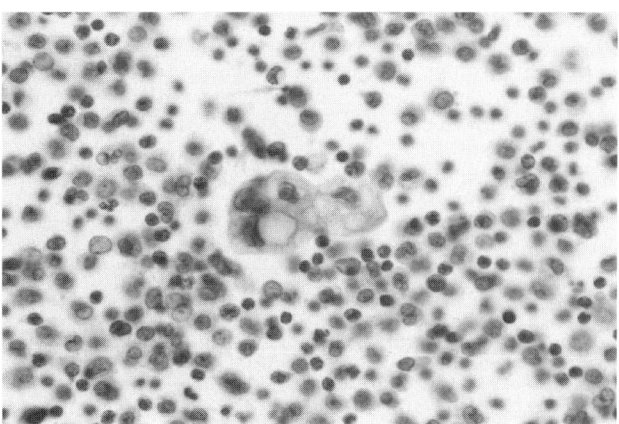

FIGURE 26.12. Positive peritoneal cytology: malignant pancreatic cells at the center. Papanicolaou stain ×400 magnification.

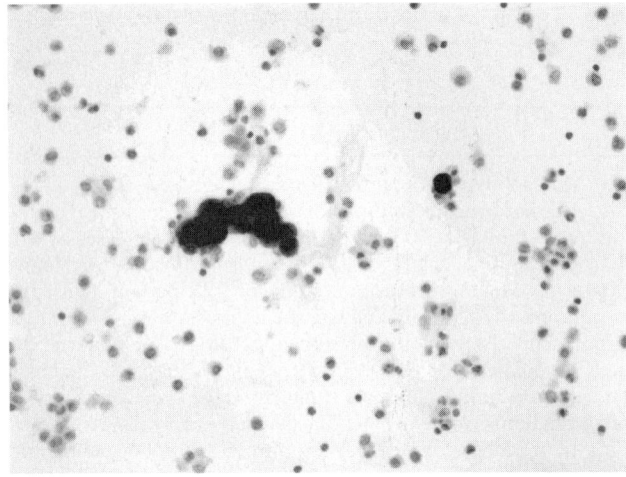

FIGURE 26.13. Immunocytology. Malignant pancreatic cells stained by monoclonal epithelial antibody ×200 magnification.

immunocytochemistry on 134 patients who had surgical resection for adenocarcinoma of the pancreas. Three groups were identified: 114 patients had negative cytology (group 1), 16 patients had positive cytology but no macroscopic peritoneal metastases (group 2), and 3 patients had positive cytology with macroscopic peritoneal metastases (group 3). They found no significant difference in the cumulative survival rate between groups 1 and 2 ($p = 0.022$) and identified two patients who survived for long periods of 40 and 58 months in group 2. They concluded that positive peritoneal cytology, although associated with advance disease, is not a contraindication for radical surgery. However, many investigators (119,176,177,179,180) will regard positive peritoneal cytology as a contraindication to radical resection in patients with resectable pancreatic carcinomas. These patients should be treated as having "M1" disease. The use of immunocytochemistry (Fig. 26.13) improves the sensitivity of standard peritoneal cytology technique and might be helpful (181,182).

CONCLUSION

Accurate staging of patients with pancreatic cancer allows for the appropriate direction of therapy, avoidance of nontherapeutic intervention, and reliable stratification of outcomes for research. Advances in technology have improved the sensitivity and predictive value of cross-sectional staging modalities such as CT and MRI to the point that abdominal US, cholangiography, and angiography are no longer required for accurate staging. The addition of laparoscopy in conjunction with LUS and peritoneal cytology decreases the nontherapeutic laparotomy rate. As more advanced patients are diagnosed preoperatively, the options for nonsurgical and minimally invasive palliation are also increasing.

References

1. Parkin DM, Pisani P, Ferlay J. Estimates of the worldwide incidence of 25 major cancers in 1990. *Int J Cancer* 1999;80(6):827–841.
2. Jemal A, Siegel R, Ward E, et al. Cancer statistics. *CA Cancer J Clin* 2006; 56:106–130.
3. Greenlee RT, Murray T, Bolden S, Wingo PA. Cancer statistics. *CA Cancer J Clin* 2000;50:7–33.
4. Conlon K, Minnard E. The value of laparoscopic staging in upper gastrointestinal malignancy. *Oncologist* 1997;2:10–17.
5. Watanapa P, Williamson R. Surgical palliation for pancreatic cancer: developments during the last two decades. *Br J Surg* 1992;79:8–20.
6. Standring S. *Gray's Anatomy.* 39th ed. Philadelphia: Elsevier Churchill Livingstone; 2005.
7. Hall-Craggs ECB. *Anatomy as a Basis for Clinical Medicine.* 2nd ed. Baltimore: Urban & Schwarzenberg; 1990.
8. Murakami G, Hirata K, Takamuro T, Mukaiya M, Hata F, Kitagawa S. Vascular anatomy of the pancreaticoduodenal region: a review. *J Hepatobiliary Pancreat Surg* 1999;6(1):55–68.
9. Bertelli E, Di Gregorio F, Mosca S, Bastianini A. The arterial blood supply of the pancreas: a review. V. The dorsal pancreatic artery. An anatomic review and a radiologic study. *Surg Radiol Anat* 1998;20(6):445–452.
10. O'Morchoe CC. Lymphatic system of the pancreas. *Microsc Res Tech* 1997; 37(5(6):456–477.
11. Geer RJ, Brennan MF. Prognostic indicators for survival after resection of pancreatic adenocarcinoma. *Am J Surg* 1993;165:68–72.
12. Sener SF, Fremgen A, Menck HR, Winchester DP. Pancreatic cancer: a report of treatment and survival trends for 100,313 patients diagnosed from 1985–1995, using the National Cancer Database. *J Am Coll Surg* 1999; 189:1–7.
13. Nordback IH, Hruban RH, Boitnott JK, Pitt HA, Cameron JL. Carcinoma of the body and tail of the pancreas. *Am J Surg* 1992;164:26–31.
14. Brennan MF, Moccia RD, Klimstra D. Management of adenocarcinoma of the body and tail of the pancreas. *Ann Surg* 1996;223:506–511.
15. Johnson CD, Schwall G, Flechtenmacher J, Trede M. Resection for adenocarcinoma of the body and tail of the pancreas. *Br J Surg* 1993;80:1177–1179.
16. Modolell I, Guarner L, Malagelada JR. Vagaries of clinical presentation of pancreatic and biliary tract cancer. *Ann Oncol* 1999;10(suppl 4):82–84.
17. Maringhini A, Ciambra M, Raimondo M, et al. Clinical presentation and ultrasonography in the diagnosis of pancreatic cancer. *Pancreas* 1993; 8(2):146–150.
18. Nix GA, Schmitz PI, Wilson JH, Van Blankenstein M, Goeneveld CF, Hofwijk R. Carcinoma of the head of the pancreas: therapeutic implications of endoscopic retrograde cholangiopancreatography findings. *Gastroenterology* 1984;87(1):37–43.
19. Dalton RR, Sarr MG, van Heerden JA, Colby TV. Carcinoma of the body and tail of the pancreas: is curative resection justified? *Surgery* 1992; 111:489–494.
20. Geer RJ, Brennan MF. Prognostic indicators for survival after resection of pancreatic adenocarcinoma. *Am J Surg* 1993;165:68–72.
21. Howard JM, Jordan GL, Jr. Cancer of the pancreas. *Curr Probl Cancer* 1977;2(3):5–52.
22. van den Bosch RP, van Eijck CH, Mulder PG, Jeekel J. Serum CA19-9 determination in the management of pancreatic cancer. *Hepatogastroenterology* 1996;43(9):710–713.
23. Forsmark CE, Lambiase L, Vogel SB. Diagnosis of pancreatic cancer and prediction of unresectability using the tumor-associated antigen CA19-9. *Pancreas* 1994;9(6):731–734.
24. Schlieman MG, Ho HS, Bold RJ. Utility of tumor markers in determining resectability of pancreatic cancer. *Arch Surg* 2003;138(9):951–955; discussion 955–956.
25. Freeny PC, Ball TJ. Endoscopic retrograde cholangiopancreatography (ERCP) and percutaneous transhepatic cholangiography (PTC) in the evaluation of suspected pancreatic carcinoma: diagnostic limitations and contemporary roles. *Cancer* 1981;47(6 suppl):1666–1678.
26. Pasanen P, Partanen K, Pikkarainen P, Alhava E, Pirinen A, Janatuinen E. Diagnostic accuracy of ultrasound, computed tomography and endoscopic retrograde cholangiopancreatography in the detection of pancreatic cancer in patients with jaundice or cholestasis. *In Vivo* 1992;6(3):297–301.
27. Tobin RS, Vogelzang RL, Gore RM, Keigley B. A comparative study of computed tomography and ERCP in pancreaticobiliary disease. *J Comput Tomogr* 1987;11(3):261–266.
28. Gilinsky NH, Bornman PC, Girdwood AH, Marks IN. Diagnostic yield of endoscopic retrograde cholangiopancreatography in carcinoma of the pancreas. *Br J Surg* 1986;73(7):539–543.
29. Freeny PC, Bilbao MK, Katon RM. "Blind" evaluation of endoscopic retrograde cholangiopancreatography (ERCP) in the diagnosis of pancreatic carcinoma: the "double duct" and other signs. *Radiology* 1976;119(2):271–274.
30. Nix GA, Van Overbeeke IC, Wilson JH, ten Kate FJ. ERCP diagnosis of tumors in the region of the head of the pancreas: analysis of criteria and computer-aided diagnosis. *Dig Dis Sci* 1988;33(5):577–586.
31. Hatfield AR, Smithies A, Wilkins R, Levi AJ. Assessment of endoscopic retrograde cholangio-pancreatography (ERCP) and pure pancreatic juice cytology in patients with pancreatic disease. *Gut* 1976;17(1):14–21.
32. Mackie CR, Cooper MJ, Lewis MH, Moosa AR. Non-operative differentiation between pancreatic cancer and chronic pancreatitis. *Ann Surg* 1979; 189(4):480–487.
33. Ralls PW, Halls J, Renner I, Juttner H. Endoscopic retrograde cholangiopancreatography (ERCP) in pancreatic disease: a reassessment of the specificity of ductal abnormalities in differentiating benign from malignant disease. *Radiology* 1980;134(2):347–352.
34. Plumley TF, Rohrmann CA, Freeny PC, Silverstein FE, Ball TJ. Double duct sign: reassessed significance in ERCP. *AJR Am J Roentgenol* 1982; 138(1):31–35.
35. Carter DC. Cancer of the head of pancreas or chronic pancreatitis? A diagnostic dilemma. *Surgery* 1992;111(6):602–603.

36. Loperfido S, Angelini G, Benedetti G, et al. Major early complications from diagnostic and therapeutic ERCP: a prospective multicenter study. *Gastrointest Endosc* 1998;48(1):1–10.

37. Halme L, Doepel M, von Numers H, Edgren J, Ahonen J. Complications of diagnostic and therapeutic ERCP. *Ann Chir Gynaecol* 1999;88(2):127–131.

38. Farrell RJ, Mahmud N, Noonan N, Kelleher D, Keeling PW. Diagnostic and therapeutic ERCP: a large single centre's experience. *Ir J Med Sci* 2001;170(3):176–180.

39. Aliperti G. Complications related to diagnostic and therapeutic endoscopic retrograde cholangiopancreatography. *Gastrointest Endosc Clin N Am* 1996;6(2):379–407.

40. Burke DR, Lewis CA, Cardella JF, et al. Quality improvement guidelines for percutaneous transhepatic cholangiography and biliary drainage. *J Vasc Interv Radiol* 2003;14(9):S243–S246.

41. Rossi RL, Traverso LW, Pimentel F. Malignant obstructive jaundice: evaluation and management. *Surg Clin North Am* 1996;76(1):63–70.

42. Kozarek RA. Endoscopy in the management of malignant obstructive jaundice. *Gastrointest Endosc Clin N Am* 1996;6(1):153–176.

43. Frick MP, Feinberg SB, Goodale RL. The value of endoscopic retrograde cholangiopancreatography in patients with suspected carcinoma of the pancreas and indeterminate computed tomographic results. *Surg Gynecol Obstet* 1982;155(2):177–182.

44. Bottger TC, Boddin J, Duber C, Heintz A, Kuchle R, Junginger T. Diagnosing and staging of pancreatic carcinoma—what is necessary? *Oncology* 1998;55(2):122–129.

45. Warshaw AL, Tepper JE, Shipley WU. Laparoscopy in the staging and planning of therapy for pancreatic cancer. *Am J Surg* 1986;151:76–80.

46. Angeli E, Venturini M, Vanzulli A, et al. Color Doppler imaging in the assessment of vascular involvement by pancreatic carcinoma. *AJR Am J Roentgenol* 1997;168(1):193–197.

47. Gress F, Savides T, Cummings O, et al. Radial scanning and linear array endosonography for staging pancreatic cancer: a prospective randomized comparison. *Gastrointest Endosc* 1997;45:138–142.

48. Yasuda K, Kiyota K, Mukai H, et al. Clinical evaluation of ultrasonic endoscopy for hepatic, pancreatic and biliary tract diseases. *Nippon Rinsho* 1984;42(10):2249–2258.

49. Rosch T, Lorenz R, Braig C, et al. Endoscopic ultrasound in pancreatic tumor diagnosis. *Gastrointest Endosc* 1991;37(3):347–352.

50. Midwinter MJ, Beveridge CJ, Wilsdon JB, Bennett MK, Baudouin CJ, Charnley RM. Correlation between spiral computed tomography, endoscopic ultrasonography and findings at operation in pancreatic and ampullary tumours. *Br J Surg* 1999;86(2):189–193.

51. Snady H, Bruckner H, Siegel J, Cooperman A, Neff R, Kiefer L. Endoscopic ultrasonographic criteria of vascular invasion by potentially resectable pancreatic tumors. *Gastrointest Endosc* 1994;40(3):326–333.

52. Santo E. Pancreatic cancer imaging: which method? *JOP* 2004;5(4):253–237. Varadarajulu S, Wallace MB. Applications of endoscopic ultrasonography in pancreatic cancer. *Cancer Control* 2004;11:15–22.

53. Chang KJ. Endoscopic ultrasound-guided fine needle aspiration in the diagnosis and staging of pancreatic tumors. *Gastrointest Endosc Clin N Am* 1995;5(4):723–734.

54. Harewood GC, Wiersema MJ. Endosonography-guided fine needle aspiration biopsy in the evaluation of pancreatic masses. *Am J Gastroenterol* 2002;97(6):1386–1391.

55. Giovannini M, Seitz JF, Monges G, Perrier H, Rabbia I. Fine-needle aspiration cytology guided by endoscopic ultrasonography: results in 141 patients. *Endoscopy* 1995;27(2):171–177.

56. Williams DB, Sahai AV, Aabakken L, et al. Endoscopic ultrasound guided fine needle aspiration biopsy: a large single centre experience. *Gut* 1999;44:720–726.

57. Fazel A, Draganov P. Interventional endoscopic ultrasound in pancreatic disease. *Curr Gastroenterol Rep* 2004;6(2):104–110.

58. Chan HH, Nishioka NS, Mino M, et al. EUS-guided photodynamic therapy of the pancreas: a pilot study. *Gastrointest Endosc* 2004;59(1):95–99.

59. Ferrucci JT. Biliopancreatic malignancy current diagnostic possibilities: an overview. *Ann Oncol* 1999;10(suppl 4):143–144.

60. Palazzo L, Roseau G, Gayet B, et al. Endoscopic ultrasonography in the diagnosis and staging of pancreatic adenocarcinoma: results of a prospective study with comparison to ultrasonography and CT scan. *Endoscopy* 1993;25(2):143–150.

61. Freeny PC, Marks WM, Ryan JA, Traverso LW. Pancreatic ductal adenocarcinoma: diagnosis and staging with dynamic CT. *Radiology* 1988;166(1 pt 1):125–133.

62. Muller MF, Meyenberger C, Bertschinger P, Schaer R, Marincek B. Pancreatic tumors: evaluation with endoscopic US, CT, and MR imaging. *Radiology* 1994;190(3):745–751.

63. Baron RL, Stanley RJ, Lee JK, et al. A prospective comparison of the evaluation of biliary obstruction using computed tomography and ultrasonography. *Radiology* 1982;145(1):91–98.

64. Hessel SJ, Siegelman SS, McNeil BJ, et al. A prospective evaluation of computed tomography and ultrasound of the pancreas. *Radiology* 1982;143(1):129–133.

65. de Roos WK, Welvaart K, Bloem JL, Hermans J. Assessment of resectability of carcinoma of the pancreatic head by ultrasonography and computed tomography: a retrospective analysis. *Eur J Surg Oncol* 1990;16(5):411–416.

66. Rosch T, Braig C, Gain T, et al. Staging of pancreatic and ampullary carcinoma by endoscopic ultrasonography: comparison with conventional sonography, computed tomography, and angiography. *Gastroenterology* 1992;102(1):188–199.

67. Bakkevold KE, Arnesjo B, Kambestad B. Carcinoma of the pancreas and papilla of Vater—assessment of resectability and factors influencing resectability in stage I carcinomas: a prospective multicentre trial in 472 patients. *Eur J Surg Oncol* 1992;18(5):494–507.

68. Freeny PC, Traverso LW, Ryan JA. Diagnosis and staging of pancreatic adenocarcinoma with dynamic computed tomography. *Am J Surg* 1993;165(5):600–606.

69. Tabuchi T, Itoh K, Ohshio G, et al. Tumor staging of pancreatic adenocarcinoma using early and late-phase helical CT. *AJR Am Roentgenol* 1999;173:375–380.

70. Hommeryer SC, Freeney PC, Crabo LG. Carcinoma of the head of the pancreas: evaluation of the pancreaticoduodenal veins with dynamic CT—potential for improved accuracy in staging. *Radiology* 1995;196:133–238.

71. Vedantham S, Lu DSK, Reber HA, Kadell B. Small peripancreatic veins: improved assessment in pancreatic cancer patients using thin-section pancreatic phase helical CT. *AJR Am J Roentgenol* 1998;170:377–383.

72. Valls C, Andia E, Sanchez A, et al. Dual-phase helical CT of pancreatic adenocarcinoma: assessment of resectability before surgery. *AJR Am J Roentgenol* 2002;178(4):821–826.

73. Calculli L, Casadei R, Amore B, et al. The usefulness of spiral computed tomography and colour-Doppler ultrasonography to predict portal-mesenteric trunk involvement in pancreatic cancer. *Radiologia Medica* 2002;104(4):307–315.

74. Zhang LY, Zhao YP. Assessment of unresectability of pancreatic carcinoma by enhanced-CT and selective angiography. *Aizheng* 2002;21(7):761–763.

75. Soriano A, Castells A, Ayuso C, et al. Preoperative staging and tumor resectability assessment of pancreatic cancer: prospective study comparing endoscopic ultrasonography, helical computed tomography, magnetic resonance imaging, and angiography. *Am J Gastroenterol* 2004;99(3):492–501.

76. Grenacher L, Klauss M, Dukic L, et al. Diagnosis and staging of pancreatic carcinoma: MRI versus multislice-CT—a prospective study. *Rofo* 2004;176(11):1624–1633.

77. McCarthy MJ, Evans J, Sagar G, Neoptolemos JP. Prediction of resectability of pancreatic malignancy by computed tomography. *Br J Surg* 1998;85:320–325.

78. Freeny PC. Computed tomography in the diagnosis and staging of cholangiocarcinoma and pancreatic carcinoma. *Ann Oncol* 1999;10(suppl 4):12–17.

79. Bluemke DA, Fishman EK. CT and MR evaluation of pancreatic cancer. *Surg Oncol Clin N Am* 1998;7:103–124.

80. Legmann P, Vignaux O, Dousset B, et al. Pancreatic tumors: comparison of dual-phase helical CT and endoscopic sonography. *AJR Am J Roentgenol* 1998;170:1315–1322.

81. Nishiharu T, Yamashita Y, Abe Y, et al. Local extension of pancreatic carcinoma: assessment with thin-section helical CT versus with breath-hold fast MR imaging—ROC analysis. *Radiology* 1999;212:445–452.

82. Phoa SS, Reeders JW, Rauws EA, De Wit L, Gouma DJ, Lameris JS. Spiral computed tomography for preoperative staging of potentially resectable carcinoma of the pancreatic head. *Br J Surg* 1999;86:789–794.

83. Diehl SJ, Lehmann KJ, Sadick M, Lachmann R, Georgi M. Pancreatic cancer: value of dual-phase helical CT in assessing resectability. *Radiology* 1998;206(2):373–378.

84. Saldinger PF, Reilly M, Reynolds K, et al. Is CT angiography sufficient for prediction of resectability of periampullary neoplasms? *J Gastrointest Surg* 2000;4:233–237.

85. Gmeinwieser J, Feuerbach S, Hohenberger W, et al. Spiral-CT in diagnosis of vascular involvement in pancreatic cancer. *Hepatogastroenterology* 1995;42(4):418–422.

86. Zeman RK, Cooper C, Zeiberg AS, et al. TNM staging of pancreatic carcinoma using helical CT. *AJR Am J Roentgenol* 1997;169(2):459–464.

87. Megibow AJ, Zhou XH, Rotterdam H, et al. Pancreatic adenocarcinoma: CT versus MR imaging in the evaluation of resectability—report of the Radiology Diagnostic Oncology Group. *Radiology* 1995;195:327–332.

88. Outwater EK and Siegelman ES. MR imaging of pancreatic disorders. *Top Magn Reson Imaging* 1996;8:265–289.

89. Mueller MF, Meyenberger C, Bertschinger P, Schaer R, Marincek B. Pancreatic tumors: evaluation with endoscopic US, CT, and MR imaging. *Radiology* 1994;190:745–751.

90. Spencer JA, Ward J, Guthrie JA, Guillou PJ, Robinson PJ. Assessment of resectability of pancreatic cancer with dynamic contrast-enhanced MR imaging: technique, surgical correlation and patient outcome. *Eur Radiol* 1998;8:23–29.

91. Vellet AD, Romano W, Bach DB, Passi RB, Taves DH, Munk PL. Adenocarcinoma of the pancreatic ducts: comparative evaluation with CT and MR imaging at 1,5T. *Radiology* 1992;183:87–95.

92. Vahldiek G, Broemel T, Klapdor R. MR-cholangiopancreaticography (MRCP) and MR-angiography: morphologic changes with magnetic resonance imaging. *Anticancer Res* 1999;19:2451–2458.

93. Trede M, Rumstadt B, Wendl K, et al. Ultrafast magnetic resonance imaging improves the staging of pancreatic tumors. *Ann Surg* 1997;226:393–405.

94. Birchard KR, Semelka RC, Hyslop WB, et al. Suspected pancreatic cancer: evaluation by dynamic gadolinium-enhanced 3D gradient-echo MRI. *AJR Am J Roentgenol* 2005;185(3):700–703.

95. Strauss LG, Conti PS. The applications of PET in clinical oncology. *J Nucl Med* 1991;32(4):623–648.

96. Hoh CK, Hawkins RA, Glaspy JA, et al. Cancer detection with whole-body PET using 2-[18F]fluoro-2-deoxy-D-glucose. *J Comput Assist Tomogr* 1993;17(4):582–589.

97. Kole AC, Plukker JT, Nieweg OE, Vaalburg W. Positron emission tomography for staging of oesophageal and gastroesophageal malignancy. *Br J Cancer* 1998;78(4):521–527.

98. Vansteenkiste JF, Stroobants SG, De Leyn PR, et al. Lymph node staging in non-small-cell lung cancer with FDG-PET scan: a prospective study on 690 lymph node stations from 68 patients. *J Clin Oncol* 1998;16(6):2142–2149.

99. Adler LP, Blair HF, Makley JT, et al. Noninvasive grading of musculoskeletal tumors using PET. *J Nucl Med* 1991;32(8):1508–1512.

100. Reske SN, Kotzerke J. FDG-PET for clinical use. Results of the 3rd German Interdisciplinary Consensus Conference, "Onko-PET III", 21 July and 19 September 2000. *Eur J Nucl Med* 2001;28(11):1707–1723.

101. Berberat P, Friess H, Kashiwagi M, Beger HG, Buchler MW. Diagnosis and staging of pancreatic cancer by positron emission tomography. *World J Surg* 1999;23(9):882–887.

102. Imdahl A, Nitzsche E, Krautmann F, et al. Evaluation of positron emission tomography with 2-[18F]fluoro-2-deoxy-D-glucose for the differentiation of chronic pancreatitis and pancreatic cancer. *Br J Surg* 1999;86(2):194–199.

103. Rajput A, Stellato TA, Faulhaber PF, Vesselle HJ, Miraldi F. The role of fluorodeoxyglucose and positron emission tomography in the evaluation of pancreatic disease. *Surgery* 1998;124(4):793–797.

104. Sperti C, Pasquali C, Decet G, Chierichetti F, Liessi G, Pedrazzoli S. F-18-fluorodeoxyglucose positron emission tomography in differentiating malignant from benign pancreatic cysts: a prospective study. *J Gastrointest Surg* 2005;9(1):22–28; discussion 28–29.

105. Sendler A, Avril N, Helmberger H, et al. Preoperative evaluation of pancreatic masses with positron emission tomography using 18F-fluorodeoxyglucose: diagnostic limitations. *World J Surg* 2000;24(9):1121–1129.

106. Kasperk RK, Riesener KP, Wilms K, Scumpelick V. Limited value of positron emission tomography in treatment of pancreatic cancer: surgeon's view. *World J Surg* 2001;25(9):1134–1139.

107. Lytras D, Connor S, Bosonnet L, et al. Positron emission tomography does not add to computed tomography for the diagnosis and staging of pancreatic cancer. *Dig Surg* 2005;22(1–2):55–61.

108. Frohlich A, Diederichs CG, Staib L, Vogel J, Beger HG, Reske SN. Detection of liver metastases from pancreatic cancer using FDG PET. *J Nucl Med* 1999;40:250–255.

109. Delbeke D, Rose DM, Chapman WC, et al. Optimal interpretation of FDG PET in the diagnosis, staging and management of pancreatic carcinoma. *J Nucl Med* 1999;40:1784–1791.

110. Inokuma T, Tamaki N, Torizuka T, et al. Evaluation of pancreatic tumors with positron emission tomography and F-18 fluorodeoxyglucose: comparison with CT and US. *Radiology* 1995;195(2):345–352.

111. Keogan MT, Tyler D, Clark L, et al. Diagnosis of pancreatic carcinoma: role of FDG PET. *AJR Am J Roentgenol* 1998;171(6):1565–1570.

112. Zimny M, Bares R, Fass J, et al. Fluorine-18 fluorodeoxyglucose positron emission tomography in the differential diagnosis of pancreatic carcinoma: a report of 106 cases. *Eur J Nucl Med* 1997;24(6):678–682.

113. Diederichs CG, Staib L, Glatting G, Beger HG, Reske SN. FDG PET: elevated plasma glucose reduces both uptake and detection rate of pancreatic malignancies. *J Nucl Med* 1998;39(6):1030–1033.

114. Maisey NR, Webb A, Flux GD, et al. FDG-PET in the prediction of survival of patients with cancer of the pancreas: a pilot study. *Br J Cancer* 2000;83(3):281–283.

115. Rose DM, Delbeke D, Beauchamp RD, et al. 18-Fluorodeoxyglucose-positron emission tomography in the management of patients with suspected pancreatic cancer. *Ann Surg* 1999;229(5):729–737.

116. Bernheim H. Organoscopy: cystoscopy of the abdominal cavity. *Ann Surg* 1911;53:764–767.

117. Cuschieri A. Laparoscopy for pancreatic cancer: does it benefit the patient? *Eur J Surg Oncol* 1988;14:41–44.

118. Warshaw AL, Gu ZY, Wittenberg J, Waltman AC. Preoperative staging and assessment of resectability of pancreatic cancer. *Arch Surg* 1990;125:230–233.

119. Jimenez RE, Warshaw AL, Rattner DW, Willett CG, McGrath D, Fernandez-del Castillo C. Impact of laparoscopic staging in the treatment of pancreatic cancer. *Arch Surg* 2000;135:409–414.

120. Reddy KR, Levi J, Livingstone A, et al. Experience with staging laparoscopy in pancreatic malignancy. *Gastrointest Endosc* 1999;49:498–503.

121. Catheline JM, Turner R, Rizk N, Barrat C, Champault G. The use of diagnostic laparoscopy supported by laparoscopic ultrasonography in the assessment of pancreatic cancer. *Surg Endosc* 1999;13:239–245.

122. Conlon KC, Dougherty E, Klimstra DS, Coit DG, Turnbull AD, Brennan MF. The value of minimal access surgery in the staging of patients with potentially resectable peripancreatic malignancy. *Ann Surg* 1996;223(2):134–140.

123. Menack MJ, Spitz JD, Arregui ME. Staging of pancreatic and ampullary cancers for resectability using laparoscopy with laparoscopic ultrasound. *Surg Endosc* 2001;15(10):1129–1134.

124. Schachter PP, Avni Y, Shimonov M, Gvirtz G, Rosen A, Czerniak A. The impact of laparoscopy and laparoscopic ultrasonography on the management of pancreatic cancer. *Arch Surg* 2000;135:1303–1307.

125. Pietrabissa A, Caramella D, Di Candio G, et al. Laparoscopy and laparoscopic ultrasonography for staging pancreatic cancer: critical appraisal. *World J Surg* 1999;23:998–1003.

126. Andren-Sandberg A, Lindberg CG, Lundsted C, Ihse I. Computed tomography and laparoscopy in the assessment of the patients with pancreatic cancer. *J Am Coll Surg* 1998;186:35–40.

127. Bemelman WA, de Wit LT, van Delden OM, et al. Diagnostic laparoscopy combined with laparoscopic ultrasonography in staging of cancer of the pancreatic head region. *Br J Surg* 1995;82:820–824.

128. Callery MP, Strasberg SM, Doherty GM, Soper NJ, Norton JA. Staging laparoscopy with laparoscopic ultrasonography: optimizing resectability in hepatobiliary and pancreatic malignancy. *J Am Coll Surg* 1997;185:33–39.

129. Fernandez-Del Castillo C, Rattner DW, Warshaw AL. Standards for pancreatic resection in the 1990s. *Arch Surg* 1995;130:295–299.

130. John TG, Wright A, Allan PL, Redhead DN, Paterson-Brown S, Carter DC, Garden OJ. Laparoscopy with laparoscopic ultrasonography in the TNM staging of pancreatic carcinoma. *World J Surg* 1999;23:870–881.

131. Friess H, Kleeff J, Silva JC, Sadowski C, Baer HU, Buchler MW. The role of diagnostic laparoscopy in pancreatic and periampullary malignancies. *J Am Coll Surg* 1998;186:675–682.

132. Holzman MD, Reintgen KL, Tyler DS, Pappas TN. The role of laparoscopy in the management of suspected pancreatic and periampullary malignancies. *J Gastrointest Surg* 1997;1:236–244.

133. Spitz FR, Abbruzzese JL, Lee JE, et al. Preoperative and postoperative chemoradiation strategies in patients treated with pancreaticoduodenectomy for adenocarcinoma of the pancreas. *J Clin Oncol* 1997;15:928–937.

134. Pisters PW, Lee JE, Vauthey JN, Charnsangavej C, Evans DB. Laparoscopy in the staging of pancreatic cancer. *Br J Surg* 2001;88(3):325–337.

135. de Rooij PD, Rogatko A, Brennan MF. Evaluation of palliative surgical procedures in unresectable pancreatic cancer. *Br J Surg* 1991;78:1053–1058.

136. Connor S, Bosonnet L, Alexakis N, et al. Serum CA19-9 measurement increases the effectiveness of staging laparoscopy in patients with suspected pancreatic malignancy. *Dig Surg* 2005;22(1–2):80–85.

137. Espat NJ, Brennan MF, Conlon KC. Patients with laparoscopically staged unresectable pancreatic adenocarcinoma do not require subsequent surgical biliary or gastric bypass. *J Am Coll Surg* 1999;188:649–655.

138. Sohn TA, Lillemoe KD, Cameron JL, Huang JJ, Pitt HA, Yeo CJ. Surgical palliation of unresectable periampullary adenocarcinoma in the 1990s. *J Am Coll Surg* 1999;188:658–666.

139. Van Dijkum EJ, de Wit LT, van Delden OM, et al. The efficacy of laparoscopic staging in patients with upper gastrointestinal tumors. *Cancer* 1997;79:1315–1319.

140. Vollmer CM, Drebin JA, Middleton WD, et al. Utility of staging laparoscopy in subsets of peripancreatic and biliary malignancies. *Ann Surg* 2002;235:1–7.

141. Barreiro CJ, Lillemoe KD, Koniaris LG, et al. Diagnostic laparoscopy for periampullary and pancreatic cancer: what is the true benefit? *J Gastrointest Surg* 2002;6(1):75–81.

142. Tilleman EHBM, Kuikena BW, Phoab SSKS, et al. Limitation of diagnostic laparoscopy for patients with a periampullary carcinoma. *Eur J Surg Oncol* 2004;30:658–662.

143. Nieveen van Dijkum EJ, de Wit LT, van Delden OM, et al. Staging laparoscopy and laparoscopic ultrasonography in more than 400 patients with upper gastrointestinal carcinoma. *J Am Coll Surg* 1999;189(5):459–465.

144. Shoup M, Winston C, Brennan MF, Bassman D, Conlon KC. Is there a role for staging laparoscopy in patients with locally advanced, unresectable pancreatic adenocarcinoma? *J Gastrointest Surg* 2004;8:1068–1071.

145. Liu RC, Traverso LW. Diagnostic laparoscopy improves staging of pancreatic cancer deemed locally unresectable by computed tomography. *Surg Endosc* 2005;19:638–642.

146. Minnard EA, Conlon KC, Hoos A, Dougherty EC, Ann LE, Brennan MF. Laparoscopic ultrasound enhances standard laparoscopy in the staging of pancreatic cancer. *Ann Surg* 1998;228(2):182–187.

147. John TG, Greig JD, Carter DC, Garden OJ. Carcinoma of the pancreatic head and periampullary region: tumor staging with laparoscopy and laparoscopic ultrasonography. *Ann Surg* 1995;221(2):156–164.

148. van Delden OM, Smits NJ, Bemelman WA, de Wit LT, Gouma DJ, Reeders JW. Comparison of laparoscopic and transabdominal ultrasonography in staging of cancer of the pancreatic head region. *J Ultrasound Med* 1996;15(3):207–212.

149. Hann LE, Conlon KC, Dougherty EC, Hilton S, Bach AM, Brennan MF. Laparoscopic sonography of peripancreatic tumors: preliminary experience. *AJR Am J Roentgenol* 1997;169(5):1257–1262.

150. Sener SF, Fremgen A, Menck HR, Winchester DP. Pancreatic cancer: a report of treatment and survival trends for 100,313 patients diagnosed from 1985–1995, using the National Cancer Database. *J Am Coll Surg* 1999;189:1–7.

151. Tan HP, Smith J, Garberoglio CA. Pancreatic adenocarcinoma: an update. *J Am Coll Surg* 1996;183:164–184.
152. Warshaw AL, Fernandez-del Castillo C. Pancreatic carcinoma. *N Engl J Med* 1992;326:455–465.
153. Yeo CJ. Pancreatic cancer: 1998 update. *J Am Coll Surg* 1998;187:429–442.
154. Andren-Sandberg A. Pain relief in pancreatic disease. *Br J Surg* 1997;84:1041–1042.
155. Deziel DJ, Wilhelmi B, Staren ED, Doolas A. Surgical palliation for ductal adenocarcinoma of the pancreas. *Ann Surg* 1996;62:585–588.
156. Lillemoe KD, Cameron JL, Hardacre JM, et al. Is prophylactic gastrojejunostomy indicated for unresectable peri-ampullary cancer? A prospective randomized trial. *Ann Surg* 1999;230:322–330.
157. Sarr MG, Cameron JL. Surgical management of unresectable carcinoma of the pancreas. *Surgery* 1982;91:123–133.
158. Singh SM, Longmire WP, Reber HA. Surgical palliation for pancreatic cancer. *Surg Clin North Am* 1989;69:599–611.
159. Watanapa P, Williamson RCN. Surgical palliation for pancreatic cancer: developments during the past two decades. *Br J Surg* 1992;79:8–20.
160. Maosheng D, Ohtsuka T, Ohuchida J, et al. Surgical bypass versus metallic stent for unresectable pancreatic cancer. *J Hepatobiliary Pancreat Surg* 2001;8:367–373.
161. Speer AG, Cotton PB, Russell RC, et al. Randomised trial of endoscopic versus percutaneous stent insertion in malignant obstructive jaundice. *Lancet* 1987;2:57–62.
162. Isla AM, Worthington T, Kakkar AK, Williamson RC. A continuing role for surgical bypass in the palliative treatment of pancreatic carcinoma. *Dig Surg* 2000;17:143–146.
163. Van Wagensveld BA, Coene PP, van Gulik TM, Rauws EA, Obertop H, Gouma DJ. Outcome of palliative biliary and gastric surgery for pancreatic head carcinoma in 126 patients. *Br J Surg* 1997;84:402–406.
164. Nieveen van Dijkum EJ, Romijn MG, Terwee CB, et al. Laparoscopic staging and subsequent palliation in patients with peripancreatic carcinoma. *Ann Surg* 2003;237:66–73.
165. Rhodes M, Nathanson L, Fielding G. Laparoscopic biliary and gastric bypass: a useful adjunct in the treatment of carcinoma of the pancreas. *Gut* 1995;36:778–780.
166. Bergamaschi R, Marvik R, Thoresen JE, Ystgaard B, Johnsen G, Myrvold HE. Open versus laparoscopic gastrojejunostomy for palliation in advanced pancreatic cancer. *Surg Laparosc Endosc* 1998;8:92–96.
167. Rothlin MA, Schob O, Weber M. Laparoscopic gastro and hepaticojejunostomy for palliation of pancreatic cancer: a case controlled study. *Surg Endosc* 1999;13:1065–1069.
168. Kuriansky J, Saenz A, Astudillo E, Cardona V, Fernandez-Cruz L. Simultaneous laparoscopic biliary and retrocolic gastric bypass in patients with unresectable carcinoma of the pancreas. *Surg Endosc* 2000;14:179–181.
169. Kazanjian KK, Reber HA, Hines OJ. Laparoscopic gastrojejunostomy for gastric outlet obstruction in pancreatic cancer. *Ann Surg* 2004;70(10):910–913.
170. Date RS, Siriwardena AK. Current status of laparoscopic biliary bypass in the management of non-resectable peri-ampullary cancer. *Pancreatology* 2005,5.325 329.
171. World Health Organization (WHO). *Cancer Pain Relief*. Geneva: WHO; 1986.
172. Abedi M, Zfass AM. Endoscopic ultrasound-guided (neurolytic) celiac plexus block. *J Clin Gastroenterol* 2001;32(5):390–393.
173. Lillemoe KD, Cameron JL, Kaufman HS, Yeo CJ, Pitt HA, Sauter PK. Chemical splanchnicectomy in patients with unresectable pancreatic cancer: a prospective randomized trial. *Ann Surg* 1993;217(5):447–455; discussion 456–457.
174. Worsey J, Ferson PF, Keenan RJ, Julian TB, Landreneau RJ. Thorascopic pancreatic denervation for pain control in unresectable pancreatic cancer. *Br J Surg* 1993;80:1051–1052.
175. Krishna S, Chang VT, Shoukas JA, Donahoo J. Video-assisted thorascopic sympathetectomy-splanchnicectomy for pancreatic cancer pain. *J Pain Symptom Manage* 2001;22:610–616.
176. Jimenez RE, Warshaw AL, Fernandez-del Castillo C. Laparoscopy and peritoneal cytology in the staging of pancreatic cancer. *J Hepatobiliary Pancreat Surg* 2000;7(1):15–20.
177. Merchant NB, Conlon KC, Saigo P, Dougherty E, Brennan MF. Positive peritoneal cytology predicts unresectability of pancreatic adenocarcinoma. *J Am Coll Surg* 1999;188(4):421–426.
178. Fernandez-del Castillo CL, Warshaw AL. Pancreatic cancer: laparoscopic staging and peritoneal cytology. *Surg Oncol Clin N Am* 1998;7(1):135–142.
179. Konishi M, Kinoshita T, Nakagohri T, Inoue K, Oda T, Takahashi S. Prognostic value of cytologic examination of peritoneal washings in pancreatic cancer. *Arch Surg* 2002;137:475–480.
180. Makary MA, Warshaw AL, Centeno BA, Willett CG, Rattner DW, Fernández-del Castillo C. Implications of peritoneal cytology for pancreatic cancer management. *Arch Surg* 1998;133:361–365.
181. Yachida S, Fukushima N, Sakamoto M, Matsuno Y, Kosuge T, Hirohashi S. Implications of peritoneal washing cytology in patients with potentially resectable pancreatic cancer. *Br J Surg* 2002;89(5):573–578.
182. Vogel I, Krüger U, Marxsen J, et al. Disseminated tumor cells in pancreatic cancer patients detected by immunocytology: a new prognostic factor. *Clin Cancer Res* 1999;5:593–599.

CHAPTER 27 ■ PATHOLOGY OF PANCREATIC CANCER

DAVID S. KLIMSTRA AND N. VOLKAN ADSAY

Although the most common neoplasm of the pancreas, infiltrating ductal adenocarcinoma ("pancreatic cancer"), constitutes more than 85% of primary pancreatic neoplasms, a wide array of other distinctive tumor types can arise in this organ (1). Most epithelial neoplasms of the pancreas exhibit differentiation along the lines of one of the three normal epithelial cell types, the ductal, acinar, or islet (endocrine) cells (1–3). The type of cellular differentiation is one of the major bases for pathological classification of pancreatic neoplasms (Table 27.1) because most entities display a specific cell phenotype as judged by their microscopic appearance or their immunohistochemical properties (3). Rarely, however, neoplasms exhibit differentiation along multiple lines, and there is a pancreatic neoplasm (solid pseudopapillary neoplasm [SPN]) for which the specific line of cellular differentiation is unknown (4). In addition to cellular differentiation, the gross configuration of the tumor (solid, cystic, intraductal, etc.) is used in the pathological subclassification. Of particular recent interest is a family of intraductal neoplasms of the pancreas that includes intraductal papillary mucinous neoplasms and other more recently described variants (5); these neoplasms represent a clinically detectable form of preinvasive neoplasia that may be cured by complete surgical resection in the majority of patients, provided they are detected before the development of invasive carcinoma. In addition, studies of intraductal papillary mucinous neoplasms provided evidence of more than one pathway for the development of invasive carcinoma in the pancreas (6,7). Since the early 2000s, more information has been accumulated regarding the clinical and pathological features of these and other less common pancreatic neoplasms, and the volume of data regarding the molecular genetics of pancreatic tumors has also grown exponentially. This chapter provides an overview of the pathological features of pancreatic neoplasms with an emphasis on diagnostic criteria, prognostic information, and natural history.

INFILTRATING DUCTAL ADENOCARCINOMA

The most common neoplasm of the pancreas is infiltrating ductal adenocarcinoma. In the United States, approximately 32,000 new cases occur each year, representing the fourth leading cause of cancer death in both men and women (8). Despite recent advances in the surgical and medical treatment of ductal adenocarcinoma, the 5-year survival rate remains <5%. Even the minority of patients who present at a sufficiently early stage to undergo surgical resection have a 5-year survival of only 12% to 15% (9,10). It is particularly sobering to note that in follow-up of 5-year survivors, a significant proportion still succumb to pancreatic cancer following late recurrences (11). Because of the high rate of unresectability and the increasing use of neoadjuvant therapy prior to surgery for those with resectable disease, the initial pathological specimen from many patients consists of core biopsies and fine-needle aspiration specimens, either from the primary tumor or from a metastasis. The distinction of ductal adenocarcinoma from chronic pancreatitis, a common coincident finding in pancreatic cancer patients, can be particularly challenging on the basis of biopsy specimens, and it is this differential diagnosis that constitutes one of the more challenging aspects of pancreatic pathology.

The gross and microscopic features of infiltrating ductal adenocarcinoma are usually quite characteristic (12–16). Approximately two-thirds of ductal adenocarcinomas arise in the head of the pancreas, with the remainder involving the body, tail, or entire gland (14,16). Multifocal invasive carcinoma is uncommon but is described. Most of the resectable ductal adenocarcinomas are relatively small (<3 cm), especially those involving the head of the gland (17,18); due to their highly aggressive nature, it is uncommon for ductal adenocarcinomas to attain large sizes in the absence of detectable distant metastases. The typical gross appearance is that of a remarkably firm, ill-defined solid mass that can merge imperceptibly with areas of fibrosing chronic pancreatitis (Fig. 27.1). Direct invasion into adjacent structures is typical, including the distal common bile duct, duodenum, ampulla of Vater or mesenteric vessels (for carcinomas of the pancreatic head), and the splenic vessels and spleen (for distally located carcinomas). In addition, extrapancreatic soft tissue invasion is frequent. Cystic change is described in ductal adenocarcinomas and may occur due to several mechanisms (19,20). In some cases, extensive central necrosis results in a degenerative cyst that can simulate the appearance of a pancreatic pseudocyst. In other cases, the carcinoma may obstruct a pancreatic duct resulting in a ductal retention cyst adjacent to the carcinoma. Finally, rare ductal adenocarcinomas contain massively dilated invasive glands that may be perceived grossly as microcystic structures (1).

The microscopic appearance of conventional ductal adenocarcinomas is that of well-formed, round to angulated glands associated with a cellular, desmoplastic stromal response (Fig. 27.2) (13,14,21,22). This "tubular pattern" of infiltrating ductal adenocarcinoma is often associated with the other histologic variants, detailed later in this chapter. The neoplastic glands may be simple or branched and may be lined by a flat layer of epithelium or have architectural complexity such as cribriforming or micropapilla formation. It is also common to find small solid clusters of cells within the stroma, and individual cells may be present and difficult to distinguish from the activated myofibroblasts that constitute the desmoplastic response. The proportion of the tumor composed of well-formed glands, as

TABLE 27.1

CLASSIFICATION OF PANCREATIC NEOPLASMS

A. Exocrine neoplasms
   1. Serous cystic neoplasms
      a) Microcystic serous cystadenoma
      b) Macrocystic serous cystadenoma
      c) Solid serous adenoma
      d) von Hippel-Lindau–associated serous cystic neoplasm
      e) Serous cystadenocarcinoma
   2. Mucinous cystic neoplasms
      a) Mucinous cystic neoplasm with low-grade dysplasia
      b) Mucinous cystic neoplasm with moderate dysplasia
      c) Mucinous cystic neoplasm with high-grade dysplasia (carcinoma in situ)
      d) Mucinous cystic neoplasm with an associated invasive carcinoma
   3. Intraductal neoplasms
      a) Intraductal papillary mucinous neoplasms
         i) Intraductal papillary mucinous neoplasm with low-grade dysplasia
         ii) Intraductal papillary mucinous neoplasm with moderate dysplasia
         iii) Intraductal papillary mucinous neoplasm with high-grade dysplasia (carcinoma in situ)
         iv) Intraductal papillary mucinous neoplasm with an associated invasive carcinoma
      b) Intraductal oncocytic papillary neoplasm
      c) Intraductal tubular neoplasms
         i) Intraductal tubular neoplasm with low-grade dysplasia
         ii) Intraductal tubular neoplasm with high-grade dysplasia (carcinoma in situ)
         iii) Intraductal tubular neoplasm with an associated invasive carcinoma
   4. Pancreatic intraepithelial neoplasia (PanIN)
      a) PanIN-1A and PanIN-1B
      b) PanIN-2
      c) PanIN-3
   5. Invasive ductal adenocarcinoma
      a) Tubular adenocarcinoma
      b) Adenosquamous carcinoma
      c) Colloid (mucinous noncystic) adenocarcinoma
      d) Hepatoid carcinoma
      e) Medullary carcinoma
      f) Signet ring cell carcinoma
      g) Undifferentiated carcinoma
         i) Anaplastic carcinoma
         ii) Sarcomatoid carcinoma
         iii) Carcinosarcoma
      h) Undifferentiated carcinoma with osteoclastlike giant cells
   6. Acinar cell neoplasms
      a) Acinar cell cystadenoma
      b) Acinar cell carcinoma
      c) Acinar cell cystadenocarcinoma
B. Endocrine neoplasms
   1. Microadenoma (<0.5 cm)
   2. Well-differentiated pancreatic endocrine neoplasm
   3. Poorly differentiated endocrine carcinoma
      a) Small cell carcinoma
      b) Large cell endocrine carcinoma
C. Epithelial neoplasms with multiple directions of differentiation
   1. Mixed acinar-endocrine carcinoma
   2. Mixed acinar-ductal carcinoma
   3. Mixed ductal-endocrine carcinoma
   4. Mixed acinar-endocrine-ductal carcinoma
   5. Pancreatoblastoma
D. Epithelial neoplasms of uncertain direction of differentiation
   1. Solid pseudopapillary neoplasm

From ref. 1.

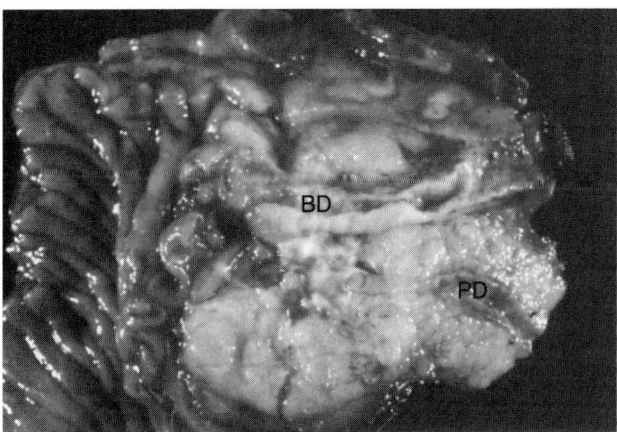

FIGURE 27.1. Gross appearance of ductal adenocarcinoma. The tumor is ill defined, solid, and sclerotic. Compression of the bile duct (BD) and pancreatic duct (PD) is seen. Lobulated pancreatic parenchyma persists but is microscopically infiltrated by carcinoma.

to cell within the individual glands. The finding of a 4:1 nuclear size variation is a helpful diagnostic feature. The highly invasive growth pattern of ductal adenocarcinoma is also evident microscopically. Even in well-differentiated examples, the individual glands extend into the uninvolved pancreatic parenchyma, and microscopic foci of carcinoma may be found well beyond the apparent gross limits of the tumor. Frequent perineural and vascular invasion is found as well as extension of carcinoma into peripancreatic adipose tissue (24). Invasion adjacent to muscular arteries is another helpful diagnostic feature because normal ducts are usually separated from the vasculature by lobules of acini. An additional characteristic feature of infiltrating ductal adenocarcinoma is the haphazard arrangement of the neoplastic glands, which contrasts with the lobular organization of ductules in atrophic chronic pancreatitis.

As the infiltrating glands encounter other structures such as the bile duct, the small bowel mucosa, or even the native uninvolved pancreatic ducts, they commonly extend along the preexisting basement membranes, with the resulting growth patterns simulating a preinvasive neoplasm of the respective structures (1).

In addition to the conventional tubular pattern, ductal adenocarcinomas may focally or diffusely exhibit a variety of other histologic patterns such as adenosquamous, anaplastic, colloid, hepatoid, medullary, signet ring cell, and undifferentiated carcinomas. Most histologic variants of ductal adenocarcinoma carry the same prognosis as conventional tubular type adenocarcinoma. Some cases contain exceptionally well-differentiated glands with abundant microvesicular (foamy) cytoplasm and relatively uniform nuclei; this has been described as the foam cell pattern of ductal adenocarcinoma (Fig. 27.3)

contrasted to solid nests and individual cells, is an important criterion for grading ductal adenocarcinomas (14,22,23), although it is common for both well-differentiated and poorly differentiated elements to coexist within an individual tumor. The neoplastic cells often contain relatively abundant cytoplasm rich in mucin. Although the nuclei of ductal adenocarcinomas may be superficially uniform, they are enlarged and usually vary in size, shape, and intracellular location from cell

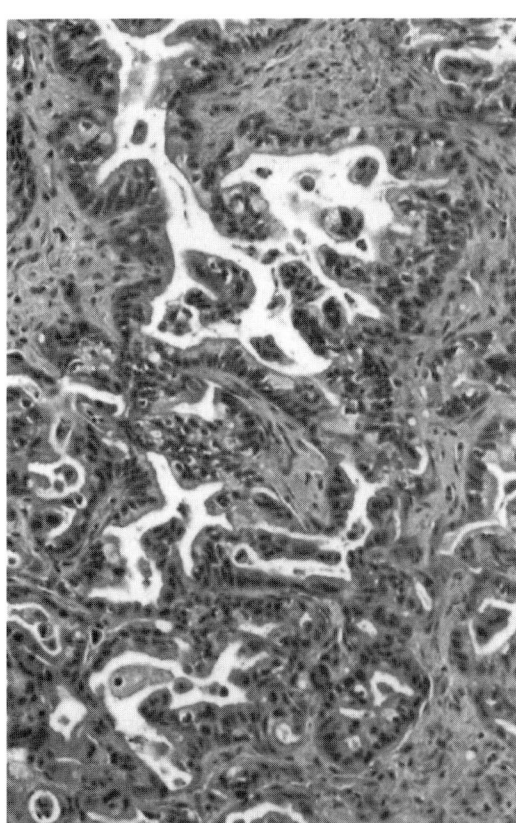

FIGURE 27.2. Moderately differentiated ductal adenocarcinoma. Neoplastic glands are complex, with irregular branches and micropapillae. Marked nuclear atypia is present. A desmoplastic stromal response is seen.

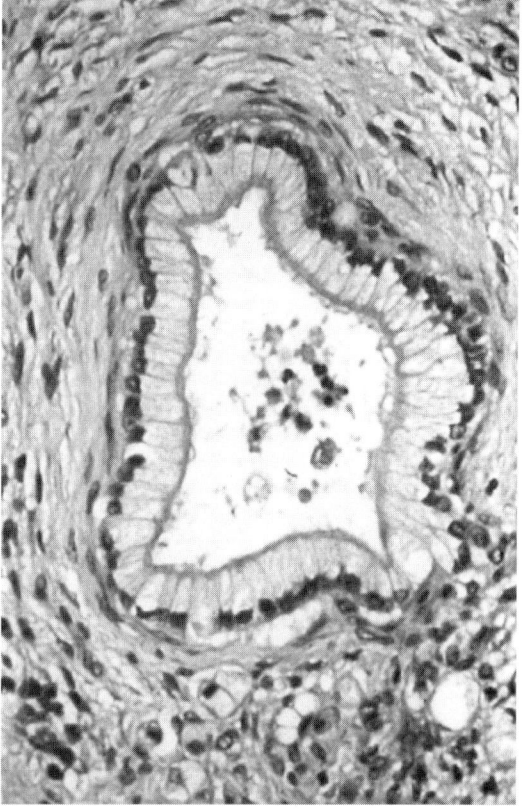

FIGURE 27.3. Well-differentiated ductal adenocarcinoma with "foam cell" pattern. The neoplastic glands are so well formed that they resemble metaplastic ducts. Abundant vesicular cytoplasm is seen, and the nuclei are uniformly basal with minimal atypia.

(25). Approximately 4% of ductal adenocarcinomas have a substantial amount of the foam cell pattern. If due attention is not paid to subtle but distinctive morphologic features, foam cell carcinoma can be nearly indistinguishable from low-grade pancreatic intraepithelial neoplasia (PanIN), particularly in limited specimens such as cytologic preparations, frozen sections, or biopsy samples. The most characteristic feature is the abundant, pale, microvesicular cytoplasm with a peculiar condensation at the apical edge, which forms a brush borderlike zone that is not seen in benign mucinous glands (Fig. 27.3). Occasionally, invasive tubular adenocarcinomas have marked ectasia of the infiltrating neoplastic glands; some authors refer to this as "large duct-type" invasive carcinoma (26). This phenomenon is particularly pronounced in regions of the tumor infiltrating the overlying duodenal muscularis propria. The cytologic findings of the lining epithelium may be deceptively bland. Large duct-type adenocarcinomas should not be mislabeled as a mucinous cystadenocarcinoma, a neoplasm with a much better prognosis. Some ductal adenocarcinomas have a pattern similar to that of diffuse gastric carcinoma (27,28). Instead of the usual tubule formation, the cells form cords and are arranged individually, often with signet ring cells.

Colloid (mucinous noncystic) carcinomas occur rarely in the pancreas (29); more than half of such cases arise in association with intraductal papillary mucinous neoplasms (IPMNs) (29,30). Colloid carcinomas consist of large extracellular lakes of mucin in which relatively minimal neoplastic epithelium is suspended (Fig. 27.4). These tumors are histologically similar to colloid carcinomas arising in the breast, colon, or other sites. Elements of conventional tubular-type ductal adenocarcinoma may occur together with the colloid carcinoma pattern, but for a carcinoma to qualify as colloid overall, at least 80% of the neoplasm must consist of extracellular mucin with suspended epithelium (29). When defined strictly, colloid carcinomas represent one of the more indolent types of invasive pancreatic adenocarcinoma (31−33). However, many cases occurring in association with IPMNs may have an invasive component limited to a few microscopic foci, raising the possibility that the favorable prognosis could be attributable to the early stage of many of the cases. A study of 17 colloid carcinomas limited to those cases having an invasive component >1 cm in size suggested otherwise, however, and the 5-year survival was 55% despite an average tumor size of 5.3 cm and regional lymph node metastases in eight cases (29). Thus, the favorable biology of colloid carcinoma seems to be an inherent property of

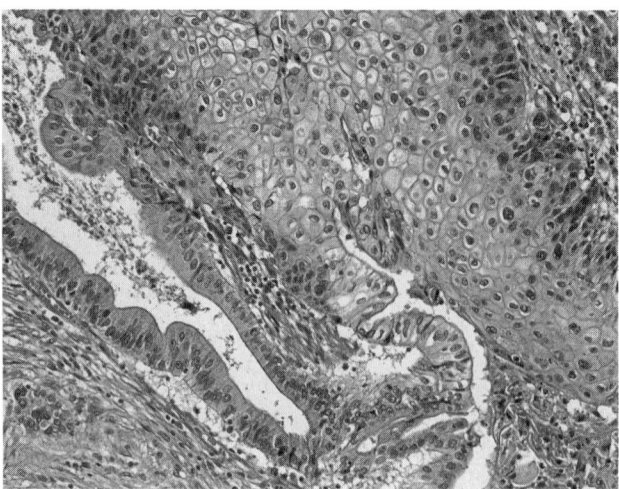

FIGURE 27.5. Adenosquamous carcinoma. Sheets of squamous cells (*right*) are juxtaposed to well-formed glands (*left*) (See also color Figure 27.5).

this histologic variant. In addition to the morphologic differences from conventional ductal adenocarcinoma, colloid carcinoma commonly has an intestinal phenotype, with immunohistochemical expression of MUC-2 and CDX2 and negative labeling for MUC-1, in contrast to tubular-type adenocarcinomas having the opposite labeling pattern for these markers (23). The genetic alterations of colloid carcinomas are similar to those of conventional ductal adenocarcinomas, but occur at a lower rate. Only one-third of colloid carcinomas harbor mutations in codon 12 of the *KRAS* oncogene, and one-fourth have *TP53* (*p53*) gene mutations (29). The expression of Smad4 (Dpc4) protein is normal in almost all cases (34).

Adenosquamous carcinomas constitute 3% to 4% of pancreatic carcinomas (35−37). In most of these lesions, a component of the tumor resembles conventional tubular adenocarcinoma. The squamous elements should arbitrarily constitute at least 30% of the neoplasm for it to qualify as an adenosquamous carcinoma (Fig. 27.5) (1). The clinical outcome of these tumors is as poor as that of ordinary (tubular) adenocarcinomas, if not worse.

Other tumors generally classified with ductal adenocarcinoma are the undifferentiated carcinomas. Several different types have been described in the pancreas. All may have associated components of tubular-type adenocarcinoma, or they may occur in pure form. Anaplastic giant cell carcinoma is a type of undifferentiated carcinoma in which the tumor cells are enormous (Fig. 27.6), with highly pleomorphic nuclei (38,39). The histologic pattern of anaplastic giant cell carcinoma of the pancreas resembles that of giant cell carcinomas of other organs such as the lung, adrenal, and liver (40). The cells are discohesive and often suspended in a sea of neutrophils, which may be present within the cytoplasm of some of the tumor cells (emperipolesis). Sarcomatoid carcinomas and carcinosarcomas are neoplasms having a spindle cell component, resembling a true sarcoma (41). In sarcomatoid carcinomas, the entire tumor is composed of spindle cells, which may retain epithelial differentiation at the immunohistochemical level. Carcinosarcomas are biphasic tumors that have an epithelial component and a separate sarcomatoid component, sometimes with heterologous stromal differentiation in the form of cartilage, bone, or striated muscle. Both components are believed to originate from epithelial precursors, however (42). All of these types of undifferentiated carcinoma are extremely rare in the pancreas, constituting <1% of its carcinomas, and prognostically are even more aggressive than conventional ductal adenocarcinomas.

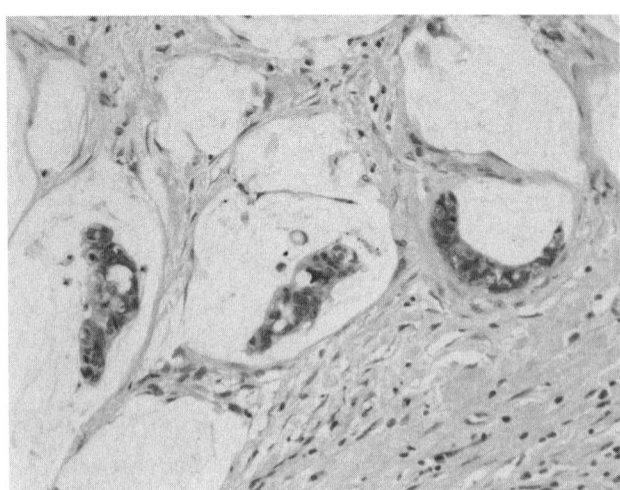

FIGURE 27.4. Colloid carcinoma. Strips of neoplastic glandular epithelium float in abundant extracellular pools of mucin (See also color Figure 27.4).

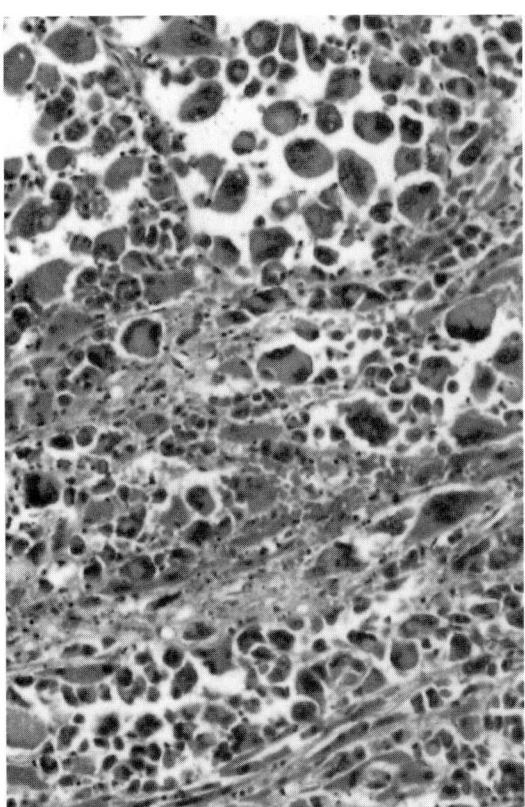

FIGURE 27.6. Anaplastic giant cell carcinoma. The tumor cells are huge and largely discohesive. No gland formation is evident. A reactive inflammatory cell infiltrate accompanies the neoplastic cells.

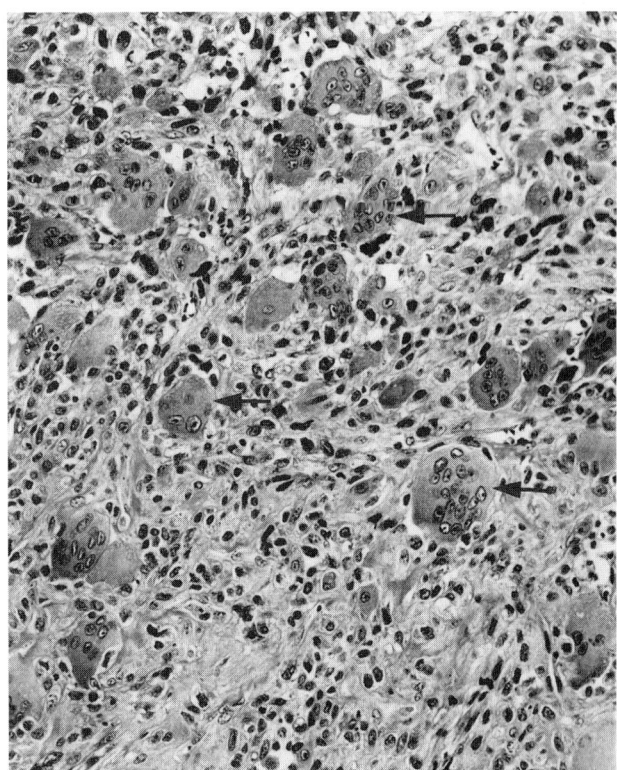

FIGURE 27.7. Undifferentiated carcinoma with osteoclastlike giant cells. The neoplastic component consists of undifferentiated plump to spindled mononuclear cells. Numerous nonneoplastic multinucleated osteoclastic giant cells are present (*arrows*).

A separate and distinctive neoplasm is the undifferentiated carcinoma with osteoclastlike giant cells. This tumor consists of a neoplastic spindle to epithelioid cell component with admixed nonneoplastic osteoclastlike giant cells (Fig. 27.7) (43–48). Undifferentiated carcinomas with osteoclastlike giant cells are remarkably similar to osteoclast-containing tumors of many diverse organs, which suggests that some property of the neoplastic component may be responsible for the accumulation of intratumoral multinucleated giant histiocytes (44), which are formed from the fusion of circulating macrophages. Although the neoplastic components generally have a mesenchymal appearance and often fail to express evidence of epithelial differentiation by immunohistochemistry, the histogenesis of most cases is still believed to be epithelial, particularly in those cases associated with an adenocarcinomatous component. The finding of *KRAS* mutations in the tumor cells supports this hypothesis (49,50). In contrast to other types of undifferentiated carcinoma, undifferentiated carcinoma with osteoclastlike giant cells may have a more favorable prognosis, although recent studies suggested that most are quite aggressive (45).

Another neoplasm, classified as a variant of ductal adenocarcinoma, is medullary carcinoma of the pancreas (51,52). The term *medullary carcinoma* is also applied to mammary and colorectal carcinomas that, despite a poorly differentiated histologic appearance, have a favorable clinical course. In the large bowel, medullary carcinomas are more frequent in patients with hereditary nonpolyposis colorectal cancer and commonly exhibit mutations in DNA-mismatch repair genes (53,54). Pancreatic medullary carcinomas are histologically similar to the mammary or colorectal counterparts (51,52). The tumors are poorly differentiated, lack gland formation, and have sheets of large cells with ill-defined borders suspended in a lymphocyte-rich stroma (Fig. 27.8). Patients more commonly

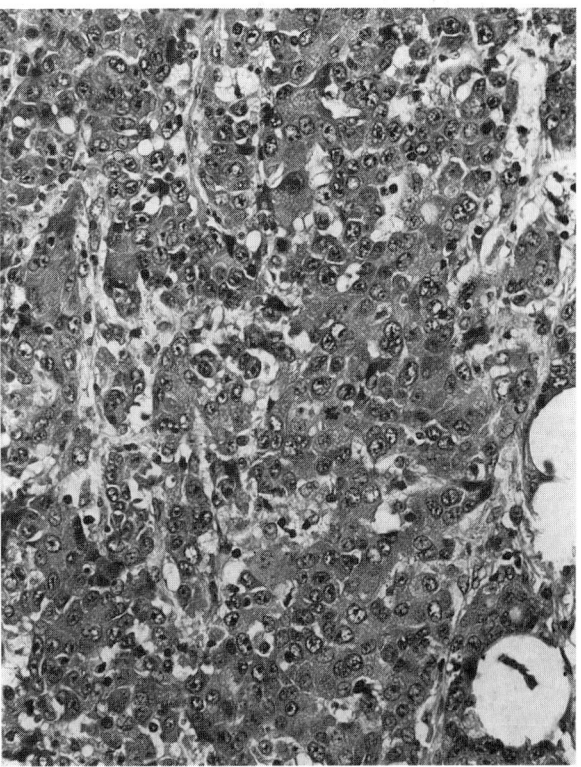

FIGURE 27.8. Medullary carcinoma. The tumor is poorly differentiated, with syncytially arranged cells lacking gland formation. A lymphocytic inflammatory infiltrate is present.

have first-degree relatives with other extrapancreatic carcinomas than do patients with conventional pancreatic adenocarcinomas, but medullary carcinomas are not prone to occur more commonly in the setting of familial pancreas cancer. Pancreatic medullary carcinomas also more commonly have inactivation of DNA-mismatch repair genes than conventional ductal adenocarcinomas, and the *KRAS* oncogene is usually wild type. The first cases reported of pancreatic medullary carcinoma included some patients with a favorable outcome (51), but experience with additional cases has suggested that the prognosis is not as favorable as for medullary carcinomas of the breast or colorectum (52).

Pancreatic Intraepithelial Neoplasia

It is common to find a variety of ductal proliferative lesions associated with infiltrating ductal adenocarcinomas (Fig. 27.9) (55). The older terminology for these lesions included descriptive terms such as mucinous metaplasia (or mucous cell hypertrophy), papillary hyperplasia, atypical hyperplasia, and carcinoma in situ (21,56). Other investigators used grades of dysplasia. Recently, based on the recognition that these lesions formed a morphologic and genetic continuum of precursor lesions to infiltrating ductal adenocarcinoma (7,55,57–62), the unifying terminology of *pancreatic intraepithelial neoplasia* (PanIN) was adopted. Grades of PanIN include PanIN-1A, PanIN-1B, PanIN-2, and PanIN-3, based on the degree of cytoarchitectural atypia (14). PanIN1 is a common incidental finding that may occur in pancreata with or without a concomitant infiltrating ductal adenocarcinoma, whereas PanIN3 is

much more closely associated with invasive carcinoma, rarely being detected in its absence. The progression of PanIN to invasive carcinoma is difficult to observe because PanINs are radiographically occult and are usually only identified in pancreatectomy specimens. However, a few rare cases of progression have been documented (57,58) that further support the precursor status of PanINs.

Most of the genetic abnormalities of infiltrating carcinoma are found at different stages in the PanIN sequence, including telomere shortening, and mutations in the *KRAS, SMAD4, CDKN2A (p16)*, and *p53* genes (33,63–66). What is most intriguing is that PanIN-1, the lesion historically regarded as simple mucinous metaplasia (tall columnar mucin-containing cells with basally located, uniform nuclei), has been found by several investigators to have *KRAS* mutations and telomere shortening (59,62,66), suggesting that it represents the earliest intraductal neoplastic alteration. This is an exciting observation, but one of uncertain practical value, for PanIN-1 is a common morphologic alteration, present in up to 45% of pancreata of older adults at autopsy (67). Nonetheless, the examination of early neoplastic lesions in the pancreas is one of the most interesting and promising avenues of study because early detection of pancreatic adenocarcinoma appears to represent the best chance for improvement in the nearly uniform lethality of this disease.

Intraductal Papillary Mucinous Neoplasms

Intraductal papillary mucinous neoplasms (IPMNs) are papillary tumors arising within the pancreatic ducts and often producing copious luminal mucin (14,31,68–70). These tumors

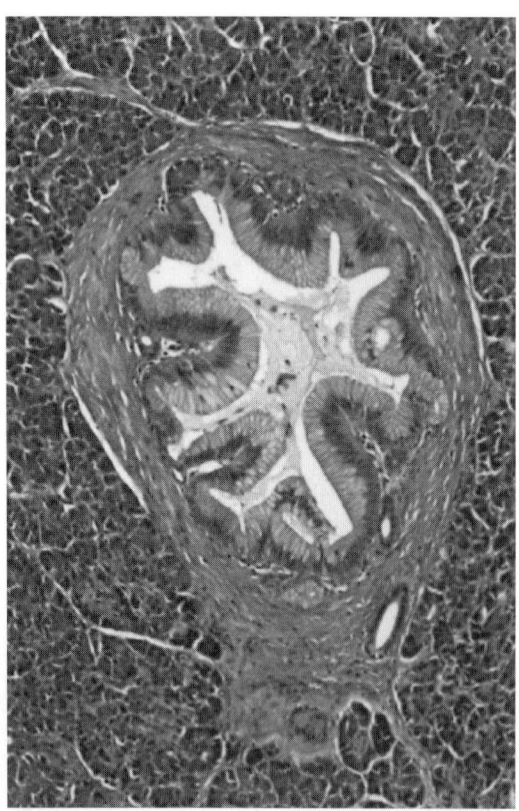
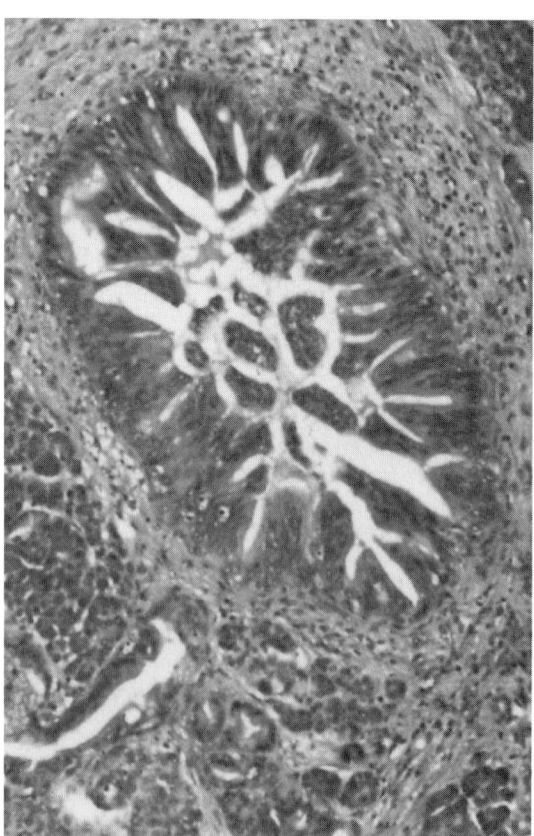

FIGURE 27.9. Pancreatic intraepithelial neoplasia (PanIN). These lesions commonly accompany infiltrating ductal adenocarcinomas. Lower-grade lesions (PanIN-1) have columnar mucin-containing cells with minimal nuclear atypia and basal pseudostratification (**A**). Complete loss of polarity, apical budding of epithelial tufts, and cytologic atypia are found in high-grade lesions (PanIN-3) (**B**).

have been recognized as a distinct subset of pancreatic neoplasms for more than 20 years, but their prevalence appears to be increasing, perhaps due to the greater use of sensitive abdominal imaging. Alternative terms for IPMNs used predominantly in earlier reports include *mucinous duct ectasia* (71–73), *papillary carcinoma, mucin-producing tumor,* or *villous adenoma of the pancreatic ducts* (74,75).

IPMNs occur in a patient population similar to that affected by ductal adenocarcinomas: adult patients, usually in the sixth to eighth decades of life (32,70,71). Men are affected more than women. The presenting symptoms are often vague and nonspecific, including abdominal pain, diarrhea, and other signs of exocrine insufficiency. Patients may have symptoms of chronic pancreatitis for many years before a diagnosis of IPMN is made. Biliary obstruction with jaundice is usually a late occurrence, often reflecting the development of invasive carcinoma.

The majority of IPMNs (75%) involve predominantly the head of the pancreas; others are centered in the tail, and 5% to 10% diffusely involve the entire gland. Preoperative imaging may be very helpful in establishing a diagnosis of IPMN (69,70,76,77). Probably because of the excessive mucin production by the intraductal neoplasm, the pancreatic ducts involved by IPMNs commonly have significant dilatation, a finding that is usually apparent on computed tomography (CT) scanning, endoscopic retrograde pancreatography (ERCP), or

magnetic resonance cholangiopancreatography (MRCP) (Fig. 27.10) (78,79). On cross-sectional imaging, the dilated ducts of IPMNs often appear as multiple separate cysts within the pancreas. This results from the fact that dilatated ducts become tortuous, so as to be cut multiple times in each plane of the CT scan. Mucinous cystic neoplasms (MCNs) instead appear as single multilocular cysts. IPMNs are separated into main duct and branch duct types, depending on whether the neoplasm is present within the major ducts or is limited to the peripheral secondary (branch) ducts (80,81). Branch duct–type IPMNs are particularly prone to resemble other cystic lesions of the pancreas because the connection to the ductal system can be difficult to recognize.

At endoscopy, the spillage of mucin from an engorged ampulla of Vater is a classic sign of IMPNs (73). Biopsy specimens taken from within the ampulla may disclose neoplastic papillary epithelium, often morphologically resembling a villous adenoma of the tubular gastrointestinal tract. Percutaneous biopsies or fine-needle aspiration procedures may also yield neoplastic epithelium and evidence of the luminal mucin accumulation (82,83). Correlating the results of biopsy procedures with the endoscopic and radiographic appearance of the lesion is important. Because the intraductal papillary proliferation may exhibit severe cytoarchitectural atypia in the absence of invasive carcinoma, the cytologic features of cells obtained from small biopsy or aspiration specimens may wrongly suggest the presence of invasive ductal adenocarcinoma if the intraductal location of the neoplastic proliferation is not apparent.

Pathologically, IPMNs vary in their gross and microscopic appearances (31,32,70,84). Depending on the extent of the tumor, diffuse ductal dilatation or localized cystic transformation of smaller ducts may be present. Some examples exhibit minimal gross evidence of papilla formation, appearing only as dilated, mucin-filled ducts (Fig. 27.11). Other cases have abundant intraductal papillae, with a velvety lining of tan papillations covering the entire luminal surface. The extent of ductal dilatation may be impressive, with some IPMNs having ducts larger than 5 cm in diameter.

Microscopically, variations are seen from region to region within a single IPMN. Some areas can have a flattened mucinous epithelium lacking significant proliferative changes. Elsewhere, well-developed uniform papillae lined by cytologically bland mucinous epithelial cells may be present. Striking cytoarchitectural atypia may also be noted, with markedly complex, arborizing papillae lined by highly dysplastic epithelium

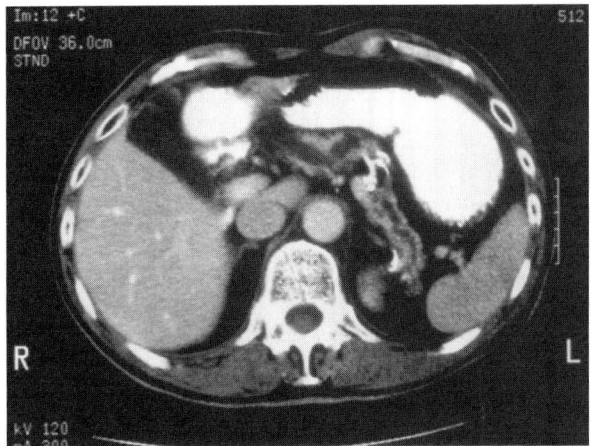

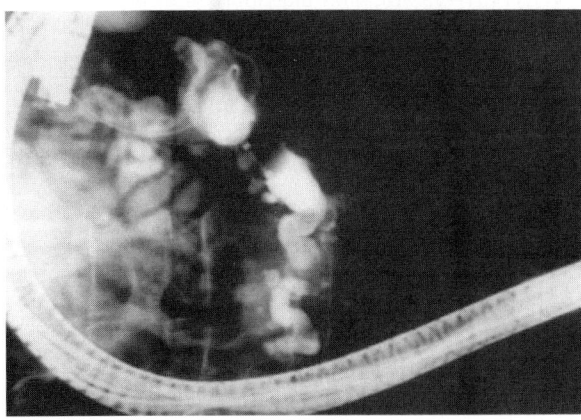

FIGURE 27.10. Radiographic appearance of intraductal papillary mucinous neoplasm. On computed tomography scan (**A**), cystic dilatation of the main pancreatic duct is noted, being most pronounced in the head but extending the length of the gland. Endoscopic retrograde pancreatography (**B**) shows the tortuous dilatated duct, with saccular dilatation of secondary ducts.

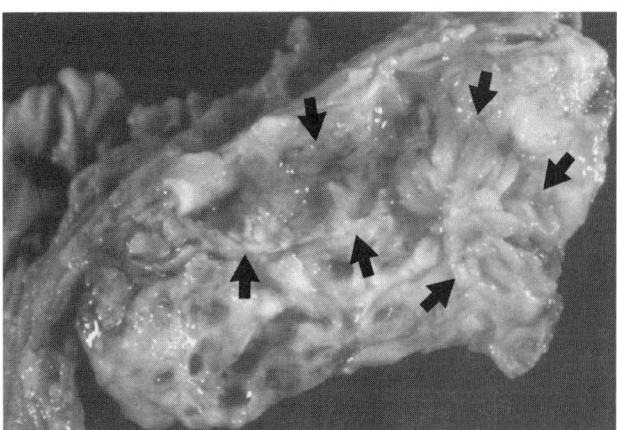

FIGURE 27.11. Gross appearance of intraductal papillary mucinous neoplasm. The main duct (*arrows*) is dilated and covered with papillary tumor. Secondary ducts are also dilated and contain glistening mucin.

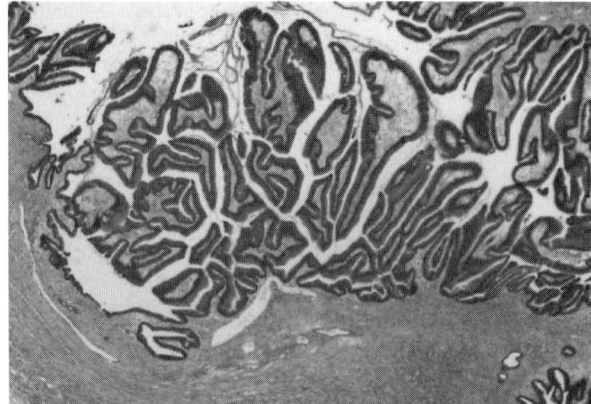

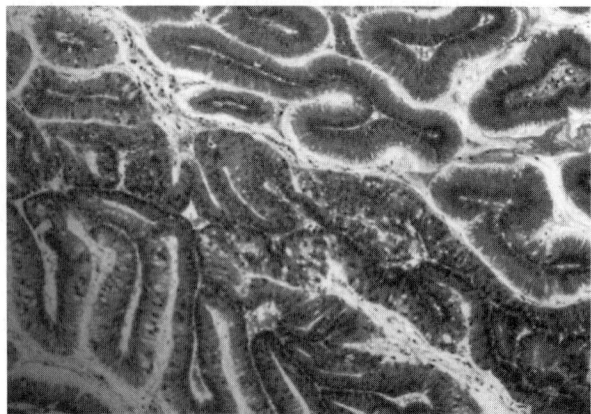

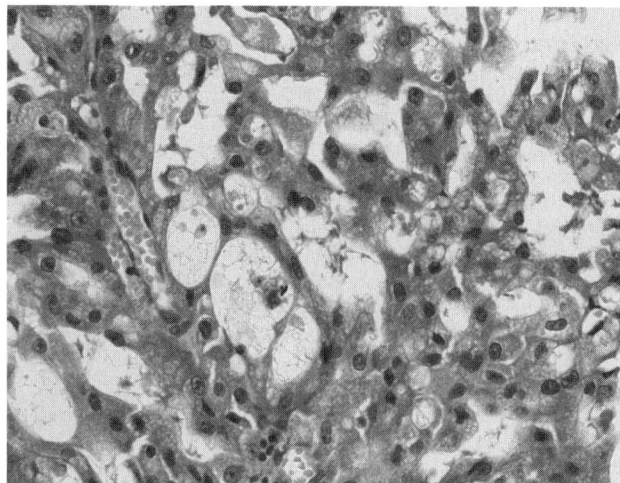

FIGURE 27.13. Intraductal oncocytic papillary neoplasm. Complex papillae are lined by large, eosinophilic cells. Intraepithelial lumina are present (See also color Figure 27.13).

FIGURE 27.12. Microscopically, intraductal papillary mucinous neoplasms have numerous long papillae projecting into the lumen of the ducts (**A**). At higher power (**B**), some regions are seen to have minimal cytoarchitectural atypia (*top*), with basal, uniform nuclei. Elsewhere (*bottom*), the papillae are complex, and loss of polarity accompanied by nuclear atypia is seen.

(Fig. 27.12). Because these features may coexist in a single case, extensive microscopic examination is suggested to detect the most severely atypical region. Different morphologic patterns of papillae occur in IPMNs (85,86). Most cases are composed of either tall columnar cells with abundant apical mucin and basally oriented nuclei, resembling gastric foveolar cells (gastric type), or villiform papillae lined by cells with pseudostratified, elongate nuclei, resembling villous adenomas of the bowel (intestinal type). Less commonly, the papillary architecture is markedly complex, with micropapillae and cribriformed structures lined by cuboidal cells with a single layer of round nuclei. These IPMNs resemble the papillary carcinomas more commonly found in the bile ducts and are referred to as pancreatobiliary-type IPMNs. In addition to having different histologic patterns, these types of IPMNs differ in immunophenotypes and are associated with different types of invasive carcinoma. Also, some intraductal papillary neoplasms are composed predominantly of oncocytic cells with abundant granular eosinophilic cytoplasm (Fig. 27.13) (87). Although these were originally reported as a separate entity (*intraductal oncocytic papillary neoplasm*), some authorities classify them as the oncocytic type of IPMN (85). Finally, a recently recognized intraductal neoplasm has minimal papilla formation and is composed of back-to-back tubules with minimal intracellular mucin; such cases are termed *intraductal tubular carcinomas* and appear to be closely related to IPMNs (88).

Grading of IPMNs is based on the highest grade of atypia identified. According to the World Health Organization (WHO), cases with minimal cytoarchitectural atypia are designated "intraductal papillary mucinous *adenoma*"; those with moderate atypia are designated "intraductal papillary mucinous *tumor, borderline*"; and those with severe cytoarchitectural atypia are designated "intraductal papillary mucinous *carcinoma*" (70). An alternative strategy calls for designating all IPMNs as "intraductal papillary mucinous neoplasm" with the degree of dysplasia graded as low grade (i.e., IPM adenoma), moderate (IPM tumor, borderline), or high grade (IPM carcinoma in situ) (1).

Approximately one-third of reported IMPNs have had an associated invasive carcinoma (Fig. 27.14) (31–33,72,80,86), although a greater proportion of noninvasive IPMNs are now being detected as more early stage neoplasms are incidentally found by imaging. Invasion may occur as isolated microscopic foci limited to the periductal stroma, or the invasive carcinoma may constitute a substantial, or even predominant, component of the tumor (89). Two histologically distinct types of invasive carcinoma occur in association with IPMNs. Approximately half of the cases resemble ordinary tubular ductal adenocarcinomas (31–33,86), with individual well-formed glands associated with a desmoplastic stromal response. This pattern is more commonly associated with the gastric- or especially the pancreatobiliary-type IPMNs (86). Interestingly, the other half are colloid (mucinous noncystic) carcinomas (14,29,86). This pattern is most commonly associated with intestinal-type IPMNs (29,31,86). When invasive carcinoma is present, both the intraductal and invasive components should be reported separately, with a description of the type and extent (stage) of the invasive component.

The biological behavior of an IPMN is generally that of an indolent neoplasm. Taken as a group, the majority of patients with IPMNs are cured by complete surgical excision (31,32). Intuitively, one would expect that IPMNs lacking an invasive component should be biologically benign, essentially representing in situ carcinomas. This generally has been true, although rare cases of patients developing metastases from IPMNs in the absence of detectable invasive carcinoma have been recorded (86). In these cases an invasive carcinoma likely did exist but was either undetected due to inadequate pathological sampling or remained unresected after partial pancreatectomy. With the exception of these rare cases, no difference in behavior is seen between completely resected IPMNs with

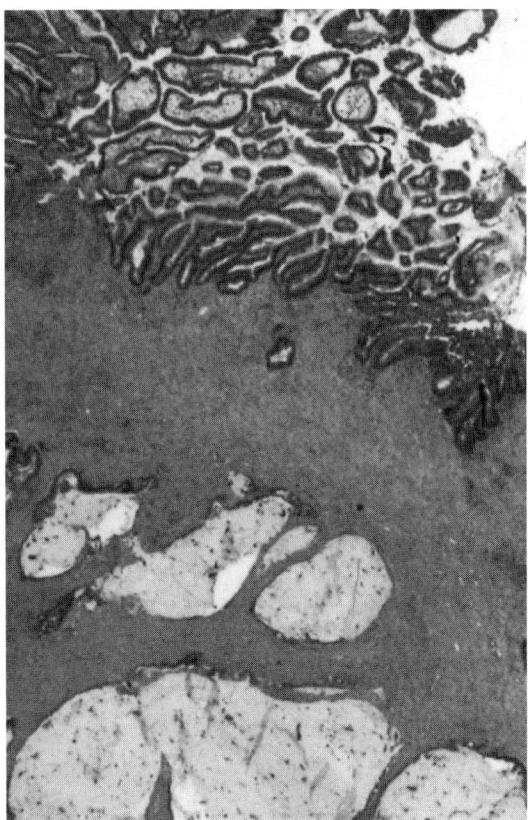

FIGURE 27.14. Invasive colloid carcinoma arising in association with an intraductal papillary mucinous neoplasm. The intraductal component (*top*) retains a papillary architecture and respects the wall of the duct. The infiltrating component (*bottom*) dissects into the stroma.

low-, moderate-, or high-grade dysplasia. A minority of patients experience intraductal recurrence (81), a phenomenon that is not rigidly linked to the histologic status of the pancreatic resection margin.

Once invasive carcinoma is present, the prognosis depends on the type and extent of the invasive component (81,86). Patients who have a significant amount of tubular-type adenocarcinoma have a poor prognosis, probably approaching that of ductal adenocarcinomas not arising in association with IPMNs. Not enough of these cases are on record, however, to define stage-related survival rates. In one study, the mean survival of patients with invasive tubular-type adenocarcinomas arising in IPMNs was 56 months after resection, substantially better than the survival for conventional ductal adenocarcinoma (86). In contrast to the tubular-type carcinomas, the colloid carcinomas arising in IPMNs have a much more favorable prognosis (5-year survival of 55% after resection) (29,31–33). This difference in survival, along with the differences in the types of IPMNs that precede the development of tubular and colloid carcinomas, suggests that two different pathways of carcinogenesis exist: one that follows the typical pathway for pancreatic ductal adenocarcinoma and the other that follows an intestinal pathway (6,7). Immunohistochemical studies of IPMNs add support to this hypothesis (6,90). Studies of MUC protein expression in pancreatic neoplasms have revealed that MUC1, which is commonly detected in conventional ductal adenocarcinomas and in high-grade PanINs, is also found in pancreatobiliary-type IPMNs and their associated tubular-type adenocarcinomas. In contrast, intestinal-type IPMNs and colloid carcinomas lack MUC1 expression but instead have MUC2, an intestinal-type mucin. The fre-

quent expression in intestinal-type IPMNs and colloid carcinomas of CDX2, a major determinant of intestinal differentiation, strengthens the intestinal analogy. CDX2 is rarely expressed in pancreatobiliary-type IPMNs, tubular-type invasive carcinomas, or PanINs.

Because IMPNs represent a clinically detectable form of intraepithelial (i.e., noninvasive) pancreatic neoplasm, they constitute a model for the optimal stage of detection of pancreatic neoplasia. Because the small duct lesions (PanINs) more commonly associated with conventional pancreatic ductal adenocarcinoma are clinically and radiographically occult, the study of IPMNs may provide valuable clues to the identification of PanINs, to the extent that the clinical, pathological, and molecular features of IPMNs resemble those of PanINs (91). Molecular abnormalities of both groups of precursor lesions are being actively studied. Mutations in the KRAS oncogene are present in the majority of IPMNs, although a somewhat smaller percentage of IPMNs have KRAS mutations as compared to PanINs and infiltrating ductal adenocarcinomas (64). Abnormalities in p53 are present in IPMNs with high-grade dysplasia (33,92,93). One molecular difference between invasive ductal adenocarcinomas and PanINs versus IPMNs lies in the status of the *SMAD4* tumor-suppressor gene. Abnormalities in *SMAD4* are present in approximately 55% of invasive carcinomas and 40% to 50% of high-grade PanINs (94), but such abnormalities are rarely detectable in IPMNs, even those associated with invasive carcinoma (34). Inactivation of *p16* occurs more commonly in IPMNs with high-grade dysplasia (95,96). The Peutz-Jeghers gene (SKT11/LKB1) is inactivated in 25% of IPMNs (97).

Mucinous Cystic Neoplasms

MCNs have many histologic similarities to IPMNs but do not arise within the native ducts (98–102). Instead, MCNs consist of a single multilocular cyst, generally located in the tail of the pancreas. MCNs generally affect young to middle-age women (101). In fact, if the tumors are defined strictly, more than 95% of patients are female. MCNs often present with nonspecific symptoms, and because they rarely arise in the head of the gland, jaundice is uncommon. MCNs are usually large (mean size of 10 cm) and appear as cysts with relatively few, large locules on ultrasonography or cross-sectional imaging (Fig. 27.15). The presence of solid areas should raise concerns about invasive carcinoma. Their appearance is generally

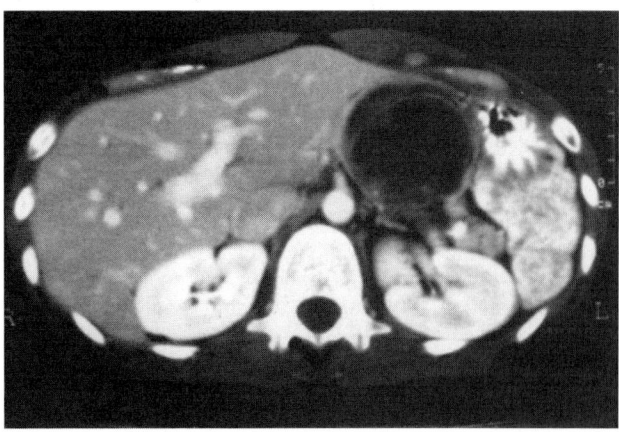

FIGURE 27.15. On computed tomography scan, a mucinous cystic neoplasm is a well-circumscribed cyst in the tail of the gland. Curved septa separate large locules.

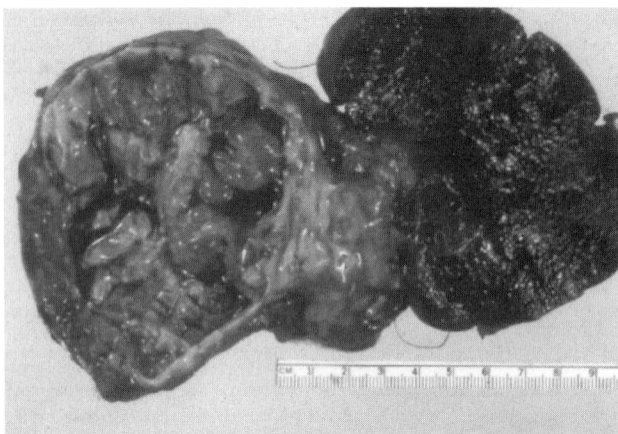

FIGURE 27.16. Grossly, this mucinous cystic neoplasm consists of a large dominant locule with smaller locules projecting into the wall. A thick fibrous capsule surrounds the lesion. No obvious solid areas are noted.

different from that of the other common cystic neoplasm of the pancreas, serous cystadenoma, which is composed of innumerable small (microscopic to 1-cm) cysts. Because serous cystic tumors are essentially always benign, much emphasis has been placed on the preoperative distinction of MCNs and other mucinous neoplasms (e.g., IPMNs) from serous cystic tumors. Biochemical analysis of fluid obtained from the cysts has been used to help identify mucinous tumors (103,104), but the technique may not be sensitive enough to conclude preoperatively that a given cystic neoplasm is definitely benign.

Pathologically, MCNs are generally surrounded by a thick fibrous capsule (Fig. 27.16). Each locule is lined by tall columnar, mucin-producing epithelium arranged in a simple or pseudostratified layer or in papillary projections (Fig. 27.17). The cytoarchitectural atypia in MCNs varies from one region of the tumor to another (98,105). For this reason, it is critical for the pathologist to sample the gross specimen thoroughly (if not entirely) to ensure that the most severe dysplasia is identified. MCNs are subclassified based on the most severely atypical region. In the WHO classification, MCNs with little or no atypia are regarded as "mucinous cyst*adenoma*"; those with moderate atypia as "mucinous cystic *neoplasm, borderline*"; and those with severe atypia as "mucinous cyst*adenocarcinoma*" (106). Alternatively, all MCNs can be designated as "mucinous cystic neoplasm" with the degree of dysplasia graded as low, moderate, or high grade (1). Not only do MCNs have the potential for high-grade dysplasia, but also invasive carcinoma may develop within them, and most data suggest that it is the presence and extent of any invasive carcinoma that determines the prognosis (102,105). Any invasive component should be reported separately because a noninvasive mucinous cystadenocarcinoma with only high-grade dysplasia in the cyst lining is unlikely to behave aggressively, in contrast to a mucinous cystadenocarcinoma that has extensive invasive carcinoma. Many types of carcinoma may arise in MCNs, including conventional tubular-type ductal adenocarcinoma, colloid carcinoma, sarcomatoid carcinoma, and undifferentiated carcinoma with osteoclastlike giant cells (47,101,107,108).

Another fascinating aspect of MCNs is their stromal component. The stroma immediately underlying the neoplastic mucinous epithelium is hypercellular and closely resembles the stroma of the ovary (Fig. 27.17) (98,102). This ovarianlike stroma is an essential feature for the diagnosis of MCNs and is useful for separating MCNs from other types of mucinous neoplasms such as IPMNs. In addition to the histologic sim-

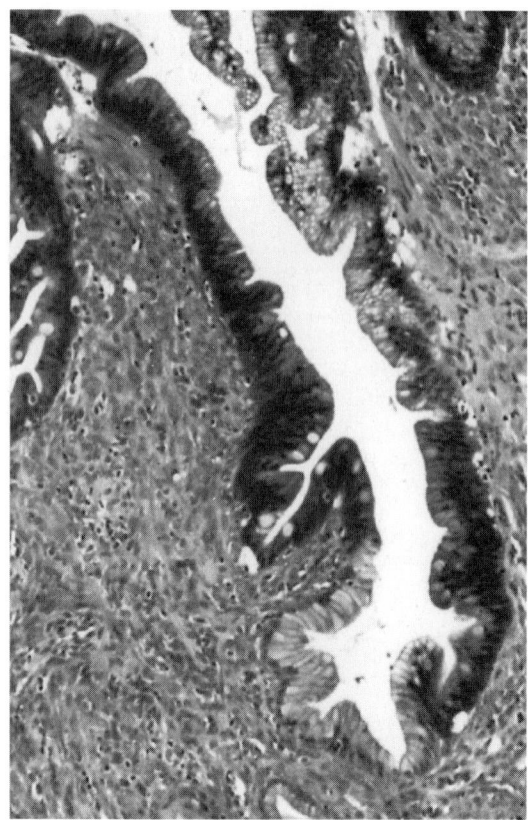

FIGURE 27.17. Microscopic appearance of mucinous cystic neoplasm. The degree of cytoarchitectural atypia varies from region to region. The subepithelial stroma is hypercellular, resembling the stroma of the ovary.

ilarity, the stroma of MCNs resembles the ovarian stroma in the expression of estrogen and progesterone receptors, as well as in the scattered presence of larger epithelioid cells that resemble steroid-rich decidualized ovarian stromal cells and that express inhibin, a marker of steroid synthesis (102,109). For these reasons, some have speculated that MCNs of the pancreas (as well as the analogous tumor of the liver, biliary cystadenoma) are derived from misplaced embryonic ovarian tissue.

The prognosis of MCNs after surgical resection is excellent, with only 10% of patients suffering recurrence or metastases (98,100,105,110). The debate about MCNs revolves around the malignant potential of those cases lacking an identifiable component of invasive carcinoma. In early work characterizing the pathological features of MCNs and separating them from other cystic tumors of the pancreas, investigators described rare cases in which recurrence or metastases developed from tumors apparently lacking invasive carcinoma (98). Based on this observation, the argument had been made that *all* MCNs should be regarded as potentially malignant, even those lacking high-grade dysplasia in the lining epithelium. Recent studies have challenged this view, however. Two large studies found that only the patients with invasive carcinoma had recurrence after complete surgical excision (102,105). These authors argued that aggressive behavior resulting from an apparently benign tumor was a reflection of inadequate sampling by the pathologist (with failure to detect small foci of invasive carcinoma) or inadequate surgery. Thus, the recommendation was made that all MCNs should be completely resected and submitted in their entirety for histologic examination, and that those lacking invasive carcinoma could be considered biologically benign (105). This concept is certainly in keeping with the model of neoplastic progression from benign through increasing degrees of dysplasia to invasive carcinoma suggested morphologically by MCNs. The daunting proposition of complete submission of neoplasms that may measure >15 to 20 cm was met with concern by some pathologists, but for very large MCNs, thorough sampling with particular attention to solid areas is probably adequate to detect foci of invasive carcinoma. A practical approach would be to submit smaller MCNs entirely and to apply the WHO terminology based on the most severe dysplasia detected. Entirely submitted MCNs lacking invasive carcinoma could then be regarded as biologically benign. In the case of larger tumors for which complete submission may be impractical, the less committal, more generic term *mucinous cystic neoplasm* may be used, with the recognition that aggressive behavior is unlikely but not entirely excluded.

Once invasive carcinoma develops in an MCN, the prognosis is related to the age of the patient, the size of the invasive component, the status of the lymph nodes, and the adequacy of resection. In one study, the 2- and 5-year survival rates were 67% and 31%, respectively (100). Importantly, when larger numbers of cases have been analyzed and compared with data for conventional ductal adenocarcinomas using the Surveillance, Epidemiology, and End Results database of the National Cancer Institute, the prognosis for mucinous cystadenocarcinomas appears to be much better than that for ductal adenocarcinomas (106). These findings suggest that the invasive carcinomas arising in MCNs may be inherently less aggressive than conventional ductal adenocarcinomas. Detailed study of the molecular differences between these tumor types has yet to be performed, although the progression to invasive carcinoma in MCNs seems to involve many of the same genetic changes as ductal adenocarcinoma (111).

Acinar Cell Carcinoma and Pancreatoblastoma

Acinar cell carcinomas (ACCs) constitute 1% to 2% of pancreatic neoplasms (112–115). They are defined as carcinomas histologically resembling nonneoplastic acinar cells and likewise exhibiting evidence of pancreatic enzyme production. In some patients, sufficient lipase is secreted into the blood to result in a syndrome of disseminated fat necrosis and polyarthralgia (113). ACCs are solid, cellular tumors with nests and small glands composed of relatively uniform cells with granular eosinophilic cytoplasm and basally polarized nuclei (Fig. 27.18). To confirm the diagnosis of ACC, enzyme production can be demonstrated using immunohistochemical markers against trypsin, chymotrypsin, or lipase (112,116,117). Alternatively, electron microscopy can be used to identify enzyme-containing zymogen granules. Variants of ACC include acinar cell cystadenocarcinoma and mixed acinar carcinomas, in which acinar elements are combined with ductal or endocrine elements (20,118,119). The prognosis of ACC (including these variants) is not dramatically better than that of ductal adenocarcinomas; the 5-year survival is only 6% (117,120). However, numerous reports have been published of patients with advanced-stage ACC surviving for 3 or more years, an uncommon occurrence in patients with ductal adenocarcinoma. Thus, an impression has emerged that ACC is somewhat less rapidly progressive than ductal adenocarcinoma.

Pancreatoblastoma is a rare neoplasm most commonly occurring in children younger than 10 years, although histologically identical tumors also occur in adults (121–123). Pancreatoblastoma is closely related to ACC but has some additional histologic features, including more pronounced lobulation, a

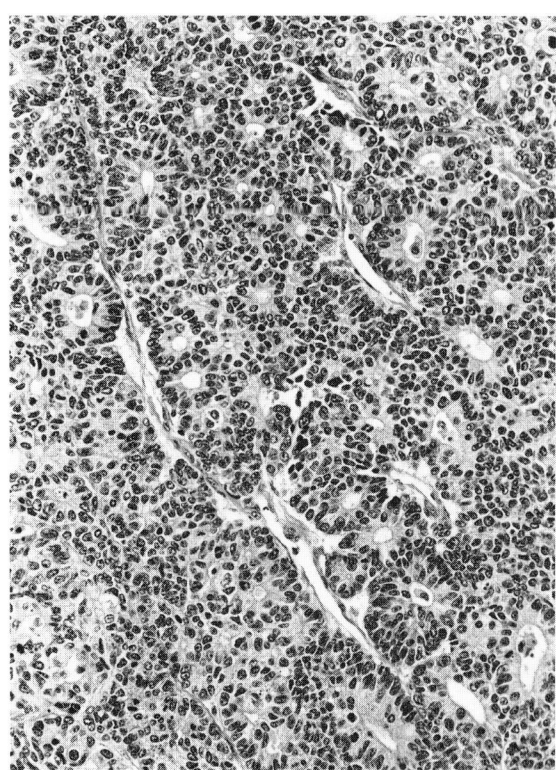

FIGURE 27.18. Acinar cell carcinoma. The tumor is highly cellular, with solid nests of cells punctuated by small acinar lumina.

cellular stromal component, and characteristic squamoid nests (Fig. 27.19), the last feature being necessary to distinguish pancreatoblastoma from ACC. By immunohistochemistry, studies of pancreatoblastomas consistently demonstrate acinar differentiation with labeling for trypsin and chymotrypsin (122,123). In addition, they commonly express chromogranin or synaptophysin as well as CA19–9 or carcinoembryonic antigen as evidence of endocrine and ductal differentiation, respectively. The prognosis of pancreatoblastomas occurring in children is relatively favorable. Although metastases occur in at least half of cases, those treated surgically prior to the

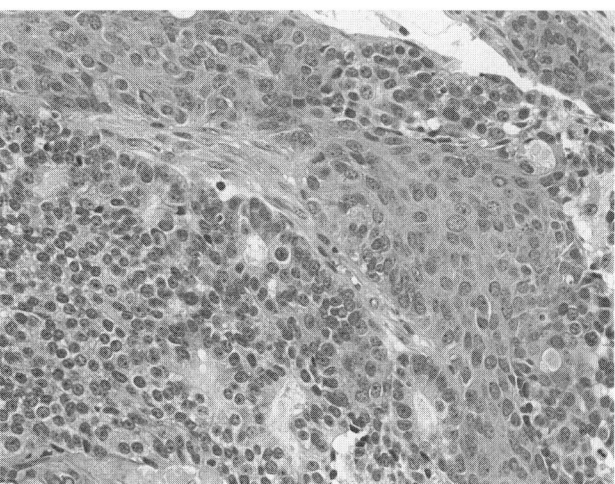

FIGURE 27.19. Pancreatoblastoma. Acinar formations and squamoid nests are present (See also color Figure 27.19).

development of metastases are often cured, and favorable responses to chemotherapy have been noted. Adults with pancreatoblastomas have a very poor prognosis.

Pancreatic Endocrine Neoplasms

Pancreatic endocrine neoplasms (PENs) are uncommon but not rare, constituting 3% to 5% of primary pancreatic tumors (1,124,125). Clinical features are discussed in detail in Chapter 48. Traditionally designated "islet cell tumors," they may occur at any age but are more common in middle-age or older adults. PENs are one of the endocrine tumors to affect patients with multiple endocrine neoplasia, type 1 (MEN1) (126,127), and they also occur in association with von Hippel-Lindau syndrome (128–130). Patients with MEN1 usually have multiple PENs, including both endocrine microadenomas (benign endocrine neoplasms measuring <0.5 cm) and at least one functional PEN. Functional PENs exhibit one of several characteristic paraneoplastic syndromes due to excessive hormone secretion. Based on the syndrome present, these tumors are designated "insulinoma," "glucagonoma," "gastrinoma," and so on (124,127,131). In contrast to these functioning or "syndromic" tumors, a sizable proportion of PENs are not associated with a clinically evident paraneoplastic syndrome (clinically nonfunctioning or "nonsyndromic" PENs), although evidence of peptide or bioamine production may be found if serologic assays or immunohistochemical studies are performed (14,125,132–134). One of the reasons for recognizing the functional nature of PENs is that a specific biological behavior has been ascribed to each different variety (135). Most important, clinically functioning insulinomas pursue an indolent clinical course in 90% of cases and are often regarded as benign. In contrast, most other functional PENs result in recurrence or metastases in 50% to 70% of cases (136). The favorable outcome of patients with insulinomas may be due in part to the small size at which these tumors are typically detected, relative to other PENs.

The pathological features of PENs are generally similar to those of other low-grade endocrine neoplasms (14,124,125,132). Grossly, the tumors are usually circumscribed, solid, and soft because they lack the fibrotic stromal reaction of ductal adenocarcinomas (Fig. 27.20). Cystic PENs also occur due to degeneration of the central portions of the tumor (137). Microscopically, PENs are hypercellular tumors with cells arranged in nests, trabecula, and ribbons (Fig. 27.21).

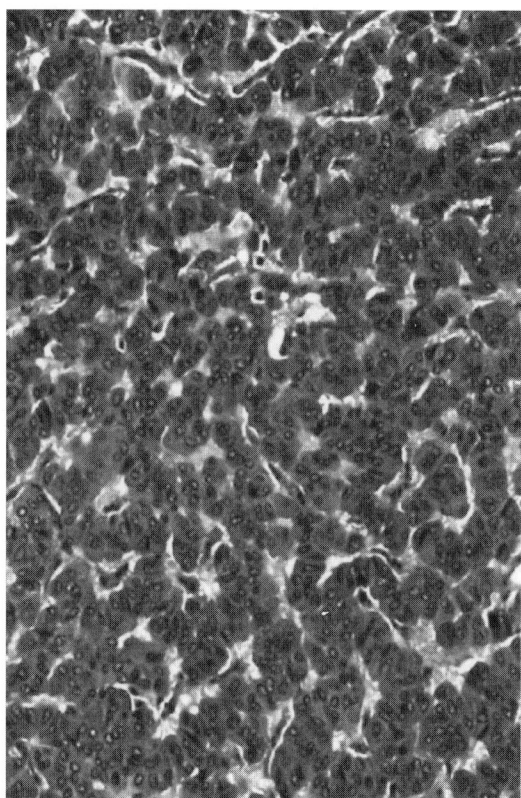

FIGURE 27.21. Microscopically, pancreatic endocrine neoplasms exhibit characteristic organoid growth patterns, trabecular in this example. The nuclei are uniform, and the chromatin is stippled.

The cytologic features are also highly characteristic, with a stippled ("salt-and-pepper") chromatin pattern and generally minimal nuclear atypia (138). Consistent with their low-grade nature, usually no necrosis is present, and mitotic figures are rare (<10 per 10 high-power microscopic fields). Relative to low-grade endocrine tumors of other organs, however, PENs may exhibit a broad spectrum of histologic appearances, and confusion with other tumor types may occur (139). Histologic variants of PENs include oncocytic (139,140), rhabdoid (141), clear cell (129,142), and pleomorphic (143), the distinction among which has not been shown to have prognostic significance. The clear cell phenotype (Fig. 27.22) is reportedly characteristic of PENs arising in patients with von Hippel-Lindau syndrome (129).

Immunohistochemistry is helpful in recognizing PENs. Most PENs are positive for general endocrine markers, including synaptophysin and chromogranin (14), the former being expressed more consistently and diffusely. Immunohistochemical positivity for specific peptides is commonly found as well, although evaluation of these markers is generally not necessary for diagnostic purposes. In functional PENs, a good correlation of peptide expression with the hormone causing the clinical syndrome is usually found. It is also common to find expression of one or more other hormones in minor cell populations, both in functional and nonfunctional PENs. Ultrastructural studies may also be used to document endocrine differentiation. Dense core neurosecretory granules are usually readily detectable, and sometimes the morphology of the granules correlates with the specific type of peptide produced by the tumor cells.

One of the most controversial aspects of PENs is the prediction of their biological behavior. Attempts to sharply separate benign and malignant PENs have been frustrating because

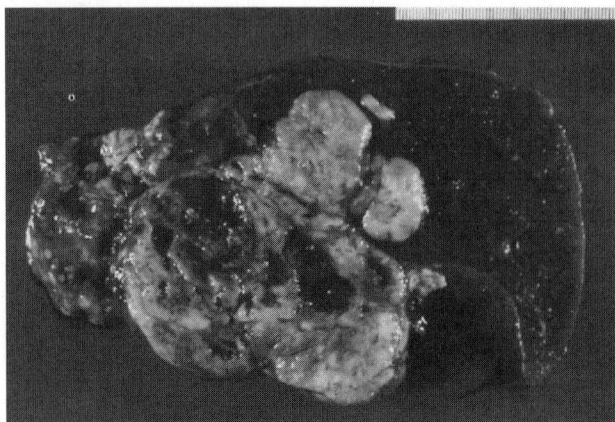

FIGURE 27.20. Gross appearance of a pancreatic endocrine neoplasm. This solid, lobulated tumor arising in the tail of the pancreas grossly invades the spleen.

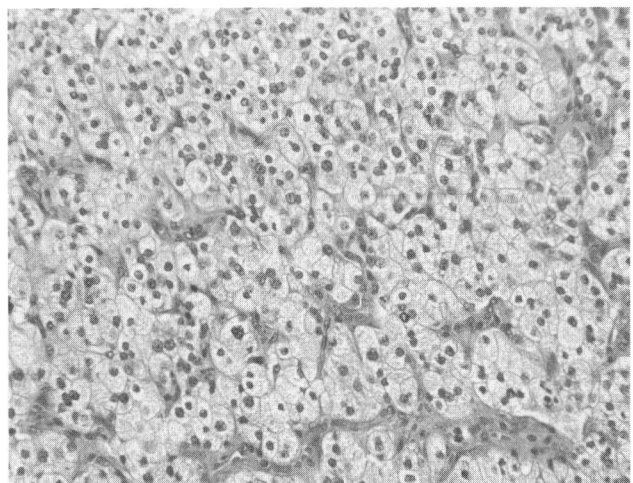

FIGURE 27.22. Clear cell pancreatic endocrine neoplasm. The cells have microvesicular, clear cytoplasm (See also color Figure 27.22).

apparently benign examples may recur after resection, whereas tumors with some aggressive features may not. The most recent WHO classification (124) divides PENs into two groups: well-differentiated endocrine tumors and well-differentiated endocrine carcinomas. According to this classification, well-differentiated endocrine tumors are confined to the pancreas (or have only local extension into peripancreatic tissues), whereas well-differentiated endocrine carcinomas have either gross local invasion or metastases. The well-differentiated endocrine tumor category is further subdivided into a "benign behavior" group (those that measure <2 cm in diameter, have <2 mitotic figures per 10 high-power fields [or have a Ki67 labeling index <2%], and lack perineural and vascular invasion) and an "uncertain behavior" group (those that either are >2 cm in diameter, have 2–10 mitotic figures per 10 high-power fields [or have a Ki67 index >2%], or have perineural or vascular invasion). In this scheme, no group of PENs is designated as benign neoplasms, but the subcategories are intended to provide an indication of the likely clinical behavior based on relatively well-characterized prognostic factors. An alternative approach divides PENs in low- and intermediate-grade groups based on the mitotic rate (> or <2 mitotic figures per 50 high-power fields) and the presence or absence of necrosis (144). Intermediate-grade PENs have a more aggressive clinical course than low-grade PENs, even when only the cases with metastases are compared.

A variety of pathological prognostic factors in PENs have been recognized (56–59). Factors that adversely correlate with clinical outcome include tumor size (>2 cm), capsular and vascular invasion, elevated mitotic rate, production of a hormone other than insulin, absence of immunohistochemical positivity for progesterone receptors, aneuploidy, and a relatively high Ki67 labeling index. Although each factor has been correlated with a worse prognosis, neither the significance of each individual factor nor whether, in the absence of specific factors, a completely resected tumor safely can be regarded as cured is yet clear. Tumors with more of these adverse prognostic factors carry a higher risk for recurrence, but whether this information would be helpful in clinical management is uncertain because effective adjuvant therapy after surgery is not currently available.

It is important to recognize a small subset of endocrine tumors occurring in the pancreas, the cytoarchitecturally poorly differentiated endocrine carcinomas (also known as high-grade neuroendocrine carcinomas) (145–149). These rare tumors most often resemble small cell carcinomas of the lung, with

a diffusely infiltrative growth pattern, numerous mitotic figures, and abundant tumor necrosis. Other cases are composed of larger cells with more abundant cytoplasm (large cell endocrine carcinoma). Some cases are associated with paraneoplastic syndromes, including hypercalcemia and Cushing syndrome (148,149). Poorly differentiated endocrine carcinomas constitute <5% of PENs. These tumors pursue an aggressive course similar to that of small cell carcinomas of other sites. Of course, the possibility of a metastasis from a pulmonary primary tumor must always be considered.

Solid Pseudopapillary Neoplasm

An uncommon but highly distinctive pancreatic neoplasm is SPN. SPNs generally occur in young female patients (mean age of 27 years), but unlike MCNs, SPNs are well described in male patients and may occur anywhere within the pancreas (4,150–152). Presenting symptoms are often nonspecific, and some cases are detected incidentally during gynecologic examinations or after trauma. The tumors are often quite large at the time they are detected and appear as relatively circumscribed solid masses with irregular degenerative cystic spaces on CT scans (Fig. 27.23). A variety of other names have been applied to SPNs, all describing the various gross and microscopic features of the tumor: solid and cystic tumor, papillary cystic tumor, and solid and papillary epithelial neoplasm (153–156).

The gross appearance of SPNs depends on the size of the tumor. Large examples have friable tan tissue with areas of hemorrhage and cystic cavities lined by ragged degenerating soft tissue (Fig. 27.24). Smaller examples may have less cystic change or none at all, sometimes appearing as circumscribed, firm, yellow-tan solid masses. Although the microscopic appearance varies in different regions of the tumor, the features are often characteristic enough to establish a diagnosis without requiring special studies. Many areas of the tumor have a solid appearance, with numerous small vessels penetrating sheets of polygonal cells. No lumen formation occurs in SPNs. Elsewhere, the characteristic pseudopapillae are formed when tumor cells at a distance from the small vessels degenerate, leaving a cuff of discohesive cells loosely clinging to each small vessel (Fig. 27.25). The pseudopapillary structures are a highly characteristic if not defining feature of SPNs. Aggregates of foamy histocytes and cholesterol clefts may be seen. Clusters of cells

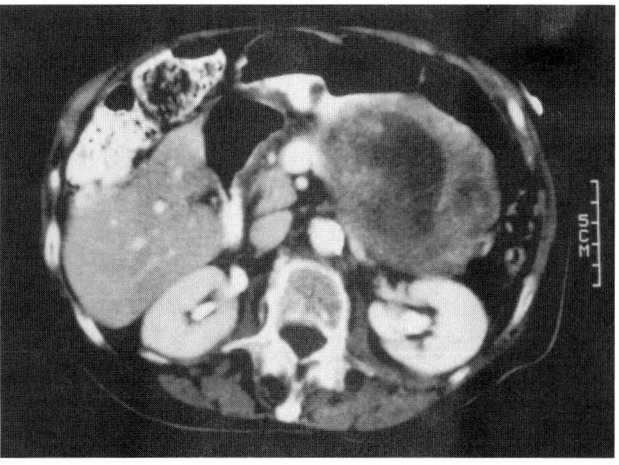

FIGURE 27.23. Solid pseudopapillary neoplasm on computed tomography scan. The tumor in the tail of the gland is large and contains a central irregular cyst.

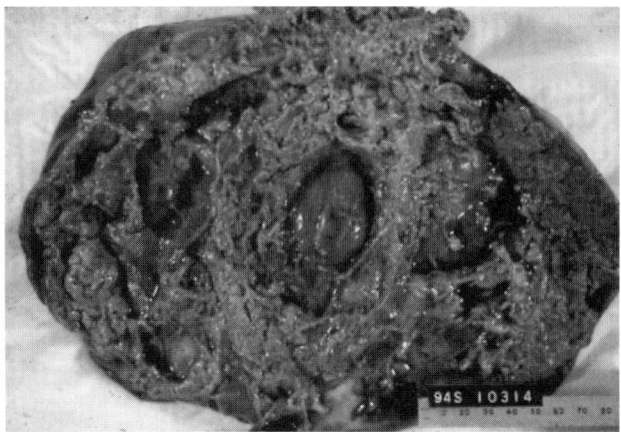

FIGURE 27.24. Gross appearance of solid pseudopapillary neoplasm. The tumor is circumscribed and very friable, with soft, ragged fragments of tumor projecting into irregular degenerative cystic cavities.

containing large eosinophilic globules rich in α_1-antitrypsin are also typically present. The nuclei have longitudinal grooves, generally with minimal atypia and infrequent mitoses. Despite the grossly and radiographically circumscribed appearance of SPNs, a common finding is areas of infiltration into the adjacent pancreatic tissue, where the tumor elicits no stromal response and where nests of tumor cells grow immediately adjacent to unremarkable pancreatic parenchyma. The characteristic pseudopapillary structures and nuclear grooves are readily appreciated on cytologic preparations from fine-needle aspiration,

findings that often allow accurate preoperative diagnosis in the appropriate clinical setting (156,157).

Attempts to define the cell lineage of SPNs have been generally unsuccessful, which explains the variety of descriptive terms applied to this tumor (4,116,158,159). Immunohistochemical studies for markers of acinar differentiation (pancreatic enzymes), endocrine differentiation (general endocrine markers), and ductal differentiation (glycoprotein markers) have detected no consistent line of differentiation (4). Specifically, pancreatic enzymes and glycoproteins are never found, and although some markers of neuroendocrine differentiation such as synaptophysin, neural cell adhesion molecule (CD56), and neuron-specific enolase may be identified in SPNs (4,160), the most specific marker, chromogranin, is never detected. In fact, keratin is expressed in only approximately one-third of cases in a focal fashion (4,150). The markers typically found include vimentin, α_1-antitrypsin, and CD10 (4,116,160). Abnormal nuclear labeling for β-catenin is also commonly found (161), and a subset of SPNs overexpress Kit (162). This immunohistochemical profile is characteristic, but none of the findings is specific for the diagnosis of SPN. Ultrastructural studies also reveal characteristic findings but do not point to a defined cell lineage. Analysis of the data suggests that convincing endocrine differentiation may characterize SPNs (160) but that they remain strikingly different from typical PENs.

SPNs are indolent malignancies, with <15% of patients experiencing recurrence or metastasis (4,150,163). When present, metastases are essentially restricted to the peritoneum and liver, with nodal disease being vanishingly rare. Most patients with metastatic disease have it at presentation. Thus far, attempts to identify histologic or clinical factors predictive of metastatic disease have been unsuccessful in typical cases of SPN. Most interestingly, patients with metastases may live for many years (if not decades) with stable disease (163). Resection of isolated liver metastases has been performed, but the stability of asymptomatic metastatic disease in some patients raises the question of whether aggressive treatment of metastases truly enhances survival. Thus, SPN is a pathologically and clinically characteristic, if not enigmatic, pancreatic tumor with very low-grade malignant potential. A recent report has documented the rare occurrence of high-grade malignant transformation of SPNs (164); the two reported cases had sheets of undifferentiated cells with a high mitotic rate, and the patients died of disease in 6 and 16 months, respectively.

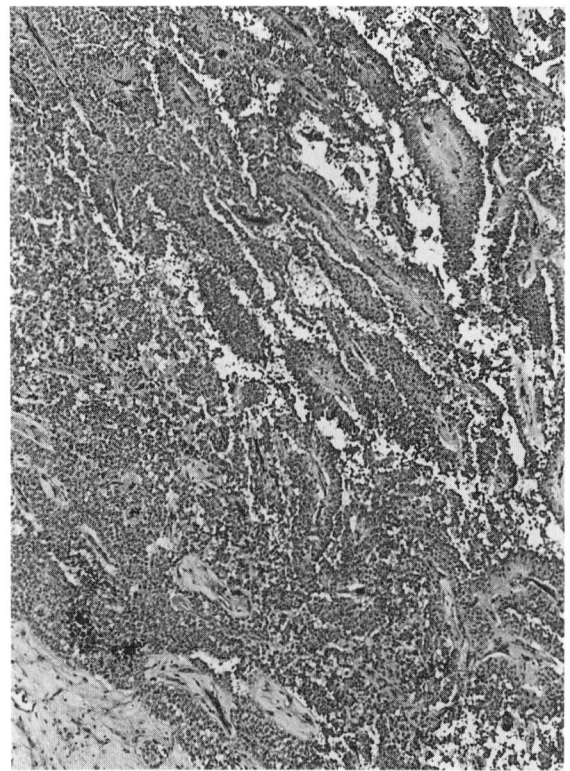

FIGURE 27.25. Microscopically, solid pseudopapillary neoplasms have hypercellular solid areas (*lower left*) giving way to degenerative pseudopapillae where the cells away from the vessels have dropped out (*upper right*).

References

1. Hruban RH, Pitman MB, Klimstra DS. Tumors of the pancreas. In: Silverberg S, ed. *Atlas of Tumor Pathology, 4th Series, Fascicle 6*. Washington, DC: American Registry of Pathology; 2007.
2. Cubilla AL, Fitzgerald PJ. Morphological patterns of primary nonendocrine human pancreas carcinoma. *Cancer Res* 1975;35(8):2234–2248.
3. Klimstra DS. Cell lineage in pancreatic neoplasms. In: Sarkar FH, Dugan MC, eds. *Pancreatic Cancer: Advances in Molecular Pathology, Diagnosis and Clinical Management*. Natick, Mass.: BioTechniques Books; 1998: 21–47.
4. Klimstra DS, Wenig BM, Heffess CS. Solid-pseudopapillary tumor of the pancreas: a typically cystic carcinoma of low malignant potential. *Semin Diagn Pathol* 2000;17(1):66–80.
5. Adsay NV, Klimstra DS. Cystic forms of typically solid pancreatic tumors. *Semin Diagn Pathol* 2000;17(1):81–88.
6. Adsay NV, Merati K, Andea A, et al. The dichotomy in the preinvasive neoplasia to invasive carcinoma sequence in the pancreas: differential expression of MUC1 and MUC2 supports the existence of two separate pathways of carcinogenesis. *Mod Pathol* 2002;15(10):1087–1095.
7. Adsay NV, Merati K, Basturk O, et al. Pathologically and biologically distinct types of epithelium in intraductal papillary mucinous neoplasms: delineation of an "intestinal" pathway of carcinogenesis in the pancreas. *Am J Surg Pathol* 2004;28(7):839–848.
8. Jemal A, Tiwari RC, Murray T, et al. Cancer statistics, 2004. *CA Cancer J Clin* 2004;54(1):8–29.

9. Fortner JG, Klimstra DS, Senie RT, Maclean BJ. Tumor size is the primary prognosticator for pancreatic cancer after regional pancreatectomy. *Ann Surg* 1996;223(2):147–153.

10. Brennan MF, Moccia RD, Klimstra D. Management of adenocarcinoma of the body and tail of the pancreas. *Ann Surg* 1996;223(5):506–511; discussion 11–12.

11. Conlon KC, Klimstra DS, Brennan MF. Long-term survival after curative resection for pancreatic ductal adenocarcinoma: clinicopathologic analysis of 5-year survivors. *Ann Surg* 1996;223(3):273–279.

12. Cubilla LA, Fitzgerald PJ. Tumors of the exocrine pancreas. In: Hartmann WH, Sobin LH, eds. *Atlas of Tumor Pathology, 2nd Series, Fascicle 19.* Washington, DC: Armed Forces Institute Pathology; 1984.

13. Hermanek P. Pathology and biology of pancreatic ductal adenocarcinoma. *Langenbecks Arch Surg* 1998;383(2):116–120.

14. Solcia E, Capella C, Kloppel G. *Atlas of Tumor Pathology, 3rd Series, Fascicle 20.* Washington, DC: Armed Forces Institute of Pathology; 1997.

15. Tannapfel A, Wittekind C, Hunefeld G. Ductal adenocarcinoma of the pancreas: histopathological features and prognosis. *Int J Pancreatol* 1992; 12(2):145–152.

16. Sener SF, Fremgen A, Menck HR, Winchester DP. Pancreatic cancer: a report of treatment and survival trends for 100,313 patients diagnosed from 1985–1995, using the National Cancer Database. *J Am Coll Surg* 1999;189(1):1–7.

17. Lillemoe KD, Kaushal S, Cameron JL, et al. Distal pancreatectomy: indications and outcomes in 235 patients. *Ann Surg* 1999;229(5):693–698.

18. Sohn TA, Yeo CJ, Cameron JL, et al. Resected adenocarcinoma of the pancreas–616 patients: results, outcomes, and prognostic indicators. *J Gastrointest Surg* 2000;4(6):567–579.

19. Adsay NV, Klimstra DS, Compton CC. Cystic lesions of the pancreas: introduction. *Semin Diagn Pathol* 2000;17(1):1–6.

20. Kosmahl M, Pauser U, Anlauf M, Kloppel G. Pancreatic ductal adenocarcinomas with cystic features: neither rare nor uniform. *Mod Pathol* 2005;18(9):1157–1164.

21. Cubilla AL, Fitzgerald PJ. Morphological patterns of primary nonendocrine human pancreas carcinoma. *Cancer Res* 1975;35:2234–2248.

22. Kloppel G, Hruban RH, Longnecker DS, Adler G, Kern S, Partanen TJ. Ductal adenocarcinoma of the pancreas. In: Hamilton SR, Aaltonen LA, eds. *Pathology and Genetics of Tumours of the Digestive System.* Lyon, France: IARC Press; 2000: 221–230.

23. Adsay NV, Basturk O, Bonnett M, et al. A proposal for a new and more practical grading scheme for pancreatic ductal adenocarcinoma. *Am J Surg Pathol* 2005;29(6):724–733.

24. Takahashi T, Ishikura H, Motohara T, et al. Perineural invasion by ductal adenocarcinoma of the pancreas. *J Surg Oncol* 1997;65(3):164–170.

25. Adsay V, Logani S, Sarkar F, Crissman J, Vaitkevicius V. Foamy gland pattern of pancreatic ductal adenocarcinoma: a deceptively benign-appearing variant. *Am J Surg Pathol* 2000;24(4):493–504.

26. Andea A, Lonardo F, Adsay V. Microscopically cystic and papillary "large-duct-type" invasive adenocarcinoma of the pancreas: a potential mimic of intraductal papillary mucinous and mucinous cystic neoplasm. *Mod Pathol* In press.

27. Adsay V, Kabbani W, Sarkar F, Visscher D. Infiltrating "lobular-type" carcinoma of the pancreas: morphologically distinctive variant of ductal adenocarcinoma of the pancreas mimicking lobular carcinoma of the breast. *Mod Pathol* 1999;12:159A.

28. McArthur CP, Fiorella R, Saran BM. Rare primary signet ring carcinoma of the pancreas. *Missouri Med* 1995;92:298–302.

29. Adsay NV, Pierson C, Sarkar F, et al. Colloid (mucinous noncystic) carcinoma of the pancreas. *Am J Surg Pathol* 2001;25(1):26–42.

30. Seidel G, Zahurak M, Iacobuzio-Donahue C, et al. Almost all infiltrating colloid carcinomas of the pancreas and periampullary region arise from in situ papillary neoplasms: a study of 39 cases. *Am J Surg Pathol* 2002;26(1):56–63.

31. Adsay NV, Longnecker DS, Klimstra DS. Pancreatic tumors with cystic dilatation of the ducts: intraductal papillary mucinous neoplasms and intraductal oncocytic papillary neoplasms. *Semin Diagn Pathol* 2000;17(1):16–30.

32. Nagai E, Ueki T, Chijiiwa K, Tanaka M, Tsuneyoshi M. Intraductal papillary mucinous neoplasms of the pancreas associated with so-called "mucinous ductal ectasia": histochemical and immunohistochemical analysis of 29 cases. *Am J Surg Pathol* 1995;19(5):576–589.

33. Sessa F, Solcia E, Capella C, et al. Intraductal papillary-mucinous tumours represent a distinct group of pancreatic neoplasms: an investigation of tumour cell differentiation and K-ras, p53 and c-erbB-2 abnormalities in 26 patients. *Virchows Arch* 1994;425(4):357–367.

34. Iacobuzio-Donahue CA, Klimstra DS, Adsay NV, et al. Dpc-4 protein is expressed in virtually all human intraductal papillary mucinous neoplasms of the pancreas: comparison with conventional ductal adenocarcinomas. *Am J Pathol* 2000;157(3):755–761.

35. Ishikawa O, Matsui Y, Aoki I, et al. Adenosquamous carcinoma of the pancreas: a clinicopathologic study and report of three cases. *Cancer* 1980;146(5):1192–1196.

36. Motojima K, Tomioka T, Kohara N, Tsunoda T, Kanematsu T. Immunohistochemical characteristics of adenosquamous carcinoma of the pancreas. *J Surg Oncol* 1992;49(1):58–62.

37. Yamaguchi K, Enjoji M. Adenosquamous carcinoma of the pancreas: a clinicopathologic study. *J Surg Oncol* 1991;47(2):109–116.

38. Tschang TP, Garza-Garza R, Kissane JM. Pleomorphic carcinoma of the pancreas: an analysis of 15 cases. *Cancer* 1977;39(5):2114–2126.

39. Watanabe M, Miura H, Inoue H, et al. Mixed osteoclastic/pleomorphic-type giant cell tumor of the pancreas with ductal adenocarcinoma: histochemical and immunohistochemical study with review of the literature. *Pancreas* 1997;15(2):201–208.

40. Urbanski SJ, Medline A. Giant cell carcinoma of pancreas with clear cell pattern in metastases. *Hum Pathol* 1982;13(11):1047–1049.

41. Alguacil-Garcia A, Weiland LH. The histologic spectrum, prognosis, and histogenesis of the sarcomatoid carcinoma of the pancreas. *Cancer* 1977;39:1181–1189.

42. Hoorens A, Prenzel K, Lemoine NR, Kloppel G. Undifferentiated carcinoma of the pancreas: analysis of intermediate filament profile and Ki-ras mutations provides evidence of a ductal origin. *J Pathol* 1998;185(1):53–60.

43. Dworak O, Wittekind C, Koerfgen HP, Gall FP. Osteoclastic giant cell tumor of the pancreas: an immunohistological study and review of the literature. *Pathol Res Pract* 1993;189(2):228–231.

44. Klimstra DS, Rosai JR. Osteoclastic giant cell tumor of the pancreas: critical commentary. *Pathol Res Pract* 1993;189:232–233.

45. Molberg KH, Heffess C, Delgado R, Albores-Saavedra J. Undifferentiated carcinoma with osteoclast-like giant cells of the pancreas and periampullary region. *Cancer* 1998;182(7):1279–1287.

46. Oehler U, Jurs M, Kloppel G, Helpap B. Osteoclast-like giant cell tumour of the pancreas presenting as a pseudocyst-like lesion. *Virchows Arch* 1997;431(3):215–218.

47. Posen JA. Giant cell tumor of the pancreas of the osteoclastic type associated with a mucous secreting cystadenocarcinoma. *Hum Pathol* 1981;12(10):944–947.

48. Trepeta RW, Mathur B, Lagin S, LiVolsi VA. Giant cell tumor ("osteoclastoma") of the pancreas: a tumor of epithelial origin. *Cancer* 1981;148(9):2022–2028.

49. Gocke CD, Dabbs DJ, Benko FA, Silverman JF. KRAS oncogene mutations suggest a common histogenetic origin for pleomorphic giant cell tumor of the pancreas, osteoclastoma of the pancreas, and pancreatic duct adenocarcinoma. *Hum Pathol* 1997;28(1):80–83.

50. Westra WH, Sturm P, Drillenburg P, et al. K-ras oncogene mutations in osteoclast-like giant cell tumors of the pancreas and liver: genetic evidence to support origin from the duct epithelium. *Am J Surg Pathol* 1998;22(10):1247–1254.

51. Goggins M, Offerhaus GJ, Hilgers W, et al. Pancreatic adenocarcinomas with DNA replication errors (RER+) are associated with wild-type K-ras and characteristic histopathology: poor differentiation, a syncytial growth pattern, and pushing borders suggest RER+. *Am J Pathol* 1998;152(6):1501–1507.

52. Wilentz RE, Goggins M, Redston M, et al. Genetic, immunohistochemical, and clinical features of medullary carcinoma of the pancreas: a newly described and characterized entity. *Am J Pathol* 2000;156(5):1641–1651.

53. Jessurun J, Romero-Guadarrama M, Manivel JC. Medullary adenocarcinoma of the colon: clinicopathologic study of 11 cases. *Hum Pathol* 1999;30(7):843–848.

54. Ruschoff J, Dietmaier W, Luttges J, et al. Poorly differentiated colonic adenocarcinoma, medullary type: clinical, phenotypic, and molecular characteristics. *Am J Pathol* 1997;150(5):1815–1825.

55. Hruban RH, Wilentz RE, Goggins M, et al. Pathology of incipient pancreatic cancer. *Ann Oncol* 1999;10(suppl 4):9–11.

56. Klimstra DS, Hameed MR, Marrero AM, Conlon KC, Brenann MF. Ductal proliferative lesions associated with infiltrating ductal adenocarcinoma of the pancreas. *Int J Pancreatol* 1994;16:224–225.

57. Brat DJ, Lillemoe KD, Yeo CJ, Warfield PB, Hruban RH. Progression of pancreatic intraductal neoplasias to infiltrating adenocarcinoma of the pancreas. *Am J Surg Pathol* 1998;22(2):163–169.

58. Brockie E, Anand A, Albores-Saavedra J. Progression of atypical ductal hyperplasia/carcinoma in situ of the pancreas to invasive adenocarcinoma. *Ann Diagn Pathol* 1998;2(5):286–292.

59. Klimstra DS, Longnecker DS. K-ras mutations in pancreatic ductal proliferative lesions. *Am J Pathol* 1994;145(6):1547–1550.

60. Moskaluk CA, Hruban RH, Kern SE. p16 and K-ras gene mutations in the intraductal precursors of human pancreatic adenocarcinoma. *Cancer Res* 1997;157(11):2140–2143.

61. Hruban RH, Wilentz RE, Kern SE. Genetic progression in the pancreatic ducts. *Am J Pathol* 2000;156(6):1821–1825.

62. Yanagisawa A, Ohtake K, Ohashi K, et al. Frequent c-Ki-ras oncogene activation in mucous cell hyperplasias of pancreas suffering from chronic inflammation. *Cancer Res* 1993;153(5):953–956.

63. Terada T, Ohta T, Sasaki M, Nakanuma Y, Kim YS. Expression of MUC apomucins in normal pancreas and pancreatic tumours. *J Pathol* 1996;180(2):160–165.

64. Z'Graggen K, Rivera JA, Compton CC, et al. Prevalence of activating K-ras mutations in the evolutionary stages of neoplasia in intraductal papillary mucinous tumors of the pancreas. *Ann Surg* 1997;226(4):491–498.

65. Hruban RH, Goggins M, Parsons J, Kern SE. Progression model for pancreatic cancer. *Clin Cancer Res* 2000;6(8):2969–2972.

66. van Heek NT, Meeker AK, Kern SE, et al. Telomere shortening is nearly universal in pancreatic intraepithelial neoplasia. *Am J Pathol* 2002;161(5):1541–1547.

67. Mukada T, Yamada S. Dysplasia and carcinoma in situ of the exocrine pancreas. *Tohoku J Exp Med* 1982;137(2):115–124.

68. Fukushima N, Mukai K, Kanai Y, et al. Intraductal papillary tumors and mucinous cystic tumors of the pancreas: clinicopathologic study of 38 cases. *Hum Pathol* 1997;28(9):1010–1017.

69. Warshaw AL. Mucinous cystic tumors and mucinous ductal ectasia of the pancreas. *Gastrointest Endosc* 1991;37(2):199–201.

70. Longnecker DS, Adler G, Hruban RH, Kloppel G. Intraductal papillary-mucinous neoplasms of the pancreas. In: Hamilton SR, Aaltonen LA, eds. *Pathology and Genetics of Tumours of the Digestive System.* Lyon, France: IARC Press; 2000:237–240.

71. Itai Y, Ohhashi K, Nagai H, et al. "Ductectatic" mucinous cystadenoma and cystadenocarcinoma of the pancreas. *Radiology* 1986;161(3):697–700.

72. Yanagisawa A, Ohashi K, Hori M, et al. Ductectatic-type mucinous cystadenoma and cystadenocarcinoma of the human pancreas: a novel clinicopathological entity. *Jpn J Cancer Res* 1993;84(4):474–479.

73. Ohta T, Nagakawa T, Akiyama T, et al. The "duct-ectatic" variant of mucinous cystic neoplasm of the pancreas: clinical and radiologic studies of seven cases. *Am J Gastroenterol* 1992;87(3):300–304.

74. Morohoshi T, Kanda M, Asanuma K, Kloppel G. Intraductal papillary neoplasms of the pancreas: a clinicopathologic study of six patients. *Cancer* 1989;1564(6):1329–1335.

75. Payan MJ, Xerri L, Moncada K, et al. Villous adenoma of the main pancreatic duct: a potentially malignant tumor?. *Am J Gastroenterol* 1990;85(4):459–463.

76. Kloppel G. Clinicopathologic view of intraductal papillary-mucinous tumor of the pancreas. *Hepatogastroenterology* 1998;45(24):1981–1985.

77. Santini D, Campione O, Salerno A, et al. Intraductal papillary-mucinous neoplasm of the pancreas: a clinicopathologic entity. *Arch Pathol Lab Med* 1995;119(3):209–213.

78. Pinson CW, Munson JL, Deveney CW. Endoscopic retrograde cholangiopancreatography in the preoperative diagnosis of pancreatic neoplasms associated with cysts. *Am J Surg* 1990;159(5):510–513.

79. Shyr YM, Su CH, Tsay SH, Lui WY. Mucin-producing neoplasms of the pancreas: intraductal papillary and mucinous cystic neoplasms. *Ann Surg* 1996;223(2):141–146.

80. Paye F, Sauvanet A, Terris B, et al. Intraductal papillary mucinous tumors of the pancreas: pancreatic resections guided by preoperative morphological assessment and intraoperative frozen section examination. *Surgery* 2000;127(5):536–544.

81. D'Angelica M, Brennan MF, Suriawinata AA, Klimstra D, Conlon KC. Intraductal papillary mucinous neoplasms of the pancreas: an analysis of clinicopathologic features and outcome. *Ann Surg* 2004;239(3):400–408.

82. Maire F, Couvelard A, Hammel P, et al. Intraductal papillary mucinous tumors of the pancreas: the preoperative value of cytologic and histopathologic diagnosis. *Gastrointest Endosc* 2003;58(5):701–706.

83. Uehara H, Nakaizumi A, Iishi H, et al. Cytologic examination of pancreatic juice for differential diagnosis of benign and malignant mucin-producing tumors of the pancreas. *Cancer* 1994;174(3):826–833.

84. Paal E, Thompson LD, Przygodzki RM, Bratthauer GL, Heffess CS. A clinicopathologic and immunohistochemical study of 22 intraductal papillary mucinous neoplasms of the pancreas, with a review of the literature. *Mod Pathol* 1999;12(5):518–528.

85. Furukawa T, Kloppel G, Volkan Adsay N, et al. Classification of types of intraductal papillary-mucinous neoplasm of the pancreas: a consensus study. *Virchows Arch* 2005;447(5):794–799.

86. Adsay NV, Conlon KC, Zee SY, Brennan MF, Klimstra DS. Intraductal papillary-mucinous neoplasms of the pancreas: an analysis of in situ and invasive carcinomas in 28 patients. *Cancer* 2002;194(1):62–77.

87. Adsay NV, Adair CF, Heffess CS, Klimstra DS. Intraductal oncocytic papillary neoplasms of the pancreas. *Am J Surg Pathol* 1996;20(8):980–994.

88. Tajiri T, Tate G, Inagaki T, et al. Intraductal tubular neoplasms of the pancreas: histogenesis and differentiation. *Pancreas* 2005;30(2):115–121.

89. Miyakawa S, Horiguchi A, Hayakawa M, et al. Intraductal papillary adenocarcinoma with mucin hypersecretion and coexistent invasive ductal carcinoma of the pancreas with apparent topographic separation. *J Gastroenterol* 1996;31(6):889–893.

90. Levi E, Klimstra DS, Andea A, Basturk O, Adsay NV. MUC1 and MUC2 in pancreatic neoplasia. *J Clin Pathol* 2004;57(5):456–462.

91. Hruban RH, Adsay NV, Albores-Saavedra J, et al. Pancreatic intraepithelial neoplasia: a new nomenclature and classification system for pancreatic duct lesions. *Am J Surg Pathol* 2001;25(5):579–586.

92. Barton CM, Staddon SL, Hughes CM, et al. Abnormalities of the p53 tumour suppressor gene in human pancreatic cancer. *Br J Cancer* 1991;64(6):1076–1082.

93. Sirivatanauksorn V, Sirivatanauksorn Y, Lemoine NR. Molecular pattern of ductal pancreatic cancer. *Langenbecks Arch Surg* 1998;383(2):105–115.

94. Wilentz RE, Iacobuzio-Donahue CA, Argani P, et al. Loss of expression of Dpc4 in pancreatic intraepithelial neoplasia: evidence that DPC4 inactivation occurs late in neoplastic progression. *Cancer Res* 2000;160(7):2002–2006.

95. Biankin AV, Biankin SA, Kench JG, et al. Aberrant p16(INK4A) and DPC4/Smad4 expression in intraductal papillary mucinous tumours of

the pancreas is associated with invasive ductal adenocarcinoma. *Gut* 2002;50(6):861–868.

96. Moore PS, Orlandini S, Zamboni G, et al. Pancreatic tumours: molecular pathways implicated in ductal cancer are involved in ampullary but not in exocrine nonductal or endocrine tumorigenesis. *Br J Cancer.* 2001;84(2):253–262.

97. Sato N, Rosty C, Jansen M, et al. STK11/LKB1 Peutz-Jeghers gene inactivation in intraductal papillary-mucinous neoplasms of the pancreas. *Am J Surg Pathol* 2001;159(6):2017–2022.

98. Compagno J, Oertel JE. Mucinous cystic neoplasms of the pancreas with overt and latent malignancy (cystadenocarcinoma and cystadenoma): a clinicopathologic study of 41 cases. *Am J Clin Pathol* 1978;69(6):573–580.

99. Fukushima N, Mukai K. Pancreatic neoplasms with abundant mucus production: emphasis on intraductal papillary-mucinous tumors and mucinous cystic tumors. *Adv Anat Pathol* 1999;6(2):65–77.

100. Thompson LD, Becker RC, Przygodzki RM, Adair CF, Heffess CS. Mucinous cystic neoplasm (mucinous cystadenocarcinoma of low-grade malignant potential) of the pancreas: a clinicopathologic study of 130 cases. *Am J Surg Pathol* 1999;23(1):1–16.

101. Wilentz RE, Albores-Saavedra J, Hruban RH. Mucinous cystic neoplasms of the pancreas. *Semin Diagn Pathol* 2000;17(1):31–42.

102. Zamboni G, Scarpa A, Bogina G, et al. Mucinous cystic tumors of the pancreas: clinicopathological features, prognosis, and relationship to other mucinous cystic tumors. *Am J Surg Pathol* 1999;23(4):410–422.

103. Alles AJ, Warshaw AL, Southern JF, Compton CC, Lewandrowski KB. Expression of CA 72-4 (TAG-72) in the fluid contents of pancreatic cysts: a new marker to distinguish malignant pancreatic cystic tumors from benign neoplasms and pseudocysts. *Ann Surg* 1994;219(2):131–134.

104. Lewandrowski KB, Southern JF, Pins MR, Compton CC, Warshaw AL. Cyst fluid analysis in the differential diagnosis of pancreatic cysts: a comparison of pseudocysts, serous cystadenomas, mucinous cystic neoplasms, and mucinous cystadenocarcinoma. *Ann Surg* 1993;217(1):41–47.

105. Wilentz RE, Albores-Saavedra J, Zahurak M, et al. Pathologic examination accurately predicts prognosis in mucinous cystic neoplasms of the pancreas. *Am J Surg Pathol* 1999;23(11):1320–1327.

106. Zamboni G, Kloppel G, Hruban RH, Longnecker DS, Adler G. Mucinous cystic neoplasms of the pancreas. In: Hamilton SR, Aaltonen LA, eds. *Pathology and Genetics of Tumours of the Digestive System.* Lyon, France: IARC Press; 2000:234–236.

107. Lane RB, Jr., Sangueza OP. Anaplastic carcinoma occurring in association with a mucinous cystic neoplasm of the pancreas. *Arch Pathol Lab Med* 1997;121(5):533–535.

108. Wenig BM, Albores-Saavedra J, Buetow PC, Heffess CS. Pancreatic mucinous cystic neoplasm with sarcomatous stroma: a report of three cases. *Am J Surg Pathol* 1997;21(1):70–80.

109. Ridder GJ, Maschek H, Flemming P, Nashan B, Klempnauer J. Ovarian-like stroma in an invasive mucinous cystadenocarcinoma of the pancreas positive for inhibin: a hint concerning its possible histogenesis. *Virchows Arch* 1998;432(5):451–454.

110. Southern JF, Warshaw AL, Lewandrowski KB. DNA ploidy analysis of mucinous cystic tumors of the pancreas: correlation of aneuploidy with malignancy and poor prognosis. *Cancer* 1996;177(1):58–62.

111. Jimenez RE, Warshaw AL, Z'Graggen K, et al. Sequential accumulation of K-ras mutations and p53 overexpression in the progression of pancreatic mucinous cystic neoplasms to malignancy. *Ann Surg* 1999;230(4):501–509.

112. Hoorens A, Lemoine NR, McLellan E, et al. Pancreatic acinar cell carcinoma: an analysis of cell lineage markers, p53 expression, and Ki-ras mutation. *Am J Pathol* 1993;143(3):685–698.

113. Klimstra DS, Heffess CS, Oertel JE, Rosai J. Acinar cell carcinoma of the pancreas: a clinicopathologic study of 28 cases. *Am J Surg Pathol* 1992;16(9):815–837.

114. Cingolani N, Shaco-Levy R, Farruggio A, Klimstra DS, Rosai J. Alpha-fetoprotein production by pancreatic tumors exhibiting acinar cell differentiation: study of five cases, one arising in a mediastinal teratoma. *Hum Pathol* 2000;31(8):938–944.

115. Klimstra DS, Longnecker D. Acinar cell carcinoma. In: Hamilton SR, Aaltonen LA, eds. *Pathology and Genetics of Tumours of the Digestive System.* Lyon, France: IARC Press; 2000:241–243.

116. Morohoshi T, Kanda M, Horie A, et al. Immunocytochemical markers of uncommon pancreatic tumors: acinar cell carcinoma, pancreatoblastoma, and solid cystic (papillary-cystic) tumor. *Cancer* 1987;1559(4):739–747.

117. Klimstra DS. Acinar cell carcinoma of the pancreas: a case associated with the lipase hypersecretion syndrome. *Pathol Case Rev* 2001;6:121–126.

118. Cantrell BB, Cubilla AL, Erlandson RA, Fortner J, Fitzgerald PJ. Acinar cell cystadenocarcinoma of human pancreas. *Cancer* 1981;1547(2):410–416.

119. Klimstra DS, Rosai J, Heffess CS. Mixed acinar-endocrine carcinomas of the pancreas. *Am J Surg Pathol* 1994;18(8):765–778.

120. Holen KD, Klimstra DS, Hummer A, et al. Clinical characteristics and outcomes from an institutional series of acinar cell carcinoma of the pancreas and related tumors. *J Clin Oncol* 2002;1520(24):4673–4678.

121. Hoorens A, Gebhard F, Kraft K, Lemoine NR, Kloppel G. Pancreatoblastoma in an adult: its separation from acinar cell carcinoma. *Virchows Arch* 1994;424(5):485–490.

122. Klimstra DS, Wenig BM, Adair CF, Heffess CS. Pancreatoblastoma: a clinicopathologic study and review of the literature. *Am J Surg Pathol* 1995;19(12):1371–1389.

123. Klimstra DS, Longnecker D. Pancreatoblastoma. In: Hamilton SR, Aaltonen LA, eds. *Pathology and Genetics of Tumours of the Digestive System.* Lyon, France: IARC Press; 2000:244–245.

124. Heitz PU, Komminoth P, Perren A, et al. Pancreatic endocrine tumours: introduction. In: DeLellis RA, Lloyd RV, Heitz PU, Eng C, eds. *Pathology and Genetics of Tumours of Endocrine Organs.* Lyon, France: IARC Press; 2004:177–182.

125. Klimstra DS, Perren A, Oberg K, et al. Pancreatic endocrine tumours: non-functioning tumours and microadenomas. In: DeLellis RA, Lloyd RV, Heitz PU, Eng C, eds. *Pathology and Genetics of Tumours of Endocrine Organs.* Lyon, France: IARC Press; 2004:201–204.

126. Debelenko LV, Zhuang Z, Emmert-Buck MR, et al. Allelic deletions on chromosome 11q13 in multiple endocrine neoplasia type 1-associated and sporadic gastrinomas and pancreatic endocrine tumors. *Cancer Res* 1997;157(11):2238–2243.

127. Donow C, Pipeleers-Marichal M, Schroder S, et al. Surgical pathology of gastrinoma: site, size, multicentricity, association with multiple endocrine neoplasia type 1, and malignancy. *Cancer* 1991;1568(6):1329–1334.

128. Hammel PR, Vilgrain V, Terris B, et al. Pancreatic involvement in von Hippel-Lindau disease. The Groupe Francophone d'Etude de la Maladie de von Hippel-Lindau. *Gastroenterology* 2000;119(4):1087–1095.

129. Hoang MP, Hruban RH, Albores-Saavedra J. Clear cell endocrine pancreatic tumor mimicking renal cell carcinoma: a distinctive neoplasm of von Hippel-Lindau disease. *Am J Surg Pathol* 2001;25(5):602–609.

130. Lubensky IA, Pack S, Ault D, et al. Multiple neuroendocrine tumors of the pancreas in von Hippel-Lindau disease patients: histopathological and molecular genetic analysis. *Am J Surg Pathol* 1998;153(1):223–231.

131. Capella C, Heitz PU, Hofler H, Solcia E, Kloppel G. Revised classification of neuroendocrine tumors of the lung, pancreas and gut. *Digestion* 1994;55(suppl 3):11–23.

132. Heitz PU, Kasper M, Polak JM, Kloppel G. Pancreatic endocrine tumors. *Hum Pathol* 1982;13(3):263–271.

133. Kruseman AC, Knijnenburg G, de la Riviere GB, Bosman FT. Morphology and immunohistochemically-defined endocrine function of pancreatic islet cell tumours. *Histopathology* 1978;2(6):389–399.

134. Liu TH, Zhu Y, Cui QC, et al. Nonfunctioning pancreatic endocrine tumors: an immunohistochemical and electron microscopic analysis of 26 cases. *Pathol Res Pract* 1992;188(1(2)):191–198.

135. Kloppel G, Heitz PU. Pancreatic endocrine tumors. *Pathol Res Pract* 1988;183(2):155–168.

136. Lam KY, Lo CY. Pancreatic endocrine tumour: a 22-year clinico-pathological experience with morphological, immunohistochemical observation and a review of the literature. *Eur J Surg Oncol* 1997;23(1):36–42.

137. Ligneau B, Lombard-Bohas C, Partensky C, et al. Cystic endocrine tumors of the pancreas: clinical, radiologic, and histopathologic features in 13 cases. *Am J Surg Pathol* 2001;25(6):752–760.

138. Collins BT, Cramer HM. Fine-needle aspiration cytology of islet cell tumors. *Diagn Cytopathol* 1996;15(1):37–45.

139. Pacchioni D, Papotti M, Macri L, Forte G, Bussolati G. Pancreatic oncocytic endocrine tumors: cytologic features of two cases. *Acta Cytol* 1996; 40(4):742–746.

140. Hussain S, Arwini A, Chetty R, Klimstra D. Oncocytic pancreatic endocrine neoplasms: a clinicopathologic and immunohistochemical analysis of 21 cases. *Mod Pathol* 2005;18:279A.

141. Perez-Montiel MD, Frankel WL, Suster S. Neuroendocrine carcinomas of the pancreas with 'Rhabdoid' features. *Am J Surg Pathol* 2003;27(5):642–649.

142. Singh R, Basturk O, Klimstra DS, et al. Lipid-rich variant of pancreatic endocrine neoplasms. *Am J Surg Pathol* 2006;30(2):194–200.

143. Zee SY, Hochwald SN, Conlon KC, Brennan MF, Klimstra DS. Pleomorphic pancreatic endocrine neoplasms: a variant commonly confused with adenocarcinoma. *Am J Surg Pathol* 2005;29(9):1194–1200.

144. Hochwald SN, Zee S, Conlon KC, et al. Prognostic factors in pancreatic endocrine neoplasms: an analysis of 136 cases with a proposal for low-grade and intermediate-grade groups. *J Clin Oncol* 2002;120(11):2633–4262.

145. O'Connor TP, Wade TP, Sunwoo YC, et al. Small cell undifferentiated carcinoma of the pancreas: report of a patient with tumor marker studies. *Cancer* 1992;1570(6):1514–1519.

146. Ordonez NG, Cleary KR, Mackay B. Small cell undifferentiated carcinoma of the pancreas. *Ultrastruct Pathol* 1997;21(5):467–474.

147. Reyes CV, Wang T. Undifferentiated small cell carcinoma of the pancreas: a report of five cases. *Cancer* 1981;1547(10):2500–2502.

148. Corrin B, Gilby ED, Jones NF, Patrick J. Oat cell carcinoma of the pancreas with ectopic ACTH secretion. *Cancer* 1973;31:1523–1527.

149. Hobbs RD, Stewart AF, Ravin ND, Carter D. Hypercalcemia in small cell carcinoma of the pancreas. *Cancer* 1984;153(7):1552–1554.

150. Adair CF, Wenig BM, Heffess CS. Solid and papillary cystic carcinoma of the pancreas: a tumor of low malignant potential [abstract]. *Int J Surg Pathol* 1995;2(suppl):326.

151. Kloppel G, Morohoshi T, John HD, et al. Solid and cystic acinar cell tumour of the pancreas: a tumour in young women with favourable prognosis. *Virchows Arch A Pathol Anat Histol* 1981;392(2):171–183.

152. Kloppel G, Luttges J, Klimstra D, Hruban R, Kern S, Adler G. Solid-pseudopapillary neoplasm. In: Hamilton SR, Aaltonen LA, eds. *Pathology and Genetics of Tumours of the Digestive System.* Lyon, France: IARC Press; 2000: 246–248.

153. Bombi JA, Milla A, Badal JM, et al. Papillary-cystic neoplasm of the pancreas: report of two cases and review of the literature. *Cancer* 1984;1554(4):780–784.

154. Balercia G, Zamboni G, Bogina G, Mariuzzi GM. Solid-cystic tumor of the pancreas: an extensive ultrastructural study of fourteen cases. *J Submicrosc Cytol Pathol* 1995;27(3):331–340.

155. Nishihara K, Nagoshi M, Tsuneyoshi M, Yamaguchi K, Hayashi I. Papillary cystic tumors of the pancreas: assessment of their malignant potential. *Cancer* 1993;171(1):82–92.

156. Oertel JE, Mendelsohn G, Compagno J. Solid and papillary epithelial neoplasms of the pancreas. *Cancer Treat Res* 1982;8:167–171.

157. Pelosi G, Iannucci A, Zamboni G, et al. Solid and cystic papillary neoplasm of the pancreas: a clinico-cytopathologic and immunocytochemical study of five new cases diagnosed by fine-needle aspiration cytology and a review of the literature. *Diagn Cytopathol* 1995;13(3):233–246.

158. Pettinato G, Manivel JC, Ravetto C, et al. Papillary cystic tumor of the pancreas: a clinicopathologic study of 20 cases with cytologic, immunohistochemical, ultrastructural, and flow cytometric observations, and a review of the literature. *Am J Clin Pathol* 1992;98(5):478–488.

159. Lieber MR, Lack EE, Roberts JR, Jr., et al. Solid and papillary epithelial neoplasm of the pancreas: an ultrastructural and immunocytochemical study of six cases. *Am J Surg Pathol* 1987;11(2):85–93.

160. Notohara K, Hamazaki S, Tsukayama C, et al. Solid-pseudopapillary tumor of the pancreas: immunohistochemical localization of neuroendocrine markers and CD10. *Am J Surg Pathol* 2000;24(10):1361–1371.

161. Abraham SC, Wu TT, Hruban RH, et al. Genetic and immunohistochemical analysis of pancreatic acinar cell carcinoma: frequent allelic loss on chromosome 11p and alterations in the APC/beta-catenin pathway. *Am J Pathol* 2002;160(3):953–962.

162. Cao D, Antonescu C, Wong G, et al. Positive immunohistochemical staining of KIT in solid-pseudopapillary neoplasms of the pancreas is not associated with KIT/PDGFRA mutations. *Mod Pathol* 2006;19(9):1157–1163.

163. Sclafani LM, Reuter VE, Coit DG, Brennan MF. The malignant nature of papillary and cystic neoplasm of the pancreas. *Cancer* 1991;168(1):153–158.

164. Tang LH, Aydin H, Brennan MF, Klimstra DS. Clinically aggressive solid pseudopapillary tumors of the pancreas: a report of two cases with components of undifferentiated carcinoma and a comparative clinicopathologic analysis of 34 conventional cases. *Am J Surg Pathol* 2005;29(4):512–519.

CHAPTER 28 ■ PANCREAS CANCER: CLINICAL MANAGEMENT

JOHN P. HOFFMAN, CHRISTOPHER G. WILLETT, AND STEVEN J. COHEN

SURGICAL CONSIDERATIONS IN THE MANAGEMENT OF PANCREATIC ADENOCARCINOMA

The clinical management of pancreatic cancer has undergone many fundamental changes since the 1970s. During that decade, few patients were offered any hope after diagnosis. Since then, however, we have seen major improvements in the safety of surgical resection, the quality of radiation therapy, and the efficacy of systemic therapy. Still, the majority of patients diagnosed with pancreatic adenocarcinoma succumb to the disease.

Once an image (transcutaneous ultrasound, computed tomography [CT] scan, or magnetic resonance imaging) shows an abnormal mass or dilatation of pancreatic and/or bile ducts (from a single stricture), the possibility of a pancreatic cancer should be recognized. From this point on, controversy exists at nearly every step in the process from suspicion of cancer to its proof to its treatment (Fig. 28.1A and B).

If jaundice is associated with a mass in the pancreatic head, the issue of biliary stent placement arises. For many years, surgeons have argued that the majority of mass lesions causing jaundice will be malignant, that inserting a needle into the tumor from the peritoneal cavity may cause tumor seeding, and that preoperative biliary stenting increases the perioperative morbidity and mortality (1–3). Counterarguments would bring up rare lesions such as lymphoma and localized pancreatitis, which can be successfully treated without resection. Furthermore, semiurgent resection solves the problem of obstructive jaundice and therefore obviates the need for preoperative stent placement. Those that provide adjuvant treatment given prior to resection (neoadjuvant therapy) require biopsy proof that the lesion is an adenocarcinoma before providing the therapy. Because neoadjuvant therapy requires a period of at least 2 to 3 months prior to surgery, biliary stenting is also usually necessary for such an approach. Although it has been shown to be problematic in some neoadjuvant series, others had few complications if the stents were changed frequently (4,5). Now that biopsies are more easily obtained by endoscopic ultrasonography and the biopsy needle does not traverse the peritoneal cavity, more surgeons are requesting preoperative biopsies, even when no neoadjuvant therapy is planned. Although pancreatic resection for masses not proven to be neoplastic has been recommended for decades in surgical teachings, the present climate of litigation promotes at least an attempt at preoperative tumor confirmation. Even with state-of-the-art ultrasonic endoscopic biopsy techniques, the fibrosis and inflammatory reaction surrounding many pancreatic adenocarcinomas may render even multiple needle biopsy attempts unsuccessful. Thus, many patients will have resections without preoperative and intraoperative biopsy confirmation of cancer.

The presence of a solid mass increases the probability of cancer. However, several forms of pancreatitis (focal pancreatitis, lymphocytoplasmic sclerosing pancreatitis, chronic pancreatitis) can present as a mass. In addition, pancreatic lymphoma, metastatic lesions, and pancreatic endocrine lesions can also present as pancreatic masses. Each may have a different treatment algorithm (see Chapter 25).

Classically, pancreatic adenocarcinoma in the head of the pancreas will demonstrate obstruction of both pancreatic and bile ducts (double duct sign). Sometimes one or the other duct will be strictured without a visible surrounding mass. These stenoses may be assessed cytologically by endoscopically mediated brushings. Endoscopic ultrasonography may show the presence of a small associated mass not well seen by other imaging modalities. Kalady et al. studied a large series of such patients in an era prior to use of endoscopic ultrasound (6). They found that tumor location (head vs. other), a history of no prior pancreatitis, and an endoscopic retrograde cholangiopancreatography showing no fibrotic changes in pancreatic duct side branches correlated with a 94% chance of a diagnosis of pancreatic cancer. The double duct sign had a positive predictive value of only 65% and a negative predictive value of 87.6% (6). It is therefore rational to proceed with resection in such cases, even after multiple preoperative and intraoperative attempts at biopsy confirmation have failed. However, the patients and their families must be made fully aware of the possible untoward consequences, both with resection (operative complications and the possibility of benign findings) and with observation (continued growth of a malignant lesion).

CYSTIC MASSES

Cystic masses form another controversial category, both from a diagnostic and a treatment perspective. Treatment is, of course, based on an estimate of the future behavior of any given lesion. Formerly, lesions were grouped by imaging characteristics into serous and mucinous lesions. Now we have a spectrum from a small, microcystic lesion to a large either single or complex cyst. We can now measure many cytologic and molecular features of the fluid and cell walls. However, there is not unanimity of opinion as to when to resect these lesions. Allen et al. from Memorial Sloan-Kettering Cancer Center have a large database of patients with cystic lesions of the pancreas who have been either observed or operated on based on radiographic and clinical criteria (size <3 cm, no solid component, no septations, and no pain) (7). This was a retrospective review of what surgeons

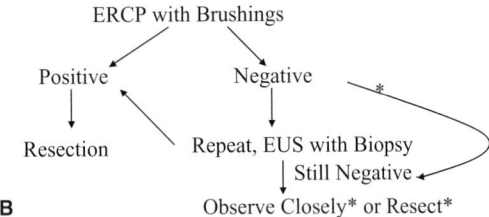

A:
Mass in Pancreas

Head of Pancreas   Body   Tail

Involving Major Vessels or Adjacent Organs

Yes   No

Laparoscopy* ──────→ Distant Metastases

No Distant Metastases

Biopsy Lesion   Resection or   Chemotherapy,
                 Biopsy*   Palliative Surgery*

If +

Preoperative   Postoperative
A Adjuvant Therapy*   Adjuvant Therapy

Stricture in Bile Duct or Pancreatic Duct (No History of Pancreatitis)

ERCP with Brushings

Positive   Negative   *

Resection   Repeat, EUS with Biopsy
             Still Negative
B
             Observe Closely* or Resect*

FIGURE 28.1. A: Algorithm for a mass in the pancreas. **B:** Algorith for a bile duct or pancreatic duct stricture. * Denotes an area of controversy. ERCP, endoscopic retrograde cholangiopancreatography; EUS, endoscopic ultrasound.

decided at this institution. The study is ongoing, but preliminary reporting indicates that there are cysts <3 cm in diameter, without symptoms, solid components, or septations that are safe to observe. Many others have been in the process of assessing endoscopically obtained cyst fluid for the discovery of tissue fragments or molecular markers of malignancy (8–10).

Once a lesion is either proven or highly suspected to be pancreatic adenocarcinoma, issues of importance in the therapy are resectability, the conduct of the resection, and adjuvant therapy. The latter is largely covered in the subsequent sections from the perspectives of radiation therapy and chemotherapy.

RESECTABILITY

Definitions of what constitutes a lesion that may be removed with safety and a reasonable probability of prolonged postoperative survival have varied since the 1970s. When surgical resection was the only method of therapy, only those lesions that were small, well away from the superior mesenteric vessels, and free of gross nodal metastases held any chance for meaningful prolonged postoperative survival. With the advent of somewhat effective adjuvant therapy, larger lesions and those impinging on the mesenteric vessels and involving regional lymph nodes can now be safely removed and occasionally achieve significant postoperative survival (11).

The 1970s definition of a resectable cancer was that of a lesion without distant or regional nodal spread and one that was not abutting the superior mesenteric vessels. An intraoperative test for resectability was the easy passage of a clamp beneath the neck of the pancreas overlying the superior mesenteric vein. Current imaging criteria for resectability include lack of distant metastases and the same lack of involvement of the superior mesenteric vein, as well as a clear fat plane surrounding the superior mesenteric artery (SMA). With the demonstration of chemotherapy and radiation therapy effects on these tumors, many have used this adjuvant therapy in a preoperative

---

TABLE 28.1

THREE RESECTABILITY CATEGORIES FOR LOCALIZED PANCREATIC ADENOCARCINOMA

RESECTABLE
No distant metastases
Clear fat plane around celiac, hepatic, and superior mesenteric arteries
No abutment of superior mesenteric vein or portal vein

BORDERLINE RESECTABLE
No distant metastases
Abutment of celiac, hepatic, or superior mesenteric arteries
Abutment, compression, or short segment occlusion of superior mesenteric or portal vein
Mesocolic, colonic, or gastric invasion

LOCALLY ADVANCED, UNRESECTABLE
No distant metastases
Encasement of superior mesenteric artery or celiac axis
Long segment occlusion of portal or superior mesenteric vein without adequate trunk on either side to accept graft

---

sequence, allowing for marginfree resections of more locally advanced pancreatic cancers (12). These locally advanced cancers are defined as borderline resectable lesions (Table 28.1). Those lesions that are considered never to be resectable, even with successful preoperative adjuvant therapy, are called locally unresectable (Table 28.1). These terms have been poorly delineated in the literature, such that the conscientious readers must be cautious as to the effects of treatment until they understand the extent of the lesions being discussed.

Laparoscopy performed as a separate preoperative procedure or done immediately prior to a planned resection may occasionally discover distant metastases not seen on imaging studies. Opinion and data differ as to its indications (13,14). As imaging becomes more discriminative and tumors become smaller, the indications for staging laparoscopy will diminish. For more advanced lesions and those arising in the tail or body of the pancreas (usually discovered at a later stage), most authors would advise preoperative laparoscopy. The scope of the procedure may also vary, from an inspection of the peritoneal surfaces only to laparoscopic liver ultrasound and dissection within the lesser omental bursa and excisional biopsy of distant nodes. See Chapter 26 for a full discussion of these issues.

SURGICAL PROCEDURES

The procedures usually performed for pancreatic cancer are pancreatoduodenectomy with or without resection of the gastric antrum and pylorus (Whipple or Kausch-Whipple procedure), distal pancreatectomy, and total pancreatectomy (Fig. 28.2). The primary indications for each procedure are the location and extent of the cancer. There have been multiple trials comparing the pylorus-preserving and antrectomy operations, but there were no strong differences in tumor control or quality of life found.

Some surgeons stress a complete dissection of tissue surrounding the SMA, whereas the majority leaves some adjacent tissue and the nerve plexi around it. There have been several surgical trials of "radical" versus "standard" lymph node and soft tissue dissection (15–17). However, the definition of what peripancreatic lymphatic and soft tissue should be included in the "standard" dissection varies. Even the smallest pancreatic

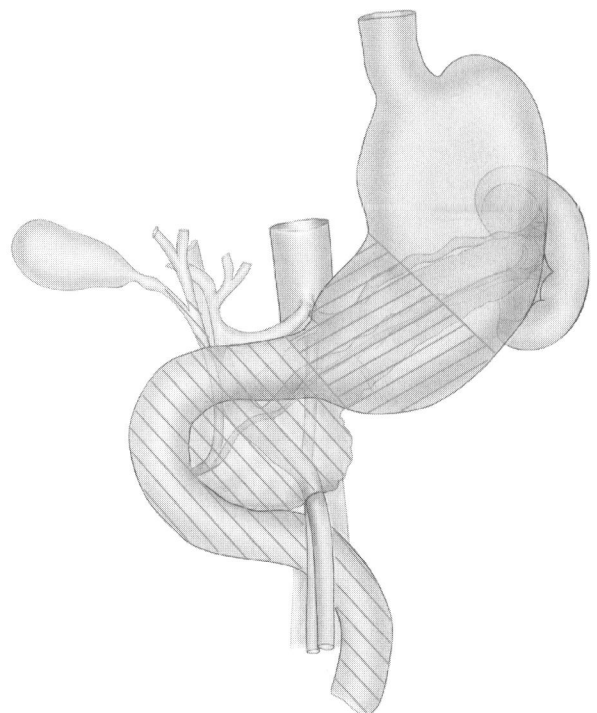

FIGURE 28.2. Tissues removed for a pylorus-preserving pancreato-duodenectomy are shown in the nearly vertical lines. The additional tissue for a classical Whipple procedure is shaded by the near horizontal lines. The gallbladder is removed in both procedures.

adenocarcinomas will not have widely free surgical margins because of the close proximity of the pancreatic head and uncinate process to the superior mesenteric vessels. Thus, it is rational to dissect at least all tissue from the tumor edge to the nearest side of the superior mesenteric vessels, and to resect all lymph nodes within 5 to 6 cm of the tumor.

What adjacent organs or tissues may be resected along with a pancreatic cancer and what is the expectation of disease control? Direct invasion of a cancer into the colon, mesocolon, adrenal gland, stomach, small bowel, or superior mesenteric vein does not render that cancer unresectable or incurable (18). However, resection of liver metastases along with primary cancers is not associated with long-term survival.

Complications of Surgery

Other than the usual morbidity and mortality of major abdominal surgery, pancreatic resection has its unique complications. Whenever the pancreas is divided, its reconnection to either the small bowel or stomach is sometimes tenuous. The incidence of leakage from the pancreatic anastomosis is increased with a soft pancreas and a small pancreatic duct, and in hospitals where the surgery is not performed frequently (19,20). There are many definitions of leakage at the pancreatic anastomosis (21). Therefore, its incidence is unclear. However, the most serious complications of intraabdominal hemorrhage and infection are usually associated with leakage at the pancreatic anastomosis. Fortunately, this is an unusual occurrence in experienced hands.

Palliative Surgery

Palliative surgery may be emergency or elective. Often, ulceration in the stomach or duodenum by a cancer may occur. This

is more common after chemotherapy and/or radiation therapy have shrunken the cancer and left a hemorrhaging vessel. Usually, these vessels can be controlled with embolization by the interventional radiologist, but occasionally the tumor and vessel need to be excised. The operation performed in these circumstances is usually an R2 resection (where gross tumor is left behind). Although this type of procedure is not recommended unless it is the only option to immediately save a life, it has occasionally been associated with long survival in a patient with a cancer sensitive to chemotherapy.

The more common emergency surgery for these tumors is bypass of an obstructed duodenum by gastrojejunostomy (22). Although most patients with peritoneal metastases from pancreatic cancer will eventually develop small bowel obstruction, it is unusual for the surgeon to be able to help them because the metastases are frequently diffuse.

Elective palliative surgery will be either to alleviate or prevent future biliary or duodenal obstruction. This would usually be in the setting of a planned resection where distant metastases were discovered, thus rendering resection irrational. Because the patient's abdominal cavity is already exposed, a bypass of the bile duct and duodenum can be performed without any extra incision. A prospective, randomized trial showed that approximately 20% of these patients will go on to have duodenal obstruction before death if no prophylactic bypass is done (23). However, most surgeons would use nonoperative means to bypass biliary or duodenal obstructions in patients with metastatic disease proven before exploratory celiotomy.

Patency of bile duct or duodenum can be accomplished by means of stents by the gastroenterologists or interventional radiologists. There have been a number of trials comparing biliary stents with surgical bypass (24). Most of these show that surgical procedures necessitate more hospitalization initially but less eventually, and produce much longer palliation without the need for stent change. Even the larger metal stents will need attention every 4 to 6 months. As this technology advances, there will probably be little need for open surgical palliative procedures. However, laparoscopically performed bypasses will probably be more competitive.

RADIATION THERAPY IN THE TREATMENT OF PANCREATIC ADENOCARCINOMA

Adjuvant Therapy

After resection of pancreatic cancer, local recurrence occurs in 50% to 90% of patients (25–28). Forty to 90% of patients develop distant metastases, most commonly in the liver and/or peritoneum. For this reason, adjuvant radiation therapy, chemotherapy, and combined radiation and chemotherapy have been studied in an effort to improve patient outcomes (Table 28.2). However, despite multiple trials, a definitive role for adjuvant therapy for resected pancreatic cancer has not been established.

Prospective Trials

The Gastrointestinal Tumor Study Group (GITSG) conducted the first prospective trial of adjuvant chemoradiotherapy for patients with resected pancreatic cancer and negative surgical margins (29). These patients were randomized to external beam radiation therapy (ERBT) to 40 Gy delivered in split-course fashion with concurrent 5-fluorouracil (5-FU) 500 mg/m^2 given as an intravenous bolus on the first 3 and last 3 days of

TABLE 28.2

PROSPECTIVE, RANDOMIZED TRIALS FOR ADJUVANT THERAPY FOR PANCREATIC CANCER

Series	No. of patients	Median Survival (mo)	2-yr Survival	5-yr Survival
GASTROINTESTINAL TUMOR STUDY GROUP (29)				
Treatment	21	21.0	43%	19%
Observation	22	10.9	18%	5%
Treatment (expanded cohort) (30)	30	18.0	46%	NA
EUROPEAN ORGANIZATION FOR RESEARCH AND TREATMENT OF CANCER (31)				
Treatment	60	17.1	37%	20%
Observation	54	12.6	23%	10%

Series	No. of patients	Survival (mo)	2-yr Survival	5-yr Survival
EUROPEAN STUDY GROUP FOR PANCREATIC CANCER-1 (32,33)				
Pooled data				
Chemotherapy	244	19.7	NA	NA
No chemotherapy	237	14.0	NA	NA
Chemoradiation	178	15.5	NA	NA
No chemoradiation	180	16.1	NA	NA
2 × 2 Factorial				
Chemotherapy	147	20.1	40%	21%
No chemotherapy	142	15.5	30%	8%
Chemoradiation	145	15.9	29%	10%
No chemoradiation	144	17.9	41%	20%

NA, not applicable.

radiation, followed by maintenance 5-FU for 2 years or until disease progression, or to observation only. This trial was stopped early secondary to slow accrual (43 patients over 8 years) and a positive interim analysis, which found that patients treated on the chemoradiotherapy arm had a positive survival benefit. Patients who received chemoradiotherapy had a longer median survival (21 months vs. 11 months) and a higher 2-year survival (43% vs. 19%). An additional 30 patients were then enrolled to receive adjuvant chemoradiation (30). These additional patients confirmed the survival outcomes seen in the original trial with median survival of 18 months and a 2-year survival of 46%. The GITSG trial was criticized for many reasons: only 9% of patients received the 2-year maintenance chemotherapy, the radiation dose was low, the number of patients was small, there was slow accrual, there was an unusually poor survival for the surgical control group, 25% of patients did not begin adjuvant therapy until more than 10 weeks after resection, and 32% of the original treatment arm had violations of the scheduled radiation therapy. Nevertheless, this trial resulted in chemoradiation therapy being accepted as appropriate adjuvant therapy in the United States.

A second study sponsored by the European Organization for Research and Treatment of Cancer sought to confirm the findings of the original GITSG study (31). In this trial, 218 patients with resected pancreas or periampullary cancers were randomly assigned to receive 40 Gy of EBRT in a split-dose fashion with concurrent continuous infusional 5-FU (25 mg/kg/day) or observation alone. This study showed no significant improvement ($p = 0.208$) in median survival (24 months vs. 19 months) or 2-year survival (51% vs. 41%). Interestingly, only 114 of the patients enrolled on trial had pancreatic cancer, the remaining patients had ampullary tumors. Subset analysis of the patients with primary pancreatic tumors showed a 2-year survival of 34% for treated patients versus 26% for the control group ($p = 0.099$). Criticisms of this trial are that there was no maintenance chemotherapy given in the treatment arm, patients with positive surgical margins were allowed on trial with no prospective assessment, the radiation dose was low, there were low numbers of patients, and 20% of patients assigned to treatment never received treatment.

The European Study Group for Pancreatic Cancer (ESPAC) then conducted the largest trial evaluating adjuvant therapy for pancreatic cancer, ESPAC-1 (32). Treating physicians were allowed to enroll their patients onto one of three parallel randomized studies:

- Chemoradiation versus no chemoradiation ($n = 69$): Chemoradiation was 20 Gy over 2 weeks with 5-FU 500 mg/m² on days 1 to 3, and then repeated after a 2-week break.
- Chemotherapy versus no chemotherapy ($n = 192$): Chemotherapy was bolus 5-FU (425 mg/m²) and leucovorin (20 mg/m²) given daily for 5 days every 28 days for 6 months.
- A 2 × 2 factorial design of 289 patients enrolled on chemoradiotherapy ($n = 73$), chemotherapy ($n = 75$), chemoradiotherapy with maintenance chemotherapy ($n = 72$), or observation ($n = 69$).

The data from the treatment groups from all three parallel trials were then pooled for analysis. There was no survival difference between the 175 patients who received adjuvant chemoradiation and the 178 patients who did not receive therapy (median survival 15.5 months vs. 16.1 months, $p = 0.24$). There was, however, a survival benefit found for the patients who received adjuvant chemotherapy ($n = 238$) compared to those who did not ($n = 235$) (median survival 19.7 months vs. 14 months, $p = 0.0005$). On further follow-up of the 289 patients selected to the 2×2 factorial design trial, the 5 year survival rate for the patients who received chemotherapy was 21% versus 8% for those who did not (33).

Like its predecessors, the ESPAC-1 trial had many criticisms:

- Physicians and patients were allowed to choose which of the three parallel trials to enroll in, creating bias.
- Patients could receive "background" chemoradiation or chemotherapy if decided by their physician. Approximately one-third of the patients enrolled on the chemotherapy versus no chemotherapy trial received "background" chemoradiation therapy or chemotherapy.
- The radiation therapy was given in a split-dose fashion, with the treating physician judging the final treatment dose (40 Gy vs. 60 Gy).

In addition, there were no uniform guidelines for radiation therapy administration across participating centers and no central quality assurance review. The investigators of this trial concluded that (a) there was no benefit from adjuvant chemoradiation therapy, and (b) there was a benefit to adjuvant chemotherapy.

Recently, a meta-analysis of randomized adjuvant therapy trials for pancreatic cancer reported an improved outcome of patients with resected tumors with positive margins receiving postoperative radiation therapy and chemotherapy (34). It was recommended that further study of chemoradiation be pursued in this subset of patients.

Single Institution Experiences

Reports of single-institution experiences with adjuvant therapy for pancreatic cancer have provided support to the benefit of adjuvant therapy. The largest of these series is from The Johns Hopkins Medical Institutions, where investigators reported the results of a retrospective analysis of 174 patients who were treated by one of the following approaches: (a) EBRT (40–45 Gy) with two 3-day courses of 5-FU at the beginning and end of radiation, followed by weekly bolus 5-FU (500 mg/m^2) for 4 months ($n = 99$); (b) EBRT (50.4–57.6 Gy) to the pancreatic bed plus prophylactic hepatic irradiation (23.4–27 Gy) given with infusional 5-FU (200 mg/m^2/day) plus leucovorin (5 mg/m^2/day) for 5 of 7 days of the week for 4 months ($n = 21$); or (c) no therapy ($n = 53$) (35). Patients who received adjuvant chemoradiation had a median survival of 20 months compared to 14 months for patients who were not treated. Two-year survival was 44% and 30%, respectively. There was no survival advantage to the more intensive adjuvant therapy. A follow-up report from this group of 616 patients with resected pancreatic cancer found adjuvant chemoradiation treatment as a strong predictor of outcome, with a hazard ratio of 0.5 (36).

In addition to the Johns Hopkins series, a few small series from the Mayo Clinic and the University of Pennsylvania have also reported survival benefit to adjuvant chemoradiation therapy (37,38). In these series, the EBRT dosed in a range of 45 to 54 Gy in combination with 5-FU–based therapy yielded a superior 5-year survival compared to no therapy (17% vs. 4% and 43% vs. 35%, respectively). A series of Medicare patients from the Surveillance, Epidemiology, and End Results database has found an improved median and 3-year survival for patients who received adjuvant chemoradiation therapy over those who did not (29 months vs. 12.5 months, 45% vs. 30%, respectively) (39). However, it must be noted that in these retrospective analyses, there is a possible bias toward the treatment of better-risk patients.

Data with the highest seen survival after adjuvant therapy for pancreatic cancer come from a phase II trial done at Virginia Mason University (40). Results from 43 of 53 enrolled patients on this study were reported in 2003. These patients were treated with EBRT to 50 Gy, with concurrent chemotherapy of 5-FU 200 mg/m^2/day continuous infusion, cisplatin 30 mg/m^2 weekly, and IFN-α 3 million units subcutaneously every other day. After completion of chemoradiation, patients received 5-FU 200 mg/m^2/day continuous infusion on weeks 10 through 15 and 18 through 23. The median survival, 2-year overall survival, and 5-year overall survival were 44 months, 58%, and 45%, respectively. With these encouraging data came significant toxicity, with 70% of patients experiencing grade 3 toxicities, and 42% of patients requiring hospitalization. The American College of Surgeons Oncology Group has recently completed a larger, multicenter, phase II trial of 100 patients to further investigate this regimen.

Current Trials

There are several ongoing large clinical trials that are attempting to further clarify the role of adjuvant therapy for pancreatic cancer. The first is Radiation Therapy Oncology Group (RTOG) and GI Intergroup Trial 9704. This is a phase III study of 519 patients with resected pancreatic cancer randomized to either 3 weeks of continuous infusional 5-FU at 250 mg/m^2/day, followed by chemoradiation (50.4 Gy in 1.8-Gy daily fractions with continuous infusional 5-FU at 250 mg/m^2/day) and then two 4-week courses of continuous infusional 5-FU at 250 mg/m^2/day with 2 weeks rest between courses to begin 3 to 5 weeks after completion of chemoradiation, or three weekly doses of gemcitabine at 1,000 mg/m^2/week, followed by the same 5-FU–based chemoradiation as in the first arm and then 3 months of gemcitabine 1,000 mg/m^2 given weekly 3 of every 4 weeks. Accrual to this trial has been completed. In Europe and Australia, ESPAC-3 has enrolled more than 500 patients of a planned 990. Originally, this study was to randomized patients with resected pancreatic cancer into one of three arms: 5-FU (425 mg/m^2) and leucovorin (20 mg/m^2) given daily for 5 days every 28 days for 6 months, gemcitabine (1,000 mg/m^2) given weekly over 30 minutes for 3 of 4 weeks for 6 months, or observation. However, with the release of the matured ESPAC-1 data confirming a survival benefit to chemotherapy over observation, the observation arm has now been dropped from this trial. Notably, radiation therapy has been excluded from this trial.

Neoadjuvant Therapy

Even after undergoing curative resection for pancreatic cancer, 80% to 85% of patients will recur. In addition, positive margins or nodal disease increases this rate of recurrence to 90% (41,42). The concept of preresectional radiation therapy for these cancers arose in the early 1980s (43,44). Chemotherapy was added to the radiation therapy in the late 1980s (45,46). The use of neoadjuvant chemoradiation offers another possible way to improve on these figures for several reasons:

- Approximately 25% of patients do not receive adjuvant therapy in a timely manner after surgery or do not receive it at all (36,47).
- Given the high recurrence rates after surgical resection, pancreatic cancer is likely a systemic disease at the time of

diagnosis in 80% to 85% of patients who appear to have resectable disease (48,49), and with neoadjuvant therapy, 20% to 40% of patients will be spared the morbidity of resection because their metastatic disease becomes clinically apparent (50).

- ■ Preoperative therapy could theoretically be less toxic and more effective because the chemotherapy and radiation would be given without the postsurgical issues of small bowel in the radiation field and decreased oxygenation and decreased drug delivery to the remaining tumor bed (51).
- ■ Many patients with borderline resectable and occasional patients with unresectable lesions may be able to be downstaged to allow for surgical resection.

Other putative but unproven advantages are the preservation of function of stomach and small bowel spared from irradiation and the decreased frequency of pancreatojejunostomy leaks (19).

Indications for preoperative adjuvant therapy vary from the clearly resectable to the borderline resectable patient. The primary proponents for preoperative therapy for clearly resectable lesions have been the pancreatic surgeons at the MD Anderson Cancer Center. Because of the previous theoretical advantages to preoperative adjuvant therapy sequencing, they prefer to use it in any patient with a biopsy-proven pancreatic adenocarcinoma. They have performed several serial phase II studies of different preoperative regimens (50). The diseasefree and overall survival rates from these regimens rival any reports from postoperative adjuvant therapy trials. However, no phase III trials of preoperative versus postoperative sequencing have been conducted. Superior results may be obtained in any phase II trial simply by patient selection. Although we have many prognostic indicators for any given cancer (size, differentiation, depth of invasion, venous or arterial abutment or invasion, presence and number of nodal metastases, type of tumor, CA19–9 status), there are undoubtedly others not yet discovered. Thus, the question of the value of any sort of neoadjuvant therapy (as opposed to postoperative adjuvant therapy) will remain unanswered until phase III testing is done.

Another indication for preoperative adjuvant therapy is in the patient with borderline resectable pancreatic cancer because such a lesion would not be able to be resected with clear margins without the preoperative therapy. In a review of patients treated at one institution by either preoperative or postoperative chemoradiotherapy, Pingpank et al. showed that preoperative therapy led to more clear surgical margins and fewer multiply positive margins than did postoperative adjuvant therapy (12). The group treated with postoperative adjuvant therapy was actually a more favorable group with respect to tumor size and resectability status. Eventually, however, this setting for preoperative therapy will probably also need to be studied in phase III trials.

Before too much progress can be made in this group of patients with borderline resectable cancers, we need to develop and adopt a complex grading system of imaging parameters that could be correlated to clinical outcomes in order to determine specific prognostic factors for each imaging characteristic (52).

5-Fluorouracil—Based Regimens

Small initial studies of neoadjuvant radiation with and without continuous infusion 5-FU established the tolerability of this regimen, but showed no improvement in survival or resectability for these patients (43,44,53–55). For this reason, further studies were done increasing the radiation dose, with differ-

ent chemotherapy regimens, and with intraoperative radiation therapy (IORT) at the time of surgery.

The Eastern Cooperative Oncology Group (ECOG) treated 53 patients with potentially resectable pancreatic cancer with 5-FU 1,000 mg/m^2/day continuous infusion on days 2 to 5 and 29 to 32 of radiation, mitomycin 10 mg/m^2 on day 2, and EBRT to 50.4 Gy[4]. Nine (17%) of the treated patients developed either local progression of disease or distant metastases and were not surgical candidates, 11 patients (21%) had metastatic disease at surgery, and complete resection was possible in 24 of the 41 patients taken to surgery. For the patients who underwent resection, the median survival was 16 months, and 10 months for the entire group. The poor survival for the patients who did undergo resection was likely due to 3 of the patients having positive peritoneal cytology, 4 having lymph node metastases, 13 having close surgical margins, and 4 needing resection of the superior mesenteric vein. In addition, more than 50% of the treated patients required hospitalization due to treatment toxicity.

At MD Anderson Cancer Center, multiple trials of neoadjuvant 5-FU—based chemoradiation have been performed. The first trial treated 28 patients with 5-FU 300 mg/m^2/day continuous infusion with concurrent EBRT to 50.4 Gy over 5.5 weeks (55). Patients who underwent surgical resection also received intraoperative radiation therapy. Twenty-five percent of patients had evidence of metastatic disease on preoperative restaging. Fifteen percent had metastatic disease that was found on laparoscopy. For the patients that underwent surgery, median survival was 18 months, and 41% had a pathological partial response to therapy. However, 33% of patients treated on this study required hospitalization for gastrointestinal toxicity from therapy. For this reason, the next trials from this group focused on rapid fractionation EBRT. A prospective trial of 35 patients treated with EBRT to 30 Gy (3 Gy per fraction for 10 fractions) with concurrent 5-FU 300 mg/m^2/day continuous infusion found grade 3 nausea and vomiting in only 9% of patients with no grade 4 toxicities (56). Twenty-seven patients were taken to surgery and 20 patients underwent resection and IORT to 10 to 15 Gy. Locoregional recurrence occurred in only 2 of the 20 resected patients. Median survival for patients who underwent surgery was 25 months with a 3-year survival of 23%.

Gemcitabine-Based Regimens

Several phase I studies have attempted to use the radiosensitization effects and the improved efficacy in advanced pancreatic cancer of gemcitabine in the neoadjuvant setting. A phase I study of twice-weekly gemcitabine in combination with EBRT to 50.4 Gy in 28 fractions for patients with localized pancreatic cancer found a maximum tolerated dose (MTD) of 50 mg/m^2 twice a week (57). Another phase I study used full-dose gemcitabine in combination with EBRT (58). The gemcitabine was given as 1,000 mg/m^2 over 30 minutes on days 1, 8, and 15 of a 28-day cycle. Radiation therapy was directed at the primary tumor alone at a starting radiation dose of 24 Gy in 1.6-Gy fractions. The MTD of the radiation was 36 Gy in 2.4-Gy fractions. The dose-limiting toxicities were vomiting and gastroduodenal ulceration. The phase II trial of this regimen enrolled 41 patients with resectable or locally advanced pancreatic cancer. Eight of the 32 evaluable patients for toxicity showed grade 3 gastrointestinal toxicity, grade 3 fatigue, and one unexplained death (59). Survival data are not yet available. Another trial of weekly gemcitabine at a dose of 400 mg/m^2 for seven doses plus concurrent ERBT to 30 Gy in 10 fractions over 2 weeks, beginning 3 days after first gemcitabine dose, has had preliminary results reported (60). Of the 86 patients treated, all received the total dose of radiation, but only 45%

received the full dose of gemcitabine. Forty-three percent of patients were hospitalized prior to surgery. However, 86% of patients went to laparotomy, with 73% undergoing a successful tumor resection, and 59% of tumor specimens had >50% tumor necrosis. The median survival was 37 months.

Gemcitabine has also been studied in combination with other chemotherapy agents and EBRT in the neoadjuvant setting. A phase I study of 19 patients with pancreatic cancer evaluated the MTD of cisplatin when given with gemcitabine at 1,000 mg/m^2 weekly with EBRT to 36 Gy given in 2.4-Gy fractions (61). Cisplatin was given on days 1 and 15 following gemcitabine. The MTD of cisplatin was 40 mg/m^2. Another trial by the MD Anderson Cancer Center group evaluated a treatment schedule of gemcitabine 750 mg/m^2 and cisplatin 30 mg/m^2 given every 14 days for four treatments, followed by four weekly doses of gemcitabine at 400 mg/m^2 concurrent with 30 Gy of EBRT given as 3-Gy fractions over 2 weeks, beginning 2 days after the first dose of gemcitabine (62). Preliminary results from 37 patients showed 67% underwent resection, with 70% of the pathological specimens showing necrosis of >50% of the tumor. This regimen, however, had significant toxicity, with 62% of patients requiring hospitalization, most due to biliary stent occlusion.

Taxane-Based Regimens

In radiobiological models, paclitaxel may result in enhanced radiosensitization through (a) synchronization of tumor cells at G2/M, a relatively radiosensitive phase of cell cycle; and (b) tumor reoxygenation after apoptotic clearance of paclitaxel-damaged cells. Pisters et al. from MD Anderson Cancer Center examined the use of paclitaxel as a radiation sensitizer in the neoadjuvant setting for pancreatic cancer (63). In this trial, 35 patients received paclitaxel 60 mg/m^2 weekly with concurrent EBRT to 30 Gy. Eighty percent underwent resection with 21% of pathology specimens showing >50% tumor necrosis. The 3-year survival for the patients who underwent preoperative therapy and resection was 28%. Hospitalization was required in 11% of patients for toxicity, primarily involving nausea and vomiting. These preliminary data show an increased toxicity without a significant improvement compared to histologic response rate or overall survival for this paclitaxel-based regimen.

Targeted Therapies/Future Directions

Future directions for neoadjuvant therapy include the incorporation of novel, targeted agents with ERBT alone or with chemoradiation, and newer radiation therapy techniques. The use of targeted therapies is based on impressive phase II data combining targeted agents with chemotherapy in the metastatic pancreatic cancer setting. A phase II trial of the vascular endothelial growth factor (VEGF) inhibitor, bevacizumab, in combination with gemcitabine for patients with advanced pancreatic cancer (64) has shown a response rate of 27% compared to 5.6% historically for gemcitabine alone (65), and a 1-year survival of 53% compared to <20%, respectively. A phase II trial of an epidermal growth factor receptor (EGFR) inhibitor, cetuximab, in combination with gemcitabine for patients with advanced pancreatic cancer has shown a 1-year survival of 33% (66). In addition, a randomized controlled phase III trial of gemcitabine ± erlotinib, another EGFR inhibitor, has shown a 23.5% increase in overall survival with the addition of erlotinib compared to gemcitabine alone (67). No trials of these agents in the neoadjuvant setting have yet been reported, but preliminary results are available in the locally advanced setting. The use of intraoperative ra-

diation therapy technique and three-dimensional conformal radiation therapy is further discussed in the locally advanced section.

Unfortunately, there are few randomized studies comparing different chemotherapy partners for radiation therapy in pancreatic cancer. In addition, results regarding resectability are difficult to compare due to differing definitions of unresectable disease. Recent efforts by the ECOG to compare gemcitabine with 5-FU−based radiation programs for potentially resectable patients (E1200) and gemcitabine alone with gemcitabine and radiation therapy (E4201) for unresectable disease both closed due to poor accrual. A small study randomized 34 patients with locally advanced disease to receive radiation therapy with either weekly gemcitabine 600 mg/m^2 ($n = 18$) or 3 days of bolus 5-FU every 2 weeks ($n = 16$) (68). Although median survival favored gemcitabine (14.5 m vs. 7.1 m, $p = 0.027$), the small sample size and significant toxicity limits firm conclusions. Thus, either 5-FU or gemcitabine (but not both) can be administered with radiation therapy for locally advanced disease or as preoperative therapy. However, the impact on the natural history of the disease is unclear and patient prognosis, if not rendered resectable, is uniformly fatal. Thus, the study of new compounds with radiation therapy is critical. A phase I study of bevacizumab with capecitabine and radiation in locally advanced pancreatic cancer documented a response rate of 20% with 4 patients able to undergo a margin negative resection. However, 4 patients had more than or equal to a grade 3 gastrointestinal ulceration with bleeding or perforation (69). An RTOG phase II study of this regimen recently reached its accrual goal. In preclinical pancreatic cancer models, cetuximab with gemcitabine and radiation resulted in greater growth inhibition than either therapy alone both in vitro and in vivo (70). In head and neck cancer, the addition of cetuximab to radiation therapy significantly improves both locoregional control and survival (71). Thus, several investigations of cetuximab with concurrent radiation therapy are underway in pancreatic cancer, including a German study of cetuximab with gemcitabine and IMRT (72) and an adjuvant ECOG study of capecitabine with cetuximab and radiation therapy.

Locally Advanced Therapy

Patients with locally advanced carcinoma of the pancreas comprise a group of patients with an intermediate prognosis between resectable and metastatic patients. These patients have pancreatic tumors that are defined as surgically unresectable but have no evidence of distant metastases. As described previously, a tumor is considered to be unresectable if it has one of the following features:

- Extensive peripancreatic lymph node involvement and/or distant metastases (typically to the liver or peritoneum)
- Encasement or occlusion of the superior mesenteric vein (SMV) or SMV/portal vein confluence
- Direct involvement of the SMA, inferior vena cava, aorta, or celiac axis

However, recent advances in surgical technique may allow for resection of selected patients with tumors involving the SMV (73). Combined treatment with radiation and chemotherapy increases median survival for patients with locally advanced cancers to approximately 9 to 13 months but rarely results in long-term survival. The therapeutic options of patients with locally advanced pancreatic cancer include EBRT with 5-FU chemotherapy, and more recently, EBRT with novel chemotherapeutic and target agents. In evaluating the results of these various therapies, it is useful to remember that a median survival of 3 to 6 months has been reported for this subset of patients undergoing palliative gastric or biliary bypass only (74).

TABLE 28.3

PROSPECTIVE, RANDOMIZED TRIALS FOR LOCALLY ADVANCED, UNRESECTABLE PANCREATIC CANCER

Series	No. of patients	Median survival (mo)	Local failure	1-yr Survival	18-mo Survival
MAYO CLINIC (75)					
EBRT (35–40 Gy/3–4 wk) only	32	6.3	NS	6%	6%
EBRT (35–40 Gy/3–4 wk) + 5-flourouracil (5-FU)	32	10.4	NS	22%	13%
GITSG (76)					
EBRT (60 Gy/10 wk) only	25	5.3	24%	10%	5%
EBRT (40 Gy/6 wk) + 5-FU	83	8.4	26%	35%	20%
EBRT (60 Gy/10 wk) + 5-FU	86	11.4	27%	46%	20%
GITSG (77)					
EBRT (60 Gy/10 wk) + 5-FU	73	8.5	58% (First site)	33%	15%
EBRT (40 Gy/4 wk) + doxorubicin	70	7.6	51% (First site)	27%	17%
GITSG (78)					
EBRT (54 Gy/6 wk) + 5-FU and SMF	22	9.7	45% (First site)	41%	18%
SMF only	21	7.4	48% (First site)	19%	0%
ECOG (79)					
EBRT (40 Gy/6 wk) + 5-FU	47	8.3	32%	26%	11%
5-FU only	44	8.2	32%	32%	21%

ERBT, external beam radiation therapy; NS, not significant; GITSG, Gastrointestinal Tumor Study Group; SMF, streptozocin, mitomycin-C, and 5-FU; ECOG; Eastern Cooperative Oncology Group.

Prospective Trials

With the exception of one trial, conventional EBRT for locally advanced pancreatic cancer has been shown to improve survival when combined with 5-FU compared to EBRT alone or chemotherapy alone (Table 28.3). The Mayo Clinic undertook an early randomized trial in the 1960s in which 64 patients with locally unresectable, nonmetastatic pancreatic adenocarcinoma received 35 to 40 Gy of EBRT with concurrent 5-FU versus the same EBRT schedule plus placebo. A significant survival advantage was seen for patients receiving EBRT with 5-FU versus EBRT only (10.4 months vs. 6.3 months) (75).

The GITSG followed with a similar study comparing EBRT alone to EBRT with concurrent and maintenance 5-FU (76). One hundred and ninety-four eligible patients with surgically confirmed unresectable and nonmetastatic pancreatic adenocarcinoma were randomized to receive 60 Gy split-course EBRT alone, 40 Gy split-course EBRT with two to three cycles of concurrent bolus 5-FU chemotherapy, or 60 Gy split-course EBRT using a similar chemotherapy regimen. Patients in the latter groups received maintenance 5-FU after EBRT completion. The EBRT alone arm was closed early as a result of an inferior survival rate. The median 1-year survival rate in the two combined modality therapy arms was 38% and 36%, respectively, versus 11% in the EBRT alone arm.

The second GITSG trial of this series randomized 157 eligible patients with unresectable disease to 60 Gy split-course EBRT with concurrent and maintenance 5-FU from the previous trial or 40 Gy continuous-course radiation with weekly concurrent doxorubicin chemotherapy, followed by maintenance doxorubicin and 5-FU (77). A significant increase in treatment-related toxicity was seen in the doxorubicin arm. However, no survival difference was observed between the two groups (median survival 37 weeks vs. 33 weeks). No clinical benefit was seen in substituting Adriamycin for 5-FU.

A follow-up GITSG trial compared chemotherapy alone to chemoradiation, again in surgically confirmed unresectable tumors (78). Forty-three patients were randomized to receive combination streptozocin, mitomycin-C, and 5-FU (SMF) chemotherapy or 54 Gy of EBRT with two cycles of concurrent bolus 5-FU chemotherapy, followed by adjuvant SMF chemotherapy. The chemoradiation arm demonstrated a significant survival advantage over the chemotherapy alone arm (1-year survival of 41% vs. 19%).

In contrast to the results of the prior studies, the ECOG reported no benefit to chemoradiation versus chemotherapy only (79). In this study, patients with unresectable, nonmetastatic pancreatic or gastric adenocarcinoma were randomized to receive either 5-FU chemotherapy alone or 40 Gy EBRT with concurrent bolus 5-FU week 1. Patients with locally recurrent disease and patients undergoing surgery with residual disease were eligible for this trial. In the 91 analyzable pancreatic patients, no survival difference was observed between the two groups (median survival 8.2 months vs. 8.3 months).

In summary, with the exception of one study, conventional EBRT combined with 5-FU chemotherapy has been shown to offer a modest survival benefit for patients with locally advanced unresectable pancreatic cancer compared to radiation alone or chemotherapy alone. The most favorable median survival duration and 2-year survival rate for EBRT plus 5-FU are approximately 10 months and 12%, respectively. Because of these results, EBRT with 5-FU–based chemotherapy has become a frequently employed therapy for these patients.

Newer Chemotherapeutic Agents

Because of the high incidence of hepatic and peritoneal metastases and poor results with standard chemoradiotherapy, current and future research efforts include evaluation of EBRT with newer systemic agents (gemcitabine and paclitaxel). Interest in these agents is based on both their systemic cytotoxic effects and their radiosensitizing properties. At present, numerous investigators are pursuing phase I and II studies combining EBRT with gemcitabine. Investigators from Wake Forest University and the University of North Carolina have recently reported the results of a phase I trial of twice-weekly gemcitabine and 50.4 Gy of concurrent upper abdominal EBRT in 19 patients with unresectable/inoperable pancreatic adenocarcinoma (80). In this study, the maximum tolerated dose of gemcitabine was 40 mg/m^2. At this dose level, gemcitabine was well tolerated. Of eight patients with a minimum follow-up of 12 months, three remain alive, and one of the three has no evidence of disease progression. Following this trial the Cancer and Leukemia Group B (CALGB) began a phase II study of this regimen for locally advanced pancreatic cancer. Data from this trial show a median overall survival for 38 patients enrolled for 8.2 months (81). Using an alternate dosing scheme, McGinn et al. investigated weekly full-dose gemcitabine combined with radiation therapy at escalating doses in a phase I trial of 37 patients with locally advanced or incompletely resected pancreatic cancer (58). These patients received two cycles of gemcitabine at 1,000 mg/m^2 on days 1, 8, and 15 of a 28-day cycle with concurrent EBRT during the first 3 weeks. An optimal dose of 36 Gy in 2.4-Gy fractions was determined and recommended for a phase II trial that has completed accrual (59).

Gemcitabine has also been studied in combination with 5-FU and radiation. ECOG performed a phase I trial of continuous infusion 5-FU at 200 mg/m^2, weekly gemcitabine at 50 to 100 mg/m^2, and 59.4 Gy of EBRT (82). The patients in this trial showed a significant amount of toxicity, with five of seven patients experiencing dose-limiting toxicities of gastric or duodenal ulcers, thrombocytopenia, or Stevens-Johnson syndrome. Because of these toxicities, the authors concluded that the combination of gemcitabine, 5-FU, and EBRT was not appropriate. However, the Massachusetts General Hospital, Dana Farber Cancer Center, and Brigham and Women's Hospital conducted a phase I/II study of continuous infusion 5-FU with weekly gemcitabine and concurrent 50.4 Gy of EBRT for locally advanced pancreatic cancer (C. Fuchs, personal communication). In this study the MTD of weekly gemcitabine was 200 mg/m^2 when given with continuous infusion 5-FU at 200 mg/m^2 and concurrent EBRT. In this study, 32 patients were treated (13 at the MTD), and the severe toxicities were limited to one patient experiencing a grade 3 gastrointestinal bleed. The reason behind this is believed to be due to the lower dose of EBRT given, smaller treatment fields, and the fact that continuous infusion 5-FU was given 5 days out of the week instead of 7 days. This dosage is now being used for investigation in a phase II, multicenter trial through CALGB.

In a phase I trial at Brown University evaluating paclitaxel and 50 Gy of EBRT for patients with unresectable pancreatic and gastric cancers, the maximum tolerated dose of weekly paclitaxel with conventional irradiation was 50 mg/m^2 (83). The response rate was 31% among 13 evaluable pancreatic cancer patients. In the Brown University phase II study employing 50 Gy of EBRT with 50 mg/m^2/week of paclitaxel, 6 (33%) of 18 evaluable pancreatic cancer patients have had a partial response; stable disease has been observed in 7 patients (39%); only 1 patient (6%) has had local tumor progression after completion of treatment; and 4 (22%) have developed distant metastases. These data have led to an RTOG phase II study evaluating paclitaxel with EBRT for patients with unresectable pancreatic cancer (84). The median survival of 109 patients on this study was 11.2 months (95% CI, 10.1–12.3) with estimated 1- and 2-year survivals of 43% and 13%, respectively. External irradiation plus concurrent weekly paclitaxel was well tolerated when given with large-field radiotherapy. The median survival is better than historical results achieved with irradiation and fluoropyrimidines. These data provided the basis for a Radiation Therapy Oncology Group trial using paclitaxel and irradiation combined with a second radiation sensitizer, gemcitabine, and a farnesyl transferase inhibitor.

Newer Radiation Techniques

Three-dimensional conformal radiation therapy is being integrated into the treatment of a variety of malignancies, including intraabdominal tumors. This CT-based treatment allows implementation of "unconventional" beam orientations, permitting coverage of the target volume with reductions in irradiation of nontarget tissues compared to conventional techniques. For example, an important technical consideration in the radiation treatment of pancreatic cancer is minimizing kidney irradiation, given the marked radiosensitivity of this organ. By optimizing beam orientation and weighting, significant reductions in renal irradiation have been achieved relative to standard techniques without significantly increasing the dose to other surrounding organs (85).

Further refinement of this approach is now being obtained by the use of intensity-modulated radiation therapy. With this new technology, inverse treatment planning can be performed, permitting computer-based treatment optimization versus a standard "trial-and-error" planning approach. In addition, a computer-controlled, nonuniform radiation treatment can be delivered to the target, permitting an even more precise and conformal dose pattern with further reductions in normal tissue irradiation. Evolution of these techniques will likely result in improved treatment tolerance and reduction of late morbidity. This is especially critical in this era of intensive chemoradiation protocols with their potential toxicity.

Targeted Therapies/Future Directions

As the biological basis of cancer is better understood, the use of cancer-specific targeted therapies is being increasingly investigated. There is preclinical evidence for either additive or synergistic effects for several of these approaches (e.g., antibodies against VEGF and EGFR), with both chemotherapy and radiation therapy making them especially promising. The RTOG is currently undertaking a phase II study combining bevacizumab, an anti-VEGF antibody with EBRT, and capecitabine in the treatment of this group of patients. Erlotinib is an oral EGFR inhibitor recently shown to improve survival in patients with metastatic pancreatic cancer when used in combination with gemcitabine versus gemcitabine alone (86). A phase I study of erlotinib, gemcitabine, and radiation therapy for patients with locally advanced pancreatic cancer has found an MTD of erlotinib 100 mg daily, gemcitabine 40 mg/m^2 biweekly, and EBRT to 50.4 Gy. Of eight patients treated, seven have stable disease, and one patient was taken for R1 resection. Another phase I study has established an MTD for the combination of erlotinib, gemcitabine, paclitaxel, and radiation therapy for patients with locally advanced pancreatic cancer (87).

Pancreatic cancer remains one of the most formidable challenges in oncology. Newer imaging modalities have improved staging, thus facilitating treatment decisions. Since the 1970s, modest improvements in median survival have been attained for patients with locally advanced tumors treated by chemoradiation protocols. However, no significant impact on long-term survival has been accomplished. Local tumor control has been improved by the use of specialized radiation techniques permitting safe dose escalation. Even with these techniques, it is not clear that a survival benefit is achieved given the proclivity of metastases in this malignancy. Trials are underway to test newer systemic agents that also act as potent radiosensitizers.

Despite the recognized limitations of current therapy, palliation can be achieved for a high percentage of patients by combined modality treatment. Quality of life should be considered a paramount end point in the care and protocol design of these patients. In patients with marginal or poor performance status, gemcitabine administration alone represents a reasonable alternative to combined modality therapy. Significant improvements in long-term survival will likely be achieved through exploitation of the basic biological anomalies of this malignancy.

SYSTEMIC THERAPY FOR PANCREATIC CANCER

Despite improvements in imaging and surgical techniques, the vast majority of the approximately 32,000 patients diagnosed with adenocarcinoma of the pancreas each year will develop metastases and die of their disease (88). Even among patients with localized disease, the majority are either unresectable or will recur after surgery (89). Thus, future advances will rely heavily on new systemic therapies. Given the modest benefit of current therapies, the enrollment of pancreatic cancer patients onto clinical trials is of utmost importance. Most of this section will focus on pancreatic adenocarcinoma, with less common histologies briefly discussed.

Metastatic Disease

Cytotoxic Therapy

Until 1997, systemic therapy was comprised of fluoropyrimidine-based regimens. Although small randomized studies demonstrated a survival benefit for 5-FU combinations compared to best supportive care (90,91), larger studies did not (92). A meta-analysis showed a benefit in median survival for 5-FU chemotherapy compared to best supportive care (6.4 months vs. 3.9 months, $p < 0.0001$) (93). However, no advantage was noted between chemotherapy combinations or against single-agent 5-FU. In the 1990s, tumor responses and improvements in pain and/or performance status were noted in advanced pancreatic cancer patients treated with the nucleoside analog gemcitabine (94,95). A phase III study reported

by Burris et al. randomized 126 patients with locally advanced or metastatic pancreatic cancer to receive weekly bolus 5-FU or gemcitabine as initial therapy (96). All patients had either a compromised functional status or minimum analgesic requirement. The principal end point was clinical benefit response, defined as improvement in pain or performance status without a decrease in other parameters. This was seen in 24% of gemcitabine patients compared to 5% of 5-FU patients ($p = 0.0022$), despite response rates of only 5% and 0%, respectively. A small improvement in median survival was noted (5.7 months vs. 4.4 months, $p = 0.0025$), and gemcitabine was approved for advanced pancreatic cancer.

As overall survival remained poor, a number of phase II studies reported modest activity with gemcitabine in combination with other chemotherapy agents, including irinotecan (97), oxaliplatin and cisplatin (98,99), fluoropyrimidines (100), docetaxel (101), paclitaxel (102), and pemetrexed (103). Unfortunately, phase III studies randomizing patients to gemcitabine ± new agent generally failed to demonstrate a survival benefit (65,104–110) (Table 28.4). Louvet et al. randomized 313 patients with advanced disease to receive either gemcitabine, 1,000 mg/m² as a weekly 30-minute infusion, or gemcitabine, 1,000 mg/m² by fixed-dose rate infusion (FDRI) over 100 minutes plus oxaliplatin, 100 mg/m² once every 2 weeks (106). The gemcitabine plus oxaliplatin arm was superior in response rate (26.8% vs. 17.3%, $p = 0.04$) and progressionfree survival (5.8 months vs. 3.7 months, $p = 0.04$), but not overall survival (median 9.0 months vs. 7.1 months, $p = 0.13$). The relative contribution of the oxaliplatin and FDRI gemcitabine is unknown. Recent work from Tempero et al. suggested that FDRI may be superior to a 30-minute infusion (111). ECOG 6201, a three-arm randomized study, compared gemcitabine 30-minute infusion to gemcitabine FDRI and gemcitabine FDRI with oxaliplatin. Results are expected shortly to clarify the role of oxaliplatin and FDRI gemcitabine in pancreatic cancer.

Several randomized studies of gemcitabine with or without a fluoropyrimidine have been reported. Berlin et al. for ECOG randomized 322 patients to weekly gemcitabine (30 minutes) with or without weekly bolus 5-FU (600 mg/m²/week) (65). Objective responses were rare in both arms (6.9% for the combination, 5.6% for gemcitabine), with no difference in median survival (6.7 months, combination vs. 5.4 months, gemcitabine; $p = 0.09$). Riess et al. evaluated the addition of infusional 5-FU to gemcitabine in 473 patients (112) and found no improvement in median survival (5.9 months, combination vs. 6.2 months, gemcitabine; $p = 0.68$). Two studies of gemcitabine ± capecitabine have been reported in abstract form. Herrmann et al. randomized 319 patients with locally

---

TABLE 28.4

SUMMARY OF RANDOMIZED STUDIES OF GEMCITABINE WITH OR WITHOUT A CYTOTOXIC AGENT

Author	n	Cytotoxic agent	Gemcitabine survival	Combination survival	p-Value
Colucci et al. (104)	107	Cisplatin	20 wk	30 wk	0.43
Heinemann et al. (105)	192	Cisplatin	6.0 mo	7.6 mo	0.12
Louvet et al. (106)	300	Oxaliplatin	7.1 mo	9.0 mo	0.13
Rocha Lima et al. (107)	360	Irinotecan	6.6 mo	6.3 mo	0.789
Oettle et al. (108)	565	Pemetrexed	6.3 mo	6.2 mo	0.85
Hermann et al. (109)	319	Capecitabine	7.3 mo	8.4 mo	0.314
Berlin et al. (65)	322	5-Flourouracil	5.4 mo	6.7 mo	0.09
Cunningham et al. (110)	533	Capecitabine	6.0 mo	7.4 mo	0.026

advanced or metastatic disease to receive weekly gemcitabine (30 minutes) alone or with capecitabine 650 mg/m^2 orally twice daily for 14/21 days (109). No difference in survival was seen between the combination and gemcitabine (8.4 months vs. 7.3 months, respectively; $p = 0.314$). Cunningham et al. randomized 533 patients to receive gemcitabine weekly with or without capecitabine, 840 mg/m^2 twice daily for 21 days every 4 weeks (110). Response rate (13% vs. 7%, $p = 0.008$), median (7.4 months vs. 6.0 months) and 1-year survival (26% vs. 19%, $p = 0.026$) favored the combination arm as of a preliminary report. Thus, 5-FU is not beneficial in advanced disease. Capecitabine may have a role, although updated results from the Cunningham et al. study are awaited before being widely adopted.

Although most studies have focused on front-line therapy for advanced disease, there is no standard second-line therapy of benefit, and survival is often measured in weeks. The camptothecin derivative rubitecan has been studied in this setting. In a phase II trial, 7% of patients had responses (113). However, a phase III study failed to document a survival benefit compared to physician's choice of therapy (median survival 108 days vs. 94 days, $p = 0.63$) (114). Multiple combinations have been evaluated. Raltitrexed with oxaliplatin resulted in a 24% response rate and a median survival of 5.2 months (115). Oxaliplatin and 5-FU in 30 previously treated patients had a response rate of 23% and median survival of 25 weeks (116). Kozuch et al. studied the combination of gemcitabine, 5-FU, irinotecan, and cisplatin in a retrospective review of 34 consecutively previously treated patients (117). Approximately one-fourth had responses, with a median survival of 10.3 months. Fine et al. treated 44 patients, one-fourth of whom had prior chemotherapy, with the combination of gemcitabine, capecitabine, and docetaxel (118). Of 10 patients with prior treatment, 4 had responses. These encouraging response rates and survivals obtained with chemotherapy combinations need to be validated in randomized studies with prospectively defined homogenous populations.

New Therapeutics—Epidermal Growth Factor Receptor and Vascular Endothelial Growth Factor (Table 28.5)

Despite small advances with cytotoxic therapy, survival remains poor. Additional progress is likely to be made through an application of underlying biology (119). EGFR and its ligands are overexpressed in pancreatic cancer (120) and are associated with poor prognosis (121). Preclinically, EGFR blockade results in tumor regression both alone and with gemcitabine (122,123). Thus, clinical trials were pursued. Erlotinib is an oral small molecule inhibitor of the EGFR tyrosine kinase. In vitro, erlotinib inhibits phosphorylation of EGFR in pancreatic cancer xenografts and potentiates gemcitabine apoptosis (124). Thus, Moore et al. randomized 569 patients with locally advanced or metastatic disease to receive weekly gemcitabine alone or with once daily erlotinib (125). Although median survival was only slightly improved with the combination (6.4 months vs. 5.9 months), 1-year survival increased from 17% to 24% ($p = 0.025$). Objective responses were rare. Rash and diarrhea were more common with the combination, although infrequently grade 3/4. As a result, erlotinib with gemcitabine was approved for the treatment of advanced pancreatic cancer and has become the standard of care. However, survival for the average patient remains dismal, and standard of care should not imply an acceptable standard. All patients with adequate performance status should be offered and strongly encouraged to enroll in an appropriate clinical trial.

Cetuximab is a chimeric monoclonal antibody approved for the treatment of advanced colorectal cancer (126). Xiong et al.

TABLE 28.5

NOVEL DRUGS AND THEIR TARGETS

Drug	Target
Cetuximab, erlotinib	EGFR
Bevacizumab	VEGF
ISIS-2503	H-Ras mRNA
Tipifarnib	Farnesyltransferase
Sorafenib (BAY 43-9006)	Raf kinase, VEGFR-2, VEGFR-3, PDGFR-β, FLT3, and c-KIT
CI-1040	MEK1/2
Temsirolimus (CCI-779)	mTOR
AZD0530	src
Imatinib mesylate, sunitinib	PDGFR, VEGFR, KIT, bcr-abl, and FLT3
PTK787/ZK 222584 (PTK/ZK)	VEGFR-1, VEGFR-2
Ipilimumab (MDX010)	CTLA-4
G17DT	Gastrin
PANVAC-VF	CEA, MUC1
ARQ501	Cell cycle checkpoint
Curcumin	Multiple, cell proliferation
Talabostat (PT-100)	Fibroblast activation protein
Flavopiridol	Cyclin-dependent kinases
Imexon	Mitochondria

EGFR, epidermal growth factor receptor; VEGF, vascular endothelial growth factor; PDGFR, platelet-derived growth factor receptor; VEGFR, vascular endothelial growth factor receptor; FLT3, Fms-like tyrosine kinase-3; MEK1/2, mitogen-activated protein kinase kinase 1/2; mTOR, mammalian target of rapamycin; CEA, carcinoembryonic antigen.

treated 41 patients with advanced pancreatic cancer and EGFR expression by immunohistochemistry with weekly gemcitabine and cetuximab (127). The response rate was 12% with a median survival of 7.1 months and encouraging 1-year survival of 31%. Nearly all patients developed skin rash, with intensity correlating with survival. A phase III front-line study of gemcitabine with or without cetuximab for advanced pancreatic cancer is ongoing. A large phase II front-line study is randomizing patients to receive irinotecan and docetaxel with or without cetuximab and is nearing its accrual goal. These results will define the role of cetuximab in advanced pancreatic cancer.

VEGF is overexpressed in pancreatic cancer (128), and its inhibition decreases pancreatic cell growth in vitro (129). VEGF signaling blockade inhibits pancreatic cancer growth in vivo, both alone and with gemcitabine (130,131). A phase II study of weekly gemcitabine plus every 2 weeks bevacizumab (10 mg/kg), an anti-VEGF monoclonal antibody, in 52 patients with metastatic pancreatic cancer demonstrated a response rate (21%), median (8.8 months), and 1-year survival (29%) that compared favorably to gemcitabine monotherapy (132). As a result, a phase III study of gemcitabine $\pm$ bevacizumab as front-line therapy is currently enrolling patients. Other phase II trials have evaluated bevacizumab with cisplatin and FDRI gemcitabine (133) and with gemcitabine and capecitabine (134). A second-line randomized phase II study of bevacizumab with or without docetaxel is ongoing. Concurrent targeting of VEGF with EGFR may add additional benefit. Inhibition of EGFR results in antiangiogenic effects on pancreatic cancer nude mice models both alone (135) and with gemcitabine (123). In other solid tumors, dual inhibition of the EGFR and VEGF pathways leads to clinical benefit (136,137). A randomized phase II study of gemcitabine with bevacizumab and either cetuximab or erlotinib is ongoing in advanced pancreatic cancer (138).

Other Targets—Signal Transduction

Although mutations in *K-Ras* are found in the majority of pancreatic cancers (139), efforts to target this pathway through farnesylation inhibition have been unsuccessful (140–142). Antisense strategies have also not resulted in clinical benefit, with a phase II study of gemcitabine plus ISIS-2503 (an inhibitor of human H-*Ras* mRNA) noting a median survival of only 6.6 months (143). Two strategies to inhibit downstream Raf involve small molecule tyrosine kinase inhibition or antisense strategies. Sorafenib (BAY 439006) is an inhibitor of the raf and VEGFR-2, VEGFR-3, and c-Kit tyrosine kinases, which inhibits pERK in vitro and growth of human pancreatic cancer xenografts in vivo (144). A phase I study of sorafenib and gemcitabine with an expanded cohort for patients with advanced pancreatic cancer (145) documented tolerability but without objective responses. Phase II studies are ongoing. Further "downstream," a phase II study targeting the MEK/ERK pathway with the small molecule inhibitor CI-1040 demonstrated no responses in pancreatic cancer patients (146), despite a partial response in a phase I study (147).

AKT is related to growth of pancreatic cancer cells (148), frequently activated to promote pathogenesis (149), and inhibition of AKT phosphorylation induces proapoptotic and antiproliferative effects in pancreatic cancer cell lines (150). However, clinical development of direct inhibitors has proven challenging. Downstream of AKT is the mammalian target of rapamycin (mTOR), whose inhibitor temsirolimus (CCI-779) blocks pancreatic cancer growth in vivo both alone and in combination with gemcitabine (151). Another target is src, which acts as an intermediary between growth factor receptor binding and downstream signaling. Inhibition of src tyrosine kinase both alone and with gemcitabine demonstrates antitumor activity in vivo (152). A phase II study of the src inhibitor AZD0530 with gemcitabine is ongoing.

Other Targets—Cell Surface Receptors

Platelet-derived growth factor receptor (PDGFR) activates downstream signaling through Src and PI3K and has proangiogenic effects. Pancreatic tumors in vitro treated with gemcitabine and imatinib, a PDGFR and c-kit tyrosine kinase inhibitor, showed increased apoptosis and growth inhibition than either therapy alone (153). Concurrent inhibition of PDGFR, EGFR, and VEGF with gemcitabine enhances tumor control and prolongs survival in vivo (154). A phase I/II study of imatinib with gemcitabine in advanced pancreatic cancer is ongoing. Sunitinib also inhibits PDGFR, VEGF receptors, and c-kit, and has antitumor activity in neuroendocrine tumors (155). Its role in pancreatic adenocarcinoma is unknown. Finally, the VEGFR-1 and VEGFR-2 tyrosine kinase inhibitor PTK787/ZK 222584 (PTK/ZK) inhibits pancreatic cancer growth in vivo and has entered phase II evaluation (130).

Other Targets—Immunotherapy

Several approaches to modulate the immune system are under investigation in pancreatic cancer. Ipilimumab (MDX-010) is a human CTLA-4 antibody that potentiates the endogenous immune response (156). Antitumor activity was noted in melanoma (157), and a single-agent study in advanced pancreatic cancer is underway. A comprehensive review of vaccine approaches was recently published (158). Several tumor antigens have been exploited, including MUC1, Ras, gastrin, and mesothelin. MUC1 is a transmembrane glycoprotein overexpressed in pancreatic cancer (159). Ramanathan et al. treated 16 resected or locally advanced patients with a 100 mer MUC1 peptide and SB-AS2 adjuvant and detected mucin-specific humoral and T-cell responses (160). An antibody targeting MUC 1 inhibits tumor growth with gemcitabine in human pancreatic cancer xenografts (161). A phase I study of an Y^{90}-labeled anti-MUC1 antibody is enrolling patients. Ras has also been targeted by vaccine approaches, with a phase I/II study of a mutant ras peptide and GM-CSF adjuvant demonstrating peptide-specific immunity in 58% of patients (162). The antigastrin immunogen G17DT was initially studied in a phase II trial in 30 patients with advanced pancreatic cancer (163). Administration was well tolerated, with approximately two-thirds of patients producing an antibody response and having improved survival (217 days vs. 121 days, $p = 0.0023$). Building on this, Gilliam et al. randomized 154 patients with advanced disease to G17DT or placebo (164). Although median survival favored G17DT (151 days vs. 82 days, $p = 0.03$), a second larger study of 383 patients did not confirm any advantage to G17DT when combined with gemcitabine (165). Another vaccine, PANVAC-VF, contains two viral vectors and genes for CEA, MUC1, and costimulatory molecules. A pooled analysis of two phase I studies reported a 32% 1-year survival, and a phase III study is ongoing (166). Finally, mesothelin is an inositol-linked cytoplasmic membrane glycoprotein that is nearly universally expressed in pancreatic cancer but not normal pancreas (167). With an autologous tumor cell vaccine approach, 3 of 14 patients who developed a delayed-type hypersensitivity response developed CD8+ T-cell responses to mesothelin, which correlated with improved survival (168). A phase I study of a chimeric monoclonal antibody against mesothelin is about to begin. Thus, vaccine approaches in pancreatic cancer are safe and may define relevant therapeutic targets for antibody targeting. However, efficacy remains unproven.

Other Targets—Miscellaneous

ARQ501 is a cell cycle checkpoint activator that has synergistic antitumor activity against pancreatic cells in culture (169) and inhibits pancreatic tumor growth in vitro (170). A minor response was noted in a phase I monotherapy study (171) and has led to a phase II study with gemcitabine. Curcumin is a food chemical that suppresses proliferation and induces apoptosis in pancreatic cell lines (172). A phase II study is ongoing. Talabostat (PT-100) inhibits the stromal protein fibroblast activation protein. Given the extensive desmoplasia surrounding pancreatic cancer and evidence of broad preclinical growth inhibition in vivo (173) a phase II study with gemcitabine for metastatic disease and a phase I study with gemcitabine and radiation therapy for locally advanced disease have been initiated. The cyclin-dependent kinase inhibitor flavopiridol enhances gemcitabine-induced apoptosis in pancreatic cancer cell lines (174) and is being tested with gemcitabine and radiation therapy. Finally, the aziridine-containing small molecule imexon induces apoptosis through mitochondrial inhibition and cell cycle arrest in pancreatic cancer cell lines (175) and has entered phase I study with gemcitabine.

Chemotherapy for Unusual Histologies

MCNs can range from borderline malignant to aggressive neoplasms. Although outcome is excellent without adenocarcinoma present or for noninvasive cancer, patients with an invasive component have a 5-year survival of 33% (176). No controlled studies of adjuvant chemotherapy have been conducted. Use of gemcitabine or 5-FU for patients with an invasive component is appropriate. ACC is a rare malignant epithelial malignancy with exocrine enzyme production.

It accounts for 1% to 2% of all pancreatic malignancies. The largest series of 39 patients suggests that clinical outcome is better than adenocarcinomas (177). Of 18 patients who received chemotherapy, two responses were noted with a cisplatin-containing and a fluoropyrimidine/irinotecan combination. Case reports describe responses to paclitaxel (178) and capecitabine (179). In the absence of prospective studies, treatment with a fluoropyrimidine-containing regimen is reasonable. Adenosquamous tumors or pure squamous cancers of the pancreas are extremely rare, accounting for <0.01% and 0.005% of pancreas tumors, respectively (180). Experience with chemotherapy is limited, although consideration of a gemcitabine and platinum combination would be reasonable. Pancreatoblastoma is an epithelial neoplasm with acinar features and squamous nests. Approximately 10% can arise in adults. Chemotherapy is more effective in pediatric patients and includes Adriamycin, cisplatin, or vincristine (181). Small cell carcinomas, lymphomas, and sarcomas of the pancreas are extremely rare, and chemotherapy recommendations are similar to those for these tumors arising in a typical location.

References

1. Heslin MJ, Brooks AD, Hochwald SN, et al. A preoperative biliary stent is associated with increased complications after pancreatoduodenectomy. Arch Surg 1998;133:149–154.
2. Saleh MM, Norregaard P, Jorgensen HL, et al. Preoperative endoscopic stent placement before pancreaticoduodenectomy: a meta-analysis of the effect on morbidity and mortality. Gastrointest Endosc 2002;56:529–534.
3. Sohn TA, Yeo CJ, Cameron JL, et al. Do preoperative biliary stents increase postpancreaticoduodenectomy complications? J Gastrointest Surg 2000;4:258–267; discussion 267–268.
4. Hoffman JP, Lipsitz S, Pisansky T, et al. Phase II trial of preoperative radiation therapy and chemotherapy for patients with localized, resectable adenocarcinoma of the pancreas: an Eastern Cooperative Oncology Group Study. J Clin Oncol 10–998;16:317–323.
5. Pisters PW, Hudec WA, Hess KR, et al. Effect of preoperative biliary decompression on pancreaticoduodenectomy-associated morbidity in 300 consecutive patients. Ann Surg 2001;234:47–55.
6. Kalady MF, Peterson B, Baillie J, et al. Pancreatic duct strictures: identifying risk of malignancy. Ann Surg Oncol 2004;11:581–588.
7. Allen PJ, Jaques DP, D'Angelica M, et al. Cystic lesions of the pancreas: selection criteria for operative and nonoperative management in 209 patients. J Gastrointest Surg 2003;7:970–977.
8. Brugge WR, Lewandrowski K, Lee-Lewandrowski E, et al. Diagnosis of pancreatic cystic neoplasms: a report of the cooperative pancreatic cyst study. Gastroenterology 2004;126:1330–1336.
9. van der Waaij LA, van Dullemen HM, Porte RJ. Cyst fluid analysis in the differential diagnosis of pancreatic cystic lesions: a pooled analysis. Gastrointest Endosc 2005;62:383–389.
10. Khalid A, McGrath KM, Zahid M, et al. The role of pancreatic cyst fluid molecular analysis in predicting cyst pathology. Clin Gastroenterol Hepatol 2005;3:967–973.
11. Tseng JF, Raut CP, Lee JE, et al. Pancreaticoduodenectomy with vascular resection: margin status and survival duration. J Gastrointest Surg 2004;8:935–949; discussion 949–950.
12. Pingpank JF, Hoffman JP, Ross EA, et al. Effect of preoperative chemoradiotherapy on surgical margin status of resected adenocarcinoma of the head of the pancreas. J Gastrointest Surg 2001;5:121–130.
13. Conlon KC, Dougherty E, Klimstra DS, et al. The value of minimal access surgery in the staging of patients with potentially resectable peripancreatic malignancy. Ann Surg 1996;223:134–140.
14. Pisters PW, Lee JE, Vauthey JN, et al. Laparoscopy in the staging of pancreatic cancer. Br J Surg 2001;88:325–337.
15. Pedrazzoli S, DiCarlo V, Dionigi R, et al. Standard versus extended lymphadenectomy associated with pancreatoduodenectomy in the surgical treatment of adenocarcinoma of the head of the pancreas: a multicenter, prospective, randomized study. Lymphadenectomy Study Group. Ann Surg 1998;228:508–517.
16. Yeo CJ, Cameron JL, Lillemoe KD, et al. Pancreaticoduodenectomy with or without distal gastrectomy and extended retroperitoneal lymphadenectomy for periampullary adenocarcinoma, part 2: randomized controlled trial evaluating survival, morbidity, and mortality. Ann Surg 2002;236:355–66; discussion 366–368.
17. Farnell MB, Pearson RK, Sarr MG, et al. A prospective randomized trial comparing standard pancreatoduodenectomy with pancreatoduodenectomy with extended lymphadenectomy in resectable pancreatic head adenocarcinoma. Surgery 2005;138:618–628; discussion 628–630.
18. Sasson AR, Hoffman JP, Ross EA, et al. En bloc resection for locally advanced cancer of the pancreas: is it worthwhile? J Gastrointest Surg 2002;6:147–57; discussion 157–158.
19. Cheng TY, Sheth K, White RR, et al. Effect of neoadjuvant chemoradiation on operative mortality and morbidity for pancreaticoduodenectomy. Ann Surg Oncol 2006;13:66–74.
20. Birkmeyer JD, Finlayson SR, Tosteson AN, et al. Effect of hospital volume on in-hospital mortality with pancreaticoduodenectomy. Surgery 1999;125:250–256.
21. Bassi C, Dervenis C, Butturini G, et al. Postoperative pancreatic fistula: an international study group (ISGPF) definition. Surgery 2005;138:8–13.
22. Arciero CA, Joseph N, Watson JC, et al. Partial stomach-partitioning gastrojejunostomy for malignant duodenal obstruction. Am J Surg 2006;191:428–432.
23. Lillemoe KD, Cameron JL, Hardacre JM, et al. Is prophylactic gastrojejunostomy indicated for unresectable periampullary cancer? A prospective randomized trial. Ann Surg 1999;230:322–328; discussion 328–330.
24. Moss AC, Morris E, Mac Mathuna P. Palliative biliary stents for obstructing pancreatic carcinoma. Cochrane Database Syst Rev 2006;CD004200.
25. Tepper J, Nardi G, Sutt H. Carcinoma of the pancreas: review of MGH experience from 1963 to 1973: analysis of surgical failure and implications for radiation therapy. Cancer 1976;37:1519–1524.
26. Griffin JF, Smalley SR, Jewell W, et al. Patterns of failure after curative resection of pancreatic carcinoma. Cancer 1990;66:56–61.
27. Ozaki H. Improvement of pancreatic cancer treatment from the Japanese experience in the 1980s. Int J Pancreatol 1992;12:5–9.
28. Westerdahl J, Andren-Sandberg A, Ihse I. Recurrence of exocrine pancreatic cancer—local or hepatic? Hepatogastroenterology 1993;40:384–387.
29. Kalser MH, Ellenberg SS. Pancreatic cancer: adjuvant combined radiation and chemotherapy following curative resection. Arch Surg 1985;120:899–903.
30. Gastrointestinal Tumor Study Group. Further evidence of effective adjuvant combined radiation and chemotherapy following curative resection of pancreatic cancer. Cancer 1987;59:2006–2010.
31. Klinkenbijl JH, Jeekel J, Sahmoud T, et al. Adjuvant radiotherapy and 5-fluorouracil after curative resection of cancer of the pancreas and periampullary region: phase III trial of the EORTC gastrointestinal tract cancer cooperative group. Ann Surg 1999;230:776–782; discussion 782–784.
32. Neoptolemos JP, Dunn JA, Stocken DD, et al. Adjuvant chemoradiotherapy and chemotherapy in resectable pancreatic cancer: a randomised controlled trial. Lancet 2001;358:1576–1585.
33. Neoptolemos JP, Stocken DD, Friess H, et al. A randomized trial of chemoradiotherapy and chemotherapy after resection of pancreatic cancer. N Engl J Med 2004;350:1200–1210.
34. Stocken DD, Buchler MW, Dervenis C, et al. Meta-analysis of randomised adjuvant therapy trials for pancreatic cancer. Br J Cancer 2005;92:1372–1381.
35. Yeo CJ, Abrams RA, Grochow LB, et al. Pancreaticoduodenectomy for pancreatic adenocarcinoma: postoperative adjuvant chemoradiation improves survival: a prospective, single-institution experience. Ann Surg 1997;225:621–633; discussion 633–636.
36. Sohn TA, Yeo CJ, Cameron JL, et al. Resected adenocarcinoma of the pancreas—616 patients: results, outcomes, and prognostic indicators. J Gastrointest Surg 2000;4:567–579.
37. Foo ML, Gunderson LL, Nagorney DM, et al. Patterns of failure in grossly resected pancreatic ductal adenocarcinoma treated with adjuvant irradiation ± 5 fluorouracil. Int J Radiat Oncol Biol Phys 1993;26:483–489.
38. Whittington R, Bryer MP, Haller DG, et al. Adjuvant therapy of resected adenocarcinoma of the pancreas. Int J Radiat Oncol Biol Phys 1991;21:1137–1143.
39. Lim JE, Chien MW, Earle CC. Prognostic factors following curative resection for pancreatic adenocarcinoma: a population-based, linked database analysis of 396 patients. Ann Surg 2003;237:74–85.
40. Picozzi VJ, Kozarek RA, Traverso LW. Interferon-based adjuvant chemoradiation therapy after pancreaticoduodenectomy for pancreatic adenocarcinoma. Am J Surg 2003;185:476–480.
41. Willett CG, Lewandrowski K, Warshaw AL, et al. Resection margins in carcinoma of the head of the pancreas: implications for radiation therapy. Ann Surg 1993;217:144–148.
42. Cameron JL, Crist DW, Sitzmann JV, et al. Factors influencing survival after pancreaticoduodenectomy for pancreatic cancer. Am J Surg 1991;161:120–124; discussion 124–125.
43. Pilepich MV, Miller HH. Preoperative irradiation in carcinoma of the pancreas. Cancer 1980;46:1945–1949.
44. Kopelson G. Curative surgery for adenocarcinoma of the pancreas/ampulla of Vater: the role of adjuvant pre or postoperative radiation therapy. Int J Radiat Oncol Biol Phys 1983;9:911–915.
45. Weese JL, Nussbaum ML, Paul AR, et al. Increased resectability of locally advanced pancreatic and periampullary carcinoma with neoadjuvant chemoradiotherapy. Int J Pancreatol 1990;7:177–185.
46. Evans DB, Byrd DR, Mansfield PF. Preoperative chemoradiotherapy for adenocarcinoma of the pancreas: rationale and technique. Am J Clin Oncol 1991;14:359–364.
47. Spitz FR, Abbruzzese JL, Lee JE, et al. Preoperative and postoperative chemoradiation strategies in patients treated with pancreaticoduodenectomy for adenocarcinoma of the pancreas. J Clin Oncol 1997;15:928–937.

48. Evans DB, Pisters PW, Lee JE, et al. Preoperative chemoradiation strategies for localized adenocarcinoma of the pancreas. *J Hepatobiliary Pancreat Surg* 1998;5:242–250.

49. Wayne JD, Abdalla EK, Wolff RA, et al. Localized adenocarcinoma of the pancreas: the rationale for preoperative chemoradiation. *Oncologist* 2002;7:34–45.

50. Raut CP, Evans DB, Crane CH, et al. Neoadjuvant therapy for resectable pancreatic cancer. *Surg Oncol Clin N Am* 2004;13:639–661.

51. White RR, Tyler DS. Neoadjuvant therapy for pancreatic cancer: the Duke experience. *Surg Oncol Clin N Am* 2004;13:675–684.

52. Loyer EM, David CL, Dubrow RA, et al. Vascular involvement in pancreatic adenocarcinoma: reassessment by thin-section CT. *Abdom Imaging* 1996;21:202–206.

53. Ishikawa O, Ohhigashi H, Teshima T, et al. Clinical and histopathological appraisal of preoperative irradiation for adenocarcinoma of the pancreato-duodenal region. *J Surg Oncol* 1989;40:143–151.

54. Jessup JM, Steele G, Jr., Mayer RJ, et al. Neoadjuvant therapy for unresectable pancreatic adenocarcinoma. *Arch Surg* 1993;128:559–564.

55. Evans DB, Rich TA, Byrd DR, et al. Preoperative chemoradiation and pancreaticoduodenectomy for adenocarcinoma of the pancreas. *Arch Surg* 1992;127:1335–1339.

56. Pisters PW, Abbruzzese JL, Janjan NA, et al. Rapid-fractionation preoperative chemoradiation, pancreaticoduodenectomy, and intraoperative radiation therapy for resectable pancreatic adenocarcinoma. *J Clin Oncol* 1998;16:3843–3850.

57. Pipas JM, Mitchell SE, Barth RJ, Jr., et al. Phase I study of twice-weekly gemcitabine and concomitant external-beam radiotherapy in patients with adenocarcinoma of the pancreas. *Int J Radiat Oncol Biol Phys* 2001;50:1317–1322.

58. McGinn CJ, Zalupski MM, Shureiqi I, et al. Phase I trial of radiation dose escalation with concurrent weekly full-dose gemcitabine in patients with advanced pancreatic cancer. *J Clin Oncol* 2001;19:4202–4208.

59. McGinn CJ, Talamonti MS, Small W, Jr., et al. A phase II trial of full-dose gemcitabine with concurrent radiation therapy in patients with resectable or unresectable non-metastatic pancreatic cancer. Proceedings of the GI ASCO; 2004.

60. Wolff RA, Evans DB, Crane CH, et al. Initial results of preoperative gemcitabine (GEM)-based chemoradiation for resectable pancreatic adenocarcinoma. Proceedings of the American Society of Clinical Oncology; 2002;21; Abstract 576.

61. Muler JH, McGinn CJ, Normolle D, et al. Phase I trial using a time-to-event continual reassessment strategy for dose escalation of cisplatin combined with gemcitabine and radiation therapy in pancreatic cancer. *J Clin Oncol* 2004;22:238–243.

62. Wolff RA, Crane CH, Xiong HQ, et al. Preliminary analysis of preoperative systemic gemcitabine (GEM) and cisplatin (CIS) followed by GEM-based chemoradiation for resectable pancreatic adenocarcinoma. *J Clin Oncol* 2004;23:16S.

63. Pisters PW, Wolff RA, Janjan NA, et al. Preoperative paclitaxel and concurrent rapid-fractionation radiation for resectable pancreatic adenocarcinoma: toxicities, histologic response rates, and event-free outcome. *J Clin Oncol* 2002;20:2537–2544.

64. Kindler H, Friberg G, Singh D, et al. Phase II trial of bevacizumab plus gemcitabine in patients with advanced pancreatic cancer. *J Clin Oncol* 2005;23:8033–8040.

65. Berlin JD, Catalano P, Thomas JP, et al. Phase III study of gemcitabine in combination with fluorouracil versus gemcitabine alone in patients with advanced pancreatic carcinoma: Eastern Cooperative Oncology Group Trial E2297. *J Clin Oncol* 2002;20:3270–3275.

66. Xiong HQ, Abbruzzese JL. Epidermal growth factor receptor-targeted therapy for pancreatic cancer. *Semin Oncol* 2002;29:31–37.

67. Moore M, Goldstein D, Hamm J, et al. Erlotinib plus gemcitabine compared to gemcitabine alone in patients with advanced pancreatic cancer: a phase III trial of the National Cancer Institute of Canada Clinical Trials Group [NCIC-CTG]. *J Clin Oncol* 2007;25:1960–1966.

68. Li CP, Chao Y, Chi KH, et al. Concurrent chemoradiotherapy treatment of locally advanced pancreatic cancer: gemcitabine versus 5-fluorouracil, a randomized controlled study. *Int J Radiat Oncol Biol Phys* 2003;57:98–104.

69. Crane CH, Ellis LM, Abbruzzese JL, et al. Phase I trial evaluating the safety of bevacizumab with concurrent radiotherapy and capecitabine in locally advanced pancreatic cancer. *J Clin Oncol* 2006;24:1145–1151.

70. Buchsbaum DJ, Bonner JA, Grizzle WE, et al. Treatment of pancreatic cancer xenografts with Erbitux (IMC-C225) anti-EGFR antibody, gemcitabine, and radiation. *Int J Radiat Oncol Biol Phys* 2002;54:1180–1193.

71. Bonner JA, Harari PM, Giralt J, et al. Radiotherapy plus cetuximab for squamous-cell carcinoma of the head and neck. *N Engl J Med* 2006;354:567–578.

72. Krempien R, Muenter MW, Huber PE, et al. Randomized phase II—study evaluating EGFR targeting therapy with cetuximab in combination with radiotherapy and chemotherapy for patients with locally advanced pancreatic cancer—PARC: study protocol [ISRCTN56652283]. *BMC Cancer* 2005;5:131.

73. Leach SD, Lee JE, Charnsangavej C, et al. Survival following pancreatico-duodenectomy with resection of the superior mesenteric-portal vein conflu-

ence for adenocarcinoma of the pancreatic head. *Br J Surg* 1998;85:611–617.

74. Gunderson LL, Haddock MG, Burch P, et al. Future role of radiotherapy as a component of treatment in biliopancreatic cancers. *Ann Oncol* 1999;10(suppl 4):291–295.

75. Moertel CG, Childs DS, Jr., Reitemeier RJ, et al. Combined 5-fluorouracil and supervoltage radiation therapy of locally unresectable gastrointestinal cancer. *Lancet* 1969;2:865–867.

76. Moertel CG, Frytak S, Hahn RG, et al. Therapy of locally unresectable pancreatic carcinoma: a randomized comparison of high dose (6000 rads) radiation alone, moderate dose radiation (4000 rads + 5-fluorouracil), and high dose radiation + 5-fluorouracil: the Gastrointestinal Tumor Study Group. *Cancer* 1981;48:1705–1710.

77. Gastrointestinal Tumor Study Group. Radiation therapy combined with Adriamycin or 5-fluorouracil for the treatment of locally unresectable pancreatic carcinoma. *Cancer* 1985;56:2563–2568.

78. Gastrointestinal Tumor Study Group. Treatment of locally unresectable carcinoma of the pancreas: comparison of combined-modality therapy (chemotherapy plus radiotherapy) to chemotherapy alone. *J Natl Cancer Inst* 1988;80:751–755.

79. Klaassen DJ, MacIntyre JM, Catton GE, et al. Treatment of locally unresectable cancer of the stomach and pancreas: a randomized comparison of 5-fluorouracil alone with radiation plus concurrent and maintenance 5-fluorouracil—an Eastern Cooperative Oncology Group study. *J Clin Oncol* 1985;3:373–378.

80. Blackstock AW, Bernard SA, Richards F, et al. Phase I trial of twice-weekly gemcitabine and concurrent radiation in patients with advanced pancreatic cancer. *J Clin Oncol* 1999;17:2208–2212.

81. Blackstock AW, Tepper JE, Niedwiecki D, et al. Cancer and leukemia group B (CALGB) 89805: phase II chemoradiation trial using gemcitabine in patients with locoregional adenocarcinoma of the pancreas. *Int J Gastrointest Cancer* 2003;34:107–116.

82. Talamonti MS, Catalano PJ, Vaughn DJ, et al. Eastern Cooperative Oncology Group Phase I trial of protracted venous infusion fluorouracil plus weekly gemcitabine with concurrent radiation therapy in patients with locally advanced pancreas cancer: a regimen with unexpected early toxicity. *J Clin Oncol* 2000;18:3384–3389.

83. Safran H, Akerman P, Cioffi W, et al. Paclitaxel and concurrent radiation therapy for locally advanced adenocarcinomas of the pancreas, stomach, and gastroesophageal junction. *Semin Radiat Oncol* 1999;9:53–57.

84. Rich T, Harris J, Abrams R, et al. Phase II study of external irradiation and weekly paclitaxel for nonmetastatic, unresectable pancreatic cancer: RTOG-98-12. *Am J Clin Oncol* 2004;27:51–56.

85. Steadham AM, Liu HH, Crane CH, et al. Optimization of beam orientations and weights for coplanar conformal beams in treating pancreatic cancer. *Med Dosim* 1999;24:265–271.

86. Kortmansky J, O'Reilly E, Minsky B, et al. A phase I trial of erlotinib, gemcitabine, and radiation for patients with locally-advanced, unresectable pancreatic cancer. Presented at: ASCO Gastrointestinal Cancers Symposium; 2005.

87. Iannitti D, Dipetrillo T, Bearnett J, et al. Erlotinib and chemoradiation followed by maintenance erlotinib for locally advanced pancreatic cancer: a phase I study. Presented at: ASCO Gastrointestinal Cancers Symposium; January 2005, San Francisco, CA.

88. Jemal A, Murray T, Ward E, et al. Cancer statistics, 2005. *CA Cancer J Clin* 2005;55:10–30.

89. Willett CG, Czito BG, Bendell JC, et al. Locally advanced pancreatic cancer. *J Clin Oncol* 2005;23:4538–4544.

90. Mallinson CN, Rake MO, Cocking JB, et al. Chemotherapy in pancreatic cancer: results of a controlled, prospective, randomised, multicentre trial. *Br Med J* 1980;281:1589–1591.

91. Palmer KR, Kerr M, Knowles G, et al. Chemotherapy prolongs survival in inoperable pancreatic carcinoma. *Br J Surg* 1994;81:882–885.

92. Frey C, Twomey P, Keehn R, et al. Randomized study of 5-FU and CCNU in pancreatic cancer: report of the Veterans Administration Surgical Adjuvant Cancer Chemotherapy Study Group. *Cancer* 1981;47:27–31.

93. Fung MC, Takayama S, Ishiguro H, et al. [Chemotherapy for advanced or metastatic pancreatic cancer: analysis of 43 randomized trials in 3 decades (1974–2002)]. *Gan To Kagaku Ryoho* 2003;30:1101–1111.

94. Casper ES, Green MR, Kelsen DP, et al. Phase II trial of gemcitabine (2,2′-difluorodeoxycytidine) in patients with adenocarcinoma of the pancreas. *Invest New Drugs* 1994;12:29–34.

95. Rothenberg ML, Moore MJ, Cripps MC, et al. A phase II trial of gemcitabine in patients with 5-FU-refractory pancreas cancer. *Ann Oncol* 1996;7:347–353.

96. Burris HA, III, Moore MJ, Andersen J, et al. Improvements in survival and clinical benefit with gemcitabine as first-line therapy for patients with advanced pancreas cancer: a randomized trial. *J Clin Oncol* 1997;15:2403–2413.

97. Wagener DJ, Verdonk HE, Dirix LY, et al. Phase II trial of CPT-11 in patients with advanced pancreatic cancer, an EORTC early clinical trials group study. *Ann Oncol* 1995;6:129–132.

98. Philip PA, Zalupski MM, Vaitkevicius VK, et al. Phase II study of gemcitabine and cisplatin in the treatment of patients with advanced pancreatic carcinoma. *Cancer* 2001;92:569–577.

99. Demols A, Peeters M, Polus M, et al. Gemcitabine and oxaliplatin

(GEMOX) in gemcitabine refractory advanced pancreatic adenocarcinoma: a phase II study. *Br J Cancer* 2006;94:481–485.

100. Stathopoulos GP, Syrigos K, Polyzos A, et al. Front-line treatment of inoperable or metastatic pancreatic cancer with gemcitabine and capecitabine: an intergroup, multicenter, phase II study. *Ann Oncol* 2004;15:224–229.

101. Shepard RC, Levy DE, Berlin JD, et al. Phase II study of gemcitabine in combination with docetaxel in patients with advanced pancreatic carcinoma (E1298): a trial of the Eastern Cooperative Oncology Group. *Oncology* 2004;66:303–309.

102. Whitehead RP, Jacobson J, Brown TD, et al. Phase II trial of paclitaxel and granulocyte colony-stimulating factor in patients with pancreatic carcinoma: a Southwest Oncology Group study. *J Clin Oncol* 1997;15:2414–9.

103. Kindler HL. The pemetrexed/gemcitabine combination in pancreatic cancer. *Cancer* 2002;95:928–932.

104. Colucci G, Giuliani F, Gebbia V, et al. Gemcitabine alone or with cisplatin for the treatment of patients with locally advanced and/or metastatic pancreatic carcinoma: a prospective, randomized phase III study of the Gruppo Oncologia dell'Italia Meridionale. *Cancer* 2002;94:902–910.

105. Heinemann V, Quietzsch D, Gieseler F, et al. A phase III trial comparing gemcitabine plus cisplatin vs. gemcitabine alone in advanced pancreatic carcinoma. Proceedings of the American Society of Clinical Oncology; 2003; abst 1003.

106. Louvet C, Labianca R, Hammel P, et al. Gemcitabine in combination with oxaliplatin compared with gemcitabine alone in locally advanced or metastatic pancreatic cancer: results of a GERCOR and GISCAD phase III trial. *J Clin Oncol* 2005;23:3509–3516.

107. Rocha Lima CM, Green MR, Rotche R, et al. Irinotecan plus gemcitabine results in no survival advantage compared with gemcitabine monotherapy in patients with locally advanced or metastatic pancreatic cancer despite increased tumor response rate. *J Clin Oncol* 2004;22:3776–3783.

108. Oettle H, Richards D, Ramanathan RK, et al. A phase III trial of pemetrexed plus gemcitabine versus gemcitabine in patients with unresectable or metastatic pancreatic cancer. *Ann Oncol* 2005;16:1639–1645.

109. Herrmann R, Bodoky G, Ruhstaller T. Gemcitabine (G) plus Capecitabine (C) versus G alone in locally advanced or metastatic pancreatic cancer: a randomized phase III study of the Swiss Group for Clinical Cancer Research (SAKK) and the Central European Cooperative Oncology Group (CECOG). Proceedings of the American Society of Clinical Oncology; 2005; abst 4010.

110. Cunningham D, Chau I, Stocken D, et al. Phase III randomised comparison of gemcitabine with gemcitabine plus capecitabine in patients with advanced pancreatic cancer. Proceedings of the ECCO 13; 2005; abst PS11.

111. Tempero M, Plunkett W, Ruiz Van Haperen V, et al. Randomized phase II comparison of dose-intense gemcitabine: thirty-minute infusion and fixed dose rate infusion in patients with pancreatic adenocarcinoma. *J Clin Oncol* 2003;21:3402–3408.

112. Riess H, Helm A, Niedergethmann M, et al. A randomised, prospective, multicenter, phase iii trial of gemcitabine, 5-fluorouracil (5-FU), folinic acid vs. gemcitabine alone in patients with advanced pancreatic cancer. Proceedings of the American Society of Clinical Oncology; 2005; abst 4009.

113. Burris HA, Rivkin S, Reynolds R, et al. Phase II trial of oral rubitecan in previously treated pancreatic cancer patients. *Oncologist* 2005;10:183–190.

114. Jacobs AD, Burris HA, Rivkin S, et al. A randomized phase III study of rubitecan (ORA) vs. best choice (BC) in 409 patients with refractory pancreatic cancer report from a North-American multi-center study. Proceedings of the American Society of Clinical Oncology; 2004; abst 4013.

115. Reni M, Pasetto L, Aprile G, et al. Raltitrexed-Eloxatin salvage chemotherapy in gemcitabine-resistant metastatic pancreatic cancer. *Br J Cancer* 2006;94:785–791.

116. Tsavaris N, Kosmas C, Skopelitis H, et al. Second-line treatment with oxaliplatin, leucovorin and 5-fluorouracil in gemcitabine-pretreated advanced pancreatic cancer: a phase II study. *Invest New Drugs* 2005;23:369–375.

117. Kozuch P, Grossbard ML, Barzdins A, et al. Irinotecan combined with gemcitabine, 5-fluorouracil, leucovorin, and cisplatin (G-FLIP) is an effective and noncrossresistant treatment for chemotherapy refractory metastatic pancreatic cancer. *Oncologist* 2001;6:488–495.

118. Fine R, Fogelman D, Sherman W, et al. The GTX regimen: a biochemically synergistic combination for advanced pancreatic cancer (PC). Proceedings of the American Society of Clinical Oncology; 2003; abst 1129.

119. Cohen SJ, Meropol NJ. Drug development in pancreatic cancer: finally, biology begets therapy. *Int J Gastrointest Cancer* 2002;32:91–106.

120. Lemoine NR, Hughes CM, Barton CM, et al. The epidermal growth factor receptor in human pancreatic cancer. *J Pathol* 1992;166:7–12.

121. Yamanaka Y, Friess H, Kobrin MS, et al. Coexpression of epidermal growth factor receptor and ligands in human pancreatic cancer is associated with enhanced tumor aggressiveness. *AntiCancer Res* 1993;13:565–569.

122. Overholser JP, Prewett MC, Hooper AT, et al. Epidermal growth factor receptor blockade by antibody IMC-C225 inhibits growth of a human pancreatic carcinoma xenograft in nude mice. *Cancer* 2000;89:74–82.

123. Bruns CJ, Harbison MT, Davis DW, et al. Epidermal growth factor receptor blockade with C225 plus gemcitabine results in regression of human pancreatic carcinoma growing orthotopically in nude mice by antiangiogenic mechanisms. *Clin Cancer Res* 2000;6:1936–1948.

124. Ng SS, Tsao MS, Nicklee T, et al. Effects of the epidermal growth factor receptor inhibitor OSI-774, Tarceva, on downstream signaling pathways

and apoptosis in human pancreatic adenocarcinoma. *Mol Cancer Ther* 2002;1:777–783.

125. Moore MJ, Goldstein D, Hamm J, et al. Erlotinib plus gemcitabine compared to gemcitabine alone in patients with advanced pancreatic cancer: a phase III trial of the National Cancer Institute of Canada Clinical Trials Group [NCIC-CTG]. Proceedings of the American Society of Clinical Oncology; 2005; abst 1.

126. Cunningham D, Humblet Y, Siena S, et al. Cetuximab monotherapy and cetuximab plus irinotecan in irinotecan-refractory metastatic colorectal cancer. *N Engl J Med* 2004;351:337–345.

127. Xiong HQ, Rosenberg A, LoBuglio A, et al. Cetuximab, a monoclonal antibody targeting the epidermal growth factor receptor, in combination with gemcitabine for advanced pancreatic cancer: a multicenter phase II trial. *J Clin Oncol* 2004;22:2610–2616.

128. Korc M. Pathways for aberrant angiogenesis in pancreatic cancer. *Mol Cancer* 2003;2:8.

129. Luo J, Guo P, Matsuda K, et al. Pancreatic cancer cell-derived vascular endothelial growth factor is biologically active in vitro and enhances tumorigenicity in vivo. *Int J Cancer* 2001;92:361–369.

130. Solorzano CC, Baker CH, Bruns CJ, et al. Inhibition of growth and metastasis of human pancreatic cancer growing in nude mice by PTK 787/ZK222584, an inhibitor of the vascular endothelial growth factor receptor tyrosine kinases. *Cancer Biother Radiopharm* 2001;16:359–370.

131. Bruns CJ, Shrader M, Harbison MT, et al. Effect of the vascular endothelial growth factor receptor-2 antibody DC101 plus gemcitabine on growth, metastasis and angiogenesis of human pancreatic cancer growing orthotopically in nude mice. *Int J Cancer* 2002;102:101–108.

132. Kindler HL, Friberg G, Singh DA, et al. Phase II trial of bevacizumab plus gemcitabine in patients with advanced pancreatic cancer. *J Clin Oncol* 2005;23:8033–8040.

133. Ko AH, Dito EA, Schillinger BJ, et al. A phase II study of gemcitabine (GEM) given at fixed-dose rate (FDR) infusion, low-dose cisplatin (CDDP), and bevacizumab (BEV) for metastatic adenocarcinoma of the pancreas (PanCa). Proceedings of the 2006 Gastrointestinal Cancers Symposium; 2006; abst 115.

134. Javle M, Iyer R, Yu J, et al. Gemcitabine, capecitabine, and bevacizumab: a phase II study for advanced pancreatic cancer (APC) patients with good performance status. Proceedings of the 2006 Gastrointestinal Cancers Symposium; 2006; abst 117.

135. Bruns CJ, Solorzano CC, Harbison MT, et al. Blockade of the epidermal growth factor receptor signaling by a novel tyrosine kinase inhibitor leads to apoptosis of endothelial cells and therapy of human pancreatic carcinoma. *Cancer Res* 2000;60:2926–2935.

136. Hainsworth JD, Sosman JA, Spigel DR, et al. Treatment of metastatic renal cell carcinoma with a combination of bevacizumab and erlotinib. *J Clin Oncol* 2005;23:7889–7896.

137. Sandler AB, Blumenschein GR, Henderson T, et al. Phase I/II trial evaluating the anti-VEGF MAb bevacizumab in combination with erlotinib, a HER1/EGFR-TK inhibitor, for patients with recurrent non-small cell lung cancer. Proceedings of the American Society of Clinical Oncology; 2004; abst 2000.

138. National Cancer Institute. Phase II randomized study of bevacizumab and gemcitabine with cetuximab versus erlotinib in patients with advanced adenocarcinoma of the pancreas. Available at: http://www.cancer.gov/search/ViewClinicalTrials.aspx?cdrid=383145&version=HealthProfessional&protocolsearchid=2266849. Accessed April 26, 2007.

139. Grunewald K, Lyons J, Frohlich A, et al. High frequency of Ki-ras codon 12 mutations in pancreatic adenocarcinomas. *Int J Cancer* 1989;43:1037–1041.

140. Cohen SJ, Ho L, Ranganathan S, et al. Phase II and pharmacodynamic study of the farnesyltransferase inhibitor R115777 as initial therapy in patients with metastatic pancreatic adenocarcinoma. *J Clin Oncol* 2003;21:1301–1306.

141. Van Cutsem E, van de Velde H, Karasek P, et al. Phase III trial of gemcitabine plus tipifarnib compared with gemcitabine plus placebo in advanced pancreatic cancer. *J Clin Oncol* 2004;22:1430–1438;

142. Rich TA, Myerson RJ, Harris J, et al. A randomized phase II trial of weekly gemcitabine (G), paclitaxel (P), and external irradiation followed by the farnesyl transferase inhibitor R115777 (NSC#702818) for locally advanced pancreatic cancer (RTOG 0020). Proceedings of the 2006 Gastrointestinal Cancers Symposium; 2006; abst 121.

143. Alberts SR, Schroeder M, Erlichman C, et al. Gemcitabine and ISIS-2503 for patients with locally advanced or metastatic pancreatic adenocarcinoma: a North Central Cancer Treatment Group phase II trial. *J Clin Oncol* 2004;22:4944–4950.

144. Wilhelm SM, Carter C, Tang L, et al. BAY 43-9006 exhibits broad spectrum oral antitumor activity and targets the RAF/MEK/ERK pathway and receptor tyrosine kinases involved in tumor progression and angiogenesis. *Cancer Res* 2004;64:7099–109.

145. Siu LL, Awada A, Takimoto CH, et al. Phase I trial of sorafenib and gemcitabine in advanced solid tumors with an expanded cohort in advanced pancreatic cancer. *Clin Cancer Res* 2006;12:144–151.

146. Rinehart J, Adjei AA, Lorusso PM, et al. Multicenter phase II study of the oral MEK inhibitor, CI-1040, in patients with advanced non-small-cell lung, breast, colon, and pancreatic cancer. *J Clin Oncol* 2004;22:4456–4462.

147. Lorusso PM, Adjei AA, Varterasian M, et al. Phase I and pharmacodynamic study of the oral MEK inhibitor CI-1040 in patients with advanced malignancies. *J Clin Oncol* 2005;23:5281–5293.

148. Yao Z, Okabayashi Y, Yutsudo Y, et al. Role of Akt in growth and survival of PANC-1 pancreatic cancer cells. *Pancreas* 2002;24:42–46.

149. Altomare DA, Tanno S, De Rienzo A, et al. Frequent activation of AKT2 kinase in human pancreatic carcinomas. *J Cell Biochem* 2003;88:470–476.

150. Li J, Zhu J, Melvin WS, et al. A structurally optimized celecoxib derivative inhibits human pancreatic cancer cell growth. *J Gastrointest Surg* 2006;10:207–214.

151. Ito D, Fujimoto K, Mori T, et al. In vivo antitumor effect of the mTOR inhibitor CCI-779 and gemcitabine in xenograft models of human pancreatic cancer. *Int J Cancer* 2006;118:2337–2343.

152. Yezhelyev MV, Koehl G, Guba M, et al. Inhibition of SRC tyrosine kinase as treatment for human pancreatic cancer growing orthotopically in nude mice. *Clin Cancer Res* 2004;10:8028–8036.

153. Hwang RF, Yokoi K, Bucana CD, et al. Inhibition of platelet-derived growth factor receptor phosphorylation by STI571 (Gleevec) reduces growth and metastasis of human pancreatic carcinoma in an orthotopic nude mouse model. *Clin Cancer Res* 2003;9:6534–6544.

154. Yokoi K, Sasaki T, Bucana CD, et al. Simultaneous inhibition of EGFR, VEGFR, and platelet-derived growth factor receptor signaling combined with gemcitabine produces therapy of human pancreatic carcinoma and prolongs survival in an orthotopic nude mouse model. *Cancer Res* 2005;65:10371–10380.

155. Kulke M, Lenz HJ, Meropol NJ, et al. A phase 2 study to evaluate the efficacy and safety of SU11248 in patients (pts) with unresectable neuroendocrine tumors (NETs). Proceedings of the American Society of Clinical Oncology; 2005; abst 4008.

156. Phan GQ, Yang JC, Sherry RM, et al. Cancer regression and autoimmunity induced by cytotoxic T lymphocyte-associated antigen 4 blockade in patients with metastatic melanoma. *Proc Natl Acad Sci U S A* 2003;100:8372–8377.

157. Ribas A, Camacho LH, Lopez-Berestein G, et al. Antitumor activity in melanoma and anti-self responses in a phase I trial with the anti-cytotoxic T lymphocyte-associated antigen 4 monoclonal antibody CP-675,206. *J Clin Oncol* 2005;23:8968–8977.

158. Laheru D, Jaffee EM. Immunotherapy for pancreatic cancer—science driving clinical progress. *Nat Rev Cancer* 2005;5:459–467.

159. Hollingsworth MA, Swanson BJ. Mucins in cancer: protection and control of the cell surface. *Nat Rev Cancer* 2004;4:45–60.

160. Ramanathan RK, Lee KM, McKolanis J, et al. Phase I study of a MUC1 vaccine composed of different doses of MUC1 peptide with SB-AS2 adjuvant in resected and locally advanced pancreatic cancer. *Cancer Immunol Immunother* 2005;54:254–264.

161. Gold DV, Modrak DE, Schutsky K, et al. Combined 90Yttrium-DOTA-labeled PAM4 antibody radioimmunotherapy and gemcitabine radiosensitization for the treatment of a human pancreatic cancer xenograft. *Int J Cancer* 2004;109:618–626.

162. Gjertsen MK, Buanes T, Rosseland AR, et al. Intradermal ras peptide vaccination with granulocyte-macrophage colony-stimulating factor as adjuvant: clinical and immunological responses in patients with pancreatic adenocarcinoma. *Int J Cancer* 2001;92:441–450.

163. Brett BT, Smith SC, Bouvier CV, et al. Phase II study of anti-gastrin-17 antibodies, raised to G17DT, in advanced pancreatic cancer. *J Clin Oncol* 2002;20:4225–4231.

164. Gilliam AD, Topuzov EG, Garin AM, et al. Randomised, double blind, placebo-controlled, multi-centre, group-sequential trial of G17DT for patients with advanced pancreatic cancer unsuitable or unwilling to take chemotherapy. Proceedings of the American Society of Clinical Oncology; 2004; abst 2511.

165. Shapiro J, Marshall J, Karasek P, et al. G17DT+gemcitabine [Gem] versus placebo+Gem in untreated subjects with locally advanced, recurrent, or metastatic adenocarcinoma of the pancreas: results of a randomized, double-blind, multinational, multicenter study. Proceedings of the American Society of Clinical Oncology; 2005; abst 4012.

166. Scheutz T, Kaufman HL, Marshall JL, et al. Extended survival in second-line pancreatic cancer after therapeutic vaccination. Proceedings of the American Society of Clinical Oncology; 2005; abst 2576.

167. Hassan R, Laszik ZG, Lerner M, et al. Mesothelin is overexpressed in pancreaticobiliary adenocarcinomas but not in normal pancreas and chronic pancreatitis. *Am J Clin Pathol* 2005;124:838–845.

168. Thomas AM, Santarsiero LM, Lutz ER, et al. Mesothelin-specific CD8(+) T cell responses provide evidence of in vivo cross-priming by antigen-presenting cells in vaccinated pancreatic cancer patients. *J Exp Med* 2004;200:297–306.

169. Li CJ, Li YZ, Pinto AV, et al. Potent inhibition of tumor survival in vivo by beta-lapachone plus Taxol: combining drugs imposes different artificial checkpoints. *Proc Natl Acad Sci U S A* 1999;96:13369–13374.

170. Ough M, Lewis A, Bey EA, et al. Efficacy of beta-lapachone in pancreatic cancer treatment: exploiting the novel, therapeutic target NQO1. *Cancer Biol Ther* 2005;4:95–102.

171. Shapiro GI, Ryan DP, Appleman LJ, et al. A phase 1 monotherapy trial of ARQ 501, a novel checkpoint pathway activator, in patients with advanced solid tumors. Proceedings of the American Association for Cancer Research; 2006; abst LB-142.

172. Li L, Aggarwal BB, Shishodia S, et al. Nuclear factor-kappaB and IkappaB kinase are constitutively active in human pancreatic cells, and their down-regulation by curcumin (diferuloylmethane) is associated with the suppression of proliferation and the induction of apoptosis. *Cancer* 2004;101:2351–2362.

173. Adams S, Miller GT, Jesson MI, et al. PT-100, a small molecule dipeptidyl peptidase inhibitor, has potent antitumor effects and augments antibody-mediated cytotoxicity via a novel immune mechanism. *Cancer Res* 2004;64:5471–5480.

174. Jung CP, Motwani MV, Schwartz GK. Flavopiridol increases sensitization to gemcitabine in human gastrointestinal cancer cell lines and correlates with down-regulation of ribonucleotide reductase M2 subunit. *Clin Cancer Res* 2001;7:2527–2536.

175. Dorr RT, Raymond MA, Landowski TH, et al. Induction of apoptosis and cell cycle arrest by imexon in human pancreatic cancer cell lines. *Int J Gastrointest Cancer* 2005;36:15–28.

176. Wilentz RE, Albores-Saavedra J, Zahurak M, et al. Pathologic examination accurately predicts prognosis in mucinous cystic neoplasms of the pancreas. *Am J Surg Pathol* 1999;23:1320–1327.

177. Holen KD, Klimstra DS, Hummer A, et al. Clinical characteristics and outcomes from an institutional series of acinar cell carcinoma of the pancreas and related tumors. *J Clin Oncol* 2002;20:4673–4678.

178. Riechelmann RP, Hoff PM, Moron RA, et al. Acinar cell carcinoma of the pancreas. *Int J Gastrointest Cancer* 2003;34:67–72.

179. Lee JL, Kim TW, Chang HM, et al. Locally advanced acinar cell carcinoma of the pancreas successfully treated by capecitabine and concurrent radiotherapy: report of two cases. *Pancreas* 2003;27:e18–e22.

180. Itani KM, Karni A, Green L. Squamous cell carcinoma of the pancreas. *J Gastrointest Surg* 1999;3:512–515.

181. Dhebri AR, Connor S, Campbell F, et al. Diagnosis, treatment and outcome of pancreatoblastoma. *Pancreatology* 2004;4:441–51; discussion 452–3.

HEPATOCELLULAR CANCER

CHAPTER 29 ■ HEPATOCELLULAR CARCINOMA: EPIDEMIOLOGY, SCREENING, AND PREVENTION

MORRIS SHERMAN

EPIDEMIOLOGY

Hepatocellular carcinoma (HCC) is the fifth most common solid tumor in the world, accounting for >500,000 deaths each year (1). Most HCC occurs as a complication of underlying chronic liver disease. Therefore, the epidemiology of HCC is largely the epidemiology of the underlying liver diseases. Furthermore, the epidemiology of HCC is changing as the epidemiology of the underlying liver diseases also changes. For example, the incidence of HCC in children in Taiwan and other places has been dramatically reduced by the introduction of neonatal hepatitis B vaccination (2). In contrast, HCC related to chronic hepatitis C is increasing in incidence, related to epidemics of hepatitis C that occurred many years ago.

China has the highest incidence of HCC in the world (~100/100,000 population) (1,3). The major risk factor in China is chronic hepatitis B infection. Similarly, in Africa, where the HCC incidence is also very high, the major risk factor is also chronic hepatitis B. In contrast, hepatitis C accounts for about 63% of the attributable risk in Europe (3). In the United States, hepatitis C is the major contributor, but the attributable risk due to alcohol is also high at about 45% (3).

North America and Western Europe are generally considered to be low incidence regions (incidence 2.6–9.8/100,000 population) (3), but the incidence of HCC is rising in these regions. Studies from cancer registries have shown a rising trend in HCC incidence and death in the United States, France, Japan, the United Kingdom, and Italy (3–7). In the United States, HCC incidence has increased from 1.4/100,000/year to 2.4/100,000/year between 1976 and 1995. The increased incidence is present among all races and is mainly due to an increase in the incidence of HCC related to hepatitis C, with much smaller increases in the incidence of HCC associated with alcohol and hepatitis B (8).

The incidence of HCC increases with age, but the age distribution varies in different local regions of the world. The pattern suggests that with urbanization, the median age of onset is shifted to older age groups. In less well-developed countries, it is not rare to find HCC in persons younger than 45 years. However, the incidence of HCC in developed countries only really starts to increase in persons older than 45 years, and it continues to increase until a person reaches his or her 70s (3). These differences may reflect a difference in the age of exposure to hepatitis viruses, exposure occurring at younger ages in high incidence countries. The incidence of HCC is higher in men than in women. The incidence ratio varies in different parts of the world but ranges from 1.3 to 3.6 (3). There are, as yet, no satisfactory explanations for this phenomenon. Studies in migrant populations have clearly shown that first-generation immigrants carry with them the high incidence of HCC that is present in their native countries. However, in the second and subsequent generations, the incidence decreases (9). This is likely a reflection of improved sanitation, improved health care, and improved health in general, resulting in a lower prevalence of underlying viral hepatitis. In North America, HCC incidence may be particularly high in specific ethnic groups. First-generation immigrants from Hong Kong, China, and Taiwan bring with them the high prevalence of chronic hepatitis B and are at risk for HCC. Immigrants from Egypt, Somalia, Vietnam, and Pakistan have a high prevalence of hepatitis C. Thus, trends in immigration will also affect HCC incidence.

Hepatitis B

That chronic hepatitis B infection is a risk factor for HCC has been known for some years. The first prospective cohort study to show this was that of Beasley et al. (10,11), who, in a now classic prospective cohort study, showed that the relative risk of HCC in a carrier versus noninfected was about 100. In that study, the annual incidence of HCC in hepatitis B carriers was 0.5%. The annual incidence increased with age, so that at age 70 the incidence was 1%. The incidence in patients with known cirrhosis was 2.5% per year. A second prospective study by Sakuma et al. (12) found the incidence of HCC in male Japanese railway workers who were hepatitis B carriers was 0.4%/year. Both populations were male and Asian, with the hepatitis B infection likely acquired at birth or in early childhood. There are no equivalent studies in Asian women, but the incidence of HCC in Asian women is about one-fourth to one-eighth of that in men. Uncontrolled prospective cohort studies in North America, where the epidemiology of hepatitis B is often different (i.e., hepatitis may be acquired later in life), have found a wide incidence of HCC in hepatitis B carriers, ranging from 0% to 0.46% (13–15). In Europe, HCC in hepatitis B carriers occurs mainly in patients with established cirrhosis (16,17). Caucasian noncirrhotic chronic carriers who are anti–HBe positive with long-term inactive viral replication have little risk of developing HCC (18–20). This may not be true for Asian noncirrhotic hepatitis B carriers, who remain at risk for HCC regardless of replication status (21–24). Similarly, the risk of HCC persists in long-term HBV carriers from Asia who lose HBsAg (25). In Caucasian hepatitis B carriers who lose surface antigen, the risk of HCC seems to decline dramatically (26).

The epidemiology of hepatitis B is changing as a result of the introduction of mass vaccination against hepatitis B. It has already been shown that the incidence of childhood HCC has been dramatically reduced following the introduction of hepatitis B vaccination (2). It is likely that as the vaccinated cohort ages the incidence of HCC in older age groups will also decrease. However, there are still many millions of individuals persistently infected with hepatitis B, who remain at risk for the development of HCC.

Hepatitis C

The risk of HCC in hepatitis C infection is largely associated with the presence of cirrhosis (27–30). In these patients, the incidence of HCC is between 2% and 8% per year. Noncirrhotic hepatitis C–infected individuals have a much lower risk of developing HCC (30). Most of the data is from clinic-based studies. However, a prospective population-based study of 12,008 men of (31) found a 20-fold increased risk of HCC compared to anti–hepatitis C virus (HCV)-negative subjects. The presence or absence of cirrhosis was not evaluated.

The epidemiology of hepatitis C is different in North America and elsewhere. In Japan, Italy, Eastern Europe, and elsewhere, an epidemic of hepatitis C infection occurred between the end of the Second World War and about 1975 to 1980. This was related to medical procedures, injections, vaccinations, transfusions, and hospitalizations, as well as the use of improperly sterilized equipment. Those infected during that era are now at least in their 50s and are entering the period of highest risk for HCC. In contrast, in the United States and Northern Europe, the epidemic of HCV infection occurred in the 1960s and 1970s related to injection drug use. Thus, the peak onset of HCC in these populations is still to come. It is predicted that the incidence of HCC will increase by about 80% over the next 20 years in the United States (32) but will more than triple elsewhere (33,34).

Cirrhosis Due to Causes Other Than Viral Hepatitis

The incidence of HCC in cirrhosis caused by diseases other than viral hepatitis is, with some exceptions, not accurately known. Most of the studies of the incidence of HCC in alcoholic cirrhosis date from before the identification of the HCV. Given that hepatitis C is relatively frequent in alcoholics, most of the reported incidence rates in these earlier studies are likely to be overestimates. Thus, it is not possible to provide precise estimates of HCC incidence in this group. Nonetheless, alcoholic cirrhosis is a well-recognized risk factor for HCC. In one study, alcoholic liver disease accounted for 32% of all HCCs (35). In an Austrian cohort with HCC, alcoholic liver disease was the risk factor in 35% of subjects (36). In the United States, the approximate hospitalization rate for HCC related to alcoholic cirrhosis is 8–9/100,000/year compared to about 7/100,000/year for hepatitis C (37). This study did not determine the incidence of HCC in alcoholic liver disease, but it does confirm that alcoholic cirrhosis is a significant risk factor for HCC, probably sufficient to warrant surveillance for HCC.

With the recognition of nonalcoholic liver disease (mainly steatohepatitis) as a cause of cirrhosis has come the suspicion that this too is a risk factor for HCC. No study to date has followed a sufficiently large group of patients for long enough to describe an incidence rate for HCC. In one cohort study of patients with HCC (38), diabetes was found in 20% as the only risk factor for HCC. The likely link is insulin resistance causing steatohepatitis, in turn causing cirrhosis. Whether these

patients were cirrhotic was not noted. Nonalcoholic fatty liver disease has also been described in cohorts of patients with HCC (39,40).

Patients with genetic hemochromatosis (GH) who have established cirrhosis have an increased risk of HCC (41–43) of about 20-fold. The standardized incidence ratio of HCC in cirrhotic GH is 92.9 (95% confidence interval, 25–238). For cirrhosis due to alpha 1-antitrypsin deficiency (44,45) or autoimmune hepatitis, there are insufficient data from cohort studies to accurately assess HCC incidence. However, there does seem to be an increased HCC risk. The incidence of HCC in stage 4 primary biliary cirrhosis is about the same as in cirrhosis due to hepatitis C (46).

SCREENING FOR HEPATOCELLULAR CARCINOMA

HCC develops silently. There is no opportunity for early detection by self-examination as with breast or skin cancer, nor does it call attention to itself by bleeding into a hollow organ, as bladder or bowel cancer might. Therefore, in the absence of screening and early detection programs, HCC presents late in the course of the disease with the onset of symptoms due to liver failure (massive replacement of liver by tumor), obstructive jaundice due to bile duct infiltration, or constitutional symptoms. At this late stage of disease, curative therapy can seldom be applied and has a low chance of success. Palliative therapy may also not be possible because of advanced hepatic failure. Furthermore, progression of disease is usually rapid with a prognosis of only a few weeks to months. Therefore, there has long been an interest in early detection of HCC, although formalization of methods of early detection and definition of the diagnostic features of early HCC have only been recently achieved.

The objective of cancer screening is to reduce the mortality from that specific cancer. Several studies have shown that screening does detect earlier disease (stage migration) (47). There are several surrogate markers of successful screening, including stage migration. Clearly, it is important to find cancers at an earlier stage, but stage migration does not necessarily correlate with a reduction in disease-specific mortality. Similarly, changes in 5-year survival may reflect changes in underlying cancer incidence rather than changes in mortality (50). Uncontrolled studies, all subject to lead-time bias, have also suggested that survival is improved after screening (48–50).

There have been two randomized controlled trials of HCC screening. Both were conducted in China. The first failed because although screening found early cancers, too many patients did not get the proposed treatment (51). The second study, a large population-based study followed patients for 5 years (52). This study used cluster randomization to allocate patients with chronic hepatitis B to a screening or no screening arm. Screening was with ultrasonography and alphafetoprotein (AFP) testing at 6-month intervals. The study found a 37% reduction in HCC-related mortality despite a compliance rate that was less than optimal. There are limitations to generalizing this study to HCC related to other liver diseases. In the study, the main therapy that was offered was resection. However, in hepatitis B, as discussed later in this chapter, HCC develops in noncirrhotic as well as cirrhotic livers, although at lower frequency. The presence of cirrhosis in diseases other than hepatitis B limits the possibility for resection. Therefore, in all other causes of HCC, fewer patients will be able to have resections. The possibility of using local ablation and liver transplantation as therapy also makes it harder to generalize these results, and although one would expect the availability of these additional forms of therapy to improve the results, the presence of cirrhosis itself will limit survival.

In addition, there have been several decision analytic models of screening for HCC (53,54). In summary, all suggest that there is benefit to HCC screening under standard baseline conditions, but the increase in life expectancy is only just above the 3-month limit considered to be acceptable. Screening for HCC may also be appropriate because the cure rate for symptomatic cancers is very low (0%–10% 5-year survival) (55–59). However, 5-year diseasefree survival of >50% has been reported for liver transplantation (60–63). The more advanced the disease, the less likely that liver transplant will eradicate it.

There are cogent reasons to undertake screening in all patients at sufficiently high risk:

- Cure is more likely with treatment of early stage disease, especially with liver transplantation.
- Advances in the ability to treat HCC are unlikely to come from treating late stage disease; therefore, it is important to find early stage disease. Ideally, patients with HCC found on screening should be entered into clinical trials of newer forms of therapy.
- A randomized controlled trial of screening versus no screening in hepatitis C and other causes of cirrhosis will likely never be undertaken because of the difficulties such a trial would involve. Thus, patient management decisions will have to be made in the absence of high-quality evidence.
- Minimally invasive therapies, such as radiofrequency ablation, can completely ablate small lesions with an appreciable frequency, which might approach 95% in very small lesions (64).

Although the broad outlines of the risk groups that might benefit from screening are well known, it is clear that not all patients need screening. For example, in male hepatitis B carriers, the risk of HCC only starts to rise significantly in persons older than 40 years (10,11). This is not to say that there is no HCC at younger ages. However, from a cost-efficacy point of view, it might be difficult to justify screening in a population with a low incidence of HCC.

Definition of the At-Risk Population

The decision to enter a patient into an HCC screening program depends on the physician's perception of the patient's risk of developing HCC. Patients at high risk are offered screening, whereas those at low risk (usually interpreted as risk equivalent to the general population risk) are not. However, risk is hard to quantitate, and most physicians equate risk with HCC incidence. There are no experimental data to indicate what level of risk or what incidence of HCC should trigger surveillance. HCC incidence in the general population is low. In contrast, in various populations with liver disease, the incidence may be as high as 8% annually. The incidence at which screening becomes worthwhile probably varies with different liver diseases. Decision analysis has been used to determine incidence rates at which screening might be effective. As a general rule in decision analysis, an intervention is considered effective if it provides an increase in longevity of about 100 days (i.e., about 3 months). If this can be achieved at a cost of less than about $50,000/year of life gained, the intervention is considered cost effective (65,66). There are now several published decision analysis/cost-efficacy models for HCC surveillance. The models differ in the nature of the theoretical population being analyzed and in the intervention being applied. Nonetheless, these models have several results in common. They all find that surveillance is cost effective, although in some cases only marginally so, and most find that the efficacy of surveillance is highly dependent on the

incidence of HCC. For example, Sarasin et al. (53) studied a theoretical cohort of patients with child's A cirrhosis and found that if the incidence of HCC was 1.5%/year, surveillance resulted in an increase in longevity of about 3 months. However, if the incidence of HCC was 6%, the increase in survival was about 9 months. This study did not include transplantation as a treatment option. Arguedas et al. (54), using a similar analysis that did include liver transplantation in a population of hepatitis C cirrhotics with normal liver function, found that surveillance with either computed tomography (CT) scanning alone or CT scanning plus ultrasound (US) became cost effective when the incidence of HCC was >1.4%. However, this study has to be interpreted cautiously because the performance characteristics of CT scanning were derived from diagnostic studies, not surveillance studies. Lin et al. (67) found that surveillance with AFP and US was cost effective regardless of HCC incidence. Thus, for patients with cirrhosis of varying etiologies, surveillance should be offered when the risk of HCC is ≥1.5%/year. Table 29.1 describes the groups of patients in which these limits are exceeded.

HCC in patients with chronic hepatitis B may develop in a noncirrhotic liver, particularly in Asian and African patients. The previous cost-efficacy analyses, which were restricted to cirrhotic populations, cannot be applied to noncirrhotic hepatitis B carriers. These patients, particularly in Asia and Africa, are also at risk for HCC. A cost-efficacy analysis of surveillance of hepatitis B carriers using US and AFP levels suggested that surveillance became cost effective once the incidence of HCC exceeded 0.2%/year (J. Collier and M. Sherman, unpublished observations, 2000). The subgroups of hepatitis B carriers in which the incidence of HCC exceeds 0.2%/year are listed in Table 29.1. These groups are discussed in more detail later in this chapter.

Screening, as used here, refers to the repeated application of diagnostic tests to asymptomatic subjects who have a defined risk of developing HCC but in whom there is no reason to believe that HCC is present. Patients who have some reason to suspect that HCC is present, such as an abnormal screening test result, are no longer candidates for screening. Instead,

---

TABLE 29.1

SURVEILLANCE IS RECOMMENDED FOR THE FOLLOWING GROUPS OF PATIENTS

HEPATITIS B CARRIERS
- Asian males older than ~40 yr
- Asian females older than ~50 yr
- Africans older than 20 yr
- All cirrhotic hepatitis B carriers, regardless of whether successfully treated
- Family history of hepatocellular carcinoma
- For other noncirrhotic hepatitis B carriers not listed, the risk of HCC varies, depending on the severity of the underlying liver disease, and current and past hepatic inflammatory activity. The need for surveillance must be individually assessed.

NON–HEPATITIS B CIRRHOTICS
- Hepatitis C
- Alcoholic cirrhosis
- Genetic hemochromatosis
- Primary biliary cirrhosis
- Alpha1-antitrypsin deficiency
- Nonalcoholic steatohepatitis

they undergo enhanced follow-up. This is the process of confirming or refuting that an abnormal screening test result is due to HCC. Enhanced follow-up is more frequent than screening and involves a wider range of diagnostic tests. Part of enhanced follow-up is a strategy to deal with equivocal diagnostic test results, and it requires an understanding of the diagnostic features of early HCC.

Screening is more than the application of a diagnostic test. Rather screening is a process that requires identification of the at-risk population, choosing the appropriate screening test(s) and the appropriate screening interval, setting recall policies for abnormal screening test results, and developing strategies for enhanced follow-up and diagnosis. Screening should be applied in a setting where screening tests are standardized and quality control is instituted to ensure that the risk of false-positive and false-negative results is minimized.

Surveillance Tests

Screening tests fall into two categories: serologic and radiologic. Of the serologic tests, the performance characteristics of AFP have been best studied (68–70). AFP levels are frequently elevated in patients with established HCC. However, when the performance characteristics of AFP as a diagnostic test are carefully evaluated, it is clear that it is not a good test for small HCCs. In tumors that secrete AFP, the concentration is related to the size of the tumor. Thus, in early HCCs found by screening, a diagnostically high AFP is unlikely. Furthermore, AFP is not specific for HCC. Titers also rise with flares of active hepatitis. Of 44 HBV carriers with elevated AFP levels detected during surveillance for HCC, only 6 were found to have HCC on further investigation, and in 18 (41%) the raised AFP was associated with an exacerbation of underlying liver disease or changes in HBV replication status (71). Recent data from the HALT-C study confirm that AFP is frequently elevated in chronic viral hepatitis, even in the absence of HCC (72). In the era of sensitive radiologic tests, when US can identify lesions <2 cm in diameter, the role of AFP is questionable. However, AFP is still diagnostically useful. In the presence of cirrhosis and a mass in the liver, the positive predictive value (PPV) for an elevated AFP (>200 ng/L) is >90% (68).

When the AFP concentration is very high in the appropriate clinical setting, the likelihood of a false positive is negligible. However, when the HCC is small, the false-negative rate of AFP will be very high (68). Receiver operating curve analysis of AFP used as a diagnostic test suggests that a value of about 20 ng/mL provides the optimal balance between sensitivity and specificity (68). However, the sensitivity is only 60% at this level (i.e., AFP surveillance would miss 40% of HCC if a value of 20 ng/mL is used as the trigger for further investigation). This is inadequately sensitive for general use. If a higher cut-off is used, a progressively smaller proportion of HCCs will be detected. For example, if the AFP cut-off is raised to 200 ng/mL, the sensitivity drops to 22%. Conversely, reducing the cut-off means that more HCCs would be identified, although at the cost of a progressive increase in the false-positive rate. This analysis was performed in a case-control study where the prevalence of HCC was artificially set at 50%. At this prevalence, the PPV of an AFP of 20 ng/mL was 84.6%. However, if the HCC prevalence rates were more like those seen in most liver clinics (i.e., about 5%), the PPV of an AFP of 20 ng/mL is only 41.5%, and even at a cut-off of 400 ng/mL, the PPV is only 60%. In cohorts undergoing surveillance, the incidence of HCC may be even <5%, depending on the criteria for entry into surveillance. For example, in noncirrhotic hepatitis B carriers infected at birth, the incidence of HCC is usually <1%.

Therefore, AFP is an inadequate screening test (73). AFP still has a role in the diagnosis of HCC because in cirrhotic patients with a mass in the liver, an AFP >200 ng/mL has a very high PPV for HCC (68). Furthermore, a persistently elevated AFP has been clearly shown to be a risk factor for HCC (74). Thus, the AFP can be used to help define patients at risk but appears to have limited utility as a screening test.

Another serologic test used to diagnose HCC is the des-gamma-carboxy prothrombin (DCP), also known as prothrombin induced by vitamin K absence or antagonist II (75–79). Most reports on the use of DCP have evaluated the use of this test in a diagnostic mode, rather than for surveillance. Although there are reports of its use in a surveillance mode, they do not yet provide sufficient justification for routine use of this marker. There are also reports that DCP is a marker for portal vein invasion by tumor (80). If confirmed, this would also suggest that DCP is not a good screening test. A screening test should be able to identify early disease, not late disease. Another test that has been reported as a screening test is the ratio of glycosylated AFP (L3 fraction) to total AFP (81–84). AFP exists in serum as a family of molecules with different degrees of glycosylation. These can be separated electrophoretically. The L3-to-total AFP ratio can be elevated in the presence of small HCC. However, as with DCP, there are data suggesting that an elevated ratio is a marker for more advanced disease (85,86).

The radiologic test most widely used for surveillance is ultrasonography. A small HCC on US may take on one of several different appearances. The smallest lesions may be echogenic because of the presence of fat in the cells. Other lesions may be hypoechoic or show a "target lesion" appearance. None of these appearances is specific. US has been reported to have a sensitivity of between 65% and 80% and a specificity >90% when used as a screening test (15,87). However, the surveillance performance characteristics have not been as well defined in nodular cirrhotic livers (88,89). These performance characteristics, although not ideal, are considerably superior to the serologic tests. The major drawback to using US for HCC surveillance is that it is extremely operator dependent. In addition, scanning is difficult in obese subjects. Ideally, ultrasonographers performing HCC surveillance should receive special training, much as is done for mammographic surveillance in some jurisdictions.

Strategies such as alternating AFP and ultrasonography at intervals have no scientific basis. The guiding principle should be to choose the best available screening test and apply it regularly. Combined use of AFP and ultrasonography increases detection rates, costs, and false-positive rates (90). AFP-only surveillance had a 5.0% false-positive rate, and US alone had a 2.9% false-positive rate, but in combination the false-positive rate was 7.5%. US alone costs about $2,000 per tumor found, whereas the combination costs about $3,000 per tumor found (90).

Some reports suggest the use of CT scanning as a screening test for HCC (91–93). This is problematic for several reasons. First, a screening test is usually not also the diagnostic test of choice. Second, the performance characteristics of CT scanning have been developed in diagnostic/staging studies and the performance characteristics of CT scanning in HCC surveillance are unknown. If CT scan is to be used as a screening test (i.e., every 6–12 months over many years), there is a significant radiation exposure to be considered. In addition, practical experience suggests that the false-positive rate will be very high.

Surveillance Interval

The surveillance interval is determined by the tumor growth rates and not by the degree of risk. This is an important concept because it means that the surveillance interval does not need to be shortened for patients at higher risk. However, it is important to make the distinction between patients undergoing surveillance (i.e., those in whom although high risk is recognized, there is no a priori reason to suspect HCC vs. those in whom surveillance tests have been abnormal and there is a concern that HCC is already present). Strictly speaking, such patients are not candidates for surveillance but should be receiving enhanced follow-up.

The ideal surveillance interval is not known. A surveillance interval of 6 to 12 months has been proposed based on tumor doubling times. The positive randomized controlled trial described previously (52) used a 6-month interval. However, a retrospective study has reported that survival is no different in patients screened at 6- or 12-month intervals (94). Another study in HCV-infected hemophiliacs without cirrhosis suggested that the likelihood of finding HCC at the single nodule stage (as opposed to multinodular HCC) was the same with 6- and 12-month surveillance intervals (95). Both studies had problematic designs. The American Association for the Study of Liver Diseases (AASLD) guidelines (96) suggest a 6- to 12-month interval. However, once an abnormal screening test has been identified and patients are entered into enhanced follow-up, the interval between evaluations should be shorter.

RECALL POLICIES

Recall policies are the policies instituted to deal with an abnormal screening test result. The first step is to define an abnormal result. Establishing what constitutes an abnormal result on a screening US is not easy. A new mass in a patient who has been undergoing surveillance previously is clearly abnormal. A mass that enlarges is also abnormal, even if it was previously considered to be benign. In nodular cirrhotic livers, early HCC can be difficult to distinguish from background nodularity. Some cirrhotic nodules can be as large as 2 cm in diameter.

Diagnosis of Hepatocellular Carcinoma

The tests used to diagnose HCC include radiology, biopsy, and AFP serology. Which tests should be used depends on the context. Some form of imaging such as CT scan or magnetic resonance imaging (MRI) is always required to determine the extent of disease. In the setting of a patient with known hepatitis B or cirrhosis of other etiology, when a mass is found incidentally or on screening US, the likelihood of it being HCC depends on its size.

The radiologic features that are typical of HCC are that the lesion exhibits hypervascularity on the arterial phase of a dynamic study (CT, MRI, or contrast US) and exhibits "washout" during the venous phase. These features are highly specific for HCC (97,98). The physiological basis for these appearances is as follows. HCC is fed by an arterial supply. Thus, during the arterial phase, the liver is supplied by arterial and portal venous blood, whereas the tumor is fed by only arterial blood. The portal venous blood in the liver dilutes the contrast agent. This does not occur in the tumor, so the tumor exhibits a higher concentration of contrast agent and appears "brighter" than the surrounding liver. During the venous phase, the liver is fed by portal blood, now containing contrast, and arterial blood, which no longer contains contrast. The tumor is fed by arterial blood, which also has no contrast agent. Thus, the liver will be "brighter" than the lesion, or, in the terminology used, the lesion will exhibit "washout" of contrast. The smaller the lesion, the less likely typical features will be found.

Only a single morphologic variant between a normal hepatocyte and a malignant cell can be identified on biopsy. This is the so-called high-grade dysplasia. However, not all high-grade dysplastic lesions will develop into HCC. The diagnosis of high-grade dysplasia and early HCC are difficult to make on needle biopsy, and often requires expert pathology interpretation. High-grade dysplasia exhibits increased cell density, some nuclear irregularity, nuclear hyperchromasia, and cytoplasmic basophilia. In contrast, well-differentiated HCC lesions exhibit widened cell plates, further increased cell density, increased nuclear-cytoplasmic ratio, frequent mitotic figures, and the absence of portal tracts, among other features.

If the AFP is >200 ng/mL in the setting of a mass in a cirrhotic liver, the likelihood of HCC is >90%, and biopsy is not required (99,100). It should be noted that biopsy of small lesions (1–2 cm in diameter) may not be reliable. First, when the lesion is so small that needle placement is problematic, it is difficult to be certain that the sample did indeed come from the lesion. Second, there is disagreement between pathologists as to the dividing line between dysplasia and well-differentiated HCC (101), and this disagreement occurs more frequently as the size of the lesion decreases. Finally, it may be difficult, if not impossible, to distinguish well-differentiated HCC from normal liver on biopsy or from normal hepatocytes on fine-needle aspiration, where the architectural features of HCC, such as widened plates, are lost.

Lesions <1 cm in diameter on US, particularly in a cirrhotic liver, have a low likelihood of being HCC (102). Malignancy is even less likely if such lesions do not show contrast uptake on dynamic imaging (103). Even if CT or MRI shows arterial vascularization, the vascularized areas may not correspond to HCC foci (104,105). However, the possibility remains high that minute hepatic nodules detected by US may become malignant over time (106,107). Therefore, these nodules need to be regularly followed up every few months in order to detect growth suggestive of malignant transformation. Lack of growth over more than 1 to 2 years suggests that the lesion is not HCC.

Lesions between 1 and 2 cm in diameter have an indeterminate likelihood of being HCC. The AASLD guidelines (96) recommend that the diagnosis of HCC can be made without biopsy in patients with chronic liver disease and cirrhosis who have a mass between 1 and 2 cm in diameter if the mass shows characteristic radiologic features on at least two dynamic imaging techniques. Lesions showing typical features on both techniques should be treated as HCC because the PPV of the clinical and radiologic findings exceeds 95% (98,99). If the two techniques give discordant results (one typical and one atypical) or if both techniques give atypical results, a biopsy is required to confirm the diagnosis. If the lesion is >2 cm in diameter, only a single dynamic study is necessary to confirm the diagnosis if the findings are typical of HCC. If the appearances are not typical, a biopsy should be done. These algorithms are demonstrated in Figs. 29.1 to 29.3. Of course, if the radiologic appearances

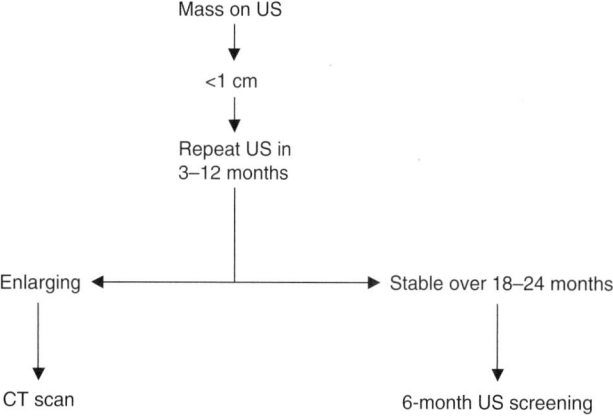

FIGURE 29.1. Investigation of a liver <1 cm in diameter.

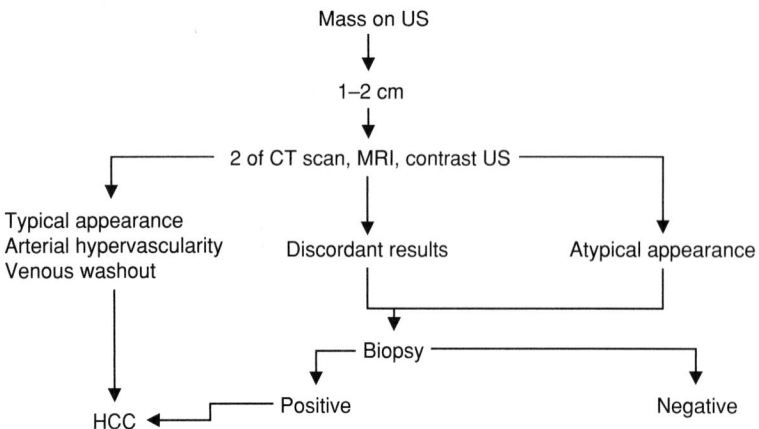

FIGURE 29.2. Investigation of a liver mass 1–2 cm in diameter.

are typical of some other diagnosis, such as hemangioma, no further investigation or follow-up is required.

Recently, a distinction has been made between "early HCC" or "carcinoma in situ" (101,107) and "small HCC" (102). Early HCC, as defined by Japanese pathologists, is generally hypovascular and has ill-defined margins. Thus, it has a somewhat vague outline on US and may be hypovascular on CT scanning. Histologically, there are few unpaired arteries, but the cells show varying grades of dysplasia. There may be invasion of the portal space by hepatocytes, but vessel invasion is absent. The pathology of these "very early HCC" lesions has been defined in resected specimens, and therefore, the natural history of these lesions is unknown. However, the presence of small foci of typical HCC within them has been noted, suggesting that these lesions are precursors of typical HCC lesions. The frequency with which these lesions develop typical HCC is unknown.

In contrast, "small HCC" have well-defined margins on US, and exhibit the typical features of HCC on CT and on histology (101,108). These lesions often show microvascular invasion, despite their small size. The presence of microvascular invasion suggests that the prognosis of these lesions after treatment is less good than for "early HCC," where vascular invasion is rare. However, this has not been proven in clinical studies. The identification of features of early HCC requires expert pathol-

ogy interpretation, but if present should result in therapy being offered. Therefore, a positive biopsy is helpful, but a negative biopsy can never be taken as conclusive. Patients with lesions 1 to 2 cm in diameter who have a negative biopsy should continue to undergo enhanced follow-up. There are no data to establish the best policy to follow at this point, but repeated biopsy or follow-up CT/MRI to detect further growth should be considered.

The smaller the lesion, the less likely there is to be microscopic vascular invasion (107). In addition, the smaller the lesion, the more likely it is that local ablation will be complete (64). It is therefore important to make the diagnosis early. However, it is equally important not to apply invasive treatment to lesions that have not developed malignant potential and can still regress. This is often a fine distinction that is not always possible to make

An additional concern about thin needle liver biopsy is the risk of bleeding and needle track seeding. Most studies that report needle track seeding do not specify the size of the lesion being biopsied. Although the rate of needle track seeding after biopsy of small lesions (<2 cm in diameter) has not been accurately measured, it is probably uncommon. The current rate of bleeding from thin needle biopsy of small HCC has not been reported, but it is probably no different than for biopsy of the liver in general.

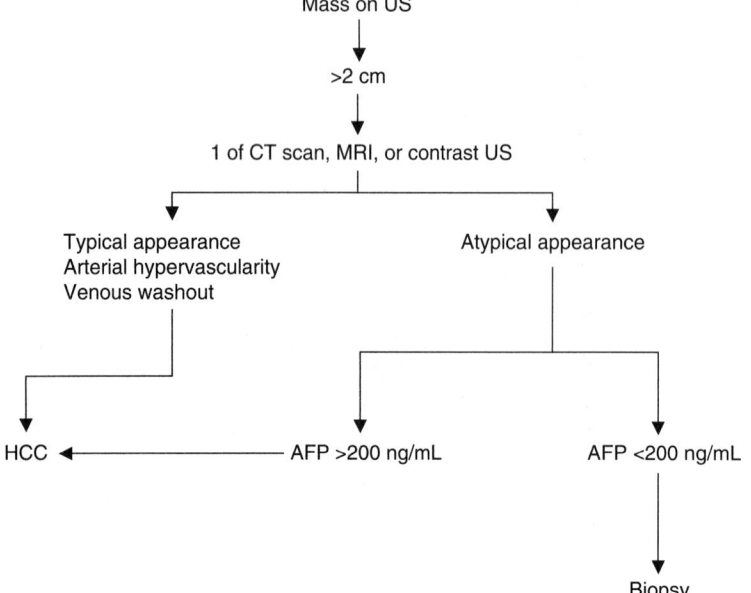

FIGURE 29.3. Investigation of a liver mass >2 cm in diameter.

FOLLOW-UP OF SUSPICIOUS LESION

Although the natural history of small lesions detected on ultrasonography is unknown, finding these lesions requires additional vigilance because it is likely that at least some of them will indeed become cancerous.

The interval between evaluations in the follow-up of suspicious lesions should be shorter than the usual screening interval. This is because in screening the objective is to find a lesion that has grown from being undetectable to being detectable. In follow-up, the objective is to reevaluate the patient at an interval that will identify a minimal amount of growth of a preexisting lesion. As with screening, there is no evidence to indicate what the interval should be, but because there is already an existing lesion, and because the consequences of too long an interval might be incurability, most experts will repeat the tests at a 3- to 4-month interval

One of the most important concepts is that a negative test result cannot, on its own, adequately rule out the presence of HCC. There is always the possibility of biopsy sampling error (biopsy) or incorrect interpretation (both pathology and radiology). Only lack of growth over a prolonged period of time indicates that a lesion is not malignant. Because small HCC may be slow growing, follow-up should be for a minimum of 18 to 24 months.

Lesions <1 cm in diameter do not require invasive diagnostic studies. If these small lesions are found on US, they should simply be monitored by the same technique (e.g., US). The interval between US examinations should be shorter than for screening (3–4 months). As long as the lesion is not growing, the US can be repeated at 3- to 4-month intervals. The required duration of this more intensive surveillance is not known but should be for at least 18 to 24 months. There is no need to do a CT scan for lesions <1 cm in diameter.

PREVENTION OF HEPATOCELLULAR CARCINOMA

There are several possible approaches to the prevention of HCC. The first is prevention of the underlying disease, the second is effective treatment of the liver disease once present, and the third approach is the use of medication to decrease the HCC risk in patients in whom the risk is perceived to be high (i.e., chemoprevention).

There is data from Taiwan that reduction in the incidence of hepatitis B will result in a decrease in HCC incidence. The initial studies were performed in children. HCC used to occur in hepatitis B–infected children in Taiwan with appreciable frequency. A large-scale study from Taiwan showed that after the introduction of neonatal hepatitis B vaccination, the rate of HCC in children younger than 12 years fell from 0.52 to 0.13 (2). It is unlikely that such a clear demonstration of the effect of control of the underlying liver disease will be shown for other causes of liver disease. Given the strong causal relationship that has been demonstrated between many liver diseases and HCC, it is highly likely that prevention of hepatitis C and alcoholic liver disease will also result in a reduction in HCC incidence rates.

It is also becoming clear that effective treatment of viral hepatitis will result in a reduction in HCC incidence. Early studies on the effect of interferon treatment of chronic hepatitis B showed a reduction in the incidence of HCC in patients who were responders to treatment (109,110). However, more recent studies have suggested that interferon therapy does not reduce the incidence of HCC (111). These studies used seroconversion from HBeAg positive to anti–HBe positive as the end point of therapy. One study (111) suggested that interferon therapy advanced seroconversion by a few years but did not increase the total number of patients who underwent seroconversion. It is now becoming apparent that the best predictor of the development of HCC is the viral load. There are several studies confirming this, including large-scale studies from Taiwan and China (112,113). Both studies enrolled about 3,500 hepatitis B carriers and followed them for more than 10 years. The relative risk of HCC increased as the baseline viral load rose. Among the highest viral loads, the relative risk of HCC was 11.6, with an incidence of 1150/100,000/year, compared to an incidence of 145/100,000/year for those with undetectable HBV DNA at baseline (113). The same study showed that subjects who had a spontaneous decline in viral load had a lower incidence of HCC than those in whom the viral load remained elevated (114). For example, in subjects who had a viral load of more than 10^5 copies/mL that persisted over the study period, the incidence of HCC was 10,108/100,000/year (just >10%). In comparison, in those in whom the viral load fell from $>10^5$ copies/mL to $<10^4$ copies/mL, the incidence was 5,882/100,000/year. This would suggest that if the viral load could be suppressed by treatment, a similar reduction in risk would be observed. Indeed, there is a single controlled study in which cirrhotic hepatitis B carriers who had active viral replication were randomized to receive either lamivudine or placebo (115). There was a significant reduction in the incidence of HCC in the treated group. Thus, the principle has been established that control of viral replication results in a decline in HCC incidence. Although it has not yet been proven, it is likely that suppression of viral load in precirrhotic patients who have active viral replication will also result in a reduction in HC incidence.

Up to 40% of patients with chronic hepatitis B will die of liver-related complications, and most of that will be due to HCC. Current treatment guidelines target only a small proportion of all hepatitis B carriers. Thus, to have a significant effect on HCC incidence, the treatment guidelines will have to be revised.

Effective treatment of chronic hepatitis C will also reduce HCC incidence. There are numerous studies, mostly from Japan, in which it has been demonstrated that patients who are sustained responders to therapy do indeed have a reduction in HCC incidence (116,117). Some of these studies also demonstrated that even those who did not have a sustained response had a reduction in HCC incidence. Studies elsewhere have not found these associations. The issue has been subject to a meta-analysis (118), which showed that there is a reduction in HCC incidence in successfully treated patients, although the reduction is not large. The meta-analysis also confirmed that even nonresponders have a reduction in HCC risk.

Successful treatment of hepatitis C results in eradication of the virus. Thus, it is likely that successfully treated precirrhotic patients will have a much reduced incidence of HCC. However, it is unlikely that this will ever be shown by prospective cohort studies given how long it will take for such a study to be completed and given that it would not be possible to have an untreated control group.

Several agents have been proposed as potentially having chemoprotective properties. These include chlorophyllin, oltipraz, and acyclic retinoids. Oltipraz inhibits the formation of aflatoxin adducts. Studies have shown that oltipraz administered to patients at high risk for HCC does indeed result in a change in concentration of various aflatoxin metabolites (119,120). There are as yet no studies demonstrating that this is correlated with a reduction in HCC incidence. Chlorophyllin also interferes with aflatoxin metabolism. Studies have shown that administration of chlorophyllin results in a reduction in the excretion of the oncogenic metabolite of aflatoxin (121,122), presumably because less of this metabolite is formed. There is a single publication showing that acyclic retinoids reduce the incidence of recurrence of HCC after initial treatment (resection) (123). These compounds have not been tested in a primary chemopreventative mode.

In summary, chemoprevention is not yet a practical consideration for the prevention of HCC.

References

1. Parkin DM, Bray F, Ferlay J, Pisani P. Estimating the world cancer burden: Globocan 2000. *Int J Cancer* 2001;94(2):153–156.
2. Chang MH, Chen CJ, Lai MS, et al. Universal hepatitis B vaccination in Taiwan and the incidence of hepatocellular carcinoma in children. Taiwan Childhood Hepatoma Study Group. *N Engl J Med* 1997;336:1906–1907.
3. Bosch FX, Ribes J, Diaz M, Cleries R. Primary liver cancer: worldwide incidence and trends. *Gastroenterology* 2004;127(5 suppl 1):S5–S16.
4. El Serag HB, Mason AC. Rising incidence of hepatocellular carcinoma in the United States. *N Engl J Med* 1999;340(10):745–750.
5. Deuffic S, Poynard T, Buffat L, Valleron AJ. Trends in primary liver cancer. *Lancet* 1998;351(9097):214–215.
6. Taylor-Robinson SD, Foster GR, Arora S, Hargreaves S, Thomas HC. Increase in primary liver cancer in the UK, 1979–94. *Lancet* 1997; 350(9085):1142–1143.
7. Stroffolini T, Andreone P, Andriulli A, et al. Characteristics of hepatocellular carcinoma in Italy. *J Hepatol* 1998;29(6):944–952.
8. El Serag HB, Mason AC. Risk factors for the rising rates of primary liver cancer in the United States. *Arch Intern Med* 2000;160(21):3227–3230.
9. Rosenblatt KA, Weiss NS, Schwartz SM. Liver cancer in Asian migrants to the United States and their descendants. *Cancer Causes Control* 1996;7:345–350.
10. Beasley RP, Hwang LY, Lin CC, Chien CS. Hepatocellular carcinoma and hepatitis B virus: a prospective study of 22 707 men in Taiwan. *Lancet* 1981;2(8256):1129–1133.
11. Beasley RP. Hepatitis B virus as the etiologic agent in hepatocellular carcinoma. *Hepatology* 1982;2(suppl):21s–26s.
12. Sakuma K, Saitoh N, Kasai M, et al. Relative risks of death due to liver disease among Japanese male adults having various statuses for hepatitis B s and e antigen/antibody in serum: a prospective study. *Hepatology* 1988;8:1642–1646.
13. Villeneuve JP, Desrochers M, Infante-Rivard C, et al. A long-term follow-up study of asymptomatic hepatitis B surface antigen-positive carriers in Montreal. *Gastroenterology* 1994;106(4):1000–1005.
14. McMahon BJ, Alberts SR, Wainwright RB, Bulkow L, Lanier AP. Hepatitis B-related sequelae: prospective study of 1400 hepatitis B surface antigen-positive Alaska native carriers. *Arch Intern Med* 1990;150:1051–1054.
15. Sherman M, Peltekian KM, Lee C. Screening for hepatocellular carcinoma in chronic carriers of hepatitis B virus: incidence and prevalence of hepatocellular carcinoma in a North American urban population. *Hepatology* 1995;22:432–438.
16. Fattovich G, Brollo L, Giustina G, et al. Natural history and prognostic factors for chronic hepatitis type B. *Gut* 1991;32(3):294–298.
17. Manno M, Camma C, Schepis F, et al. Natural history of chronic HBV carriers in northern Italy: morbidity and mortality after 30 years. *Gastroenterology* 2004;127(3):756–763.
18. de Franchis R, Meucci G, Vecchi M, et al. The natural history of asymptomatic hepatitis B surface antigen carriers. *Ann Intern Med* 1993;118:191–194.
19. Sanchez-Tapias JM, Costa J, Mas A, Bruguera M, Rodes J. Influence of hepatitis B virus genotype on the long-term outcome of chronic hepatitis B in Western patients. *Gastroenterology* 2002;123(6):1848–1856.
20. Fattovich G. Natural history of hepatitis B. *J Hepatol* 2003;39(suppl 1): S50–S58.
21. Hsu YS, Chien RN, Yeh CT, et al. Long-term outcome after spontaneous HBeAg seroconversion in patients with chronic hepatitis B. *Hepatology* 2002;35(6):1522–1527.
22. Yang HI, Lu SN, Liaw YF, et al. Hepatitis B e antigen and the risk of hepatocellular carcinoma. *N Engl J Med* 2002;347(3):168–174.
23. Evans AA, Chen G, Ross EA, Shen FM, Lin WY, London WT. Eight-year follow-up of the 90,000-person Haimen City cohort: I. Hepatocellular carcinoma mortality, risk factors, and gender differences. *Cancer Epidemiol Biomarkers Prev* 2002;11:369–376.
24. Yuen MF, Wong DK, Sablon E, et al. HBsAg seroclearance in chronic hepatitis B in the Chinese: virological, histological, and clinical aspects. *Hepatology* 2004;39(6):1694–1701.
25. Huo TI, Wu JC, Lee PC, et al. Sero-clearance of hepatitis B surface antigen in chronic carriers does not necessarily imply a good prognosis. *Hepatology* 1998;28(1):231–236.
26. Fattovich G, Giustina G, Sanchez-Tapias J, et al. Delayed clearance of serum HBsAg in compensated cirrhosis B: relation to interferon alpha therapy and disease prognosis. European Concerted Action on Viral Hepatitis (EUROHEP) [see comments]. *Am J Gastroenterol* 1998;93(6):896–900.
27. Fattovich G, Giustina G, Degos F, et al. Morbidity and mortality in compensated cirrhosis type C: a retrospective follow-up study of 384 patients. *Gastroenterology* 1997;112(2):463–472.
28. Niederau C, Lange S, Heintges T, et al. Prognosis of chronic hepatitis C: results of a large, prospective cohort study. *Hepatology* 1998;28(6):1687–1695.
29. Degos F, Christidis C, Ganne-Carrie N, et al. Hepatitis C virus related cirrhosis: time to occurrence of hepatocellular carcinoma and death. *Gut* 2000;47(1):131–136.
30. Roudot-Thoraval F, Bastie A, Pawlotsky JM, Dhumeaux D. Epidemiological factors affecting the severity of hepatitis C virus-related liver disease: a French survey of 6,664 patients. The Study Group for the Prevalence and the Epidemiology of Hepatitis C Virus. *Hepatology* 1997;26:485–490.
31. Sun CA, Wu DM, Lin CC, et al. Incidence and cofactors of hepatitis C virus-related hepatocellular carcinoma: a prospective study of 12,008 men in Taiwan. *Am J Epidemiol* 2003;157(8):674–682.
32. Davis GL, Albright JE, Cook SF, Rosenberg DM. Projecting future complications of chronic hepatitis C in the United States. *Liver Transpl* 2003;9:331–338.
33. Law MG, Dore GJ, Bath N, et al. Modelling hepatitis C virus incidence, prevalence and long-term sequelae in Australia, 2001. *Int J Epidemiol* 2003;32:717–724.
34. Sypsa V, Touloumi G, Papatheodoridis GV, et al. Future trends of HCV-related cirrhosis and hepatocellular carcinoma under the currently available treatments. *J Viral Hepat* 2005;12:543–550.
35. Hassan MM, Hwang LY, Hatten CJ, et al. Risk factors for hepatocellular carcinoma: synergism of alcohol with viral hepatitis and diabetes mellitus. *Hepatology* 2002;36(5):1206–1213.
36. Schoniger-Hekele M, Muller C, Kutilek M, Oesterreicher C, Ferenci P, Gangl A. Hepatocellular carcinoma in Austria: aetiological and clinical characteristics at presentation. *Eur J Gastroenterol Hepatol* 2000;12(8): 941–948.
37. El Serag HB, Mason AC. Risk factors for the rising rates of primary liver cancer in the United States. *Arch Intern Med* 2000;160(21):3227–3230.
38. Adami HO, Chow WH, Nyren O, et al. Excess risk of primary liver cancer in patients with diabetes mellitus. *J Natl Cancer Inst* 1996;88(20):1472–1477.
39. Bugianesi E, Leone N, Vanni E, et al. Expanding the natural history of nonalcoholic steatohepatitis: from cryptogenic cirrhosis to hepatocellular carcinoma. *Gastroenterology* 2002;123(1):134–140.
40. Shimada M, Hashimoto E, Taniai M, et al. Hepatocellular carcinoma in patients with non-alcoholic steatohepatitis. *J Hepatol* 2002;37(1):154–160.
41. Elmberg M, Hultcrantz R, Ekbom A, et al. Cancer risk in patients with hereditary hemochromatosis and in their first-degree relatives. *Gastroenterology* 2003;125:1733–1741.
42. Hsing AW, McLaughlin JK, Olsen JH, Mellemkjar L, Wacholder S, Fraumeni JF, Jr. Cancer risk following primary hemochromatosis: a population-based cohort study in Denmark. *Int J Cancer* 1995;60(2):160–162.
43. Fracanzani AL, Conte D, Fraquelli M, et al. Increased cancer risk in a cohort of 230 patients with hereditary hemochromatosis in comparison to matched control patients with non-iron-related chronic liver disease. *Hepatology* 2001;33(3):647–651.
44. Elzouki AN, Eriksson S. Risk of hepatobiliary disease in adults with severe alpha 1-antitrypsin deficiency (PiZZ): is chronic viral hepatitis B or C an additional risk factor for cirrhosis and hepatocellular carcinoma? *Eur J Gastroenterol Hepatol* 1996;8(10):989–994.
45. Eriksson S, Carlson J, Velez R. Risk of cirrhosis and primary liver cancer in alpha 1-antitrypsin deficiency. *N Engl J Med* 1986;314(12):736–739.
46. Caballeria L, Pares A, Castells A, Gines A, Bru C, Rodes J. Hepatocellular carcinoma in primary biliary cirrhosis: similar incidence to that in hepatitis C virus-related cirrhosis. *Am J Gastroenterol* 2001;96(4):1160–1163.
47. Welch HG, Schwartz LM, Woloshin S. Do increased 5-year survival rates in prostate cancer indicate better outcomes? *JAMA* 2000;284(16):2053–2055.
48. McMahon BJ, Bulkow L, Harpster A, et al. Screening for hepatocellular carcinoma in Alaska natives infected with chronic hepatitis B: a 16-year population-based study. *Hepatology* 2000;32(4 pt 1):842–846.
49. Wong LL, Limm WM, Severino R, Wong LM. Improved survival with screening for hepatocellular carcinoma. *Liver Transpl* 2000;6(3):320–325.
50. Oka H, Kurioka N, Kim K, et al. Prospective study of early detection of hepatocellular carcinoma in patients with cirrhosis. *Hepatology* 1990;12(4 pt 1):680–687.
51. Chen JG, Parkin DM, Chen QG, et al. Screening for liver cancer: results of a randomised controlled trial in Qidong, China. *J Med Screen* 2003; 10(4):204–209.
52. Zhang BH, Yang BH, Tang ZY. Randomized controlled trial of screening for hepatocellular carcinoma. *J Cancer Res Clin Oncol* 2004;130(7):417–422.
53. Sarasin FP, Giostra E, Hadengue A. Cost-effectiveness of screening for detection of small hepatocellular carcinoma in western patients with Child-Pugh class A cirrhosis. *Am J Med* 1996;101(4):422–434.
54. Arguedas MR, Chen VK, Eloubeidi MA, Fallon MB. Screening for hepatocellular carcinoma in patients with hepatitis C cirrhosis: a cost-utility analysis. *Am J Gastroenterol* 2003;98:679–690.
55. Calvet X, Bruix J, Bru C, et al. Natural history of hepatocellular carcinoma in Spain: five year's experience in 249 cases. *J Hepatol* 1990;10:311–317.

56. Lerose R, Molinari R, Rocchi E, Manenti F, Villa E. Prognostic features and survival of hepatocellular carcinoma in Italy: impact of stage of disease. *Eur J Cancer* 200;37:239–245.

57. Colleoni M, Bajetta E, Nelli P, et al. Prognostic factors in patients affected by hepatocellular carcinoma treated with systemic chemotherapy: the experience of the National Cancer Institute of Milan. *Ann Oncol* 1993;4: 489–493.

58. Di Carlo V, Ferrari G, Castoldi R, et al. Surgical treatment and prognostic variables of hepatocellular carcinoma in 122 cirrhotics. *Hepatogastroenterology* 1995;42:222–229.

59. Zavaglia C, De Carlis L, Alberti AB, et al. Predictors of long-term survival after liver transplantation for hepatocellular carcinoma. *Am J Gastroenterol* 2005;100(12):2708–2716.

60. Zavaglia C, De Carlis L, Alberti AB, et al. Predictors of long-term survival after liver transplantation for hepatocellular carcinoma. *Am J Gastroenterol* 2005;100:2708–2716.

61. Island ER, Pomposelli J, Pomfret EA, Gordon FD, Lewis WD, Jenkins RL. Twenty-year experience with liver transplantation for hepatocellular carcinoma. *Arch Surg* 2005;140:353–358.

62. Yao FY, Ferrell L, Bass NM, et al. Liver transplantation for hepatocellular carcinoma: expansion of the tumor size limits does not adversely impact survival. *Hepatology* 2001;33:1394–1403.

63. Mazzaferro V, Regalia E, Doci R, et al. Liver transplantation for the treatment of small hepatocellular carcinomas in patients with cirrhosis. *N Engl J Med* 1996;334:693–699.

64. Sala M, Llovet JM, Vilana R, et al. Initial response to percutaneous ablation predicts survival in patients with hepatocellular carcinoma. *Hepatology* 2004;40(6):1352–1360.

65. Laupacis A, Feeny D, Detsky AS, Tugwell PX. How attractive does a new technology have to be to warrant adoption and utilization? Tentative guidelines for using clinical and economic evaluations. *CMAJ* 1992;146:473–481.

66. Naimark D, Naglie G, Detsky AS. The meaning of life expectancy: what is a clinically significant gain? *J Gen Intern Med* 1994;9(12):702–707.

67. Lin OS, Keeffe EB, Sanders GD, Owens DK. Cost-effectiveness of screening for hepatocellular carcinoma in patients with cirrhosis due to chronic hepatitis C. *Aliment Pharmacol Ther* 2004;19:1159–1172.

68. Trevisani F, D'Intino PE, Morselli-Labate AM, et al. Serum alpha-fetoprotein for diagnosis of hepatocellular carcinoma in patients with chronic liver disease: influence of HBsAg and anti-HCV status. *J Hepatol* 2001;34(4):570–575.

69. Pateron D, Ganne N, Trinchet JC, et al. Prospective study of screening for hepatocellular carcinoma in Caucasian patients with cirrhosis [see comments]. *J Hepatol* 1994;20(1):65–71.

70. Zoli M, Magalotti D, Bianchi G, Gueli C, Marchesini G, Pisi E. Efficacy of a surveillance program for early detection of hepatocellular carcinoma. *Cancer* 1996;78(5):977–985.

71. Di Bisceglie AM, Hoofnagle JH. Elevations in serum alpha-fetoprotein levels in patients with chronic hepatitis B. *Cancer* 1989;64:2117–2120.

72. Di Bisceglie AM, Sterling RK, Chung RT, et al. Serum alpha-fetoprotein levels in patients with advanced hepatitis C: results from the HALT-C trial. *J Hepatol* 2005;43:434–441.

73. Sherman M. Alphafetoprotein: an obituary. *J Hepatol* 2001;34:603–605.

74. Oka H, Tamori A, Kuroki T, Kobayashi K, Yamamoto S. Prospective study of alpha-fetoprotein in cirrhotic patients monitored for development of hepatocellular carcinoma. *Hepatology* 1994;19:61–66.

75. Izuno K, Fujiyama S, Yamasaki K, Sato M, Sato T. Early detection of hepatocellular carcinoma associated with cirrhosis by combined assay of des-gamma-carboxy prothrombin and alpha-fetoprotein: a prospective study. *Hepatogastroenterology* 1995;42:387–393.

76. Grazi GL, Mazziotti A, Legnani C, et al. The role of tumor markers in the diagnosis of hepatocellular carcinoma, with special reference to the des-gamma-carboxy prothrombin. *Liver Transpl Surg* 1995;1:249–255.

77. Tsai SL, Huang GT, Yang PM, Sheu JC, Sung JL, Chen DS. Plasma des-gamma-carboxyprothrombin in the early stage of hepatocellular carcinoma. *Hepatology* 1990;11:481–488.

78. Suehiro T, Sugimachi K, Matsumata T, Itasaka H, Taketomi A, Maeda T. Protein induced by vitamin K absence or antagonist II as a prognostic marker in hepatocellular carcinoma: comparison with alpha-fetoprotein. *Cancer* 1994;73:2464–2471.

79. Marrero JA, Su GL, Wei W, et al. Des-gamma-carboxyprothrombin can differentiate hepatocellular carcinoma from nonmalignant chronic liver disease in American patients. *Hepatology* 2003;37:1114–1121.

80. Koike Y, Shiratori Y, Sato S, et al. Des-gamma-carboxy prothrombin as a useful predisposing factor for the development of portal venous invasion in patients with hepatocellular carcinoma: a prospective analysis of 227 patients. *Cancer* 2001;91:561–569.

81. Kumada T, Nakano S, Takeda I, et al. Clinical utility of *Lens culinaris* agglutinin-reactive alpha-fetoprotein in small hepatocellular carcinoma: special reference to imaging diagnosis. *J Hepatol* 1999;30:125–130.

82. Sato Y, Nakata K, Kato Y, et al. Early recognition of hepatocellular carcinoma based on altered profiles of alpha-fetoprotein. *N Engl J Med* 1993;328:1802–1806.

83. Shiraki K, Takase K, Tameda Y, Hamada M, Kosaka Y, Nakano T. A clinical study of lectin-reactive alpha-fetoprotein as an early indicator of hepatocellular carcinoma in the follow-up of cirrhotic patients. *Hepatology* 1995;22:802–807.

84. Taketa K, Endo Y, Sekiya C, et al. A collaborative study for the evaluation of lectin-reactive alpha-fetoproteins in early detection of hepatocellular carcinoma. *Cancer Res* 1993;53:5419–5423.

85. Hayashi K, Kumada T, Nakano S, et al. Usefulness of measurement of *Lens culinaris* agglutinin-reactive fraction of alpha-fetoprotein as a marker of prognosis and recurrence of small hepatocellular carcinoma. *Am J Gastroenterol* 1999;94(10):3028–3033.

86. Okuda K, Tanaka M, Kanazawa N, et al. Evaluation of curability and prediction of prognosis after surgical treatment for hepatocellular carcinoma by *Lens culinaris* agglutinin-reactive alpha-fetoprotein. *Int J Oncol* 1999;14(2):265–271.

87. Chen TH, Chen CJ, Yen MF, et al. Ultrasound screening and risk factors for death from hepatocellular carcinoma in a high risk group in Taiwan. *Int J Cancer* 2002;98(2):257–261.

88. Larcos G, Sorokopud H, Berry G, Farrell GC. Sonographic screening for hepatocellular carcinoma in patients with chronic hepatitis or cirrhosis: an evaluation. *AJR Am J Roentgenol* 1998;171(2):433–435.

89. Lencioni R, Menu Y. Ultrasound and doppler ultrasound of hepatocellular carcinoma. In: Bartolozzi C, Lencioni R, eds. *Liver Malignancies: Diagnostic and Interventional Radiology*. Berlin: Springer-Verlag; 1999;5:47070.

90. Zhang B, Yang B. Combined alpha fetoprotein testing and ultrasonography as a screening test for primary liver cancer. *J Med Screen* 1999;6:108–110.

91. Kobayashi K, Sugimoto T, Makino H, et al. Screening methods for early detection of hepatocellular carcinoma. *Hepatology* 1985;5(6):1100–1105.

92. Takayasu K, Moriyama N, Muramatsu Y, et al. The diagnosis of small hepatocellular carcinomas: efficacy of various imaging procedures in 100 patients. *AJR Am J Roentgenol* 1990;155(1):49–54.

93. Miller WJ, Baron RL, Dodd GD, III, Federle MP. Malignancies in patients with cirrhosis: CT sensitivity and specificity in 200 consecutive transplant patients. *Radiology* 1994;193(3):645–650.

94. Trevisani F, De NS, Rapaccini G, et al. Semiannual and annual surveillance of cirrhotic patients for hepatocellular carcinoma: effects on cancer stage and patient survival (Italian experience). *Am J Gastroenterol* 2002;97(3):734–744.

95. Santagostino E, Colombo M, Rivi M, et al. A 6-month versus a 12-month surveillance for hepatocellular carcinoma in 559 hemophiliacs infected with the hepatitis C virus. *Blood* 2003;102(1):78–82.

96. Bruix J, Sherman M. Management of hepatocellular carcinoma. Practice Guidelines Committee, American Association for the Study of Liver Diseases. *Hepatology* 2005;42:1208–1236.

97. Roncalli M, Roz E, Coggi G, et al. The vascular profile of regenerative and dysplastic nodules of the cirrhotic liver: implications for diagnosis and classification. *Hepatology* 1999;30:1174–1178.

98. Iannaccone R, Laghi A, Catalano C, et al. Hepatocellular carcinoma: role of unenhanced and delayed phase multi-detector row helical CT in patients with cirrhosis. *Radiology* 2005;234:460–467.

99. Levy I, Greig PD, Gallinger S, Langer B, Sherman M. Resection of hepatocellular carcinoma without preoperative tumor biopsy. *Ann Surg* 2001;234(2):206–209.

100. Torzilli G, Minagawa M, Takayama T, et al. Accurate preoperative evaluation of liver mass lesions without fine-needle biopsy. *Hepatology* 1999;30(4):889–893.

101. Kojiro M. Focus on dysplastic nodules and early hepatocellular carcinoma: an Eastern point of view. *Liver Transpl* 2004;10(2 suppl 1):S3–S8.

102. Nakashima T, Kojiro M. *Hepatocellular Carcinoma*. Tokyo: Springer Verlag; 1987.

103. Iwasaki M, Furuse J, Yoshino M, Ryu M, Moriyama N, Mukai K. Sonographic appearances of small hepatic nodules without tumor stain on contrast-enhanced computed tomography and angiography. *J Clin Ultrasound* 1998;26(6):303–307.

104. Burrel M, Llovet JM, Ayuso C, et al. MRI angiography is superior to helical CT for detection of HCC prior to liver transplantation: an explant correlation. *Hepatology* 2003;38(4):1034–1042.

105. Jeong YY, Mitchell DG, Kamishima T. Small (<20 mm) enhancing hepatic nodules seen on arterial phase MR imaging of the cirrhotic liver: clinical implications. *AJR Am J Roentgenol* 2002;178(6):1327–1334.

106. Fracanzani AL, Burdick L, Borzio M, et al. Contrast-enhanced doppler ultrasonography in the diagnosis of hepatocellular carcinoma and premalignant lesions in patients with cirrhosis. *Hepatology* 2001;34(6):1109–1112.

107. Takayama T, Makuuchi M, Hirohashi S, et al. Malignant transformation of adenomatous hyperplasia to hepatocellular carcinoma. *Lancet* 1990;336(8724):1150–1153.

108. Nakashima Y, Nakashima O, Tanaka M, Okuda K, Nakashima M, Kojiro M. Portal vein invasion and intrahepatic micrometastasis in small hepatocellular carcinoma by gross type. *Hepatol Res* 2003;26(2):142–147.

109. Niederau C, Heintges T, Lange S, et al. Long-term follow-up of HBeAg-positive patients treated with interferon alfa for chronic hepatitis B. *N Engl J Med* 1996;334:1422–1427.

110. Lin SM, Sheen IS, Chien RN, Chu CM, Liaw YF. Long-term beneficial effect of interferon therapy in patients with chronic hepatitis B virus infection. *Hepatology* 1999;29:971–975.

111. Yuen MF, Hui CK, Cheng CC, Wu CH, Lai YP, Lai CL. Long-term follow-up of interferon alfa treatment in Chinese patients with chronic hepatitis B infection: the effect on hepatitis B e antigen seroconversion and the

development of cirrhosis-related complications. *Hepatology* 2001;34:139–145.

112. Evans AA, Fabre RE, Chen G, Pasternack L, Iloeje UH. Hepatitis B viral load is associated with the development of hepatocellular carcinoma [abstract]. *Hepatology* 2004;40(suppl 1):602A.

113. Chen CJ, Yang HI, Su J, et al. Risk of hepatocellular carcinoma across a biological gradient of serum hepatitis B virus DNA level. *JAMA* 2006;295:65–73.

114. Iloeje UH, Yang HI, Su J, et al. Viral load is a strong predictor of hepatocellular carcinoma risk in people chronically infected with hepatitis B virus and with normal serum alanine aminotransferases [abstract]. *J Hepatol* 2005;42(suppl 2):179.

115. Liaw YF, Sung JJ, Chow WC, et al. Lamivudine for patients with chronic hepatitis B and advanced liver disease. *N Engl J Med* 2004;351:1521–1531.

116. Shiratori Y, Ito Y, Yokosuka O, et al. Antiviral therapy for cirrhotic hepatitis C: association with reduced hepatocellular carcinoma development and improved survival. *Ann Intern Med* 2005;142:105–114.

117. Hino K, Kitase A, Satoh Y, et al. Interferon retreatment reduces or delays the incidence of hepatocellular carcinoma in patients with chronic hepatitis C. *J Viral Hepat* 2002;9:370–376.

118. Camma C, Giunta M, Andreone P, Craxi A. Interferon and prevention of hepatocellular carcinoma in viral cirrhosis: an evidence-based approach. *J Hepatol* 2001;34:593–602.

119. Wang JS, Shen X, He X, et al. Protective alterations in phase 1 and 2 metabolism of aflatoxin B1 by oltipraz in residents of Qidong, People's Republic of China. *J Natl Cancer Inst* 1999;91:347–354.

120. Kensler TW, He X, Otieno M, et al. Oltipraz chemoprevention trial in Qidong, People's Republic of China: modulation of serum aflatoxin albumin adduct biomarkers. *Cancer Epidemiol Biomarkers Prev* 1998;7:127–134.

121. Egner PA, Munoz A, Kensler TW. Chemoprevention with chlorophyllin in individuals exposed to dietary aflatoxin. *Mutat Res* 2003;523–524:209–216.

122. Egner PA, Wang JB, Zhu YR, et al. Chlorophyllin intervention reduces aflatoxin-DNA adducts in individuals at high risk for liver cancer. *Proc Natl Acad Sci U S A* 2001;98(25):14601–14606.

123. Muto Y, Moriwaki H, Ninomiya M, et al. Prevention of second primary tumors by an acyclic retinoid, polyprenoic acid, in patients with hepatocellular carcinoma. Hepatoma Prevention Study Group. *N Engl J Med* 1996;334:1561–1567.

CHAPTER 30 ■ HEPATOCELLULAR CARCINOMA: MOLECULAR BIOLOGY AND GENETICS

MICHAEL C. KEW

INTRODUCTION

Hepatocellular carcinoma (HCC) is the most common primary malignant tumor of the liver and is regarded as one of the major malignant diseases in the world today. Among the reasons for this view are its high incidence, limited treatment options, and grave prognosis. HCC is either the most common tumor or among the three most common tumors in many of the most populous regions of the world, and it is fifth in overall frequency (1). It ranks third in annual cancer mortality rates (1), being responsible for >500,000 deaths each year. Attesting to the poor prognosis of HCC is the observation that in Black African and Chinese populations, which have the highest incidences of the tumor, the annual mortality rate from HCC is virtually the same as its annual incidence (2). Another reason for the importance of the tumor is that, unlike most types of malignant disease in humans, the majority of the risk factors for HCC have been identified, allowing substantial progress to be made in its primary prevention.

The incidence of HCC differs considerably in different geographic regions (1–3), as do the major causes of the tumor. In industrialized Western countries, usually with a low but sometimes an intermediate incidence of HCC, the major etiologic associations are alcoholic cirrhosis and chronic hepatitis C virus (HCV) infection; in Japan, with a high incidence of the tumor, chronic HCV infection is the predominant risk factor; and in eastern and Southeast Asia and sub-Saharan Africa, regions that have the highest incidences of HCC, chronic hepatitis B virus (HBV) infection, sometimes in association with heavy dietary exposure to the mycotoxin, aflatoxin B_1 (AFB$_1$), is responsible for approximately 80% of HCCs. HBV and HCV, between them, account for 70% to 85% of global HCC. Less frequent causes of the tumor, such as obesity/diabetes/nonalcoholic steatohepatitis (NASH), some of the inherited metabolic diseases, dietary iron overload in the African, and membranous obstruction of the inferior vena cava, may also occur predominantly in certain populations or regions.

HCC is proving to be heterogenous in its molecular genesis, with appreciable differences depending on the cause of the tumor. Moreover, the multiple and complex pathogenetic mechanisms involved, how they interact, and the sequence in which they occur are still poorly understood. The absence of a unifying explanation for hepatocarcinogenesis at a molecular level is limiting attempts both at designing effective treatments and at secondary and tertiary prevention of the tumor.

Regardless of the etiologic agent or agents involved, hepatocarcinogenesis is a complicated multistep process with the essential components being DNA mutations or damage and dysregulated hepatocyte proliferation in the face of reduced cell death. As a result of the linear and progressive process, increasingly more aberrant monoclonal populations of hepatocytes evolve and progress ultimately to a fully malignant phenotype. Several oncogenic mechanisms are involved, including loss of tumor-suppressor gene function, protooncogene activation, direct and indirect viral effects, changes in DNA methylation, failed DNA repair, telomerase activation, and angiogenesis. These events interact with host factors, such as immune responses and the hormonal milieu, in initiating and furthering the transition from normal to malignant hepatocytes. Local invasion and metastasis are related events.

Current knowledge of the molecular genesis of HCC is reviewed in relation to the more common or important causal associations of the tumor.

MOLECULAR GENESIS OF HEPATOCELLULAR CARCINOMA

Chronic Necroinflammatory Hepatic Disease

With almost all known causes of HCC—namely, chronic hepatitis virus infections, habitual alcohol consumption, diabetes/obesity/NASH, hereditary hemochromatosis and African dietary iron overload, α-1-antitrypsin deficiency, glycogen storage disease, hereditary tyrosinemia, hypercitrillinemia, Wilson disease, primary biliary cirrhosis, and membranous obstruction of the inferior vena cava—and in most geographic regions, the majority of the tumors occur in association with chronic necroinflammatory hepatic disease, commonly in the form of cirrhosis (4,5), occasionally chronic hepatitis (4,5), and rarely reversed hepatic lobulation complicating hepatic venous outflow obstruction (6). Moreover, all forms of cirrhosis, whatever their cause, may be complicated by the development of HCC (4,5,7). The tumor is also the major cause of liver-related deaths in patients with compensated cirrhosis (4,8). Chronic necroinflammatory hepatic disease is therefore the most common etiologic association of HCC worldwide.

Although chronic necroinflammatory hepatic disease may act alone in hepatocarcinogenesis, far more often it acts in concert with other known or not yet identified causes of the tumor, as shown by the observation that the frequency with which

HCC complicates cirrhosis ranges from as high as 30% with chronic HCV infection to as low as 4% with Wilson disease and primary biliary cirrhosis (4). Apart from the additional risk factors' inherent potential to induce malignant transformation, they are usually also the cause of the chronic hepatic inflammation and necrosis.

Constitutive (unrestrained) proliferation of hepatocytes is one of two essential components of hepatocellular carcinogenesis (9), the other being a series of mutations or changes at the genetic or epigenetic level. Cell cycle activation in the genesis of the tumor can be directly triggered by overexpression of a single gene or combinations of genes, or be initiated indirectly by compensatory proliferation of hepatocytes in response to injury (9). Hepatocytes are normally in a quiescent state, with a very low turnover rate (the estimated half-life of hepatocytes is 6 months [10]), but they react to loss of liver cells with an extraordinarily vigorous proliferative response (11,12). This response is normally short lived and tightly controlled, and does not lead to malignant transformation. Proliferation of hepatocytes is regulated by a number of factors, including nuclear factor-κB (NF-κB), transforming growth factor-α (TGF-α), insulinlike growth factor-2 (IGF-2), hepatocyte growth factor (HGF), and HGF receptor met (13–15). Transcriptional activation of these factors by proinflammatory mediators such as tumor necrosis factor-α (TNF-α), chemokines, and interleukins released during the inflammatory process regulates proliferation (13,14) and has, in addition, an antiapoptotic effect through upregulation of antiapoptotic target genes (15). With continuous hepatocyte proliferation, regardless of the initiating cause, the regulated proliferation, at some point and for reasons as yet poorly understood, may become unrestrained (9). A proliferative response with a change in the hepatocyte from a quiescent to a constitutively replicating cell is obligatory for the initiating activity in hepatocarcinogenesis (9,16).

Chronic necroinflammatory hepatic disease, irrespective of its cause, is characterized by continuous or intermittent necrosis of hepatocytes followed by regenerative proliferation that can, in certain circumstances, trigger the conversion of regulated proliferation to unconstrained proliferation. Rates of proliferation always exceed rates of apoptosis (13) so constitutive hepatocyte proliferation, in association with the accumulation over time of a number of DNA mutations or changes, results in the formation of hyperplastic hepatocyte nodules that progress to dysplastic nodules and finally to HCC (9). The exact timing of the original genetic or epigenetic change in relation to the onset of constitutive hepatocyte proliferation is uncertain, but thereafter the accumulation of successive mutations or damage occurs during the ongoing proliferation.

Existing quiescent hepatocytes are the cells mainly responsible for proliferation (9,12). Indeed, these cells have a proliferative potential that may exceed that of stem cells. They also appear to escape the senescence expected after several rounds of replication (17). Only uncommonly do oval cells (bipotential liver cells able to differentiate into either hepatocytes or bile duct epithelium cells) directly give rise to tumor cells, although it is possible that hepatocytes originating from oval cells could be at greater risk of oncogenic transformation than other hepatocytes (9).

By increasing the hepatocyte turnover rate, chronic necroinflammatory hepatic disease greatly enhances the risk of a cell being initiated and progressing to a malignant phenotype. At least three putative mechanisms are involved. Resting hepatocytes do not undergo mutation (18). However, spontaneous mutation or exogenously induced DNA damage or mutation may occur when quiescent hepatocytes enter the cell cycle (18) and are therefore prone to occur during hepatocyte proliferation. A variety of DNA repair mechanisms normally protect cells from mutations and damage (19). However, an accelerated rate of hepatocyte turnover allows less time for mutated, damaged, or rearranged DNA to be repaired before the cell divides again, thereby "fixing" the abnormal DNA in the daughter cells. For this and a number of other reasons, the failure of DNA repair processes facilitates the accumulation over time of a series of mutations. Progressive accumulation of mutations, rather than a single critical mutation, is an essential prerequisite for cancer formation (20,21). If cells harboring these mutations escape elimination by apoptosis or the host's immune response, they may over time become fully transformed. Unconstrained hepatocyte proliferation also provides an opportunity for the selective growth advantage of initiated cells to be exercised and allows clonal expansion of these cells, a crucial step in tumor promotion and progression (20,21).

Another contributor to the persistence and growth advantage of initiated cells is reactivation of telomerase, a ribonucleoprotein enzyme that prevents the shortening of telomeres (22). During progression of chronic hepatitis to cirrhosis, progressive shortening of telomeres occurs as a result of multiple cycles of cell injury, death, and regeneration, leading to premature senescence of hepatocytes (22). Telomere shortening beyond a critical length causes a proliferative block, manifesting as chromosomal instability, end-to-end fusions, and cell death (22). Hepatocarcinogenesis is characterized by the evolution of clones of hepatocytes with increased telomerase expression and an immortalized phenotype (22). Thus, almost all HCCs show reactivation of telomerase activity.

Concurrently with these various oncogenic mechanisms, the development of hepatic fibrosis distorts the lobular architecture of the liver, modifying normal cell-to-cell and cell-to-extracellular matrix interactions, which may contribute to loss of cell growth control (23). Furthermore, changes in the microcirculation of the liver, secondary to the disturbed architecture, may impair DNA repair processes and channel oncogenic substances to selected groups of hepatocytes (24,25).

In addition to providing the stimulus to constitutive proliferation of hepatocytes, chronic necroinflammatory hepatic disease can cause the mutations and DNA damage that are also required for oncogenesis. Oxidative stress induced by overproduction of reactive oxygen species (ROS) and reactive nitrogen species, in tandem with an unregulated increased hepatocyte turnover rate, plays an important role in the initiation and progression of carcinogenesis (26,27). Chronic necroinflammatory hepatic disease generates ROS (26,27). Putative mechanisms of free radical–induced hepatocyte damage and malignant transformation are the mutagenic properties of the radicals and their effect on lipid peroxidation. Different forms of oxidative damage cause different mutations, including chromosomal translocation, and modify gene expression in different ways. DNA strand breaks may also be induced (28). Deoxyguanosine residues in DNA are hydroxylated at the C8 position by hydroxyl radical or singlet oxygen to form 8-hydroxy-2-deoxyguanosine (8-OH-dG). Misreading of 8-OH-dG results in guanine (G) to thymine (T) transversions that may be important in carcinogenesis (29). Peroxidative decomposition of membrane polyunsaturated fatty acids releases reactive aldehyde metabolites, such as malondialdehyde (MDA), which may impair cellular functions, including nucleotide and protein synthesis, and damage intracellular organelles (30,31). The proteins affected include transcriptional regulators, such as *fos*, *jun*, and NF-κB, as well as components required for the activation of the antioxidant response element. Another biogenic aldehyde derivative, 4-hydroxy-2'-nonenol (4 HNE), interacts with DNA to form exocyclic guanine products, as shown by the significantly increased 4-HNE-deoxyguanine product in hepatic tissue in HCC (32).

The other recognized etiologic associations of HCC may either act in association with chronic necroinflammatory hepatic disease or independently.

Chronic Hepatitis B Virus Infection

HBV was one of the first viruses to be causally linked to a human tumor, and it is now believed to be, with tobacco, the most important environmental carcinogen to which humans are exposed. Of the estimated 350 million carriers of this virus in the world today (about 5% of the global population) or as many as one-fourth, will develop HCC. HBV infection acquired early in life is likely to become chronic and is implicated in the development of the great majority of HCCs that occur with high frequency in Chinese and Black African populations. However, the virus plays a far lesser causal role in industrialized countries. HBV is estimated to be responsible for approximately 53% of global HCC (1). The different genotypes of the virus have different hepatocarcinogenic potentials. In Far Eastern countries, where genotypes B and C predominate, a greater risk of tumor formation has been found with genotype C, and in southern Africa, where genotype A constitutes approximately 75% of the isolates, the risk of HCC development is 4.2 times higher with this genotype (33).

An effective and safe vaccine against HBV has been available for some years, and universal immunization of newborns in those countries in which the virus is endemic has already resulted in striking decreases in the carrier rates. Furthermore, in those endemic countries where universal immunization has been practiced for the longest times, HCC rates among children have already declined by as much as 70%. HBV vaccine can legitimately be regarded as the first "anticancer vaccine."

Many, perhaps even most, HBV-related HCCs coexist with cirrhosis and a few with chronic hepatitis, indicating that chronic necroinflammatory hepatic disease resulting from the host's immune response to the ongoing presence of the virus plays a key role in the pathogenesis of the tumor. HCC develops in 2% to 7% of patients with HBV-induced cirrhosis each year, but less often in those without cirrhosis. Given the seminal role of constitutive proliferation of hepatocytes in hepatocarcinogenesis, even in those patients with normal or near normal livers at the time of presentation of the tumor, a period of ongoing hepatocyte necrosis and regeneration may have occurred earlier, initiating the unconstrained proliferation of those cells that later became transformed. The necroinflammation could subsequently have resolved with little or no residual histologic changes. Chronic necroinflammatory hepatic disease is thus often an integral component of the hepatocarcinogenic potential of HBV.

Support for this belief is provided by the consequences of introducing HBV preS/S gene into transgenic mice. These mice overproduce large envelope (preS1) protein, which accumulates in the endoplasmic reticulum (ER) of hepatocytes, resulting in severe injury to the cells and initiating a response characterized by inflammation, oxidative DNA damage, regenerative hyperplasia, transcriptional deregulation and aneuploidy, and progressing ultimately to neoplasia (34). These findings imply that severe and prolonged hepatocyte injury, caused by the presence of the viral protein, ultimately lead to malignant transformation. The same series of events could be triggered by a relatively inefficient immune response by the host to the presence of HBV, resulting in some infected hepatocytes undergoing necrosis without downregulating overall HBV gene expression (35,36).

Possible pathogenetic mechanisms of HCC developing in a cirrhotic liver have already been mentioned, but additional mechanisms peculiar to HBV-associated HCC exist. HBV DNA does not integrate into cellular DNA in resting hepatocytes (34). However, the frequent cell divisions that occur in chronic necroinflammatory disease create the opportunity for HBV DNA to be inserted into host DNA. Moreover, oxidative DNA damage caused by chronic virally induced inflammation induces both DNA strand breaks and DNA instability that further increase the likelihood of integration events (37). In addition, enhanced intracellular activity of topoisomerase 1, a nicking/closing enzyme that reduces tension between the strands of DNA in supercoiled DNA resulting from hepatocyte proliferation, may predispose to insertion of HBV DNA by cleaving the viral genome at specific motifs, linearizing the circular DNA, and promoting its integration into chromosomal DNA (38).

Substantial evidence has accumulated that HBV has inherent potential to induce malignant transformation in addition to its ability to cause hepatic inflammation and necrosis. Observations that both woodchucks chronically infected with woodchuck hepatitis virus (WHV), which shares with HBV membership of the *Hepadnaviridae*, and transgenic mice into which the HBV x (HBx) gene with its regulatory sequences had been introduced develop HCC in the absence of cirrhosis support an inherent carcinogenic potential of the virus (39,40). Multiple factors appear to contribute to this potential, but the role of each and how they interact remains uncertain. The finding that HBV DNA was integrated into chromosomal DNA in the great majority of HBV-related HCCs (41,42) pointed to a number of putative mechanisms. HBV does not contain a recognized oncogene, but the presence of HBV DNA integrants in cellular DNA is consistent with the mechanism described for nonacutely transforming viruses, namely, insertional mutagenesis. This mechanism may take a number of forms.

Deletion, translocation, duplication, or amplification of chromosomal DNA in the sequences flanking integrated viral DNA occur far more often in HBV-related HCC than in HCC attributable to other risk factors (43,44). These changes may result in increased genomic instability, as well as in loss of tumor-suppressor genes, changes in the physical relation between protooncogenes or tumor-suppressor genes and their regulatory sequences that may perturb the expression of these genes in such a way as to contribute to malignant transformation, or the translocation of a protooncogene into a constitutively expressed gene.

HBV DNA integration precedes the development of HCC (45). Insertion occurs at one or, far more often, multiple sites. Viral DNA may integrate as a single linear sequence (almost always with some nucleotides missing from one or both ends of the insert [42]), but more usually it comprises contiguous fragments of viral sequences rearranged as a result of the oxidative damage caused by the chronic necroinflammatory hepatic disease (37,40,42). Insertion into host DNA appears to take place at random sites (although repeat Alu or satellite III DNA sequences are often targeted). However, allelic losses occur more often in certain chromosomes (1p,4q,6q, 8p,9p,13q,16p,16q,17q), and essentially the same chromosomes harbor changes in DNA copy numbers (46), suggesting that these regions contain genes often involved in hepatocarcinogenesis. Early data suggested that insertion of HBV DNA into chromosomal DNA at a site that may directly induce transformation (i.e., *cis* activation) was rare (47). However, more recent studies have shown HBV DNA to be integrated not infrequently in genes encoding for proteins that are important in the control of cell signaling, proliferation, and viability (48,49). Moreover, the telomerase gene has been shown to be targeted, and this might also be true of genes regulating calcium homeostasis and mitogen-activated protein kinase (MAPK)–dependent signaling, some of which have not previously been known to be involved in malignant transformation (48).

A *cis*-acting mechanism does, however, appear to be important in WHV-induced HCC in woodchucks. In 50% of infected animals, integration of WHV DNA occurs in the vicinity of N-*myc*-2 retroposon or *MYC*, considerably enhancing transcriptional activity of the promoters of these genes (50). Moreover, transgenic mice in which the WHV *MYC* gene, in tandem with upstream WHV DNA, has been incorporated into the germline, develop HCC (51).

The most common sites of HBV DNA insertion in the virus are in the cohesive overlap region between direct repeat sequences1 and 2 (DR1 and DR2) (52). This clustering suggests that intermediates of HBV replication serve as the substrates for integration (53). Strand invasion of chromosomal DNA by single-stranded linear HBV DNA is believed to initiate recombination.

Trans-activation by HBV proteins of cellular genes remote from the site of integration, thereby influencing cellular proliferation and differentiation, or apoptosis, is a more frequent mechanism of inherent oncogenesis (47,50,54). This effect could be mediated through signal conduction pathways. Two HBV genes, HBx and the preS2/S when 3' truncated during or after integration, have been shown to have transactivating capability (54).

Several lines of evidence support a role in the transformation process for deregulated HBx protein expression from integrated fragments of HBV DNA (55). Because the gene is close to the preferred insertion sites of HBV, it is the region of the genome most often included in integrants (56), and a selective accumulation of HBx gene transcripts has been reported in HBV-related HCC. Moreover, integrated HBx, even when truncated, frequently encodes functionally active transactivator proteins and may overexpress these proteins (56). Viral sequences encompassing the RNA encapsidation signal (which overlaps HBx) might also have intrinsic recombinogenic activity by virtue of binding to a putative recombinogenic cellular protein (57). The possible hepatocarcinogenic role for HBx protein is supported by a number of in vitro and animal model studies (51).

HBx protein does not contain any structural motifs that indicate a capacity to bind DNA directly. The 17-kDa protein is mainly a cytoplasmic protein, although there is also evidence for nuclear localization. HBx protein constitutively activates transcription from HBV enhancers and promoters, as well as from promoters of a number of cellular genes involved in the control of cell growth and proliferation, including protooncogenes, growth factors, and cytokines (58–61). Activation of transcription is mediated by modulating cell signaling pathways within the cytoplasm. The pathways activated include MAPK, the *Janus* family tyrosine kinase (JAK)/signal transducer and activators of transcription (STAT), Src, protein kinase C (PKC), activator protein-2 (AP-2), and *jun*-N-terminal kinase (58,59). Activation of JAK/STAT and Src signaling, as well as IGF-2 and TGF-α promoters, has been associated with increased hepatocyte proliferation (13,51,62). There is also evidence for transcriptional activation of the *ras/raf* signaling pathway leading to the activation of several oncogenes, including *FOS*, *MYC*, and *JUN*. Transcriptional activation of other genes, including those encoding for adhesion (intracellular adhesion molecule-1 [ICAM-1]) and HLAII molecules, is mediated by NF-κB, activator protein-1 (AP-1), and cAMP response element-binding (CREB) protein (60,61). In addition, HBx has been shown to inhibit the activity of some serine protease inhibitors and components of the proteasome complex (63), and might thus modulate the degradation and turnover of some cellular proteins involved in transcription or regulation of cell cycle progression, or both. HBx protein also binds directly to a number of transcription factors in the nucleus, such as activating transcription factor-2 (ATF-2), CREB, and p53 (58). In addition, HBx protein interacts at this site with transcription factors and elements of the basal transcription machinery transcription factor IIB, TATA box-binding protein (TBP), and RNA polymerase II subunit retinol-binding protein 5 (RBP5) (64,65).

Among the growth regulatory proteins whose functions are known to be perturbed by the HBx protein are p53, damage-specific DNA-binding protein 1 (DDB1), and the signal-mediated nuclear export receptor Crm1. The p53 tumor-suppressor gene maintains chromosomal integrity by arresting the cell cycle in G_1 and regulating the DNA damage-control response, thereby permitting repair of damaged DNA (66). If repair is not possible, apoptosis is induced. HBx protein binds to specific sequences in the C-terminal end of p53 protein, preventing its entry into the nucleus and abrogating its sequence-specific DNA binding and transcriptional activity (67,68). p53 Protein transcriptionally activates a tumor-suppressor gene product PTEN (phosphatase and tensin homology deleted on chromosome 10). Inactivation of p53 and PTEN proteins by HBx protein results in increased levels of hypoxia-induced factor-1α (HIF-1α) and vascular endothelial growth factor (VEGF), both of which are important for the survival and neovascularization of early stage tumors (69).

Inactivation of p53 protein may interfere with p53-dependent DNA repair (70–73). HBx protein may also compromise p53 protein function and DNA repair in other ways, thereby leading to the accumulation of potentially transforming mutations and microsatellite instability (19,70–76). The protein inhibits binding of the DNA repair proteins, XBP and XPD, to p53 protein, thereby compromising the efficiency of the DNA repair. It also directly interferes with DNA repair by complexing with the DNA repair protein, hepatitis Bx–associated protein, XAP-1, which normally binds to damaged DNA in the first step of nucleotide excision repair, as well as binding to damaged DNA.

The nuclear protein encoded by the p53 gene modulates transcription of a number of genes by binding to specific DNA sequences and to other cellular factors such as mouse double mutant 2 (MDM2), TBP, and Wilm tumor-1 (WT-1) (66). Missense mutations are common in the p53 gene, and these can cause loss of tumor-suppressor function or gain in oncogenic function (66). There is no evidence that the transversion of guanine (G) to thymine (T) at codon 249 of p53 (249^{ser}p53), induced by heavy dietary exposure to AFB$_1$, specifically interacts with the HBx protein in oncogenesis.

In addition to its inhibitory effect on p53-induced apoptosis (74,76), HBx protein inhibits caspase-3–dependent apoptosis (75). The presence of the protein may also sensitize cells to programmed cell death induced by TNF-α, an effect mediated by prolonged stimulation by N-*myc* transcription and the stress-mediated MAPK pathway (74). HBx protein transactivates the retinoblastoma (Rb) gene promoter, increasing expression of Rb protein, thereby resulting in cell cycle progression (77) and suppression of apoptosis (78). Another oncogenic pathway deregulated in HCC is the Wnt/β-catenin pathway. HBx protein transcriptionally upregulates the expression of β-catenin and may cause mutations of this gene (79).

Deletions in the C-terminal portion of HBx gene have been identified in HCC cells (80). Such deletions may enhance HBx protein-transforming capacity.

The PreS/S gene is also frequently included in HBV DNA integrants and might contribute to oncogenesis (55). PreS/S protein is exclusively cytoplasmic in location, and its transactivating effects are mediated by modulating PKC signal transduction; interaction with several transcription factors, such as NF-κB and AP1; and sequence-specific binding to DNA (81–83). Target genes for inactivation include *MYC*, *FOS*, *HRAS* oncogenes and the inflammation-associated cytokine IL-6 (84,85). Mutations in the transactivator region of presS/S gene may also contribute to escape of the virus from the host's defence mechanisms. In addition, PreS mutants may result in the accumulation of abnormal S proteins in the ER and induce ER stress, possibly contributing to hepatocarcinogenesis (86). These mutants also upregulate cyclin A expression and induce hepatocyte proliferation (87).

TGF-α is overexpressed in malignant hepatocytes in which HBsAg or HBV DNA is detected (88). Some of these liver cells have a morphology consistent with that of oval cells, implying that this growth factor, driven by HBV, might favor expansion of progenitor cells. PreS1 protein may be responsible for transactivation of TGF-α and another growth factor, IGF-2.

Chronic Hepatitis C Virus Infection

In approximately 80% of individuals acutely infected with HCV, the infection persists, and about 30% ultimately develop cirrhosis. Around 170 million people worldwide are estimated to be chronically infected with this virus. Those who develop HCC have usually been infected for 20 to 40 years and almost invariably have underlying cirrhosis, with most of the remainder having advanced hepatic fibrosis or chronic hepatitis. The risk of developing HCC in those with HCV-induced cirrhosis is 1% to 7% per annum, with a lower risk in those with chronic hepatitis. HCV is the predominant cause of the tumor in Japan, Italy, and Spain, and in other industrialized countries, alcoholic cirrhosis and HCV are the main risk factors. HCV-related HCC is increasing in frequency in a number of countries, including Japan and the United States. The reservoir of HCV infection in the general population of industrialized Western countries raises concerns that there is likely to be an increasing incidence of cirrhosis and HCC in these countries in the coming decades. HCV and HBV, between them, are responsible for 70% to 85% of global HCC. Successful treatment of chronic HCV infection with antiviral agents decreases the risk of tumor development. A vaccine against HCV is not yet available and is unlikely to become available in the near future.

Relatively little is known about the molecular genesis of HCV-induced HCC. This is explained, in part, by the almost invariable association between HCV-induced cirrhosis and the tumor that led to the early assumption that the virus caused chronic necroinflammatory hepatic disease, which in turn was responsible for the malignant transformation. In addition, the lack of a reliable tissue culture system or a small animal model of HCV infection made it difficult to investigate possible mechanisms of HCV hepatocarcinogenicity. Evidence is, however, accumulating that the virus also has inherent carcinogenic potential. HCV differs from HBV in that its replicative intermediates do not integrate into cellular DNA. In common with HBV, the genome of HCV does not contain a known oncogene. The virus has, however, been shown to replicate in HCC tissue (89), and the tumor develops in transgenic mice carrying the HCV core gene alone or the complete HCV genome (90). The evidence available suggests that HCV, like HBV, promotes tumorigenesis by upregulating genes that promote hepatocyte growth and survival and downregulating genes that act as tumor suppressors and negative growth-regulatory molecules (47). The core and NS5A genes have thus far been shown to be involved in hepatocarcinogenesis. Moreover, some similarities in the oncogenic mechanisms attributed to HBx protein and the HCV core and, to a lesser extent, NS5A proteins are beginning to emerge.

A close association exists between chronic HCV infection and oxidative stress (91,92). ROS are produced by the virally induced hepatic inflammation and by expression of the core and NS5A proteins (91,93). The ROS generated are highly reactive and attack biomolecules such as DNA, lipids, and proteins. In transfection studies in tissue culture, HCV core protein has been localized to the mitochondria, where it appears to induce production of ROS (94). Mitochondrial DNA is far more susceptible to mutation caused by ROS than is nuclear DNA (95). NS5A protein also generates oxidative stress, as well as activating NF-κB and STAT-3 (93). In the presence of hepatic steatosis, a feature of HCV-induced chronic liver disease, production of ROS is further enhanced as a result, in part, of viral gene expression.

Oxidative stress may exert synergistic effects with altered intracellular signaling pathways, including indirect activation of TNF-α, raf-1-kinase, and NF-κB pathways or B-cell lymphoma-2 (Bcl-2) expression, resulting in inhibition of TNF-α– and fas-mediated apoptosis (96,97). HCV core protein is specifically incriminated in this effect, but NS5A may also be involved. Induction of nitric oxide (NO) by inducible NO synthase by viral DNA may contribute to hepatocyte injury in chronic HCV infection (91,98). Nitric oxide also reduces the frequency of apoptosis by inhibiting caspases (99).

The p21$^{waf1/cip1}$ protein, a universal inhibitor of cyclin-dependent kinases, is upregulated by HCV-induced chronic hepatic inflammation and fibrosis, and this may play a role in oncogenic transformation. Other possible ways in which the hepatocarcinogenic effect of HCV may be explained include the high mutation rates in infected hepatocytes, including those in the mitochondria (100). Mutations of the p53, β-catenin, and other protooncogenes and tumor-suppressor genes are common (96). In addition, HCV core protein increases endogenous P4-mediated IGF-2 expression by phosphorylation and DNA binding of two cis-acting elements, the transcription factor Sp1 and early growth response1 (Egr1) binding sites (92), thereby increasing the rate of hepatocyte proliferation (51). Core protein activation of NF-κB is enhanced by NS5A expression in cell culture experiments (101). Core protein also inhibits the tumor-suppressor protein promyelocytic leukaemia isoform IV (PML-IV)–induced apoptosis and interferes with the coactivator function of PML-IV for proapoptotic p53 genes (102). Furthermore, it regulates expression of the DEAD box RNA helicase, DDX3, which has cell growth regulatory functions (103).

NS5A protein protects hepatocytes from TNF-α– and p53-induced apoptosis, the latter by sequestering the protein in the cytoplasm (104). There is also a direct link between HCV RNA replication and cellular expression of the Rb tumor-suppressor gene (105). Expression of Rb is downregulated posttranslationally in hepatocytes containing replicating HCV RNA, and NS5B RNA-dependent RNA polymerase is responsible for this effect (106). Hypermethylation of the promoter of p16^{ink4A} tumor-suppressor gene, with the resulting loss of its function, may be an early event in HCV-induced hepatocarcinogenesis (107).

Coinfection with HBV and HCV probably increases the risk of HCC, at a superadditive rather than at a multiplicative level (108). One way in which this may be achieved is by the increased incidence and severity of cirrhosis with coinfection with the two viruses. Proof of synergism between the inherent carcinogenic potentials of the two viruses will have to await a clearer understanding of the pathogenetic mechanisms involved with the individual viruses (108).

Alcohol

In 80% to 95% of patients with HCC in industrialized countries, the tumor develops in a cirrhotic liver (4,6). Habitual alcohol abuse or chronic hepatitis C virus infection, or the two together, are the cause of the cirrhosis in the great majority of these patients. No further increase in the risk of HCC occurs in patients with cirrhosis from causes other than alcohol if alcohol abuse becomes an additional risk factor (109,110). Furthermore, HCC rarely develops in alcoholics in the absence of chronic necroinflammatory hepatic disease (109,110). Studies in experimental animals support the belief that alcohol is not directly carcinogenic (111) but may act as a cocarcinogen or a tumor promoter, a belief in keeping with the observation that

HCC develops only in a minority of patients with alcoholic cirrhosis. A direct correlation between alcohol consumption and the development of HCC thus remains tenuous, although a causal association between alcoholic cirrhosis and HCC is undoubted.

Despite an increased understanding of the metabolism and actions of alcohol, the mechanisms by which alcohol causes hepatocyte injury and the reasons for progression from the resulting chronic necroinflammatory hepatic disease, and cirrhosis in particular, to HCC are not yet clearly defined. A number of mechanisms may be involved. Acetaldehyde, the product of ethanol metabolism by alcohol dehydrogenase, causes cellular damage and generates free radicals that bind to numerous cellular targets, including components of cell signaling pathways and DNA (112,113). DNA damage and oxidative stress result in cirrhosis and ultimately HCC. Oxidative stress produces dysregulation of gene expression and cell signaling cascades, which manifest in unregulated hepatocyte proliferation (114). Acetaldehyde also depletes the antioxidant, glutathione; decreases the methylation of cytosine; impairs DNA repair; and affects sister chromatid exchange, all of which may contribute to its carcinogenic effects (115,116). Acetaldehyde also potentiates the promitogenic Gi protein-MAPK signaling cascade (117). Polymorphisms of alcohol dehydrogenase and aldehyde dehydrogenase, which metabolizes acetaldehyde, have been shown not to influence the risk of HCC development with heavy alcohol consumption but to modify the risk at lower levels of intake (118).

Alcohol ingestion also induces oxidative stress in hepatocytes by mechanisms other than the formation of acetaldehyde. Cytochrome p450 2E1 (CYP2E1) is induced by alcohol (119). Although most ingested alcohol is oxidized by alcohol dehydrogenase, CYP2E1 assumes a more important role with higher levels of intake and with chronic consumption of alcohol (118,119). This enzyme facilitates the absorption of procarcinogens and their activation to carcinogens, as well as generates ROS. Induction of CYP2E1 may therefore result in DNA damage and mutations, or be involved in dysregulation of gene expression and cellular signaling cascades, manifesting in upregulated cell proliferation (118). Another result of oxidative stress is the peroxidative decomposition of membrane polyunsaturated fatty acids, such as arachidonate, and the β-cleavage of lipid hydroperoxides (119). The resulting biogenic aldehydes, particularly 4-HNE and MDA, are electrophilic and can interact with DNA or protein nucleophiles that specifically target the p53 tumor-suppressor gene (120). Iron accumulates in the liver in alcoholic liver disease for reasons not yet fully clarified (121), and this contributes to the oxidative stress (122,123). The combined prooxidant potential of alcohol and iron is at least additive and may be synergistic.

Alcohol abuse also results in interference with DNA methylation, which is an important epigenetic mechanism affecting the transcriptional regulation of genes involved in the development of HCC. This effect on hepatic methylation capacity is the result of its detrimental influence on the intake, absorption, and metabolism of vitamins responsible for methyl group synthesis and transfer (124). The latter also result in reduced levels of important antioxidants, methionine, S-adenosylmethionine, and glutathione, which have consequences with respect to hepatocarcinogenesis. In addition, promoter hypermethylation silences cyclooxygenase-2 and regulates growth in HCC (125). The ingestion and metabolism of alcohol reduces hepatic retinoic acid levels, and may thereby enhance cell proliferation and malignant transformation via upregulation of AP-1 gene expression (112).

Abuse of alcohol and cigarette smoking has synergistic hepatocarcinogenic effects (125,126). Apart from the accelerated hepatocyte turnover rate resulting from alcohol-induced cell injury that increases the likelihood of DNA damage by carcinogens in the cigarette smoke normally metabolized by the liver, CYP2E1 induction by alcohol may enhance the carcinogenicity of these compounds (127). Alcohol also has interactive hepatocarcinogenic effects with HCV (128) and, to a lesser extent, HBV (129). A number of mechanisms may be involved, but the additive effect on the development and severity of chronic necroinflammatory disease caused by two agents as opposed to a single agent is probably the major cause.

Aflatoxin B1

Aflatoxins are a family of difuranocoumarin derivatives produced by *Aspergillus flavus* and *Aspergillus parasiticus*. These fungi occur throughout the world but are more prevalent in poor resource countries with warm, humid climates. Heavy dietary exposure to aflatoxins is a major risk factor for HCC in parts of sub-Saharan Africa, China, and Taiwan. AFB_1 is the most potent of the aflatoxins as an experimental hepatocarcinogen and is the major component of aflatoxin mixtures found in human foodstuffs. Foods most often contaminated are corn, peanuts, various other nuts, rice, fermented soybeans, and soy sauce. The International Agency for Research on Cancer classifies AFB_1 as a definite human carcinogen.

The liver is the primary site of biotransformation of ingested AFB_1. Phase I cytochrome p450 enzymes (CYP1A2 and CYP3A4) oxidize the innocuous parent molecule to highly reactive intermediates, of which the most electrophilic is AFB_1-*exo*-8,9-epoxide (130). Phase II detoxification is accomplished by glutathione-S-transferase–mediated conjugation to glutathione. If AFB_1-*exo*-8,9-epoxide accumulates as a result either of excessive dietary intake of AFB_1 or decreased efficiency of phase II detoxification, the unstable intermediate soon binds with high affinity to guanine bases to form promutagenic covalent DNA adducts, the most prevalent of which is 8,9-dihydro-8-(N7-guanyl)-9-hydroxyaflatoxin B_1 (AFB_1-N7-Gua) (131). The positively charged imidazole ring of the adduct promotes depurination, forming an abasic site, or can be converted into AFB_1-formamidopyrimidine adducts (AFB_1-FAPY) by the opening of the imidazole ring of the adduct (132,133). Both AFB_1-*exo*-8,9 epoxide and AFB_1-FAPY give rise to G-to-T transversions (133), although the latter is far more potent in this regard (131). These two substances are the prime causes of both the genotoxicity and the mutagenicity of AFB_1. Studies of a possible effect of polymorphisms of glutathione-S-transferase on the risk of AFB_1-induced HCC have produced inconclusive results (134). Glutathione-S-transferase P1 is transcriptionally silenced by promoter hypermethylation in 20% to 85% of HCCs (135), and a statistically significant association has been reported between promoter hypermethylation of glutathione-S-transferase P1 and levels of AFB_1-DNA adducts in Taiwanese patients with HCC (135). In addition, O(6)-methylguanine-DNA methyltransferase (MGMT), a repair protein that specifically removes promutagenic alkyl groups from the O(6) position of guanine in DNA, is transcriptionally silenced by promoter hypermethylation (136). A significant association was found between MGMT promoter hypermethylation and high levels of AFB_1-DNA adducts in HCC tissue (136).

Patients with HCC show a strongly positive correlation between heavy dietary exposure to AFB_1 and the presence of a G-to-T transversion (arginine to serine) at the third base of codon 249 of the p53 tumor-suppressor gene (249^{ser}p53) (137,138), a region corresponding to the DNA-binding domain of the p53 protein (139,140). This association is supported by experimental studies (141). The mutation coincides with homozygous deletions in chromosome 16q and instability at the fragile site FRA16D (142). Whether the codon 249 site is an exceptional target for mutations or whether this mutation is selected for once it occurs remains to be determined. p53 Protein modulates multiple cellular functions, including gene transcription, DNA synthesis and repair, cell cycle arrest, senescence, and apoptosis (143). The biological effects of the 249^{ser}p53 mutation are not fully understood, but the mutation may abrogate these functions, transform cells in culture, and progress to cancer formation (144). AFB_1-FAPY lesions are preferentially repaired by nucleotide excision repair (145), which is compromised by inactivation of the p53 tumor-suppressor gene.

Other ways in which dietary exposure to AFB_1 might contribute to hepatocarcinogenesis have been suggested. A possible role for mutations of the β-catenin gene and the Wnt signaling pathway has been reported from China (146) but not from southern Africa (147). Another possible mechanism arises from the effect that the 249^{ser}p53 mutation has on increasing transcription of IGF-2 (148). This factor, together with the HBx protein and TNF-α inhibit apoptosis, providing an opportunity for the persistence of transformed hepatocytes. Aberrant methylation of the CpG island promoters of the ras association domain (RASSF) gene isoform 1A is a frequent occurrence in hepatocarcinogenesis, and an association has been described between the methylation status of RASSF1A and p16 and the level of AFB_1-DNA adducts in HCC tissues (149). CYP2E1 induction by AFB_1 may enhance the carcinogenicity of compounds inhaled from cigarette smoking, offering one explanation for the synergistic hepatocarcinogenic effects between smoking and AFB_1 ingestion (150).

Epidemiologic data have produced compelling evidence of a synergistic interaction between AFB_1 and HBV in hepatocarcinogenesis (151), and studies in transgenic mice and other animal models have confirmed the interaction (152,153). Several possible explanations have been offered. The increased hepatocyte necrosis and regeneration induced by chronic HBV infection increases the probability of AFB_1-induced mutations and the clonal expansion of cells containing these mutations (20). Cytochrome p450 enzymes may be induced, either by the chronic hepatitis attributable to the virus or by the presence of the virus itself (154,155), increasing the generation of electrophilic and mutagenic AFB_1 intermediates. In addition, increased hepatocyte proliferation reduces glutathione-S-transferase production, further increasing the opportunity for adduct formation (156–158). HBx protein expressed from integrated HBV DNA binds to p53, sequestering it in the cytoplasm, and inhibiting its sequence-specific DNA binding and transcriptional activity (159,160). In this way, the protein interferes with p53-dependent apoptosis (159,160) and nucleotide excision repair of the mutations caused by aflatoxin-induced DNA adducts, resulting in their persistence (161). DNA repair is also compromised by the rapid cell turnover rate in chronic hepatitis. The transcription of p21$^{waf1/cif1}$, which normally induces cell cycle arrest at the G_1-S checkpoint, is repressed by HBx protein when p53 protein is not functional or is functional at a low level (162). Finally, the chronic necroinflammatory hepatic disease resulting from HBV infection generates oxidative stress that is mutagenic (163).

Obesity/Diabetes Mellitus/Nonalcoholic Steatohepatitis

Obesity and diabetes mellitus, together with other overweight-related metabolic disturbances—dyslipidemia and insulin resistance—and arterial hypertension are causes of NASH and cirrhosis. NASH is now believed to be the most common cause of cryptogenic cirrhosis, at least in industrial-ized countries (164). Obesity, diabetes, and NASH have recently been shown to be complicated by the development of HCC (165). Other unrecognized risk factors such as hepatitis virus infections or excessive alcohol consumption may explain the association in some instances, but in the majority, obesity/diabetes/NASH is suspected to be the cause. Because obesity and diabetes predispose to NASH, the hepatocarcinogenic potential of NASH has come under focus. One way in which NASH may cause HCC is by its progression to cirrhosis. Certainly, no patients with HCC have been described with NASH without cirrhosis or in subjects with steatosis but no NASH (165).

NASH, in association with cirrhosis, may cause malignant transformation by the generation of ROS resulting in oxidative damage and lipid peroxidation (166,167). Other ways are by stimulating hepatocyte proliferation through disturbances in the expression of growth factors and cytokines and effects on apoptosis (168,169).

Insulin resistance and compensatory hyperinsulinemia are cardinal features of obesity and diabetes, and they may contribute to malignant transformation. Insulin is a potent activator of hepatocyte proliferation through its signaling pathways, the insulin receptor, and insulin growth factor-1 (IGF-1) (170,171). Both insulin receptor and IGF-1 act as dominant cellular mitogens for HCC (154). On binding to the insulin receptor, insulin activates antiapoptotic mediators such as NF-κB and TNF-α, thus reducing loss of cells by apoptosis (172). A key molecule in insulin signaling, insulin receptor substrate-1 (IRS-1), is overexpressed in HCC cell lines and tumor tissue and may have transforming properties (173). Inactivation of IRS-1 reverses the malignant phenotype of HCC cells, mainly by inhibiting IGF-1–mediated signal transduction pathways (174).

The IGF axis has important autocrine, paracrine, and endocrine roles in the promotion of growth. IGF-1 stimulates hepatic cell proliferation (175), including in preneoplastic foci (176). It also inhibits apoptosis (175,176). IGF-2 overexpression increases cell proliferative activity and is associated with the development of HCC (177). IGF-1 receptor is also involved in the process of malignant transformation (178): It is required for optimal growth (179), inhibits apoptosis, and is key to the establishment and maintenance of the transformed phenotype (180,181). Free radical production and oxidative stress may be involved in the generation of these changes (182).

In ob/ob obese mice, activation of signaling pathways involved in hepatocyte proliferation and the induction of several antiapoptotic mechanisms have been observed, suggesting that fat-laden hepatocytes display an increased proliferative activity and decreased apoptosis (182). Decreased expression of methionine adenosyltransferase1A (MAT1A) and induction of MAT-2A cause oxidative stress and induction of genes involved in cell proliferation (183,184).

The metabolism of long-chain fatty acids produces oxidative stress, which in turn induces DNA damage and an altered profile of key genes involved in cell proliferation (fos, jun, NF-κB, p53) (185). In obesity and diabetes, increased fatty acid and fat overload might activate peroxisome proliferator-activated receptor-α (PPARα), which in turn activates growth regulatory genes and produces neoplastic transformation (186,187).

Hepatic fibrosis, independent of etiology, results from activation of hepatic stellate cells leading to collagen deposition and disruption of normal metabolic functions of the liver. Hepatic stellate cells play a critical role in disease progression by regulating extracellular matrix deposition and homeostasis. Overexpression of platelet-derived growth factor-C causes activation of hepatic stellate cells, resulting in fibrosis in a pattern resembling that seen in alcoholic and nonalcoholic fatty liver disease, steatosis, and HCC (188).

Hepatic Iron Overload (Hereditary Hemochromatosis and Dietary Iron Overload)

Although essential for the growth of cells, iron is toxic in excessive amounts. The liver is especially subject to this toxic effect because it is the major site of iron storage. Hereditary hemochromatosis (HH) is an autosomal recessive metabolic disorder often complicated by portal fibrosis, cirrhosis, and HCC. HCC accounts for as much as 45% of deaths in HH, with a relative risk for the tumor calculated to be >200. The major mutant responsible for HH results in the substitution of tyrosine for cysteine at amino acid 282 (C282Y) of the $\alpha 3$ loop of the HFE protein. Dietary iron overload (previously called Bantu visceral siderosis) occurs in rural areas of sub-Saharan Africa, affecting as many as 15% of adult males (189). Increased hepatic iron concentrations, which may be as high as those found in HH, result from the consumption of large volumes of iron-rich beer that is home-brewed in iron drums. During the fermentation process, the pH of the ferment falls to a low level, leaching iron from the container into the beverage. This iron is in an ionized, highly bioavailable form. Genetic predisposition has been postulated to interact with the high dietary iron intake in causing African iron overload, but no mutation has yet been identified. Portal fibrosis and cirrhosis complicate dietary iron overload less often than they do in HH. Dietary iron overload was initially believed not to be complicated by HCC, but recent reports have documented an association (190,191). Cirrhosis is present in the vast majority of patients with HH and in a smaller proportion of those with dietary iron overload who develop HCC, and chronic necroinflammatory hepatic disease undoubtedly plays a major role in the malignant transformation that complicates these conditions. However, evidence is emerging that excess hepatic iron may also be inherently hepatocarcinogenic. Included in this evidence are reports of HCC developing in the absence of cirrhosis in a few patients with other iron-loading conditions such as thalassemia, sideroblastic anemias, and spherocytosis, as well as the recent finding of the development of ironfree preneoplastic foci and HCC in the absence of cirrhosis or portal fibrosis in albino Wistar rats fed an iron-supplemented but otherwise carcinogenfree diet (192).

The mechanisms responsible for a direct hepatocarcinogenic effect of iron have yet to be fully defined, although oxidative stress appears to be one mechanism (193). Intracellular free iron is a catalyst for the formation of ROS and, as a result, may cause oxidative damage to hepatocytes, DNA, protein, and lipids (194,195). The resulting chronic necroinflammatory hepatic disease in turn generates more ROS and additional oxidative damage. Putative mechanisms for free radical–induced malignant transformation include the mutagenic properties of the radicals and their effect on lipid peroxidation. Serum 8-OH-dG levels correlate well with serum iron levels, and a link between 8-OH-dG and MDA has been demonstrated in HCC (196). Both MDA and 4-HNE are genotoxic and cytotoxic (197,198). 8-OH-2-dG also correlates with the rate of DNA unwinding and strand breaks in liver tissue (199). An association between DNA unwinding and the risk of HCC formation in HH has been described (200).

ROS may also cause oxidative damage to polyunsaturated fatty acids of membrane phospholipids releasing cytotoxic and reactive aldehyde derivatives. These may impair cellular functions, including nucleotide and protein synthesis (201). Iron is involved in the initiation of this free radical chain reaction by causing decomposition of hydrogen peroxide to form the highly reactive hydroxyl radical in the Fenton reaction. ROS are also activated by ferrous and ferric compounds (202).

Increased LPO is believed to be an important contributor to hepatocarcinogenesis in iron overload. In addition to participating in the initiation and propagation steps of lipid peroxidation, iron is believed to be involved in β-cleavage of the lipid hydroperoxides giving rise to biogenic aldehydes that interact with DNA to form exocyclic guanine products, which have been shown to be increased in a rat model of hepatocarcinogenesis (203). Overexpression of NO and NO synthase-2 has been reported in preneoplastic hepatic regenerative nodules and to induce mutations and DNA damage in vitro and in animal models (203).

Experimental evidence in animals has shown that cyclin D1, a protein involved in G_{1-2} phase of the cell cycle, is overexpressed in the iron-overloaded liver. This could contribute to cell cycle abnormalities and might play a role in iron-induced hepatocarcinogenesis (204).

INHERITED METABOLIC DISEASES

α-1-Antitrypsin Deficiency

Homozygous PIZZ α-1-antitrypsin (α1-ATZ) deficiency is the most common metabolic liver disease in children. α-1-AT is the archetype of the serine protease (Serpin) supergene family. This glycoprotein is an acute phase reactant with the principal function of inhibiting neutrophil elastase. The histopathological hallmark of the disease is the presence of PAS-positive, diastase-resistant globules of the glycoprotein in hepatocytes. α-1-ATZ results from a glutamate to lysine mutation at amino acid 342, which alters the conformation of the resulting protein in such a way that it is retained in the ER of hepatocytes (205). This triggers a series of events that are eventually hepatotoxic and oncogenic. Considerable variation exists in the phenotypic expression of liver disease among homozygotes for the Z allele (206). Clinically significant liver disease, in the form of cirrhosis and HCC, develops in only about 10% of homozygotes, and then usually in adulthood (206). These observations support the belief that genetic modifiers and/or environmental factors that influence the intracellular disposal of the mutant glycoprotein, or the signal transduction pathways that are activated, predispose a subgroup of homozygotes to liver injury. The mechanisms by which retention of the aggregated protein leads to malignant transformation are not fully understood, although the predilection for HCC in homozygotes for the Z allele is significantly greater than that attributable to cirrhosis alone (207).

The mechanism responsible for the accumulation of α-1-ATZ in the ER of hepatocytes is uncertain. A small fraction only of the accumulated α-1-ATZ undergoes retrograde translocation to the cytosol, although how this is achieved is not certain. Both the ubiquitin-dependent and the ubiquitin-independent proteasomal systems may be involved (208), and there is also evidence for nonproteasomal degradation pathways (209,210), including macroautophagy. Accumulation of α-1-ATZ in the ER specifically activates the intense autophagic response (210). As a result of its retention, some of the α-1-ATZ undergoes polymerization by a novel "loop sheet" insertion mechanism (211), and the polymerogenic properties may prove to be critical determinants in the pathobiology of the liver disease (205). Autophagy may be particularly important as a means of degrading insoluble polymers or aggregates.

Accumulation of α-1-ATZ may result in mitochondrial damage. Whether this is the result of the ER stress or of an overexuberant autophagic response is uncertain (205). ER retention of α-1-ATZ may also elicit signal transduction pathways in the unfolded protein response and the ER overload pathway. In cell line and transgenic mouse models, transcription of NF-κB and the ER overload pathway are activated when α-1-ATZ accumulates in the ER (212). Activation of

NF-κB has been shown to play a key role in inflammation-associated carcinogenesis (212). ER retention may also lead to cleavage/activation of the ER caspases (213) and BAP31, a ubiquitous integral membrane protein of the ER that appears to mediate proapoptotic signals from the ER to mitochondria (213).

Using BrdU labeling, hepatocellular proliferation was shown in transgenic mice with α-1-ATZ deficiency. However, almost all BrdU-positive cells were devoid of globules, and few of the globule-containing cells were BrdU positive (212), indicating that the globule-devoid hepatocytes had a proliferative advantage. The globule-containing cells show no histologic or TUNEL staining evidence of apoptosis. It has been suggested that the globule-containing cells have activated ER and mitochondrial caspases, NF-κB and autophagy, with a relative block in proliferation, but they are not apoptotic (213). However, many of the hepatocytes do not contain globules, and these increase in number over time. Those hepatocytes with lesser amounts of α-1-ATZ and devoid of globules have a proliferative advantage in the presence of hepatocyte injury and inflammation. The globule-containing hepatocytes are believed to chronically stimulate in trans the relatively undamaged hepatocytes. Rudnick and Perlmutter believed that HCC ultimately arises in these α-1-AT–negative areas (203).

Hereditary Tyrosinemia Type 1

Hereditary tyrosinemia type I (HTI) is an autosomal recessive metabolic disorder caused by a deficiency of fumaryl acetoacetate hydrolase (FAH), the final enzyme in the tyrosine catabolism pathway. Deficiency of FAH results in the accumulation of metabolites that are highly toxic because of their alkylating potential (214). One of these metabolites, fumaryl acetoacetate, has been shown to have mutagenic activity and to induce cell cycle arrest at G_2/M and apoptosis (215,216). Patients with the chronic form of HTI are at high risk for the development of cirrhosis and HCC. Administration of 2-(2-nitro-4-trifluoromethylbenzoyl[-1,3-cyclohexanedione]) (NTBC) corrects the tyrosinemia phenotype but does not prevent tumor formation (217).

The gene encoding the FAH protein has been mapped to chromosome 15q23–25. A large number of mutations have been identified in the gene in HTI patients (202). In one patient and a mouse model, FAH expression in liver sections revealed a mosaic pattern of expression: no FAH was found in the tumor or in dysplastic regions, but expression did occur in nontumorous regions (218). This pattern correlated with the presence of a putative missense mutation, glutamine to arginine at amino acid 279, which acted as a splicing mutation, inhibiting the expression of FAH mRNA and the corresponding protein. Another mutation described in these patients is a splice mutant IVS12+5g––>a (219).

Glycogen Storage Diseases

Glycogen storage diseases are a group of inherited metabolic disorders characterized by the accumulation of glycogen in the liver and other tissues, and frequently complicated by hepatic adenoma formation and less often by HCC. HCC has been reported to occur in types Ia, III, IV, and V1 of the disease. Patients with glycogen storage disease 1a usually present with HCC between 8 and 20 years after hepatic adenoma is diagnosed (220–222). In type III, hepatic fibrosis and cirrhosis, rather than adenomas, precede HCC formation (223).

Type Ia (von Gierke disease), the most common type, is caused by a deficiency of glucose-6-phosphatase resulting from mutation of the glucose-6-phosphatase C (G6PC) gene, which encodes the phosphatase of the microsomal glucose-6-phosphatase system (220–222). Many mutations have been described in these patients, although a homozygous G727T mutation is commonly present in Japanese patients (220), and HCC develops in between 22% and 75% of these patients (221). In type III disease, the affected enzyme is amylo-1,6-glucosidase, 4-α-glucanotransferase, which is responsible for the debranching of the glycogen molecule during catabolism. A number of mutations have been described in these patients (223). Type 1V is caused by a deficiency of the glycogen branching enzyme (224).

Hypercitrullinemia

Hypercitrullinemia is a rare hereditary metabolic disease caused by a deficiency of citrin, a liver-type mitochondrial aspartate-glutamate carrier encoded by the SLC25A13 gene on chromosome 7q21.3, which gives rise to a decreased activity of argininosuccinate synthetase (225,226). Three types of mutations have been described, but only type II, which occurs in adults, is associated with the development of cirrhosis and HCC (225,227,228). Type II hypercitrullinemia occurs particularly in Japan (225,226). In this form of the disease, the argininosuccinate synthetase is reduced in liver tissue only. There is no mutation of the gene and the level of mRNA of the enzyme is normal. The decreased levels are believed to result from increased degradation of the enzyme or inhibited translation of its mRNA (228). The molecular mechanism responsible for malignant transformation is not known (209). Possible explanations include promotion of hepatocyte proliferation by citrulline and enhancement of DNA synthesis by polyamine (229).

Wilson Disease

Copper is an essential component of many enzymes and is required for such diverse processes as oxidative metabolism, free radical detoxification, neurotransmitter synthesis, and maturation of connective tissue. The metal is required in trace amounts only and is toxic in higher concentrations. Excess copper is normally eliminated through the biliary system. Wilson disease is a rare autosomal recessive disorder characterized by impaired biliary copper excretion and defective incorporation of the metal into ceruloplasmin, resulting in progressive accumulation of copper in hepatocytes and other tissues. The copper overload causes pathological changes in the liver and neurologic tissue. Chronic active hepatitis, cirrhosis, and fulminant hepatic failure are the three main complications of copper accumulation in the liver (230,231). HCC is a very rare and late complication (230,231)—so much so that it has been suggested that excess hepatic copper might have a protective effect against cancer development.

The gene responsible for Wilson disease encodes a cation-transporting P-type ATPase (230,231). The gene product, designated ATP7B, is localized to the late endosomes and functions in copper secretion from the late endosomes into plasma, coupled with ceruloplasmin synthesis and copper transport to the lysosomes, from which it is subsequently secreted into bile. A great many mutations of the Wilson gene have been described (232), but most occur in a few families or individuals only. They include missense, frame-shift, nonsense, and splice-site mutations. The most common mutation, histidine to glutamine at codon 1069, is present in 70% of Polish, 60% of Austrian, and 10% to 40% of other European and North American patients but is rare in Asian, Indian, and Sardinian patients (232).

The His1069gln protein does not localize in the late endosomes but is degraded in proteasomes and forms aggresomes in the microtubule organizing center (233). Aggresomes are probably responsible for the Mallory bodies seen in Wilson disease. They may explain the damage to hepatocytes and the development of HCC.

In addition, copper is required as a cofactor for mediators of angiogenesis, such as fibroblast growth factor-1, matrix metalloproteinase, and angiogenin (234,235).

Acute Intermittent Porphyria

Acute intermittent pophyria is an inherited disorder of heme metabolism characterized by the accumulation of the porpyhrin precursors, Δ-aminolevulnic acid (ALA) and porphobilinogen, in plasma and organs. The majority of the patients have a guanine-to-adenine (G593A) substitution in codon 198 of the porphobilinogen deaminase gene (236). ALA generates ROS and induces dose-dependent damage to nuclear and mitochondrial DNA, including strand breaks, proteins, and subcellular structures (237).

Cigarette Smoking

The evidence for cigarette smoking as a risk factor for HCC is conflicting, although an evaluation of the available data indicates a weakly positive association (238), and the International Agency for Research on Cancer has classified it as causal. Polycyclic aromatic hydrocarbons present in cigarette smoke are metabolically activated by cytochrome p450 into electrophilic reactants that covalently bind to DNA to form adducts, and this may play a role in hepatocarcinogenesis (238). Polymorphisms of N-acetyltransferase may also contribute to smoking-related hepatocarcinogenesis (239). There may be a synergistic interaction between smoking and chronic HCV and smoking and alcohol abuse in the development of the tumor (125).

References

1. Parkin DM, Bray FI, Devesa SS. Cancer burden in the year 2000: the global picture. *Eur J Cancer* 2001;37(suppl 8):S4–S66.
2. Parkin DM, Muir CS, Whelan SL, et al., eds. *Cancer Incidence in Five Continents.* Vol 6. Lyon, France: International Agency for Research on Cancer; 1997.
3. Bosch FX, Ribes J, Diaz M, et al. Primary liver cancer: wordwide incidence and trends. *Gastroenterology* 2004;127:S5–S16.
4. Fattovich G, Stroffolini T, Zagni I, et al. Hepatocellular carcinoma in cirrhosis: incidence and risk factors. *Gastroenterology* 2004;127:S35–S50.
5. Kew MC, Popper H. Relationship between hepatocellular carcinoma and cirrhosis. *Semin Liver Dis* 1984;1:59–67.
6. Kew MC, Hodkinson HJ. Membranous obstruction of the inferior vena cava and its causal relation to hepatocellular carcinoma. *Liv Int* 2006;26:1–7.
7. Kew MC. Role of cirrhosis in hepatocarcinogenesis. In: Bannasch P, Keppler D, Weber G, eds. *Liver Cell Carcinoma.* Dordrecht: Kluwer Academic Press; 1989:37–46.
8. Sangiovanni A, Del Ninno E, Fasani P, et al. Increased survival of cirrhotic patients with hepatocellular carcinoma detected during surveillance. *Gastroenterology* 2004;53:744–749.
9. Fausto N. Mouse liver tumorigenesis: models, mechanisms, and relevance to human disease. *Semin Liver Dis* 1999;19:243–252.
10. Michalopoulos GK, DeFrancis MC. Liver regeneration. *J Hepatol* 2000;32:19–31.
11. Rhim JA, Sandgren EP, Palmiter R, et al. Replacement of diseased mouse liver with xenogeneic hepatocytes. *Proc Natl Acad Sci U S A* 1995;92:4942–4946.
12. Overturf K, al Dhalimy M, Ou CN, et al. Serial transplantation reveals the stem cell-like regenerative potential of adult mice hepatocytes. *Am J Pathol* 1997;151:1273–1280.
13. Grisham JW. Molecular genetic alterations in hepatocellular neoplasms: hepatocellular adenoma, hepatocellular carcinoma and hepatoblastoma. In: Coleman WB, Tsongalis JG, eds. *Molecular Basis of Human Cancer.* Totawa, N.J.: Humana Press; 2001:269–346.
14. Taub R. Blocking NF-κB in the liver: the good and bad news. *Hepatology* 1998;27:1445–1446.
15. Kucharczak J, Simmons MJ, Fan Y, et al. To be or not to be: NF-κB is the answer—role of Rel/NF-κB in the regulation of apoptosis. *Oncogene* 2003;22:8961–8982.
16. Fausto N. Hepatocytes break the rules of senescence in serial transplantation studies. Is there a limit to their replicative capacity? *Am J Pathol* 1997;151:1187–1189.
17. Rabes HM, Muller L, Hartmann A, et al. Cell cycle-dependent initiation of ATP-ase populations in adult rat liver by a single dose of N-methyl-N-nitrosourea. *Cancer Res* 1986;46:465–478.
18. Cayana E, Tsuda H, Sarma DCR, et al. Initiation of chemical carcinogenesis requires cell proliferation. *Nature* 1978;275:60–62.
19. Ishikawa T, Ide F, Qin X, et al. Importance of DNA repair in carcinogenesis: evidence from transgenic and gene targeting studies. *Mutat Res* 2001;477:41–49.
20. Thorgeirsson SS, Grisham JW. Molecular pathogenesis of human hepatocellular carcinoma. *Nat Genet* 2002;31:339–346.
21. Sugimara T. Multistep carcinogenesis. *Science* 1992;258:603–607.
22. Farazi PA, Glickman J, Jiang S, et al. Differential impact of telomere dysfunction on initiation and progression of hepatocellular carcinoma. *Cancer Res* 2003;63:5021–5027.
23. Davis BH, Kresina TF. Hepatic fibrogenesis. *Clin Lab Med* 1996;16:361–375.
24. Rappaport AM, MacPhee PJ, Fisher MM, et al. The scarring of the liver acini (cirrhosis): tridimensional and microcirculatory considerations. *Virchows Arch (Pathol Anat)* 1983;402(2):107–137.
25. Craig JR, Klatt EC, Yu M. Role of cirrhosis and the development of HCC: evidence from histologic studies and large population studies. In: Tabor E, DiBisceglie AM, Purcell RH, eds. *Etiology, Pathology, and Treatment of Hepatocellular Carcinoma in North America.* Houston, Tex.: Gulf Publishing Co.; 1991:177–190.
26. Poli G, Albino E, Dianzani MU. The role of lipid peroxidation in liver damage. *Chem Phys Lipids* 1987;45:117–142.
27. Wiseman H, Halliwell B. Damage to DNA by reactive oxygen and nitrogen species: role in inflammatory disease and progression to cancer. *Biochem J* 1996;313:17–29.
28. Dolle MET, Giese H, Hopkins CL, et al. Rapid accumulation of genome rearrangements in liver but not in brain of old mice. *Nat Genet* 1997;17:431–434.
29. Cheng KC, Cahill DS, Kasai H, et al. 8-Hydroxyl guanine, an abundant form of oxidative DNA damage, causes G-T and A-C substitutions. *J Biol Chem* 1992;267:166–172.
30. Trush MA, Kensler TW. An overview of the relationship between oxidative stress and chemical carcinogenesis. *Free Radic Biol Med* 1991;10:201–209.
31. Cheeseman KH. Lipid peroxidation and cancer. In: Halliwell B, Arouma AI, eds. *DNA and Free Radicles.* London: Ellis Horwood; 1993:109–144.
32. Chung FL, Nath RG, Ocanda J, et al. Deoxyguanine adducts of 4-hydroxy-2-nonenol are endogenous DNA lesions in rodents and humans: detection and potential sources. *Cancer Res* 2000;60:1507–1511.
33. Kew MC, Kramvis A, Yu MC, et al. Increased hepatocarcinogenic potential of of hepatitis B virus genotype A in Bantu-speaking sub-Saharan Africans. *J Med Virol* 2005;75:513–521.
34. Chisari FV, Klopchin K, Moriyama T, et al. Molecular pathogenesis of hepatocellular carcinoma in hepatitis B virus transgenic mice. *Cell* 1989;59:1145–1156.
35. Nakamoto Y, Guidotti LG, Kuhlen CV, et al. Immune pathogenesis of hepatocellular carcinoma. *J Exp Med* 1998;188:341–350.
36. Chisari FV. Viruses, immunity, and cancer: lessons from hepatitis B. *Am J Pathol* 2000;156:1118–1132.
37. Dandri M, Burda MR, Burkle A, et al. Increase in de novo HBV DNA integrations in response to oxidative DNA damage or inhibition of poly (ADP)-ribosylation. *Hepatology* 2002;35:217–223.
38. Wang HP, Rogler CE. Topoisomerase 1 mediated integration of hepadnavirus DNA in vitro. *J Virol* 1991;65:2381–2392.
39. Popper H, Roth L, Purcell RH, et al. Hepatocarcinogenicity of the woodchuck hepatitis virus. *Proc Natl Acad Sci U S A* 1987;84:866–870.
40. Kim CM, Koike K, Saito I, et al. HBx gene of hepatitis B virus induces liver cancer in transgenic mice. *Nature* 1991;351:317–320.
41. Shafritz DA, Kew MC. Identification of integrated hepatitis B virus DNA sequences in human hepatocellular carcinomas. *Hepatology* 1981;1:1–8.
42. Matsubara K, Tokino T. Integration of hepatitis B virus DNA and its implications for hepatocarcinogenesis. *Mol Biol Med* 1980;7:243–260.
43. Laurent-Puig P, Legoix P, Bluteau O, et al. Genetic alterations associated with hepatocellular carcinomas define distinct pathways of hepatocarcinogenesis. *Gastroenterology* 2001;120:1763–1773.
44. Takado S, Gotoh Y, Hayashi S, et al. Structural rearrangement of integrated hepatitis B virus DNA as well as cellular flanking DNA is present in chronically infected hepatic tissues. *J Virol* 1990;64:822–828.
45. Dandri M, Burda MR, Burkie, A, et al. Increase in de novo HBV DNA integrations in response to oxidative DNA damage or inhibition of poly(ADPribosyl)ation. *Hepatology* 2002;35:217–233.
46. Rogler CE, Chisari FV. Cellular and molecular mechanisms of hepatocarcinogenesis. *Semin Liv Dis* 1992;12:265–278.
47. Buendia MA. Genetics of hepatocellular carcinoma. *Semin Cancer Biol* 2000;10:185–200.

48. Robinson WS. Molecular events in the pathogenesis of hepadnavirus-associated hepatocellular carcinoma. *Ann Rev Med* 1994;45:297–323.

49. Paterlini-Brechot P, Saigo K, Murakami Y, et al. Hepatitis B virus-related insertional mutagenesis occurs frequently in human liver cancers and recurrently targets human telomerase gene. *Oncogene* 2003;22:3911–3916.

50. Minami M, Daimon Y, Mori K, et al. Hepatitis B virus-related insertional mutagenesis in chronic hepatitis B patients as an early drastic genetic change leading to hepatocarcinogenesis. *Oncogene* 2005;24:4340–4348.

51. Fourel J, Trepo C, Bouguelereret L, et al. Frequent activation of n-myc genes by hepadnavirus insertion in woodchuck liver tumors. *Nature* 1990;347:294–298.

52. Etiemble J, Degott C, Renard CA, et al. Liver-specific expression and high oncogenic efficiency of a c-myc transgene activated by woodchuck hepatitis virus insertion. *Nature* 1990;347:294–298.

53. Caselmann WH. Trans-activation of cellular genes by hepatitis B virus proteins: a possible mechanism of hepatocarcinogenesis. *Adv Virus Res* 1996;47:253–302.

54. Shih C, Burke K, Chou MJ, et al. Tight clustering of human hepatitis B virus integration sights near a triple stranded region. *J Virol* 1987;61:3491–3498.

55. Schluter V, Meyer M, Hofschneider OPH, et al. Integrated hepatitis B virus x and truncated preS/S sequences derived from human hepatomas encode functionally active transactivators. *Oncogene* 1994;9:3335–3344.

56. Paterlini P, Poussin K, Kew MC, et al. Selective accumulation of the X transcript of the hepatitis B virus in patients negative for hepatitis B surface antigen with hepatocellular carcinoma. *Hepatology* 1995;21:313–321.

57. Aoki H, Kajino K, Arakawa Y, et al. Molecular cloning of a rat chromosome putative recombinogenic sequence homologous to the hepatitis B virus encapsidation signal. *Proc Natl Acad Sci U S A* 1996;93:7300–7304.

58. Rosner MT. Hepatitis B virus x gene product: a promiscuous transcriptional activator. *J Med Virol* 1992;36:101–117.

59. Feitelson MA. Parallel genetic and epigenetic changes in the pathogenesis of hepatitis B virus-associated hepatocellular carcinoma. *Cancer Lett* 2005;20:1–11.

60. Hildt E, Munz B, Saher G, et al. The preS 2 activator MHBs(t) of hepatitis B virus activates c-raf-1/ERK2 signalling in transgenic mice. *EMBO J* 2005;21:525–535.

61. MacQuire HF, Hoeffler JP, Siddiqi A. HBZx protein alters the DNA binding specificity of CREB and ATF-2 by protein–protein interactions. *Science* 1991;252:842–844.

62. Kim JH, Rho HM. Activation of the human transforming growth factor-α (TGF-α) gene by the hepatitis B viral X protein through AP-2 sites. *Mol Cell Biochem* 2002;231:155–161.

63. Zhang Z, Torii N, Furusaka A, et al. Structural and functional characterization of interaction between hepatitis B virus x protein and the proteasome complex. *J Biol Chem* 2000;275:15157–15165.

64. Qadri I, MacGuire HF, Siddiqui A. Hepatitis B virus transactivator protein x interacts with TATA-binding protein. *Proc Natl Acad Sci U S A* 1995;92:1003–1007.

65. Haviv I, Shamay M, Doitsch G, et al. Hepatitis B virus x protein targets TFIIB in transcription co-activation. *Mol Cell Biol* 1998;18:1562–1569.

66. Shimamura A, Fisher DE. p53 in life and death. *Clin Cancer Res* 1996;2:235–240.

67. Truant T, Antunovic J, Greenblatt J, et al. Direct interaction of the hepatitis B virus x protein with p53 protein leads to the inhibition by HBx of p53 response element-directed transactivation. *J Virol* 1995;69:1851–1859.

68. Wang XW, Forrester K, Yeh MA, et al. Hepatitis B virus protein inhibits p53 sequence-specific DNA binding, transcriptional activity, and associated transcription factor ERCC3. *Proc Natl Acad Sci U S A* 1994;91:2230–2234.

69. Huang J, Kontos CD. PTEN modulates vascular endothelial growth factor-mediated signalling and angiogenic effects. *J Biol Chem* 2002;277:10760–10766.

70. Lee TH, Elledge SJ, Butel JS. Hepatitis B virus x protein interacts with a probable cellular DNA repair protein. *J Virol* 1995;69:1107–1114.

71. Wood RW. Nucleotide excision repair in mammalian cells. *J Biol Chem* 1997;272:23465–23468.

72. Capovilla A, Carmona S, Arbuthnot P. Hepatitis B virus x protein binds damaged DNA and sensitises liver cells to ultraviolet irradiation. *Biochem Biophys Res Commun* 1997;232:255–260.

73. Becker SA, Lee T, Butel JS, et al. Hepatitis B virus x protein interferes with cellular DNA repair. *J Virol* 1998;72:266–272.

74. Elmore LW, Hancock AR, Chang SF, et al. Hepatitis B virus x protein and p53 tumor suppressor interactions in the modulation of apoptosis. *Proc Natl Acad Sci U S A* 1997;94:14707–14712.

75. Gottlob K, Fulco M, Levrero M, et al. The hepatitis B virus x protein inhibits caspase 3 activity. *J Biol Chem* 1998;273:33347–33353.

76. Su F, Schneider RJ. Hepatitis B virus HBx protein sensitises cells to apoptotic killing by tumor necrosis factor-α. *Proc Natl Acad Sci U S A* 1997;94:8744–8749.

77. Farshid M, Jedjar S, Mitchell F, et al. Effect of hepatitis B x protein on the expression of retinoblastoma gene product. *Arch Virol* 1997;41:125–129.

78. Haas-Kogen DA, Kogan SC, Levi D, et al. Inhibition of apoptosis by the retinoblastoma gene product. *EMBO J* 1995;14:461–473.

79. Miyoshi Y, Iwao K, Nagasawa, et al. Activation of the β-catenin gene in primary hepatocellular carcinoma by somatic alterations involving exon 3. *Cancer Res* 1998;58:2524–2527.

80. Tu H, Bonura C, Giannini C, et al. Biological impact of natural COOH-terminal deletions of hepatitis B virus x protein in hepatocellular carcinoma tissues. *Cancer Res* 2001;61:7803–7810.

81. Kekule AS, Lauer U, Meyer M, et al. The preS2/S region of integrated hepatitis B virus DNA encodes a transcriptional transactivator. *Nature* 1990;343:457–461.

82. Hildt E, Saher G, Bruss V, et al. The hepatitis B virus large surface protein (LHBs) is a transcriptional activator. *Virology* 1996;225:235–239.

83. Alka S, Hemlata D, Vaishali C, et al. Hepatitis B virus surface transactivator with DNA binding properties. *J Med Virol* 2000;61:1–10.

84. Meyer M, Caselmann WH, Schluter V, et al. Hepatitis B virus transactivator MHBst: activation of NF-κB, selective inhibition by anti-oxidants and integral membrane localization. *EMBO J* 1992;11:2991–3001.

85. Lauer U, Weiss L, Lipp M, et al. The hepatitios B virus presS/St transactivator utilizes AP-1 and other transcription factors for transactivation. *Hepatology* 1994;19:23–31.

86. Wang HC, Wu HC, Chen CF et al. Different types of ground glass hepatocytes in chronic hepatitis B virus infection contain specific preS mutants that may induce endoplasmic reticulum stress. *Am J Pathol* 2003;163:2441–2449.

87. Wang HC, Chang WT, Chang WW, et al Hepatitis B virus pre-S2 mutant upregulates cyclin A expression ani induces nodular regeneration of hepatocytes. *Hepatology* 2005;41:761–770.

88. Hsia CC, Axiotis CA, DiBisceglie AM, et al. Transforming growth factor-α in human hepatocellular carcinoma and co-expression with hepatitis B surface antigen in adjacent liver. *Cancer* 1992;70:1049–1056.

89. Gerber MA, Shieh YSC, Shieh KS, et al. Detection of replicative hepatitis C virus sequences in hepatocellular carcinoma. *Am J Pathol* 1992;141:1271–1277.

90. Moriya K, Fujie H, Shintani Y, et al. The core protein of hepatitis C virus induced hepatocellular carcinoma in transgenic mice. *Nat Med* 1998;4:1065–1067.

91. Koike K, Miyoshi H. Oxidative stress and hepatitis C viral infection. *Hepatol Res* 2006;34:65–73.

92. Lieber CS. Role of oxidative stress and anti-oxidant therapy in alcoholic and non-alcoholic liver diseases. *Adv Pharmacol* 1997;38:601–628.

93. Gong G, Waris G, Tanveer R, et al. Human hepatitis C virus NS5A protein alters intracellular calcium levels, induces oxidative stress, and activates STAT-3 and NF-αB. *Proc Natl Acad Sci U S A* 2001;98:9599–9604.

94. Okuda M, Li K, Beard MR, et al. Mitochondrial injury, oxidative stress, and anti-oxidant gene expression are induced by hepatitis C virus core protein. *Gastroenterology* 2002;122:366–375.

95. Nishikawa M, Nishiguchi S, Shiomi S, et al. Somatic mutation of mitochondrial DNA in cancerous and noncancerous liver tissue in individuals with hepatocellular carcinoma. *Cancer Res* 2001;61:1843–1845.

96. Marusawa H, Hijikata M, Chiba T, et al. Hepatitis C virus core protein inhibits *Fas*- and tumor necrosis factor-α-mediated apoptosis via NF-κB activation. *J Virol* 1999;73:4713–4720.

97. Otsuka NM, Kato N, Taniguchi H. Hepatitis C virus core protein inhibits apoptosis via enhanced Bcl-xL expression. *Virology* 2001;296:84–93.

98. Mihim S, Fayyazi A, Ramadori G. Hepatic expression of inducible nitric oxide synthase transcripts in chronic hepatitis C virus infection: relation to hepatic viral load and liver injury. *Hepatology* 1997;26:451–458.

99. Melillo G, Musso T, Sica LS, et al. A hypoxia-responsive element mediates a novel pathway of activation of inducible nitric oxide synthase promoter. *J Exp Med* 1995;182:1683–1693.

100. Machida K, Cheng KT, Sung VM, et al. Hepatitis C virus induces a mutator phenotype: enhanced mutations of immunoglobulin and proto-oncogenes. *Proc Natl Acad Sci U S A* 2004;101:4262–4267.

101. Lee Yi, Lee S, Lee Y, et al. Hepatitis C core protein transactivates insulin-like growth factor II gene transcription through acting concurrently on Egr1 and Sp1 sites. *Virology* 2001;88:733–739.

102. Liao QJ, Timani KA, Shr XL, et al. Hepatitis C virus non-structural S5 protein can enhance full-length core protein-induced nuclear factor-κB activation. *World J Gastroenterol* 2005;11:6433–6439.

103. Herzer K, Weyer S, Gutenberg J. Hepatitis C virus core gene inhibits tumor suppressor protein promyelocytic leukaemia function in human hepatoma cells. *Cancer Res* 2005;65:10830–10837.

104. Chang PC, Chi CW, Chau GY, et al. DDX3, a DEAD box RNA helicase, is deregulated in hepatitis virus-associated hepatocellular carcinoma and is involved in cell growth control. *Oncogene* 2005;25:1991–2003.

105. Majumder M, Ghosh AK, Steele R, et al. Hepatitis C virus NS5A protein impairs tumor necrosis-α-mediated hepatocyte apoptosis, but not anti-FAS antibody, in transgenic mice. *Virology* 2002;294:94–105.

106. Munukata T, Nakamura M, Liang Y, et al. Down-regulation of the retinoblastoma tumor suppressor by hepatitis C virus NS5B RNA-dependent RNA polymerase. *Proc Natl Acad Sci U S A* 2005;102:18159–18164.

107. Kaneto H, Sasaki S, Yamamoto Y, et al. Detection of hypermethylation of p16ink4A gene promoter in chronic hepatitis and cirrhosis associated with hepatitis B or C. *Gut* 2001;48:372–377.

108. Kew MC. Interaction between hepatitis B and C viruses in hepatocarcinogenesis. *J Viral Hepat* 2006;13:145–149.

109. Kuper H, Ye W, Broome U, et al. The risk of liver and bile duct cancer in

patients with chronic viral hepatitis, alcoholism, or cirrhosis. *Hepatology* 2001;34:714–718.

110. Del Olmo JA, Serra MA, Rodriguex F, et al. Incidence and risk factors for hepatocellular carcinoma in 967 patients with cirrhosis. *J Cancer Res Clin Oncol* 1998;124:560–564.

111. Seitz HK, Poeschl G, Simanowski UA. Alcohol and cancer. In: Galanter M, ed. *Recent Developments in Alcoholism.* New York: Plenum Press; 1998: 67–95.

112. Stickel F, Schuppan D, Hahn EG, et al. Cocarcinogenic effects of alcohol in hepatocarcinogenesis. *Gut* 2002;51:132–139.

113. Arteel GE. Oxidants and antioxidants in alcohol-induced liver disease. *Gastroenterology* 2003;124:778–790.

114. Obe G, Ristow H. Mutagenic, cancerogenic and teratogenic effects of alcohol. *Mutat Res* 1979;65:229–259.

115. Lieber CS, DeCarli LM, Hepatic microsomal ethanol-oxidizing systems: in vitro characteristics and adaptive properties. *J Biol Chem* 1970;245:2505–2512.

116. Sakamoto T, Hara M, Higaki Y, et al. Influence of alcohol consumption and gene polymorphisms of ADH2 and ALDH2 on hepatocellular carcinoma in a Japanese population. *Int J Cancer* 2006;118:1501–1507.

117. Caro AA, Cederbaum AI. Oxidative stress, toxicology, and pharmacology of CYP2E1. *Ann Rev Pharmacol Toxicol* 2004;44:9–18.

118. McKillop IH, Schrum LW. Alcohol and liver cancer. *Alcohol* 2005;35:195–203.

119. Petersen DR. Alcohol, iron-associated oxidative stress, and cancer. *Alcohol* 2005;35:243–249.

120. Klaunig JE, Kamendelis LMK. The role of oxidative stress in carcinogenesis. *Ann Rev Pharmacol Toxicol* 2004;44:239–267.

121. Tavill AS, Qadri AM. Alcohol and iron. *Semin Liver Dis* 2004;24:317–325.

122. Tsukamoto H, Horne W, Kamimura S, et al. Experimental liver cirrhosis induced by alcohol and iron. *J Clin Invest* 1995;96:620–630.

123. Gloria L, Cravo M, Camilo ME, et al. Nutritional deficiencies in chronic alcoholics: relation to dietary intake and alcohol consumption. *Am J Gastroenterol* 1997;92:485–489.

124. Murata H, Tsuji S, Tsuji M, et al. Promoter hypermethylation silences cyclooxygenase-2 and regulates growth of human hepatocellular carcinoma cells. *Lab Invest* 2004;84:1050–1059.

125. Austin A. The role of tobacco use and alcohol consumption in the etiology of hepatocellular carcinoma. In: Tabor E, DiBiscegie AM, Purcell R, eds. *Etiology, Pathology, and Treatment of Hepatocellular Carcinoma in North America.* Houston, Tex.: Gulf Publishing Co.; 1991:57–76.

126. Mukaiya M, Nishi M, Miyake H, et al. Chronic liver diseases for the risk of hepatocellular carcinoma: a case/control study in Japan. *Hepatogastroenterology* 1998;45:2328–2332.

127. Staretz ME, Murphy SE, Patten CJ, et al. Comparative comparison of the tobacco-related carcinogens benz[a]pyrene, 4-(methylnitrosoamino)-1-(3-pyridyl)-1-butanone, 4-(methylnitrosamino)-1-(3-pyridyl)-1-(butanol and N′nitrosonornicotine in human hepatic microsomes. *Drug Metab Dispos* 1997;25:154–162.

128. Fong TL, Kanel GC, Conrad A, et al. Clinical significance of concomitant hepatitis C infection in patients with alcoholic liver disease. *Hepatology* 1994;19:554–557.

129. Onishi K, Iida S, Iwama S, et al. The effect of habitual alcohol intake on the development of cirrhosis and hepatocellular carcinoma; relation to hepatitis B surface antigen carriage. *Cancer* 1982;49:672–677.

130. Guengerich FP. Forging the links between metabolism and carcinogenesis. *Mutat Res* 2001;488:195–209.

131. Smela ME, Hamm ML, Henderson PT, et al. Aflatoxin B₁ formamidopyrimidine adducts play a major role in causing the types of mutations observed in human hepatocellular carcinoma. *Proc Natl Acad Sci U S A* 2002;99:6655–6660.

132. Alekseyev YO, Hamm ML, Essigmann JM. Aflatoxin B₁ formamidopyrimidine adducts are preferentially repaired by the nucleotide excision repair pathway in vivo. *Carcinogenesis* 2004;25:1045–1051.

133. Bailey EA, Iyer RS, Stone MP, et al. Mutational properties of the primary aflatoxin B₁-DNA adduct. *Proc Natl Acad Sci U S A* 1996;93:1535–1539.

134. McGlynn KA, Hunter K, LeVoyer T, et al. Susceptibility to aflatoxin B₁–related primary hepatocellular carcinoma in mice and humans. *Cancer Res* 2003;63:4594–4601.

135. Zhang YJ, Chen Y, Ahsan H, et al. Silencing of glutathione-S-transferase by promoter hypermethylation and its relationship to environmental chemical carcinogens in hepatocellular carcinoma. *Cancer Lett* 2005;221:135–143.

136. Zhang YJ, Chen Y, Ahsan H, et al. Inactivation of the DNA repair gene o5-methylguanine-DNA methyl transferase by promoter hypermethylation and its relationship to aflatoxin B₁-DNA adducts and p53 mutation in hepatocellular carcinoma. *Int J Cancer* 2003;103:440–444.

137. Ozturk M, Bressac B, Pusieux A, et al. A p53 mutational hotspot in primary liver cancer is geographically localised to high aflatoxin areas of the world. *Lancet* 1991;338:1356–1359.

138. Qian GS, Ross RK, Yu MC, et al. A follow-up study of urinary markers of aflatoxin exposure and liver cancer risk in Shanghai, People's Republic of China. *Cancer Epidemiol Biomark Prev* 1994;3:3–10.

139. Hsu IC, Metcalf RA, Sun T, et al. Mutational hotspot in the p53 gene in human hepatocellular carcinomas. *Nature* 1991;350:427–428.

140. Bressac B, Kew MC, Wands J, et al. Selective G to T mutations of p53 in hepatocellular carcinoma from southern Africa. *Nature* 1991;350: 429–431.

141. Aguilar F, Hussain P, Cerutti P. Aflatoxin B1 induces the transversion of G to T in codon 249 of the p53 tumor suppressor gene in human hepatocytes. *Proc Natl Acad Sci U S A* 1993;90:8586–8590.

142. Yakicier MC, Legoix P, Vaury C, et al. Identification of homozygous deletions at chromosome 16q23 in aflatoxin B₁ exposed hepatocellular carcinoma. *Oncogene* 2001;20:5232–5238.

143. Kern SE, Pietenpol JA, Thiagalingam S, et al. Oncogenic forms of p53 inhibit p53-regulated gene expression. *Science* 1992;256:827–830.

144. Ghebranious N, Knoll B, Wu H, et al. Characterization of murine p53ser246 equivalent to the human p53ᵍᵉʳ240 associated with hepatocellular carcinoma and aflatoxin exposure. *Mol Carcinogen* 1995;13:104–111.

145. Alekseyev YO, Hamm ML, Essigmann JM. Aflatoxin B₁ formamidopyrimidine adducts are preferentuially repaired by the nucleotide excision repair pathway in vivo. *Carcinogenesis* 2004;6:1045–1051.

146. Devereux TR, Stern MC, Flake GP, et al. CTNNB1 mutations and β-cata protein accumulation in human hepatocellular carcinomas associated with high exposures to aflatoxin B1. *Mol Carcinog* 2001;31:68–73.

147. Elmilek H, Paterson AC, Kew MC. β-catenin mutation and expression, 249ᵍᵉʳp53 mutation and hepatitis B virus infection in southern African Blacks. *J Surg Oncol* 2005;98:258–263.

148. Lee YI, Lee S, Das GC, et al. Activation of the insulin-like growth transcription by aflatoxin B1-induced p53 mutant is caused by the activation of transcription complexes: implications for a gain-of-function during the formation of hepatocellular carcinoma. *Oncogene* 2000;3:3717–3726.

149. Zhang YJ, Ashan H, Chen Y, et al. High frequency of promoter hypermethylation of RASSF1A and p16 and its relationship to aflatoxin B₁–DNA adduct levels in human hepatocellular carcinoma. *Mol Carcinog* 2002; 35:85–92.

150. Bulatao-Jaime J, Almero EM, Castro CA. A case/control dietary study of primary liver cancer risk from aflatoxin exposure. *Int J Epidemiol* 1982; 11:112–119.

151. Kew MC. Synergistic interaction between aflatoxin B₁ and hepatitis B virus in hepatocarcinogenesis. *Liver Int* 2003;23:1–5.

152. Dragani T, Manenti G, Farza al. Transgenic mice containing hepatitis B virus sequences are more susceptible to carcinogen-induced hepatocarcinogenesis. *Carcinogenesis* 1990;11:953–956.

153. Sell S, Hunt JM, Dunsford HA, et al. Synergy between hepatitis B virus expression and chemical hepatocarcinogenesis in transgenic mice. *Cancer Res* 1991;51:1278–1285.

154. Gemechu-Hatewu M, Platt KL, Oesch F, et al. Metabolic activation of aflatoxin B1 to aflatoxin B1-8,9-epoxide in woodchuck undergoing chronic active hepatitis. *Int J Cancer* 1997;73:587–591.

155. Chemin I, Ohgaki H, Chisari FV, Wild CP. Altered expression of hepatic carcinogen metabolizing enzymes with liver injury in HBV transgenic mouse lineages expressing various amounts of hepatitis B surface antigen. *Liver* 1999;19:81–87.

156. Sun C-A, Wang L-Y, Chen C-J, et al. Genetic polymorphisms of glutathione-S-transferases M1 and T1 associated with susceptibility to aflatoxin-related carcinogenesis among chronic hepatitis B carriers: a nested case-control study in Taiwan. *Carcinogenesis* 2001;22:1289–1294.

157. McGlynn KA, Rosvold EA, Lustbader ED, et al. Susceptibility to hepatocellular carcinoma is associated with genetic variation in the enzymatic detoxification of aflatoxin B₁. *Proc Natl Acad Sci U S A* 1995;92:2384–2387.

158. Shupe S, Shell S. Low hepatic glutathione-S-transferase and increased hepatic DNA adduction contribute to the increased tumorigenicity of aflatoxin B1 in newborn and partially hepatectomized mice. *Toxicol Lett* 2004;148:1–9.

159. Ahn JI, Jung EY, Kwun HJ, et al. Dual effects of hepatitis B virus x protein on the regulation of cell cycle depending on the status of cellular p53. *J Gen Virol* 2002;83:2765–2772.

160. Jia L, Wang XW, Harris CC. Hepatitis B virus x protein inhibits nucleotide excision repair. *Int J Cancer* 1999;80:875–879.

161. Huo TI, Wang HW, Forgues M, et al. Hepatitis B virus mutants derived from human hepatocellular carcinoma retain the ability to abrogate p53-induced apoptosis. *Oncogene* 2001;20:3620–3628.

162. Hussain SP, Aguilar F, Amstad P, et al. Oxy-radical-induced mutagenesis of hot spot codons 248 and 249 of the human p53 gene. *Oncogene* 1994;9:2277–2281.

163. Liu RH, Jacob JR, Hotchkiss JH, et al. Woodchuck hepatitis virus surface antigen induces nitric oxide synthesis in hepatocytes: possible role in hepatocarcinogenesis. *Carcinogenesis* 1994;15:2875–2877.

164. Poonawala A, Nair SP, Thuluwath PJ. Prevalence of obesity and diabetes in patients with cryptogenic cirrhosis: a case-control study. *Hepatology* 2000;32:689–692.

165. Ratziu V, Poynard T. Hepatocellular carcinoma in NAFLD. In: Farrell GC, George J, de la Hall P, McCullough AJ, eds. *Fatty Liver Disease: NASH and Related Disorders.* Oxford: Blackwell; 2005:276–288.

166. Roskams T, Yang SQ, Koteish A, et al. Oxidative stress and oval cell accumulation in mice and humans with alcoholic and non-alcoholic fatty liver disease. *Am J Pathol* 2003;163:1301–1311.

167. Hu W, Feng Z, Eveleigh J, et al. The major lipid peroxidation product, trans-4-hydroxy-2-nonenol, preferentially forms adducts at codon 249 of

human p53 gene, a unique mutational hotspot in hepatocellular carcinoma. *Carcinogenesis* 2002;23:1781–1789.

168. Rashid A, Wu TC, Huang CC, et al. Mitochondrial proteins that regulate apoptosis and necrosis in mouse fatty liver. *Hepatology* 1999;29:1131–1138.

169. Yu S, Rao S, Reddy JK. Perioxisome proliferator-activated receptors, fatty acid oxidation, steatohepatitis and hepatocarcinogenesis. *Curr Mol Med* 2003;3:561–572.

170. McGowan JR, Strain AJ, Bucher NL. DNA synthesis in primary cultures of adult rat primary hepatocytes in a defined medium: effects of epidermal growth factor, insulin, glucagons, and cyclic AMP. *J Cell Physiol* 1981; 108:353–363.

171. Macauley VM. Insulin-like growth factors and cancer. *Br J Cancer* 1992; 65:311–320.

172. Bertrand F, Desbois-Mouthon C, Cadoret A, et al. Insulin antiapoptotic signalling involves insulin activation of the NF-κB dependent survival genes encoding tumor necrosis factor receptor-associated factor 2 and manganese–superoxide dismutase. *J Biol Chem* 1999;274:30596–30602.

173. Tanaka S, Wands JR. A carboxy-terminal-truncated insulin receptor substrate-1 dominant negative protein reverses the human hepatocellular carcinoma malignant phenotyope. *J Clin Invest* 1996;98:2100–2108.

174. Koch KS, Shapiro P, Skelly H, et al. Rat hepatocyte proliferation is stimulated by insulin-like peptides in defined medium. *Biochem Biophys Res Commmun* 1982;109:1054–1060.

175. Sell C, Baserga R, Rubin R. IGF-1 and IGF-1R prevent etoposide-induced apoptosis. *Cancer Res* 1995;55:303–306.

176. Lin SB, Hsieh SH, Hsu HL, et al. Antisense oligodeoxynucleotides of IGF-2 selectively inhibit growth of human hepatoma cells overproducing IGF-2. *J Biochem (Tokyo)* 1997;122:717–722.

177. Rubbin R, Baserga R. Insulin-like growth factor receptor: its role in cell proliferation, apoptosis, and tumorigenicity. *Lab Invest* 1995;73:311–331.

178. Baserga R. The insulin-like growth factor-1 receptor: a key to tumor growth. *Cancer Res* 1995;55:249–252.

179. Miura CM, Surmacz E, Burgaud JL, et al. Different effects on mitogenesis and transformation of a mutation at tyrosine 1251 of the insulin-like-1 receptor. *J Biol Chem* 1995;270:22639–22644.

180. Resnikoff M, Burgaud JL, Rotman HL, et al. Correlation between apoptosis, tumorigenesis, and levels of insulin-like growth factor-1 receptor. *Cancer Res* 1995;55:3739–3741.

181. Ito T, Sasaki Y, Wands JR. Overexpression of human insulin receptor substrate-1 induces cellular transformation with activation of mitogen-activated protein kinases. *Mol Cell Biol* 1996;16:943–951.

182. Yang S, Lin HZ, Hwang J, et al. Hepatic hyperplasia in non-cirrhotic fatty livers: is obesity-related hepatic steatosis a premalignant condition? *Cancer Res* 2001;61:5016–5023.

183. Cai J, Mao Z, Hwang JJ, et al. Differential expression of methione adenyltransferase genes influence the crate of of growth of human hepatocellular carcinonma cells. *Cancer Res* 1998;58:1444–1450.

184. Martinez-Chantar ML, Marcia-Trjevijano ER, Latasa MU, et al. Methionene adenyltransferase-2β subunit gene expression provides a proliferative advantage in human hepatoma. *Gastroenterology* 2003;124: 940–948.

185. Ockner RK, Kaikus RM, Bass NM. Fatty acid metabolism and the pathogenesis of hepatocellular carcinoma: review and hypothesis. *Hepatology* 1993;18:669–676.

186. Bass NM. Three for the price of one knockout: a mouse model of a congenital perioxysomal disorder, steatohepatitis and hepatocarcinogenesis. *Hepatology* 1999;29:606–608.

187. Gonzalez FJ, Peters JM, Cattley RC. Mechanism of action of the nongenotoxic perioxysome proliferators: role of the perioxysome proliferators-activator receptor α. *J Natl Cancer Inst* 1998;90:1702–1709.

188. Campbell JS, Hughes SD, Gilbertson DG, et al. Platelet-derived growth factor C induces liver fibrosis, steatosis, and hepatocellular carcinoma. *Proc Natl Acad Sci U S A* 2005;102:3389–3394.

189. Gordeuk VR. African iron overload. *Semin Hematol* 2002;39:263–269.

190. Moyo VM, Makunike R, Gangaidzo IT, et al. African iron overload and hepatocellular carcinoma. *Eur J Hematol* 1998;60:28–34.

191. Mandishona E, MacPhail PA, Gordeuk VR, et al. Dietary iron overload as a risk factor for hepatocellular carcinoma in Black Africans. *Hepatology* 1998;27:1563–1566.

192. Asare GA, Paterson AC, Kew MC, et al. Development of altered hepatic foci, iron-free preneoplastic nodules and hepatocellular carcinoma without cirrhosis in Wistar rats fed a diet high in iron. *J Pathol* 2006;208:82–90.

193. Young IS, Trouton TG, Torney JJ, et al. Antioxidant status and lipid peroxidation in hereditary hemochromatosis. *Free Radic Biol Med* 1994;16: 393–397.

194. Hagen TM, Huang S, Curnuttle J, et al. Extensive oxidative DNA damage in hepatocytes of transgenic mice with chronic active hepatitis destined to develop hepatocellular carcinoma. *Proc Natl Acad Sci U S A* 1994;91:12808–12812.

195. Jungst C, Cheng B, Gehrke R, et al. Oxidative damage is increased in human liver tissue adjacent to hepatocellular carcinoma. *Hepatology* 2004; 39:1663–1672.

196. Ichiba M, Maeta Y, Mukoyama T, et al. Expression of 8-hydroxy-2′-deoxyguanosine in chronic liver disease and hepatocellular carcinoma. *Liver Int* 2003;23:1781–1789.

197. Cheng KC, Cahill DS, Kasai H, et al. 8-Hydroxyl guanine, an abundant form of oxidative DNA damage, causes G-T and A-C substitutions. *J Biol Chem* 1992;267:166–172.

198. Dabbagh AJ, Mannion T, Lynch SM, et al. The effect of iron overload on rat plasma and liver oxidant status: in vivo. *Biochem J* 1994;300:799–803.

199. Asare GA, Mossanda KS, Kew MC, et al. Hepatocellular carcinoma caused by iron overload: a possible mechanism of direct hepatocarcinogenicity. *Toxicology* 2006;219:41–52.

200. Niederau C, Fischer R, Sonnenberg A, et al. Survival and causes of death in cirrhotic and non-cirrhotic patients with primary hemochromatosis. *N Engl J Med* 1985;313:1256–1262.

201. Cheeseman KH. Lipid peroxidation in cancer. In: Halliwell B, Arouma AI, eds. *DNA and Free Radicals*. London: Ellis Horwood; 1993: 109–144.

202. Cadenzas E. Biochemistry of oxygen toxicity. *Ann Rev Biochem* 1989; 58:79–110.

203. Marrogi AJ, Khan MA, van Gijssel HE, et al. Oxidative stress and p53 mutations in the carcinogenesis of iron-overload-associated hepatocellular carcinopma. *J Natl Cancer Inst* 2001;93:1652–1655.

204. Troadec MB, Courseland B, Détivaud L, et al. Iron overload promotes cyclinD1 expression and alters cell cycle in mouse hepatocytes. *J Hepatol* 2006;44:391–399.

205. Rudick DA, Perlmutter DH. α-1-Antitrypsin deficiency: a new paradigm for hepatocellular carcinoma in genetic liver disease. *Hepatology* 2005;42:514–521.

206. Sveger T. The natural history of liver disease in α-1-antitrypisin deviant children. *Acta Pediatr Scand* 1988;77:847–851.

207. Eriksson S, Carlson J, Velez R. Risk of cirrhosis and primary liver cancer in α-1-antitrypsin deficiency. *N Engl J Med* 1986;314:736–739.

208. Teckman JH, Gilmore T, Perlmutter DH. Role of ubiquitin in proteasomal degradation of mutant α-1-antitrypsin Z in the endopiasmic reticulum. *Am J Physiol* 2000;297:G39–GF48.

209. Cabral CM, Choudhury P, Liu Y, et al. Processing by endoplasmic reticulum mannosidases partitions a secretion-impaired glycoprotein into distinct disposal pathways. *J Biol Chem* 2000;275:25015–25022.

210. Teckman JH, Perlmutter DH. Retention of mutant α-1-antitrypsin Z in the endoplasmic reticulum is associated with an autophagic response. *Am J Physiol* 2000;279:G961–G974.

211. Lomas DA, Mahadeva R. α-1-Antitrypsin polymerization and the serpinopathies: pathobiology and prospects for therapy. *J Clin Invest* 2002; 110:1585–1590.

212. Pilarsky KI, Porat RM, Stein I, et al. NF-βB functions as a tumor promoter in inflammation-associated cancer. *Nature* 2004;431:461–466.

213. Rudnick DA, Liao Y, An JK, et al. Analyses of hepatocellular proliferation in a mouse model of α-1-antitrypsin deficiency. *Hepatology* 2004;39:1048–1055.

214. St. Louis M, Tanquay RM. Mutations in the fumaryl acetoaceteate hydrolase gene causing hereditary tyrosinemia type 1: overview. *Hum Mutat* 1997;2:291–299.

215. Jorquera R, Tanguay RM. The mutagenicity of the tyrosine metabolite, fumaryl acetoacetate, is enhanced by glutathione depletion. *Biochem Biophys Res Commun* 1997;232:42–48.

216. Jorquera R, Tanguay RM. Cyclin-B dependent kinase and caspase-1 activation precedes mitochondrial dysfunction in fumaryl acetoacetate-induced apoptosis. *FASEB J* 1999;15:2284–2298.

217. Luijerink MC, Jacobs SMM, van Beurden EACM, et al. Extensive changes in liver gene expression induced by hereditary tyrosinemia type 1 are not normalized by treatment with 2-(2-nitro-4-trifluoromethylbenzoyl)-1,3-cyclohexanediole (NTBC). *J Hepatol* 2003;39:901–909.

218. Dreumont N, Poudrier JA, Bergeron A, et al. A missense mutation in the fumarylacetoacetate hydrolase gene, responsible for hereditary tyrosinemia, acts a splicing mutation. *BMC Genet* 2001;2:9–15.

219. Poudrier J, Lettre F, Scriver CR, et al. Different clinical forms of hereditary tyrosinemia (typeI) in patients with identical genotypes. *Mol Gene Metab* 1998;64:119–125.

220. Matern D, Seydewitz HH, Bali D, et al. Glycogen storage disease type I: diagnosis and phenotype/genotype correlation. *Eur J Pediatr* 2002;161: S10–S19.

221. Franco LM, Krishnamurthy V, Bali D, et al. Hepatocellular carcinoma in glycogen storage disease type 1a: a case series. *J Inherit Metab Dis* 2005; 28:153–163.

222. Nakamura T, Ozawa T, Kawasaki T, et al. Glucose-6-phosphatase gene mutations in 20 adult Japanese patients with glycogen storage disease type Ia with reference to hepatic tumors. *J Gastroenterol Hepatol* 2001; 16:1402–1408.

223. Zhuang TF, Qiu ZO, Wei M, et al. Mutation analysis of glycogen debrancher enzyme gene in five Chinese patients with glycogen storage disease type III. *Zhonghua Er Ke Za Zhi* 2005;43:85–88.

224. De Moor RA, Schweizer JJ, van Hoek B, et al. Hepatocellular carcinoma in glycogen storage disease type 1V. *Arch Dis Child* 2000;82:479–480.

225. Ito T, Shiraki K, Sekoguchi K, et al. Hepatocellular carcinoma associated with adult-type citrullinemia. *Dig Dis Sci* 2000;45:2203–2206.

226. Lu YB, Kobayashi K, Ushikai M, et al. Frequency and distribution in East Asia of 12 mutations identified in the SLC25A13Gene of Japanese patients with citrin deficiency. *J Hum Genet* 2005;50:338–346.

227. Ito T, Shiraki K, Sekoguchi K, et al. Hepatocellular carcinoma associated with adult-type citrullinemia. *Dig Dis Sci* 2000;45:2203–2206.

228. Hagiwara N, Sekjima Y, Takei Y, et al. Hepatocellular carcinoma in a case of adult-onset type II cirtrullinemia. *Intern Med* 2003;42:978–982.

229. Kobayashi K, Shaheen N, Kumashira R, et al. A search for the primary abnormality in adult-onset type II citrullinemia. *Am J Hum Genet* 1993;53:1024–1030.

230. Walshe JM, Waldenstrom E, Sams V, et al. Abdominal malignancies in patients with Wilson's disease. *Q J Med* 2003;96:656–662.

231. Bull PC, Thomas GR, Rommens JM, et al. The Wilson disease gene is a putative copper transporting P-type ATPase similar to the Menkes gene. *Nat Genet* 1993;5:327–337.

232. Riordan SM, Williams R. The Wilson's gene and phenotypic diversity. *J Hepatol* 2001;120:165–171.

233. Harada M, Sakisaka S, Terado K, et al. A mutation of the Wilson disease protein, ATP7BB, is degraded in the proteasomes and forms protein aggregates. *Gastroenterology* 2001;120:967–974.

234. Iwadate H, Ohira H, Suzuki T, et al. Hepatocellular carcinoma associated with Wilson's disease. *Intern Med* 2004;43:1042–1045.

235. Kimura H, Nakajima T, Kagawa K, et al. Angiogenesis in hepatocellular carcinoma. *Liver* 1998;18:14–19.

236. Bjersing L, Andersson C, Liythner F. Hepatocellular carcinoma in patients from northern Sweden with acute intermittent porphyria. *Cancer Epidemiol Biomarkers Prev* 1996;5:393–397.

237. Onuki J, Chen Y, Texeira PC, et al. Mitochondrial and nuclear damage induced by 5-aminolevullinic acid. *Arch Biochem Biophys* 2004;15:178–187.

238. Chen Sy, Wang IY, Luan RM, et al. Polycyclic aromatic hydrocarbon-DNA adducts in liver tissues of hepatocellular carcinoma patients and controls. *Int J Cancer* 2002;99:14–21.

239. Farker K, Schotte U, Scheele J, et al. Impact of N-acetyltransferase polymorphism in hepatocellular carcinoma. *Exp Toxicol Pathol* 2003;54:387–391.

CHAPTER 31 ■ HEPATOCELLULAR CANCER: PATHOLOGY

GREGORY Y. LAUWERS AND VIKRAM DESHPANDE

An increasing incidence of hepatocellular carcinoma (HCC) in Western countries, secondary to HCV hepatitis and other factors, including obesity, has been paralleled by advances in hepatic imaging and surgery. Detected either during monitoring of patients at risk or secondary to symptoms, the resection of an increased number of cases has resulted in an abundance of pathological material. Consequently, over the past few years, there has been a steady stream of information related to the histologic characteristics of HCCs, their pattern of spread, the risk factors for recurrence, and long-term prognosis. Another growing field has been related to the diagnosis of early HCC. Understanding by histopathologists, surgeons, hepatologists, and oncologists of the nuances of the diagnosis of early HCC, as well as the importance of detailed pathological analysis of a hepatectomy specimen, is crucial to developing an appropriate therapeutic algorithm.

MACROSCOPIC FEATURES OF HEPATOCELLULAR CARCINOMA

Despite early reports to the contrary, the gross morphologic characteristics in HCC do not seem to be affected by the geographic origins of the patients (1–3). Essentially, variations in the morphologic appearance of HCC depend on the size of the tumor and the quality of the surrounding liver, namely, the presence or absence of cirrhosis. Western series have emphasized that between 42% and 51% of HCCs arise in noncirrhotic livers (4,5). However, some of the "noncirrhotic" cases may be better characterized as being associated with limited fibrosis.

Differences in the multiplicity of tumors, incidence of encapsulation, and rate of venous invasion have been reported in these tumors. Also, HCCs in noncirrhotic livers grow faster and are larger than those in cirrhotic livers (6,7).

In cirrhotic livers, small HCCs are usually well demarcated and surrounded by a fibrous capsule, whereas advanced tumors are expansive multinodular masses, frequently accompanied by intrahepatic metastases (8). Conversely, HCCs arising in noncirrhotic livers tend to present as single large massive tumors that may infiltrate both lobes (5,6).

The size of HCCs is an important risk factor for intrahepatic and extrahepatic spread (9–11). Tumors measuring <5 cm are less likely to develop intrahepatic metastasis, portal vein tumor thrombosis, or hematogenous metastasis (9,11,12). However, the rate of intrahepatic metastasis rises dramatically (96% vs. 60% of cases) and the incidence of portal vein thrombosis almost doubles (75% vs. 40% of cases) when HCCs grow larger than 5 cm in size (9,10).

Irrespective of the pattern of growth, most HCCs are soft neoplasms often displaying hemorrhage and necrotic foci. Their color ranges from tan-gray to green, the intensity of the latter reflecting the degree of bile production (13). Presence of a capsule is a function of the tumor's size and is found around 46% of HCCs measuring <2 cm in diameter, seen in 84% of tumors between 2 and 5 cm, and in only 45% of HCCs >5 cm in diameter (14). The presence of a capsule is an important characteristic because it is associated with improved survival, lower intrahepatic recurrence rate, and reduced incidence of local venous invasion (4,15). Whether tumor encapsulation is more frequent in patients without cirrhosis remains debated (2,4,16).

Macroscopic Classification

The growth pattern of HCCs has some importance because the different types are associated with various risks of intrahepatic and extrahepatic spread (9). The classification of Eggel, published a century ago and based on autopsy cases, is still widely used (17). In this scheme, HCCs are divided into three categories: nodular, massive, and diffuse types. The *nodular* type is composed of tumor nodules scattered within the cirrhotic parenchyma. The *massive* type consists of a circumscribed, huge tumor mass occupying most or all of a hepatic lobe. This type, commonly observed in patients without cirrhosis, arises frequently in the right lobe and can be surrounded by satellite nodules. The relatively rare *diffuse* type is characterized by innumerable indistinct small tumor nodules. However, nowadays, the smaller resected HCCs, do not readily fit into Eggel's classification. This has led to the development of new classifications, none of them widely accepted (1,18). The most notable change is the one proposed by the Liver Cancer Study Group of Japan, by which the nodular type is divided into three categories: the single nodular type, the single nodular type with perinodular tumor growth, and the confluent multinodular type (13) (Fig. 31.1). Other classification schemes have included subtypes such as the small HCC (<2 cm) and the rare pedunculated HCC (19).

Other Significant Gross Features of Hepatocellular Carcinomas

Multicentricity of Hepatocellular Carcinoma

Multicentricity, an important predictor of late intrahepatic recurrence after hepatectomy, is noted in 16% to 74% of resected HCCs (9,14,20–23). These results, however, pertain essentially to patients with cirrhosis and contrast sharply with HCCs arising in noncirrhotic livers, in which the rate of

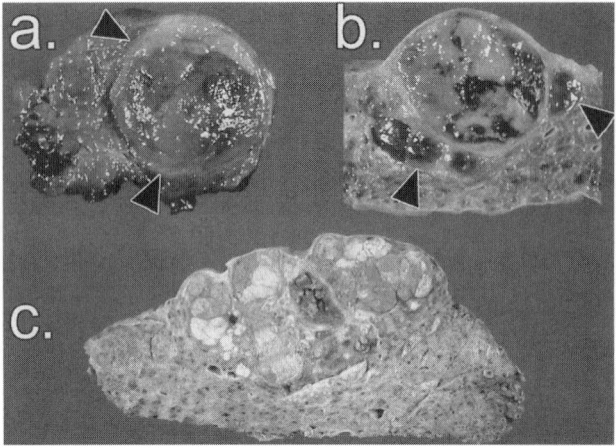

FIGURE 31.1. Macroscopic appearances of hepatocellular carcinoma (HCC). These examples display the three subtypes of nodular HCC. **A:** Encapsulated HCC, single nodular type. Note the fibrous capsule (*arrowheads*). **B:** Encapsulated HCC, single nodular type, with extranodular growths (*arrowheads*). **C:** Large HCC, confluent multinodular type.

multifocal tumors is only 12% (6). Two mechanisms account for the multiplicity of HCCs: the metachronous development of tumors through the mechanism of multicentric carcinogenesis, and metastatic intrahepatic spread via the portal system (24,25). Lesions are considered metastatic in nature

- If they demonstrate a portal vein tumor thrombus or grow contiguously with a thrombus
- If multiple small satellite lesions surround a larger main tumor
- If a single tumor is present near the main tumor but is significantly smaller in size and exhibits the same histology (24)

Intravascular and Biliary Growth

Tumor thrombi in the portal vein system represent the source of intrahepatic metastases of HCC. Major portal vessel thrombosis portends a poor prognosis, with most such patients experiencing recurrence within 1 year and death within 2 years after the resection (12,26). Less frequently, tumor thrombi may form within hepatic veins, sometimes extending into the inferior vena cava and eventually the right atrium (27).

Tumor invasion into the hepatic duct, common bile duct, or both is rare but is associated with notably worse prognosis (19). It sometimes poses a preoperative diagnostic challenge, with most patients presenting with obstructive jaundice or hemobilia frequently and incorrectly diagnosed as having a cholangiocarcinoma or choledocholithiasis (28).

MICROSCOPIC FEATURES OF HEPATOCELLULAR CARCINOMA

Neoplastic hepatocytes exhibit various degrees of hepatocellular differentiation. They are usually polygonal with abundant eosinophilic and granular cytoplasm surrounded by distinct cell membranes. Characteristically, the nucleus is round and vesicular with a distinct nucleolus. Various intracytoplasmic inclusions can be observed, including glycogen, fat, bile, fibrinogen (pale bodies), Mallory bodies (accumulation of keratin and p62 stress protein) and intracellular hyaline bodies (accumulations of p62 stress protein), alpha-fetoprotein (AFP), giant lysosomes, or α_1-antitrypsin (29,30).

A trabecular arrangement mimicking normal hepatic cords is the basic architectural growth pattern of HCCs. However, the histologic appearance is variable, with several variations on this basic theme.

Histologic Patterns

The World Health Organization classification recognizes five major histologic patterns. Except for the fibrolamellar pattern, their significance is more of diagnostic value than indicative of prognosis (29). The four other subtypes, frequently found simultaneously, are *trabecular*, *pseudoglandular* (acinar), *compact*, and *scirrhous*.

The trabecular and pseudoglandular architectural patterns are commonly encountered in well to moderately differentiated HCCs. The trabeculae, which can vary widely in thickness from a few cells thick (microtrabecular) to more than a dozen cells (macrotrabecular), are separated by sinusoidlike spaces lined by flat endothelial cells (Fig. 31.2). In the acinar (or pseudoglandular) variant, the cells are arranged in a rosettelike fashion with a central bile canaliculus (Fig. 31.3). In the solid type, a variant of macrotrabecular architecture, the sinusoids are compressed and obscured by the broad and compact trabeculae. Finally, the scirrhous pattern is characterized by abundant fibrous stroma separating cords of tumor cells. This pattern is often seen as a secondary change after radiation, chemotherapy, or infarction. Various degrees of the scirrhous pattern are found without any previous treatment in approximately 4% of cases (13,29).

Histologic Grading of Hepatocellular Carcinomas

The most commonly used grading scheme, developed by Edmondson and Steiner in 1954, is a four-tier system based on the degree of differentiation of the neoplastic cells (31). *Grade I* is composed of well-differentiated neoplastic hepatocytes arranged in thin trabeculae. In such cases, distinguishing HCC from small cell dysplasia is frequently difficult, particularly in needle biopsy specimens (Fig. 31.4). In *grade II*, the cells are larger and more atypical, sometimes organized in an acinar pattern. In *grade III*, architectural and cytologic anaplasia is prominent, but the tumor is still readily identified as hepatocytic in origin (Fig. 31.4). In *grade IV*, the neoplastic cells are markedly anaplastic and not easily identified as hepatocytic origin.

An alternate four-tier histologic grading scheme is advocated by the Liver Cancer Study Group of Japan (13). In this system, *well-differentiated HCCs*, most measuring <2 cm in diameter, are characterized by increased cellular density with irregular microtrabeculae, focal acinar formation, and frequent fatty change (Fig. 31.4). Cellular and nuclear atypia are distinctly absent. This carcinoma would correspond to the grade I carcinoma of the Edmondson-Steiner classification. In *moderately differentiated HCCs*, atypical hepatocytes have a trabecular arrangement, but a pseudoglandular pattern can also be observed (Fig. 31.3). Cytologically, the neoplastic hepatocytes have abundant eosinophilic cytoplasm with round nuclei and distinct nucleoli. The nucleus-to-cytoplasm ratio is equal to that of the normal hepatocytes. This type corresponds to grade II and III carcinoma of the Edmondson-Steiner scheme and is common among advanced HCCs.

A solid growth pattern characterizes the *poorly differentiated HCCs*. The neoplastic hepatocytes have an increased

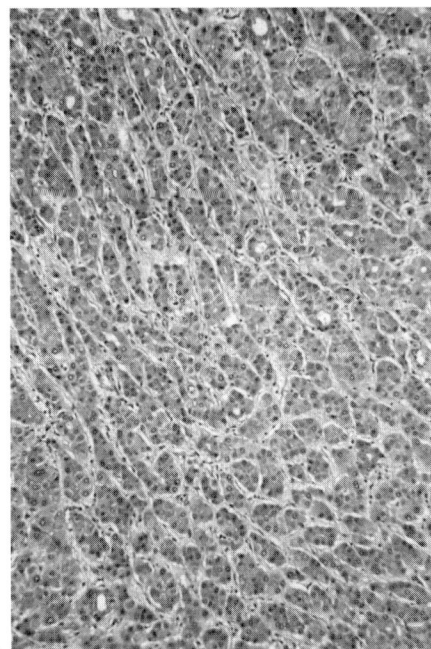
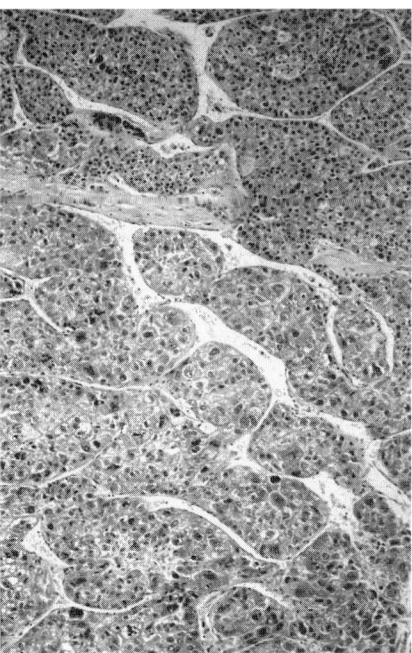

FIGURE 31.2. Histologic patterns of hepatocellular carcinoma. **A:** The microtrabecular pattern is characterized by malignant hepatocytes organized in thin cords mimicking the normal hepatic architecture. **B:** The macrotrabecular growth pattern is composed of wider anastomosing cords.

nucleus-to-cytoplasm ratio and show pleomorphism, including mononucleated or multinucleated giant cells, or both. This category corresponds to Edmondson-Steiner grades III to IV.

In *undifferentiated HCCs*, the cells are characterized by scant cytoplasm with short spindle-shaped or round nuclei and grow in a solid or medullary pattern. These correspond to grade IV carcinoma of the Edmondson-Steiner classification.

Although they are widely used, the prognostic value of these systems is debated. Some series report better prognosis for low-grade HCC, whereas others deny a correlation between poor prognosis and high histologic grade (4,32). Also, Edmondson-Steiner grading was not found to be a predictor of intrahepatic recurrence by some, whereas a high histologic grade has been estimated by others to be a strong predictor of portal vein invasion (15,33). Whether the presence of cirrhosis influences the histologic grade is also debated. According to one series, the odds of having a high-grade HCC is almost double for patients with a cirrhotic liver compared to that of patients without cirrhosis (4).

Cytologic Subtypes

The *clear cell variant* of HCC is composed of well to moderately differentiated tumor cells with a clear cytoplasm resulting from excessive intracytoplasmic deposits of glycogen (29). A tumor can be entirely of the clear cell type, or this variant may represent only a limited portion of an otherwise typical HCC. Its reportedly favorable prognosis has not been confirmed (34,35). In practice, clear cell HCC should be distinguished from metastatic clear cell variants of renal cell and adrenocortical carcinomas. In most cases, immunohistochemistry can provide the appropriate diagnosis.

Pleomorphic HCCs are characterized by marked variations in shape and size of the neoplastic hepatocytes and their nuclei. Seemingly benign giant cells (osteoclast type) or highly anaplastic bizarre cells can be observed (29). *Spindle* (or sarcomatoid) tumor cells are either focal or represent most of the tumor (29) (Fig. 31.5). Arterial chemotherapy has been implicated in this phenotypic transformation (27). The diagnosis of this variant can be challenging because it may resemble fibrosarcoma, leiomyosarcoma, and malignant fibrous histiocytoma. Distinction of this variant from a sarcoma is largely dependent on the identification of foci morphologically typical for HCCs. Cytokeratin (CK) immunoreactivity, although supportive of this variant, is not universally present, being reported in 62% of cases in one series (36).

Vascular Invasion

Because HCCs have a rich vascular stroma, microscopic portal vein or hepatic vein invasion can be expected to be a frequent finding. Even among candidates for liver transplantation (either single small HCCs of <5 cm or no more than three tumors all ≤3 cm), 33% of patients were shown to have microvascular invasion (37). Risk factors for portal vein invasion include tumor diameter >3 cm, high histologic grade, tumor multiplicity,

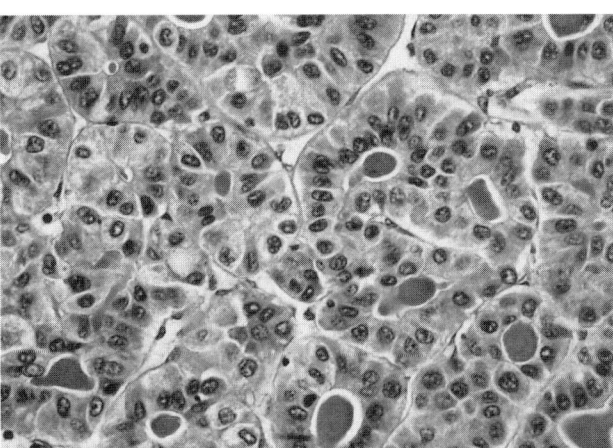

FIGURE 31.3. The pseudoglandular (acinar) pattern of hepatocellular carcinoma. The neoplastic hepatocytes are moderately atypical (grade II). Bile plugs are identified in the lumen.

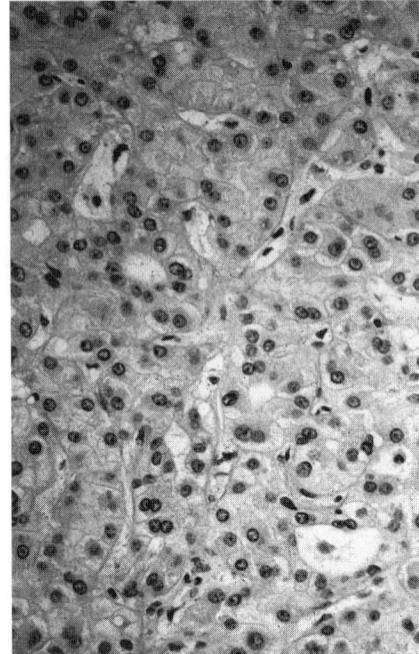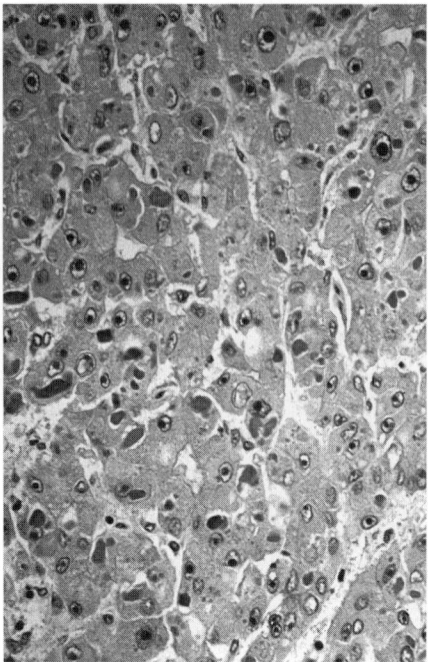

A

B

FIGURE 31.4. Cytologic subtypes of hepatocellular carcinoma. **A:** Grade I (well differentiated). The well-differentiated neoplastic hepatocytes show minimal cytologic and architectural atypia. Note the central acinar structure. **B:** Grade III (moderately differentiated). The tumor cells, arranged in ill-formed trabeculae, have large vesicular nuclei with prominent nucleoli.

and mitotic rate >4 per 10 high-power fields (33,37). Whether venous invasion is more frequent in patients with cirrhosis than in those without is debated (4,33). Overall, it is an important prognostic indicator with patients with no vascular invasion experiencing a longer overall and diseasefree survival in part because intrahepatic metastases occur through portal vein invasion (23,32,38,39).

SPECIAL VARIANTS OF HEPATOCELLULAR CARCINOMA

Several histologic types present unique features worth reporting.

Fibrolamellar Carcinoma

The fibrolamellar variant is rare, accounting for <5% of cases overall but about 13% of all patients younger than 40 years. Besides being usually diagnosed in adolescents and young adults, a previously unrecognized predilection for women and Caucasians has been noted (29,40–42). Frequently amenable to surgical extirpation, the survival of fibrolamellar carcinoma is longer than that for usual HCCs. Overall 5-year survival is estimated at between 35% and 76% for patients undergoing hepatic resection (43–46). However, a recent series pointed out that with frequent vascular invasion (36%) and lymph node metastases (50%), late recurrences are common, and the 5-year recurrencefree survival was only 18% (45). Fibrolamellar carcinomas are firm, sharply demarcated, and lack a fibrous capsule. Most frequently single, they range in size from 7 to 20 cm (41). On gross examination, they are usually devoid of hemorrhage and necrosis but display a central fibrous scar in 10% to 15% of cases. The surrounding parenchyma is frequently unremarkable, with cirrhosis reported in <5% of cases (41). The characteristic histologic features include large polygonal and deeply eosinophilic tumor cells embedded in hyalinized connective tissue arranged in a lamellar fashion (29,41) (Fig. 31.6). The cells present single round vesicular nuclei and prominent nucleoli. The eosinophilia is caused by the intracytoplasmic accumulation of swollen mitochondria (29,41). The cells may also contain α_1-antitrypsin, seen as proteinaceous cytoplasmic inclusions, and fibrinogen containing

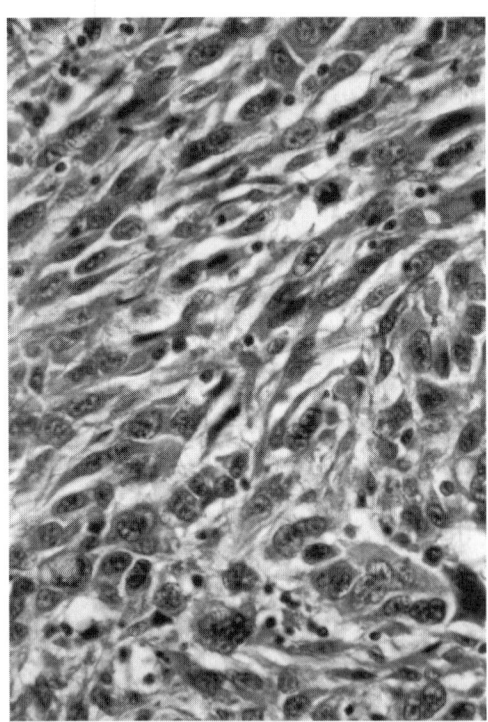

FIGURE 31.5. Spindle (sarcomatoid) variant of hepatocellular carcinoma (HCC). This type is composed of spindle neoplastic cells mimicking a sarcoma. Usually, areas of transition with traditional HCC are found. Immunohistochemical detection of cytokeratin is successful in approximately 60% of cases.

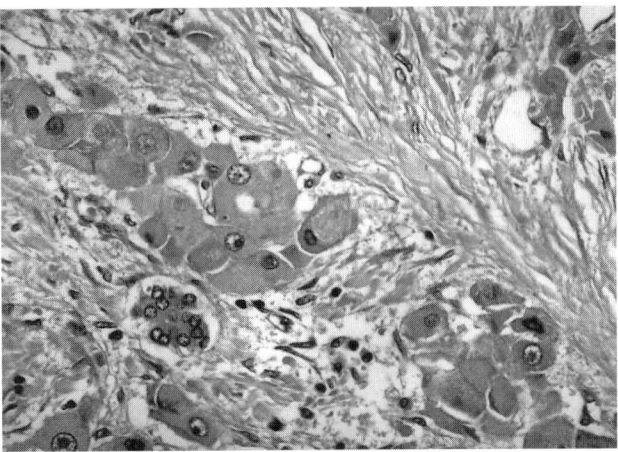

FIGURE 31.6. Fibrolamellar hepatocellular carcinoma. An abundant granular cytoplasm and vesicular nuclei with prominent nucleoli characterize the tumor cells. Note the typical lamellar fibrosis in which the tumor cells are embedded.

pale bodies, recognized as pale ground-glass cytoplasmic inclusions (29,41).

Combined Hepatocellular Carcinoma and Cholangiocarcinoma

Combined HCC and cholangiocarcinomas (combined HCC-CC) are defined as tumors containing admixed, unequivocal elements of HCC and CC (29). Two types, the HCC-predominant type (the most frequent) and the CC-predominant type, are recognized (47). These neoplasms should be distinguished from separate HCC and CC synchronously arising in the liver. Although parts of these tumors may show bile production, intercellular bile canaliculi, or a trabecular growth pattern characteristic of HCC, the CC component is recognized by the presence of glandular structure lined by cells resembling the biliary epithelium, intracellular mucin production, MUC-1 reactivity, or positive CK 7 and 19 immunoreactivity (47–50). Also, parathyroid hormone–related immunoreactivity, a marker of classical CC, can be noted in the areas of cholangiocellular differentiation (51). Characteristically, AFP levels are low, whereas an increase in serum carcinoembryonic antigen (CEA) and carbohydrate antigen 19-9 can be detected (47,52). Cirrhosis is associated with most cases of the HCC-predominant type (55% of cases) and only occasionally with the CC-predominant type (13% of cases) (47). Notably, combined neoplasms may be more common in patients with genetic hemochromatosis. Reflecting the common embryologic origin of hepatocytes and cholangiocytes, two mechanisms of histogenesis have been hypothesized: (a) the CC component could differentiate from an initial pure HCC, and (b) an intermediate "stem cell" cell could give rise to both HCC and a CC components (47,48,53). Support for the latter hypothesis includes include the presence of hepatic progenitor cells, as well as the detection of hepatocellular (albumin RNA) and biliary markers (keratin profile) in combined HCC (53,54).

Sclerosing Hepatic Carcinoma

Sclerosing HCCs represent a heterogeneous group of tumors not sanctioned by the World Health Organization classification (29,55). A common and unifying clinical feature found in the majority of patients is hypercalcemia with hypophosphaturia (55). These tumors present as large white-tan, firm, well-circumscribed masses with scalloping borders, a pattern reminiscent of metastatic carcinoma and CC. Most cases occurred in patients without cirrhosis who are generally older than patients with typical HCC. Some of these tumors display characteristic features of HCC, whereas others have features suggestive of a biliary lineage. Others might be classified as combined HCC-CCs (55). In 60% of cases, the neoplastic cells resemble those of the usual HCCs (sclerosing HCC) and blend with benign hepatocytes at the periphery of the tumor. The cytologic similarities are less obvious in the center of the mass; however, where, embedded in the abundant fibrous stroma, the tumor cells may form pseudoductules and resemble cholangioles, and are difficult to distinguish from metastatic carcinoma and cholangiocarcinoma (55). Sclerosing hepatic carcinomas are less frequently associated with elevated serum AFP levels than other types of HCCs but may be associated with hypercalcemia and elevated levels of parathyroid hormone–related protein (55). The latter has been demonstrated in tumor cells by immunohistochemistry (56).

Unusual Histologic Types of Hepatocellular Carcinoma

Only histologic types of hepatocellular carcinoma that pose diagnostic problems are touched on in this section. For example, a rare medullary-type variant of HCC has been recorded. The patients, most of whom are cirrhotic, present with tumor composed of large amphophilic cells arranged in a solid growth pattern with a rich lymphoplasmacytic stroma (57). Although this tumor type is associated with Epstein-Barr virus in other organs, except for a single example, this association does not extend to HCCs (58). Recently, a diagnostically challenging and rare form of combined HCC with an intermixed aggressive neuroendocrine component has also been described (59).

Precursor Lesions

The multistep sequence of macroregenerative nodules, low- and high-grade dysplastic nodules, and well-differentiated HCC is largely accepted as the morphologic chronologic process preceding the development of HCCs in cirrhotic livers.

Macroregenerative nodules are distinctly larger than most cirrhotic nodules. They variably measure between 0.5 and 1.5 cm and although well circumscribed are not encapsulated (60). Most large regenerative nodules are indistinguishable from smaller cirrhotic nodules, but others may display aberrant and *dysplastic*, architectural, and cytologic features. Initially, these features are focal, but eventually these dysplastic hepatocytes replace the surrounding areas. When the entire nodule is occupied, they are referred to as a *dysplastic nodule* (of either low or high grade) (61). However, histologic differences between simple macroregenerative and dysplastic nodules are not always clear, and they present diagnostic challenges, especially on needle biopsies. Architecturally, *dysplasia* refers to the presence of uniformly thick cell plates (three or more cells thick), microacinar formation, increased number of unpaired arteries, and maplike clonal growth (62). Cytologically, liver cell dysplasia refers to putative preneoplastic changes. Large cell changes refer to cellular enlargement with nuclear pleomorphism and frequent multinucleation (63). In the small cell variant, nuclear atypia is subtle, with densely packed, smaller-than-normal hepatocytes, thickening of the nuclear membrane, higher nucleus-to-cytoplasm ratios, and rare mitoses (64). However, the exact significance of these changes (particularly large cell type) is

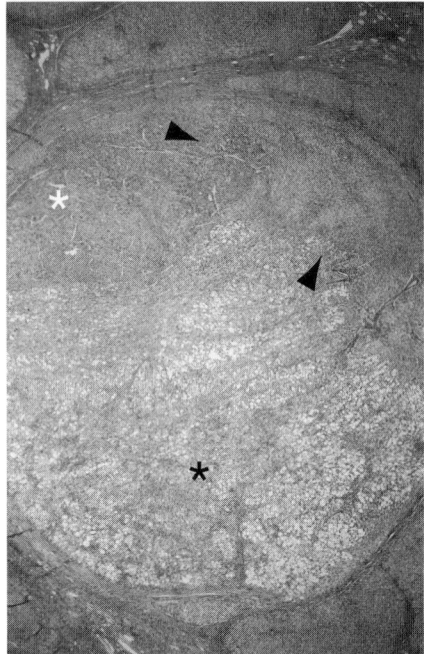
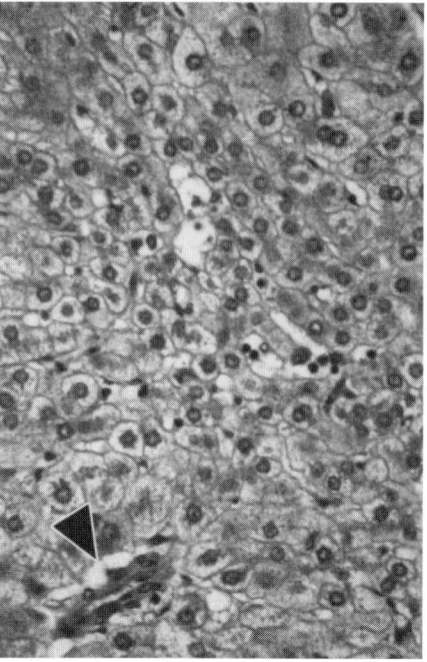

FIGURE 31.7. Transformation of a dysplastic nodule. **A:** The residual dysplastic area is noted in the right upper quadrant (*arrowheads*). Macrotrabecular hepatocellular carcinoma (HCC) (*white star*) and compact HCC with massive fat accumulation (*black star*) replace the rest of the nodule. **B:** The residual small cell dysplastic changes (small cell dysplasia). Increased nuclear density and the naked artery (*arrowhead*) are useful diagnostic features.

debated, and whether they represent a direct precursor of HCC remains unclear (65–68).

Early HCCs may develop within dysplastic nodules, initially preserving a seemingly normal cytologic and architectural pattern (Fig. 31.7). These lesions measure <2 cm in diameter, and although sometimes surrounded by an ill-defined fibrous condensation, most have only a vaguely nodular morphology (13,69). The majority of these HCCs are extremely well differentiated, with little cellular and structural atypia, and thus present diagnostic challenges on biopsy material (13,61,70). Histologically, they are characterized by subtle changes, including increased cell density associated with increased nucleus-to-cytoplasm ratio. Cytoplasmic changes, including increased eosinophilia, fatty or clear cell changes, or both, as well as ironfree foci, can also be noted (13,61,70,71). Architecturally, an irregular thin trabecular pattern, as well as acinar or pseudoglandular patterns or both, can be seen (13,61,70). Another notable feature is the increased number of unpaired muscularized arteries (71). Vascular invasion is rare, but "stromal invasion" of portal spaces can be observed (69,70). As they grow, dedifferentiation of these well-differentiated tumors occurs, and approximately 40% of HCCs measuring between 1 and 3 cm in diameter consist of more than two patterns of varying differentiation (47). The dedifferentiated component usually arises as a *nodule-in-nodule* fashion. In this process, the higher-grade component arises in the center and proliferates expansively, whereas the peripheral well-differentiated rim is compressed and eventually replaced (47,61,70,72) (Fig. 31.7).

CYTOLOGY

Fine-needle aspiration biopsy (FNAB) can be an effective tool in the diagnosis of HCC, with a sensitivity ranging from 67% to 93% (73). However, difficulties arise in distinguishing benign hepatocellular nodules from low-grade HCC. The most specific cytologic criteria of well-differentiated HCC are as follows:

- Numerous stripped atypical nuclei
- Macronucleoli
- Increased mitoses
- Multinucleation (74)

Architectural criteria helpful in smear material are as follows:

- Widened trabeculae
- Well-defined capillaries traversing tissue fragments
- Islands of hepatocytes rimmed by endothelial cells (Fig. 31.8)

Cellblocks prepared from FNABs are particularly important because they improve the specificity of the diagnosis by allowing a better evaluation of architecture and being amenable to special stains, which can be helpful in equivocal cases (75,76).

Diagnosing FNABs from less differentiated HCCs can also be a difficult exercise because they may show features that overlap with metastatic carcinomas. In a study from the College of American Pathologists, FNABs from HCC were misclassified

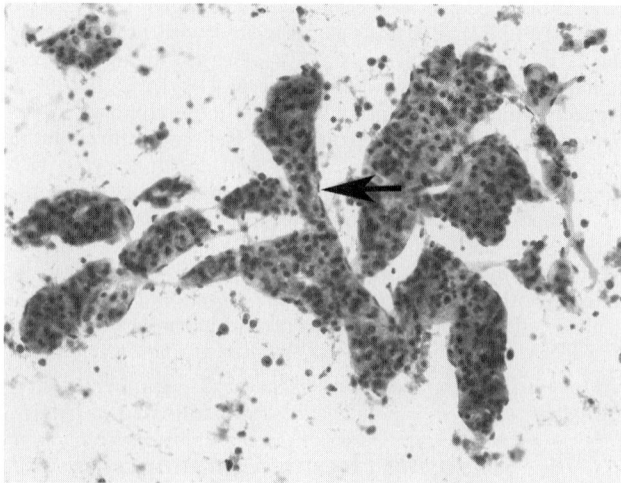

FIGURE 31.8. Cytomorphologic features of HCC with a macrotrabecular pattern encased by a rim of endothelial cells (*arrow*) (See also color Figure 31.8).

in 26% of the examinations (77). Thus, although FNAB can diagnose HCC efficiently, the availability of concurrent cellblock material is of cardinal importance in improving the sensitivity and specificity of this test.

ANCILLARY STUDIES

Occasionally, routine microscopic evaluation of hepatic masses needs to be supplemented by special studies in order to confirm a diagnosis of HCC, distinguishing it from a metastatic adenocarcinoma or, less frequently, a peripheral cholangiocarcinoma. These ancillary aids can also be of great help in distinguishing well-differentiated HCC from benign hepatocellular proliferations such as hepatocellular adenomas. Techniques used have included immunohistochemistry, conventional cytogenetics, fluorescent in situ hybridization, and comparative genomic hybridization (78,79). A plethora of markers have been tested over time, and several of these techniques are not readily available at most diagnostic laboratories. Because an exhaustive review of all markers is beyond the scope of this chapter, only a few of them, either well established or promising, are discussed herein in the context of the usual clinical dilemmas.

Hepatocellular Carcinoma versus Metastatic Adenocarcinoma and Cholangiocarcinoma

Mucin

Although it is generally accepted that HCC tumor cells do not produce mucin, it has been noted rarely in the lumen of the pseudoglandular (acinar) variant (31). However, the intracytoplasmic demonstration of mucin by mucicarmine stain generally rules out this diagnosis, and raises a differential diagnosis of metastatic adenocarcinoma and cholangiocarcinoma. Recently, emphasis has been placed on MUC antibodies against glycoproteins components of mucin. Hepatocellular carcinomas are uniformly negative for mucin core proteins, including MUC-1, MUC-2, and MUC-5AC. Conversely, MUC-1 and MUC-5AC are positive in 73% and 45% of cholangiocarcinomas, respectively, as well as in gastrointestinal cancers likely to metastasize to the liver (80). If definite immunohistochemical evidence of hepatocytic and cholangiocytic differentiation are observed in the same lesion, then a diagnosis of combined HCC-CC is warranted.

Albumin

Albumin, which is exclusively synthesized by hepatocytes, is a highly specific marker of hepatocytic lineage (81), making this protein the ideal tool for distinguishing HCC from a metastatic adenocarcinoma. Unfortunately, immunohistochemistry is not well suited for its detection because of the abundance of the protein in the serum. In situ hybridization is a better technique, with albumin mRNA demonstrated in up to 96% of HCC (81). However, this methodology is not readily available in all laboratories.

Polyclonal Carcinoembryonic Antigen and CD10

In addition to resembling normal hepatocytes morphologically, HCCs have a biliary canalicular network, albeit disorganized. Both polyclonal CEA and CD10 delineate this pattern due to cross-reaction with glycoprotein I, and hence offer evidence of hepatocellular differentiation, when present (82,83). However, poorly differentiated HCC, which are most likely to cause diagnostic difficulties, are occasionally negative for this immunohistochemical marker (82,83).

Alpha-Fetoprotein

Alpha-fetoprotein is an oncofetal glycoprotein of low sensitivity that stains about 15% to 60% of HCCs (84–86), which makes it an unreliable marker of hepatocellular differentiation. However, its specificity is close to 100%, after exclusion of rare lesions such as yolk sac tumors (87–89).

Hepatocyte Paraffin 1

Hepatocyte paraffin 1 (HepPar1) is a highly sensitive marker of both benign and neoplastic hepatocellular proliferations (90–92). Its sensitivity is reported to be about 91%, with only 4% of nonhepatic tumors staining positively (92). However, poorly differentiated HCCs can be negative, and occasional metastatic adenocarcinomas have been reported to be immunoreactive (92). Notably, metastatic adenocarcinomas with hepatoid differentiation are uniformly negative for HepPar 1 (93).

Cytokeratin

Hepatocellular carcinomas tend to recapitulate the keratin profile of hepatocytes and are typically positive for low-molecular-weight keratins, including CAM 5.2 and CK 8 and 18. Conversely, cholangiocarcinomas stain positively for keratins 7 and 19, whereas HCCs are typically negative for these keratins. However, overlap in CK phenotype between HCC and CCs (reflecting their common progenitor cells) and metastatic tumor (depending on the organ of origin) limit their diagnostic applicability (87–89).

CD 34

Refer to the "CD 34" section that follows.

Markers for Distinguishing Benign From Malignant Hepatic Tumors

Reticulin

A well-differentiated HCC may masquerade as a hepatocellular adenoma, particularly on needle biopsy specimens. However, adenomas show a dense framework of reticulin fibers deposited along the hepatic sinusoids. In contrast, HCCs are usually

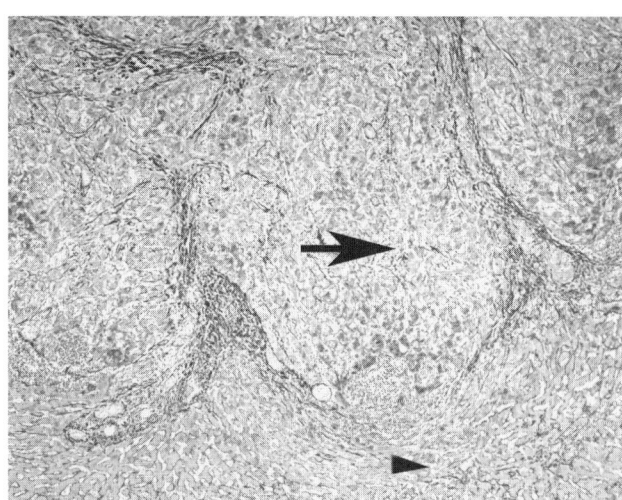

FIGURE 31.9. Reticulin stain demonstrating partial loss of reticulin fibers (*arrow*). The adjacent benign hepatic parenchyma shows a normal and preserved reticulin framework (*arrowhead*) (See also color Figure 31.9).

characterized by the loss of this framework and/or the presence of thickened hepatic plates (Fig. 31.9), although the changes may be subtle in very well-differentiated lesions (94).

CD 34

CD 34, a marker of endothelial cells, is not normally expressed by hepatic sinusoidal cells. However, "capillarization" of sinusoids, as expressed by various degrees of CD34 immunoreactivity, has been noted in hepatic adenoma, cirrhotic liver, adenomatous hyperplasia, and HCC (78,95,96). Diffuse sinusoidal reactivity would support a diagnosis of HCC (76) and can help differentiate dysplastic nodules and early HCCs from macroregenerative nodules (97). However, there is considerable overlap in the staining profiles of hepatocellular proliferations (benign and malignant), and therefore caution is necessary in making a distinction based on this immunohistochemical stain. Of note, one series reported the lack of CD34 immunoreactivity in a series of metastatic carcinomas to the liver, suggesting a role in this situation (98).

In closing, these markers are best used to support a methodic histologic evaluation and do not supersede it. Immunohistochemical panels combining HepPar 1 with polyclonal CEA and CD10 provide the highest yield in differentiating HCCs from other neoplasms.

References

1. Okuda K, Peters RL, Simson IW. Gross anatomic features of hepatocellular carcinoma from three disparate geographic areas: proposal of new classification. *Cancer* 1984;54:2165–2173.
2. Kemeny F, Vadrot J, Wu A, Smadja C, Meakins JL, Franco D. Morphological and histological features of resected hepatocellular carcinoma in cirrhotic patients in the West. *Hepatology* 1989;9:253–257.
3. Kojiro M, Nakashima O, Kiyomatsu K, et al. *Comparative Study of HCC Between Japan and Spain.* Amsterdam: Excerpta Medica; 1990.
4. Nzeako UC, Goodman ZD, Ishak KG. Hepatocellular carcinoma in cirrhotic and noncirrhotic livers: a clinico-histopathologic study of 804 North American patients. *Am J Clin Pathol* 1996;105:65–75.
5. Smalley SR, Moertel CG, Hilton JF, et al. Hepatoma in the noncirrhotic liver. *Cancer* 1988;62:1414–1424.
6. Bismuth H, Chiche L, Castaing D. Surgical treatment of hepatocellular carcinomas in noncirrhotic liver: experience with 68 liver resections. *World J Surg* 1995;19:35–41.
7. Kishi K, Shikata T, Hirohashi S, Hasegawa H, Yamazaki S, Makuuchi M. Hepatocellular carcinoma: a clinical and pathologic analysis of 57 hepatectomy cases. *Cancer* 1983;51:542–548.
8. Lauwers GY, Vauthey JN. Pathological aspects of hepatocellular carcinoma: a critical review of prognostic factors. *Hepatogastroenterology* 1998;45(suppl 3):1197–1202.
9. Yuki K, Hirohashi S, Sakamoto M, Kanai T, Shimosato Y. Growth and spread of hepatocellular carcinoma: a review of 240 consecutive autopsy cases. *Cancer* 1990;66:2174–2179.
10. Adachi E, Maeda T, Matsumata T, et al. Risk factors for intrahepatic recurrence in human small hepatocellular carcinoma. *Gastroenterology* 1995;108:768–775.
11. Japan LCSGo. Primary liver cancer in Japan: clinicopathologic features and results of surgical treatment. *Ann Surg* 1989;211:277–287.
12. Izumi R, Shimizu K, Ii T, et al. Prognostic factors of hepatocellular carcinoma in patients undergoing hepatic resection. *Gastroenterology* 1994;106:720–727.
13. Japan LCSGo. *The General Rules for the Clinical and Pathological Study of Primary Liver Cancer.* Tokyo: Kanehira & Co.; 1997.
14. Nagao T, Inoue S, Goto S, et al. Hepatic resection for hepatocellular carcinoma: clinical features and long-term prognosis. *Ann Surg* 1987;205:33–40.
15. Arii S, Tanaka J, Yamazoe Y, et al. Predictive factors for intrahepatic recurrence of hepatocellular carcinoma after partial hepatectomy. *Cancer* 1992;69:913–919.
16. Ng IO, Lai EC, Ng MM, Fan ST. Tumor encapsulation in hepatocellular carcinoma: a pathologic study of 189 cases. *Cancer* 1992;70:45–49.
17. Eggel H. Uber das primare carcinom der leber. *Beitr Pathol Ann* 1901;30:506–604.
18. Kanai T, Hirohashi S, Upton MP, et al. Pathology of small hepatocellular carcinoma: a proposal for a new gross classification. *Cancer* 1987;60:810–819.
19. Nakashima T, Kojiro M. Pathologic characteristics of hepatocellular carcinoma. *Semin Liver Dis* 1986;6:259–266.
20. Nagao T, Inoue S, Yoshimi F, et al. Postoperative recurrence of hepatocellular carcinoma. *Ann Surg* 1990;211:28–33.
21. Lai EC, You KT, Ng IO, Shek TW. The pathological basis of resection margin for hepatocellular carcinoma. *World J Surg* 1993;17:786–790; discussion 791.
22. Imamura H, Matsuyama Y, Tanaka E, et al. Risk factors contributing to early and late phase intrahepatic recurrence of hepatocellular carcinoma after hepatectomy. *J Hepatol* 2003;38:200–207.
23. Lauwers GY, Terris B, Balis UJ, et al. Prognostic histologic indicators of curatively resected hepatocellular carcinomas: a multi-institutional analysis of 425 patients with definition of a histologic prognostic index. *Am J Surg Pathol* 2002;26:25–34.
24. Sakamoto M, Hirohashi S, Tsuda H, Shimosato Y, Makuuchi M, Hosoda Y. Multicentric independent development of hepatocellular carcinoma revealed by analysis of hepatitis B virus integration pattern. *Am J Surg Pathol* 1989;13:1064–1067.
25. Toyosaka A, Okamoto E, Mitsunobu M, Oriyama T, Nakao N, Miura K. Pathologic and radiographic studies of intrahepatic metastasis in hepatocellular carcinoma: the role of efferent vessels. *HPB Surg* 1996;10:97–103; discussion 103–104.
26. Ikai I, Yamaoka Y, Yamamoto Y, et al. Surgical intervention for patients with stage IV-A hepatocellular carcinoma without lymph node metastasis: proposal as a standard therapy. *Ann Surg* 1998;227:433–439.
27. Kojiro M, Sugihara S, Kakizoe S, Nakashima O, Kiyomatsu K. Hepatocellular carcinoma with sarcomatous change: a special reference to the relationship with anticancer therapy. *Cancer Chemother Pharmacol* 1989;23(suppl):S4–S8.
28. Kojiro M, Kawabata K, Kawano Y, Shirai F, Takemoto N, Nakashima T. Hepatocellular carcinoma presenting as intrabile duct tumor growth: a clinicopathologic study of 24 cases. *Cancer* 1982;49:2144–2147.
29. Ishak KG, Anthony PP, Sobin L. *Histological Typing of Tumours in the Liver.* Berlin: Springer-Verlag; 1994.
30. Denk H, Stumptner C, Fuchsbichler A, et al. Are the Mallory bodies and intracellular hyaline bodies in neoplastic and non-neoplastic hepatocytes related? *J Pathol* 2006;208:653–661.
31. Edmondson HA, Steiner PE. Primary carcinoma of the liver: a study of 100 cases among 48,900 necropsies. *Cancer* 1954;7:462–503.
32. Haratake J, Takeda S, Kasai T, Nakano S, Tokui N. Predictable factors for estimating prognosis of patients after resection of hepatocellular carcinoma. *Cancer* 1993;72:1178–1183.
33. Adachi E, Maeda T, Kajiyama K, et al. Factors correlated with portal venous invasion by hepatocellular carcinoma: univariate and multivariate analyses of 232 resected cases without preoperative treatments. *Cancer* 1996;77:2022–2031.
34. Lai CL, Wu PC, Lam KC, Todd D. Histologic prognostic indicators in hepatocellular carcinoma. *Cancer* 1979;44:1677–1683.
35. Yang SH, Watanabe J, Nakashima O, Kojiro M. Clinicopathologic study on clear cell hepatocellular carcinoma. *Pathol Int* 1996;46:503–509.
36. Maeda T, Adachi E, Kajiyama K, Takenaka K, Sugimachi K, Tsuneyoshi M. Spindle cell hepatocellular carcinoma: a clinicopathological and immunohistochemical analysis of 15 cases. *Cancer* 1996;77:51–57.
37. Esnaola NF, Lauwers GY, Mirza NQ, et al. Predictors of microvascular invasion in patients with hepatocellular carcinoma who are candidates for orthotopic liver transplantation. *J Gastrointest Surg* 2002;6:224–232; discussion 232.
38. Vauthey JN, Klimstra D, Franceschi D, et al. Factors affecting long-term outcome after hepatic resection for hepatocellular carcinoma. *Am J Surg* 1995;169:28–34; discussion 34–25.
39. Nigam A, Zhurak M, Boitnott JK, et al. Factors affecting survival in Western patients following curative resection for hepatocellular carcinoma [abstract]. *Gastroenterology* 1995;108:A1235.
40. Craig JR, Peters RL, Edmondson HA, Omata M. Fibrolamellar carcinoma of the liver: a tumor of adolescents and young adults with distinctive clinicopathologic features. *Cancer* 1980;46:372–379.
41. Berman MA, Burnham JA, Sheahan DG. Fibrolamellar carcinoma of the liver: an immunohistochemical study of nineteen cases and a review of the literature. *Hum Pathol* 1988;19:784–794.
42. El-Serag HB, Davila JA. Is fibrolamellar carcinoma different from hepatocellular carcinoma? A US population-based study. *Hepatology* 2004;39:798–803.
43. Ringe B, Wittekind C, Weimann A, Tusch G, Pichlmayr R. Results of hepatic resection and transplantation for fibrolamellar carcinoma. *Surg Gynecol Obstet* 1992;175:299–305.
44. Soreide O, Czerniak A, Bradpiece H, Bloom S, Blumgart L. Characteristics of fibrolamellar hepatocellular carcinoma: a study of nine cases and a review of the literature. *Am J Surg* 1986;151:518–523.
45. Stipa F, Yoon SS, Liau KH, et al. Outcome of patients with fibrolamellar hepatocellular carcinoma. *Cancer* 2006;106:1331–1338.
46. Kakar S, Burgart LJ, Batts KP, Garcia J, Jain D, Ferrell LD. Clinicopathologic features and survival in fibrolamellar carcinoma: comparison with conventional hepatocellular carcinoma with and without cirrhosis. *Mod Pathol* 2005;18:1417–1423.
47. Kojiro M. *Pathology of Hepatocellular Carcinoma.* New York, NY: Churchill Livingstone; 1997.
48. Goodman ZD, Ishak KG, Langloss JM, Sesterhenn IA, Rabin L. Combined

hepatocellular-cholangiocarcinoma: a histologic and immunohistochemical study. *Cancer* 1985;55:124–135.

49. Maeda T, Adachi E, Kajiyama K, Sugimachi K, Tsuneyoshi M. Combined hepatocellular and cholangiocarcinoma: proposed criteria according to cytokeratin expression and analysis of clinicopathologic features. *Hum Pathol* 1995;26:956–964.

50. Morcos M, Dubois S, Bralet MP, Belghiti J, Degott C, Terris B. Primary liver carcinoma in genetic hemochromatosis reveals a broad histologic spectrum. *Am J Clin Pathol* 2001;116:738–743.

51. Roskams T, Willems M, Campos RV, Drucker DJ, Yap SH, Desmet VJ. Parathyroid hormone-related peptide expression in primary and metastatic liver tumours. *Histopathology* 1993;23:519–525.

52. Nakamura S, Suzuki S, Sakaguchi T, et al. Surgical treatment of patients with mixed hepatocellular carcinoma and cholangiocarcinoma. *Cancer* 1996;78:1671–1676.

53. Theise ND, Yao JL, Harada K, et al. Hepatic 'stem cell' malignancies in adults: four cases. *Histopathology* 2003;43:263–271.

54. Tickoo SK, Zee SY, Obiekwe S, et al. Combined hepatocellular-cholangiocarcinoma: a histopathologic, immunohistochemical, and in situ hybridization study. *Am J Surg Pathol* 2002;26:989–997.

55. Omata M, Peters RL, Tatter D. Sclerosing hepatic carcinoma: relationship to hypercalcemia. *Liver* 1981;1:33–49.

56. Albar JP, De Miguel F, Esbrit P, Miranda R, Fernandez-Flores A, Sarasa JL. Immunohistochemical detection of parathyroid hormone-related protein in a rare variant of hepatic neoplasm (sclerosing hepatic carcinoma). *Hum Pathol* 1996;27:728–731.

57. Zimmermann A, Kappeler A, Friess H, Buchler MW. Hepatocellular carcinoma with an unusual medullary-like histology and signs of regression ("medullary-like hepatocellular carcinoma"). *Dig Liver Dis* 2002;34:748–753.

58. Si MW, Thorson JA, Lauwers GY, DalCin P, Furman J. Hepatocellular lymphoepithelioma-like carcinoma associated with Epstein Barr virus: a hitherto unrecognized entity. *Diagn Mol Pathol* 2004;13:183–189.

59. Yamaguchi R, Nakashima O, Ogata T, Hanada K, Kumabe T, Kojiro M. Hepatocellular carcinoma with an unusual neuroendocrine component. *Pathol Int* 2004;54:861–865.

60. Earls JP, Theise ND, Weinreb JC, et al. Terminology of nodular hepatocellular lesions. International Working Party. *Hepatology* 1995;22:983–993.

61. Kondo Y, Niwa Y, Akikusa B, Takazawa H, Okabayashi A. A histopathologic study of early hepatocellular carcinoma. *Cancer* 1983;52:687–692.

62. Borzio M, Fargion S, Borzio F, et al. Impact of large regenerative, low grade and high grade dysplastic nodules in hepatocellular carcinoma development. *J Hepatol* 2003;39:208–214.

63. Anthony PP, Vogel CL, Barker LF. Liver cell dysplasia: a premalignant condition. *J Clin Pathol* 1973;26:217–223.

64. Watanabe S, Okita K, Harada T, et al. Morphologic studies of the liver cell dysplasia. *Cancer* 1983;51:2197–2205.

65. Lee RG, Tsamandas AC, Demetris AJ. Large cell change (liver cell dysplasia) and hepatocellular carcinoma in cirrhosis: matched case-control study, pathological analysis, and pathogenetic hypothesis. *Hepatology* 1997;26:1415–1422.

66. Borzio M, Borzio F, Croce A, et al. Ultrasonography-detected macroregenerative nodules in cirrhosis: a prospective study. *Gastroenterology* 1997;112:1617–1623.

67. Theise ND, Schwartz M, Miller C, Thung SN. Macroregenerative nodules and hepatocellular carcinoma in forty-four sequential adult liver explants with cirrhosis. *Hepatology* 1992;16:949–955.

68. Terasaki S, Kaneko S, Kobayashi K, Nonomura A, Nakanuma Y. Histological features predicting malignant transformation of nonmalignant hepatocellular nodules: a prospective study. *Gastroenterology* 1998;115:1216–1222.

69. Kojiro M. Focus on dysplastic nodules and early hepatocellular carcinoma: an Eastern point of view. *Liver Transpl* 2004;10:S3–S8.

70. Sakamoto M, Hirohashi S, Shimosato Y. Early stages of multistep hepatocarcinogenesis: adenomatous hyperplasia and early hepatocellular carcinoma. *Hum Pathol* 1991;22:172–178.

71. Roncalli M. Hepatocellular nodules in cirrhosis: focus on diagnostic criteria on liver biopsy: a Western experience. *Liver Transpl* 2004;10:S9–S15.

72. Arakawa M, Kage M, Sugihara S, Nakashima T, Suenaga M, Okuda K. Emergence of malignant lesions within an adenomatous hyperplastic nodule in a cirrhotic liver: observations in five cases. *Gastroenterology* 1986;91:198–208.

73. Jain D. Diagnosis of hepatocellular carcinoma: fine needle aspiration cytology or needle core biopsy. *J Clin Gastroenterol* 2002;35:S101–S108.

74. de Boer WB, Segal A, Frost FA, Sterrett GF. Cytodiagnosis of well differentiated hepatocellular carcinoma: can indeterminate diagnoses be reduced? *Cancer* 1999;87:270–277.

75. Saad RS, Luckasevic TM, Noga CM, Johnson DR, Silverman JF, Liu YL. Diagnostic value of HepPar1, pCEA, CD10, and CD34 expression in separating hepatocellular carcinoma from metastatic carcinoma in fine-needle aspiration cytology. *Diagn Cytopathol* 2004;30:1–6.

76. de Boer WB, Segal A, Frost FA, Sterrett GF. Can CD34 discriminate between benign and malignant hepatocytic lesions in fine-needle aspirates and thin core biopsies? *Cancer* 2000;90:273–278.

77. Renshaw AA, Haja J, Wilbur DC, Miller TR. Fine-needle aspirates of adenocarcinoma/metastatic carcinoma that resemble hepatocellular carcinoma: correlating cytologic features and performance in the College of American Pathologists Nongynecologic Cytology Program. *Arch Pathol Lab Med* 2005;129:1217–1221.

78. Wilkens L, Bredt M, Flemming P, et al. Comparative genomic hybridization (CGH) and fluorescence in situ hybridization (FISH) in the diagnosis of hepatocellular carcinoma. *J Hepatobiliary Pancreat Surg* 2002;9:304–311.

79. Chen ZM, Crone KG, Watson MA, Pfeifer JD, Wang HL. Identification of a unique gene expression signature that differentiates hepatocellular adenoma from well-differentiated hepatocellular carcinoma. *Am J Surg Pathol* 2005;29:1600–1608.

80. Lau SK, Weiss LM, Chu PG. Differential expression of MUC1, MUC2, and MUC5AC in carcinomas of various sites: an immunohistochemical study. *Am J Clin Pathol* 2004;122:61–69.

81. Krishna M, Lloyd RV, Batts KP. Detection of albumin messenger RNA in hepatic and extrahepatic neoplasms: a marker of hepatocellular differentiation. *Am J Surg Pathol* 1997;21:147–152.

82. Ma CK, Zarbo RJ, Frierson HF, Jr., Lee MW. Comparative immunohistochemical study of primary and metastatic carcinomas of the liver. *Am J Clin Pathol* 1993;99:551–557.

83. Borscheri N, Roessner A, Rocken C. Canalicular immunostaining of neprilysin (CD10) as a diagnostic marker for hepatocellular carcinomas. *Am J Surg Pathol* 2001;25:1297–1303.

84. Kondo Y. Histologic features of hepatocellular carcinoma and allied disorders. *Pathol Annu* 1985;20(pt 2):405–430.

85. Thung SN, Gerber MA, Sarno E, Popper H. Distribution of five antigens in hepatocellular carcinoma. *Lab Invest* 1979;41:101–105.

86. Fucich LF, Cheles MK, Thung SN, Gerber MA, Marrogi AJ. Primary vs metastatic hepatic carcinoma: an immunohistochemical study of 34 cases. *Arch Pathol Lab Med* 1994;118:927–930.

87. Hurlimann J, Gardiol D. Immunohistochemistry in the differential diagnosis of liver carcinomas. *Am J Surg Pathol* 1991;15:280–288.

88. Johnson DE, Herndier BG, Medeiros LJ, Warnke RA, Rouse RV. The diagnostic utility of the keratin profiles of hepatocellular carcinoma and cholangiocarcinoma. *Am J Surg Pathol* 1988;12:187–197.

89. Minervini MI, Demetris AJ, Lee RG, Carr BI, Madariaga J, Nalesnik MA. Utilization of hepatocyte-specific antibody in the immunocytochemical evaluation of liver tumors. *Mod Pathol* 1997;10:686–692.

90. Kakar S, Muir T, Murphy LM, Lloyd RV, Burgart LJ. Immunoreactivity of Hep Par 1 in hepatic and extrahepatic tumors and its correlation with albumin in situ hybridization in hepatocellular carcinoma. *Am J Clin Pathol* 2003;119:361–366.

91. Fan Z, van de Rijn M, Montgomery K, Rouse RV. Hep par 1 antibody stain for the differential diagnosis of hepatocellular carcinoma: 676 tumors tested using tissue microarrays and conventional tissue sections. *Mod Pathol* 2003;16:137–144.

92. Lugli A, Tornillo L, Mirlacher M, Bundi M, Sauter G, Terracciano LM. Hepatocyte paraffin 1 expression in human normal and neoplastic tissues: tissue microarray analysis on 3,940 tissue samples. *Am J Clin Pathol* 2004;122:721–727.

93. Terracciano LM, Glatz K, Mhawech P, et al. Hepatoid adenocarcinoma with liver metastasis mimicking hepatocellular carcinoma: an immunohistochemical and molecular study of eight cases. *Am J Surg Pathol* 2003;27:1302–1312.

94. Bergman S, Graeme-Cook F, Pitman MB. The usefulness of the reticulin stain in the differential diagnosis of liver nodules on fine-needle aspiration biopsy cell block preparations. *Mod Pathol* 1997;10:1258–1264.

95. Scott FR, el-Refaie A, More L, Scheuer PJ, Dhillon AP. Hepatocellular carcinoma arising in an adenoma: value of QBend 10 immunostaining in diagnosis of liver cell carcinoma. *Histopathology* 1996;28:472–474.

96. Kimura H, Nakajima T, Kagawa K, et al. Angiogenesis in hepatocellular carcinoma as evaluated by CD34 immunohistochemistry. *Liver* 1998;18:14–19.

97. Frachon S, Gouysse G, Dumortier J, et al. Endothelial cell marker expression in dysplastic lesions of the liver: an immunohistochemical study. *J Hepatol* 2001;34:850–857.

98. Gottschalk-Sabag S, Ron N, Glick T. Use of CD34 and factor VIII to diagnose hepatocellular carcinoma on fine needle aspirates. *Acta Cytol* 1998;42:691–696.

CHAPTER 32 ■ HEPATOCELLULAR CANCER: ANATOMY AND STAGING

CHRISTOPHER J. GANNON AND STEVEN A. CURLEY

INTRODUCTION

Hepatocellular carcinoma (HCC) is a common malignancy worldwide, with more than 500,000 cases presenting annually (1). Although this prevalence is not mirrored in the population of the United States, the incidence of HCC continues to increase, with more than 19,000 estimated new cases expected in 2007 in the United States. Unfortunately, this disease remains highly lethal, with more than 17,000 deaths anticipated that same year (2). Chronic liver disease is the common underlying cause of HCC.

Worldwide, chronic viral hepatitis is primarily responsible for hepatic dysfunction and cirrhosis. In Western countries, other factors such as excessive, chronic alcohol consumption may have an impact on the carcinogenesis of HCC. Hepatitis B virus (HBV) is already a well-documented entity responsible for the underlying hepatic injury found in patients with HCC. Similarly, chronic infection with hepatitis C virus (HCV) has been shown to be a powerful etiologic element (3). Despite the international prevalence and increasing incidence within the United States, successful therapy is limited to patients with early stage disease and is typically dependent on clinical factors as well as the anatomy of the cancer. As a result, multiple staging systems for HCC have been developed. We discuss the systems that have gained wide acceptance through clinical verification.

ANATOMY

A thorough understanding of the anatomy of the liver is necessary to assess patients as candidates for surgical resection or other local therapies. The vasculature of the liver has robust inflow with the hepatic artery, a branch of the celiac artery, and the portal vein, venous blood from the intestinal tract. Consistent nomenclature is also paramount to improve understanding among caregivers and to clarify the sometimes divergent literature.

The liver lies in the right upper quadrant of the abdomen, nestled underneath the rib cage. It is completely surrounded by a peritoneal membrane, known as Glisson capsule. This investing sheath also envelopes the portal vascular structures as they enter the liver. In contrast, hepatic veins are not covered by Glisson capsule. The liver receives a dual blood supply from both the hepatic artery and portal vein. The portal vein supplies approximately 75% of the blood supply, with the hepatic artery providing the remainder. The liver is drained predominantly by three major veins: the left, middle, and right hepatic veins. The remaining drainage occurs through several small veins that directly enter the vena cava from the posterior aspect of the liver.

For surgical approaches to hepatic tumors, it is important to recognize the variability of the extrahepatic arterial anatomy (4,5). In the majority of patients, the common hepatic artery arises from the celiac trunk giving off the gastroduodenal artery, followed by a right gastric artery. The proper hepatic artery gives rise to the cystic artery followed by the right and left hepatic arteries. However, the cystic artery frequently arises from the right hepatic artery and rarely may arise from the left hepatic artery. Anatomical variants include a replaced right hepatic artery (right hepatic artery arising off the superior mesenteric artery) and a replaced left hepatic artery (left hepatic artery arising from the left gastric artery). The importance of these variants in hepatic surgery is in recognizing their presence so as to prevent inadvertent injury. Other anatomical variants exist, including accessory vessels (a vessel that exists in conjunction with a vessel with a more standard origin) and variations in the cystic artery anatomy.

An understanding of biliary anatomy and its variations is essential to perform surgery for hepatic neoplasms successfully. The proximal right hepatic duct is largely intrahepatic, while the proximal left hepatic duct is extrahepatic and runs perpendicular to the common hepatic duct to the level of the round ligament. At the round ligament, the left hepatic duct is formed by confluence of ducts from segment IV and segments II/III. The confluence of the left and right hepatic ducts is cephalad and ventral to the portal vein bifurcation. The hepatic bile duct confluence gives rise to the common hepatic duct, the portion of the duct between the confluence and the cystic duct entrance. The common bile duct extends from the cystic duct to the ampulla of Vater. The blood supply to the extrahepatic bile duct arises from the right hepatic artery superiorly and from the gastroduodenal artery inferiorly, and runs longitudinally along its course.

One of the greatest advances in hepatic surgery is the understanding of the segmental anatomy of the liver. The Couinaud system for liver segmental nomenclature is widely accepted (6,7). The liver is divided into longitudinal planes drawn through each hepatic vein to the vena cava and a transverse plane at the level of the main portal bifurcation (Fig. 32.1). The plane of the middle hepatic vein and the primary bifurcation of the portal vein divide the liver into a right and left lobe, this runs from the inferior vena cava to the tip of the gallbladder fossa (also know as the Cantlie line or portal fissure). The secondary portal bifurcations on the right and left give rise to four sectors (also sometimes called segments or sections). The segments are then numbered clockwise in a frontal plane, beginning with the first segment, historically called the caudate lobe. On the right side, this produces the anterior and posterior sectors that are split by the plane of the right hepatic vein. The tertiary branches on the right supply four segments, two in each sector. On the left, the ascending branch gives off recurrent

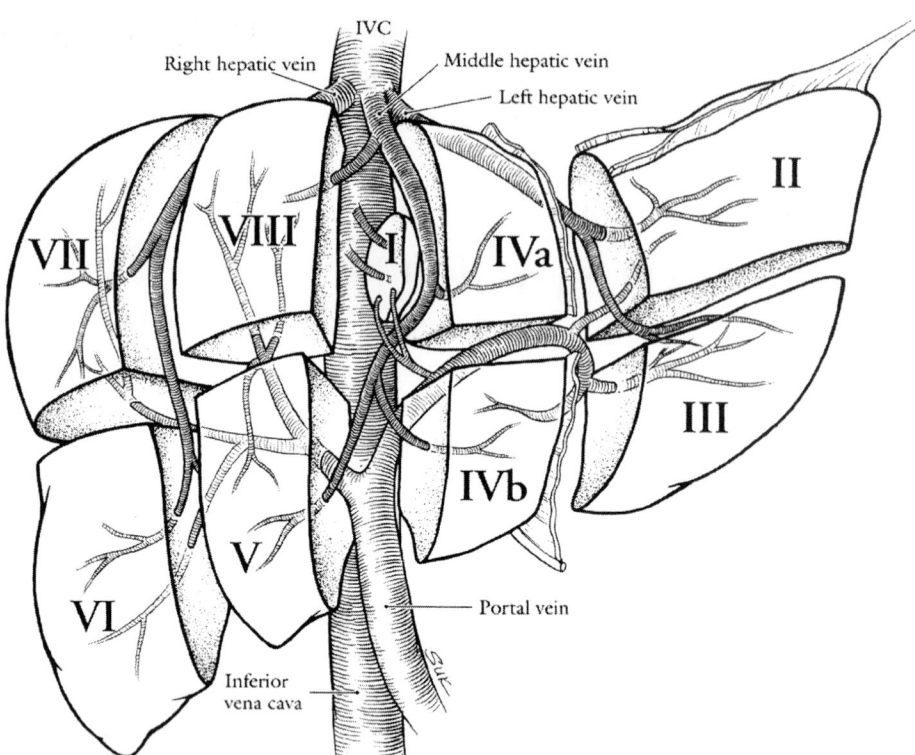

FIGURE 32.1. Anatomy of the liver with Couinaud's segments.

branches to the medial sector (8), whereas the left lateral sector is supplied by separate branches supplying segments II and III. Segment I, the caudate lobe, receives blood supply from both the left and right portal pedicles; bile ducts from segment I also drain into the right and left hepatic ducts.

The application of surgical segmental anatomy to axial radiologic imaging (computed tomography [CT] or magnetic resonance imaging [MRI] studies) is critical in evaluating the resection potential of hepatic tumors. Reading axial studies should begin with the identification of the hepatic vein insertions into the vena cava and the plane of the portal bifurcation. Any segments cephalad to the portal vein bifurcation are VII, VIII, IVA, or II. Those caudal to the portal vein bifurcation are VI, V, IVB, and III.

STAGING—CLINICAL SYSTEMS

Most patients with HCC present with advanced disease and thus are not candidates for curative therapy. A significant proportion of the remaining patients have coexistent, severe liver disease, including cirrhosis and chronic active hepatitis, and they may not have adequate functional hepatic reserve to tolerate hepatic resection. As a result, there are multiple clinical staging systems for HCC. These systems represent attempts to standardize the initial therapy for HCC. Selection of the most appropriate candidates for surgical resection, liver transplant, or definitive tumor ablative therapy is the ultimate goal. The most widely accepted clinical staging systems include Okuda, Barcelona Clinic Liver Cancer (BCLC), Cancer of the Liver Italian Program (CLIP), and Model for End-Stage Liver Disease (MELD).

Okuda Staging System

A group of Japanese patients with HCC was used to devise this system. It takes into account physiological liver function parameters and tumor characteristics. Liver function parameters include measurement of serum albumin and bilirubin. The other two parameters are the presence of ascites and the tumor size or volume in relation to the hepatic parenchyma (Table 32.1). Each criterion is marked as either positive or negative, depending on the value. A serum albumin of <3 g/dL is "+". A serum bilirubin >3 mg/dL is "+". Clinically detectable ascites is "+". Tumor size of >50% of the largest cross-sectional area of the liver is "+".

The Okuda stage is determined by the number of positive criterion. The Okuda stage I patient has no positive findings, Okuda stage II has one or two positives, and Okuda stage III has three or four positives. In the original series of 850 patients describing the clinical scheme for staging, patients with Okuda stage I disease who underwent resection displayed a median survival of 25.6 months, whereas Okuda stage II patients treated with hepatic resection had a 12.2-month median survival. Medically treated Okuda stage I patients fared worse with median survival of 9.4 months. Compared to no treatment, Okuda stage II and III patients fared better with medical therapy (stage II: 1.6 vs. 3.5 months, stage III: 0.7 vs.

TABLE 32.1

OKUDA STAGING SYSTEM

Criteria	Scores	
	0	1
Size of tumor	<50% of liver	>50% of liver
Ascites	Absent	Present
Albumin (g/dL)	≥3.0	<3.0
Bilirubin (mg/dL)	<3.0	>3.0

Stage I, score = 0; stage II, score = 1 or 2; stage III, score = 3 or 4.

1.6 months). A majority of these patients presented with advanced disease (>80%), either based on tumor or hepatic function (9). This staging system has been found to be most reliable and reproducible in advanced cases of HCC (10,11).

The Okuda system does not provide stratification for small (<2 cm) tumor size, tumor multifocality, or vascular invasion. Each element has individually been shown to carry significant prognostic value in early HCC (12–14). Another criticism of the Okuda system is the heterogeneity of the initial study group. Patients eligible for resection are a more homogenous group based on the clinical parameters used in this system and important differences are not elucidated by the Okuda system. As a result, the Okuda staging system is not typically employed to determine patient eligibility for treatment with curative intent.

Barcelona Clinic Liver Cancer

Developed as a clinical staging system, the BCLC uses variables from tumor stage, liver function (including Child-Pugh classification) (Table 32.2), patient performance status, and symptoms to derive a stage applicable to a treatment algorithm. Early HCC is classified as stage A in the BCLC. This stage includes small solitary tumors and small multinodular tumors in patients with good hepatic reserve and good performance status. Depending on the specific details of each patient's clinical situation, treatment recommendations shift for different groups within stage A BCLC (Table 32.3). Stage B patients are considered to have large, multifocal disease in a background of good performance status and at least moderate hepatic reserve. The BCLC group recommends chemoembolization alone for stage B. Stage C, also called advanced HCC in this system, represents patients with vascular invasion and/or extrahepatic disease in the setting of diminishing performance status and moderate hepatic reserve. Patients with stage C are offered either a clinical trial with novel agents or supportive care by the authors of the BCLC. Terminal stage HCC, as defined by BCLC, is stage D, and denotes any patient with poor performance status and poor hepatic reserve (Child-Pugh C). These patients are offered symptomatic, supportive care (15,16).

At least two retrospective studies have shown the BCLC staging classification to provide better prognostic data than the other systems outlined in this chapter. Marrero et al. reported a retrospective review of 239 patients from the United States with cirrhosis and HCC. They found in their mix of heterogenous patients that BCLC staging had the best interstage survival predictability with low intrastage variability (17). A similar retrospective study in European patients by Cillo et al. also found BCLC to have better interstage discriminatory survival predictions. This was especially true for the early HCC surgically resected patients (BCLC stage A1) who had a 74% 5-year survival rate. Disappointingly, 5-year survival plummeted to 17% for the remainder of stage A patients (A2–4) (18).

The BCLC staging system takes into account the performance status of the patient. This is not included in other systems and has been shown to be an independent predictor of survival in patients with HCC (17). This additional analytic factor may strengthen the overall schema of BCLC, but in general the system is relatively more difficult to apply than the other systems outlined here. In addition, BCLC currently lacks a prospective validation study.

Cancer of the Liver Italian Program

The CLIP score was designed to be a prognostic indicator more sensitive than the Okuda staging system. The CLIP score, similar to the Okuda system, was specifically designed to assess patients with HCC. The score is easily calculated. It includes both tumor characteristics and functional hepatic indicators.

TABLE 32.2

CHILD-PUGH STAGE CLASSIFICATION

Parameters	Points		
	1	2	3
Albumin (g/dL)	>3.5	2.8–3.5	<2.8
Bilirubin (mg/dL)	<2	2–3	>3
Prothrombin time (s prolonged)	1–3	4–6	>6
Encephalopathy	None	Controlled	Dense
Ascites	None	Controlled	Refractory

Pugh score: 5–6 points = child's A: good hepatic reserve; 7–9 points = child's B: moderate hepatic reserve; 10–15 points = child's C: low hepatic reserve.

TABLE 32.3

BARCELONA CLINIC LIVER CANCER STAGING SYSTEM

Stage	Performance status	Tumor stage	Liver function
Stage A (early HCC)			
A1	0	Single, <5 cm	No portal HTN; normal bilirubin
A2	0	Single, <5 cm	Portal HTN; normal bilirubin
A3	0	Single, <5 cm	Portal HTN; elevated bilirubin
A4	0	Up to 3, <3 cm	Child-Pugh Class A–B
Stage B (intermediate HCC)	0	Large, multinodular	Child-Pugh Class A–B
Stage C (advanced HCC)	1–2	Vascular invasion or extrahepatic disease	Child-Pugh Class A–B
Stage D (terminal HCC)	3–4	Any of above	Child-Pugh Class C

HCC, hepatocellular carcinoma; HTN, hypertension.
At least one of the conditions needs to be met for Stage D.

TABLE 32.4

CANCER OF THE LIVER ITALIAN PROGRAM (CLIP) SCORING SYSTEM

	Points		
Criteria	0	1	2
Child-Pugh stage	A	B	C
Tumor morphology	Solitary and extent ≤50% of liver	Multinodular and extent ≤50%	Massive or extent >50%
AFP (ng/mL)	<400	≥400	
Portal vein thrombosis	Absent	Present	

AFP, alpha-fetoprotein.
CLIP score calculated by adding points from the four criteria.

The original series retrospectively reviewed 435 Italian patients with HCC and cirrhosis. From these data, the CLIP scoring system was developed to include Child-Pugh stage (Table 32.2), tumor morphology and extent, presence/absence of portal vein tumor thrombus, and serum alpha-fetoprotein (AFP) level (Table 32.4).

The 5-year survival for patients with HCC correlates with the CLIP score (i.e., the lower the score, the better the survival rate) (19–21). The prospective validation study by CLIP confirmed the prognostic capability of the CLIP categories 0, 1, 2, 3, and 4 by demonstrating median survival of 36, 22, 9, 7, and 3 months, respectively. The CLIP score is also more accurate than the Okuda staging system in predicting prognoses for patients with early HCC. When calculated at the time of HCC diagnosis, the CLIP score can be used to inform both clinician and patient about prognosis and delineate therapeutic options.

Despite advances over prior clinical staging systems, there are limitations to its usefulness. Specifically, the tumor morphology category does not stratify for small tumors. Indeed, a CLIP score of 0 can still include a tumor >5 cm in diameter with evidence of vascular invasion. In the literature that confirms the efficacy of the CLIP score, a majority of patients had unresectable HCC and <50% of these patients were treated with a local-regional therapy. As a result, several authors have investigated other staging systems that have more utility than CLIP when selecting treatment strategies that include hepatic resection (11,22).

Model for End-Stage Liver Disease

Originally developed to estimate mortality risk in cirrhotic patients undergoing transjugular intrahepatic portosystemic shunt procedures, the MELD score is a continuous points system using objective criteria. The MELD score is calculated with three serum levels: bilirubin, international normalized ration (INR), and creatinine. These values are then placed in a calculation to derive the MELD score:

$$\text{MELD score} = 10\ \{0.957\ \text{Ln (serum creatinine [mg/dL])}$$
$$+\ 0.378\ \text{Ln (total bilirubin [mg/dL])}$$
$$+\ 1.12\ \text{Ln (INR)} + 0.643\}$$

This number is then rounded to the nearest integer. Maximum score is 40. The higher the score, the higher the risk of mortality due to progressive hepatic disease (23).

MELD has been validated both prospectively and retrospectively as an efficient predictor of mortality for patients with end-stage liver disease (23,24). The success of this score led to its adoption by the United Network for Organ Sharing (UNOS) as an equitable means to allocate cadaver livers. MELD eliminates the opportunity for subjective bias when listing a patient for hepatic transplant.

Prior to adoption of MELD by UNOS, patients with HCC had unacceptable waiting times for cadaveric liver transplantation. After UNOS adopted MELD as its listing criteria, patients with HCC often had a low MELD score that caused them to wait even longer for transplantation. This prompted the arbitrary assignment of MELD scores to patients with HCC and cirrhosis. Patients with American Joint Committee on Cancer (AJCC) stage I disease (discussed in the next section) were given a MELD score of 24; AJCC stage II disease was given a score of 29. These numbers were selected on the basis that HCC patients progressing beyond stage II were no longer candidates for transplantation. Therefore, HCC beyond stage II could be equated with death in non-HCC patients with chronic liver disease. This allocation policy increased HCC patients transplanted, decreased waiting time for HCC patients, and had no impact on the early survival (1 year).

To date, there is little data published regarding the use of MELD scores to guide treatment of HCC patients. Teh et al. from the Mayo Clinic recently reported their experience implementing MELD scores retrospectively to cirrhotic patients with HCC treated with hepatic resection. They described a significant increase in perioperative mortality for MELD ≥9. Indeed, all perioperative deaths in this group of 82 patients occurred with a MELD score >9 (25). Due to the limitations of this retrospective study, it is unclear whether MELD scoring can clinically discriminate between these two groups (>8 and <8). Strict selectivity of only the healthiest patients has been shown to provide the best outcomes but may not provide a significant number of patients with viable therapeutic options (low number of available cadaver livers and ineffectiveness of systemic therapy).

PATHOLOGY-BASED STAGING SYSTEMS

Japan Integrated Staging Score

HCC is a much more common entity in Japan when compared to the United States. As discussed previously, the clinical staging systems often lack appropriate sensitivity for small HCC and potentially resectable tumors. Led by the Liver Cancer Study Group of Japan (LCSGJ), a pathology-based system was developed in an attempt to address this shortfall. Japan

TABLE 32.5

LIVER CANCER STUDY GROUP OF JAPAN DEFINITION AND CRITERIA OF THE TNM CLASSIFICATION FOR HEPATOCELLULAR CANCER

Factors	Solitary tumor/tumor size <2 cm/ absence of vessel invasion (portal vein, hepatic vein, bile duct)
T1	Tumor fulfills all three factors
T2	Tumor fulfills two factors
T3	Tumor fulfills one factor
T4	Tumor fulfills no factors
N	Regional nodes
Stage I	T1N0M0
Stage II	T2N0M0
Stage III	T3N0M0
Stage IV-A	T4N0M0 or T1–4, N1M0
Stage IV-B	T1–4, N0 or 1, M1

TNM, tumor, node, metastasis.

Integrated Staging (JIS) uses LCSGJ TNM (tumor, node, metastasis) staging in combination with Child-Pugh classification to determine a score.

LCSGJ Tumor (T) staging is an assessment of three factors of each patient's tumor and is markedly different from AJCC tumor staging. The greater number of factors met, the lower the T stage. The factors are inclusively (a) presence of solitary tumor, (b) tumor size <2 cm, and (c) no vessel invasion (portal vein, hepatic vein, or bile duct) (Table 32.5). A tumor with all three factors is T1, two factors equal T2, one factor is T3, and lack of any favorable factors is T4. In the JIS, the tumor scores of 0, 1, 2, and 3 are given to T stage 1, 2, 3, and 4, respectively.

Child-Pugh classification is assigned a JIS score of 0, 1, and 2 for C-P A, B, and C, respectively. JIS score can than range from a best prognosis of 0 to a worst of 5 (Table 32.6). Several studies have validated the JIS score as a useful prognostic indicator for early stage HCC with reports of 5-year cumulative survival for stage 0, 1, and 2 reaching 80%, 60%, and 42%, respectively (22,26,27). In the populations studied, the JIS score reveals promising prognostic capabilities for early HCC and consistent results for advanced HCC. To date, there are no data available to validate this system in a Western patient group.

TABLE 32.6

CALCULATION OF JAPAN INTEGRATED STAGING SCORE

	Score			
	0	1	2	3
LCSGJ TNM	I	II	III	IV
Child-Pugh classification	A	B	C	

LCSGJ, Liver Cancer Study Group of Japan; TNM, tumor, node, metastasis.
Score calculated adding TNM score and Child-Pugh score.

American Joint Committee on Cancer/International Union Against Cancer Staging System

The AJCC/Internation Union Against Cancer (UICC) pathological staging system is perhaps the most commonly used tool for prognostic assessment after resection and for planning of adjuvant therapy. This system employs a TNM classification to stratify patients according to predicted survival following resection. A recent change was made in the T classification in order to better stratify patients according to prognosis.

The new AJCC/UICC T staging is based on a multicenter review of 557 patients by Vauthey et al. (28). In evaluating the previous T-stage stratification, patients classified as T1 and T2 tumors according to prior AJCC system had similar 5-year survivals. Similarly, patients with bilobar tumors (prior AJCC T4) and those classified by prior AJCC as T3 had matching survival. Given this poor prognostic separation, the investigators evaluated independent risk factors for mortality.

There were several independent predictors of mortality. Tumor size >5 cm purported a significantly worse prognosis for solitary tumors <5 cm. Confirming other reports, both major vascular and microscopic vascular invasion are significant pathological predictors of poor survival (13,29,30). Another independent predictor was the presence of more than one tumor within the hepatic parenchyma. Finally, the presence of severe fibrosis or cirrhosis increased the mortality rate.

As a result of these findings, the new AJCC/UICC tumor (T) staging was developed (Table 32.7). Any solitary tumor, regardless of size, without vascular invasion is now classified as T1. Because survival of patients with more than one tumor, as long as none were >5 cm, was statistically equal to patients with solitary tumors and vascular invasion, these groups now comprise T2. Multiple tumors with any individual tumor >5 cm or with invasion of a major branch of the hepatic or portal veins is now classified as T3. T4 is now simplified to tumors of any size with direct invasion of adjacent organs, excluding the gallbladder (31).

Another addition to this staging system is a separate consideration of fibrosis of the adjacent, nontumor-bearing hepatic parenchyma (Table 32.7). The presence of severe fibrosis (F1) was found to have a significant negative effect on long-term survival in each simplified T stage of the new AJCC/UICC system (28). Perioperative risk is more accurately assessed by grading the severity of the underlying fibrosis (32). Ishak et al. developed a grading of hepatic fibrosis that is independent of hepatitis activity: Ishak 0–2, no or minimal fibrosis; Ishak 3–4, incomplete bridging fibrosis; and Ishak 5–6, complete fibrosis and nodules (33). This grading system is the one that was adopted by the AJCC/UICC. An Ishak score of 5–6 is graded as F1. Any lower Ishak score is graded as F0. Although fibrosis is listed with the AJCC/UICC classification scheme, it is not considered in the staging system.

SUMMARY

The myriad of scoring and staging systems employed for HCC denote the overall poor outcome of patients diagnosed with this disease and clinicians' attempts to select the best candidates for surgical resection, ablative therapy, or hepatic transplantation. Patients with advanced disease as graded by any of the previous systems lack significant long-term survival, and the systemic and regional therapies applied provide survival advantages measured in weeks, not months or years. Employment of either AJCC/UICC or JIS pathology-based systems provides validated prognostic information for patients being considered for potentially curative therapy. The clinical staging

TABLE 32.7

AJCC/UICC TNM, HISTOLOGIC GRADE, AND FIBROSIS SCORE CLASSIFICATION SCHEME FOR HEPATOCELLULAR CANCER

PRIMARY TUMOR (T)

TX	Primary tumor cannot be assessed
T0	No evidence of primary tumor
T1	Solitary tumor without vascular invasion
T2	Solitary tumor with vascular invasion or multiple tumors none >5 cm
T3	Multiple tumors >5 cm or tumor involving a major branch of the portal or hepatic vein(s)
T4	Tumor(s) with direct invasion of adjacent organs other than the gallbladder or with perforation of visceral peritoneum

REGIONAL LYMPH NODES (N)

NX	Regional lymph nodes cannot be assessed
N0	No regional lymph node metastasis
N1	Regional lymph node metastasis

DISTANT METASTASIS (M)

MX	Distant metastasis cannot be assessed
M0	No distant metastasis
M1	Distant metastasis

STAGE GROUPING

Stage I	T1	N0	M0
Stage II	T2	N0	M0
Stage IIIA	T3	N0	M0
Stage IIIB	T4	N0	M0
Stage IIIC	Any T	N1	M0
Stage IV	Any T	Any N	M1

HISTOLOGIC GRADE

GX	Grade cannot be assessed
G1	Well differentiated
G2	Moderately differentiated
G3	Poorly differentiated
G4	Undifferentiated

FIBROSIS SCORE (F)

F0	Fibrosis score 0–4 (no fibrosis to moderate fibrosis)
F1	Fibrosis score 5–6 (severe fibrosis to cirrhosis)

AJCC, American Joint Committee on Cancer; UICC, International Union Against Cancer; TNM, tumor, node, metastasis.
Reprinted from Green F, Page D, Fleming I, et al., eds. *AJCC Cancer Staging Handbook*. 6th ed. New York, NY: Springer; 2002:145–153, with permission.

systems have varying degrees of validation in heterogenous patient populations, a majority of which have advanced disease. The MELD score holds promise as another prognostic tool when evaluating for hepatic resection or transplantation. However, differences between MELD scores have not been definitively validated with regard to the long-term outcome of patients treated with resection or transplantation.

References

1. Bosch F. Global epidemiology of hepatocellular carcinoma. In: Tabor E, ed. *Liver Cancer*. New York, NY: Churchill Livingstone; 1997:13–28.
2. Jemal A, Murray T, Ward E, et al. Cancer statistics, 2007. *CA Cancer J Clin* 2007;57(1):10–30.
3. El-Serag HB, Mason AC. Rising incidence of hepatocellular carcinoma in the United States. *N Engl J Med* 1999;340(10):745–750.
4. Gruttadauria S, Foglieni CS, Luca A, Lauro A, Doria C, Marino IR. Hepatic artery anomalies: anatomy review. *Liver Transpl* 2002;8(10):981.
5. Jones RM, Hardy KJ. The hepatic artery: a reminder of surgical anatomy. *J R Coll Surg Edinb* 2001;46(3):168–170.
6. Couinaud C. *Etudes Anatomiques et Chirurgales*. Paris: Mason; 1957.
7. Strasberg SM, Belghiti J, Clavien P-A, et al. The Brisbane 2000 terminology of liver anatomy and resections. *HPB Surg* 2000;2:333–339.
8. Botero AC, Strasberg SM. Division of the left hemiliver in man—segments, sectors, or sections. *Liver Transpl Surg* 1998;4(3):226–231.
9. Okuda K, Ohtsuki T, Obata H, et al. Natural history of hepatocellular carcinoma and prognosis in relation to treatment: study of 850 patients. *Cancer* 1985;56(4):918–928.
10. Pawlik TM, Scoggins CR, Thomas MB, Vauthey JN. Advances in the surgical management of liver malignancies. *Cancer J* 2004;10(2):74–87.
11. Huang YH, Chen CH, Chang TT, et al. Evaluation of predictive value of CLIP, Okuda, TNM and JIS staging systems for hepatocellular carcinoma patients undergoing surgery. *J Gastroenterol Hepatol* 2005;20(5):765–771.
12. Poon RT, Fan ST, Ng IO, Lo CM, Liu CL, Wong J. Different risk factors and prognosis for early and late intrahepatic recurrence after resection of hepatocellular carcinoma. *Cancer* 2000;89(3):500–507.
13. Kondo K, Chijiiwa K, Makino I, et al. Risk factors for early death after liver resection in patients with solitary hepatocellular carcinoma. *J Hepatobiliary Pancreat Surg* 2005;12(5):399–404.
14. Ercolani G, Grazi GL, Ravaioli M, et al. Liver resection for hepatocellular

carcinoma on cirrhosis: univariate and multivariate analysis of risk factors for intrahepatic recurrence. *Ann Surg* 2003;237(4):536–543.

15. Llovet JM. Updated treatment approach to hepatocellular carcinoma. *J Gastroenterol* 2005;40(3):225–235.

16. Bruix J, Llovet JM. Prognostic prediction and treatment strategy in hepatocellular carcinoma. *Hepatology* 2002;35(3):519–524.

17. Marrero JA, Fontana RJ, Barrat A, et al. Prognosis of hepatocellular carcinoma: comparison of 7 staging systems in an American cohort. *Hepatology* 2005;41(4):707–716.

18. Cillo U, Bassanello M, Vitale A, et al. The critical issue of hepatocellular carcinoma prognostic classification: which is the best tool available? *J Hepatol* 2004;40(1):124–131.

19. Prospective validation of the CLIP score: a new prognostic system for patients with cirrhosis and hepatocellular carcinoma. The Cancer of the Liver Italian Program (CLIP) Investigators. *Hepatology* 2000;31(4):840–845.

20. A new prognostic system for hepatocellular carcinoma: a retrospective study of 435 patients: the Cancer of the Liver Italian Program (CLIP) investigators. *Hepatology* 1998;28(3):751–755.

21. Farinati F, Rinaldi M, Gianni S, Naccarato R. How should patients with hepatocellular carcinoma be staged? Validation of a new prognostic system. *Cancer* 2000;89(11):2266–2273.

22. Kudo M, Chung H, Osaki Y. Prognostic staging system for hepatocellular carcinoma (CLIP score): its value and limitations, and a proposal for a new staging system, the Japan Integrated Staging Score (JIS score). *J Gastroenterol* 2003;38(3):207–215.

23. Wiesner R, Edwards E, Freeman R, et al. Model for end-stage liver disease (MELD) and allocation of donor livers. *Gastroenterology* 2003;124(1):91–96.

24. Wiesner RH, McDiarmid SV, Kamath PS, et al. MELD and PELD: application of survival models to liver allocation. *Liver Transpl* 2001;7(7):567–580.

25. Teh SH, Christein J, Donohue J, et al. Hepatic resection of hepatocellular carcinoma in patients with cirrhosis: model of end-stage liver disease (MELD) score predicts perioperative mortality. *J Gastrointest Surg* 2005;9(9):1207–1215.

26. Nanashima A, Omagari K, Tobinaga S, et al. Comparative study of survival of patients with hepatocellular carcinoma predicted by different staging systems using multivariate analysis. *Eur J Surg Oncol* 2005;31(8):882–890.

27. Kudo M, Chung H, Haji S, et al. Validation of a new prognostic staging system for hepatocellular carcinoma: the JIS score compared with the CLIP score. *Hepatology* 2004;40(6):1396–1405.

28. Vauthey JN, Lauwers GY, Esnaola NF, et al. Simplified staging for hepatocellular carcinoma. *J Clin Oncol* 2002;20(6):1527–1536.

29. Capussotti L, Muratore A, Amisano M, Polastri R, Bouzari H, Massucco P. Liver resection for hepatocellular carcinoma on cirrhosis: analysis of mortality, morbidity and survival—a European single center experience. *Eur J Surg Oncol* 2005;31(9):986–993.

30. Ikai I, Yamamoto Y, Yamamoto N, et al. Results of hepatic resection for hepatocellular carcinoma invading major portal and/or hepatic veins. *Surg Oncol Clin N Am* 2003;12(1):65–75, ix.

31. Greene F. *AJCC Cancer Staging Handbook*. 6th ed. New York, NY: Springer; 2002:145–153.

32. Farges O, Malassagne B, Flejou JF, Balzan S, Sauvanet A, Belghiti J. Risk of major liver resection in patients with underlying chronic liver disease: a reappraisal. *Ann Surg* 1999;229(2):210–215.

33. Ishak K, Baptista A, Bianchi L, et al. Histological grading and staging of chronic hepatitis. *J Hepatol* 1995;22(6):696–699.

CHAPTER 33 ■ HEPATOCELLULAR CANCER: CLINICAL MANAGEMENT

ALAN P. VENOOK, RONNIE T. P. POON, DERRICK WONG, AND THEODORE LAWRENCE

Primary hepatocellular carcinoma (HCC) is among the most common cancers of solid organs. Worldwide, this cancer occurs in more than 1 million individuals yearly and results in an almost equal number of deaths. The reason that most patients die is partly because of the insidious nature of the growth of this cancer, which usually does not present with clinical findings until late in the course of disease. Furthermore, this cancer occurs most commonly in patients with cirrhosis, which makes surgical and ablative treatments difficult. Nevertheless, the past decade has seen significant improvements in the surgical, ablative, chemotherapeutic, and radiotherapeutic options for treatment of HCC. Recent advances in therapies are summarized, with an emphasis on current standard practice and ongoing controversies.

CLINICAL PRESENTATION

Most cases of HCC present at an advanced stage, well beyond the reach of curative therapies. This is due to the relatively asymptomatic nature of small HCCs. Until such time as significant liver function compromise occurs, either because of tumor invasion into major vasculature (1–3) or significant replacement of the liver by tumor, the few symptoms that occur are often vague and nonspecific. When tumors are large, local symptoms are common and usually include a dull, right upper quadrant ache that is often referred to the shoulder. The liver, tumor, or both are often palpable as hard and irregular. General symptoms, including anorexia, nausea, lethargy, fever, and weight loss, may be due to both the malignancy and the cirrhosis. The triad of right upper quadrant pain, mass, and weight loss is a common presentation (4–6).

Symptoms of hepatic decompensation are a potential presentation of HCC and include encephalopathy, jaundice (4,7–9), or bleeding from esophageal varices (3). In fact, jaundice occurs in up to one-half of all patients. When patients present with jaundice, distinguishing jaundice due to hepatic parenchymal insufficiency (4,7–9) from that due to biliary obstruction (4,10–15) is extremely important. Jaundice due to liver failure has no therapy, and survival is on the order of weeks, whereas that due to biliary obstruction can usually be palliated and may even be treated with curative intent (12,13,16–20).

Rare cases of HCC (<5%) can present with paraneoplastic syndromes due to hormonal or immune effects of the tumors (21). The most important of these are hypoglycemia and hypercalcemia. When hypercalcemia is present, it must be distinguished from the hypercalcemia seen with widespread bony metastases. A bone scan will distinguish these two clinical scenarios, which have different prognostic implications.

A rare but devastating presentation of HCC is spontaneous rupture, which occurs in approximately 2% of patients (22–27). Patients present with acute abdominal and hemodynamic instability. An abdominal scan demonstrating hepatic mass and hemoperitoneum confirms the diagnosis (26,28,29). Patients with a history of chronic hepatitis or cirrhosis presenting with an abdominal catastrophe should be suspected of having a ruptured hepatoma. Diagnosis by cross-sectional scanning or by paracentesis may lead to lifesaving angiography and embolization, which are now preferred to exploratory laparotomy.

Definitive diagnosis of HCC can usually be established noninvasively using a combination of history, physical examination, imaging, and blood tests. In a patient with chronic hepatitis or cirrhosis, the findings of a liver mass and a serum alpha-fetoprotein (AFP) level of >500 ng/dL are diagnostic. In a patient with a potentially resectable liver mass and a nondiagnostic AFP level, most surgeons would proceed to potentially curative resection if imaging is suggestive of cancer and no other primary sites of tumors that may have metastasized to the liver are found. Most would avoid a percutaneous liver biopsy, which may be complicated by hemorrhage, tumor rupture, tumor spillage, and seeding of the needle tract (30).

In patients with nondiagnostic AFP levels who are not candidates for curative therapy, fine-needle aspiration for cytologic evaluation is performed (31) if patients are candidates for palliative therapy. Patients who are not candidates for palliative therapy do not need to undergo biopsy.

POTENTIALLY CURATIVE TREATMENTS

A wide variety of methods are used for treatment of HCC (Table 33.1). Of these, the only therapies with curative potential are partial hepatectomy and total hepatectomy with liver transplantation. Partial hepatectomy has the greatest applicability and is summarized first.

Partial Hepatectomy

Partial hepatectomy is the most common procedure performed for HCC with curative intent. In the United States, a substantial number of patients with HCC have no associated cirrhosis (32). In a noncirrhotic liver, routine recovery can be expected even after resection of more than two-thirds of functional parenchyma because of the remarkable regenerative capacity of the liver (33). At most major centers, partial hepatectomy in patients without cirrhosis has been refined to allow operative mortalities well below 5% (32,34–40) (Table 33.2). Patients generally stay <10 days in hospital and return to normal, functional lifestyles. Such resections are associated with a 5-year survival of one-third of patients (Table 33.3) (32,37,39–52).

TABLE 33.1

TREATMENT OPTIONS FOR HEPATOCELLULAR CARCINOMA

Potentially curative options
  Partial hepatectomy
  Total hepatectomy with orthotopic liver transplantation
Palliative treatments
  Systemic therapies
    Chemotherapy
    Targeted biological therapy
    Hormonal therapy
    Immunotherapy
  Regional therapies
    Hepatic artery transcatheter treatments
      Transarterial chemotherapy
      Transarterial embolization
      Transarterial chemoembolization
      Transarterial radioembolization
    Ablative/cytoreductive therapies
      Ethanol injection
      Cryosurgery
      Radiofrequency ablation
      Palliative resection
    External beam radiation
Supportive care

TABLE 33.2

OPERATIVE MORTALITY AFTER PARTIAL HEPATECTOMY AS RELATED TO LIVER CIRRHOSIS

Study	No. of patients	Mortality (%)
PATIENTS WITHOUT CIRRHOSIS		
Wu et al. (34)	55	2
Tsuzuki et al. (35)	39	3
Chen et al. (36)	65	2
Nagasue et al. (37)	52	6
Vauthey et al. (38)	70	1
Bismuth et al. (39)	68	3
Fong et al. (32)	54	4
Shimada et al. (40)	65	2
PATIENTS WITH CIRRHOSIS		
Liver Study Group of Japan (53)	153	30
Nagao et al. (54)	72	19
Wu et al. (34)	126	12
Kanematsu et al. (55)	50	12
Franco et al. (42)	72	7
Tsuzuki et al. (35)	119	13
Chen et al. (36)	55	7
Nagasue et al. (37)	177	12
Capussotti et al. (57)	33	6
Vauthey et al. (38)	30	14
Fuster et al. (56)	48	4
Fong et al. (32)	100	5
Shimada et al. (40)	451	3

Thus, when HCC occurs in patients without cirrhosis, partial hepatectomy is justified both by the low risk and by the potential for long-term survival and cure.

Partial hepatectomy in patients with cirrhosis is associated with a higher risk. Even in centers with extensive experience in liver resection, partial hepatectomy in patients with cirrhosis was, until recently, associated with a mortality of 10% or more (Table 33.2) (34,35,37,38,53–55). This was the major impetus for exploring total hepatectomy and liver transplantation as treatment for HCC. Nevertheless, partial hepatectomy clearly provided good long-term outcome, provided the patient survived the operation. Patients with cirrhosis who survived the surgical procedure had a 5-year survival of approximately 30% (Table 33.3) (34,38,53,55). Since the 1990s, improvements in patient selection, operative conduct, and perioperative care have significantly decreased the operative mortality associated with partial hepatectomy in patients with cirrhosis (Table 33.2). The mortality at many centers has been reduced to <5% (32,40,42,50,56,57). Some centers have reported <2% mortality in their most recent experience (58). Given the shortage of organs for transplantation, partial hepatectomy should be considered as the curative treatment of choice for eligible patients (see "Patient Selection for Partial Hepactectomy" section).

A solitary HCC with a diameter of <5 cm is regarded by some as the best candidate for resection because of the increased risk of additional nodules or vascular invasion and, consequently, incomplete resection with larger HCCs (59,60). However, it has been shown that patients with a large solitary HCC (Fig. 33.1) are suitable candidates for successful resection, and reasonable long-term survival results can be achieved (61,62). The presence of multiple tumor nodules or vascular invasion in major intrahepatic venous branches may be associated with worse prognosis. However, surgical resection is still considered the best treatment in terms of long-term survival (63,64). Bilobar HCC used to be a contraindication for resection, but a recent study suggested that patients with a predominant mass in one lobe and one or two small tumor nodules in the other lobe may benefit from combined resection of the predominant tumor and ablation or chemoembolization for the contralateral nodules (65).

Patient Selection for Partial Hepatectomy

Partial resection with curative intent can be performed for patients with disease confined to the liver, patients with adequate hepatic functional reserve, and patients with disease anatomically disposed so as to allow adequate residual liver after resection.

A most important factor influencing outcome of patients with HCC is baseline liver functional status. The majority of patients have cirrhosis of the liver. This associated cirrhosis greatly increases the risks of any therapy (66,67), but particularly those of partial hepatectomy. The cirrhotic liver is rigid and hard, and consequently difficult to handle. The accompanying portal hypertension, varices, thrombocytopenia, and coagulopathy seen in patients with cirrhosis further increase the risk of operative hemorrhage. After surgery, the portal hypertension is exaggerated and commonly results in ascites and sometimes in variceal bleeding. The cirrhotic liver may also have difficulty regenerating, which results in liver failure. Assessment of the severity of cirrhosis is therefore paramount in patient selection. Various serum measures of liver function have been suggested as useful predictors of perioperative outcome, including elevations in serum bilirubin (68) and serum alanine aminotransferase (69), low platelet count, and prolonged prothrombin time (70).

Staging for hepatocellular carcinoma has been extensively reviewed in the preceding chapter (see Chapter 32). In brief, several staging systems have been used, including the Child-Pugh classification of liver functional derangement. The Child-Pugh classification is based on the levels of serum bilirubin and serum albumin, coagulation profile, presence or absence

TABLE 33.3

SURVIVAL RATES AFTER LIVER RESECTION FOR HEPATOCELLULAR CARCINOMA

Study	No. of patients	Survival (%)				
		1 yr	2 yr	3 yr	5 yr	10 yr
Okuda et al. (41)	98	62	43	34	—	—
Franco et al. (42)	72	68	55	51	—	—
Yamanaka et al. (43)	295	76	—	44	31	—
Fong and Blumgart (44)	2,174	67	—	40	29	—
Ringe et al. (45)	131	68	54	42	36	—
Sasaki et al. (46)	186	—	—	—	44	—
Nagasue et al. (37)	229	80	—	51.3	26	19
Takenaka et al. (47)	229	89	—	76	76	—
Suenaga et al. (48)	134	100	—	88	68	—
Bismuth et al. (39)	68	74	—	52	40	26
Lai et al. (49)	343	60	—	33	24	—
Kawasaki et al. (50)	112	92	—	79	—	—
Takenaka et al. (51)	280	88	—	70	50	—
Makuuchi et al. (92)	352	—	—	—	47	—
Lise et al. (93)	100	—	—	—	38	—
Fan et al. (91)	211	—	—	—	37	—
Fong et al. (32)	154	80	—	51	39	—
Hanazaki et al. (52)	386	—	—	51	35	11
Shimada et al. (40)	516	85	80	70	42	18
Grazi et al. (94)	264	—	—	63	41	—
Capusotti et al. (95)	216	—	—	51	34	—

of ascites and encephalopathy, and nutritional status (71,72). In general, only Child-Pugh class A patients are suitable for a major hepatectomy removing three or more segments of the liver. Child-Pugh class B patients may be suitable for minor hepatectomy, whereas Child-Pugh class C cirrhosis is generally a contraindication for resection. The bilirubin and albumin levels reflect the excretory function and synthetic function of the liver, respectively. Platelet count is also important because it reflects the severity of portal hypertension. In some centers, special tests of excretory function of the liver, such as indocyanine green clearance test and galactose elimination capacity, are used to further refine the assessment of liver function (73,74). However, these specific liver function tests reflect the

function of the whole liver, while the risk of postoperative liver failure depends on the liver function reserve of the remnant liver.

The volume of the remnant liver can be assessed by CT volumetry to provide a guideline as to the safety of major hepatic resection (75). Extended right or left hepatic resection can be performed even in the presence of cirrhosis, provided patients are carefully selected in terms of liver function reserve (62a). In patients with inadequate remnant liver volume for a right or extended right hepatectomy, preoperative portal vein embolization can be employed to induce hypertrophy of the liver remnant before resection (Fig. 33.2). The role of portal vein embolization in the cirrhotic liver remains unclear. However, one

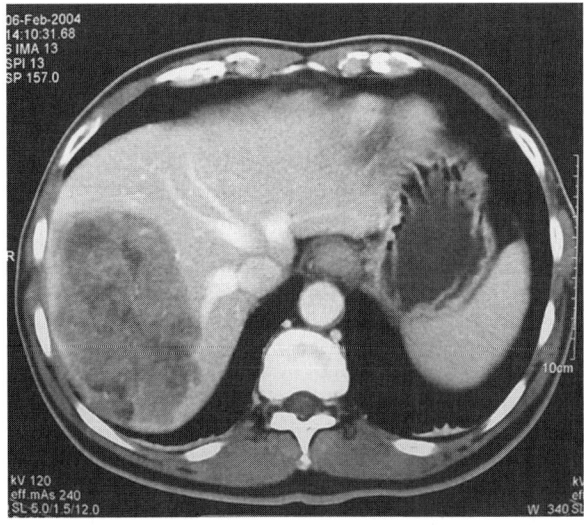

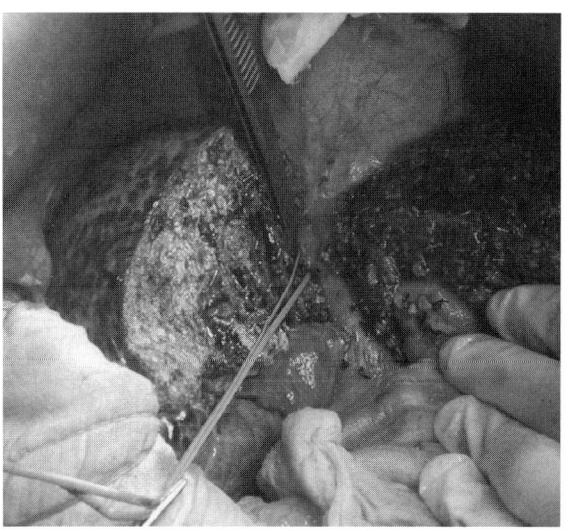

FIGURE 33.1. A cirrhotic patient with a large HCC (9 cm) (**A**) in the right lobe of the liver underwent right hepatectomy (**B**). The patient has remained diseasefree for 3 years (See also color Figure 33.1b).

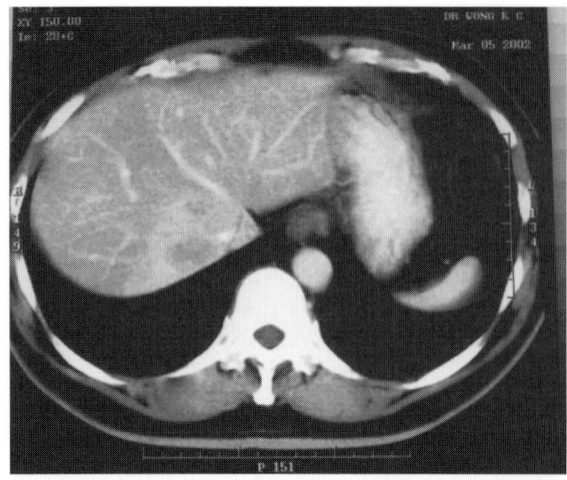
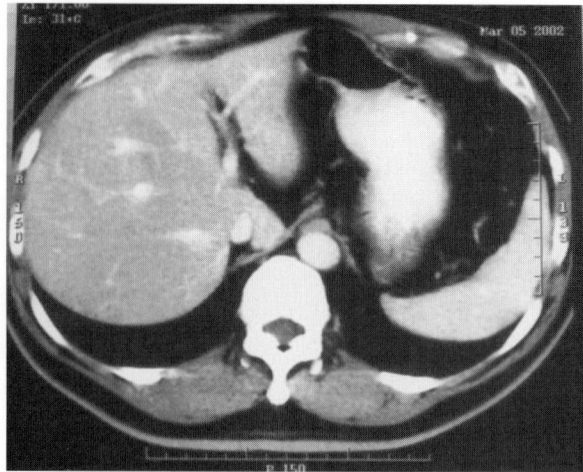
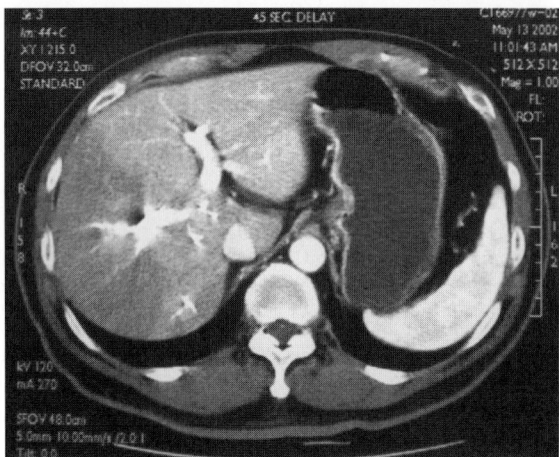

FIGURE 33.2. A: A patient with a HCC situated at posterior right lobe closely related to right and middle hepatic veins (*arrow*), requiring an extended right hepatectomy. **B:** The left lobe liver remnant volume was only 272 cc by CT volumetry, after right portal vein embolization. **C:** Satisfactory atrophy of the right lobe and hypertrophy of the left lobe were observed, with left lobe volume increased to 358 cc. Extended right hepatectomy was performed subsequently without complication.

prospective nonrandomized study suggested that preoperative right portal vein embolization induced significant hypertrophy in some patients with liver fibrosis or mild cirrhosis, and it reduced the incidence of postoperative complications compared with cases of right hepatectomy without preoperative portal vein embolization (76).

A number of changes in operative conduct have combined to improve perioperative outcome. A willingness to use inflow occlusion during resection is now seen. This technique of temporarily occluding the hepatic artery and portal vein during liver resection by clamping the gastrohepatic ligament significantly decreases blood loss during hepatectomy (77). In the past, surgeons have been reluctant to use this technique in patients with cirrhosis for fear that cirrhotic parenchyma will not tolerate even transient ischemia. Recent physiological studies have proven these fears to be unfounded. That the cirrhotic liver can tolerate warm ischemia for longer than 30 minutes is now well documented (78,79). Safety has also increased with acceptance of the use of limited, nonanatomical resections in treating patients with cirrhosis. For patients with no cirrhosis, most major centers adhere to the anatomical boundaries of the various segments during liver resection for cancer because these anatomical procedures provide better tumor clearance than nonanatomical resections (80). The anatomy of the liver is shown in Chapter 32. In the cirrhotic liver, however, the smallest resection that will remove all gross tumor is gener-

ally used at most centers, with tumor clearance sacrificed for operative safety.

Patients with extrahepatic metastases are excluded from partial hepatectomy. The search for extrahepatic disease must therefore be thorough and must include the locations at greatest risk for metastases, including the lungs, peritoneum, adrenal glands, and bone. The chest should be examined by chest radiography. Computed tomography (CT) or magnetic resonance imaging (MRI) should be used to evaluate the other sites. Bone scans should be obtained if the patient has symptoms or if hypercalcemia is noted.

A helical contrast CT is the most important study to evaluate the tumor status (Fig. 33.1). In addition to assessment of tumor size and number, it provides important information regarding the relationship of the tumor to major intrahepatic portal pedicles and hepatic vein, and it also detects any major vascular invasion. HCC has a great propensity for vascular invasion and extension, and tumor thrombus in the portal vein, hepatic vein, or vena cava is therefore not unusual. Presence of tumor within the vena cava or main portal vein indicates uniformly poor prognosis. MRI is an alternative that provides similar information.

Angiography was widely used in the past to diagnose HCC, but its use is now limited to selected patients with uncertain diagnosis of HCC by CT scan because the modern three-phase CT scan can demonstrate the arterial enhancement and portal venous washout that are typical of HCC. Some have advocated routine angiography and injection of lipiodol, a lipid that preferentially lodges within tumors, for delineation of extent of disease (81). Although angiographic techniques are highly sensitive for the presence of tumor and should be used in patients with suspected small tumors not seen by conventional cross-sectional imaging, they should not be used routinely. Helical CT or MRI suffices for staging in the majority of patients.

Patient selection should also take into account determinants of long-term prognosis. No patient should be put at risk if improvement in outcome would not be provided by the therapy. Patients with intravascular extension of tumor have very poor outcomes. Even though tumor thrombus can be treated with liver resection and thrombus extraction, the risk of disseminated disease is extremely high, and few are cured (82). Most surgeons would therefore consider tumor thrombus involving the vena cava or main portal vein to be a relative contraindication for liver resection.

As the number of long-term survivors after partial hepatectomy has been documented to increase, many factors that in years past were believed to be contraindications to surgical resection have not been substantiated by the data. Presence of multiple lesions does not seem to preclude long-term survival (37,38). Presentation with jaundice does not preclude long-term survival after surgical resection, provided the jaundice is due to intraductal extension of tumor (35). Synchronous direct invasion of adjacent organs such as the diaphragm by HCC is potentially curable, provided the area of direct organ invasion is also resectable (83,84).

In general, those selected for partial hepatectomy are those with no cirrhosis or well-compensated cirrhosis, who have HCC confined to the liver or with resectable direct extension into an adjacent organ. Up to 80% of noncancerous liver parenchyma can be resected in patients without cirrhosis, and anatomical resections are favored in this patient population. In patients with cirrhosis, resections are performed if resection of <20% to 25% of noncancerous parenchyma is necessary for complete extirpation of tumors (37,38,85–87).

Current Results of Hepatic Resection

With advances in surgical techniques and perioperative management, near-zero hospital mortality rate after resection of HCC can be achieved in experienced centers (88,89). In most major centers, an operative mortality rate of <5% is the current standard. However, the morbidity rate remains high at about 30% to 40%, even in experienced centers (88,89). Life-threatening complications such as liver failure, intraabdominal hemorrhage, bile leakage, and intraabdominal sepsis are less frequent today, but wound infection and pulmonary complications remain common (88). These complications may be reduced with the use of laparoscopic approach for liver resection, which is applicable in selected patients with small HCCs in the anterior segments or left lateral segments of the liver (90).

Improvement in the long-term survival results after resection of HCC has also been observed over the past decade (90a). The 5-year survival after resection of HCC in recent large series is in the range of 35% to 50% (Table 33.3) (51,91–95). The recent improvement in survival may be attributed to early diagnosis of HCC and reduction in perioperative blood transfusion. Perioperative transfusion has been found to have an adverse impact on the long-term survival after resection of HCC, perhaps by an inhibitory effect on the immune system that leads to increased risk of recurrence. Hence, the surgeon can play an important role in improving the long-term prognosis of patients after resection of HCC by minimizing intraoperative blood loss and avoiding perioperative transfusion (91).

The long-term prognosis after resection of HCC has been hampered by a high incidence of postoperative recurrence due to metastatic lesions or multicentric recurrences in the liver remnant (96). Adverse tumor factors such as the presence of macroscopic or microscopic vascular invasion are the most important risk factors of recurrence, suggesting that microscopic metastasis is an important cause of recurrence. The presence of cirrhosis also adversely affects the long-term prognosis, not only because it leads to worse liver function but also because it predisposes to increased risk of multicentric recurrence. However, aggressive treatment of recurrent tumors by reresection or nonsurgical modalities, such as transarterial chemoembolization and percutaneous ablation therapy, can result in prolonged survival, even after the development of recurrent tumors (96a). Postoperative adjuvant systemic or regional chemotherapy has thus far failed to prevent recurrence in prospective clinical trials (96). A recent study has shown that apart from providing the prospect of long-term survival, hepatic resection also improves the quality of life of patients with HCC (96b). It is likely that hepatic resection will play an increasingly important role in the management of HCC with the documented safety of the operation and increasing diagnosis of small HCCs in the setting of wider screening for HCC among chronic hepatitis and cirrhotic patients.

Adjuvant Therapy

Two-thirds of patients experience recurrence after partial hepatectomy for HCC, which indicates the presence of microscopic disease undetected at the time of liver resection (97–99). This explains the active investigation for effective adjuvant therapy for treatment of such residual disease. Use of adjuvant therapy has been hindered by the poor efficacy of chemotherapeutic agents against this cancer cell type and the extended period needed for complete recovery of patients with cirrhosis, which makes administration of potentially toxic agents difficult. This may explain the poor results seen in adjuvant chemotherapy or chemoembolization trials. In one study in which 61 patients with resected HCC were randomly assigned to receive no further therapy or postoperative hepatic infusion of lipiodol and cisplatin with systemic epirubicin hydrochloride, the treated patients had a higher recurrence rate and a worse outcome (100). Another study in which 57 patients with resected HCC were randomly assigned to receive hepatic arterial infusional and systemic epirubicin or no adjuvant treatment found no difference in survival (101). In three different trials of chemoembolization, survival has been worse for those treated after resection (102–104). One study in which 49 patients with resected HCC were randomized to low-dose epirubicin and mitomycin or no adjuvant treatment did find a trend toward improvement in diseasefree survival and overall survival, but it did not reach statistical significance (105). A more recent meta-analysis of three randomized control trials, which compared resection alone versus resection followed by intraarterial and/or systemic chemotherapy in HCC patients, found no difference in diseasefree survival or overall survival (106). In cirrhotic patients, postoperative chemotherapy was associated with a worse outcome. To date, no study has shown any systemic chemotherapy or chemoembolization to improve survival after partial hepatectomy for HCC.

Four randomized trials of adjuvant therapy after resection for HCC have shown positive results. The first involved radioembolization using transarterial delivery of lipiodol tagged with iodine 131 (^{131}I). In a prospective, randomized trial, patients who received no adjuvant therapy were compared with those who were treated with 50 mCi of transarterial ^{131}I-lipiodol within 6 weeks of liver resection (107). The study was halted at an interim time because the preliminary data, compiled after the accrual of 43 patients, demonstrated a significant improvement in survival in the patients who received treatment. The 3-year survival rates for the treated group and the control group were 85% and 46%, respectively. Toxicity was mild, although patients were hospitalized until the radiation had dissipated. These results are quite remarkable but require validation in a multicenter trial to confirm the feasibility of performing such radioembolization at multiple centers.

A second positive study involved the use of the retinoid derivative polyprenoic acid. This chemopreventive agent has been shown to inhibit hepatocarcinogenesis in rodents (108). In a placebo-controlled randomized trial examining patients after curative resection or percutaneous ethanol injection (PEI) for HCC, treatment with polyprenoic acid reduced tumor recurrence. Currently, this compound is not available in the United States.

A third study demonstrating an impact on HCC recurrence with adjuvant therapy involved interferon. In this small Japanese trial that randomized 30 patients who had undergone resection of their hepatitis C–associated HCC to 88 weeks of tapering interferon-alpha therapy or no adjuvant therapy, patients on the treatment arm had a significantly lower disease recurrence rate than those in the control group ($P = 0.037$) (109).

Finally, immunotherapy has also shown potential as an adjuvant treatment. In a randomized trial of 150 patients with resected HCC, immunotherapy via infusion of autologous lymphocytes activated with recombinant interleukin-2 and CD3 antibody was associated a longer time to recurrence and a higher 5-year diseasefree survival rate than observation (110).

The sample sizes in these adjuvant studies are small, but their positive results offer strong encouragement for further evaluation of these adjuvant therapies in well-designed multicenter randomized phase III trials to determine their efficacy and feasibility. Until such studies are undertaken and completed, postoperative adjuvant therapy following partial hepatectomy remains an investigational approach.

Liver Transplantation

Indications

In the 1980s, when liver transplantation was at the initial phase of development, advanced unresectable HCC was a common indication for transplantation. However, the results of transplantation for advanced HCC turned out to be disappointing, with a 5-year survival rate of around 20% (111). The reason for the poor survival results was the high incidence of recurrent tumors, presumably due to the presence of circulating tumor cells associated with large HCCs.

Experience of liver transplantation over the past decade has shown that tumor size and vascular invasion were the two most important factors in determining the survival results after transplantation for HCC. Recent studies have indicated that for solitary HCC <5 cm or for three or less tumor nodules each of size <3 cm, the long-term survival rate was comparable to that after resection, and the diseasefree survival rate was superior to that after resection (66,112–115). It is now well accepted that child's C cirrhotic patients with HCC <5 cm or more than three tumor nodules each of size <3 cm and without radiologic evidence of venous invasion or distant metastasis should be treated by transplantation because hepatic resection is usually contraindicated in this group of patients with poor hepatic function (116,117). These so-called Milan criteria have become widely accepted as the selection criteria for liver transplantation for HCC (112). Recently, Yao et al. (118) suggested the expanded criteria of solitary tumor ≤6.5 cm or three or less nodules with the largest lesion ≤4.5 cm and total tumor diameter ≤8 cm for liver transplantation. Their study showed that the long-term survival after transplantation for such patients was similar to that of liver transplantation for HCCs

within the Milan criteria. In that study, patients with HCC fulfilling the expanded criteria had a 5-year survival of 75.2%. Although the expanded criteria have been supported by other studies (119), there is inadequate data in the literature to validate the long-term survival results seen using the expanded criteria. Furthermore, it has to be noted that Yao's criteria were based on pathological examination of explants rather than preoperative radiologic imaging, which often underestimates the size of the tumor compared with measurement of tumor size in the explants. Currently, most centers worldwide still adopt Milan criteria in the selection of patients for liver transplantation.

Current Results of Liver Transplantation

Table 33.4 shows the results of liver transplantation for HCC within the Milan criteria in patients with Child-Pugh class C liver cirrhosis (112,117,120–123). With the improvement in surgical techniques and better immunosuppressants to reduce the risk of graft rejection, the hospital mortality rate is <5% in major centers. The possibility of long-term survival and cure after transplantation for patients with HCC is well documented (66,112,124–134). The best results are seen in patients with fibrolamellar HCC. Favorable results are also seen in patients with small tumors, particularly when these are found incidentally within the explanted liver during transplantation for noncancerous indications. Overall, the 5-year survival rate is about 60% to 75%, while the 5-year diseasefree survival rate is about 60% to 70%.

The most important adverse prognostic factors of liver transplantation for HCC are adverse tumor factors such as the presence of microscopic vascular invasion and histopathological grading (123,135). Although the incidence of tumor recurrence is much lower after liver transplantation compared with partial hepatic resection, tumor recurrence is an important cause of long-term mortality after liver transplantation. Currently, there is no effective adjuvant therapy to reduce the risk of tumor recurrence. Although some authors suggested that preoperative transarterial chemoembolization may reduce the risk of tumor recurrence, the role of pretransplant chemoembolization remains uncertain because there are no data from prospective randomized trials (136).

Role of Liver Transplantation for Child's A Cirrhotic Patients with Early Hepatocellular Carcinoma

Whether child's A cirrhotic patients with preserved liver function and a small HCC <5 cm in diameter should be treated with transplantation or resection is a controversial issue. Some authors recommended liver transplantation for small HCC even in child's A patients because of the superior diseasefree survival results after transplantation (113,114). Others argued that hepatic resection should be the first-line therapy for such patients because of the similar overall survival results of the two treatments and the shortage of organ donors (120,137,138). Recently, a few retrospective studies have directly compared liver resection and transplantation for these patients. Bigourdan et al. (139) reported significantly better survival results after liver transplantation than after hepatic resection. However, a closer look at the data of the study revealed that there was significant selection bias in favor of the liver transplantation group, which had smaller tumors, a higher proportion of solitary tumor, a lower incidence of vascular invasion, and a lower proportion of alcoholic cirrhosis. Shabahang et al. (140) reported similar operative mortality and survival results after resection and transplantation for HCC in child's A cirrhotic patients, but hepatic resection was associated with faster recovery. More recently, Margarit et al. (141) reported similar survival results after resection and transplantation in child's A cirrhotic patients,

TABLE 33.4

RESULTS OF LIVER TRANSPLANTATION FOR HEPATOCELLULAR CARCINOMA

Study	No. of patients	Operative mortality (%)	Survival (%)			
			1 yr	3 yr	5 yr	10 yr
O'Grady et al. (124)	50	23	40	—	—	—
Ringe et al. (125)	52	15	—	37	—	—
Yokoyama et al. (126)	80	13	64	45	45	—
Iwatsuki et al. (127)	71	NR	—	43	—	—
Pichlmayr et al. (128)	87	24	—	—	20	—
Bismuth et al. (66)	60	5	—	49	—	—
Dalgic et al. (129)	39	NR	56	32	26	—
Farmer et al. (130)	44	17	71	42	—	—
Selby et al. (131)	105	NR	66	39	36	—
Schwartz et al. (133)	57	0	72	57	—	—
Iwatsuki et al. (134)	344	NR	73	59	49	—
RESULTS OF LIVER TRANSPLANTATION WITHIN THE MILAN CRITERIA						
Mazzaferro et al. (112)	48	6	—	—	75 at 4 yr	—
Otto et al. (120)	102	—	—	63	—	—
Llovet et al. (121)	58 (<5 cm)	13.8	—	—	74	—
Bismuth et al. (117)	105	3	—	—	58	—
Figueras et al. (122)	307	—	—	67	63	44
Jonas et al. (123)	120	1.7	90	—	71	60

NR, not reported.

whereas postoperative mortality was higher and hospital stay was longer in the transplantation group.

Because of the severe shortage of liver grafts worldwide, liver transplantation is not immediately applicable to most patients with HCC. A significant proportion of HCC patients listed for liver transplantation may drop out of the waiting list because of tumor progression. Dropout rates of 15% to 33% have been reported even in countries where waiting time for deceased donor graft is relatively short (121,142–144). This is the most critical limitation of the approach of primary transplantation for early HCC in patients with child's A cirrhosis, to whom the option of liver resection may be more appealing because it is immediately applicable. A study showed that on an intention-to-treat analysis, the 5-year survival rate of resection of patients with early HCC <5 cm in diameter among the best candidates without portal hypertension was significantly better than those listed for liver transplantation (121). The main argument in favor of liver transplantation is the better long-term diseasefree survival results compared with liver resection. However, specific long-term complications of liver transplantation such as recurrent viral hepatitis, graft rejection, and infection or second malignancies as a result of immunosuppression may lead to mortalities. This explains the similar overall 5-year survival rates after liver transplantation and resection in some studies, despite a higher tumor recurrence rate in the resected group.

With the current severe shortage of organ donors, most centers still consider hepatic resection as the first-line treatment in patients with resectable HCC and preserved liver function. It has been recently suggested that resection followed by salvage transplantation for intrahepatic recurrence or deterioration of liver function may be a more effective strategy for patients with small HCC and preserved liver function when the waiting time for cadaveric graft is long (145). Studies have suggested that 70% to 80% of recurrent tumor after resection of early HCC <5 cm in diameter may still be transplantable according to the Milan criteria (145a,146). However, the benefit of such an approach has been controversial from recent studies. Adam et al. (147) reported an operative mortality rate of 28.6% after salvage transplantation in 17 patients, compared with that of 2.1% after primary transplantation in 195 patients. They reported worse 5-year posttransplant survival after salvage transplantation compared with primary transplantation (41% vs. 61%), which was partly attributable to the much higher operative mortality rate in the former group. In contrast, Belghiti et al. (148) reported no significant difference in operative mortality and posttransplant survival after salvage transplantation for recurrent HCC after resection and primary transplantation. Both studies included only a small series of patients, and further studies are needed to evaluate the benefit and feasibility of this approach.

Role of Live Donor Liver Transplantation for Hepatocellular Carcinoma

Because of the shortage of cadaveric liver grafts, adult live donor liver transplantation has been developed in recent years (149). Live donor graft is a dedicated graft to a related recipient, and it can significantly reduce the waiting time. It appears to be a particularly appealing alternative for patients with transplantable HCC because it reduces the chance of dropout from the transplantation waiting list as a result of tumor progression. Hence, the indications for live donor liver transplantation have been extended to include HCC. A study has demonstrated that live donor transplantation could significantly improve the chance of long-term survival compared to patients listed for cadaveric transplantation (150). However, in that study, about half of the HCC patients who were initially considered for live donor liver transplantation eventually could not have a live donor graft for various reasons. Hence, live donor transplantation cannot completely resolve the issue of graft shortage.

Recently, some authors have proposed to extend the criteria for transplantation using live donor liver transplantation (151). However, the long-term survival of patients with HCC beyond the Milan criteria was significantly worse than that of patients with HCC confined to the Milan criteria in that study. The benefit of live donor liver transplantation for HCC patients has to be balanced against a risk of about 0.5% mortality in the live donor undergoing right lobe donor hepatectomy (152). The ethical consideration in live donor liver transplantation remains an unsettled issue. Furthermore, there is some concern over the theoretical effect of the regeneration of the partial liver graft in stimulating the growth of microscopic metastasis, although there are not enough clinical data on this issue. Before these issues are settled, the selection criteria for HCC patients to undergo live donor liver transplantation should be similar to that of cadaveric liver transplantation. It is likely that the role of live donor liver transplantation for HCC will continue to evolve with further development of this treatment modality and availability of more long-term survival data.

Palliative Treatment Modalities

The majority of patients presenting with HCC have disease not treatable by partial hepatectomy or transplantation. If the disease is nevertheless confined completely or largely to the liver, ablative therapies such as ethanol injection, embolization, cryotherapy, radiofrequency ablation (RFA), or radiotherapy can be performed, often with effective control of local disease. The most common scenario, however, is widely disseminated disease, for which systemic therapies are the most attractive.

Ablative Therapies

Indications

Faced with a small HCC in a cirrhotic patient who is not a candidate for resection because of inadequate liver function reserve, the clinician has the option of local ablative therapy if liver transplantation is not available or contraindicated due to advanced age and comorbid illnesses. The biology of HCC makes this tumor suitable for treatment by ablative therapies. This tumor usually occurs in patients with cirrhosis of the liver; therefore, any method that destroys tumor while minimizing destruction of noncancerous liver parenchyma could be advantageous. Currently, most centers consider patients with HCC ≤5 cm and up to three nodules as the best candidates for ablative therapies, although some centers are more aggressive in ablating larger tumors. Although there is some preliminary evidence suggesting that ablative therapies may achieve similar survival results compared to surgical resection (153,154), the evidence is not yet strong enough to recommend local ablation as the first-line therapy for patients with a resectable small HCC. Local ablative therapies are also useful in treating recurrent HCC after previous resection, which occurs mostly in the liver remnant (96a). Local ablative therapy may also be employed as a bridging therapy for control of tumors before a liver graft is available, even if liver transplantation is contemplated (155).

In addition, growth of tumor at sites incompletely ablated can frequently be noted in sufficient time for repeated, effective therapy. The three methods of ablation used most often are alcohol injection, cryoablation, and RFA. The data supporting each, as well as the technical limitations and guidelines for use, are reviewed in the following sections.

Percutaneous Ethanol Injection

Percutaneous ethanol injection (PEI) has the longest record of use for ablation in HCC and was introduced in the early 1980s for treatment of liver cancers. Absolute ethanol is injected directly into the tumor under ultrasound guidance to induce co-agulative necrosis of tumor cells, with minimal injury to the surrounding liver. Tumor cells are killed by cellular dehydration, coagulative necrosis, and vascular thrombosis. The extent of necrosis is related to the size of the tumor, with small nodules <3 cm being more likely to have complete necrosis (156). Alcohol injection can also be performed during open surgery or via laparoscopy. This ablative technique is quite effective in covering areas of tumor because the hard cirrhotic liver limits diffusion of alcohol beyond the soft HCC. Alcohol injected within the tumor usually diffuses quite well throughout the tumor. PEI is well tolerated by patients and is usually performed under local anesthesia. The side effects include pain, fever, a transient rise in liver enzyme levels, and a transient rise in circulating alcohol levels. More serious side effects, such as bleeding, tumor rupture, needle tract tumor implantation (157), and death are rare.

In general, the indication for ethanol injection therapy is limited to less than three nodules of tumor <3 cm each in size (156). Patients with Child-Pugh class A or good Child-Pugh class B liver functional status are the best candidates for treatment, because the ascites seen in patients with more severe derangements of liver function increases the risk of bleeding. The ascites prevents the abdominal wall from tamponading the bleeding from the sites of injection. Tumors at the dome of the liver are also difficult to treat because of overlying lung and risks of pneumothorax.

PEI has had a superb record of safety and effectiveness in the treatment of small HCCs. Large nonrandomized studies have reported 3-year survival rates of 55% to 77% (157–160). Five-year survival in trials with sufficient follow-up has been as high as 33% to 40% (157,161). These favorable results have prompted comparisons of PEI with partial hepatectomy or total hepatectomy and transplantation. In a nonrandomized case study comparing PEI with partial hepatectomy in the treatment of small (<4 cm) HCCs, 1- and 4-year survival rates were comparable, but the recurrence rate was higher for patients treated with PEI (159). A recent randomized trial suggested that ethanol injection therapy may achieve survival similar to that of resection for small HCC ≤3 cm (153). In this trial, 38 patients received PEI, and 38 patients received surgical resection. There was no significant difference in complication rates and tumor recurrence rates. The actuarial 5-year survival after ethanol injection was 46% and after resection was 81.8%, although the difference was not statistically significant.

The authors use PEI as the ablative method of choice for HCCs that are small (<3 cm) and limited in number (less than three) in patients with Child-Pugh class A or B cirrhosis in whom surgery is not advisable or resection is not possible. Patients must be followed closely, because repeated treatments are usually necessary when viable tumor is again demonstrated. Trials comparing use of this technique with hepatectomy or transplantation for treatment of small, resectable lesions are sorely needed.

Thermal Ablative Therapies

Other modalities of local ablative therapies include cryotherapy and thermotherapy using microwave, laser, or radiofrequency wave (161a).

Cryoablation. Cryotherapy is effective in ablation of liver tumors, but it is associated with a high complication rate and can lead to cryoshock phenomenon characterized by multiorgan failure in a small proportion of patients (62). Hence, its popularity has decreased with the availability of thermotherapy. Cryoablation can be performed relatively easily for destruction of liver tumors due to the wide availability of vacuum-sealed cryoablation probes that are cooled by liquid nitrogen or argon. Either during an open operation or via laparoscopy, these probes can be introduced into tumors under ultrasonographic guidance. The tumor can then be frozen until the ice ball is >2 cm beyond the tumor margin. Thawing the tumor and repeating the freezing further improves effectiveness of such cryoablations.

A number of series have been published demonstrating the effectiveness of such a process in destroying tumors (162,163). The major advantage of such cryoablation over PEI is the relatively larger size of tumor that can be treated effectively by cryoablation. Tumors of ≥5 cm can be treated by cryoablation, whereas PEI is generally useful only for tumors <3 cm. The major disadvantages are clearly the need for general anesthesia and laparoscopy/laparotomy, as well as the high complication rate (62). Patients who are not candidates for surgery are therefore not candidates for cryoablation. Recently, small cryoprobes have become available that may allow percutaneous cryoablation of tumors. Such less invasive methods of delivering cryoablation are under active investigation. Although cryotherapy remains an option, these technical issues make it much less preferred compared to RFA.

Radiofrequency Ablation. Recent interest has been focused on RFA, which is able to achieve tumor necrosis with a single treatment session for most cases of small HCC. RFA can be performed through percutaneous, laparoscopic, or open approaches. The choice of treatment approach should be individualized according to the size and location of the tumor and patients' comorbid conditions. The percutaneous approach is the least invasive route for RFA. Patients with one to three tumor nodules each ≤3 cm in diameter located in the periphery of the liver are the best candidates for percutaneous RFA under ultrasonographic, computed tomography, or magnetic resonance imaging guidance (Fig. 33.3). RFA by the laparoscopic approach is advantageous in its use of laparoscopic ultrasonography, which has higher accuracy in detecting intrahepatic tumor metastases than transcutaneous ultrasonography. It also provides a survey of the peritoneal cavity to exclude extrahepatic metastases. Patients' recovery can be hastened because of the reduced wound pain compared with open surgery. In addition, laparoscopic RFA permits the ablation of liver tumors in close contact with the surrounding organs, such as bowel, kidney, gallbladder, and diaphragm, for which percutaneous RFA carries the risk of bowel perforation or visceral damage. However, the applicability of laparoscopic RFA is limited for tumors situated at the right posterior lobe of the liver due to the difficulty in maneuvering the laparoscopic ultrasound probe to provide accurate guidance. RFA using an open surgical approach is indicated in patients with large tumors (>5 cm in diameter), multiple tumor nodules, and history of previous abdominal surgery precluding the use of laparoscopic approach.

So that more effective ablation can be carried out to minimize the chance of residual tumor at the treatment site, there is a higher degree of freedom for introduction of the RF needle into the tumor in open RFA compared with other approaches.

Table 33.5 shows the results of RFA for HCC reported in the literature (164–172). RFA is associated with a mortality rate of ≤1% in most series, and the morbidity rate is <15% in most series. In a review by Mulier et al. (173), the mortality and morbidity rates of 3,670 patients after RFA were 0.5% and 8.9%, respectively. The open approach of RFA and the presence of cirrhosis or hyperbilirubinemia are associated with a higher risk of morbidity (150,173a,173b). The survival results of RFA for HCC reported in the literature are also summarized in Table 33.5. There are few studies with long-term follow-up of patients documenting the survival results of RFA up to 5 years. Rossi et al. (164) reported the results of RFA in 39 patients with HCC and 11 patients with liver metastases. With a median follow-up of 22.6 months, the cumulative median survival was 44 months, and the 1-, 3-, and 5-year survival rates were 94%, 68%, and 40%, respectively. Another study by Buscarini et al. (169) compared the use of conventional and multitined expandable RF electrodes in treating 88 patients with HCC. The overall 5-year survival rate was 33%, but the 5-year diseasefree survival rate was only 3%. The local recurrence rate was higher in patients treated by conventional electrodes (29%) than in those treated by multitined, expandable electrodes (14%). The local recurrence after RFA for HCC ranged from 3.6% to 15%, and the overall recurrence rate was 40% to 50% in most reported series with follow-up >12 months (Table 33.5).

Recently, two randomized controlled trials have demonstrated that RFA is superior to ethanol injection in that it requires fewer treatment sessions, and it achieves a higher complete ablation rate, lower tumor progression rate, and higher overall survival rate (174,175). In one of the randomized trials, complete tumor necrosis rate was 96% after RFA and 88% after ethanol injection, and the 3-year survival was 74% after RFA and 50% after ethanol injection (174). More recently, a randomized controlled trial comparing RFA in 71 patients and surgical resection in 88 patients for solitary HCC ≤5 cm has been reported (154). This study demonstrated that RFA can achieve similar long-term survival compared with partial hepatectomy, with 4-year survival rates of 67.9% and 64%, respectively, and 4-year diseasefree survival rates of 46.4% and 51.6%, respectively. However, the sample size of this trial is relatively small. In contrast, a prospective but nonrandomized trial comparing percutaneous RFA and resection showed that

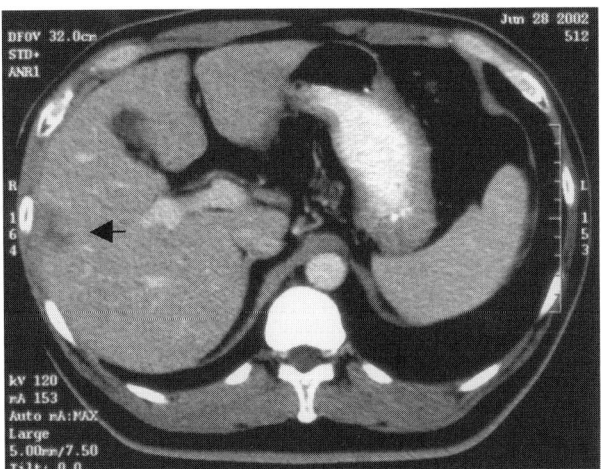
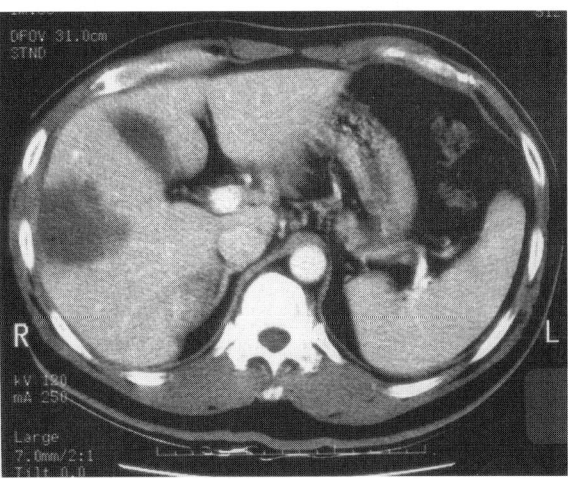

FIGURE 33.3. A small peripheral HCC (**A**) (*arrow*) treated by percutaneous RFA under ultrasound guidance and complete ablation with good margin was demonstrated in CT scan 1 month after RFA (**B**).

TABLE 33.5

SURVIVAL OUTCOME OF RADIOFREQUENCY ABLATION (RFA) FOR HEPATOCELLULAR CARCINOMA (HCC)

Study	No. of patients	Tumor type (no. of patients)	Route of RFA (no. of patients)	Needle type	Mean follow-up (mo)	Complete ablation	Morbidity	Mortality	Recurrence rate[a]	Survival
Rossi (164)	50	HCC (39) Liver met. (11)	Percut.	Conventional	22.6	95%	0%	0%	41%	1 yr: 94% 2 yr: 86% 5 yr: 40%
Rossi (165)	37	HCC (23) Liver met. (14)	Percut.	Expandable	12	91%	0%	0%	40%	1 yr: 91%
Curley (166)	110	HCC	Percut. (76) Lap. (31) Open (3)	Expandable	19	100%	12.7%	0%	45.5% (3.6%)	2 yr: 71.8%
Nicoli (167)	47	HCC	Percut. (33) Open (14)	Expandable	11.8	—	0%	0%	—	2 yr: 83%
Bowles (168)	76	HCC (25) Liver met. (51)	Percut. (57) Lap. (8) Open (34)	Expandable	15	—	7%	1%	(9%)	2 yr: 50%
Buscarini (169)	39 49	HCC HCC	Percut. Percut.	Conventional Expandable	34	100%	2%	—	(29%) (14%)	5 yr: 33%
Guglielmi (170)	53	HCC	Percut.	Expandable	18	100%	20.7%	0%	28.3%	2 yr: 63% 3 yr: 45%
Giovannini (171)	56	HCC	Percut.	Internally-cooled	14	92.8%	3.5%	0%	17.8% (7%)	1 yr: 96.2% 2 yr: 94.2%
Vivarelli (172)	79	HCC	Percut.	Expandable	15.6	87%	—	0%	48.1% (15%)	1 yr: 78% 3 yr: 33%

[a]Figure in parentheses indicates local recurrence rate.
Liver met., liver metastases; percut., percutaneous; lap., laparoscopic; —, data not available.

RFA resulted in lower 3-year overall and diseasefree survival rates compared with resection, and the survival advantage of resection was more evident for Child-Pugh class A patients and for single tumors of >3 cm in diameter (172). Further randomized trials with large sample size are needed before a definite conclusion can be arrived at regarding whether RFA can replace hepatic resection as the first-line treatment for small HCC ≤5 cm.

In summary, for ablative therapies, PEI or RFA are favored over cryotherapy. If a patient has a small tumor and is not a candidate for surgery, either RFA or PEI can be used (176,177). Patients tolerate either procedure quite well. RFA theoretically carries a lower risk of bleeding because the needle track can be coagulated during withdrawal of the RFA electrode, although this has not been substantiated by data. PEI is less expensive, however, and has had a longer record of use. A direct trial comparing these techniques is clearly in order.

Radiation Therapy

Initial attempts to use whole liver radiation to treat primary hepatobiliary cancer were unsuccessful (178,179). For instance, in one series, only 1 of 31 patients with unresectable disease who underwent radiation survived longer than 1 year. The most important reason for this lack of success is the low tolerance of the liver to whole organ radiation. Indeed, the radiation tolerance of the whole liver may tend to be lower for patients with primary HCC than for those with metastatic cancer to the liver because many patients with primary disease have some degree of underlying cirrhosis.

Attempts have been made to increase the effectiveness of whole liver radiation in the treatment of patients with unresectable hepatoma by the addition of intravenous chemotherapy (180,181) and ^{131}I antiferritin monoclonal antibody therapy (182,183). The conclusions from these and other studies (184) are (a) ^{131}I antiferritin increases toxicity without benefit, and (b) hepatic arterial cisplatin, when combined with radiation, may be superior to doxorubicin plus 5-fluorouracil delivered either intravenously (180) or via the hepatic artery. The finding that hepatic arterial cisplatin and radiation can produce an objective response rate of 43% and lead to a median survival of 7.5 months in a relatively large group of patients suggests that this combination has some activity (184).

In contrast to the relative ineffectiveness of whole liver radiation when used alone, focal liver radiation can produce regression of primary hepatobiliary cancers. At least four techniques have been assessed: use of microspheres embedded with ^{90}Y, use of ^{131}I-labeled ethiodized oil, and external beam radiation with either protons or photons. In ^{90}Y therapy, yttrium 89 (^{89}Y) oxide is incorporated into a stable glass matrix. When bombarded with neutrons, ^{89}Y is converted to ^{90}Y, a pure beta emitter with a half-life of 64.5 hours and average electron energy of 2.23 MeV, which produces an electron range of approximately 2.5 cm. Two kinds of microspheres are now in use: resin spheres and glass spheres. Resin microspheres are approximately 30 μM in diameter, compared to about 25 μM for the glass spheres, but the glass can be labeled to a higher specific activity. The microspheres have been infused into the hepatic artery as a form of regional therapy for well-vascularized tumors. Resin microspheres are approved for the treatment of colorectal cancer metastatic to the liver, based on a randomized trial showing that spheres plus hepatic arterial floxuridine is superior to hepatic arterial floxuridine alone (184a; reviewed in 184b). The glass spheres were studied briefly in the United States and Canada, then became unavailable, and are now available again for use under a humanitarian device exemption for the treatment of patients with hepatocellular cancer. Objective response rates have ranged from 0% to 25% (185–

187; reviewed in 188). Note that ^{90}Y doses (50–150 Gy) cannot be compared directly with the more familiar doses of external beam radiation because the former are calculated by assuming full decay with all radiation homogeneously deposited within the liver. More important, the low-dose-rate irradiation (<0.2 Gy/hour) delivered by ^{90}Y has far less effect than the same physical dose delivered by standard external beam treatment (>2 Gy/minute). Prospective trials of glass microspheres are lacking, making the role of this therapy difficult to determine. In addition, a better understanding of the dosimetry of this technique (189), as well as of the technical factors involved (e.g., pulmonary shunting, which can lead to radiation pneumonitis [190] or variant arterial supply to the stomach, which can produce gastric ulcers), is required before the use of microspheres can become routine.

Another method of delivering focal liver radiation is through hepatic arterial administration of ^{131}I ethiodized oil. Ethiodized oil has been used extensively for chemoembolization for HCC (discussed below). For focal radiation delivery, it is formulated with radioactive iodine to deliver localized radiation using the beta (electron) component of the ^{131}I emissions (191,192). Randomized trials led by French investigators compared radiotherapy using ^{131}I-labeled ethiodized oil with chemoembolization (193) and with supportive care for patients with portal vein thrombosis (194). In the former study, 129 patients were randomly assigned to receive either 60 mCi of ^{131}I-labeled ethiodized oil or chemoembolization with cisplatin (70 mg). No difference was seen in overall survival between the two groups (median survival was approximately 40 weeks), but toxicity was significantly less in patients on the ethiodized oil arm. In the second study, 27 patients were randomly assigned to receive either 60 mCi of ^{131}I-labeled ethiodized oil or a control treatment (e.g., tamoxifen). The ethiodized oil group showed a statistically significantly greater median survival (of approximately 6 months vs. 2 months for the control group). Although these findings suggest that ^{131}I-labeled ethiodized oil has activity against HCC, this small study does not permit a firm conclusion to be drawn. Furthermore, as is the case for ^{90}Y, little is known about dosimetry in tumor and normal tissue. ^{131}I-labeled ethiodized oil is not yet available for use in the United States.

Traditional external beam photon techniques, either alone (195) or in combination with chemoembolization (196), have produced objective responses in patients with unresectable HCCs. Standard photon techniques, however, often require the treatment of large volumes of normal liver. In contrast, conformal three-dimensional (3-D) treatment planning using beams not confined to the axial plane can substantially reduce irradiation of normal liver (197). Phase I and II trials investigating the use of 3-D conformal external beam irradiation combined with fluorodeoxyuridine delivered via the hepatic artery have demonstrated that high-dose focal radiation can produce a 60% response rate. More recent results support the hypothesis that the dose delivered is an important prognostic factor in both local control and survival for patients with primary hepatobiliary cancers. In this study, dose was prescribed (to a maximum of 90 Gy) according to the fraction of normal liver that was spared based on a normal tissue complication probability (NTCP) model. Patients who could receive >70 Gy had a median survival in excess of 17 months, which approaches that achieved by surgical resection. In a multivariate analysis, dose was a prognostic factor independent of tumor size (198).

An important step in defining the limits of external beam radiation was to develop a model to describe the dependence of liver tolerance on the combination of dose and volume. Recent investigations have suggested that a quantitative model can be derived to predict radiation-induced liver disease (199). An NTCP model with parameters calculated from patient data has been used prospectively to prescribe a dose that would subject each patient to a predetermined complication risk. Twenty-one patients have completed treatment on such a protocol. The mean dose delivered was 56.6 ± 2.3 Gy (range: 40.5–81.0 Gy). One of 21 patients developed radiation-induced liver disease. The observed complication rate of 4.8% (95% confidence interval, 0%–23.8%) did not differ significantly from the predicted 8.8% NTCP (based on dose delivered). These results suggest that an NTCP model can be used prospectively to safely deliver far higher doses of radiation to patients with intrahepatic cancer than with previous approaches (198,200). The widespread adoption of 3-D conformal planning systems should permit these concepts to be tested in multiinstitutional trials.

An increasing number of investigators are exploring the use of stereotactic body radiation for the treatment of primary hepatocellular cancer and colorectal cancer metastatic to the liver. In one such study, 37 patients were treated in a prospective phase I/II trial with single fractions up to 26 Gy without reaching dose-limiting toxicity. The maximum lesion size was 5 cm, with a median of about 3 cm. The actuarial lesion control was 81% at 18 months, which approximates that produced by RFA. To deliver this treatment safely, they took great care to immobilize patients and localize lesions so as to limit the amount of normal liver treated and to avoid the intestine (201). This area continues to undergo technical improvements (201a).

Finally, another method of delivering highly conformal radiation is with protons. Investigators in Japan have demonstrated response rates similar to those reported earlier using 3-D conformal radiation (202). Interestingly, high-dose focal radiation using either photons (203) or protons (204) can produce hypertrophy in the unirradiated liver, which resembles the effect of partial hepatectomy.

In summary, whole liver radiation alone has little efficacy in the treatment of HCC. High-dose fractionated focal radiation, especially using external beam photons or protons, can produce objective responses in the majority of patients with unresectable lesions. In addition, stereotactic body radiation appears to produce control rates equivalent to those of invasive local ablative techniques. However, the relative merit of these techniques compared to that of other nonsurgical approaches described in this chapter has not been assessed in randomized trials.

Systemic Therapies

The medical management of HCC is complicated because two diseases coexist in most patients: cancer and liver disease. Often, the HCC becomes apparent only when a patient's liver function deteriorates. In that case, supportive care is often the only option. When liver function is still normal or nearly normal, however, numerous nonsurgical therapies are available that may be tried.

Further confusing the assessment of the relative efficacies of these various treatments is the marked variability in the natural histories of patients with HCC, depending on the cause and extent of underlying liver disease, the stage at diagnosis, and other comorbidities. For example, results of a given treatment in a study conducted in Hong Kong, where nearly every patient with HCC has underlying hepatitis B virus (HBV) infection, may not be applicable to patients in Japan, where hepatitis C virus (HCV) infection is the dominant underlying cause of liver cirrhosis.

With those caveats, results of numerous medical treatment options for HCC that have been studied are discussed in the following sections. These range from systemic chemotherapy, using a single agent or a combination of agents, to treatment with interferons and targeted biological agents. Regional treatments, including hepatic intraarterial chemotherapy and tumor embolization with chemotherapy, have also been investigated.

Chemotherapy

For a number of reasons, systemic chemotherapy may appear to be or may be ineffective against HCC. Inherent drug resistance may be present because hepatocytes constitutively express the multidrug resistance gene. This gene has been shown to confer drug resistance to doxorubicin hydrochloride in HCC cell lines (205). The underlying hepatic dysfunction may also be problematic, requiring dosage adjustments of chemotherapeutics to avoid excessive drug toxicity. Drug delivery to the tumor may be compromised due to portal hypertension or blood shunting. Finally, assessment of response may be inaccurate in some cases, because radiographic changes associated with tumor shrinkage may not be apparent in the inelastic, rock-hard cirrhotic liver.

Whether for these or other reasons, systemic chemotherapy has been tested and shown to be minimally effective or ineffective in HCC. Nearly every commercially available chemotherapeutic agent has been studied in treatment of this disease, and none has demonstrated meaningful activity. Based on historical data, doxorubicin is generally considered to be the first-line treatment. A report in 1978 suggested an objective response rate of 32% with single-agent doxorubicin (206), but subsequent studies have failed to confirm this level of activity and have demonstrated substantial toxicity (207,208) (Table 33.6).

As with all solid tumors, combination chemotherapy has also been studied extensively. For the most part, multidrug treatment has resulted in magnified toxicity without any apparent clinical benefit (207–209). A report from Hong Kong, however, shows surprising activity of an aggressive chemotherapy and immunotherapy regimen in HBV-associated HCC (210). According to personal communication of a case report later published (211), these investigators combined cisplatin, doxorubicin, and 5-fluorouracil with interferon-α (PIAF) in treatment of patients with inoperable HCC and found an objective response rate of 26%; one-third of those responding had documented pathological complete responses at surgery. A subsequent larger series of 149 patients with predominantly HBV-associated HCC treated with the same regimen found a lower response rate of 16.8% and a complete response rate of only 2% (212). Significant factors that predicted a response to treatment include absence of cirrhosis and low total bilirubin. The toxicity was substantial but not insurmountable. Based on these early results, the PIAF combination was compared to doxorubicin in a randomized phase III trial of 188 patients with unresectable HCC. Unfortunately, however, there was no significant difference in response rates and overall survival between the two arms (213). Therefore, while associated with increased toxicity, combination regimens have not shown any additional survival benefit over single-agent chemotherapy in HCC.

Interferon Therapy

The inclusion of interferon treatment in HCC trials is not uncommon. The original rationale—that HCC is a virally mediated disease and interferon may have antiviral properties—was speculative when these trials were first initiated. Subsequent data, however, confirmed that interferon-α is effective in normalizing transaminases and clearing HCV infection in approximately 20% of patients with chronic hepatitis C (214,215) and, in those patients, may prevent or delay the subsequent development of HCC. Moreover, a recent trial suggested that interferon-α may reduce HCC recurrence after medical ablation therapy for primary tumors (216).

TABLE 33.6

SELECTED RANDOMIZED TRIALS OF CHEMOTHERAPY FOR TREATMENT OF HEPATOCELLULAR CARCINOMA

Study and location	No. of patients	Treatment arms	Results
Choi et al. (207), Hong Kong	39	Doxorubicin hydrochloride vs. 5-FU/methotrexate sodium/ cyclophosphate/vincristine sulfate	13.0 wk vs 6.5 wk survival (No change)
Falkson et al. (209), South Africa and United States	192	Doxorubicin hydrochloride vs. 5-FU/MeCCNU vs. 5-FU/streptozocin 5-FU/MeCCNU/doxorubicin hydrochloride	5-FU/MeCCNU 28 wk vs. Doxorubicin 12 wk
Yeo et al. (213), Hong Kong and United Kingdom	188	Cisplatin/IFN-α 2b/doxorubicin/5-FU vs. Doxorubicin hydrochloride	8.67 mon vs. 6.83 mon (p = 0.83)
Lai et al. (208), Hong Kong	60	Doxorubicin hydrochloride vs. Supportive care	10.6 wk vs. 7.5 wk (p = .036)

5-FU, 5-fluorouracil; MeCCNU, methylchlorethylcyclohexylnitrosurea (semustine).

Unfortunately, interferon-α has not consistently demonstrated substantial efficacy in treating HCC patients (Table 33.7). Phase II trials suggest only marginal tumor response activity with interferon-α as a single agent (217), and combining it with 5-fluorouracil (217a,218,219) or doxorubicin (220) does not make it any more efficacious. One study using the combination of mitoxantrone hydrochloride and interferon-α (221) did not suggest any additive effect with interferon-α. Again, the PIAF regimen described previously combining interferon-α with three chemotherapy drugs, although effective in early phase trials (212), ultimately did not demonstrate a survival advantage in the randomized phase III setting (213). Two studies hint at some benefit for interferon-α compared to doxorubicin (222) or to supportive care (223), but this reflects the dismal outcome for the HCC patients in these series who did not receive interferon (median survival of 4.8 and 7.5 weeks), rather than a dramatic improvement in survival in the treated group. The minimal efficacy of interferon-α was confirmed in a more recent randomized trial, where it showed substantial toxicity and no improvement in 1- or 2-year survival rate compared to symptomatic treatment (224).

Hormonal Therapy

HCC is far more common in men than it is in women, and the natural history of the cancer seems to be more aggressive in men as well. Furthermore, epidemiologic evidence exists tying the use of sex and anabolic steroids to the development of HCC. These clinical observations have prompted a search for evidence of hormone receptors in HCC and of the potential effectiveness of agents targeting these receptors for treatment. Glucocorticoid and hormonal receptors were first identified in HCC specimen homogenates, which led to a small trial of the use of progestational hormones to treat the disease. Tumor regression was noted in a few patients (225).

TABLE 33.7

TRIALS OF IFN-α FOR TREATMENT OF HEPATOCELLULAR CARCINOMA

Study and location	No. of patients	Treatment	Results
GITSG (217), United States	30	IFN-α2b	Objective response = 2/30 Median survival = 22 wk
Kardinal et al. (220), United States	31	IFN-α2b + doxorubicin hydrochloride	Response = 3% Median survival = 10 mo
Stuart et al. (219), United States	10	IFN-α2b + 5-FU	Responses = 0 Median survival = 10 mo
Lai et al. (222), Hong Kong	75	IFN-α (two doses) vs. doxorubicin hydrochloride	Median survival = 4.8 wk vs. 8.3 wk (NS)
Lai et al. (223), Hong Kong	71	IFN-α vs. observation	Median survival = 14.5 wk vs. 7.5 wk (p = 0.0471)
Llovet et al. (224), Spain	58	IFN-α2b vs. supportive care	1-yr survival rate = 58% v. 38% (NS)
Patt et al. (218), United States	28	IFN-α + 5-FU	Response rate = 18%

INF-α, interferon-α; GITSG, Gastrointestinal Tumor Study Group; 5-FU, 5-fluorouracil; NS, not significant.

By far, the hormonal agent most often studied in clinical trials is the weak estrogen tamoxifen citrate. Unfortunately, no objective responses have been shown with tamoxifen (226), and most randomized trials comparing tamoxifen with (227–229) or without chemotherapy (230,231) to placebo or observation have found no significant difference in survival between the treatment and control arms. Even in studies in which a significant survival difference was seen, the median survival was <10 months (232–234). These results are typified by a recent large randomized phase III trial of 420 patients with unresectable HCC that found no survival difference between tamoxifen and best supportive care and a median survival of <5 months in both arms (235). Based on these data, there appears to be no role for hormonal treatment thus far in HCC.

REGIONAL CHEMOTHERAPY

Rationale

The fact that the blood supply to the liver can be isolated and that the liver plays the dominant role in metabolizing agents make regional drug delivery to the liver intriguing. The pharmacologic principles behind this approach have been well described (236). Depending on the features of the chemotherapeutic agent used, delivery to the liver via the hepatic artery may confer a substantial regional advantage for the drug compared to its systemic administration. The selective tumor uptake of drugs appears to be greater with hepatic arterial delivery than through the portal venous route (237). This may be especially appealing for agents with marginal activity if a dose–response curve exists, so that higher drug concentrations are potentially more effective. Based on these considerations, the fluoropyrimidines, especially floxuridine, appear to be the ideal agents for this treatment modality.

This approach has been studied extensively in patients with colorectal liver metastases. Numerous phase II and III trials have addressed the relative utility of fluoropyrimidines administered systemically and regionally (238). So far, hepatic intraarterial (HIA) therapy has not been shown to be clearly superior to systemic treatments in these patients, although data suggest an improvement in patients who receive HIA adjuvant chemotherapy after metastasectomy for colorectal liver tumors (239). A recent Cancer and Leukemia Group B (CALGB) trial (CALGB 9481) comparing HIA chemotherapy to systemic chemotherapy in patients with liver-only colorectal metastases confirmed a better outcome for the regional therapy arm, although this may no longer be applicable in these patients with the availability of numerous new chemotherapeutics and biologics since the study was conducted (240). Although HCC behaves even more as a regional malignancy than metastatic colorectal cancer, the frequent coexistence of underlying liver disease or cirrhosis complicates the local delivery of agents. The safe and ongoing delivery of HIA therapy depends on careful tracking of liver function test results, which may be confusing in patients with baseline abnormalities in those parameters. Also, patients with severe underlying liver disease and cancer may be prone to substantial arteriovenous shunting (190), which negates some of the regional advantages of HIA delivery by distributing agents to the lung. Nonetheless, the theoretic considerations have prompted efforts to administer agents via the hepatic artery to HCC patients.

In an attempt to further augment the regional advantage described previously, numerous investigators coadminister lipiodol via the hepatic artery. Lipiodol is an ethyl ester of the fatty acid of poppy seed oil containing 38% iodine by weight. It is the contrast agent used for lymphangiograms and concentrates in neoplastic lesions in the liver after hepatic arterial administration. It appears to aid in detecting the presence of satellite lesions in patients being considered for surgical resection of HCC (241) and is used to carry lipophilic chemotherapeutics, but it does not appear to be an embolizing substance. It can also be radiolabeled with ^{131}I for the delivery of internal radiation treatment (107).

Results

A number of phase II trials of HIA chemotherapy for HCC have been conducted. The combination of floxuridine and mitomycin C delivered via an implanted pump into the hepatic artery of patients with HCC or cholangiocarcinoma resulted in four partial responses in HCC (242). Toxicity was mild, with only one patient developing hepatobiliary problems. The median survival for all patients in the series was 14.5 months.

Other investigators have combined fluoropyrimidines and anthracyclines in the same patient population. In one study, combinations of etoposide, doxorubicin, and cisplatin, or of etoposide, cisplatin, and 5-fluorouracil, were given via a percutaneous catheter into the common or proper hepatic artery (243). A 50% objective partial response rate was seen in these studies, although substantial hepatic and systemic toxicity was observed.

In the largest series reported on the HIA administration of floxuridine, leucovorin calcium, doxorubicin, and cisplatin (244), treatment was administered through either a percutaneous catheter or an implanted pump over 4 days per cycle. The objective response rate in the 31 patients included in the series was 41%, but marked toxicity occurred. Although response did not appear to be correlated with the cause of the underlying liver disease, patients with viral hepatitis lived only a median of 7.5 months, much less than the median survival of those without viral liver disease. Toxicity was also far greater in patients with hepatitis-associated HCC.

The results of these studies cannot be generalized, however. Surgery to implant delivery devices is technically difficult, even in the absence of cirrhosis or HCC (245), and the risks in patients with portal hypertension make this a safe and reasonable approach for only a minority of HCC patients (246). Percutaneous catheterization of the hepatic artery is less intrusive but is also associated with formidable bleeding and infectious risks. Therefore, the response rate and survival data for HCC patients seen in the HIA series may reflect rigorous patient selection as much as the impact of the HIA therapy.

Chemoembolization

The hepatic artery supplies 80% of the blood to tumors in the liver, whereas normal liver tissue receives the majority of its blood supply from the portal vein (247). This explains the selective tumor drug uptake of agents that has been demonstrated with HIA delivery compared with delivery via the portal vein for floxuridine, for example (237). This feature also makes tumor vasculature an inviting target because occlusion of the hepatic arterial supply could induce selective tumor ischemia without affecting the remaining uninvolved liver. Ligation of the hepatic artery can be done surgically and may induce some tumor ischemia, but the benefit is at best transient (248) because collateral vessels rapidly develop within the liver (249). Vascular interruption performed in conjunction with HIA chemotherapy can increase regional drug distribution and dwell time at the tumor, and this has been verified with numerous agents, including mitomycin C and cisplatin (250,251).

This combined approach is called *chemoembolization*. It is done by a percutaneous approach, in which distal hepatic arterial vessels are occluded. The embolization can be performed with numerous materials (252–254), including the following:

- Gelatin sponge
- Collagen
- Polyvinyl alcohol
- Starch microspheres
- Autologous clot
- Glass microspheres
- Yttrium 90 (^{90}Y) resin microspheres

These substances have varying durations of occlusion, size, weight, and flow characteristics, which lead to differences in intrahepatic distribution, extrahepatic shunting, and local and systemic toxicity. The optimal features of an embolizing particle or material are unknown.

The numerous studies assessing chemoembolization are impossible to compare. The populations of patients treated range from patients with single encapsulated lesions and well-preserved hepatic function to patients with multifocal HCC and highly compromised liver reserve. Furthermore, the exact methods (chemotherapy, particle, contrast agent) and techniques (selective HIA administration, whole liver treatment) vary greatly from one institution to another. With this disclaimer in mind, the objective response rate in terms of tumor shrinkage is approximately 50%. Necrosis of the tumor, as demonstrated by liquefaction on imaging studies (252), occurs more often than actual tumor shrinkage. Little effort has been made to assess the impact this tumor liquefaction or chemoembolization in general has on the quality of life of HCC patients.

A few randomized trials of chemoembolization have been performed. The first by Pelletier et al. found no significant difference in 6- and 12-month survival rates between patients with unresectable HCC who received symptomatic treatment and those who received chemoembolization with doxorubicin and Gelfoam powder (255). Another was a multicenter trial by the Barcelona Clinic Liver Cancer Group that compared repeated arterial embolization with gelatin sponge, repeated chemoembolization with doxorubicin and gelatin sponge, and conservative treatment in patients with unresectable HCC (255a). Chemoembolization induced an objective response for at least 6 months in one-third of the patients and was associated with significantly higher 1- and 2-year survival rates than conservative treatment.

Different underlying etiologies of cirrhosis may result in HCCs with different characteristics, including how they respond to ischemia or chemotherapy. The majority of patients in the two aforementioned randomized studies with chemoembolization had chronic hepatitis C. How applicable their results are to HCC patients with cirrhosis due to other etiologies, such as chronic hepatitis B or alcohol, are unclear. Therefore, despite the large number of published series, the role of chemoembolization in the management of patients with unresectable HCC remains undefined.

When chemoembolization is believed to be indicated, a number of relative or absolute exclusion criteria are used in patient selection. Patients with occlusion of the main portal vein cannot safely undergo chemoembolization, although some interventional radiologists will consider superselective chemoembolization to the tumor alone if only branches of the portal vein are thrombosed. In general, patients with ascites, pancytopenia, a recent history of variceal bleeding, hyperbilirubinemia, or other manifestations of poorly compensated liver failure are at substantial risk from chemoembolization.

Chemoembolization is often incorporated into multimodality treatment plans in patients with HCC, both before resec-

tion or while under evaluation for orthotopic liver transplantation (OLT). The treatment was first used with the rationale that it could both delay tumor progression while patients were on the waiting list and diminish the dissemination of cancer cells at the time of liver mobilization and explant (82). Two series (112,136) that used strict eligibility criteria to select candidates—fewer than four tumors, negativity for hepatitis B surface antigen, no tumor > 5 cm—have demonstrated an overall survival in OLT patients receiving preoperative chemoembolization for HCC that is comparable to that of liver transplantation patients without underlying HCC. A third retrospective study of 168 patients with HCC stratified by tumor stage found a significant improvement in 5-year recurrencefree survival in patients with either T2 or T3 stage disease who received locoregional therapy prior to OLT compared to those who did not receive any preoperative therapy (256). The locoregional therapy in this study included chemoembolization (70.9%), ablation (either PEI or RFA, 14.6%), or a combination of chemoembolization and ablation (14.6%).

Nevertheless, no randomized data exist for the use of chemoembolization in OLT candidates, so one cannot conclude that chemoembolization contributed to the excellent patient outcomes. Furthermore, the 80% to 90% tumorfree survival rates seen in these series are for patients who were on the waiting list for only a few months. Given the relative unavailability of livers and the increasing incidence of HCV-related chronic liver disease, the average patient today waits nearly 2 years for an OLT, so these data may not be applicable for current decision making.

Lipiodol Chemoembolization

Lipiodol, which does not appear to occlude vessels but may enhance drug delivery, is a common component of many chemoembolization protocols. Unlike the chemoembolization techniques described previously, lipiodol chemoembolization has been investigated in excellent, randomized studies. The first compared chemoembolization (with lipiodol, cisplatin, and gelatin sponge) to best supportive care for patients with locally advanced HCC in the setting of preserved hepatic function and patency of the main portal vein (257). In the absence of clinical deterioration or progressive cancer, patients received lipiodol chemoembolization at 2-month intervals for four cycles. Objective responses were seen in the treated patients, but actuarial predictions led to an early closure of the study because no survival benefit could be predicted. The multiple lipiodol chemoembolizations led to the frequent development of acute hepatic failure and raised the question of toxic complications.

A similar prospective study treated control patients with tamoxifen and assessed the potential additive value of lipiodol chemoembolization administered every 3 months (258). The patient characteristics were comparable to those in the first study, and although the number of patients was smaller than in the previous study, the findings were quite similar. No apparent survival benefit was seen in the group undergoing lipiodol chemoembolization, and 51% of patients had signs of accelerated hepatic dysfunction after the lipiodol chemoembolization.

A third randomized trial conducted in Hong Kong compared previously untreated patients with unresectable HCC who received symptomatic treatment to those who were treated with chemoembolization using varying doses of an emulsion of cisplatin in lipiodol, depending on tumor size at every 2- to 3-month intervals until disease progression (258a). Most patients had chronic hepatitis B, and the study excluded patients who had poor liver function and poor performance status. The chemoembolization group in this trial had a 39% objective response rate and significantly higher 1-, 2-, and 3-year survival rates than the control group. Similar to the previous studies, worsening hepatic dysfunction and deaths from liver failure occurred more frequently in the chemoembolization group, but the liver functions of survivors were not significantly different in both groups.

The negative results in the former two randomized studies and the increased incidence of hepatic failure seen in the treatment groups in these trials may reflect ill-advised chemoembolization strategies, particularly the use of recurrent treatments in patients with underlying liver disease. That interpretation is consistent with a retrospective analysis comparing historical subsets of patients, one treated with planned periodic chemoembolizations and the second treated at the time of radiographic progression (259). That analysis concluded that patients treated selectively appeared to do better than those receiving treatments at predetermined intervals even in the absence of progressive disease. In any case, the randomized studies appear to support modest and selective use of lipiodol chemoembolization in treating patients with unresectable HCC.

Lipiodol chemoembolization has also been proposed in the preoperative setting for patients with resectable HCC, with the goals of decreasing tumor vascularity or enabling the residual liver to hypertrophy. Whether such an outcome can be realized has never been clear, and no randomized studies addressing this potential role have been conducted. Certainly, this approach has not been analyzed to determine if any survival advantage is associated with the preoperative treatment. Lipiodol chemoembolization is safe and feasible in this setting (260), although one retrospective study suggested an increase in postoperative complications related to gallbladder ischemia (261).

The role of preoperative lipiodol chemoembolization in liver transplant has also been explored. One retrospective series looked at liver transplant patients and found that clinical response to lipiodol chemoembolization predicted an improved diseasefree survival (261a). In contrast, a different retrospective study comparing outcomes for 21 patients with HCC who underwent pretransplant lipiodol chemoembolization with outcomes for 21 historical control patients who went straight to transplantation found no apparent benefit from the preoperative treatment (262).

In summary, the role of chemoembolization with or without lipiodol in patients with HCC would appear to be limited. Randomized studies have been conducted and have failed to demonstrate significant benefit, and quality-of-life issues have not been adequately addressed. Although the regional delivery of agents to the liver for the treatment of HCC makes perfect sense, the results do not meet the hypothetical promise that modeling would have predicted.

Novel Systemic Therapies

Given the repeatedly discouraging results discussed previously for systemic chemotherapy, hormonal manipulations, and regional chemotherapy with or without lipiodol or embolization, an appropriate conclusion is that the nonsurgical weapons being deployed are simply inadequate in the face of the complexity of HCC. A survey of the features—both clinical and molecular—of HCC, however, raises a number of potential possibilities for new treatment strategies. The pharmacologic principles outlined previously should apply to novel agents and to classic chemotherapeutic agents, which opens up a range of possibilities for new drugs or biologics.

Experimental efforts to deliver regional treatment to the liver include magnetic targeting of agents into the liver and prodrug formulation for selective activation within the liver.

Novel systemic chemotherapeutic agents currently under investigation include new cytotoxic drugs such as nolatrexed and

T138067. Nolatrexed dihydrochloride (Thymitaq, AG337; Eximias Pharmaceutical, Berwyn, PA) is a novel thymidylate synthase inhibitor that was rationally designed using structure-based modeling techniques. In an early phase study, HCC patients treated with nolatrexed had an 8% partial response rate, an 8% minor response rate, and a 54% stable disease rate (263). In a subsequent randomized phase II trial, nolatrexed treatment did not result in any objective responses but was associated with a 52% significant improvement in median survival compared to doxorubicin (264). As in the case of previous drugs, however, these early encouraging results have not translated into success in the phase III setting. In the largest randomized phase III trial ever completed in HCC comparing nolatrexed to doxorubicin in 446 patients, preliminary results recently presented in abstract form showed no difference in objective response rate (1.4% vs. 4.0%, respectively) and progressionfree survival between the two arms (265). T138067 (Amgen, Thousand Oaks, CA) is a new cytotoxic agent that irreversibly inhibits the mitotic spindle component, β-tubulin, which blocks mitosis and eventually leads to apoptotic cell death. In a randomized phase III trial, T138067 did not improve survival in patients with unresectable HCC compared to doxorubicin (266).

Other novel systemic antitumor strategies being explored in HCC include enzymatic depletion of arginine, a nonessential amino acid for humans. Normal human cells synthesize arginine using the enzymes argininosuccinate synthase (ASS) and argininosuccinate lyase. Some human cancers, including various HCC cell lines, do not express ASS and thus die without exogenous arginine. These HCC cell lines have been shown to be killed in vitro and in vivo by the arginine-degrading enzyme arginine deaminase. In a phase I/II trial of 19 patients with unresectable HCC, a pegylated form of arginine deaminase induced two complete responses, seven partial responses, and seven stable disease (266a). The 19 patients had a median survival of 410 days with 4 patients alive for longer than 680 days. These provocative early results provide strong encouragement for the further study of this agent in the multicenter randomized phase III setting.

As in other malignancies, much attention in HCC has been focused on exploring targeted biologic therapies. Hepatocarcinogenesis is complex and its mechanisms are largely unknown, but many carcinogenic pathways are aberrant to some degree in HCC. These molecular aberrations involve growth factors and their receptors; angiogenic factors; intracellular signaling proteins such as those in the Ras/Raf/MAP-kinase and PTEN/Akt pathways; cell cycle control proteins such as cyclins and cyclin-dependent kinases; tumor suppressors such as PTEN, p53, and Rb; proteases and matrix metalloproteinases that play an important role in tumor cell invasion and metastasis; and cyclooxygenase (267). Strategies targeting these aberrant proteins involve the use of small molecule inhibitors, monoclonal antibodies, and antisense oligonucleotides. Evidence supporting the development of these agents comes mostly from preclinical studies where the drugs are found to inhibit tumor cell growth but occasionally from clinical reports of significant response of HCC tumors to these drugs. Such is the case with a recent report published in the *Journal of Clinical Oncology* of a patient with refractory HCC who had a near-complete response to treatment with the cyclooxygenase inhibitor celecoxib (268).

Much of the development of targeted therapy, however, is still in its infancy, with the exception of those involving angiogenesis and growth factor signaling pathways. Numerous lines of evidence have linked tumor growth and metastases with angiogenesis (269). Of the identified angiogenic factors, vascular endothelial growth factor (VEGF) is the most potent and specific, and has been identified as a crucial regulator of both normal and pathological angiogenesis (270).

VEGF has been shown to play an important role in tumor growth. HCC is commonly viewed as a very vascular tumor. Increased levels of VEGF and high microvessel density have been found in HCC (271–273). Clinically, high VEGF expression has been associated with poorer survival in liver cancer (274). A number of agents that interfere with VEGF signaling are currently being investigated in cancer treatment, including the monoclonal antibody bevacizumab (275,276) and the small molecule inhibitor sorafenib (277,278). Bevacizumab (Avastin; Genentech, South San Francisco, CA) is currently approved for the treatment of colorectal cancer and has also been effective in treating lung cancer (276). Early trials indicate that bevacizumab can be given safely in HCC and is associated with modest clinical activity (279,280). Further phase II trials are now ongoing. Sorafenib (BAY-439006; Bayer Corp., Lever-kusen, Germany) is a small molecule multitargeted VEGF and Raf kinase inhibitor that has recently been approved for the treatment of advanced renal cell carcinoma. A randomized phase III trial comparing doxorubicin with or without sorafenib in patients with advanced HCC is currently accruing.

Epidermal growth factor receptor (EGFR) plays an important role in the development and progression of human malignancies and has been a relevant target for chemotherapeutics (281). HCC has been shown to frequently overexpress EGFR (282). Therapeutic agents targeting EGFR include small molecules such as erlotinib (Tarceva; OSI Pharmaceuticals, New York, NY) that inhibit its intracellular kinase domain and monoclonal antibodies such as cetuximab (Erbitux; Bristol-Myers Squibb, New York, NY) that bind its extracellular receptor domain. Erlotinib is approved for the treatment of lung cancer, whereas cetuximab is approved for the second-line treatment of metastatic colorectal cancer. Two recent trials suggest some clinical benefit (25% and 35% progressionfree survival at 4 and 6 months, respectively) for the use of erlotinib in patients with HCC; toxicity was acceptable (283,284). Phase II trials evaluating erlotinib and cetuximab in patients with unresectable HCC are currently underway.

Receptor-targeted therapy in the form of a somatostatin analog has also been explored in HCC. Somatostatin receptors have been identified in various nonneuroendocrine tumors, including breast, kidney, colon, ovary, and HCC (285,286). A case report has shown evidence of marked AFP reduction in a patient with advanced HCC treated with the long-acting somatostatin analog lanreotide (287). This strategy was tested in a randomized study comparing treatment with daily subcutaneous administration of the somatostatin analog octreotide to placebo. An improvement in median survival (13 months vs. 4 months, respectively), accompanied by decreases in AFP levels, was noted with the use of somatostatin (288). However, in early data from a recent randomized phase III trial comparing long-acting octreotide to placebo in 272 patients with unresectable HCC, there was no significant difference in median survival between the treatment and control groups (289).

Another intriguing systemic therapy being evaluated in HCC is 3-hydroxy-3-methylglutaryl coenzyme A (HMG-CoA) reductase inhibition. Mevalonic acid, produced by HMG-CoA reductase, has been found to regulate cell growth independent of cholesterogenesis (290). In a randomized trial of HCC patients pretreated with a combination of arterial embolization and 5-fluorouracil chemotherapy, the HMG-CoA reductase inhibitor, pravastatin, was found to double the median survival compared to control (291).

HCC is also a target of gene therapy strategies. In particular, the replacement of absent p53 tumor-suppressor function, which results from a common mutation in HCC, is in clinical trials with the HIA administration of a viral vector constructed to carry the p53 gene (292).

Finally, due to the ineffectiveness of systemic therapies for unresectable HCC, many patients have explored the use of alternative therapies, such as traditional Chinese medicine. In unpublished case reports, patients with unresectable HCC have had near-complete responses to treatment with oral extracts of the mushroom *Ganoderma lucidum* (lingzhi, Reishi) that is frequently used in traditional Chinese medicine. These remarkable observations warrant further investigation.

In general, HCC has thus far been refractory to essentially all systemic treatments. Cytotoxic chemotherapies have not only been ineffective, but toxicities also make their use difficult, if not entirely prohibitive, in the cirrhotic patient population. New strategies are sorely needed. Future advancement of systemic therapies in this disease rests on understanding the biology and molecular mechanisms of hepatocarcinogenesis. Potentially relevant pathways currently under investigation include VEGF and other angiogenic mechanisms, as well as intracellular signaling cascades such as the EGFR, MAPK, protein kinase C, and Ras pathways (267). Drugs that specifically target these mechanisms of hepatocarcinogenesis may not only be efficacious but may also prove to be much less toxic than cytotoxic chemotherapy, which is extremely important in patients with significant liver dysfunction. Therefore, present and future investigative efforts should be focused on understanding and targeting molecular mechanisms of hepatocarcinogenesis if any headway is to be made in the systemic treatment of this disease.

References

1. Ho J, Wu PC, Kung TM. An autopsy study of hepatocellular carcinoma in Hong Kong. *Pathology* 1981;13(3):409–416.
2. Ng WD, Chan YT, Ho KK, Kong CK. Injection sclerotherapy for bleeding esophageal varices in cirrhotic patients with hepatocellular carcinoma. *Gastrointest Endosc* 1989;35(1):69–70.
3. Yeo W, Sung JY, Ward SC, et al. A prospective study of upper gastrointestinal hemorrhage in patients with hepatocellular carcinoma. *Dig Dis Sci* 1995;40(12):2516–2521.
4. Ihde DC, Sherlock P, Winawer SJ, Fortner JG. Clinical manifestations of hepatoma: a review of 6 years' experience at a cancer hospital. *Am J Med* 1974;56(1):83–91.
5. Lai CL, Lam KC, Wong KP, Wu PC, Todd D. Clinical features of hepatocellular carcinoma: review of 211 patients in Hong Kong. *Cancer* 1981;47(11):2746–2455.
6. Shiu W, Dewar G, Leung N, et al. Hepatocellular carcinoma in Hong Kong: clinical study on 340 cases. *Oncology* 1990;47(3):241–245.
7. Edmondson HA, Steiner PE. Primary carcinoma of the liver: a study of 100 cases among 48,900 necropsies. *Cancer* 1954;7(3):462–503.
8. Kappel DA, Miller DR. Primary hepatic carcinoma: a review of thirty-seven patients. *Am J Surg* 1972;124(6):798–802.
9. Kew MC, Geddes EW. Hepatocellular carcinoma in rural southern African blacks. *Medicine (Baltimore)* 1982;61(2):98–108.
10. Lin TY. Tumors of the liver. Part I. Primary malignant tumors. In: Bockus H, ed. *Gastroenterology*. Philadelphia, Pa.: WB Saunders; 1976:522–534.
11. Okuda K. Clinical aspects of hepatocellular carcinoma-an analysis of 134 cases. In: Okuda K, Peters F, eds. *Hepatocellular Carcinoma*. New York, NY: Wiley; 1976:387–436.
12. Kojiro M, Kawabata K, Kawano Y, Shirai F, Takemoto N, Nakashima T. Hepatocellular carcinoma presenting as intrabile duct tumor growth: a clinicopathologic study of 24 cases. *Cancer* 1982;49(10):2144–2147.
13. Lee NW, Wong KP, Siu KF, Wong J. Cholangiography in hepatocellular carcinoma with obstructive jaundice. *Clin Radiol* 1984;35(2):119–123.
14. Lai EC, Ng IO, Ng MM, et al. Long-term results of resection for large hepatocellular carcinoma: a multivariate analysis of clinicopathological features. *Hepatology* 1990;11(5):815–818.
15. Lau WY, Leung KL, Leung TW, et al. Obstructive jaundice secondary to hepatocellular carcinoma. *Surg Oncol* 1995;4(6):303–308.
16. Afroudakis A, Bhuta SM, Ranganath KA, Kaplowitz N. Obstructive jaundice caused by hepatocellular carcinoma: report of three cases. *Am J Dig Dis* 1978;23(7):609–617.
17. Van Sonnenberg E, Ferucci J. Bile duct obstruction in hepatocellular carcinoma (hepatoma)—clinical and cholangiographical characteristics: report of 6 cases and a review of the literature. *Radiology* 1979;130:7–13.
18. Roslyn JJ, Kuchenbecker S, Longmire WP, Tompkins RK. Floating tumor debris: a cause of intermittent biliary obstruction. *Arch Surg* 1984;119(11):1312–1315.
19. Wu CS, Wu SS, Chen PC, et al. Cholangiography of icteric type hepatoma. *Am J Gastroenterol* 1994;89(5):774–777.
20. Lau W, Leung K, Leung TW, et al. A logical approach to hepatocellular carcinoma presenting with jaundice. *Ann Surg* 1997;225(3):281–285.

21. Kew MC, Dusheiko GM. Paraneoplastic manifestations of hepatocellular carcinoma. In: Berk PD, Chalmers TC, eds. *Frontiers in Liver Disease.* New York, NY: Thieme-Stratton; 1981:305–319.
22. Spontaneous rupture of the liver. *BMJ* 1976;2:1278–1279.
23. Nagasue N, Inokuchi K. Spontaneous and traumatic rupture of hepatoma. *Br J Surg* 1979;66(4):248–250.
24. Chearanai O, Plengvanit U, Asavanich C, Damrongsak D, Sindhvananda K, Boonyapisit S. Spontaneous rupture of primary hepatoma: report of 63 cases with particular reference to the pathogenesis and rationale treatment by hepatic artery ligation. *Cancer* 1983;51(8):1532–1536.
25. Chen MF, Hwang TL, Jeng LB, Jan YY, Wang CS. Surgical treatment for spontaneous rupture of hepatocellular carcinoma. *Surg Gynecol Obstet* 1988;167(2):99–102.
26. Dewar GA, Griffin SM, Ku KW, Lau WY, Li AK. Management of bleeding liver tumours in Hong Kong. *Br J Surg* 1991;78(4):463–466.
27. Kew MC, Dos Santos HA, Sherlock S. Diagnosis of primary cancer of the liver. *Br Med J* 1971;4(784):408–411.
28. Ong GB, Taw JL. Spontaneous rupture of hepatocellular carcinoma. *Br Med J* 1972;4(833):146–149.
29. Miyamoto M, Sudo T, Kuyama T. Spontaneous rupture of hepatocellular carcinoma: a review of 172 Japanese cases. *Am J Gastroenterol* 1991;86(1):67–71.
30. Lau JWY, Leow CK. Surgical management (including liver transplantation). In: Leong A, Leiw CT, Lau JWY, eds. *Hepatocellular Carcinoma: Diagnosis, Investigation and Management.* London: Arnold; 1999:147–172.
31. Caturelli E, Bisceglia M, Fusilli S, Squillante MM, Castelvetere M, Siena DA. Cytological vs microhistological diagnosis of hepatocellular carcinoma: comparative accuracies in the same fine-needle biopsy specimen. *Dig Dis Sci* 1996;41(12):2326–2331.
32. Fong Y, Sun RL, Jarnagin W, Blumgart LH. An analysis of 412 cases of hepatocellular carcinoma at a Western center. *Ann Surg* 1999;229(6):790–799; discussion 799-800.
33. Bismuth H, Houssin D, Mazmanian G. Postoperative liver insufficiency: prevention and management. *World J Surg* 1983;7(4):505–510.
34. Wu MC, Chen H, Zhang XH, Yao XP, Yang JM. Primary hepatic carcinoma resection over 18 years. *Chin Med J (Engl)* 1980;93(10):723–728.
35. Tsuzuki T, Sugioka A, Ueda M, et al. Hepatic resection for hepatocellular carcinoma. *Surgery* 1990;107(5):511–520.
36. Chen MF, Hwang TL, Jeng LB, Jan YY, Wang CS, Chou FF. Hepatic resection in 120 patients with hepatocellular carcinoma. *Arch Surg* 1989;124(9):1025–1028.
37. Nagasue N, Kohno H, Chang YC, et al. Liver resection for hepatocellular carcinoma: results of 229 consecutive patients during 11 years. *Ann Surg* 1993;217(4):375–384.
38. Vauthey JN, Klimstra D, Franceschi D, et al. Factors affecting long-term outcome after hepatic resection for hepatocellular carcinoma. *Am J Surg* 1995;169(1):28–34; discussion -5.
39. Bismuth H, Chiche L, Castaing D. Surgical treatment of hepatocellular carcinomas in noncirrhotic liver: experience with 68 liver resections. *World J Surg* 1995;19(1):35–41.
40. Shimada M, Rikimaru T, Sugimachi K, et al. The importance of hepatic resection for hepatocellular carcinoma originating from nonfibrotic liver. *J Am Coll Surg* 2000;191(5):531–537.
41. Okuda K, Obata H, Nakajima Y, Ohtsuki T, Okazaki N, Ohnishi K. Prognosis of primary hepatocellular carcinoma. *Hepatology* 1984;4(1 suppl):3S–6S.
42. Franco D, Capussotti L, Smadja C, et al. Resection of hepatocellular carcinomas: results in 72 European patients with cirrhosis. *Gastroenterology* 1990;98(3):733–738.
43. Yamanaka N, Okamoto E, Toyosaka A, et al. Prognostic factors after hepatectomy for hepatocellular carcinomas: a univariate and multivariate analysis. *Cancer* 1990;65(5):1104–1110.
44. Fong Y, Blumgart LH. Liver resection for cancer. In: Zakim D, Boyer T, eds. *Hepatology: A Textbook of Liver Disease.* Philadelphia, Pa.: WB Saunders; 1996.
45. Ringe B, Pichlmayr R, Wittekind C, Tusch G. Surgical treatment of hepatocellular carcinoma: experience with liver resection and transplantation in 198 patients. *World J Surg* 1991;15(2):270–285.
46. Sasaki Y, Imaoka S, Masutani S, et al. Influence of coexisting cirrhosis on long-term prognosis after surgery in patients with hepatocellular carcinoma. *Surgery* 1992;112(3):515–521.
47. Takenaka K, Shimada M, Higashi H, et al. Liver resection for hepatocellular carcinoma in the elderly. *Arch Surg* 1994;129(8):846–850.
48. Suenaga M, Sugiura H, Kokuba Y, Uehara S, Kurumiya T. Repeated hepatic resection for recurrent hepatocellular carcinoma in eighteen cases. *Surgery* 1994;115(4):452–457.
49. Lai EC, Fan ST, Lo CM, Chu KM, Liu CL, Wong J. Hepatic resection for hepatocellular carcinoma: an audit of 343 patients. *Ann Surg* 1995;221(3):291–298.
50. Kawasaki S, Makuuchi M, Miyagawa S, et al. Results of hepatic resection for hepatocellular carcinoma. *World J Surg* 1995;19(1):31–34.
51. Takenaka K, Kawahara N, Yamamoto K, et al. Results of 280 liver resections for hepatocellular carcinoma. *Arch Surg* 1996;131(1):71–76.
52. Hanazaki K, Kajikawa S, Shimozawa N, et al. Survival and recurrence after hepatic resection of 386 consecutive patients with hepatocellular carcinoma. *J Am Coll Surg* 2000;191(4):381–388.
53. Okuda K, the Liver Study Group of Japan. Primary liver cancer in Japan. *Cancer* 1980;71:19–25.
54. Nagao T, Inoue S, Goto S, et al. Hepatic resection for hepatocellular carcinoma: clinical features and long-term prognosis. *Ann Surg* 1987;205(1):33–40.
55. Kanematsu T, Takenaka K, Matsumata T, Furuta T, Sugimachi K, Inokuchi K. Limited hepatic resection effective for selected cirrhotic patients with primary liver cancer. *Ann Surg* 1984;199(1):51–56.
56. Fuster J, Garcia-Valdecasas JC, Grande L, et al. Hepatocellular carcinoma and cirrhosis: results of surgical treatment in a European series. *Ann Surg* 1996;223(3):297–302.
57. Capussotti L, Borgonovo G, Bouzari H, Smadja C, Grange D, Franco D. Results of major hepatectomy for large primary liver cancer in patients with cirrhosis. *Br J Surg* 1994;81(3):427–431.
58. Fan ST, Lai EC, Lo CM, Ng IO, Wong J. Hospital mortality of major hepatectomy for hepatocellular carcinoma associated with cirrhosis. *Arch Surg* 1995;130(2):198–203.
59. Akriviadis EA, Llovet JM, Efremidis SC, et al. Hepatocellular carcinoma. *Br J Surg* 1998;85(10):1319–1331.
60. Bruix J, Llovet JM. Prognostic prediction and treatment strategy in hepatocellular carcinoma. *Hepatology* 2002;35(3):519–524.
61. Regimbeau JM, Farges O, Shen BY, Sauvanet A, Belghiti J. Is surgery for large hepatocellular carcinoma justified? *J Hepatol* 1999;31(6):1062–1068.
62. Poon RT, Fan ST, Wong J. Selection criteria for hepatic resection in patients with large hepatocellular carcinoma larger than 10 cm in diameter. *J Am Coll Surg* 2002;194(5):592–602.
62a. Poon RT, Fan ST, Lo CM, et al. Extended hepatic resection for hepatocellular carcinoma in patients with cirrhosis: is it justified? *Ann Surg* 2002;236(5):602–611.
63. Ng KK, Vauthey JN, Pawlik TM, et al. Is hepatic resection for large or multinodular hepatocellular carcinoma justified? Results from a multi-institutional database. *Ann Surg Oncol* 2005;12(5):364–373.
64. Pawlik TM, Poon RT, Abdalla EK, et al. Hepatectomy for hepatocellular carcinoma with major portal or hepatic vein invasion: results of a multicenter study. *Surgery* 2005;137(4):403–410.
65. Liu CL, Fan ST, Lo CM, Ng IO, Poon RT, Wong J. Hepatic resection for bilobar hepatocellular carcinoma: is it justified? *Arch Surg* 2003;138(1):100–104.
66. Bismuth H, Chiche L, Adam R, Castaing D, Diamond T, Dennison A. Liver resection versus transplantation for hepatocellular carcinoma in cirrhotic patients. *Ann Surg* 1993;218(2):145–151.
67. Bismuth H, Morino M, Sherlock D, et al. Primary treatment of hepatocellular carcinoma by arterial chemoembolization. *Am J Surg* 1992;163(4):387–394.
68. Hasegawa H, Yamazaki S, Makuuchi M, et al. Hepatectomies pour hepatocarcinome sur goie cirrhotique: schemes desionnels et principes de reanimation peri-operatoir : experience de 204 cas. *J Chir* 1987;124:425–431.
69. Noun R, Jagot P, Farges O, Sauvanet A, Belghiti J. High preoperative serum alanine transferase levels: effect on the risk of liver resection in child grade A cirrhotic patients. *World J Surg* 1997;21(4):390–394; discussion 5.
70. Lau WY, Leow CK, Li AKC. Hepatocellular carcinoma—current management and treatment. *Gastrointest Cancer* 1996;2:35–42.
71. Child CG, Turcotte JG. Surgery and portal hypertension. In: Child CG, ed. *The Liver and Portal Hypertension.* Philadelphia, Pa.: WB Saunders; 1964: 50–62.
72. Pugh RN, Murray-Lyon IM, Dawson JL, Pietroni MC, Williams R. Transection of the oesophagus for bleeding oesophageal varices. *Br J Surg* 1973; 60(8):646–649.
73. Lau H, Man K, Fan ST, Yu WC, Lo CM, Wong J. Evaluation of preoperative hepatic function in patients with hepatocellular carcinoma undergoing hepatectomy. *Br J Surg* 1997;84(9):1255–1259.
74. Redaelli CA, Dufour JF, Wagner M, et al. Preoperative galactose elimination capacity predicts complications and survival after hepatic resection. *Ann Surg* 2002;235(1):77–85.
75. Kubota K, Makuuchi M, Kusaka K, et al. Measurement of liver volume and hepatic functional reserve as a guide to decision-making in resectional surgery for hepatic tumors. *Hepatology* 1997;26(5):1176–1181.
76. Farges O, Belghiti J, Kianmanesh R, et al. Portal vein embolization before right hepatectomy: prospective clinical trial. *Ann Surg* 2003;237(2):208–217.
77. Melendez JA, Arslan V, Fischer ME, et al. Perioperative outcomes of major hepatic resections under low central venous pressure anesthesia: blood loss, blood transfusion, and the risk of postoperative renal dysfunction. *J Am Coll Surg* 1998;187(6):620–625.
78. Kim YI, Nakashima K, Tada I, Kawano K, Kobayashi M. Prolonged normothermic ischaemia of human cirrhotic liver during hepatectomy: a preliminary report. *Br J Surg* 1993;80(12):1566–1570.
79. Man K, Fan ST, Ng IO, Lo CM, Liu CL, Wong J. Prospective evaluation of Pringle maneuver in hepatectomy for liver tumors by a randomized study. *Ann Surg* 1997;226(6):704–711; discussion 11–13.

80. DeMatteo RP, Palese C, Jarnagin WR, Sun RL, Blumgart LH, Fong Y. Anatomic segmental hepatic resection is superior to wedge resection as an oncologic operation for colorectal liver metastases. *J Gastrointest Surg* 2000;4(2):178–184.

81. Lau WY, Arnold M, Leung NW, et al. Hepatic intra-arterial lipiodol ultrasound guided biopsy in the management of hepatocellular carcinoma. *Surg Oncol* 1993;2(2):119–124.

82. Yamanaka N, Okamoto E, Fujihara S, et al. Do the tumor cells of hepatocellular carcinomas dislodge into the portal venous stream during hepatic resection? *Cancer* 1992;70(9):2263–2267.

83. Sitzmann JV, Abrams R. Improved survival for hepatocellular cancer with combination surgery and multimodality treatment. *Ann Surg* 1993;217(2):149–154.

84. Lau WY, Leung KL, Leung TW, Liew CT, Chan M, Li AK. Resection of hepatocellular carcinoma with diaphragmatic invasion. *Br J Surg* 1995;82(2):264–266.

85. Nagasue N, Yukaya H, Ogawa Y, Kohno H, Nakamura T. Human liver regeneration after major hepatic resection: a study of normal liver and livers with chronic hepatitis and cirrhosis. *Ann Surg* 1987;206(1):30–39.

86. Takenaka K, Kanematsu T, Fukuzawa K, Sugimachi K. Can hepatic failure after surgery for hepatocellular carcinoma in cirrhotic patients be prevented? *World J Surg* 1990;14(1):123–127.

87. Tanabe G, Sakamoto M, Akazawa K, et al. Intraoperative risk factors associated with hepatic resection. *Br J Surg* 1995;82(9):1262–1265.

88. Fan ST, Lo CM, Liu CL, et al. Hepatectomy for hepatocellular carcinoma: toward zero hospital deaths. *Ann Surg* 1999;229(3):322–330.

89. Torzilli G, Makuuchi M, Inoue K, et al. No-mortality liver resection for hepatocellular carcinoma in cirrhotic and noncirrhotic patients: is there a way? A prospective analysis of our approach. *Arch Surg* 1999;134(9):984–992.

90. Ker CG, Chen HY, Juan CC, et al. Laparoscopic subsegmentectomy for hepatocellular carcinoma with cirrhosis. *Hepatogastroenterology* 2000;47(35):1260–1263.

90a. Poon RT, Fan ST, Lo CM, et al. Improving survival results after resection of hepatocellular carcinoma: a prospective study of 377 patients over 10 years. *Ann Surg* 2001;234(1):63–70.

91. Fan ST, Ng IO, Poon RT, Lo CM, Liu CL, Wong J. Hepatectomy for hepatocellular carcinoma: the surgeon's role in long-term survival. *Arch Surg* 1999;134(10):1124–1130.

92. Makuuchi M, Takayama T, Kubota K, et al. Hepatic resection for hepatocellular carcinoma—Japanese experience. *Hepatogastroenterology* 1998;45(suppl 3):1267–1274.

93. Lise M, Bacchetti S, Da Pian P, Nitti D, Pilati PL, Pigato P. Prognostic factors affecting long term outcome after liver resection for hepatocellular carcinoma: results in a series of 100 Italian patients. *Cancer* 1998;82(6):1028–1036.

94. Grazi GL, Ercolani G, Pierangeli F, et al. Improved results of liver resection for hepatocellular carcinoma on cirrhosis give the procedure added value. *Ann Surg* 2001;234(1):71–78.

95. Capussotti L, Muratore A, Amisano M, Polastri R, Bouzari H, Massucco P. Liver resection for hepatocellular carcinoma on cirrhosis: analysis of mortality, morbidity and survival—a European single center experience. *Eur J Surg Oncol* 2005;31(9):986–993.

96. Tung-Ping Poon R, Fan ST, Wong J. Risk factors, prevention, and management of postoperative recurrence after resection of hepatocellular carcinoma. *Ann Surg* 2000;232(1):10–24.

96a. Poon RT, Fan ST, Lo CM, Liu CL, Wong J. Intrahepatic recurrence after curative resection of hepatocellular carcinoma: long-term results of treatment and prognostic factors. *Ann Surg* 1999;229(2):216–222.

96b. Poon RT, Fan ST, Yu WC, Lam BK, Chan FY, Wong J. A prospective longitudinal study of quality of life after resection of hepatocellular carcinoma. *Arch Surg* 2001;136(6):693–699.

97. Friedman MA. Primary hepatocellular cancer—present results and future prospects. *Int J Radiat Oncol Biol Phys* 1983;9(12):1841–1850.

98. Okuda K, Ohtsuki T, Obata H, et al. Natural history of hepatocellular carcinoma and prognosis in relation to treatment: study with 850 patients. *Cancer* 1985;56(4):918–928.

99. Dewar GA, Griffin SM, Ku KW, et al. Hepatocellular carcinoma. *Ann Intern Med* 1991;108:390–401.

100. Lai EC, Choi TK, Tong SW, Ong GB, Wong J. Treatment of unresectable hepatocellular carcinoma: results of a randomized controlled trial. *World J Surg* 1986;10(3):501–509.

101. Carr BI, Zajko A, Bron K, Orons P, Sammon J, Baron R. Phase II study of Spherex (degradable starch microspheres) injected into the hepatic artery in conjunction with doxorubicin and cisplatin in the treatment of advanced-stage hepatocellular carcinoma: interim analysis. *Semin Oncol* 1997;24(2 suppl 6):S6–97–S6–9.

102. Lai EC, Lo CM, Fan ST, Liu CL, Wong J. Postoperative adjuvant chemotherapy after curative resection of hepatocellular carcinoma: a randomized controlled trial. *Arch Surg* 1998;133(2):183–188.

103. Izumi R, Shimizu K, Iyobe T, et al. Postoperative adjuvant hepatic arterial infusion of lipiodol containing anticancer drugs in patients with hepatocellular carcinoma. *Hepatology* 1994;20(2):295–301.

104. Wu CC, Ho YZ, Ho WL, Wu TC, Liu TJ, P'Eng FK. Preoperative transcatheter arterial chemoembolization for resectable large hepatocellular carcinoma: a reappraisal. *Br J Surg* 1995;82(1):122–126.

105. Huang YH, Wu JC, Lui WY, et al. Prospective case-controlled trial of adjuvant chemotherapy after resection of hepatocellular carcinoma. *World J Surg* 2000;24(5):551–555.

106. Ono T, Yamanoi A, Nazmy El Assal O, Kohno H, Nagasue N. Adjuvant chemotherapy after resection of hepatocellular carcinoma causes deterioration of long–term prognosis in cirrhotic patients: metaanalysis of three randomized controlled trials. *Cancer* 2001;91(12):2378–2385.

107. Lau WY, Leung TW, Ho SK, et al. Adjuvant intra-arterial iodine-131-labelled lipiodol for resectable hepatocellular carcinoma: a prospective randomised trial. *Lancet* 1999;353(9155):797–801.

108. Muto Y, Moriwaki H, Ninomiya M, et al. Prevention of second primary tumors by an acyclic retinoid, polyprenoic acid, in patients with hepatocellular carcinoma. Hepatoma Prevention Study Group. *N Engl J Med* 1996;334(24):1561–1567.

109. Kubo S, Nishiguchi S, Hirohashi K, et al. Effects of long-term postoperative interferon-alpha therapy on intrahepatic recurrence after resection of hepatitis C virus-related hepatocellular carcinoma: a randomized, controlled trial. *Ann Intern Med* 2001;134(10):963–967.

110. Takayama T, Sekine T, Makuuchi M, et al. Adoptive immunotherapy to lower postsurgical recurrence rates of hepatocellular carcinoma: a randomised trial. *Lancet* 2000;356(9232):802–807.

111. Penn I. Hepatic transplantation for primary and metastatic cancers of the liver. *Surgery* 1991;110(4):726–734; discussion 34–35.

112. Mazzaferro V, Regalia E, Doci R, et al. Liver transplantation for the treatment of small hepatocellular carcinomas in patients with cirrhosis. *N Engl J Med* 1996;334(11):693–699.

113. Dmitrewski J, El-Gazzaz G, McMaster P. Hepatocellular cancer: resection or transplantation. *J Hepatobiliary Pancreat Surg* 1998;5(1):18–23.

114. Michel J, Suc B, Montpeyroux F, et al. Liver resection or transplantation for hepatocellular carcinoma? Retrospective analysis of 215 patients with cirrhosis. *J Hepatol* 1997;26(6):1274–1280.

115. Figueras J, Jaurrieta E, Valls C, et al. Resection or transplantation for hepatocellular carcinoma in cirrhotic patients: outcomes based on indicated treatment strategy. *J Am Coll Surg* 2000;190(5):580–587.

116. Mor E, Kaspa RT, Sheiner P, Schwartz M. Treatment of hepatocellular carcinoma associated with cirrhosis in the era of liver transplantation. *Ann Intern Med* 1998;129(8):643–653.

117. Bismuth H, Majno PE, Adam R. Liver transplantation for hepatocellular carcinoma. *Semin Liver Dis* 1999;19(3):311–322.

118. Yao FY, Ferrell L, Bass NM, et al. Liver transplantation for hepatocellular carcinoma: expansion of the tumor size limits does not adversely impact survival. *Hepatology* 2001;33(6):1394–1403.

119. Fernandez JA, Robles R, Marin C, et al. Can we expand the indications for liver transplantation among hepatocellular carcinoma patients with increased tumor size? *Transplant Proc* 2003;35(5):1818–1820.

120. Otto G, Heuschen U, Hofmann WJ, Krumm G, Hinz U, Herfarth C. Survival and recurrence after liver transplantation versus liver resection for hepatocellular carcinoma: a retrospective analysis. *Ann Surg* 1998;227(3):424–432.

121. Llovet JM, Fuster J, Bruix J. Intention-to-treat analysis of surgical treatment for early hepatocellular carcinoma: resection versus transplantation. *Hepatology* 1999;30(6):1434–1440.

122. Figueras J, Ibanez L, Ramos E, et al. Selection criteria for liver transplantation in early-stage hepatocellular carcinoma with cirrhosis: results of a multicenter study. *Liver Transpl* 2001;7(10):877–883.

123. Jonas S, Bechstein WO, Steinmuller T, et al. Vascular invasion and histopathologic grading determine outcome after liver transplantation for hepatocellular carcinoma in cirrhosis. *Hepatology* 2001;33(5):1080–1086.

124. O'Grady JG, Polson RJ, Rolles K, Calne RY, Williams R. Liver transplantation for malignant disease: results in 93 consecutive patients. *Ann Surg* 1988;207(4):373–379.

125. Ringe B, Wittekind C, Bechstein WO, Bunzendahl H, Pichlmayr R. The role of liver transplantation in hepatobiliary malignancy: a retrospective analysis of 95 patients with particular regard to tumor stage and recurrence. *Ann Surg* 1989;209(1):88–98.

126. Yokoyama I, Todo S, Iwatsuki S, Starzl TE. Liver transplantation in the treatment of primary liver cancer. *Hepatogastroenterology* 1990;37(2):188–193.

127. Iwatsuki S, Starzl TE, Sheahan DG, et al. Hepatic resection versus transplantation for hepatocellular carcinoma. *Ann Surg* 1991;214(3):221–228; discussion 8–9.

128. Pichlmayr R, Weimann A, Steinhoff G, Ringe B. Liver transplantation for hepatocellular carcinoma: clinical results and future aspects. *Cancer Chemother Pharmacol* 1992;31(suppl):S157–S161.

129. Dalgic A, Mirza DF, Gunson BK, et al. Role of total hepatectomy and transplantation in hepatocellular carcinoma. *Transplant Proc* 1994;26(6):3564–3565.

130. Farmer DG, Rosove MH, Shaked A, Busuttil RW. Current treatment modalities for hepatocellular carcinoma. *Ann Surg* 1994;219(3):236–247.

131. Selby R, Kadry Z, Carr B, Tzakis A, Madariaga JR, Iwatsuki S. Liver transplantation for hepatocellular carcinoma. *World J Surg* 1995;19(1):53–58.

132. Kishi K, Shikata T, Hirohashi S, Hasegawa H, Yamazaki S, Makuuchi M. Hepatocellular carcinoma: a clinical and pathologic analysis of 57 hepatectomy cases. *Cancer* 1983;51(3):542–548.

133. Schwartz ME, Sung M, Mor E, et al. A multidisciplinary approach to hepatocellular carcinoma in patients with cirrhosis. *J Am Coll Surg* 1995; 180(5):596–603.

134. Iwatsuki S, Dvorchik I, Marsh JW, et al. Liver transplantation for hepatocellular carcinoma: a proposal of a prognostic scoring system. *J Am Coll Surg* 2000;191(4):389–394.

135. Klintmalm GB. Liver transplantation for hepatocellular carcinoma: a registry report of the impact of tumor characteristics on outcome. *Ann Surg* 1998;228(4):479–490.

136. Venook AP, Ferrell LD, Roberts JP, et al. Liver transplantation for hepatocellular carcinoma: results with preoperative chemoembolization. *Liver Transpl Surg* 1995;1(4):242–248.

137. Pichlmayr R, Weimann A, Oldhafer KJ, Schlitt HJ, Tusch G, Raab R. Appraisal of transplantation for malignant tumours of the liver with special reference to early stage hepatocellular carcinoma. *Eur J Surg Oncol* 1998;24(1):60–67.

138. Yamamoto J, Iwatsuki S, Kosuge T, et al. Should hepatomas be treated with hepatic resection or transplantation? *Cancer* 1999;86(7):1151–1158.

139. Bigourdan JM, Jaeck D, Meyer N, et al. Small hepatocellular carcinoma in child A cirrhotic patients: hepatic resection versus transplantation. *Liver Transpl* 2003;9(5):513–520.

140. Shabahang M, Franceschi D, Yamashiki N, et al. Comparison of hepatic resection and hepatic transplantation in the treatment of hepatocellular carcinoma among cirrhotic patients. *Ann Surg Oncol* 2002;9(9):881–886.

141. Margarit C, Escartin A, Castells L, Vargas V, Allende E, Bilbao I. Resection for hepatocellular carcinoma is a good option in Child-Turcotte-Pugh class A patients with cirrhosis who are eligible for liver transplantation. *Liver Transpl* 2005;11(10):1242–1251.

142. Yao FY, Bass NM, Nikolai B, et al. Liver transplantation for hepatocellular carcinoma: analysis of survival according to the intention-to-treat principle and dropout from the waiting list. *Liver Transpl* 2002;8(10): 873–883.

143. Maddala YK, Stadheim L, Andrews JC, et al. Drop-out rates of patients with hepatocellular cancer listed for liver transplantation: outcome with chemoembolization. *Liver Transpl* 2004;10(3):449–455.

144. Pierie JP, Muzikansky A, Tanabe KK, Ott MJ. The outcome of surgical resection versus assignment to the liver transplant waiting list for hepatocellular carcinoma. *Ann Surg Oncol* 2005;12(7):552–560.

145. Manjo PE, Sarasin FP, Mentha G, Hadengue A. Primary liver resection and salvage transplantation or primary liver transplantation in patients with single, small hepatocellular carcinoma and preserved liver function: an outcome-oriented decision analysis. *Hepatology* 2000;31(4):899–906.

145a. Poon RT, Fan ST, Lo CM, Liu CL, Wong J. Long-term survival and pattern of recurrence after resection of small hepatocellular carcinoma in patients with preserved liver function: implications for a strategy of salvage transplantation. *Ann Surg* 2002;235(3):373–382.

146. Cha CH, Ruo L, Fong Y, et al. Resection of hepatocellular carcinoma in patients otherwise eligible for transplantation. *Ann Surg* 2003;238(3):315–321; discussion 21–23.

147. Adam R, Azoulay D, Castaing D, et al. Liver resection as a bridge to transplantation for hepatocellular carcinoma on cirrhosis: a reasonable strategy? *Ann Surg* 2003;238(4):508–518; discussion 18–19.

148. Belghiti J, Cortes A, Abdalla EK, et al. Resection prior to liver transplantation for hepatocellular carcinoma. *Ann Surg* 2003;238(6):885–892; discussion 92–93.

149. Fan ST, Lo CM, Liu CL. Technical refinement in adult-to-adult living donor liver transplantation using right lobe graft. *Ann Surg* 2000;231(1): 126–131.

150. Lo CM, Fan ST, Liu CL, Chan SC, Wong J. The role and limitation of living donor liver transplantation for hepatocellular carcinoma. *Liver Transpl* 2004;10(3):440–447.

151. Kaihara S, Kiuchi T, Ueda M, et al. Living-donor liver transplantation for hepatocellular carcinoma. *Transplantation* 2003;75(3 suppl):S37–S40.

152. Brown RS, Jr., Russo MW, Lai M, et al. A survey of liver transplantation from living adult donors in the United States. *N Engl J Med* 2003;348(9):818–825.

153. Huang GT, Lee PH, Tsang YM, et al. Percutaneous ethanol injection versus surgical resection for the treatment of small hepatocellular carcinoma: a prospective study. *Ann Surg* 2005;242(1):36–42.

154. Chen MS, Li JQ, Zheng Y, et al. A prospective randomized trial comparing percutaneous local ablative therapy and partial hepatectomy for small hepatocellular carcinoma. *Ann Surg* 2006;243(3):321–328.

155. Fontana RJ, Hamidullah H, Nghiem H, et al. Percutaneous radiofrequency thermal ablation of hepatocellular carcinoma: a safe and effective bridge to liver transplantation. *Liver Transpl* 2002;8(12):1165–1174.

156. Vilana R, Bruix J, Bru C, Ayuso C, Sole M, Rodes J. Tumor size determines the efficacy of percutaneous ethanol injection for the treatment of small hepatocellular carcinoma. *Hepatology* 1992;16(2):353–357.

157. Ebara M, Ohto M, Sugiura N, et al. Percutaneous ethanol injection for the treatment of small hepatocellular carcinoma: study of 95 patients. *J Gastroenterol Hepatol* 1990;5(6):616–626.

158. Livraghi T, Bolondi L, Lazzaroni S, et al. Percutaneous ethanol injection in the treatment of hepatocellular carcinoma in cirrhosis: a study on 207 patients. *Cancer* 1992;69(4):925–929.

159. Yu JS, Burwick JA, Dranoff G, Breakefield XO. Gene therapy for metastatic brain tumors by vaccination with granulocyte-macrophage colony-stimulating factor-transduced tumor cells. *Hum Gene Ther* 1997;8(9):1065–1072.

160. Isobe H, Sakai H, Imari Y, Ikeda M, Shiomichi S, Nawata H. Intratumor ethanol injection therapy for solitary minute hepatocellular carcinoma: a study of 37 patients. *J Clin Gastroenterol* 1994;18(2):122–126.

161. Livraghi T, Lazzaroni S, Meloni F, Torzilli G, Vettori C. Intralesional ethanol in the treatment of unresectable liver cancer. *World J Surg* 1995; 19(6):801–806.

161a. Poon RT, Fan ST, Tsang FH, Wong J. Locoregional therapies for hepatocellular carcinoma: a critical review from the surgeon's perspective. *Ann Surg* 2002;235(4):466–486.

162. Zhou XD. Improved cryosurgery for primary liver cancer. *Zhonghua Zhong Liu Za Zhi* 1992;14(1):61–63.

163. Tang ZY, Yu YQ, Zhou XD, et al. Cytoreduction and sequential resection: a hope for unresectable primary liver cancer. *J Surg Oncol* 1991;47(1):27–31.

164. Rossi S, Di Stasi M, Buscarini E, et al. Percutaneous RF interstitial thermal ablation in the treatment of hepatic cancer. *AJR Am J Roentgenol* 1996;167(3):759–768.

165. Rossi S, Buscarini E, Garbagnati F, et al. Percutaneous treatment of small hepatic tumors by an expandable RF needle electrode. *AJR Am J Roentgenol* 1998;170(4):1015–1022.

166. Curley SA, Izzo F, Ellis LM, Nicolas Vauthey J, Vallone P. Radiofrequency ablation of hepatocellular cancer in 110 patients with cirrhosis. *Ann Surg* 2000;232(3):381–391.

167. Nicoli N, Casaril A, Marchiori L, et al. Intraoperative and percutaneous radiofrequency thermal ablation in the treatment of hepatocellular carcinoma. *Chir Ital* 2000;52(1):29–40.

168. Bowles BJ, Machi J, Limm WM, et al. Safety and efficacy of radiofrequency thermal ablation in advanced liver tumors. *Arch Surg* 2001;136(8):864–869.

169. Buscarini L, Buscarini E, DiStasi M, Vallisa D, Quaretti P, Rocca A. Percutaneous radiofrequency ablation of small hepatocellular carcinoma: long-term results. *Eur Radiol* 2001;11(6):914–921.

170. Guglielmi A, Ruzzenente A, Battocchia A, Tonon A, Fracastoro G, Cordiano C. Radiofrequency ablation of hepatocellular carcinoma in cirrhotic patients. *Hepatogastroenterology* 2003;50(50):480–484.

171. Giovannini M, Moutardier V, Danisi C, Bories E, Pesenti C, Delpero JR. Treatment of hepatocellular carcinoma using percutaneous radiofrequency thermoablation: results and outcomes in 56 patients. *J Gastrointest Surg* 2003;7(6):791–796.

172. Vivarelli M, Guglielmi A, Ruzzenente A, et al. Surgical resection versus percutaneous radiofrequency ablation in the treatment of hepatocellular carcinoma on cirrhotic liver. *Ann Surg* 2004;240(1):102–107.

173. Mulier S, Mulier P, Ni Y, et al. Complications of radiofrequency coagulation of liver tumours. *Br J Surg* 2002;89(10):1206–1222.

173a. Poon RT, Ng KK, Lam CM, et al. Learning curve for radiofrequency ablation of liver tumors: prospective analysis of initial 100 patients in a tertiary institution. *Ann Surg* 2004;239(4):441–449.

173b. Curley SA, Marra P, Beaty K, et al. Early and late complications after radiofrequency ablation of malignant liver tumors in 608 patients. *Ann Surg* 2004;239(4):450–458.

174. Lin SM, Lin CJ, Lin CC, Hsu CW, Chen YC. Radiofrequency ablation improves prognosis compared with ethanol injection for hepatocellular carcinoma < or = 4 cm. *Gastroenterology* 2004;127(6):1714–1723.

175. Shiina S, Teratani T, Obi S, et al. A randomized controlled trial of radiofrequency ablation with ethanol injection for small hepatocellular carcinoma. *Gastroenterology* 2005;129(1):122–130.

176. Goldberg SN, Hahn PF, Tanabe KK, et al. Percutaneous radiofrequency tissue ablation: does perfusion-mediated tissue cooling limit coagulation necrosis? *J Vasc Interv Radiol* 1998;9(1 pt 1):101–111.

177. Livraghi T, Goldberg SN, Monti F, et al. Saline-enhanced radio-frequency tissue ablation in the treatment of liver metastases. *Radiology* 1997; 202(1):205–210.

178. el-Domeiri AA, Huvos AG, Goldsmith HS, Foote FW, Jr. Primary malignant tumors of the liver. *Cancer* 1971;27(1):7–11.

179. Phillips R, Murikami K. Primary neoplasms of the liver: results of radiation therapy. *Cancer* 1960;13:714–720.

180. Cochrane AM, Murray-Lyon IM, Brinkley DM, Williams R. Quadruple chemotherapy versus radiotherapy in treatment of primary hepatocellular carcinoma. *Cancer* 1977;40(2):609–614.

181. Friedman IH, Mehler G, Ginzburg L. Pyloroduodenal obstruction due to carcinoma of the gallbladder. *Am J Gastroenterol* 1969;52(3):224–230.

182. Abrams RA, Pajak TF, Haulk TL, Flam M, Asbell SO. Survival results among patients with alpha-fetoprotein-positive, unresectable hepatocellular carcinoma: analysis of three sequential treatments of the RTOG and Johns Hopkins Oncology Center. *Cancer J Sci Am* 1998;4(3):178–184.

183. Order S, Pajak T, Leibel S, et al. A randomized prospective trial comparing full dose chemotherapy to 131I antiferritin: an RTOG study. *Int J Radiat Oncol Biol Phys* 1991;20(5):953–963.

184. Abrams RA, Cardinale RM, Enger C, et al. Influence of prognostic groupings and treatment results in the management of unresectable hepatoma: experience with cisplatinum-based chemoradiotherapy in 76 patients. *Int J Radiat Oncol Biol Phys* 1997;39(5):1077–1085.

184a. Gray B, Van Hazel G, Hope M, et al. Randomized trial of SIR-Spheres plus chemotherapy vs. chemotherapy alone for treating patients with liver metastases from primary large bowel cancer. *Ann Oncol* 2001;12(12):1711–1720.

184b. Kennedy AS, Coldwell D, Nutting C, et al. Resin (90)Y-microsphere brachytherapy for unresectable colorectal liver metastases: modern USA experience. *Inter J of Rad Oncol Biol Phys* 2006;65(2):412–425.

185. Shepherd FA, Rotstein LE, Houle S, Yip TC, Paul K, Sniderman KW. A phase I dose escalation trial of yttrium-90 microspheres in the treatment of primary hepatocellular carcinoma. *Cancer* 1992;70(9):2250–2254.

186. Tian JH, Xu BX, Zhang JM, Dong BW, Liang P, Wang XD. Ultrasound-guided internal radiotherapy using yttrium-90-glass microspheres for liver malignancies. *J Nucl Med* 1996;37(6):958–963.

187. Lau WY, Ho S, Leung TW, et al. Selective internal radiation therapy for nonresectable hepatocellular carcinoma with intraarterial infusion of 90yttrium microspheres. *Int J Radiat Oncol Biol Phys* 1998;40(3):583–592.

188. Ho S, Lau WY, Leung TW, Johnson PJ. Internal radiation therapy for patients with primary or metastatic hepatic cancer: a review. *Cancer* 1998;83(9):1894–1907.

189. Ho S, Lau WY, Leung TW, Chan M, Johnson PJ, Li AK. Clinical evaluation of the partition model for estimating radiation doses from yttrium-90 microspheres in the treatment of hepatic cancer. *Eur J Nucl Med* 1997;24(3):293–298.

190. Leung TW, Lau WY, Ho SK, et al. Radiation pneumonitis after selective internal radiation treatment with intraarterial 90yttrium-microspheres for inoperable hepatic tumors. *Int J Radiat Oncol Biol Phys* 1995;33(4):919–924.

191. Leung WT, Lau WY, Ho S, et al. Selective internal radiation therapy with intra-arterial iodine-131-lipiodol in inoperable hepatocellular carcinoma. *J Nucl Med* 1994;35(8):1313–1318.

192. Raoul JL, Retagne JF, Caucanus JP, et al. Internal radiation therapy for hepatocellular carcinoma. Results of a French multicenter phase II trial of transarterial injection of iodine 131-labeled lipiodol. *Cancer* 1992;69(2):346–352.

193. Raoul JL, Guyader D, Bretagne JF, et al. Prospective randomized trial of chemoembolization versus intra-arterial injection of 131I-labeled-iodized oil in the treatment of hepatocellular carcinoma. *Hepatology* 1997;26(5):1156–1161.

194. Raoul JL, Guyader D, Bretagne JF, et al. Randomized controlled trial for hepatocellular carcinoma with portal vein thrombosis: intra-arterial iodine-131-iodized oil versus medical support. *J Nucl Med* 1994;35(11):1782–1787.

195. Matsuura M, Nakajima N, Arai K, Ito K. The usefulness of radiation therapy for hepatocellular carcinoma. *Hepatogastroenterology* 1998;45(21):791–796.

196. Seong J, Keum KC, Han KH, et al. Combined transcatheter arterial chemoembolization and local radiotherapy of unresectable hepatocellular carcinoma. *Int J Radiat Oncol Biol Phys* 1999;43(2):393–397.

197. Ten Haken RK, Lawrence TS, McShan DL, Tesser RJ, Fraass BA, Lichter AS. Technical considerations in the use of 3-D beam arrangements in the abdomen. *Radiother Oncol* 1991;22(1):19–28.

198. Ben-Josef E, Normolle D, Ensminger WD, et al. Phase II trial of high-dose conformal radiation therapy with concurrent hepatic artery floxuridine for unresectable intrahepatic malignancies. *J Clin Oncol* 2005;23(34):8739–8747.

199. Dawson LA, Normolle D, Balter J, et al. Analysis of radiation-induced liver disease using the Lyman NTCP model. *Int J Radiat Oncol Biol Phys* 2002;53:810–821.

200. McGinn CJ, Ten Haken RK, Ensminger WD, Walker S, Wang S, Lawrence TS. Treatment of intrahepatic cancers with radiation doses based on a normal tissue complication probability model. *J Clin Oncol* 1998;16(6):2246–2252.

201. Herfarth KK, Debus J, Lohr F, et al. Stereotactic single-dose radiation therapy of liver tumors: results of a phase I/II trial. *J Clin Oncol* 2001;19(1):164–170.

201a. Shioyama Y, NaKamura K, Anai S, et al. Stereotactic radiotherapy for lung and liver tumors using a body cast system: setup accuracy and preliminary clinical outcome. *Radiation Medicine* 2005;23(6):407–413.

202. Chiba T, Tokuuye K, Matsuzaki Y, et al. Proton beam therapy for hepatocellular carcinoma: a retrospective review of 162 patients. *Clin Cancer Res* 2005;11(10):3799–3805.

203. Yamasaki SA, Marn CS, Francis IR, Robertson JM, Lawrence TS. High-dose localized radiation therapy for treatment of hepatic malignant tumors: CT findings and their relation to radiation hepatitis. *AJR Am J Roentgenol* 1995;165(1):79–84.

204. Ohara K, Okumura T, Tsuji H, et al. Radiation tolerance of cirrhotic livers in relation to the preserved functional capacity: analysis of patients with hepatocellular carcinoma treated by focused proton beam radiotherapy. *Int J Radiat Oncol Biol Phys* 1997;38(2):367–372.

205. Park JG, Lee SK, Hong IG, et al. MDR1 gene expression: its effect on drug resistance to doxorubicin in human hepatocellular carcinoma cell lines. *J Natl Cancer Inst* 1994;86(9):700–705.

206. Johnson PJ, Williams R, Thomas H, Sherlock S, Murray-Lyon IM. Induction of remission in hepatocellular carcinoma with doxorubicin. *Lancet* 1978;1(8072):1006–1009.

207. Choi TK, Lee NW, Wong J. Chemotherapy for advanced hepatocellular carcinoma: Adriamycin versus quadruple chemotherapy. *Cancer* 1984;53(3):401–405.

208. Lai CL, Wu PC, Chan GC, Lok AS, Lin HJ. Doxorubicin versus no antitumor therapy in inoperable hepatocellular carcinoma: a prospective randomized trial. *Cancer* 1988;62(3):479–483.

209. Falkson G, MacIntyre JM, Moertel CG, Johnson LA, Scherman RC. Primary liver cancer: an Eastern Cooperative Oncology Group Trial. *Cancer* 1984;54(6):970–977.

210. Leung TW, Patt YZ, Lau WY, et al. Complete pathological remission is possible with systemic combination chemotherapy for inoperable hepatocellular carcinoma. *Clin Cancer Res* 1999;5(7):1676–1681.

211. Patt YZ, Hoque A, Roh M, et al. Durable clinical and pathologic response of hepatocellular carcinoma to systemic and hepatic arterial administration of Platinol, recombinant interferon alpha 2B, doxorubicin, and 5-fluorouracil: a communication. *Am J Clin Oncol* 1999;22(2):209–213.

212. Leung TW, Tang AM, Zee B, et al. Factors predicting response and survival in 149 patients with unresectable hepatocellular carcinoma treated by combination cisplatin, interferon-alpha, doxorubicin and 5-fluorouracil chemotherapy. *Cancer* 2002;94(2):421–427.

213. Yeo W, Mok TS, Zee B, et al. A randomized phase III study of doxorubicin versus cisplatin/interferon alpha-2b/doxorubicin/fluorouracil (PIAF) combination chemotherapy for unresectable hepatocellular carcinoma. *J Natl Cancer Inst* 2005;97(20):1532–1538.

214. Nishiguchi S, Kuroki T, Nakatani S, et al. Randomised trial of effects of interferon-alpha on incidence of hepatocellular carcinoma in chronic active hepatitis C with cirrhosis. *Lancet* 1995;346(8982):1051–1055.

215. Mazzella G, Accogli E, Sottili S, et al. Alpha interferon treatment may prevent hepatocellular carcinoma in HCV-related liver cirrhosis. *J Hepatol* 1996;24(2):141–147.

216. Lin SM, Lin CJ, Hsu CW, et al. Prospective randomized controlled study of interferon-alpha in preventing hepatocellular carcinoma recurrence after medical ablation therapy for primary tumors. *Cancer* 2004;100(2):376–382.

217. The Gastrointestinal Tumor Study Group. A prospective trial of recombinant human interferon alpha 2B in previously untreated patients with hepatocellular carcinoma. *Cancer* 1990;66(1):135–139.

217a. Patt YZ, Hassan MM, Lozano RD, et al. Phase II trial of systemic continuous fluorouracil and subcutaneous recombinant interferon Alfa-2b for treatment of hepatocellular carcinoma. *J Clin Oncol* 2003;21(3):421–427.

218. Patt YZ, Yoffe B, Charnsangavej C, et al. Low serum alpha-fetoprotein level in patients with hepatocellular carcinoma as a predictor of response to 5-FU and interferon-alpha-2b. *Cancer* 1993;72(9):2574–2582.

219. Stuart K, Tessitore J, Huberman M. 5-Fluorouracil and alpha-interferon in hepatocellular carcinoma. *Am J Clin Oncol* 1996;19(2):136–139.

220. Kardinal CG, Moertel CG, Wieand HS, et al. Combined doxorubicin and alpha-interferon therapy of advanced hepatocellular carcinoma. *Cancer* 1993;71(7):2187–2190.

221. Colleoni M, Buzzoni R, Bajetta E, et al. A phase II study of mitoxantrone combined with beta-interferon in unresectable hepatocellular carcinoma. *Cancer* 1993;72(11):3196–3201.

222. Lai CL, Wu PC, Lok AS, et al. Recombinant alpha 2 interferon is superior to doxorubicin for inoperable hepatocellular carcinoma: a prospective randomised trial. *Br J Cancer* 1989;60(6):928–933.

223. Lai CL, Lau JY, Wu PC, et al. Recombinant interferon-alpha in inoperable hepatocellular carcinoma: a randomized controlled trial. *Hepatology* 1993;17(3):389–394.

224. Llovet JM, Sala M, Castells L, et al. Randomized controlled trial of interferon treatment for advanced hepatocellular carcinoma. *Hepatology* 2000;31(1):54–58.

225. Friedman MA, Demanes DJ, Hoffman PG, Jr. Hepatomas: hormone receptors and therapy. *Am J Med* 1982;73(3):362–366.

226. Engstrom PF, Levin B, Moertel CG, Schutt A. A phase II trial of tamoxifen in hepatocellular carcinoma. *Cancer* 1990;65(12):2641–2643.

227. Melia WM, Johnson PJ, Williams R. Controlled clinical trial of doxorubicin and tamoxifen versus doxorubicin alone in hepatocellular carcinoma. *Cancer Treat Rep* 1987;71(12):1213–1216.

228. Uchino J, Une Y, Sato Y, Gondo H, Nakajima Y, Sato N. Chemohormonal therapy of unresectable hepatocellular carcinoma. *Am J Clin Oncol* 1993;16(3):206–209.

229. Grimaldi C, Bleiberg H, Gay F, et al. Evaluation of antiandrogen therapy in unresectable hepatocellular carcinoma: results of a European Organization for Research and Treatment of Cancer multicentric double-blind trial. *J Clin Oncol* 1998;16(2):411–417.

230. Riestra S, Rodriguez M, Delgado M, et al. Tamoxifen does not improve survival of patients with advanced hepatocellular carcinoma. *J Clin Gastroenterol* 1998;26(3):200–203.

231. Castells A, Bruix J, Bru C, et al. Treatment of hepatocellular carcinoma with tamoxifen: a double-blind placebo-controlled trial in 120 patients. *Gastroenterology* 1995;109(3):917–922.

232. Farinati F, De Maria N, Fornasiero A, et al. Prospective controlled trial with antiestrogen drug tamoxifen in patients with unresectable hepatocellular carcinoma. *Dig Dis Sci* 1992;37(5):659–662.

233. Martinez Cerezo FJ, Tomas A, Donoso L, et al. Controlled trial of tamoxifen in patients with advanced hepatocellular carcinoma. *J Hepatol* 1994;20(6):702–706.

234. Manesis EK, Giannoulis G, Zoumboulis P, Vafiadou I, Hadziyannis SJ. Treatment of hepatocellular carcinoma with combined suppression and inhibition of sex hormones: a randomized, controlled trial. *Hepatology* 1995;21(6):1535–1542.

235. Barbare JC, Bouche O, Bonnetain F, et al. Randomized controlled trial of tamoxifen in advanced hepatocellular carcinoma. *J Clin Oncol* 2005; 23(19):4338–4346.

236. Collins JM. Pharmacologic rationale for regional drug delivery. *J Clin Arch* 1984;2(5):498–504.

237. Sigurdson ER, Ridge JA, Kemeny N, Daly JM. Tumor and liver drug uptake following hepatic artery and portal vein infusion. *J Clin Oncol* 1987; 5(11):1836–1840.

238. Venook AP. Update on hepatic intra-arterial chemotherapy. *Oncology* (Huntingt) 1997;11(7):947–957; discussion 61–62, 64, 70.

239. Kemeny N, Huang Y, Cohen AM, et al. Hepatic arterial infusion of chemotherapy after resection of hepatic metastases from colorectal cancer. *New Eng J Med* 1999;341(27):2039–2048.

240. Kemeny NE, Niedzwiecki D, Hollis DR, et al. Hepatic arterial infusion versus systemic therapy for hepatic metastases from colorectal cancer: a randomized trial of efficacy, quality of life, and molecular markers (CALGB 9481). *J Clin Oncol* 2006;24(9):1395–1403.

241. Ngan H. Lipiodol computerized tomography: how sensitive and specific is the technique in the diagnosis of hepatocellular carcinoma? *Br J Radiol* 1990;63(754):771–775.

242. Atiq OT, Kemeny N, Niedzwiecki D, Botet J. Treatment of unresectable primary liver cancer with intrahepatic fluorodeoxyuridine and mitomycin C through an implantable pump. *Cancer* 1992;69(4):920–924.

243. Yodono H, Sasaki T, Tarusawa K, Midorikawa H, Saito Y, Takekawa SD. Arterial infusion chemotherapy for advanced hepatocellular carcinoma using EPF and EAP therapies. *Cancer Chemother Pharmacol* 1992; 31(suppl):S89–S92.

244. Patt YZ, Charnsangavej C, Yoffe B, et al. Hepatic arterial infusion of floxuridine, leucovorin, doxorubicin, and cisplatin for hepatocellular carcinoma: effects of hepatitis B and C viral infection on drug toxicity and patient survival. *J Clin Oncol* 1994;12(6):1204–1211.

245. Campbell KA, Burns RC, Sitzmann JV, Lipsett PA, Grochow LB, Niederhuber JE. Regional chemotherapy devices: effect of experience and anatomy on complications. *J Clin Oncol* 1993;11(5):822–826.

246. Doci R, Bignami P, Bozzetti F, et al. Intrahepatic chemotherapy for unresectable hepatocellular carcinoma. *Cancer* 1988;61(10):1983–1987.

247. Breedis C, Young G. The blood supply of neoplasms in the liver. *Am J Pathol* 1954;30(5):969–977.

248. Sparks FC, Mosher MB, Hallauer WC, et al. Hepatic artery ligation and postoperative chemotherapy for hepatic metastases: clinical and pathophysiological results. *Cancer* 1975;35(4):1074–1082.

249. Charnsangavej C, Chuang VP, Wallace S, Soo CS, Bowers T. Angiographic classification of hepatic arterial collaterals. *Radiology* 1982;144(3):485–494.

250. Andersson M, Aronsen KF, Balch C, et al. Pharmacokinetics of intra-arterial mitomycin C with or without degradable starch microspheres (DSM) in the treatment of non-resectable liver cancer. *Acta Oncol* 1989;28(2):219–222.

251. Civalleri D, Esposito M, Fulco RA, et al. Liver and tumor uptake and plasma pharmacokinetic of arterial cisplatin administered with and without starch microspheres in patients with liver metastases. *Cancer* 1991;68(5):988–994.

252. Venook AP, Stagg RJ, Lewis BJ, et al. Chemoembolization for hepatocellular carcinoma. *J Clin Oncol* 1990;8(6):1108–1114.

253. Daly PF, Lyon RC, Straka EJ, Cohen JS. 31P-NMR spectroscopy of human cancer cells proliferating in a basement membrane gel. *FASEB J* 1988; 2(10):2596–2604.

254. Ho S, Lau WY, Leung TW, et al. Tumour-to-normal uptake ratio of 90Y microspheres in hepatic cancer assessed with 99Tcm macroaggregated albumin. *Br J Radiol* 1997;70(836):823–828.

255. Pelletier G, Roche A, Ink O, et al. A randomized trial of hepatic arterial chemoembolization in patients with unresectable hepatocellular carcinoma. *J Hepatol* 1990;11(2):181–184.

255a. Llovet JM, Real MI, Montana X, et al. Arterial embolisation or chemoembolisation versus symptomatic treatment in patients with unresectable hepatocellular carcinoma: a randomized controlled trial. *Lancet* 2002;359(9319):1734–1739.

256. Yao FY, Kinkhabwala M, LaBerge JM, et al. The impact of pre-operative loco-regional therapy on outcome after liver transplantation for hepatocellular carcinoma. *Am J Transplant* 2005;5(4 pt 1):795–804.

257. A comparison of lipiodol chemoembolization and conservative treatment for unresectable hepatocellular carcinoma. Groupe d'Etude et de Traitement du Carcinome Hepatocellulaire. *N Engl J Med* 1995;332(19):1256–1261.

258. Pelletier G, Ducreux M, Gay F, et al. Treatment of unresectable hepatocellular carcinoma with lipiodol chemoembolization: a multicenter randomized trial. Groupe CHC. *J Hepatol* 1998;29(1):129–134.

258a. Lo CM, Ngan H, Tso WK, et al. Randomized controlled trial of transarterial lipiodol chemoembolization for unresectable hepatocellular carcinoma. *Hepatology* 2002;35(5):1164–1171.

259. Ernst O, Sergent G, Mizrahi D, Delemazure O, Paris JC, L'Hermine C. Treatment of hepatocellular carcinoma by transcatheter arterial chemoembolization: comparison of planned periodic chemoembolization and chemoembolization based on tumor response. *AJR Am J Roentgenol* 1999;172(1):59–64.

260. Harada T, Matsuo K, Inoue T, Tamesue S, Nakamura H. Is preoperative hepatic arterial chemoembolization safe and effective for hepatocellular carcinoma? *Ann Surg* 1996;224(1):4–9.

261. Paye F, Jagot P, Vilgrain V, Farges O, Borie D, Belghiti J. Preoperative chemoembolization of hepatocellular carcinoma: a comparative study. *Arch Surg* 1998;133(7):767–772.

261a. Majno PE, Adam R, Bismuth H, et al. Influence of preoperative transarterial lipiodol chemoembolization on resection and transplantation for hepatocellular carcinoma in patients with cirrhosis. *Ann Surg* 1997;226(6):688–701; discussion 3.

262. Oldhafer KJ, Chavan A, Fruhauf NR, et al. Arterial chemoembolization before liver transplantation in patients with hepatocellular carcinoma: marked tumor necrosis, but no survival benefit? *J Hepatol* 1998;29(6):953–959.

263. Stuart K, Tessitore J, Rudy J, Clendennin N, Johnston A. A Phase II trial of nolatrexed dihydrochloride in patients with advanced hepatocellular carcinoma. *Cancer* 1999;86(3):410–414.

264. Mok TS, Leung TW, Lee SD, et al. A multi-centre randomized phase II study of nolatrexed versus doxorubicin in treatment of Chinese patients with advanced hepatocellular carcinoma. *Cancer Chemother Pharmacol* 1999;44(4):307–311.

265. Porta C, Ruff P, Feld R. Results of a phase III, randomized controlled study, the largest ever completed in hepatocellular carcinoma (HCC), comparing the survival of patients with unresectable HCC treated with nolatrexed (NOL) or doxorubicin (DOX) [abstract]. Am Soc Clin Onc Gastrointestinal Cancers Symposium, San Francisco, CA 2006: 97.

266. Posey J, Johnson P, Mok T. Results of a phase 2/3 open-label, randomized trial of T138067 versus doxorubicin (DOX) in chemotherapy-naïve, unresectable hepatocellular carcinoma (HCC) [abstract]. *Proc Am Soc Clin Oncol* 2005;23(16S):4035.

266a. Izzo F, Marra P, Beneduce G, et al. Pegylated arginine deaminase treatment of patients with unresectable hepatocellular carcinoma: results from phase I/II studies. *J Clin Oncol* 2004;22(10):1815–1822.

267. Thomas MB, Abbruzzese JL. Opportunities for targeted therapies in hepatocellular carcinoma. *J Clin Oncol* 2005;23(31):8093–8108.

268. Malka D, Pacault V, De Baere T, Ducreux M, Boige V. Antitumoral effect of celecoxib in hepatocellular carcinoma. *J Clin Oncol* 2005;23(21):4805–4806.

269. Folkman J. *Antiangiogenic Therapy.* 5th ed. Philadelphia, Pa.: Lippincott-Raven; 1997.

270. Ferrara N, Davis-Smyth T. The biology of vascular endothelial growth factor. *Endocr Rev* 1997;18(1):4–25.

271. Suzuki K, Hayashi N, Miyamoto Y, et al. Expression of vascular permeability factor/vascular endothelial growth factor in human hepatocellular carcinoma. *Cancer Res* 1996;56(13):3004–3009.

272. Miura H, Miyazaki T, Kuroda M, et al. Increased expression of vascular endothelial growth factor in human hepatocellular carcinoma. *J Hepatol* 1997;27(5):854–861.

273. Yao DF, Wu XH, Zhu Y, et al. Quantitative analysis of vascular endothelial growth factor, microvascular density and their clinicopathologic features in human hepatocellular carcinoma. *Hepatobiliary Pancreat Dis Int* 2005;4(2):220–226.

274. Jeng KS, Sheen IS, Wang YC, et al. Prognostic significance of preoperative circulating vascular endothelial growth factor messenger RNA expression in resectable hepatocellular carcinoma: a prospective study. *World J Gastroenterol* 2004;10(5):643–648.

275. Hurwitz H, Fehrenbacher L, Novotny W, et al. Bevacizumab plus irinotecan, fluorouracil, and leucovorin for metastatic colorectal cancer. *N Engl J Med* 2004;350(23):2335–2342.

276. Sandler AB, Gray R, Brahmer J. Randomized phase II/III trial of paclitaxel (P) plus carboplatin (C) with or without bevacizumab (NSC #704865) in patients with advanced non-squamous non-small cell lung cancer (NSCLC): an Eastern Cooperative Oncology Group (ECOG) Trial-E4599 [abstract]. *Proc Am Soc Clin Oncol* 2005; 23(16S):4.

277. Steinbild S, Baas F, Gmehling D. Phase I study of BAY 43–9006 (sorafenib), a Raf kinase and VEGFR inhibitor, combined with irinotecan (CPT-11) in advanced solid tumors [abstract]. *Proc Am Soc Clin Oncol* 2005;23(16S):3115.

278. Escudier B, Szczylik C, Eisen T. Randomized phase III trial of the Raf kinase and VEGFR inhibitor sorafenib (BAY 43–9006) in patients with advanced renal cell carcinoma (RCC) [abstract]. *Proc Am Soc Clin Oncol* 2005;23(16S):LBA4510.

279. Britten CD, Finn RS, Gomes AS. A pilot study of IV bevacizumab in hepatocellular cancer patients undergoing chemoembolization. *Proc Am Soc Clin Oncol* 2005;23(16S):4138.

280. Zhu AX, Sahani D, Norden-Zfoni A. A phase II study of gemcitabine, oxaliplatin in combination with bevacizumab (GEMOX-B) in patients with hepatocellular carcinoma [abstract]. *Proc Am Soc Clin Oncol* 2005; 23(16S):4120.

281. Mendelsohn J, Baselga J. Status of epidermal growth factor receptor

antagonists in the biology and treatment of cancer. *J Clin Oncol* 2003; 21(14):2787–2799.

282. Tabor E. Tumor suppressor genes, growth factor genes, and oncogenes in hepatitis B virus-associated hepatocellular carcinoma. *J Med Virol* 1994; 42(4):357–365.

283. Thomas MB, Dutta A, Brown T. A phase II open-label study of OSI-774 (NSC 718781) in unresectable hepatocellular carcinoma [abstract]. *Proc Am Soc Clin Oncol* 2005;23(16S):4038.

284. Philip PA, Mahoney M, Thomas J. Phase II Trial of erlotinib (OSI-774) in patients with hepatocellular or biliary cancer [abstract]. *Proc Am Soc Clin Oncol* 2004;22(14S):4025.

285. Reubi JC, Kvols L, Krenning E, Lamberts SW. Distribution of somatostatin receptors in normal and tumor tissue. *Metabolism* 1990;39(9 suppl 2):78–81.

286. Lamberts SW, Krenning EP, Reubi JC. The role of somatostatin and its analogs in the diagnosis and treatment of tumors. *Endocr Rev* 1991;12(4): 450–482.

287. Raderer M, Hejna MH, Kurtaran A, et al. Successful treatment of an advanced hepatocellular carcinoma with the long-acting somatostatin analog lanreotide. *Am J Gastroenterol* 1999;94(1):278–279.

288. Kouroumalis E, Skordilis P, Thermos K, Vasilaki A, Moschandrea J, Manousos ON. Treatment of hepatocellular carcinoma with octreotide: a randomised controlled study. *Gut* 1998;42(3):442–447.

289. Barbare JC, Bouché O, Bonnetain F. Treatment of advanced hepatocellular carcinoma with long-acting octreotide: preliminary results of a randomized placebo-controlled trial (FFCD-ANGH 2001–01 CHOC) [abstract]. *Proc Am Soc Clin Oncol* 2005;23(16S):4036.

290. Goldstein JL, Brown MS. Regulation of the mevalonate pathway. *Nature* 1990;343(6257):425–430.

291. Kawata S, Yamasaki E, Nagase T, et al. Effect of pravastatin on survival in patients with advanced hepatocellular carcinoma: a randomized controlled trial. *Br J Cancer* 2001;84(7):886–891.

292. Bookstein R, Demers W, Gregory R, Maneval D, Park J, Wills K. p53 gene therapy in vivo of hepatocellular and liver metastatic colorectal cancer. *Semin Oncol* 1996;23(1):66–77.

CANCER OF THE BILIARY TREE

CHAPTER 34 ■ CANCER OF THE GALLBLADDER AND BILIARY TREE: EPIDEMIOLOGY

MICHAEL J. HALL, JULIAN A. ABRAMS, AND ALFRED I. NEUGUT

Carcinomas of the biliary tract are an uncommon form of gastrointestinal malignancy with an aggressive and often lethal outcome. The *International Classification of Diseases for Oncology* includes tumors arising in the gallbladder, extrahepatic bile ducts, and the ampulla of Vater under the category of carcinomas of the biliary tract (1). Biliary tract cancers rank sixth in incidence among gastrointestinal cancers. The incidence of these tumors varies among countries, with an annual incidence in the United States of approximately 7,500 cases (2). This group of cancers results in 3,300 deaths per year, or approximately 0.6% of cancer deaths. These tumors are nearly all adenocarcinomas and have a poor prognosis, with <5% of all patients with gallbladder cancer alive after 5 years (3). Pathological stage remains the best prognostic indicator; the outcome declines with increasing stage of disease. The U.S. National Cancer Database reported that patients younger than 60 years with gallbladder cancer were more frequently diagnosed with advanced, stage IV disease (4).

Specific risk factors are known for both gallbladder cancer and bile duct cancer, and many hypotheses have been put forward as well. Most interesting and important in the United States is cholelithiasis, which is closely tied to gallbladder cancer and associated to a lesser degree with bile duct cancer. As a result, gallbladder cancer is closely related to risk factors associated with gallstones, such as female gender (2,5) and age, whereas other biliary tract cancers have a slightly higher incidence among men (6). These possible etiologic factors have been suggested by clinical observation, autopsy results, and epidemiologic studies, and are described in detail in this chapter. The role of molecular biology is also being defined, and the potential impact of surveillance, screening, and prevention on the incidence and survival of biliary tract cancers is being investigated.

DESCRIPTIVE EPIDEMIOLOGY

Geographic Variation

Cancers of the gallbladder, extrahepatic bile duct, and ampulla of Vater have distinct demographic patterns and should be described as distinct disease entities (7). Cancer of or near the ampulla of Vater (ampullary cancer) arises from the region of the small bowel where the main pancreatic duct and the common bile duct unite and exit the duodenal wall (8). More than 50% of malignant duodenal lesions are found in this area. Although ampullary cancer is sometimes grouped with malignancies of

pancreatic origin, this tumor type has several features that distinguish it from pancreatic adenocarcinoma, most notably a better prognosis (9,10). Ampullary cancer is the least common of the biliary tree tumors and has a worldwide distribution. Its risk profile is to some degree independent of the other biliary tumors, as evidenced by the low rates of ampullary cancer in populations with traditionally very high rates of gallbladder cancer, such as the Australian Maori (10). Geographic clustering of ampullary cancer has been reported in at least one study from Japan (11).

Primary cancers of the bile ducts (cholangiocarcinomas) may arise from the epithelial lining of either the intrahepatic or the extrahepatic bile ducts (12). Carcinoma of the gallbladder also primarily arises from the gallbladder epithelium, although other histologic types with varying geographic distributions and survival outcomes (e.g., cystadenocarcinoma, squamous cell carcinoma, papillary carcinoma) also exist. Both cholangiocarcinoma and gallbladder cancer demonstrate wide geographic variation in frequency, suggesting environmental causes as one potential factor in their etiology. For example, incidence rates of these two tumors show remarkable regional variation in Asia, with some of the greatest extremes seen in Thailand and China. A comparison of the annual incidence rates for gallbladder cancer in international cancer registries shows differences of up to a factor of 25 (13). At least part of the geographic differences in gallbladder cancer, more so than cholangiocarcinoma, may relate to variation in the prevalence of gallstones in different ethnic groups (14).

Gallbladder cancer is rare in most Caucasian populations but is among the most frequently observed cancers in the native populations of North and South America and in the Maori of New Zealand. High rates are seen in the cancer registries of South American countries, such as Colombia; Eastern European countries, such as Poland and Hungary; and Israel (especially among Jews of European origin), where rates as high as 13.8 per 100,000 for women and 7.5 per 100,000 for men have been reported (15). Low rates are seen in the Middle and Far East, except in some high-risk areas; in the United Kingdom; and in the United States. Many regions of the world have reported declining rates of gallbladder cancer in recent years, including much of South America, Canada, Europe, and Poland. In China, where significant differences in incidence between mountain areas and flatlands have been previously reported (16), changes in gallbladder cancer incidence have been mixed, with Tianjin and Shanghai reporting increases, and Hong Kong decreases (17) (Table 34.1).

Within the United States, biliary tree cancers remain an exceedingly rare diagnosis, with <10,000 new cases reported per

TABLE 34.1

ANNUAL AGE-STANDARDIZED INCIDENCE RATES
(PER 100,000) FOR GALLBLADDER CANCER BY
GENDER IN SELECTED CANCER REGISTRIES,
1987–1997

Location	Female	Male	Ratio
ASIA			
China (Hong Kong)	2.7	3.4	0.8
China (Quidong)	0.6	0.8	0.7
Japan (Nagasaki)	8.1	8.4	0.9
Japan (Osaka)	5.7	6.3	0.9
EUROPE			
Italy (Torino)	4.0	3.8	1.0
Norway	1.4	1.3	1.0
Poland	6.3	3.6	1.7
Scotland	1.5	1.4	1.0
Spain (Granada)	5.2	2.8	1.8
AMERICAS			
Canada (Ontario)	1.9	1.8	1.0
Canada (Alberta)	1.8	1.5	1.2
Colombia	7.3	3.1	2.3
Costa Rica	4.2	1.8	2.3
U.S. SEER (black)	1.5	1.4	1.0
U.S. SEER (white)	1.6	1.4	1.1

SEER, Surveillance, Epidemiology, and End Result.
From International Agency for Research on Cancer. Available at:
http://www-dep.iarc.fr. Accessed May 7, 2007.

year (2). Extrahepatic cholangiocarcinoma incidence has been decreasing in recent years (18), whereas intrahepatic cancers, more commonly found in peoples of Asian decent, have been increasing in the United States and other Western nations (12). Gallbladder cancer rates are high among Native Americans, in whom the overall rate of cancer is low, and in the Mexican American population (19). Recent data from the National Cancer Institute Surveillance, Epidemiology, and End Result (SEER) program shows more than threefold higher rates of gallbladder cancer among Native American/Alaskan Native males than among Caucasian or African American counterparts (20). These rates closely parallel those of gallstone disease.

Gender

Ampullary carcinoma is approximately 1.4 to 1.5 times more common in men than in women (9). This ratio is similar for cholangiocarcinoma (20). Carcinoma of the gallbladder in contradistinction is one of the few forms of cancer that does not arise in a gender-specific organ but that nonetheless occurs more commonly in women than in men (2,17,20). The female-to-male ratio in the United States is approximately 1.7 to 1 across all races, with higher female-to-male ratios seen in Native American/Alaskan Native (2.0–1) and Hispanic subgroups (1.9–1) (2,20).

Age

Cancers of the biliary tree are primarily diseases of the elderly. Diagnosis and mortality for all types of biliary tract cancer are closely associated with age (2,4). The incidence of ampullary cancer and cholangiocarcinoma increases with age, with a mean age of diagnosis of approximately 63 years and 65 years, respectively (19). The trend of increasing incidence of intrahepatic cholangiocarcinoma appears to be greatest in older individuals (12). Like other epithelial cancers, gallbladder cancer rates also increase with age. The mean age at diagnosis of gallbladder carcinoma is 65 years (19).

Race

Ampullary cancers have been described in a variety of racial and ethnic subgroups, but no studies have specifically examined the association of race with the incidence of this tumor. The rate of cholangiocarcinoma in Caucasian Americans is about 1.3 times that in African Americans. In particular, rates in Caucasian women and African American men appear to be increasing (20). Age-adjusted incidence rates of intrahepatic cholangiocarcinoma are equal among Caucasians and African Americans, whereas overall rates of extrahepatic cholangiocarcinoma are lower for African Americans (12).

In the United States, racial/ethnic groups with higher incidence rates of cholelithiasis, such as Native Americans and Hispanic Americans, have a higher incidence rate of gallbladder cancer as well. These data may reflect either environmental or genetic differences among the populations studied. In a case-control study of 131 patients with gallbladder cancer and 2,399 subjects without gallbladder cancer from three racial groups—Caucasian, African American, and southwestern Native American (14)—a significant relationship was seen between gallstones and gallbladder cancer. The overall estimated relative risk (RR) was 4.4 (95% confidence interval [CI], 2.6–7.3), but the estimated RR was much higher for the Native American group at 20.9 (95% CI, 8.1–54).

Updated incidence rates (per 100,000) published by the SEER program are shown in Table 34.2. Hispanic Americans have a high risk of developing carcinoma of the gallbladder (5,21), but this is not true for all Hispanic Americans. For example, in New Mexico, Texas, and California, where the ancestry of this group comprises European Spanish and Native

TABLE 34.2

INCIDENCE RATES (PER 100,000) FOR GALLBLADDER
AND BILIARY TREE CANCER BY GENDER AND
RACIAL/ETHNIC GROUP AND SUBSITE, 2001

	Male	Female
GALLBLADDER		
All races	0.8	1.4
Asian/Pacific Islander	1.1	1.7
Black	0.9	1.6
Hispanic	1.5	2.9
White	0.8	1.4
OTHER BILIARY TRACT		
All races	1.9	1.3
Asian/Pacific Islander	2.7	1.9
Black	1.5	1.1
Hispanic	2.5	1.9
White	1.9	1.2

From http://www.seer.cancer.gov/csr

Americans, the risk of gallbladder cancer is higher (22). Other Hispanic groups, such as Cubans and Puerto Ricans, have gallbladder cancer incidence rates no different from those of the general U.S. population (23).

Time Trends

Temporal changes in incidence have been observed for the biliary tree tumors. A recent 20-year population-based series (1976–1995) reported an increasing incidence of ampullary cancer in France (9). Based on SEER data, the incidence of cholangiocarcinoma has also steadily increased over the past 20 years in the United States and may be secondary to increases in intrahepatic cholangiocarcinoma (12). Overall gallbladder cancer incidence and mortality rates have continued to decrease in the United States, although rates in black females have slowly trended upward (7).

Changes in the management of benign biliary disease may impact cancer rates. Benign gallbladder disease increases the risk of cancer in all regions of the biliary tract (24,25). Cholecystectomy is now frequently undertaken for benign gallbladder disease, in part as a prophylactic measure against subsequent malignancy. This has become more widespread with the use of laparoscopic cholecystectomy, and increases in cholecystectomy rates in the United States have been documented (26,27). This is one possible explanation for the reduced mortality from gallbladder cancer that has been observed in the United States and Europe (28). In a more recent Italian series, only 20% of gallbladder cancers identified histologically after laparoscopic cholecystectomy were suspected preoperatively or intraoperatively, indicating that many gallbladder tumors are likely removed serendipitously (29). Interestingly, the risk of cholangiocarcinoma is also reduced after cholecystectomy (30).

RISK FACTORS

A number of etiologic factors have been described for gallbladder cancer and cancer of the bile ducts (Table 34.3).

Cholelithiasis

Gallbladder carcinoma has been shown to be strongly associated with cholelithiasis. Numerous studies have shown an increased risk of gallbladder cancer in individuals with cholelithiasis (31–33). Gallstones are found in up to 90% of patients with gallbladder cancer (33). It is not clear whether there is a causal relationship between gallstones and the development of carcinoma of the gallbladder or whether the two conditions share similar risk factors. The epidemiology of cholelithiasis runs parallel to that of gallbladder cancer. The highest incidence of gallbladder cancer is seen in those areas with the highest prevalence of gallstones, especially in the indigenous populations of Chile, Bolivia, Ecuador, Mexico, and Native Americans of the southwestern United States (34). It has been hypothesized that inflammation due to the presence of gallstones probably contributes to the stepwise progression from epithelial dysplasia to carcinoma in situ to invasive carcinoma of the gallbladder (35).

Patients with gallstones have been shown to have an increased risk of gallbladder cancer. A hospital-based case-control study, with a review of medical records of 69 patients with primary biliary tract cancer, found a significant association between cholelithiasis and biliary tract cancers (odds ratio [OR], 19.5; 95% CI, 6.4–59.4) (36). A multicenter case-control study by Zatonski et al. (37) found that patients with gallbladder cancer had an OR of 4.4 (95% CI, 2.6–7.5) for having a history of symptomatic cholelithiasis or choledocholithiasis. In addition, studies of patients undergoing cholecystectomy for cholelithiasis have shown a postoperative incidental finding of gallbladder cancer in 0.3% to 3% of cases (38–40). Larger gallstones appear to correlate with an increased risk of gallbladder cancer as compared to smaller stones. A study by Diehl (41) demonstrated an odds ratio of 10.1 (95% CI, 2.6–39.7) for the development of gallbladder cancer in individuals with gallstones >3.0 cm in diameter. A cross-sectional study of 1,676 patients undergoing cholecystectomy calculated an odds ratio of 9.2 (95% CI, 2.3–37) for gallbladder cancer in subjects with gallstones >3 cm compared to subjects with gallstones <1 cm in diameter (42).

Although the evidence is limited, there may also be an association between cholelithiasis and increased risk of cholangiocarcinoma. A retrospective review from two hospitals in Taiwan showed that up to 67% of patients with cholangiocarcinoma had a history of cholelithiasis (43). The presence of intrahepatic stones has also been observed in 5.7% to 17.5% of cholangiocarcinoma cases in a Japanese series (44). In such instances, the bile duct epithelium generally shows chronic proliferative cholangitis and epithelial hyperplasia (45).

Cholecystitis/Porcelain Gallbladder

In approximately 1% of patients who undergo cholecystectomy for cholecystitis, an undiagnosed gallbladder cancer is present. In a single center retrospective review of 80 patients older than 60 years who were admitted with acute cholecystitis, 0.9% were found to have gallbladder cancer (46). Premalignant changes include epithelial hyperplasia, dysplasia, and frank carcinoma. These changes have been identified in 13.5%, 8.3%, and 3.5%, respectively, of patients undergoing cholecystectomy for cholelithiasis or cholecystitis (47). In a Japanese series,

TABLE 34.3

POSTULATED RISK FACTORS FOR GALLBLADDER CANCER AND CHOLANGIOCARCINOMA

Gallbladder cancer	Cholangiocarcinoma
Cholelithiasis	PSC
Chronic cholecystitis	Choledochal cysts
Porcelain gallbladder	Partial gastrectomy
Choledochal cysts	Parasitic infections
Anomalous junction of the pancreaticobiliary duct	*Clonorchis sinensis*
	Opisthorchis viverrini
Adenomatous gallbladder polyps	Thorotrast exposure
Bacterial colonization *Helicobacter* spp. *Salmonella typhi*	Bacterial colonization *Helicobacter* spp.
Partial gastrectomy	Drugs
Occupational exposures	Isoniazid
Obesity	Methyldopa
Tobacco	Occupational exposures
Female gender (prolonged estrogen exposure[a])	Obesity
Diabetes mellitus[a]	Tobacco
Primary sclerosing cholangitis (PSC)[a]	Cholelithiasis[a]
	Ulcerative colitis[a]

[a]Possible risk factors.

14% of patients who underwent cholecystectomy for chronic cholecystitis had evidence of either severe dysplasia or carcinoma in situ (48).

Patients with long-standing cholecystitis can develop calcification of the gallbladder wall, a condition known as porcelain gallbladder. Several older series have demonstrated a strong association between porcelain gallbladder and gallbladder cancer, with a cumulative incidence ranging between 12.5% and 61.0% (49,50). A more recent retrospective review, however, failed to identify any cases of carcinoma in patients with porcelain gallbladder (51).

Primary Sclerosing Cholangitis

Cholangiocarcinoma, both intrahepatic and extrahepatic, has been reported as a complication of sclerosing cholangitis. Lifetime risks of developing carcinoma have been reported as between 10% and 30%, although the majority of reports estimate a risk closer to 10% (52–54). Undiagnosed cholangiocarcinoma in association with primary sclerosing cholangitis (PSC) has been found at the time of orthotopic liver transplantation (55,56). The time from diagnosis of PSC to the development of cholangiocarcinoma ranges from 1 to 25 years, with more than one-third of the cases being detected within 2 years of the initial diagnosis (53,57). This short interval is likely due to the lack of symptoms associated with early PSC. There may be an increased risk of gallbladder cancer in patients with PSC. In a series of 121 patients with PSC, 3 were found to have gallbladder cancer (58). Whether the observed cases were related to PSC itself or to the presence of gallstones is unclear.

Secondary sclerosing cholangitis, which clinically mimics PSC, is due to an underlying insult, such as chronic biliary obstruction due to stones or ischemic biliary strictures. Individuals with this condition also can progress to cirrhosis. Although the natural history of secondary sclerosing cholangitis is not fully known, there have not been any reports to date of cholangiocarcinoma developing in the setting of secondary sclerosing cholangitis (59).

Inflammatory Bowel Disease

Bile duct carcinoma has been documented as a complication of inflammatory bowel disease, albeit much less frequently than carcinomas affecting the colon. This may be in part due to the strong association between PSC and ulcerative colitis, and the presence of serum antibodies in patients with both conditions that cross-react with bile ducts (60,61). The incidence of bile duct cancer was 1 in 246 patients with ulcerative colitis in one series (62), with one-fifth of cases occurring in intrahepatic bile ducts, and 2 in 200 patients at The Johns Hopkins Hospital (63). In a series at the Mayo Clinic, the average age at diagnosis of bile duct cancer for patients with ulcerative colitis was 38 years and occurred at a mean follow-up of 19 years after the diagnosis of ulcerative colitis (64). The risk of bile duct cancer does not appear to be affected by proctocolectomy (63).

Preexisting Adenomatous Lesions

Benign neoplasms of the extrahepatic bile ducts are relatively uncommon. In a histopathological study of 43 cases of carcinoma of the extrahepatic ducts, adenomatous residue was found in 9 cases (21.4%). This frequency was comparable to that seen in carcinoma of the colon and rectum (65), in which most carcinomas arise from preexisting adenomas. The frequency of preexisting adenomas was also similar for carcinoma of the gallbladder (66), and in the ampulla of Vater, adenomatous residue was found in 18 or 22 carcinomas (81.8%) (67).

Adenomatous gallbladder polyps are a predisposing factor for the development of carcinoma and gallbladder polyps are not uncommon. Malignant polyps tend to be found in older patients and in individuals with larger polyps. In a study from Japan, 194,767 subjects had an abdominal ultrasound as part of routine health screening. The prevalence of gallbladder polyps in this population was 5.6%. In addition, the presence of polyps ≥1 cm in diameter was found to be associated with a significantly increased risk of gallbladder cancer (68). In a retrospective study of 100 patients who underwent cholecystectomy and were found to have polypoid lesions of the gallbladder, 73% of the patients with malignant polyps were older than 60 years, and 88% of the malignant polyps were ≥1 cm in diameter (69). Small polyps (<1 cm) are unlikely to be malignant. In a study evaluating gallstone prevalence by ultrasound in diabetics and matched controls, 6.7% of the diabetics were found to have gallbladder polyps. More than 90% of these polyps were <1 cm in diameter, and very few of these polyps changed in size over the 5-year follow-up period (70). It appears that patients with PSC have a much higher risk of malignant gallbladder polyps. Buckles et al. (71) performed a retrospective case series from the Mayo Clinic and found that, in patients with PSC who underwent cholecystectomy for polypoid lesions of the gallbladder, 57% of the gallbladders had adenocarcinoma, and one-third of the benign gallbladder lesions had associated epithelial cell dysplasia.

Patients with familial adenomatous polyposis (FAP) have a risk of ampullary adenocarcinoma that is estimated to be 100 times that of the general population (72). An association is also found between adenomatous polyps of the gallbladder seen with Peutz-Jeghers syndrome (PJS) and gallbladder cancer (73,74).

Choledochal Cysts and Anatomical Abnormalities

Patients with choledochal cysts have an increased incidence of both gallbladder and bile duct carcinoma. Choledochal cysts are preexisting lesions that is present in 9–24% of bile duct cancers. Cholangiocarcinomas in the presence of choledochal cysts tend to develop at an earlier age than sporadic cholangiocarcinoma (75,76). The incidence of cholangiocarcinoma in individuals with choledochal cysts increases with age, and the mean age of diagnosis of cholangiocarcinoma is in the fourth decade of life (77). Premalignant changes, such as epithelial metaplasia, are also seen with increasing frequency with older age in these cysts (78). Choledochal cysts are more prevalent in females (4:1) and in Asia (79). The Todani classification system (75) is used to differentiate these cysts on an anatomical basis. Type I cysts (fusiform dilation of the extrahepatic duct) and type IV cysts (combined intra- and extrahepatic dilation or multiple extrahepatic dilations) have the highest risk of malignant transformation (80). Although the majority of cancers arise from within the cysts, malignant transformation can occur anywhere in the biliary tree.

Gallbladder cancer has also been seen in the setting of an anomalous junction of the pancreaticobiliary duct (AJPD) (15), at times in association with a choledochal cyst (81). A study of 1,876 consecutive patients in China who underwent endoscopic retrograde cholangiopancreatography (ERCP), 10 patients were identified as having AJPD, and 7 of these had gallbladder cancer. The odds ratio for having AJPD in patients with gallbladder cancer in that study was 50.7 (95% CI, 12.7–202.3) (82). In another study of 126 patients with gallbladder cancer who had previously undergone cholangiography, the prevalence of AJDP was 18% (83). Whether the increased risk of cancer is a result of the anomalous junction and subsequent bile stasis and carcinogen retention within the biliary tree, the regurgitation of pancreatic juice or chronic inflammation is unclear.

Partial or Total Gastrectomy

The incidence of biliary tract cancer is increased after partial gastrectomy. This may relate to the increased occurrence of gallstones after gastrectomy (84). In a prospective study of 48 gastric cancer patients who underwent partial or total gastrectomy, 18% subsequently went on to develop gallstones (85). After distal gastrectomy, patients have prolonged gallbladder bile emptying into the duodenum (86). Alternatively, the increased risk of biliary cancer may be due to the presence of N-nitroso compounds that are formed in the gastric remnant after partial gastrectomy (87). In a study evaluating risk factors for the development of gallstones after gastrectomy, total gastrectomy (vs. partial), reconstruction with duodenal exclusion (vs. nonexclusion), and lymph node dissection in the hepatoduodenal ligament were all identified as risk factors for the subsequent development of gallstones (88).

Parasitic Infections

Numerous studies have examined the relationship between chronic bacterial or parasitic infections and cancers of the biliary tree and gallbladder.

An established association exists between the occurrence of biliary tract cancer and the presence of liver flukes. *Clonorchis sinensis* was once endemic in Korea, Japan, China, and Vietnam. It is now much less prevalent, and, as a result, cholangiocarcinoma has become relatively infrequent in more recent years. Previously, Belamaric identified cellular changes suggestive of infection with *C. sinensis* in 18 of 19 patients with cholangiocarcinoma at autopsy, compared with only one-third of control patients (89).

Opisthorchis viverrini is a liver fluke found in northeast Thailand, where the prevalence of infection remains high. The first reports of the role of *O. viverrini* in the induction of cholangiocarcinoma came from reports of the coincidence of the two diseases in the same area and in the same individuals (90).

The incidence of cholangiocarcinoma varies at least 12-fold in the five regions of Thailand, correlating strongly with the prevalence of *O. viverrini* infection as measured by antibody titer in the general population (91). The risk associated with *O. viverrini* infection also appeared to be higher in men than in women, which is consistent with the higher incidence of cholangiocarcinoma among men in areas where *O. viverrini* is endemic, despite similar infection prevalence for the two genders. A similar association between the intensity of *O. viverrini* infection and the risk of cholangiocarcinoma has also been reported within northeast Thailand (92–94).

Several mechanisms of liver fluke–induced carcinogenesis have been proposed. Some evidence suggests a role for nitrosation and nitrosamines, which occur as a result of fluke infestation, as the mechanism of carcinogenesis in cholangiocarcinoma, and in other situations in which the development of cancer is a result of long-term infectious processes (91). The possibility of an immunologic mechanism has also been postulated on the basis of a correlation of an *O. viverrini*–specific antibody and ultrasonographic changes in the biliary tract in an endemic area; however, this association is indirect (95).

Bacterial Infections

An association has been noted between gallbladder and bile duct cancers and the presence of hepatic *Helicobacter* species (especially *Helicobacter bilis*) in the biliary tree of these patients. In a Japanese study of patients with hepatobiliary cancer, *Helicobacter* spp. DNA was found in the biliary epithelium of 53% of patients with hepatobiliary cancer compared to 16% of the patients with benign biliary diseases ($p = 0.03$) (96). A study by Matsukura et al. (97) showed that 79% to 87% of patients with bile duct or gallbladder cancer tested positive for *H. bilis* in the bile. It is possible that the presence of the *Helicobacter* spp. may result in gallstone formation and subsequent chronic inflammation, thus increasing the risk of development of biliary cancer. Fox et al. (98) demonstrated a high incidence of *Helicobacter* colonization in the bile and gallbladder tissue of patients with chronic cholecystitis. In a mouse model of cholesterol gallstone development, 80% of mice infected with hepatic *Helicobacter* spp. and fed a lithogenic diet developed gallstones after 8 weeks, compared to only 10% of uninfected mice fed a lithogenic diet (99).

Chronic typhoid carriers harbor typhoid bacilli in their gallbladders. A retrospective cohort study comparing 471 chronic typhoid carriers with matched controls over a 50-year period found mortality from "hepatobiliary cancers" (including some cases of gallbladder cancer) to be six times higher in carriers than in controls (100). Other studies in Chile, Bolivia, and India support the association between gallbladder cancer and the combination of chronic infection with *Salmonella typhi* and cholelithiasis (101,102). Csendes et al. (103), however, did not find an association between bile typhoid colonization and biliary cancer.

Thorotrast Exposure and Drug Therapy

Thorotrast is a colloidal preparation of thorium dioxide, a radioactive α-particle emitter, which was widely used as a radiopaque contrast medium between 1930 and 1955. It had many routes of administration, including intravenous, which resulted in 70% uptake by the liver. Carcinomas of the biliary tract, as well as hepatocellular carcinoma and hepatic angiosarcoma, have been described many years after exposure (104,105). Drugs that have been implicated in the pathogenesis of carcinoma of the bile ducts include isoniazid (106) and methyldopa (107).

Occupational Exposures

Toxic metabolites are frequently cleared by biliary excretion. This mechanism may account in part for numerous associations between occupation and cancers of the biliary tract (108). Processes vital to normal cellular function, including successful DNA replication, cell division, and programmed cell death (apoptosis), may all be targets of exogenous agents introduced into the biliary tree milieu through hepatic detoxification and elimination.

Epidemiologic studies have identified a number of putative biliary duct toxins. In a small case series, two biliary tree cancers (ampullary cancer and cholangiocarcinoma) and a third rare neoplasm (pancreatic adenocarcinoma) were reported in young men (all younger than 45 years) heavily exposed to trichlorinated hydrocarbon solvents (109). Neither of two American case-control studies found that extrahepatic bile duct cancer or gallbladder cancer was linked to a specific occupation, industry, or selected occupational exposure (24,101). Nonetheless, a number of industrial exposures, including chlorinated biphenyls, certain industrial dyes, asbestos, and cutting oil mist, have been associated with a risk of cholangiocarcinoma (15,110).

A variety of exposures have also been associated with gallbladder cancer. In aggregate data from Sweden, an increased risk of gallbladder cancer was seen for men employed in petroleum refineries, paper mills, chemical processing, and shoemaking, and for both men and women employed in textile mills (111). Increased risks in textile workers have also been noted in a retrospective Canadian series (112). A more recent 20-year prospective study of Lithuanian laborers estimated a standardized incidence ratio (SIR) of 3.2 for gallbladder cancer among longtime textile workers (113). Uranium and radon exposure (114), as well as exposure to mineral oil transformer fluid (115) and organic solvents (116), have also been implicated in gallbladder and bile duct tumors.

Autopsy series have suggested an association between cancer of the biliary tree with work in particular industries (automotive, dry cleaning, chemical) (117–119). These cases of biliary tract cancer also tended to occur in younger patients, and the likelihood of metachronous or synchronous second primary malignant tumors at other sites was increased. A suggestion has been seen of an increased risk of gallbladder cancer in those exposed to asbestos (120,121).

Obesity

An association with body mass index (BMI) has been observed for ampullary cancers, cancers of the bile ducts, and cancers of the gallbladder (101,111). A large retrospective cohort study that followed more than 4 million U.S. veterans from 1969 to 1996 found that obesity was significantly associated with both ampullary and gallbladder cancer (122). Other studies have supported these findings, with excess body weight found to lead to an increase in the risk of both gallbladder and biliary tree cancers (123). A recent prospective population-based study of more than 900,000 American men and women also found an increased RR of death from gallbladder cancer in obese men (RR 1.76, 1.06–2.94) and obese women (RR 2.13, 1.56–2.90) (124). Higher rates of gallbladder cancer among Hispanic Americans may reflect higher rates of obesity in this population (125). These findings are in contrast to those of one case-control study in Japan, in which a lean build was linked with an increased risk of development of bile duct cancers (126); however, a more recent Japanese population-based prospective cohort study found that higher BMI was significantly associated with cancer of the gallbladder in women (127).

Obese persons have elevated risks of gallstones and benign gallbladder disease (128), and benign biliary disease and gallstones are risk factors for gallbladder and biliary tree cancers. Therefore, the fact that increased body weight may correlate with an increased risk of biliary cancers is not surprising. Although obese persons who undergo weight loss may exacerbate their risk of benign gallbladder disease (129), intentional weight loss may lower the long-term risk of obesity-related cancer (130). A recent meta-analysis estimated that excess body mass accounts for 5% of all European cancers (3% in men, 6% in women), with 25% of all gallbladder cancer estimated to be attributable to excess body weight (131).

Reproductive Factors

Across racial and ethnic lines, women have higher rates of benign and malignant gallbladder disease compared to men. Reproductive factors, such as age at menarche, age at first birth, parity, oral contraceptive use, and hormone replacement therapy, have been postulated as possible factors in disease risk. In a case-control study of risk factors for extrahepatic bile duct

cancers in Los Angeles County, no clear patterns of association were observed for a number of reproductive factors (24), although three smaller case-control studies showed a significant association between oral contraceptive use and extrahepatic bile duct cancers in women younger than 60 years (132), as well as younger age at menarche, early age at first pregnancy, greater parity, prolonged fertility (133), and use of hormone replacement therapy (134). The World Health Organization Collaborative Study of Neoplasia and Steroid Contraceptives compared 58 patients with gallbladder cancer to 355 control patients in six countries and found no association between oral contraceptive use and gallbladder cancer (135).

Two large international case-control studies have examined the epidemiology of gallbladder cancer. In the first, menopausal status and use of hormone replacement therapy were shown to have no impact on risk, whereas oral contraceptive use was suggestive of increasing risk of gallbladder cancer only among controls without gallstones (OR 3.8, 0.7–23) (101). In the second study, risk of gallbladder cancer was found to increase with increasing parity and to decrease with older age at first childbirth; no effect was seen for age at menopause, use of oral contraceptives, or use of hormone replacement therapy (37).

In summary, the etiology of the increased risk of gallbladder cancer in women appears multifactorial. As with breast cancer, a prolonged period of estrogen exposure secondary to prolonged fertility and/or hormone replacement may increase risk, although the protective effects seen from increasing parity in breast cancer are not evident. The risk associated with greater parity in gallbladder cancer may be related to gallbladder stasis during pregnancy, which is believed to promote the formation of gallstones and bile duct sludge (136). The role of oral contraceptive use in gallbladder cancer remains controversial, particularly in view of the new lower-dose estrogen and progesterone formulations that are available.

Diet

Due to the vast geographic distribution of gallbladder and biliary tree disease, dietary factors contributing to risk differ considerably, depending on the region of the world examined. Consumption of raw fish in areas of Thailand endemic for *O. viverrini* and *C. sinensis* infection is associated with an increased incidence of cholangiocarcinoma (137). In Japan, an increased risk of gallbladder cancer has been associated with increased intake of oily foods, while consumption of animal proteins and fats, as well as fruits and vegetables, offered a protective effect (126). A Dutch case-control study also found that increased vegetable consumption lowered the risk of biliary tumors, while sweetened desserts and drinks increased risk (133). A recent study from Italy found a protective effect from whole grain cereal consumption (28). Finally, an American case-control study (Los Angeles County, CA), which examined 80 individual food items in seven food groups, found no relationship of dietary intake to risk of gallbladder cancer (24).

Two international collaborative case-control studies have examined diet and gallbladder cancer risk. One found only a weak association between coffee consumption and risk of gallbladder cancer (19); a second identified total carbohydrate intake as the strongest dietary predictor of risk. Increased vitamin B6 (pyridoxine) and vitamin E also reduced risk significantly, while increased fat intake, vitamin C, and fiber were all protective (37).

Diabetes

A history of diabetes mellitus has been associated with an increased risk of a number of gastrointestinal cancers (138).

More recently, a large United States—based prospective cohort of 467,922 men and 588,321 women followed for 16 years estimated a RR of gallbladder cancer of 1.46 (0.92—2.30) in men and a RR of 1.19 (0.77—1.83) in women, with extensive multivariate adjustment for age, BMI, smoking history, alcohol use, physical activity, dietary factors, and hormone replacement (139).

Tobacco Smoking

Cigarette smoking and other forms of tobacco use have been associated with a wide range of disease, including cancers of the gastrointestinal tract and biliary tree. Various forms of smoking (cigars/pipes/cigarettes) have been associated with both ampullary cancer and extrahepatic cholangiocarcinoma, with risk magnified in men and women smoking more than 50 pack-years (24). At least three studies have demonstrated an increased risk of biliary tree disease related to smoking. A population-based case-control study conducted by the International Agency for Research on Cancer found that the RR of cholangiocarcinoma was 2.82 (1.01—7.87) for nonfiltered cigarette smokers (25). A hospital-based case-control study also found an association between cigarette smoking and gallbladder cancer (36), whereas a third study specifically using individuals with benign gallstone disease as controls also identified smoking as a risk for gallbladder cancer, although this result did not achieve statistical significance (140). These findings are in contrast to those of an earlier study in which reduced risk of cholangiocarcinoma was seen with cigarette smoking (132), although controls in this study were other cancers that have clear associations with smoking. A Dutch population-based case-control study (133) and an international case-control study (101) have shown no association between cigarette smoking and biliary tree cancer or gallbladder cancer.

Alcohol Ingestion

Alcohol consumption has not been clearly associated with a risk of benign biliary disease or biliary cancer (128,141,142). One case-control study found that alcohol drinkers had a 10% to 40% reduction in the risk of ampullary cancer and cholangiocarcinoma compared to nondrinkers, although these results did not reach statistical significance (24). Other case-control studies have reported no association of alcohol to cholangiocarcinoma (132) or biliary tree cancers (133). A prospective study of American-born men of Japanese ancestry found that individuals who developed biliary tract cancers consumed more alcohol (mainly beer) than those who remained cancer free (141). A more recent prospective study in Sweden found that individuals employed in occupations with higher rates of alcohol consumption (journalists, cooks/stewards) had higher incidence of gallbladder cancer ([SIR 2.72, 1.35—4.57] and [SIR 3.17, 1.51—5.45], respectively) (143).

Familial Predisposition

Biliary tree cancers are exceedingly rare tumors, making familial inheritance of these cancers challenging to study. A portion of biliary cancers is related to a familial predisposition for cancer, although most are likely sporadic or due to environmental causes. One case-control study estimated the RR of gallbladder cancer associated with a positive family history of gallbladder cancer as 13.9 (1.2—163.9) (144). Certain premalignant biliary tumors have been documented as part of familial cancer syndromes. Ampullary and periampullary adenomas are strongly associated with clinical FAP and germline mutations of the APC gene on chromosome 5q21. The presence and severity of ampullary neoplasia segregate within affected families, although no genotype–phenotype correlation relating the causative APC mutation to ampullary polyp frequency or severity has been found (72,145). An association of ampullary cancer and the attenuated form of FAP has also been documented in one case report (146). An increased incidence of ampullary and biliary cancers is seen in individuals from Lynch syndrome/hereditary nonpolyposis colorectal cancer (HNPCC) families. In a large prospective Finnish study, the incidence of biliary tree tumors was ninefold greater (SIR 9.1, 1.1—33) in members of genetically diagnosed HNPCC families, with lifetime risk of biliary cancer estimated at 18% in individuals with HNPCC (147). It is currently unknown whether mutations in any particular mismatch repair enzyme (MLH1, MSH2, MSH6) confer a higher risk of biliary tumors compared to the others.

Excess biliary tree tumors, particularly gallbladder cancer, may also be associated with germline mutations in the ATM gene on chromosome 11q22 (the gene implicated in ataxia-telangiectasia) (148), as well as the BRCA1 (carrier RR 1.87, 0.59—5.88) (149) and BRCA2 genes (RR 4.97, 1.50—16.52) (150). Germline mutation of the STK11/LKB1 gene associated with PJS may lead to an increased risk for biliary cancer because somatic mutations of this gene have been identified in 4% to 6% of sporadic biliary tumors (151). Interestingly, the risk of biliary tract cancers may be even greater in the subset (30%) of families who phenotypically have PJS but in whom a germline STK11/LKB1 mutation cannot be detected, suggesting the presence of an as-yet unidentified cancer predisposition gene (152).

A family history of nonmalignant medical disorders may also predispose families to biliary tree tumors. Family history of gallstone disease has been associated with an increased risk of biliary tumors (101,126). PSC may also run in families with inflammatory bowel disease (153). A Swedish study of 604 PSC patients followed over 28 years described an incidence of 13% for cholangiocarcinoma (154). Familial predisposition to gallstones and subsequent gallbladder cancer may involve a genetic defect in cholesterol and bile acid metabolism (155), whereas the etiology of PSC-related cholangiocarcinoma is unknown.

Association with Cancers of Other Sites

Cancers of the biliary tree occur simultaneously with cancers at other sites. Cancers that have been described in association with biliary tract tumors include prostate cancer (156), ovarian cancer (157), breast cancer (158), and other gastrointestinal cancers (159). Many of these are likely associated with identified (FAP, HNPCC) and as-yet unidentified familial cancer syndromes.

Four recent studies have used large cancer databases to investigate associations of biliary tract cancers and cancers at other sites. Su et al. evaluated associations between biliary tract cancer and other cancers using SEER data. No association was found between biliary tract cancer and either estrogen-related cancers of the breast and uterine corpus or smoking-related upper aerodigestive tract cancers. An inverse relationship was noted between the risk of gallbladder cancer and the risk of prostate cancer, but a positive relationship was seen with the risk of cervical cancer (160). The SEER database has also been used to show an association between ampullary cancer and colorectal cancer (161). A study of the Swedish Family Cancer Database found that gallbladder cancer was associated with pancreatic cancer, cholangiocarcinoma with ovarian cancer, and ampullary cancer with thyroid cancer (162). Finally, an investigation of collaborative European data from the Cancer

Incidence in Five Continents found correlations between gallbladder cancer and hepatocellular, colon, and pancreas cancers, while, like in the SEER analysis of Su et al., prostate cancer was negatively correlated to gallbladder cancer (163).

MOLECULAR BIOLOGY

Despite the anatomical proximity of the biliary tree structures, molecular carcinogenesis is somewhat different for each organ site. Although oncogenes and tumor suppressors, such as K-ras and p53, are associated with tumorigenesis in a wide range of cancers, they are only a small part of the complex evolution of a normal cell to a malignant cell.

A number of molecular events have been associated with ampullary cancer. Although ampullary cancer incidence is increased in individuals with germline *APC* mutations, somatic mutations of the *APC* gene have also been identified in sporadic ampullary cancers (164). As in other gastrointestinal tumors, high frequency of K-ras (10%–40%) (37,165) and p53 (30%–50%) (164) mutations have been reported, with K-ras mutations commonly found in carcinomas and adenomas (37), suggesting that mutations in K-ras are an early molecular event in ampullary carcinogenesis. In contradistinction, evidence suggests that *TP53* mutations occur late in ampullary carcinogenesis and are associated with more advanced tumors (those with lymph node invasion and/or metastatic disease) (37). DNA-mismatch repair defects in ampullary cancers have also been described (164).

The role of K-ras activation and p53 dysregulation has also been investigated in cholangiocarcinoma. Reported frequency of K-ras mutations varies widely in cholangiocarcinoma. K-ras mutations are reported to be less common in intrahepatic cholangiocarcinoma (range 4.6%–22.5%) compared to hilar or extrahepatic disease, where they are found in 75% and 30% of tumors, respectively (166–168). *TP53* mutations have been found in approximately 30% of cholangiocarcinomas (10.7–37.5) (167,169,170). At least two groups have reported an increased frequency of microsatellite instability in cholangiocarcinomas (4.7% [167] and 18.2% [170]).

As in ampullary and bile duct tumors, K-ras and *TP53* dysregulation are believed to be central elements in gallbladder carcinogenesis. Here, a well-described progression of somatic mutations in the gallbladder epithelium is predicted to be necessary for malignant transformation, as summarized by Wistuba and Gazdar (171). K-ras mutations have been reported in gallbladder cancers, but for the most part they appear to be rare in Western patients and cholelithiasis-related gallbladder cancers (172). Overexpression of p53 protein and *TP53* gene mutations may be related to increasing cytologic atypia (173) and tumor invasiveness (174). Gallbladder carcinomas from patients in two high-prevalence areas (Niigata, Japan, and Santiago, Chile) were analyzed for acquired mutations in exons 5 to 8 of the *TP53* tumor-suppressor gene (175). Of 42 tumors, 22 (52.4%) had alterations identified by polymerase chain reaction amplification and direct sequencing; on immunohistochemical analysis, 55 of 84 cases (65.5%) showed overexpression of p53 protein, which suggests that *TP53* mutations are important in gallbladder carcinogenesis.

COX-2 overexpression has been found in a number of tumor types, including breast and colorectal cancer. Through the constitutive production of prostaglandins, COX-2 enzyme activation leads to blood vessel proliferation and unregulated tumor growth. Elevated COX-2 activity plays a role in biliary tree tumor pathogenesis. COX-2 overexpression has been noted in gallbladder cancer, with more advanced tumors (T3 and T4) having a significantly increased level of COX-2 mRNA expression compared to T1 and T2 lesions. In advanced lesions, COX-2 expression was also upregulated in the adjacent stromal tissue, with the stroma demonstrating high prostaglandin PGE2 (a product of COX-2 activity) (176). The same group has demonstrated a correlation between COX-2 upregulation and more aggressive disease (177).

SCREENING

Both gallbladder cancer and cholangiocarcinoma carry a poor prognosis unless detected at an early stage. Therefore, it is important to identify individuals at high risk for developing biliary cancers and intervene prophylactically in a timely manner.

Various serum and bile markers have been evaluated for the early detection of both gallbladder cancer and cholangiocarcinoma. Thus far, CA 19-9 has been shown to be the most useful marker for the detection of early neoplasia in biliary tumors. Serum CA 19-9 has been shown to have a sensitivity of 53% to 92% and a specificity of 50% to 98%. Unfortunately, different studies have used different cut-off values. Other drawbacks of this test are false positives seen with pancreatic cancer, as well as benign biliary obstruction with hyperbilirubinemia and false negatives in patients who are Lewis blood antigen negative (∼7% of the population) (178). The addition of serum carcinoembryonic antigen (CEA) and bile levels of CA 19-9 and CEA have shown similar results but in combination do not appear to improve the diagnostic accuracy of serum CA 19-9 alone. Other markers, such as CA 242 and CA 125, appear to have high specificity but relatively low sensitivity, which limits their utility as screening tests. In the future, analysis of bile aspirates for genetic mutations, such as K-*ras*, p53, and p16, may prove useful in the early detection of biliary cancers (178).

Gallbladder polyps are generally followed by transabdominal ultrasound for change in size. Transabdominal ultrasound has traditionally not been accurate in the differentiation between benign and malignant small polyps (<2 cm). In addition, many patients with polyps have concomitant gallstones, which produce acoustic shadowing that limits the evaluation of the gallbladder. Endoscopic ultrasound (EUS) appears to have improved diagnostic capability for small polyps (179). EUS scoring systems have been proposed to differentiate benign from malignant polyps (180,181), but these have yet to be prospectively validated.

The early detection of cholangiocarcinoma in PSC with extrahepatic strictures is often challenging. ERCP with cholangiogram alone has a diagnostic accuracy of 60% to 80% for differentiating benign from malignant strictures (182). The recent addition of intraductal ultrasound can improve the diagnostic accuracy to up to 90% (183). Unfortunately, obtaining a tissue diagnosis is still elusive, and brush cytology and intraductal biopsy of strictures have a 35% to 45% diagnostic yield (182). In the future, techniques such as molecular analysis of cytology specimens or direct imaging with fluorescence cholangioscopy may prove to be useful screening tools for the detection of early cholangiocarcinoma.

PREVENTION

Individuals at high risk for the development of gallbladder cancer or cholangiocarcinoma should have prophylactic surgery to prevent the development of cancer (Table 34.4). However, there have been no studies prospectively validating cholecystectomy as prophylaxis against gallbladder cancer. Available data support cholecystectomy for individuals with gallstones >3 cm in diameter, porcelain gallbladder, gallbladder polyps >1 cm in diameter, and any size gallbladder polyp causing biliary colic. Gallstones may increase the risk of gallbladder cancer in patients with PSC, (58) and a study by Buckles et al. (71)

TABLE 34.4

INDICATIONS FOR CHOLECYSTECTOMY WITH OR WITHOUT BILIARY RESECTION FOR THE PREVENTION OF GALLBLADDER CANCER OR CHOLANGIOCARCINOMA

RECOMMENDED
Gallstones >3 cm
Gallbladder polyps >1 cm
Biliary colic due to gallbladder polyps of any size
Porcelain gallbladder
Choledochal cysts (with biliary resection)
Anomalous junction of the pancreaticobiliary duct (± biliary resection)

OPTIONAL
Primary sclerosing cholangitis
High prevalence background with any size gallstones

demonstrated a high incidence of adenocarcinoma in gallbladder polyps in PSC patients. A majority of patients with PSC also have ulcerative colitis; if colectomy is required, it may be reasonable to perform cholecystectomy at the same time. There may be a role for screening all individuals from high-risk geographic regions and ethnic backgrounds for gallstones, and then performing cholecystectomy in those with stones of any size. However, appropriate cost–benefit analyses should be performed prior to adopting such a strategy.

Most children with choledochal cysts, which can now be detected with magnetic resonance cholangiopancreatography, subsequently undergo complete biliary resection (184). Occasionally, these anatomical abnormalities are not detected until adulthood, and biliary resection should be performed at the time of diagnosis. If the patient is a poor surgical candidate, then serum CA 19-9 should be serially measured to evaluate for the development of cholangiocarcinoma. Individuals with an anomalous junction of the pancreaticobiliary duct are at markedly increased risk for developing both gallbladder and bile duct cancer. Cholecystectomy and excision of the biliary tree is recommended for patients with AJPD, although there is evidence that cholecystectomy alone may be adequate for patients with AJPD and no common bile duct dilation (167,185).

There has been little research evaluating chemopreventive agents for biliary cancers. Liu et al. (186) conducted a case-control study of aspirin use in subjects with biliary cancer, benign gallstone disease, and healthy controls. Aspirin use was associated with significantly reduced odds of gallbladder cancer (OR, 0.37; 95% CI, 0.17–0.88) and a nonsignificant reduction in odds of extrahepatic bile duct and ampullary cancers. In vitro and in vivo laboratory studies have demonstrated that COX-2 inhibitors promote apoptosis in gallbladder cancer and cholangiocarcinoma cells (187–189). Individuals with FAP generally undergo total proctocolectomy at the time of diagnosis. However, not everyone undergoes surgery, and COX-2 inhibitors have been shown to reduce the number of adenomatous colon polyps in patients with FAP (190). Aspirin and other COX-2 inhibitors may likewise prevent ampullary adenomas, although this has not been formally studied. Ursodeoxycholic acid (UDCA) is a compound derived from bile, and in vitro studies have shown that UDCA inhibits the proliferation of colon cancer cells (191,192). UDCA also has antiinflammatory effects and is used in the treatment of primary biliary cirrhosis to slow the progression of liver fibrosis. Future research is warranted to examine UDCA as a chemopreventive agent for biliary cancers.

References

1. Percy C, van Holten V, Muir C, eds. International Classification of Diseases for Oncology. 2nd ed. Geneva: World Health Organization; 1990.
2. Jemal A, Murray T, Ward E, et al. Cancer statistics, 2005. CA Cancer J Clin 2005;55(1):10–30. [erratum: CA Cancer J Clin 2005;55(4):259].
3. Dixon E, Vollmer CM, Jr., Sahajpal A, et al. An aggressive surgical approach leads to improved survival in patients with gallbladder cancer: a 12-year study at a North American Center. Ann Surg 2005;241(3):385–394.
4. Donohue JH, Stewart AK, Menck HR. The National Cancer Data Base report on carcinoma of the gallbladder, 1989–1995. Cancer 1998;83(12): 2618–2628.
5. Abi-Rached B, Neugut AI. Diagnostic and management issues in gallbladder carcinoma. Oncology (Huntingt) 1995;9(1):19–24; discussion 24.
6. Lazaridis KN, Gores GJ. Cholangiocarcinoma. Gastroenterology 2005; 128(6):1655–67.
7. Devesa SS, Grauman MA, Blot WJ, Pennello G, Hoover RN, Fraumeni JF Jr. Atlas of Cancer Mortality in the United States, 1950–94. Washington, DC: U.S. Government Printing Office; 1999.
8. Ross RK, Hartnett NM, Bernstein L, Henderson BE. Epidemiology of adenocarcinomas of the small intestine: is bile a small bowel carcinogen? Br J Cancer 1991;63(1):143–145.
9. Benhamiche AM, Jouve JL, Manfredi S, Prost P, Isambert N, Faivre J. Cancer of the ampulla of Vater: results of a 20-year population-based study. Eur J Gastroenterol Hepatol 2000;12(1):75–79.
10. Koea J, Phillips A, Lawes C, Rodgers M, Windsor J, McCall J. Gall bladder cancer, extrahepatic bile duct cancer and ampullary carcinoma in New Zealand: demographics, pathology and survival. ANZ J Surg 2002;72(12):857–861.
11. Kato I, Kuroishi T, Tominaga S. Descriptive epidemiology of subsites of cancers of the liver, biliary tract and pancreas in Japan. Jpn J Clin Oncol 1990;20(3):232–237.
12. Shaib Y, El-Serag HB. The epidemiology of cholangiocarcinoma. Semin Liver Dis 2004;24(2):115–125.
13. Diehl AK. Epidemiology of gallbladder cancer: a synthesis of recent data. J Natl Cancer Inst 1980;65(6):1209–1214.
14. Lowenfels AB, Lindstrom CG, Conway MJ, Hastings PR. Gallstones and risk of gallbladder cancer. J Natl Cancer Inst 1985;75(1):77–80.
15. Pitt HA, Dooley WC, Yeo CJ, Cameron JL. Malignancies of the biliary tree. Curr Probl Surg 1995;32(1):1–90.
16. Zou S, Zhang L, Zen G, Chen J, Xia S. Clinical epidemiologic characteristics of 430 cases of gallbladder cancer. Chin Med J 1998;111(5):391–393. [erratum: Chin Med J (Engl) 1998;111(10):902].
17. www.iarc.org.
18. Khan SA, Taylor-Robinson SD, Toledano MB, Beck A, Elliott P, Thomas HC. Changing international trends in mortality rates for liver, biliary and pancreatic tumours. J Hepatol 2002;37(6):806–813.
19. Strom BL, Hibberd PL, Soper KA, Stolley PD, Nelson WL. International variations in epidemiology of cancers of the extrahepatic biliary tract. Cancer Res 1985;45(10):5165–5168.
20. www.seer.org.
21. Menck HR, Mack TM. Incidence of biliary tract cancer in Los Angeles. Natl Cancer Inst Monogr 1982;62:95–99.
22. Morris DL, Buechley RW, Key CR, Morgan MV. Gallbladder disease and gallbladder cancer among American Indians in tricultural New Mexico. Cancer 1978;42(5):2472–2477.
23. Martinez I, Torres R, Frias Z. Cancer incidence in the United States and Puerto Rico. Cancer Res 1975;35(11 pt 2):3265–3271.
24. Chow WH, McLaughlin JK, Menck HR, Mack TM. Risk factors for extrahepatic bile duct cancers: Los Angeles County, California (USA). Cancer Causes Control 1994;5(3):267–272.
25. Ghadirian P, Simard A, Baillargeon J. A population-based case-control study of cancer of the bile ducts and gallbladder in Quebec, Canada. Revue Epidemiol Sante Publique 1993;41(2):107–112.
26. Legorreta AP, Silber JH, Costantino GN, Kobylinski RW, Zatz SL. Increased cholecystectomy rate after the introduction of laparoscopic cholecystectomy [see comment]. JAMA 1993;270(12):1429–1432.
27. Diehl AK. Laparoscopic cholecystectomy: too much of a good thing? [comment]. JAMA 1993;270(12):1469–1470.
28. Levi F, Lucchini F, Negri E, La Vecchia C. The recent decline in gallbladder cancer mortality in Europe. Eur J Cancer Prev 2003;12(4):265–267.
29. Darabos N, Stare R. Gallbladder cancer: laparoscopic and classic cholecystectomy. Surg Endosc 2004;18(1):144–147.
30. Lambe M, Trichopoulos D, Hsieh CC, Ekbom A, Adami HO, Pavia M. Parity and cancers of the gall bladder and the extrahepatic bile ducts. Int J Cancer 1993;54(6):941–944.
31. Nervi F, Duarte I, Gomez G, et al. Frequency of gallbladder cancer in Chile, a high-risk area. Int J Cancer 1988;41(5):657–660.
32. Lowenfels AB, Maisonneuve P, Boyle P, Zatonski WA. Epidemiology of gallbladder cancer. Hepatogastroenterology 1999;46(27):1529–1532.
33. Misra S, Chaturvedi A, Misra NC, Sharma ID. Carcinoma of the gallbladder. Lancet Oncol 2003;4(3):167–176.
34. Lazcano-Ponce EC, Miquel JF, Munoz N, et al. Epidemiology and molecular pathology of gallbladder cancer. CA Cancer J Clin 2001;51(6):349–364.

35. Nagorney DM, McPherson GA. Carcinoma of the gallbladder and extrahepatic bile ducts. *Semin Oncol* 1988;15(2):106–115.

36. Khan ZR, Neugut AI, Ahsan H, Chabot JA. Risk factors for biliary tract cancers. *Am J Gastroenterol* 1999;94(1):149–152.

37. Zatonski WA, Lowenfels AB, Boyle P, et al. Epidemiologic aspects of gallbladder cancer: a case-control study of the SEARCH Program of the International Agency for Research on Cancer. *J Natl Cancer Inst* 1997;89(15):1132–1138.

38. Silecchia G, Raparelli L, Jover Navalon JM, et al. Laparoscopic cholecystectomy and incidental carcinoma of the extrahepatic biliary tree. *JSLS* 2002;6(4):339–344.

39. Vitetta L, Sali A, Little P, Mrazek L. Gallstones and gall bladder carcinoma. *Aust N Z J Surg* 2000;70(9):667–673.

40. Mori T, Souda S, Hashimoto J, Yoshikawa Y, Ohshima M. Unsuspected gallbladder cancer diagnosed by laparoscopic cholecystectomy: a clinicopathological study. *Surg Today* 1997;27(8):710–713.

41. Diehl AK. Gallstone size and the risk of gallbladder cancer. *JAMA* 1983;250(17):2323–2326.

42. Lowenfels AB, Walker AM, Althaus DP, Townsend G, Domellof L. Gallstone growth, size, and risk of gallbladder cancer: an interracial study. *Int J Epidemiol* 1989;18(1):50–54.

43. Su WC, Chan KK, Lin XZ, et al. A clinical study of 130 patients with biliary tract cancers and periampullary tumors. *Oncology* 1996;53(6):488–493.

44. Parkin DM, Ohshima H, Srivatanakul P, Vatanasapt V. Cholangiocarcinoma: epidemiology, mechanisms of carcinogenesis and prevention. *Cancer Epidemiol Biomarkers Prev* 1993;2(6):537–544.

45. Nakanuma Y, Terada T, Tanaka Y, Ohta G. Are hepatolithiasis and cholangiocarcinoma aetiologically related? A morphological study of 12 cases of hepatolithiasis associated with cholangiocarcinoma. *Virchows Arch A Pathol Anat Histopathol* 1985;406(1):45–58.

46. Liu KJ, Richter HM, Cho MJ, Jarad J, Nadimpalli V, Donahue PE. Carcinoma involving the gallbladder in elderly patients presenting with acute cholecystitis. *Surgery* 1997;122(4):748–754; discussion 754–756.

47. Black WC. The morphogenesis of gallbladder carcinoma. In: Fenoglio CM, Wolff M, ed. *Progress in Surgical Pathology*. New York, NY: Masson; 1980:207–220.

48. Kanoh K, Shimura T, Tsutsumi S, et al. Significance of contracted cholecystitis lesions as high risk for gallbladder carcinogenesis. *Cancer Lett* 2001;169(1):7–14.

49. Berk RN, Armbuster TG, Saltzstein SL. Carcinoma in the porcelain gallbladder. *Radiology* 1973;106(1):29–31.

50. Polk HC, Jr. Carcinoma and the calcified gall bladder. *Gastroenterology* 1966;50(4):582–585.

51. Towfigh S, McFadden DW, Cortina GR, et al. Porcelain gallbladder is not associated with gallbladder carcinoma. *Am Surg* 2001;67(1):7–10.

52. Kornfeld D, Ekbom A, Ihre T. Survival and risk of cholangiocarcinoma in patients with primary sclerosing cholangitis: a population-based study. *Scand J Gastroenterol* 1997;32(10):1042–1045.

53. Broome U, Olsson R, Loof L, et al. Natural history and prognostic factors in 305 Swedish patients with primary sclerosing cholangitis. *Gut* 1996;38(4):610–615.

54. Farges O, Malassagne B, Sebagh M, Bismuth H. Primary sclerosing cholangitis: liver transplantation or biliary surgery. *Surgery* 1995;117(2):146–155.

55. Rosen CB, Nagorney DM. Cholangiocarcinoma complicating primary sclerosing cholangitis. *Semin Liver Dis* 1991;11(1):26–30.

56. Abu-Elmagd KM, Malinchoc M, Dickson ER, et al. Efficacy of hepatic transplantation in patients with primary sclerosing cholangitis. *Surg Gynecol Obstet* 1993;177(4):335–344.

57. Rosen CB, Nagorney DM, Wiesner RH, Coffey RJ, Jr., LaRusso NF. Cholangiocarcinoma complicating primary sclerosing cholangitis. *Ann Surg* 1991;213(1):21–25.

58. Brandt DJ, MacCarty RL, Charboneau JW, LaRusso NF, Wiesner RH, Ludwig J. Gallbladder disease in patients with primary sclerosing cholangitis. *AJR Am J Roentgenol* 1988;150(3):571–574.

59. Gossard AA, Angulo P, Lindor KD. Secondary sclerosing cholangitis: a comparison to primary sclerosing cholangitis. *Am J Gastroenterol* 2005;100(6):1330–1333.

60. Chapman RW, Cottone M, Selby WS, Shepherd HA, Sherlock S, Jewell DP. Serum autoantibodies, ulcerative colitis and primary sclerosing cholangitis. *Gut* 1986;27(1):86–91.

61. Mandal A, Dasgupta A, Jeffers L, et al. Autoantibodies in sclerosing cholangitis against a shared peptide in biliary and colon epithelium. *Gastroenterology* 1994;106(1):185–192.

62. Ritchie JK, Allan RN, Macartney J, Thompson H, Hawley PR, Cooke WT. Biliary tract carcinoma associated with ulcerative colitis. *Q J Med* 1974;43(170):263–279.

63. Lupinetti M, Mehigan D, Cameron JL. Hepatobiliary complications of ulcerative colitis. *Am J Surg* 1980;139(1):113–118.

64. Akwari OE, Van Heerden JA, Foulk WT, Baggenstoss AH. Cancer of the bile ducts associated with ulcerative colitis. *Ann Surg* 1975;181(3):303–309.

65. Kozuka S. Premalignancy of the mucosal polyp in the large intestine: I. Histologic gradation of the polyp on the basis of epithelial pseudostratification and glandular branching. *Dis Colon Rectum* 1975;18(6):483–493.

66. Kozuka S, Tsubone N, Yasui A, Hachisuka K. Relation of adenoma to carcinoma in the gallbladder. *Cancer* 1982;50(10):2226–2234.

67. Kozuka S, Tsubone M, Yamaguchi A, Hachisuka K. Adenomatous residue in cancerous papilla of Vater. *Gut* 1981;22(12):1031–1034.

68. Okamoto M, Okamoto H, Kitahara F, et al. Ultrasonographic evidence of association of polyps and stones with gallbladder cancer. *Am J Gastroenterol* 1999;94(2):446–450.

69. Terzi C, Sokmen S, Seckin S, Albayrak L, Ugurlu M. Polypoid lesions of the gallbladder: report of 100 cases with special reference to operative indications. *Surgery* 2000;127(6):622–627.

70. Collett JA, Allan RB, Chisholm RJ, Wilson IR, Burt MJ, Chapman BA. Gallbladder polyps: prospective study. *J Ultrasound Med* 1998;17(4):207–211.

71. Buckles DC, Lindor KD, Larusso NF, Petrovic LM, Gores GJ. In primary sclerosing cholangitis, gallbladder polyps are frequently malignant. *Am J Gastroenterol* 2002;97(5):1138–1142.

72. Offerhaus GJ, Giardiello FM, Krush AJ, et al. The risk of upper gastrointestinal cancer in familial adenomatous polyposis. *Gastroenterology* 1992;102(6):1980–1982.

73. Wada K, Tanaka M, Yamaguchi K, Wada K. Carcinoma and polyps of the gallbladder associated with Peutz-Jeghers syndrome. *Dig Dis Sci* 1987;32(8):943–946.

74. Vogel T, Schumacher V, Saleh A, Trojan J, Moslein G. Extraintestinal polyps in Peutz-Jeghers syndrome: presentation of four cases and review of the literature. Deutsche Peutz–Jeghers Studiengruppe. *Int J Colorectal Dis* 2000;15(2):118–123.

75. Todani T, Tabuchi K, Watanabe Y, Kobayashi T. Carcinoma arising in the wall of congenital bile duct cysts. *Cancer* 1979;44(3):1134–1141.

76. Tsuchiya R, Harada N, Ito T, Furukawa M, Yoshihiro I. Malignant tumors in choledochal cysts. *Ann Surg* 1977;186(1):22–28.

77. Soreide K, Korner H, Havnen J, Soreide JA. Bile duct cysts in adults. *Br J Surg* 2004;91(12):1538–1548.

78. Komi N, Tamura T, Tsuge S, Miyoshi Y, Udaka H, Takehara H. Relation of patient age to premalignant alterations in choledochal cyst epithelium: histochemical and immunohistochemical studies. *J Pediatr Surg* 1986;21(5):430–433.

79. Wiseman K, Buczkowski AK, Chung SW, Francoeur J, Schaeffer D, Scudamore CH. Epidemiology, presentation, diagnosis, and outcomes of choledochal cysts in adults in an urban environment. *Am J Surg* 2005;189(5):527–531; discussion 531.

80. Kobayashi S, Asano T, Yamasaki M, Kenmochi T, Nakagohri T, Ochiai T. Risk of bile duct carcinogenesis after excision of extrahepatic bile ducts in pancreaticobiliary maljunction. *Surgery* 1999;126(5):939–944.

81. Chijiiwa K, Kimura H, Tanaka M. Malignant potential of the gallbladder in patients with anomalous pancreaticobiliary ductal junction: the difference in risk between patients with and without choledochal cyst. *Int Surg* 1995;80(1):61–64.

82. Hu B, Gong B, Zhou DY. Association of anomalous pancreaticobiliary ductal junction with gallbladder carcinoma in Chinese patients: an ERCP study. *Gastrointest Endosc* 2003;57(4):541–545.

83. Elnemr A, Ohta T, Kayahara M, et al. Anomalous pancreaticobiliary ductal junction without bile duct dilatation in gallbladder cancer. *Hepatogastroenterology* 2001;48(38):382–386.

84. Tersmette AC, Offerhaus GJ, Giardiello FM, Tersmette KW, Vandenbroucke JP, Tytgat GN. Occurrence of non-gastric cancer in the digestive tract after remote partial gastrectomy: analysis of an Amsterdam cohort. *Int J Cancer* 1990;46(5):792–795.

85. Inoue K, Fuchigami A, Higashide S, et al. Gallbladder sludge and stone formation in relation to contractile function after gastrectomy: a prospective study. *Ann Surg* 1992;215(1):19–26.

86. Hamasaki T, Hamanaka Y, Adachi A, Suzuki T. Evaluation of gallbladder function before and after gastrectomy using a double-isotope method. *Dig Dis Sci* 1995;40(4):722–729.

87. Caygill C, Hill M, Kirkham J, Northfield TC. Increased risk of biliary tract cancer following gastric surgery. *Br J Cancer* 1988;57(4):434–436.

88. Kobayashi T, Hisanaga M, Kanehiro H, Yamada Y, Ko S, Nakajima Y. Analysis of risk factors for the development of gallstones after gastrectomy. *Br J Surg* 2005;92(11):1399–1403.

89. Belamaric J. Intrahepatic bile duct carcinoma and C. sinensis infection in Hong Kong. *Cancer* 1973;31(2):468–473.

90. Bunyaratvej S, Meenakanit V, Tantachamrun T, Srinawat P, Susilaworn P, Chongchitnan N. Nationwide survey of major liver diseases in Thailand analysis of 3 305 biopsies as to year-end 1978. *J Med Assoc Thai* 1981;64(9):432–439.

91. Srivatanakul P, Ohshima H, Khlat M, et al. Opisthorchis viverrini infestation and endogenous nitrosamines as risk factors for cholangiocarcinoma in Thailand. *Int J Cancer* 1991;48(6):821–825.

92. Vatanasapt V, Uttaravichien T, Mairiang EO, Pairojkul C, Chartbanchachai W, Haswell-Elkins M. Cholangiocarcinoma in north-east Thailand. *Lancet* 1990;335(8681):116–117.

93. Elkins DB, Haswell-Elkins MR, Mairiang E, et al. A high frequency of hepatobiliary disease and suspected cholangiocarcinoma associated with heavy Opisthorchis viverrini infection in a small community in north-east Thailand. *Trans R Soc Trop Med Hyg* 1990;84(5):715–719.

94. Mairiang E, Elkins DB, Mairiang P, et al. Relationship between intensity of Opisthorchis viverrini infection and hepatobiliary disease detected by ultrasonography. *J Gastroenterol Hepatol* 1992;7(1):17–21.

95. Haswell-Elkins MR, Sithithaworn P, Mairiang E, et al. Immune responsiveness and parasite-specific antibody levels in human hepatobiliary disease associated with *Opisthorchis viverrini* infection. *Clin Exp Immunol* 1991;84(2):213–218.

96. Fukuda K, Kuroki T, Tajima Y, et al. Comparative analysis of *Helicobacter* DNAs and biliary pathology in patients with and without hepatobiliary cancer. *Carcinogenesis* 2002;23(11):1927–1931.

97. Matsukura N, Yokomuro S, Yamada S, et al. Association between *Helicobacter bilis* in bile and biliary tract malignancies; *H. bilis* in bile from Japanese and Thai patients with benign and malignant diseases in the biliary tract. *Jpn J Cancer Res* 2002;93(7):842–847.

98. Fox JG, Dewhirst FE, Shen Z, et al. Hepatic Helicobacter species identified in bile and gallbladder tissue from Chileans with chronic cholecystitis. *Gastroenterology* 1998;114(4):755–763.

99. Maurer KJ, Ihrig MM, Rogers AB, et al. Identification of cholelithogenic enterohepatic *Helicobacter* species and their role in murine cholesterol gallstone formation. *Gastroenterology* 2005;128(4):1023–1033.

100. Welton JC, Marr JS, Friedman SM. Association between hepatobiliary cancer and typhoid carrier state. *Lancet* 1979;1(8120):791–794.

101. Strom BL, Soloway RD, Rios-Dalenz JL, Rodriguez-Martinez HA, West SL, Kinman JL, et al. Risk factors for gallbladder cancer: an international collaborative case-control study. *Cancer* 1995;76(10):1747–1756.

102. Dutta U, Garg PK, Kumar R, Tandon RK. Typhoid carriers among patients with gallstones are at increased risk for carcinoma of the gallbladder. *Am J Gastroenterol* 2000;95(3):784–787.

103. Csendes A, Becerra M, Burdiles P, Demian I, Bancalari K, Csendes P. Bacteriological studies of bile from the gallbladder in patients with carcinoma of the gallbladder, cholelithiasis, common bile duct stones and no gallstones disease. *Eur J Surg* 1994;160(6–7):363–367.

104. Kato I, Kido C. Increased risk of death in thorotrast-exposed patients during the late follow-up period. *Jpn J Cancer Res* 1987;78(11):1187–1192.

105. Kiyosawa K, Imai H, Sodeyama T, et al. Comparison of anamnestic history, alcohol intake and smoking, nutritional status, and liver dysfunction between thorotrast patients who developed primary liver cancer and those who did not. *Environ Res* 1989;49(2):166–172.

106. Lowenfels AB, Norman J. Isoniazid and bile duct cancer. *JAMA* 1978;240(5):434–5.

107. Broden G, Bengtsson L. Biliary carcinoma associated with methyldopa therapy. *Acta Chir Scand Suppl* 1980;500:7–12.

108. Neugut AI, Wylie P, Brandt-Rauf PW. Occupational cancers of the gastrointestinal tract. II. Pancreas, liver, and biliary tract. *Occup Med* 1987;2(1):137–153.

109. Zarchy TM. Chlorinated hydrocarbon solvents and biliary-pancreatic cancer: report of three cases. *Am J Ind Med* 1996;30(3):341–342.

110. Kazerouni N, Thomas TL, Petralia SA, Hayes RB. Mortality among workers exposed to cutting oil mist: update of previous reports. *Am J Ind Med* 2000;38(4):410–416.

111. Malker HS, McLaughlin JK, Malker BK, et al. Biliary tract cancer and occupation in Sweden. *Br J Ind Med* 1986;43(4):257–262.

112. Goldberg MS, Theriault G. Retrospective cohort study of workers of a synthetic textiles plant in Quebec: II. Colorectal cancer mortality and incidence. *Am J Ind Med* 1994;25(6):909–922.

113. Kuzmickiene I, Didziapetris R, Stukonis M. Cancer incidence in the workers cohort of textile manufacturing factory in Alytus, Lithuania. *J Occup Environ Med* 2004;46(2):147–153.

114. Tomasek L, Darby SC, Swerdlow AJ, Placek V, Kunz E. Radon exposure and cancers other than lung cancer among uranium miners in West Bohemia [see comment]. *Lancet* 1993;341(8850):919–923.

115. Yassi A, Tate RB, Routledge M. Cancer incidence and mortality in workers employed at a transformer manufacturing plant: update to a cohort study. *Am J Ind Med* 2003;44(1):58–62.

116. Lynge E, Anttila A, Hemminki K. Organic solvents and cancer. *Cancer Causes Control* 1997;8(3):406–419.

117. Blair A. Mortality among workers in the metal polishing and plating industry, 1951–1969. *J Occup Med* 1980;22(3):158–162.

118. Blair A, Decoufle P, Grauman D. Causes of death among laundry and dry cleaning workers. *Am J Public Health* 1979;69(5):508–511.

119. Bond GG, Reeve GR, Ott MG, Waxweiler RJ. Mortality among a sample of chemical company employees. *Am J Ind Med* 1985;7(2):109–121.

120. Kanarek MS. Epidemiological studies on ingested mineral fibres: gastric and other cancers. *IARC Sci Publ* 1989;(90):428–437.

121. Moran EM. Epidemiological factors of cancer in California. *J Environ Pathol Toxicol Oncol* 1992;11(5–6):303–307.

122. Samanic C, Gridley G, Chow WH, Lubin J, Hoover RN, Fraumeni JF, Jr. Obesity and cancer risk among white and black United States veterans. *Cancer Causes Control* 2004;15(1):35–43.

123. Zatonski WA, La Vecchia C, Przewozniak K, Maisonneuve P, Lowenfels AB, Boyle P. Risk factors for gallbladder cancer: a Polish case-control study. *Int J Cancer* 1992;51(5):707–711.

124. Calle EE, Rodriguez C, Walker-Thurmond K, Thun MJ. Overweight, obesity, and mortality from cancer in a prospectively studied cohort of U.S. adults [see comment]. *N Engl J Med* 2003;348(17):1625–1638.

125. O'Brien K, Cokkinides V, Jemal A, et al. Cancer statistics for Hispanics, 2003. *CA Cancer J Clin* 2003;53(4):208–226. [erratum: *CA Cancer J Clin* 2003;53(5):314.]

126. Kato K, Akai S, Tominaga S, Kato I. A case-control study of biliary tract cancer in Niigata Prefecture, Japan. *Jpn J Cancer Res* 1989;80(10):932–938.

127. Kuriyama S, Tsubono Y, Hozawa A, et al. Obesity and risk of cancer in Japan. *Int J Cancer* 2005;113(1):148–157.

128. Maclure KM, Hayes KC, Colditz GA, Stampfer MJ, Speizer FE, Willett WC. Weight, diet, and the risk of symptomatic gallstones in middle-aged women [see comment]. *N Engl J Med* 1989;321(9):563–569.

129. Syngal S, Coakley EH, Willett WC, Byers T, Williamson DF, Colditz GA. Long-term weight patterns and risk for cholecystectomy in women. *Ann Intern Med* 1999;130(6):471–477.

130. Parker ED, Folsom AR. Intentional weight loss and incidence of obesity-related cancers: the Iowa Women's Health Study. *Int J Obes Relat Metab Disord* 2003;27(12):1447–1452.

131. Bergstrom A, Pisani P, Tenet V, Wolk A, Adami HO. Overweight as an avoidable cause of cancer in Europe. *Int J Cancer* 2001;91(3):421–430. [erratum: *Int J Cancer* 2001;92(6):927.]

132. Yen S, Hsieh CC, MacMahon B. Extrahepatic bile duct cancer and smoking, beverage consumption, past medical history, and oral-contraceptive use. *Cancer* 1987;59(12):2112–2116.

133. Moerman CJ, Berns MP, Bueno de Mesquita HB, Runia S. Reproductive history and cancer of the biliary tract in women. *Int J Cancer* 1994;57(2):146–153.

134. Tavani A, Negri E, La Vecchia C. Menstrual and reproductive factors and biliary tract cancers. *Eur J Cancer Prev* 1996;5(4):241–247.

135. Anonymous. Combined oral contraceptives and gallbladder cancer: the WHO Collaborative Study of Neoplasia and Steroid Contraceptives. *Int J Epidemiol* 1989;18(2):309–314.

136. Everson GT, McKinley C, Lawson M, Johnson M, Kern F, Jr. Gallbladder function in the human female: effect of the ovulatory cycle, pregnancy, and contraceptive steroids. *Gastroenterology* 1982;82(4):711–719.

137. Watanapa P, Watanapa WB. Liver fluke-associated cholangiocarcinoma. *Br J Surg* 2002;89(8):962–970.

138. Adami HO, Chow WH, Nyren O, et al. Excess risk of primary liver cancer in patients with diabetes mellitus [see comment]. *J Natl Cancer Inst* 1996;88(20):1472–1477.

139. Coughlin SS, Calle EE, Teras LR, Petrelli J, Thun MJ. Diabetes mellitus as a predictor of cancer mortality in a large cohort of US adults. *Am J Epidemiol* 2004;159(12):1160–1167.

140. Scott TE, Carroll M, Cogliano FD, Smith BF, Lamorte WW. A case-control assessment of risk factors for gallbladder carcinoma. *Digest Dis Sci* 1999;44(8):1619–1625.

141. Kato I, Nomura A, Stemmermann GN, Chyou PH. Prospective study of clinical gallbladder disease and its association with obesity, physical activity, and other factors. *Digest Dis Sci* 1992;37(5):784–790.

142. Scragg RK, McMichael AJ, Baghurst PA. Diet, alcohol, and relative weight in gall stone disease: a case-control study. *Br Med J (Clin Res Ed)* 1984;288(6424):1113–1119.

143. Ji J, Couto E, Hemminki K. Incidence differences for gallbladder cancer between occupational groups suggest an etiological role for alcohol. *Int J Cancer* 2005;116(3):492–493.

144. Fernandez E, La Vecchia C, D'Avanzo B, Negri E, Franceschi S. Family history and the risk of liver, gallbladder, and pancreatic cancer. *Cancer Epidemiol Biomarkers Prev* 1994;3(3):209–212.

145. Sanabria JR, Croxford R, Berk TC, Cohen Z, Bapat BV, Gallinger S. Familial segregation in the occurrence and severity of periampullary neoplasms in familial adenomatous polyposis. *Am J Surg* 1996;171(1):136–140; discussion 140–141.

146. Trimbath JD, Griffin C, Romans K, Giardiello FM. Attenuated familial adenomatous polyposis presenting as ampullary adenocarcinoma. *Gut* 2003;52(6):903–904.

147. Aarnio M, Sankila R, Pukkala E, et al. Cancer risk in mutation carriers of DNA-mismatch-repair genes [see comment]. *Int J Cancer* 1999;81(2):214–218.

148. Swift M, Morrell D, Massey RB, Chase CL. Incidence of cancer in 161 families affected by ataxia-telangiectasia [see comment]. *N Engl J Med* 1991;325(26):1831–1836.

149. Thompson D, Easton DF, Breast Cancer Linkage C. Cancer incidence in BRCA1 mutation carriers [see comment]. *J Natl Cancer Inst* 2002;94(18):1358–1365.

150. Anonymous. Cancer risks in BRCA2 mutation carriers. The Breast Cancer Linkage Consortium. *J Natl Cancer Inst* 1999;91(15):1310–1316.

151. Su GH, Hruban RH, Bansal RK, et al. Germline and somatic mutations of the STK11/LKB1 Peutz-Jeghers gene in pancreatic and biliary cancers. *Am J Pathol* 1999;154(6):1835–1840.

152. Olschwang S, Boisson C, Thomas G. Peutz-Jeghers families unlinked to STK11/LKB1 gene mutations are highly predisposed to primitive biliary adenocarcinoma. *J Med Genet* 2001;38(6):356–360.

153. Bergquist A, Lindberg G, Saarinen S, Broome U. Increased prevalence of primary sclerosing cholangitis among first-degree relatives. *J Hepatol* 2005;42(2):252–256.

154. Bergquist A, Ekbom A, Olsson R, Kornfeldt D, Loof L, Danielsson A, et al. Hepatic and extrahepatic malignancies in primary sclerosing cholangitis [see comment]. *J Hepatol* 2002;36(3):321–327.

155. Pullinger CR, Eng C, Salen G, et al. Human cholesterol 7alpha-hydroxylase (CYP7A1) deficiency has a hypercholesterolemic phenotype [see comment]. *J Clin Invest* 2002;110(1):109–117.

156. Kleinerman RA, Liebermann JV, Li FP. Second cancer following cancer of the male genital system in Connecticut, 1935–82. *Natl Cancer Inst Monogr* 1985;68:139–147.

157. Lynge E, Jensen OM, Carstensen B. Second cancer following cancer of the digestive system in Denmark, 1943–80. *Natl Cancer Inst Monogr* 1985;68:277–308.

158. Ewertz M, Mouridsen HT. Second cancer following cancer of the female breast in Denmark, 1943–80. *Natl Cancer Inst Monogr* 1985;68:325–329.

159. Hoar SK, Wilson J, Blot WJ, McLaughlin JK, Winn DM, Kantor AF. Second cancer following cancer of the digestive system in Connecticut, 1935–1982. *Natl Cancer Inst Monogr* 1985;68:49–82.

160. Su Y, Ahsan H, Neugut AI. The association between biliary tract cancers and cancers of other sites. *Am J Gastroenterol* 1999;94(8):2256–2262.

161. Das A, Neugut AI, Cooper GS, Chak A. Association of ampullary and colorectal malignancies. *Cancer* 2004;100(3):524–530.

162. Hemminki K, Li X. Familial liver and gall bladder cancer: a nationwide epidemiological study from Sweden. *Gut* 2003;52(4):592–596.

163. Moore MA, Park CB, Tsuda H. European registry comparisons provide evidence of shared risk factors for renal, colon and gallbladder cancer development. *Eur J Cancer Prev* 1999;8(2):137–146.

164. Achille A, Scupoli MT, Magalini AR, et al. APC gene mutations and allelic losses in sporadic ampullary tumours: evidence of genetic difference from tumours associated with familial adenomatous polyposis. *Int J Cancer* 1996;68(3):305–312.

165. Ebert MP, Hoffmann J, Schneider-Stock R, et al. Analysis of K-ras gene mutations in rare pancreatic and ampullary tumours. *Eur J Gastroenterol Hepatol* 1998;10(12):1025–1029.

166. Rijken AM, van Gulik TM, Polak MM, Sturm PD, Gouma DJ, Offerhaus GJ. Diagnostic and prognostic value of incidence of K-ras codon 12 mutations in resected distal bile duct carcinoma. *J Surg Oncol* 1998;68(3):187–192.

167. Kusano T, Isa T, Tsukasa K, Sasaki M, Ohtsubo M, Furukawa M. Long-term results after cholecystectomy alone for patients with pancreaticobiliary maljunction without bile duct dilatation. *Int Surg* 2002;87(2):107–113.

168. Suto T, Habano W, Sugai T, et al. Aberrations of the K-ras, p53, and APC genes in extrahepatic bile duct cancer. *J Surg Oncol* 2000;73(3):158–163.

169. Kang YK, Kim WH, Lee HW, Lee HK, Kim YI. Mutation of p53 and K-ras, and loss of heterozygosity of APC in intrahepatic cholangiocarcinoma. *Lab Invest* 1999;79(4):477–483.

170. Momoi H, Itoh T, Nozaki Y, et al. Microsatellite instability and alternative genetic pathway in intrahepatic cholangiocarcinoma. *J Hepatol* 2001;35(2):235–244.

171. Wistuba II, Gazdar AF. Gallbladder cancer: lessons from a rare tumour. *Nat Rev Cancer* 2004;4(9):695–706.

172. Wistuba II, Sugio K, Hung J, et al. Allele-specific mutations involved in the pathogenesis of endemic gallbladder carcinoma in Chile. *Cancer Res* 1995;55(12):2511–2515.

173. Itoi T, Watanabe H, Yoshida M, Ajioka Y, Nishikura K, Saito T. Correlation of p53 protein expression with gene mutation in gall-bladder carcinomas. *Pathology Int* 1997;47(8):525–530.

174. Roa I, Villaseca M, Araya JC, et al. DNA ploidy pattern and tumor suppressor gene p53 expression in gallbladder carcinoma. *Cancer Epidemiol Biomarkers Prev* 1997;6(7):547–550.

175. Yokoyama N, Hitomi J, Watanabe H, et al. Mutations of p53 in gallbladder carcinomas in high-incidence areas of Japan and Chile. *Cancer Epidemiol Biomarkers Prev* 1998;7(4):297–301.

176. Asano T, Shoda J, Ueda T, et al. Expressions of cyclooxygenase-2 and prostaglandin E-receptors in carcinoma of the gallbladder: crucial role of arachidonate metabolism in tumor growth and progression. *Clin Cancer Res* 2002;8(4):1157–1167.

177. Ghosh M, Kamma H, Kawamoto T, et al. MUC 1 core protein as a marker of gallbladder malignancy. *Eur J Surg Oncol* 2005;31(8):891–896.

178. Nehls O, Gregor M, Klump B. Serum and bile markers for cholangiocarcinoma. *Semin Liver Dis* 2004;24(2):139–154.

179. Sugiyama M, Atomi Y, Yamato T. Endoscopic ultrasonography for differential diagnosis of polypoid gall bladder lesions: analysis in surgical and follow up series. *Gut* 2000;46(2):250–254.

180. Sadamoto Y, Oda S, Tanaka M, et al. A useful approach to the differential diagnosis of small polypoid lesions of the gallbladder, utilizing an endoscopic ultrasound scoring system. *Endoscopy* 2002;34(12):959–965.

181. Choi WB, Lee SK, Kim MH, et al. A new strategy to predict the neoplastic polyps of the gallbladder based on a scoring system using EUS. *Gastrointest Endosc* 2000;52(3):372–379.

182. Brugge WR. Endoscopic techniques to diagnose and manage biliary tumors. *J Clin Oncol* 2005;23(20):4561–4565.

183. Stavropoulos S, Larghi A, Verna E, Battezzati P, Stevens P. Intraductal ultrasound for the evaluation of patients with biliary strictures and no abdominal mass on computed tomography. *Endoscopy* 2005;37(8):715–721.

184. Park do H, Kim MH, Lee SK, Lee SS, Choi JS, Lee YS, et al. Can MRCP replace the diagnostic role of ERCP for patients with choledochal cysts? *Gastrointest Endosc* 2005;62(3):360–366.

185. Kobayashi S, Asano T, Yamasaki M, Kenmochi T, Saigo K, Ochiai T. Prophylactic excision of the gallbladder and bile duct for patients with pancreaticobiliary maljunction. *Arch Surg* 2001;136(7):759–763.

186. Liu E, Sakoda LC, Gao YT, et al. Aspirin use and risk of biliary tract cancer: a population-based study in Shanghai, China. *Cancer Epidemiol Biomarkers Prev* 2005;14(5):1315–1318.

187. Tsuneoka N, Tajima Y, Kitazato A, et al. Chemopreventive effect of a cyclooxygenase-2-specific inhibitor (etodolac) on chemically induced biliary carcinogenesis in hamsters. *Carcinogenesis* 2005;26(2):465–469.

188. Lai GH, Zhang Z, Sirica AE. Celecoxib acts in a cyclooxygenase-2-independent manner and in synergy with emodin to suppress rat cholangiocarcinoma growth in vitro through a mechanism involving enhanced Akt inactivation and increased activation of caspases-9 and -3. *Mol Cancer Ther* 2003;2(3):265–271.

189. Tsuchida A, Itoi T, Kasuya K, et al. Inhibitory effect of meloxicam, a cyclooxygenase-2 inhibitor, on N-nitrosobis (2-oxopropyl) amine induced biliary carcinogenesis in Syrian hamsters. *Carcinogenesis* 2005;26(11):1922–1928.

190. Steinbach G, Lynch PM, Phillips RK, et al. The effect of celecoxib, a cyclooxygenase-2 inhibitor, in familial adenomatous polyposis. *N Engl J Med* 2000;342(26):1946–1952.

191. Im E, Martinez JD. Ursodeoxycholic acid (UDCA) can inhibit deoxycholic acid (DCA)-induced apoptosis via modulation of EGFR/Raf-1/ERK signaling in human colon cancer cells. *J Nutr* 2004;134(2):483–486.

192. Choi YH, Im EO, Suh H, Jin Y, Yoo YH, Kim ND. Apoptosis and modulation of cell cycle control by synthetic derivatives of ursodeoxycholic acid and chenodeoxycholic acid in human prostate cancer cells. *Cancer Lett* 2003;199(2):157–167.

CHAPTER 35 ■ PATHOLOGY OF BILIARY TRACT CANCER

N. VOLKAN ADSAY AND DAVID S. KLIMSTRA

INTRODUCTION

The components of the biliary tract, that is, the gallbladder, extrahepatic biliary tree, and intrahepatic bile ducts, have fairly similar histologic characteristics; therefore, the pathological classification of the neoplasms arising in these three sites is also similar (1–3). In contrast, the risk factors for these neoplasms, which include clinical findings, treatment indications, and biological behavior, may vary. For instance, although adenocarcinomas of the proximal bile ducts have a strong association with primary sclerosing cholangitis (4,5) or anomalous pancreatobiliary duct junction (6,7), gallstones (8) are the main risk factor for gallbladder adenocarcinomas, and parasites (9) are well-established instigators of intrahepatic (peripheral) cholangiocarcinomas. This variability is also partially reflected in molecular alterations, which, although not specific for the histologic subtype of the tumor, may impact the management and prognosis. The various presentations of biliary tract adenocarcinomas also influence the mode by which a specimen is obtained for pathological examination. Many gallbladder adenocarcinomas present with findings of cholecystitis and, thus, are often removed via "routine" cholecystectomy procedures in primary care facilities; in contrast, extrahepatic bile duct lesions are seldom biopsied or resected without a strong suspicion of carcinoma, and this is usually performed in a tertiary care center.

Tumors of the biliary tree are relatively rare, but they are also often problematic diagnostically at both the clinical and the histologic levels. In addition to the rarity of these tumors, which translates to lack of familiarity for most medical disciplines, there are other factors that render biliary tumors problematic:

- The extrahepatic biliary tract has complex anatomy in which different tissue types converge in a small area.
- This region is relatively inaccessible, which makes it difficult for screening and diagnosis.
- Inflammatory conditions of this region closely mimic neoplasia; for example, primary sclerosing cholangitis often forms a cancerlike stricture.
- There are well-documented causal relationships between chronic inflammatory conditions (8,10) and carcinoma in the biliary tract, further complicating diagnosis.

In this chapter, the pathological aspects of biliary neoplasia are discussed, with emphasis being placed on the main malignant tumor type, adenocarcinoma. The topic is discussed by approaching the biliary system as a whole, with brief mention of the site-specific characteristics.

ADENOCARCINOMA OF PANCREATOBILIARY TYPE

The vast majority of biliary tumors are adenocarcinomas. In the gallbladder, this neoplasm is designated "gallbladder adenocarcinoma"; in the intrahepatic bile ducts, "cholangiocarcinoma"; and in the extrahepatic biliary ducts, "adenocarcinoma of the extrahepatic bile ducts." The vast majority of adenocarcinomas are of the generic histologic type referred to as *pancreatobiliary* because of their morphologic, immunophenotypic, and prognostic similarities to pancreatic ductal adenocarcinomas.

Adenocarcinomas of the biliary tract are seen predominantly in elderly patients. The association of biliary adenocarcinomas with prior chronic inflammation has been well established, mostly by epidemiologic data showing a high incidence of gallbladder cancer in populations with a high incidence of gallstones or cholecystitis, such as Native Americans (8). Also, the risk of carcinoma is high in patients with primary sclerosing cholangitis (6,7) (and, thus, with ulcerative colitis [10]). The association of intrahepatic cholangiocarcinomas with parasites (9) and of extrahepatic adenocarcinomas with choledochal cyst (11) is also presumably a reflection of inflammation-associated carcinoma.

Macroscopic Features and Growth Patterns

Biliary carcinomas have traditionally been divided into four types based on their macroscopic growth pattern: scirrhous constricting, diffusely infiltrative, polypoid, and nodular (12–15). The constricting and diffusely infiltrative patterns may be difficult to differentiate from chronic inflammatory conditions, especially primary sclerosing cholangitis. Polypoid growth is typically found in papillary or well-differentiated carcinomas, which are associated with a better prognosis. The nodular and scirrhous types have a propensity to infiltrate surrounding tissues and are therefore difficult to resect. The diffusely infiltrating type tends to spread linearly along the ducts. There are significant histologic overlaps among these different growth patterns, and their utility in tumor classification is limited.

On cut sections, the infiltrating component of adenocarcinomas are scirrhous (scarlike), with a firm, white, gritty appearance due to the abundance of desmoplastic stroma (fibrotic tissue reaction associated with infiltrating carcinoma). Necrosis can be seen in larger tumors. Ulceration is common in gallbladder carcinomas (Fig. 35.1). Intraluminal components of biliary carcinomas, especially those with a polypoid gross appearance, may appear more friable, soft, and tan, reflecting the

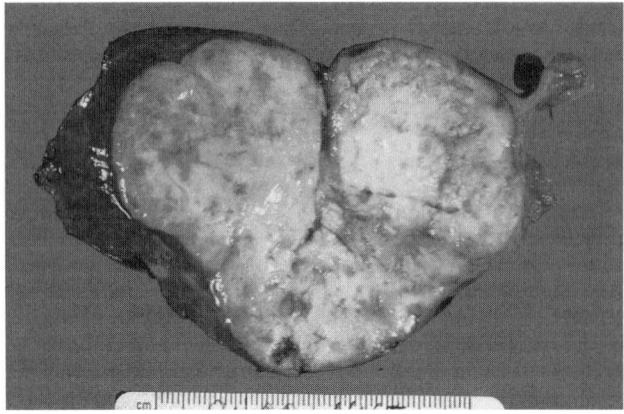

FIGURE 35.1. Adenocarcinomas of the biliary tract are usually characterized by a scirrhous, gray-white, firm cut surface. Extension into the liver, as seen here, may cause more sharply demarcated appearance (See also color Figure 35.1).

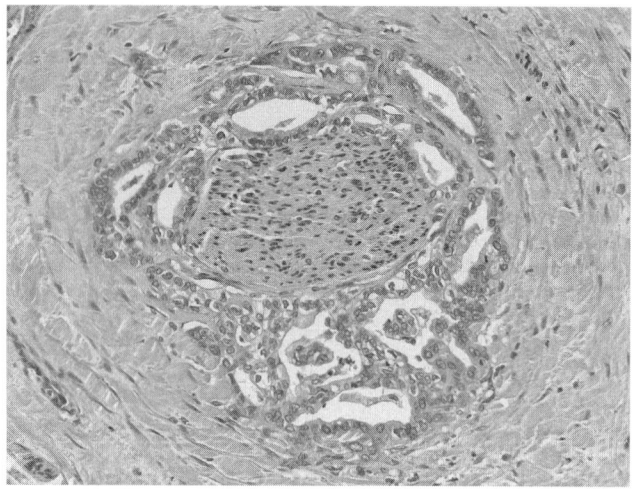

FIGURE 35.3. Adenocarcinoma, perineural invasion. Relatively well-differentiated adenocarcinoma wrapping around a nerve is a common finding in biliary adenocarcinomas (See also color Figure 35.3).

presence of papillary elements growing into the lumen. Due to the relatively thin wall of the gallbladder and major bile ducts, it is common for small (<1.0 cm) carcinomas to invade deeply into, or through the wall to, adjacent soft tissues, liver, or pancreas. Often the gross limits of the carcinoma are difficult to determine, and the tumor may merge with adjacent areas of inflammation and fibrosis; thus, it can be difficult to grossly assess the margins of surgical resection, necessitating frozen section analysis.

Peripheral cholangiocarcinomas and the intrahepatic extension of extrahepatic biliary carcinomas may appear deceptively well demarcated. This allows for easier identification of the boundaries of these carcinomas in hepatic resections. In contrast, carcinomas invading the hilar soft tissue typically have ill-defined borders that are difficult to appreciate. Gallbladder carcinomas are often associated with gallstones. In cases of porcelain gallbladder (16), the wall of the gallbladder may be entirely calcified.

Microscopic Aspects

Most biliary adenocarcinomas are of the pancreatobiliary type, characterized by relatively small clusters of cells, often with

gland formation, and associated with a desmoplastic or fibrotic stroma (1–3) (Fig. 35.2). The glands are often well formed, are lined by cuboidal cells, and show dilated lumina. Often the nuclear grade is unexpectedly high for the degree of glandular differentiation. The cytoplasm may be acidophilic and granular in some cases or pale to clear in others. A variable amount of intracytoplasmic and intraluminal mucin is present; in some, it is readily evident by routine histologic examination, and in others, demonstrable by special stains. Abundant stromal mucin deposition (mucinous or colloid adenocarcinoma) is only seen in rare cases and usually as a focal finding.

Biliary adenocarcinomas have a highly insidious pattern of spread. Perineural (Fig. 35.3) and vascular invasion (Fig. 35.4) are common, and malignant glands may have a deceptively benign appearance even when they invade these structures. In fact, the distinction of a well-differentiated adenocarcinoma from a benign reactive process in this region is one of the more challenging differential diagnoses in surgical pathology.

Tumors that infiltrate the adjacent liver may acquire a more trabecular pattern, presumably by growing along the sinusoidal framework of the liver parenchyma. Entrapped reactive bile ductules and hepatocytes are often present within the tumor, and may create a diagnostic problem in biopsy specimens.

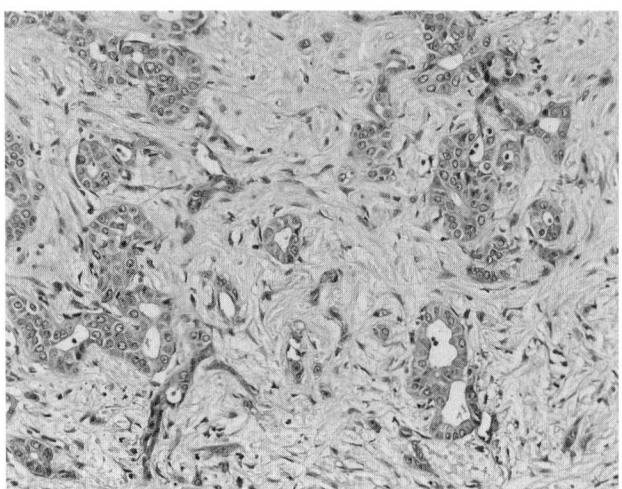

FIGURE 35.2. Adenocarcinoma (pancreatobiliary type). Small glandular units lined by cuboidal cells. They are often embedded in a dense, desmoplastic stroma (See also color Figure 35.2).

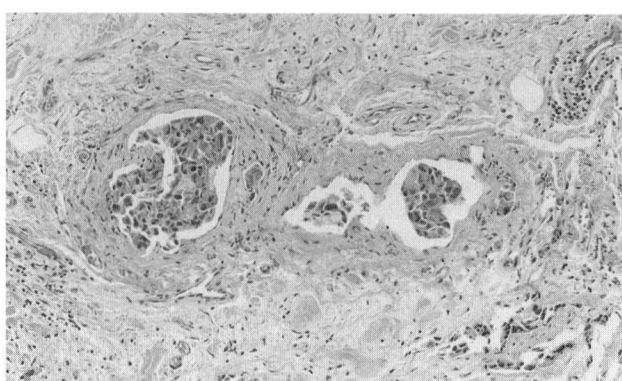

FIGURE 35.4. Adenocarcinoma, vascular invasion. Vascular invasion is commonly detected in adenocarcinomas of biliary tract (See also color Figure 35.4).

Site-Specific Aspects

The distinctive clinical characteristics of adenocarcinomas occurring in the different regions of the biliary tract are discussed in other chapters of this book, so only a few issues pertinent to pathological aspects are mentioned here. For therapeutic and prognostic purposes, tumors of the extrahepatic biliary tract are separated by their anatomical distribution into upper third (above the cystic duct junction, including both hepatic ducts, the common hepatic duct, and the cystic duct), middle third (upper half of the common bile duct [CBD]) and lower third (distal half of the CBD) (12,14,17,18). The majority of carcinomas in the upper third tend to be the scirrhous-constricting and diffusely infiltrative types. More recent studies have shown that many originate within 5 mm of the cystic duct junction or within the cystic duct itself. Hilar carcinoma located at the confluence of the right and left hepatic ducts, sometimes referred to as a Klatskin tumor (17,19), has distinctive clinical features. Klatskin tumors usually grow into the liver rather than distally toward duodenum (20). The component that invades the liver is often well demarcated. Carcinomas in the middle third tend to be of the "nodular-sclerosing" type (thickened along a long segment, with a narrow lumen and inflammatory changes in the surrounding tissues) and hence are difficult to differentiate from sclerosing cholangitis. They have a very high propensity for perineural invasion and spread radially into the periductal connective tissue, making curative resection difficult (21). Those carcinomas in the distal third have the best prognosis, partly due to their resectability by pancreatoduodenectomy, and partly due to the fact that some, especially those close to the ampullary region, are composed predominantly of noninvasive papillary elements (1–3).

Pathological Differential Diagnosis

The difficulty at the clinical level of distinguishing biliary adenocarcinomas from benign inflammatory conditions such as sclerosing cholangitis is also valid, perhaps to a greater degree, at the microscopic level (22,23). Reactive changes in the biliary ductules in the wall of the bile ducts can mimic adenocarcinoma. Conversely, biliary adenocarcinomas can be deceptively benign appearing, composed of well-formed glandular elements lined by fairly organized, cytologically bland glandular cells (Fig. 35.5). The distinction of reactive changes in the surface epithelium from dysplasia often proves to be even more challenging, especially because any injury of biliary epithelium

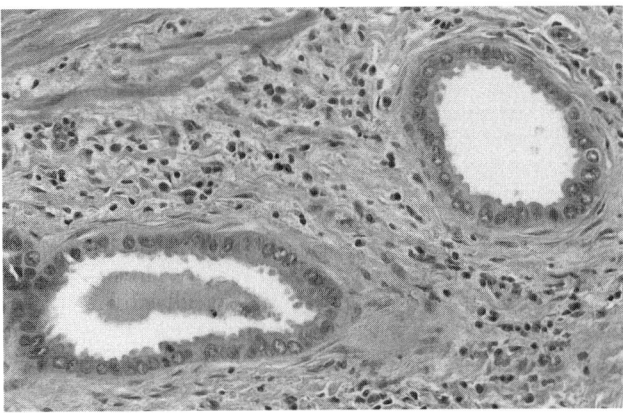

FIGURE 35.5. Adenocarcinoma, well differentiated. In many cases, neoplastic cells exhibit bland cytologic features and well-defined glandular structures, creating a deceptively benign appearance (See also color Figure 35.5).

(including instrumentation and stent placement) has a tendency to induce marked cytologic changes that mimic those of dysplastic cells. Marked nuclear enlargement, nuclear irregularities, hyperchromasia, loss of polarity, mitotic figures, apoptotic cells, and intraluminal necrosis are findings in favor of a neoplastic process; however, overlaps are common, and sometimes this distinction may not be possible on the basis of biopsies or frozen sections. This differential diagnosis is even more difficult in cytologic specimens, obtained by fine-needle aspiration or endoscopic brushing. The latter poses significant problems for the pathologist, both in terms of the amount of the specimen and the degree of subjectivity in identifying the cytologic features of malignancy versus reactive atypia.

As discussed previously, most biliary adenocarcinomas of different sites are also referred to collectively as "pancreatobiliary" due to striking morphologic and biological similarities. For this reason, based on microscopic findings alone, it is impossible to determine from which part of the biliary tract such a tumor has arisen or whether it may be of pancreatic ductal origin. Carcinomas of other foregut derivative organs, in particular those of the gastroesophageal region, are also quite similar to pancreatobiliary-type adenocarcinomas.

Peripheral cholangiocarcinomas can also be difficult to distinguish from primary hepatocellular carcinomas. The presence of true glandular elements, mucin and sclerotic stroma, are common findings in biliary carcinomas and are typically lacking in hepatocellular carcinoma. In contrast, hepatocellular carcinomas may have intracellular bile. Other distinctive features of hepatocellular carcinomas, including the solid and trabecular growth pattern, centrally located nuclei with prominent nucleoli, and abundant eosinophilic cytoplasm are usually enough to make the distinction. Further complicating this differential diagnosis are "mixed" carcinomas in which cholangiolar and hepatocellular differentiation coexist.

Carcinomas of the CBD may be difficult to distinguish from ampullary, pancreatic, and duodenal neoplasms because the tumors of these sites readily infiltrate neighboring structures due to their close proximity. In such cases, determination of the primary site depends on locating the center of the tumor, and this can often be best achieved by close correlation of the radiographic and gross findings. In addition, if present, in situ (or preinvasive) neoplasia may be a clue for the site of origin, although early neoplastic changes in the pancreas (pancreatic intraepithelial neoplasia) are extremely common and may be present even when the primary carcinoma is in the bile duct. In this complex region, it is important to evaluate the origin of the carcinoma (by site) separately from the type of the carcinoma; for example, ampullary carcinomas may be of pancreatobiliary type. However, intestinal-type carcinomas in this region are more likely to be either ampullary or duodenal in origin.

Biliary carcinomas metastatic to other sites may mimic the primary tumors of those organs. In particular, metastases to the ovary are often cystic and can be mistaken for primary ovarian mucinous cystic neoplasms (24), and pulmonary metastases can resemble mucinous bronchioloalveolar carcinomas. Metastases to the liver periphery from hilar biliary carcinomas can be nearly impossible to distinguish from metastatic pancreatic ductal adenocarcinoma.

Immunohistochemical and Molecular Characteristics

Biliary adenocarcinomas typically express CEA, CA19–9, MUC1, MUC5AC, CK19, and CK7 (1–3). On occasion, these markers can be helpful in the differential diagnosis from other malignancies that do not express these markers (e. g., hepatocellular carcinoma). However, none of these stains is specific enough to be useful in the distinction of biliary adenocarcinomas from adenocarcinomas of other organs. However, some metastases to the liver express specific markers not found in biliary adenocarcinoma, such as thyroid transcription factor-1 (TTF-1) in pulmonary adenocarcinomas, prostate-specific antigen (PSA) in prostatic primaries, and hormone receptors in mammary or Müllerian carcinomas. Mutations at codon-12 of the KRAS oncogene, which are seen in >90% of pancreatic ductal adenocarcinomas, are much less common in biliary adenocarcinomas (25), and the incidence of KRAS mutation appears to decrease from distal to proximal along the biliary tree. Similarly, loss of DPC4 is also less common in biliary than in pancreatic adenocarcinomas (26). More than half of the cases have abnormal expression of p53. Loss of heterozygosity at chromosomes 8p, 9q, and 18q, and amplification of c-erbB-2 is also reported in more than half. Again, none of the genetic alterations of biliary adenocarcinomas are sufficiently specific to be useful diagnostically.

OTHER TYPES OF CARCINOMAS IN THE BILIARY TRACT

There are other types of adenocarcinomas in the gallbladder and biliary tract that are histologically distinct from the pancreatobiliary-type adenocarcinomas (1–3,27).

Intestinal-type adenocarcinomas are morphologically similar to their counterparts in the tubular gastrointestinal tract. *Signet ring cell* carcinomas (27), characterized by a diffusely infiltrative pattern of individual cells (often with signet ring morphology) or a cordlike growth pattern, may also occur in the biliary tract. *Mucinous adenocarcinomas* (27), with extensive mucin production associated with stromal mucin deposition, may be seen in some cases, usually admixed with conventional-type adenocarcinomas. Some studies suggest that the prognosis of mucinous adenocarcinomas may be better (19). *Adenosquamous carcinomas* (28) are rare tumors in which a mixture of glandular and squamous differentiation is seen in variable amounts. *Clear cell carcinomas* (29) (Fig. 35.6) are described in which the morphologic features resemble those of renal cell carcinoma.

Mixed cholangiocarcinoma-hepatocellular carcinoma (30,31) is a rare tumor that arises in the liver periphery and has both areas of cholangiocarcinoma and hepatocellular differentiation

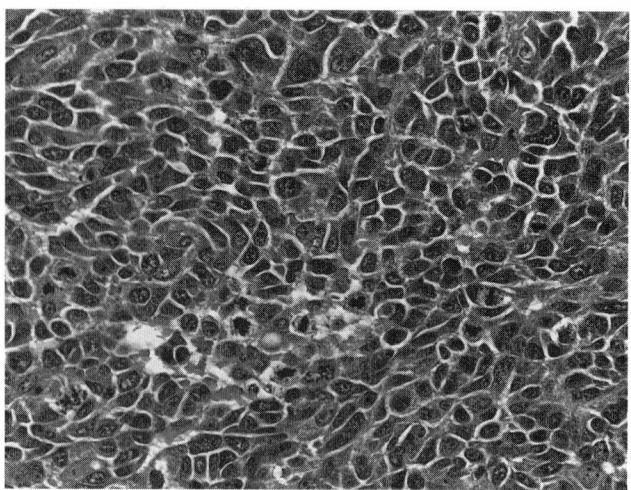

FIGURE 35.7. Adenocarcinoma, poorly differentiated. This carcinoma is characterized by a diffuse, sheetlike growth pattern of large cells. Characteristics of ordinary carcinomas such as gland formation or papillae are not evident (See also color Figure 35.7).

in variable degrees. The literature on this tumor type has some conflicting information due to the lack of a uniform definition. It appears that its behavior is similar to that of pure cholangiocarcinomas.

There are also other biliary carcinomas that lack gland, mucin, or papilla formation, and are thus not adenocarcinomas. *Undifferentiated* and *sarcomatoid* carcinomas (32–34) probably represent the least differentiated end of the spectrum of adenocarcinomas, in which glandular differentiation is no longer detectable (Fig. 35.7). In sarcomatoid carcinomas, the cells acquire mesenchymal characteristics, including spindle-shaped cells, and in some cases, even heterologous elements such as bone and cartilage. In the absence of a more epithelioid or glandular component or an in situ carcinoma, these tumors may be difficult to distinguish from true sarcomas. Some undifferentiated carcinomas are associated with abundant non-neoplastic multinucleated giant cells to the extent that they are referred to as *undifferentiated carcinoma with osteoclasticlike giant cells* (35–37). It has been well documented that these giant cells are of histiocytic origin, and the malignant cells in this tumor are the spindle cells in the background.

High-grade neuroendocrine carcinoma (*small cell carcinoma*) (38,39) also occurs in the region of biliary tree, predominantly in the gallbladder or distal CBD. Small cell carcinomas are defined by the same histologic criteria applied to their counterparts in the lung, which include a high nucleus-to-cytoplasm ratio, molding of nuclei, a diffuse chromatin pattern, and absence of nucleoli. Neuroendocrine markers such as chromogranin, synaptophysin, and neural cell adhesion molecule are often detectable by immunohistochemistry. *Large cell neuroendocrine carcinomas* may also occur in this region (40).

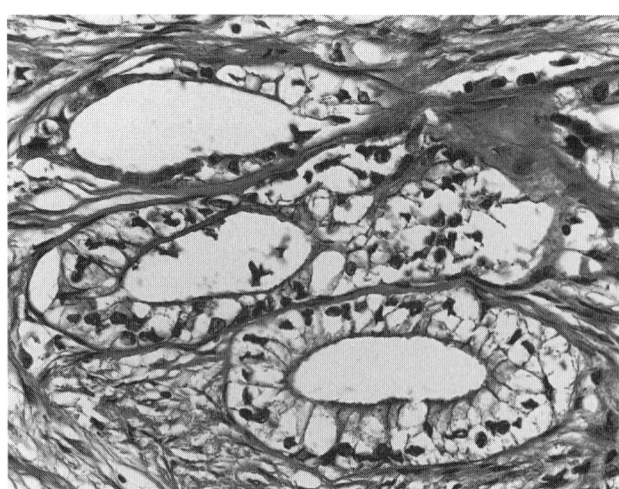

FIGURE 35.6. Adenocarcinoma, clear cell pattern. Variations that can be seen in the morphologic phenotype of adenocarcinomas include the clear cell pattern (See also color Figure 35.6).

CLINICALLY RELEVANT PATHOLOGICAL PARAMETERS IN BILIARY RESECTIONS

1. *Tumor type:* Whether the tumor is a conventional pancreatobiliary-type adenocarcinoma or another type of neoplasm is important (41). For instance, papillary carcinoma with focal microinvasion has a significantly better prognosis, whereas undifferentiated carcinoma has a worse outcome.

2. *Invasive versus noninvasive components:* For carcinomas with predominantly intraluminal growth (noninvasive papillary carcinoma), the extent of the noninvasive and invasive components should be considered separately. In fact, cases of biliary adenocarcinomas associated with an unusually protracted clinical course are often predominantly noninvasive papillary carcinomas.

3. *Assessment of surgical margins:* Proper orientation of the specimen with identification of the margins by the surgical team (using sutures or dyes) often proves helpful for accurate evaluation of the surgical margins, especially in complex specimens. The status of the resection margins is an important factor predictive of recurrence (42).

4. *Pathological stage:* The size and depth of the tumor are the most important aspects of pathological staging of biliary carcinomas (43). There are, however, pitfalls in establishing the depth of the tumor in some parts of the biliary tract, where, unlike other sites such as the tubular gastrointestinal tract, the layers that constitute the duct walls are not distinct. In particular, in parts of CBD, the interface of the mucosa with the muscular layer, as well as the interface of the muscle with the perimuscular tissue, is highly irregular, which may hinder the accurate evaluation of tumor depth (44).

5. *Grading:* The grading scheme advocated by the World Health Organization (15) is based on the percent of the tumor showing glandular differentiation (tubule formation). If >95% of the tumor is composed of tubules, it is well differentiated; 40% to 95% is moderately differentiated, and 5% to 39% is poorly differentiated. Those without any glandular differentiation are regarded as undifferentiated.

6. *Perineural and vascular invasion:* Although the prognostic significance of perineural and vascular invasion has not been fully established, these are nevertheless regarded as components of the pathological evaluation, especially in resection specimens. Perineural invasion is particularly common in biliary adenocarcinomas.

PREINVASIVE NEOPLASIA

Throughout the biliary tract, there are different types of preinvasive (intraepithelial) neoplastic lesions that can be classified based on their configuration as either flat or exophytic. The terminology for these lesions varies somewhat with the anatomical location, but there are many similarities, both in the histologic patterns and in the accumulation of genetic defects that accompanies the morphologic progression from low- to high-grade intraepithelial neoplasia. In general, flat lesions are designated *dysplasia* or *carcinoma in situ,* whereas the exophytic lesions are termed *adenoma* (tubular or papillary), *papilloma,* or *noninvasive papillary carcinoma.*

In the gallbladder, dysplasia can be detected incidentally in cholecystectomies performed for cholelithiasis and cholecystitis. Most of these are microscopic foci of low-grade dysplasia; however, high-grade dysplasia has also been reported in up to 3.5% of routine cholecystectomy specimens (45,46) in populations at high risk to develop gallbladder carcinoma. Dysplasia is also seen commonly in the mucosa adjacent to invasive biliary carcinomas, and on occasion, as an incidental finding in specimens obtained for other reasons (45,47–50). Generally, dysplasia is a grossly and radiographically invisible process that is characterized by cytoarchitectural atypia, including nuclear enlargement, irregularities, loss of polarity, and mitotic activity (Fig. 35.8). Based on the degree of atypia, dysplasia is graded as low grade and high grade, the latter also being referred to as

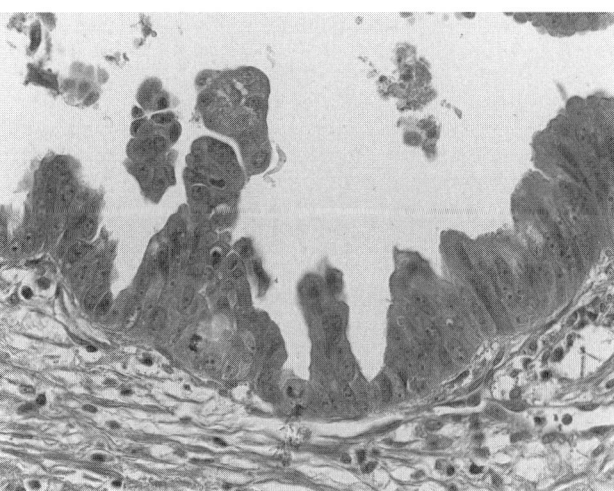

FIGURE 35.8. Dysplasia, high grade. There is nuclear stratification, marked nuclear enlargement, pleomorphism, and hyperchromasia. Mitotic figures are also present (See also color Figure 35.8).

carcinoma *in situ.* It should be kept in mind, however, that the diagnostic criteria for dysplasia are highly subjective, and as discussed previously, reactive atypia in the biliary epithelium is difficult to distinguish microscopically from dysplasia. In contrast, in patients with invasive carcinoma, dysplasia may be difficult to distinguish from retrograde mucosal involvement by invasive carcinoma, a phenomenon that is referred to as "cancerization" or "colonization" of the surface epithelium. For these reasons, the true frequency of dysplasia in biliary tract is difficult to determine.

In the gallbladder sphere in which it is best recognized and studied, dysplasia associated with invasive carcinoma appears to have no bearing on the prognosis. Low-grade dysplasia detected incidentally, usually by histologic examination of routine cholecystectomy specimens, also appears to be clinically silent and has no documented clinical consequences. However, high-grade dysplasia seen in isolation (i.e., without invasive carcinoma) appears to have some clinical implications. Data from the Surveillance, Epidemiology, and End Results program of National Cancer Institute show that one-third of the patients with carcinoma in situ of the gallbladder died of carcinoma after 10 years (although all were alive at 5 years), suggesting that either a small invasive carcinoma was missed or the patients developed a second malignancy elsewhere in the biliary system (51). Extrapolating from these observations, a "field effect" phenomenon may occur in some cases, and patients with gallbladder high-grade dysplasia (especially when extensive) should probably have some surveillance to screen for subsequent invasive carcinoma elsewhere in the biliary tract. It is also important for pathologists to examine the entire gallbladder histologically when foci of dysplasia are identified to search for a grossly inapparent invasive carcinoma.

Biliary carcinomas may also arise from exophytic mass-forming preinvasive neoplasms. Benign exophytic neoplasms (*adenomas* and *papillomas*) in the biliary tree occur predominantly in the gallbladder (51–53). Most gallbladder adenomas are composed of tightly packed, cytologically bland pyloric-type glands and are referred to as *tubular* or *pyloric gland adenomas* (54); this type is rarely seen in the bile ducts.

Carcinomatous transformation is highly uncommon in pyloric gland adenomas, although high-grade dysplasia may be present. In contrast, exophytic neoplasms that resemble the adenomas of the gastrointestinal tract (*intestinal-type adenomas;* Fig. 35.9) or papillary neoplasms with nonspecific lineage

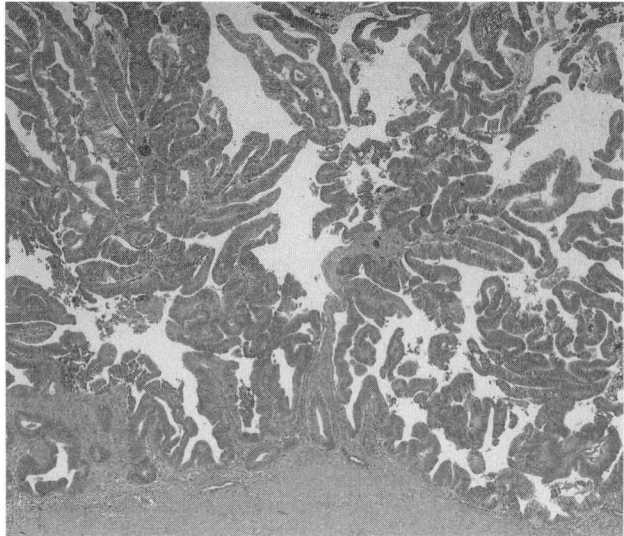

FIGURE 35.9. Adenoma, intestinal type. Just like in colonic villous adenomas, these have villous architecture with pseudostratified, cigar-shaped nuclei (See also color Figure 35.9).

may occur both in the gallbladder and in the bile ducts, and may harbor (or progress to) invasive carcinoma. In fact, most papillary neoplasms of the bile ducts have significant cytoarchitectural atypia and are designated *papillary carcinoma* (51). Multicentric papillary neoplasms within the biliary tree are designated *papillomatosis* (55–57), but again this rare condition often displays sufficient atypia to warrant a diagnosis of multicentric papillary carcinoma when current diagnostic criteria are applied.

As in other organs, there is a spectrum in the extent of carcinomatous transformation that can occur in exophytic biliary neoplasms, ranging from microfocal high-grade dysplasia to macroscopically visible foci of invasive carcinoma. The terminology applied to this spectrum may be problematic. When a portion of the exophytic tumor retains the features of a benign adenoma, it is reasonable to regard the process as malignant transformation of an adenoma. However, as mentioned previously, when the entire exophytic tumor shows significant cytologic or architectural atypia, it is regarded as a papillary carcinoma; those lacking an associated invasive component should be so designated (*noninvasive papillary carcinoma* in the gallbladder or *intraductal papillary carcinoma* in the bile ducts). Conversely, in some patients with invasive adenocarcinomas, a residual papillary carcinoma component is identifiable. In fact, many adenocarcinomas with a polypoid gross appearance belong to this latter group. Noninvasive papillary carcinomas have an excellent prognosis if they can be completely resected, and those cases with minimal invasive carcinoma also have a favorable prognosis (51). Once there is a significant amount of invasive carcinoma, however, the prognosis approaches that of biliary adenocarcinomas that do not arise from papillary precursors.

Some of the clinical and pathological characteristics of these exophytic intraepithelial biliary neoplasms are so similar to those of *pancreatic intraductal papillary mucinous neoplasms* (IPMNs) that some authors have begun to refer to these tumors as *biliary IPMNs* (58–62). Although some of the features of pancreatic IPMNs are likely to be applicable to their biliary counterparts, there are also significant differences in the frequency and types of associated invasive carcinomas, as well as the morphology and staining characteristics of the papillary components.

HEPATOBILIARY CYSTIC NEOPLASMS

Hepatobiliary cystic neoplasms (63,64), which are analogous to mucinous cystic neoplasms of the pancreas, can also be regarded as a type of mass-forming preinvasive neoplasm. They form multilocular cystic lesions that occur predominantly in adult women, and they exhibit pathognomonic hormone receptor expressing ovarianlike stroma (65). The lining epithelium is composed of cuboidal to columnar cells, sometimes with abundant apical mucin. Polypoid projections may be identified in the cyst lumen. Although most hepatobiliary cystic neoplasms show benign cytoarchitectural features (i.e., hepatobiliary cystadenoma), some may harbor in situ or invasive carcinoma (hepatobiliary cystadenocarcinoma). Carcinoma can be focal, and for this reason, thorough histologic examination is warranted.

CARCINOID TUMOR

Carcinoid tumors, which are well-differentiated endocrine neoplasms, may occur in any part of the biliary tract; however, they tend to be more common in the gallbladder and CBD (66,67). They are seen predominantly in young or middle-age adults and are usually nonfunctioning, the patients presenting with biliary obstruction. Some are multiple or may be part of a syndrome that involves endocrine tumors of other organs. Rare examples may be associated with von Hippel-Lindau syndrome (68). Grossly, carcinoids form relatively well-demarcated nodules that may have a mucosa-covered polypoid component. They are fleshy, soft, and homogeneous on cut sections. Microscopically, they are characterized by distinct nests of cells with round uniform nuclei, "salt-and-pepper chromatin," and abundant cytoplasm (Fig. 35.10). The proliferative rate is low. Rarely, the cytoplasm may exhibit clear cell, oncocytic, or signet ring–like changes, and a goblet cell variant has also been described. The nests are separated by a fibrovascular stroma; carcinoid tumors are well vascularized. By immunohistochemistry, they express general endocrine markers such as chromogranin and synaptophysin. In general, carcinoids are low-grade malignant neoplasms with an indolent clinical course. Those rare carcinoids that are admixed with adenocarcinoma (composite adenocarcinoma-carcinoid) (69) behave more like adenocarcinomas.

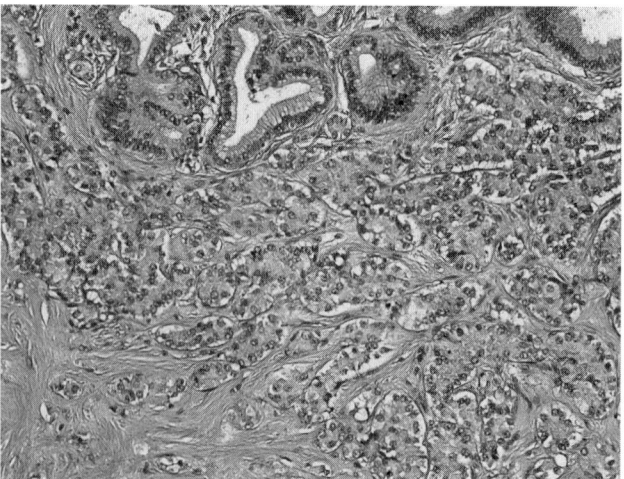

FIGURE 35.10. Carcinoids in the biliary tract have the typical morphologic characteristics of carcinoids elsewhere, exhibiting distinct nests of cells with round and uniform nuclei, endocrine chromatin pattern, and a fair amount of cytoplasm (See also color Figure 35.10).

Focal neuroendocrine differentiation and carcinoidlike patterns may be seen in other neoplasms of the biliary tract that should not be classified as carcinoid tumors. Rarely, paraganglioma (70), a tumor also displaying neuroendocrine differentiation, may occur in the biliary tract.

SARCOMA

Among the extremely rare mesenchymal tumors of the biliary tree (1–3), the one that warrants specific attention because it is relatively well characterized in this region is *embryonal (botryoid) rhabdomyosarcoma* (71,72). These are seen predominantly in young children (3–4 years old) and constitute 1% of all rhabdomyosarcomas. The tumor consists of aggregates of soft, mucosa-covered polyps filling the lumen. The most common site is the CBD. Beneath the surface layer of flattened biliary epithelium is a dense zone of primitive spindle cells that represent the so-called cambium layer. Cytoplasmic cross-striations may be seen. Skeletal muscle differentiation is demonstrable by immunohistochemical stains for actin, desmin, or myoD1. Although the prognosis is poor, multimodality therapy has resulted in long-term survival in some cases. Metastases occur in 40%, but death is usually caused by the local effects of the tumor.

Virtually every malignant mesenchymal neoplasm has been documented to occur in the biliary tract, including malignant peripheral nerve sheath tumor, leiomyosarcoma, Kaposi sarcoma, angiosarcoma, malignant fibrous histiocytoma, and others (1–3). It should be kept in mind that before a case is classified as sarcoma, the possibility of a sarcomatoid carcinoma, discussed previously, should be carefully considered.

SECONDARY TUMORS AND HEMATOPOIETIC MALIGNANCIES

The biliary tree may be involved by a variety of tumors originating in other organs, especially the pancreas, stomach, colon, kidney, and breast, either by metastasis or by direct invasion (1–3). Among these, metastatic renal cell carcinoma is notorious for mimicking a primary tumor because it may form polypoid lesions, and the history of the primary tumor may be remote. Similarly, melanomas may form polypoid lesions and mimic primary tumors, and often the history of melanoma (Fig. 35.11) may be absent or vague.

The biliary tree may also be involved by hematopoietic malignancies (lymphoma, myeloma, or leukemia) as part of systemic disease; rarely, this may be the initial presentation (1–3). Primary lymphomas of mucosa-associated type have also been reported (73).

PSEUDOTUMORS

In addition to sclerosing cholangitis, discussed previously, a few other nonneoplastic conditions of the biliary tract may mimic carcinomas clinically. Rarely, heterotopic tissue, particularly pancreatic tissue (74), may form a mass. Traumatic (or "amputation") neuroma (75), which is an exuberant regenerative proliferation of transected nerves, may form a tumorlike nodule, typically in the cystic duct stump after cholecystectomy. These tumorlike lesions may present with obstruction-related signs and symptoms, sometimes several years after surgery. Occasionally, a condition referred to as "eosinophilic cholangitis" may form a pseudotumor. Whether such cases represent a distinct subset of "autoimmune" sclerotic processes (i.e., related to sclerosing cholangitis) remains to be determined. Biliary strictures simulating carcinomas may occur in the extrahepatic

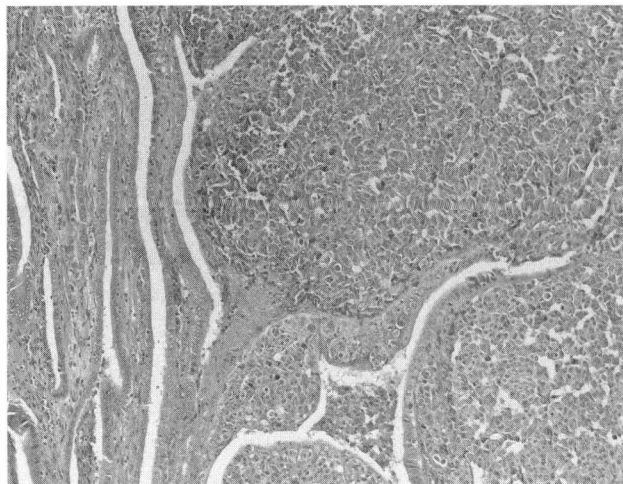

FIGURE 35.11. Sheets of pigmented melanoma cells filling the lamina propria (See also color Figure 35.11).

bile ducts of patients with autoimmune (lymphoplasmacytic sclerosing) pancreatitis.

There are certain types of tumorlike lesions that occur rather frequently in the gallbladder but not often in the remainder of the biliary tree. Rarely, these lesions may be mistaken as cancer. Nonneoplastic polyps of various kinds, including cholesterolosis, lymphoid polyps, inflammatory (fibrous or granulation tissue) polyps, and hamartomatous polyps (53), may present as "tumors." Cystic change in Aschoff-Rokitansky sinuses and adenomyomas (76) also form pseudotumors in the gallbladder; however, these are not seen in the bile ducts.

References

1. Adsay NV. Gallbladder, extrahepatic biliary tree and ampulla. In: Mills SE, Greenson JK, Carter D, et al., eds. *Sternberg's Diagnostic Surgical Pathology.* Vol 2. Philadelphia, Pa.: Lippincott Williams & Wilkins; 2004: 1775–1829.
2. Albores-Saavedra J, Henson DE, Klimstra DS. *Tumors of the Gallbladder, Extrahepatic Bile Ducts and Ampulla of Vater.* Washington, DC: Armed Forces Institute of Pathology; 2000.
3. Lack EE. Gall bladder and extrahepatic biliary tract. In: *Pathology of the Pancreas, Gallbladder, Extrahepatic Biliary Tract and Ampullary Region.* New York, NY: Oxford University Press; 2003: 3–391.
4. Morowitz DA, Glagov S, Dordal E, Kirsner JB. Carcinoma of the biliary tract complicating chronic ulcerative colitis. *Cancer* 1971;27(2):356–361.
5. Mir-Madjlessi SH, Farmer RG, Sivak MV, Jr. Bile duct carcinoma in patients with ulcerative colitis: relationship to sclerosing cholangitis: report of six cases and review of the literature. *Dig Dis Sci* 1987;32(2):145–154.
6. Morohosi T, Kunimura T, Kanda M, et al. Multiple carcinomas associated with anomalous arrangement of the biliary and pancreatic duct system: a report of two cases with a literature survey. *Acta Pathol Jpn* 1990;60:755–763.
7. Chijiiwa K, Tanaka M, Nakayama F. Adenocarcinoma of the gallbladder associated with anomalous pancreaticobiliary ductal junction. *Am Surg* 1993;59:430–434.
8. Sheth S, Bedford A, Chopra S. Primary gallbladder cancer: recognition of risk factors and the role of prophylactic cholecystectomy. *Am J Gastroenterol* 2000;95(6):1402–1410.
9. Carriaga MT, Henson DE. Liver, gallbladder, extrahepatic bile ducts, and pancreas. *Cancer* 1995;75:175–190.
10. Herzog K, Goldblum JR. Gallbladder adenocarcinoma, acalculous chronic lymphoplasmacytic cholecystitis, ulcerative colitis. *Mod Pathol* 1996;9:194–198.
11. Komi N, Tamura T, Miyoshi Y, Kunitomo K, Udaka H, Takehara H. Nationwide survey of cases of choledochal cyst: analysis of coexistent anomalies, complications and surgical treatment in 645 cases. *Surg Gastroenterol* 1984;3:69–73.
12. Van Heerden JA, Judd ES, Dockerty MB. Carcinoma of the extrahepatic bile ducts: a clinicopathologic study. *Am J Surg* 1967;113(1):49–56.
13. Todoroki T, Okamura T, Fukao K, et al. Gross appearance of carcinoma of the main hepatic duct and its prognosis. *Surg Gynecol Obstet* 1980;150(1):33–40.

14. Weinbren K, Mutum SS. Pathological aspects of cholangiocarcinoma. *J Pathol* 1983;139:217–238.

15. Albores–Saavedra J, Scoazec JC, Wittekind C, et al. Tumors of the gallbladder and extrahepatic bile ducts. In: Hamilton SR, Aaltonen LA, eds. *World Health Organization Classification of Tumors. Pathology and Genetics of Tumors of the Digestive System.* Lyon: IARC Press; 2000;204–220.

16. Stephen AE, Berger DL. Carcinoma in the porcelain gallbladder: a relationship revisited. *Surgery* 2001;129(6):699–703.

17. Klatskin G. Adenocarcinoma of the hepatic duct as its bifurcation within the porta hepatis: an unusual tumor with distinctive clinical and pathological features. *Am J Med* 1965;38:241–256.

18. Tompkins RK, Thomas D, Wile A, Longmire WP, Jr. Prognosis factors in bile duct carcinoma: analysis of 96 cases. *Ann Surg* 1981;194:447–457.

19. Bosma A. Surgical pathology of cholangiocarcinoma of the liver hilus (Klatskin tumor). *Semin Liver Dis* 1990;10:85–90.

20. Hayashi S, Miyazaki M, Kondo Y, Nakajima N. Invasive growth patterns of hepatic hilar ductal carcinoma: a histologic analysis of 18 surgical cases. *Cancer* 1994;73:2922–2929.

21. Bhuiya MR, Nimura Y, Kamiya J, Kondo S, Nagino M, Hayakawa N. Clinicopathologic factors influencing survival of patients with bile duct carcinoma: multivariate statistical analysis. *World J Surg* 1993;17(5):653–657.

22. Ludwig J. Surgical pathology of the syndrome of primary sclerosing cholangitis. *Am J Surg Pathol* 1989;13(1):43–49.

23. Ludwig T, Wahlstrom HE, Batts KP, Wiesner RH. Papillary bile duct dysplasia in primary sclerosing cholangitis. *Gastroenterology* 1992;102:2134–2138.

24. Young RH, Hart WR. Metastases from carcinomas of the pancreas simulating primary mucinous tumors of the ovary: a report of seven cases. *Am J Surg Pathol* 1989;13(9):748–756.

25. Rashid A, Ueki T, Gao YT, et al. K–ras mutation, p53 overexpression, and microsatellite instability in biliary tract cancers: a population–based study in China. *Clin Cancer Res* 2002;8(10):3156–3163.

26. Argani P, Shaukat A, Kaushal M, et al. Differing rates of loss of DPC4 expression and of p53 overexpression among carcinomas of the proximal and distal bile ducts. *Cancer* 2001;91(7):1332–1341.

27. Albores–Saavedra J, Molberg K, Henson DE. Unusual malignant epithelial tumors of the gallbladder. *Semin Diagn Pathol* 1996;13:326–338.

28. Nishihara K, Nagai E, Izumi Y, Yamaguchi K, Tsuneyoshi M. Adenosquamous carcinoma of the gallbladder: a clinicopathological, immunohistochemical and flow–cytometric study of twenty cases. *Jpn J Cancer Res* 1994;85(4):389–399.

29. Vardaman C, Albores–Saavedra J. Clear cell carcinomas of the gallbladder and extrahepatic bile ducts. *Am J Surg Pathol* 1995;19(1):91–99.

30. Goodman ZD, Ishak KG, Langloss JM, Sesterhenn IA, Rabin L. Combined hepatocellular–cholangiocarcinoma: a histologic and immunohistochemical study. *Cancer* 1985;55(1):124–135.

31. Jarnagin WR, Weber S, Tickoo SK, et al. Combined hepatocellular and cholangiocarcinoma: demographic, clinical, and prognostic factors. *Cancer* 2002;94(7):2040–2046.

32. Appelman HD, Coopersmith N. Pleomorphic spindle–cell carcinoma of the gallbladder: relation to sarcoma of the gallbladder. *Cancer* 1970;25:535–541.

33. Suster S, Huszar M, Herczeg E, Bubis JJ. Adenosquamous carcinoma of the gallbladder with spindle cell features: a light microscopic and immunocytochemical study of a case. *Histopathology* 1987;11(2):209–214.

34. Nishihara K, Tsuneyoshi M. Undifferentiated spindle cell carcinoma of the gallbladder: a clinicopathologic, immunohistochemical, and flow cytometric study of 11 cases. *Hum Pathol* 1993;24:1298–1305.

35. Husek K. [Anaplastic osteoclastic carcinoma of the gallbladder]. *Cesk Patol* 1990;26(3):138–141.

36. Haratake J, Yamada H, Horie A, Inokuma T. Giant cell tumor–like cholangiocarcinoma associated with systemic cholelithiasis. *Cancer* 1992;69(10):2444–2448.

37. Ito M, Hsu CT, Naito S, et al. Osteoclast–like giant cell tumour of the gallbladder. *Virchows Arch A Pathol Anat Histopathol* 1992;420(4):359–366.

38. Maitra A, Shaukat A, Tascilar M, Hruban RH, Offerhaus GJ, Albores–Saavedra J. Small cell carcinoma of the gallbladder: a clinicopathologic, immunohistochemical, and molecular pathology study of 12 cases. *Am J Surg Pathol* 2001;25(5):595–601.

39. van der Wal AC, van Leeuwen DJ, Walford N. Small cell neuroendocrine (oat cell) tumour of the common bile duct. *Histopathology* 1990;16:398–400.

40. Papotti M, Cassoni P, Sapino A, Passarino G, Krueger JE, Albores–Saavedra J. Large cell neuroendocrine carcinoma of the gallbladder: report of two cases. *Am J Surg Pathol* 2000;24(10):1424–1428.

41. Bivins BA, Meeker WR, Griffen WO, Jr. Importance of histologic classification of carcinoma of the gallbladder. *Am Surg* 1975;41(3):121–124.

42. Weber SM, Jarnagin WR, Klimstra D, DeMatteo RP, Fong Y, Blumgart LH. Intrahepatic cholangiocarcinoma: resectability, recurrence pattern, and outcomes. *J Am Coll Surg* 2001;193(4):384–391.

43. Greene FL, Page DL, Fleming DI, et al. Extrahepatic bile ducts. In: *AJCC Cancer Staging Manual.* 6th ed. New York, NY: Springer–Verlag; 2002;155–171.

44. Hong SM, Kim MJ, Cho H, et al. Superficial vs deep pancreatic parenchymal invasion in the extrahepatic bile duct carcinomas: a significant prognostic factor. *Mod Pathol* 2005;18(7):969–975.

45. Ojeda VJ, Shilkin KB, Walters MNI. Premalignant epithelial lesions of the gallbladder: a prospective study of 120 cholecystectomy specimens. *Pathology* 1985;17:451–454.

46. Chan KW. Review of 253 cases of significant pathology in 7,910 cholecystectomies in Hong Kong. *Pathology* 1988;20(1):20–23.

47. Albores–Saavedra J, Alcantara–Vazques A, Curz–Ortiz H, Herrera–Goepfert R. The precursor lesions of invasive gallbladder carcinoma: hyperplasia, atypical hyperplasia and carcinoma in situ. *Cancer* 1980;45:919–927.

48. Laitio M. Histogenesis of epithelial neoplasms of the gallbladder. I. Dysplasia. *Pathol Res Pract* 1983;178:51–56.

49. Suzuki M, Takahashi T, Ouchi K, Matsuno S. The development and extension of hepatohilar bile duct carcinoma: a three–dimensional tumor mapping in the intrahepatic biliary tree visualized with the aid of a graphics computer system. *Cancer* 1989;64:658–666.

50. Yamagiwa H. Mucosal dysplasia of the gallbladder: isolated and adjacent lesions to carcinoma. *Jpn J Cancer Res* 1989;80:238–243.

51. Albores–Saavedra J, Murakata L, Krueger JE, Henson DE. Noninvasive and minimally invasive papillary carcinomas of the extrahepatic bile ducts. *Cancer* 2000;89(3):508–515.

52. Christensen AH, Ishak KG. Benign tumors and pseudotumors of the gallbladder: report of 180 cases. *Arch Pathol* 1970;90:423–432.

53. Albores–Saavedra J, Vardaman CJ, Vuitch F. Non–neoplastic polypoid lesions and adenomas of the gallbladder. In: Rosen PP, Fechner RE, eds. *Pathology Annual.* Norwalk, Conn.: Appleton and Lange; 1993: 145–177.

54. O'Shea M, Fletcher HS, Lara JF. Villous adenoma of the extrahepatic biliary tract: a rare entity. *Am J Surg* 2002;68(10):889–891.

55. Gouma DJ, Mutum SS, Benjamin IS, Blumgart LH. Intrahepatic biliary papillomatosis. *Br J Surg* 1984;71(1):72–74.

56. Sagar PM, Omar M, Macrie J. Extrahepatic biliary papillomatosis occurring after removal of a dysplastic gall bladder. *HPB Surg* 1993;6(3):219–221.

57. Taguchi J, Yasunaga M, Kojiro M, Arita T, Nakayama T, Simokobe T. Intrahepatic and extrahepatic biliary papillomatosis. *Arch Pathol Lab Med* 1993;117:944–947.

58. Kim HJ, Kim MH, Lee SK, et al. Mucin–hypersecreting bile duct tumor characterized by iking homology with an intraductal papillary mucinous tumor (IPMT) of the pancreas. *Endoscopy* 2000;32(5):389–393.

59. Chen TC, Nakanuma Y, Zen Y, et al. Intraductal papillary neoplasia of the liver associated with hepatolithiasis. *Hepatology* 2001;34(4 pt 1):651–658.

60. Tamada S, Goto M, Nomoto M, et al. Expression of MUC1 and MUC2 mucins in extrahepatic bile duct carcinomas: its relationship with tumor progression and prognosis. *Pathol Int* 2002;52(11):713–723.

61. Abraham SC, Lee JH, Hruban RH, Argani P, Furth EE, Wu TT. Molecular and immunohistochemical analysis of intraductal papillary neoplasms of the biliary tract. *Hum Pathol* 2003;34(9):902–910.

62. Shibahara H, Tamada S, Goto M, et al. Pathologic features of mucin–producing bile duct tumors: two histopathologic categories as counterparts of pancreatic intraductal papillary–mucinous neoplasms. *Am J Surg Pathol* 2004;28(3):327–338.

63. Wheeler DA, Edmondson HA. Cystadenoma with mesenchymal stroma (CMS) in the liver and bile ducts: a clinicopathologic study of 17 cases, 4 with malignant change. *Cancer* 1985;56(6):1434–1445.

64. Devaney K, Goodman ZD, Ishak KG. Hepatobiliary cystadenoma and cystadenocarcinoma: a light microscope and immunohistochemical study of 70 patients. *Am J Surg Pathol* 1994;18:1078–1091.

65. Grayson W, Teare J, Myburgh JA, Paterson AC. Immunohistochemical demonstration of progesterone receptor in hepatobiliary cystadenoma with mesenchymal stroma. *Histopathology* 1996;29(5):461–463.

66. Barron–Rodriguez LP, Manivel JC, Mendez–Sanchez N, Jessurun J. Carcinoid tumor of the common bile duct: evidence for its origin in metaplastic endocrine cells. *Am J Gastroenterol* 1991;86(8):1073–1076.

67. Modlin IM, Sandor A. An analysis of 8305 cases of carcinoid tumors. *Cancer* 1997;79(4):813–829.

68. Sinkre PA, Murakata L, Rabin L, Hoang MP, Albores–Saavedra J. Clear cell carcinoid tumor of the gallbladder: another distinctive manifestation of von Hippel–Lindau disease. *Am J Surg Pathol* 2001;25(10):1334–1339.

69. Olinici CD, Vasiu R. Composite endocrine cell, typical adenocarcinoma and signet ring carcinoma of the gallbladder. *Rom J Morphol Embryol* 1991;37(3–4):171–173.

70. Caceres M, Mosquera LF, Shih JA, O'Leary JP. Paraganglioma of the bile duct. *South Med J* 2001;94(5):515–518.

71. Davis GL, Kissane JM, Ishak KG. Embryonal rhabdomyosarcoma (sarcoma botryoides) of the biliary tree: report of five cases and a review of the literature. *Cancer* 1969;24(2):333–342.

72. Lack EE, Perez–Atayde AR, Schuster SR. Botryoid rhabdomyosarcoma of the biliary tract. *Am J Surg Pathol* 1981;5(7):643–652.

73. Tsuchiya T, Shimokawa I, Higami Y, et al. Primary low–grade MALT lymphoma of the gallbladder. *Pathol Int* 2001;51(12):965–969.

74. Inceoglu R, Dosluoglu HH, Kullu S, Ahiskali R, Doslu FA. An unusual cause of hydropic gallbladder and biliary colic—heterotopic pancreatic tissue in the cystic duct: report of a case and review of the literature. *Surg Today* 1993;23(6):532–534.

75. Sano T, Hirose T, Kagawa N, Hizawa K, Saito K. Polypoid traumatic neuroma of the gallbladder. *Arch Pathol Lab Med* 1985;109(6):574–576.

76. Jutras JA, Levesque HP. Adenomyoma and adenomyomatosis of gallbladder: radiologic and pathologic correlations. *Radiol Clin North Am* 1966;4:483–500.

CHAPTER 36 ■ CANCERS OF THE BILIARY TREE: ANATOMY AND STAGING

ATTILA NAKEEB AND HENRY A. PITT

Biliary tract cancers affect more than 7,500 Americans each year, with an incidence of 4 cases per 100,000 residents in the United States. Biliary malignancies are composed of cancers of the bile ducts (cholangiocarcinomas) and gallbladder cancers. Cholangiocarcinomas are further subdivided by anatomic location into (i) intrahepatic, (ii) perihilar, and (iii) distal tumors (1). Biliary malignancies are often asymptomatic until late in the course of the disease. As a result, these tumors often present in an advanced stage. A margin-negative (R_0) surgical resection provides the only opportunity for long-term survival. Both the late diagnosis and the complex operative techniques required for potentially curative resection contribute to the challenge of managing patients with biliary malignancies. A thorough understanding of hepatobiliary anatomy and both clinical and pathological tumor staging are essential for determining the most appropriate treatment for patients with biliary malignancies.

HEPATIC ANATOMY

A precise knowledge of the anatomy of the liver and biliary tract and of their relationship to associated blood vessels is essential for the performance of safe hepatobiliary surgery. Surgeons must have a complete understanding of the general anatomy of the liver, biliary tree, portal veins, and hepatic arteries. In addition, a detailed understanding of each individual patient's anatomy is necessary because anatomic variants in the liver vasculature and biliary tree are common (2).

Segmental Anatomy

The most widely accepted nomenclature is based on Couinaud's description of the discrete anatomic segments of the liver (Fig. 36.1). The eight segments of a liver can be determined using surface anatomy and location of the three main hepatic veins, the portal pedicle bifurcation into right and left, and the umbilical fissure and falciform ligament. The right and left halves of the liver are delineated by a plane through the middle hepatic vein and the inferior vena cava (IVC). Segments II, III, and IV lie to the left of this plane and form the left half of the liver. Segments V, VI, VII, and VIII lie to the right of this plane and form the right half of the liver. Segment I, or the caudate lobe, is morphologically distinct from the two halves of the liver and emanates from a process of liver lying posterior to the portal pedicle and anterior to the IVC. Whereas the right and left halves of the liver derive their blood supply from the corresponding right and left portal veins and hepatic arteries, segment I derives its blood supply from both. Additionally, the right half of the liver has venous drainage through the right and middle hepatic veins, and the left half of the liver through the left and middle hepatic veins. Segment I, however, drains directly via small branches into the IVC.

The right half of the liver can be further subdivided using a plane through the right hepatic vein and the IVC. Liver anterior to this plane forms its right anterior section, and liver posterior to this plane forms the right posterior section. The right anterior section of the liver comprises segment V (inferior to the portal bifurcation) and segment VIII (superior to the portal bifurcation). The right posterior section of the liver comprises segment VI (inferior to the portal bifurcation) and segment VII (superior to the portal bifurcation). The left half of the liver can be further subdivided using a plane through the umbilical fissure and falciform ligament. Liver medial to this plane forms the left medial section of the liver or segment IV, and liver lateral to this plane forms the left lateral section of the liver. The left lateral section of the liver is further subdivided into segment II (which is superior to the left hepatic vein) and segment III (which is inferior to the left hepatic vein).

Hepatic Veins

Three major hepatic veins carry blood from the liver to the IVC. Most patients have a single, large right hepatic vein that joins the right anterior wall of the IVC and a middle and left hepatic vein that converge into a common trunk 1 to 2 cm from the IVC and enter the left anterior wall of the IVC. In approximately one third of patients, the three main hepatic veins join the IVC via three distinct trunks. Usually, multiple accessory right hepatic veins empty from the right half of the liver directly into the IVC as it courses posterior to the liver.

Portal Veins

The superior mesenteric and splenic veins join posterior to the neck of the pancreas to form the main portal vein. It receives pyloric and coronary vein branches as it courses cephalad and obliquely to the right to form the most posterior structure within the hepatoduodenal ligament (portal triad). In the hilus of the liver, the main portal vein bifurcates into a short oblique right portal vein and a longer, more transverse, and more superficial left portal vein (Fig. 36.2). These branches then enter the parenchyma and become invested along with the other components of the portal triad by extensions of Glisson's capsule. Both the right and left portal veins give off small branches to dually supply segment I. The right portal vein usually enters the hepatic parenchyma immediately and is quick to divide into a right anterior portal vein supplying segments V and VIII and a right posterior portal vein supplying segments VI and VII. The left portal vein may remain near the surface of the left half of the liver in the hilar plate for a significant distance as it courses

483

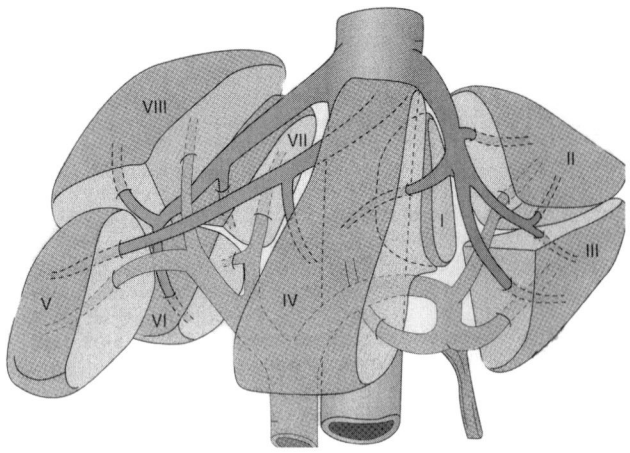

FIGURE 36.1. Segmental anatomy of the liver. (Reprinted with permission from Schulick RD. Hepatobiliary anatomy. In: Mullholand MW, Lillemoe KD, Doherty GM, Maier RV, Upchirch GR, eds. *Greenfield's Surgery: Scientific Principles & Practice,* 4th ed. Philadelphia: Lippincott Williams & Wilkins; 2006:892–908.)

to the umbilical fissure to give off medial branches to segment IV and lateral branches to segments II and III.

Hepatic Arteries

There is much variability in the hepatic arterial supply to the liver. The most common anatomy (Fig. 36.3) is a common hepatic artery that arises from the celiac trunk and courses near the superior border of the neck of the pancreas. After the origins of the gastroduodenal and right gastric arteries, the proper hepatic artery courses in the hepatoduodenal ligament in front of the portal vein and to the left of the common hepatic duct. The proper hepatic artery usually bifurcates into right and left hepatic arteries outside the liver. The right hepatic artery usually courses posterior to the common hepatic duct but anterior to the right portal vein to supply the right liver. The left hepatic artery usually remains extrahepatic until near the base of the umbilical fissure, where it enters the liver to give off branches

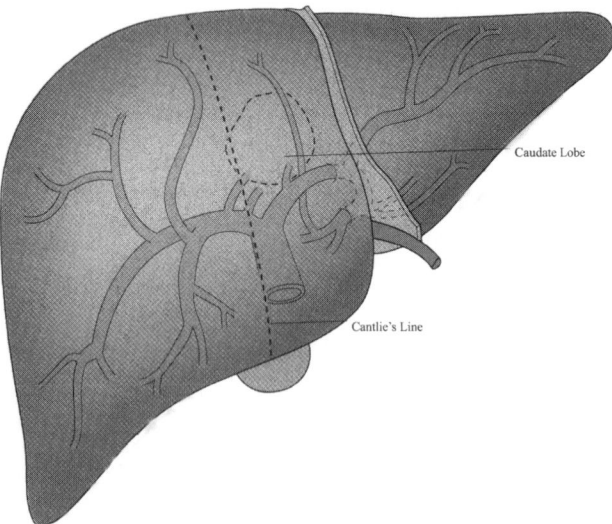

FIGURE 36.2. Intrahepatic anatomy of the portal vein. (Reprinted with permission from Schulick RD. Hepatobiliary anatomy. In: Mullholand MW, Lillemoe KD, Doherty GM, Maier RV, Upchirch GR, eds. *Greenfield's Surgery: Scientific Principles & Practice,* 4th ed. Philadelphia: Lippincott Williams & Wilkins; 2006:892–908.)

to segments II, III, and IV. Classical hepatic arterial anatomy is found in only approximately 50% to 60% of patients. A replaced or accessory right hepatic artery may arise off of the superior mesenteric artery near its origin and course posteriorly or through the head of the pancreas to lie along the right posterior border of the hepatoduodenal ligament. A replaced or accessory left hepatic artery may arise off of the left gastric artery and course transversely toward the base of the umbilical fissure in the lesser omentum. In general, within the hepatic parenchyma, the hepatic arterial branches course closely with bile duct branches and fairly closely with portal venous branches.

Biliary Tree

Intrahepatic Bile Ducts. The right and left livers are drained by the right and left hepatic ducts, respectively, whereas the caudate (Segment I) is drained by several small ducts joining the bifurcation and the first several centimeters of both hepatic ducts. The intrahepatic ducts are tributaries of the corresponding hepatic ducts, which penetrate the liver invaginating Glisson's capsule at the hilus (Fig. 36.4). Bile ducts are usually located above the corresponding portal branches, whereas hepatic arterial branches run inferiorly to the veins. The left hepatic duct directly drains the bile ducts to segments II, III, and IV, which constitute the left liver. The right hepatic duct drains the bile ducts from segments V, VI, VII, and VIII, which constitute the right liver. Usually, the bile ducts from segments V and VIII join to first form the anterior sectoral duct, and the bile ducts from segments VI and VII join to first form the posterior sectoral duct prior to forming the right hepatic duct.

Gallbladder. The gallbladder is a reservoir for bile located on the undersurface of the liver at the confluence of the right and left halves of the liver. It is separated from the hepatic parenchyma by a cystic plate, which is composed of connective tissue applied to Glisson's capsule. The gallbladder may be deeply imbedded into the liver or occasionally presents on a mesenteric attachment, but usually lies in a gallbladder fossa. The gallbladder varies in size and consists of a fundus, a body, and an infundibulum. The tip of the fundus usually reaches the free edge of the liver and is closely applied to the cystic plate. The infundibulum of the gallbladder makes an angle with the body and may obscure the common hepatic duct constituting a danger point during cholecystectomy. The cystic duct arises from the infundibulum of the gallbladder and extends to join the common hepatic duct. The lumen measures between 1 and 3 mm in diameter, and its length varies depending on the type of union with the common hepatic duct. Calot's triangle is bounded by the common hepatic duct on the left, the cystic duct inferiorly, and the cystic artery superiorly. Arterial blood reaches the gallbladder via the cystic artery, which usually originates from the right hepatic artery. The cystic artery may also originate from the left hepatic, common hepatic, gastroduodenal, or superior mesenteric artery. The cystic artery is usually located parallel and medial to the cystic duct, but its course varies with its origin. The cystic artery divides into superficial and deep branches before entering the gallbladder. The venous drainage of the gallbladder is directly into the liver parenchyma or into the common bile duct plexus. Lymphatic drainage from the gallbladder occurs in a predictable fashion and correlates with the pattern of lymph node metastases seen in gallbladder cancer. Lymph flow from the gallbladder initially drains to the cystic duct node and then descends along the common bile duct to pericholedochal lymph nodes. Flow then proceeds to nodes posterior to the head of the pancreas and then to interaortocaval lymph nodes. Secondary routes of lymphatic drainage include the retroportal and right celiac lymph nodes.

Common Bile Duct. The cystic and common hepatic ducts join to form the common bile duct. The common bile duct is

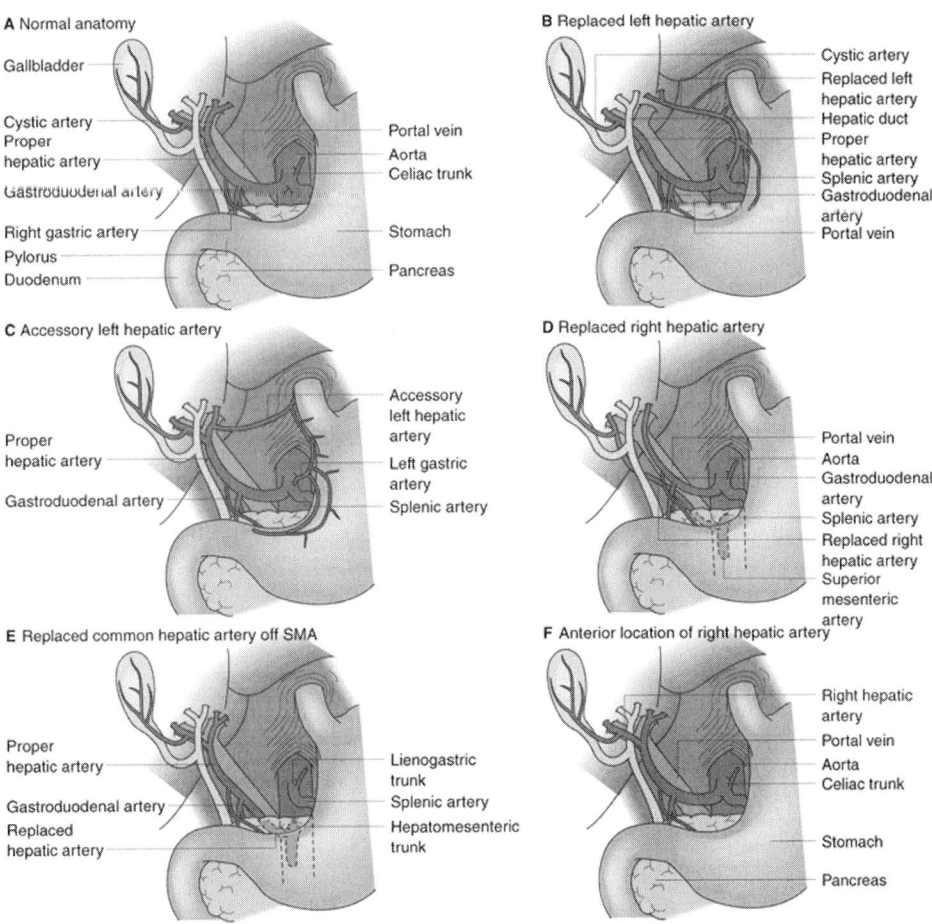

FIGURE 36.3. Hepatic artery anatomy and common variations. (Reprinted with permission from Schulick RD. Hepatobiliary anatomy. In: Mullholand MW, Lillemoe KD, Doherty GM, Maier RV, Upchirch GR, eds. *Greenfield's Surgery: Scientific Principles & Practice*, 4th ed. Philadelphia: Lippincott Williams & Wilkins; 2006:892–908.)

approximately 8 to 10 cm in length and 0.4 to 0.8 cm in diameter. The common bile duct can be divided into three anatomic segments: supraduodenal, retroduodenal, and intrapancreatic. The supraduodenal segment resides in the hepatoduodenal ligament lateral to the hepatic artery and anterior to the portal vein. The course of the retroduodenal segment is posterior to the first portion of the duodenum, anterior to the IVC, and lateral to the portal vein. The pancreatic portion of the duct lies within a tunnel or groove on the posterior aspect of the pancreas. The common bile duct then enters the medial wall of the duodenum, courses tangentially through the submucosal layer for 1 to 2 cm, and terminates in the major papilla in the second portion of the duodenum (Fig. 36.4). The distal portion of the duct is encircled by smooth muscle that forms the sphincter of Oddi. The common bile duct may enter the duodenum directly (25%) or join the pancreatic duct (75%) to form a common channel, termed the ampulla of Vater.

The blood supply of the common bile duct is segmental in nature and consists of branches from the cystic, hepatic, and gastroduodenal arteries. These meet to form collateral vessels that run in the 3 and 9 o'clock positions. The venous drainage forms a plexus on the anterior surface of the common bile duct that enters the portal system. The lymphatic drainage follows the course of the hepatic artery to the celiac nodes.

CLINICOPATHOLOGIC STAGING OF GALLBLADDER CANCER

Gallbladder cancer most often presents with right upper quadrant abdominal pain often mimicking other more common biliary and nonbiliary disorders. Weight loss, jaundice, and an abdominal mass are less common symptoms. Unfortunately, the nonspecific nature of these symptoms often leads to a delay in the diagnosis. Specific symptoms usually develop only after invasion or obstruction of nearby structures has occurred.

Pathologic Staging

Accurate pathologic staging of biliary malignancies is important for providing prognostic information to patients and for comparing the results of various therapeutic trials. The American Joint Committee on Cancer (AJCC) staging for gallbladder cancer is shown in Table 36.1 (3). This system, based on the TNM classification, takes into account the extent of the primary tumor (T), the presence or absence of regional lymph node involvement (N), and the presence or absence of distant metastatic disease (M).

Only 10% of gallbladder cancers are confined to the gallbladder wall at diagnosis, with liver involvement found in 59%, lymph node involvement in 45%, infiltration of the common hepatic duct in 35%, perineural involvement in 42%, and involvement of other organs in 45% of patients. Hepatic and other hematogenous metastases were detected in 34% and 20% of patients, respectively (4).

The appropriate management and overall prognosis for gallbladder cancer are strongly dependent on tumor stage and are discussed in detail in the following chapter. For stage I tumors, simple cholecystectomy may be the only treatment that is required. Unfortunately, tumors that are limited to the gallbladder's mucosa represent only about 5% of all gallbladder cancers. Stage II tumors require an "extended cholecystectomy," which includes segmental resection of the adjacent liver bed

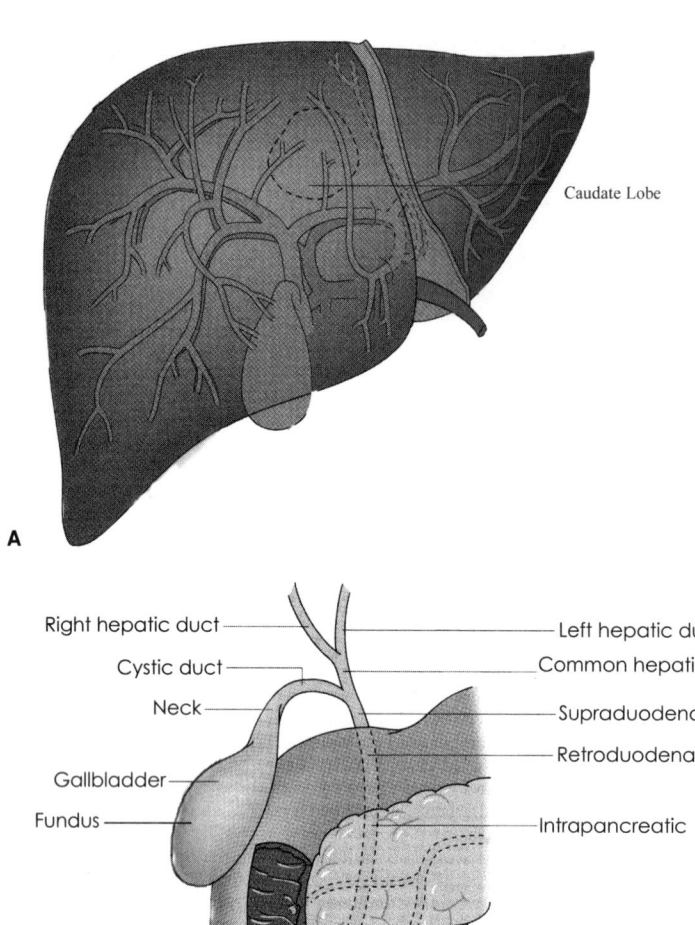

Caudate Lobe

A

Right hepatic duct — Left hepatic duct

Cystic duct — Common hepatic duct

Neck — Supraduodenal

— Retroduodenal

Gallbladder —

Fundus — Intrapancreatic

Ampulla of Vater — Intramural

B

FIGURE 36.4. (A) Intrahepatic bile duct anatomy. (B) Anatomy of the extrahepatic biliary tree. (Reprinted with permission from Schulick RD. Hepatobiliary anatomy. In: Mullholand MW, Lillemoe KD, Doherty GM, Maier RV, Upchirch GR, eds. *Greenfield's Surgery: Scientific Principles & Practice*, 4th ed. Philadelphia: Lippincott Williams & Wilkins; 2006:892–908.)

and a regional lymph node dissection including all periportal, retropancreatic, and celiac lymph nodes. For stage II tumors, which represent approximately 10% of gallbladder cancers, an extended cholecystectomy may improve survival from 30% to 40% with simple cholecystectomy to 70% to 85% with the more aggressive approach (5–12). This major improvement in survival with extended cholecystectomy is achieved with minimal morbidity and a low mortality. Stage III and IV patients are not considered resectable and are treated with chemotherapy and/or radiation therapy.

Radiologic Evaluation

Ultrasound, computed tomography (CT), and magnetic resonance (MR) can all be used in the diagnosis of gallbladder cancer. Their techniques are reviewed in more detail in the following chapter but are briefly summarized here. Any of these techniques can be used to demonstrate replacement of the gallbladder by tumor; invasion into the liver or adjacent structures such as the colon, duodenum, or extrahepatic bile ducts; and involvement of the hepatic arteries or portal veins.

Initial assessment of patients with biliary tract symptoms often includes a right upper quadrant ultrasound. Early carcinoma may present as a fixed mass not associated with acoustic shadowing or a complex mass filling the lumen with localized

thickening of the gallbladder wall. Often, it is difficult to differentiate between cholecystitis and early carcinoma because thickening of the gallbladder wall is a feature of both diseases (13). If the tumor is advanced, ultrasonography shows a loss of the interface between the gallbladder and liver. This feature is indicative of tumor invasion. Ultrasound can reveal other associated signs such as the presence of cholelithiasis, porcelain gallbladder, invasion of neighboring structures or hepatic metastases, vascular invasion, biliary dilatation, adenopathies, and ascites (14). In advanced stages of the disease, when most patients are diagnosed, ultrasound has a sensitivity of 85% and an accuracy of 80% for the diagnosis of gallbladder cancer (15), but it has limitations in the diagnosis of involved lymph nodes and staging of disease (16). With the recent advent of color doppler ultrasonography, it is now possible to differentiate between biliary sludge and carcinoma by studying fine vessel patterns (17). Endoscopic ultrasonography (EUS) has also been used for diagnostic evaluation. This technique, which may greatly improve the diagnosis of gallbladder carcinoma, can better predict the depth of tumor involvement and can be combined with fine needle aspiration (FNA) biopsy (15,18).

CT scanning is commonly performed in the preoperative staging of gallbladder cancer (Fig. 36.5). It can be used to assess the primary tumor, involvement of the adjacent liver and or surrounding structures, regional lymph nodes, and distant metastatic disease to the liver or peritoneal cavity (19–21).

TABLE 36.1

AMERICAN JOINT COMMITTEE ON CANCER (AJCC) STAGING SYSTEM FOR GALLBLADDER CANCER

Primary tumor (T)
- TX: Primary tumor cannot be assessed
- T0: No evidence of primary tumor
- Tis: Carcinoma *in situ*
- T1: Tumor invades lamina propria or muscle layer
  - T1a: Tumor invades lamina propria
  - T1b: Tumor invades the muscle layer
- T2: Tumor invades the perimuscular connective tissue; no extension beyond the serosa or into the liver
- T3: Tumor perforates the serosa (visceral peritoneum) and/or directly invades the liver and/or one other adjacent organ or structure, such as the stomach, duodenum, colon, pancreas, omentum, or extrahepatic bile ducts
- T4: Tumor invades main portal vein or hepatic artery or invades multiple extrahepatic organs or structures

Regional lymph nodes (N)
- NX: Regional lymph nodes cannot be assessed
- N0: No regional lymph node metastasis
- N1: Regional lymph node metastasis

Distant metastasis (M)
- MX: Distant metastasis cannot be assessed
- M0: No distant metastasis
- M1: Distant metastasis

AJCC stage groupings

Stage			
Stage 0	Tis, N0, M0		
Stage IA	T1, N0, M0		
Stage IB	T2, N0, M0		
Stage IIA	T3, N0, M0		
Stage IIB	T1, N1, M0		
	T2, N1, M0		
	T3, N1, M0		
Stage III	T4, any N, M0		
Stage IV	Any T, any N, M1		

Gallbladder carcinomas can be identified by the presence of a polypoidal mass protruding into the lumen or completely filling it, or a focal or diffuse thickening of the gallbladder wall. Another common finding is the presence of a mass in the gallbladder fossa, with the gallbladder itself being indiscernible.

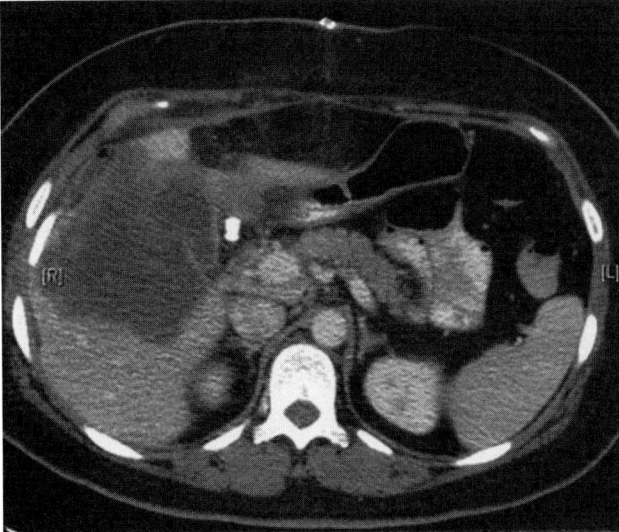

FIGURE 36.5. Computed tomography of abdomen showing a gallbladder cancer with extensive invasion of the liver.

The tumor is usually heterogeneous, containing hyperdense areas due to necrosis and unequal uptake, which is preferentially peripheral with necrotic (low uptake) areas (21). Dual-phase spiral CT studies can show early uptake in the arterial phase, with either peripheral or heterogeneous enhancement. When calculi are seen, they are surrounded by the mass, and in most cases at least part of the uninvolved gallbladder can be observed (21,22).

Regional lymph nodes that are involved with tumors usually have an anteroposterior diameter of >1 cm, are ring-shaped, and demonstrate a heterogeneous enhancement after intravenous contrast administration (23,24). Using these criteria, the sensitivity for detection of the different lymph node chains ranges from 18% for interaortocaval nodes to 78% for the celiac chain. In contrast, the specificity and positive predictive values range between 83% and 100%. Therefore, although CT does not localize all regional lymph nodes involved by the tumor, their size and uptake are useful to indicate possible lymphatic involvement (23).

Biliary invasion can occur by direct spread of the lesion along the hepatoduodenal ligament or by compression from portal lymphadenopathy. Abdominal CT can detect the presence of bile duct involvement by the demonstration of biliary dilation, although false negatives are possible because of minimal invasion with no evident dilatation. Invasion of the duodenum, colon, or the head of the pancreas should be established to assist in treatment planning. Even high resolution spiral CT may fail to demonstrate peritoneal carcinomatosis or liver metastasis <0.5 cm. There are few published studies on the usefulness of CT for staging gallbladder cancer. A retrospective study of 59 patients by Ohtani et al. (25) correlated surgical and pathological findings with presurgical CT results, applying three different protocols with conventional equipment. The sensitivity of CT to detect lymph node metastasis was between 36% and 47% (positive predictive value 94%, negative predictive value 92%). The sensitivity for determining hepatic infiltration of <2 cm was 65% and for liver infiltration >2 cm it was 100%. The sensitivity of CT for determining extrahepatic spread to adjacent organs was lower (extrahepatic bile duct 50%; duodenum, colon, or pancreas 57%). No cases of peritoneal or omentum infiltration were detected in their series. The authors concluded that the sensitivity of CT to detect the extension of gallbladder cancer is low to moderate, although its high positive predictive value means that it is useful to determine resectability and to assist in treatment planning, especially in advanced cases.

MR imaging (MRI) provides information similar to that provided by a high-quality CT scan. Gallbladder cancer appears on MR as a hypo- or isointense mass or wall thickening in T1 in relation to the liver and is usually hyperintense and poorly defined in T2 sequences (26). Assessment of the invasion of neighboring organs and lymph node metastasis is facilitated by the combination of enhanced sequences in T2 with fat suppression, dynamic postgadolinium T1-weighted images in arterial phase and T1 with fat suppression in equilibrium phase, 2 minutes after contrast administration (27). An irregular interface between tumor and parenchyma in T1 in early phase assists assessment of the extent of the primary tumor. Detection of metastases is based, as with CT, on a size of >1 cm and ring-shaped or heterogeneous uptake of involved nodes (14).

Endoscopic retrograde cholangiography (ERC) or percutaneous transhepatic cholangiography (PTC) also may be helpful in staging patients with gallbladder cancer who present with jaundice. A typical finding is a long stricture of the common hepatic duct. This finding alone suggests a more advanced tumor that may be associated with metastatic disease or vascular encasement. A small percentage of patients will have extensive biliary involvement either proximally or distally which may preclude resection.

If radiologic studies suggest that the tumor may be resectable, preoperative establishment of a tissue diagnosis is not required. In contrast, the presence of liver or peritoneal metastases, encasement of the main portal vein or common hepatic artery, or extensive hepatic invasion suggests that the tumor will not be resectable. In these circumstances, establishment of a tissue diagnosis by percutaneous ultrasound- or CT-guided biopsy or biopsy of the biliary tract at the time of endoscopic or percutaneous biliary stent placement is indicated.

In selected patients, EUS with FNA and cytology may establish the diagnosis and/or determine lymph node involvement or vascular encasement. However, the routine use of EUS in these patients is not indicated. Unfortunately, positron emission tomography (PET) even with PET/CT has not proven to be more accurate than CT or MRI in staging these patients. Similarly, the routine use of chest CT or bone scans is not cost-effective. In contrast, the Memorial Sloan-Kettering group has demonstrated that approximately two thirds of patients with T-3 and 80% of patients with T-4 gallbladder cancers will have liver and/or peritoneal metastases (8–10). Thus, the yield of staging laparoscopy is very high in patients with larger gallbladder cancers, and this procedure will often establish a tissue diagnosis and avoid an unnecessary laparotomy (28,29).

CLINICOPATHOLOGIC STAGING OF CHOLANGIOCARCINOMA

Cholangiocarcinoma can occur anywhere along the intrahepatic or extrahepatic biliary tree. Cholangiocarcinoma almost always presents with painless jaundice, and this diagnosis should be considered in every case of obstructive jaundice. The diagnostic evaluation and clinical management of a bile duct cancer are in large part determined by the anatomic location; therefore, cholangiocarcinomas are best classified into three broad anatomic groups: (i) intrahepatic, (ii) perihilar, and (iii) distal (1).

The hepatic duct bifurcation is the most frequently involved site, and approximately 60% to 80% of cholangiocarcinomas are found in the perihilar region. In 1965, Klatskin (30) reported 13 patients with cancers involving the perihilar region, which subsequently has been called Klatskin's tumor. Bismuth and Corlette (31) further classified tumors of the hepatic duct bifurcation by the extent of ductal involvement (Fig. 36.6). In

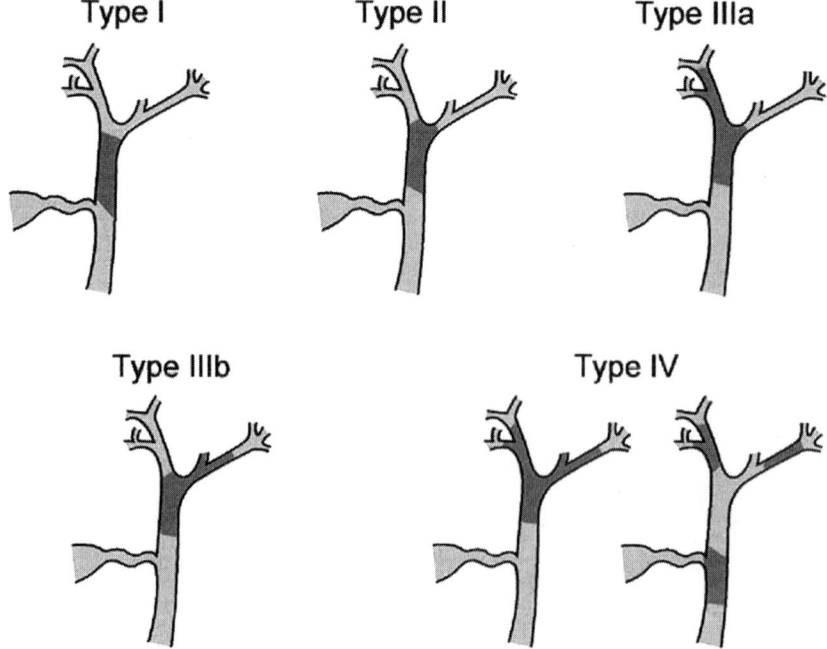

FIGURE 36.6. Bismuth classification of perihilar bile duct cancers.

TABLE 36.2

AMERICAN JOINT COMMITTEE ON CANCER (AJCC) STAGING SYSTEM FOR EXTRAHEPATIC BILE DUCT CANCER

Primary tumor (T)
- TX: Primary tumor cannot be assessed
- T0: No evidence of primary tumor
- Tis: Carcinoma *in situ*
- T1: Tumor confined to the bile duct histologically
- T2: Tumor invades beyond the wall of the bile duct
- T3: Tumor invades the liver, gallbladder, pancreas, and/or unilateral branches of the portal vein (right or left) or hepatic artery (right or left)
- T4: Tumor invades any of the following: main portal vein or its branches bilaterally, common hepatic artery, or other adjacent structures, such as the colon, stomach, duodenum, or abdominal wall

Regional lymph nodes (N)
- NX: Regional lymph nodes cannot be assessed
- N0: No regional lymph node metastasis
- N1: Regional lymph node metastasis

Distant metastasis (M)
- MX: Distant metastasis cannot be assessed
- M0: No distant metastasis
- M1: Distant metastasis

AJCC stage groupings

Stage	
Stage 0	Tis, N0, M0
Stage IA	T1, N0, M0
Stage IB	T2, N0, M0
Stage IIA	T3, N0, M0
Stage IIB	T1, N1, M0
	T2, N1, M0
	T3, N1, M0
Stage III	T4, any N, M0
Stage IV	Any T, any N, M1

Adapted from Extrahepatic bile ducts. In: American Joint Committee on Cancer. *AJCC Cancer Staging Manual,* 6th ed. New York: Springer; 2002:145–150.

this system, Type I tumors are confined to the common hepatic duct, and Type II tumors involve the hepatic duct bifurcation including both the main right and left hepatic ducts. Type IIIa and IIIb tumors extend into the right and left secondary intrahepatic ducts, respectively, and Type IV tumors involve the secondary intrahepatic duct on both sides.

Distal tumors are the second most common and are usually treated like pancreatic cancer with pancreatoduodenectomy. Purely intrahepatic cholangiocarcinomas occur with the lowest frequency and are managed like hepatocellular carcinomas with liver resection. Surgical resection with negative margins is the most important factor in achieving long-term survival, and several recent innovative approaches have led to an increase in the number of patients reaching this goal.

Pathologic Staging

The AJCC staging for cholangiocarcinoma is shown in Table 36.2 (3). This system, based on the TNM classification, takes into account the extent of the primary tumor (T), the presence or absence of regional lymph node involvement (N), and the presence or absence of distant metastatic disease (M). Currently, there is no clinical staging system available that stratifies patients preoperatively into subgroups based on potential for resection. The Bismuth–Corlette classification stratifies patients based only on the extent of biliary involvement by tumor, and the AJCC staging system is based largely on pathologic criteria and has little applicability for preoperative staging. Neither is useful for predicting resectability and survival. Recently, the Memorial Sloan-Kettering group has proposed a preoperative staging system, using data from preoperative imaging studies, based on biliary ductal involvement, vascular involvement, and lobar atrophy (32,33). This clinical T staging system (Table 36.3) accounts fully for local tumor extent and correlates closely with resectability and survival.

Radiologic Evaluation

The goals of the radiologic evaluation of the jaundiced patient include: (i) the confirmation of clinically suspected extrahepatic biliary obstruction by the demonstration of a dilated biliary tree, (ii) the identification of the cause and site of extrahepatic biliary obstruction, and (iii) the selection of patients in whom surgical or interventional radiologic or endoscopic treatment is indicated.

Imaging studies play a critical role in evaluating patients with biliary obstruction, and because resection is the only effective treatment, such studies should be directed at fully assessing the extent of disease. In patients with hilar cholangiocarcinoma, evaluation must address four critical components of resectability: level and extent of tumor within the biliary tree, vascular invasion, hepatic lobar atrophy, and distant metastatic disease.

The initial radiographic study in the jaundiced patient consists of either an abdominal ultrasound or CT scan. Intrahepatic tumors are easily visualized on CT and appear as a liver

TABLE 36.3

CLINICAL T STAGE CRITERIA FOR HILAR CHOLANGIOCARCINOMA

Clinical stage	Criteria
T1	Tumor involving biliary confluence ± unilateral extension to 2° biliary radicles
T2	Tumor involving biliary confluence ± unilateral extension to 2° biliary radicles and ipsilateral portal vein involvement ± ipsilateral hepatic lobar atrophy
T3	Tumor involving biliary confluence + bilateral extension to 2° biliary radicles, unilateral extension to 2° biliary radicles with contralateral portal vein involvement, unilateral extension to 2° biliary radicles with contralateral hepatic lobar atrophy, or main portal vein involvement

Adapted from Jarnagin WR, Fong Y, DeMatteo RP, et al. Staging, resectability, and outcome in 225 patients with hilar cholangiocarcinoma. *Ann Surg.* 2001;234:507–519.

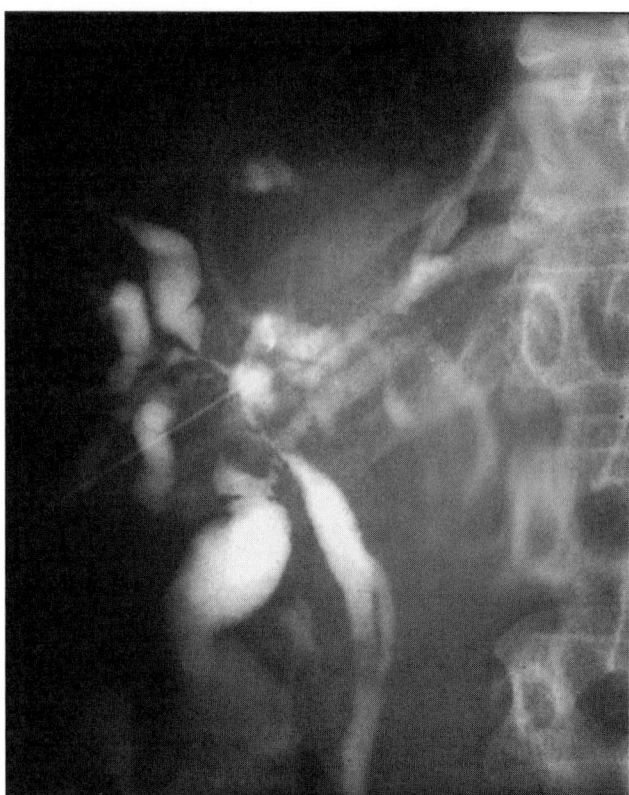

FIGURE 36.7. Percutaneous transhepatic cholangiogram of a perihilar cholangiocarcinoma.

mass with or without biliary ductal dilation. A perihilar cholangiocarcinoma will give a picture of a dilated intrahepatic biliary tree, a normal or collapsed gallbladder and extrahepatic biliary tree, and a normal pancreas. Distal bile duct tumors lead to dilation of both the intra- and extrahepatic biliary tree and gallbladder with or without a pancreatic head mass.

The primary tumor mass in patients with perihilar and distal tumors can be difficult to visualize on ultrasound and standard CT scan. Improvements in these imaging techniques have increased their utility in defining the extent of biliary tract tumors. Duplex ultrasonography identified masses in 87% of 39 patients with perihilar cholangiocarcinoma (34). The extent of bile duct involvement was accurately determined in 86% of the tumors, and portal vein involvement by tumor was identified with a sensitivity of 86%. Thin section spiral CT has produced comparable results with an overall sensitivity for detecting ductal thickening or a mass approaching 100%; however, identification of the level of biliary obstruction was possible in only in 63% of patients (35).

Accurate and complete delineation of the anatomy of the biliary tree is important in determining the appropriate treatment for patients with cholangiocarcinoma. Cholangiography in patients with perihilar or distal tumors can be accomplished through either the PTC (Fig. 36.7) or the ERC routes or noninvasively with MR cholangiopancreatography (MRCP). The most proximal extent of the tumor is the most important feature in determining resectability. MRCP provides visualization of the intrahepatic biliary tree comparable to percutaneous cholangiography and better than endoscopic cholangiography in patients with cholangiocarcinoma (36). In a series of 73 patients with biliary obstruction, MRCP correctly identified the etiology (benign vs. malignant), and level of biliary obstruction in 90% and 96% of patients, respectively (37). MRCP also has the added advantage of obtaining two-dimensional (2D) images to further define an obstructing lesion. Guthrie et al. (38) demonstrated a mass or ductal thickening in all 24 patients with hilar cholangiocarcinoma using T2-weighted spin-echo MRI.

If preoperative or palliative biliary drainage is planned for patients with perihilar tumors, PTC is favored over ERC because it defines the proximal extent of tumor involvement most reliably (39). This approach also allows for the placement of percutaneous transhepatic catheters. The advantages of transhepatic catheter placement include (i) assistance in the technical aspects of hilar dissection by allowing palpation of the catheter within the biliary tree at the time of exploration, and (ii) facilitation of intraoperative silastic transhepatic stent placement. Currently available randomized studies do not support the practice of placing preoperative transhepatic catheters in an effort to reduce operative mortality, and preoperative biliary drainage has been associated with an increase in perioperative infectious complications (40). However, if a liver resection and/or preoperative portal vein or hepatic arterial embolization is contemplated, preoperative drainage may be justified.

Endoscopic cholangiography may provide additional information in patients with distal tumors. However, comparable diagnostic information can be obtained noninvasively with MRCP (36,37). Distal cholangiocarcinomas are often associated with obstruction of the distal common bile duct and a patent pancreatic duct, whereas both the common bile duct and pancreatic duct are usually obstructed in carcinoma of the head of the pancreas. The cholangiogram may be unremarkable in patients with intrahepatic cholangiocarcinoma.

Angiography has been used to further define vascular involvement, especially in patients with perihilar tumors. Findings of hepatic arterial or portal venous encasement are present in one-third of patients with hilar cholangiocarcinoma on angiography. Three-dimensional reconstructions of the arterial anatomy from a spiral CT scan can now provide information about arterial and venous encasement. MRI can also provide information on vascular involvement with the use of gadolinium enhancement. In a series of 24 patients with perihilar tumors, occluded portal vein branches were demonstrated in 10 patients and tumor-encased branches in two patients (38). MRI may be the preferred investigation for preoperative staging for cholangiocarcinoma and for avoiding any invasive procedures in patients in whom preoperative biliary drainage is not indicated. MRCP will identify the tumor and the level of biliary obstruction and may reveal obstructed, isolated ducts not appreciated at endoscopic or percutaneous study. MRCP also provides information regarding the hilar vascular structures, lobar atrophy, and nodal or distant metastases (38,41,42). Lobar atrophy is an often-overlooked finding in patients with hilar cholangiocarcinoma. However, its importance in determining resectability cannot be overemphasized, because it often influences therapy. Longstanding biliary obstruction may cause moderate atrophy, whereas concomitant portal venous compromise induces rapid and severe atrophy of the involved segments. On cross-sectional imaging, atrophy is characterized by a small, often hypoperfused lobe with crowding of the dilated intrahepatic ducts. Thus, the finding of lobar atrophy implies portal venous involvement and mandates hepatic resection, if the tumor is resectable (31).

After the preoperative evaluation is completed, a determination of resectability is made. CT or MRI scan findings signifying unresectable disease include peripheral hepatic metastases or extrahepatic disease. Extensive bilobar involvement in patients with intrahepatic tumors also precludes resection. Findings on traditional or MRI cholangiography suggestive of unresectable disease in patients with perihilar cholangiocarcinoma include proximal extension of tumor into second order bile ducts in both hepatic lobes. The angiographic or MRI findings of tumor encasement or occlusion of the proper hepatic artery, main portal vein, or both right and left portal venous branches or hepatic arterial branches are also considered contraindications to resection by most groups.

Efforts to establish a tissue diagnosis including percutaneous FNA biopsy, brush and scrape biopsy, and cytological examination of bile have all been used (43). If surgery is contemplated, a preoperative tissue diagnosis is not essential. Prolonged efforts to obtain a preoperative tissue diagnosis are NOT indicated unless the patient is not an operative candidate. Bile obtained from a percutaneous catheter will demonstrate malignant cells in approximately 30% of cases. This yield may be improved to approximately 40% by brush cytological techniques through transhepatic stents at the time of endoscopic procedures and to 67% by percutaneous FNA. EUS has also been used to guide FNA of distal lesions or enlarged lymph nodes. The use of cholangioscopy through percutaneous tube tracts may be used to guide biopsies and determine the extent of the tumor. However, even with these efforts, up to one-third of patients with cholangiocarcinoma will have negative biopsy and/or cytologic results. If the tumor is localized and resectable, efforts to establish a tissue diagnosis before resection are usually unnecessary.

Preoperative portal vein and hepatic arterial embolization are both being used increasingly in patients requiring resection of >60% of the hepatic parenchyma (44,45). In these approaches, preoperative embolization of the hepatic lobe containing the extensive cholangiocarcinoma leads to atrophy of the lobe to be resected and hypertrophy of the segments to be preserved at surgery. Most commonly, embolization of the right portal vein or right hepatic artery is followed 2 to 3 weeks later by right trisegmentectomy once segments II and III have hypertrophied to >30% of their original volume. This approach may lower the morbidity and mortality from hepatic failure following extensive hepatic resection in jaundiced patients with hilar cholangiocarcinoma.

Finally, the role of laparoscopy in staging these patients needs to be further evaluated. At The Johns Hopkins Hospital, approximately 45% of patients with perihilar cholangiocarcinoma have been found at exploration to have intraperitoneal or liver metastases (15%) or extensive tumor involvement of the porta hepatis (30%) precluding resection (1). In comparison, only 10% of patients with distal cholangiocarcinoma will have unresectable lesions at operative exploration. The incidence of liver and peritoneal metastases is much higher in patients with gallbladder cancer. For patients with peritoneal carcinomatosis who would benefit little from operative intervention, laparoscopy may avoid the morbidity and longer hospital stay following laparotomy. Jarnagin et al. (46) recently demonstrated an increase in the percentage of patients undergoing potentially curative resections for primary hepatobiliary malignancies from 67% to 83% in a nonrandomized series of patients managed with laparotomy without laparoscopy or routine staging laparoscopy prior to laparotomy, respectively. Laparoscopy was sensitive at detecting peritoneal metastases (90%) or additional hepatic tumors (83%), but often failed to detect vascular or extensive biliary involvement.

SUMMARY

Complete surgical resection remains the only curative treatment for malignancies of the biliary tract. A thorough knowledge of both standard hepatobiliary anatomy and the relationship of an individual patient's tumor to his own anatomy is essential to determining which patients are ultimately resectable. As improvements in noninvasive imaging including spiral CT, duplex ultrasonography, MRI and, perhaps, PET improve, our ability to stage patients with biliary malignancies will also improve.

References

1. Nakeeb A, Pitt H, Sohn T, et al. Cholangiocarcinoma: a spectrum of intrahepatic, perihilar, and distal tumors. *Ann Surg.* 1996;224:463–473.
2. Schulick RD. Hepatobiliary anatomy. In: Mullholand MW, Lillemoe KD, Doherty GM, Maier RV, Upchirch GR, eds. *Greefield's Surgery Scientific Principles & Practice*, 4th ed. Philadelphia: Lippincott Williams & Wilkins; 2006:892–908.
3. American Joint Committee on Cancer (AJCC). *AJCC Cancer Staging.* New York: Springer-Verlag; 2005:1–150.
4. Boerma EJ. Towards an oncological resection of gallbladder cancer. *Eur J Surg Oncol.* 1994;20:537–544.
5. Shirai Y, Yoshida K, Tsukada K, et al. Radical surgery for gallbladder carcinoma: long-term results. *Ann Surg.* 1992;216:565–568.
6. Todoroki T, Kawamoto T, Takahashi H, et al. Treatment of gallbladder cancer by radical resection. *Br J Surg.* 1999;86:622–627.
7. Kondo S, Nimura Y, Hayakawa N, et al. Extensive surgery for carcinoma of the gallbladder. *Br J Surg.* 2002;89:179–184.
8. Bartlett DL, Fong Y, Fortner JG, et al. Long-term results after resection for gallbladder cancer: implications for staging and management. *Ann Surg.* 1996;224:639–646.
9. Fong Y, Jarnagin W, Blumgart LH. Gallbladder cancer: comparison of patients presenting initially for definitive operation with those presenting after prior noncurative intervention. *Ann Surg.* 2000;232:557–569.
10. Shoup M, Fong Y. Surgical indications and extent of resection in gallbladder cancer. *Surg Oncol Clin North Am.* 2002;11:985–994.
11. Dixon E, Vollmer CM, Sahajpal A, et al. An aggressive surgical approach leads to improved survival in patients with gallbladder cancer: a 12-year study at a North American center. *Ann Surg.* 2005;241:385–394.
12. Shih SP, Schulick RD, Cameron JL, et al. Gallbladder cancer: the role of laparoscopy and radical resection. *Ann Surg.* 2007;245:893–901.
13. Hederstrom E, Forsberg L. Ultrasonography in carcinoma of the gallbladder: diagnostic difficulties and pitfalls. *Acta Radiol.* 1987;28:715–721.
14. Antonio Rodriguez-Fernandez A, Gomez-Rio M, Medina-Benitez A, et al. Application of modern imaging methods in diagnosis of gallbladder cancer. *J Surg Oncol.* 2006;93:650–664.
15. Chijiiwa K, Sumiyoshi K, Nakayama F. Impact of recent advances in hepatobiliary imaging techniques on the preoperative diagnosis of carcinoma of the gallbladder. *World J Surg.* 1991;15:332–337.
16. Bach AM, Loring LA, Hann LE, et al. Gallbladder cancer: can ultrasonography evaluate extent of disease? *J Ultrasound Med.* 1998;17:303–309.
17. Ueno N, Tomiyama T, Tano S, et al. Diagnosis of gallbladder carcinoma with color doppler ultrasonography. *Am J Gastroenterol.* 1996;91:1647–1649.
18. Azuma T, Yoshikawa T, Araida T, Takasaki K. Differential diagnosis of polypoid lesions of the gallbladder by endoscopic ultrasonography. *Am J Surg.* 2001;181:65–70.
19. Franquet T, Montes M, Ruiz de Azua Y, et al. Primary gallbladder carcinoma: imaging findings in 50 patients with pathologic correlation. *Gastrointest Radiol.* 1991;16:143–148.

20. Tsuchiya Y. Early carcinoma of the gallbladder: macroscopic features and US findings. *Radiology*. 1991;179:171–175.
21. Kumar A, Aggarwal S. Carcinoma of the gallbladder: CT findings in 50 cases. *Abdom Imaging*. 1994;19:304–308.
22. Kumaran V, Gulati S, Paul B, et al. The role of dual-phase helical CT in assessing resectability of carcinoma of the gallbladder. *Eur Radiol*. 2002;12:1993–1999.
23. Ohtani T, Shirai Y, Tsukada K, et al. Carcinoma of the gallbladder: CT evaluation of lymphatic spread. *Radiology*. 1993;189:875–880.
24. Efremidis SC, Vougiouklis N, Zafiriadou E, et al. Pathways of lymph node involvement in upper abdominal malignancies: evaluation with high-resolution CT. *Eur Radiol*. 1999;9:868–874.
25. Ohtani T, Shirai Y, Tsukada K, et al. Spread of gallbladder carcinoma: CT evaluation with pathologic correlation. *Abdom Imaging*. 1996;21:195–220.
26. Sagoh T, Itoh K, Togashi K, et al. Gallbladder carcinoma: evaluation with MR imaging. *Radiology*. 1990;174:131–136.
27. Till RB, Semelka RC, Reinhold C. Gallbladder and biliary system. In: Semelka RC, ed. *Abdominal-Pelvic MRI*. New York: Wiley-Liss; 2002:319–371.
28. Vollmer CM, Drebin JA, Middleton WD, et al. Utility of staging laparoscopy in subsets of peripancreatic and biliary malignancies. *Ann Surg*. 2002;235:1–7.
29. Weber JC, Navarra G, Jiao LR, et al. New technique for liver resection using heat coagulative necrosis. *Ann Surg*. 2002;236:560–563.
30. Klatskin G. Adenocarcinoma of the hepatic duct at its bifurcation within the porta hepatis: an unusual tumor with distinctive clinical and pathologic features. *Am J Med*. 1965;38:241–256.
31. Bismuth H, Corlette MB. Cholangioenteric anastomosis in carcinoma of the hilus of the liver. *Surg Gynecol Obst* 1975;140:170–178.
32. Burke EC, Jarnagin WR, Hochwald SN, et al. Hilar cholangiocarcinoma: patterns of spread, the importance of hepatic resection for curative operation, and a presurgical clinical staging system. *Ann Surg*. 1998;228:385–394.
33. Jarnagin WR, Fong Y, DeMatteo RP, et al. Staging, resectability, and outcome in 225 patients with hilar cholangiocarcinoma. *Ann Surg*. 2001;234:507–519.
34. Hann LE, Greatrex KV, Bach AM, et al. Cholangiocarcinoma at the hepatic hilus: sonographic findings. *AJR Am J Roentgenol*. 1997;168:985–989.
35. Han JK, Choi BI, Kim TK, et al. Hilar cholangiocarcinoma: thin-section spiral CT findings with cholangiographic correlation. *Radiographics*. 1997;17:1475–1485.
36. Lomanto D, Pavone P, Laghi A, et al. Magnetic resonance cholangiopancreatography in the diagnosis of biliopancreatic disease. *Am J Surg*. 1997;174:33–38.
37. Magnuson TH, Bender JS, Duncan MD, et al. Utility of magnetic resonance cholangiography in the evaluation of biliary obstruction. *J Am Coll Surg*. 1999;189:63–71.
38. Guthrie JA, Ward J, Robinson PJ. Hilar cholangiocarcinomas T2-weighted spin-echo and gadolinium-enhanced FLASH MR imaging. *Radiology*. 1996;201:347–351.
39. Pitt HA, Dooley WC, Yeo CJ, et al. Malignancies of the biliary tree. *Curr Probl Surg*. 1995;32:1–90.
40. Hochwald SN, Burke EC, Jarnagin WR, et al. Association of preoperative biliary stenting with increased postoperative infectious complications in proximal cholangiocarcinoma. *Arch Surg*. 1999;34:261–266.
41. Lee MG, Lee HJ, Kim MH, et al. Extrahepatic biliary diseases: 3D MR cholangiopancreatography compared with endoscopic retrograde cholangiopancreatography. *Radiology*. 1997;202:663–669.
42. Schwartz LH, Coakley FV, Sun Y, et al. Neoplastic pancreaticobiliary duct obstruction: evaluation with breathhold MR cholangiopancreatography. *AJR Am J Roentgenol*. 1998;170:1491–1495.
43. Desa LA, Akosa AB, Lazzara S, et al. Cytodiagnosis in the management of extrahepatic biliary stricture. *Gut*. 1991;32:1188–1191.
44. Kawasaki S, Makuuchi M, Miyagawa S. Radical operation after portal embolization for tumors of the hilar bile duct. *J Am Coll Surg*. 1994;178:480–486.
45. Vogl TJ, Balzer JO, Dette K, et al. Initially unresectable hilar cholangiocarcinoma hepatic regeneration after transarterial embolization. *Radiology*. 1998;208:217–222.
46. Jarnagin WR, Bodniewicz J, Dougherty E, et al. A prospective analysis of staging laparoscopy in patients with primary and secondary hepatobiliary malignancies. *J Gastrointest Surg*. 2000;4:34–43.

CHAPTER 37 ■ CANCERS OF THE BILIARY TREE: CLINICAL MANAGEMENT

KEITH D. LILLEMOE, RICHARD D. SCHULICK, ANDREW S. KENNEDY, AND JOEL PICUS

Carcinomas of the biliary tree, including the gallbladder and bile duct, represent a significant clinical challenge. They are often asymptomatic early in their course, usually present at an advanced stage, and frequently are not amenable to curative therapy. In both gallbladder and bile duct cancers, the surgical and oncologic management has not been clearly defined, and survival even after curative resection remains poor. Furthermore, biliary obstruction may complicate both the initial and terminal management of both diseases. Biliary obstruction may cause the life-threatening complications of cholangitis and progressive liver dysfunction, and commonly causes anorexia and pruritus. Adequate decompression of the biliary tree must be obtained, even in the face of unresectable disease. This chapter focuses on the management of gallbladder and bile duct carcinoma by addressing the diagnostic, operative, adjuvant, and palliative measures in these diseases.

GALLBLADDER CARCINOMA

Clinical Presentation

Gallbladder carcinoma is the fifth most common cancer of the gastrointestinal tract and is the most common cancer of the biliary tree (1). The clinical presentation of gallbladder carcinoma ranges from that of an incidental finding after cholecystectomy for symptomatic gallstones to a rapidly progressive disease offering little opportunity to provide treatment of therapeutic benefit. Unfortunately, many patients in the United States present with advanced disease at the time of diagnosis.

Gallbladder carcinoma is a disease of the elderly population and is three to four times more common in women than in men. Symptoms of gallbladder carcinoma are similar to those of benign gallbladder disease, including biliary colic and acute cholecystitis. Right upper quadrant abdominal pain is the most common symptom and is present in >80% of patients. The pain is often continuous rather than the colicky pain typical of gallstone disease. Nonspecific symptoms such as nausea, intolerance of fatty foods, anorexia, weight loss, fever, and chills are also common. In more advanced cases, the gallbladder malignancy obstructs the biliary system, which results in obstructive jaundice. Physical findings in these cases include right upper quadrant tenderness, a palpable mass, hepatomegaly, and ascites. Laboratory studies are generally nonspecific unless biliary tract obstruction has developed. Levels of common tumor markers such as carcinoembryonic antigen and carbohydrate antigen 19-9 may be elevated but are not reliably useful for diagnosis.

Diagnosis

Gallbladder carcinoma is not diagnosed preoperatively in the majority of cases due to the nonspecific presentation and lack of reliable diagnostic criteria. Most patients present with symptoms suggestive of benign gallstone disease, and ultrasonography is the usual initial diagnostic procedure. Because gallstones are present in >90% of patients with gallbladder carcinoma, the ultrasonographic findings often suggest benign cholelithiasis as the cause of the patient's symptoms. A thickening of the gallbladder or a polypoid or fungating mass protruding into the gallbladder lumen, or both, should raise suspicion of a gallbladder neoplasm (Fig. 37.1). Less subtle findings of liver invasion, lymphadenopathy, or blood vessel invasion are seen in more advanced cases.

Computed tomography (CT) is more sensitive than ultrasonography in identifying a gallbladder carcinoma and better delineates a gallbladder mass (Fig. 37.2A), lymphadenopathy (Fig. 37.2B), and invasion of adjacent organs. In addition, CT can demonstrate the presence of liver metastases and ascites. The sensitivity and specificity of contrast-enhanced CT in diagnosing neoplastic lesions of the gallbladder is close to 90% (2). CT is also valuable in defining major vascular invasion of portal structures (portal vein and hepatic artery), which may indicate unresectability. Improvements in magnetic resonance imaging, including the development of magnetic resonance cholangiopancreatography (MRCP), have enabled its use as a single noninvasive imaging modality that allows complete assessment of the hepatic parenchyma (Fig. 37.3A), biliary tree (Fig. 37.3B), vasculature, and lymph nodes. Endoscopic ultrasonography has been reported to be useful for diagnosis and staging of gallbladder cancer (3). This technique has been found to be particularly useful in distinguishing early- and advanced-stage tumors by demonstrating tumor invasion and lymph node metastasis. Finally, positron emission tomography with fluorine-18–labeled fluorodeoxyglucose (FDG–PET) scanning has been shown to demonstrate uptake in patients with gallbladder cancer assisting in both diagnosis and staging (4).

Cholangiography has generally been used for patients with gallbladder carcinoma and obstructive jaundice. Either endoscopic retrograde cholangiography or percutaneous transhepatic cholangiography (PTC) can be useful in identifying the area of obstruction. The typical finding in a patient with gallbladder carcinoma is a long stricture involving the common hepatic duct (Fig. 37.4). Although biliary stents can be placed by either the endoscopic or percutaneous route, percutaneous catheters are a more reliable means to relieve the biliary obstruction and may be helpful in operative management. As stated previously, MRCP techniques can provide similar, high-quality imaging

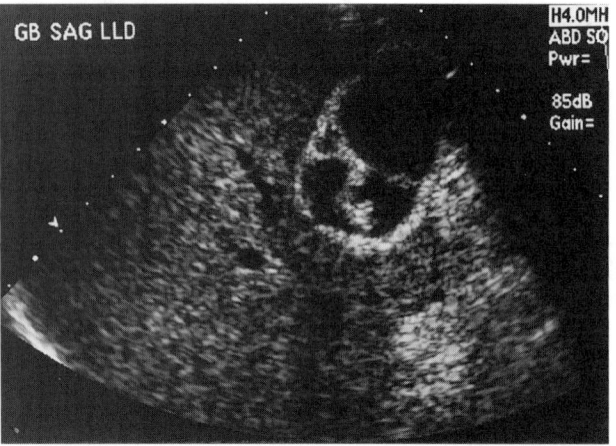

FIGURE 37.1. Ultrasonographic image of a gallbladder carcinoma demonstrating a thickened wall with a polypoid mass protruding into the lumen.

of the biliary tree, and their use has eliminated the need for invasive cholangiography in many patients.

Management

The management of gallbladder carcinoma depends largely on the mode and the stage of presentation. The disease generally presents in one of three ways: (i) as an incidental finding during or after cholecystectomy for suspected benign disease, (ii) as a suspected or confirmed lesion that appears resectable based on preoperative evaluation, or (iii) as an advanced intra-abdominal malignancy. Each of these specific presentations generally requires a different management strategy. In general, an aggressive attitude favoring surgical resection is appropriate because it offers the only chance for cure. The appropriate extent of surgical resection for each stage of disease is controversial and highly debated. Alfred Blalock wrote in 1924, "in malignancy of the gallbladder, when a diagnosis can be made without exploration, no operation should be performed, inasmuch as it only shortens the patient's life" (5). Although the

ability to diagnose gallbladder carcinoma has improved over the last 75 years, Blalock's point still remains valid for many patients, and palliation is often the primary goal of treatment.

Surgical Resection

The role of surgery for gallbladder carcinoma depends on the mode of tumor presentation and the extent of disease. The discovery of gallbladder carcinoma during or after laparoscopic cholecystectomy is a common scenario, as many patients present with signs and symptoms similar to those of benign gallstone disease. If preoperative studies suggest gallbladder carcinoma, laparoscopic cholecystectomy should be avoided. Should gallbladder carcinoma be found at the time of laparoscopic cholecystectomy, biopsy of the gallbladder mass should be avoided, and conversion to an open laparotomy should be considered unless liver metastases or carcinomatosis is identified. Tumor dissemination is the major concern related to laparoscopic cholecystectomy. Diffuse peritoneal tumor spread associated with disruption of the gallbladder wall and bile spillage as well as cancer recurrence at trochar sites have been well documented (6,7).

If gallbladder cancer is diagnosed on pathologic examination after laparoscopic cholecystectomy, further therapy is dependent on the pathologic findings. Patients with T1 N0 M0 (stage IA) gallbladder carcinoma, with disease confined to the lamina propria or muscle layer, generally do not require more than a simple cholecystectomy as long as the cystic duct margin is negative. Furthermore, T1 tumors have not yet invaded the subserosal layer, which contains the lymphatics, and therefore lymphadenectomy is not required. Most surgeons believe that the morbidity and mortality of an extended resection are not justified for disease at this early stage as the 5-year survival for stage IA disease in most series exceeds 85% (8–12). In contrast, most centers advocate a more extensive resection for T2, which invades the muscle layer of the gallbladder wall (stage IB) (8,13–17). Table 37.1 summarizes the results of a series of studies on the surgical resection of T1 N0 M0 (stage IA) gallbladder cancer.

Patients with disease of higher T stage have a significant chance of having lymph node metastasis. A series at the Memorial Sloan-Kettering Cancer Center reported the incidence of lymph node involvement with T2 lesions to be 33% (14). In

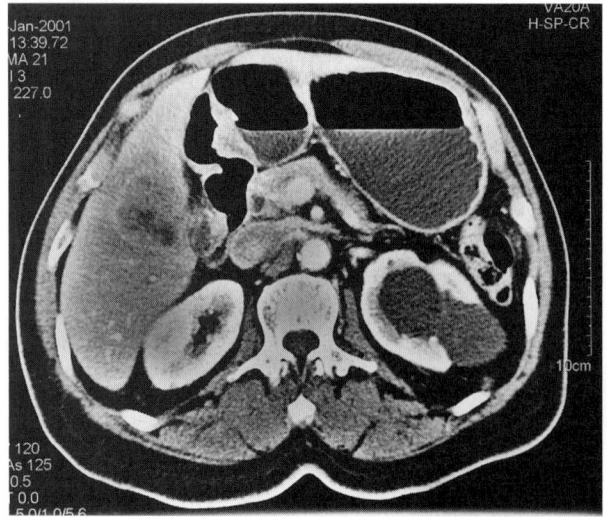
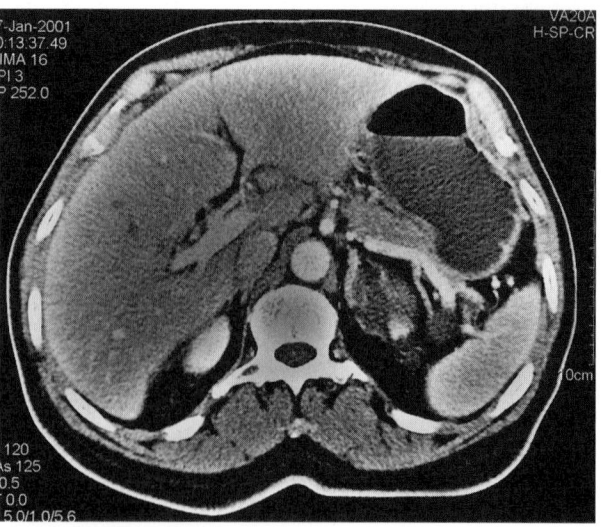

FIGURE 37.2. A: Computed tomographic (CT) image of a gallbladder carcinoma demonstrating invasion into the liver. B: CT image of a gallbladder carcinoma with diffuse portal lymphadenopathy.

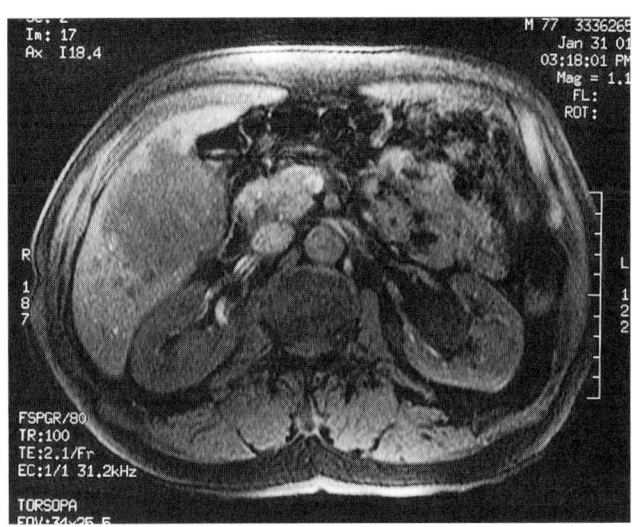
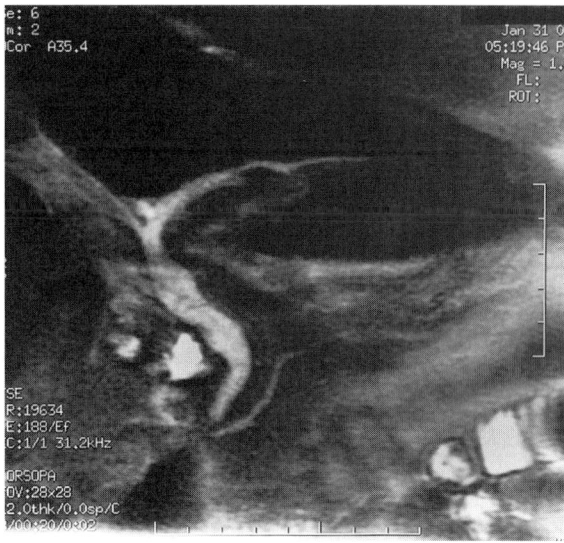

FIGURE 37.3. **A:** Magnetic resonance image of a gallbladder carcinoma demonstrating invasion into the liver. **B:** Magnetic resonance cholangiopancreatographic image with visualization of the common bile duct, pancreatic duct, and both hepatic ducts.

the same series, the incidence of lymph node involvement with T3 lesions was 58% and with T4 lesions was 69%. The management of T2 and T3 lesions is generally accepted to include extended or radical cholecystectomy consisting of *en bloc* resection of the gallbladder and wedge excision of liver segments IV and V with at least a 3- to 4-cm margin of normal parenchyma. Some centers advocate more radical liver resections, including extended lobectomies for the bulkier lesions and for cases in which differentiation of tumor from inflammation is difficult at the second operation. Regional lymphadenectomy, including

resection of all choledochal, periportal, hilar, and high pancreatic lymph nodes, should be performed. Bile duct resection and reconstruction may be necessary depending on the location of the tumor with respect to the junction of the cystic duct and common duct, and to facilitate lymph node dissection. Most groups also recommend resection of all laparoscopic trochar sites.

In patients in whom the gallbladder cancer is detected preoperatively, ample evidence supports more radical excision for T2 and T3 tumors. Patients with T2 lesions undergoing simple cholecystectomy have had reported 5-year survivals of 36% to 40% (15,18), whereas patients with T2 lesions undergoing wide resection and lymphadenectomy have had reported 5-year survivals of 83% to 100% (13,15,18). Proponents of wide resection and lymphadenectomy for T3 lesions point out that distinguishing T2 from T3 tumors at the time of surgery is often difficult and that resection of the liver allows the best chance for tumor clearance.

With T4 lesions, the enthusiasm to perform wide resection and lymphadenectomy is somewhat more tempered. Conventional clinical judgment is that the prognosis is poor in these patients regardless of treatment, and the morbidity of an extensive operation is not justified. The group at Memorial Sloan-Kettering Cancer Center, however, has demonstrated long-term survival in patients with T4 N0 M0 lesions who underwent wide resection usually including at least liver segments 4b and 5, and in may cases extended right hepatectomy (segments 4,5,6,7, and 8) lymphadenectomy (14). In this series, 27 patients who underwent resection for T4 disease were described. The 5-year survival rate in this group of patients was 28%, and five patients actually survived beyond 5 years. These results suggest that resection may be justified, especially if no gross nodal involvement is apparent at the time of operation.

The results of a number of series studying radical resection for gallbladder carcinoma are shown in Table 37.2. These series demonstrate that radical resections for gallbladder carcinoma can be performed with low mortality rates in the range of 0% to 4% (12–20). They also demonstrate that radical resections for gallbladder carcinoma can lead to long-term survival. Representative of modern Western results, a review at Memorial Sloan-Kettering Cancer Center examining 410 patients who

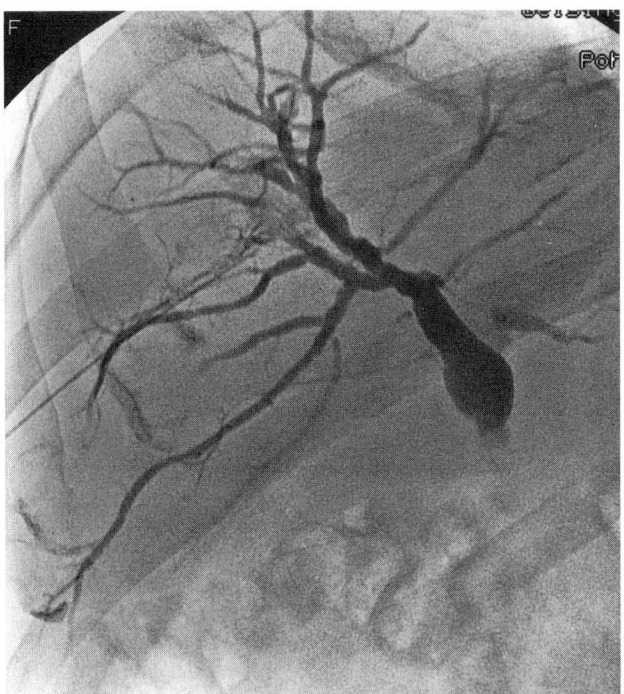

FIGURE 37.4. Percutaneous transhepatic cholangiogram of a gallbladder carcinoma that obstructs the common hepatic duct.

TABLE 37.1

RESULTS OF SURGICAL RESECTION OF T1 N0 M0 (STAGE IA) GALLBLADDER CANCER

Authors, year (ref)	Number	Procedure	5-year survival
Shirai et al., 1992 (8)	56	Simple cholecystectomy	100%
Yamaguchi and Tsuneyoshi, 1992 (9)	6	Simple cholecystectomy	100%
Donohue et al., 1990 (10)	9	Simple cholecystectomy (89%)	89%
Matsumoto et al., 1992 (13)		Simple cholecystectomy	100%
De Aretxabala et al., 1997 (11)	32	Simple cholecystectomy (69%)	94%
Yoshida et al., 2000 (12)	13	Simple cholecystectomy	91%

presented over a 14-year period found that only 102 patients were able to undergo potentially curative resection (14). Fifty-one patients had inoperable disease, 135 patients underwent noncurative cholecystectomy, and 92 patients underwent exploration and biopsy only. Median survival for patients undergoing resection was 26 months, and 5-year survival was 38%. Patients who did not undergo resection had a mean survival of 5.4 months and a 5-year survival of only 4%. In patients undergoing resection, the factors that most influenced survival based on multivariate analysis included T stage and N stage. Patients with T2 tumors had a more favorable outcome than those with T3 or T4 tumors, but advanced T stage did not preclude long-term survival. Patients with nodal metastasis had a poor outcome. Of 36 patients with node-positive disease after tumor resection for curative intent, only 2 survived more than 5 years, and both eventually died of disease.

This study also analyzed results with respect to long-term survival after curative resection involving two operations versus one; that is, results among patients who underwent an inadequate first operation (cholecystectomy only) and then had a second definitive procedure. The long-term survival after curative resection was no different for patients who had one operation and for those who had two. These data indicate that reoperative radical surgery in carefully selected patients is associated with the same long-term outcome as primary radical surgery. This finding was confirmed by a recent report from The Johns Hopkins Hospital (17).

TABLE 37.2

RESULTS OF RADICAL SURGICAL RESECTION FOR LOCALLY ADVANCED GALLBLADDER CANCER

Authors, year (ref)	Number	Operative mortality (%)	5-Year survival (%)
Donohue et al., 1990 (10)	42	2	33
Shirai et al., 1992 (15)	40	0	65
Bartlett et al., 1996 (18)	23	0	51
Fong et al., 2000 (14)	102	4	38
Shih et al., 2007 (17)	50	4	47

Palliation

The major indication for palliation of gallbladder carcinoma is biliary obstruction caused either by direct extension of the tumor into the extrahepatic biliary tree or by compression produced by lymph node metastasis. If unresectable local disease is found at the time of laparotomy, a biliary bypass (hepaticojejunostomy) can be performed to alleviate extrahepatic biliary obstruction. If, however, disseminated disease is found at laparotomy (or laparoscopy) or if the patient is found to have unresectable disease based on preoperative evaluation, palliative biliary drainage can be performed by either percutaneous or endoscopic stent placement. Metallic expandable Wallstents (Boston Scientific Corp., Natick, MA) placed by either percutaneous or endoscopic techniques can provide permanent internal palliation of biliary obstruction in patients with life expectancy limited to a few months (Fig. 37.5).

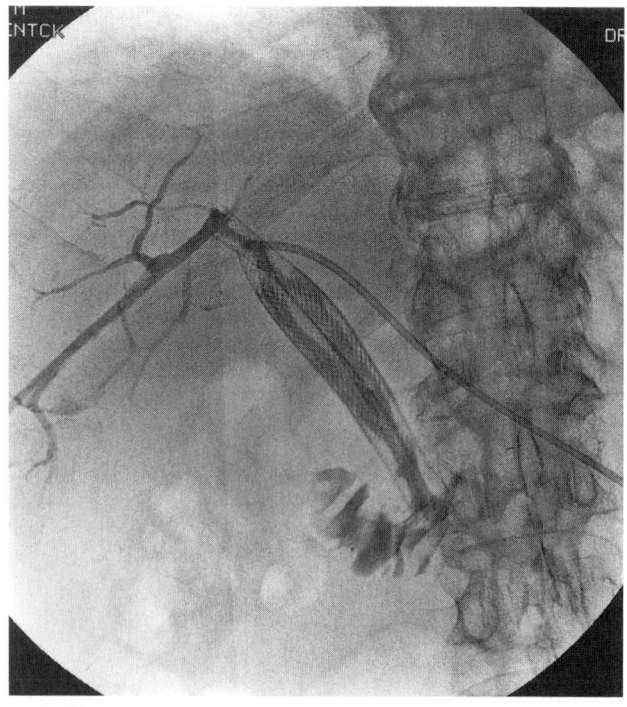

FIGURE 37.5. Metallic expandable Wallstents placed by a percutaneous technique to palliate obstruction of the extrahepatic bile ducts by a gallbladder carcinoma.

Adjuvant Therapy

The role of adjuvant chemotherapy and radiotherapy for gallbladder carcinoma has been poorly defined because the available literature is derived from small, single-institution experiences in which heterogeneous treatment methods were used. The small percentage of patients with gallbladder carcinoma undergoing curative surgery, the failure to accrue patients under protocol, and the incomplete reporting of technical treatment data, histology, and tumor extent in these studies contribute to this problem. Finally, these reports are often strongly biased by patient selection, which makes interpretation even more difficult. The rationale for the use of adjuvant chemoradiation for gallbladder carcinoma is that minimal tumor-free margins are often achieved even after radical surgery. Therefore, radiotherapy is added to control microscopic residual deposits of carcinoma in the tumor bed and regional lymph nodes. Chemotherapy is added as both a radiation sensitizer as well as for potential systemic effects.

Approaches to delivering radiotherapy to the gallbladder fossa have varied from standard external beam radiotherapy using multiple-field arrangements and low daily fractions, to intraoperative external beam radiotherapy and brachytherapy (21–24). Typically, external beam radiation for gallbladder cancer treats the tumor bed, with a 2- to 3-cm margin around the primary tumor and the regional lymph node drainage basin. Often, this treatment incorporates the porta hepatis, a portion of the liver, celiac axis, regional periaortic nodes, and pancreaticoduodenal nodes. The typical delivered dose of 45 Gy is unlikely to control gross disease, so approaches using brachytherapy and intraoperative radiotherapy (IORT) have been attempted (25–27). Due to intolerance of the liver, kidneys, spinal cord, and C loop of the duodenum, doses above 54 Gy are prohibited. IORT or brachytherapy can exclude these structures from the high-dose region and enable delivery of doses above 50 Gy. Unfortunately, the data on these techniques are limited.

A few recent reports are available describing experience with adjuvant therapy for resected gallbladder cancer. Czito et al. (28) reported a single-institution retrospective experience of primary adenocarcinoma of the gallbladder. Twenty-two patients with primary and nonmetastatic gallbladder cancer were treated with radiation therapy after surgical resection over a 23-year period. The median radiation dose was 45 Gy. Eighteen patients received concurrent 5-fluorouracil (5-FU) chemotherapy. Median follow-up was 1.7 years in all patients and 3.9 years in survivors. The 5-year actuarial overall survival, disease-free survival, metastases-free survival, and local-regional control of all 22 patients were 37%, 33%, 36%, and 59%, respectively. Median survival for all patients was 1.9 years. The conclusion of the authors was that 5-FU concurrent with radiotherapy in the adjuvant setting was helpful in nonmetastatic gallbladder carcinoma patients. Houry et al. (29) performed a meta-analysis of all publications on radiotherapy for gallbladder carcinoma between 1974 and 2000. The best benefit was obtained when only microscopic residual disease was found. Higher doses of radiation were recommended especially delivered as an intraoperative "boost" (15 Gy). Postoperative adjuvant external radiotherapy (45 to 50 Gy) was found to slightly improve survival time.

Itoh et al. (30) described the adjuvant treatment of 18 patients with gallbladder carcinoma using radiotherapy alone. The 5-year survival was 56% with multivariate analysis, confirming that the best results were found in patients with R0 (76%) versus R2 (0%) and that radiotherapy had a positive effect on survival.

Neoadjuvant Radiotherapy

Due to the locally advanced stage of many gallbladder cancers at presentation, some investigators have attempted to downsize these tumors with neoadjuvant therapy in hopes of enabling surgical resection. Aretxabala et al. (31) have reported on the use of preoperative external beam radiotherapy with chemotherapy in a phase II trial. Twenty-seven eligible patients unexpectedly found to have localized gallbladder cancer were enrolled to receive chemoradiation before definitive tumor bed and regional node resection. They received 45 Gy of external beam radiation at 1.8 Gy per fraction concurrent with two cycles of short-term continuous 5-FU infusion (days 1 through 5 and 28 through 32). Eighteen patients accepted preoperative treatment, and 15 patients completed reoperation. Surgical resection was possible in 13 cases, and three patients were found to have biopsy-proven residual disease. The median follow-up was 4 months. Seven patients were alive at last follow-up, with local failure proven in only one patient, who succumbed to disease. Uno et al. (32) attempted to downstage disease in 22 patients with unresectable gallbladder adenocarcinoma with preoperative external beam radiotherapy. Only five patients eventually underwent resection for cure; five others underwent palliative bypass; and in 12 patients, tumors remained unresectable or demonstrated metastases. Patients responding to radiotherapy had a significantly longer survival ($p = .0008$) than did patients who did not respond. Overall survival was 36% at 1 year and 14% at 2 years.

Czito et al. used radiation with concurrent eniluracil in a phase I study of gallbladder, cholangiocarcinoma, and pancreatic tumors. After 45 Gy, a field reduction was made and a 5.4-Gy boost completed (33). Oral eniluracil/5-FU mimics a continuous infusion of 5-FU via a safe oral preparation. Eniluracil inactivates dihydropyrimidine dehydrogenase (DPD), enabling sustained plasma levels of 5-FU. Patients were considered for surgery 4 weeks after chemoradiation. A total of 13 patients were enrolled with encouraging downstaging found at surgery, and one patient had a pathologic complete response. The authors concluded that this regimen was safe and potentially effective in the neoadjuvant setting and that the maximum tolerated dose was not achieved.

Palliative Therapy

The reports describing chemotherapy and/or radiotherapy in patients undergoing biopsy only for unresectable gallbladder cancer are highly biased by patient selection, include small numbers of heterogeneously treated patients, and have an extended period of patient accrual. Most series suggest a survival of >2 months after biopsy only (24) and up to 6 months after palliative surgery with bypass (34). In multiple series (21,23,24,26,35–38), the addition of palliative chemotherapy and/or radiotherapy after biopsy only has led to an increase in median survival to approximately 4 months (range, 1 to 20 months). Palliative radiotherapy after surgical bypass has yielded median survival times of >8 months (range, 1 to 15 months) in patients fit to undergo this combination (23,36).

In addition to modestly improving survival times in these treated patients, radiation for advanced-stage gallbladder carcinoma has some effect in palliating pain, pruritus, jaundice, early satiety, and other locoregional symptoms. The reports cited have suggested a 50% to 90% improvement in symptoms with radiotherapy. Balanced against this are the time, expense, and potential complications involved in this therapy. Fortunately, few complications have been reported with doses of <54 Gy using radiotherapy alone, although the acute treatment side effects that often accompany upper abdominal radiotherapy, such as nausea, vomiting, weight loss, and diarrhea, may be underreported.

The major cytotoxic chemotherapy in use for the palliative treatment of gallbladder cancer remains 5-FU. In the last several years, several modifications of 5-FU–based therapy have become available, or have been in development. Most notable among these are the development of oral formulations, such as capecitabine. Such treatments allow less frequent visits, and may allow better preservation of quality of life. Whether such treatments will lead to equivalent tumor suppression as the parent compound may never be known, given the complexity of conducting phase III trials with such an uncommon tumor.

Other drugs that have some activity in this disease include drugs such as cisplatin and doxorubicin. Again, published literature concerning these drugs is limited and is closer to anecdotal in nature. Also concerning these groups of drugs is their propensity for increased toxicity, which has limited their widespread use in this group of patients. In this particular setting, the use of combination therapy has not been shown to dramatically increase clinical responses.

A newer analog of cisplatin is oxaliplatin. This compound has a broader spectrum of action, as it shows substantial activity in other gastrointestinal malignancies, including colon cancer, where cisplatin is inactive. In addition, it has less nephrotoxicity, allowing a wider use. It preserves a high level of synergy with 5-FU–based chemotherapies. Several trials have been reported with the activity of this drug given in conjunction with either 5-FU or capecitabine.

Some of the newer chemotherapy compounds that have begun to show activity in closely related tumors are entering trials for the treatment of biliary tract tumors. One of the first of these drugs is gemcitabine. The original U.S. Food and Drug Administration (FDA) approval for this drug was for the treatment of pancreatic cancer, based on both some degree of clinical benefit and some improvement in quality of life, as compared to 5-FU–based therapy (39). Given the similarity of this cancer to biliary tract cancers, phase II trials in bilary tract cancers were performed using gemcitabine as a single agent, as well as in combination with capecitabine. A response rate of 36% was seen in one small trial using gemcitabine as a single agent (40). In a more recent trial, gemcitabine was combined with capecitabine; 45 patients were treated. The response rate was 31%, with a median progression-free survival of 2 months. The investigators suggested that enough activity had been seen to warrant a phase III trial (41). Targeted agents have begun their trial in bilary tract tumors. The epidermal growth factor receptor (EGFR) tyrosine kinase inhibitor erlotinib was studied in a group of 42 patients with bilary tract cancers. EGFR expression was found in 29 of 36 patients in whom immunohistochemistry was performed. Three of 40 patients with evaluable disease had objective tumor response (42).

CHOLANGIOCARCINOMA

Cholangiocarcinoma is a rare cancer that arises from the biliary epithelium and occurs at a frequency of 2 per 100,000 people in the United States and in Western Europe. It represents approximately 3% of gastrointestinal malignancies, but there are considerable worldwide differences in incidence (43). Cholangiocarcinoma can occur anywhere along the biliary ductal system. The most pragmatic way to classify these tumors is by dividing them into intrahepatic, perihilar, and distal lesions, based on their likely surgical management if they are resectable. At tertiary referral centers, the majority of patients with cholangiocarcinoma have perihilar tumors (40% to 60%), followed by distal tumors (30% to 40%), and the least common intrahepatic tumors (approximately 10%) (44,45). Perihilar cholangiocarcinoma is managed by excision of extrahepatic biliary tree and typically extended right hepatectomy or sometimes extended left hepatectomy. Distal cholangiocarcinoma is managed by pancreaticoduodenectomy and intrahepatic cholangiocarcinoma by partial hepatectomy.

Clinical Presentation

The clinical presentation of cholangiocarcinoma depends primarily on the location of the tumor. The great majority of cases of cholangiocarcinoma occur in patients between the ages of 50 and 80 years. There is a slight male predominance. Most cases of cholangiocarcinoma develop in patients thought to have normal livers (46). However, in approximately 10% of cases, cholangiocarcinoma is preceded by a chronic inflammatory disease process of the bile ducts that might induce progressive changes in the biliary epithelium that culminate in cancer. Diseases with strong association include sclerosing cholangitis, opisthorchosis viverrini infection, thorotrast, choledochal cysts, hepatolithiasis, and liver cirrhosis. Diseases with possible association include Clonorchis sinensis infection, viral hepatitis (hepatitis C virus [HCV] and hepatitis B virus [HBV]), and alcohol consumption (43).

Patients with perihilar or distal cholangiocarcinoma typically present with relatively painless obstructive jaundice commonly associated with pruritus, fatigue, anorexia, and weight loss. Cholangitis is not typically a common presentation in these patients and usually only occurs after instrumentation and introduction of bacteria to the obstructed biliary system. If the point of biliary obstruction is distal to the cystic duct, the gallbladder may become enlarged and possibly palpable (Courvoisier's sign). Patients with intrahepatic cholangiocarcinoma usually do not present until the mass becomes large enough to cause discomfort and usually without the signs and symptoms of obstructive jaundice. These patients may also have fatigue, anorexia, and weight loss. Patients with intrahepatic cholangiocarcinoma can also be discovered incidentally from imaging studies whereupon a workup for a primary source with presumed metastatic disease is initiated. When no other primary source is found, the diagnosis of intrahepatic cholangiocarcinoma is usually made by exclusion. The physical examination is normal in most patients with cholangiocarcinoma except for the presence of jaundice in patients with perihilar and distal tumors, a palpable gallbladder in patients with distal tumors, and occasionally a palpable mass in patients with intrahepatic tumors.

Diagnosis

At the time of presentation, most patients with perihilar or distal cholangiocarcinoma have an elevated serum bilirubin associated with a significant elevation in serum alkaline phosphatase and mild elevation in serum transaminase levels. Patients with a prolonged disease course may have hypoalbuminemia representing malnutrition, depressed hepatic synthetic function, or both. Prolongation of the prothrombin time may also be seen due to deficiencies in vitamin K absorption. Serum carcinoembryonic antigen or carbohydrate antigen 19-9 levels may be elevated, but typically serum α-fetoprotein levels are normal (47).

Evaluation of patients with obstructive jaundice begins usually with noninvasive imaging such as ultrasonography or CT. The findings on these examinations are dependent on the location of the tumor. Imaging of an intrahepatic cholangiocarcinoma may simply demonstrate an intrahepatic mass or sometimes subtle dilation of the peripheral intrahepatic bile ducts proximal to the lesion (Fig. 37.6A). Imaging of a perihilar cholangiocarcinoma characteristically demonstrates a dilated

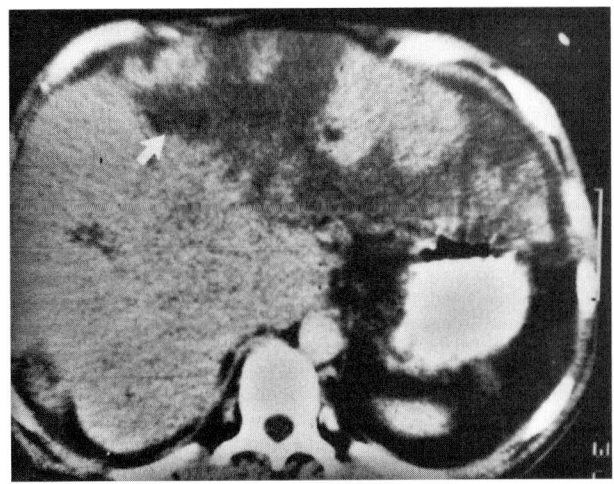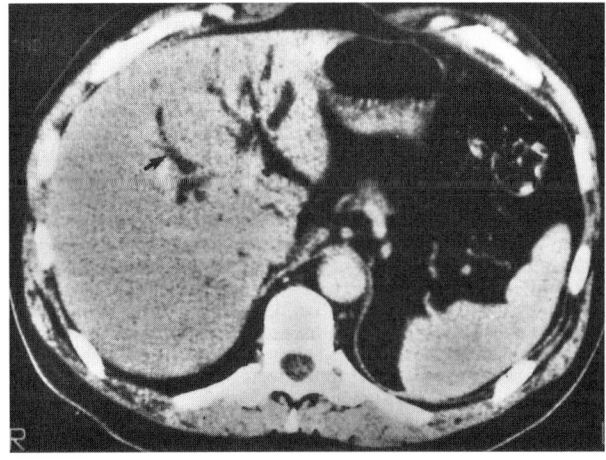

FIGURE 37.6. A: Computed tomographic (CT) image of extensive intrahepatic cholangiocarcinoma (*arrow*), mainly on the *left*. **B:** CT image of a perihilar cholangiocarcinoma demonstrating dilatated intrahepatic ducts (*arrow*). (From Pitt HA, Dooley WC, Yeo CJ, et al. Malignancies of the biliary tree. *Curr Probl Surg.* 1995;32:1–100, with permission.)

intrahepatic biliary system and a collapsed distal bile duct and gallbladder (Fig. 37.6B). Imaging of distal cholangiocarcinoma usually demonstrates a dilated intrahepatic and extrahepatic biliary system and may be difficult to distinguish from the other periampullary carcinomas. A mass is not commonly seen in patients with a distal cholangiocarcinoma (unlike pancreatic cancer). Over the last 10 to 15 years, MRCP has become more commonly used to image the biliary tree (Fig. 37.7). The technique is particularly useful in noninvasively defining the biliary anatomy and the extent of the cancer. Complete sequencing of the liver, peritoneal cavity, and angiography sequences may also define the existence of metastases and major vascular involvement.

Although the quality of MRCP is quite good, invasive cholangiographic techniques are still often used. Endoscopic retrograde cholangiopancreatography (ERCP) (Fig. 37.8) and PTC (Fig. 37.9) are both useful in defining bile duct tumors. Additionally, at the time of either procedure, stents may be placed

to relieve biliary obstruction. Patients with perihilar cholangiocarcinoma are better visualized and stented with PTC, whereas patients with distal lesions can easily be visualized and stented with either technique. Some centers, mostly in Japan, choose to map out the extent of disease by performing methodical mappings of the biliary ductal system by multiple biopsies through percutaneous transhepatic drains (PTDs) prior to resection.

Management

The management of cholangiocarcinoma, as of gallbladder cancer, is dependent on the extent of disease. Resectability requires the absence of metastatic disease and local invasion of major vascular structures, and the potential ability to obtain a negative surgical margin. Whether or not to perform

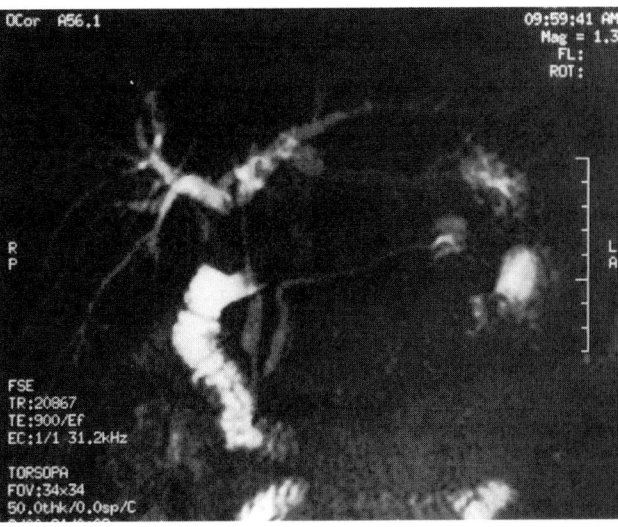

FIGURE 37.7. Magnetic resonance cholangiopancreatographic image of a perihilar cholangiocarcinoma demonstrating obstruction at the bifurcation of the hepatic ducts.

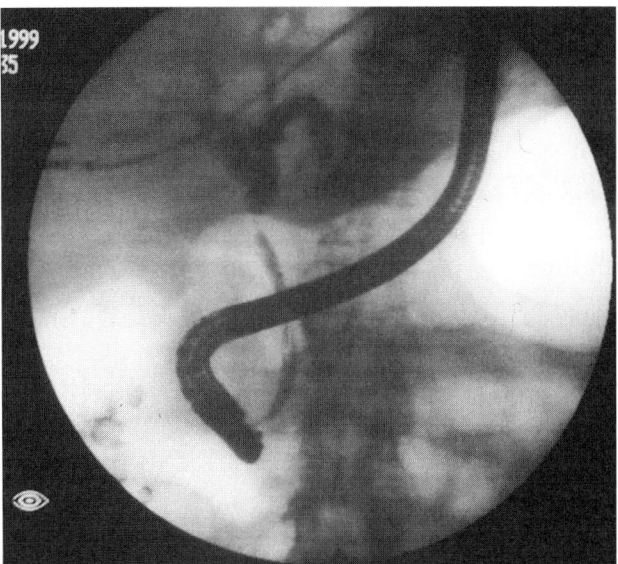

FIGURE 37.8. Endoscopic retrograde cholangiopancreatographic image of a perihilar cholangiocarcinoma demonstrating obstruction just below the bifurcation of the hepatic ducts.

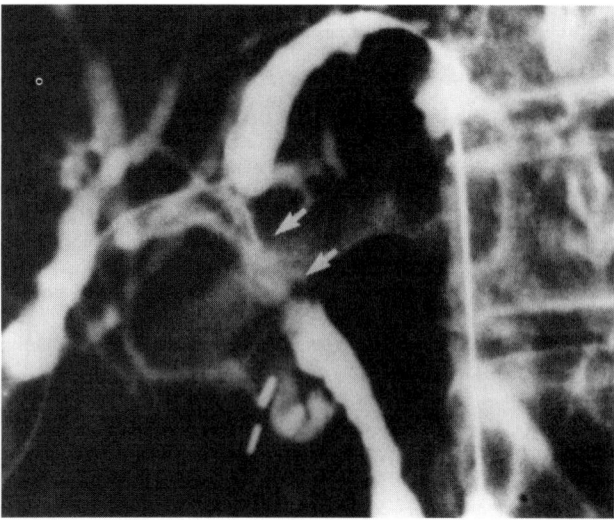

FIGURE 37.9. Percutaneous transhepatic cholangiogram of a patient with long-standing primary sclerosing cholangitis who developed a cholangiocarcinoma in the common hepatic duct (*arrows*). (From Pitt HA, Dooley WC, Yeo CJ, et al. Malignancies of the biliary tree. *Curr Probl Surg.* 1995;32:1–100, with permission.)

The technical steps to resection of a cholangiocarcinoma vary significantly and depend on the location of the lesions and the extent of involvement of surrounding structures. Intrahepatic cholangiocarcinoma confined to the biliary system and liver proximal to the bifurcation are best managed by standard liver resection techniques. Distal cholangiocarcinoma, if resectable, is managed with pancreaticoduodenectomy. The treatment of a cholangiocarcinoma involving the perihilar area depends on the exact biliary anatomy, the extent of proximal and distal involvement, the vascular anatomy and involvement, and predicted volumes of the future liver remnant after hepatectomy. These issues will be treated in more detail in the following sections.

Some groups advocate staging laparoscopy to evaluate for metastatic disease that may be missed on preoperative imaging studies. In general, these groups show a modest ability to prevent unnecessary laparotomy and the benefit was realized in only certain high risk subsets of patients (50–52). Laparoscopy was better at picking up unresectable disease secondary to carcinomatosis or liver metastases rather than blood vessel involvement. Another approach is to perform a limited laparotomy in which the peritoneal cavity is evaluated and a cholecystectomy can be performed should metastatic disease be found.

preoperative transhepatic biliary decompression and drainage varies greatly from center to center. Proponents of preoperative drainage cite the ability to better evaluate the biliary anatomy by direct cholangiography, the ability to perform endoluminal biopsies, relief of patients' symptoms of jaundice, and the ability to incorporate the percutaneous biliary drains in the reconstruction to decompress the biliary tree during healing. Opponents of preoperative drainage prefer to avoid the increased infectious complications that have been documented in multiple studies secondary to seeding the biliary tree with bacteria, as well as the less common but sometimes devastating problems of bleeding, fistulization, and pancreatitis (48,49). They also are very comfortable with the rapidly improving noninvasive imaging techniques such as magnetic resonance imaging and high-resolution, three-dimensional CT. The use of preoperative biliary decompression with stents does not greatly change the technical aspects of removing a cholangiocarcinoma. It may, however, obscure the ability to palpate the transition from cancerous bile duct to uninvolved bile duct in hilar lesions, as the stents themselves may cause an inflammatory response.

Intrahepatic Cholangiocarcinoma

Intrahepatic cholangiocarcinoma is the least common of the three locations. The surgical management of intrahepatic cholangiocarcinoma focuses on partial hepatectomy, the extent of which is dictated by the location and hepatic parenchyma involved. If the tumor approaches the hilum, then it may be best managed (and classified) as a perihilar lesion. Typically, intrahepatic cholangiocarcinoma presents as a large lesion as they generally do not cause obstructive jaundice as perihilar and distal lesions do. Aggressive surgical resection offers the only hope for long-term survival. Table 37.3 summarizes recently published series of patients undergoing resection of intrahepatic cholangiocarcinoma (44,53–59). The overall 5-year survival rates for the patients reported in these series ranged from 17% to 40%, with most above 30%. The 5-year survival rates for patients undergoing margin-negative resection reported in these series ranged from 44% to 63%. These resections were accomplished with acceptable operative mortality rates in the 0% to 7% range.

TABLE 37.3

RESULTS OF SURGICAL RESECTION OF INTRAHEPATIC CHOLANGIOCARCINOMA

Authors, year (ref)	Number	5-year survival R0 resection	5-year survival all	Operative mortality
Pichlmayr et al., 1995 (53)	32	NR	17%	6%
Jan et al., 1996 (54)	41	44%	27%	0%
Casavilla et al., 1997 (55)	34	NR	31%	7%
Madariaga et al., 1998 (56)	34	51%	35%	6%
Valverde et al., 1999 (57)	30	NR	22%	3%
Inoue et al., 2000 (58)	52	55%	36%	2%
Weber et al., 2001 (59)	33	NR	31%	3%
de Oliviera et al., 2007 (44)	34	63%	40%	2%

NR, not reported.

Perihilar Cholangiocarcinoma

Perihilar cholangiocarcinoma is the most common location for bile duct cancer. It represents a significant technical challenge due to the close proximity to major vascular structures and to the liver and arborization of the right and left biliary tree. Most centers will approach these lesions with extended right hepatectomy, and less commonly with extended left or central hepatectomy. Many centers can correlate the ability to obtain a margin-negative resection and long-term survival (at least indirectly) with the performance of an appropriate hepatectomy.

The typical resection for perihilar cholangiocarcinoma proceeds as follows. The distal common bile duct cephalad to the head of the pancreas is isolated and divided. A frozen sec-

tion should be checked to confirm that this margin is clear of tumor. The gallbladder is dissected off of the gallbladder fossa, and the cystic artery is divided. The divided distal common bile duct is next dissected away from the portal vein and hepatic artery, resecting the associated lymphatic tissue in continuity. The hilus of the liver is next dissected by lowering the hilar plate (Fig. 37.10A). The perihilar cholangiocarcinoma and bile duct bifurcation are next dissected out. The bridge of liver tissue between segments II and IV overlying the round ligament is divided to increase the exposure to the base of the umbilical fissure. The left bile duct can be dissected out at the base of the umbilical fissure and divided after placement of stay sutures. A frozen section of the left hepatic duct margin is taken to confirm clearance of the tumor (Fig. 37.10B). If the left bile duct margin is negative and the main portal vein and hepatic artery

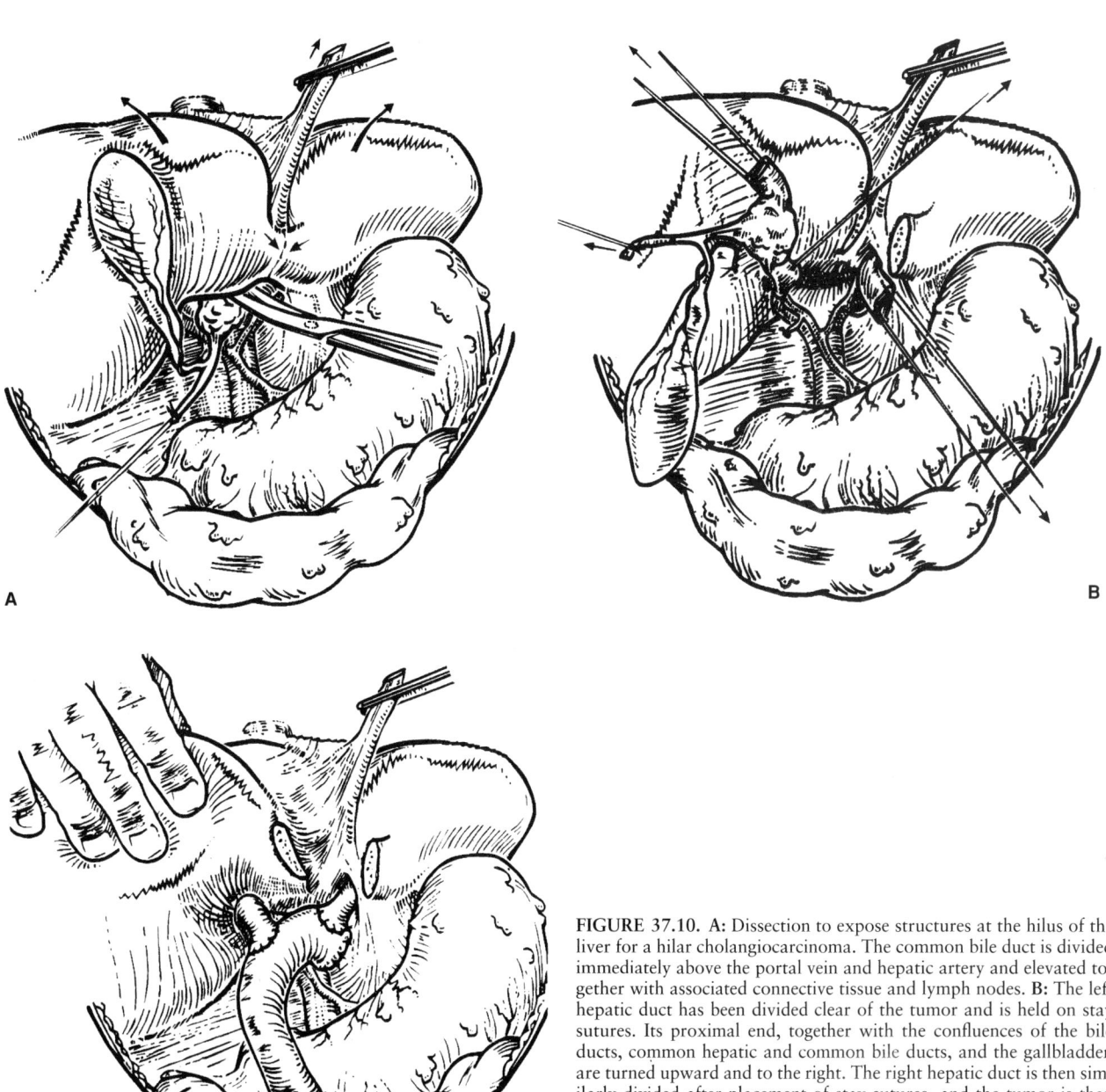

FIGURE 37.10. A: Dissection to expose structures at the hilus of the liver for a hilar cholangiocarcinoma. The common bile duct is divided immediately above the portal vein and hepatic artery and elevated together with associated connective tissue and lymph nodes. **B:** The left hepatic duct has been divided clear of the tumor and is held on stay sutures. Its proximal end, together with the confluences of the bile ducts, common hepatic and common bile ducts, and the gallbladder, are turned upward and to the right. The right hepatic duct is then similarly divided after placement of stay sutures, and the tumor is then removed. **C:** The right and left hepatic ducts are anastomosed to a retrocolic Roux-en-Y loop of jejunum. (From Jarnagin WR, Saldinger PF, Blumgart LH. Cancer of the bile ducts: the hepatic ducts and common bile ducts. In: Blumgart LH, Fong Y, eds. *Surgery of the Liver and Biliary Tract*, 3rd ed. London: WB Saunders, 2000:1017–1058, with permission.)

TABLE 37.4

RESULTS OF SURGICAL RESECTION OF PERIHILAR CHOLANGIOCARCINOMA

Authors, year (ref)	Number	5-year survival R0 resection	5-year survival all	Operative mortality
Sugiura et al., 1994 (60)	83	33%	20%	8%
Su et al., 1996 (61)	49	34%	15%	10%
Nagino et al., 1998 (62)	138	26%	NR	10%
Miyazaki et al., 1998 (63)	76	40%	26%	15%
Madariaga et al., 1998 (56)	28	25%	9%	14%
Kosuge et al., 1999 (64)	65	52%	35%	9%
Neuhaus et al., 1999 (65)	95	37%	22%	6%
Jarnagin et al., 2001 (66)	80	30%	NR	10%
Rea et al., 2004 (67)	46	30%	26%	9%
Nishio et al., 2005 (68)	301	27%	22%	8%
Dianant et al., 2006 (69)	99	33%	27%	15%
Wahab et al., 2006 (70)	73	NR	13%	11%
de Oliveira et al., 2007 (44)	173	30%	10%	5%

NR, not reported.

including their bifurcations are clear, then an extended right hepatectomy can be performed. This can be done by dividing the right hepatic artery, right portal vein, and right hepatic vein and transecting the parenchyma. If the left bile duct margin is positive, then an attempt at extended left hepatectomy can be made. In general, the anatomy of the liver, bile ducts, and vasculature are less favorable for extended left hepatectomy because (i) the main right bile duct is very short and intrahepatic; (ii) the right hepatic artery bifurcates from the hepatic artery, usually courses directly under the bile duct bifurcation, and is frequently involved; and (iii) the plane of hepatic parenchymal resection is much larger than for a right sided resection. However, in some patients, the cancer will infiltrate the left biliary system much more than the right, and an extended left hepatectomy is appropriate. In very select cases where the cholangiocarcinoma only involves below the bifurcation and does not extend above, adequate clearance can be obtained on both sides, and preservation of hepatic parenchyma would benefit the patient, a central hepatectomy may be considered. For biliary reconstruction, a suitable Roux-en-Y loop of jejunum is prepared and brought up in retrocolic fashion. Anastomosis of the bile duct(s) to the jejunum is accomplished using a single layer of 4-0 absorbable suture (Fig. 37.10C). There is significant variation in biliary anatomy, and it is not uncommon to have to perform more than one anastomosis to either the right or left biliary system.

Table 37.4 summarizes recently published series of patients undergoing resection of perihilar cholangiocarcinoma (44,57,60–70). Most high volume centers that treat patients with hilar cholangiocarcinoma routinely perform partial hepatectomy to resect these lesions. These series report a 5-year survival rate between 25% and 52% for those patients who underwent a margin-negative resection. The overall 5-year survival rate in all patients operated on in the series was between 9% and 35%, with operative mortality rates between 5% and 15%.

Local recurrence within the hilar resection bed is a significant problem after removal of a perihilar cholangiocarcinoma. To decrease local recurrence, some groups are advocating routine removal of segment I (caudate). The caudate and caudate process that connects it to the liver typically lie just posterior to the bifurcation of the bile ducts and portal veins. There are usually multiple small caudate bile ducts that drain into the main biliary tree very close to the bifurcation (71). One study demonstrated that, in 44 of 46 consecutively treated patients,

caudate ducts were involved with tumor (69). Partial hepatectomy with caudate resection *en bloc* should be considered to obtain adequate negative margins. This concept has been advanced further by Neuhaus et al. (65), who have advocated routine resection of the portal vein bifurcation *en bloc* with the specimen including the caudate with portal vein reconstruction between the main and left portal veins. This theoretically will clear all tissues at risk surrounding the periportal bile duct.

Distal Cholangiocarcinoma

Distal cholangiocarcinoma is the second most common site of disease. These cancers are resected with pancreaticoduodenectomy, as are other malignancies of the periampullary region. The technical aspects of a pancreaticoduodenectomy are described in detail elsewhere in this text. The Johns Hopkins Hospital has recently reported a series of 239 patients undergoing pancreaticoduodenectomy for distal cholangiocarcinoma (44). These patients were resected with acceptable morbidity rates including a pancreatic leak rate of 13%, a wound infection rate of 11%, and a delayed gastric emptying rate of 10%. The operative mortality rate in this group of patients was 3%. The margin-negative resection rate was 78%, and the lymph node–positive rate was 60%. Overall, the 5-year survival rate of resected patients was 23% (27% in patients who underwent margin-negative resection).

Liver Transplantation

Orthotopic liver transplantation has been used to treat both resectable and unresectable perihilar cholangiocarcinoma; however, the high incidence of lymph node and distant metastases associated with this disease has limited the success. Abdel Pichlmayr et al. (70) reported on a series of 249 patients with perihilar cholangiocarcinoma in which 125 patients underwent resection and 25 patients underwent liver transplantation. Resection yielded equivalent or superior survival rates for all stages of disease. The authors concluded that resection is the treatment of choice for perihilar cholangiocarcinoma but noted that liver transplantation may be considered in selected patients. Several centers have adopted a neoadjuvant approach to better select appropriate patients who will more likely benefit from this very aggressive liver transplantation approach (74).

Although there is some experience with liver transplantation for perihilar cholangiocarcinoma, it should not be considered a standard form of therapy for this disease.

Adjuvant Therapy

Local failure is a significant problem after complete surgical resection in cholangiocarcinoma. Unfortunately, many patients are not able to have a complete resection, and even when a pathologically proven negative margin is obtained, surgical margins are minimal. Therefore, considering adjuvant radiotherapy to sterilize the surgical margins is reasonable. Most studies (21,25,36,75–88) have included a mixture of patients with completely resected, partially resected, and unresected disease (Table 37.5). No prospective randomized trials have compared resection alone with surgery plus adjuvant chemoradiation; however, in many institutions the treatment policy has been to refer patients with positive margins for external beam radiotherapy after resection.

Some of the most quoted series on this topic come from The Johns Hopkins Hospital (77,80,81), where a large cohort of patients have been offered radiotherapy. Although no statistically significant survival advantage was found with adjuvant radiotherapy, all three patients surviving longer than 5 years had received radiotherapy. No significant advantage was seen in median survival; however, this was a heterogeneous group, with 8 of the 14 patients receiving brachytherapy boosts in addition to external beam radiation (80). Kamada et al. reported on 59 patients who received postoperative external beam irradiation and brachytherapy on a consistent basis for positive margins. Their median survival of 21.5 months is among the best reported (76). These authors reported that median survival was significantly longer with the addition of brachytherapy than with external beam radiation alone. This finding suggests that radiotherapy given in adequate doses may sterilize microscopically positive margins and improve survival. Kraybill et al. (21) reported on a series of patients undergoing curative resection that received postoperative radiation and found a 10% 5-year survival rate versus no survival in a group of similar patients who could not undergo surgical resection. Conversely, at least one report has shown that dose escalation of external beam therapy with brachytherapy can be detrimental to survival. Gonzalez et al. (85) reported on 71 patients treated with curative surgery, followed by 40- to 45-Gy external beam radiotherapy and a 10-Gy boost with brachytherapy. A decrement in survival was seen with total doses of radiotherapy >55 Gy. In a series at Thomas Jefferson University Hospital (89), 24 patients were treated with external beam radiotherapy, brachytherapy, and concurrent chemotherapy with 5-FU or a combination of 5-FU, doxorubicin, and mitomycin C. A significant increase in survival was seen (48% at 2 years), and median survival was 25 months for those patients receiving 66 to 70 Gy versus 6 months for patients receiving <55 Gy for unresected tumors. Overall, 19 of the 24 patients receiving radiotherapy for unresectable cholangiocarcinoma received 5-FU or 5-FU plus doxorubicin and mitomycin C, and a trend was seen toward improved survival with the addition of chemotherapy. Others have also shown a radiation dose response in cholangiocarcinoma; however, those studies did not systematically combine 5-FU with radiation (21,90–93).

Foo et al. (94) updated results obtained at the Mayo Clinic using external beam radiotherapy and bolus 5-FU concurrently with brachytherapy. A trend was seen toward increased survival with radiotherapy combined with 5-FU, with 2 of 9 patients treated with 5-FU among the 5-year disease-free survivors. The investigators reported a 22% 5-year survival rate for patients receiving combined-modality therapy versus 9% for those receiving only radiotherapy. The Eastern Coopera-

tive Oncology Group (79) conducted a dose-finding phase I trial in which 5-FU was given by protracted venous infusion concurrently with radiation to 59.4 Gy at 1.8 Gy per day, with three or four fields treated daily. They determined the optimal 5-FU dose to be 250 mg/m^2, which was associated with a 12-month mean survival, and 1- and 2-year actuarial survival of 48% and 14%, respectively.

Serefini et al. (95) reported a retrospective review of 192 patients with hepatobiliary tumors treated between 1988 and 1999. Cholangiocarcinoma was found in 90 patients. Surgery alone for 50 patients was compared to the 38 patients who did receive chemoradiotherapy. Mean survival of resected patients with adjuvant CT/(chemo radiation) was 42 ± 37.0 months and without CT/chemo radiation it was 29 ± 24.5 months ($p = .07$). Mean survival of patients with distal tumors receiving or not receiving CT/chemo radiation was 41 ± 21.8 versus 25 ± 20.1 months, respectively ($p = .04$). The authors concluded that adjuvant chemoradiation appeared to improve survival after resection for cholangiocarcinoma ($p = .07$) particularly for distal tumors ($p = .04$).

Neoadjuvant Therapy

In an attempt to "downstage" cholangiocarcinoma, some centers have reported series of neoadjuvant therapy. Urego et al. (96) have reported on the largest series of induction radiotherapy combined with chemotherapy, which was followed by either complete resection alone or resection with orthotopic liver transplantation. They noted a 38% complete response rate to induction radiotherapy with concurrent continuous infusion of 5-FU. Median survival and 5-year survival were impressive: A median survival was 20 months, and the 5-year survival rate was 53% for those patients with negative margins at resection. Even those patients with positive margins had a 24% 5-year survival rate. In addition, in a number of patients, tumors that were considered unresectable before neoadjuvant therapy were successfully downstaged, and survival was greater than expected with definitive radiotherapy and bypass or surgical debulking. Of interest was this reversal of sequencing from that described in a previous study (35) involving 55 patients, which used postoperative external beam radiotherapy with chemotherapy. Median survival increased from 12 months to 20 months with the transposition of chemoradiation to the preoperative period.

McMaster et al. (97) reported on nine patients who received external beam radiotherapy and chemotherapy concurrently to downstage extrahepatic cholangiocarcinomas. They reported a 33% complete response rate and median survival of 22.2 months. Five-year survival for the entire cohort was 30%. Gunderson et al. (75) described the Mayo Clinic treatment approach, which used preoperative external beam radiotherapy and 5-FU chemotherapy, and brachytherapy before resection and liver transplantation. That series reported nine patients with a median survival longer than 60 months and 100% 5-year survival.

Heimbach et al. (74) treated unresectable, stage I and II perihilar cholangiocarcinoma with external beam irradiation, brachytherapy, and 5-FU and/or oral capecitabine prior to liver transplantation. Fifty-six patients underwent treatment between 1993 and 2003. Operative staging was completed in 48 patients, with 14 having findings precluding transplantation. Eventually 28 patients underwent transplantation. Three patients died from perioperative complications, and 4 developed recurrent disease 22 to 63 months after transplantation. Actuarial patient survival was 54% at 5 years for all 56 patients, 64% for 48 operatively staged patients, and 84% for 34 patients with negative staging operations. Actuarial survival was 88% at 1 year and 82% 5 years after transplantation.

TABLE 37.5

ADJUVANT RADIATION THERAPY FOR CHOLANGIOCARCINOMA

Study	Treatment	No. of patients	EBRT (Gy)	Brachytherapy (Gy)	Median survival (mo)	1 y	2 y	3 y	5 y	Comments
Pitt et al., 1995 (80)	Surg	31	None	None	20	—	—	—	—	Survival differences not significant, 87% vs. 71% + margins
	Surg + XRT	14	46	13	14	—	—	—	—	
Cameron et al., 1990 (81)	Surg	15	None	None	None	60.0	43.0	21.0	—	3 patients survived >5 y, all in XRT group
Kamada et al., 1996 (76)	Surg + XRT	38	50–60	20	NS	70.0	31.0	21.0	—	
	Surg + XRT	59	30–50	30–50	21.5	73.0	31.0	18.0	—	
Kraybill et al., 1994 (21)	Surg (negative margin) + XRT	12	48	NS	11	—	—	—	10	
Verbeek et al., 1991 (82)	XRT alone	31	48	NS	NS	—	—	—	0	
	Surg	22	—	—	8	—	—	—	—	p = .001
	Surg + XRT	29	45	10	27	—	—	—	—	p = .001
Gonzalez et al. (EORTC), 1990 (83)	Surg	17	—	—	8.3	—	—	—	—	p = .0005
	Surg + XRT	38	42–55	10–40	19	—	—	—	—	p = .0005
Mahe et al. (Lyon), 1991 (36) — All patients	Surg + XRT	26	—	—	22	—	48.0	32.0	—	
Microscopic +	Surg + XRT	14	45	10–15	27.5	86.0	62.0	55.0	—	p = .045
Gross +	Surg + XRT	12	45	10–15	13	57.0	30.0	10.0	—	p = .045
Veeze-Kuijpers et al., 1989 (84) — Microscopic +	Surg + XRT	11	30–40+	15	15	65.0	36.0	36.0	—	p = .06
Unresectable	XRT alone	31	40	25	8	40.0	18.0	6.0	—	
Gonzalez et al., 1999 (85)	Surg + XRT	71	40–45	10	24	84.0	—	37.0	24.0	
Schoenthaler et al., 1994 (86) — Curative cases	Surg	15	None	None	16	—	—	—	—	
	Surg + XRT	35	54	NS	16	—	—	—	—	
	Surg + CTX	18	60	NS	23	—	—	—	—	
Serefini et al., 2001 (95)	Surg	50			29					
	Surg + CTX+XRT	38			42					

CTX, chemotherapy; EBRT, external beam radiation therapy; EORTC, European Organization for Research and Treatment of Cancer; Gross +, gross metastases present; Microscopic +, microscopic metastasis present; NS, not stated; Surg, surgery; XRT, radiation therapy.

Palliation

When advanced local disease or obvious extrahepatic metastases are identified preoperatively or at the time of laparotomy, therapy is directed toward the relief of biliary obstruction and the associated symptoms such as itching and cholangitis. A number of therapeutic maneuvers can be performed to accomplish biliary decompression. Percutaneous transhepatic intubation is the most common palliative modality used. If unresectability is determined at operation, palliative options include the use of transhepatic drains or the performance of an operative bilioenteric bypass.

When PTDs are placed, they drain internally into the small bowel, as well as externally into bile drainage bags. This external drainage system can be internalized later by the placement of metallic Wallstents and removal of the transhepatic drain. The advantage of Wallstents is that they do not require any catheter care on the part of the patient and they have a relatively good duration of patency. After adequate drainage, resolution of jaundice and associated symptoms usually occurs rapidly. If cholangitis is absent, the entire liver does not need to be drained, as only 30% of the functioning hepatic mass needs decompression for relief of jaundice. Failure of jaundice to resolve after adequate drainage may indicate vascular compromise to the liver.

Some centers advocate the use of an intrahepatic bilioenteric bypass to the segment III hepatic duct. In a series of 20 patients undergoing segment III bilioenteric bypass, no operative mortality occurred, and the 1-year patency rate of the bypass was 80% (98). The investigators reported excellent palliation and the elimination of the need for frequent stent changes.

Primary Radiotherapy

Early attempts to use radiotherapy to treat unresectable cholangiocarcinomas were limited by the lack of modern-day imaging, low radiation energies that could not produce deeply penetrating photons, and very limited treatment-planning capabilities for external beam radiation and brachytherapy. Even with these limitations, authors (79,99) have reported that the use of external beam radiotherapy in a dose range of 20 to 60 Gy produced a median survival of 10 to 15 months. Moreover, even in these early studies, a dose-response relationship was noted, with increased survival seen in patients receiving >40 Gy. Also of interest was the fact that the majority of patients in these reports received 5-FU chemotherapy after completion of radiation.

Palliation of unresectable cholangiocarcinoma with radiotherapy is challenging for patients who are not good candidates for external beam radiotherapy. These patients often present with jaundice and pain. Biliary infection and obstruction are relieved with intravenous antibiotics combined with drainage. The data for brachytherapy suggest an improvement in palliation and survival compared with drainage alone. Obviously, patient selection is a major factor, and no prospective trials have been carried out, but all published reports indicate some benefit to additional therapy (99–101).

The overall goal for these patients is immediate and long-lasting palliation and improvement in quality of life. Some series suggested that doses of 40 to 50 Gy, given with iridium dosed at 0.5 to 1.0 cm from the lumen, significantly increased survival, length of stent patency, and palliation when compared to stenting alone. In a retrospective review, Chakravarti et al. (101) reported 100% palliation with stent placement and brachytherapy in 18 patients with cholangiocarcinoma. Between 30 and 50 Gy was delivered with iridium in patients who were not candidates for external beam radiotherapy. Outcomes for 14 patients with similar age and sex distribution who underwent surgical resection at the same institutions were also compared. Long-term survival in the group receiving stent plus brachytherapy, as expected, was inferior to that in the group able to undergo resection, but was not significantly so over time. The 13-month median survival for the brachytherapy group was not significantly different from the 14-month median survival for the surgery group. The actuarial survival was considerably different for the two groups, however: 70% for the surgery group and 53% for the brachytherapy group at 1 year, and 31% for the surgery group and 20% for the brachytherapy group at 2 years.

Golfieri et al. (102) reported a single-institution experience of multimodality palliative care of Klatskin-type cholangiocarcinoma. Evaluation of outcome, mean survival, and quality of life was performed in patients with unresectable hilar cholangiocarcinoma treated with surgical palliation, biliary stenting, or brachytherapy alone. Twenty-six patients with hilar cholangiocarcinoma were studied: 16 patients were enrolled in the multimodality protocol (bilateral biliary drainage; iridium-192 brachytherapy; plastic endoprosthesis or metallic stent positioning and external radiotherapy plus systemic chemotherapy), 5 patients underwent surgical palliation, and 5 patients received percutaneous decompression alone. Nine patients completed the protocol, and 7 patients were treated with brachytherapy followed by biliary stenting alone. The multimodality approach obtained mean survival (10 months) similar to that for surgery and higher than that of the brachytherapy and metallic stenting groups (6 and 2.75 months, respectively). The average hospital stay (15 days) was lower than that of the surgical group (20 days).

Schleicher et al. (103) combined external beam radiation and intraluminal brachytherapy for unresectable proximal cholangiocarcinomas. Thirty patients were treated with external beam radiotherapy (median dose 30 Gy) and a high-dose-rate brachytherapy boost (median dose 40 Gy) delivered in four of five fractions; 15 patients received brachytherapy alone, and 9 patients received external beam radiotherapy (no brachytherapy) with 5-FU. As anticipated, higher radiation doses (i.e., brachytherapy boost) improved the effect of external beam radiotherapy by increasing survival from a median of 3.9 months in the nonbrachytherapy group to 9.1 months in the brachytherapy group. The dose effect was significant >30 Gy, and in those patients without jaundice at the beginning of radiotherapy ($p < .05$).

In summary, cancers of the bilary tree are uncommon tumors with a poor prognosis. Their heterogenous presentation has further limited prospective studies. Complete surgical resection offers the only chance for long stem survival. Combined modality therapy may modestly improve outcome.

References

1. Jermal A, Siegel R, Ward E, et al. Cancer statistics. *CA Cancer J Clin.* 2007;57:43–66.
2. Shinka H, Kimura W, Muto T. Surgical indications for small polypoid lesions of the gallbladder. *Am J Surg.* 1998;175:114–117.
3. Sugiyama M, Xie XY, Atomi Y, Saito M. Differential diagnosis of small polypoid lesions of the gallbladder: the value of endoscopic ultrasonography. *Ann Surg.* 1999;229:498–507.
4. Koh T, Taniguchi H, Yamaquchi A, et al. Differential diagnosis of gallbladder cancer using positron emission tomography with fluorine-18–labeled fluorodeoxyglucose (FDG-PET). *J Surg Oncol.* 2003;84:74–81.
5. Blalock AA. A statistical analysis of 888 cases of biliary tract disease. *Johns Hopkins Hosp Bull* 1924;35:391–409.
6. Lundberg O, Kristoffersson A. Port site metastases from gallbladder cancer after laparoscopic cholecystectomy. Results of a Swedish survey and review of published reports. *Eur J Surg.* 1999;165:215–222.
7. Duchi K, Mikuni J, Kakagawa Y. Laparoscopic cholecystectomy for gallbladder carcinoma: results of a Japanese surgery of 498 patients. *J Hepatobiliary Pancreat Surg.* 2002;9:256–260.

8. Shirai Y, Yoshida K, Tsukuda K, et al. Early carcinoma of the gallbladder. *Eur J Surg.* 1992;158:545–548.

9. Yamaguchi K, Tsuneyoshi M. Subclinical gallbladder carcinoma. *Am J Surg.* 1992;163:382–386.

10. Donohue JH, Nagorney DM, Grant CS, et al. Carcinoma of the gallbladder. *Arch Surg.* 1990;125:237–241.

11. De Aretxabala X, Roa IS, Burgos LA, et al. Curative resection in potentially resectable tumors of the gallbladder. *Eur J Surg.* 1997;163:419–426.

12. Yoshida T, Matsumoto T, Sasaki A, et al. Laparoscopic cholecystectomy in the treatment of patients with gallbladder cancer. *J Am Coll Surg.* 2000;191:158–163.

13. Matsumoto Y, Fujii H, Aoyama H, et al. Surgical treatment of primary carcinoma of the gallbladder based on the histologic analysis of 48 surgical specimens. *Am J Surg.* 1992;163:239–245.

14. Fong Y, Jarnagin W, Blumgart L. Gallbladder cancer: comparison of patients presenting initially for definitive operation with those presenting after prior noncurative intervention. *Ann Surg.* 2000;232:557–569.

15. Shirai Y, Yoshida K, Tsukada K, et al. Inapparent carcinoma of the gallbladder: an appraisal of a radical second operation after simple cholecystectomy. *Ann Surg.* 1992;215:326–331.

16. Dixon E, Vollmer C, Sahajpal U, et al. An aggressive surgical approach leads to improved survival in patients with gallbladder cancer. *Ann Surg.* 2005;241:385–394.

17. Shih SP, Schulick RD, Cameron JL, et al. Gallbladder cancer: the role of laparoscopy and radical resection. *Ann Surg.* 2007;245:893–901.

18. Bartlett DL, Fong Y, Fortner JG, et al. Long-term results after resection for gallbladder cancer. *Ann Surg.* 1996;224:639–646.

19. Shirai Y, Yoshida K, Tsukada K, et al. Radical surgery for gallbladder carcinoma. Long-term results. *Ann Surg.* 1992;216:565–568.

20. Chijiiwa K, Tanaka M. Carcinoma of the gallbladder: an appraisal of surgical resection. *Surgery.* 1994;115:751–756.

21. Kraybill WG, Lee H, Picus J, et al. Multidisciplinary treatment of biliary tract cancers. *J Surg Oncol.* 1994;55:239–245.

22. Fields JN, Emami B. Carcinoma of the extrahepatic biliary system–results of primary and adjuvant radiotherapy. *Int J Radiat Oncology Biol Phys.* 1987;13:331–338.

23. Houry S, Schlienger M, Huguier M, et al. Gallbladder carcinoma: role of radiation therapy. *Br J Surg.* 1989;76:448–450.

24. Houry S, Haccart V, Huguier M, et al. Gallbladder cancer: role of radiation therapy. *Hepatogastroenterology.* 1999;46:1578–1584.

25. Todoroki T, Iwasaki Y, Okamura T, et al. Intraoperative radiotherapy for advanced carcinoma of the biliary system. *Cancer.* 1980;46:2179–2184.

26. Todoroki T, Kawamoto T, Otsuka M, et al. Benefits of combining radiotherapy with aggressive resection for stage IV gallbladder cancer. *Hepatogastroenterology.* 1999;46:1585–1591.

27. Kurisu K, Hishikawa Y, Taniguchi M, et al. High dose rate intraluminal brachytherapy for post-operative residual tumor of gallbladder carcinoma: a case report. *Radiat Med.* 1991;9:241–243.

28. Czito BG, Hurwitz HI, Clough RW, et al. Adjuvant external-beam radiotherapy with concurrent chemotherapy after resection of primary gallbladder carcinoma: a 23-year experience. *Int J Radiat Oncol Biol Phys.* 2005;62:1030–1034.

29. Houry S, Barrier A, Huguier M. Irradiation therapy for gallbladder carcinoma: recent advances. *J Hepatobiliary Pancreat Surg.* 2001;8:518–524.

30. Itoh H, Nishijima K, Kurosaka Y, et al. Magnitude of combination therapy of radical resection and external beam radiotherapy for patient with carcinomas of the extrahepatic bile duct and gallbladder. *Dig Dis Sci.* 2005;50:2231–2242.

31. Aretxabala XD, Roa I, Burgos L, et al. Preoperative chemoradiotherapy in the treatment of gallbladder cancer. *Am Surg.* 1999;65:241–246.

32. Uno T, Itami J, Aruga M, et al. Primary carcinoma of the gallbladder: role of external beam radiation therapy in patients with locally advanced tumor. *Strahlenther Onkol.* 1996;172:496–500.

33. Czito BG, Hong TJ, Cohen DP, et al. A phase I study of enilaracil/5-FU in combination with radiation therapy for potentially resectable and/or unresectable cancer of the pancreas and biliary tract. *Cancer Invest.* 2006;24: 9–17.

34. Douglass HO, Tepper J, Leichman L. Neoplasms of the gallbladder. In: Holland JF, Frei E, Bast RC, et al., eds. *Cancer Medicine,* 3rd ed. Philadelphia: Lea & Febiger; 1993:1448–1454.

35. Flickenger JC, Epstein AH, Iwatsuki S, et al. Radiation therapy for primary carcinoma of the extrahepatic biliary system. *Cancer.* 1991;68:289–294.

36. Mahe M, Romestaing P, Talon B, et al. Radiation therapy in extrahepatic bile duct carcinoma. *Radiother Oncol.* 1991;21:121–127.

37. Silk YN, Douglass HO, Nava HR, et al. Carcinoma of the gallbladder. The Roswell Park experience. *Ann Surg.* 1989;210:751–757.

38. Okamoto A, Tsuruta K, Ishiwata J, et al. Treatment of T3 and T4 carcinomas of the gallbladder. *Int Surg.* 1996;81:130–135.

39. Burris HA, Moore MJ, Andersen J, et al. Improvements in survival and clinical benefit with gemcitabine as first-line therapy for patients with advanced pancreatic cancer: a randomized trial. *J Clin Oncol.* 1997;15:2403–2413.

40. Gallardo JO, Rubio B, Fodor M, et al. A phase II study of gemcitabine in gallbladder carcinoma. *Ann Oncol.* 2001;12:1403–1406.

41. Knox JJ, Hedley D, Oza A, et al. Combining gemcitabine and capecitabine in patients with advanced biliary cancer: a phase II trial. *J Clin Oncol.* 2005;23:2332–2338.

42. Phillip PA, Mahoney MR, Allmer C, et al. Phase II study of erlotinib in patients with advanced biliary cancer. *J Clin Oncol.* 2006;24:3069–3074.

43. Shaib Y, El-Serag HB. The epidemiology of cholangiocarcinoma. *Semin Liver Dis.* 2004;24:115–125.

44. deOliveira ML, Cunningham SC, Cameron JL, et al. Cholangiocarcinoma: 31-year experience with 564 patients at a single institution. *Ann Surg.* 2007;245:755–762.

45. D'Angelica MI, Jarnagin WR, Blumgart LH. Resectable hilar cholangiocarcinoma: surgical treatment and long-term outcome. *Surg Today.* 2004;34:885–890.

46. Nakanuma Y, Mashiso H, Tadashi T. Clinical and pathologic features of cholangiocarcinoma. In: Okuda K, Tabor E, eds. *Liver Cancer.* New York: Churchill Livingstone; 1997:279–290.

47. Qin XL, Wang ZR, Shi JS, et al. Utility of serum CA19-9 in diagnosis of cholangiocarcinoma: in comparison with CEA. *World J Gastroenterol.* 2004;10:427–432.

48. Hochwald SN, Burke EC, Jarnagin WR, Fong Y, Blumgart LH. Association of preoperative biliary stenting with increased postoperative infectious complications in proximal cholangiocarcinoma. *Arch Surg.* 1999;134:261–266.

49. Howard TJ, Yu J, Greene RB, et al. Influence of bactibilia after preoperative biliary stenting on postoperative infectious complications. *J Gastrointest Surg.* 2006;10:523–531.

50. Goere D, Wagholikar GD, Pessaux P, et al. Utility of staging laparoscopy in subsets of biliary cancers : laparoscopy is a powerful diagnostic tool in patients with intrahepatic and gallbladder carcinoma. *Surg Endosc.* 2006;20:721–725.

51. Connor S, Barron E, Wigmore SJ, et al. The utility of laparoscopic assessment in the preoperative staging of suspected hilar cholangiocarcinoma. *J Gastrointest Surg.* 2005;9:476–480.

52. Corvera CU, Weber SM, Jarnagin WR. Role of laparoscopy in the evaluation of biliary tract cancer. *Surg Oncol Clin N Am.* 2002;11:877–891.

53. Pichlmayr R, Lamesch P, Weimann A, et al. Surgical treatment of cholangiocellular carcinoma. *World J Surg.* 1995;19:83–88.

54. Jan YY, Jeng LB, Hwang TL, et al. Factors influencing survival after hepatectomy for peripheral cholangiocarcinoma. *Hepatogastroenterology.* 1996;43:614–619.

55. Casavilla FA, Marsh JW, Iwatsuki S, et al. Hepatic resection and transplantation for peripheral cholangiocarcinoma. *J Am Coll Surg.* 1997;185:429–436.

56. Madariaga JR, Iwatsuki S, Todo S, et al. Liver resection for hilar and peripheral cholangiocarcinomas: a study of 62 cases. *Ann Surg.* 1998;227: 70–79.

57. Valverde A, Bonhomme N, Farges O, et al. Resection of intrahepatic cholangiocarcinoma: a Western experience. *J Hepatobiliary Pancreat Surg.* 1999;6:122–127.

58. Inoue K, Makuuchi M, Takayama T, et al. Long-term survival and prognostic factors in the surgical treatment of mass-forming type cholangiocarcinoma. *Surgery.* 2000;127:498–505.

59. Weber SM, Jarnagin WR, Klimstra D, et al. Intrahepatic cholangiocarcinoma: resectability, recurrence pattern, and outcomes. *J Am Coll Surg.* 2001;193:384–391.

60. Sugiura Y, Nakamura S, Iida S, et al. Extensive resection of the bile ducts combined with liver resection for cancer of the main hepatic duct junction: a cooperative study of the Keio Bile Duct Cancer Study Group. *Surgery.* 1994;115:445–451.

61. Su CH, Tsay SH, Wu CC, et al. Factors influencing postoperative morbidity, mortality, and survival after resection for hilar cholangiocarcinoma. *Ann Surg.* 1996;223:384–394.

62. Nagino M, Nimura Y, Kamiya J, et al. Segmental liver resections for hilar cholangiocarcinoma. *Hepatogastroenterology.* 1998;45:7–13.

63. Miyazaki M, Ito H, Nakagawa K, et al. Aggressive surgical approaches to hilar cholangiocarcinoma: hepatic or local resection? *Surgery.* 1998;123:131–136.

64. Kosuge T, Yamamoto J, Shimada K, et al. Improved surgical results for hilar cholangiocarcinoma with procedures including major hepatic resection. *Ann Surg.* 1999;230:663–671.

65. Neuhaus P, Jonas S, Bechstein WO, et al. Extended resections for hilar cholangiocarcinoma. *Ann Surg.* 1999;230:808–818.

66. Jarnagin WR, Fong Y, DeMatteo RP, et al. Staging, resectability, and outcome in 225 patients with hilar cholangiocarcinoma. *Ann Surg.* 2001;234:507–517.

67. Rea DJ, Munoz-Juarez M, Farnell MB, et al. Major hepatic resection for hilar cholangiocarcinoma: analysis of 46 patients. *Arch Surg.* 2004;139: 514–523.

68. Nishio H, Nagino M, Nimura Y. Surgical management of hilar cholangiocarcinoma: the Nagoya experience. *HPB.* 2006;7:259–262.

69. Dinant S, Gerhards MF, Rauws EA, et al. Improved outcome of resection of hilar cholangiocarcinoma (Klatskin tumor). *Ann Surg Oncol.* 2006;13:872–880.

70. Abdel Wahab M, Fathy O, Elghwalby N, et al. Resectability and prognostic factors after resection of hilar cholangiocarcinoma. *Hepatogastroenterology.* 2006;53:5–10.

71. Mizumoto R, Suzuki H. Surgical anatomy of the hepatic hilum with special reference to the caudate lobe. *World J Surg.* 1988;12:2–10.

72. Nimura Y, Hayakawa N, Kamiya J, et al. Hepatic segmentectomy with

caudate lobe resection for bile duct carcinoma of the hepatic hilus. *World J Surg.* 1990;14:535–543.

73. Pichlmayr R, Weimann A, Klempnauer J, et al. Surgical treatment in proximal bile duct cancer. A single-center experience. *Ann Surg.* 1996;224:628–638.

74. Heimbach JK, Gores GJ, Nagorney DM, Rosen CB. Liver transplantation for perihilar cholangiocarcinoma after aggressive neoadjuvant therapy: a new paradigm for liver and biliary malignancies? *Surgery.* 2006;140:331–334.

75. Gunderson LL, Haddock MG, Foo ML, et al. Conformal irradiation for hepatobiliary malignancies. *Ann Oncol.* 1999;10:S221–S225.

76. Kamada T, Saitou H, Takamura A, et al. The role of radiotherapy in the management of extrahepatic bile duct cancer: an analysis of 145 consecutive patients treated with intraluminal and/or external beam radiotherapy. *Int J Radiat Oncol Biol Phys.* 1996;34:767–774.

77. Abrams RA, Grochow LB, Chakravarth A, et al. Intensified adjuvant therapy for pancreatic and periampullary adenocarcinoma: survival results and observations regarding patterns of failure, radiotherapy dose and CA19-9 levels. *Int J Radiat Oncol Biol Phys.* 1999;44:1039–1046.

78. Gunderson LL, Haddock MG, Burch P, et al. Future role of radiotherapy as a component of treatment in biliopancreatic cancers. *Ann Oncol.* 1999;10:S291–S295.

79. Whittington R, Neuberg D, Tester WJ, et al. Protracted intravenous fluorouracil infusion with radiation therapy in the management of localized pancreaticobiliary carcinoma: a phase I Eastern Cooperative Oncology Group trial. *J Clin Oncol.* 1995;13:227–232.

80. Pitt HA, Nakeeb A, Abrams RA, et al. Perihilar cholangiocarcinoma. *Ann Surg.* 1995;221:788–798.

81. Cameron JL, Pitt HA, Zinner MJ, et al. Management of proximal cholangiocarcinomas by surgical resection and radiotherapy. *Am J Surg.* 1990;159:91–98.

82. Verbeek PCM, van Leeuwen DJ, van Der Heyde MN, et al. Does additive radiotherapy after hilar resection improve survival of cholangiocarcinoma? *Ann Chir.* 1991;45:350–354.

83. Gonzalez DG, Gerard JP, Maners AW, et al. Results of radiation therapy in carcinoma of the proximal bile duct (Klatskin tumor). *Semin Liver Dis.* 1990;10:131–140.

84. Veeze-Kuijpers B, Meerwaldt JH, Lameris JS, et al. The role of radiotherapy in the treatment of bile duct carcinoma. *Int J Radiat Oncol Biol Phys.* 1989;18:63–67.

85. Gonzalez DG, Gouma DJ, Rauws EAJ, et al. Role of radiotherapy, in particular intraluminal brachytherapy, in the treatment of proximal bile duct carcinoma. *Ann Oncol.* 1999;18:S215–S220.

86. Schoenthaler R, Phillips TL, Castro J, et al. Carcinoma of the extrahepatic bile ducts. The University of California at San Francisco experience. *Ann Surg.* 1994;219:267–274.

87. Kopelson G, Galdabini J, Warshaw AL, et al. Patterns of failure after curative surgery for extra-hepatic biliary tract carcinoma: implications for adjuvant therapy. *Int J Radiat Oncol Biol Phys.* 1981;7:413–417.

88. Kopelson G, Gunderson LL. Primary and adjuvant radiation therapy in gallbladder and extrahepatic biliary tract carcinoma. *J Clin Gastroenterol.* 1983;5:43–50.

89. Alden ME, Mohiuddin M. The impact of radiation dose in combined external beam and intraluminal IR-192 brachytherapy for bile duct cancer. *Int J Radiat Oncol Biol Phys.* 1994;28:945–951.

90. Mittal B, Deutsch M, Iwatsuki S. Primary cancers of extrahepatic biliary passages. *Int J Radiat Oncol Biol Phys.* 1985;11:849–854.

91. Milella M, Salvetti M, Cerrotta A, et al. Interventional radiology and radiotherapy for inoperable cholangiocarcinoma of the extrahepatic bile ducts. *Tumori.* 1998;84:467–471.

92. Hayes JK, Sapozink MD, Miller FJ. Definitive radiation therapy in bile duct carcinoma. *Int J Radiat Oncol Biol Phys.* 1988;15:735–744.

93. Meyers WC, Jones RS. Internal radiation for bile duct cancer. *World J Surg.* 1988;12:99–104.

94. Foo ML, Gunderson LL, Bender CE, et al. External radiation therapy and transcatheter iridium in the treatment of extrahepatic bile duct carcinoma. *Int J Radiat Oncol Biol Phys.* 1997;39:929–935.

95. Serefini FM, Sachs D, Bloomston M, et al. Location, not staging, of cholangiocarcinoma determines the role for adjuvant chemoradiation therapy. *Am Surg.* 2001;67:839–843.

96. Urego M, Flickinger JC, Carr BI. Radiotherapy and multimodality management of cholangiocarcinoma. *Int J Radiat Oncol Biol Phys.* 1999;44:121–126.

97. McMaster KM, Tuttle TM, Leach SD, et al. Neoadjuvant chemoradiation for extrahepatic cholangiocarcinoma. *Am J Surg.* 1997;174:605–609.

98. Jarnigan WR, Burke E, Power C, et al. Intrahepatic biliary enteric bypass provides effective palliation in selected patients with malignant obstruction at the hepatic duct confluence. *Am J Surg.* 1998;175:453–460.

99. Leung JG, Kuan R. Intraluminal brachytherapy in the treatment of bile duct carcinomas. *Australas Radiol.* 1997;41:151–154.

100. Grove MK, Hermann RE, Vogt DP, et al. Role of radiation after operative palliation in cancer of the proximal bile ducts. *Am J Surg.* 1991;161:454–458.

101. Chakravarti A, Madre-Bell R, Constable WC, et al. Ir-192 brachytherapy vs. radical surgery in the management of primary extrahepatic bile duct adenocarcinoma. *Appl Radiol.* 1999;28:22–26.

102. GolfieriGR, Giampalma E, Renzulli M, et al. Unresectable hilar cholangiocarcinoma: multimodality approach with percutaneous treatment associated with radiotherapy and chemotherapy. *In Vivo.* 2006;20:757–760.

103. Schleicher UM, Staatz G, Alzen G, et al. Combined external beam and intraluminal radiotherapy for irresectable Klatskin tumors. *Strahlenther Onkol.* 2002;178:682–687.

COLORECTAL CANCER

CHAPTER 38 ■ ENVIRONMENTAL AND LIFESTYLE ISSUES IN COLORECTAL CANCER

ELIZABETH T. JACOBS, PATRICIA A. THOMPSON, AND MARÍA ELENA MARTÍNEZ

INTRODUCTION

Worldwide, colorectal cancer accounted for 1 million new cases and 500,000 deaths in 2002 (1). Rates of this malignancy vary by country. Although cancer of the colorectum is rare in developing countries, this malignancy is the second most frequently diagnosed in developed countries. Wide geographic variation in colorectal cancer incidence and mortality rates is believed to be due to lifestyle/environmental factors. Migrant studies, which compare individuals who move from countries with low rates to those with high rates, also suggest that lifestyle/environmental factors influence the development of colorectal cancer. Furthermore, incidence rates of this disease are increasing in some countries with formerly low rates, which also suggest that lifestyle/environmental factors are involved in their etiology.

The presentation that follows begins with a review of the descriptive epidemiology, followed by a summary of results of analytic epidemiologic studies. Prior to the discussion of the published work, a review of study designs is provided to familiarize the reader with these concepts. The summary further focuses on epidemiologic studies pertaining to obesity, physical activity, hormone replacement therapy (HRT), tobacco, nonsteroidal antiinflammatory drugs (NSAIDs), and diet.

DESCRIPTIVE EPIDEMIOLOGY

Incidence and Mortality Rates Worldwide

In general, the incidence of colorectal cancer is rising worldwide, although there are a few exceptions. However, mortality rates are not rising as rapidly as incidence rates and have dropped significantly in Canada, the United States, and some European countries, which is possibly the result of improved survival.

Countries in Asia and Oceania show a 10-fold range in variation in colorectal cancer incidence. Among these countries, the largest rise in incidence has been seen in Japan, where incidence increased at a rate of 20% to 30% per 5-year period from 1970 to 1985 (2). Of interest, rates among Japanese living in Hawaii are also rising. Overall, in most of the countries of Asia and Oceania, there have been increases among Japanese and Chinese populations, whereas no significant change or declines were seen among the low-risk populations of India. As well, incidence rates in Australia have been rising by 12% to 14% every 5 years, although no such rise in mortality rates has been shown (2).

Fig. 38.1 shows wide international geographic variations in mortality rates for colorectal cancer. Rates of this malignancy have increased by approximately 25% since 1965 in Japan. In the eastern countries of Czechoslovakia, Hungary, Poland, and Yugoslavia, mortality rates have also been increasing steadily. Fig. 38.1 also shows that the male-to-female ratio for colorectal cancer in high-risk areas is higher than that in low-risk areas. Another interesting fact related to international variation in colorectal cancer involves the geographic distribution for cancers of the colon and rectum. In locations considered to be high risk, the ratio of colon to rectal cancer incidence is approximately 2:1 or more, whereas in low-risk regions, the ratio is close to one.

Incidence and Mortality Rates in the Americas and the United States

Incidence rates of colorectal cancer have been rising steadily in areas of Central and South America (2). In the United States, however, decreases in colorectal cancer incidence rates began in the mid-1980s, and have occurred among both males and females. Incidence rates of colorectal cancer decreased by an average of 1.8% per year between 1998 and 2002 (3). Based on 1998 to 2002 data, incidence rates in the United States are 65.9 per 100,000 for colon and 47.9 per 100,000 for rectal cancer.

In 2006, of the estimated 148,610 new colorectal cases that will occur in the United States, 55,170 will die of this disease (3). Colorectal cancer incidence rates increase with age, with 86% of cases occurring in people 55 years and older. In North America, mortality rates from this cancer have been falling significantly. In the United States, annual age-standardized colorectal cancer mortality rates peaked in the 1940s and have steadily fallen since the 1950s (3). The age-standardized mortality rate between 1998 and 2002 was 24.7 per 100,000 for colon and 17.4 per 100,000 for rectal cancer (3).

In the United States, differences in colorectal cancer incidence and mortality rates among various racial/ethnic groups are evident (3). Incidence rates of this disease are highest among blacks (72.5/100,000 in males and 56.0/100,000 in females), intermediate among non-Hispanic whites (NHWs) (61.7/100,000 in males and 45.3/100,000 in females), and lower among Hispanics (48.3/100,000 in males and 32.3/100,000 in females) and Native Americans/Alaskan Natives (36.7/100,000 in males and 32.2/100,000 in females). Fig. 38.2 shows that the highest mortality rates are found among blacks. The age-standardized mortality rate for black men from 1998 to 2002 was 34.0 per 100,000; the rate for black women was 24.1 per 100,000. In addition, when compared to other nonwhite populations, black men and women are twice as likely to die of colorectal cancer. These data clearly indicate that the greatest racial/ethnic disparity is shown for mortality rates in

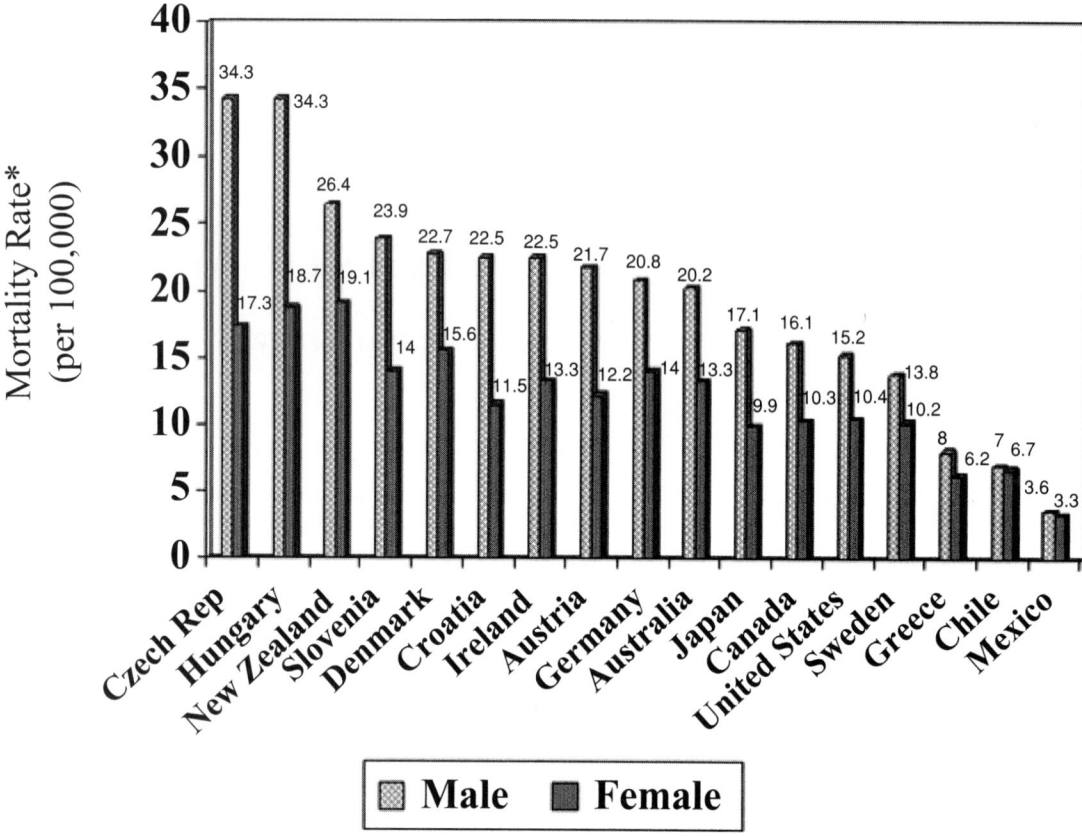

FIGURE 38.1. Mortality rates (per 100,000) of colorectal cancer for selected countries around the world. *Rates are age-adjusted to the World Health Organization world standard population.

blacks. Although incidence and mortality rates of colorectal cancer are lower in Asian/Pacific Islanders, Hispanics, and Native Americans/Alaskan Natives, it will be important to monitor future trends because there are suggestions in the literature that they are on the rise in some of these racial/ethnic groups. Data from the New Mexico Tumor Registry showed that colon cancer rates increased 3.6% per year among Hispanics between 1969 and 1994 (4). Furthermore, although a decline in inci-

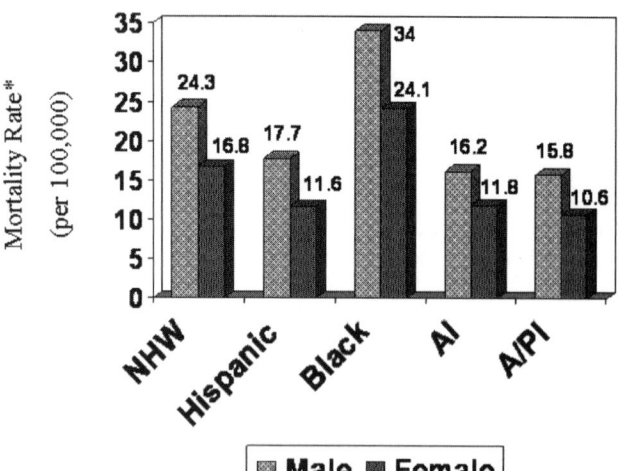

FIGURE 38.2. Mortality rates (per 100,000) of colorectal cancer by age and race/ethnicity in the United States, 1998 to 2002. *Rates are age-adjusted to the 2000 U.S. standard population. NHW, non-Hispanic white; AI, American Indian (Native American); A/PI, Asian/Pacific Islander.

dence rates was shown among Hispanics in California (5), the data show that this decline is not as pronounced as that for NHWs or other racial/ethnic groups.

Survival

Between the 1970s and 1990s, 5-year colorectal cancer survival rates in the United States have increased from 50% to 63% in NHWs (6), with current survival rates being at 64% (3). The global picture, however, clearly shows that survival is lower in countries outside the United States: 41% in Europe, 42% in India, and 32% in China (7). Data for survival in the United States also indicate significant racial/ethnic group disparities, where less pronounced increases in survival are observed for certain groups compared to NHWs (8). For example, comparing survival rates from 1975 to 1987 to those in 1988 to 1997, rates among NHW males increased by 10%, and those for black males increased by 9%; however, this change was only 7.4% for Hispanics and 6.4% for Hawaiian natives. For females, changes in survival for the same period of time were 9.2% for NHWs, 6.5% for Hispanics, 5.9% for blacks, and 4.6% for Native Americans/Alaskan Natives, and these actually decreased by 1.3% for Hawaiian natives.

In the United States, additional disparities by racial/ethnic group also present for stage of disease at diagnosis, which clearly affects survival. For example, 16% of colorectal cancer cases are diagnosed with distant disease among NHWs, whereas 20% of Hispanics present with distant disease, which is similar to what is observed for African Americans (9). Furthermore, as noted by Clegg et al. (8), although the proportion of individuals who present with distant disease at diagnosis has decreased among NHW and African Americans, this has actually increased among Hispanics and Native

Americans/Alaskan Natives. These data show that the proportion of Hispanics who presented with distant colorectal cancer increased from 19.8 to 20.3 from 1975 to 1987 to 1988 to 1997; among Native Americans/Alaskan Natives, the increase was more pronounced, from 19.8 to 24.4. More recently published data show similar findings. Using 11 Surveillance, Epidemiology, and End Results cancer registries, Chien et al. (10) showed various racial/ethnic disparities in risk of advanced stage colorectal cancer. One of the strengths of this study is the ability of the investigators to subdivide specific racial/ethnic groups, such as Hispanics, into the various subpopulations. For example, compared to NHWs, men and women of Mexican descent were significantly more likely to present with stage III or IV disease.

Migrant Studies

Wide geographic differences in colorectal cancer rates have been believed to be due in part to environmental factors, namely, dietary intake. Migrant studies have supported these hypotheses, given that individuals moving from countries with low rates to countries with higher rates of colorectal cancer show increased risks similar or close to those of the host country (2,11–15); however, there are some exceptions (16,17). In some instances, the rates of migrants from low-incidence countries exceed those of the host country (11,12,14). For example, colon cancer rates in Japanese living in the United States are currently higher than those of whites. High rates are seen in Caucasian populations of northern European origin, and these high rates continue to be shown with migration. Conversely, where lower rates are seen (i.e., southern Europe, Asia, and Africa), these rates tend to rise with migration to higher rate areas. It has also been shown in recent studies that it is important to take into account length of stay in the host country (13,18). Migrant studies have suggested that colorectal cancer is particularly sensitive to changes in lifestyle/environmental factors. Incidence rates reach those of the host country within one or two generations, sometimes even within the migrating generation, arguing strongly for a nongenetic, environmental etiology.

COLORECTAL ADENOMAS

Most colorectal cancers arise from adenomas (19). Because adenomas are usually asymptomatic, they may not be detected until years after onset; thus, the appropriate measure of their frequency is prevalence (e.g., prevalence at the time of endoscopy or autopsy). The prevalence of adenomas increases with age and is greater in men than in women (20). Results of autopsy studies and screening studies of average-risk populations have found that 20% to 60% of individuals have adenomas (20), with the lowest prevalence rates observed in areas of Finland, the Philippines, Mexico, Colombia, Iran, and South Africa (21). Compared to colorectal cancer end points, relatively fewer epidemiologic studies have been conducted using the adenoma as an end point. It is not entirely clear whether lifestyle factors influence adenoma and carcinoma in a differential manner; however, given the complexity of this disease, it is possible that some factors have greater influence in early stages and others in later stages.

Epidemiologic Study Designs

Ecologic or Correlational Studies

The association between colorectal cancer and environmental factors, such as dietary intake, can be assessed using ecologic aggregations by examining correlations between the lifestyle/environmental factor and the corresponding incidence or mortality rates. Such correlational studies, commonly conducted to assess dietary etiology by using per capita consumption data, can be based on comparisons among nations or among administrative units within a single country. It is difficult to draw strong conclusions about cancer etiology based on these studies; nations showing substantial variation in cancer incidence may exhibit, in addition to diverse dietary patterns, differences in nondietary environmental factors. For example, rates of colon cancer are strongly correlated with national per capita disappearance of animal fat and meat, with correlation coefficients ranging between 0.8 and 0.9 (22,23). However, it is difficult to attribute these rates with a high degree of certainty to one or more dietary variables. The primary problem of these correlational studies is that many potential determinants of the cancer of interest, other than the dietary factor under consideration, may vary between areas with high and low incidence rates. Indeed, the number of significant correlates of colon cancer risk may exceed the number of countries under study. These correlates confound one another. Such confounding factors can include genetic predisposition, other dietary factors, and other environmental or lifestyle practices. For this reason, ecologic studies have traditionally been considered the weakest form of epidemiologic evidence.

Analytical Epidemiologic Studies

In case-control studies, information about lifestyle and other factors prior to disease onset is obtained from patients with cancer and compared to those without cancer. Compared to ecologic studies, results from case-control studies may provide stronger evidence given that information on confounding factors can be taken into account. A primary advantage of case-control studies is that these can be conducted over a relatively short period of time, which decreases their cost. An important drawback of case-control studies is the potential for selection or recall bias. Selection bias occurs if an inappropriate control group is selected or if the cases or controls that refuse to participate have characteristics that may bias the results. Recall bias could occur if study participants with a specific cancer remember and report their diet differently from control participants. The possibility of interviewer-induced reporting bias is a consideration, especially if the interviewer is not blinded to the case status of the study participant. Another limitation of such studies is that only dietary factors that are etiologically relevant relatively shortly before the diagnosis of cancer can be practically studied because in the majority of the studies, only diet in the previous year or few years can be assessed. For a disease such as colorectal cancer, in which risk factors from the more distant past appear to be relevant, dietary intake beyond a few years prior to diagnosis may be more relevant; however, difficulty in measuring and validating such dietary intake must be taken into account.

Cohort studies involve identifying a study sample and monitoring the incidence and/or mortality of disease over time as well as exposure to potential risk factors. In these studies, the assessment of exposure factors is obtained before the development of the disease. Thus, the possibility for recall bias that afflicts case-control studies is eliminated. However, a potential drawback related to cohort studies is the loss to follow-up of participants. If disease incidence or specific risk factor exposures are related to a loss to follow-up, then estimates of risk may be biased positively or negatively. Noteworthy associations may not be detected. Cohort studies are generally considered to be expensive; however, inasmuch as several disease end points and intermediate end points can be ascertained in a cohort, these studies can be quite cost effective. When assessing the multicausal nature of various cancers, studies that examine various etiologic factors and outcomes in one data set are of immense value. For example, studies such as the Nurses' Health Study (NHS) and the Health Professionals Follow-up Study (HPFS) ascertain risk factor data periodically throughout the follow-up period. This allows for the consideration of variation in the risk factor of interest during follow-up. An additional advantage of prospective studies is that biochemical markers can be used, with samples collected prior to the onset of disease. In case-control studies, it is not possible to determine whether the marker reflects true variation in prediagnostic intake or a change related to malignancy.

Lifestyle and Environmental Factors

Notwithstanding the importance of genetic influences, several lines of evidence support the substantial role of lifestyle/environmental factors in the etiology of colorectal cancer. Unlike other malignancies, risk of colorectal cancer appears to be influenced by a variety of modifiable factors, ranging from those that are relatively easy to quantify (i.e., tobacco exposure) to those whose assessment is much more challenging and complex (i.e., dietary intake, physical activity, and environmental/occupational exposures). This section presents lifestyle and environmental risk factors that are currently believed to have an important role in the development of colorectal neoplasia.

Obesity

The majority of epidemiologic studies supports a role for obesity as a risk factor for colorectal adenoma (24–27), cancers (25,28–33), and colon cancer mortality (29,34). These observations suggest a continuous action of the adverse effects of obesity along the adenoma to carcinoma continuum. In general, the effect of obesity on colorectal cancer risk has been stronger for cancers arising in the colon, for those occurring in men (30,35–40), and for cancers in the proximal colon (30,33). In the Physician's Health Study (PHS), a large cohort of male health professionals, the relative risk (RR) for colon cancer was 1.48 among men in the upper quintile of body mass index (BMI) compared to those in the lowest quintile ($p = 0.02$) (25). In NHS, a large cohort study of women, a BMI >29 kg/m^2 was associated with a RR of 1.45 (95% CI, 1.02–2.07) when compared to a BMI <21 kg/m^2 (41). Further recent findings from the prospective Framingham Cohort study, where waist circumference and waist-to-hip ratio (WHR) measures were available, suggest that measures of central adiposity may be more informative for risk of colon cancer than measures of BMI (30). In the Framingham study, a large waist circumference was associated with a RR for colon cancer of 4.4 for middle-age adults and 3.0 for older sedentary adults (30). Earlier data from the HPFS reported similar findings where stronger associations were observed with measures of waist circumference (RR, 2.6) and WHR (RR, 3.5) than for BMI (25).

Studies among women have been less consistent, with the majority of studies reporting weak or null associations between measures of BMI and colon cancer risk and strong effect modification by menopausal status (39). The use of waist circumference as a measure of central obesity may improve the precision of point estimates for colon cancer risk among women (30,41–43). Stronger effects of high BMI on colorectal cancer among premenopausal versus postmenopausal women (39,44) has led to the suggestion of effect modification by menopausal status. The consistent reporting of protective effects of hormone replacement therapy for colorectal cancers in postmenopausal women (see "Hormone Replacement Therapy" section), and attenuation of colorectal cancer risk among heavier older women may indicate a physiological shift from obesity as a risk-enhancing to a risk-reducing factor as women age. Although exposure to higher levels of growth-promoting effects of insulinlike growth factor 1 are proposed as an explanation of the menopause-specific effects of obesity on colorectal cancer risk (39), further study is needed to delineate the mechanism for the observed attenuation of risk for colorectal cancers among heavier, older women.

Physical Activity

Results of prospective (41,45–55) and retrospective (56–77) studies support an inverse association between physical activity and risk of colon but not rectal cancer (46,50,51,53,56, 69,78,79). The results are consistent, whether assessing active versus nonactive or sedentary versus active individuals. In a prospective study of female nurses (41), leisure-time physical activity and body size were assessed in relation to the subsequent development of colon cancer. Women in the upper quintile of physical activity exhibited approximately half the colon cancer risk of inactive women (RR, 0.54; 95% CI, 0.33–0.90). These findings are supported by results of other published studies, including those of the HPFS (25). When physical activity and BMI are assessed jointly, the highest risk of colon cancer occurs among those who are both physically inactive and have high BMI levels (25,30,80). The joint adverse effect of obesity and sedentary behavior is demonstrated for both men and women (30).

Despite the wide variation in physical assessment methodology among studies, including type of activity (leisure-time or occupational) and method of assessment, considerable consistency between studies is found. Based on a comprehensive review of the literature, Colditz et al. (81) reported a dose–response protective effect of physical activity on colon cancer with approximately a 50% reduction in incidence of colon cancer among individuals with the highest level of physical activity. In addition, a recent meta-analysis of 19 cohort studies (82) supports an approximate 30% significant reduction in the risk of colon cancer in physically active males and females with no protective effect of physical activity on rectal cancers.

The proposed biological mechanisms for the effect of physical activity on colon carcinogenesis are numerous and not necessarily mutually exclusive. The protective action of aspirin and other NSAIDs in the colon suggest that proinflammatory prostaglandins play an important role in the development of colon cancer (83–86). Martínez et al. (87) found a strong inverse association between physical activity and rectal mucosal PGE^2 concentrations. These results suggest that one potential biological mechanism by which physical activity alters the risk of colon cancer is through direct effects on local PGE^2 and other prostanoid synthesis.

Other mechanisms proposed to explain the protective effect of physical activity in the colon include decreased bowel transit time with concomitant reduction in exposure to dietary carcinogens, lower bile acid secretion, and maintenance of insulin sensitivity and glucoregulatory function (88). Chronic insulin exposure or hyperinsulinemia coupled with impaired insulin sensitivity is perhaps the best supported of the mechanisms and provides a strong link between the main colon cancer risk factors of age, inflammation, physical inactivity, and central adiposity (89).

Hormone Replacement Therapy

Although studies on reproductive factors and colorectal cancer risk have provided conflicting results, HRT use has been consistently associated with a decreased risk of colon cancer with weaker or null effects in the rectum in the majority of case-control and cohort studies (45,90–104). In the NHS (105), current postmenopausal HRT use was associated with a decreased risk of colorectal cancer; the relationship with any past use was weaker and absent 5 years after hormone use was stopped. These findings, along with two additional large prospective studies (106,107), support an inverse association between colon cancer and estrogen use in postmenopausal women. A large multicenter case-control study (108) also indicated that women who had ever used HRT had a lower colon cancer risk (OR, 0.82; 95% CI, 0.67–0.99), with recent use associated with approximately 30% reduction in risk (OR, 0.71; 95% CI, 0.56–0.89). Results of another large case-control study (109) also found an inverse association between HRT and colorectal cancer, particularly among recent users (RR, 0.54; 95% CI, 0.36–0.81). Overall, the results of recent studies show inverse associations ranging from 0.5 to 0.8 for HRT use. A meta-analysis of 18 studies conducted to assess the role of HRT and colorectal cancer (91) found an overall 20% reduction in risk for colon cancer associated with every use of HRT (RR = 0.80; 95% CI = 0.74–0.86). These results were not appreciably different for rectal cancers (RR, 0.81; 95% CI, 0.72–0.92). Furthermore, the association with colorectal cancer was strongest among current HRT users (RR, 0.66; 95% CI, 0.59–0.74).

More recently, evidence from the published findings of the large randomized clinical trial of HRT conducted in older postmenopausal women by the Women's Health Initiative (WHI) supports previous findings from case-control and cohort studies for a protective effect of HRT in the colon. Among women taking combination HRT (estrogen combined with progestin), the WHI reported 43 cases of invasive colorectal cancers in the treatment group and 72 in the placebo group (HR, 0.56; 95% CI, 0.38–0.81) (110). In contrast, among all users of estrogen only, there were no differences in incidence of colorectal cancers when compared to placebo in unpublished early reports (111). Notable for women taking combination HRT therapy, among those developing colorectal cancers, the disease was significantly more likely to present with lymph node or regional/distant metastasis compared to placebo; features associated with poor outcomes (110). The significant association of combination HRT with advanced disease at diagnosis was unexplained, but its observation early in the trial suggest either a promoting effect of the hormonal exposure on the growth of existing malignancies or perhaps a masking effect of early symptoms of disease and delayed diagnosis. Taken together, the evidence is highly compelling for HRT use as beneficial for the prevention of colon cancers, with some caution warranted for active surveillance among users (110,112). Given potential limitations of the WHI randomized trial study population, most notably the older age of subjects at initiation of HRT use, additional studies to estimate the overall benefit of HRT in younger postmenopausal women is warranted.

Tobacco

Although tobacco has not been clearly implicated as a cause of colorectal malignancies, a higher risk of adenomatous polyps has been consistently observed among smokers in numerous studies (113). A long induction period between smoking and risk of colorectal cancer was hypothesized based on results from two large cohort studies (114,115). Subsequently, the vast majority of published studies have reported positive associations between cigarette smoking and colorectal cancer (45,116–125), although several studies did not support an association (126–129). Of note, some of the nonsupportive studies were conducted in Sweden (127,128), suggesting that some factor, possibly genetic, in Swedes may counter the impact of smoking. In an earlier review of the published data,

Giovannucci and Martínez (113) suggested that the evidence earlier in the decade tended not to support the hypothesis that smoking influenced colorectal carcinogenesis because a sufficient lag period had not elapsed between smoking and colorectal cancer risk. With the assumption that an increased risk emerges only about four decades after smoking initiation, a pattern consistent with a positive association emerges. The consistent finding of a positive association between smoking and the risk of adenomas probably results from a presumably much shorter induction period for these lesions. Based on this earlier review of the literature, Giovannucci and Martínez (113) concluded that overall evidence supports the hypothesis that tobacco smoke is an initiator of colorectal carcinogenesis and that the induction period is very long, possibly up to four decades.

A more recent review of the literature conducted by Giovannucci (130) indicates that data published since the 1990s strongly supports the association between tobacco and colorectal neoplasia. For colorectal adenoma, there is a high degree of consistency in the findings across studies reporting an association with tobacco smoke, with risk estimates ranging between 2 and 5. In a review of colorectal cancer studies conducted after 1970, which would allow for long-term exposure, all 10 studies conducted in the United States support an association with tobacco smoke. Given that women in the United States took up smoking later than men in the United States, a sufficient induction period would only be observed after 1990. As a result, a review of studies published after 1990 also shows that all five of these support this association; data from recent studies outside the United States also show positive associations. In his review, Giovannucci advocates for the inclusion of colorectal cancer in the list of tobacco-associated malignancies. Due to the hypothesized potential causal nature of this association, population-attributable risk estimates have been provided in the literature, which range from 11% for colon cancer in women (118) to 22% of rectal cancer in men (131). This implies that if the association between tobacco and colorectal cancer is causal, 11% to 22% for these malignancies are attributable to this particular exposure.

Nonsteroidal Anti-inflammatory Drugs

As reviewed by Thun et al. (132), a lot of support exists for a protective effect of NSAID use and COX-2 inhibitors on colorectal neoplasia. Evidence in favor of an inverse association between NSAID use (e. g., aspirin, indomethacin, ibuprofen, piroxicam) and colorectal cancer stems from epidemiologic (133–137), animal (138–141), and intervention studies among individuals with familial adenomatous polyposis (142–144). In addition, patients with rheumatoid arthritis, who generally have higher use of NSAIDs, have lower incidence and mortality rates of gastrointestinal malignancies (145,146). Supporting evidence is also derived from observational studies of NSAIDs and colorectal adenomas (127,137–139).

Results of epidemiologic studies are consistent with an approximately 50% reduction in colorectal cancer risk associated with use of aspirin or other NSAIDs, although in one study a positive association was observed (147). In the NHS, a statistically significant reduction of colorectal cancer in women after 20 years of consistent (two or more tablets per week) aspirin use was observed (RR, 0.56; 95% CI, 0.36–0.90; $p = 0.008$) (137). Similarly, a prospective study in male health professionals reported relative risks of comparable magnitude (136). Perhaps the strongest evidence of a protective effect of NSAIDs for sporadic colorectal neoplasia was provided by a randomized, double-blind clinical trial conducted by Baron et al. (148). Results from this study revealed a significantly reduced risk for colorectal adenoma in those randomized to receive 81 mg/day of aspirin compared to the placebo group, although no effect was found for an aspirin dose of 325 mg/day (148).

Despite these encouraging results, the use of COX-2 inhibitors for chemoprevention of colorectal neoplasia in the general public is unlikely in the near future. The Vioxx Gastrointestinal Outcomes Research trial, designed to test the effects of rofecoxib on gastrointestinal outcomes, reported significant increases in adverse cardiovascular events related to the use of rofecoxib (149). This led to the termination of several other ongoing trials of COX-2 inhibitors and colorectal neoplasia. Therefore, despite a wealth of information indicating protection from colorectal adenoma and cancer by COX-2 inhibitors, the future use of these compounds as preventive agents for sporadic colorectal adenoma and cancer is uncertain.

Diet

It has been frequently cited that up to 90% of cancer is environmentally related (150,151). Diet constitutes one of the most obviously differential population parameters in that it involves a daily exposure that is highly adaptable to a new environment. The epidemiologic and experimental evidence that dietary pattern is an important causal determinant of colorectal tumors is compelling. However, controversy exists regarding the specific nutrients, foods, or combinations of these that are causally related to the development of colorectal cancer. Specifically, hypotheses that were prevalent a decade or two ago remain controversial despite intensive investigation.

Long-term diet is usually the exposure of interest for epidemiologic studies of cancer. An assessment that takes into account day-to-day variation in dietary intake is essential when choosing an appropriate assessment method. Therefore, dietary instruments that measure only 1 or a few days can result in substantial misclassification of an individual's true long-term intake. The inability to reduce this error can result in an attenuation of relative risks, that is, to lower the strength of the associations (152,153). High intraindividual variation of micronutrient intake is possible given wide differences of individual nutrient concentration in certain foods (154). In the same context, fruit and vegetables may only be abundant during a certain part of the year, resulting in additional variation. Cultural and socioeconomic influences may also play a role in the variation of dietary intake. Given these complexities, it is important to note that all dietary assessment methods are prone to measurement error that may arise from various sources. Consequently, individuals may be classified in the wrong intake categories. This misclassification in turn weakens observed associations.

As noted previously, long-term dietary intake is of relevance in epidemiologic studies of cancer. As a result, the food frequency questionnaire (FFQ) approach has been the preferred instrument of assessment. Rather than obtaining a more precise but likely unrepresentative estimate of short-term dietary intake, the FFQ seeks to measure average, long-term intake. Most FFQs focus on the preceding year (or the year prior to diagnosis of cancer for case-control studies) as the period of exposure. The basic components of the FFQ include a food list and a frequency response section. Other questionnaires also incorporate a section related to usual portion size. Because FFQs are relatively easy to administer, they are considered to be extremely practical in epidemiologic settings. Unlike other dietary instruments such as diet records, processing of large numbers of FFQs is feasible and relatively inexpensive.

However, FFQs are not without weaknesses for studies of diet and cancer. Major criticisms of this method include the inability of study participants to recall long-term food intake patterns, poor validity of instruments, and inability to detect diet–cancer relationships as compared to dietary biomarkers

or food records (155). Suggestions for improvements to FFQs include measurement of dietary behavior as well as food intake, and collection of real-time information via computers (155).

Energy Intake

The assessment of the relationship between energy intake and colon cancer presents a challenge because total energy is correlated with both "good" and "bad" nutrients (e. g., folate, calcium, red meat) and nonnutrient factors (e. g., physical activity, obesity), which themselves have been implicated in colon cancer risk. Variation in energy intake among individuals within a population is influenced largely by level of physical activity, metabolic efficiency, and body size (156). Therefore, the confounding effects of these factors on total energy intake should be taken into account when examining the role of dietary factors on the risk of developing colorectal cancer.

Results of most published case-control studies have shown a positive association between total energy intake and risk of colon cancer (56,59,65,157–166). Howe et al. (167) conducted a pooled analysis of 13 case-control studies and found that total energy intake was associated with a higher risk of colon cancer, regardless of whether the energy source was fat, protein, or carbohydrate. Slattery et al. (80) reported similar findings based on three case-control studies and suggested that total energy intake is more important than the specific energy sources. In contrast to the findings of case-control studies, cohort studies have shown no relationship or even a slight inverse association between total energy intake and risk of colon cancer (168–173). In one of these studies (173), a statistically significant RR of 0.62 was reported between high energy intake and colorectal cancer.

Compatible with the emerging hyperinsulinemia hypothesis in colorectal cancer risk (174), more recent dietary intake studies have investigated the importance of dietary glycemic load (GL) as a risk factor for colorectal cancer. Using the glycemic index (GI) as an estimate of the postprandial blood glucose response to a food item (175), along with carbohydrate content and frequency of intake, high glycemic diets have been positively associated with increased risk of colorectal cancer in some (80,176,177), but not all (178,179), studies. For example, in an analysis of the Women's Health Study, a RR of 2.85 (95% CI, 1.40–5.80) was observed for colorectal cancer risk among women in the highest quintile of energy-adjusted GL compared to women in the lowest GL quintile (177). The association remained even after adjusting for BMI and level of physical activity. In contrast, the results of another large prospective study of women showed no association between GL and risk of colorectal cancer (178). In a recent analysis on the role of the quality and quantity of carbohydrates on colorectal cancer risk in both men and women, Michaud et al. examined the association between dietary carbohydrate, sucrose, fructose, GI, and GL in both the NHS and the HPFS (179). No association with colorectal cancer risk was observed with GL or GI in women, and only a modest association was observed among men in the highest quintile of dietary GL (RR, 1.35; 95% CI, 0.98–1.79); furthermore, risk was greatest among men with comparatively higher BMI measurements (25 kg/m^2).

The reason for the discrepancy between findings from cohort and case-control studies regarding energy intake, high glycemic diets, and colon cancer is unclear. Methodologic biases, such as differential recall or reporting of past diet, selective participation, or survival in case-control studies, as well as difficulty in accounting for confounding and lack of direct measures of exposure, all likely contribute to unstable estimates of risk. In summary, the majority of current evidence supports a state of chronic positive energy balance, regardless of macronutrient source, as a risk factor in colorectal cancers, with risks estimated to be on the order of 30% to 40% higher in chronically exposed individuals.

Red Meat and Cooking Methods

Rates of colorectal cancer are strongly correlated with national per capita disappearance of animal fat and meat, with correlation coefficients ranging between 0.8 and 0.9 (22,23). A sharp increase in colorectal cancer incidence rates in Japan in the decades following World War II coincided with an increase in fat and meat intake (180,181). Inconsistencies, however, have been cited (182), including the high meat intake and low rates in Greece, as well as decreasing meat intake with corresponding increasing rates in Australia and the United Kingdom, although at least one recent study has detected positive associations between red meat intake and colorectal cancer rates in Australia (183).

Results of analytic epidemiologic studies also support the association between animal fat and colon cancer; most case-control studies have shown a positive association with intake of animal or saturated fat (56,157−160,162−164,184) or red meat (62,185−190), with some exceptions (166,191−193). In a pooled analysis of 13 case-control studies, there was little or no evidence of an effect of total fat on colorectal cancer risk (194). Prospective cohort studies of colorectal cancer have shown inconsistent findings for the association of fat or red meat consumption and colon cancer (52,168,169,183, 195−202), although other cohort studies have shown statistically significant or suggestive positive associations for intake of processed meats and risk of colorectal cancer (171−173, 183,201). Regular consumption of well-done or fried meats has been associated with increased risk for colorectal cancer in some studies (60,185,203,204), although there are some inconsistencies (205,206). In a review of the literature published in 2002, 10 of 30 case-control studies revealed significant associations between red meat and colorectal cancer, although the effect varied by gender and cancer site, whereas 3 of 15 cohort studies detected increased risk for colorectal cancer with consumption of red meat (207). Since the publication of that review, results from large prospective studies have shown positive associations for red meat and rectal cancer (183,201), as well as cancer of the distal colorectum (198).

The mechanisms responsible for the effect of red meat on colorectal carcinogenesis are uncertain and include its role as a source of total or saturated fat, carcinogens, or iron (which can act as an antioxidant catalyst). In addition, results of some studies suggest that risk of colorectal cancer or adenoma may be increased among meat eaters who consume meat with a heavily browned surface but not increased among those who consume meat with a medium or lightly browned surface (185,190,199,204,208). More than two decades ago, Sugimura et al. (209) found that charred parts of broiled meat were mutagenic. When meat is cooked, particularly at high temperatures for a long period of time, mutagenic heterocyclic aromatic amines (HAAs) are formed (210−212). Since the 1990s, several HAAs have been isolated from cooked meat (210). However, previous studies have been unable to directly assess the carcinogenic effect of these compounds in humans due to inadequate dietary questionnaires. Although HAAs are considered to be both mutagenic and carcinogenic, little is known about the carcinogenic potencies of a mixture of several HAAs. The role of a possible synergistic effect of a combination of HAAs generated in cooked foods deserves special attention (213). In addition, because bioactivation and detoxification of HAAs appear to be genetically determined, it is of considerable importance that the associations of HAAs and colorectal cancer risk take this into consideration. Metabolism of HAAs varies among individuals and has been shown to depend on polymorphisms in genes involved in converting HAAs to their electrophilic metabolites or on polymorphisms in genes that detoxify the activated metabolites. Specifically, N-acetyl transferases (NATs) are known to be involved in the metabolism of several aromatic amines and HAAs. Variability in metabolism of HAAs by NAT1 and NAT2 appears to be related to susceptibility to mutagenesis and carcinogenesis by these agents. Therefore, it is possible that rapid acetylation is important only in individuals who consume a diet high in meats that are significant sources of HAAs, thus demonstrating the importance of gene−environment interactions. In general, the studies that have found that rapid NAT2 increased risk of colon cancer, observed the strongest associations among those in the upper categories of meat consumption (214−216); however, there are some inconsistencies (200). Smoking may also influence the risk related to red meat intake via pathways involving the phase I enzymes that activate HAAs (217).

Selenium

The trace element selenium has received increasing attention as a possible cancer preventive substance. The main dietary sources of selenium in the United States are meats and grains (218). However, given the wide variability of selenium concentrations in the soil, assessment of intake is problematic, making epidemiologic studies difficult to conduct. The correlations for selenium and colorectal cancer, although plausible, are mainly derived from ecologic data; these data show higher cancer mortality rates in low-selenium areas (219) compared to those of high regions. Epidemiologically, perhaps the strongest support for chemopreventive effects of selenium has come from a large, randomized, double-blind, placebo-controlled trial that involved supplementation with 200 μg of selenium per day for prevention of nonmelanoma skin cancer (220). Although selenium supplementation did not reduce skin cancer risk as compared to placebo in this trial, secondary analyses of the data showed a statistically significant 58% reduction in colorectal cancer incidence among participants randomized to the selenium-supplemented group (220); albeit the results were attenuated and no longer significant after additional years of follow-up (221). Furthermore, there is evidence that only those that were in the lowest tertile of baseline blood selenium levels in this trial may have benefited from supplementation (221). Several other epidemiologic investigations of the relationship between selenium and colon and/or rectal neoplasia have shown an inverse association (222−229), although others have reported null results (230,231). Several mechanisms for anticarcinogenic effects of selenium have been proposed. These include increased protection from oxidative damage (232), enhanced immune function (233), and induction of apoptosis (234).

Further clinical trials to investigate the relationship between selenium intake and colorectal neoplasia are currently ongoing. The inclusion of several genes related to selenium metabolism and function in these studies should help clarify the mechanism of action, and possibly help identify populations that would most benefit from selenium supplementation.

Vitamin D and Calcium

Calcium and vitamin D have been investigated in relation to risk reduction for colorectal neoplasia for several decades, with a lot of recent attention focused on vitamin D. Both exhibit biologically plausible pathways for prevention of colorectal cancer and are so closely interrelated (Fig. 38.3) that they are considered in the same section of this chapter.

Vitamin D. Vitamin D is a secosteroid hormone that can be obtained from dietary sources such as fatty fish or fortified dairy products, or it can be synthesized endogenously from 7-dehydrocholesterol in the skin after exposure to ultraviolet irradiation from the sun. The most abundant circulating

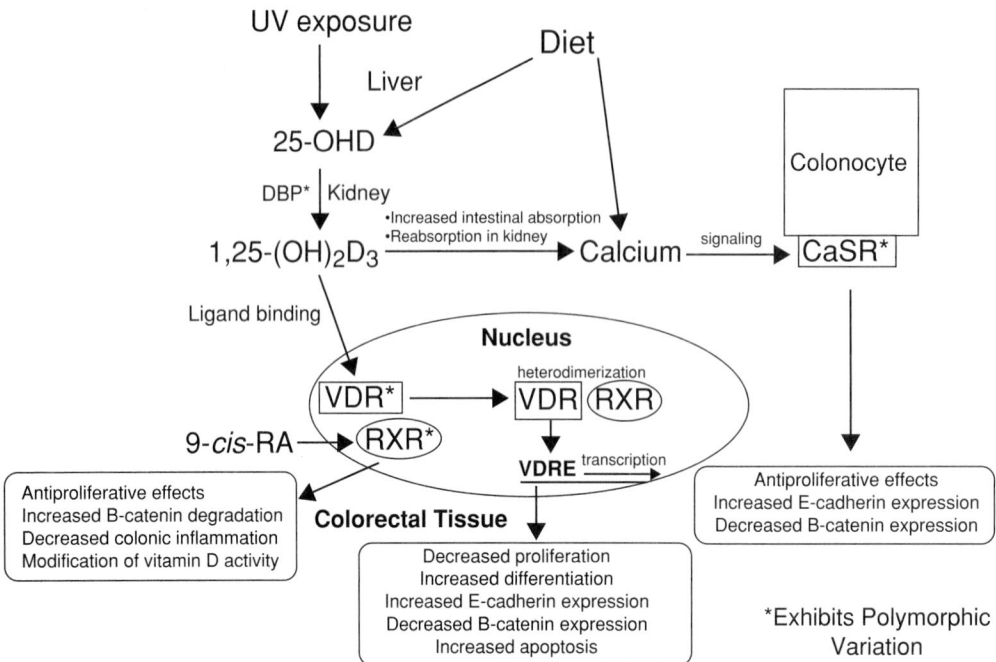

FIGURE 38.3. The intricate relationship between the effects of vitamin D, calcium, and 9-*cis*-retinoic acid (9-*cis*-RA) on tissues of the colorectum. UV, ultraviolet; 25-OHD, 25-dihydroxyvitamin D; DBP, vitamin D–binding protein; 1,25-(OH)$_2$D$_3$, 1,25-dihydroxyvitamin D$_3$; VDR, vitamin D receptor; RXR, retinoid X receptor, VDRE, vitamin D response element; CaSR, calcium-sensing receptor. *Source:* Reprinted from ref. 333, with permission.

vitamin D metabolite is 25-hydroxycholecalciferol (25-OHD), which can be used as a reliable marker for vitamin D status (235). In the kidney, 25-OHD is hydroxylated at the one-carbon position to form 1,25-dihydroxycholecalciferol [1,25-(OH)$_2$D$_3$] (235). This potent metabolite of vitamin D can exert transcriptional effects on target genes after binding with the nuclear VDR, a member of the steroid nuclear receptor superfamily (236). Although the classical role for vitamin D is the regulation of calcium homeostasis in the kidney and the intestine, there has recently been great interest in the potential use of vitamin D as a chemopreventive and/or chemotherapeutic agent. Ecologic studies indicate that colorectal cancer shares a geographic distribution with the primary disease of vitamin D deficiency, rickets (237). Among Caucasian men in the United States, death rates for colon cancer are significantly higher in northeastern regions compared to southern areas; these northeastern regions exhibit a 5-month "vitamin D winter," where exposure to sunlight is minimal and thus endogenous production of vitamin D is limited (237). Epidemiologic and clinical researchers have further investigated the potential association between vitamin D and risk of colorectal neoplasia. Low serum levels of 25-OHD were found to be significantly associated with risk of both colorectal adenoma (238) and cancer (239) in two cohort studies. Prospective studies have found an inverse nonsignificant association between dietary intake of vitamin D and colorectal adenomas or cancer (240–242), whereas some case-control studies have found no relationship (243,244). Prospective studies are less susceptible to study design-related biases, and the consistency of results from these investigations is remarkable. The apparent contradictions between case-control and prospective studies may also be partly the result of vitamin D assessment. Because vitamin D can be produced endogenously, it is important to include blood levels of vitamin D as an exposure measure in epidemiologic studies in addition to dietary data (245), although assays of vitamin D metabolites can be quite challenging and costly (245). The proposed

mechanisms of action for vitamin D with regard to colorectal neoplasia include its prodifferentiating and antiproliferative effects (246,247), possibly via G$_0$/G$_1$ cell cycle arrest (248,249), and induction of apoptosis (250,251).

Calcium. The mineral calcium has many metabolic roles in the human body, including its classical structural role in maintenance of the skeleton and teeth, as well as in signal transduction, muscle contraction, transmission of nerve impulses, and blood clotting. The major dietary sources of calcium in the United States are dairy products and grains (252). Calcium intake can be measured with dietary questionnaires, but estimations should include consideration of bioavailability of calcium from different food products and supplemental sources (245). After ingestion, calcium absorption can occur via an active transport process (transcellular) that requires the action of 1,25-(OH)$_2$D$_3$, or by passive diffusion (paracellular), a vitamin D-independent process. The vast majority of calcium absorption (77%–92%) relies on the transcellular pathway, and thus on the activity of 1,25-(OH)$_2$D$_3$ (253). Therefore, it is difficult to separately establish the potential effects of these two nutrients on health and disease, and it is of clear importance to evaluate the effects of these nutrients on disease risk simultaneously. As discussed previously, vitamin D has recently been investigated in relation to cancer risk, while a role for calcium in colorectal neoplasia has also been studied. There are several proposed mechanisms of action for calcium and the prevention of colorectal neoplasia, including the binding of bile acids (254,255), decreased fecal water cytotoxicity (256), inhibition of cellular proliferation (256,257), or induction of apoptosis.

Within clinical and epidemiologic studies, both dietary and supplemental calcium intake have been shown to be associated with a decreased risk of developing colorectal neoplasia. In a clinical trial conducted by Baron et al. (258), subjects assigned to daily supplementation with calcium carbonate had a significantly reduced risk of adenoma recurrence compared to the placebo group. In addition, there was an indication that the risk of developing a large adenoma might be decreased by the supplement (258). Further analyses of this clinical trial revealed that higher serum 25-OHD levels were associated with a protective effect for those in the calcium-supplemented group, although not for those in the placebo group (259), lending further support to the importance of the biological intricacies of these two nutrients in colorectal neoplasia (260). Published epidemiologic literature on the potential association between calcium and colorectal neoplasia is considerable. Martínez and Willett (261) reviewed the epidemiologic data published at the time and concluded that although calcium is not associated with a substantially decreased risk of colorectal neoplasia, a moderately protective calcium effect cannot be excluded, and that larger studies with repeated data measurements are required to elucidate this relationship. In addition, data from prospective studies in the literature from 1998 onward have shown a significantly decreased risk of either adenoma recurrence (241,258) or colorectal cancer (262–264) with increasing calcium intake. Because the effect of calcium may be more marked in the distal colon than in the proximal region (262), further clarification by colonic site is necessary, in addition to elucidation of any dose–response for calcium intake. On the whole, it appears that calcium does have a protective effect, but the magnitude and specificity of the effect is not yet clear and requires further study.

The most recent contribution to the calcium/vitamin D and colorectal neoplasia literature results from the WHI (265). In this randomized, double-blind placebo-controlled trial of 36,282 women, participants were assigned to a supplement of 500 mg of calcium carbonate plus 200 IU of vitamin D_3 twice daily or a placebo. The results showed that the intervention had no appreciable effect on colorectal cancer (OR, 1.08; 95% CI, 0.86–1.34). However, participants in the WHI had a mean daily intake of 1,151 mg of calcium and 367 IU of vitamin D (265). Given that any protective effect of calcium for colorectal cancer may plateau at 700 mg/day (262), it is possible that the WHI participants could not attain additional benefit from further supplementation from calcium. Thus, the WHI did not test an intervention in the setting of suboptimal calcium intake, which could explain the lack of efficacy in the findings. Furthermore, recent publications have suggested that intakes of vitamin D well in excess of the 400 IU/day administered in the WHI are necessary for optimal health (266). Of note, a nested case-control investigation of baseline 25-OHD levels within the WHI indicated that there was significant risk for colorectal cancer among those with lower serum 25-OHD (265). Therefore, although vitamin D appears to have a role in the development of colorectal neoplasia, supplementation at higher levels may be necessary. Further studies are ongoing to determine the optimal doses of calcium and vitamin D that are required for chemoprevention of colorectal adenomas and cancer.

Folate and One-Carbon Metabolism

Folate is a water-soluble B vitamin that functions as a coenzyme in single-carbon transfer in nucleic and amino acid metabolism. Low levels of this nutrient in the diet or blood have been shown to be associated with higher risk of colorectal cancer. A recent meta-analysis of the epidemiologic literature based on cohort studies showed a significant 25% lower risk of developing colorectal cancer among individuals in the highest compared to those in the lowest category of dietary folate (267). Although it has been proposed that supplemental sources of folate might confer greater protection than dietary sources due to the higher bioavailability of the synthetic form of folate found in supplements (268), results of the meta-analysis did not support this hypothesis. Inverse associations between blood folate and

colorectal neoplasia (i.e., cancer and adenoma) have also been shown (269–271). In further support of the protective effect of folate on colorectal neoplasia are the studies supporting its role in reducing risk of adenoma recurrence among individuals who have undergone polypectomy (271,272). Of interest, Martínez et al. (272) showed that higher plasma levels were associated with lower risk of adenoma recurrence primarily among individuals who did not report use of multivitamin supplements, which are a rich source of folic acid (272). The investigators further hypothesize that multivitamin supplements or supplemental folate primarily benefits individuals with low plasma folate levels. This finding has potential implications in the interpretation of results of recently completed trials of folic acid in the prevention of colorectal adenoma recurrence. Furthermore, as also noted in this publication (272), because fortification of the food supply has taken place in the United States and other countries, future intervention studies might need to be conducted in countries where such programs do not exist.

Mechanisms responsible for the protective effect of folate on risk of colorectal cancer are not entirely understood and may involve disturbances in DNA synthesis, methylation, and repair (273–275). Because folate is the primary methyl donor in cellular metabolism (276), markers of folate status are important factors in the etiology of DNA synthesis (277), possibly increasing spontaneous mutation rates (278), DNA methylation and DNA repair (279–281), and chromosome aberrations (281,282). It has also been hypothesized (283) that the increased risk associated with low folate levels is related to intracellular methylation defects. Animal studies also support a role for folate, where colon carcinogenesis is shown to be enhanced by dietary folate deficiency (284); however, these have generally dealt with highly deficient folate diets.

Studies involving associations of genetic polymorphisms in enzymes involved in the folate metabolic pathway could also be considered as supportive of a causal role between folate and colorectal neoplasia. In particular, a high degree of consistency exists in the published data supporting an association between colorectal cancer and a genetic polymorphism in the methylenetetrahydrofolate reductase (*MTHFR*) gene (285,286), a critical enzyme involved in the production of the form of folate that supplies the methyl group for methionine synthesis (287). *MTHFR* is involved in the irreversible conversion of 5,10-methylenetetrahydrofolate (5,10-MTHF) to 5-methyltetrahydrofolate (5-MTHF), which is the most abundant form of folate found in circulation. The C to T transition at base pair 677 results in low MTHFR enzyme activity. Furthermore, individuals with the *TT* genotype have lower plasma folate levels compared to those with the wild-type (*CC*) genotype (288). Studies that have assessed the effect modification between *MTHFR* and folate status show that the highest risk of colorectal neoplasia is found among individuals with low folate intake and the *MTHFR TT* variant (289–294). In addition, an interaction between the *MTHFR TT* variant and alcohol consumption, a folate antagonist, in relation to colorectal adenomas has been demonstrated (295). Based on these findings, the authors suggest that individuals with the homozygous *TT* variant appear to be particularly sensitive to folate and alcohol such that those with high folate levels and low alcohol consumption have low risk of colorectal neoplasia but those with low folate and high alcohol intakes are at high risk.

Additional dietary factors involved in one-carbon metabolism and the folate-colorectal neoplasia pathway include methionine and other B vitamins. Furthermore, as previously noted, because alcohol is a folate antagonist (296), its role in the pathway is also critical. Published data support the modifying effect of folate and methionine on the alcohol and colorectal neoplasia relationship (283,285,286,297). The importance of one-carbon metabolism in the context of colorectal neoplasia has to do with the critical role of this pathway in nucleotide synthesis and DNA methylation. Methionine, which can be directly converted to S-adenosylmethionine (298), has been shown to be inversely associated with risk of colon cancer or adenoma (63,171–173,196,283,299–303).

Data on the association between vitamins B_6 and B_{12} and the risk of colorectal neoplasia are sparse and inconsistent (244,286,304,305). However, results of two recent studies support an inverse association between B_6 and colorectal cancer and adenoma (271,306). Vitamin B_6 is involved in the regeneration of 5,10-MTHF, which is involved in the conversion of uracil to thymidylate; deficiencies in 5,10-MTHF can result in misincorporation of uracil instead of thymidylate in DNA, which in turn can lead to chromosomal instability (307). In one of these studies (306), significantly lower risk of developing colorectal cancer and adenoma was shown among individuals with higher plasma levels of pyridoxal 5′-phosphate, the circulating form of vitamin B_6, compared to those with lower levels. In the second study (271), higher intake of vitamin B_6 was associated with lower risk of colorectal adenoma recurrence.

The role of folate and other factors involved in one-carbon metabolism in the etiology of colorectal neoplasia will no doubt continue to be investigated. Existing literature so far underscores the importance of considering complex interactions and biological pathways when assessing cancer risk. Furthermore, results of recently completed trials of the effect of folic acid on adenoma recurrence might help further elucidate this active area of research. However, these will have to be interpreted within the context of the study design used to test the hypothesis and the implementation of folic acid fortification of the food supply.

Fiber and Fiber Sources

In 1971, Burkitt proposed that high fiber intake could be protective for colon cancer, based on the very low rates of this malignancy observed in Africa, where high quantities of fiber were consumed (308). Since then, there has been much investigation into the potential protective effect of fiber on colorectal neoplasia, and several mechanisms have been proposed to describe this association. These include inhibition of nitrosamine formation, provision of substrate for formation of antineoplastic agents, dilution and binding of carcinogens, alteration of hormone metabolism, antioxidant effects, and the induction of detoxification enzymes by cruciferous vegetables (309).

Early epidemiologic studies found that high consumption of fruit and vegetables was associated with a decreased risk of colorectal cancer (162–164,184,186,188–191,195,310–315). This evidence, however, is largely based on data from case-control studies. Trock et al. (316) conducted a pooled analysis of six case-control studies and found a high intake of vegetables was associated with an OR for colon cancer of 0.48 (95% CI, 0.41–0.57) and a weaker inverse association with fiber (OR, 0.58 for upper vs. lower categories). More recent results of published epidemiologic studies of fruits, vegetables, and colorectal neoplasia have been more equivocal, with some prospective or clinical studies showing protection (317,318), but several others not (319–325).

Foods high in fiber have also been shown to be inversely associated with colon cancer risk in most (56,59,62,65,162,166, 184,191,312,326), but not all (157,160,164,170,193), studies. A pooled analysis of 13 case-control studies (327) found a lower risk associated with higher fiber intake (OR, 0.53 for upper vs. lower quintile). In contrast, large prospective studies have shown weak or nonexistent inverse associations for fiber and risk of colon cancer. Furthermore, the results of two large, randomized clinical trials failed to show protection from recurrent adenomas with increased fiber and/or decreased fat in the diet (328,329). In the Polyp Prevention Trial (PPT), there

was no reduction in risk of colorectal adenoma recurrence with consumption of a low-fat, high-fiber diet (329). In the Wheat Bran Fiber (WBF) trial, there was no difference in the rate of recurrent adenomatous polyps between those randomized to consume a high-fiber supplement as compared to those in the low-fiber group (328). Furthermore, the results of a large pooling project that included data from a total of 13 prospective cohort studies failed to find a significant protective effect of fiber in analyses adjusted for other risk factors (330). Conversely, two recent reports from large, prospective investigations found that increased fiber intake was significantly associated with reduced risk for colorectal adenomas (318) and cancer (317). Thus, the true relationship between fiber and colorectal neoplasia remains elusive, but there are several possible explanations for the apparently conflicting results observed in these investigations. These include errors in exposure measurement, the presence of unaddressed confounding factors, and variable outcome measurements. In addition, there may be gender differences in the response to fiber, as shown when the study populations of the PPT and the WBF were combined and assessed for a fiber effect on colorectal adenoma recurrence (331). A reduced risk for adenoma recurrence was observed for men in the pooled population (OR, 0.81; 95% CI, 0.67–0.98), but not for women (OR, 1.13; 95% CI, 0.87–1.48) (331). Overall, the relationship between fiber intake and risk for colorectal neoplasia remains equivocal, despite the completion of several large studies. However, because fiber appears to be a safe and potentially chemopreventive agent, there seems to be little risk in adding more fiber to the diet.

FUTURE RESEARCH

The understanding of the environmental and lifestyle factors involved in the development of colorectal neoplasia continues to improve via extensive epidemiologic and laboratory investigations. Improvements in the understanding of the molecular events underlying this disease continue at a rapid pace. As the molecular biology of this disease becomes better understood and discoveries of modifiable factors continue to be made, there is potential for also understanding important mechanisms by which these factors may influence risk.

Traditionally, epidemiologic research has focused on studies related to the etiology of cancer, referred to as primary prevention, and much work has been done in this area. In secondary prevention, the main focus is on early detection of disease so neoplastic development is halted during the stage of the precursor lesion. At present, the best hope for colorectal cancer prevention is secondary: identification and ablation of adenomatous polyps through the use of colonoscopic examinations. However, given that only approximately 33% of the U. S. population 50 years of age and older reported screening by sigmoidoscopy (332), primary prevention continues to remain an important avenue for decreasing the public health burden of this malignancy. In tertiary prevention, the goal is the reduction of the risk of unfavorable clinical outcomes, such as recurrence or death. The assessment of lifestyle and environmental factors in studies of secondary and tertiary prevention can be of valuable importance in understanding the disease process. Nesting these analyses in ongoing and completed chemoprevention and treatment trials will be of extreme importance in this effort.

To date, physical inactivity is considered to be the most consistent risk factor for colon cancer. In addition, a low intake of folate, possibly in combination with excess alcohol consumption, and smoking early in life are likely to increase risk. Additional dietary and nutritional factors, such as energy intake; red meat consumption; and calcium, vitamin D, and selenium intake are potentially important. The role of fiber in colorectal neoplasia remains equivocal even after the completion of large clinical and prospective cohort studies.

Future studies will continue to link certain lifestyle characteristics to specific genetic alterations, potentially enhancing our ability to reach firm conclusions from epidemiologic investigations where one or more dietary and lifestyle factors are likely to have a major impact on colorectal cancer. However, even with technologies such as genomics and proteomics, many challenges lie ahead for identifying useful genetic modifiers of environmental effects on the colorectum. The use of pathway approaches for studying the effects of multiple genes and their interactions with lifestyle characteristics may help clarify some of these relationships; however, reliable statistical methods for analyzing these pathways are still in developmental stages.

References

1. Parkin DM, Bray F, Ferlay J, Pisani P. Global cancer statistics, 2002. *CA Cancer J Clin* 2005;55:74–108.
2. World Health Organization, International Agency for Research on Cancer. *Trends in Cancer Incidence and Mortality*. IARC Scientific Publication No. 121. Lyon, France: 1993.
3. Jemal A, Siegel R, Ward E, et al. Cancer statistics, 2006. *CA Cancer J Clin* 2006;56:106–130.
4. Chao A, Gilliland FD, Hunt WC, Bulterys M, Becker TM, Key CR. Increasing incidence of colon and rectal cancer among Hispanics and American Indians in New Mexico (United States), 1969–94. *Cancer Causes Control* 1998;9:137–144.
5. Cress RD, Morris CR, Wolfe BM. Cancer of the colon and rectum in California: trends in incidence by race/ethnicity, stage, and subsite. *Prev Med* 2000;31:447–453.
6. Greenlee RT, Murray T, Bolden S, Wingo PA. Cancer statistics, 2000. *CA Cancer J Clin* 2000;50:7–33.
7. Parkin DM, Pisani P, Ferlay J. Global cancer statistics. *CA Cancer J Clin* 1999;49:33–64.
8. Clegg LX, Li FP, Hankey BF, Chu K, Edwards BK. Cancer survival among US whites and minorities: a SEER (Surveillance, Epidemiology, and End Results) program population-based study. *Arch Intern Med* 2002;162:1985–1993.
9. American Cancer Society. *Arizona Cancer Facts and Figures 2004–2005: A Sourcebook for Planning and Implementing Programs for Cancer Prevention and Control*. Phoenix, Ariz.: American Cancer Society, Great West Division, Inc.; 2005. Available at: http://www.org/downloads/COM/AZ%20Facts%20and%20Figuresletter.pdf.Accessed May 8, 2007.
10. Chien C, Morimoto LM, Tom J, Li CI. Differences in colorectal carcinoma stage and survival by race and ethnicity. *Cancer* 2005;104:629–639.
11. Mallin K, Anderson K. Cancer mortality in Illinois Mexican and Puerto Rican immigrants, 1979–1984. *Int J Cancer* 1988;41:670–676.
12. Stemmermann GN, Nomura AMY, Chyou P-H, Kato I, Kuroishi T. Cancer incidence in Hawaiian Japanese: migrants from Okinawa compared with those from other prefectures. *Jpn J Cancer Res* 1991;82:1366–1370.
13. Tyczynski J, Tarkowski W, Parkin DM, Zatonski W. Cancer mortality among Polish migrants to Australia. *Eur J Cancer* 1994;30A:478–484.
14. Nilsson B, Gustavson-Kadaka E, Totstein S, Hakulinen T, Rahu M, Aareleid T. Cancer incidence in Estonian migrants to Sweden. *Int J Cancer* 1993;55:190–195.
15. Grulich AE, McCredie M, Coates M. Cancer incidence in Asian migrants to New South Wales, Australia. *Br J Cancer* 1995;71:400–408.
16. Khlat M. Cancer in Mediterranean migrants—based on studies in France and Australia. *Cancer Causes Control* 1995;6:525–531.
17. Swerdlow AJ, Marmot MG, Grulich AE, Head J. Cancer mortality in Indian and British ethnic immigrants from the Indian subcontinent to England and Wales. *Br J Cancer* 1995;72:1312–1319.
18. Iscovich J, Howe GR. Cancer incidence patterns (1972–91). *Cancer Causes Control* 1998;9:29–36.
19. Morson BC. Evolution of cancer of the colon and rectum. *Cancer* 1974;34(suppl):845–849.
20. Markowitz AJ, Winawer SJ. Management of colorectal polyps. *CA Cancer J Clin* 1997;47:93–112.
21. Peipins LA, Sandler RS. Epidemiology of colorectal adenomas. *Epidemiol Rev* 1994;16:273–297.
22. Armstrong B, Doll R. Environmental factors and cancer incidence and mortality in different countries, with special reference to dietary practices. *Int J Cancer* 1975;15:617–631.
23. Rose DP, Boyar AP, Wynder EL. International comparisons of mortality rates for cancer of the breast, ovary, prostate, and colon, and per capita food consumption. *Cancer* 1986;58:2263–2271.
24. Shinchi K, Kono S, Honjo S, et al. Obesity and adenomatous polyps of the sigmoid colon. *Jpn J Cancer Res* 1994;85:479–484.
25. Giovannucci E, Ascherio A, Rimm EB, Colditz GA, Stampfer MJ, Willett WC. Physical activity, obesity, and risk of colon cancer and adenoma in men. *Ann Intern Med* 1995;122:327–334.
26. Kono S, Handa K, Hayabuchi H, et al. Obesity, weight gain and risk of colon adenomas in Japanese men. *Jpn J Cancer Res* 1999;90:805–811.
27. Terry MB, Neugut AI, Bostick RM, et al. Risk factors for advanced colorectal adenomas: a pooled analysis. *Cancer Epidemiol Biomarkers Prev* 2002;11:622–629.
28. Moller H, Mellemgaard A, Lindvig K, Olsen JH. Obesity and cancer risk: a Danish record-linkage study. *Eur J Cancer* 1994;30A:344–350.
29. Murphy TK, Calle EE, Rodriguez C, Kahn HS, Thun MJ. Body mass index and colon cancer mortality in a large prospective study. *Am J Epidemiol* 2000;152:847–854.
30. Moore LL, Bradlee ML, Singer MR, et al. BMI and waist circumference as predictors of lifetime colon cancer risk in Framingham Study adults. *Int J Obes Relat Metab Disord* 2004;28:559–567.
31. Rapp K, Schroeder J, Klenk J, et al. Obesity and incidence of cancer: a large cohort study of over 145,000 adults in Austria. *Br J Cancer* 2005;93:1062–1067.
32. Giovannucci E, Colditz GA, Stampfer MJ, Willett WC. Physical activity, obesity, and risk of colorectal adenoma in women (United States). *Cancer Causes Control* 1996;7:253–263.
33. Lin J, Zhang SM, Cook NR, Rexrode KM, Lee IM, Buring JE. Body mass index and risk of colorectal cancer in women (United States). *Cancer Causes Control* 2004;15:581–589.
34. Lew EA, Garfinkel L. Variations in mortality by weight among 750,000 men and women. *J Chronic Dis* 1979;32:563–576.
35. Phillips RL, Snowdon DA. Dietary relationships with fatal colorectal cancer among Seventh–Day Adventists. *J Natl Cancer Inst* 1985;74:307–317.
36. Shike M. Body weight and colon cancer. *Am J Clin Nutr* 1996;63:442S–444S.
37. Russo A, Franceschi S, La Vecchia C, et al. Body size and colorectal–cancer risk. *Int J Cancer* 1998;78:161–165.
38. Terry P, Giovannucci E, Bergkvist L, Holmberg L, Wolk A. Body weight and colorectal cancer risk in a cohort of Swedish women: relation varies by age and cancer site. *Br J Cancer* 2001;85:346–349.
39. Terry PD, Miller AB, Rohan TE. Obesity and colorectal cancer risk in women. *Gut* 2001;51:191–194.
40. Slattery ML, Ballard-Barbash R, Edwards S, Caan BJ, Potter JD. Body mass index and colon cancer: an evaluation of the modifying effects of estrogen (United States). *Cancer Causes Control* 2003;14:75–84.
41. Martinez ME, Giovannucci E, Spiegelman D, Hunter DJ, Willett WC, Colditz GA. Leisure–time physical activity, body size, and colon cancer in women. Nurses' Health Study Research Group. *J Natl Cancer Inst* 1997;89:948–955.
42. Macinnis RJ, English DR, Hopper JL, Gertig DM, Haydon AM, Giles GG. Body size and composition and colon cancer risk in women. *Int J Cancer* 2006;118:1496–1500.
43. Caan BJ, Coates AO, Slattery ML, Potter JD, Quesenberry CP, Jr., Edwards SM. Body size and the risk of colon cancer in a large case-control study. *Int J Obes Relat Metab Disord* 1998;22:178–184.
44. Hou L, Ji BT, Blair A, et al. Body mass index and colon cancer risk in Chinese people: menopause as an effect modifier. *Eur J Cancer* 2006;42:84–90.
45. Wu AH, Paganini-Hill A, Ross RK, Henderson BE. Alcohol, physical activity and other risk factors for colorectal cancer: a prospective study. *Br J Cancer* 1987;55:687–694.
46. Lee I, Paffenbarger R, Hsieh C. Physical activity and risk of developing colorectal cancer among college alumni. *J Natl Cancer Inst* 1991;83:1324–1329.
47. Thun MJ, Calle EE, Namboodiri MM, et al. Risk factors for fatal colon cancer in a large prospective study. *J Natl Cancer Inst* 1992;84:1491–1500.
48. Ballard–Barbash R, Schatzkin A, Albanes D, et al. Physical activity and risk of large bowel cancer in the Framingham Study. *Cancer Res* 1990;50:3610–3613.
49. Albanes D, Blair A, Taylor PR. Physical activity and risk of cancer in the NHANES I population. *Am J Public Health* 1989;79:744–750.
50. Severson RK, Nomura AMY, Grove JS, Stemmerman GN. A prospective analysis of physical activity and cancer. *Am J Epidemiol* 1989;130:522–529.
51. Lynge E, Thygesen L. Use of surveillance system for occupational cancer: data from the Danish national system. *Int J Epidemiol* 1988;17:493–500.
52. Gerhardsson de Verdier M, Floderus B, Norell SE. Physical activity and colon cancer risk. *Int J Epidemiol* 1988;17:743–746.
53. Paffenbarger RSJ, Hyde RT, Wing AL. Physical activity and incidence of cancer in diverse populations: a preliminary report. *Am J Clin Nutr* 1987;45(suppl):312–317.
54. Gerhardsson l, Norell S, Kiviranta H, Pedersen N, Ahlbom A. Sedentary jobs and colon cancer. *Am J Epidemiol* 1986;123:775–780.
55. Thune I, Lung E. Physical activity and risk of colorectal cancer in men and women. *Br J Cancer* 1996;73:1134–1140.
56. Whittemore AS, Wu-Williams AH, Lee M, et al. Diet, physical activity and colorectal cancer among Chinese in North America and China. *J Natl Cancer Inst* 1990;82:915–926.
57. Kune G, Kune S, Wason L. Body weight and physical activity as predictors of colorectal cancer risk. *Nutr Cancer* 1990;13:9–17.

58. Markowitz S, Morabia A, Garibaldi K, Wynder E. Effect of occupational and recreational activity on the risk of colorectal cancer among males: a case-control study. *Int J Epidemiol* 1992;21:1057–1062.

59. Slattery ML, Schumacher MC, Smith KR, West DW, Abd–Elghany N. Physical activity, diet, and risk of colon cancer in Utah. *Am J Epidemiol* 1988;128:989–999.

60. Peters RK, Garabrandt DH, Yu MC, Mack TM. A case-control study of occupational and dietary factors in colorectal cancer in young men by subsite. *Cancer Res* 1989;49:5459–5468.

61. Brownson RC, Zahm SH, Chang JC, Blair A. Occupational risk of colon cancer: an analysis of anatomic subsite. *Am J Epidemiol* 1989;130:675–687.

62. Benito E, Obrador A, Stiggelbout A, et al. A population-based case-control study of colorectal cancer in Majorca. I. Dietary factors. *Int J Cancer* 1990;45:69–76.

63. Kato I, Tominaga S, Matsuura A, Yoshii Y, Shirarai M, Kobayashi S. A comparative case-control study of colorectal cancer and adenoma. *Jpn J Cancer* 1990;82:915–926.

64. Kato I, Tominaga S, Ikari A. A case-control study of male colorectal cancer in Aichi Prefecture, Japan: with special reference to occupational activity level, drinking habits and family history. *Jpn J Cancer Res* 1990;81:115–121.

65. Gerhardsson de Verdier M, Hagman U, Steineck G, et al. Diet, body mass and colorectal cancer: a case-referent study. *Int J Cancer* 1990;46:832–838.

66. Fredriksson M, Bengtsson NO, Hardell L, Axelson O. Colon cancer, physical activity, and occupational exposure. *Cancer* 1989;63:1838–1842.

67. Fraser G, Pearce N. Occupational physical activity and risk of cancer of the colon and rectum in New Zealand males. *Cancer Causes Control* 1993;4:45–50.

68. Slattery M, Abd-Elghany N, Kerber R, Schumacher M. Physical activity and colon cancer: a comparison of various indicators of physical activity to evaluate the association. *Epidemiology* 1990;1:481–485.

69. Longnecker M, Gerhardsson de Verdier M, Frumkin H, Carpenter C. A case-control study of physical activity in relation to risk of cancer of the right colon and rectum. *Int J Epidemiol* 1995;24:42–50.

70. Chow WH, Dosemeci M, Zheng W, et al. Physical activity and occupational risk of colon cancer in Shanghai, China. *Int J Epidemiol* 1993;22:23–29.

71. Arbman G, Axelson O, Fredriksson M, Nilsson E, Sjodahl R. Do occupational factors influence the risk of colon and rectal cancer in different ways? *Cancer* 1993;72:22543–22549.

72. Gerhardsson de Verdier M, Steineck G, Hagman U, Rieger A, Norrell S. Physical activity and colon cancer: a case–referent study in Stockholm. *Int J Cancer* 1990;46:985–999.

73. Vineis P, Ciccone G, Magnino A. Asbestos exposure, physical activity, and colon cancer: a case–control study. *Tumori* 1993;79:301–303.

74. Vlajinac H, Jarebinski M, Adanja B. Relationship of some biosocial factors to colon cancer in Belgrade. *Neoplasma* 1987;34:503–507.

75. Dosemeci M, Hayes R, Vetter R, et al. Occupational physical activity, socioeconomic status, and risk of 15 cancer sites in Turkey. *Cancer Causes Control* 1993;4:313–321.

76. Marcus P, Newcomb P, Storer B. Early adulthood physical activity and colon cancer risk among Wisconsin women. *Cancer Epidemiol Biomarkers Prev* 1994;3:641–644.

77. White E, Jacobs EJ, Daling JR. Physical activity in relation to colon cancer in middle–aged men and women. *Am J Epidemiol* 1996;144:42–50.

78. Vena JE, Graham S, Zielezny M, Swanson MK, Barnes RE, Nolan J. Lifetime occupational exercise and colon cancer. *Am J Epidemiol* 1985;122:357–365.

79. Garabrant DH, Peters JM, Mack TM, Berstein L. Job activity and colon cancer risk. *Am J Epidemiol* 1984;119:1005–1014.

80. Slattery M, Potter J, Caan B, et al. Energy balance and colon cancer—beyond physical activity. *Cancer Res* 1997;57:75–80.

81. Colditz GA, Cannuscio CC, Frazier AL. Physical activity and reduced risk of colon cancer: implications for prevention. *Cancer Causes Control* 1997;8:649–667.

82. Samad AK, Taylor RS, Marshall T, Chapman MA. A meta-analysis of the association of physical activity with reduced risk of colorectal cancer. *Colorectal Dis* 2005;7:204–213.

83. Karmali RA. Prostaglandins and cancer. *CA Cancer J Clin* 1983;33:322–332.

84. Bennett A, Del Tacca M. Prostaglandins in human colonic carcinoma. *Gut* 1975;16:409.

85. Bennett A, Del Tacca M, Stamford IF, Zebro T. Prostaglandins from tumours of human large bowel. *Br J Cancer* 1977;35:881–884.

86. Jaffe BM, Parker CW, Philpott GW. Immunochemical measurement of prostaglandin or prostaglandin-like activity from normal and neoplastic cultured tissue. *Surg Forum* 1971;22:90–92.

87. Martinez ME, Heddens D, Earnest DL, et al. Physical activity, body mass index, and PGE2 levels in rectal mucosa. *J Natl Cancer Inst* 1999;91:950–953.

88. Bartram HP, Wynder EL. Physical activity and colon cancer risk? Physiological considerations. *Am J Gastroenterol* 1989;84:109–112.

89. Frezza EE, Wachtel M, Chiriva-Internati M. Influence of obesity on the risk of developing colon cancer. *Gut* 2006;55:285–291.

90. Chute CG, Willett WC, Colditz GA, Stampfer MJ, Rosner B, Speizer FE. A prospective study of reproductive history and exogenous estrogens on the risk of colorectal cancer in women. *Epidemiology* 1991;2:201–207.

91. Davis FG, Furner SE, Persky V, Koch M. The influence of parity and exogenous female hormones on the risk of colorectal cancer. *Int J Cancer* 1989;43:587–590.

92. Furner SE, Davis GD, Nelson RL, Haenszel W. A case-control study of large bowel cancer and hormone exposure in women. *Cancer Res* 1989;49:4936–4940.

93. Gerhardsson de Verdier M, London S. Reproductive factors, exogenous female hormones, and colorectal cancer by subsite. *Cancer Causes Control* 1992;3:355–360.

94. Jacobs EJ, White E, Weiss NS. Exogenous hormones, reproductive history, and colon cancer. *Cancer Causes Control* 1995;5:359–366.

95. Calle EE, Miracle-McMahill HL, Thun MJ, Heath CW. Estrogen replacement therapy and risk of fatal colon cancer in a prospective cohort of postmenopausal women. *J Natl Cancer Inst* 1995;87:517–523.

96. Dietz AT, Newcomb PA, Marcus PM, Strer BE. The association of body size and large bowel cancer risk in Wisconsin (United States) women. *Cancer Causes Control* 1995;6:30–36.

97. Newcomb PA, Storer BE. Postmenopausal hormone use and risk of large bowel cancer. *J Natl Cancer Inst* 1995;87:1967–1071.

98. Folsom AR, Mink PJ, Sellers TA, Hong CP, Zheng W, Potter JD. Hormone replacement therapy and morbidity and mortality in a prospective study of postmenopausal women. *Am J Public Health* 1995;1995:1128–1132.

99. Fernandez E, La Vecchia C, A'Avanzo B, Franceschi S, Negri E, Parazzini F. Oral contraceptives, hormone replacement therapy and the risk of colorectal cancer. *Br J Cancer* 1996;73:1431–1436.

100. Weiss NS, Daling JR, Chow WH. Incidence of cancer of the large bowel in women in relation to reproductive and hormonal factors. *J Natl Cancer Inst* 1981;67:57–60.

101. Risch HA, Howe GR. Menopausal hormone use and colorectal cancer in Saskatchewan: a record linkage cohort study. *Cancer Epidemiol Biomarkers Prev* 1995;4:21–28.

102. Peters RK, Pike MC, Chang WWL, Mack MT. Reproductive factors and colon cancer. *Br J Cancer* 1990;61:741–748.

103. Troisi R, Schairer C, Chow W-H, Schatzkin A, Brinton LA, Fraumeni JF. A prospective study of menopausal hormones and risk of colorectal cancer. *Cancer Causes Control* 1997;8:130–138.

104. Kampman E, Potter JD, Slattery ML, Caan BJ, Edwards S. Hormone replacement therapy, reproductive history, and colon cancer: a multicenter, case–control study in the United States. *Cancer Causes Control* 1997;8:146–158.

105. Grodstein F, Martinez ME, Platz EA, et al. Postmenopausal hormone use and risk of colorectal cancer and adenoma. *Ann Intern Med* 1998;128:705–712.

106. Howell M. The association between colorectal cancer and breast cancer. *J Chronic Dis* 1976;29:243–261.

107. Boyle P, Robertson C. Breast cancer and colon cancer incidence in females in Scotland, 1960–1984. *J Natl Cancer Inst* 1987;79:1175–1179.

108. La Vecchia C, Decarli A. Correlations between cancer mortality rates from various Italian regions. *Tumori* 1985;71:441–448.

109. Issa JP, Ottaviano YL, Celano P, Hamilton SR, Davidson NE, Baylin SB. Methylation of the estrogen receptor CpG island links aging and neoplasia in human colon. *Nat Genet* 1994;7:536–540.

110. Chlebowski RT, Wactawski-Wende J, Ritenbaugh C, et al. Estrogen plus progestin and colorectal cancer in postmenopausal women. *N Engl J Med* 2004;350:991–1004.

111. Hulley SB, Grady D. The WHI estrogen-alone trial—do things look any better? *JAMA* 2004;291:1769–1771.

112. Nelson HD, Humphrey LL, Nygren P, Teutsch SM, Allan JD. Postmenopausal hormone replacement therapy: scientific review. *JAMA* 2002;288:872–881.

113. Giovannucci E, Martz ME. Tobacco, colorectal cancer, and adenomas: a review of the evidence. *J Natl Cancer Inst* 1996;88:1717–1730.

114. Giovannucci E, Rimm EB, Stampfer MJ, et al. A prospective study of cigarette smoking and risk of colorectal adenoma and colorectal cancer in U.S. men. *J Natl Cancer Inst* 1994;86:183–191.

115. Giovannucci E, Colditz GA, Stampfer MJ, et al. A prospective study of cigarette smoking and risk of colorectal adenoma and colorectal cancer in U.S. women. *J Natl Cancer Inst* 1994;86:192–199.

116. Slattery ML, West DW, Robison LM, et al. Tobacco, alcohol, coffee, and caffeine as risk factors for colon cancer in a low–risk population. *Epidemiology* 1990;1:141–145.

117. Heineman EF, Zahm SH, McLaughlin JK, Vaught JB. Increased risk of colorectal cancer among smokers: results of a 26-year follow-up of US veterans and a review. *Int J Cancer* 1995;59:728–738.

118. Newcomb PA, Storer BE, Marcus PM. Cigarette smoking in relation to risk of large bowel cancer in women. *Cancer Res* 1995;55:4906–4909

119. Slattery ML, Potter JD, Friedman GD, Ma K-N, Edwards S. Tobacco use and colon cancer. *Int J Cancer* 1997;70:259–264.

120. Hsing AW, McLaughlin JK, Chow W-H, et al. Risk factors for colorectal cancer in a prospective study among U.S. white men. *Int J Cancer* 1998;77:549–553.

121. Knekt P, Hakama M, Jrvinen R, Pukkala E, Helivaara M. Smoking and risk of colorectal cancer. *Br J Cancer* 1998;78:136–139.

122. Le Marchand L, Wilkens LR, Kolonel LN, Hankin JH, Lyu L-C. Associations of sedentary lifestyle, obesity, smoking, alcohol use, and diabetes with the risk of colorectal cancer. *Cancer Res* 1997;57:4787–4794.

123. Yamada K, Araki S, Tamura M, et al. Case-control study of colorectal carcinoma in situ and cancer in relation to cigarette smoking and alcohol use (Japan). *Cancer Causes Control* 1997;8:780–785.

124. Chyou P-H, Nomura AMY, Stemmermann GN. A prospective study of colon and rectal cancer among Hawaii Japanese men. *Ann Epidemiol* 1996; 6;276–282.

125. Freedman AN, Michalek AM, Marshall JR, et al. The relationship between smoking exposure and p53 overexpression in colorectal cancer. *Genet Epidemiol* 1995;12:333.

126. Baron JA, Gerhardsson de Verdier M, Ekbom A. Coffee, tea, tobacco, and cancer of the large bowel. *Cancer Epidemiol Biomarkers Prev* 1994;3:565–570.

127. Nordlund LA, Carstensen JM, Pershagen G. Cancer incidence in female smokers: a 26-year follow-up. *Int J Cancer* 1997;73:625–628.

128. Nyrén O, Bergström R, Nyström L, et al. Smoking and colorectal cancer: a 20-year follow-up study of Swedish construction workers. *J Natl Cancer Inst* 1996;88:1302–1307.

129. Tavani A, Pregnolato A, La Vecchia C, Negri E, Talamini R, Franceschi S. Coffee and tea intake and risk of cancers of the colon and rectum: a study of 3,530 cases and 7,057 controls. *Int J Cancer* 1997;73:193–197.

130. Giovannucci E. An updated review of the epidemiological evidence that cigarette smoking increases risk of colorectal cancer. *Cancer Epidemiol Biomarkers Prev* 2001;10:725–731.

131. Heineman EF, Zahm SH, McLaughlin JK, Vaught JB. Increased risk of colorectal cancer among smokers: results of a 26-year follow-up of US veterans and a review. *Int J Cancer* 1994;59:728–738.

132. Thun MJ, Henley SJ, Patrono C. Nonsteroidal anti-inflammatory drugs as anticancer agents: mechanistic, pharmacologic, and clinical issues. *J Natl Cancer Inst* 2002;94:252–266.

133. Kune GA, Kune S, Watson LF. Colorectal cancer risk, chronic illnesses, operations, and medications: case control results from the Melbourne Colorectal Cancer Study. *Cancer Res* 1988;48:4399–4404.

134. Rosenberg L, Palmer JR, Zauber AG, Warshauer ME, Stolley PD, Shapiro SA. A hypothesis: nonsteroidal anti-inflammatory drugs reduce the incidence of large-bowel cancer. *J Natl Cancer Inst* 1991;83:355–358.

135. Thun MJ, Namboodiri MM, Heath CW. Aspirin use and reduced risk of fatal colon cancer. *N Engl J Med* 1991;325:1593–1596.

136. Giovannucci E, Rimm EB, Stampfer MJ, Colditz GA, Ascherio A, Willett WC. Aspirin use and the risk of colorectal cancer and adenoma in male health professionals. *Ann Intern Med* 1994;121:241–246.

137. Giovannucci E, Egan KM, Hunter DJ, et al. Aspirin use and risk of colorectal cancer in women. *N Engl J Med* 1995;333:609–614.

138. Narisawa T, Sato M, Tani M, Kudo T, Takahashi T, Goto A. Inhibition of development of methylnitrosourea-induced rat colon tumors by indomethacin. *Cancer Res* 1981;41:1954–1957.

139. Pollard M, Luckert PH. Effect of piroxicam in primary intestinal tumors induced in rats by N-methylnitrosourea. *Cancer Lett* 1984;25:117–121.

140. Reddy BS, Maruyama H, Kelloff G. Dose related inhibition of colon *Carcinogenesis* by dietary piroxicam, a nonsteroidal antiinflammatory drug, during different stages of rat colon tumor development. *Cancer Res* 1987;47:534–536.

141. Moorghen M, Ince P, Finney KJ, Sunter JP, Appleton DR, Watson AJ. A protective effect of sulindac against chemically-induced primary colonic tumors in mice. *J Pathol* 1988;156:341–347.

142. Rigau J, Pique JM, Rubio E, Planas R, Tarrech JM, Bordas JM. Effect of long-term sulindac therapy on colonic polyposis. *Ann Intern Med* 1991; 115:952–954.

143. Labayle D, Fischer D, Vielh P, et al. Sulindac causes regression of rectal polyps in familial adenomatous polyposis. *Gastroenterology* 1991;101:635–639.

144. Giardiello FM, Hamilton SR, Krush AJ, et al. Treatment of colonic and rectal adenomas with sulindac in familial adenomatous polyposis. *N Engl J Med* 1993;328:1313–1316.

145. Laasko M, Mutru O, Isomaki H, Koota K. Cancer mortality in patients with rheumatoid arthritis. *J Rheumatol* 1986;13:522–526.

146. Gridley G, McLaughlin JK, Ekbom A, et al. Incidence of cancer among patients with rheumatoid arthritis. *J Natl Cancer Inst* 1993;85:307–311.

147. Paganini-Hill A, Chao A, Ross RK, Henderson BE. Aspirin use and chronic diseases: a cohort study of the elderly. *Br Med J* 1989;299:1247–1250.

148. Baron JA, Cole B, Sander RS, et al. A randomized trial of aspirin as a chemo-preventive agent against colorectal adenomas. *N Engl J Med* 2003;348:891–899.

149. Fitzgerald GA. Coxibs and cardiovascular disease. *N Engl J Med* 2004; 351:1709–1711.

150. Wynder EL, Gori GB. Contribution of the environment to cancer incidence: an epidemiologic exercise. *J Natl Cancer Inst* 1977;58:825–832.

151. Doll R, Peto R. The causes of cancer: quantitative estimates of avoidable risks of cancer in the United States today. *J Natl Cancer Inst* 1981;66:1191–1308.

152. Marshall JR, Hastrup JL. Mismeasurement and resonance of strong confounders: uncorrelated errors. *Am J Epidemiol* 1996;143:1069–1078.

153. Marshall JR, Hastrup JL, Ross JS. Mismeasurement and the resonance of strong confounders: correlated errors. *Am J Epidemiol* 1999;150:88–96.

154. Willett WC, Sampson L, Stampfer MJ, et al. Reproducibility and validity of a semiquantitative food frequency questionnaire. *Am J Epidemiol* 1985; 122:51–65.

155. Kristal AR, Peters U, Potter JD. Is it time to abandon the food frequency questionnaire? *Cancer Epidemiol Biomarkers Prev* 2005;14:2826–2828.

156. Willett WC, Stampfer MJ. Total energy intake: implications for epidemiologic analyses. *Am J Epidemiol* 1986;124:17–27.

157. Jain M, Cook GM, Davis FG, Grace MG, Howe GR, Miller AB. A case-control study of diet and colorectal cancer. *Int J Cancer* 1980;26:757–760.

158. Bristol JB, Emmett PM, Heaton KW, Williamson RC. Sugar, fat, and the risk of colorectal cancer. *Br Med J (Clin Res Ed)* 1985;291:1467–1470.

159. Potter JD, McMichael AJ. Diet and cancer of the colon and rectum: a case-control study. *J Natl Cancer Inst* 1986;76:557–569.

160. Lyon JL, Mahoney AW, West DW, et al. Energy intake: its relationship to colon cancer risk. *J Natl Cancer Inst* 1987;78:853–861.

161. Kune S, Kune GA, Watson LF. Case-control study of dietary etiologic factors: the Melbourne Colorectal Cancer Study. *Nutr Cancer* 1987;9:21–42.

162. Graham S, Marshall J, Haughey B, et al. Dietary epidemiology of cancer of the colon in western New York. *Am J Epidemiol* 1988;128:490–503.

163. West DW, Slattery ML, Robison LM, et al. Dietary intake and colon cancer: sex and anatomic site-specific associations. *Am J Epidemiol* 1989;130:883–94.

164. Peters RK, Pike MC, Garabrandt D, Mack TM. Diet and colon cancer in Los Angeles County, California. *Cancer Causes Control* 1992;3:457–473.

165. Iscovich JM, L'Abbe KA, Caastellerto R, et al. Colon cancer in Argentina. II. Risk from fiber, fat and nutrients. *Int J Cancer* 1992;51:858–861.

166. Meyer F, White E. Alcohol and nutrients in relation to colon cancer in middle-aged adults. *Am J Epidemiol* 1993;138:225–236.

167. Howe GR. Meeting Presentation. Advances in the biology and therapy of colorectal cancer. Presented at: Thirty-Seventh Annual Clinical Conference and Twenty-Sixth Annual Special Pathology Program; 1993; Houston, Tex.

168. Stemmermann GN, Nomura AM, Heilbrun LK. Dietary fat and the risk of colorectal cancer. *Cancer Res* 1984;44:4633–4637.

169. Garland C, Shekelle RB, Barrett-Conner E, Criqui MH, Rossof AH, Paul O. Dietary vitamin D and calcium and risk of colorectal cancer: a 19-year prospective study in men. *Lancet* 1985;i:307–309.

170. Willett WC, Stampfer MJ, Colditz GA, Rosner BA, Speizer FE. Relation of meat, fat, and fiber intake to the risk of colon cancer in a prospective study among women. *N Engl J Med* 1990;323:1664–1672.

171. Giovannucci E, Rimm EB, Stampfer MJ, Colditz GA, Ascherio A, Willett WC. Intake of fat, meat, and fiber in relation to risk of colon cancer in men. *Cancer Res* 1994;54:2390–2397.

172. Goldbohm RA, van den Brandt PA, van't Veer P, et al. A prospective cohort study on the relation between meat consumption and the risk of colon cancer. *Cancer Res* 1994;54:718–723.

173. Bostick RM, Potter JD, Kushi LH, et al. Sugar, meat, and fat intake, and non-dietary risk factors for colon cancer incidence in Iowa women (United States). *Cancer Causes Control* 1994;5:38–52.

174. Kaaks R, Lukanova A. Energy balance and cancer: the role of insulin and insulin-like growth factor-I. *Proc Nutr Soc* 2001;60:91–106.

175. Foster-Powell K, Holt SH, Brand-Miller JC. International table of glycemic index and glycemic load values: 2002. *Am J Clin Nutr* 2002;76:5–56.

176. Franceschi S, Dal Maso L, Augustin L, et al. Dietary glycemic load and colorectal cancer risk. *Ann Oncol* 2001;12:173–178.

177. Higginbotham S, Zhang ZF, Lee IM, et al. Dietary glycemic load and risk of colorectal cancer in the Women's Health Study. *J Natl Cancer Inst* 2004; 96:229–233.

178. Terry PD, Jain M, Miller AB, Howe GR, Rohan TE. Glycemic load, carbohydrate intake, and risk of colorectal cancer in women: a prospective cohort study. *J Natl Cancer Inst* 2003;95:914–916.

179. Michaud DS, Fuchs CS, Liu S, Willett WC, Colditz GA, Giovannucci E. Dietary glycemic load, carbohydrate, sugar, and colorectal cancer risk in men and women. *Cancer Epidemiol Biomarkers Prev* 2005;14:138–147.

180. Aoki K, Hayakawa N, Kurihara M, Suzuki S. *Death Rates for Malignant Neoplasms for Selected Sites by Sex and Five-Year Age Group in 33 Countries, 1953–57 to 1983–87.* International Union Against Cancer. Nagoya, Japan: University of Nagoya Coop Press; 1992.

181. Kono S. Secular trend of colon cancer incidence and mortality in relation to fat and meat intake in Japan. *Eur J Cancer Prev* 2004;13:127–132.

182. Truswell AS. Report of an expert workshop on meat intake and colorectal cancer risk convened in December 1998 in Adelaide, South Australia. *Eur J Cancer Prev* 1999;8:175–178.

183. English DR, MacInnis RJ, Hodge AM, Hopper JL, Haydon AM, Giles GG. Red meat, chicken, and fish consumption and risk of colorectal cancer. *Cancer Epidemiol Biomarkers Prev* 2004;13:1509–1514.

184. Kune GA, Kune S, Watson LF. The nutritional causes of colorectal cancer: an introduction to the Melbourne study. *Nutr Cancer* 1987;9:5–56.

185. Gerhardsson de Verdier M, Hagman U, Peters RK, Steineck G. Meat, cooking methods and colorectal cancer: a case-referent study in Stockholm. *Int J Cancer* 1991;49:520–525.

186. Manousos O, Day NE, Trichopoulos D, Gerovassilis F, Tzonou A, Polychronopoulou A. Diet and colorectal cancer: a case-control study in Greece. *Int J Cancer* 1983;32:1–5.

187. La Vecchia C, Negri E, Decarli A, et al. A case-control study of diet and colorectal cancer in northern Italy. *Int J Cancer* 1988;41:492–498.

188. Miller AB, Howe GR, Jain M, Craib KJ, Harrison L. Food items and food groups as risk factors in a case-control study of diet and colo-rectal cancer. *Int J Cancer* 1983;32:155–161.

189. Young TB, Wolf TB. Case-control study of proximal and distal colon cancer and diet in Wisconsin. *Int J Cancer* 1988;42:167–175.

190. Lee HP, Gourley L, Duffy SW, Esteve J, Lee J, Day NE. Colorectal cancer and diet in an Asian population—a case-control study among Singapore Chinese. *Int J Cancer* 1989;43:1007–1016.

191. Macquart-Moulin G, Riboli E, Cornee J, Charnay B, Berthezene P, Day N. Case-control study on colorectal cancer and diet in Marseilles. *Int J Cancer* 1986;38:183–191.

192. Berta JL, Coste T, Rautureau J, Guilloud-Bataille M, Pequignot G. Diet and rectocolonic cancers: results of a case-control study. *Gastroenterol Clin Biol* 1985;9:348–353.

193. Tuyns AJ, Haelterman M, Kaaks R. Colorectal cancer and the intake of nutrients: oligosaccharides are a risk factor, fats are not: a case-control study in Belgium. *Nutr Cancer* 1987;10:181–196.

194. Howe GR, Aronson KJ, Beito E, et al. The relationship between dietary fat intake and risk of colorectal cancer: evidence from the combined analysis of 13 case control studies. *Cancer Causes Control* 1997;8:215–228.

195. Bjelke E. Epidemiology of colorectal cancer, with emphasis on diet. In: Davis W, Harrup KR, Stathopoulos G, eds. *Human Cancer: Its Characterization and Treatment.* Congress Series No. 484. Amsterdam: Excerpta Medica; 1980: 158–174.

196. Hirayama T. A large-scale study on cancer risks by diet—with special reference to the risk reducing effects of green-yellow vegetable consumption. In: Hayashi Y, Magao M, Sugimura T, et al., eds. *Diet, Nutrition, and Cancer.* Tokyo: Japan Scientific Societies Press; 1986:41–53.

197. Phillips RL, Snowdon DA. Association of meat and coffee use with cancers of the large bowel, breast, and prostate among Seventh-Day Adventists: preliminary results. *Cancer Res* 1983;43(suppl):2403S–2408S.

198. Larsson SC, Rafter J, Holmberg L, Bergkvist L, Wolk A. Red meat consumption and risk of cancers of the proximal colon, distal colon and rectum: the Swedish Mammography Cohort. *Int J Cancer* 2005;113:829–834.

199. Sinha R, Peters U, Cross AJ, et al. Meat, meat cooking methods and preservation, and risk for colorectal adenoma. *Cancer Res* 2005;65:8034–8041.

200. Kampman E, Slattery ML, Bigler J, et al. Meat consumption, genetic susceptibility, and colon cancer risk: a large multi-center case-control study. *Cancer Epidemiol Biomarkers Prev* 1999;8:15–24.

201. Chao A, Thun MJ, Connell CJ, et al. Meat consumption and risk of colorectal cancer. *JAMA* 2005;293:172–182.

202. Nowell S, Coles B, Sinha R, et al. Analysis of total meat intake and exposure to individual heterocyclic amines in a case-control study of colorectal cancer: contribution of metabolic variation to risk. *Mutat Res* 2002;506–507:175–185.

203. Schiffman MH, Felton JS. Re: "Fried foods and risk of colon cancer." *Am J Epidemiol* 1990;131:376–378.

204. Murtaugh MA, Ma KN, Sweeney C, Caan BJ, Slattery ML. Meat consumption patterns and preparation, genetic variants of metabolic enzymes, and their association with rectal cancer in men and women. *J Nutr* 2004;134:776–784.

205. Lyon JL, Mahoney AW. Fried foods and risk of colon cancer. *Am J Epidemiol* 1988;128:1000–1006.

206. Muscat JE, Wynder EL. The consumption of well-done meat and the risk of colorectal cancer. *Am J Public Health* 1994;84:856–858.

207. Truswell AS. Meat consumption and cancer of the large bowel. *Eur J Clin Nutr* 2002;56(suppl 1):S19–S24.

208. Sinha R, Chow WH, Kulldorf M, et al. Well-done, grilled red meat increases the risk of colorectal adenoma. *Cancer Res* 1999;59:4320–4324.

209. Sugimura T, Nagao M, Kawachi T, et al. Mutagen-carcinogens in food, with special reference to highly mutagenic pyrolytic products in broiled foods. In: Hiatt HH, Watson JD, Winsten JA, eds. *Origins of Human Cancer.* New York, NY: Cold Spring Harbor Laboratory; 1977: 11561–11577.

210. Wakabayashi K, Nagao M, Esumi H, Sugimura T. Food-derived mutagens and carcinogens. *Cancer Res* 1992;52:2092s–2098s.

211. Sugimura T, Sato S. Mutagens-carcinogens in foods. *Cancer Res* 1983; 43:2415S–2421S.

212. Sugimura T, Sato S. Past, present, and future of mutagens in cooked foods [review]. *Environ Health Perspect* 1986;67:5–10.

213. Hasegawa R, Miyata E, Futakuchi M, et al. Synergistic enhancement of hepatic foci development by combined treatment of rats with 10 heterocyclic amines at low doses. *Carcinogenesis* 1994;15:1037–1041.

214. Lang NP, Butler MA, Massengill J, al. e. Rapid metabolic phenotypes for acetyltransferase and cytochrome P450A2 and putative exposure to foodborne heterocyclic amines increase the risk for colorectal cancer or polyps. *Cancer Epidemiol Biomarkers Prev* 1994;3:675–682.

215. Wohlleb JC, Hunter CF, Blass B, Kadlubar FF, Chu DZ, Lang NP. Aromatic amine acetyltransferase as a marker for colorectal cancer: environmental and demographic associations. *Int J Cancer* 1990;46:22–30.

216. Welfare MR, Cooper J, Bassendine MF, Daly AK. Relationship between acetylator status, smoking, diet and colorectal cancer risk in the north-east of England. *Carcinogenesis* 1994;15:1351–1354.

217. Le Marchand L, Hankin JH, Pierce LM, et al. Well-done red meat, metabolic phenotypes and colorectal cancer in Hawaii. *Mutat Res* 2002; 506–507:205–214.

218. Pennington JA, Young BE. Total diet study nutritional elements, 1982–1989. *J Am Diet Assoc* 1991;91:179–183.

219. Nelson RL. Dietary minerals and colon *Carcinogenesis* [review]. Anti*Cancer Res* 1987;7:259.

220. Clark L, Combs G, et al. Effects of selenium supplementation for cancer prevention for cancer prevention in patients with carcinoma of the skin: a randomized controlled trial. *JAMA* 1996;276:1957–1963.

221. Duffield-Lillico AJ, Reid ME, Turnbull BW, et al. Baseline characteristics and the effect of selenium supplementation on cancer incidence in a randomized clinical trial: a summary report of the Nutrition Prevention of Cancer Trial. *Cancer Epidemiol Biomarkers Prev* 2002;11:630–639.

222. Willett WC, Polk BF, Morris JS, et al. Prediagnostic serum selenium and risk of cancer. *Lancet* 1983;2:130–134.

223. Clark LC, Hixson LJ, Combs GF, Jr., Reid ME, Turnbull BW, Sampliner RE. Plasma selenium concentration predicts the prevalence of colorectal adenomatous polyps. *Cancer Epidemiol Biomarkers Prev* 1993;2:41–46.

224. Dworkin BM, Rosenthal WS, Mittelman A, Weiss L, Applebee-Brady L, Arlin Z. Selenium status and the polyp-cancer sequence: a colonoscopically controlled study. *Am J Gastroenterol* 1988;83:748–751.

225. Russo MW, Murray SC, Wurzelmann JI, Woosley JT, Sandler RS. Plasma selenium levels and the risk of colorectal adenomas. *Nutr Cancer* 1997;28:125–129.

226. Psathakis D, Wedemeyer N, Oevermann E, Krug F, Siegers CP, Bruch HP. Blood selenium and glutathione peroxidase status in patients with colorectal cancer. *Dis Colon Rectum* 1998;41:328–335.

227. Fernandez-Banares F, Cabre E, Esteve M, et al. Serum selenium and risk of large size colorectal adenomas in a geographical area with a low selenium status. *Am J Gastroenterol* 2002;97:2013–2108.

228. Ghadirian P, Maisonneuve P, Perret C, et al. A case-control study of toenail selenium and cancer of the breast, colon, and prostate. *Cancer Detect Prev* 2000;24:305–313.

229. Jacobs ET, Jiang R, Alberts DS, et al. Selenium and colorectal adenoma: results of a pooled analysis. *J Natl Cancer Inst* 2004;96:1669–1675.

230. Early DS, Hill K, Burk R, Palmer I. Selenoprotein levels in patients with colorectal adenomas and cancer. *Am J Gastroenterol* 2002;97:745–748.

231. Nelson RL, Davis FG, Sutter E, et al. Serum selenium and colonic neoplastic risk. *Dis Colon Rectum* 1995;38:1306–1310.

232. Combs GF, Jr., Gray WP. Chemopreventive agents: selenium. *Pharmacol Ther* 1998;79:179–192.

233. McKenzie RC, Rafferty TS, Beckett GJ. Selenium: an essential element for immune function. *Immunol Today* 1998;19:342–345.

234. Samaha HS, Hamid R, el-Bayoumy K, Rao CV, Reddy BS. The role of apoptosis in the modulation of colon *Carcinogenesis* by dietary fat and by the organoselenium compound 1,4-phenylenebis(methylene)selenocyanate. *Cancer Epidemiol Biomarkers Prev* 1997;6:699–704.

235. Holick M.Vitamin D. In: Shils ME, Shike M, Ross AC, eds. *Modern Nutrition in Health and Disease.* Baltimore, Md.: Williams & Wilkins; 1999: 329–345.

236. Haussler MR, Whitfield GK, Haussler CA, et al. The nuclear vitamin D receptor: biological and molecular regulatory properties revealed. *J Bone Miner Res* 1998;13:325–349.

237. Garland CF, Garland FC, Gorham ED. Calcium and vitamin D: their potential roles in colon and breast cancer prevention. *Ann N Y Acad Sci* 1999;889:107–119.

238. Peters U, McGlynn KA, Chatterjee N, et al. Vitamin D, calcium, and vitamin D receptor polymorphism in colorectal adenomas. *Cancer Epidemiol Biomarkers Prev* 2001;10:1267–1274.

239. Tangrea J, Helzlsouer K, Pietinen P, et al. Serum levels of vitamin D metabolites and the subsequent risk of colon and rectal cancer in Finnish men. *Cancer Causes Control* 1997;8:615–625.

240. Martinez ME, Marshall JR, Sampliner R, Wilkinson J, Alberts DS. Calcium, vitamin D, and risk of adenoma recurrence (United States). *Cancer Causes Control* 2002;13:213–220.

241. Martinez ME, Giovannucci EL, Colditz GA, et al. Calcium, vitamin D, and the occurrence of colorectal cancer among women. *J Natl Cancer Inst* 1996;88:1375–1382.

242. Bostick RM, Potter JD, Sellers TA, McKenzie DR, Kushi H, Folsom AR. Relation of calcium, vitamin D, and dairy food intake to incidence of colon cancer in older women. *Am J Epidemiol* 1993;137:1302–1317.

243. Kampman E, Giovannucci E, van't Veer P, et al. Calcium, vitamin D, dairy foods, and the occurrence of colorectal adenomas among men and women in two prospective studies. *Am J Epidemiol* 1994;139:16–29.

244. Ferraroni M, La Vecchia C, D'Avanzo B, Negri E, Franceschi S, Decarli A. Selected micronutrient intake and the risk of colorectal cancer. *Br J Cancer* 1994;70:1150–1155.

245. Heaney RP. *Nutrition and Risk for Osteoporosis.* New York, NY: Academic Press; 1996.

246. Giuliano AR, Franceschi RT, Wood RJ. Characterization of the vitamin D receptor from the Caco-2 human colon carcinoma cell line: effect of cellular differentiation. *Arch Biochem Biophys* 1991;285:261–269.

247. Shabahang M, Buras RR, Davoodi F, Schumaker LM, Nauta RJ, Evans SR. 1,25-Dihydroxyvitamin D3 receptor as a marker of human colon carcinoma cell line differentiation and growth inhibition. *Cancer Res* 1993;53:3712–3718.

248. Wang QM, Jones JB, Studzinski GP. Cyclin-dependent kinase inhibitor p27 as a mediator of the G1-S phase block induced by 1,25-dihydroxyvitamin D3 in HL60 cells. *Cancer Res* 1996;56:264–267.

249. Sheikh MS, Rochefort H, Garcia M. Overexpression of p21WAF1/CIP1 induces growth arrest, giant cell formation and apoptosis in human breast carcinoma cell lines. *Oncogene* 1995;11:1899–1905.

250. Elstner E, Linker-Israeli M, Umiel T, et al. Combination of a potent 20-epi-vitamin D3 analogue (KH 1060) with 9-cis-retinoic acid irreversibly inhibits clonal growth, decreases bcl-2 expression, and induces apoptosis in HL-60 leukemic cells. *Cancer Res* 1996;56:3570–3576.

251. Donohue MM, Demay MB. Rickets in VDR null mice is secondary to decreased apoptosis of hypertrophic chondrocytes. *Endocrinology* 2002; 143:3691–3694.

252. Weaver CM. Calcium. In: Shils ME, Shike M, Ross AC, eds. *Modern Nutrition in Health and Disease.* Baltimore, Md.: Williams & Wilkins; 1999: 141–167.

253. McCormick CC. Passive diffusion does not play a major role in the absorption of dietary calcium in normal adults. *J Nutr* 2002;132:3428–3430.

254. Newmark HL, Wargovich MJ, Bruce WR. Colon cancer and dietary fat, phosphate, and calcium: a hypothesis. *J Natl Cancer Inst* 1984;72:1323–1325.

255. Nagengast FM, Grubben MJ, van Munster IP. Role of bile acids in colorectal carcinogenesis. *Eur J Cancer* 1995;31A:1067–1070.

256. Lipkin M, Newmark H. Effect of added dietary calcium on colonic epithelial-cell proliferation in subjects at high risk for familial colonic cancer. *N Engl J Med* 1985;313:1381–1384.

257. Pence BC. Role of calcium in colon cancer prevention: experimental and clinical studies. *Mutat Res* 1993;290:87–95.

258. Baron JA, Beach M, Mandel JS, et al. Calcium supplements for the prevention of colorectal adenomas. *N Engl J Med* 1999;340:101–107.

259. Grau MV, Baron JA, Sandler RS, et al. Vitamin D, calcium supplementation, and colorectal adenomas: results of a randomized trial. *J Natl Cancer Inst* 2003;95:1765–1771.

260. Jacobs ET, Martinez ME, Alberts DS. Research and public health implications of the intricate relationship between calcium and vitamin D in the prevention of colorectal neoplasia. *J Natl Cancer Inst* 2003;95:1736–1737.

261. Martz ME, Willett WC. Calcium, vitamin D, and colorectal cancer: a review of the epidemiologic evidence. *Cancer Epidemiol Biomarkers Prev* 1998;7:163–168.

262. Wu K, Willett WC, Fuchs CS, Colditz GA, Giovannucci EL. Calcium intake and risk of colon cancer in women and men. *J Natl Cancer Inst* 2002;94:437–446.

263. Marcus PM, Newcomb PA. The association of calcium and vitamin D, and colon and rectal cancer in Wisconsin women. *Int J Epidemiol* 1998;27:788–793.

264. Kampman E, Slattery ML, Caan B, Potter JD. Calcium, vitamin D, sunshine exposure, dairy products and colon cancer risk (United States). *Cancer Causes Control* 2000;11:459–466.

265. Wactawski-Wende J, Kotchen JM, Anderson GL, et al. Calcium plus vitamin D supplementation and the risk of colorectal cancer. *N Engl J Med* 2006;354:684–696.

266. Hollis BW. Circulating 25-hydroxyvitamin D levels indicative of vitamin D sufficiency: implications for establishing a new effective dietary intake recommendation for vitamin D. *J Nutr* 2005;135:317–322.

267. Sanjoaquin MA, Allen N, Couto E, Roddam AW, Key TJ. Folate intake and colorectal cancer risk: a meta-analytical approach. *Int J Cancer* 2005;113:825–828.

268. Gregory JF. The bioavailability of folate. In: Bailey LB, ed. *Folate in Health and Disease.* New York, NY: Marcel Dekker; 1995: 195–235.

269. Glynn SA, Albanes D, Pietinen P, et al. Colorectal cancer and folate status: a nested case-control study among male smokers. *Cancer Epidemiol Biomarkers Prev* 1996;5:487–494.

270. Kato I, Dnistrian AM, Schwartz M, et al. Serum folate, homocysteine and colorectal cancer risk in women: a nested case-control study. *Br J Cancer* 1999;79:1917–1921.

271. Martinez ME, Henning SM, Alberts DS. Folate and colorectal neoplasia: relationship between plasma and dietary markers of folate and adenoma recurrence. *Am J Clin Nutr* 2004;79:691–697

272. Martínez ME, Jiang R, Henning SM, et al. Folate fortification of the US food supply, plasma folate, homocysteine, and colorectal adenoma recurrence. *Int J Cancer* 2006; 119(6)1440–1446.

273. Choi SW, Mason JB. Folate status: effects on pathways of colorectal carcinogenesis. *J Nutr* 2002;132:2413S–2418S.

274. Kim YI. Folate and carcinogenesis: evidence, mechanisms, and implications. *J Nutr Biochem* 1999;10:66–88.

275. Duthie SJ. Folic acid deficiency and cancer: mechanisms of DNA instability. *Br Med Bull* 1999;55:578–592.

276. Hoffman RM. Altered methionine metabolism and transmethylation in cancer. *Anticancer Res* 1985;5:1–30.

277. Wickramasinghe S, Fida S. Bone marrow cells from vitamin B12- and folate-deficient patients misincorporate uracil into DNA. *Blood* 1994;83:1656–1661.

278. Weinberg G, Ullman B, Martin D, Jr. Mutator phenotypes in mammalian cell mutants with distinct biochemical defects and abnormal deoxyribonucleoside triphosphate pools. *Proc Natl Acad Sci U S A* 1981;78:2447–2451.

279. Hunting D, Dresler S. Dependence of UV-induced DNA excision repair in deoxyribonucleoside triphosphate concentrations in permeable human fibroblasts: a model for the inhibition of repair by hydroxyurea. *Carcinogenesis (Lond)* 1985;6:1525–1528.

280. James S, Basnakian A, Miller B. In vitro folate deficiency induces deoxynucleotide pool imbalance, apoptosis, and mutagenesis in Chinese hamster ovary cells. *Cancer Res* 1994;54:5075–5080.

281. Fenech M, Rinaldi J. The relationship between micronuclei in human lymphocytes and plasma levels of vitamin C, vitamin E, vitamin B12 and folic acid. *Carcinogenesis* 1994;15:1405–1411.

282. Sutherland G. The role of nucleotides in human fragile site expression. *Mutat Res* 1988;200:207–213.

283. Giovannucci E, Stampfer MJ, Colditz GA, et al. Folate, methionine, and alcohol intake and risk of colorectal adenoma. *J Natl Cancer Inst* 1993;85:875–884.

284. Cravo ML, Mason JB, Dayal Y, et al. Folate deficiency enhances the development of colonic neoplasia in dimethylhydrazine-treated rats. *Cancer Res* 1992;52:5002–5006.

285. Chen J, Giovannucci E, Kelsey K, et al. A methylenetetrahydrofolate reductase polymorphism and the risk of colorectal cancer. *Cancer Res* 1996; 56:4862–4864.

286. Ma J, Stampfer MJ, Giovannucci E, et al. Methylenetetrahydrofolate reductase polymorphism, dietary interactions and risk of colorectal cancer. *Cancer Res* 1997;57:1098–1102.

287. Kutzbach C, Stokstad E. Mammalian methylenetetrahydrofolate reductase: partial purification, properties, and inhibition by S-adenosylmethionine. *Biochem Biophys Acta* 1971;250:459–477.

288. Jacques PF, Bostom AG, Williams RR, et al. Relation between folate status, a common mutation in methylenetetrahydrofolate reductase, and plasma homocysteine concentrations. *Circulation* 1996;93:7–9.

289. Chen J, Giovannucci E, Kelsey K, et al. A methylenetetrahydrofolate reductase polymorphism and the risk of colorectal cancer. *Cancer Res* 1996;56: 4862–4864.

290. Ma J, Stampfer MJ, Giovannucci E, et al. Methylenetetrahydrofolate reductase polymorphism, dietary interactions, and risk of colorectal cancer. *Cancer Res* 1997;57:1098–1102.

291. Slattery ML, Potter JD, Samowitz W, Schaffer D, Leppert M. Methylenetetrahydrofolate reductase, diet, and risk of colon cancer. *Cancer Epidemiol Biomarkers Prev* 1999;8:513–518.

292. Le Marchand L, Donlon T, Hankin JH, Kolonel LN, Wilkens LR, Seidenfeld J. B-vitamin intake, metabolic genes, and colorectal cancer risk (United States). *Cancer Causes Control* 2002;13:239–248.

293. Ulrich CM, Kampman E, Bigler J, et al. Colorectal adenomas and the C677T MTHFR polymorphism: evidence for gene-environment interaction? *Cancer Epidemiol Biomarkers Prev* 1999;8:659–668.

294. Levine AJ, Siegmund KD, Ervin CM, et al. The methylenetetrahydrofolate reductase 677C→T polymorphism and distal colorectal adenoma risk. *Cancer Epidemiol Biomarkers Prev* 2000;9:657–663.

295. Giovannucci E, Chen J, Smith-Warner SA, et al. Methylenetetrahydrofolate reductase, alcohol dehydrogenase, diet, and risk of colorectal adenomas. *Cancer Epidemiol Biomarkers Prev* 2003;12:970–979.

296. Hillman RS, Steinberg SE. The effects of alcohol on folate metabolism. *Annu Rev Med* 1982;33:345–354.

297. Giovannucci E, Rimm EB, Ascherio A, Stampfer MJ, Colditz GA, Willett WC. Alcohol, low-methionine-low-folate diets, and risk of colon cancer in men. *J Natl Cancer Inst* 1995;87:265–273.

298. Finkelstein J, Cello J, Kyle W. Ethanol-induced changes in methionine metabolism in rat livers. *Biochem Biophys Res Commun* 1974;61:525–531.

299. Willett WC, Stampfer MJ, Colditz GA, Rosner BA, Speizer FE. Relation of meat, fat and fiber intake to colon cancer risk in a prospective study among women [abstract]. *Am J Epidemiol* 1989;130:820.

300. Giovannucci E, Stampfer MJ, Colditz GA, Rimm EB, Willett WC. Relationship of diet to risk of colorectal adenoma in men. *J Natl Cancer Inst* 1992;84:91–98.

301. Benito E, Cabeza E, Moreno V, Obrador A, Bosch F. Diet and colorectal adenomas: a case-control study in Majorca. *Int J Cancer* 1993;55:213–219.

302. Neugut A, Garbowski G, Lee W, et al. Dietary risk factors for the incidence and recurrence of colorectal adenomatous polyps: a case-control study. *Ann Int Med* 1993;118:91–95.

303. Sandler R, Lyles C, Peipins L, McAuliffe C, Woosley J, Kupper L. Diet and risk of colorectal adenomas: macronutrients, cholesterol and fiber. *J Natl Cancer Inst* 1993;85:884–891.

304. Wainfan E, Dizik M, Stender M, Christman JK. Rapid appearance of hypomethylated DNA in livers of rats fed cancer-promoting, methyl-deficient diets. *Cancer Res* 1989;49:4094–4097.

305. Konings EJM, Goldbohm RA, Brants HAM, Saris WHM, van den Brandt PA. Intake of dietary folate vitamers and risk of colorectal carcinoma: results from The Netherlands Cohort Study. *Cancer* 2002;95:1421–1433.

306. Wei EK, Giovannucci E, Selhub J, Fuchs CS, Hankinson SE, Ma J. Plasma vitamin B6 and the risk of colorectal cancer and adenoma in women. *J Natl Cancer Inst* 2005;97:684–692.

307. Wickramasinghe SN, Fida S. Misincorporation of uracil into the DNA of folate- and B12-deficient HL60 cells. *Eur J Haematol* 1993;50:127–132.

308. Burkitt DP. Epidemiology of cancer of the colon and rectum. *Cancer* 1971; 28:3–13.

309. Steinmetz KA, Potter JD. A review of vegetables, fruit and cancer. I. Epidemiology. *Cancer Causes Control* 1991;2:325–357.

310. Phillips RL. Role of life-style and dietary habits in risk of cancer among Seventh-Day Adventists. *Cancer Res* 1975;35:3513–3522.

311. Mayne ST, Janerich DT, Greenwald P, et al. Dietary beta carotene and lung cancer risk in U.S. nonsmokers. *J Natl Cancer Inst* 1994;86:33–38.

312. Modan B, Barell V, Lubin F, Modan M, Greenberg RA. Low-fiber intake as an etiologic factor in cancer of the colon. *J Natl Cancer Inst* 1975;55:15–18.

313. Tuyns AJ, Kaaks R, Haelterman M. Colorectal cancer and the consumption of foods: a case-control study of Belgium. *Nutr Cancer* 1988;11:189–204.

314. Steinmetz KA, Kushi LH, Bostick RM, Folsom AR, Potter JD. Vegetables, fruit, and colon cancer in the Iowa Women's Health Study. *Am J Epidemiol* 1994;139:1–15.

315. Benito E, Stiggelbout A, Bosch FX, et al. Nutritional factors in colorectal cancer risk: a case-control study in Majorca. *Int J Cancer* 1991;49:161–167.

316. Trock B, Lanza E, Greenwald P. Dietary fiber, vegetables, and colon cancer: critical review and meta-analyses of the epidemiologic evidence. *J Natl Cancer Inst* 1990;82:650–661.

317. Bingham SA, Day NE, Luben R, et al. Dietary fibre in food and protection against colorectal cancer in the European Prospective Investigation into Cancer and Nutrition (EPIC): an observational study. *Lancet* 2003;361:1496–1501.

318. Peters U, Sinha R, Chatterjee N, et al. Dietary fibre and colorectal adenoma in a colorectal cancer early detection programme. *Lancet* 2003;361:1491–1495.

319. Mai V, Flood A, Peters U, Lacey JV, Jr. , Schairer C, Schatzkin A. Dietary fibre and risk of colorectal cancer in the Breast Cancer Detection Demonstration Project (BCDDP) follow-up cohort. *Int J Epidemiol* 2003;32:234–239.

320. Jacobs ET, Giuliano AR, Roe DJ, Guillen-Rodriguez JM, Alberts DS, Martinez ME. Baseline dietary fiber intake and colorectal adenoma recurrence in the wheat bran fiber randomized trial. *J Natl Cancer Inst* 2002;94:1620–1625.

321. Terry P, Giovannucci E, Michels KB, et al. Fruit, vegetables, dietary fiber, and risk of colorectal cancer. *J Natl Cancer Inst* 2001;93:525–533.

322. Fuchs CS, Giovannucci EL, Colditz GA, et al. Dietary fiber and the risk of colorectal cancer and adenoma in women. *N Engl J Med* 1999;340:169–176.

323. Pietinen P, Malila N, Virtanen M, et al. Diet and risk of colorectal cancer in a cohort of Finnish men. *Cancer Causes Control* 1999;10:387–396.

324. Lin J, Zhang SM, Cook NR, et al. Dietary intakes of fruit, vegetables, and fiber, and risk of colorectal cancer in a prospective cohort of women (United States). *Cancer Causes Control* 2005;16:225–233.

325. Robertson DJ, Sandler RS, Haile R, et al. Fat, fiber, meat and the risk of colorectal adenomas. *Am J Gastroenterol* 2005;100:2789–2795.

326. Zaridze D, Filipchenko V, Kustov V, et al. Diet and colorectal cancer: results of two case-control studies in Russia. *Eur J Cancer* 1993;29A:112–115.

327. Howe GR, Benito E, Castelleto R, et al. Dietary intake of fiber and decreased risk of cancers of the colon and rectum: evidence from the combined analysis of 13 case-control studies. *J Natl Cancer Inst* 1992;84:1887–1896.

328. Alberts DS, Martinez ME, Roe DJ, et al. Lack of effect of a high-fiber cereal supplement on the recurrence of colorectal adenomas. Phoenix Colon Cancer Prevention Physicians' Network. *N Engl J Med* 2000;342:1156–1162.

329. Schatzkin A, Lanza E, Corle D, et al. Lack of effect of a low-fat, high-fiber diet on the recurrence of colorectal adenomas. Polyp Prevention Trial Study Group. *N Engl J Med* 2000;342:1149–1155.

330. Park Y, Hunter DJ, Spiegelman D, et al. Dietary fiber intake and risk of colorectal cancer: a pooled analysis of prospective cohort studies. *JAMA* 2005;294:2849–2857.

331. Jacobs ET, Lanza E, Alberts DS, et al. Fiber, sex, and colorectal adenoma: results of a pooled analysis. *Am J Clin Nutr* 2006;83:343–349.

332. Vernon SW. Participation in colorectal cancer screening: a review. *J Natl Cancer Inst* 1997;89:1406–1422.

333. Jacobs ET, Haussler MR, Martinez ME. Vitamin D activity and colorectal neoplasia: a pathway approach to epidemiologic studies. *Cancer Epidemiol Biomarkers Prev* 2005;14:2061–2063.

CHAPTER 39 ■ COLORECTAL CANCER: SCREENING AND SURVEILLANCE

BERNARD LEVIN

Colorectal cancer is the second most common cancer and the second most common cause of cancer death in the United States for both men and women (1). In women, it is responsible for approximately 11% of all new cancer cases and 11% of cancer deaths; in men, it is 10% for both measures. In 2006, the American Cancer Society estimated that approximately 153,000 new cases were diagnosed and that the disease had claimed 53,000 lives (1).

More than any other characteristic, age and its advancement signal risk, as demonstrated by the data in Table 39.1 (2). Colorectal cancer incidence and mortality rates have been declining since approximately 1985 (Fig. 39.1), but overall incidence and mortality continue to be higher in African Americans than in their white counterparts. Furthermore, the declines in incidence found for the overall population are not found to the same degree in the African American population (Fig. 39.2). Declines in the overall U. S. mortality rate have been attributed to greater surveillance of those at risk, improved diagnostic techniques, broadening use of effective adjuvant therapy, and, recently, better therapy for metastatic disease (2). Statistically significant gains have been made in 5-year survival rates for colon cancer and rectal cancer since 1992 for all races, according to the 1975 to 2003 statistics of the National Cancer Institute Surveillance, Epidemiology, and End Results (SEER) program (2).

Internationally, colorectal cancer incidence is highest in Japan, Australia and New Zealand, western Europe, and northern Europe, which indicates its more common occurrence in developed nations (3). Survival estimates are better on average than those for cancers at less common sites, and they are highest in North America (65%), Western Europe (54%), eastern Europe (34%), and India (30%) (3). The rising incidence in Asian countries, of which Japan is a notable example (4), is attributed to adoption of Western lifestyles, especially diet, although other unknown factors cannot yet be excluded.

In the United States, the declining overall incidence and mortality rates, as well as the upward trend in colorectal cancer 5-year survival rates, are positive signs. Educational campaigns through the media with the endorsement of government and professional organizations may further improve early detection rates and expand gains for all groups (5). Advances in molecular genetics have given families at high risk of colorectal cancer powerful lifesaving tools to enhance screening, early detection, and prevention of cancer (6,7).

Widespread screening for colorectal neoplasia over the next decade could lead to a 50% reduction in annual colorectal cancer death rate (8,9). The following sections examine the screening process and recommended colorectal screening tests; discuss their appropriate use among populations of average, moderate, and high risk; and consider current screening participation and how it could be improved.

SCREENING

Screening for colorectal cancer has the goal of reducing morbidity and mortality from colorectal cancer. Risk categories are (a) average-risk individuals are those age 50 years and older in a Western or "westernizing" country, and (b) higher-risk individuals with a family history or a personal history of colorectal neoplasia or chronic inflammatory bowel disease. These latter individuals require more intensive surveillance. The screening process should embody the characteristics shown in Table 39.2.

The long-recognized standard examinations for colorectal cancer screening have included digital rectal examination, fecal occult blood test (FOBT), sigmoidoscopy, double-contrast barium enema, and colonoscopy. Of these five, digital rectal examination is generally no longer recommended because alone it has not proven effective in colorectal cancer screening. The 7- to 8-cm reach of the examining finger could detect at best only 10% of colorectal cancers. Nonetheless, digital rectal examination remains a part of sigmoidoscopy, colonoscopy, and barium enema examinations and may be considered a component of comprehensive preventive health care (10).

Fecal Occult Blood Testing

Types of Fecal Occult Blood Tests: Guaiac and Immunochemical Tests

FOBTs are based on two principal techniques: chemical tests and immunochemical tests. The major features of these tests are described in Table 39.3. Key usage and performance issues related to different types of FOBTs are described in Tables 39.4 and 39.5.

Effectiveness

FOBT is the most rigorously and extensively studied method used to detect colorectal cancer in asymptomatic persons (11). Bleeding occurs from cancer and large adenomas but probably not from small adenomas; hence, sensitivity of the test for detection of these lesions is limited. Researchers have demonstrated that FOBTs, whether performed annually or biennially, reduce mortality from colorectal cancer (12,13). The tests used are the six sample-based home FOBTs and not the digital office test. The latter has been shown to be significantly inferior (14).

TABLE 39.1

COLORECTAL CANCER INCIDENCE AND MORTALITY RATE FOR SELECTED GROUPS

Incidence and mortality rate	Men (per 100,000)	Women (per 100,000)
INCIDENCE BY AGE (yr)	All Races	All Races
All ages	60.4	44.2
30–34	4.5	4.1
35–39	8.2	7.7
40–44	16.1	15.0
45–49	30.3	26.2
50–54	62.0	47.2
55–59	96.0	66.9
60–64	149.7	98.6
65–69	225.7	153.3
70–74	290.7	201.0
75–79	386.5	264.8
80–84	428.4	315.5
MORTALITY RATE BY AGE (yr)		
30–34	0.9	0.9
35–39	2.1	1.9
40–44	4.1	3.3
45–49	8.8	6.7
50–54	16.5	11.8
55–59	27.6	18.4
60–64	46.9	30.4
65–69	75.1	45.5
70–74	103.4	67.0
75–79	143.4	97.8
80–84	197.2	135.7
INCIDENCE RATES BY RACE		
All Races	60.8	44.8
White	60.4	44.0
Black	72.8	55.0
American Indian	42.1	32.9
Hispanic	47.5	32.9
MORTALITY		
All Races	23.5	16.4
White	22.9	15.9
Black	32.7	22.9
American Indian	20.6	14.3
Hispanic	17.0	11.1

Data from SEER Age Adjusted Incidence Rates by 'Expanded' Race for Colon and Rectum Cancer, All Ages, Both Sexes–SEER 13 Registries for 1995–2004, Age-Adjusted to the 2000 US Std Population.

Annual screening, using a guaiac-based method (Hemoccult) according to the Minnesota Trial, reduced mortality by 33% (15). In a meta-analysis of mortality results from randomized controlled trials, Hewitson et al. (12) found the reduction to be 16% overall (relative risk [RR], 0.84; confidence interval [CI], 0.77–0.92) (Fig. 39.3) and 23% when adjusted for screening attendance (11).

The success of FOBT in reducing colorectal cancer mortality is enhanced by other benefits, including a lowering of incidence due to removal of adenomatous polyps after detection (15) and a potential reduction in surgical intervention because of earlier detection of disease. The FOBT is both effective and cost efficient; has a long record of testing in the United States and abroad; and has been recommended by government, professional organizations, and patient advocacy groups.

The major shortcoming of FOBT—its high false-positive rate—is viewed as something of a virtue by some, inasmuch as more rigorous testing follows the initial false-positive findings, and true cases are subsequently detected (Table 39.3 provides sensitivity and specificity measures) (11,16). Others find intolerable the unnecessary risks and stresses that patients wrongly identified must endure with colonoscopy (12). In contrast, a negative FOBT could falsely reassure patients and lead to delayed response to the development of colorectal symptoms (17).

There has been considerable recent interest in the use of fecal immunochemical tests (FITs). FITs use antibodies specific for human globin and thus are not affected by dietary hemoglobin or peroxidase. A variety of stool sampling methods have been developed, including the use of a wooden spatula,

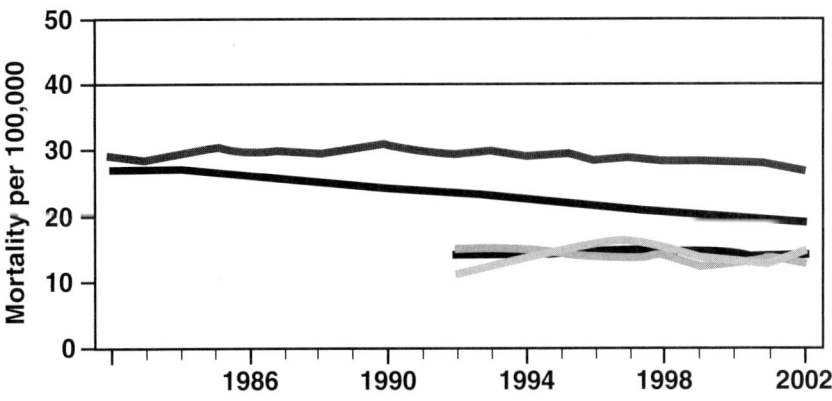

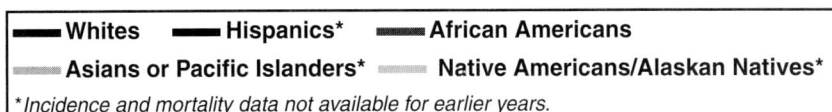

FIGURE 39.1. U.S. colorectal cancer mortality. *Source:* Adapted from Surveillance, Epidemiology, and End Results (SEER) Program and NCHS, 2006. (See also color Figure 39.1)

probe, or brush. Using a predetermined standard threshold of hemoglobin to indicate a positive test, laboratory development of a quantitative method is preferable to a qualitative result. The test output is a continuous variable that offers the option of adjusting the threshold to suit the objective. The U.S. Food and Drug Administration approved the use of an FIT in 2001. Subsequently, the American Cancer Society recommended using FITs instead of guaiac-based FOBT because of ease of use and better sensitivity and specificity (18). Smith et al. compared a sensitive guaiac FOBT (Hemoccult II Sensa, Beckman-Coulter, Fullerton, CA) with a brush-sampling FIT (Insure, Enterix, Inc, Edison, NJ) in both a screening cohort ($n = 2,351$) and a symptomatic diagnostic group ($n = 161$). Combining results for both cohorts, the FIT returned a true-positive result notably more often in cancer ($n = 24$, 87.5% vs. 54.2%) or significant adenomas ($n = 61$, 42.6% vs. 23.0%). In the screening cohort, the false-positive rate for any neoplasia was marginally higher than the guaiac FOBT (3.4% vs. 2.5%, 95% CI of difference), whereas positive predictive values were 41.9% and 40.4%, respectively (19). Levi et al. (19) compared colonoscopy with hemoglobin content of three bowel

movements in 1,000 patients, some asymptomatic but at increased risk for colorectal neoplasia and some symptomatic, using an FIT (OC-MICRO, Eiken Chemical Co., Tokyo, Japan). Colonoscopy identified clinically significant neoplasia in 91 patients (cancer in 17 patients and advanced adenomas in 74 patients). Using three FITs and a hemoglobin threshold of 75 mg/mL, sensitivity and specificity were 94.1% (95% CI, 82.9%–100%) and 87.5% (85.4%–89.6%), respectively, for cancer and 67% (CI, 57.4%–76.7%) and 91.4% (CI, 89.6%–93.2%), respectively, for any clinically significant neoplasia (20). These data may not be completely applicable to an average-risk screening population, but the methodology may well be suited to enhance the effectiveness of our current strategies (20).

TABLE 39.2

SCREENING PROCESS

- **Invite** participation in a screening program by targeting those at risk for colorectal cancer:
  - Use a personalized approach within a health care environment.
  - Use a mass population approach with wide coverage of the population.
- For those with **high-risk factors** (colorectal symptoms, family history, or personal history of relevant colorectal disease), provide access to an individualized prevention strategy.
- Provide a **safe, effective, acceptable,** and **affordable** screening test in one of two main ways:
  - Two-step process: perform a simple test such as a fecal occult blood test to establish risk and select who moves on to colonoscopy.
  - One-step process: perform a colonoscopy.
- Facilitate **compliance** with any necessary diagnostic and therapeutic follow-up.
- Offer **rescreening** at the appropriate interval, having more accurately identified risk status.
- **Monitor** adequacy of participation, quality of tests and clinical procedures, and outcomes of the program.

Adapted from ref. 80.

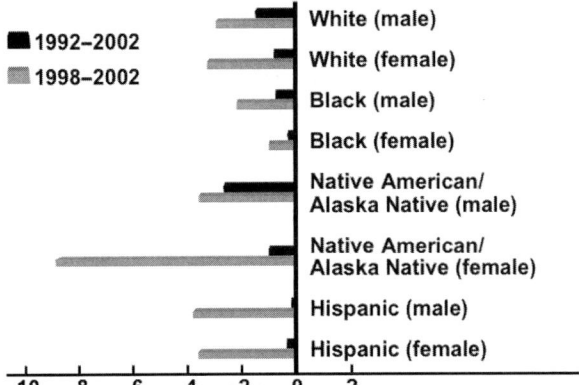

FIGURE 39.2. Annual percentage changes in Surveillance, Epidemiology, and End Results (SEER) incidence rates for colon and rectum cancer for 1992 to 2000 and 1998 to 2002. *Source:* Adapted from Surveillance, Epidemiology, and End Results (SEER) Program, 2005.

TABLE 39.3

SENSITIVITY AND SPECIFICITY RANGES FOR FOUR COLORECTAL CANCER SCREENING EXAMINATIONS

Test	Sensitivity			Specificity		
	Small adenomas	Large adenomas	Cancer	Small adenomas	Large adenomas	Cancer
Fecal occult blood test	—	—	40.00–80.00	—	—	90.00–94.00
Flexible sigmoidoscopy	73.30–88.00	88.00–98.00	88.00–98.00	92.00–92.00	92.00–94.00	92.00–96.00
Double-contrast barium enema imaging	52.00–82.00	73.00–91.00	78.00–90.00	60.00–83.30	69.70–91.80	97.50–99.80
Colonoscopy	73.00–84.00	85.00–90.00	90.00–96.70	96.00–98.00	96.00–98.00	96.00–100.00

Data from ref. 11.

Flexible Sigmoidoscopy

Offering greater reliability than FOBT and incorporating visualization and removal of potentially life-threatening adenomatous polyps is flexible sigmoidoscopy (FSIG), although its impact is limited to the left side of the colon and the rectosigmoid. Sensitivity varies from 73.3% for small polyps to 96.7% for cancer and large polyps; specificity ranges from 92% for small polyps to 94% for cancer and large polyps (Table 39.3).

The place of sigmoidoscopy in screening was first secured through case-control studies and through research indicating that removal of adenomatous polyps reduces risk of colorectal cancer (21,22). The investigators found that sigmoidoscopy screening reduced colorectal cancer mortality from disease detectable by the procedure by 70% to 80%. A prospective controlled study published in 1999 found that FSIG (followed on discovery of polyps by colonoscopy with polypectomy) had significantly reduced the incidence of colorectal cancer among those screened ($p = 0.02$); 10 persons in the control group, but only 2 in the screened group, had colorectal cancer during 13 years of study (RR, 0.2; 95% CI, 0.03–0.95). Interestingly, the overall mortality rate from all causes was found to

be higher in the screened group (14%) than in the unscreened group (9%), which prompted the researchers to call for more study of overall mortality in screening (23). The United States, through the National Cancer Institute, and the United Kingdom hope to resolve lingering questions about the appropriate use of FSIG in screening by undertaking prospective studies. The National Cancer Institute's Prostate, Lung, Colorectal, and Ovarian Cancer Screening Trial is seeking to document the mortality reduction achieved by screening for these cancers, including that for FSIG, by conducting randomized controlled studies that encompass almost 150,000 subjects at 74 centers across the United States. A report from the PLCO Trial on the baseline screening examination included 64,658 subjects (83.5% of those randomized). The yields per 1,000 screened were as follows: for colorectal cancer, 1.1 to 2.5 in women and 2.4 to 5.6 in men; for advanced adenoma, 18.0 to 30.4 in women and 36.1 to 49.1 in men; and for colorectal cancer or any adenoma, 50.6 to 79.6 in women and 101.9 to 128.6 in men. Approximately, 77% (130/169) of colorectal adenocarcinomas were stage I or II at diagnosis (24).

In the United Kingdom, researchers are evaluating effects of a single FSIG examination in 120,000 participants over

TABLE 39.4

USAGE AND PERFORMANCE ISSUES FOR DIFFERENT TYPES OF FECAL OCCULT BLOOD TESTS (FOBTs)

Type of FOBT	Diet restrictions	Drug interference	Site of detectable occult bleeding	Specificity for neoplasia	Sensitivity for cancer
Chemical (guaiac)	Required: red meats; possibly certain raw plant foods[a]	Vitamin C, possibly NSAIDs[b]	Rectum > colon > stomach (in decreasing order of sensitivity)	90%–98%, depending on test brand, sensitivity, and usage	35%–80%, one-time testing. More than 90% with repeated testing
Immunochemical (FIT)	None required	None	Colon and rectum	Around 95%, depending on what sensitivity level is accepted[c]	70%–90%, but data are limited

FIT, fecal immunochemical test; NSAID, nonsteroidal antiinflammatory drug.
[a]Delaying development of 72 hr minimizes interference from plant foods and avoids need for their restriction. Red meats must be restricted when using a more sensitive guaiac FOBT.
[b]Low-dose aspirin is not a problem, but therapeutic doses for rheumatic disorders may be so.
[c]The tests generally provide a qualitative result, but newer immunochromatographic tests may be quantifiable.
From ref. 79.

TABLE 39.5

COMPARISON OF COLORECTAL CANCER SCREENING RECOMMENDATIONS FOR AVERAGE-RISK ADULTS 50 YEARS OR OLDER

Test	American Cancer Society	American College of Gastroenterology	Multi-Society Task Force	U.S. Preventive Services Task Force
Fecal occult blood test (FOBT)	Annually plus flexible sigmoidoscopy (FSIG) every 5 yr	As alternative to colonoscopy: FOBT annually plus FSIG every 5 yr	Annually	Annually
	OR			
Sigmoidoscopy	FSIG every 5 yr plus FOBT annually	As alternative to colonoscopy: FSIG every 5 yr plus FOBT annually	FSIG every 5 yr	FSIG or rigid sigmoidoscopy recommended but insufficient evidence to recommend periodicity
	OR			
Combination of FOBT and sigmoidoscopy	FOBT annually plus FSIG every 5 yr	As alternative to colonoscopy: FOBT annually plus FSIG every 5 yr	FOBT annually plus FSIG every 5 yr	Both "effective" but "insufficient evidence to determine which of these methods is preferable or whether the combination … produces greater benefits than either test alone"
	OR			
Double-contrast barium enema (DCBE) with radiographic studies[a]	Every 5–10 yr	"Where individual radiologists take a strong interest in DCBE and have established a pattern of high quality DCBE as estimated by local clinicians," DCBE may be substituted for FSIG as an alternative strategy	Every 5 years	"Insufficient evidence" to recommend for or against routine screening
	OR			
Colonoscopy	Every 10 yr	Every 10 yr	Every 10 yr	"Insufficient evidence" to recommend for or against routine screening

[a]See footnote in Table 39.3 regarding findings of Winawer and the National Polyp Study Work Group (16).
Data from American Cancer Society. *Cancer Facts & Figures—2007*. Atlanta, Ga.: American Cancer Society; 2007; Smith RA, Cokkinides V, Eyre HJ. American Cancer Society guidelines for early detection of cancer, 2006. *CA Cancer J Clin* 2006;56:11–25; Winawer SJ, Fletcher RH, Rex DK , et al. Colorectal cancer screening and surveillance: clinical guidelines and rationale—update based on new evidence. *Gastroenterology* 2003;124:544–560; U.S. Preventive Task Force. *Guide to Clinical Preventive Services*. 2nd ed. Baltimore, Md.: Williams & Wilkins; 2002.

15 years (25,26). In the United Kingdom, the baseline findings of a multicenter trial showed that of approximately 40,000 patients screened, distal adenomas were detected in 12%, and distal cancers were detected in 0.3% (27).

Obstacles to more widespread use of FSIG include lack of training and low reimbursement rates. Training of nonphysicians may facilitate more widespread use of this technique, particularly in high-volume centers (28). Limitations of FSIG include its confinement to the length of the scope, which permits detection of 65% to 75% of adenomatous polyps and 40% to 65% of colorectal cancers (29–31). Also, the proportion of cancers located in the right colon proximal to the splenic flexure appears to be increasing for unknown reasons (32). Attendant risks of the procedure include bowel perforation, which occurs in approximately 1 of every 5,000 procedures, and complications associated with biopsy and polypectomy. Projected

increases in the population needing this examination have also driven the expansion in those performing the procedure beyond physicians (33).

To visualize a greater proportion of the colon, one must turn to double-contrast barium enema imaging, computed tomography (CT) colonography, or colonoscopy.

Double-Contrast Barium Enema Imaging

Double-contrast barium enema testing, like sigmoidoscopy, initially claimed its place in colorectal cancer screening not because well-defined prospective studies produced clear evidence of its effectiveness but because of recognition that early detection and removal of adenomas could avert cancerous transformation. Sensitivity and specificity measures for double-contrast

Review: Screening for colorectal cancer using the faecal occult blood test, Hemoccult

Comparison: 01 All Hemoccult Screening Groups Versus Control Groups

Outcome: 01 Colorectal cancer mortality (Fixed)

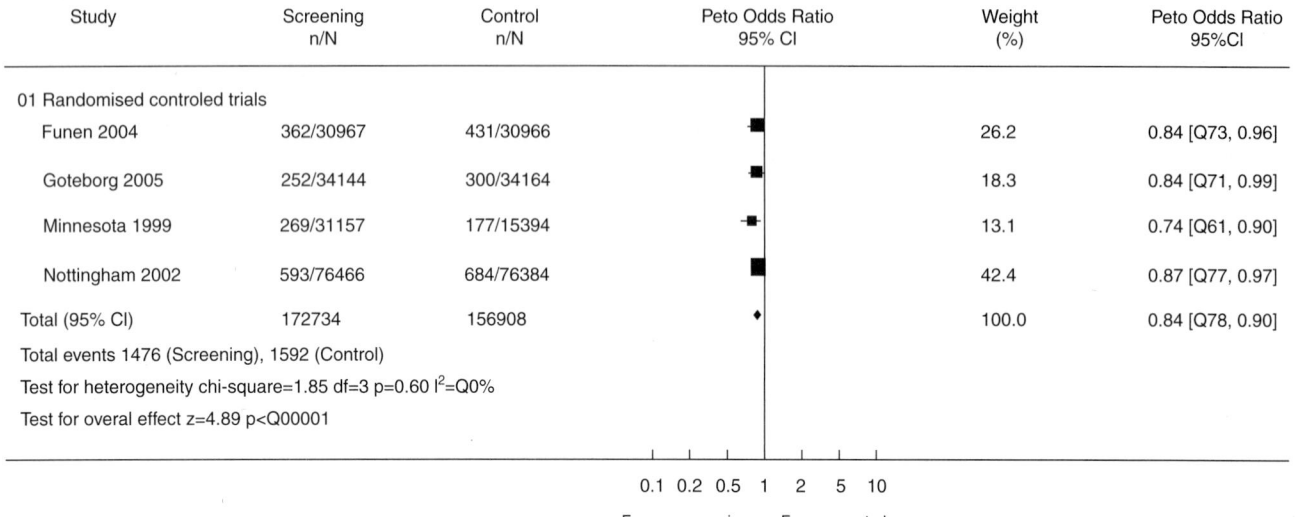

Study	Screening n/N	Control n/N	Peto Odds Ratio 95% CI	Weight (%)	Peto Odds Ratio 95%CI
01 Randomised controled trials					
Funen 2004	362/30967	431/30966		26.2	0.84 [Q73, 0.96]
Goteborg 2005	252/34144	300/34164		18.3	0.84 [Q71, 0.99]
Minnesota 1999	269/31157	177/15394		13.1	0.74 [Q61, 0.90]
Nottingham 2002	593/76466	684/76384		42.4	0.87 [Q77, 0.97]
Total (95% CI)	172734	156908		100.0	0.84 [Q78, 0.90]

Total events 1476 (Screening), 1592 (Control)

Test for heterogeneity chi-square=1.85 df=3 p=0.60 I^2=Q0%

Test for overall effect z=4.89 p<Q00001

```
0.1  0.2  0.5   1    2    5   10
```

Favours screening   Favours control

FIGURE 39.3. Screening for colorectal cancer using the fecal occult blood test. *Source:* From *Hemoccult (Review)*. Copyright © 2007 The Cochrane Collaboration. Published by John Wiley & Sons, Ltd.

barium enema imaging were found to be an improvement over those of FOBT and FSIG (Table 39.3), but new data indicate that barium enema testing deserves less confidence than previously believed (34).

Many studies of double-contrast barium enema imaging have been performed using patients referred for testing because of symptoms or findings on other tests indicative of disease; therefore, the selected population and alerted radiologists may combine to produce upwardly biased measures of sensitivity. Sensitivity measures in these studies ranged from 85% to 95% for polyps. Measures of specificity in these tests are fewer and for polyps and cancer range from 90% to 98% (35). A prospective, blinded study escaped some of the shortcomings of previous research in its evaluation of double-contrast barium enema imaging as a method of surveillance after colonoscopic polypectomy (34). Efforts were made throughout the study to achieve uniformity of practice and protocol adherence. Researchers used only agreed-on cleansing regimens, and radiologic and endoscopic examiners had similar levels of experience. The findings of the study were that colonoscopy was superior to barium enema imaging in detecting adenomas and that rate of detection with barium enema imaging was correlated with adenoma size. In 242 paired examinations in which adenomas were detected by colonoscopy, barium enema imaging detected one or more polyps in 94 (39%). The proportion of adenomas detected by barium enema imaging varied at statistically significant different levels (p = 0.009) according to the size of the largest adenoma: of 155 adenomas of ≤0.5 cm detected by colonoscopy, 49 (32%) were detected by barium enema imaging; of 64 adenomas 0.6 to 1.0 cm in size, 34 (53%) were detected by barium enema imaging; and of 23 adenomas >1.0 cm, 11 (48%) were detected by barium enema imaging. The researchers concluded that the clinical shift toward colonoscopy as the preferred examination is supported by their findings.

Double-contrast barium enema testing also cannot match the ability of colonoscopy to remove polyps for pathologi-cal evaluation. This makes the risks associated with double-contrast barium enema testing fewer than those associated with sigmoidoscopy and colonoscopy but limits its versatility and efficiency in comparison.

With the introduction of CT colonography, it is likely that the use of barium enema for screening purposes will disappear over the next 5 years.

Colonoscopy

Colonoscopy provides visualization of the entire rectum and colon, and affords the efficiency of being a screening, diagnostic, and therapeutic tool. Although few studies have evaluated its ability to reduce the incidence or mortality of colorectal cancer in those at average risk, its role in FOBT trials indicates its usefulness and associates it with the reduced mortality in those who were screened. New studies continued to delineate it more precisely in relation to other tests. As mentioned previously, the National Polyp Study Work Group, in a study relying on 862 paired examinations, found that the proportion of examinations in which adenomatous polyps were detected by barium enema was significantly related to the size of the adenomas (p = 0.009). The rate was 32% for colonoscopic examinations in which the largest adenomas detected were ≤0.5 cm, 53% for those in which the largest adenomas were 0.6 to 1.0 cm, and 48% for those in which the largest adenomas exceeded 1.0 cm in diameter (34). Other work also dramatically highlights the ability of colonoscopy to detect what other tests cannot. In a study of 3,121 asymptomatic patients undergoing complete examination of the colon, Lieberman et al. found that 52% of 128 patients with advanced proximal neoplasia had no distal adenomas. If these patients had undergone sigmoidoscopy alone, these adenomas would have remained undetected (36). Published simultaneously was another study with approximately one-third fewer subjects and similar findings (37). Researchers reported that an even greater percentage of asymptomatic persons undergoing screening (62%) had advanced proximal lesions without any distal lesions or only hyperplastic polyps, whose presence, under current guidelines, would not have prompted further study. These studies confirm what is known—that sigmoidoscopy cannot detect what is beyond the scope of the test—and serve as a reminder that translating what is known about the limits of each test into reasonable screening recommendations requires not only knowledge of the tests' capabilities but also a better understanding of the nature of adenomas.

Benefits are also ascribed to the use of colonoscopy as a screening tool because of its similarity to sigmoidoscopy, for which direct evidence exists regarding colorectal cancer mortality reduction. The sensitivity of colonoscopy ranges from 78.5% to 96.7%, and for cancers and both large and small polyps, its specificity is 98% (38) (Table 39.3).

Although it is commonly believed that colonoscopic polypectomy lowers the incidence of subsequent colorectal cancers by 50% to 90%, this view has been challenged by recent data. A case-control study in the Veterans' Administration System showed only a 50% reduction in incidence associated with colonoscopy (39–42), it showed that colonoscopy and polypectomy provided incomplete protection from development of subsequent colorectal cancer. A study of 35,000 patients in Manitoba showed that the reduction in colorectal cancer incidence in the first 5 years after the negative colonoscopy was <50% (43). However, the risk of developing colorectal cancer remains decreased for more than 10 years following a negative colonoscopy.

The techniques used in colonoscopy are also important factors in adenoma detection. In one 12-member group of gastroenterologists, the range of adenoma varied 10-fold between the highest and lowest performer. As compared with colonoscopists with mean withdrawal times of less than 6 minutes, those with mean withdrawal times of 6 minutes or more had higher rates of detection of any neoplasia (28.3% vs. 11.8%, p <0.001) and of advanced neoplasia (6.4% vs. 2.6%, p = 0.005) (44). It also has been shown that in tandem colonoscopy studies, 15% to 27% of adenomas were missed by a single colonoscopy and 6% of adenomas 1 cm or larger were missed (45).

Recently, there have been a variety of attempts to modify the insertion shaft of the colonoscope to render the colonoscopic examination easier and safer for patients and endoscopists. Two examples are described. The Aer-O-Scope is a self-propelling, self-navigating endoscope that propels itself using a low-pressure technology (46). The Neo Guide System uses a computer to minimize large loops from forming in the colon by the use of an algorithm for continuous real-time tracking through the colon (47). These and other methods may enhance the wider availability of colonoscopy and possibly its use by nonphysicians under supervision.

The benefit of colonoscopy must also be measured against risk of perforation and procedure-related deaths. Cardiovascular events, including arrhythmias, are also listed among complications, and lower tolerance and clinically significant respiratory depression as a complication may occur in older patients. In a study of 16,318 individuals 40 years of age or older undergoing colonoscopy between 1994 and 2002, the rate of serious complications was 5.0/1,000 (95% CI, 4.0–6.2/1,000 colonoscopies). Serious complications occurred in 0.8/1,000 colonoscopies without biopsy or polypectomy and in 7.0/1,000 colonoscopies with biopsy or polypectomy. Perforations occurred in 0.9/1,000 colonoscopies (CI, 0.5–1.5/1,000 colonoscopies), 0.6/1,000 without biopsy or polypectomy and 1.1/1,000 with biopsy or polypectomy. Ten deaths (one attributable to colonoscopy) occurred within 30 days of the colonoscopy (48).

Virtual Colonoscopy (Computed Tomographic Colonography)

Virtual colonoscopy, also known as CT colonography, refers to examination of computer-generated images of the colon constructed from data obtained from an abdominal CT examination. These images simulate the effect of an optical colonoscopy. A bowel preparation is required to cleanse the bowel before the examination, and the colon is insufflated with carbon dioxide by insertion of a rectal tube.

The performance of virtual colonoscopy depends heavily on the size of the target lesion. The accuracy of detection is also a reflection of the experience and training of the radiologist, as well as his or her familiarity with both two- and three-dimensional (3-D) reconstruction techniques.

An example of the high quality of examination that can be attained by close attention to all details of the examination is illustrated by the study of Pickhardt et al. (49). A total of 1,233 asymptomatic adults (mean age 57.8 years) underwent same-day CT and optical colonoscopy. Radiologists used the 3-D endoluminal display for the initial detection of polyps on CT colonography. For the initial examination of each colonic segment, the colonoscopists were unaware of the findings on virtual colonoscopy, which were revealed to them before any subsequent reexamination. The sensitivity and specificity of virtual colonoscopy and the sensitivity of optical colonoscopy were calculated with the use of the findings of the final, unblended optical colonoscopy as the reference standard. The sensitivity of virtual colonoscopy for adenomatous polyps was 93.8% for polyps at least 10 mm in diameter, 93.9% for polyps at least 8 mm in diameter, and 88.7% for polyps at least 6 mm in diameter. The sensitivity of optical colonoscopy for adenomatous polyps was 87.5%, 91.5%, and 92.3% for the three sizes of polyps, respectively. The specificity of virtual colonoscopy was 96% for polyps at least 10 mm in diameter, 92.2% for polyps at least 8 mm in diameter, and 79.6% for polyps at least 6 mm in diameter. Such data raise the possibility that virtual colonoscopy performed with excellent techniques compares favorably with optical colonoscopy. The methodology for performing virtual colonoscopy is evolving rapidly, and results from a national trial comparing virtual colonoscopy with optical colonoscopy will be published in 2007 (American College of Radiology Imaging Network [ACRIN] Study 6664). Technical improvements involving interpretation methodology such as computer-aided diagnosis, 3-D imaging, and limited bowel preparation are under development in centers throughout the world.

The appropriate management of patients with lesions ≤9 mm detected on virtual colonoscopy is still under discussion. At present, at least in the United States, it seems likely that endoscopists will be inclined to perform colonoscopy on most individuals with polypoid lesions found on virtual colonoscopy, irrespective of size. Extracolonic abnormalities may be found commonly on CT colonography. In several series, extracolonic abnormalities have ranged from 15% to 63% of asymptomatic patients (50). The extent to which workup of these incidental findings provides clinical benefit or harms is unknown (51).

Molecular Screening of Stool

Mutations in oncogenes and tumor-suppressor genes have been identified that are associated with the progression from normal mucosa to adenomatous polyps to colorectal carcinomas. Neoplastic epithelial cells containing these genetic abnormalities are constantly shed into the lumen. Polymerase chain reaction technology enables the separation of human DNA from bacterial DNA in the stool.

Because the molecular changes in colorectal neoplasia are heterogeneous, multiple DNA alterations must be targeted to enhance sensitivity. Also, it is important for each assay within a marker panel to have high specificity to avoid false-positive results. A more recent study using colonoscopy as a reference standard assessed in a prospective screening trial the performance of a panel of 21 DNA targets in 4,404 average-risk asymptomatic individuals. Sensitivity for colorectal cancer was 52%, and sensitivity for colorectal cancer or advanced adenoma was 18%. Specificity was 95% (52). Techniques for stool DNA analysis are evolving; for example, in a more recent study using two markers in combination viz. DIA (a marker of DNA integrity) and a marker of vimentin methylation, sensitivity for colorectal cancer was 87.5% with 82.0% sensitivity (53).

Considerable scientific and economic interest continues for the development of an accurate, easy-to-use, affordable molecular test for the early detection of both advanced adenomas and early colorectal cancer. Because of the reduction in subsequent development of cancer associated with the identification and removal of adenomas, the adenoma should be a prime target for these efforts (54).

DETERMINATION OF LEVEL OF RISK

Using these screening tests appropriately requires identifying characteristics that may increase risk of colorectal cancer and matching level of risk to overall test performance. Combining tests, adjusting testing intervals, and accelerating initiation of testing are ways of securing effective screening regimens for specific populations. Risk of colorectal cancer is determined by age, family history, and whether the individual or family members have hereditary diseases that are associated with an increased risk of colorectal cancer. Risk is rated as average, moderate, or high, 70% to 80% of the general population is believed to be at average risk, 15% to 20% at moderate risk, and 5% to 10% at high risk of colorectal cancer.

Average Risk

All asymptomatic persons who are 50 years of age are considered to be at average risk, provided their medical history contains no familial or personal evidence of colorectal, ovarian, or uterine cancer or of other diseases known to increase risk of colorectal cancer. In this population, the only factor indicating risk is age. The individual's medical status, the community's screening resources, and the quality of services available shape choice. Options for screening those at average risk have been developed. Recommendations from the American Cancer Society, the American College of Gastroenterology, the panel convened by the U.S. Multi-Society Task Force, and the U.S. Preventive Services Task Force are included in Table 39.3.

Moderate Risk

Those considered to be at moderate risk of colorectal cancer are also asymptomatic, but they have a personal medical history of adenomatous polyps, colorectal cancer, or ovarian or uterine cancer. Others classified as having moderate risk include those with a family history of adenomatous polyps or colorectal cancer. The finding or diagnosis of adenomas or colorectal cancer must have occurred in a first-degree relative younger than 60 years at diagnosis or in two first-degree relatives at any age. This population requires stepped-up screening that is initiated earlier, performed more frequently, and conducted with the most reliable and thorough tests. Table 39.6 stratifies this population and the population at high risk, identifies appropriate initial screening procedures, and recommends subsequent screening methods and intervals of testing. It is a schema adapted from one published by the American Cancer Society (55,56).

High Risk

Persons considered at high risk are those with a personal medical history of inflammatory bowel disease or a family history of familial adenomatous polyposis or hereditary nonpolyposis colon cancer (HNPCC) (Table 39.6). Causes of inflammatory bowel disease (Crohn disease and ulcerative colitis) remain

---

TABLE 39.6

Colon cancer screening recommendations for people with familial or inherited risk

Familial risk category	Screening recommendations
First-degree relative affected with colorectal cancer or an adenomatous polyp at age ≥60 yr, or two second-degree relatives affected with colorectal cancer	Same as average risk but starting at age 40 yr
Two or more first-degree relatives[a] with colon cancer, or a single first-degree relative with colon cancer or adenomatous polyps diagnosed at an age <60 yr	Colonoscopy every 5 years, beginning at age 40 yr or 10 yr younger than the earliest diagnosis in the family, whichever comes first
One second-degree or any third-degree relative[b,c] with colorectal cancer	Same as average risk
Gene carrier or at risk for familial adenomatous polyposis[d]	Sigmoidoscopy annually, beginning at age 10–12 yr[e]
Gene carrier or at risk for hereditary nonpolyposis colon cancer	Colonoscopy, every 1–2 yr, beginning at age 20–25 yr or 10 yr younger than the earliest case in the family, whichever comes first

[a]First-degree relatives include patients, siblings, and children.
[b]Second-degree relatives include grandparents, aunts, and uncles.
[c]Third-degree relatives include great-grandparents and cousins.
[d]Includes the subcategories of familial adenomatous polyposis, Gardner syndrome, some Turcot syndrome families, and AAPC.
[e]In AAPC, colonoscopy should be used instead of sigmoidoscopy because of the preponderance of proximal colonic adenomas. Colonoscopy screening in AAPC should probably begin in the late teens or early 20s.

unknown, but a review of the literature indicates that research predominantly continues to associate it with an increased risk of colon cancer (57). Screening recommendation intervals are linked to the site of the colitis; pancolitis requires an earlier initiation of annual or biennial colonoscopic screening than colitis on the left side.

Familial adenomatous polyposis is characterized by the presence of 100 or more colorectal adenomatous polyps, which are believed to progress naturally to colorectal cancer, typically by the time the patient is 40 years of age. Diagnosis is usually made when patients are in their late teen years, but familial adenomatous polyposis may be detected as early as 10 years or as late as age 60. Surveillance begins early, and cancer control decisions may be made after molecular testing and correlation with the clinical phenotype (58).

Early identification of patients with HNPCC is important because colorectal cancer in these families is also characterized by early onset of colorectal cancer, which occurs usually 5 to 10 years before screening would typically begin. Formerly, an HNPCC family was defined as one in which colorectal cancer had been diagnosed in three relatives from two or more generations, with one being the first-degree relative of the other two and at least one case occurring before age 50 without gastrointestinal polyposis. Molecular genetics is now used to identify an increasing variety of DNA-mismatch repair gene mutations linked to HNPCC (59). Genetic counseling, including cancer syndrome natural history and genetics, DNA testing risk and benefits, and open discussion, precedes intensified screening in these high-risk families. Participation can result in a significant reduction in colorectal cancer incidence and mortality, a reduction largely attributable to the removal of adenomas during screening (60).

ANALYSIS OF COST EFFECTIVENESS

Analysis of cost effectiveness must, by necessity, make many assumptions about sensitivity and specificity, adenoma-to-carcinoma progression rate, screening interval, costs of the tests themselves, and costs of treatment, and must factor in a discount rate (usually 5% annually) to arrive at the best estimate of cost over time and to avoid bias. Much of the sensitivity and specificity data regarding tests other than FOBT are from studies of populations at more than average risk, so questions about their applicability must be acknowledged. Cost estimates can vary widely. Consider the range of $285 to $1,000 for colonoscopy (36). Furthermore, estimating what tests a patient might choose, what interval he or she might follow, and what combinations of tests might be created could produce an overwhelming number of possibilities. Necessary speculation about the time required for an adenoma to progress to carcinoma further complicates the equation.

Despite these multiple factors, sufficient evidence was available concerning the cost effectiveness of screening to convince the U.S. Congress that making screening a benefit of Medicare, the national health insurance, was appropriate. That meant agreeing that paying to screen Medicare beneficiaries to prevent cancer or treat a cancer early when it was curable was more cost effective than paying the costs associated with the consequences of not screening. In January 1998, the U.S. Health Care Financing Administration expanded Medicare coverage to include routine colorectal cancer screening. Coverage for those at average risk includes FOBT annually complemented by sigmoidoscopy every 4 years. Coverage for those at high risk includes colonoscopy every 2 years, but providers may substitute double-contrast barium enema imaging if they submit a request in writing.

Unit costs used in calculations in one study (61) were based on Medicare reimbursements and included the following, with acknowledgment that the cost could range as high as twice that given: FOBT, $10; FSIG, $80; screening double-contrast barium enema imaging, $131; and screening colonoscopy, $285. Citing the Kaiser Health Plan, the study reported midrange reimbursement for colonoscopy to be $834 in northern California. Diagnostic colonoscopy with polypectomy was higher than colonoscopy alone (Medicare, $434; Kaiser, $1,048). FOBT, the least expensive of the tests, but the one used most frequently, was studied in Britain and found to be cost effective in biennial screening (62). Researchers found it to be of equal or superior cost effectiveness to analogous screening in the U.K. breast cancer screening program.

Theuer et al. (63) studied 16 strategies for screening, including

- Annual FOBT
- Flexible sigmoidoscopy every 3, 5, or 10 years
- Colonoscopy every 3, 5, or 10 years
- Annual FOBT and FSIG every 3, 5, or 10 years
- Annual FOBT and double-contrast barium enema imaging every 3, 5, or 10 years

They concluded that screening fell below the benchmark for cost effectiveness of $40,000 per added year of life. Annual mammographic screening for breast cancer is believed to cost approximately $34,500 per year of life gained (64).

Even the most expensive test, colonoscopy, is believed to be cost effective in comparison with other screening test regimens (61). One must remember that no data yet characterize the safety, feasibility, and acceptability of widespread colonoscopic screening. Speculation about the risks of coronary artery events related to colonoscopy has been fueled by findings in two colorectal cancer screening study populations of an offsetting of reductions in mortality from colorectal cancer screening by an increase in cardiovascular-related deaths and an increase in noncolorectal cancer mortality in a third (65). These findings argue for caution in choice of both initial and subsequent screening tests, especially in placing patients with detected adenomas on a colonoscopic surveillance schedule that has unquantified coronary consequences.

It is also when colonoscopy must be repeated in surveillance and continues indefinitely that costs rise in a screening program using primarily FOBT and FSIG. Atkin and Whynes (66) argued that overtreatment is bound to be the outcome of a strategy that aims to prevent cancer by detecting adenomas. Recent guidelines based on risk provide a rational basis for follow-up surveillance (67).

Despite the intricacies of cost analysis, organizations have found it possible to offer meaningful schedules of examinations that can be performed at costs that government and some insurers are willing to say are cost effective; however, if individuals fail to undergo the tests, it matters little how sensitive they are or how cost effective they prove. Now that so much groundwork has been laid, all are eager to see reductions in the mortality, morbidity, and economic loss imposed by colorectal cancer, reductions that are the expected fruits of appropriate screening.

IMPROVEMENT OF SCREENING PARTICIPATION

Improving compliance with colorectal cancer screening recommendations, although always important, becomes even more vital as the proportion of citizens 50 years of age and older—those identified as being most likely to benefit from screening—grows and as life expectancy continues to increase. Startling in its implications for colorectal screening is the striking demographic statistic of the "baby boomer" cohort that every day adds 10,000 more Americans who are 50 years of age. The aging trend is global and is expected to change the proportion of the population age 65 or older from 390 million (6.6%) in 1997 to 800 million (10%) in 2025 (68). These people will also be living longer: Average life expectancy worldwide, having risen from 48 years in 1955 to 65 years in 1995, will reach 73 years in 2025 (68).

The Behavioral Risk Factor Surveillance System (BRFSS) is a population-based random telephone survey conducted in all 50 states, the District of Columbia, and Puerto Rico. Results from the 2004 BRFSS Survey were compared with results from 2002. In 2004, 57.3% of adults age ≥ 50 years reported having an FOBT within 1 year preceding the survey and/or a lower gastrointestinal (GI) endoscopy within 10 years preceding the survey. The proportion of persons age ≥ 50 years who had received FOBT within 1 year preceding the survey declined to 18.7% in 2004 from 21.8% in 2002. However, the proportion who reported receiving a lower GI endoscopy within the 10 years preceding the survey increased to 50.6% in 2004 from 45.2% in 2002. The number of states in the United States where $\geq 60\%$ of the population have been screened for colorectal cancer nearly doubled from 8 in 2002 to 15 in 2004. Although this increase in reported use of colorectal cancer tests is encouraging, use of screening tests for colorectal cancer continues to lag behind use of mammography and Papanicolaou (Pap) smear tests for breast and cervical cancer, respectively (60). Whites are more likely than African Americans to undergo screening. Non-Hispanics were more likely to have undergone either test than were Hispanics. Higher education and higher income were both predictors of compliance.

Barriers preventing patients from complying with screening recommendations may include ignorance of or confusion over screening recommendations, problems with access to health care, cost, fear of discomfort, and embarrassment (11,60,69). Providers may face the barriers of lack of skill, lack of time for patient counseling, and lack of knowledge of up-to-date research findings and screening guidelines (70–72).

Cost can certainly affect access to health care and may be a significant barrier, not only to the most expensive examination (colonoscopy) but also for less expensive procedures such as FSIG when it is presented as part of a combination strategy with FOBT (11,69). After receiving only descriptive test information about FOBT and FSIG, the most popular strategies were FOBT alone (45%) or both tests (38%). Fewer patients preferred FSIG (13%). After receiving information about test performance, more subjects preferred both tests (47%), and fewer subjects preferred FOBT alone (36%) ($p = 0.12$). With hypothetical out-of-pocket costs to be incurred, the proportion preferring FOBT alone increased to 53%, whereas those preferring both tests decreased to 31% ($p < 0.001$). Some of those who changed their preference reported changing their minds not because of cost but because FOBT was easier to perform and could be done alone. Patients, insurers, and physicians working in a capitated system may favor a less expensive test over colonoscopy (11,69).

Initiatives for drawing more people to colorectal screening should include targeting of those who are less likely to participate, including women who may have the perception that colorectal cancer is a man's disease and women of low income (71,72). Recommendations from physicians could encourage compliance among these groups (60,72). Physician counseling, a catalyst for change, may be integrated into primary care routine practice and sustained by progress reports at subsequent visits. Burke et al. (73) suggested that women may be receptive to colorectal cancer preventive counseling because

- They may be more amenable to colorectal screening because of familiarity with Pap and mammography screening.

- They are often the health promotion leaders in the family.
- They have power as agents of change in special populations such as the medically underserved, the elderly, and those of low socioeconomic status.

Public and physician education programs can make a difference. Research evaluating the effects of mass media on health services utilization (74) and studies of successful public relations efforts demonstrate that mass media can make an impact on use of health services, whether as a result of planned campaigns or ordinary day-to-day coverage. A wide range of organizations, coalitions, and individuals representing nonprofit groups have in the past few years been attempting to wield influence through the mass media in favor of better colorectal cancer screening practices. One education program encompassed a multiyear colon cancer awareness campaign that reached millions of men and women with patient brochures, appearances on television by celebrities such as Katie Couric, and cooperative publishing efforts with a popular woman's magazine. Couric, a nationally recognized television show host, joined with the Entertainment Industry Foundation to cofound the National Colorectal Cancer Research Alliance to promote screening and research. Relying on celebrities to attract attention to the screening message and money to the cause, the National Colorectal Cancer Research Alliance organized the message to the public and funded cutting-edge research. Another coalition, the National Colorectal Cancer Roundtable, founded by the American Cancer Society and the Centers for Disease Control and Prevention, works to promote screening for colorectal cancer nationally and regionally, and thereby lower morbidity and mortality of the disease.

Pignone et al. (69) reported that patient preferences are not strongly tied to a single test. Other investigators (61) also suggested that having a spectrum of tests was advantageous in encouraging screening participation and that, when presented with choices, patients' selections varied (75). Additional research such as that of Schoen et al. (76) concerning patient satisfaction with FSIG will help both physicians and patients put aside assumptions and will aid in making recommendations for screening that are based on research findings.

Finally, just as failure to undergo screening can have medical consequences for the patient, failure to offer screening may have legal consequences for the physician (77). Because factors usually used as a gauge of malpractice risk—for example, scope or incidence of the problem, potential for serious consequences, preventability of consequences, and clarity of the relevant standard of care—are evident in colorectal cancer screening, the risk of malpractice may be significant. Recommendations for lowering risk include offering to provide screening or referring the patient for screening on the applicable schedule and ensuring that the patient is reasonably educated about it. Ways to fulfill the obligation to the patient and perhaps improve compliance while documenting the patient's response include using an information sheet with recommendations, writing a message about the importance of screening, providing check boxes to indicate request for or declining of tests, and providing signature (patient and physician/nurse) and date lines. One copy stays in the chart; the other is given to the patient. Other less effective options are annual practice letters and chart progress notes.

CONCLUSION

Many advances in research, screening, cooperative planning, and organizational initiatives indicate new opportunities for reducing the morbidity and mortality of colorectal cancer (78). Increases in 5-year survival rates; the issuance of screening guidelines that offer more consistency with each other and greater choice; the government's willingness to fund screening in its national health care program; and the efforts of professional, educational, and patient advocacy groups to endorse screening will all help nurture further growth of screening. These—together with discovery of new molecular bases for colorectal cancer and development of new, more acceptable methods of screening—should further fuel enthusiasm among physicians and the public for continuing efforts against colorectal cancer.

References

1. Jemal A, Siegel R, Ward E, et al. Cancer statistics, 2007. *CA Cancer J Clin* 2007;57:43–66.
2. Ries LAG, Harkins D, Krapcho M, et al., eds. *SEER Cancer Statistics Review, 1975–2003*. Bethesda, Md.: National Cancer Institute; 2006. Available at: http://seer.cancer.gov/csr/1975_2003. Accessed May 7, 2007.
3. Parkin DM. International variation. *Oncogene* 2004;23:6329–6340.
4. Minami Y, Nishino Y, Tsubono Y, et al. Increase of colon and rectal cancer incidence rates in Japan: trends in incidence rates in Miyagi Prefecture, 1959–1997. *J Epidemiol* 2006;16:240–248.
5. Gross CP, Anderson MS, Krumholz HM, et al. Relation between Medicare screening reimbursement and stage at diagnosis for older patients with colon cancer. *JAMA* 2006;296:2815–2822.
6. Ricciardiello L, Boland CR. Lynch syndrome (hereditary non-polyposis colorectal cancer): current concepts and approaches to management. *Curr Gastroenterol Rep* 2005;7:412–420.
7. Moshkowitz M, Arber N. Emerging technologies in colorectal cancer screening. *Surg Oncol Clin N Am* 2005;13:723–746.
8. Nicholson FB, Barro JL, Atkin W, et al. Population screening for colorectal cancer. *Aliment Pharmacol Ther* 2005;22:1069–1077.
9. National Cancer Institute. Conquering colorectal cancer: a blueprint for the future. Report of the Colorectal Cancer Progress Review Group. Available at: http://planning.cancer.gov/cprgreport/execsumm.htm. Accessed July 17, 2001.
10. Winawer SJ. Surveillance overview. In: Cohen AM, Winawer SJ, eds. *Cancer of the Colon, Rectum, and Anus*. New York, NY: McGraw-Hill; 1995:279–290.
11. Winawer SJ, Fletcher RH, Miller L, et al. Colorectal cancer screening: clinical guidelines and rationale. *Gastroenterology* 1997;12:594–642.
12. Hewitson P, Glasziou P, Irwig L, et al. Screening for colorectal cancer using the faecal occult blood test, Hemoccult. In: *The Cochrane Database of Systematic Reviews*. Issue 1. Oxford: UK: Cochrane Database; 2006.
13. Mandel JS, Bond JH, Church TR, et al. Reducing mortality from colorectal cancer by screening for fecal occult blood. Minnesota Colon Cancer Control Study. *N Engl J Med* 1993;328:1365–1371.
14. Collins JF, Lieberman DA, Durbin TE, et al. Accuracy of screening for fecal occult blood on a single stool sample obtained by digital rectal examination: a comparison with recommended sampling practice. *Ann Intern Med* 2005;142:81–85.
15. Mandel JS, Church TR, Bond JH, et al. The effect of fecal occult-blood screening on the incidence of colorectal cancer. *N Engl J Med* 2000;343:1603–1607.
16. Young GP, Macrae FA, St. John DJB. Clinical methods for early detection: basis, use, and evaluation. In: Young GP, Rozen P, Levin B, eds. *Prevention and Early Detection of Colorectal Cancer*. Philadelphia, Pa.: WB Saunders; 1996:241–270.
17. Smith RA, Cokkinides V, Eyre HJ. American Cancer Society guidelines for early detection of cancer, 2003. *CA Cancer J Clin* 2003;53:27–43.
18. Smith A, Young GP, Cole SR, et al. Comparison of a brush-sampling fecal immunochemical test for hemoglobin with a sensitive guaiac-based fecal occult blood test in detection of colorectal neoplasia. *Cancer* 2006;107:2152–2159.
19. Levi Z, Rozen P, Harari R, et al. A quantitative immunochemical fecal occult blood test for colorectal neoplasia. *Ann Intern Med* 2007;146:244–255.
20. Imperiale TF. Quantitative immunochemical fecal occult blood tests: is it time to go back to the future? *Ann Intern Med* 2007;146:309–311.
21. Selby JV, Friedman GD, Quesenberry CP, Jr., et al. A case-control study of screening sigmoidoscopy and mortality from colorectal cancer. *N Engl J Med* 1992;326:653–657.
22. Newcomb PA, Norfleet RG, Storer BE. Screening sigmoidoscopy and colorectal cancer mortality. *J Natl Cancer Inst* 1992;84:1572–1575.
23. Thiis-Evensen E, Hoff GS, Sauar J, et al. Population-based surveillance by colonoscopy: effect on the incidence of colorectal cancer. Telemark Polyp Study I. *Scand J Gastroenterol* 1999;34:414–420.
24. Weissfeld JL, Schoen RE, Pinsky PF, et al. Flexible sigmoidoscopy in the PLCO Cancer Screening Trial: results from the baseline screening examination of a randomized trial. *J Natl Cancer Inst* 2005;97:989–997.
25. Atkin W, Edwards R, Wardle J, et al. UK randomised trial of "once only" flexible sigmoidoscopy screening: baseline results. *Endoscopy* 1999;31(suppl 1):E1.
26. Whynes DK, Frew EJ, Edwards R, Atkin WS. Costs of flexible sigmoidoscopy screening for colorectal cancer in the United Kingdom. *Int J Technol Assess Health Care* 2003;19(2):384–395.
27. UK Flexible Sigmoidoscopy Screening Trial Investigators. Single flexible sigmoidoscopy screening to prevent colorectal cancer: baseline findings of a U.K. multicenter randomized trial. *Lancet* 2002;359:1291.
28. Wong RC. Screening flexible sigmoidoscopy by nonphysician endoscopists: it's here to stay, but is it the right test to do? *Gastrointest Endosc* 1999;49:262–264.
29. Muller AD, Sonnenberg A. Prevention of colorectal cancer by flexible endoscopy and polypectomy: a case control study of 32,702 veterans. *Ann Intern Med* 1995;123:904–910.
30. Tedesco JP, Wave JD, Avella JR, et al. Diagnostic implications of the spatial distribution of colonic mass lesions (polyps and cancers): a prospective colonoscopic study. *Gastrointest Endosc* 1980;26:95–97.
31. Shinya H, Wolff WI. Morphology, anatomic distribution and cancer potential of colonic polyps: an analysis of 7000 polyps endoscopically removed. *Ann Surg* 1979;190:679–683.
32. Beart RW, Jr., Steele GD, Jr., Menck HR, et al. Management and survival of patients with adenocarcinoma of the colon and rectum: a national survey of the Commission on Cancer. *J Am Coll Surg* 1995;181:225–236.
33. Schoenfeld P, Piorkowski M, Allaire J, et al. Flexible sigmoidoscopy by nurses: state of the art 1999. *Gastroenterol Nurs* 1999;22:254–261.
34. Winawer SJ, Stewart ET, Zauber AG, et al., for the National Polyp Study Work Group. A comparison of colonoscopy and double-contrast barium enema for surveillance after polypectomy. *N Engl J Med* 2000;342:1766–1772.
35. Glick S, Wagner JL, Johnson CD. Cost-effectiveness of double-contrast barium enema in screening for colorectal cancer. *Am J Radiol* 1998;170:629–636.
36. Lieberman DA, Weiss DG, Bond JH, et al., for Veterans Affairs Cooperative Study Group 380. Use of colonoscopy to screen asymptomatic adults for colorectal cancer. *N Engl J Med* 2000;343:162–168.
37. Imperiale TF, Wagner DR, Lin CY, et al. Risk of advanced proximal neoplasms in asymptomatic adults according to the distal colorectal findings. *N Engl J Med* 2000;343(3):169–174.
38. Markowitz AJ, Winawer SJ. Screening and surveillance for colorectal cancer. *Semin Oncol* 1999;26:485–498.
39. Muller AD, Sonneby A. Prevention of colorectal cancer by flexible endoscopy and polypectomy: a case-control study of 32,702 veterans. *Ann Intern Med* 1995;123:904–910.
40. Alberts DS, Martinez ME, Doe DJ, et al. Lack of effect of a high fiber cereal on the recurrence of colorectal adenomas. *N Engl J Med* 2000;342:1156–1162.
41. Schatzkin A, Lanza F, Corle DJ, et al. Lack of effect of a low-fat, high fiber diet on the recurrence of colorectal adenomas. *N Engl J Med* 2000;342:1149–1155.
42. Robertson DJ, Greenbey FR, Bead M, et al. Colorectal cancer in patients under close colonoscopic surveillance. *Gastroenterology* 2005;129:34–41.
43. Singh H, Turner D, Xue L, et al. Risk of developing colorectal cancer following a negative colonoscopy examination: evidence for a 10-year interval between colonoscopies. *JAMA* 2006;295:2366–2373.
44. Barclay RL, Vicari JJ, Doughty AS, Johanson JF, Greenlaw RL. Colonoscopic withdrawal times and adenoma detection during screening colonoscopy. *N Engl J Med* 2006;355:2533–2541.
45. Hixson LJ, Fennerty MB, Sampliner RI, et al. Prospective blinded trial of the colonoscopic miss-rate of large colorectal polyps. *Gastrointest Endosc* 1991;37:125–127.
46. Vucelic B, Rex D, Pulanic R, et al. The Aer-O-Scope: proof of concept of a pneumatic, skill-independent, self-propelling, self-navigating colonoscope. *Gastroenterology* 2006;130:672–677.
47. Eickhoff A, Van Dam J, Jakobs R, et al. Computer-associated colonoscopy (The NeoGuide Endoscopy System): results of the first human clinical trial. *Am J Gastroenterol* 2007;102:261–266.
48. Levin TR, Zhau W, Conell C, et al. Complications of colonoscopy in an integrated health care delivery system. *Ann Intern Med* 2006;145:880–886.
49. Pickhardt PJ, Choi JR, Hwang I, et al. Computed tomographic virtual colonoscopy to screen for colorectal neoplasia in asymptomatic adults. *N Engl J Med* 2003;349:2191–2200.
50. Glueker TM, Johnson CD, Wilson LA, et al. Extracolonic findings at CT colonography: evaluation of prevalence and cost in a screening population. *Gastroenterology* 2003;124:911–916.
51. Hur C, Chung DC, Schoen RE, Gazelle GS. The management of small polyps found by virtual colonoscopy: results of a decision analysis. *Clin Gastroenterol Hepatol* 2007;5:237–244.
52. Imperiale TF, Ransohoff DF, Itzkowitz SH, et al. Fecal DNA versus fecal occult blood for colorectal cancer screening in an average risk population. *N Engl J Med* 2004;351:2704–2714.
53. Itzkowitz S, Jandof L, Brand R, et al. Improved performance of a non-invasive fecal DNA test to screen for colorectal cancer. *Gastroenterology* 2006;130:51862A.
54. Levin B. Molecular screening testing for colorectal cancer. *Clin Cancer Res* 2006;17:5014–5017.
55. Smith RA, Cokkinides V, Eyre HJ. American Cancer Society guidelines for early detection of cancer, 2006. *CA Cancer J Clin* 2006;56:11–25.
56. Levin B. Colorectal prevention and early detection. In: *The American Cancer Society Atlas of Clinical Oncology: Colon, Rectal, Anal*. Hamilton, Ontario, Canada: BC Decker; 2001.
57. Bernstein CN. Neoplasia in inflammatory bowel diseases: surveillance and management strategies. *Curr Gastroenterol Rep* 2006;8:513–518.

58. Guillem JG, Wood WC, Moley JF, et al. ASCO/SSO review of current role of risk-reducing surgery in common hereditary cancer syndromes. *J Clin Oncol* 2006;24:4642–4660.

59. Lindor NM, Peterson GM, Hadley DW, et al. Recommendations for the care of individuals with an inherited predisposition to Lynch syndrome: a systematic review. *JAMA* 2006;296:1507–1517.

60. Increased use of colorectal cancer tests—United States 2002 and 2004. *MMWR Morb Mortal Wkly Rep* 2006;55:308–311.

61. Maciosek MV, Solberg LI, Coffield AB, et al. Colorectal cancer screening: health impact and cost effectiveness. *Am J Prev Med* 2006;55:308–311.

62. Whynes DK, Nielson AR, Walker AR, et al. Faecal occult blood screening for colorectal cancer: is it cost-effective? *Health Econ* 1998;7:21–29.

63. Theuer CP, Wagner JL, Taylor TH, et al. Racial and ethnic colorectal cancer patterns affect the cost-effectiveness of colorectal cancer screening in the United States. *Gastroenterology* 2001;120:1043–1046.

64. Levin B. Colorectal cancer: population screening and surveillance. In: McDonald JWD, Burroughs AK, Feagan BG, eds. *Evidence Based Gastroenterology and Hepatology*. London: BMJ Publishing Group; 2004:255–263.

65. Atkin WS. Screening for colorectal cancer: the heart of the matter. *Gut* 1999;45:480–481.

66. Atkin WS, Whynes DK. Improving the cost-effectiveness of colorectal cancer screening. *J Natl Cancer Inst* 2000;92:513–514.

67. Winawer SJ, Zauber AG, Fletcher RH, et al. Guidelines for colonoscopy surveillance after polypectomy: a consensus update by the American Cancer Society and the US Multi-Society Task Force on Colorectal Cancer. *Gastroenterology* 2006;130:1872–1885.

68. World Health Organization (WHO). *The World Health Report: 1998: Life in the 21st Century—A Vision for All: Executive Summary*. Geneva: WHO; 1998. Available at: http://whqlibdoc.who.int/hq/1998/WHO_WHR_98.1.pdf. Accessed May 7, 2007.

69. Pignone M, Bucholtz D, Harris R. Patient preferences for colon cancer screening. *J Gen Intern Med* 1999;14:432–437.

70. Donovan JM, Syngal S. Colorectal cancer in women: an underappreciated but preventable risk. *J Womens Health* 1998;7:45–48.

71. Woolf SH. Overcoming the barriers to change: screening for colorectal cancer. *Am Fam Physician* 2000;61:1621–1622, 1628.

72. Paskett ED, Tatum C, Rushing J, et al. Racial differences in knowledge, attitudes, and cancer screening practices among a triracial rural population. *Cancer* 2004;101:2650–2659.

73. Burke W, Beeker C, Kraft JM, et al. Engaging women's interest in colorectal cancer screening: a public health strategy. *J Womens Health Gend Based Med* 2000;9:363–371.

74. Grilli R, Freemantle N, Minozzi S, et al. Mass media interventions: effects on health services utilisation (Cochrane Review). In: *The Cochrane Library*. Issue 1. Oxford: Update Software; 2000.

75. Leard L, Savides T, Ganiats T. Patient preferences for colorectal cancer screening. *J Fam Pract* 1997;45:211–218.

76. Schoen RE, Weissfeld JL, Bowen NJ, et al. Patient satisfaction with screening flexible sigmoidoscopy. *Arch Intern Med* 2000;160:1790–1796.

77. Feld AD. Medicolegal implications of colon cancer screening. *Gastrointest Endosc Clin N Am* 2002;12:171–179.

78. Levin B, Ades TB, Brooks D, et al. *American Cancer Society's Complete Guide to Colorectal Cancer*. Atlanta, GA: American Cancer Society; 2005.

79. Winawer SJ, Fletcher RH, Rex DK, et al. Colorectal cancer screening and surveillance: clinical guidelines and rationale—update based on new evidence. *Gastroenterology* 2003;124:544–560.

80. Rozen P, Blanchard J, Campbell D, et al. Implementing colorectal cancer screening: group 2 report. ESGE/UEGF Colorectal Cancer-Public Awareness Campaign. The Public/Professional Interface Workshop: Oslo, Norway, June 20–22, 2003. *Endoscopy* 2004;36:354–358 .

CHAPTER 40 ■ COLORECTAL CANCER: MOLECULAR BIOLOGY AND GENETICS

WILLIAM M. GRADY

INTRODUCTION

Colorectal cancer (CRC) develops as a result of the progressive accumulation of genetic and epigenetic alterations that lead to the transformation of normal colorectal epithelium to colorectal adenocarcinoma. The loss of genomic stability is a key molecular and pathophysiological step in this process, and it serves to create a permissive environment for the occurrence of alterations in tumor-suppressor genes and oncogenes. Alterations in these genes, which include *APC, CTNNB1, KRAS, BRAF, SMAD4, TP53, PIK3CA,* and *TGFBR2,* appear to promote colorectal tumorigenesis by perturbing the function of signaling pathways, such as the transforming growth factor-beta (TGF-ß) and phosphatidylinositol 3-kinase (PI3K) signaling pathways, or by affecting genes that regulate genomic stability, such as the mismatch repair (MMR) genes.

The process of colorectal carcinogenesis, which has been termed the *polyp-carcinoma sequence,* is believed to typically occur over 10 to 15 years and involves concurrent histologic and molecular changes. The subsequent effect of these genetic and epigenetic alterations on the cell and molecular biology of the cancer cells in which they occur is the acquisition of key biological characteristics that are central to the malignant phenotype (1). From the analysis of the molecular genetics of CRC, it has become clear that the formation of CRC involves a multistage process that is currently characterized based on genomic instability (i.e., the loss of the ability to maintain the wild-type DNA coding sequence and repair DNA mutations). In the background of genomic instability, genetic and epigenetic alterations accumulate and cooperate with each other to drive the initiation and progression of CRC (2–4).

CRC appears to be most commonly initiated by alterations that affect the Wingless/Wnt signaling pathway. The initiated CRC then progresses as a result of the accumulation of sequential genetic or epigenetic events that either activate oncogenes or inactivate tumor-suppressor genes that are involved in other signaling pathways, such as the RAS-RAF-MAPK pathway, TGF-ß pathway, and the PI3K-AKT pathway (5,6). Some of the alterations that have been convincingly shown to promote colorectal carcinogenesis affect *KRAS, TP53,* the gene for p53, and elements of the TGF-ß signaling pathway, such as *TGFBR2* and *SMAD4* (Fig. 40.1). The identification of these alterations has provided potential targets for the development of new therapies for the prevention and/or treatment of colorectal tumors throughout their progression from normal epithelium to adenocarcinoma.

POLYP-CARCINOMA SEQUENCE

The evolution of normal epithelial cells to adenocarcinoma usually follows a predictable progression of histologic changes and concurrent genetic and epigenetic changes. These gene mutations and epigenetic alterations provide a growth advantage and lead to the clonal expansion of the altered cells. This process leads to the progression of adenomas to adenocarcinomas by the serial acquisition of genetic and epigenetic alterations that produce clonal heterogeneity followed by Darwinian evolution at the cellular level. Until more recently, it was believed that only conventional tubular and tubulovillous adenomatous polyps had the potential to undergo malignant transformation; however, it now also appears that a subset of CRCs can evolve from sessile serrated adenomas (7). Moreover, a subset of hyperplastic polyps appears to be the precursor lesions for at least some of the serrated polyps, and this subset of hyperplastic polyps appears to have the potential to transform into adenocarcinomas through a hyperplastic polyp-serrated adenoma-adenocarcinoma progression sequence (7–9). CRCs arising through a hyperplastic polyp-serrated adenoma-CRC pathway appear to have a unique molecular and histologic pathway through which they arise (9). The serrated polyps commonly display a form of genomic instability termed microsatellite instability (MSI) and commonly carry mutations in BRAF (both are discussed in detail later) (9).

GENOMIC INSTABILITY

Genomic instability, which is the loss of the ability of the cell to maintain the fidelity of the DNA, is a fundamental aspect of the tumorigenesis process. Early neoplastic lesions, including colorectal adenomas, demonstrate activation of the ATR-ATM DNA damage checkpoint system (e.g., phosphorylated ATM-Thr68, ATR-Ser1981, and H2AX), and it is believed that activation of this system serves as a barrier to transformation whose loss contributes to the progression of adenomas to adenocarcinomas by promoting genomic instability, increased cell proliferation, and cell survival (10). The loss of genomic instability also likely contributes to increased clonal diversity, which has been shown to correlate with the progression of cancer, possibly through promoting Darwinian adaptation to intracellular and extracellular environmental changes (11–13).

At least three forms of genomic instability have been identified in CRC: (a) MSI, (b) chromosome instability (CIN) (i.e., aneusomy, gains and losses of chromosomal regions), and (c) chromosomal translocations (14). The etiology of CIN has

539

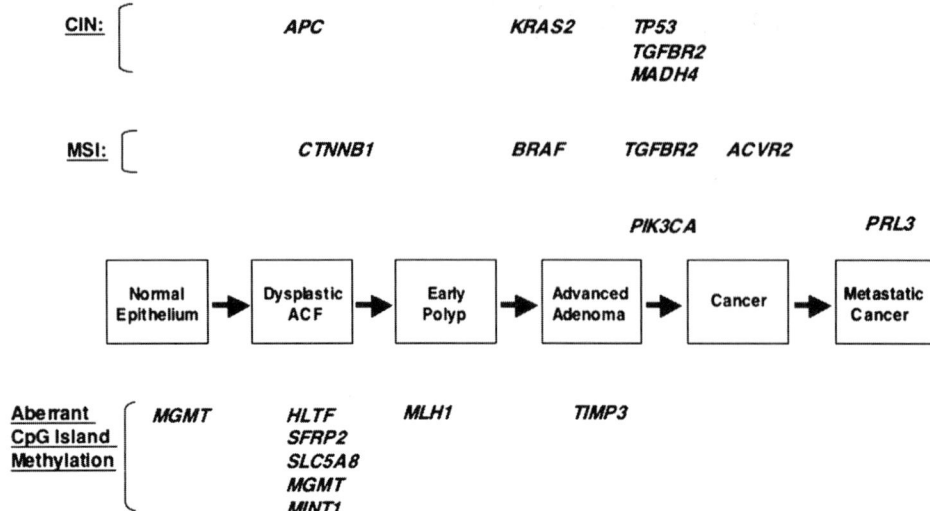

FIGURE 40.1. Schematic diagram of the polyp-carcinoma progression sequence. Each recognized histologic step in the process is depicted as a box. Above the histologic sequence is a list of genes that are commonly altered in the setting of two recognized forms of genomic instability that occur in colorectal cancer, chromosomal instability (CIN), and microsatellite instability (MSI). Below the histologic sequence is a list of genes that have been demonstrated to be aberrantly methylated in colorectal cancer. The genes are listed above or below the histologic steps in which they have been identified and presumably occur during the polyp-cancer sequence.

only been identified in a small subset of CRCs; however, MSI is known to result from inactivating mutations or from the aberrant methylation of genes in the DNA-MMR family, which repairs DNA base pair mismatches that arise during DNA replication. The timing of the loss of genomic stability, either CIN or MSI, during the initiation and progression of CRC appears to be after adenoma formation but before progression to frank malignancy. In fact, both CIN and MSI can be detected in colorectal adenomas (15–21). Shih et al. demonstrated that >90% of early adenomas (1–3 mm in size) exhibit allelic imbalance of at least one of four chromosomes tested (15). A stepwise increase in the average number of copy alterations using comparative genomic hybridization has been observed when comparing adenomas with low-grade dysplasia, to adenomas with high-grade dysplasia, and then to adenocarcinomas (20,22). Adenomas with intramucosal carcinoma carry approximately twice as many chromosomal gains and losses compared to tubular adenomas (10.5 vs. 4.6 abnormalities), and losses in 8p21-pter, 15q11–q21, 17p12–13, and 18q12–21 and gains in 8q23-qter, 13q14–31, and 20q13 associate with adenomas with intramucosal carcinoma and adenocarcinomas (22). Despite the accumulation of data demonstrating the presence of genomic instability in early colorectal tumors, the causative role of genomic instability in cancer remains a source of considerable controversy (3,14). Nonetheless, genomic instability is an attractive target for anticancer therapies because it is nearly ubiquitous in CRC and is a unique characteristic of cancer cells that is not present in normal epithelial cells. The feasibility of targeting genomic instability for anticancer treatments has been shown in in vitro systems (23).

CHROMOSOME INSTABILITY

CIN is the most common type of genomic instability observed in CRC. It occurs in approximately 85% of colorectal tumors. However, despite the high frequency of CIN in CRC and the fact that aneuploidy has long been appreciated as a hallmark of cancer, the understanding of the basis for this state of chromosomal disarray is rudimentary. It is still controversial whether aneuploidy is simply a state that occurs nonspecifically during tumor formation, which the tumor cells can tolerate because of independence from the normal mechanisms that control cell growth and death, or whether it reflects an active process of chromosomal instability that is itself an important element in a tumor's development. The recognition that CRCs display recurrent and tumor-specific chromosome abnormalities implies that this process is not random or simply accessory and likely

means that chromosomal instability plays a role in tumor progression by increasing clonal diversity that can contribute to tumor progression by enhancing opportunities for Darwinian evolution in the tumors (12,14,22).

Mechanisms for Chromosomal Instability

A major challenge in this area of investigation is the complexity of the mechanisms that regulate chromosomal stability and the current superficial level of understanding of the processes involved in maintenance of genomic stability. In *Saccharomyces cerevisiae*, more than 100 genes have been shown to cause a CIN phenotype when mutated (24,25). These genes regulate a variety of cellular processes, including chromosome condensation, sister-chromatid cohesion, kinetochore structure, kinetochore function, microtubule formation, and cell cycle checkpoint regulation. Nonetheless, despite this complexity, progress has been made in identifying a genetic etiology for aneuploidy, and presumably CIN, in a subset of CRCs. Since the late 1990s, mutations or amplification of genes known to cause experimental forms of CIN have been identified in cancer, including *BUB1, ATM, ATR, BRCA1, BRCA2, STK15, PLK1,* and *CDC4* (26–32). More recently, Wang et al. used computational analysis to identify more than 1,000 possible genes that could cause genomic instability based on their homology to genes in yeast and *Drosophila melanogaster*. They identified somatic mutations in a subset of these genes in cancers, but the role of these genes in causing CIN is still to be determined (33).

Other potential candidate genes that mediate CIN have been identified in subsets of CRCs. Somatic mutations in *hCDC4*, which is also known as *Fbw7* or *Archipelago*, were found in 11.5% of human CRCs (N = 22/190) and in 4/58 adenomas (34). CDC4 is an evolutionarily conserved E3 ubiquitin ligase that regulates the G1-S checkpoint by targeting proteins for destruction by the SCF complex of proteins. After identifying CDC4 mutations in a subset of CRCs, the functional consequence of CDC4 inactivation was demonstrated by disrupting both alleles through homologous recombination and in the karyotypically stable CRC cell lines HCT116 and DLD1. The inactivation of CDC4 resulted in nuclear atypia, an increased frequency of multipolar spindles, and CIN. Notably, this effect was dependent on an increase in cyclin E, which is a substrate of CDC4 (34,35). The significance of deregulation of the CDC4-cyclin E pathway has been substantiated in other systems and has shown that the inhibition of degradation of cyclin E in mice leads to tumors that display genomic instability and that Fbxw7/hCDC4 cooperates with p53 to suppress tumor formation (36,37). It appears that Cdc4 is regulated by p53 and is one of the downstream effectors of p53-mediated regulation of genome stability, especially in the setting of genomic stress. Notably, Cdc4 may affect genome stability not only through the regulation of cyclin E, but also through the regulation of Notch and/or JUN (37). In aggregate, these data provide further support for an underlying genetic basis for CIN and for the hypothesis that deregulation of mechanisms that mediate DNA fidelity lead to complex consequences that ultimately induce CIN.

DNA-Mismatch Repair Pathway/Inactivation of Mismatch Repair Genes

Genomic instability arises because of inactivation or inhibition of the normal mechanisms the cell uses to maintain its DNA fidelity. Defects in two of the systems that regulate DNA fidelity, the MMR system and base excision repair (BER), have been identified in independent subsets of CRC. The DNA MMR system consists of a complex of proteins that recognizes and repairs base pair mismatches that occur during DNA replication. Inactivation of the MMR system occurs in 1% to 2% of CRCs due to germline mutations in members of the MMR system, *MLH1*, *MSH2*, *PMS2*, and *MSH6*, and is the cause of the CRC family syndrome, hereditary nonpolyposis colon cancer (HNPCC) (38,39). In addition to HNPCC-related colon cancers, 15% of sporadic CRCs have an inactivated MMR system due to the aberrant methylation of *MLH1* (40). MSI occurs as the consequence of inactivation of the MMR system and is recognized by frameshift mutations in microsatellite repeats located throughout the genome. Because many CRCs demonstrate frameshift mutations at a small percentage of microsatellite repeats, the designation of a colorectal adenocarcinoma as showing MSI depends on the detection of >30% unstable loci from a panel of 5 to 10 loci that were selected at a National Cancer Institute (NCI) consensus conference (41).

Study of the biochemistry of the MMR proteins has revealed that recognition of the base–base mismatches and insertion/deletion loops is performed by a heterodimer of either MSH2 and MSH6 or MSH2 and MSH3. Of interest, the MSH2-MSH3 heterodimer preferentially recognizes insertion/deletion loops and thus cannot compensate for loss of MSH6. Consequently, cancers arising with a loss of MSH6 function display MSI only in mononucleotide repeats and may display an attenuated form of MSI called MSI-low, which is recognized clinically by having 10% to 29% unstable loci in the NCI consensus panel noted previously (42). The MLH1, PMS2, and PMS1 proteins appear to operate primarily in performing the repair of the base–base mismatches and insertion/deletion loops. A heterodimer of MLH1-PMS2 operates as a "molecular matchmaker" and is involved in executing the repair of the mismatches in conjunction with DNA-polymerase ∂ and the replication factors proliferating cell nuclear antigen, replication protein A, and replication factor C, as well as the 5′ → 3′ exo/endonucleases EXO1 and FEN1 and other unidentified 3′ → 5′ exonucleases and helicases (42,43).

The MSI that results from loss of MMR activity affects mono-, di-, and trinucleotide tracts predominantly. However, cell lines from these tumors also show up to a 1,000-fold increased mutation rate at expressed gene sequences, and in particular, show instability of short sequence repeats with expressed sequences (44). Genes that possess such "microsatellitelike" repeats in their coding regions appear to be the targets relevant to carcinogenesis. This pathway to tumor formation appears to be distinct from that seen in CRCs that are microsatellite stable (MSS) (45). Genes that are targeted for

mutation in this pathway include the TGF-ß receptor type II tumor-suppressor gene (*TGFBR2*), the activin receptor type II gene (*ACVR2*), and *BAX* (46,47). Importantly, MSI and the subsequent target gene mutations appear to occur throughout the adenoma-to-carcinoma progression. The timing of many of these events during tumor formation remains to be determined, but preliminary studies have shown they occur at distinct phases of tumor progression (17). Thus, MSI appears to create a favorable state for accumulating mutations in vulnerable genes that promote tumorigenesis, and these alterations ultimately lead to the generation of CRC.

The relationship between the MSI pathway and other genetic alterations frequently found in CRC is only partially understood. The most notable association is between mutant *BRAF V600E* and sporadic MSI CRC (48). *BRAF V600E* mutations associate with sporadic MSI tumors that carry aberrantly methylated *MLH1*, but not MSI CRCs arising in the setting of HNPCC (48,49). Alteration of the Wnt/Wingless pathway can be observed in tumors irrespective of MSI (50). Mutations in *APC* and *CTNNB1* can be found in 21% and 43% of MSI tumors, respectively (51,52). In addition, the incidence of *KRAS* mutations appears to be as high as 22% to 31%, which is similar to the incidence observed in MSS CRCs (53,54). Mutations in *TP53* are less frequent in MSI cancers than in MSS cancers. The mutation incidence in MSI CRCs ranges between 0% and 40%, whereas the incidence in MSS tumors is between 31% and 67% (51,53,55,56). Of interest, monoallelic and biallelic *BAX* mutations and the aberrant methylation of $p14^{ARF}$ are found frequently in MSI CRCs and may serve to replace the role of mutant *TP53* in colorectal carcinogenesis (57,58). Thus, the microsatellite mutator pathway appears to be initiated through changes in the Wnt/Wingless pathway and shares some alterations with the MSS CRC pathway. However, other events, such as *TP53* and *TGFBR2* mutations, occur at different frequencies in the MSI versus the MSS pathway.

The impact of genomic instability and particularly microsatellite instability on the clinical behavior of CRCs has been intensely investigated but remains only partly understood to date. Several retrospective studies have shown mixed results regarding the effect of MSI on prognosis. Watanabe et al. found that 18q loss of heterozygosity (LOH) correlated with a reduction in 5-year survival from 74% to 50% in stage III CRC patients and that *TGFBR2 BAT-RII* mutations correlated with improved 5-year survival in tumors with MSI, 74% versus 46% (59). In addition, a systematic review of MSI revealed that there was a combined hazard ratio estimate for overall survival associated with MSI of 0.65 (95% CI, 0.59–0.71) (60).

Base Excision Repair Defects

Inactivation of a second "DNA caretaker" mechanism, the BER system, is found in a subset of CRC cell lines and is a cause of an autosomal recessive form of adenomatous polyposis called the MYH adenomatous polyposis (MAP) syndrome (61). Germline mutations in *MYH*, which encode for a protein involved in base excision repair, is the cause of adenomatous polyposis in up to 5% to 10% of individuals who have an adenomatous polyposis syndrome. *MYH* germline mutations were discovered as a cause of adenomatous polyposis when investigators identified an excessive number of somatic G:C→A:T mutations in neoplasms of people with adenomatous polyposis but who had no detectable germline mutations in *APC* (62–64). This type of mutation is commonly a consequence of oxidative damage to DNA that results in 8-oxo-7,8-dihydro2′deoxyguanosine (8-oxodG), which is one of the most stable deleterious products of oxidative DNA damage (61,65). The BER system is responsible for repairing this form of DNA damage, which led these investigators to assess candidate genes involved in this process, *OGG1*, *MTHF1*, and *MYH*. This assessment revealed biallelic germline mutations in a subset of people with adenomatous polyposis who did not have germline mutations in *APC*. The most common mutations are Tyr165Cys and Gly382Asp, which account for 82% of the mutant alleles detected to date (64). Despite the role of germline mutations in *MYH* as a cause of a CRC family syndrome, somatic *MYH* mutations are not common in sporadic CRC. A study of 1042 unselected CRC patients in Finland revealed no somatic *MYH* mutations (61,66). Of interest, the tumors arising in the setting of biallelic *MYH* germline mutations do not show differences in the frequency of *TP53*, *SMAD4*, or *TGFBR2* mutations but do show an absence of MSI or CIN, suggesting that they follow a unique molecular pathogenesis compared to sporadic CRC (67). The discovery of *MYH* germline mutations in people with a hereditary CRC syndrome provides more evidence for the importance of genomic instability in cancer formation.

TELOMERES AND TELOMERASE

Telomeres are special chromatin structures at the ends of linear chromosomes that are believed to play a fundamentally important role in protecting these regions from degradation and recombination. The regulation of telomeres is tightly associated with the regulation of senescence. In vertebrates, telomeres are composed of tandem repeats of the TTAGGG sequence and are bound by specific proteins (68). Conventional DNA polymerases are not able to completely synthesize chromosomal ends, resulting in the gradual shortening of telomeres with successive rounds of cell divisions until a critical short length is reached that elicits the activation of cellular checkpoints similar to those activated by DNA damage (69). In human cells, this telomere shortening culminates in activation of the Hayflick limit and the cessation of cell divisions. However, if p53 or Rb is inactivated, then the cells can continue to divide and will go through a period of massive cell death termed "cellular crisis." Cells that survive crisis appear to activate mechanisms to maintain the telomeres, and they do this most frequently by increasing the expression of telomerase, a specialized ribonucleoprotein complex that consists of a catalytic telomerase reverse transcriptase (TERT) and an RNA subunit encoded by *TERC*. Most human cancers express telomerase, and it appears that during the evolution of normal cells to cancer cells that the cells progress through a period of severe telomere dysfunction before regaining mechanisms to maintain telomere length (70). Now, data from experiments from *Ter*$^{-/-}$ mice suggest that this period of telomere dysfunction may cause marked CIN that promotes the formation of cancer cells (69). Consistent with this model, human colon cancers show a peak in the anaphase bridge index, which is a measure of the number of metaphases that contain anaphase bridges, in early high-grade dysplastic lesions and less in more advanced carcinoma stages (71). However, the identification of chromosomal abnormalities in early colon adenomas, at a stage that precedes telomere dysfunction, suggests that telomere dysfunction cannot be the only potential mechanism that induces genomic instability in colon cancer and that its role in tumor formation may depend on the nature of concurrent genetic alterations in the tumor cells. In support of this model, *mTerc*$^{-/-}$; Min (*Apc*$^{-/+}$), mice form fewer macroadenomas than mice with wild-type *mTerc*, but *mTerc*$^{-/-}$; *Tp53*$^{-/-}$ mice show a high level of genomic instability similar to that seen in human cancers and reduced tumor latency in late generation mice (69,72,73). Thus, it appears that telomere dysfunction may also contribute to genomic instability seen in cancer, although more definitive evidence of its role in human cancer remains to be shown.

EPIGENTIC ALTERATIONS

DNA methylation is present throughout the majority of the genome and is maintained in relatively stable patterns that are established during development (74). In humans, approximately 70% of CpG dinucleotides carry this epigenetic modification. However, there are regions called CpG islands that are enriched for CpG dinucleotides, which are present in the 5′ region of approximately 50% to 60% of genes and are normally maintained in an unmethylated state. In cancers, many of these CpG islands become aberrantly methylated, and this aberrant methylation can be accompanied by transcriptional repression (75,76).

The significance of these epigenetic alterations in the pathogenesis of cancer has been a point of significant controversy (77,78). Nonetheless, there is now sufficient data to demonstrate that the aberrant methylation of at least some of these genes, such as *MLH1*, can be pathogenetic in cancer (40,79,80). Aberrant methylation of *MLH1* occurs in approximately 80% of sporadic MSI CRCs, and the restoration of *MLH1* expression and function by demethylating the *MLH1* promoter in MSI CRC cell lines strongly suggests that such aberrant methylation is a cause rather than a consequence of colorectal carcinogenesis (40,79,80). Moreover, it is likely that the aberrant hypermethylation of 5′ CpG dinucleotides that has been demonstrated to silence a variety of tumor-suppressor genes in CRC, including *CDKN2A/p16*, *MGMT*, *p14*^{ARF}, and *HLTF*, may be similarly pathogenetic in CRC (75,79–83). Of specific note, methylation of *CDKN2A/p16*, a canonical tumor-suppressor gene, is detected in 40% of CRCs (82) and has been found in not only CRC but also in colorectal adenomas, as have other aberrantly methylated genes (84,85). This observation, as well as the detection of aberrantly methylated genes (e.g. *HLTF SLC5A8*, *MGMT*, *MINT1*, and *MINT31*) in aberrant crypt foci, demonstrates that aberrant promoter methylation is occurring early in the adenoma sequence, although it does not confirm that the aberrant methylation is a primary rather than a secondary event in the tumorigenesis process (86–88). More broadly, early work has suggested that CRCs that hypermethylate *MLH1* and/or *CDKN2A/p16* may belong to a distinct subclass of CRCs, termed the CpG island methylator phenotype (CIMP), that demonstrate genomewide aberrant methylation of gene promoters and that may arise by distinct and unique mechanisms (82,83,89).

Also worthy of note is recent progress in our understanding of mechanisms through which DNA methylation may affect transcription. DNA methylation may impair transcription by direct inhibition between methylated promoters and transcription factors, such as AP-2, CREB, E2F, CBF, and NF-KB (74,90). CpG island methylation can also mediate transcriptional silencing by recruiting methyl-binding proteins, MeCP2, MBD2, and MBD3, that recognize methylated sequence and recruit histone deacetylases (HDACs). The HDACs then induce changes in chromatin structure that impede the access of transcription factors to the promoter (75,90). Indeed, the posttranslational modification state of the histones, which includes modifications such as acetylation of histone 3 (H3) at lysines 9 (K9) and 18 (K18), acetylation of histone 4 at lysine 12 (K12), dimethylation of histone 4 at arginine 3 (di-me R3), and dimethylation of histone 3 at lysine 4, among others, appears to regulate the chromatin state in a transcriptionally active (euchromatin) or transcriptionally repressed state (heterochromatin) through a "histone code" (91). This "histone code" is altered from the normal state in cancer and appears to cooperate with aberrant methylation to alter the expression of tumor-suppressor genes in cancer (92,93). It is noteworthy that the relationship between DNA methylation and posttranslational modification of histones is complex and only partially understood at this time. Studies have shown that changes in the methylation state of H3-lysine 9 and H3-lysine 4 precede changes in DNA methylation, suggesting that the histone modification state and chromatin structure may cause the DNA methylation changes as opposed to the DNA methylation directing alterations in the histones as noted previously (74).

GENETIC ALTERATIONS

Wingless/Wnt Signaling Pathway

APC

The role of genetic alterations in CRC formation was initially suggested by the CRC family syndrome familial adenomatous polyposis (FAP). FAP is a hereditary CRC predisposition syndrome that is characterized by the development of hundreds of intestinal adenomatous polyps. The gene responsible for this syndrome, adenomatous polyposis coli (*APC*) was identified as the result of the discovery of an interstitial deletion on chromosome 5q in a patient affected with FAP and from classical linkage analysis of families affected by FAP (94–96). The *APC* gene has 15 exons and encodes a large protein (310 kDa, 2,843 amino acids) that possesses multiple functional domains that mediate oligomerization and bind to a variety of intracellular proteins, including ß-catenin, γ-catenin, glycogen synthase kinase (GSK)-3ß, axin, tubulin, end-binding protein 1, and homolog of discs large (4). Germline mutations in *APC* result in FAP or one of its variants, Gardner syndrome, attenuated FAP, and Turcott syndrome (97–99).

APC is mutated in up to 70% of all sporadic colorectal adenocarcinomas, and these mutations are present beginning in the earliest stages of CRC formation and precede the other alterations observed during CRC formation (Table 40.1)

(52,100–103). In fact, aberrant crypt foci, a presumptive precursor lesion to CRC, have been found to harbor *APC* mutations (104,105). The mutations observed in sporadic CRC occur most frequently in the 5′ end of exon 15 between amino acid residues 1280 and 1500 (106). Mutations in this region can affect the domains between amino acid residues 1020–1169 and 1324–2075, which have been implicated in ß-catenin interactions. These mutations can also affect the SAMP (Ser-Ala-Met-Pro) domains located between amino acids 1324–2075 and thus disrupt APC's interaction with axin (107–109). The vast majority of *APC* mutations (>90%) result in premature stop codons and truncated gene products (110). As mentioned previously, these mutations are often accompanied by chromosomal deletion of the residual wild-type allele, but biallelic inactivation of *APC* can also occur by second somatic mutations and possibly by aberrant methylation (111,112).

One of the central tumor-promoting effects of these mutations is to lead to overactivation of the Wingless/Wnt signaling pathway with the subsequent expression of genes that favor cell growth (Fig. 40.2). The disruption of the association of APC with ß-catenin leads to overactivation of the Wnt signaling pathway, which leads to the transcription of genes that favor tumor formation, such as *MYC* or *MMP7* (100,113). Normally, GSK-3ß forms a complex with APC, ß-catenin, and axin, and phosphorylates these proteins. The phosphorylation of ß-catenin by GSK-3ß targets it for ubiquitin-mediated proteasomal degradation. Truncating *APC* mutations prevent this process from occurring and cause an increase in the amount of cytoplasmic ß-catenin, which can then translocate to the nucleus and interact with other transcription factors such as T-cell factor/lymphoid enhancing factor (Tcf/Lef). TCF-4 is the predominant TCF family member expressed in colonic epithelium. Consistent with the concept that increased Wnt-ß-catenin pathway activity is a central tumor-promoting effect of *APC* mutations, oncogenic mutations in the ß-catenin gene (*CTNNB1*) have been observed in some CRCs, as has methylation of *SFRP2* and *SFRP4*, members of a family of

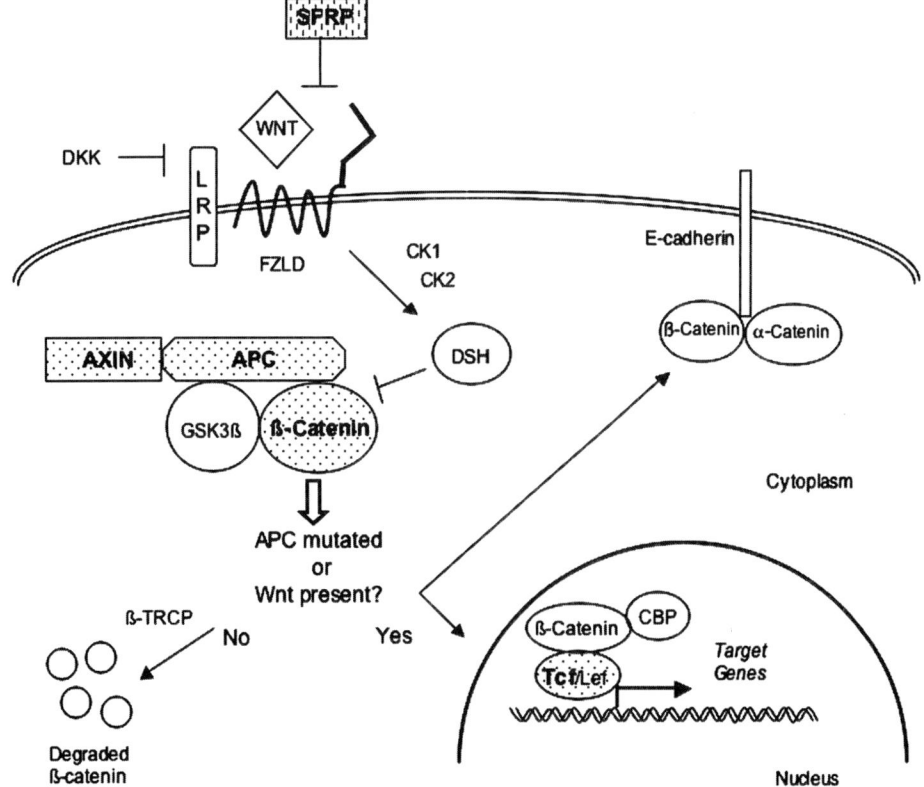

FIGURE 40.2. Diagram of the Wnt signaling pathway depicting the consequence of *APC* mutation on activation of the pathway. Axin, APC, β-Catenin, TCF$_4$ have been shown to be mutated in CRC. SFRP aand DKK have been shown to be aberrantly methylated. DKK, dikkopf; LRP,; FZLD, Frizzled; DSH, dishelved.

TABLE 40.1

ALTERED GENES IN COLORECTAL CANCER

Gene	Affected pathway/ function	Alteration	Frequency in CRCs (approximate)	Germline mutations	Comments/additional reference
APC	Wingless/Wnt	Mutation	70%	Yes	
CTNNB1	Wingless/Wnt	Mutation	2%	No	More common in microsatellite instability (MSI) cancers
AXIN2	Wingless/Wnt	Mutation	Uncommon	Yes	(238,239)
SFRP1	Wingless/Wnt	Methylation	90%	No	(114)
SFRP2	Wingless/Wnt	Methylation	85%	No	(114)
KRAS	Ras-Raf pathway	Mutation	40%	No	
BRAF	Ras-Raf pathway	Mutation	30% MSI/5% microsatellite stability (MSS) colorectal cancers (CRCs)	No	*V600E* is mutation hot spot in *BRAF*
PIK3CA	PI3K signaling pathway	Mutation	30%	No	
PIK3R1	PI3K signaling pathway	Mutation	5%	No	
PTEN	PI3K signaling pathway	Mutation	Uncommon	Yes	Germline mutation is cause of Cowden syndrome
TP53		Mutation	>50%	Yes	Germline mutations cause Li-Fraumeni syndrome, which may be cause of some cases of early onset CRC (12)
P14ARF		Methylation	20%	No	
TGFBR2	Tumor growth factor-beta (TGF-ß) signaling pathway	Mutation	25%–30%	Yes[a]	Mutations more common in MSI CRCs
TGFBR1	TGF-ß signaling pathway	Polymorphism	Rare somatic mutations	Yes[b]	TGFBR1*6A[b] polymorphism associated with cancer risk (240)
SMAD4	TGF-ß and bone morphogenetic protein (BMP) signaling pathway	Mutation	16%	Yes	Germline mutation is cause of juvenile polyposis syndrome
SMAD2	TGF-ß signaling pathway	Mutation	2%	No	
ACVR2	Activin/TGF-ß signaling pathway	Mutation	60%–90% of MSI CRCs	No	More common in MSI cancers
BMPR1A	BMP signaling pathway	Mutation	—	Yes	Mutation is uncommon in sporadic CRCs
MYH	Base excision repair	Mutation	Rare somatic mutations	Yes	Cause of 5%–10% of adenomatous polyposis cases
MLH1	Mismatch repair (MMR)	Methylation	10% of sporadic cases	Yes	Most common gene affected in hereditary nonpolyposis colon cancer (HNPCC)
MSH2	MMR	Mutation	Uncommon	Yes	Cause of HNPCC
MSH6	MMR	Mutation	Rare somatic mutations	Yes	Cause of HNPCC
PMS2	MMR	Mutation	Rare somatic mutations	Yes	Cause of HNPCC

[a]*TGFBR2* germline mutation is a cause of a Marfanlike syndrome, but not a cause of cancer family syndrome (241).
[b]TGFBR1*6A is a common variant of TGFBR1 that has a deletion of 3 GCG repeats coding for alanine within a 9 alanine (9A) repeat sequence of TGFBR1 (TGFBR1*9A) exon 1 resulting in a six alanine repeat (TGFBR1*6A). TGFBR1*6A is less effective at mediating TGF-β growth inhibition.

secreted Wnt antagonists called secretory frizzled related proteins (114–116).

The clinical effects of *APC* mutations are best understood in the context of FAP in which the location of the mutations associates with the severity of the phenotype and the occurrence of extraintestinal tumors, such as desmoid tumors (54,117–119). Polymorphisms in the *APC* gene that associate with a slight increased risk of colorectal have also been identified, and include *I1307K* and *E1317Q* polymorphisms. *APC* I1307K occurs exclusively in people of Ashkenazi Jewish descent and results in a twofold increased risk of colorectal adenomas and adenocarcinomas compared to the general population (120,121). The *I1307K* polymorphism results from a transition from T to A at nucleotide 3920 in the *APC* gene and appears to create a region of hypermutability.

ß-Catenin (*CTNNB1*)

ß-Catenin is a member of the APC/ß-catenin/Tcf/Lef pathway that plays a role in the formation of a subset of CRCs. ß-Catenin is a homolog of armadillo, and its expression is increased by activation of the Wnt signaling pathway (122–124). APC interacts with ß-catenin and forms a macromolecular complex with it and GSK-3ß. ß-Catenin is consequently directed toward degradation as a result of phosphorylation by GSK-3ß (125–127). Mutations of *CTNNB1* or *APC* often render ß-catenin insensitive to APC/ß-catenin/GSK-3ß—mediated degradation (128,129). One of the functions of ß-catenin is to bind members of the Tcf family of transcription factors and activate gene transcription. Accordingly, cancers with *APC* or *CTNNB1* mutations have increased ß-catenin/Tcf-mediated transcription, which leads to the inappropriate expression of genes such as *CCND1* (the gene for cyclin D1) and *MYC* (130,131). The majority of these mutations are in a portion of exon 3 encoding for the GSK-3ß phosphorylation consensus region of ß-catenin. These mutations are often missense mutations in the highly conserved aspartic acid 32 and presumably impair the ability of GSK-3ß to phosphorylate ß-catenin (132). Caca et al. found *CTNNB1* mutations in the NH2-terminal phosphorylation sites of ß-catenin and found increased Tcf/Lef transcriptional activity in association with this mutation (133). Mutations that abolish ß-catenin binding with E-cadherin have also been identified and have been shown to impair cell adhesion (134,135). Like *APC* mutations, *CTNNB1* mutations have an essential role in early colorectal tumor formation. Mouse models with conditional *Ctnnb1* alleles that lead to the stabilization of ß-catenin in the intestinal tract result in a phenotype similar to mice that have germline mutations in *Apc*, providing functional evidence that *CTNNB1* mutations contribute to the formation of adenomas (136). Of interest, though, the incidence of *CTNNB1* mutations decreases from 12.5% in benign adenomas to 1.4% in invasive cancers, suggesting that *CTNNB1* mutations do not favor the progression of adenomas to adenocarcinomas (137).

KRAS, BRAF, and RAS-RAF-MAPK Signaling Pathway

One of the most prominent protooncogenes in colorectal carcinogenesis is a member of the *RAS* family of genes, *KRAS*. The *RAS* oncogenes, which include *HRAS, NRAS,* and *KRAS,* were initially discovered as the transforming genes of the Harvey and Kirsten murine sarcoma viruses (Ha-MSV, Ki-MSV) (138,139). *KRAS* is the most commonly mutated *RAS* family member in CRC, although *NRAS* mutations are also observed in a small percentage of CRCs (140).

The *RAS* family genes encode a highly conserved family of 21-kDa proteins that are involved in signal transduction. One major function of the ras protein family is to couple growth factors to the Raf-mitogen—activated protein (MAP) kinase kinase-MAP kinase signal transduction pathway, which leads to the nuclear expression of early response genes (141). *KRAS* consists of four exons that produce either a 188 or 189 amino acid peptide, depending on whether the fourth exon is alternatively spliced (142). The protein encoded by *KRAS* has three domains that mediate the following processes:

- Binding to guanosine triphosphate (GTP) or guanosine diphosphate (GDP)

- Attachment of the protein to the inner side of the plasma membrane after posttranslational modification (isoprenylation) of the carboxy terminus
- Interaction with cellular targets

Inactive KRAS binds GDP and, on activation, GDP is exchanged for GTP. The activated KRAS then interacts with downstream signaling molecules to propagate cell proliferation. The activated KRAS is normally immediately deactivated by intrinsic GTP hydrolysis. Oncogenic mutations of *KRAS* disrupt the GTPase activity of KRAS and allow it to remain in an activated state (142). In fact, the most common mutations observed in human cancers involve codons 12, 13, and 61, which correspond to areas in the GTP/GDP-binding domains in the KRAS protein. The consequence of these mutations is that approximately 30% of the KRAS protein is in the GTP-bound state as compared to <0.3% in cells with wild-type *KRAS* (143). The increased fraction of activated KRAS leads to activation of the RAS-RAF-MAPK signaling pathway, which promotes cell proliferation and increased survival as well as other protumorigenic effects (144,145) (Fig. 40.3).

Mutation of *KRAS* and *KRAS* amplification has been observed in a large percentage of gastrointestinal tract tumors, including CRCs. As in other tumors, the *KRAS* mutations observed in CRC almost always affect codons 12, 13, and 61. *KRAS* mutations can be detected in 37% to 41% of CRCs. Codon 12 is the most commonly mutated codon in CRC and usually undergoes a missense mutation (103,146–148). The *KRAS* mutations appear to occur after *APC* mutations in the temporal events of the polyp-to-cancer progression sequence and are associated with advanced adenomatous lesions (103). Evidence for this model comes from the observation that small adenomas with *APC* mutations carry *KRAS* mutations in approximately 20% of the tumors, whereas approximately 50% of more advanced adenomas have been found to have *KRAS* mutations (101,149). Thus, alterations of *KRAS* appear to promote CRC formation early in the adenoma-carcinoma sequence by mediating adenoma growth. Of interest, though, they are not necessary for the malignant conversion of adenomas to adenocarcinomas.

More recently, mutations in *BRAF*, which is a kinase that is activated by KRAS, have also been recognized. *BRAF* mutations can be found in 27% to 31% of MSI CRCs and 5% of MSS CRCs and can be detected in ACFs, adenomas, and adenocarcinomas (32,150,151). Eighty percent of the mutations are *V600E* mutations, which are only found in MSI cancers and lead to activation of the ERK and NFκB pathways (152). *BRAF* mutations appear to be mutually exclusive from *KRAS* mutations, suggesting that mutations in either gene affect tumor formation by activating the RAS-RAF-MAPK pathway. *BRAF* mutations also appear to occur rarely in MSI CRCs that occur in the setting of HNPCC and are tightly associated with CIMP CRCs, suggesting that there may be two distinct molecular pathways for the formation of sporadic MSI CRCs (48,49,89,153).

p53 (*TP53*)

The p53 protein was initially identified as a protein forming a stable complex with the SV40 large T antigen and suspected to be an oncogene (154). Subsequent studies demonstrated that *TP53* is located at 17p13.1 and is mutated in 50% of primary human tumors, including tumors of the gastrointestinal tract (155). Currently, p53 is appreciated to be a transcription factor that is involved in maintaining genomic stability through the control of cell cycle progression and induction of apoptosis in response to genotoxic stress (155). The protein encoded by p53 has been structurally divided into four domains:

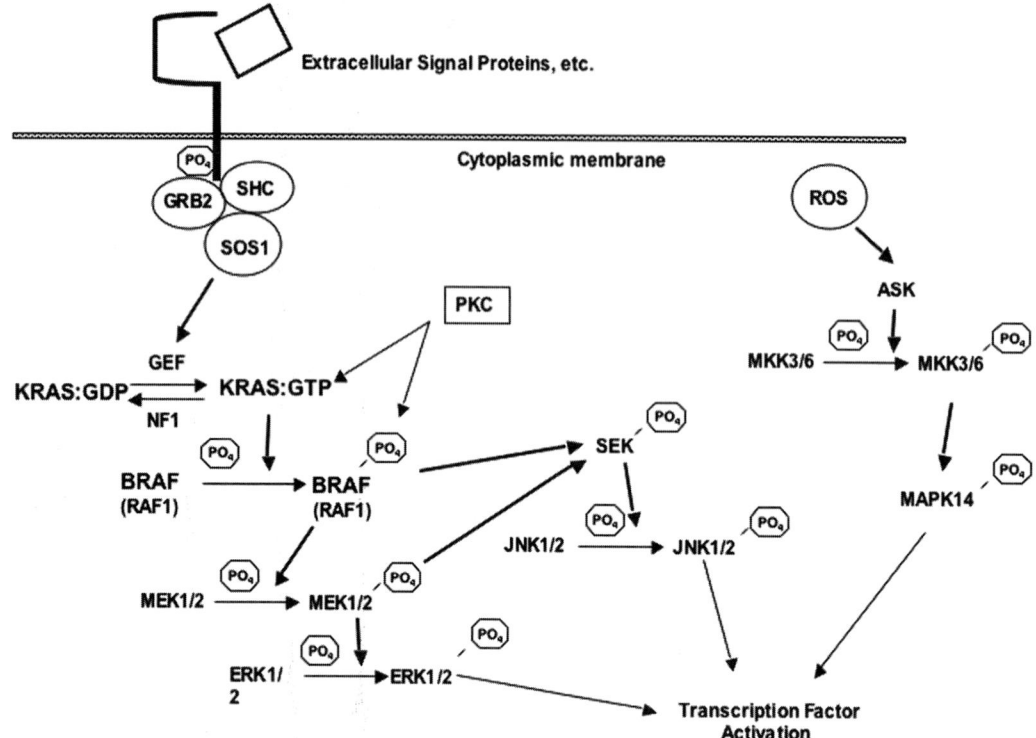

FIGURE 40.3. Diagram of the Ras-Raf-MAPK signaling pathway demonstrating the location of Ras and Raf, the most commonly mutated members of this signaling pathway in colorectal cancer, in the signaling cascade. ROS, reactive oxygen species; ASK, apoptosis signal-regulating kinase; MKK, MAPK kinase; PKC, protein kinase C; SOS, son of sevenless.

- An acidic amino-terminal domain (codons 1–43) required for transcriptional activation
- A central core sequence-specific DNA-binding domain (codons 100–300)
- A tetramerization domain (codons 324–355)
- A C-terminal regulatory domain (codons 363–393) rich in basic amino acids and believed to regulate the core DNA-binding domain (155)

The spectrum of mutations in *TP53* seen in CRC appears similar to that seen in other tumors with mutations of *TP53* clustering at four hot spots in highly conserved regions (domains II–V). *TP53* is mutated in >50% of colorectal adenocarcinomas and the mutations localize primarily to exons 5 to 8 (103,156). The mutations found to occur commonly in colorectal carcinoma are G:C to A:T transitions at CpG dinucleotide repeats and in general interfere with the DNA-binding activity of the protein (157,158). The mutation of *TP53* in CRC is commonly accompanied by allelic loss at 17p, consistent with its role as a tumor-suppressor gene (159). In CRCs, *TP53* mutations have not been observed in colorectal adenomas but rather appear to be late events in the colorectal adenoma-carcinoma sequence that may mediate the transition from adenoma to carcinoma (103). Furthermore, mutation of *TP53* coupled with LOH of the wild-type allele was found to coincide with the appearance of carcinoma in an adenoma providing further evidence of its role in the transition to malignancy (159–162).

p53 normally serves to regulate cell growth and division in the context of genotoxic stress. It is expressed at very low levels in cells until it is activated by poorly understood mechanisms by DNA damage resulting from gamma irradiation, ultraviolet irradiation, or chemotherapeutic agents (163). Its activation results in the transcription of genes that directly regulate cell cycle progression and apoptosis. These genes include *p21*$^{WAF1/CIP1}$*, GADD45, MDM2, 14–3-3-σ, BAX, B99,*

TSP1, KILLER/DR5, FAS/APO1, CYCLIN G, and others (155). Expression of many of these genes effectively halts DNA replication and induces DNA repair (164–167). This function of p53 to recognize DNA damage and induce cell cycle arrest and DNA repair or apoptosis has led to p53 being called the "guardian of the genome" (163). Thus, *TP53* normally acts as a tumor-suppressor gene by inducing genes that can cause cell cycle arrest or apoptosis, and also by inhibiting angiogenesis through the induction of *TSP1* (168,169). Mutant p53 protein can block these functions through forming oligomers with wild-type p53, causing diminished DNA-binding specificity (170). Furthermore, the majority of p53 mutations occur in the sequence-specific DNA-binding region and serve to interfere with binding to the consensus sequence, 5′-PuPuPuC(A/T)-3′ (171).

With regard to *TP53* mutation status as a prognostic or predictive marker for CRC response to treatment, there are conflicting results in the literature. *TP53* mutations are common in CRC and are believed to play a fundamental role in deregulating the cell cycle and inducing resistance to apoptosis in CRC. The overexpression of p53 as measured by immunohistochemistry has been interpreted to indicate the presence of mutant p53 protein because the mutant forms of p53 have prolonged protein half-lives. Using this method or DNA mutation analysis for assessing *TP53* mutations, mutant p53 has not consistently shown any prognostic or predictive value in CRC (172,173). It is possible that the prognostic value of *TP53* mutations will only be appreciated when specific *TP53* mutations are correlated with the clinical outcomes.

PI3K Pathway

The PI3Ks are a family of lipid kinases that regulates the activity of kinases such as AKT and p70S6K, which ultimately affects cell proliferation, apoptosis, and cell motility, hallmark biological functions that are commonly deregulated in cancer (174). Multiple isoforms of PI3K can be identified in mammalian cells and can be divided into three classes, including notably the class I PI3Ks, which is composed of a p110 catalytic subunit and a regulatory adapter subunit. The class I PI3K members share homologous domains that include the lipid kinase domain, the helical domain, the C2 domain, a Ras-binding domain, and a NH2-terminal domain that interacts with the regulatory subunit (175). More recently, large-scale mutational analysis studies of members of the PI3K signaling pathway have identified mutations that activate this pathway in a large proportion of CRCs (5,176). Gain-of-function mutations in *PIK3CA*, the p110α catalytic subunit of PI3K, have been found in 32% of CRCs (176). Seventy-five percent of the *PIK3CA* mutations occur in two small clusters in the regions encoding the helical and kinase domains of the protein, which are highly evolutionarily conserved. One of the most common mutations, H1074R, has been shown to increase lipid kinase activity in in vitro studies and a broader screen of other mutation hot spots identified in CRCs, including E542K and E454K, as well as five other *PIK3CA* mutations, revealed that these mutations increased lipid kinase activity of PIK3CA (176,177). Analysis of 76 colorectal adenomas and 199 CRCs detected *PIK3CA* mutations only in advanced adenomas or CRCs, suggesting that these mutations influence the transition of the adenomas to adenocarcinomas (176). In addition to mutations in *PIK3CA*, mutations in other members of the PI3K pathway have been detected in a series of 180 CRCs, including mitogen-activated protein-kinase kinase-4 (*MKK4/JNKK1*), myosin light-chain kinase-2 (*MYLK2*), phosphoinositide-dependent protein kinase-1 (*PDK1*), p21-activated kinase 4 (*PAK4*), v-akt murine thymoma viral oncogene homolog-2 kinase (*AKT2*), MAP/microtubule affinity-regulating kinase 3 (*MARK3*), cell division cycle-7 kinase (*CDC7*), and a hypothetical casein kinase (*PDIK1L*), insulin-related receptor (*INSRR*), and v-Erb-B erythroblastic leukemia viral oncogene homolog *ERBB4* (5). Amplification of insulin-receptor substrate *IRS2* was also detected in a subset of CRCs.

In addition, inactivating mutations in *PTEN*, a lipid dual-specificity phosphatase, and in *PIK3R1*, the p85α regulatory subunit of PI3K, have been demonstrated in 5% and 2% of CRCs, respectively (174,178). Remarkably, mutations that affect the PI3K pathway can be detected in nearly 40% of CRCs, and these mutations are nearly mutually exclusive, suggesting that they have equivalent tumorigenic effects through the activation of the PI3K pathway and that this pathway is an attractive therapeutic target (5).

TGF-ß Superfamily and Signaling Pathways

TGF-ß is a multifunctional cytokine that can induce growth inhibition, apoptosis, and differentiation in intestinal epithelial cells (179,180). Evidence of the role of TGF-ß in CRC formation first came from studies that demonstrated CRC cell lines were resistant to the normal growth inhibitory effects of TGF-ß (181). Furthermore, this pathway is deregulated in approximately 75% of CRC cell lines, suggesting that it is an important tumor-suppressor pathway in CRC (182). TGF-ß mediates its effects on cells through a heteromeric receptor complex that consists of type I (TGFBR1) and type II (TGFBR2) components (Fig. 40.4). TGFBR1 and TGFBR2 are serine-threonine kinases that phosphorylate downstream signaling proteins on activation (183). The receptor complex is activated by TGF-ß binding to the TGFBR2 component of the receptor complex, causing formation of the heteromeric R1–R2 receptor complex. The activated TGFBR2 component then phosphorylates the TGFBR1 component in the GS box of TGFBR1, a glycine-serine–rich region of the receptor. TGFBR1 then propagates the signal from the receptor through the phosphorylation of downstream proteins, including the Smad proteins, Smad2 and Smad3, and non-Smad proteins, such as PI3K, p38MAPK, and RhoA (179,184). The Smad pathway is the most extensively characterized post TGF-ß receptor pathway, and for the majority of the non-Smad pathways, it is not clear whether the activation of the pathway is a direct or indirect effect of

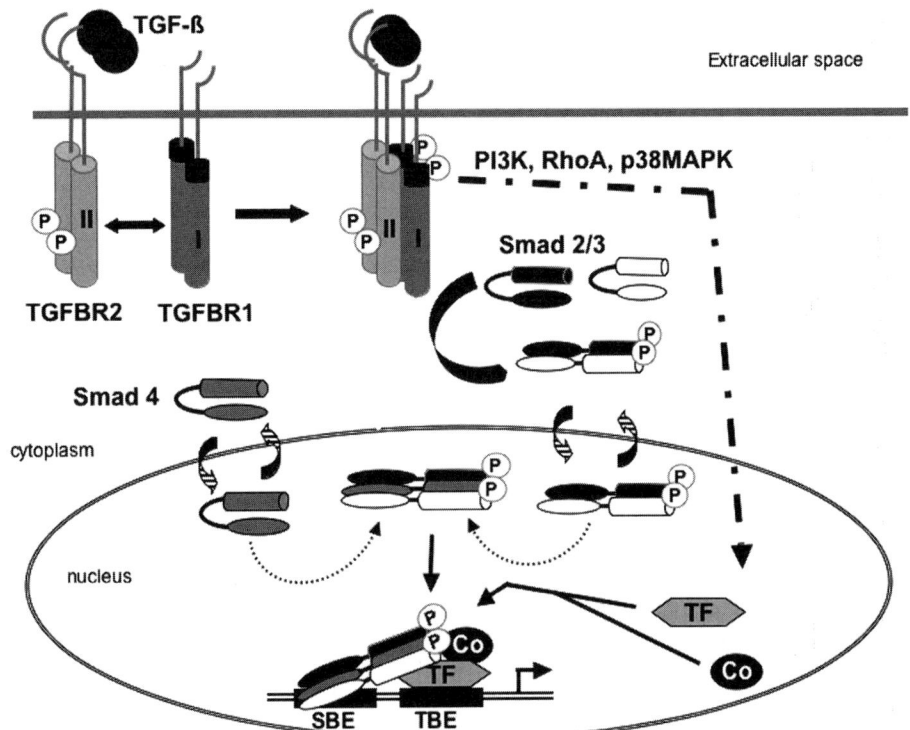

FIGURE 40.4. Diagram of the transforming growth factor ß signaling pathway. The Smad pathway is shown in detail because it is the most extensively characterized. The non-Smad pathways include p38MAPK, PI3K, RhoA, and JNK, among others. The protein–protein interactions that mediate TGF-ß–induced activation of these pathways are not known at this time. TF, transcription factor; Co, coactivator; P, phosphate group.

TGF-ß receptor activation. With regard to the Smad pathway, once the activated TGFBR1 phosphorylates Smad2, Smad2, and Smad3 form a heteromeric complex, which can also include Smad4, and translocate to the nucleus (183,185). In the nucleus, they modulate transcription of specific genes through cis-regulatory Smad-binding sequences and through binding with other transcription factors such as p300/CBP, TFE3, Ski, and JUN (100,186,187).

The downstream transcriptional targets of the TGF-ß signaling pathway are involved in the regulation of a variety of cell functions, including cell proliferation, extracellular matrix production, and immune surveillance. These functions are not only an integral part of tissue homeostasis but also logical targets for dysregulation in colorectal carcinogenesis. Elements involved in growth regulation that have been clearly shown to be controlled in part by TGF-ß include the cyclin-associated proteins cyclin D1, cdk4, p21, p27, p15, and Rb (188–193). MYC is also a downstream target of TGF-ß and has been shown to be transcriptionally repressed in MvLu1 cells after treatment with TGF-β1 (192,194). In addition to the cyclin-associated proteins, the extracellular matrix proteins and regulators of extracellular matrix proteins, fibronectin, tenascin, and plasminogen activator inhibitor 1, also appear to be regulated by TGF-ß (195,196).

The disruption of the normal extracellular matrix production may play a role in tumor invasion. In support of this concept, TGFBR2 mutations in MSI colorectal adenomas are only detected in areas of high-grade dysplasia or in adenomas with concurrent adenocarcinoma, suggesting that TGFBR2 inactivation promotes the malignant transition of colorectal adenomas to adenocarcinomas (17). Furthermore, an in vivo mouse model that is knocked out for Tgfbr2 in the colorectum ($Fabp^{4xat-132}$ Cre; $Tgfbr2^{flx/flx}$) does not develop spontaneous colorectal neoplasms commonly but shows a significant increase in adenocarcinomas compared to control mice after treatment with a rodent colorectal carcinogen, azoxymethane (197).

TGFBR2

A common mechanism through which CRCs acquire TGF-ß resistance is through genetic alterations of the *TGFBR2* gene. Functionally significant alterations of *TGFBR2* have been identified in up to 30% of CRCs, and the mutational inactivation of TGFBR2 is the most common mechanism identified to date for inactivating the TGF-ß signaling pathway in CRC (46,182). No alterations in *TGFBR1* or the type III TGF-ß receptor (*TGFBR3)* have been observed in studies of TGF-ß–resistant CRC cell lines, suggesting that mutational inactivation of *TGFBR2* is a particularly favorable event that leads to tumor formation. Markowitz et al. demonstrated that mutational inactivation of *TGFBR2* is an extremely common event in MSI CRCs because *TGFBR2* has a microsatellite-like region in exon 3 that consists of a 10 base pair polyadenine tract, making it particularly susceptible to mutation in the setting of MSI (46,198,199). The mutation in this region, which has been named *BAT-RII* (big adenine tract in TGF-ß receptor type II), is a frameshift mutation that results in the insertion or deletion of one or two adenines between nucleotides 709 and 718, introducing nonsense mutations that encode a truncated TGFBR2 protein lacking the intracellular serine-threonine kinase domain (46). In a series of 110 MSI CRCs, 100 were found to carry *BAT-RII* mutations, and in almost all of these cases, the mutations were biallelic consistent with the tumor-suppressor function of TGFBR2 (198). *TGFBR2*'s role as a tumor-suppressor gene in CRC has been further elucidated by studies in mouse models. Deletion of a conditional Tgfbr2 allele in the colorectal epithelium substantially promotes the formation of colorectal adenocarcinomas

in the azoxymethane mouse model of CRC (197). Further support for *TGFBR2*'s role as a tumor-suppressor gene in CRC in general was provided by the demonstration of *TGFBR2* mutations in CRC cell lines that are MSS. *TGFBR2* mutations have been found in 15% ($n = 3/14$) of TGF-ß–resistant MSS CRC cell lines. These mutations are not frameshift mutations in *BAT-RII* but are inactivating missense mutations in the kinase domain or putative binding domain of *TGFBR2* (182). In aggregate, the overall incidence of *TGFBR2* mutation in both MSS and MSI CRCs appears to be 30% (182). Interestingly, in a study of CRC cell lines, the incidence of TGF-ß resistance was found to be 55%, despite frequently having wild-type *TGFBR1* and *TGFBR2* (182). These cancers have presumably inactivated the TGF-ß signaling pathway through genetic or epigenetic alterations in postreceptor defects further underscoring the significance of the TGF-ß signaling pathway in CRC formation.

SMAD2 and SMAD4

LOH occurs commonly at 5q, 18q, and 17p in CRC and suggests that there are tumor-suppressor genes at these loci. LOH of chromosome 18q occurs in approximately 70% of colorectal adenocarcinomas. The incidence of 18q LOH is only about 10% in early stage colorectal adenomas and 30% in later stage, larger adenomas, demonstrating that the incidence of LOH involving 18q increases through the adenoma-carcinoma sequence (103,156). A region of deletion on 18q that is shared among CRCs that demonstrate allelic loss involving a contiguous segment of 18q has been observed and is the locus of a number of tumor-suppressor genes implicated in CRC formation, including *DCC*, *SMAD2*, and *SMAD4*. These genes have been shown to be mutated in CRCs (200–202). Other genes that are candidate tumor-suppressor genes and map at 18q21-qter include *BCL-2*, gastrin-releasing peptide, and the cellular homolog of *YES-1*; however, none of these have been shown to be altered in CRCs (203).

The most likely tumor-suppressor genes that are the targets of 18q LOH are *SMAD2*, *SMAD4*, and *DCC*. The Smad proteins are a family of proteins that serve as intracellular mediators to regulate TGF-ß superfamily signaling. The Smad proteins compose an evolutionarily conserved signaling pathway that has been demonstrated in *Caenorhabditis elegans*, *D. melanogaster*, *Xenopus*, and humans. These proteins are characterized by two regions that are homologous to the *Drosophila* ortholog, Mad, and that are located at the N- and C-termini of the protein. These regions are termed the Mad-homology domains MH1 and MH2, respectively, and are connected by a less well-conserved, proline-rich linker domain. Numerous studies have identified three major classes of Smad proteins:

- The receptor-regulated Smads (R-Smads), which are direct targets of the TGF-ß receptor family type I kinases and include Smads1, 2, 3, and 5
- The common Smads (Co-Smads: Smad4), which form heteromeric complexes with the R-Smads and propagate the TGF-ß–mediated signal
- The inhibitory Smads (I-Smads: Smad6 and Smad7), which antagonize TGF-ß signaling through the Smad pathway

Ligand binding to the TGF-ß receptor complex results in TGF-ß receptor type I–mediated phosphorylation of Smad2 and Smad3 on two serine residues in a conserved –SS(M/V)S motif located at the C-terminus of the R-Smads (204,205). Phosphorylation of these serine residues is required for downstream signaling pathway activation (206,207).

In light of the known tumor-suppressor effects of the TGF-ß signaling pathway and the role Smad proteins play in propagating this signal, it is not surprising that alterations of some of the SMAD genes have been found in CRC. Mutational inactivation of *SMAD2* and *SMAD4* has been observed in a high percentage of pancreatic cancers and in 5% to 16% of CRCs (202,208–210). *SMAD4* alterations have been found in up to 16% of CRCs (209). The effect of these mutations on colorectal carcinogenesis is being investigated in a number of different animal models. One murine model, a compound heterozygote *Smad4*$^{-/+}$/*Apc*$^{\Delta 716}$, develops CRC unlike the *Apc*$^{\Delta 716}$ mouse, which only develops small intestinal adenomas (211). This model suggests that *SMAD4* inactivation may play a role in the progression of CRCs as opposed to their initiation. However, in some contexts, *SMAD4* mutations also appear to initiate tumor formation. Elderly *Smad4*$^{-/+}$ mice develop gastric and intestinal juvenile polyps and invasive gastric cancer; however, they do not develop CRC (212,213). Furthermore, germline mutations in *SMAD4* have been found in approximately one-third of individuals with juvenile polyposis syndrome (JPS), an autosomal dominant syndrome characterized by gastrointestinal hamartomatous polyps and an increased risk of gastrointestinal cancer, consistent with the concept that haploid insufficiency of *SMAD4* may contribute to tumor initiation (214–216). Importantly, though, the polyps observed in JPS and the invasive cancers in the *Smad4*$^{-/+}$ mouse have been shown to have allelic loss of *SMAD4*, supporting the idea that biallelic inactivation of *SMAD4* is needed for cancer formation (213,217). Taken together, these studies suggest that *SMAD4* is a tumor-suppressor gene in CRC and is one of the targets of 18q LOH. However, given the frequency of 18q LOH versus detected *SMAD4* mutations or deletions, there are likely other tumor-suppressor loci on 18q21.

Although also located at 18q21 and presumably a target for inactivation in colorectal carcinogenesis, mutations in *SMAD2* occur infrequently in CRC and have been found in only 0% to 5% of cancers (202,210,218). The other *SMAD* genes are not frequently altered in CRC, despite the fact that *SMAD3* and *SMAD6* are located on chromosome 15q 21–22, which is a frequent site of allelic loss in CRC (210,219,220). Interestingly, and in contrast to the studies of human CRC, Graff et al. observed a high frequency of invasive colorectal carcinoma in *Smad3*$^{-/-}$ mice (221). In conclusion, *SMAD* mutations appear to play a role in tumor formation in a subset of CRCs but are not as common as *TGFBR2* mutations. This observation raises the possibility that there are non-Smad TGF-ß signaling pathways that play an important role in the tumor-suppressor activity of *TGFBR2*.

The effect of 18q LOH and thus presumably inactivation of the tumor-suppressor genes at this locus on the clinical behavior of colorectal carcinomas has been subjected to intense scrutiny with inconclusive results to date. Several different groups have assayed for LOH of 18q using microsatellite markers in stage II CRC and have found either no association with the clinical behavior of the cancer or an association with more aggressive cancer behavior (203,222–225). The reason for the discrepancy is unclear but may be related to different microsatellite loci assessed in each study, and thus the specific region of 18q that was assessed by each investigator. Adding to this confusion, *SMAD4* diploidy and *TGFBR2 BAT-RII* mutations have been shown to associate with improved survival after adjuvant chemotherapy (59,226).

TGF-ß Superfamily Receptors: ACVR2 and BMPR1A

The TGF-ß superfamily includes not only TGF-ß 1, TGF-TGF-ß 2, and TGF-ß 3, but also the bone morphogenetic proteins (BMPs), activin, nodal, growth and differentiation factors, and inhibin. The identification of germline mutations in signaling elements of the BMP signaling pathway in individuals with juvenile polyposis, a hereditary CRC syndrome, and somatic mu-

tations in the activin receptor in CRCs has globally implicated deregulation of the TGF-ß superfamily in the pathogenesis of CRC. Germline mutations in *SMAD4* and *BMPR1A*, a type I receptor for the BMPs, in families with JPS has implicated inactivation of BMP signaling in this subset of hereditary CRCs. Nonsense and missense germline mutations in *BMPR1A* in JPS families, 44–47delTGTT, 715C>T, 812G>A, and 961delC affecting exons 1, 7, 7, and 8, respectively, have been identified (227). Mutations in *SMAD4* account for 5% to 62% of cases, and published mutations to date include deletions (1244–1247delAGAC), missense mutations, and frameshift mutations in exons 5, 6, 8, 9, 10, and 11 (228). These mutations are usually predicted to cause a truncated protein product and often occur in the highly conserved MH2 domain of the protein (228). The 1244–1247delAGAC mutation has been identified in multiple unrelated families and appears to be a mutation hot spot in the gene (229).

The BMPs are disulfide-linked dimeric proteins that number at least 15 in total and include BMP-2, BMP-4, and BMP-7 (OP-1). They have a wide range of biological activities, including the regulation of morphogenesis of various tissues and organs during development, as well as the regulation of growth, differentiation, chemotaxis, and apoptosis in monocytes, epithelial cells, mesenchymal cells, and neuronal cells (230). The BMPs transduce their signals through a heteromeric receptor that consists of a type I and type II receptor. BMPR1A is one of two different type I BMP receptors (BMPR1A and BMPR1B). It serves to predominantly bind BMP-4, BMP-2, and other BMPs, and transduces their signals when partnered with a BMP type II receptor. As with the TGF-ß receptor, the best understood post-BMP receptor pathway is the Smad pathway. The R-Smads, Smads 1 and 5, partner with Smad4 (Co-Smad) to transduce BMP-mediated signals from the BMP receptors (230). Thus, the identification of both *BMPR1A* and *SMAD4* germline mutations in JPS families strongly implicates BMP signaling disruption in the pathogenesis of this syndrome. Furthermore, mice that overexpress Noggin, a soluble antagonist for the BMPs, or a dominant-negative *Bmpr1a* in the intestinal epithelium display ectopic crypt formation and a phenotype reminiscent of JPS (231,232).

With regard to activin, activin is a secreted dimeric ligand, composed of either Activin ßA and/or Activin ßB, that activates intracellular signaling pathways that include the SMAD2/3-SMAD4 pathway via a heteromeric receptor that is composed of a type I receptor (ACVRL1, ActRIA, or ActRIB) and a type II receptor (ACVR2 or ACVR2B) (233). Mutations in *ACVR2* have been found to occur in 58% to 90% of MSI CRCs as the result of a polyadenine tract in the coding region of the gene (58,234). The identification of mutations that affect activin, TGF-ß, and BMP signaling implicate at least three members of the TGF-ß family as members of tumor-suppressor pathways in CRC.

Genes Associated With Colorectal Metastases

One of the clear challenges in cancer biology is the identification of genes that contribute to the metastatic and lethal cancer phenotype. Intense investigation in this area has led to the identification of promising candidate genes that may influence the metastatic potential of the primary CRC. PRL3, a phosphatase, was found overexpressed in 12 of 12 CRC liver metastases, but not in matched CRC primaries from the same patients (235). Moreover, in 3 of 12 cases, PRL3 overexpression was accompanied by marked *PRL3* gene amplification, suggesting that PRL3 overexpression is a primary genetic event selected for during metastasis. Osteopontin is a protein that also appears to have potential to predict the metastatic potential of CRC. Osteopontin was identified through a global screen using expression arrays and is 15-fold overexpressed in primary CRCs and 27-fold overexpressed in liver metastases (236). Osteopontin is a phosphoglycoprotein that can bind to several integrins and CD44, and has been shown to contribute to the malignant phenotype in breast cancer (236,237). To date, neither PRL3 nor osteopontin has been shown to have the ability to predict the metastatic potential of CRC in a prospective clinical trial.

CONCLUSION

Investigation of the molecular pathogenesis of CRC has yielded many insights into the mechanisms driving the tumorigenesis process and to the identification of many potential therapeutic targets. Key insights from the assessment of the molecular genetics and epigenetics of CRC include the multistep nature of carcinogenesis, the central role of tumor-suppressor pathways, the role of DNA repair genes and genomic stability in cancer formation, and the role of TGF-ß signaling in tumor suppression. Nonetheless, many challenges remain. The molecular genesis of the metastatic phenotype that directly accounts for cancer lethality remains unknown. A mechanistic understanding of the basis of chromosomal instability, aneuploidy, and aberrant methylation of the cancer genome has yet to be achieved. In addition, the translation of molecular genetics to new diagnostic, prognostic, and therapeutic modalities appears promising but has yet to have a major impact on the clinical management of CRC. The hope for the future is that this field of inquiry will yield the important answers to these and other key questions.

References

1. Hanahan D, Weinberg RA. The hallmarks of cancer. *Cell* 2000;100:57–70.
2. Fearon E, Vogelstein B. A genetic model for colorectal tumorigenesis. *Cell* 1990;61:759–767.
3. Lengauer C, Kinzler K, Vogelstein B. Genetic instabilities in human cancers. *Nature* 1998;396:643–649.
4. Kinzler K, Vogelstein B. Lessons from hereditary colorectal cancer. *Cell* 1996;87:159–170.
5. Parsons DW, Wang TL, Samuels Y, et al. Colorectal cancer: mutations in a signalling pathway. *Nature* 2005;436:792.
6. Bardelli A, Parsons DW, Silliman N, et al. Mutational analysis of the tyrosine kinome in colorectal cancers. *Science* 2003;300:949.
7. Goldstein NS. Serrated pathway and APC (conventional)-type colorectal polyps: molecular-morphologic correlations, genetic pathways, and implications for classification. *Am J Clin Pathol* 2006;125:146–153.
8. Kambara T, Simms LA, Whitehall VL, et al. BRAF mutation is associated with DNA methylation in serrated polyps and cancers of the colorectum. *Gut* 2004;53:1137–1144.
9. Jass JR. Hyperplastic polyps and colorectal cancer: is there a link? *Clin Gastroenterol Hepatol* 2004;2:1–8.
10. Bartkova J, Horejsi Z, Koed K, et al. DNA damage response as a candidate anti-cancer barrier in early human tumorigenesis. *Nature* 2005;434:864–870.
11. Maley CC, Galipeau PC, Li X, et al. The combination of genetic instability and clonal expansion predicts progression to esophageal adenocarcinoma. *Cancer Res* 2004;64:7629–7633.
12. Maley CC, Galipeau PC, Finley JC, et al. Genetic clonal diversity predicts progression to esophageal adenocarcinoma. *Nat Genet* 2006;38:468–473.
13. Kops GJ, Foltz DR, Cleveland DW. Lethality to human cancer cells through massive chromosome loss by inhibition of the mitotic checkpoint. *Proc Natl Acad Sci U S A* 2004;101:8699–8704.
14. Grady WM. Genomic instability and colon cancer. *Cancer Metastasis Rev* 2004;23:11–27.
15. Shih IM, Zhou W, Goodman SN, et al. Evidence that genetic instability occurs at an early stage of colorectal tumorigenesis. *Cancer Res* 2001;61:818–822.
16. Aaltonen L, Peltomaki P, Mecklin J-P, et al. Replication errors in benign and malignant tumors from hereditary nonpolyposis colorectal cancer patients. *Cancer Res* 1994;54:1645–1648.
17. Grady W, Rajput A, Myeroff L, et al. Mutation of the type II transforming growth factor-ß receptor is coincident with the transformation of human colon adenomas to malignant carcinomas. *Cancer Res* 1998;58:3101–3104.
18. Jacoby R, Marshall D, Kailas S, et al. Genetic instability associated with adenoma to carcinoma progression in hereditary nonpolyposis colon cancer. *Gastroenterology* 1995;109:73–82.
19. Bomme L, Bardi G, Pandis N, et al. Cytogenetic analysis of colorectal adenomas: karyotypic comparisons of synchronous tumors. *Cancer Genet Cytogenet* 1998;106:66–71.
20. Ried T, Heselmeyer-Haddad K, Blegen H, et al. Genomic changes defining the genesis, progression, and malignancy potential in solid human tumors: a phenotype/genotype correlation. *Genes Chromosomes Cancer* 1999;25:195–204.
21. Rooney P, Murray G, Steven son D, et al. Comparative genomic hybridization and chromosomal instability in solid tumors. *Br J Cancer* 1999;80:862–873.
22. Hermsen M, Postma C, Baak J, et al. Colorectal adenoma to carcinoma progression follows multiple pathways of chromosomal instability. *Gastroenterology* 2002;123:1109–1119.
23. Chen WD, Eshleman JR, Aminoshariae MR, et al. Cytotoxicity and mutagenicity of frameshift-inducing agent ICR191 in mismatch repair-deficient colon cancer cells. *J Natl Cancer Inst* 2000;92:480–485.
24. Kolodner RD, Putman CD, Myung K. Maintenance of genome stability in *Saccharomyces cerevisiae*. *Science* 2002;297:552–557.
25. Jin D, Spencer F, Jeang K. Human T cell leukemia virus type 1 oncoprotein Tax targets the human mitotic checkpoint protein MAD1. *Cell* 1998;93:81–91.
26. Cahill D, Lengauer C, Yu J, et al. Mutations of mitotic checkpoint genes in human cancers. *Nature* 1998;392:300–303.
27. Rotman G, Shiloh Y. ATM: from gene to function. *Hum Mol Genet* 1998;7:1555–1563.
28. Smith L. Duplication of ATR inhibits MyoD, induces aneuploidy and eliminates radiation-induced G1 arrest. *Nat Genet* 1998;19:39–46.
29. Zhang H, Tombline G, Weber B. BRCA1, BRCA2, and DNA damage response: collision or collusion. *Cell* 1998;92:433–436.
30. Zhou H, Kuang J, Zhong L, et al. Tumour amplified kinase STK15/BTAK induces centrosome amplification, aneuploidy and transformation. *Nature Genet* 1998;20:189–193.
31. Bischoff JR, Anderson L, Zhu Y, et al. A homologue of *Drosophila aurora* kinase is oncogenic and amplified in human colorectal cancers. *EMBO J* 1998;17:3052–3065.
32. Rajagopalan H, Bardelli A, Lengauer C, et al. Tumorigenesis: RAF/RAS oncogenes and mismatch-repair status. *Nature* 2002;418:934.
33. Wang Z, Cummins JM, Shen D, et al. Three classes of genes mutated in colorectal cancers with chromosomal instability. *Cancer Res* 2004;64:2998–3001.
34. Rajagopalan H, Jallepalli PV, Rago C, et al. Inactivation of hCDC4 can cause chromosomal instability. *Nature* 2004;428:77–81.
35. Rajagopalan H, Lengauer C. hCDC4 and genetic instability in cancer. *Cell Cycle* 2004;3:693–694.
36. Loeb KR, Kostner H, Firpo E, et al. A mouse model for cyclin E-dependent genetic instability and tumorigenesis. *Cancer Cell* 2005;8:35–47.
37. Perez-Losada J, Mao JH, Balmain A. Control of genomic instability and epithelial tumor development by the p53-Fbxw7/Cdc4 pathway. *Cancer Res* 2005;65:6488–6492.
38. Lynch HT, de la Chapelle A. Genetic susceptibility to non-polyposis colorectal cancer. *J Med Genet* 1999;36:801–818.
39. Hampel H, Frankel WL, Martin E, et al. Screening for the Lynch syndrome (hereditary nonpolyposis colorectal cancer). *N Engl J Med* 2005;352:1851–1860.
40. Kane M, Loda M, Gaida G, et al. Methylation of the *hMLH1* promoter correlates with lack of expression of hMLH1 in sporadic colon tumors and mismatch repair-defective human tumor cell lines. *Cancer Res* 1997;57:808–811.
41. Boland C, Thibodeau S, Hamilton S, et al. National Cancer Institute workshop on microsatellite instability for cancer detection and familial predisposition: development of international criteria for the determination of microsatellite instability in colorectal cancer. *Cancer Res* 1998;58:5248–5257.
42. Jiricny J. Replication errors: cha(lle)nging the genome. *EMBO J* 1998;17:6427–6436.
43. Kolodner RD, Marsischky GT. Eukaryotic DNA mismatch repair. *Curr Opin Genet Dev* 1999;9:89–96.
44. Eshleman J, Lang E, Bowerfind G, et al. Increased mutation rate at the *hprt* locus accompanies microsatellite instability in colon cancer. *Oncogene* 1995;10:33–37.
45. Yamamoto H, Sawai H, Weber T, et al. Somatic frameshift mutations in DNA mismatch repair and proapoptosis genes in hereditary nonpolyposis colorectal cancer. *Cancer Res* 1998;58:997–1003.
46. Markowitz S, Wang J, Myeroff L, et al. Inactivation of the type II TGF-ß receptor in colon cancer cells with microsatellite instability. *Science* 1995;268:1336–1338.
47. Hempen PM, Zhang L, Bansal RK, et al. Evidence of selection for clones having genetic inactivation of the activin A type II receptor (ACVR2) gene in gastrointestinal cancers. *Cancer Res* 2003;63:994–999.
48. Deng G, Bell I, Crawley S, et al. BRAF mutation is frequently present in sporadic colorectal cancer with methylated hMLH1, but not in hereditary nonpolyposis colorectal cancer. *Clin Cancer Res* 2004;10:191–195.
49. Domingo E, Laiho P, Ollikainen M, et al. BRAF screening as a low-cost effective strategy for simplifying HNPCC genetic testing. *J Med Genet* 2004;41:664–668.

50. Huang J, Papadopoulos N, McKinley A, et al. APC mutations in colorectal tumors with mismatch repair deficiency. *Proc Natl Acad Sci U S A* 1996;93:9049–9054.
51. Konishi M, Kikuchi-Yanoshita R, Tanaka K, et al. Molecular nature of colon tumors in hereditary nonpolyposis colon cancer, familial polyposis, and sporadic colon cancer. *Gastroenterology* 1996;111:307–317.
52. Miyaki M, Iijima T, Kimura J, et al. Frequent mutation of beta–catenin and APC genes in primary colorectal tumors from patients with hereditary nonpolyposis colorectal cancer. *Cancer Res* 1999;59:4506–1509.
53. Fujiwara T, Stolker JM, Watanabe T, et al. Accumulated clonal genetic alterations in familial and sporadic colorectal carcinomas with widespread instability in microsatellite sequences. *Am J Pathol* 1998;153:1063–1078.
54. Olschwang S, Tiret A, Laurent-Puig P, et al. Restriction of ocular fundus lesions to a specific subgroup of APC mutations in adenomatous polyposis coli patients. *Cell* 1993;75:959–968.
55. Eshleman J, Casey G, Kochera M, et al. Chromosome number and structure both are markedly stable in RER colorectal cancers and are not destabilized by mutation of p53. *Oncogene* 1998;17:719–725.
56. Olschwang S, Hamelin R, Laurent-Puig P, et al. Alternative genetic pathways in colorectal carcinogenesis. *Proc Natl Acad Sci U S A* 1997;94: 12122–12127.
57. Shen L, Kondo Y, Hamilton SR, et al. P14 methylation in human colon cancer is associated with microsatellite instability and wild-type p53. *Gastroenterology* 2003;124:626–633.
58. Mori Y, Yin J, Rashid A, et al. Instabilotyping: comprehensive identification of frameshift mutations caused by coding region microsatellite instability. *Cancer Res* 2001;61:6046–6049.
59. Watanabe T, Wu TT, Catalano PJ, et al. Molecular predictors of survival after adjuvant chemotherapy for colon cancer. *N Engl J Med* 2001;344:1196–1206.
60. Popat S, Hubner R, Houlston RS. Systematic review of microsatellite instability and colorectal cancer prognosis. *J Clin Oncol* 2005;23:609–618.
61. Chow E, Thirlwell C, Macrae F, et al. Colorectal cancer and inherited mutations in base-excision repair. *Lancet Oncol* 2004;5:600–606.
62. Al-Tassan N, Chmiel NH, Maynard J, et al. Inherited variants of MYH associated with somatic G:C→T:A mutations in colorectal tumors. *Nat Genet* 2002;30:227–232.
63. Sampson JR, Dolwani S, Jones S, et al. Autosomal recessive colorectal adenomatous polyposis due to inherited mutations of MYH. *Lancet* 2003;362:39–41.
64. Sieber OM, Lipton L, Crabtree M, et al. Multiple colorectal adenomas, classic adenomatous polyposis, and germ-line mutations in MYH. *N Engl J Med* 2003;348:791–799.
65. Olinski R, Zastawny T, Budzbon J, et al. DNA base modifications in chromatin of human cancerous tissues. *FEBS Lett* 1992;309:193–198.
66. Halford SE, Rowan AJ, Lipton L, et al. Germline mutations but not somatic changes at the MYH locus contribute to the pathogenesis of unselected colorectal cancers. *Am J Pathol* 2003;162:1545–1548.
67. Lipton L, Halford SE, Johnson V, et al. Carcinogenesis in MYH-associated polyposis follows a distinct genetic pathway. *Cancer Res* 2003;63:7595–7599.
68. Blasco MA. Telomeres and human disease: ageing, cancer and beyond. *Nat Rev Genet* 2005;6:611–622.
69. Maser RS, DePinho RA. Connecting chromosomes, crisis, and cancer. *Science* 2002;297:565–569.
70. Kim NW, Piatyszek MA, Prowse KR, et al. Specific association of human telomerase activity with immortal cells and cancer. *Science* 1994;266:2011–2015.
71. Rudolph KL, Millard M, Bosenberg MW, et al. Telomere dysfunction and evolution of intestinal carcinoma in mice and humans. *Nat Genet* 2001;28:155–159.
72. O'Hagan RC, Chang S, Maser RS, et al. Telomere dysfunction provokes regional amplification and deletion in cancer genomes. *Cancer Cell* 2002;2:149–155.
73. Artandi SE, Chang S, Lee SL, et al. Telomere dysfunction promotes non-reciprocal translocations and epithelial cancers in mice. *Nature* 2000;406:641–645.
74. Kondo Y, Issa JP. Epigenetic changes in colorectal cancer. *Cancer Metastasis Rev* 2004;23:29–39.
75. Baylin SB, Herman JG. DNA hypermethylation in tumorigenesis: epigenetics joins genetics. *Trends Genet* 2000;16:168–174.
76. Jones P, Laird P. Cancer epigenetics comes of age. *Nature Genet* 1999;21:163–167.
77. Jubb AM, Bell SM, Quirke P. Methylation and colorectal cancer. *J Pathol* 2001;195:111–134.
78. Baylin SB, Bestor TH. Altered methylation patterns in cancer cell genomes: cause or consequence. *Cancer Cell* 2002;1:299–305.
79. Herman J, Umar A, Polyak K, et al. Incidence and functional consequences of *hMLH1* promoter hypermethylation in colorectal carcinoma. *Proc Natl Acad Sci U S A* 1998;95:6870–6875.
80. Veigl M, Kasturi L, Olechnowicz J, et al. Biallelic inactivation of *hMLH1* by epigenetic gene silencing, a novel mechanism causing human MSI cancers. *Proc Natl Acad Sci U S A* 1998;95:8698–8702.
81. Herman JG, Merlo A, Mao L, et al. Inactivation of the CDKN2/p16/MTS1 gene is frequently associated with aberrant DNA methylation in all common human cancers. *Cancer Res* 1995;55:4525–4530.
82. Toyota M, Ho C, Ahuja N, et al. Identification of differentially methylated sequences in colorectal cancer by methylated CpG island amplification. *Cancer Res* 1999;59:2307–2312.
83. Toyota M, Ahuja N, Ohe-Toyota M, et al. CpG island methylator phenotype in colorectal cancer. *Proc Natl Acad Sci U S A* 1999;96:8681–8686.
84. Rashid A, Shen L, Morris JS, et al. CpG island methylation in colorectal adenomas. *Am J Pathol* 2001;159:1129–1135.
85. Petko Z, Ghiassi M, Shuber A, et al. Aberrantly methylated CDKN2A, MGMT, and MLH1 in colon polyps and in fecal DNA from patients with colorectal polyps. *Clin Cancer Res* 2005;11:1203–1209.
86. Li H, Myeroff L, Smiraglia D, et al. SLC5A8, a sodium transporter, is a tumor suppressor gene silenced by methylation in human colon aberrant crypt foci and cancers. *Proc Natl Acad Sci U S A* 2003;100:8412–8417.
87. Chan AO, Broaddus RR, Houlihan PS, et al. CpG island methylation in aberrant crypt foci of the colorectum. *Am J Pathol* 2002;160:1823–1830.
88. Moinova HR, Chen WD, Shen L, et al. HLTF gene silencing in human colon cancer. *Proc Natl Acad Sci U S A* 2002;99:4562–4567.
89. Samowitz WS, Albertsen H, Herrick J, et al. Evaluation of a large, population-based sample supports a CpG island methylator phenotype in colon cancer. *Gastroenterology* 2005;129:837–845.
90. Deng G, Chen A, Pong E, et al. Methylation in hMLH1 promoter interferes with its binding to transcription factor CBF and inhibits gene expression. *Oncogene* 2001;20:7120–7127.
91. Jenuwein T, Allis CD. Translating the histone code. *Science* 2001;293:1074–1080.
92. Seligson DB, Horvath S, Shi T, et al. Global histone modification patterns predict risk of prostate cancer recurrence. *Nature* 2005;435:1262–1266.
93. Fraga MF, Esteller M. Towards the human cancer epigenome: a first draft of histone modifications. *Cell Cycle* 2005;4:1377–1381.
94. Herrera L, Kakati S, Gibas L, et al. Gardner syndrome in a man with an interstitial deletion of 5q. *Am J Med Genet* 1986;25:473–476.
95. Groden J, Thliveris A, Samowitz W, et al. Identification and characterization of the familial adenomatous polyposis coli gene. *Cell* 1991;66:589–600.
96. Nishisho I, Nakamura Y, Miyoshi Y, et al. Mutations of chromosome 5q21 genes in FAP and colorectal cancer patients. *Science* 1991;253:665–669.
97. Spirio L, Otterud B, Stauffer D, et al. Linkage of a variant or attenuated form of adenomatous polyposis coli to the adenomatous polyposis coli (APC) locus. *Am J Hum Genet* 1992;51:92–100.
98. Soravia C, Berk T, Madlensky L, et al. Genotype-phenotype correlations in attenuated adenomatous polyposis coli. *Am J Hum Genet* 1998;62:1290–1301.
99. Foulkes WD. A tale of four syndromes: familial adenomatous polyposis, Gardner syndrome, attenuated APC and Turcot syndrome. *Q J Med* 1995;88:853–863.
100. Chung D. The genetic basis of colorectal cancer: insights into critical pathways of tumorigenesis. *Gastroenterology* 2000;119:854–865.
101. Powell SM, Zilz N, Beazer-Barclay Y, et al. APC mutations occur early during colorectal tumorigenesis. *Nature* 1992;359:235–237.
102. Miyoshi Y, Nagase H, Ando H, et al. Somatic mutations of the APC gene in colorectal tumors: mutation cluster region in the APC gene. *Hum Mol Genet* 1992;1:229–233.
103. Vogelstein B, Fearon ER, Hamilton SR, et al. Genetic alterations during colorectal-tumor development. *N Engl J Med* 1988;319:525–532.
104. Jen J, Powell SM, Papadopoulos N, et al. Molecular determinants of dysplasia in colorectal lesions. *Cancer Res* 1994;54:5523–5526.
105. Smith AJ, Stern HS, Penner M, et al. Somatic APC and K-ras codon 12 mutations in aberrant crypt foci from human colons. *Cancer Res* 1994;54:5527–5530.
106. Miyaki M, Konishi M, Kikuchi-Yanoshita R, et al. Characteristics of somatic mutation of the adenomatous polyposis coli gene in colorectal tumors. *Cancer Res* 1994;54:3011–3020.
107. Su LK, Vogelstein B, Kinzler KW. Association of the APC tumor suppressor protein with catenins. *Science* 1993;262:1734–1737.
108. Rubinfeld B, Souza B, Albert I, et al. Association of the APC gene product with beta-catenin. *Science* 1993;262:1731–1734.
109. Behrens J, Jerchow BA, Wurtele M, et al. Functional interaction of an axin homolog, conductin, with beta- catenin, APC, and GSK3beta. *Science* 1998;280:596–599.
110. Powell SM, Petersen GM, Krush AJ, et al. Molecular diagnosis of familial adenomatous polyposis [see comments]. *N Engl J Med* 1993;329:1982–1987.
111. Sakamoto Y, Kitazawa R, Maeda S, et al. Methylation of CpG loci in 5′-flanking region alters steady-state expression of adenomatous polyposis coli gene in colon cancer cell lines. *J Cell Biochem* 2001;80:415–423.
112. Spirio LN, Samowitz W, Robertson J, et al. Alleles of APC modulate the frequency and classes of mutations that lead to colon polyps. *Nat Genet* 1998;20:385–388.
113. Crawford HC, Fingleton BM, Rudolph-Owen LA, et al. The metalloproteinase matrilysin is a target of beta-catenin transactivation in intestinal tumors. *Oncogene* 1999;18:2883–2891.
114. Suzuki H, Watkins DN, Jair KW, et al. Epigenetic inactivation of SFRP genes allows constitutive WNT signaling in colorectal cancer. *Nat Genet* 2004;36:417–422.

115. Sparks AB, Morin PJ, Vogelstein B, et al. Mutational analysis of the APC/beta-catenin/Tcf pathway in colorectal cancer. *Cancer Res* 1998;58:1130–1134.

116. Kitaeva M, Grogan L, Williams J, et al. Mutations in *β*-catenin are uncommon in colorectal cancer occurring in occasional replication error-positive tumors. *Cancer Res* 1997;57:4478–4481.

117. Caspari R, Olschwang S, Friedl W, et al. Familial adenomatous polyposis: desmoid tumours and lack of ophthalmic lesions (CHRPE) associated with APC mutations beyond codon 1444. *Hum Mol Genet* 1995;4:337–340.

118. Spirio L, Olschwang S, Groden J, et al. Alleles of the APC gene: an attenuated form of familial polyposis. *Cell* 1993;75:951–957.

119. Gardner RJ, Kool D, Edkins E, et al. The clinical correlates of a 3' truncating mutation (codons 1982–1983) in the adenomatous polyposis coli gene. *Gastroenterology* 1997;113:326–331.

120. Laken SJ, Petersen GM, Gruber SB, et al. Familial colorectal cancer in Ashkenazim due to a hypermutable tract in APC. *Nat Genet* 1997;17:79–83.

121. Lothe RA, Hektoen M, Johnsen H, et al. The APC gene I1307K variant is rare in Norwegian patients with familial and sporadic colorectal or breast cancer. *Cancer Res* 1998;58:2923–2924.

122. Hulsken J, Birchmeier W, Behrens J. E-cadherin and APC compete for the interaction with beta-catenin and the cytoskeleton. *J Cell Biol* 1994;127:2061–2069.

123. Aberle H, Butz S, Stappert J, et al. Assembly of the cadherin-catenin complex in vitro with recombinant proteins. *J Cell Sci* 1994;107:3655–3663.

124. Moon RT, Brown JD, Yang-Snyder JA, et al. Structurally related receptors and antagonists compete for secreted Wnt ligands. *Cell* 1997;88:725–728.

125. Rubinfeld B, Albert I, Porfiri E, et al. Loss of beta-catenin regulation by the APC tumor suppressor protein correlates with loss of structure due to common somatic mutations of the gene. *Cancer Res* 1997;57:4624–4630.

126. Munemitsu S, Albert I, Souza B, et al. Regulation of intracellular beta-catenin levels by the adenomatous polyposis coli (APC) tumor-suppressor protein. *Proc Natl Acad Sci U S A* 1995;92:3046–3050.

127. Munemitsu S, Albert I, Rubinfeld B, et al. Deletion of an amino-terminal sequence beta-catenin in vivo and promotes hyperphosphorylation of the adenomatous polyposis coli tumor suppressor protein. *Mol Cell Biol* 1996;16:4088–4094.

128. Morin PJ, Sparks AB, Korinek V, et al. Activation of beta-catenin-Tcf signaling in colon cancer by mutations in beta-catenin or APC [see comments]. *Science* 1997;275:1787–1790.

129. Rubinfeld B, Robbins P, El-Gamil M, et al. Stabilization of beta-catenin by genetic defects in melanoma cell lines [see comments]. *Science* 1997;275:1790–1792.

130. Shtutman M, Zhurinsky J, Simcha I, et al. The cyclin D1 gene is a target of the beta-catenin/LEF-1 pathway. *Proc Natl Acad Sci U S A* 1999;96:5522–5527.

131. He TC, Sparks AB, Rago C, et al. Identification of c-MYC as a target of the APC pathway [see comments]. *Science* 1998;281:1509–1512.

132. Park WS, Oh RR, Park JY, et al. Frequent somatic mutations of the beta-catenin gene in intestinal-type gastric cancer. *Cancer Res* 1999;59:4257–4260.

133. Caca K, Kolligs FT, Ji X, et al. Beta- and gamma-catenin mutations, but not E-cadherin inactivation, underlie T-cell factor/lymphoid enhancer factor transcriptional deregulation in gastric and pancreatic cancer. *Cell Growth Differ* 1999;10:369–376.

134. Kawanishi J, Kato J, Sasaki K, et al. Loss of E-cadherin-dependent cell-cell adhesion due to mutation of the beta-catenin gene in a human cancer cell line, HSC-39. *Mol Cell Biol* 1995;15:1175–1181.

135. Luber B, Candidus S, Handschuh G, et al. Tumor-derived mutated E-cadherin influences beta-catenin localization and increases susceptibility to actin cytoskeletal changes induced by pervanadate. *Cell Adhes Commun* 2000;7:391–408.

136. Harada N, Tamai Y, Ishikawa T, et al. Intestinal polyposis in mice with a dominant stable mutation of the beta-catenin gene. *EMBO J* 1999;18:5931–5942.

137. Samowitz WS, Powers MD, Spirio LN, et al. Beta-catenin mutations are more frequent in small colorectal adenomas than in larger adenomas and invasive carcinomas. *Cancer Res* 1999;59:1442–1444.

138. Harvey J. An unidentified virus which causes the rapid production of tumors in mice. *Nature* 1964;204:1104–1105.

139. Kirsten W, Mayer L. Morphologic responses to a murine erythroblastosis virus. *J Natl Cancer Inst* 1967;39:311–335.

140. Fearon ER. Molecular abnormalities in colon and rectal cancer. In: Mendelsohn J, Howley P, Israel M, Liotta L, eds. *The Molecular Basis of Cancer.* Philadelphia, Pa.: WB Saunders; 1995:340–357.

141. Bokoch GM, Der CJ. Emerging concepts in the Ras superfamily of GTP-binding proteins. *FASEB J* 1993;7:750–759.

142. Barbacid M. ras Genes. *Annu Rev Biochem* 1987;56:779–827.

143. Scheele JS, Rhee JM, Boss GR. Determination of absolute amounts of GDP and GTP bound to Ras in mammalian cells: comparison of parental and Ras-overproducing NIH 3T3 fibroblasts. *Proc Natl Acad Sci U S A* 1995;92:1097–1100.

144. Janda E, Lehmann K, Killisch I, et al. Ras and TGF[beta] cooperatively regulate epithelial cell plasticity and metastasis: dissection of Ras signaling pathways. *J Cell Biol* 2002;156:299–313.

145. Fang JY, Richardson BC. The MAPK signalling pathways and colorectal cancer. *Lancet Oncol* 2005;6:322–327.

146. Forrester K, Almoguera C, Han K, et al. Detection of high incidence of K-ras *Oncogenes* during human colon tumorigenesis. *Nature* 1987;327:298–303.

147. Bos JL, Fearon ER, Hamilton SR, et al. Prevalence of ras gene mutations in human colorectal cancers. *Nature* 1987;327:293–297.

148. Arber N, Shapira I, Ratan J, et al. Activation of c-K-ras mutations in human gastrointestinal tumors. *Gastroenterology* 2000;118:1045–1050.

149. Tsao J, Shibata D. Further evidence that one of the earliest alterations in colorectal carcinogenesis involves APC. *Am J Pathol* 1994;145:531–534.

150. Lubomierski N, Plotz G, Wormek M, et al. BRAF mutations in colorectal carcinoma suggest two entities of microsatellite-unstable tumors. *Cancer* 2005;104:952–961.

151. Beach R, Chan AO, Wu TT, et al. BRAF mutations in aberrant crypt foci and hyperplastic polyposis. *Am J Pathol* 2005;166:1069–1075.

152. Ikenoue T, Hikiba Y, Kanai F, et al. Different effects of point mutations within the B-Raf glycine-rich loop in colorectal tumors on mitogen-activated protein/extracellular signal-regulated kinase kinase/extracellular signal-regulated kinase and nuclear factor kappaB pathway and cellular transformation. *Cancer Res* 2004;64:3428–3435.

153. Wang L, Cunningham JM, Winters JL, et al. BRAF mutations in colon cancer are not likely attributable to defective DNA mismatch repair. *Cancer Res* 2003;63:5209–5212.

154. Ochiai A, Hirohashi S. Multiple genetic alterations in gastric cancer. In: Sugimura T, Sasako M, eds. *Gastric Cancer.* New York, NY: Oxford University Press; 1997:87–99.

155. Somasundaram K. Tumor suppressor p53: regulation and function. *Front Biosci* 2000;5:D424-D437.

156. Vogelstein B, Fearon ER, Kern SE, et al. Allelotype of colorectal carcinomas. *Science* 1989;244:207–211.

157. Hollstein M, Sidransky D, Vogelstein B, et al. p53 Mutations in human cancers. *Science* 1991;253:49–53.

158. Ko LJ, Prives C. p53: Puzzle and paradigm. *Genes Dev* 1996;10:1054–1072.

159. Baker SJ, Preisinger AC, Jessup JM, et al. p53 gene mutations occur in combination with 17p allelic deletions as late events in colorectal tumorigenesis. *Cancer Res* 1990;50:7717–7722.

160. Kikuchi-Yanoshita R, Konishi M, Ito S, et al. Genetic changes of both p53 alleles associated with the conversion from colorectal adenoma to early carcinoma in familial adenomatous polyposis and non-familial adenomatous polyposis patients. *Cancer Res* 1992;52:3965–3971.

161. Boland CR, Sato J, Appelman HD, et al. Microallelotyping defines the sequence and tempo of allelic losses at tumour suppressor gene loci during colorectal cancer progression. *Nat Med* 1995;1:902–909.

162. Ohue M, Tomita N, Monden T, et al. A frequent alteration of p53 gene in carcinoma in adenoma of colon. *Cancer Res* 1994;54:4798–4804.

163. Lane DP. Cancer: a death in the life of p53 [news; comment]. *Nature* 1993;362:786–787.

164. el-Deiry WS, Harper JW, O'Connor PM, et al. WAF1/CIP1 is induced in p53-mediated G1 arrest and apoptosis. *Cancer Res* 1994;54:1169–1174.

165. el-Deiry WS, Tokino T, Velculescu VE, et al. WAF1, a potential mediator of p53 tumor suppression. *Cell* 1993;75:817–825.

166. Smith ML, Chen IT, Zhan Q, et al. Interaction of the p53-regulated protein Gadd45 with proliferating cell nuclear antigen [see comments]. *Science* 1994;266:1376–1380.

167. Lin D, Shields MT, Ullrich SJ, et al. Growth arrest induced by wild-type p53 protein blocks cells prior to or near the restriction point in late G1 phase. *Proc Natl Acad Sci U S A* 1992;89:9210–9214.

168. Levine AJ. p53, The cellular gatekeeper for growth and division. *Cell* 1997;88:323–331.

169. Dameron KM, Volpert OV, Tainsky MA, et al. Control of angiogenesis in fibroblasts by p53 regulation of thrombospondin-1. *Science* 1994;265:1582–1584.

170. Howe JR, Guillem JG. The genetics of colorectal cancer. *Surg Clin North Am* 1997;77:175–195.

171. el-Deiry WS, Kern SE, Pietenpol JA, et al. Definition of a consensus binding site for p53. *Nat Genet* 1992;1:45–49.

172. Allegra CJ, Parr AL, Wold LE, et al. Investigation of the prognostic and predictive value of thymidylate synthase, p53, and Ki-67 in patients with locally advanced colon cancer. *J Clin Oncol* 2002;20:1735–1743.

173. Grem JL. Intratumoral molecular or genetic markers as predictors of clinical outcome with chemotherapy in colorectal cancer. *Semin Oncol* 2005;32:120–127.

174. Vivanco I, Sawyers CL. The phosphatidylinositol 3-Kinase AKT pathway in human cancer. *Nat Rev Cancer* 2002;2:489–501.

175. Djordjevic S, Driscoll PC. Structural insight into substrate specificity and regulatory mechanisms of phosphoinositide 3-kinases. *Trends Biochem Sci* 2002;27:426–432.

176. Samuels Y, Wang Z, Bardelli A, et al. High frequency of mutations of the PIK3CA gene in human cancers. *Science* 2004;304:554.

177. Ikenoue T, Kanai F, Hikiba Y, et al. Functional analysis of PIK3CA gene mutations in human colorectal cancer. *Cancer Res* 2005;65:4562–4567.

178. Philp AJ, Campbell IG, Leet C, et al. The phosphatidylinositol 3'-kinase p85alpha gene is an oncogene in human ovarian and colon tumors. *Cancer Res* 2001;61:7426–7429.

179. Markowitz S, Roberts A. Tumor suppressor activity of the TGF-ß pathway in human cancers. *Cytokine Growth Factor Rev* 1996;7:93–102.
180. Fynan TM, Reiss M. Resistance to inhibition of cell growth by transforming growth factor-beta and its role in oncogenesis. *Crit Rev Oncog* 1993;4:493–540.
181. Hoosein N, McKnight M, Levine A, et al. Differential sensitivity of subclasses of human colon carcinoma cell lines to the growth inhibitory effects of transforming growth factor-ß 1. *Exp Cell Res* 1989;181:442–453.
182. Grady W, Myeroff L, Swinler S, et al. Mutational inactivation of transforming growth factor *β* receptor type II in microsatellite stable colon cancers. *Cancer Res* 1999;59:320–324.
183. Massague J. TGF-ß signaling: receptors, transducers, and mad proteins. *Cell* 1996;85:947–950.
184. Wakefield LM, Roberts AB. TGF-beta signaling: positive and negative effects on tumorigenesis. *Curr Opin Genet Dev* 2002;12:22–29.
185. Wrana J, Pawson T. Signal transduction. Mad about SMADs [news; comment]. *Nature* 1997;388:28–29.
186. Luo K, Stroschein SL, Wang W, et al. The Ski oncoprotein interacts with the Smad proteins to repress TGFbeta signaling. *Genes Dev* 1999;13:2196–2206.
187. Hua X, Liu X, Ansari DO, et al. Synergistic cooperation of TFE3 and Smad proteins in TGF-beta-induced transcription of the plasminogen activator inhibitor-1 gene. *Genes Dev* 1998;12:3084–3095.
188. Grady WM, Willis JE, Trobridge P, et al. Proliferation and Cdk4 expression in microsatellite unstable colon cancers with TGFBR2 mutations. *Int J Cancer* 2006; 118:600–608.
189. Geng Y, Weinberg RA. Transforming growth factor beta effects on expression of G1 cyclins and cyclin-dependent protein kinases. *Proc Natl Acad Sci U S A* 1993;90:10315–10319.
190. Howe PH, Draetta G, Leof EB. Transforming growth factor beta 1 inhibition of p34cdc2 phosphorylation and histone H1 kinase activity is associated with G1/S-phase growth arrest. *Mol Cell Biol* 1991;11:1185–1194.
191. Ewen ME, Sluss HK, Whitehouse LL, et al. TGF beta inhibition of Cdk4 synthesis is linked to *Cell Cycle* arrest. *Cell* 1993;74:1009–1020.
192. Alexandrow M, Moses H. Transforming growth factor ß and *Cell Cycle* regulation. *Cancer Res* 1995;55:1452–1457.
193. Hannon G, Beach D. p15INK4B is a potential effector of TGF-ß-induced *Cell Cycle* arrest. *Nature* 1994;371:257–261.
194. Moses H, Yang E, Pietonpol J. TGF-ß stimulation and inhibition of cell proliferation: new mechanistic insights. *Cell* 1990;63:245–247.
195. Keeton MR, Curriden SA, van Zonneveld AJ, et al. Identification of regulatory sequences in the type 1 plasminogen activator inhibitor gene responsive to transforming growth factor beta. *J Biol Chem* 1991;266:23048–23052.
196. Zhao Y. Transforming growth factor-beta (TGF-beta) type I and type II receptors are both required for TGF-beta-mediated extracellular matrix production in lung fibroblasts. *Mol Cell Endocrinol* 1999;150:91–97.
197. Biswas S, Chytil A, Washington K, et al. Transforming growth factor {beta} receptor type II inactivation promotes the establishment and progression of colon cancer. *Cancer Res* 2004;64:4687–4692.
198. Parsons R, Myeroff L, Liu B, et al. Microsatellite instability and mutations of the transforming growth factor ß type II receptor gene in colorectal cancer. *Cancer Res* 1995;55:5548–5550.
199. Myeroff L, Parsons R, Kim S-J, et al. A transforming growth factor ß receptor type II gene mutation common in colon and gastric but rare in endometrial cancers with microsatellite instability. *Cancer Res* 1995;55:5545–5547.
200. Fearon ER, Cho KR, Nigro JM, et al. Identification of a chromosome 18q gene that is altered in colorectal cancers. *Science* 1990;247:49–56.
201. Nagatake M, Takagi Y, Osada H, et al. Somatic in vivo alterations of the DPC4 gene at 18q21 in human lung cancers. *Cancer Res* 1996;56:2718–2720.
202. Eppert K, Scherer S, Ozcelik H, et al. MADR2 maps to 18q21 and encodes a TGFß -regulated MAD-related protein that is functionally mutated in colorectal cancer. *Cell* 1996;86:543–552.
203. Martinez-Lopez E, Abad A, Font A, et al. Allelic loss on chromosome 18q as a prognostic marker in stage II colorectal cancer [see comments]. *Gastroenterology* 1998;114:1180–1187.
204. Kretzschmar M, Liu F, Hata A, et al. The TGF-beta family mediator Smad1 is phosphorylated directly and activated functionally by the BMP receptor kinase. *Genes Dev* 1997;11:984–995.
205. Zhang Y, Feng X-H, Wu R-Y, et al. Receptor-associated Mad homologues synergize as effectors of the TGF-ß response. *Nature* 1996;383:168–172.
206. Souchelnytskyi S, Tamaki K, Engstrom U, et al. Phosphorylation of Ser465 and Ser467 in the C terminus of Smad2 mediates interaction with Smad4 and is required for transforming growth factor-beta signaling. *J Biol Chem* 1997;272:28107–28115.
207. Abdollah S, Macias-Silva M, Tsukazaki T, et al. TbetaRI phosphorylation of Smad2 on Ser465 and Ser467 is required for Smad2-Smad4 complex formation and signaling. *J Biol Chem* 1997;272:27678–27685.
208. Hahn S, Schutte M, Shamsul Hoque A, et al. DPC4, a candidate tumor suppressor gene at human chromosome 18q21.1. *Science* 1996;271:350–353.
209. Takagi Y, Kohmura H, Futamura M, et al. Somatic alterations of

the DPC4 gene in human colorectal cancers in vivo. *Gastroenterology* 1996;111:1369–1372.
210. Riggins G, Thiagalingam S, Rozenblum E, et al. *Mad*-related genes in the human. *Nat Genet* 1996;13:347–349.
211. Takaku K, Oshima M, Miyoshi H, et al. Intestinal tumorigenesis in compound mutant mice of both *Dpc4* (*Smad4*) and *Apc* genes. *Cell* 1998;92:645–656.
212. Takaku K, Miyoshi H, Matsunaga A, et al. Gastric and duodenal polyps in *Smad4* (*Dpc4*) knockout mice. *Cancer Res* 1999;59:6113–6117.
213. Xu X, Brodie SG, Yang X, et al. Haploid loss of the tumor suppressor Smad4/Dpc4 initiates gastric polyposis and cancer in mice. *Oncogene* 2000;19:1868–1874.
214. Howe JR, Roth S, Ringold JC, et al. Mutations in the SMAD4/DPC4 gene in juvenile polyposis [see comments]. *Science* 1998;280:1086–1088.
215. Friedl W, Kruse R, Uhlhaas S, et al. Frequent 4-bp deletion in exon 9 of the SMAD4/MADH4 gene in familial juvenile polyposis patients. *Genes Chromosomes Cancer* 1999;25:403–406.
216. Roth S, Sistonen P, Salovaara R, et al. SMAD genes in juvenile polyposis. *Genes Chromosomes Cancer* 1999;26:54–61.
217. Woodford-Richens K, Williamson J, Bevan S, et al. Allelic loss at SMAD4 in polyps from juvenile polyposis patients and use of fluorescence in situ hybridization to demonstrate clonal origin of the epithelium. *Cancer Res* 2000;60:2477–2482.
218. Takenoshita S, Tani M, Mogi A, et al. Mutation analysis of the Smad2 gene in human colon cancers using genomic DNA and intron primers. *Carcinogenesis* 1998;19:803–807.
219. Park WS, Park JY, Oh RR, et al. A distinct tumor suppressor gene locus on chromosome 15q21.1 in sporadic form of colorectal cancer. *Cancer Res* 2000;60:70–73.
220. Arai T, Akiyama Y, Okabe S, et al. Genomic structure of the human Smad3 gene and its infrequent alterations in colorectal cancers. *Cancer Lett* 1998;122:157–163.
221. Zhu Y, Richardson JA, Parada LF, et al. Smad3 mutant mice develop metastatic colorectal cancer. *Cell* 1998;94:703–714.
222. Carethers JM, Hawn MT, Greenson JK, et al. Prognostic significance of allelic lost at chromosome 18q21 for stage II colorectal cancer. *Gastroenterology* 1998;114:1188–1195.
223. Jen J, Kim H, Piantadosi S, et al. Allelic loss of chromosome 18q and prognosis in colorectal cancer. *N Engl J Med* 1994;331:213–221.
224. Laurent-Puig P, Olschwang S, Delattre O, et al. Survival and acquired genetic alterations in colorectal cancer. *Gastroenterology* 1992;102:1136–1141.
225. Zhou W, Goodman SN, Galizia G, et al. Counting alleles to predict recurrence of early-stage colorectal cancers. *Lancet* 2002;359:219–225.
226. Boulay JL, Mild G, Lowy A, et al. SMAD4 is a predictive marker for 5-fluorouracil-based chemotherapy in patients with colorectal cancer. *Br J Cancer* 2002;87:630–634.
227. Howe JR, Bair JL, Sayed MG, et al. Germline mutations of the gene encoding bone morphogenetic protein receptor 1A in juvenile polyposis. *Nat Genet* 2001;28:184–187.
228. Friedl W, Uhlhaas S, Schulmann K, et al. Juvenile polyposis: massive gastric polyposis is more common in MADH4 mutation carriers than in BMPR1A mutation carriers. *Hum Genet* 2002;111:108–111.
229. Howe JR, Shellnut J, Wagner B, et al. Common deletion of SMAD4 in juvenile polyposis is a mutational hotspot. *Am J Hum Genet* 2002;70:1357–1362.
230. Kawabata M, Imamura T, Miyazono K. Signal transduction by bone morphogenetic proteins. *Cytokine Growth Factor Rev* 1998;9:49–61.
231. He XC, Zhang J, Tong WG, et al. BMP signaling inhibits intestinal stem cell self-renewal through suppression of Wnt-beta-catenin signaling. *Nat Genet* 2004;36:1117–1121.
232. Haramis AP, Begthel H, van den Born M, et al. De novo crypt formation and juvenile polyposis on BMP inhibition in mouse intestine. *Science* 2004;303:1684–1686.
233. de Caestecker M. The transforming growth factor-beta superfamily of receptors. *Cytokine Growth Factor Rev* 2004;15:1–11.
234. Deacu E, Mori Y, Sato F, et al. Activin type II receptor restoration in ACVR2-deficient colon cancer cells induces transforming growth factor-beta response pathway genes. *Cancer Res* 2004;64:7690–7696.
235. Saha S, Bardelli A, Buckhaults P, et al. A phosphatase associated with metastasis of colorectal cancer. *Science* 2001;294:1343–1346.
236. Yeatman TJ, Chambers AF. Osteopontin and colon cancer progression. *Clin Exp Metastasis* 2003;20:85–90.
237. Furger KA, Menon RK, Tuckl AB, et al. The functional and clinical roles of osteopontin in cancer and metastasis. *Curr Mol Med* 2001;1:621–632.
238. Liu W, Dong X, Mai M, et al. Mutations in AXIN2 cause colorectal cancer with defective mismatch repair by activating beta-catenin/TCF signalling. *Nat Genet* 2000;26:146–147.
239. Lammi L, Arte S, Somer M, et al. Mutations in AXIN2 cause familial tooth agenesis and predispose to colorectal cancer. *Am J Hum Genet* 2004;71:1043–1050.
240. Pasche B, Knobloch TJ, Bian Y, et al. Somatic acquisition and signaling of TGFBR1*6A in cancer. *JAMA* 2005;294:1634–1646.
241. Mizuguchi T, Collod-Beroud G, Akiyama T, et al. Heterozygous TGFBR2 mutations in Marfan syndrome. *Nat Genet* 2004;36:855–860.

CHAPTER 41 ■ COLORECTAL CANCER: PATHOLOGY

THOMAS C. SMYRK

Multiple molecular pathways may contribute to colon carcinogenesis, and colorectal carcinoma may be a more heterogeneous disease than is generally acknowledged. Nevertheless, one morphologic continuum—the dysplasia-carcinoma sequence—can encompass the histologic range of malignant and premalignant epithelial changes, and it is reasonable to discuss colorectal carcinoma as a single pathological entity. This chapter reviews the known precursor lesions, describes the histology of colorectal carcinoma, and discusses specific features associated with one molecular subtype (i.e., microsatellite instability-high [MSI-H] carcinoma).

PRECURSOR LESIONS

Aberrant crypt foci (ACF) are the earliest grossly visible precursors to adenocarcinoma (1). They can be identified in situ with the aid of magnifying endoscopy and methylene blue staining (2). Based on the combination of endoscopic appearance and histology, three types of ACF have been characterized: (a) nondysplastic, nonhyperplastic; (b) nondysplastic, hyperplastic; and (c) dysplastic. The first have round or oval lumens when viewed endoscopically; hyperplastic ACF have slitlike lumens and dysplastic ACF have compressed or indistinct lumens with a thickened epithelial lining. The histologic appearance of ACF parallels the gross changes, ranging from normal to hyperplastic to dysplastic. The number of dysplastic ACF progressively increases from normal controls to adenoma patients to cancer patients, suggesting that dysplastic ACF are precursors to adenoma (2). The most important application for ACF at this time is as an end point in chemoprevention studies (3).

Adenomas are grossly visible collections of dysplastic crypts. Macroscopically, adenomas can be elevated, flat, or depressed. Elevated adenomas range from pedunculated polyps on a stalk to sessile lesions. Flat or depressed adenomas can be recognized by mucosal reddening or changes in texture. Whatever the gross morphology, adenoma is defined by the presence of intraepithelial neoplasia, and recognizable by hypercellularity, enlarged hyperchromatic nuclei, and varying degrees of nuclear stratification (Fig. 41.1). The intraepithelial neoplasia can be classified as low-grade or high-grade, depending on the degree of architectural complexity and nuclear stratification, pleomorphism, and loss of polarity. The term tubular adenoma is applied when dysplastic glandular structures are present on at least 80% of the luminal surface. If more than 80% of the surface is covered by villiform-to-ridgelike structures, the lesion is termed a *villous adenoma*. Tubulovillous adenomas have a mixture of tubular and villous architecture. There is a general relationship between size, villosity, and the presence of high-grade dysplasia and invasive carcinoma. The frequency of high-grade dysplasia increases with adenoma size and is highest in villous adenomas (4).

Serrated adenoma (SA) has serrated crypts similar to those seen in hyperplastic polyp, but the crypts are lined by dysplastic epithelium (5) (Fig. 41.2). By convention, the entire lesion should have this appearance in order to be classified as SA. Once believed to be a variant of adenoma, SA is now placed in the general category of serrated polyps (Table 41.1) (6).

Sessile serrated adenoma (SSA) resembles hyperplastic polyp in that it contains serrated crypts, but there are subtle architectural differences (7). Dilation and lateral branching at the crypt base are the easiest to recognize; there is also abnormal maturation in the crypt base, serration at the crypt base, small foci of nuclear crowding and pseudostratification in the crypt walls and in the surface epithelium, and focal eosinophilic change in epithelial cytoplasm (Fig. 41.3). The use of the term "SSA" has been criticized because the lesion generally contains no overt cytologic dysplasia. Other proposed terms include sessile serrated polyp and sessile serrated lesion, but the defenders of SSA argue that cytologic dysplasia is not required for a diagnosis of adenoma in other sites (hepatic adenoma, adrenal cortical adenoma) and that the lesion does have architectural dysplasia. When cytologic dysplasia does develop in SSA, the dysplastic focus often has loss of expression for the mismatch repair protein MLH1 (Fig. 41.4), and when invasive carcinoma develops, it is often MSI-H. In fact, SSA may be the precursor lesion for most or all MSI-H colorectal carcinoma (6).

Sessile serrated adenomas tend to arise in the right colon. They can become large; most are >0.5 cm, and plaques 2 to 3 cm in diameter are not unusual. Current recommendations are preliminary but include complete endoscopic removal or regular endoscopic surveillance with biopsy if the lesion cannot be removed. If overt dysplasia develops in an SSA, then resection should be considered. Repeat endoscopy at an interval similar to that for patients with adenoma is recommended even for patients with a completely removed SSA (6).

COLORECTAL CARCINOMA

Macroscopic Features

The macroscopic features of colorectal carcinoma depend in part on the extent of disease progression, but gross tumor configuration can be broadly categorized as exophytic or flat. Flat cancers may be ulcerative or infiltrative. Right-sided tumors tend to form exophytic masses more often than left-sided ones, and infiltrative growth is typical of signet ring cell carcinoma. Exophytic growth has been associated with lower stage (8) and lower risk for hematogenous metastasis (9). In 1939, Grinnell

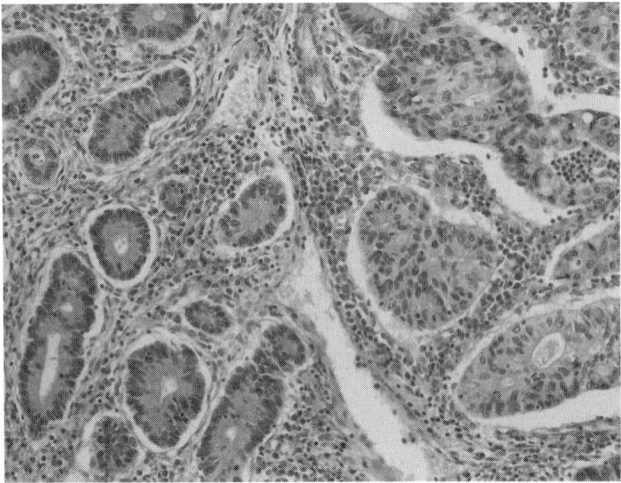

FIGURE 41.1. Adenoma, featuring crowded elongated nuclei. A transition to high-grade dysplasia is evidenced by cribriform architecture, loss of nuclear polarity, and increased variability in nuclear size and shape.

reported 83% survival for patients with tumors projecting into the bowel lumen, compared to 45% for those with tumors classified as intermediate and 38% for those with infiltrative tumors (10). An exophytic growth pattern was identified as a significant favorable prognostic feature in more recent studies as well (11,12). Whether exophytic or infiltrative, tumors that encircle more than three-fourths of the bowel circumference are associated with adverse outcome (13), and obstruction is a

TABLE 41.1
SERRATED POLYPS OF THE COLORECTUM
Hyperplastic polyp Sessile serrated adenoma Serrated adenoma Mixed serrated polyp (e.g., mixed sessile serrated   adenoma-tubular adenoma)

clinical marker of poor prognosis (14–17). In practice, overlapping growth patterns and variability in observer interpretation of macroscopic configuration limit the usefulness of this parameter. A consensus statement from the College of American Pathology (CAP), citing these difficulties, made no recommendation as to reporting guidelines for tumor configuration (18). Still, studies continue to report better outcomes for polypoid carcinoma (19). A reasonable suggestion is that pathologists attempt to characterize configuration as exophytic (polypoid), ulcerative, or infiltrative, and, for annular tumors, estimate the percentage of bowel circumference involved.

Histologic Subtypes

The current World Health Organization (WHO) classification recognizes the following histologic categories:

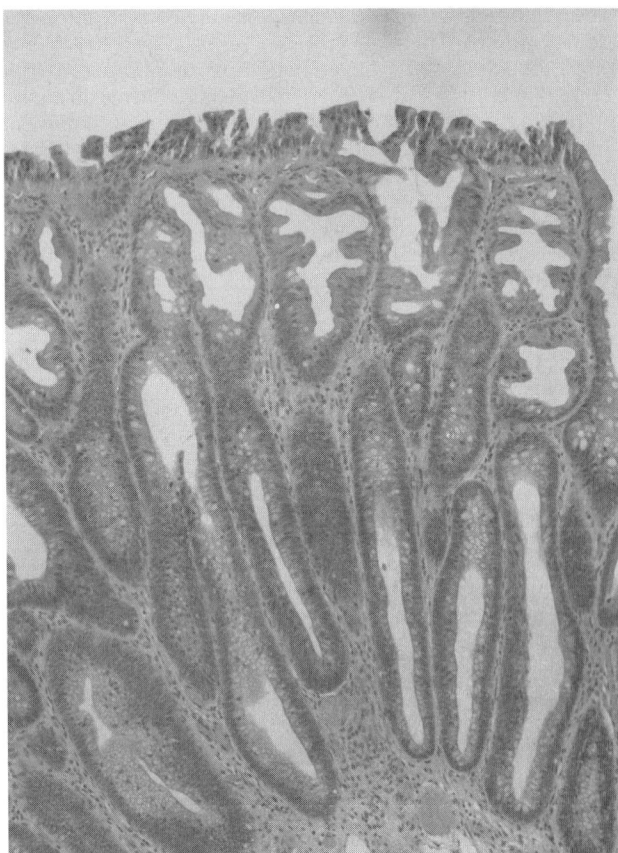

FIGURE 41.2. Serrated adenoma. The crypts have serrated outlines but are lined by dysplastic cells.

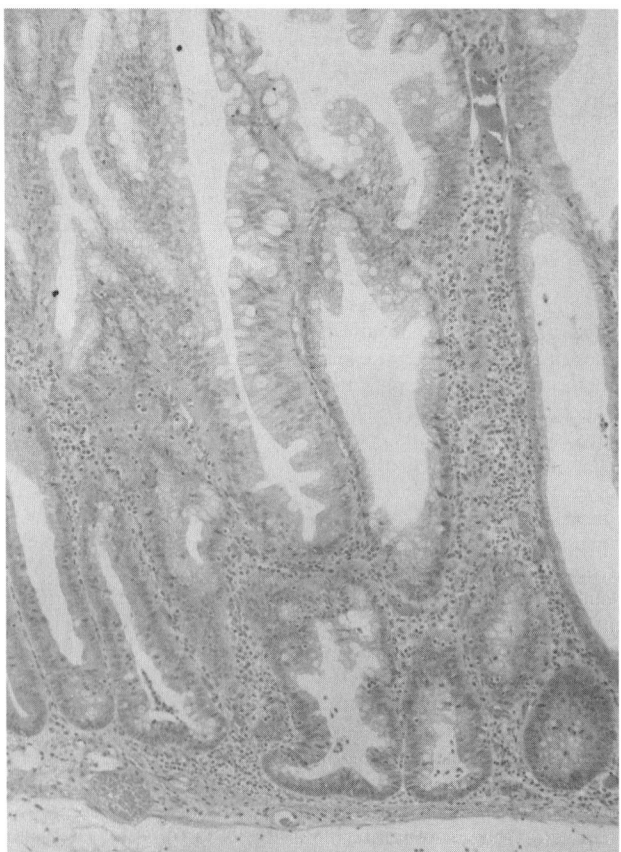

FIGURE 41.3. Sessile serrated adenoma. Serrated crypts with abnormal architecture but without overt dysplasia. Lateral extension at the crypt base is the most helpful diagnostic feature.

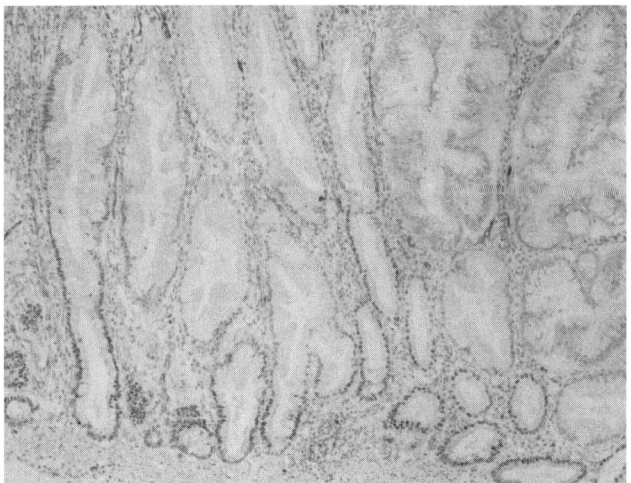

FIGURE 41.4. Transition to dysplasia in a sessile serrated adenoma, accompanied by loss of nuclear MLH1 expression. Immunohistochemistry for MLH1, counterstained by hematoxylin.

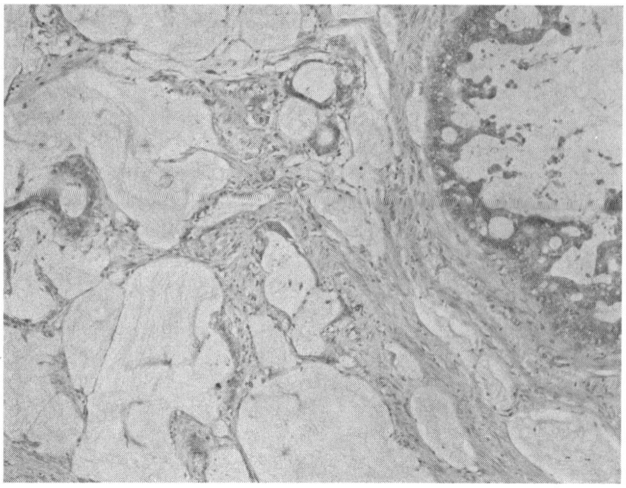

FIGURE 41.5. Mucinous carcinoma, diagnosed when extracellular mucin accounts for >50% of tumor volume.

adenocarcinoma, mucinous adenocarcinoma, signet ring cell carcinoma, squamous and adenosquamous carcinoma, small cell carcinoma, medullary carcinoma, and undifferentiated carcinoma (20).

Most colorectal carcinomas (85%–90%) are adenocarcinomas without special morphologic features. They are gland-forming tumors with variability in gland size and shape. The lining cells are tall and columnar in better-differentiated tumors, becoming more cuboidal with decreasing degrees of differentiation. There is a corresponding change in nuclear morphology, ranging from oval and fairly regular to round and pleomorphic. The gland lumens are often filled with debris, producing the "dirty necrosis" that is a helpful diagnostic clue in both primary and metastatic lesions.

The differential diagnosis of colorectal cancer includes other primary colon tumors (carcinoid, malignant lymphoma, epithelioid variants of gastrointestinal stromal tumor), tumors invading the colon by direct extension (prostate, endometrium, ovary), and metastases from other organs. The presence of gland-forming areas, confirmed by a stain for mucin if necessary, is usually sufficient to eliminate carcinoid, lymphoma, and stromal tumor from consideration, but the undifferentiated medullary subtype of colon cancer can mimic all three of these. Clinical information is, of course, helpful in recognizing noncolonic tumors involving the colon by direct extension or metastasis, but the diagnosis can be suspected when mural growth predominates over mucosal growth.

Although immunohistochemistry is rarely necessary to confirm the diagnosis of colorectal carcinoma, there is a characteristic immunohistochemical profile. More than 95% of colorectal cancers are positive for CDX2 protein, produced by a homeobox gene encoding an intestine-specific transcription factor (21). The protein is not specific for colorectal carcinoma, being immunodetected in 25% to 70% of adenocarcinomas from elsewhere in the gut and in most neuroendocrine tumors of gastrointestinal origin. Most colorectal cancers express CK20 and are negative for CK7, but one should be careful about requiring that profile for the diagnosis; poorly differentiated or undifferentiated carcinoma can be negative for both CK20 and CK7 (5% of total cases), and it is not unusual to see some immunopositivity for CK7, particularly in rectal cancers (22).

Mucinous adenocarcinomas account for 10% of colorectal cancers. A tumor is classified as mucinous if more than 50% of its volume consists of mucin (Fig. 41.5). The prognostic sig-

nificance of mucinous histology has been debated. Of seven studies published in the 1990s, four found no prognostic significance associated with this histology (16,23–25), two found adverse effect by univariate analysis but not multivariate analysis (26,27), and one found mucinous histology to be predictive of recurrence in patients younger than 45 years (28). The CAP consensus is that mucinous differentiation is not proven to be a statistically significant factor independent of histologic grade (18). Substantial mucin production is a feature of cancers with MSI; mucinous carcinoma is about twice as likely as usual adenocarcinoma to be MSI-H (30% vs. 15%) (29). MSI-H mucinous adenocarcinoma has a better outcome than microsatellite stable mucinous adenocarcinoma (29), so studies that do not subclassify mucinous adenocarcinoma by MSI status may be skewed, depending on the prevalence of MSI-H cancers in the study set.

Signet ring cell carcinomas comprise approximately 2% of colorectal cancers. The characteristic cell has an intracytoplasmic mucin-containing vacuole that pushes the nucleus to the periphery (Fig. 41.6). More than 50% of the tumor should be made up of signet cells for a diagnosis of signet ring cell

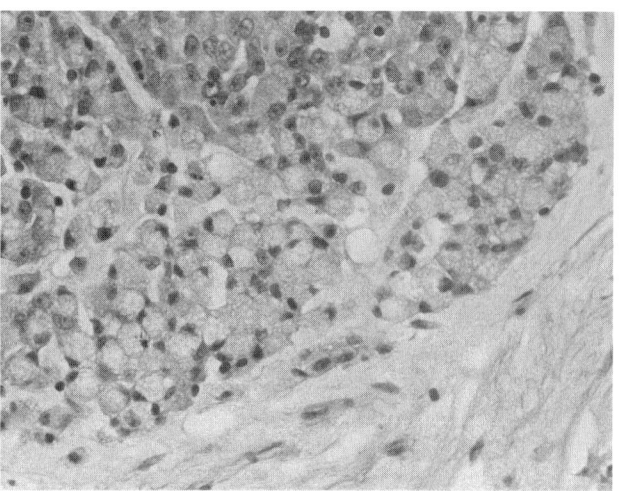

FIGURE 41.6. Signet ring cell carcinoma. Intracytoplasmic vacuoles push the nucleus to one side.

carcinoma (20), although molecular studies demonstrate that tumors with a minor signet cell component are similar to those more abundant signet cells in terms of BRAF mutations, MSI and other molecular markers (30). The tumor is rare enough that signet ring cell histology (and the infiltrative gross tumor configuration that typically accompanies it) should prompt consideration for metastasis from gastric carcinoma or lobular carcinoma of the breast. Most descriptions of primary signet ring cell carcinoma emphasize its poor prognosis (31,32), but the literature is mixed, and a small study by Giacchero et al. (nine cases of signet ring cell carcinoma) found no effect on stage-adjusted survival (33). About 30% of signet ring cell carcinomas are MSI-H, which could confound survival data when that factor is not accounted for. In one study, however, MSI status did not affect outcome within signet ring cell carcinoma patients (34). It has been suggested that 30% of patients with signet ring cell carcinoma have ulcerative colitis (35), so differences in the molecular pathogenesis and natural history of carcinoma in that setting could also confound outcome studies.

Squamous cell carcinoma of the colorectum is very rare. Keratin and intercellular bridges must be identified to make the diagnosis, and no glandular areas should be present. Because squamous carcinoma is common in the anal canal, no continuity must exist between the tumor and the anal canal. In addition, no evidence should be seen of primary squamous carcinoma at a site that could be a source of metastasis to the colon. In a 1979 review, Williams et al. found less than 30 reported cases meeting these criteria (36). More recently, a single-institution review of 4,561 colorectal cancers discovered two acceptable cases of squamous carcinoma (37).

Adenosquamous carcinoma is diagnosed when a gland-forming carcinoma has areas of squamous differentiation. No agreement exists regarding the amount of squamous epithelium required for the diagnosis, but the WHO text advises that "there should be more than just small foci of squamous differentiation" (20). Two cases of adenosquamous carcinoma reported by Cerezo et al. behaved aggressively, with distant metastases from the squamous component (38), but no definitive statement is possible about the natural history of this histologic type.

Small cell carcinomas account for <1% of colorectal cancers. The tumor is identical to its counterpart in the lung, forming sheets of malignant cells with round, dark nuclei and little or no visible cytoplasm (Fig. 41.7). Wick argued convincingly

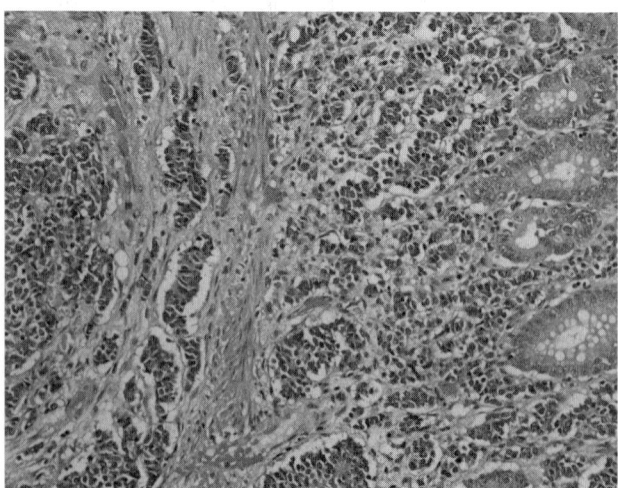

FIGURE 41.7. Small cell carcinoma. In this example, undifferentiated cells appear to drop off the bottom of a tubular adenoma, which is toward the right.

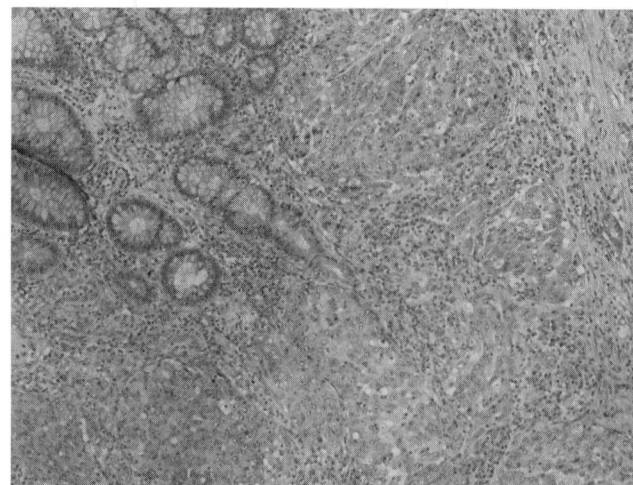

FIGURE 41.8. Medullary carcinoma. Sheets of cells occur, each cell having a round, vesicular nucleus and a prominent nucleus.

for the replacement of the term *small cell carcinoma* (in any organ) with *neuroendocrine carcinoma, grade 3* (39). By any name, this is an aggressive tumor notorious for early hematogenous spread. Of 38 patients with small cell carcinomas of the large intestine reported by the Armed Forces Institute of Pathology, 71% had liver metastases and 64% were dead at 5 months (40). A remarkable feature of small cell carcinoma is the frequent presence of an overlying adenoma, with abrupt transition from the innocuous-appearing adenoma to the aggressive carcinoma (41).

Medullary carcinoma forms a solid pattern of cells with round nuclei and a prominent nucleolus (42,43) (Fig. 41.8). There is little variability in nuclear size and shape. Many lymphocytes are immediately adjacent to tumor cells ("tumor-infiltrating lymphocytes") (44). Despite its rather ominous appearance, descriptive reports suggest that this tumor is relatively indolent (42,43,45). Medullary carcinoma is almost always MSI-H; this histologic pattern has been described in both the hereditary setting (hereditary nonpolyposis colorectal carcinoma) (46) and in sporadic MSI-H colorectal carcinoma (47).

Undifferentiated carcinoma is defined as a malignant epithelial tumor without glandular structure or other features to indicate differentiation. Small cell carcinoma should not be included in this category, despite its confusing synonym "small cell undifferentiated carcinoma."

Staging

Tumor stage is the most powerful predictor of prognosis for colorectal cancer. Accurate assignment of stage requires judicious sampling of tumor to assess depth of invasion and a careful search for lymph nodes. In the fresh state, colon cancer is often too friable to be serially sectioned at the intervals necessary to adequately document depth of invasion. Thus, resected bowel with tumor should be opened and fixed in formalin for several hours before dissection. (If fresh tumor is required for ancillary studies, a piece of tissue can usually be removed without disturbing the relevant anatomical relationships.) After fixation, the tumor should be serially sectioned at intervals of 0.5 cm, and samples demonstrating the areas of deepest invasion submitted for microscopic examination.

Lockhart-Mummery, a surgeon at St. Mark's Hospital in London, proposed the first staging system for rectal cancer (48). The name of Dukes will forever be associated with his

TABLE 41.2

TUMOR (T) DEFINITIONS FOR THE TUMOR, NODE, METASTASIS (TNM) STAGING SYSTEM

TX	Primary tumor cannot be assessed
T0	No evidence of primary tumor
Tis	Carcinoma in situ or invasion of lamina propria
T1	Tumor invades submucosa
T2	Tumor invades muscularis propria
T3	Tumor invades through the muscularis propria into the subserosa or into nonperitonealized pericolic or perirectal tissue
T4	Tumor directly invades other organs (T4a) or perforates the visceral peritoneum (T4b)

modification of Lockhart-Mummery's system (49) and the various modifications that followed (50–52). Dukes' system is easy to apply, but the existence of so many competing classifications sometimes produces confusion (53,54). The tumor, node, metastasis (TNM) staging system of the American Joint Committee on Cancer (AJCC) is the standard and is used here (55).

The T category, referring to the local extent of untreated primary tumor, is delineated in Table 41.2. When the T status has been evaluated pathologically, it is designated pT. The Tis category sometimes causes confusion. Carcinoma in situ and intraepithelial carcinoma are synonyms; both refer to malignant cells that have not yet escaped the gland basement membrane. (High-grade dysplasia is another synonym for the same situation.) The term *intramucosal carcinoma* signifies that malignant cells invade lamina propria or extend into muscularis mucosae but do not reach the submucosa. Although the recommendation is that Tis tumors be specified as either intraepithelial or intramucosal carcinoma, neither lesion has potential for lymph node metastasis, and both lesions can be considered cured by complete removal and are thus included in a single grouping. Tumors that penetrate the muscularis mucosae and invade submucosa are pT1.

Evaluation of depth of invasion is usually not difficult in a well-oriented sample of tumor, but differentiation between T2 and T3 can require some care: If even one muscle fiber is present between tumor and perimuscular soft tissue, the tumor is classified as T2. Invasive tumor typically elicits a fibroblastic response ("desmoplastic stroma") that can obscure the anatomical landmarks. A special stain (trichrome) helps differentiate between muscle and collagen in difficult cases. When there is doubt as to the level of invasion, the general rule is to choose the less advanced category (56).

The T3 category includes all tumors that invade through the muscularis propria but do not reach the serosa or infiltrate an adjacent structure. It is recommended (but not required) that the depth of extramural soft tissue invasion be measured. Deeper invasion, particularly invasion exceeding 5 mm, is associated with worse prognosis, regardless of lymph node status (56). Extramural nodules discontinuous from the main mass are counted as invasion if they have irregular contours, whereas smooth-contoured nodules are classified as replaced lymph nodes. Extramural extension of tumor that is unequivocally in angiolymphatic spaces does not by itself make a tumor T3. The AJCC staging manual suggests that all irregular extramural nodules might represent venous invasion and recommends classifying them as pV1 in addition to the appropriate T category. (Irregular extramural tumor nodules seem to predict poor outcome (57,58), which offers some support for the idea that they are in fact foci of venous invasion.)

The T4 category is an important one that requires careful dissection and sampling for proper evaluation. Serosal penetration (T4b) has strong prognostic significance (16,59,60). In a meticulous prospective study, Shepherd et al. described three types of peritoneal involvement: (a) mesothelial hyperplasia with tumor close to, but not involving, the serosal surface; (b) tumor present at the serosal surface with inflammatory reaction; and (c) free tumor cells on the serosal surface (59). Some form of peritoneal involvement was detected in 59% of 412 patients, and all three forms had adverse effect on survival, with the most unfavorable finding being free tumor cells on the serosal surface.

Lymph node dissection can be undertaken on fresh or fixed tissue. All lymph nodes that appear grossly negative should be completely submitted for histologic examination. Grossly positive nodes may be partially sampled to confirm involvement. Numerous studies have indicated that 12 to 18 lymph nodes must be examined before node-negative status is validated (60–64). If the first review of material yields less than 12 nodes and all nodes are negative, the pathologist should return to the specimen and search for more lymph nodes. In this situation, a visual enhancement method such as the addition of acetic acid to the formalin fixative can prove helpful.

For the most part, lymph nodes retrieved from resection specimens can be considered regional nodes, but any lymph nodes submitted from outside the anatomical site of the tumor should be examined separately. Metastases in regional nodes are classified as pN disease, whereas all other nodal metastases are classified as pM1. Labeling nodes as "peritumoral," "proximal to tumor," and "distal to tumor" has no value. The importance of the highest apical lymph node seems to be less emphasized now than in the past. One of Dukes' early modifications to his staging system divided the C category (node positive) into C1, with involvement limited to regional lymph nodes, and C2, with nodal spread at the point of ligature of the blood vessels (58). Apical node involvement has been shown to predict poor outcome in some subsequent studies. Malassagne et al. recorded 5-year survival rates of 17% and 45% for patients with and without metastasis to the apical node (65), but the apical node is not specifically mentioned in the latest AJCC staging manual (55).

Current practice is to prepare one hematoxylin and eosin–stained slide from a sampled lymph node. This means that only one or two $5\text{-}\mu\text{m}$ slices from each 5- to 8-mm-thick piece of tissue submitted for microscopic examination are reviewed. The potential for missed micrometastases is obvious, and in fact, an increased yield of positive nodes has been obtained by cutting an additional section (66), using immunohistochemical studies to highlight epithelial cells (67), or using molecular technology to identify tumor RNA or DNA in lymph nodes (68). Although one such study demonstrated an adverse outcome in patients with metastases discovered by immunohistochemistry (69), the data are currently considered insufficient to recommend these ancillary methods (18). Isolated tumor cells in lymph nodes (deposits measuring <0.2 mm or deposits detected only by special techniques) are classified as pN0. Deposits of 0.2 to 2 mm are described as micrometastasis and are classified as pN1.

The pathology report should always state the total number of lymph nodes examined and the number of positive nodes. The TNM staging system categorizes cases with metastases in one to three nodes as pN1, whereas cases with four or more nodes involved by metastatic tumor are designated pN2.

The M1 category includes metastases to nonregional lymph nodes, any distant organ, or the peritoneum of any abdominal structure. Positive peritoneal cytology is also considered pM1 disease. Not classified as M1 disease are isolated tumor cells found in the bone marrow or tumor deposits in the mucosa or submucosa of adjacent bowel.

Surgical Margins

Assessment of surgical margins requires careful gross examination and an understanding of the anatomical relationships between bowel and peritoneum. All segments of resected colorectum have a proximal and distal mucosal margin (or a distal margin of perianal skin in abdominal-perineal resections of the rectum). The distance between tumor and mucosal margins should be measured and reported in all cases. Colorectal cancer tends to be well circumscribed, with little submucosal spread beyond grossly visible tumor borders (70), meaning that microscopic examination of margins more than 5 cm from tumor is probably not necessary. Margins closer than 5 cm should be sampled, and the distance between tumor and margin reported.

Some large bowel cancers have a radial margin as well. A radial margin is created when the surgeon removes a tumor that has invaded nonperitonealized tissue. The ascending and descending colon have peritoneum only on their anterior surface. The upper third of the rectum has peritoneum on the front and on both sides, the middle third has peritoneum only on the anterior surface, and the lower third has no peritoneal covering. Even the segments of bowel that are completely covered by peritoneum (e.g., transverse colon) can have a radial margin if tumor infiltrates through muscularis propria on the mesenteric side. A radial margin should be assessed for all cancers infiltrating nonperitonealized tissue. This assessment involves inking the soft tissue margin, dissecting the area, and sampling appropriate tissue for microscopic examination.

A positive radial margin is predictive of local recurrence after surgical resection of rectal carcinoma (71). In fact, multivariate analysis indicates that tumor involvement of the radial margin is the most critical factor in this regard. Adam et al. calculated a hazard ratio for local recurrence of 12.23 (95% confidence interval [CI], 4.32–34.6) for patients with margin involvement, compared to 3.31 (95% CI, 1.15–4.56) for those with positive lymph nodes (72). Radial margins tend to be neglected in pathology reports, particularly for nonrectal cancers. The surgeon can help ensure proper reporting by being aware of radial margins and marking areas of concern.

Evaluation of surgical margins is mandatory after local excision of rectal carcinoma. Large sessile adenomas and early carcinomas of the rectum are often treated by transanal endoscopic microsurgery, which allows full-thickness excision of lesion and rectal wall, followed by repair of the defect. The specimen should be pinned before fixation to minimize tissue contraction and surgical margins marked with ink. After fixation, all tissue should be submitted for microscopic examination. In addition to careful evaluation of surgical margins, the pathology report should describe gross tumor configuration, tumor grade, depth of invasion, and the presence or absence of angiolymphatic invasion (73).

Surgical margins are also a critical part of evaluating colorectal adenoma with invasive adenocarcinoma. The pathologist can help guide therapy by evaluating the histologic parameters that have been shown to predict outcome in endoscopic polypectomy specimens. If the base of the polyp can be identified, it should be inked. (If ink is not used, some thermal artifact is usually present at the polypectomy margin to help with microscopic evaluation.) The polyp should be serially sectioned perpendicularly to the polypectomy margin and submitted in its entirety for microscopic examination. The histologic features of importance are tumor grade, the status of resection margin, and the presence or absence of angiolymphatic invasion. If the invasive tumor is poorly differentiated *or* extends to within 1 mm of the polypectomy margin *or* shows angiolymphatic invasion, then surgical resection of the colon is indicated (74). These rules apply to pedunculated polyps that can be ad-

equately removed endoscopically; invasion in a sessile polyp is an indication for surgical resection.

HISTOLOGIC GRADE

Histologic grade predicts prognosis. Behind that simple statement is confusion and controversy, some of it ongoing. Still being debated are these questions: Should grade be based on tubule pattern, nuclear morphology, or a combination of both? Should grade be based on the dominant pattern or on the worst area? Should the tubule pattern at the invasive edge of tumor be ignored, noted, or paid particular attention? How many grades should be used—two, three, or four?

The absence of uniform criteria explains in part the staggering degree of observer variation reported in some studies. Blenkinsopp et al. (75) reviewed histopathology reports on 2,046 patients from 22 different institutions. The overall breakdown of grades (26% well differentiated, 58% moderately differentiated, and 16% poorly differentiated) paralleled the 20/60/20 split reported in the classic paper of Dukes and Bussey (76), but the proportion placed in each grade by different observers varied from 3% to 93% for good differentiation, 8% to 82% for moderate differentiation, and 5% to 30% for poor differentiation.

The literature on the importance of histologic grade has been mixed, with some studies finding it prognostically significant in multivariate analysis (25,77,78), others finding significance in univariate analysis (79,80), and others finding no significance at all (17). Perhaps the most consistent finding is that poor differentiation is an adverse prognostic indicator (60,81,82). This observation (together with the lure of improved interobserver consistency) forms the basis for the CAP recommendation that a two-tiered grading system be used (18).

Although nuclear morphology has been used in some grading systems (83), grading based on tubule pattern is emerging as the method of choice. Nests and cords of cells with poorly formed gland spaces or solid islands and sheets of cells without any gland formation constitute the poorly differentiated end of the tubule spectrum (Fig. 41.8).

The question of whether grade should be based on the dominant pattern or the worst area is still unresolved. The CAP consensus statement favors using the overall impression so if <50% of the tumor forms tubules, it is classified as high grade. Studies continue to appear, however, that find usefulness in scoring the worst area (82,84).

Histologic Growth Pattern

The advancing edge of tumor can be characterized as pushing or infiltrative, depending on whether the tumor–stroma interface is well demarcated or irregular. This feature is rarely described in pathology reports, even though several studies have associated infiltrative growth with adverse outcome (25,79,85,86). An infiltrative growth pattern can be suspected grossly when the border of the tumor is difficult to define. Microscopically, infiltrating growth features dissection of host tissue by small glands or irregular clusters. Approximately 30% of colorectal cancers demonstrate infiltrative growth, but there is interobserver variation, which may partly explain its underutilization.

Tumor Budding

Another way to characterize invasiveness at the tumor margin is termed "tumor budding." Tumor buds—isolated single cells or small groups of cells at the advancing edge of

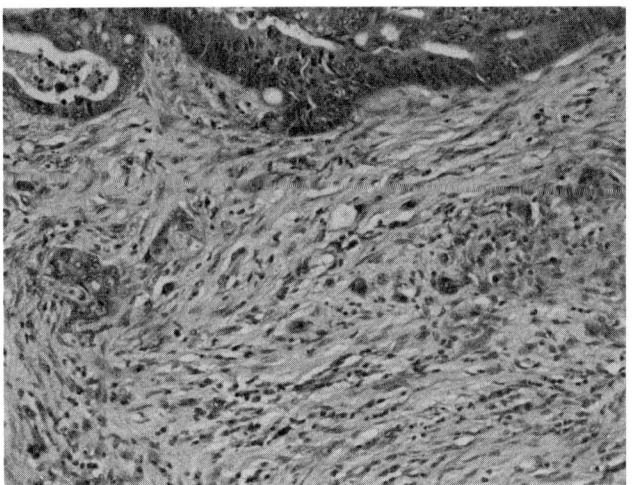

FIGURE 41.9. Tumor budding. Single cells and small groups of cells spread in advance of the tumor edge.

tumor—have been identified as predictors of aggressive behavior (87,88) (Fig. 41.9) A recent review of 638 rectal cancers found high-grade budding (10 or more foci in a microscopic field of ×250) in 30% of patients; the 5-year survival in that group was 41%, compared to 84% in those with low-grade budding (p <0.0001) (89). The authors found tumor budding to be a highly reproducible parameter (kappa coefficient 0.84), and multivariate analysis showed tumor budding was a significant independent variable (89).

Blood Vessel and Lymphatic Invasion

Blood vessel and lymphatic invasion are discussed together because elastic stains are needed to definitively separate small veins from lymphatics, and special stains are not recommended for routine practice (18). Small vessels containing tumor can be designated in the pathology report as angiolymphatic vessels.

Angiolymphatic invasion correlates with risk for hematogenous spread (90) and is an adverse prognostic factor (3-year survival was 30% for patients with invasive cancers vs. 62% for those with noninvasive cancers in one study) (91). Invasion of extramural veins is a particularly strong adverse prognosticator (92,93).

Perineural Invasion

The presence or absence of perineural invasion should be noted and reported in all cases of colorectal cancer. The prevalence of perineural invasion increases with tumor grade and stage. Spratt and Spjut reported lower survival in patients with perineural invasion (94), a finding reproduced by others (92). Perineural invasion in rectal cancer has been implicated as an independent prognostic variable in multivariate analysis (95).

Desmoplastic Stromal Response

Desmoplasia is a characteristic response to many invasive tumors, and some degree of desmoplasia is associated with nearly all colorectal carcinomas. Activated fibroblasts produce collagenous matrix, while tumor cells produce matrix-degrading enzymes, resulting in a continuous process of remodeling. It has been proposed that a dense collagenous stroma might act as a barrier to tumor spread, although stroma formation seems to be a promoter or at a least marker of invasiveness in other gastrointestinal tumors (96,97). At least one study has found improved survival in colorectal cancer when desmoplasia was scored as present rather than absent (60% vs. 35% 5-year survival) (98). This finding accords with the work of Ueno et al., who found better survival in patients whose rectal cancers were associated with fine or broad bands of collagen, as opposed to myxoid stroma (99).

HOST IMMUNE RESPONSE

Interest in host immune response to tumor dates at least to Spratt and Spjut, who found lower survival for patients whose tumors lacked an inflammatory response at the periphery (94). Interest has intensified recently with the recognition that cancers with MSI prompt an exaggerated host lymphoid response.

Host immune response can be separated into three categories. The first is peritumoral lymphocyte response, recognized as a dense band or cap of lymphocytes at the edge of tumor islands (Fig. 41.10A). This pattern has been identified as a favorable sign in multiple studies (100–103).

More recently, Graham and Appelman noted an association between prognosis and the presence of lymphoid aggregates at the tumor periphery (104) (Fig. 41.10B). They designated the nodular lymphoid response as "Crohnlike lymphoid reaction." Ten-year survival was 9% for patients harboring cancers without a Crohnlike reaction versus 39% for those with a pronounced reaction. The finding was validated by Harrison et al., who identified Crohnlike reaction as an independent predictor of favorable prognosis by multivariate analysis in a study of 344 right-sided colon cancers (105).

The third pattern of host lymphoid response is intimate mixing of tumor cells and lymphocytes. The lymphocytes in this setting are referred to as tumor-infiltrating lymphocytes (TILs) (Fig. 41.10C). TILs are indicative of favorable prognosis in malignant melanoma (106), and a similar benefit appears to accrue in colorectal cancer (107). TILs are strongly associated with MSI; in fact, when present in large numbers (more than four per high-power microscopic field), TILs are almost 100% specific for MSI (47). The CAP consensus statement recommends reporting TILs separately from other forms of host lymphoid response, scored as positive (more than four TILs per high-power field) or negative (18).

MICROSATELLITE INSTABILITY-HIGH CARCINOMA

Ten to 15% of all colorectal cancers show the phenotype of MSI-H (108–110). This phenotype reflects defective DNA-mismatch repair, which can result from either a germline mutation or somatic inactivation of a mismatch repair gene. Patients carrying a germline mutation have the syndrome hereditary nonpolyposis colorectal carcinoma (HNPCC). The genes implicated thus far in the inherited condition are MLH1 (responsible for 45%–50% of HNPCC), MSH2 (35%–40%), MSH6 (10%), and PMS2 (rare) (111). Somatic derangement of mismatch repair function results from inactivation of the hMLH1 promotor site by hypermethylation, a phenomenon more common in females and in the elderly population (112).

MSI-H colorectal cancer has a characteristic clinicopathological profile. The tumors typically arise proximal to the splenic flexure. Mucinous, signet ring cell, and medullary histology are all more common in this setting, and morphologic evidence of host lymphoid response to tumor is often present (43,45,113). Despite their rather aggressive-looking histology,

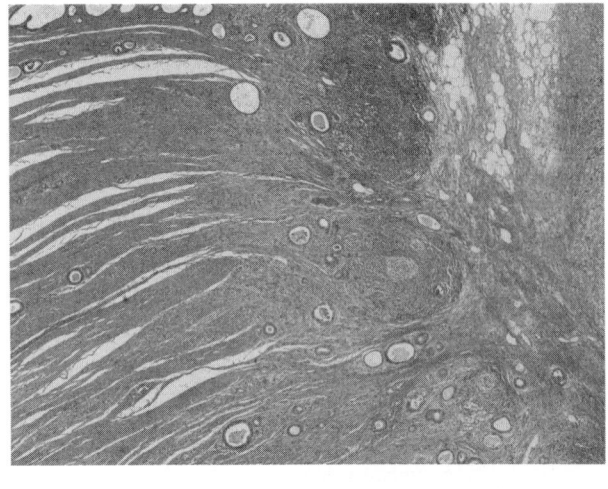

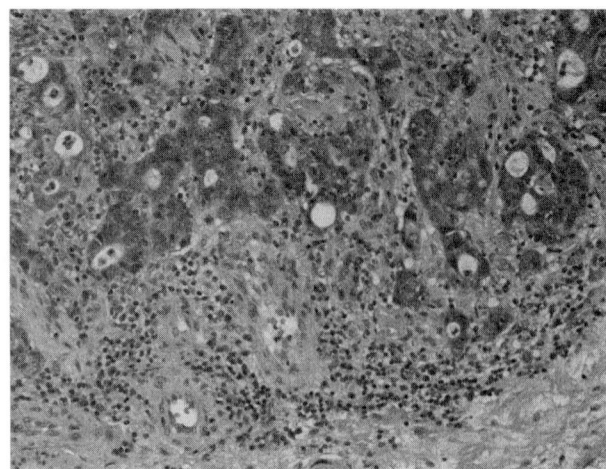

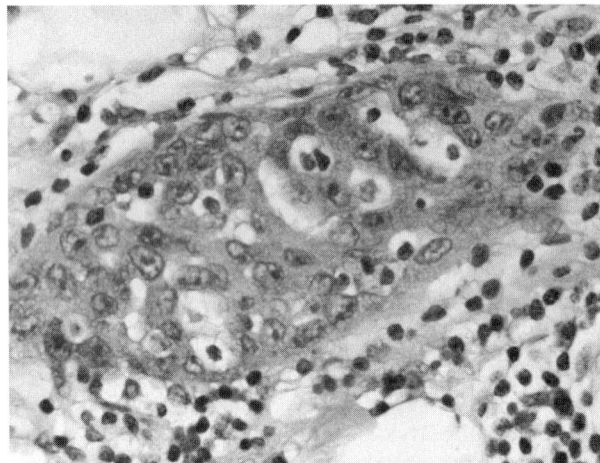

FIGURE 41.10. Host lymphoid response to tumor, in the form of peritumoral lymphocytes (**A**), lymphoid aggregates (Crohnlike reaction) (**B**), and tumor-infiltrating lymphocytes (**C**).

MSI-H cancers have a better prognosis than other cancers of like stage (114–121). Furthermore, there is some evidence that MSI-H responds to chemotherapy differently than microsatellite stable carcinoma, and that adjuvant therapy based on 5-fluorouracil may not be advisable for this subset of colorectal carcinoma (121,122).

Thus, there are three reasons why it might be of interest to recognize a given colorectal carcinoma as MSI-H: to help identify the syndrome of HNPCC, to predict prognosis, and to guide therapy. The gold standard is MSI testing. It can be performed on paraffin-embedded tissue, but it requires microdissection to enrich for both tumor and normal cell populations, followed by amplification of a panel of DNA markers. This test is offered by many clinical labs, but it is labor intensive and costly ($500–$1,000).

There are commercially available antibodies directed against the protein product of MLH1, MSH2, MSH6, and PMS2. They work very well in paraffin-embedded tissue. Loss of protein expression is the abnormal result (Fig. 41.4). Interpretation of immunohistochemistry is aided by the invariable presence of normal cells (lymphocytes, stromal cells, benign mucosa) to serve as an internal control. There is essentially complete correlation between loss of protein expression and the MSI-H phenotype; that is, loss of protein expression is 100% specific for MSI. (It should be noted here that heterodimeric relationships in the mismatch repair process mean that loss of MLH1 function is invariably accompanied by loss of PMS2, and loss of MSH2 is accompanied by loss of MSH6 [123]. Thus, there are four possible "positive" results: [a] immunonegative results for MLH1 and PMS2, implicating MLH1

as the defective or inoperative gene; [b] loss of MSH2 and MSH6, implicating MSH2; [c] loss of MSH6 alone, implicating MSH6; and [d] loss of PMS2 alone, implicating PMS2.) The question of sensitivity is more complicated; in the sporadic setting, loss of MLH1 expression is 100% sensitive for MSI-H because the phenotype results from inactivation of MLH1 by hypermethylation at the promotor. In approximately 3% of HNPCC-related cancers, MSI testing will show MSI-H, but all immunohistochemical studies will show intact protein expression (124). This could reflect involvement of additional mismatch repair genes or, more likely, the fact that some mutations of MLH1 or MSH2 produce detectable protein despite being biologically nonfunctioning (125).

Immunohistochemistry can be used as a complement to or a surrogate for MSI testing, depending on the clinical situation. If one desires to know the MSI status of a colon cancer from an elderly patient without a family history suggestive of HNPCC, a single immunohistochemical study (MLH1) is sufficient to answer the question. A more common clinical situation is colon cancer in a patient whose age and/or family history raises concern for HNPCC. Here, immunohistochemical studies can serve as a valuable first-line screen (126,127), with testing for MSI necessary only in those instances in which protein expression is intact and clinical suspicion remains high. Note that neither microsatellite analysis nor immunohistochemical studies are directly assessing the patient's germline. One advantage of immunohistochemistry, however, is that loss of expression does allow one to focus genetic testing on a specific gene. Furthermore, because sporadic hypermethylation affects only MLH1, loss of expression involving MSH2, MSH6, or PMS2 strongly suggests a germline mutation. Loss of MLH1 expression is not informative regarding germline status; some authors recommend methylation analysis of the MLH1 promoter as a second-line test in this setting, with absence of methylation predictive of a germline mutation (128).

References

1. Bird RP. Observation and qualification of aberrant crypts in the murine colon treated with a colon carcinogen: preliminary findings. *Cancer Lett* 1987;37:147–151.
2. Takayama T, Katsuki S, Takahashi Y, et al. Aberrant crypt foci of the colon as precursors of adenoma and cancer. *N Engl J Med* 1998;339:1277–1284.
3. Takayama T, Miyanishi K, Hayashi T, et al. Aberrant crypt foci: detection, gene abnormalities, and clinical usefulness. *Clin Gastroenterol Hepatol* 2005;3:542–545.
4. Muto T, Bussey HJR, Morson BC. The evolution of cancer of the colon and rectum. *Cancer* 1975;36:2251–2258.
5. Longacre TA, Fenoglio-Preiser CF. Mixed hyperplastic adenomatous polyps/serrated adenomas: a distinct form of colorectal neoplasia. *Am J Surg Pathol* 1990;14:524–537.
6. Snover DC, Jass JR, Fenoglio-Preiser C, Batts KP. Serrated polyps of the large intestine: a morphologic and molecular review of an evolving concept. *Am J Clin Pathol* 2005;124:380–391.
7. Torlakovic E, Snover DC. Serrated adenomatous polyposis in humans. *Gastroenterology* 1996;110:748–755.
8. Cohen AM, Wood WC, Gunderson LL, et al. Pathological studies in rectal cancer. *Cancer* 1980;45:2965–2968.
9. Sontag SJ, Durczak C, Aranha GV, et al. Fecal occult blood screening for colorectal cancer in a Veterans Administration hospital. *Am J Surg* 1983;145:89–94.
10. Grinnell RS. The grading and prognosis of carcinoma of the colon and rectum. *Ann Surg* 1939;109:500–503.
11. Steinberg SM, Barkin JS, Kaplan RS, et al. Prognostic indicators of colon tumors: the Gastrointestinal Tumor Group experience. *Cancer* 1986;57:1866–1870.
12. George SMC, Makinen MJ, Jernvall P, Makela J, Vihko P, Karttunen TJ. Classification of advanced colorectal carcinomas by tumor edge morphology. *Cancer* 2000;89:1901–1909.
13. Whittaker M, Goligher JC. The prognosis after surgical treatment for carcinoma of the rectum. *Br J Surg* 1976;63:384–388.
14. Griffin MR, Bergstralh EJ, Coffey RJ, et al. Predictors of survival after curative resection of carcinoma of the colon and rectum. *Cancer* 1987;60:2318–2324.
15. Wolmark N, Wieand HS, Rockette HE, et al. The prognostic significance of tumor location and bowel obstruction in Dukes B and C colorectal cancer: findings from the NSABP clinical trials. *Ann Surg* 1983;198:743–752.
16. Chapuis PH, Dent OF, Fisher R, et al. A multivariate analysis of clinical and pathological variables in prognosis after resection of large bowel cancer. *Br J Surg* 1985;72:698–702.
17. Crucitti F, Sofo L, Doglietto GB, et al. Prognostic factors in colorectal cancer: current status and new trends. *J Surg Oncol Suppl* 1991;2:76–82.
18. Compton CC, Fielding LP, Burgart LJ, et al. Prognostic factors in colorectal cancer. College of American Pathologists consensus statement 1999. *Arch Pathol Lab Med* 2000;124:979–994.
19. Nasir A, Boulware D, Kaiser HE, et al. Flat and polypoid adenocarcinomas of the colorectum: a comparative histomorphologic analysis of 47 cases. *Hum Pathol* 2004;35:604–611.
20. Hamilton SR, Aaltonen LA. *Tumours of the Digestive System. Pathology and Genetics. World Health Organization Classification of Tumours.* Lyons, France: IARC Press; 2000.
21. Werling RW, Yaziji H, Bacchi CE, Gown AM. CDX2, a highly sensitive and specific marker of adenocarcinomas of intestinal origin: an immunohistochemical survey of 476 primary and metastatic carcinomas. *Am J Surg Pathol* 2003;27:303–310.
22. Zhang PJ, Shah M, Spiegel GW, Brooks JJ. Cytokeratin 7 immunoreactivity in rectal adenocarcinomas. *Appl Immunohistochem Mol Morphol* 2003;11:306–310.
23. Cohen AM, Tremiterra S, Candela F, et al. Prognosis of node-positive colon cancer. *Cancer* 1991;67:1859–1861.
24. Green J, Timmcke A, Mitchell W, et al. Mucinous carcinoma–just another colon cancer? *Dis Colon Rectum* 1993;36:49–54.
25. Roncucci L, Fante R, Losi L, et al. Survival for colon and rectal cancer in a population-based cancer registry. *Eur J Cancer* 1996;32:295–302.
26. Harrison JC, Dean PJ, El-Zeky F, et al. From Dukes through Jass: pathological prognostic indicators in rectal cancer. *Hum Pathol* 1994;25:498–505.
27. Secco G, Fardelli R, Campora E, et al. Primary mucinous adenocarcinomas and signet-ring carcinomas of colon and rectum. *Oncology* 1994;51:30–34.
28. Heys SD, Scherif A, Bagley JS, et al. Prognostic factors in survival of patients aged less than forty-five years with colorectal cancer. *Br J Surg* 1994;81:685–688.
29. Kakar S, Aksoy S, Burgart LJ, Smyrk TC. Mucinous carcinoma of the colon: correlation of loss of mismatch repair enzymes with clinicopathologic features and survival. *Mod Pathol* 2004;17:696–700.
30. Ogino S, Brahmandam M, Cantor M, et al. Distinct molecular features of colorectal carcinoma with signet ring cell component and colorectal carcinoma with mucinous component. *Mod Pathol* 2006;19:59–68.
31. Almagro UA. Primary signet-ring carcinoma of the colon. *Cancer* 1983;52:1453–1457.
32. Lui IO, Kung IM, Lee IM, et al. Primary colorectal signet-ring carcinoma in young patients. *Pathology* 1985;17:31–35.
33. Giacchero A, Aste H, Baracchini P, et al. Primary signet-ring carcinoma of the large bowel. *Cancer* 1985;56:2723–2726.
34. Kakar S, Smyrk TC. Signet ring cell carcinoma of the colorectum: correlations between microsatellite instability: clinicopathologic features and survival. *Mod Pathol* 2005;18:244–249.
35. Ojeda VJ, Mitchell KM, Walters MN, et al. Primary colorectal linitis plastica type of carcinoma. *Pathology* 1982;14:181–189.
36. Williams GT, Blackshaw AJ, Morson BC. Squamous carcinoma of the colorectum and its genesis. *J Pathol* 1979;129:139–147.
37. Juturi JV, Francis B, Koontz PW, et al. Squamous-cell carcinoma of the colon responsive to combination chemotherapy: report of two cases and review of the literature. *Dis Colon Rectum* 1999;42:102–109.
38. Cerezo L, Alvarez M, Edwards O, et al. Adenosquamous carcinoma of the colon. *Dis Colon Rectum* 1985;28:597–603.
39. Wick MR. Neuroendocrine neoplasia: current concepts [editorial]. *Am J Clin Pathol* 2000;113:331–335.
40. Burke AB, Shekita KM, Sobin LH. Small cell carcinomas of the large intestine. *Am J Clin Pathol* 1991;95:315–321.
41. Mills SE, Allen MS, Jr., Cohen AR. Small-cell undifferentiated carcinoma of the colon: a clinicopathological study of five cases and their association with colonic adenomas. *Am J Surg Pathol* 1983;7:643–651.
42. Ruschoff J, Dietmaier W, Luttger J, et al. Poorly differentiated colonic adenocarcinoma, medullary type: clinical, phenotypic and molecular characteristics. *Am J Pathol* 1997;150:1815–1825.
43. Lanza G, Fafa R, Matteuzzi M, et al. Medullary-type poorly differentiated adenocarcinoma of the large bowel: a distinct clinicopathologic entity characterized by microsatellite instability and improved survival. *J Clin Oncol* 1999;17:2429–2438.
44. Smyrk TC, Watson P, Kaul K, Lynch HT. Tumor-infiltrating lymphocytes are a marker for microsatellite instability in colorectal carcinoma. *Cancer* 2001;91:2417–2422.
45. Wick MR, Vitsky JL, Ritter JH, Swanson PE, Mills SE. Sporadic medullary carcinoma of the colon: a clinicopathologic comparison with nonhereditary poorly differentiated enteric type adenocarcinoma and neuroendocrine colorectal carcinoma. *Am J Clin Pathol* 2005;123:56–65.
46. Jass J, Smyrk TC, Stewart SM, et al. Pathology of hereditary nonpolyposis colon cancer. *Anticancer Res* 1994;14:1631–1634.
47. Jass JR, Do K-A, Simms LA, et al. Morphology of sporadic colorectal cancer with DNA replication errors. *Gut* 1998;42:673–679.
48. Lockhart-Mummery JP. Two hundred cases of cancer of the rectum treated by perineal excision. *Br J Surg* 1927;14:110–124.
49. Dukes CE. The classification of cancer of the rectum. *J Pathol* 1932;35:323–332.
50. Simpson WC, Mayo CW. The mural penetration of the carcinoma cell in the colon: anatomic and clinical study. *Surg Gynecol Obstet* 1939;68:872–877.
51. Astler VB, Coller FA. The prognostic significance of direct extension of carcinoma of the colon and rectum. *Ann Surg* 1954;139:846–851.
52. Turnbull RB, Jr., Kyle K, Watson FR, et al. Cancer of the colon: the influence of the no-touch isolation technique on survival rates. *Ann Surg* 1967;166:420–427.
53. Kyriakos M. The president's cancer, the Dukes classification, and confusion. *Arch Pathol Lab Med* 1985;109:1063–1066.
54. Hutter RVP, Sobin LH. A universal staging system for cancer of the colon and rectum: let there be light. *Arch Pathol Lab Med* 1986;110:367–368.
55. Greene FL, Page DL, Fleming ID, et al., eds. *AJCC Cancer Staging Manual.* 6th ed. New York, NY: Springer; 2002.
56. Wittekind C, Greene FL, Henson DE, eds. *TMN Supplement: A Commentary on Uniform Use.* 3rd ed. New York, NY: Wiley-Liss; 2003.
57. Goldstein NS, Turner JR. Pericolonic tumor deposits in patients with T3N+M0 colon adenocarcinomas: markers of reduced disease free survival and intra-abdominal metastases and their implications for TNM classification. *Cancer* 2000;88:2228–2238.
58. Gabriel WB, Dukes C, Bussey HJR. Lymphatic spread in cancer of the rectum. *Br J Surg* 1935;23:395–413.
59. Shepherd NA, Baxter KJ, Love SB. The prognostic importance of peritoneal involvement in colon cancer: a prospective evaluation. *Gastroenterology* 1997;112:1096–1102.
60. Newland RC, Dent OF, Lyttle MN, et al. Pathologic determinants of survival associated with colorectal cancer with lymph node metastases: a multivariate analysis of 579 patients. *Cancer* 1994;73:2076–2082.
61. Ratto C, Sofo L, Ippoliti M, et al. Accurate lymph-node detection in colorectal specimens resected for cancer is of prognostic significance. *Dis Colon Rectum* 1999;42:143–158.
62. Goldstein NS. Lymph node recoveries from 2427 pT3 colorectal resection specimens spanning 45 years: recommendations for a minimum number of

recovered lymph nodes based on predictive probabilities. *Am J Surg Pathol* 2002;26:179–189.

63. Tepper JE, O'Connell MJ, Niedzwiecki D, et al. Impact of number of nodes retrieved on outcome in patients with rectal cancer. *J Clin Oncol* 2001;19:157–163.

64. Swanson RS, Compton CC, Stewart AK, Bland KI. The prognosis of T3N0 colon cancer is dependent upon the number of lymph nodes examined. *Ann Surg Oncol* 2003;10:65–71.

65. Malassagne B, Valeur P, Serra J, et al. Relationship of apical lymph node involvement to survival in resected colon carcinoma. *Dis Colon Rectum* 1993;36:645–653.

66. Wilkinson EJ, Hause L. Probability in lymph node sectioning. *Cancer* 1974;33:1269–1274.

67. Cutait R, Alves VA, Lopes LC, et al. Restaging of colorectal cancer based on the identification of lymph node micrometastases through immunoperoxidase staining of CEA and cytokeratins. *Dis Colon Rectum* 1991;34:917–920.

68. Sanchez-Cespedes M, Esteller M, Hibi K, et al. Molecular detection of neoplastic cells in lymph nodes of metastatic colorectal cancer patients predicts recurrence. *Clin Cancer Res* 1999;5:2450–2454.

69. Greenson JK, Isenhart CE, Rice R, et al. Identification of occult micrometastases in pericolic lymph nodes of Dukes' B colorectal cancer patients using monoclonal antibodies against cytokeratin and CC49: correlation with long-term survival. *Cancer* 1994;73:563–569.

70. Williams NS, Dixon MF, Johnston D. Reappraisal of the 5 centimetre rule of distal excision for carcinoma of the rectum: a study of distal intramural spread and of patient's survival. *Br J Surg* 1983;70:150–154.

71. Quirke P, Durdy P, Dixon MF, et al. Local recurrence of rectal adenocarcinoma due to inadequate surgical resection. *Lancet* 1986;2:996–999.

72. Adam IJ, Mohamdee MO, Martin IG, et al. Role of the circumferential margin involvement in the local recurrence of rectal cancer. *Lancet* 1994;344:707–711.

73. Tanaka S, Yokota T, Saito D, et al. Clinicopathologic features of early rectal carcinoma and indications for endoscopic treatment. *Dis Colon Rectum* 1995;38:959–963.

74. Haggitt RC, Glotzbach RE, Soffer EE, et al. Prognostic factors in colorectal carcinomas arising in adenomas: implications for lesions removed by endoscopic polypectomy. *Gastroenterology* 1985;89:328–336.

75. Blenkinsopp WK, Stewart-Brown S, Blesovsky L, et al. Histopathology reporting in large bowel cancer. *J Clin Pathol* 1981;34:509–513.

76. Dukes CE, Bussey HJR. The spread of rectal cancer and its effect on prognosis. *Br J Cancer* 1958;12:309–312.

77. Wiggers T, Arends JW, Volovics A. Regression analysis of prognostic factors in colorectal cancer after curative resections. *Dis Colon Rectum* 1988;31:33–41.

78. Jessup JM, McGinnis LS, Steele GD, Jr., et al. The National Cancer Data Base report on colon cancer. *Cancer* 1996;78:918–926.

79. Jass JR, Atkin WS, Cuzick J, et al. The grading of rectal cancer: historical perspectives in a multivariate analysis of 447 cases. *Histopathology* 1986;10:437–439.

80. Ropponen K, Eskelinen M, Kosma VM, et al. Comparison of classic and quantitative prognostic factors in colorectal cancer. *Anticancer Res* 1996;16:3875–3882.

81. Fisher ER, Sass R, Palekar A, et al. Dukes' classification revisited: findings from the National Surgical Adjuvant Breast and Bowel Projects (protocol R-01). *Cancer* 1989;64:2354–2360.

82. Purdie CA, Piris J. Histopathological grade, mucinous differentiation and DNA ploidy in relation to prognosis in colorectal carcinoma. *Histopathology* 2000;36:121–126.

83. Association of Directors of Anatomic and Surgical Pathology. Recommendations for the reporting of resected large intestinal carcinomas. *Am J Clin Pathol* 1996;106:12–15.

84. Goldstein NS, Hart J. Histologic features associated with lymph node metastasis in stage T1 and superficial T2 rectal adenocarcinomas in abdominoperineal resection specimens: identifying a subset of patients for whom treatment with adjuvant therapy or completion abdominoperineal resection should be considered after local excision. *Am J Clin Pathol* 1999;111:51–58.

85. Jass JR, Love SB, Northover JMA. A new prognostic classification of rectal cancer. *Lancet* 1987;1:1303–1306.

86. Shepherd NA, Saraga EP, Love SB, et al. Prognostic factors in colonic cancer. *Histopathology* 1989;14:613–620.

87. Morodomi T, Isomoto H, Shirouzu K, Kakegawa K, Irie K, Morimatsu M. An index for estimating the probability of lymph node metastasis in rectal cancers. *Cancer* 1989;63:539–543.

88. Hase K, Shatney C, Johnson D, Trollope M, Vierra M. Prognostic value of tumor budding in patients with colorectal cancer. *Dis Colon Rectum* 1993;36:627–635.

89. Ueno H, Murphy J, Jass JR, Mochizuki H, Talbot IC. Tumour budding as an index to estimate the potential of aggressiveness in rectal cancer. *Histopathology* 2002;40:127–132.

90. Inoue T, Mori M, Shimono R, et al. Vascular invasion of colorectal carcinoma readily visible with certain stains. *Dis Colon Rectum* 1992;35:34–39.

91. Krasna MJ, Flanobaum L, Cody RP, et al. Vascular and neural invasion in colorectal cancer. *Cancer* 1988;61:1018–1023.

92. Talbot IC, Ritchie S, Leighton MH, et al. The clinical significance of invasion of veins by rectal cancer. *Br J Surg* 1980;67:439–442.

93. Minsky BD, Mies C, Recht A, et al. Resectable adenocarcinoma of the rectosigmoid and rectum: II. The influence of blood vessel invasion. *Cancer* 1988;61:1417–1424.

94. Spratt JS, Jr., Spjut HJ. Prevalence and prognosis of individual clinical and pathologic variables associated with colorectal carcinoma. *Cancer* 1967;20:1976–1985.

95. Knudsen JB, Nilsson T, Sprechler M, et al. Venous and nerve invasion as prognostic factors in postoperative survival of patients with resectable cancer of the rectum. *Dis Colon Rectum* 1983;26:613–617.

96. Iacobuzio-Donahue CA, Ryu B, Hruban RH, et al. Exploring the host desmoplastic response to pancreatic carcinoma: gene expression of stromal and neoplastic cells at the site of primary invasion. *Am J Pathol* 2002;160:91–99.

97. Koliopanos A, Friess H, di Mola FF, et al. Connective tissue growth factor gene expression alters tumor progression in esophageal cancer. *World J Surg* 2002;26:420–427.

98. Caporale A, Vestri AR, Benvenuto E, et al. Is desmoplasia a protective factor for survival in patients with colorectal carcinoma? *Clin Gastroenterol Hepatol* 2005;3:370–375.

99. Ueno H, Jones A, Jass JR, Talbot IC. Clinicopathological significance of the 'keloid-like' collagen and myxoid stroma in advanced rectal cancer. *Histopathology* 2002;40(4):327–334.

100. Murray D, Hreno A, Dutton J, et al. Prognosis in colon cancer: a pathologic reassessment. *Arch Surg* 1975;110:908–913.

101. Pihl E, Malahy MA, Khankhanian N, et al. Immunomorphological features of prognostic significance in Dukes' class B colorectal carcinoma. *Cancer Res* 1977;37:4145–4149.

102. Jass JR, Morson BC. Reporting colorectal cancer. *J Clin Pathol* 1987;40:1016–1023.

103. Halvorsen TB, Seim E. Association between invasiveness, inflammatory reaction, desmoplasia and survival in colorectal cancer. *J Clin Pathol* 1989;42:162–166.

104. Graham DM, Appelman HD. Crohn's-like lymphoid reaction and colorectal carcinoma: a potential histologic prognosticator. *Mod Pathol* 1990;3:332–335.

105. Harrison JC, Dean PJ, el-Zeky F, et al. Impact of the Crohn's-like lymphoid reaction on staging of right-sided colon cancer: results of multivariate analysis. *Hum Pathol* 1995;26:31–38.

106. Clemente CG, Mihm MC, Bufalino R, et al. Prognostic value of tumor infiltrating lymphocytes in the vertical growth phase of primary cutaneous melanoma. *Cancer* 1996;77:1303–1310.

107. Naito Y, Saito K, Shiiba K, et al. CD8 + T cells infiltrated within cancer cell nests as a prognostic factor in human colorectal cancer. *Cancer Res* 1998;58:3491–3494.

108. Ionov Y, Peinado MA, Malkhosyan S, et al. Ubiquitous somatic mutations in simple repeated sequences reveal a new mechanism for colonic carcinogenesis. *Nature* 1993;363:558–561.

109. Salovaara R, Loukola A, Kristo P, et al. Population-based molecular detection of hereditary nonpolyposis colorectal cancer. *J Clin Oncol* 2000;18:2193–2200.

110. Slattery ML, Curtin K, Anderson K, et al. Associations between cigarette smoking, lifestyle factors and microsatellite instability in colon tumors. *J Natl Cancer Inst* 2000;92:1831–1836.

111. Peltomaki P. Deficient DNA mismatch repair: a common etiologic factor for colon cancer. *Hum Mol Genet* 2001;10:735–740.

112. Kaker S, Burgart LJ, Thibodeau SN, et al. Frequency of loss of hMLH1 expression in colorectal carcinoma increases with advancing age. *Cancer* 2003;97:1421–1427.

113. Kim H, Jen J, Vogelstein B, et al. Clinical and pathological characteristics of sporadic colon carcinomas with DNA replication errors in microsatellite sequences. *Am J Pathol* 1994;145:148–156.

114. Jernvall P, Makinen MJ, Karttunen TJ, et al. Microsatellite instability: impact on cancer progression in proximal and distal colorectal cancers. *Eur J Cancer* 1999;35:197–201.

115. Senba S, Konishi F, Okamoto T, et al. Clinicopathologic and genetic features of nonfamilial colorectal carcinomas with DNA replication errors. *Cancer* 1998;82:279–285.

116. Salahshor S, Kressner U, Fischer H, et al. Microsatellite instability in sporadic colorectal cancer is not an independent prognostic factor. *Br J Cancer* 1999;81:190–193.

117. Liang JT, Chang KJ, Chen JC, et al. Clinicopathologic and carcinogenetic appraisal for DNA replication errors in sporadic T3N0M0 stage colorectal cancer after curative resection. *Hepatogastroenterology* 1999;46:883–890.

118. Cawkwell L, Gray S, Murgatroyd H, et al. Choice of management strategy for colorectal cancer based on a diagnostic immunohistochemical test for defective mismatch repair. *Gut* 1999;45:409–415.

119. Gryfe R, Kim H, Hsieh ETK, et al. Tumor microsatellite instability and clinical outcome in young patients with colorectal cancer. *N Engl J Med* 2000;342:69–77.

120. Elsaleh H, Joseph D, Grieu F, et al. Association of tumour site and sex with survival benefit from adjuvant chemotherapy in colorectal cancer. *Lancet* 2000;355:1745–1750.

121. Ribic CM, Sargent DJ, Moore MJ, et al. Tumor microsatellite instability status as a predictor of benefit from fluorouracil-based adjuvant chemotherapy for colon cancer. *N Engl J Med* 2003;349:247–257.

122. Carethers JM, Chauhan DP, Fink D, et al. Mismatch repair proficiency and in vitro response to 5-fluorouracil. *Gastroenterology* 1999;117:123–131.

123. Gruber SB. New developments in Lynch syndrome (hereditary nonpolyposis colorectal cancer) and mismatch repair gene testing. *Gastroenterology* 2006;130:577–587.

124. Gill S, Lindor N, Burgart LJ, et al. Isolated loss of PMS2 expression in colorectal cancers: frequency, patient age and familial aggregation. *Clin Cancer Res* 2005;11:6466–6471.

125. Wahlberg S, Schmeits J, Thomas G, et al. Evaluation of microsatellite instability and immunohistochemistry for the prediction of germ-line MSH2 and MLH1 mutations in hereditary nonpolyposis colon cancer families. *Cancer Res* 2002;62:3485–3492.

126. Jover R, Paya A, Alenda C, et al. Defective mismatch-repair colorectal cancer: clinicopathologic characteristics and usefulness of immunohistochemical analysis for diagnosis. *Am J Clin Pathol* 2004;122:389–394.

127. Chai SM, Zeps N, Shearwood AM, et al. Screening for defective DNA mismatch repair in stage II and III colorectal cancer patients. *Clin Gastroenterol Hepatol* 2004;2:1017–1025.

128. Bouzourene H, Taminelli L, Chauber P, et al. A cost-effective algorithm for hereditary nonpolyposis colorectal cancer detection. *Am J Clin Pathol* 2006;125:823–831.

CHAPTER 42 ■ COLORECTAL CANCER: ANATOMY AND STAGING

IAN D. CHIN AND BOGDAN C. PAUN

To treat colon and rectal cancer, some basic essential knowledge is necessary. Detailed anatomy, embryology, and histology enable surgeons and oncologists to treat patients effectively and research new therapies. The use of modern technologies allows clinicians to accurately stage patients with colorectal cancers and to focus appropriate therapies to increase survival and reduce recurrence. Staging systems help researchers communicate effectively to compare various experimental studies to provide summary analyses.

EMBRYOLOGY, ANATOMY, AND HISTOLOGY OF THE COLON AND RECTUM

Knowledge of anatomy of the colon and rectum is vitally important not only for consideration of surgical technique but also for the understanding of the patterns of spread and behavior of cancer. We therefore include in this chapter a brief overview of the colon and rectal anatomy, and the reader is well advised to search more comprehensive sources for additional information (1–3). Short sections on embryology and histology are also included.

Embryology

By the third week of development, the primitive gut is formed from the endoderm of the yolk sac. It can be divided into the foregut, midgut, and hindgut. After the fourth week, the midgut expands faster than the abdominal cavity. The midgut is pushed into the umbilical cord as a herniated segment that extends from about the distal third of the duodenum to the proximal one-third of the transverse colon (4). This whole segment is supplied by the superior mesenteric artery, which initially forms a 90-degree axis of counterclockwise rotation. During the 10th week of development, the midgut returns to the abdomen, proximal loop first, with a further 180 degrees of counterclockwise rotation. The proximal loop passes below the mesentery of the distal loop (transverse colon). The cecum starts developing as a local enlargement in the loop posterior to the superior mesenteric artery during the period of gut herniation. The distal colon (i.e., distal one-third of transverse colon, descending colon, sigmoid colon, and rectum) is derived from the hindgut and, therefore, receives its blood supply from the inferior mesenteric artery.

The proximal anal canal, together with the rectum, is formed by the hindgut and is of endodermal origin. The distal anal canal is formed from an ingrowth of the anal pit, which is of ectodermal origin. For anatomists, the dentate line is the border between the anus and the rectum. For surgeons, the top of the muscular anal canal (anorectal ring) separates the anus from the rectum (1).

Anatomy of the Large Intestine

The large intestine extends from the terminal ileum to the dentate line in the anal canal with a length that is variable and is reported to be between 1.3 and 1.8 m (1). The diameter, which can vary with distension, gradually decreases from 7.5 cm in the cecum to 2.5 cm in the sigmoid, to expand again in the rectal vault. The colon has both inner circular and outer longitudinal muscle fibers, but some of the longitudinal fibers coalesce in three bands called the *teniae coli* separated by 120 degrees along the circumference. The *teniae* are not only thicker, but they are shorter than the intervening colonic wall. This gives rise to sacculations called *haustrae* separated by invaginations of the colonic wall called *plicae semilunares*. The *plicae* go partway along the colonic circumference and give it its characteristic radiologic appearance. The colon also has small fat appendages on the serosal side called *appendices epiploicae*.

The large bowel may be divided into several sections: cecum, ascending colon, transverse colon, descending colon, sigmoid colon, and rectum. The cecum has the largest diameter and thinnest wall. It may be quite free and completely covered with peritoneum to migrate into the pelvis, or it may be fixed to the posterior abdominal wall or iliac fossa. The appendix is a long diverticulum originating on the posterior-medial aspect of the cecum at the confluence of the three *teniae*. At the junction of the cecum and the ascending colon, the ileocecal valve is a protrusion of ileum in the medial aspect of the large bowel with a circular muscle layer that gives it a papillary appearance. The ascending colon is usually retroperitoneal (covered with peritoneum on its anterior and lateral surface but devoid of it posteriorly) and extends to the hepatic flexure. The hepatic flexure lies between the right lobe of the liver and the gallbladder anteriorly and the right kidney and duodenum posteriorly. The transverse colon extends from the hepatic flexure to the splenic flexure, at which points it is relatively fixed. It is invested with peritoneum and may hang in a V shape to below the umbilicus. It is adherent on its anterior surface with the greater omentum. The descending colon starts at the high splenic flexure and courses as a retroperitoneal structure to the pelvic brim. The sigmoid colon is a free intraperitoneal section of large bowel of variable length attached by its mesentery to the left pelvic wall and continues as the rectum where *teniae coli* coalesce.

The location of the rectosigmoid junction is controversial but is probably not as important for cancer management as the distance of the cancer from the anal canal. The proximal third of the rectum is entirely covered by peritoneum, with more fat interposing itself between the rectum and peritoneum as the rectum goes down in the pelvis. The middle third of the rectum is covered by peritoneum anteriorly. The lowermost portion of the rectum is entirely extraperitoneal. The rectum does not have a mesentery per se, but the term "mesorectum" has gained widespread use as the name for the fat surrounding the rectum containing vessels and lymphatics. It is thicker posteriorly and surrounded by a layer of endopelvic fascia. Anteriorly, the mesorectum has a fascia propria that is separate from the Denonvillier fascia covering the posterior surface of the prostate, seminal vesicles and neck of the bladder; this plane between the fascia propria and Denonvillier fascia is the anatomic dissection plane of mesorectal excision (5). Posteriorly, the mesorectum is again covered by a fascia propria that is in close apposition, but separate from, the presacral fascia (6). Laterally, the mesorectal fascia is associated with the pelvic sidewall. Older textbooks suggest that there are lateral ligaments containing the middle rectal vessels. Total mesorectal excision shows that these ligaments are really loose connective tissue, and the middle rectal vessels are usually small and close to the pelvic floor (7). In fact, the mesorectum is circumferentially enclosed in a sheath of fascia propria. When dissection is carried along this layer, the veins and nerves in the pelvis may be preserved (8).

Vascular Supply and Lymphatics

The superior mesenteric artery supplies constant blood flow to the cecum and ascending colon through the ileocolic artery. The right colic artery is variable and even absent in 30% of people

(9). The transverse colon is supplied through branches of the middle colic artery (Fig. 42.1). The first branch of the inferior mesenteric artery, the left colic artery, supplies the descending colon and may form several anastomosing arches at the splenic flexure with branches of the superior mesenteric artery that are often grouped under the name of arc of Riolan. The inferior mesenteric artery also gives rise to the sigmoid artery (or arteries) that supplies the sigmoid colon and to the superior rectal artery that supplies proximal rectum (10). The rectum is also supplied by the middle rectal arteries that are small and inconstant (11), and by the inferior rectal arteries that are branches of the pudendal artery. The arteries supplying the colon form vascular arcades that anastomose and give rise to a continuous marginal artery (of Drummond). The venous drainage follows the general pattern of the arteries, such that on the right (cecum, ascending, and transverse colons) the veins join to form the superior mesenteric vein that drains in the portal vein. On the left (descending and sigmoid colons and upper rectum), the veins join to form the inferior mesenteric vein that drains into either the superior mesenteric vein or the splenic vein. The lower rectum drains into the internal iliac veins.

Lymph nodes are classified as epicolic (subserosal), paracolic (close to the marginal artery), intermediate (along the main arteries), and principal (root of mesentery and aortic). They usually course along with the arteries and do not form additional communications. For a good oncologic resection, it is important to include all lymphatics that may be involved by cancer, so the principle is to remove an entire section of large bowel supplied by a large, named artery with its mesentery (9).

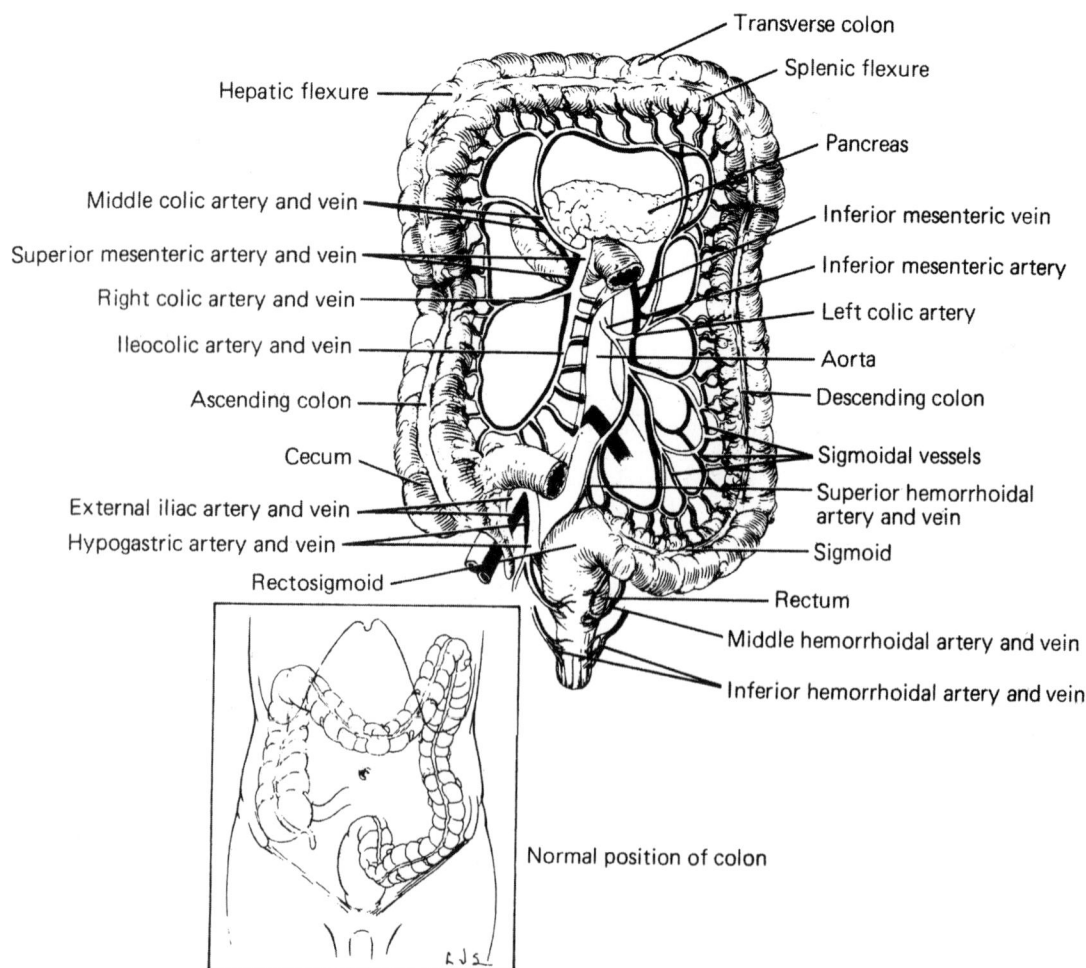

FIGURE 42.1. The vascular supply of the large bowel. The transverse colon is reflected upward. Inset shows normal position of colon within abdominal cavity. *Source:* From ref. 13.

The lymphatic drainage of the anorectal region is more complicated because of its triple vascular supply (12). The superior rectal lymph nodes first drain most of the proximal rectum to an intermediate group at the bifurcation of the superior rectal artery and then to periaortic lymph nodes. The middle rectal nodes drain to the internal iliac chains, and some inferior nodes drain through the levator ani muscle to the internal pudendal nodes. The anal canal below the dentate line is drained exclusively to the inguinal lymph nodes, while the anal canal above has dual drainage to both the inguinal lymph nodes and the internal iliac nodes.

Histology

The large bowel has the same layers as the rest of the gut: serosa, muscularis propria, submucosa, and mucosa (14). The visceral peritoneum functions as the serosa of the large bowel and is present only on the sections that are not retroperitoneal. There is some loose connective tissue and fat between the outer serosa and the inner muscularis propria, which has an outer longitudinal muscle layer (forming the *teniae*) and an inner circular muscle layer. The submucosa is another layer of loose connective tissue containing veins, lymphatics, and small arteries. The mucosa has an inner muscularis mucosa that has a thin layer of inner circular and outer longitudinal muscle fibers, and an epithelial lining consisting of simple columnar epithelium with interspersed goblet cells. Unlike the small bowel, the large bowel does not have villi, but has an endothelium, composed of columnar cells, that is flat with crypts.

STAGING OF COLON AND RECTAL CANCERS

Currently, colorectal cancer (CRC) is staged primarily by pathological assessment of the resected specimen (15). Staging the cancer provides information as to the likely behavior of the cancer and will, therefore, guide further management. Staging also provides a common language in cancer research and is essential to the advancement of knowledge in oncology. Numerous predictors have been found for CRC, including local behavior of the tumor, surgical adequacy, and molecular characteristics of the tumor, but these have not been incorporated into the mainstream staging systems or used as standard guides for therapeutic intervention. Several imaging modalities are used to estimate the pathological stage of CRC preoperatively, which include computed tomography (CT), magnetic resonance imaging (MRI), and endorectal ultrasound (ERUS). The development of several neoadjuvant therapies, especially for rectal cancer, has provided a great impetus to improving and introducing these imaging modalities into widespread use (16). The introduction of novel imaging techniques, such as positron emission tomography (PET), or novel predictors of outcome, such as molecular markers, may revolutionize colon cancer care and improve outcome.

Pathological Staging

The first staging system, based on depth of penetration, was reported in 1926 by Lockhart-Mummery. He followed 200 consecutive patients with rectal cancer and reported survival data for three classes (A, B, or C) (17). At the Mayo Clinic, Rankin and Broders believed that the local spread of rectal cancer was less important as an outcome measure in nonmetastatic disease than the microscopic behavior of the cancer cells and proposed a staging system based on the grade (1—4) of tumor (18). In 1932, Cuthbert Dukes, at St. Mark's Hospital in London,

suggested an improvement on the Lockhart-Mummery staging system (19) and defined rectal cancers as Dukes A if confined to the rectal wall, Dukes B if spread by direct extension to extrarectal tissue, and Dukes C if the regional lymph nodes were involved. He reported a 3-year survival of 80%, 73%, and 97% for the Dukes A, B, and C stages, respectively. Dukes also looked at the grades of cancers according to Broders' method and indeed found a correlation between higher grades and decreased survival. The majority of his patients were in the intermediate-grade 2 category, and there was a relationship between his stages and the grades of the cancers; therefore, Dukes concluded that grading alone would be a less useful method of staging. Later, the group at Mayo accepted the principle of the Dukes system but insisted that the grade of tumor be added for prognostic accuracy and be used as well (20).

Several modifications of the Dukes staging followed, including that of Dukes himself in 1935 that came after more detailed study of the lymphatic spread of the cancer (21). They reported on 100 cases, 62 of which were C cases, and included 24 beautiful drawings of the lymphatic spread in abdominoperineal specimens. It was found that the cancers spread to the lymph nodes in an orderly and predictable manner first to the perirectal nodes and then to the nodes higher up on the superior rectal artery, without downward or lateral spread, unless all lymph channels were blocked. They suggested that cases with involved lymph nodes close to the bowel wall should be designated C1, and those with nodes higher up on the rectal artery be C2. In 1949, Kirklin, Dockerty, and Waugh (22) modified the Dukes staging as follows:

A   Cancer limited to mucosa
B1 Cancer into, but not through, muscularis propria
B2 Cancer through muscularis propria
C   Any depth with lymph node involvement and showed penetration of the peritoneal reflection did not impact outcome

Astler and Coller took it one step further and proposed another modification to the Dukes staging, which is still in widespread use today, by further subdividing the C stage into C1—limited to bowel wall with positive nodes and C2—through muscularis propria with positive nodes (23). Furthermore, they applied this system to both colon and rectal carcinomas and showed a gradually decreasing 5-year survival from 100% to 22% for stage A to C2, respectively.

A clinicopathological system of staging (A—tumor confined to bowel wall, B—tumor extension to pericolic fat, C—lymph node involvement, and D—cancers with liver, lung, bone, or peritoneal metastases, or cancers that were not resectable because of parietal or adjacent organ involvement) was suggested in 1967 in a paper advocating the *no-touch isolation* technique of colon cancer resection (24). This was validated and compared to the old Dukes and Astler-Coller modification to show that it more closely correlated with survival (25).

Tumor, Node, Metastasis Staging

The numerous ABC staging systems and their modifications became confusing and were slowly replaced with the tumor, node, metastasis (TNM) staging system. It is quite complex and is constantly being updated, which makes for both its greatest strength and its greatest disadvantage. The initial TNM system was established in the 1940s by Dr. Pierre Denoix and then developed under the auspices of the Union Internacional Contra la Cancrum (26). The American Joint Committee on Cancer (AJCC) was established in 1959 and started publishing separate definitions for the TNM classes. The two systems were unified in 1987, and the latest iteration of classifications was published in 2002 (15).

TABLE 42.1

TUMOR, NODE, METASTASIS CLASSIFICATION FOR ADENOCARCINOMA OF THE COLON OR RECTUM

	Description
PRIMARY TUMOR (T)	
Tx	Primary tumor cannot be assessed
T0	No evidence of primary tumor
Tis	Carcinoma in situ: intraepithelial or invasion of lamina propria
T1	Tumor invades submucosa
T2	Tumor invades muscularis propria
T3	Tumor invades through the muscularis propria into the subserosa, or into nonperitonealized pericolic or perirectal tissues
T4	Tumor invades directly into other organs or structures, and/or perforates visceral peritoneum
LYMPH NODES (N)	
Nx	Regional lymph nodes cannot be assessed
N0	No regional lymph node metastasis
N1	Metastasis in 1–3 regional lymph nodes
N2	Metastasis in ≥4 regional lymph nodes
DISTANT METASTASIS (M)	
Mx	Distant metastasis cannot be assessed
M0	No distant metastasis
M1	Distant metastasis

Stage grouping					
Stage	**T**	**N**	**M**	**Dukes**	**MAC**[a]
0	Tis	N0	M0	—	—
I	T1	N0	M0	A	A
	T2	N0	M0	A	B1
IIA	T3	N0	M0	B	B2
IIB	T4	N0	M0	B	B3
IIIA	T1–T2	N1	M0	C	C1
IIIB	T3–T4	N1	M0	C	C2/C3
IIIC	Any T	N2	M0	C	C1/C2/C3
IV	Any T	Any N	M1	—	D

[a]MAC, modified Astler-Coller classification.
Adapted from ref. 15.

The TNM system may be used for both clinical and pathological staging, although the latter may be designated by the prefix *p*. It classifies tumor according to the variables of tumor invasion, lymph node involvement, and distal metastasis, but although it mentions other variables such as grade, resection margin, lymphovascular invasion, and molecular markers, it does not include them in the staging system (Table 42.1).

Surgical Resection Margins

The completeness of surgical extirpation of colon and rectal cancer is of utmost importance in effecting a cure. This is assessed by examining the margins of the resected specimen; the resection is classified as Ro if it is clear, R1 if there is microscopic evidence of tumor cells at the margin, and R2 if there is gross evidence of tumor at the margin. The proximal resection margin of colon and rectal cancers is never really of concern during surgical excision. Distally, the margin is also generous for colon cancers but becomes of great concern when dealing with rectal cancers because sphincter preservation is an important goal.

Initially, abdominal perineal resection (APR) was widely practiced. As surgical techniques improved, more sphincter-saving procedures were used, and the caveat of a 5-cm distal resection margin was employed (27). Research and technical advancements made possible low anastomoses and allowed sphincter-saving resections of rectal cancers very close to the anus with <5-cm margins. This renewed interest in the area and the original observations of Dukes (21) that rectal cancers rarely spread distally were confirmed (28) by showing advanced cancers that block the proximal lymphatics will allow distal lymphatic spread. This was confirmed by examining resected APR specimens and measuring the distal histologic spread of cancer cells. The cancer-specific survival did not seem to be adversely affected by distal margins of 2 cm (29) or even 1 cm (30). However, decreased survival and increased recurrence rates were found when the distal margin was <0.8 cm. Patients with advanced rectal cancers that had undergone preoperative chemoradiation also did not seem to benefit from a distal margin >1 cm (31). These findings were confirmed in a group of 270 patients in whom a margin of <1 cm was not an adverse prognostic factor (32). Some groups can get even closer to the anal canal by removing the internal sphincter en bloc with the tumor (33,34). However, opinion is not uniform, and some studies suggest longer mural distal margin and longer distal mesorectal margin (3 [35] or 4 [36] cm).

Historically, only the proximal and distal margins of cancers were reported. Faced with variable and high rates of local recurrence, several studies started reporting on the circumferential margin (37–39). A positive circumferential margin is defined as tumor within 1 mm of the cut surface, and it was found to predict much higher rates of local recurrence and poorer survival rates. Not all cases of local recurrence occurred in patients with positive circumferential margin, and reports of discontinuous tumor spread in the mesorectum seemed to be the explanation (40). Based on this observation, Heald and Ryall introduced the concept of total mesorectal excision (TME) for rectal cancer (the entire mesorectum is removed within its fascial envelope) and showed the extremely low local recurrence rate of 3.7% at 5 years using this technique (41). Using TME, all lymphatic-bearing tissue around the rectum is removed, and only the most advanced cancers involve the circumferential margin. Therefore, a positive margin is a predictor of poor overall outcome rather than local recurrence (42). Involvement of the radial margin continues to be a poor predictor of outcome in patients that receive postoperative radiation (43) or preoperative chemoradiation (44).

Lymph Node Metastases

Presence of lymph node metastases in CRC is an important predictor of outcome as recognized by the TNM classification. There is an inverse relationship between the number of involved lymph nodes and the 5-year survival. The best single dichotomization is obtained by dividing patients into three or less and four or more lymph nodes (45). Furthermore, lymph node metastases in the pathological specimen are the main determinants of the need for postoperative chemotherapy. The number of lymph nodes that are retrieved from the specimen is highly variable, depending on the surgical technique and on the method of handling the specimen. This affects the sensitivity of detection of metastases. By using careful pathological dissection, more lymph nodes may be retrieved, upstaging the tumor, allowing the benefit of chemotherapy, and improving outcome (46). Traditional dissection in the gross lab, usually done with a pair of scissors by sight and palpation, is the easiest, inexpensive, and most commonly employed method. Some groups have good results with this method (47), although in usual clinical practice the results are less than ideal (48). More elaborate lymph node retrieval techniques, such as fat clearance, are expensive and time consuming, but invariably obtain more lymph nodes and may upstage the tumor (49). Most laboratories cannot routinely employ these techniques. A minimum number of examined lymph nodes retrieved to accurately stage the tumor needs to be employed; the latest edition of the *AJCC Cancer Staging Manual* recommends that 7 to 14 nodes need to be recovered, which is a change from the 12-node requirement of the previous edition.

Two new techniques have been developed to improve the lymph node metastasis detection rate: ultrastaging and sentinel lymph node (SLN) mapping. Usually, lymph nodes are embedded after being retrieved and several sections are assessed on hematoxylin and eosin (H&E) staining. Using more specialized staining techniques (ultrastaging), small nests of cancer cells (micrometastases) that would not otherwise be detected on standard H&E staining can be seen. The significance of these micrometastases is difficult to determine because the literature in this area is still immature. Several studies have examined negative H&E-stained lymph nodes using an ultrastaging method to subclassify cancers into separate groups with different survival rates. Immunohistochemical staining for carcinoembryonic antigen (CEA) (50) and anticytokeratin (51) failed to show a difference. However, using a CEA-specific nested reverse-transcriptase polymerase chain reaction (RT-PCR) resulted in a 40% 5-year survival difference (52). Another study, using immunohistochemical staining for CEA and CK20, also showed a 5-year survival difference (53).

Another technique used to reduce the sampling error for lymph nodes is SLN mapping, which is based on the experience of melanoma and breast cancer (54). This technique commonly uses isosulfan blue dye injected around the tumor in vivo to detect the first lymph nodes draining the tumor bed within 10 to 15 minutes. Because these nodes are few and most likely to harbor cancer cells, they can be serially sectioned (every 20–40 μm) and studied with H&E, immunohistochemical staining, or RT-PCR technique, which would improve diagnostic accuracy. SLN mapping has been shown to be feasible, without greatly adding to operating time or adding to morbidity (55), but the technique suffers from an unclear definition for positive nodes (on H&E staining or ultrastaging) and from a false-negative rate of 4% to 5% (56) (on ultrastaging). Some of the results of SLN mapping are good, with 32% of colon and 17% of rectal cancers being upstaged (57). It is unclear at this point whether decisions about adjuvant chemotherapy may be made based on ultrastaging, SLN mapping, or a combination of the two.

Other Prognostic Factors

As mentioned previously, the tumor grade can be used as an indicator of future metastases and survival (18,58). Although there may be a problem with interobserver variability, the terms "low grade" and "high grade" may be used instead of the four classes of Broders to reduce reporting variability. The grading of rectal cancer may be used to judge the adequacy of local excision (i.e., high-grade cancer needing further surgery) (59,60) because it predicts probability of lymph node metastasis.

Invasion of nerves and lymphatic or blood vessels has been associated with a poor prognosis. Neural invasion seems to be associated with increased local recurrence (61,62) and decreased survival (63). It is often difficult to differentiate between lymphatic and venous channels because invasion in both cases appears as cancer cells within endothelial-lined spaces. So, they are described together as lymphovascular invasion (64). Lymphovascular invasion is associated with increased local recurrence (59,62), lymph node metastases (65) and distant recurrence (61), and decreased survival (63,66). Presence of lymphovascular invasion decreases the survival of node-negative disease to almost the survival of node-positive disease in rectal cancer.

Molecular Markers

Numerous tumor markers have been studied extensively in an effort to improve our prognostic ability and better target therapy. Although many are promising, none have really entered into common clinical practice or have yet been proven effective as part of an adjuvant therapy trial. Nevertheless, it is important to have some general knowledge of the advances made.

p53 is a tumor-suppressor gene on chromosome 17 that undergoes mutation commonly in CRC (~50%). Loss of the function of *p53* interferes with DNA repair and apoptosis, leading to cell proliferation and genomic instability. The mutated gene has a longer half-life and can be detected by immunohistochemistry. Nuclear overexpression of *p53* actually indicates mutation in the gene. Some studies have shown that *p53* overexpression leads to decreased survival (67–70), whereas others have not shown such an effect (71,72). *p53* overexpression may be associated with tumor sensitivity to radiation (73), although not consistently (74), and may be used as an indication for chemotherapy for stage II CRC (75). *K-ras* is an oncogene that encodes for a small protein believed to be involved in transduction of extracellular mitogenic signals. Mutations in this gene are found less commonly (~25%–30%) in CRCs than *p53* mutations. Detection of *K-ras* mutation may improve the prognostic accuracy of detection of *p53* mutations (69,76). Vascular endothelial growth factor (VEGF) is associated with angiogenesis, and its presence in stage II CRC is associated with increased recurrence (77). Indeed, a monoclonal antibody against VEGF, bevacizumab, has now been shown to be effective in metastatic colon cancer (78). Thymidylate synthase (TS) is an enzyme that catalyzes the methylation of dUMP to dTMP and is a critical target for 5-fluorouracil. CRCs that overexpress this enzyme tend to be resistant to 5-fluorouracil–based chemotherapy (79). Patients with stage III CRC that have increased polymorphism of the TS gene have worse survival (80). Similarly, patients with lymph node metastases that have high levels of TS expression also have a worse survival when receiving chemotherapy (81). Multiple other molecular markers have been associated with decreased survival in CRC, including cyclooxygenase-2 (82) and cyclin A (83).

Microsatellite instability (MSI) represents multiple errors in repetitive DNA sequences (microsatellites) that indicate a defect in the DNA-mismatch repair system and a genomic instability. MSI is present in most cases of cancers associated with the Lynch syndrome and can be used to screen for this syndrome (84). MSI is only present in about 15% of sporadic CRCs (85). In fact, MSI represents only one of the pathways of CRC; the other being chromosomal instability, characterized by allelic losses, amplifications, and translocations. Presence of MSI in CRCs is associated with improved survival and decreased tendency to metastasize (86,87). Low MSI cancers show decreased survival relative to the microsatellite stable, stage III CRCs (88). In contrast, it seems that colon cancers that have low MSI or microsatellite stability benefit from fluorouracil-based chemotherapy, whereas the MSI cancers receive no further benefit in terms of survival (89,90).

A brief overview of the literature on molecular markers for CRC is included to get an impression of what is available. Although, individually, none of these markers have yet proven to be effective, there is a real possibility that in the near future a combination of these factors could be used in combination with the classic pathological staging to better prognosticate and guide chemotherapy regimens in CRC.

Preoperative Staging

Historically, CRC was treated primarily with surgery, and the information obtained from pathology was used to guide further treatment. That is still a valid approach, especially for colon cancer. However there are an increasing number of situations in which preoperative information about CRC is useful and can potentially alter therapy. In rectal cancer, preoperative short course radiation has been shown to decrease local recurrence, especially in advanced lesions (91). Preoperative chemoradiation has been shown to induce downstaging that may improve local control and survival (92). Also, for advanced lesions (T3/4) preoperative chemoradiation may improve the rate of sphincter-saving procedures and improve local control with reduced toxicity (93). Because of these new studies that have radically changed practice, it is crucial to have a good idea of the stage of rectal cancer to best plan the appropriate therapy. Once neoadjuvant therapy is used, then pathologic staging becomes highly unreliable, and accurate preoperative staging may be the only prognostic information available. The argument for preoperative staging of colon cancer is not as convincing as that for rectal cancer, but there are situations in which the presence of metastatic or locally advanced disease may alter therapy. If

there is extensive metastatic disease with short life expectancy and/or comorbid diseases, then alternative procedures may be better than an extensive resection. The recent introduction of laparoscopic resection of CRC is contraindicated in cases with locally advanced disease (94), which makes it important to know the local stage preoperatively.

Colorectal Cancer

As is often the case in medicine, a complete history is crucial because it will offer clues about the disease process itself and will afford important details about the general health of the patient that will affect the choice of treatment. The symptom of pain in CRC is uncommon and usually represents advanced local disease with invasion of surrounding structures, nerve invasion, or nerve impingement. Pain of the anterior abdominal wall, buttock, or leg represent invasion of the abdominal wall, obturator nerves, or sciatic nerves, respectively. Obstructive symptoms, such as distension, vomiting, pain, and/or obstipation, may indicate complete or impending obstruction, whereas symptoms of sepsis or recurrent urinary tract infection may represent perforation or fistula formation.

Physical examination, although not as useful as the history, will provide some information as to the general health of the patient and the stage of the CRC. A palpable abdominal mass is a rare finding in CRC and usually represents a large, bulky tumor. This, however, is not a reliable predictor of stage. Evidence of metastatic disease may be found if the liver is found to be enlarged and/or nodular, or if there is evidence of lymphadenopathy. The importance of digital rectal examination (DRE) in rectal cancer cannot be overemphasized and is an important part of the physical exam.

Complete endoscopic examination of the colon is a necessary preoperative workup of CRC because it provides important information about the primary lesion, tissue confirmation, and also assesses for synchronous lesions. Synchronous lesions (lesions found in the large bowel within 12 months of finding the CRC) may be found in 33% of patients if one counts all colorectal neoplasms and in 6% of patients if one considers only CRC (95). Although these numbers vary according to the population under study, the information obtained at endoscopy has the potential of altering the surgical plan in as many as 11% of patients (96). Laboratory tests are routinely ordered, but their use is limited. Hematologic and biochemistry studies are performed more for general medical assessment than for staging purposes, and liver enzyme/function tests are of little use. High serum CEA levels have been correlated with poor prognosis in node-negative cancers (97), and rising CEA levels are associated with short survival in patients with recurrent CRC (98). Although controversial, some studies have shown that intensive follow-up after resection of CRC using a regimen including CEA levels leads to earlier detection of recurrence, higher rate of curative re-resection, and higher survival rates (99). Other factors, such as elevated lactate dehydrogenase level or white blood count, have been associated with poorer prognosis (100). A search for metastatic disease is performed preoperatively. The liver, as the most common site of CRC metastasis, and the lungs are the sites routinely investigated. Other sites, such as brain or bone, are not automatically investigated unless symptoms warrant. Ultrasound (US) of the abdomen is a cheap, noninvasive way for detecting liver metastases, but it is operator dependent, limited by the patient's body habitus, limited to imaging the liver, and may lack specificity (101). Computed tomography (CT) scanning is an effective method of detecting liver metastases and may actually provide information with respect to local extension; it has a sensitivity of 51% to 73% and a specificity of 94% to 99% for detecting liver metastases (102,103). These numbers are probably better with the newer CT scanners that are now available and with the use of contrast agents. The greatest advantages of CT are that it is relatively cheap, fast, and widely available, and that it provides a wealth of information other than just presence of liver metastases. Preoperative use of CT scanning in CRC provides useful additional information in 37% of cases, changes management in 19% of cases (104), and is a cost-effective strategy (105). CT is likely to miss microscopic invasion of the serosa, normal-size nodes replaced by tumor, small peritoneal implants, and small liver metastases (106).

Whole-body MRI may be more sensitive than CT at detecting hepatic metastases (103), but it is less sensitive than CT at detecting peritoneal deposits, is more expensive, and has limited availability. If hepatic lesions are present on routine CT, then US may be used to determine if they are solid or cystic, whereas MRI and hepatic-directed CT may help in sorting hemangiomas from metastatic disease. Nevertheless, preoperative methods of detecting metastatic disease, like dedicated liver CT, are not completely reliable in accurately predicting the burden of disease: only 65% of patients with solitary liver metastasis seen on CT have an accurate diagnosis, most of the rest having more extensive disease at intraoperative assessment with intraoperative ultrasound (107).

Lung metastases are less common than liver metastases (~10% of CRC patients) and are limited to the lung in only about 2% to 4% of patients (108). Patients with isolated lung metastases from CRC have a better prognosis than corresponding patients with liver involvement (100), and about half of them are amenable to metastasectomy. There is scant evidence as to the best screening method to apply in looking for lung CRC metastasis, but it seems reasonable to use chest plain radiography routinely and CT scan only to better define lesions found on chest radiography (109). Chest x-rays may be used postoperatively to look for evidence of distant recurrence as part of an intense surveillance program, but that does not seem to benefit the patients at all (110).

Colon Cancer

The preoperative staging of colon cancer does not require more interventions than have been discussed. For patients slated to undergo laparoscopic resection or for those with possible adjacent organ involvement on routine CT, it may be necessary to obtain better local staging for preoperative planning. The development of miniprobe ultrasonography that can be used through the colonoscope channel has allowed endoscopists to more accurately predict depth of cancer invasion. Preliminary studies show an accuracy of 87% to 94% for wall infiltration and 82% to 84% for lymph node involvement (111–113), but this technique has limited availability and great cost. It remains to be seen whether it will find a niche in the laparoscopic management of CRC or if endoscopic resection of the cancer is contemplated.

Rectal Cancer

Rectal cancer management and staging is a specialized area within CRC treatment. Multiple specific modalities are available. Although rectal cancers are inconveniently located from a surgical point of view, they are well placed to allow access to various probes, the most available and earliest of which is the finger. DRE is easy and cheap, can be done on all cancers within approximately 10 cm of the anal verge, and can offer a wealth of information. It can reveal the location (distance from anal verge, position on the circumference of the bowel), size, and relationship to the anal sphincters of the rectal cancer. It can also give a rough idea of the depth of tumor invasion: Freely mobile tumors are likely T1/T2 and tethered lesions are T3, whereas fixed lesions likely invade adjacent structures. Mason outlined this method of staging rectal cancers in two elegantly written articles (114,115), and it is still useful today, although

it has a steep learning curve and is not overly reliable at best. DRE has an accuracy of 68% for predicting depth of tumor penetration (116), cannot determine lymph node involvement, and seems to be more accurate for tumors >2 cm (117).

All rectal cancers should have rigid proctoscopic examination to accurately measure distance from anal verge. The proctoscopic examination, together with the information from the DRE, is used to determine whether a sphincter-preserving procedure is possible rather than an abdominal perineal resection.

ERUS has emerged as the best modality of preoperative assessment for rectal cancers. It can accurately detect depth of cancer invasion and can also detect lymph node metastases. It is considerably more accurate than DRE (116,117). ERUS has several drawbacks, including being highly operator dependent and having limited availability, but despite this it is the mainstay of rectal cancer management. MRI with endorectal coil and multislice CT also have a role in staging rectal cancers.

ENDORECTAL ULTRASOUND

ERUS may be done using a standard US machine to which a specialized probe is adapted. The endorectal probe has a transducer that sends and receives US waves. The transducer is covered by a water-filled balloon that is inserted into the rectum through a proctoscope. Insertion of the probe into the rectum allows close contact with the structures to be visualized, resulting in much greater resolution. The layers of the rectal wall have different acoustic impedance and can be clearly identified as concentric circles. The frequency range of ERUS is usually between 5 to 10 MHz. The focal length may be changed, by varying the frequency, to visualize structures at different depths. Some probes detect through an arc of 120 degrees, whereas some others see through the entire 360 degrees, which is preferable. The image is displayed in two dimensions, but newer machines have three-dimensional reconstruction capabilities (118).

ERUS identifies the anatomical layers of the rectal wall that are represented by a series of five alternating hyperechoic (white) and hypoechoic (black) concentric rings (Fig. 42.2). These five distinct ultrasonic layers, beginning from the luminal aspect, correspond to the balloon interface with the mucosa, the mucosa and muscularis mucosa, the submucosa (or interface between the mucosa and the muscularis), the muscularis propria, and the interface between the muscularis propria and perirectal fat. Rectal carcinomas appear as hypoechoic

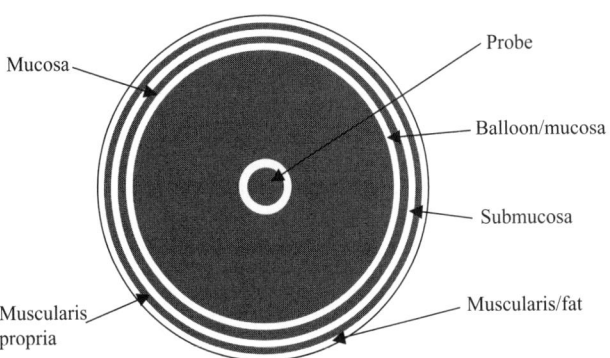

FIGURE 42.2. Diagram of a normal endorectal ultrasound image. Diagram is not to scale because the layers of the bowel wall are often thinner and in closer apposition in reality. White lines represent zones of transition between respective adjacent layers from which ultrasound energy is reflected rather than actual structures. Surrounding perirectal fat is not represented, but it usually shows as heterogeneous signal intensity.

TABLE 42.2

SYSTEM OF CLASSIFYING RECTAL TUMORS FOR ENDORECTAL ULTRASOUND

Designation	Depth of involvement
*u*T0	Benign lesions confined to mucosa
*u*T1	Invasive tumors confined to mucosa and submucosa
*u*T2	Lesions penetrate muscularis propria but are confined to rectal wall
*u*T3	Tumors penetrate the entire thickness of rectal wall and invade perirectal fat
*u*T4	Lesions penetrate an adjacent organ or pelvic side wall
*u*N0	Undetectable or benign-appearing lymph nodes
*u*N1	Malignant-appearing lymph nodes

masses with tumor extension causing disruption of subsequent layers.

Hildebrandt and Feifel introduced a system of classification of tumors for US that is based on the TNM system and is now in wide use (1). The prefix *u* denotes US staging, as opposed to the prefix *p* that denotes pathological staging (Table 42.2).

*u*T0 lesions are noninvasive and confined to the rectal mucosa with villous adenomas being the best examples. Sonographically, the mucosal layer (first black line) is expanded, but the submucosal layer (middle white line) remains intact. Due to sampling error, endoscopic biopsies of villous tumors may miss foci of malignancy. However, ERUS can detect a malignant focus within a villous adenoma by demonstrating invasion (disruption) of the submucosal layer, although initial reports showed poor sensitivity (120). More recently, a meta-analysis of reports of biopsy-proven rectal adenomas examined using ERUS, showed that almost one-fourth of them are actually cancers and that ERUS was able to establish the correct preoperative diagnosis in 81% of such lesions (121). However, ERUS incorrectly upstaged benign lesions in 12% of cases, probably leading to more extensive extirpative surgery. False positives are more likely for lesions that have already had snare polypectomy (because the residual scar obliterates tissue planes) and when the adenoma is close to the anal canal. It is recommended, therefore, that ERUS be done before any polypectomy and that higher frequency probes be used. In patients that have an unexpected diagnosis of adenocarcinoma on pathology of a snared polyp, ERUS only has an accuracy of 50% of detecting residual tumor (122), illustrating again the difficulty of doing US post polypectomy.

*u*T1 lesions are early invasive cancers that have not yet penetrated into the muscularis propria. These are characterized by thickening of the mucosal black band and an irregularity of the submucosa (middle white line) on ERUS. Stippling or thickening of the submucosal line may be seen, but there is no definite disruption, which indicates involvement of the muscularis propria (*u*T2). Local transanal excision of T1 lesions is an acceptable treatment because there is a low risk of lymph node metastasis if other favorable criteria are present (well-differentiated or moderately differentiated tumor, no lymphovascular invasion). The risk of lymph node metastasis for T1 lesions with favorable prognostic factors is as low as 7% (123), which, considering the morbidity and mortality of radical surgery, makes local excision entirely appropriate. Lymph node metastases occur in 15% to 20% of T2 tumors, which

warrants more extensive resection in all but the most debilitated patients or patients who refuse colostomy. It is important, therefore, for ERUS to accurately identify T1 lesions and differentiate them from T2 lesions. ERUS has an easier time to differentiate between T1/T2 lesions rather than T2/T3 lesions with a positive predictive value of 82% for *u*T1 but a positive predictive value of only 63% for T2 lesions (124).

*u*T3 carcinomas penetrate the full thickness of the rectal wall into the perirectal fat and display disruption of the outermost hyperechoic ring. There is usually a preservation of some perirectal fat between the cancer and adjacent organs with some hypoechoic tissue seen outside the cancer. If there is loss of this layer and loss of a hyperechoic interface between the cancer and adjacent organs, then the tumor is classified as *u*T4. Both *u*T3 and *u*T4 lesions are usually treated with preoperative chemoradiation followed by surgery. However, if able to distinguish between the two, some centers have treated *u*T3 rectal lesions with short-course radiation. T4 lesions are accurately staged by ERUS with a positive predictive value of 93% and a negative predictive value of 99%, with numbers that are slightly worse for T3 lesions (124).

ERUS also assesses the lymph nodes in the mesorectum and gives an idea of the nodal status of the tumor (125). Normal, nonenlarged lymph nodes are generally not detectable by US. Patients with no visible lymph nodes by ERUS have a low probability of having lymph node metastases (126). Enlarged lymph nodes may be either inflamed, in which case they appear as hyperechoic with ill-defined borders, or malignant, appearing hypoechoic, with sharp borders and similar echogenic pattern to the primary lesion (127). Lymph nodes with mixed echogenic patterns should be considered metastatic (126). Malignant lymph nodes also tend to be more circular rather than oval and are more commonly found adjacent to the primary cancer or in the mesorectum proximal to the primary cancer. There is no definitive size threshold that determines that the node has a metastasis, but the larger the node the more likely that it is harboring a focus of cancer. Lesions that are >5 mm in size and are hypoechoic have an 88% probability of having carcinoma in them (128). Fat clearance studies show that many metastases are in lymph nodes <5 mm in diameter (129); unfortunately, ERUS, like other imaging modality, has a difficult time identifying these. False-negative results are usually due to small nodes harboring metastases and false-positive results are due to the presence of swollen reactive nodes (130). Blood vessels may mimic lymph nodes as they branch and change direction, but Doppler US will distinguish between the two. Tongues of tumor tissue from the primary lesion may appear to be lymph nodes, but careful scanning will identify this.

The accuracy of ERUS is difficult to estimate because there are numerous reports available with different results. This probably represents differences in the populations under study, and the experience of the ultrasonographers. Earlier reports on ERUS show an accuracy of 81% to 94% for depth of wall invasion, with both understaging and overstaging in the range of 5% to 10%, and with accuracy of lymph node metastasis detection of 58% to 80% (131–133). More recently a study from Minnesota, with a large population of patients with rectal tumors, indicates lower accuracy rates for ERUS than previously reported: 69% accuracy for rectal wall invasion, with 18% of tumors overstaged and 13% understaged (134); accuracy of lymph node assessment was 64%. A recent systematic review estimated accuracy of ERUS (135):for muscularis propria invasion sensitivity was 94% and specificity 86%, for peri-rectal tissue invasion sensitivity was 90% and specificity 75% and for lymph node involvement sensitivity was 67% and specificity 78%. This systematic review included all studies since 1985 that had at least 50 patients and adjusted for year of publication and quality of study.

ERUS is highly operator dependent, and there is a significant learning curve. Reliability and reproducibility depend on the experience and expertise of the ultrasonographer, and accuracy has been shown to improve with experience (136). Preoperative therapy with radiation (137) or chemoradiation (138–140) downstages tumors and makes ERUS unreliable. Radiation therapy results in a 10% to 20% rate of pathological cure with no evidence of tumor at final pathology. The tumor is replaced by pools of mucin, fibrosis, and inflammation, which are indistinguishable from carcinoma sonographically. Re-evaluation of rectal tumors after radiation or chemoradiation by ERUS, CT, or MRI (141) is inaccurate, unreliable, and not recommended.

Other Imaging Modalities for Rectal Cancer

Conventional CT has been evaluated in the assessment of rectal tumors and compared with ERUS. Whereas earlier studies (142,143) showed a high staging accuracy for CT, later studies did not support the previous good results (144–146). This is probably because the earlier studies had populations of patients with relatively advanced cancers, where CT is good at overall staging. CT does not have the resolution to distinguish between the layers of the rectal wall and cannot assess the depth of rectal wall invasion. Furthermore, CT cannot distinguish between inflammatory nodes and cancer-containing nodes. For local staging of rectal cancer and for lymph node status assessment, conventional CT is considerably inferior to ERUS (135). The introduction of the multidetector CT (MDCT) has allowed multiplanar reformatting of much higher resolution, which is hoped to be of higher benefit for rectal cancer. Some preliminary studies of MDCT have shown a much greater accuracy for the local staging of rectal cancer than previously reported for conventional CT (147,148), on the order of 90%.

Conventional MRI, just like CT, does not have enough resolution in the pelvis to be useful for local staging of rectal cancer (149), but the use of a specialized endorectal coil allows MRI enough spatial resolution for improved anatomical detail. MRI with endorectal coil can visualize all five layers of the rectal wall and determine the depth of invasion of rectal cancers (150) and, therefore, has application in the local staging of rectal cancers. The MRI, and especially the endorectal coil, are not widely available. Patients with strictures of the rectum are unable to be studied because insertion of the coil is not possible. The initial reports were promising (151–154), but it remained unclear whether MRI with endorectal coil was better than ERUS. Some reports favored MRI (155,156), whereas others favored ERUS (157). The meta-analysis mentioned in the ERUS section of this chapter (135) shows that MRI with endorectal coil is inferior to ERUS in determining the depth of tumor wall invasion by a small margin, but is probably similar at determining the lymph node status. The differences in the literature with respect to this assessment probably represent differences in the expertise with the two techniques. MRI, with endorectal coil or with phased array coils, most often fails to differentiate between T2 and T3 lesions because it has a hard time differentiating between inflammatory/fibrosing changes in the perirectal fat and malignant invasion in the perirectal fat (158). MRI with endorectal coil may be used in the local staging of rectal cancer as an alternative to ERUS, depending on availability, but it is slightly inferior to ERUS and more expensive.

More recent research in MRI and CT use for rectal cancer has focused on the circumferential margin. Rectal cancers can be classified into two categories with respect to therapy: cancers that can be adequately treated by TME with little or no neoadjuvant therapy (T1, T2, early T3) and locally advanced cancers that need chemoradiation prior to TME (advanced T3 and T4). ERUS excels in differentiating T1 from T2/T3 cancers, but it cannot identify locally advanced T3 cancers because it cannot detect the mesorectal fascia. If the relationship between the mesorectal fascia and the closest tumor margin can be reliably identified, then the indication for preoperative therapy could be better defined. MRI with phased-array coil can predict circumferential margin at surgery involvement with high accuracy (159) but tends to overestimate cancer invasion, especially for low lying lesions of the rectum (160). MRI has a sensitivity of 80% and a specificity of 84% in detecting mesorectal envelope involvement (161). Although interesting, this application of imaging needs further study because there are no preoperative therapy studies that use MRI.

Positron Emission Tomography Scanning

Positron emission tomography (PET) is a new technology that has wide applications in oncology and is beginning to find more uses in the management of CRC. PET is a nuclear medicine technique that uses a radioactively labeled glucose analog, $[^{18}F]$2-fluoro-2-deoxy-D-glucose (FDG), to detect tissue with increased glucose uptake and metabolism that usually represents malignancy. FDG lacks a hydroxyl group, which means it is not normally metabolized inside cells. FDG is not membrane permeable, which means it accumulates intracellularly. Technical advancements allow whole body scanning and promise faster acquisition, but this technology is still expensive and has limited availability (162). PET is a physiological test with limited resolution, and it needs correlation with conventional imaging (i.e., CT) for anatomical localization. One of the latest innovations (PET-CT) allows for simultaneous acquisition of PET and CT images, which can then be exactly superimposed (163); needless to say, this is even more expensive and less available.

The most accepted use for PET is in the early detection of recurrent disease, either local or metastatic. Patients with recurrences may still have curative rescue surgery that may result in improved survival. Only patients with nondisseminated disease are eligible for such therapy. PET appears to offer additional useful information in patients with normal conventional imaging and rising CEA levels (164) or just a suspicion of recurrence (162,165). PET is useful in detecting hepatic metastases (166). Contrast-enhanced MRI is better at detecting lesions <1 cm, and it retains its usefulness in a previously irradiated field (167). PET-CT has a higher sensitivity and specificity than PET alone, although the difference may not be that large (163,168). It is difficult to quantify the usefulness or accuracy of PET because the studies available are preselected case series. It is undoubtedly true that PET does provide additional information that may change therapy. This was recognized in the United States, where Medicare approved PET for the detection and localization of recurrent colorectal cancer in patients with rising CEA levels and indeterminate conventional radiology (169). It is still not proven that PET improves survival in CRC patients suspected of recurrence.

Another application of PET is the assessment of response to preoperative therapy in rectal cancer to aid in prognosis and, possibly, in modifying the therapy itself. The theory is that tumors that respond to therapy will have less tumor mass and metabolic activity, and show a decreased PET uptake. This application is easily assessed by obtaining a PET before and after the preoperative therapy, comparing the uptakes semiquantitatively, and correlating the decrease in PET signal with the final pathological specimen. PET seems to accurately identify responders to chemoradiation in locally advanced rectal cancer (170,171), although the accuracy seems less when rectal cancers of all stages are investigated (172,173). PET assessment of response to chemoradiation seems to predict long-term outcomes (170) and offers the additional advantage of occasionally detecting unsuspected liver metastases, which may alter therapy (174). The use of PET for prognosis in rectal cancer is interesting but seems to be a strange application for such an expensive technology because it cannot hope to compete with pathology in terms of prognostication. Furthermore, although there is some correlation between PET inactivity and finding complete pathological response, it is unlikely that anybody will forego surgery based on the PET findings.

CONCLUSION

The role of preoperative staging is to assess the cancer and its spread to decide on a treatment plan based on the stage of the disease. We advocate preoperative evaluation of patients with colon cancer by history and physical examination, chest x-ray, abdominal CT scan, and colonoscopy with biopsy. Contrast enemas may be performed if the colonoscopic examination is incomplete or unsatisfactory. The identification of synchronous lesions in the colon is important because all endoscopically removable polyps should be cleared before surgery and their pathology determined. Furthermore, any synchronous cancers need to be identified to plan the extent of resection.

Abdominal CT is recommended to evaluate for metastatic disease and contiguous organ involvement. Abdominal US, liver-directed helical CT, and MRI are used selectively to characterize suspicious liver lesions. Although the presence of metastatic disease in the liver usually does not alter the initial operative approach, there are selected instances in which this may be the case. For example, identification of a solitary, left lateral segment hepatic metastasis on preoperative CT may allow for discussion, consent, and performance of a synchronous liver and colon resection in the rare patient; at the least, it would allow the presence of a hepatobiliary surgeon at the time of operation to evaluate the possibility of future metastasectomy. Any suspicious lesions on chest x-ray are assessed by chest CT.

For rectal cancer, the treatment plan is largely based on the preoperative stage of the carcinoma. Our recommendation for the preoperative evaluation of rectal cancer patients includes the same workup as discussed for patients with colon cancer, with the important addition of ERUS or MRI, depending on availability of equipment and expertise. Preoperative ERUS is the most accurate means of assessing the local stage of a rectal carcinoma and is the best guide for choosing the preoperative treatment plan. The other important factor determining the choice of management for rectal cancer is the level or location of the carcinoma in relation to the anal sphincter complex.

Postoperative staging is based on the pathological specimen using the TNM classification. In the specific cases of rectal cancers that receive neoadjuvant therapy, the preoperative radiologic studies are extremely important. The TNM staging predicts the outcome of surgical management and guides the use of oncologic management.

References

1. Skandalakis JE, Kingsnorth AN, Colborn GL, et al. Large intestine and anorectum. In: Skandalakis JE, Colborn GL, Weidman TA, et al., eds. *Skandalakis' Surgical Anatomy: The Embryologic and Anatomic Basis of Modern Surgery*. Athens, Greece: Paschalidis Medical Publications; 2004;861–918.
2. Wexner SD, Jorge JMN. Anatomy and embryology of the anus rectum and colon. In: Corman ML, ed. *Colon and Rectal Surgery*. 5th ed. Philadelphia, Pa.: Lippincott Williams & Wilkins; 2005;1–30.
3. Netter FH. *Atlas of Human Anatomy*. Summit, NJ: CIBA-GEIGY Corporation; 1989;231–384.
4. Skandalakis JE, Gray SW, Ricketts R. The colon and rectum. In: Skandalakis JE, Gray SW, eds. *Embryology for Surgeons: The Embryologic Basis for the Treatment of Congenital Anomalies*. Baltimore, Md.: Williams & Wilkins; 1994;187–216.
5. Lindsey I, Warren BF, Mortensen NJ. Denonvillier's fascia lies anterior to the fascia propria and rectal dissection plane in total mesorectal excision. *Dis Colon Rectum* 2005;48:37–42.
6. Heald RJ, Moran BJ. Embryology and anatomy of the rectum. *Semin Surg Oncol* 1998;15:66–71.
7. Jones OM, Smeulders N, Wiseman O, Miller R. Lateral ligaments of the rectum: an anatomical study. *Br J Surg* 1999;86:487–489.
8. Chapuis P, Bokey L, Fahrer M, et al. Mobilization of the rectum: anatomic concepts and the bookshelf revisited. *Dis Colon Rectum* 2002;45:1–9.
9. Yada H, Sawai K, Taniguchi H, et al. Analysis of vascular anatomy and lymph node metastases warrants segmental bowel resection for colon cancer. *World J Surg* 1997;21:109–115.
10. VanDamme JPJ. Behavioral anatomy of the abdominal arteries. *Surg Clin North Am* 1993;73:699–725.
11. DiDio LJ, Diaz-Franco C, Schemainda R, et al. Morphology of the middle rectal arteries: a study of 30 cadaveric dissections. *Surg Radiol Anat* 1986;8:229–236.
12. Godlewski G. Prudhomme M. Embryology and anatomy of the anorectum: basis of surgery. *Surg Clin North Am* 2000;80:319–343.
13. Way LW, Doherty GM, eds. *Current Surgical Diagnosis and Treatment*. 11th ed. New York, NY: McGraw-Hill; 2003.
14. Williams PL, Warwick R, Dyson M, Bannister LH, eds. *Gray's Anatomy*. 37th ed. New York, NY: Churchill Livingstone; 1989.
15. Greene FL, Page DL, Fleming ID, et al., eds. *AJCC Cancer Staging Manual*. 6th ed. New York, NY: Springer; 2002.
16. Mayer A, Fuchsjäger M. Preoperative staging of rectal cancer. *Eur J Radiol* 2003;47:89–97.
17. Lockhart-Mummery JP. Two hundred cases of cancer of the rectum treated by perineal excision. *Br J Surg* 1926;14:110–124.
18. Rankin FW, Broders AC. Factors influencing prognosis in carcinoma of the rectum. *Surg Gynecol Obstet* 1928;46:660–667.
19. Dukes CE. The classification of cancer of the rectum. *J Pathol* 1932;35:395–413.
20. Simpson WC, Mayo CW. The mural penetration of the carcinoma cell in the colon: anatomic and clinical study. *Surg Gynecol Obstet* 1939;68:872–877.
21. Gabriel WB, Dukes C, Bussey HJR. Lymphatic spread in cancer of the rectum. *Br J Surg* 1935;23:395–413.
22. Kirklin JW, Dockerty MB, Waugh JM. The role of the peritoneal reflection in the prognosis of carcinoma of the rectum and sigmoid colon. *Surg Gynecol Obstet* 1939;88:326–331.
23. Astler VB, Coller FA. The prognostic significance of direct extension of carcinoma of the colon and rectum. *Ann Surg* 1954;139:846–851.
24. Turnbull RB, Kyle K, Watson FR, Spratt J. Cancer of the colon: the influence of the no-touch isolation technic on survival rates. *Ann Surg* 1967;166:420–427.
25. Chapuis PH, Fisher R, Dent OF, Newland RC, Pheils MT. The relationship between different staging methods and survival in colorectal carcinoma. *Dis Colon Rectum* 1985;28:158–161.
26. Sobin LH. TNM: principles, history and relation to other prognostic factors. *Cancer* 2001;91:1589–1592.
27. Whittaker M, Goligher JC. The prognosis after surgical treatment for carcinoma of the rectum. *Br J Surg* 1976;63:384–388.
28. Madsen M, Christiansen J. Distal intramural spread of rectal carcinomas. *Dis Colon Rectum* 1986;29:279–282.
29. Pollett WG, Nicholls RJ. The relationship between the extent of distal clearance and survival and local recurrence rates after curative anterior resection for carcinoma of the rectum. *Ann Surg* 1983;198:159–163.
30. Vernava AM, Moran M. A prospective evaluation of distal margins in carcinoma of the rectum. *Surg Gynecol Obstet* 1992;175:333–336.
31. Moore HG, Riedel E, Minsky BD, et al. Adequacy of 1-cm distal margin after restorative rectal cancer resection with sharp mesorectal excision and preoperative combined-modality therapy. *Ann Surg Oncol* 2003;10:80–85.
32. Law WL, Chu KW. Local recurrence following total mesorectal excision with double-stapling anastomosis for rectal cancers: analysis of risk factors. *World J Surg* 2002;26:1272–1276.
33. Rullier E, Laurent C, Bretagnol F, et al. Sphincter-saving resection for all rectal carcinomas: the end of the 2-cm distal rule. *Ann Surg* 2005;241:465–469.
34. Tiret E, Poupardin B, McNamara D, et al. Ultralow anterior resection with intersphincteric dissection—what is the limit of safe sphincter preservation? *Colorectal Dis* 2003;5:454–457.
35. Ono C, Yoshinaga K, Enomoto M, Sugihara K. Discontinuous rectal cancer spread in the mesorectum and the optimal distal clearance margin in situ. *Dis Colon Rectum* 2002;45:744–749.
36. Zhao G, Zhou Z, Lei W, et al. Pathological study of distal mesorectal cancer spread to determine a proper distal resection margin. *World J Gastroenterol* 2005;11:319–322.
37. Quirke P, Durdey P, Dixon MF, Williams NS. Local recurrence of rectal adenocarcinoma due to inadequate surgical resection: histopathological study of lateral tumor spread and surgical excision. *Lancet* 1986;2:996–999.
38. Adam IJ, Mohamdee MO, Martin IG, et al. Role of circumferential margin involvement in the local recurrence of rectal cancer. *Lancet* 1994;344:707–711.
39. De Haas-Kock DFM, Baeten CGMI, Jager JJ, et al. Prognostic significance of radial margins of clearance in rectal cancer. *Br J Surg* 1996;83:781–785.

40. Heald RJ, Husband EM, Ryall RDH. The mesorectum in rectal cancer surgery—the clue to pelvic recurrence? *Br J Surg* 1982;69:613–616.

41. Heald RJ, Ryall RDH. Recurrence and survival after total mesorectal excision for rectal cancer. *Lancet* 1986;1:1479–1482.

42. Hall NR, Finan PJ, Al-Jaberi T, et al. Circumferential margin involvement after mesorectal excision of rectal cancer with curative intent: predictor of survival but not local recurrence? *Dis Colon Rectum* 1998;41:979–983.

43. Marijnen CAM, Nagtegaal ID, Kapiteijn E, et al. Radiotherapy does not compensate for positive resection margins in rectal cancer patients: report of a multicenter randomized trial. *Int J Radiat Oncol Biol Phys* 2003;55:1311–1320.

44. Luna-Pérez P, Bustos-Cholico E, Alvarado I, et al. Prognostic significance of circumferential margin involvement in rectal adenocarcinoma treated with preoperative chemoradiation and low anterior resection. *J Surg Oncol* 2005;90:20–25.

45. Cohen AM, Tremiterra S, Candela F, et al. Prognosis of node-positive colon cancer. *Cancer* 1991;67:1859–1861.

46. Ratto C, Sofo L, Ippoliti M, et al. Accurate lymph-node detection in colorectal specimens resected for cancer is of prognostic significance. *Dis Colon Rectum* 1999;42:143–158.

47. Mainprize KS, Hewavisinthe J, Savage A, et al. How many lymph nodes to stage colorectal carcinoma?. *J Clin Pathol* 1998;51:165–166.

48. Maurel J, Launoy G, Grosclaude P, et al. Lymph node harvest reporting in patients with carcinoma of the large bowel: a French population-based study. *Cancer* 1998;82:1482–1486.

49. Scott KWM, Grace RH. Detection of lymph node metastasis in colorectal carcinoma before and after fat clearance. *Br J Surg* 1989;76:1165–1167.

50. Cutait R, Alves VAF, Lopes LC, et al. Restaging of colorectal cancer based on the identification of lymph node micrometastases through immunoperoxidase staining of CEA and cytokeratins. *Dis Colon Rectum* 1991;34:917–920.

51. Choi H, Choi Y, Hong S. Incidence and prognostic implication of isolated tumor cells in lymph nodes from patients with Dukes B colorectal carcinoma. *Dis Colon Rectum* 2002;45:750–756.

52. Liefers G, Cleton-Jansen A, Van de Velde C, et al. Micrometastases and survival in stage II colorectal cancer. *N Engl J Med* 1998;339:223–228.

53. Rosenberg R, Friedrich J, Gertler R. Prognostic evaluation and review of immunohistochemically detected disseminated tumor cells in peritumoral lymph nodes of patients with pN0 colorectal cancer. *Int J Colorectal Dis* 2004;19:430–437.

54. Saha S, Wiese D, Badin J, Beutler T. Technical details of sentinel lymph node mapping in colorectal cancer and its impact on staging. *Ann Surg Oncol* 2000;7:120–124.

55. Mulsow J, Winter DC, O'Keane JC, O'Connell PR. Sentinel lymph node mapping in colorectal cancer. *Br J Surg* 2003;90:659–667.

56. Stojadinovic A, Allen PJ, Protic M, et al. Colon sentinel lymph node mapping: practical surgical applications. *J Am Coll Surg* 2005;201:297–313.

57. Saha S, Dan AG, Viehl CT, et al. Sentinel lymph node mapping in colon and rectal cancer: its impact on staging, limitations, and pitfalls. *Cancer Treat Res* 2005;127:105–122.

58. Broders AC. The grading of carcinoma. *Minn Med* 1925;8:726–730.

59. Blumberg D, Paty PB, Picon AI, et al. Stage I rectal cancer: identification of high-risk patients. *J Am Coll Surg* 1998;186:574–580.

60. Minsky BD, Rich T, Recht A, et al. Selection criteria for local excision with or without adjuvant radiation therapy for rectal cancer. *Cancer* 1989;63:1421–1429.

61. Horn A, Dahl O, Morild I. Venous and neural invasion as predictors of recurrence in rectal adenocarcinoma. *Dis Colon Rectum* 1991;34:798–804.

62. Ross A, Rusnak C, Weinerman B, et al. Recurrence and survival after surgical management of rectal cancer. *Am J Surg* 1999;177:392–395.

63. Moreira LF, Kenmotsu M, Gochi A, et al. Lymphovascular and neural invasion in low-lying rectal carcinoma. *Cancer Detect Prev* 1999;23:123–128.

64. Minsky B, Mies C. The clinical significance of vascular invasion in colorectal cancer. *Dis Colon Rectum* 1989;32:794–803.

65. Brodsky JT, Richard GK, Cohen AM, Minsky BD. Variables correlated with risk of lymph node metastasis in early rectal cancer. *Cancer* 1992;69:322–326.

66. Meguerditchian A, Bairati I, Lagacé R, et al. Prognostic significance of lymphovascular invasion in surgically cured rectal carcinoma. *Am J Surg* 2005;189:707–713.

67. Zeng Z, Sarkis A, Zhang Z. p53 overexpression: an independent predictor of survival in lymph-node positive colorectal cancer patients. *J Clin Oncol* 1994;12:2043–2050.

68. Kressner U, Inganäs M, Byding S, et al. Prognostic value of p53 genetic changes in colorectal cancer. *J Clin Oncol* 1999;17:593–599.

69. Tortola S, Marcuello E, Gonzalez I, et al. p53 and K-ras gene mutations correlate with tumor aggressiveness but are not of routine prognostic value in colorectal cancer. *J Clin Oncol* 1999;18:1375–1381.

70. Westra JL, Schaapveld M, Hollema H, de Boer JP. Determination of TP53 mutation is more relevant that microsatellite instability status for the prediction of disease-free survival in adjuvant-treated stage III colon cancer patients. *J Clin Oncol* 2005;23:5635–5643.

71. Børresen-Dale A, Lothe RA, Meling GI, et al. TP53 and long-term prognosis in colorectal cancer: mutations in the L3 zinc-binding domain predict poor survival. *Clin Cancer Res* 1998;4:203–210.

72. Samowitz WS, Curtin K, Ma K, et al. Prognostic significance of p53 mutations in colon cancer at the population level. *Int J Cancer* 2002;99:597–602.

73. Adell G, Sun X, Stål O, et al. p53 status: an indicator for the effect of preoperative radiotherapy of rectal cancer. *Radiother Oncol* 1999;51:169–174.

74. Nehls O, Klump B, Holzman K, Lammering G. Influence of p53 status on prognosis in preoperatively irradiated rectal carcinoma. *Cancer* 1999;85:2541–2548.

75. Tang R, Wang J, Fan C, Tsao K. p53 is an independent pre-treatment markers for long-term survival in stage II and III colorectal cancers: an analysis of interaction between genetic markers and fluorouracil-based adjuvant therapy. *Cancer Lett* 2004;210:101–109.

76. Bell SM, Scott N, Cross D, Sagar P. Prognostic value of p53 overexpression and c-Ki-ras gene mutations in colorectal cancer. *Gastroenterology* 1993;104:57–64.

77. Cascinu S, Staccioli MP, Gasparini G, Giordani P. Expression of vascular endothelial growth factor can predict event-free survival in stage II colon cancer. *Clin Cancer Res* 2000;6:2803–2807.

78. Hurwitz H, Fehrenbacher L, Novotny W, Cartwright T. Bevacizumab plus irinotecan, fluorouracil, and leucovorin for metastatic colorectal cancer. *N Engl J Med* 2004;350:2335–2342.

79. Johnston PG, Lenz H, Leichman CG, et al. Thymidylate synthase gene and protein expression correlate and are associated with response to 5-fluorouracil in human colorectal and gastric tumors. *Cancer Res* 1995;44:1407–1412.

80. Suh KW, Kim JH, Kim YB, et al. Thymidylate synthase gene polymorphism as a prognostic factor for colon cancer. *J Gastrointest Surg* 2005;9:336–342.

81. Öhrling K, Edler D, Hallström M, et al. Detection of thymidylate synthase expression in lymph node metastases of colorectal cancer can improve the prognostic information. *J Clin Oncol* 2005;23:5628–5634.

82. Soumaoro LT, Uetake H, Higuchi T, et al. Cyclooxygenase-2 expression: a significant prognostic indicator for patients with colorectal cancer. *Clin Cancer Res* 2004;10:8465–8471.

83. Bahnassy AA, Zekri AN, El-Houssini S, El-Shehaby AMR. Cyclin A and cyclin D1 as significant prognostic markers in colorectal cancer patients. *BMC Gastroenterol* 2004;4:22.

84. Hampel H, Frankel WL, Martin E, Arnold M. Screening for the Lynch syndrome. *N Engl J Med* 2005;352:1851–1860.

85. Niv Y. Biologic behavior of microsatellite-unstable colorectal cancer and treatment with 5-fluorouracil. *Israel Medical Association Journal* 2005;7:520–524.

86. Gryfe R, Kim H, Hsieh ETK, Aronson MD. Tumor microsatellite instability and clinical outcome in young patients with colorectal cancer. *N Engl J Med* 2000;342:69–77.

87. Watanabe T, Wu T, Catalano PJ, Ueki T. Molecular predictors of survival after adjuvant chemotherapy for colon cancer. *N Engl J Med* 2001;344:1196–1206.

88. Kohonen-Corish MRJ, Daniel JJ, Chan C, Lin BPC. Low microsatellite instability is associated with poor prognosis in stage C colon cancer. *J Clin Oncol* 2005;23:2318–2324.

89. Carethers JM, Smith EJ, Behling CA, Nguyen L. Use of 5-fluorouracil and survival in patients with microsatellite-unstable colorectal cancer. *Gastroenterology* 2004;126:394–401.

90. Ribic C, Sargent DJ, Moore MJ, Thibodeau SN. Tumor microsatellite-instability status as a predictor of benefit from fluorouracil-based adjuvant chemotherapy for colon cancer. *N Engl J Med* 2003;349:247–257.

91. Kapiteijn E, Marijnen CAM, Nagtegaal ID. Preoperative radiotherapy combined with total mesorectal excision for resectable rectal cancer. *N Engl J Med* 2001;345:638–646.

92. Bosset JF, Calais G, Mineur L, Maingon P. Enhanced tumoricidal effect of chemotherapy with preoperative radiotherapy for rectal cancer: preliminary results—EORTC 22921. *J Clin Oncol* 2005;23:5620–5627.

93. Sauer R, Becker H, Hohenberger W, Rödel C. Preoperative versus postoperative chemoradiotherapy for rectal cancer. *N Engl J Med* 2004;351:1731–1740.

94. Nelson H, Sargent DJ, Wieand S, et al. A comparison of laparoscopically assisted and open colectomy for colon cancer. *N Engl J Med* 2004;350:2050–2059.

95. Pinol V, Andreu M, Castells A, et al. Synchronous colorectal neoplasms in patients with colorectal cancer: predisposing individual and familial factors. *Dis Colon Rectum* 2004;47:1192–1200.

96. Arenas RB, Fichera A, Mhoon D, et al. Incidence and therapeutic implications of synchronous colonic pathology in colorectal adenocarcinoma. *Surgery* 1997;122:706–710.

97. Harrison LE, Gillem JG, Paty P, et al. Preoperative carcinoembryonic antigen predicts outcomes in node-negative colon cancer patients: a multivariate analysis of 572 patients. *J Am Coll Surg* 1997;185:59–64.

98. Korenaga D, Saeki H, Mawatari K, et al. Serum carcinoembryonic antigen concentration doubling time correlates with tumor biology and life expectancy in patients with recurrent gastrointestinal carcinoma. *Arch Surg* 1997;132:188–194.

99. Pietra N, Sarli L, Costi R, et al. Role of follow-up in management of local recurrences of colorectal cancer: a prospective, randomized study. *Dis Colon Rectum* 1998;41:1127–1133.

100. Kemeny N, Braun DW. Prognostic factors in advanced colorectal carcinoma: importance of lactic dehydrogenase level, performance status, and white blood cell count. *Am J Med* 1983;74:786–794.

101. Heriot AG, Grundy A, Kumar D. Preoperative staging of rectal carcinoma. *Br J Surg* 1999;86:17–28.

102. Freeny PC, Marks WM, Ryan JA, Bolen JW. Colorectal carcinoma evaluation with CT: preoperative staging and detection of postoperative recurrence. *Radiology* 1986;158:347–353.

103. Stark DD, Wittenberg J, Butch RJ, Ferrucci JT. Hepatic metastases: randomized, controlled comparison of detection with MRI imaging and CT. *Radiology* 1987;165:399–406.

104. Barton JB, Langdale LA, Cummins JS, Stelzner M. The utility of routine preoperative computed tomography scanning in the management of veterans with colon cancer. *Am J Surg* 2002;183:499–503.

105. Mauchley DC, Lynge DC, Langdale LA, Stelzner MG. Clinical utility and cost-effectiveness of routine preoperative computed tomography scanning in patients with colon cancer. *Am J Surg* 2005;189:512–517.

106. Balthazar EJ, Megibow AJ, Hilnick D, Naidich DP. Carcinoma of the colon: detection and preoperative staging by CT. *AJR Am J Roentgenol* 1988;150:301–306.

107. Wallace JR, Christians KK, Quiroz FA, et al. Ablation of liver metastasis: is preoperative imaging sufficiently accurate? *J Gastrointest Surg* 2001;5:98–107

108. Moore KH, McCaughan BC. Surgical resection for pulmonary metastases from colorectal cancer. *ANZ J Surg* 2001;71:143–146.

109. Griffiths EA, Browell DA, Cunliffe WJ. Evaluation of a pre-operative staging protocol in the management of colorectal carcinoma. *Colorectal Dis* 2005;7:35–42.

110. Schoemaker D, Black R, Giles L, et al. Yearly colonoscopy, liver CT, and chest radiography do not influence 5-year survival of colorectal patients. *Gastroenterology* 1998;114:7–14.

111. Saitoh Y, Obara T, Einami K, Nomura M. Efficacy of high-frequency ultrasound probes for the preoperative staging of invasion depth in flat and depressed colorectal tumors. *Gastrointest Endosc* 1996;44:34–39.

112. Hnerhein M, Handke T, Ulmer C, Schlag PM. Impact of miniprobe ultrasonography on planning of minimally invasive surgery for gastric and colonic tumors. *Surg Endosc* 2004;18:601–605.

113. Stergiou N, Haji-Kermani N, Schneider C, et al. Staging of colonic neoplasms by colonoscopic miniprobe ultrasonography. *Int J Colorectal Dis* 2003;18:445–449.

114. Mason AY. Rectal cancer: the spectrum of selective surgery. *Proc Roy Soc Med* 1976;69:237–244.

115. Mason AY. Role of local surgery in carcinoma of the rectum. *Proc Roy Soc Med* 1976;69:869–872.

116. Beynon J, Mortesen NJM, Foy DMA, et al. Pre-operative assessment of local invasion in rectal cancer: digital examination, endoluminal sonography or computed tomography? *Br J Surg* 1986;73:1015–1017.

117. Rafaelsen SR, Kronborg O, Fenger C. Digital rectal examination and transrectal ultrasonography in staging rectal cancer. *Acta Radiol* 1994;35:300–304.

118. Rieger N, Tjandra J, Solomon M. Endoanal and endorectal ultrasound: applications in colorectal surgery. *ANZ J Surg* 2004;74:671–675.

119. Hildebrandt U, Feifel G. Preoperative staging of rectal cancer by intrarectal ultrasound. *Dis Colon Rectum* 1985;28:42–46.

120. Adams WJ, Wong WD. Endorectal ultrasonic detection of malignancy within the rectal villous lesions. *Dis Colon Rectum* 1995;38:1093–1096.

121. Worrell S, Horvath K, Blakemore T, et al. Endorectal ultrasound detection of focal carcinoma within rectal adenomas. *Am J Surg* 2004;187:625–629.

122. Garcia-Aguilar J, Hernández de Anda E, Rothenberger DA, et al. Endorectal ultrasound in the management of patients with malignant rectal polyps. *Dis Colon Rectum* 2005;48:910–917.

123. Blumberg D, Paty PB, Guillem JG, et al. All patients with small intramural rectal cancers are at risk for lymph node metastasis. *Dis Colon Rectum* 1999;42:881–885.

124. Mackay SG, Pager CK, Joseph D, et al. Assessment of the accuracy of transrectal ultrasonography in anorectal neoplasia. *Br J Surg* 2003;90:346–350.

125. Beynon J, Mortensen NJM, Foy DMA, et al. Preoperative assessment of mesorectal lymph node involvement in rectal cancer. *Br J Surg* 1989;76:276–279.

126. Hildebrandt U, Klein T, Feifel G, et al. Endosonography of pararectal lymph nodes: in vitro and in vivo evaluation. *Dis Colon Rectum* 1990;33:863–868.

127. Tio TL, Tytgat GNJ. Endoscopic ultrasonography in analyzing periintestinal lymph node abnormality. *Scand J Gastroenterol* 1986;21:158–163.

128. Sunouchi K, Sakaguchi M, Higuchi Y, et al. Limitations of endorectal ultrasonography: what does a low echoic lesion more than 5 mm in size correspond to histologically? *Dis Colon Rectum* 1998;41:761–764.

129. Herrera-Ornelas L, Justiniano J, Castillo N, et al. Metastases in small lymph nodes from colon cancer. *Arch Surg* 1987;122:1253–1256.

130. Akasu T, Sugihara K, Moriya K, et al. Limitations and pitfalls of transrectal ultrasonography for staging of rectal cancer. *Dis Colon Rectum* 1997;40:S10-S15.

131. Phang PT, Wong WD. The use of endoluminal ultrasound for malignant and benign anorectal diseases. *Curr Opin Gastroenterol* 1997;13:47–53.

132. Glaser F, Schlag P, Herfarth C. Endorectal ultrasonography for the assessment of invasion of rectal tumors and lymph node involvement. *Br J Surg* 1990;77:883–887.

133. Katsura Y, Yamada K, Ishizawa T, et al. Endorectal ultrasonography for the assessment of wall invasion and lymph node metastasis in rectal cancer. *Dis Colon Rectum* 1992;35:362–368.

134. Garcia-Aguilar J, Pollack J, Lee SH, et al. Accuracy of endorectal ultrasonography in preoperative staging of rectal tumors. *Dis Colon Rectum* 2002;45:10–15.

135. Bipat S, Glas AS, Slors FJM, et al. Rectal cancer: local staging and assessment of lymph node involvement with endoluminal US, CT and MR imaging—a meta-analysis. *Radiology* 2004;232:773–783.

136. Orrom WJ, Wong WD, Rothenberger DA, et al. Endorectal ultrasound in the preoperative staging of rectal tumors: a learning experience. *Dis Colon Rectum* 1990;33:654–659.

137. Fleshman JW, Myerson RJ, Fry RD, et al. Accuracy of transrectal ultrasound in predicting pathologic stage of rectal cancer before and after preoperative radiation therapy. *Dis Colon Rectum* 1992;35:823–829.

138. Bernini A, Deen KI, Madoff RD, et al. Preoperative adjuvant radiation with chemotherapy for rectal cancer: its impact on stage of disease and the role of endorectal ultrasound. *Ann Surg Oncol* 1996;3:131–135.

139. Meade PG, Blatchford GJ, Thorson AG, et al. Preoperative chemoradiation downstages locally advanced ultrasound-staged rectal cancer. *Am J Surg* 1995;170:609–613.

140. Williamson PR, Hellinger MD, Larach SW, et al. Endorectal ultrasound of T3 and T4 rectal cancers after preoperative chemoradiation. *Dis Colon Rectum* 1996;39:45–49.

141. Kahn H, Alexander A, Rakinic J, et al. Preoperative staging of irradiated rectal cancers using digital rectal examination, computed tomography, endorectal ultrasound, and magnetic resonance imaging does not accurately predict T0, N0 pathology. *Dis Colon Rectum* 1997;40:140–144.

142. Holdsworth PJ, Johnston D, Chalmers AG, Chennells P. Endoluminal ultrasound and computed tomography in the staging of rectal cancer. *Br J Surg* 1988;75:1019–1022.

143. Thoeni RF, Moss AA, Schnyder P, et al. Detection and staging of primary rectal and rectosigmoid cancer by computed tomography. *Radiology* 1981;141:135–138.

144. Waizer A, Zitron S, Ben-Baruch D, et al. Comparative study for preoperative staging of rectal cancer. *Dis Colon Rectum* 1989;32:53–56.

145. Rifkin MD, Ehrlich SM, Marks G. Staging of rectal carcinoma: prospective comparison of endorectal US and CT. *Radiology* 1989;170:319–322.

146. Goldman S, Arvidsson H, Norming U, et al. Transrectal ultrasound and computed tomography in preoperative staging of lower rectal adenocarcinoma. *Gastrointest Radiol* 1991;16:259–263.

147. Kulinna C, Eibel R, Matzek W, Bonel H. Staging of rectal cancer: diagnostic potential of multiplanar reconstructions with MDCT. *AJR Am J Roentgenol* 2004;183:421–427.

148. Kulinna C, Scheidler J, Strauss T, Bonel H. Local staging of rectal cancer: assessment with double-contrast multislice computed tomography and transrectal ultrasound. *J Comput Assist Tomogr* 2004;28:123–130.

149. Starck M, Bohe M, Fork FT, et al. Endoluminal ultrasound and low-field magnetic resonance imaging are superior to clinical examination in the preoperative staging of rectal cancer. *Eur J Surg* 1995;161:841–845.

150. Chan T, Kressel HY, Milestone B, et al. Rectal carcinoma: staging at MR imaging with endorectal surface coil: work in progress. *Radiology* 1991;181:461–467.

151. Schnall MD, Furth EE, Rosato EF, et al. Rectal tumor stage: correlation of endorectal MR imaging and pathologic findings. *Radiology* 1994;190:709–714.

152. McNicholas MMJ, Joyce WP, Dolan J, et al. Magnetic resonance imaging of rectal carcinoma: a prospective study. *Br J Surg* 1994;81:911–914.

153. Joosten FBM, Jansen JBMJ, Joosten HJM, et al. Staging of rectal carcinoma using MR double surface coil, MR endorectal coil, and intrarectal ultrasound: correlation with histopathologic findings. *J Comput Assist Tomogr* 1995;19:752–758.

154. Blomqvist L, Holm T, Rubio C, et al. Rectal tumors—MR imaging with endorectal and/or phased-array coils, and histopathological staging of giant sections. *Acta Radiol* 1997;38:437–444.

155. Zagoria RJ, Schlarb CA, Ott DJ, Bechtold RE. Assessment of rectal tumor infiltration utilizing endorectal MR imaging and comparison with endoscopic rectal sonography. *J Surg Oncol* 1997;64:312–317.

156. Brown G, Davies S, Williams GT, Bourne MW. Effectiveness of pre operative staging in rectal cancer: digital rectal examination, endoluminal ultrasound or magnetic resonance imaging? *Br J Cancer* 2004;91:23–29.

157. Meyenberger C, Huch Böni RA, Bertschinger P, et al. Endoscopic ultrasound and endorectal magnetic resonance imaging: a prospective, comparative study for preoperative staging and follow-up of rectal cancer. *Endoscopy* 1995;27:469–479.

158. Beets-Tan RGH. MRI in rectal cancer: the T stage and circumferential resection margin. *Colorectal Dis* 2003;5:392–395.

159. Beets-Tan RGH, Beets GL, Vliegen RFA, Kessels AGH. Accuracy of magnetic resonance imaging in prediction of tumour-free resection margin in rectal cancer surgery. *Lancet* 2001;357:497–504.

160. Peschaud F, Cuenod CA, Benoist S, Juli C. Accuracy of magnetic resonance imaging in rectal cancer depends on location of the tumor. *Dis Colon Rectum* 2005;48:1603–1609.

161. Mathur P, Smith JJ, Ramsey C, Owen M. Comparison of CT and MRI in the pre-operative staging of rectal adenocarcinoma and prediction of circumferential resection margin involvement by MRI. *Colorectal Dis* 2003;5:396–401.

162. Flamen P, Stroobants S, Cutsem EV, Dupont P. Additional value of whole-body positron emission tomography with fluorine-18-2-fluoro-2-deoxy-D-glucose in recurrent colorectal cancer. *J Clin Oncol* 1999;17:894–901.

163. Even-Sapir E, Parag Y, Lerman H, Gutman M. Detection of recurrence in patients with rectal cancer. PET/CT after abdominoperineal or anterior resection. *Radiology* 2004;232:815–822.

164. Flanaga FL, Dehdashti F, Ogunbiyi OA, et al. Utility of FDG-PET for investigating unexplained plasma CEA elevation in patients with colorectal cancer. *Ann Surg* 1998;227:319–323.

165. Staib L, Schirrmeister H, Reske SN, et al. Is 18F-fluorodeoxyglucose positron emission tomography in recurrent colorectal cancer a contribution to surgical decision making? *Am J Surg* 2000;180:1–5.

166. Sahani DV, Kalva SP, Fischman AJ, et al. Detection of liver metastases from adenocarcinoma of the colon and pancreas: comparison of mangafodipir trisodium-enhanced liver MRI and whole-body PDG PET. *AJR. Am J Roentgenol* 2004;185:239–246.

167. Moore HG, Akhurst T, Larson SM, et al. A case-controlled study of 18-fluorodeoxyglucose positron emission tomography in the detection of pelvic recurrence in previously irradiated rectal cancer patients. *J Am Coll Surg* 2003;197:22–28.

168. Fukunaga H, Sekimoto M, Ikeda M, Higuchi I. Fusion image of positron emission tomography and computed tomography for the diagnosis of local recurrence of rectal cancer. *Ann Surg Oncol* 2005;12:1–9.

169. Dobos N, Rubesin SE. Radiologic imaging modalities in the diagnosis and management of colorectal cancer. *Hematol Oncol Clin North Am* 2002;16:875–895.

170. Guillem JG, Puig-La Calle J, Akhurst T, et al. Prospective assessment of primary rectal cancer response to preoperative radiation and chemotherapy using 18-fluorodeoxyglucose positron emission tomography. *Dis Colon Rectum* 2000;43:18–24.

171. Amthauer H, Denecke T, Rau B, Hildebrandt B. Response prediction by FDG-PET after neoadjuvant radiochemotherapy and combined regional hyperthermia of rectal cancer: correlation with endorectal ultrasound and histopathology. *Eur J Nucl Med Mol Imaging* 2004;31:811–819.

172. Carpici C, Rubello D, Chierichetti F, Crepaldi G. Restaging after neoadjuvant chemoradiotherapy for rectal adenocarcinoma: role of F18-FDG PET. *Biomed Pharmacother* 2004;58:451–457.

173. Calvo FA, Domper M, Matute R, Martínez-Lázaro R. 18F-FDG positron emission tomography staging and restaging in rectal cancer treated with preoperative chemoradiation. *Int J Radiat Oncol Biol Phys* 2004;58:528–535.

174. Heriot AG, Hicks RJ, Drummond EGP, Keck J. Does positron emission tomography change management in primary rectal cancer? A prospective assessment. *Dis Colon Rectum* 2004;47:451–458.

CHAPTER 43 ■ COLON CANCER: MANAGEMENT OF LOCOREGIONAL DISEASE

ERIC VAN CUTSEM, ANDRE D'HOORE, CAROLINE DE VLEESCHOUWER, JOCHEN DECAESTECKER, AND FREDDY PENNINCKX

Colon cancer is one of the leading causes of cancer-related deaths in the Western world. Every year, it is estimated that approximately 1 million new cases of colorectal cancer (CRC) are diagnosed. CRC is responsible for an estimated 400,000 to 500,000 deaths worldwide every year.

Seventy to 75% of patients with colon cancer present with localized disease. In these patients, surgery can be curative, but relapses after complete resection are frequent despite curative surgery leading to morbidity and eventual mortality. Colon cancer is a disease in which systemic failure is of primary importance. Metastases can occur at several sites: The liver, the peritoneum, and the lungs are the most frequent sites of metastatic disease, although other organs can also be affected. Locoregional recurrence occurs, although less frequently than metastases, and is more frequent in patients with tumor invasion of surrounding tissues (T4 tumor), tumor-associated perforation, or obstruction. Adjuvant strategies are therefore focused on preventing metastatic disease after surgical resection of the primary tumor.

Colon cancer is not uniformly fatal, and there are large differences in survival, depending on the stage of the disease. The pathological stage is currently the most important determinant of prognosis and is discussed in detail in Chapter 42. The classification system described by Dukes no longer fulfils the requirements of modern tumor staging. It does not take into account distant metastases, the number of lymph nodes involved, and carcinomas limited to the submucosa. The tumor, node, metastasis (TNM) classification of the American Joint Committee on Cancer (AJCC) is currently recommended. The updated sixth edition stratifies colon cancer stages II and III further by use of the T stage and the N stage (Table 43.1) (1,2).

Recently, survival rates have been published from the Surveillance, Epidemiology, and End Results U.S. National Cancer Registry from January 1, 1991 through December 31, 2000, based on data from 119,363 patients according to the new AJCC sixth edition staging (3). Overall, 5-year colon cancer–specific survival for this entire cohort was 65.2% (3). Five-year colon cancer–specific survival by stage was 93.2% for stage I, 84.7% for stage IIa, 72.2% for stage IIb, 83.4% for stage IIIa, 64.1% for stage IIIb, 44.3% for stage IIIc, and 8.1% for stage IV cancer. Another large analysis based on the U.S. National Cancer Database showed a 5-year survival rate of 59.8% for stage IIIa, 42.0% for stage IIIb, and 27.3% for stage IIIc colon cancer in 50,042 patients from 1987 to 1993 (4).

The initial diagnosis of colon adenocarcinoma is made by colonoscopic examination and biopsies of the tumor. The diagnosis and staging is discussed in detail in Chapter 42.

SURGERY FOR COLON CANCER

Surgery is the mainstay of treatment for patients with colon adenocarcinoma and has a curative intent in patients with locoregional disease. The goal of surgical treatment is a wide resection of the primary tumor with all locoregional lymph nodes that follow the arterial blood supply of the colonic segment. The essential role of the surgeon has been recognized, and in the absence of standardized operation techniques, the surgeon is an important variable influencing the oncologic outcome. Most patients will undergo elective surgery, and mechanical bowel cleaning has historically been considered an essential component of the preoperative preparation of the patient. This has, however, recently been questioned (5), and the evidence that suggests that luminal cleaning is not essential to allow a safe colonic anastomosis is growing. Occasionally, emergency resection is required in patients with colonic obstruction. In patients with an imminent blowout of the caecum, either an on-table lavage or a subtotal colectomy can be performed. In critically ill patients, a Hartmann-type resection can be the best option.

Clinical T4 tumors directly invading other structures and organs require a more complex "en bloc" resection to obtain an adequate resection margin. Local inoperability in colon cancer is rare and relates to direct invasion of the tumor of the corpus of the pancreas or extensive regional lymph node spread into the mesentery of the small bowel. Exceptionally, a neoadjuvant preoperative chemotherapy or chemoradiotherapy may be considered so the resection can be performed with greater chance of clear margins and/or organ preservation. A "temporary" ileocolic bypass can be performed to avoid bowel obstruction during this treatment.

It is seldom that the medical condition of the patient can prohibit a surgical intervention.

The standard curative colon resection for adenocarcinoma is based on resection with adequate proximal and distal margins and a regional lymphadenectomy. About 10 cm of the proximal and distal colon is to be resected in order to reduce the risk of leaving paracolic nodes. Preoperative colonoscopy with tattooing is recommended in small, early lesions in order to facilitate intraoperative localization and decision

TABLE 43.1

STAGES AS DEFINED BY THE AMERICAN JOINT COMMITTEE ON CANCER
IN RELATION TO SURVIVAL

Staging system	T stage	N stage	M stage	5-Year survival (%)
I	T1 or T2	N0	M0	93.2[a]
IIa	T3	N0	M0	84.7[a]
IIb	T4	N0	M0	72.2[a]
IIIa	T1 or T2	N1	M0	83.4[a]–59.8[b]
IIIb	T3 or T4	N1	M0	64.1[a]–42.0[b]
IIIc	Any T	N2	M0	44.3[a]–27.3[b]
IV	Any T	Any N	M1	8.1[a]

T1, tumor invades submucosa; T2, tumor invades muscularis propria; N0, no regional lymph node
metastasis; M0, no distant metastasis; T3, tumor invades through the muscularis propria into the
subserosa or into nonperitonealized pericolic tissues; T4, tumor directly invades other organs or structures
and/or perforates visceral peritoneum; N1, metastasis to one to three regional lymph nodes; N2,
metastasis to four or more regional lymph nodes; M1, distant metastasis.
[a] According to the Surveillance, Epidemiology, and End Results database (3).
[b] According to the U.S. National Cancer Database (4).
Adapted from refs. 1–4.

making. The regional lymphadenectomy is based on the arterial blood supply to the particular portion of the colon. A "no touch" mobilization and high (central) ligation of the vessels of the tumor-bearing colon segment are part of the surgical standards. Surgeons who advocate the "no touch" technique ligate the lymphovascular structures prior to mobilization. A lesion in the right colon requires removal of mesentery with ileocolic and right colic arteries with the right branch of the middle colic artery. Transverse colon lesions require resection of the mesentery with the middle colic artery. In advanced stages, lymph nodes can be found at the base of the gastroepiploic vessels, and a radical omentectomy seems to be indicated in these cases. Lesions in the descending colon require removal of the left colic artery, as well as the left branch of the middle colic artery and its associated mesentery. Sigmoid colon lesions require removal of the superior rectal artery and sigmoid branches with a colorectal anastomosis (anterior resection). The presence of a lesion at watershed areas of vascular supply (lesions at the hepatic or splenic flexure) can therefore indicate more extensive resections. New evidence points at the importance to obtain a broad and intact "mesocolic" resection to avoid locoregional recurrence (in agreement with the concept of total mesorectal resection in rectal cancer) (Figs. 43.1–43.4).

Occasionally, the presence of synchronous colon cancers or multiple colon adenomas that cannot be resected endoscopically, or information consistent with the hereditary nonpolyposis colon cancer syndrome, will indicate a subtotal or total colectomy with ileorectal anastomosis. Prophylactic oophorectomy seems to be of no survival benefit; only infiltrated or grossly abnormal ovaries have to be removed.

The appropriate extent of colonic resection and lymphadenectomy has been controversial. The rationale for an

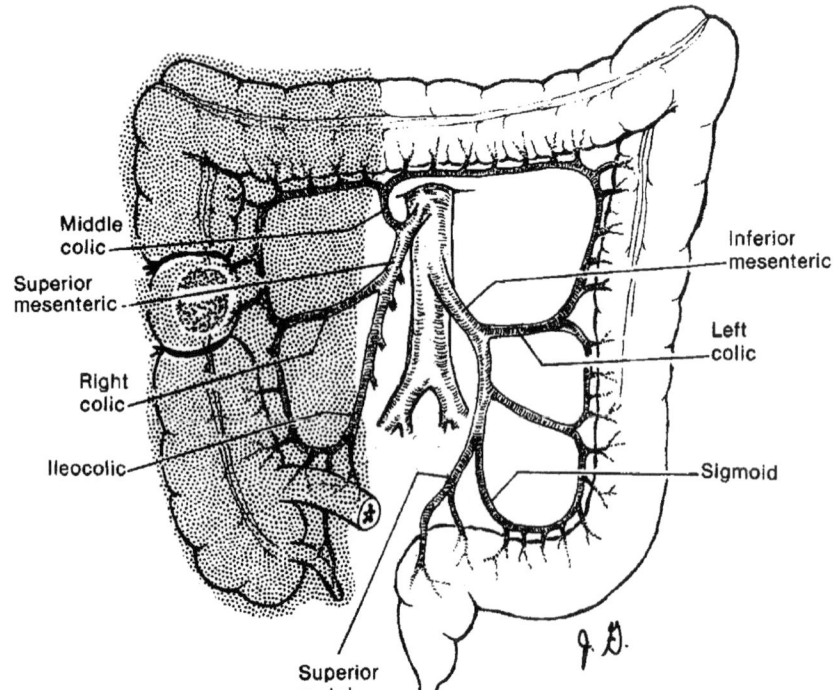

Middle colic
Superior mesenteric
Right colic
Ileocolic
Inferior mesenteric
Left colic
Sigmoid
Superior rectal

FIGURE 43.1. Right hemicolectomy. Reprinted with permission from Sharma S, Saltz LB, Ota DM, Chawla AK, Haller DG, and Willett CG. Colon cancer: management of locoregional disease. In: Kelsen DP, Daly JM, Kern SE, Levin B, and Tepper JE, eds. *Gastrointestinal oncology: principles and practice.* Philadelphia: Lippincott Williams & Wilkins, 2002;755–780.

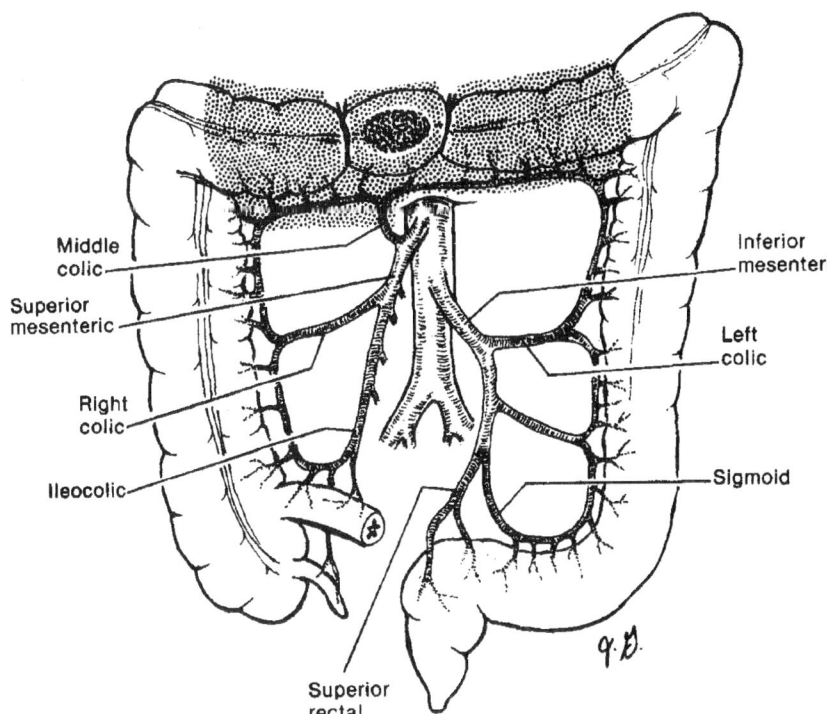

FIGURE 43.2. Transverse colectomy. Reprinted with permission from Sharma S, Saltz LB, Ota DM, Chawla AK, Haller DG, and Willett CG. Colon cancer: management of locoregional disease. In: Kelsen DP, Daly JM, Kern SE, Levin B, and Tepper JE, eds. *Gastrointestinal oncology: principles and practice.* Philadelphia: Lippincott Williams & Wilkins, 2002;755–780.

extended lymphadenectomy is that a wider dissection removes more lymph nodes with possible metastatic deposits and thereby increases the chances of cure. Although randomized trials comparing extended with limited lymphadenectomy have not shown that an extended lymphadenectomy improves the prognosis compared to a limited resection, there is a general agreement that a large number of lymph nodes should be recovered. It is often agreed that at least 12 lymph nodes should be removed. In the Intergroup Trial INT-0089 of adjuvant chemotherapy for high-risk patients with stage II and

stage III colon cancer, a secondary analysis demonstrated that examining more nodes was associated with increase of survival in both node-negative and node-positive patients (6). In this study, the median number of nodes removed at colectomy was 11 (range 1–87). This is similar to the lymph node yield in colectomy specimen after "standardized resection" reported in randomized trials comparing open and laparoscopic resections for colon cancer: 11.1–11.1 (7), 12.1–11.1 (8), 12–12 (9), and 10–10 (10). However, using a mathematical model based on data from the Intergroup Trial INT-0089, it was

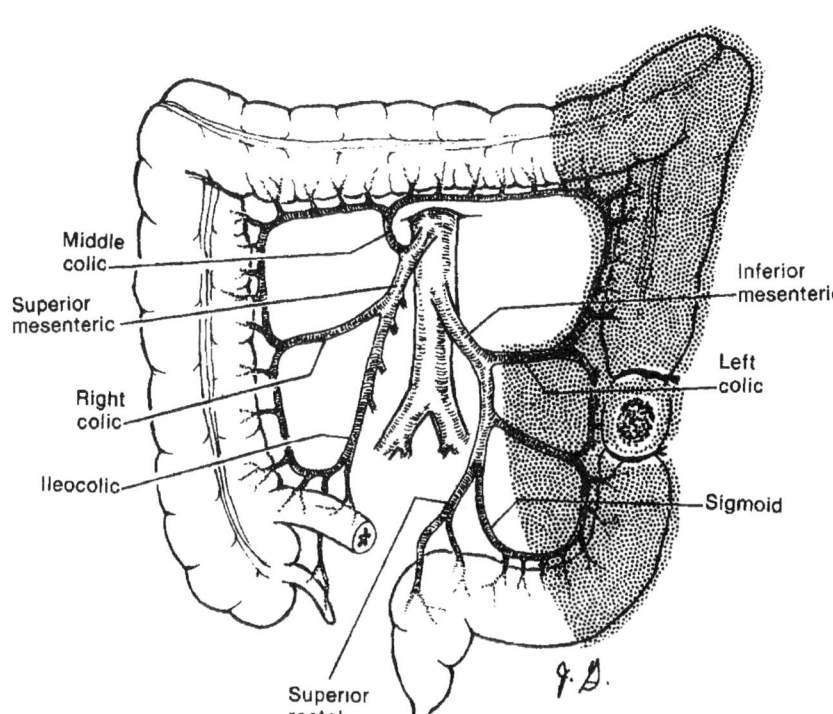

FIGURE 43.3. Left colectomy. Reprinted with permission from Sharma S, Saltz LB, Ota DM, Chawla AK, Haller DG, and Willett CG. Colon cancer: management of locoregional disease. In: Kelsen DP, Daly JM, Kern SE, Levin B, and Tepper JE, eds. *Gastrointestinal oncology: principles and practice.* Philadelphia: Lippincott Williams & Wilkins, 2002;755–780.

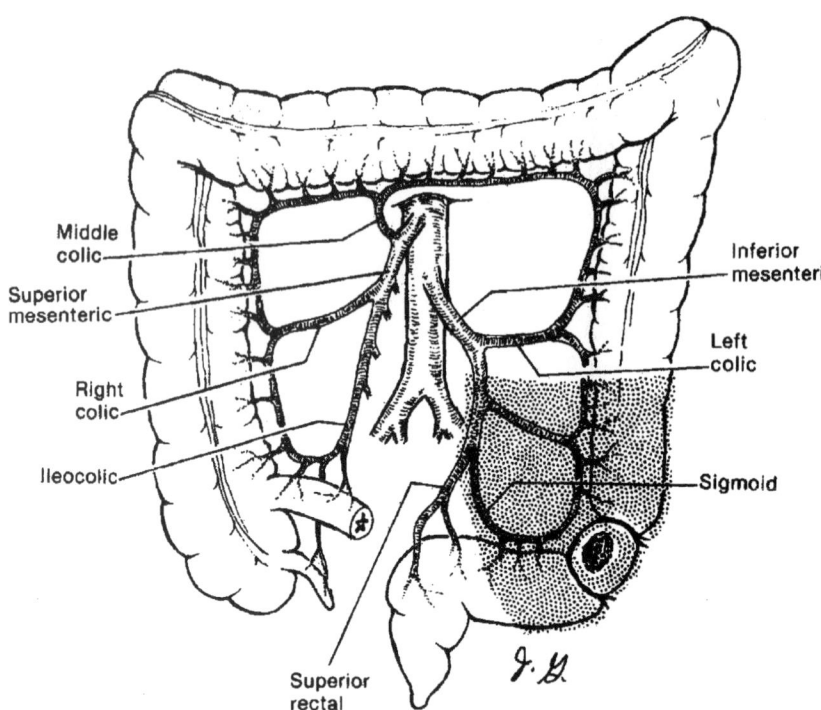

FIGURE 43.4. Sigmoid colectomy. Reprinted with permission from Sharma S, Saltz LB, Ota DM, Chawla AK, Haller DG, and Willett CG. Colon cancer: management of locoregional disease. In: Kelsen DP, Daly JM, Kern SE, Levin B, and Tepper JE, eds. *Gastrointestinal oncology: principles and practice*. Philadelphia: Lippincott Williams & Wilkins, 2002;755–780.

suggested that more than 40 nodes would need to be examined in a patient with an early stage (T1/T2) cancer for the probability to be 85% that the patient is node negative. With 18 nodes, the probability was only 25% of being truly node negative. For T3 and T4 tumors, 40 and 30 nodes, respectively, would need to be examined to achieve an 85% probability of being node negative. When 18 lymph nodes are examined, the probability of being truly node negative is >25% for T3 tumors and >50% for T4 tumors. On the basis of this analysis, a strong effort must be made to improve the surgical technique and our methods of pathological analysis (11). Special techniques such as fat clearance or submission of the entire mesenteric tissue for pathological examination after manual node dissection have been evaluated. These techniques are labor intensive and do not seem to upstage a clinically relevant number of hematoxylin and eosin node-negative patients (12). Also, sentinel lymph node (SLN) mapping has been applied and found to be safe and feasible in colon cancer after appropriate training (13,14). It has the advantage of a more focused pathological examination of the nodes that are identified as sentinel lymph nodes by using techniques such as immunohistochemistry and polymerase chain reaction (PCR). As many as 18% to 25% of patients have been upstaged from stage II to stage III after metastatic disease was detected in the sentinel node (15,16).

A 25% recurrence rate in patients with node-negative CRC suggests that current staging practices are inadequate. With an adequate surgical technique, this may be related to understaging. Thus, micrometastases or free tumor cells have been searched and identified in blood, bone marrow, and lymph nodes (LNs). Micrometastases in LNs are defined as >0.2 mm but <2 mm, and isolated tumor cells as <0.2 mm. In some institutions, all patients with isolated tumor cells and micrometastasis are receiving adjuvant chemotherapy. Instead of performing the rather expensive, labor-intensive, and time-consuming multiple sections with immunohistochemical staining or PCR on all LNs in the operative specimen, a more focused analysis of the SLNs has been applied in colon cancer. SLNs are defined as the first LNs along the direct lymphatic pathway from the primary tumor. They are identified by injecting vital blue dye close to the tumor site. Lymphatic mapping with SLN identi-

fication has been shown to be reproducible after appropriate training (13). It does not, however, replace standard pathological examination of the locoregional LNs.

The SLN concept aims to enable a pathologist to analyze more meticulously one or a few LNs harboring the highest risk of metastatic disease (14). SLN assessment has been applied for colonic cancer and resulted in a high rate of node identification and pathological upgrading. There is, however, no conformity regarding the procedure (in vivo and ex vivo staining), and there is too little evidence to allow its recommendation.

Blood loss should be minimized during surgery with meticulous attention to hemostasis in order to avoid the immunosuppressive effect associated with transfusions and to not increase the risk of recurrence.

Location of Laparoscopic Colonic Cancer Resection

The interest in the use of minimally invasive surgical techniques to treat benign disease of the gastrointestinal tract has been extended to colonic neoplasms. The early enthusiasm was tempered by cautionary reports on high occurrences of port-site metastases. A small series presenting an alarming 21% incidence of port-site metastases in 1994 initiated a virtually worldwide moratorium of laparoscopic colectomy for cancer outside the ongoing prospective randomized trials. More basic research was begun to elucidate the problem because there was a potential danger that the CO_2 pneumoperitoneum served as a potential vector for exfoliated tumor cells, which then could be trapped within the small wounds of the trocar sites. It became progressively clear that port-site metastasis was a dramatic side effect of the learning curve. The actual port-site recurrence rate is <1% and comparable with the rate of wound recurrences noted after open surgery. Recent evidence from randomized controlled trials indicates no oncosurgical disadvantage of laparoscopic colon cancer resection compared to an open resection.

In 2002, the first results of a prospective randomized trial in 219 patients with colon cancer (the so-called Barcelona Trial) were published and generated a lot of interest and enthusiasm. The oncologic outcome not only seemed comparable to the open approach but also a significant reduction in local recurrence and an improved diseasefree survival (DFS) in stage III patients was found (7). These findings fit well with data from experimental studies, suggesting that a decrease in perioperative immunosuppression, as a result of a laparoscopic approach, could lead to a decrease in tumor spread. In 2004, the 3-year results of a U.S. multicenter prospective randomized trial on laparoscopic versus open surgery (COST Trial: Clinical Outcomes of Surgical Therapy Study Group) in 872 patients with adenocarcinoma of the colon showed a similar DFS and tumor recurrence rate in all stages (9). A prospective randomized trial from Hong Kong focused on the outcome of 403 patients with rectosigmoid adenocarcinoma and found no difference in survival or in DFS (8). The conversion rate of laparoscopy to open laparotomy varies between 11% and 23% in the randomized controlled trials and is most often related to tumor characteristics. The postoperative morbidity is lower in the laparoscopic group, mainly related to a lower rate of wound complications and complications in older and compromised patients. Laparoscopic colectomy is associated with decreased postoperative pain, faster ileus resolution, shorter hospitalization, and improved cosmesis when compared with open colectomy. The postoperative mortality is similar in both groups. Hospital stay is shorter in the laparoscopic group. Thus, the laparoscopic technique has become a valid alternative to open laparotomy for resection of colon cancer. The previously mentioned trials have been criticized because evidence-based principles of fast track (open) surgery were not described or implemented, inducing a potential bias in early outcome results (17). Limitations of the laparoscopic approach include the technical requirements of advanced laparoscopic skills and training, increased operative time, and equipment costs. Surgeons performing laparoscopic colectomy should be adequately experienced and certified to ensure successful outcomes. Despite these limitations, patient recovery benefits may offset the increased operative costs and result in improved cost effectiveness overall.

ADJUVANT TREATMENT

The standard adjuvant treatment of colon cancer consists of chemotherapy. Although certain patients with colon cancer are at higher risk for local recurrence, the administration of postoperative radiotherapy or chemoradiotherapy has not been studied systematically in randomized studies. The published reports suggesting a benefit of postoperative radiotherapy or chemoradiotherapy in selected cases are nonrandomized single-institution retrospective analyses.

Although stage II and III colon cancers have significantly different recurrence and survival rates, most randomized studies to date have recruited both stage II and III patients, often with preplanned subgroup analyses, in an attempt to determine the efficacy of chemotherapy by stage. In stage I colon cancer, adjuvant chemotherapy is not indicated in view of the good prognosis of patients with stage I colon cancer.

Adjuvant Chemotherapy for Stage III Colon Cancer

Since the mid-1990s, it is generally recommended to treat patients with stage III or lymph node-positive colon cancer with adjuvant chemotherapy. It has indeed been shown that adjuvant chemotherapy decreases the relapse rate and improves the

survival in stage III colon cancer. It has been reported that the number of patients treated with adjuvant chemotherapy increased in the United States from 39% in 1991 to 64% in 2002 (18). This analysis also demonstrates that the use of adjuvant chemotherapy was not homogeneously incorporated in every patient population, at least in the first period of observation (18). Patients older than 80 years were less frequently treated with adjuvant chemotherapy, patients with more invasive tumors and a greater number of involved lymph nodes were more likely to receive adjuvant therapy, and women received adjuvant therapy less frequently than men. The perception of greater potential risk because of comorbidities among elderly patients and the perceived greater potential benefit of adjuvant therapy among patients with more aggressive disease help explain the first two observations, but there is no clear reason for the gender differences observed (19). The central issue regarding adjuvant chemotherapy is the difficulty in assessing its real benefit for an individual patient. The recommendation is generally based on the proof of efficacy in a selected population at risk for disease recurrence. The decision-making process is always complex. The physician's understanding of the potential benefit is influenced by his or her own prejudice and the patient's confidence is influenced by beliefs and fear. Factors such as comorbidities, socioeconomic status, and low adherence to therapy are among the well-described causes for not using adjuvant chemotherapy. Ongoing studies of molecular markers for CRC should help determine which patients benefit most from adjuvant therapy.

Important progress has been made in our knowledge on the options for adjuvant chemotherapy and on the outcome of patients with colon cancer treated with postoperative chemotherapy.

5-Fluorouracil/Levamisole for 1 Year

The intergroup trial (INT-0035) was the first large-scale study to demonstrate a significant effect of postoperative adjuvant treatment in patients with stage III colon cancer. This trial randomized 1,296 patients with stage II and III cancer (929 with stage III cancer) to one of the three arms:

- Surgery alone
- Surgery plus 12 months of levamisole
- Surgery plus 12 months of 5-fluorouracil (5-FU) and levamisole

The study showed a 15% absolute reduction ($\pm 40\%$ relative reduction) in the risk of recurrence and a 16% absolute reduction (33% relative reduction) in the overall death rate with a combination of surgery plus 5-FU/levamisole in patients with stage III colon cancer (20,21). The Netherlands Adjuvant Colorectal Cancer Project (NACCP) also demonstrated efficacy of 5-FU/levamisole compared to no adjuvant treatment in a randomized trial of patients with stage II and III CRC (22). The 5-year survival rate was significantly higher in the adjuvant treatment arm: 68% versus 58%.

5-FU/Folinic Acid for 6 Months

A number of studies in the 1990s have shown the efficacy of 5-FU modulated by folinic acid (FA) when compared with no postoperative treatment. The Canadian and European consortium trial (International Multicentre Pooled Analysis of Colorectal Cancer Trials [IMPACT]) is a combined analysis of the three trials that compared adjuvant treatment with high-dose 5-FU/FA with no treatment in nearly 1,500 patients. In this study, a 22% relative risk reduction in mortality at 3 years in Dukes' C patients has been reported (23). An Italian study that was similar in design, but smaller, showed a 39% reduction in mortality for the patients treated with 5-FU/FA (24). A North Central Cancer Treatment Group

(NCCTG) trial established the efficacy of 6 months adjuvant therapy with 5-FU/low-dose FA compared with observation after surgery: 74% versus 63% of patients were alive at 5 years (25). The National Surgical Adjuvant Breast and Bowel Project (NSABP) protocol C-03 indicated a DFS (73% vs. 64%) and overall survival (84% vs. 77%) advantage for 5-FU/FA compared with MOF (methyl-CCNU, Oncovin, 5-FU) at 3 years for patients with Dukes' stage B and C colon cancer (26). The control arm in this study (MOF) had previously shown a borderline survival advantage over surgery alone in the adjuvant setting.

Three large adjuvant American trials were later presented in which several thousand patients were treated. In a randomized study by the NCCTG and the National Cancer Institute of Canada, there was no additional benefit associated with the administration of a full year of chemotherapy compared with only 6 months of treatment with the same regimen (27). In the same study, if only 6 months of chemotherapy were administered, the patient's survival was significantly inferior with 5-FU plus levamisole compared with the three-drug combination of 5-FU, levamisole, and FA (27). The INT 0089 Trial demonstrated no additional benefit from the addition of levamisole to 5-FU/FA and showed no difference in DFS and survival when 5-FU/FA was administered for 6 to 8 months compared to 5-FU/levamisole for 12 months (28). The NSABP C-04 study demonstrated similar results for 1 year of treatment with 5-FU/levamisole, 5-FU/FA, and 5-FU/FA/levamisole (29). The German group showed a superior survival for 5-FU/FA compared to 5-FU/levamisole for 12 months in Dukes' C patients: 88.9 versus 78.6 months (30).

Taking into account the increased toxicity of the three-drug combination compared with the combination of 5-FU/FA, an adjuvant treatment with 5-FU/FA for 6 to 8 months became the generally accepted standard option in the mid-1990s (31,32).

Regimens of 5-FU: Infused versus Bolus Regimens

Most of the initial studies in the 1990s were done with bolus regimens of 5-FU/FA: the Roswell Park regimen that consists of a weekly administration of FA (500 mg/m^2) plus 5-FU (500 mg/m^2) during 6 weeks followed by 2 weeks of rest for four cycles and the NCCTG/Mayo Clinic regimen that consists of FA (20 mg/m^2) + 5-FU (425 mg/m^2) days 1 to 5 repeated every 4 to 5 weeks for 6 to 7 months. In a large randomized trial (Quasar 1 study), the Quick and Simple and Reliable (Quasar) Collaborative Group in the United Kingdom showed no difference between a high and low dose of FA in combination with 5-FU and no benefit of adding levamisole to the combination of 5-FU/FA (33).

The French Gercor group studied the role of an infused regimen of 5-FU/FA, the so-called LV5FU2 or de Gramont regimen (34). This schedule consists of FA 200 mg/m^2 over 2 hours followed by bolus 5-FU 400 mg/m^2 and infused 5-FU 600 mg/m^2 over 22 hours on days 1 and 2 and repeated every 2 weeks. In a 2 × 2 factorial design, 905 patients with stage II/III colon cancer were randomized to LV5FU2 or bolus 5-FU/FA (5-FU 400 mg/m^2 and FA 200 mg/m^2 days 1−5, repeated every 28 days). In addition, patients were randomized to a total duration of 24 or 36 weeks of chemotherapy. The study showed no significant differences in DFS and overall survival between the two groups. Rates of grade 3/4 diarrhea, neutropenia, and mucositis were significantly lower in the LV5FU2 arm compared to a bolus 5-FU/FA regimen (34,35). Based on this trial and on the superiority and better tolerance of the infused regimens compared to bolus regimens in patients with metastatic colon cancer, many clinicians consider the LV5FU2 a more optimal option compared to the bolus regimens of 5-FU/FA in the adjuvant treatment of colon cancer.

The Pan-European Trial Adjuvant Colon Cancer (PETACC)-2 Trial is investigating this question in more detail in stage III colon cancer. Sixteen hundred and three patients have been randomized between a bolus and an infused 5-FU/FA regimen. No difference in efficacy was shown between the bolus and infused regimen. However, the bolus regimen was more toxic (36).

A UK trial compared a protracted infusion of 5-FU 300 mg/m^2 daily for 12 weeks to a bolus regimen (Mayo Clinic regimen) for 6 months in 801 patients with Dukes' B and C colon and rectal cancer. There was no difference in relapsefree survival (RFS). A trend toward an improved 5-year survival in the infused 5-FU arm was found: 75.7 versus 71.5% ($p = 0.08$) (37). This trial, however, does not change the concept of the duration of treatment because rectal and colon cancer patients were both included and because the small sample size precluded final conclusions.

New Drugs

Oral Fluoropyrimidines. Several studies have investigated the activity of the oral fluoropyrimidines in the adjuvant treatment of colon cancer. In a meta-analysis of three randomized Japanese trials in 5,233 patients with stage I, II, or III CRC oral adjuvant chemotherapy (oral 5-FU, Uracil ftorafur (UFT), or carmofur; some patients also received mitomycin C) was compared with observation. DFS was better for patients treated with oral fluoropyrimidines: The hazard ratio (HR) was 0.85 ($p = 0.001$). Overall survival was also superior in patients receiving an oral fluoropyrimidine: The HR was 0.89 ($p = 0.04$) (38).

The X-Act study randomized 1,987 patients with resected stage III colon cancer between capecitabine 2,500 mg/m^2 days 1 to 14 every 21 days and bolus 5-FU/FA for 6 months. DFS at 3 years in the capecitabine group was at least equivalent to that in the 5-FU/FA group: $p < 0.001$ for the comparison of the upper limit of the HR with the noninferiority margin of 1.20. Capecitabine improved RFS (HR, 0.86; 95% CI, 0.74−0.99; $p = 0.04$) and was associated with significantly fewer adverse events than 5-FU/FA (Table 43.2) (39). The 3-year survival was 81.3% versus 77.6% for capecitabine versus 5-FU/FA (HR, 0.84; 95% CI, 0.69−1.01; $p = 0.07$).

The NSABP C-06 trial compared adjuvant IV 5-FU/FA (Roswell Park regimen for three cycles) with UFT/FA (300 mg/m^2/day and folinic acid 90 mg/day days 1−28, each 35 days for five cycles) in 1,608 patients with stage II or III colon cancer. No difference in 5-year DFS (66.9% vs. 68.3%) or 5-year overall survival (78.7% vs. 78.7%) has been demonstrated between the two arms (Table 43.2). Both regimens also had similar toxicity profiles (40).

These studies clearly support the hypothesis that the oral fluoropyrimidines are at least as effective as IV 5-FU/FA in the adjuvant treatment of stage III colon cancer. In view of the data: improved RR in metastatic CRC, the more global availability of capecitabine, the more optimally designed trial in the adjuvant treatment and improved tolerance compared to 5-FU/FA, capecitabine is the preferred oral fluoropyrimidine.

Oxaliplatin. The effect of adding oxaliplatin to 5-FU/FA in patients with stage II and III colon cancer was investigated in two large randomized trials.

In the MOSAIC trial, 2,246 patients with stage II and III colon cancer were randomized to 6 months treatment with LV5FU2 (de Gramont schedule) or FOLFOX-4 (identical 5-FU/FA + oxaliplatin 85 mg/m^2 on day 1 of every cycle). Forty percent of patients had stage II colon cancer and 60% stage III. The primary end point was the 3-year DFS and was defined as time from randomization to relapse or death; second CRCs were considered as relapses, whereas noncolorectal tumors were disregarded in the analyses. After a median

TABLE 43.2

ORAL FLUOROPYRIMIDINES IN THE ADJUVANT TREATMENT OF COLON CANCER

		Regimen	Diseasefree survival			Relapsefree survival			Survival		
			3 year	HR	p	3 year	HR	p	3 year	HR	p
X-Act (39)	Stage III N = 1,987	5-FU/FA capecitabine	60.6 64.2	0.87 (0.75−1.00)	0.05	61.9 65.5	0.86 (0.74−0.99)	0.04	77.6 81.3	0.84 (0.69−1.01)	0.07
			5 year			5 year			5 year		
NSABP C-06 (40)	Stage II/III N = 1,608	5-FU/FA UFT/FA	68.3 66.9		0.79	76.4 74.5		0.52	78.7 78.7		0.88

HR, hazard ratio; 5-FU, 5-fluorouracil; FA, folinic acid; UFT, uracil ftorafur.

follow-up of 56.2 months, the DFS was significantly higher in the FOLFOX-4 arm (76.4%) compared to the LV5FU2 arm (69.8%). The HR for DFS was 0.77 (95% CI, 0.65−0.90; p <0.001). A statistically significant reduction of the relapse rate was found in the subgroup of stage III colon cancer patients: HR, 0.75 (95% CI, 0.62−0.89), with an absolute difference of 8.6%. A trend, but no significant difference in the subgroup of stage II group colon cancer patients, was found: HR, 0.82 (95% CI, 0.60−1.13), with an absolute difference of 3.5% (Table 43.3). The survival difference in the total patient population (stage II and III) at 4 years did not yet reach significance: 84.9% versus 82.8% (HR, 0.91; 95% CI, 0.75−1.11) (41,42). After a follow-up of 6 years the overall survival was 78.6% in the FOLFOX-4 group compared to 76.0% in the

LV5FU2 group (HR 0.85; 95% CI 0.72 − 1.01; p = 0.057). The survival difference was, however, statistically significant different in the stage III group I favour of the FOLFOX-4 group: 73.0% compared to 68.6% (HR 0.80; 95% CI 0.66 − 0.98; p = 0.029). In the stage II group there was no difference in survival: 86.9% compared to 86.8% respectively (updated presentation at ASCO 2007 by A De Gramont). In general, FOLFOX-4 was well tolerated. The all-cause mortality on the trial was 0.5% in both arms. Grade 3/4 neutropenia occurred in 41% in FOLFOX-4 versus 5% in the LV5FU2 arm. Peripheral neuropathy occurred in 92% of the patients who received oxaliplatin. In total, 12% developed grade 3 neuropathy; however, this grade 3 persisted for 12 months in only 1.2% and for 24 months in 0.5%. Grade 2 neuropathy was present in 4%

TABLE 43.3

COMBINATION CHEMOTHERAPY IN THE ADJUVANT TREATMENT OF COLON CANCER

Trial	Stage	N	Regimen	Diseasefree survival[a] (%)		HR/p value
				3 year	5 year	
OXALIPLATIN						
MOSAIC (41,42)	II/III	2,246	LV5FU2 FOLFOX-4	72.9 78.2	67.4 73.3	0.77; p <0.001[c]
	III[b]	1,347	LV5FU2 FOLFOX-4	65.3 72.2	58.9 66.4	0.76; p <0.005[c]
NSABP C-07 (43)	II/III	2,492	Bolus 5-FU/FA FLOX	71.6 76.5		0.79; p = 0.004
	III[b]	1,774	Bolus 5-FU/FA FLOX	65.5 72.2		0.77; NA
IRINOTECAN						
CALGB-C89803 (45)	III	1,264	Bolus 5-FU/FA IFL	69 66	61 59	NA; p = 0.85
ACCORD 2 (47)	High risk III	400	LV5FU2 IF	60 51		1.19; NS
PETACC 3 (48)	III	2,111	LV5FU2 IF	60.3 63.3		0.89; 0.091
	II/III[b]	3,005	LV5FU2 IF	66.8 69.6		0.88; 0.050

HR, hazard ratio; LV5FU2, de Gramont regimen; FOLFOX-4, oxaliplatin + de Gramont regimen; 5-FU/FA, 5-fluorouracil/folinic acid; FLOX, oxaliplatin + bolus 5-FU/FA; NA, not applicable; IFL, irinotecan + bolus 5-FU/FA; NS, nonsignificant; IF, irinotecan + de Gramont regimen.
[a]Diseasefree survival (DFS)—definitions and follow-up times are different in various trials.
[b]Secondary endpoint.
[c]HR for DFS at 3 year.

at 12 months and 3% at 24 months and grade 1 neuropathy in 22% at 12 months and 14% at 24 months, showing an improvement over time in patients who developed peripheral neuropathy (42).

In the NSABP C-07 trial, 2,492 patients were randomized to a bolus regimen of 5-FU/FA (Roswell Park regimen for three cycles) or bolus 5-FU/FA + oxaliplatin (FLOX regimen = identical 5-FU/FA regimen plus oxaliplatin 85 mg/m² on days 1, 15, and 29 of each cycle) (43). Twenty-nine percent of patients had stage II colon cancer and 71% stage III. The primary end point was 3-year DFS, defined as recurrence, second primary colon cancer, new cancers of any type, or death from any cause. The 3-year DFS was improved for patients treated with FLOX compared to 5-FU/FA: 76.5% versus 71.6%. The HR for DFS was 0.79 (95% CI, 0.67–0.93; $p = 0.004$). Survival data are not yet available. In total, 85.4% of patients treated with FLOX suffered from neuropathy during treatment and 29.4% at 12 months after stopping treatment. Eight percent of patients had grade 3 neuropathy during treatment and 0.5% at 12 months after ending treatment. The number of patients with gastrointestinal toxicity was relatively high in both arms. In total, 1.2% died during FLOX treatment and 1.1% during 5-FU/FA (43) (Table 43.3).

This NSABP trial is important because it confirms the increased activity of oxaliplatin when added to 5-FU/FA in the adjuvant treatment of colon cancer. However, it does not change the concept of the type of 5-FU/FA regimen. In general, it is accepted that infused regimens of 5-FU/FA are a more optimal way of administering 5-FU/FA than bolus regimens. The experience in metastatic CRC and also in the French Gercor adjuvant of bolus 5-FU/FA versus infused 5-FU/FA supports this choice.

In the XELOXA trial, 1,886 patients were randomized between a bolus regimen of 5-FU/FA (Mayo Clinic regimen or Roswell Park regimen) for 6 months and the combination capecitabine and oxaliplatin. Efficacy results will be available at the earliest at the end of 2007. Toxicity results showed that the combination of capecitabine and oxaliplatin has a manageable safety profile in the adjuvant treatment of colon cancer (44).

Irinotecan. Three randomized trials have been reported with 5-FU/FA ± irinotecan in the adjuvant treatment of colon cancer.

The U.S. CALGB 89803 randomized patients with stage III colon cancer to bolus 5-FU/FA (Roswell Park regimen) or bolus 5-FU/FA + irinotecan (IFL = 5-FU 500 mg/m², FA 20 mg/m², and irinotecan 125 mg/m² weekly for 4 weeks on and 2 weeks off for a total of 30 weeks) (45). The trial closed due to the findings of a higher treatment-related death rate in patients treated with IFL (46). A total of 1,264 patients were enrolled, and after a median follow-up of 4.8 years, no difference in DFS or in overall survival was observed (45) (Table 43.3). Therefore, the IFL regimen is not an option in the adjuvant treatment of stage III colon cancer.

The French ACCORD 2 trial compared the LV5FU2 regimen with LV5FU2 + irinotecan 180 mg/m² (IF regimen) on day 1 of every cycle for 6 months in high-risk stage III colon cancer. High-risk stage III colon cancer was defined as N2 or N1/N2 detected by occlusion or perforation. The DFS was not improved with irinotecan: 60% (95% CI, 52.7–66.5) for LV5FU2 and 51% in the IF arm (95% CI, 43.6–57.7). The HR was 1.19 (95% CI, 0.9–1.59), and the toxicity was higher in the IF arm (47) (Table 43.3).

In the PETACC-3 trial, 3,005 patients with stage II and III colon cancer were randomized to infused 5-FU/FA ± irinotecan. In total, 894 patients had stage II, and 2,111 had stage III colon cancer. The primary end point was the 3-year DFS for patients treated with LV5FU2 ± irinotecan in stage III colon cancer patients. The DFS was defined as relapse, death from any cause, second primary colon cancer, or second primary cancer other than colon cancer. Secondary end points were DFS in

the pooled stage II/III population, RFS (= DFS with the exclusion of second primary other cancer) in stage III colon cancer, survival, and safety. There was an imbalance between the two arms: 17% had T4 tumors in the IF and 13% in the LV5FU2 arm ($p = 0.006$) because there was no stratification for T stage. At a relatively short follow-up of 38 months, the primary end point of the trial was not met. The 3-year DFS for stage III colon cancer was 63.3% in the IF arm versus 60.3% in the LV5FU2 arm. The HR for 3-year DFS was 0.89 (95% CI, 0.77–1.11; $p = 0.091$). The DFS for the pooled stage II and III population, a secondary end point, was borderline significant: 69.6% versus 66.8%. The HR for stage II/III was 0.88 (95% CI, 0.77–1.00; $p = 0.05$) (Table 43.3). The RFS for stage III patients was 66% versus 62.2%. The HR for 3-year RFS was 0.86 (95% CI, 0.75–1.00; $p = 0.045$) (48). Toxicity was slightly higher in the IF arm than in the LV5FU2 arm but was manageable. The 60-day mortality was <0.5% in both arms, and the mortality within 30 days of the last treatment was <1% in both arms (48). In view of these results, irinotecan is not indicated in the adjuvant treatment of colon cancer.

Monoclonal Antibodies

Edrecolomab is a murine IgG2 monoclonal antibody to the glycoprotein antigen 17-1A (or epithelial cell adhesion molecule [EpCAM]). An initial small randomized study in stage III CRC showed a lower relapse rate for patients treated with edrecolomab compared to observation after surgery alone (49). A large randomized study in 2,761 patients with stage III colon cancer failed to show an improved outcome for patients treated with 5-FU/FA + edrecolomab compared to 5-FU/FA: The 3-year survival was 74.7% in the edrocolomab/5-FU/FA arm versus 76.1% in the 5-FU/FA alone arm (HR, 0.94; 95% CI, 0.71–1.15; $p = 0.53$). Patients treated with edrecolomab alone had a lower DFS compared to patients with 5-FU/FA: 53% versus 65.5% (HR, 0.62; 95% CI, 0.53–0.73; $p < 0.0001$) (50).

Cetuximab is a chimeric monoclonal antibody targeting the epidermal growth factor receptor (EGFR) that is active in irinotecan-refractory EGFR-expressing metastatic CRC when given alone or in combination with irinotecan. In the first-line treatment of metastatic CRC, nonrandomized phase 2 studies showed promising results when cetuximab is combined with FOLFOX or FOLFIRI regimens in EGFR-expressing tumors and a large randomized phase 3 trial of FOLFIRI ± cetuximab has shown an increased progressionfree survival for the combination arm with cetuximab. Large studies are therefore ongoing in the United States and Europe in the adjuvant treatment of colon cancer evaluating FOLFOX ± cetuximab (protocols N0147 and PETACC 8) (Table 43.4).

Bevacizumab is a humanized monoclonal antibody that targets the vascular endothelial growth factor (VEGF), a growth factor essential for tumor angiogenesis. Randomized studies have shown the increased efficacy when bevacizumab is combined with irinotecan/5-FU/FA, oxaliplatin/5-FU/FA, and 5-FU/FA in the first-line treatment of metastatic CRC and with oxaliplatin/5-FU/FA in the second-line treatment of metastatic CRC. Three large studies in the adjuvant treatment of stage II/III colon cancer are ongoing. The NSABP C-08 protocol plans to randomize ~2,500 patients to 5-FU/FA/oxaliplatin ± bevacizumab. The Avant trial plans to randomize 3,450 patients with high-risk stage II and stage III colon cancer between 5-FU/FA/oxaliplatin with 5-FU/FA/oxaliplatin + bevacizumab and the combination capecitabine/oxaliplatin + bevacizumab. The Quasar 2 trial plans to randomize 2,240 patients with stage III and high-risk stage II colon cancer between capecitabine for 6 months and capecitabine plus bevacizumab (respectively 6 and 12 months) (Table 43.5).

The studies with cetuximab and bevacizumab are designed to further significantly improve the 3-year DFS in patients operated for stage II or III colon cancer.

TABLE 43.4

ONGOING TRIALS OF 5-FU/FA/OXALIPLATIN ± CETUXIMAB IN STAGE III COLON CANCER

Trial	n	Cancer	Treatment
PETACC-8	2,000	Stage III colon	FOLFOX-4 ± cetuximab
Intergroup 0147	2,300	Stage III colon	FOLFOX-6 ± cetuximab

5-FU/FA, 5-fluorouracil/folinic acid.

Intraportal or Intraperitoneal Chemotherapy

Several studies have investigated the role of immediately postoperative administration of chemotherapy either intraperitoneal or intraportal. Although a few studies showed a small benefit for patients treated with regional chemotherapy, larger randomized studies could not show an improved outcome for patients treated with systemic 5-FU–based chemotherapy in combination with intraportal or intraperitoneal chemotherapy (51).

Adjuvant Chemotherapy for Stage II Colon Cancer

The approach in stage II colon is certainly more controversial due to the lack of a large number of prospective randomized trials. Most of the data were derived from prospectively defined subgroup analyses of large trials, including stage II and III colon cancer patients. A pooled analysis of five randomized trials (IMPACT) failed to show a statistically significant benefit of adjuvant 5-FU/FA when compared with surgery alone in the subsets of patients with stage II disease. The 5-year survival estimates were not statistically different from patients treated with surgery alone (52). The NSABP concluded that patients with stage II colon cancer derive a similar benefit than patients with stage III colon cancer from a pooled analysis of Dukes' B and C patients (53). In this analysis, 1,565 (41%) patients were Dukes' B. However, the original trials differed substantially in the treatment regimens (53).

The best systematic review published examined 37 trials and 11 meta-analyses comparing chemotherapy with observation in stage II colon cancer. In this meta-analysis including 4,187 patients with stage II colon cancer, a trend toward a reduced mortality in patients receiving 5-FU–based chemotherapy compared to observation was found (HR, 0.87; 95% CI, 0.75–1.01; $p = 0.07$) (54).

Buyse and Piedbois provided a statistical perspective on the benefit of adjuvant therapy in stage II patients (55). They attributed the lack of a demonstrable survival benefit to the insufficient number of patients in previously reported trials, the relatively good prognosis of patients with stage II disease, and the competing non–cancer-related deaths in this population. They further described different approaches to evaluate the benefits of adjuvant therapy in stage II disease. The first approach is to consider the overall effect of therapy regardless of stage because there are no known a priori biological reasons for stage II tumors to be different from stage III tumors or to respond differently to adjuvant treatment. The second approach was to estimate the benefit in a meta-analysis of only stage II patients. One problem with this approach is the lack of consistent information provided on the stage II subsets in the trials analyzed; furthermore, the percentage of patients with stage II disease in each trial has been relatively small. The third approach is to perform tests of interaction between treatment effect and stage. Although this is the most sensitive approach, it requires adequate information and requires a high number of patients to demonstrate the benefit of therapy. In conclusion, although it seems likely that the same relative benefit results from adjuvant therapy in both stage II and stage III patients, the number of patients assessed in most individual studies is too small to detect and quantify absolute survival benefits from adjuvant therapy in stage II colon cancer.

Therefore, American Society of Clinical Oncology recommendations published in 2004 concluded the following:

[D]irect evidence from randomized controlled trials does not support the routine use of adjuvant chemotherapy for patients with stage II colon cancer. Patients and oncologists who accept the relative benefit in stage III disease as adequate indirect evidence of benefit for stage II disease are justified in considering the use of adjuvant chemotherapy, particularly for those patients with high-risk stage II disease. The ultimate clinical decision should be based on discussions with the patient about the nature of the evidence supporting treatment, the anticipated morbidity of treatment, the

TABLE 43.5

ONGOING TRIALS OF FLUOROPYRIMIDINE/OXALIPLATIN-BASED CHEMOTHERAPY ± BEVACIZUMAB IN HIGH-RISK STAGE II/STAGE III COLON CANCER

Trial	n	Cancer	Treatment
AVANT	3,450	High-risk stage II/III colon	FOLFOX-4 FOLFOX-4 + bevacizumab XELOX + bevacizumab
NSABP C-08	2,700	Stage II/III colon	FOLFOX-6 ± bevacizumab
QUASAR 2	2,240	High-risk stage II/III colon	Capecitabine ± bevacizumab

presence of high-risk prognostic features, on individual prognosis and patient preferences. (56)

Two recent randomized trials have reported specifically on the role of adjuvant therapy in patients with Dukes' B colon cancer. The Dutch NACPP study reported a similar benefit of 1 year of 5-FU/levamisole in patients with stage II colon cancer compared to patients with stage III colon cancer. In this trial, 1,029 patients with stage II or III (45% stage II) colon or rectal cancer were randomized between observation or 5-FU/levamisole. An increase in 5-year survival was reported in stage II colon cancer patients: 70% to 78% (22).

The data of the Quasar 2 trial have been presented more recently, showing a small but significant survival benefit from 5-FU−based chemotherapy (mainly 5-FU/FA) compared to surgery alone in patients with colon cancer with uncertain indication for adjuvant treatment. In this trial, 3,228 patients were randomized between observation and 5-FU modulated by high- or low-dose leucovorin with or without levamisole. Ninety-one percent had stage II CRC, and 71% had colon tumors (57). There was a reduced risk of recurrence with chemotherapy (HR, 0.78; 95% CI, 0.67−0.91; $p = 0.001$) and an improved 5-year survival in patients randomized to chemotherapy (HR, 0.83; 95% CI, 0.71−0.97; $p = 0.02$) (57). The Mosaic investigators also showed in a subgroup analysis that there was a trend toward an improved DFS in the subgroup of stage II colon cancer patients of FOLFOX compared to LV5FU2. However, the trial was not powered to show a statistical difference (41,42,58).

The most optimal and ideal situation is therefore to select patients who will derive most from an adjuvant treatment (31). The best ways to select patients are not known. The concept of the high-risk stage II colon cancer patients has therefore been introduced. Patients with a T4 tumor; with a tumor with vascular, lymphatic vessel, or perineural invasion; with a poorly differentiated adenocarcinoma; with a tumor presenting with obstruction; or with a perforating tumor, or patients with a high preoperative CEA level are at a higher risk for recurrence than patients without these characteristics (31,56). More prospective trials are therefore needed that focus on the predictive and prospective role of molecular markers in stage II colon cancer (31,59).

Molecular Markers

Risk stratification on the basis of histopathological TNM stage has been well documented and is the basis for adjuvant chemotherapy in colon cancer. In addition to the presence or absence of lymph node metastases, the number of histologically examined nodes is generally accepted as a prognostic factor, especially in stage II colon cancer (6). Tumor grade and histologic subtype are also prognostic factors: High-grade (poorly differentiated or undifferentiated) tumors and signet ring cell carcinomas have a worse prognosis than low-grade tumors and tumors without signet ring cells (3).

To better determine the prognosis of patients with colon cancer and to determine groups of patients that are most likely to benefit from an adjuvant treatment, better molecular characterization of the tumors is absolutely necessary. Several molecular markers have already demonstrated clinical efficacy as a prognostic marker: loss of heterozygosity (LOH), microsatellite instability (MSI), TGFβ RII mutation, and thymidylate synthase (TS). However, the role in the prediction of the benefit of adjuvant chemotherapy is unclear today. These and other molecular markers should therefore be evaluated in prospective randomized studies so they can contribute to the determination of an optimal adjuvant strategy in the future. Although several of the large randomized studies discussed in this chapter evaluated molecular markers (e.g., the PETACC 3 trial collected ~1,500 tumor blocks for the determination of TS, p53, DPD, telomerase, MSI, LOH, and other markers), many failed to do so.

End Points

In most of the trials evaluating the new agents, DFS was the primary endpoint. The correlation between 3-year DFS and 5-year survival in adjuvant colon trials has been studied in a large analysis (6). In this analysis of 18 trials, including more than 20,000 patients, a strong correlation between 3-year DFS and 5-year survival was shown. A small attenuation in the survival benefit was observed between these parameters. In almost all trials, the presence of a statistically significant DFS advantage at 3 years persisted at 5 years. This analysis, however, did not include oxaliplatin- or irinotecan-containing trials. It is therefore currently unknown whether this analysis and correlation is also applicable to the newer studies evaluating the newer agents.

Another important issue is the lack of uniformity of the definitions of DFS and RFS across the trials, as well as the lack of heterogeneity of the studied patient populations (e.g., stage III alone or stage II and III in the various trials) (60). The definitions of DFS are clearly not identical in all new trials. However, whether this impacts the results of the trials is unclear (61). Therefore, a plea for uniform definitions of endpoints and definitions of DFS and RFS in the adjuvant treatment of colon cancer is made.

Challenges in the Adjuvant Treatment of Colon Cancer

Many challenges and open questions, however, remain in the adjuvant treatment of colon cancer:

- The demonstration of a survival benefit with oxaliplatin/5-FU/FA in high risk stage II patients
- The understanding of the initial rather disappointing results of irinotecan in the adjuvant treatment of colon cancer, while it is active in metastatic CRC
- The demonstration of the role of capecitabine in combination regimens
- The demonstration of the activity of the novel targeted agents, such as bevacizumab and cetuximab
- The design of trials with uniform criteria and definitions of endpoints in adjuvant trials
- The integration of molecular markers in a prognostic classification and in a treatment algorithm
- The better selection of patients who benefit and who do not benefit from an adjuvant treatment
- The evaluation of shorter treatment duration in order to minimize the cumulative toxicity of oxaliplatin
- The demonstration of a larger impact of treatment in stage II
- The better selection of high-risk versus low-risk stage II colon cancer

CONCLUSION

A clear progress has been made in the adjuvant treatment of colon cancer. It is generally accepted that patients with stage III colon cancer, who are fit to receive an adjuvant treatment, should be offered adjuvant chemotherapy. A clinically meaningful and statistically significant reduction in the recurrence rate and improvement in the survival have been shown with adjuvant chemotherapy. For many years, the standard approach was 6 months of 5-FU/FA. It has been shown more recently that capecitabine is at least as active as IV 5-FU/FA in stage III colon cancer and is less toxic than 5-FU/FA and can therefore replace IV 5-FU/FA. The addition of oxaliplatin to 5-FU/FA improves the DFS in stage II and stage III colon cancer and the survival in stage III colon cancer. Long-term survival results are not yet available. Based on the results of the MOSAIC and NSABP C-07 trials, an adjuvant treatment of 6 months of FOLFOX can be recommended for patients with stage III colon cancer, who are fit to undergo this chemotherapy. The benefit of chemotherapy in stage II colon cancer is more limited and remains more controversial. A strategy of selecting patients for adjuvant chemotherapy based on risk factors is therefore often proposed in stage II colon cancer.

References

1. American Joint Committee on Cancer (AJCC). Missions and objectives. Available at: http://www.cancerstaging.org. Accessed May 15, 2007.
2. American Joint Committee on Cancer (AJCC). AJCC Cancer Staging Manual. 6th ed. New York, NY: Springer; 2002.
3. O'Connell J, Maggard M, Ko C. Colon cancer survival rates with the new American Joint Committee on Cancer sixth edition staging. J Natl Cancer Inst 2004;96:1420–1425.
4. Greene F, Stewart A, Norton H. A new TNM staging strategy for node-positive (stage III) colon cancer: an analysis of 50,042 patients. Ann Surg 2002;236:416–421.
5. Zmora O, Mahajna A, Bar-Zakai B, Rosin D. Colon and rectal surgery without mechanical bowel preparation: a randomised prospective trial. Ann Surg 2003;237:363–367.
6. Le Voyer T, Sigurdson E, Hanlon A, et al. Colon cancer survival is associated with increasing number of lymph nodes analyzed: a secondary survey of intergroup trial INT-0089. J Clin Oncol 2003;21:2912–2919.
7. Lacy A, Garcia-Valdecasas J, Delgado S, et al. Laparoscopy-assisted colectomy versus open colectomy for treatment of non-metastatic colon cancer: a randomised trial. Lancet 2002;359:2224–2229.
8. Leung KL, Kwok SP, Lam SC, Lee JF. Laparoscopic resection of rectosigmoid carcinoma: prospective randomised trial. Lancet 2004;363:1187–1192.
9. Clinical Outcomes of Surgical Therapy Study Group. A comparison of laparoscopically assisted and open colectomy for colon cancer. N Engl J Med 2004;350:2050–2059.
10. Veldkamp R, Kuhry E, Hop WC, Jeekel J. COlon cancer Laparoscopic or Open Resection Study Group (COLOR). Laparoscopic surgery versus open surgery for colon cancer: short-term outcomes of a randomised trial. Lancet Oncol 2005;6(7):477–484.
11. Joseph NE, Sigurdson ER, Hanlon AL, Wang H. Accuracy of determining nodal negativity in colorectal cancer on the basis of the number of nodes retrieved on resection. Ann Surg Oncol 2003;10(3):213–218.
12. Kim YM, Suh JH, Cha HJ, Jang SJ. Additional lymph node examination from entire submission of residual mesenteric tissue in colorectal cancer specimens may not add clinical and pathologic relevance. Hum Pathol 2007;Feb 14 [Epub ahead of print].
13. Bilchik AJ, DiNome M, Saha S, Turner RR. Prospective multicenter trial of staging adequacy in colon cancer: preliminary results. Arch Surg 2006;141(6):527–533; discussion 533–534.
14. Saha S, Dan A, Beutler T, et al. Sentinel lymph node mapping technique in colon cancer. Semin Oncol 2004;31:374–381.
15. Bendavid Y, Latulippe JF, Younan RJ, et al. Phase I study on sentinel lymph node mapping in colon cancer: a preliminary report. J Surg Oncol 2002;79:81–84.
16. Tsioulias GJ, Wood TF, Morton DL, et al. Lymphatic mapping and focused analysis of sentinel lymph nodes upstage gastrointestinal neoplasms. Arch Surg 2000;135:926–932.
17. Kehlet H, Kennedy RH. Laparoscopic colonic surgery—mission accomplished or work in progress? Colorectal Dis 2006;8:514–517.
18. Jessup J, Stewart A, Greene FL, et al. Adjuvant chemotherapy for stage III colon cancer: implications of race/ethnicity, age, and differentiation. JAMA 2005;294(21):2703–2711.
19. Van Cutsem E, Costa F. Progress in the adjuvant treatment of colon cancer: has it influenced clinical practice? JAMA 2005;294(21):2758–2760.
20. Moertel CG, Fleming TR, Macdonald JS, et al. Levamisole and fluorouracil for adjuvant therapy of resected colon carcinoma. N Engl J Med 1990;322:352–358.
21. Moertel CG, Fleming TR, Macdonald JS, et al. Intergroup study of fluorouracil plus levamisole as adjuvant therapy for stage II/Dukes' B2 colon cancer. J Clin Oncol 1995;13:2936–2943.
22. Taal B, Van Tinteren G, Zoetmulder F on behalf of the NCAPP. Adjuvant 5FU plus levamisole in colonic or rectal cancer: improved survival in stage II and III. Br J Cancer 2001;85:1437–1443.
23. International Multicentre Pooled Analysis of Colorectal Cancer Trials (IMPACT). Efficacy of adjuvant fluorouracil and folinic acid in colon cancer. Lancet 1995;345:939–944.
24. Francini G, Petrioli R, Lorenzini L, et al. Folinic acid and 5-fluorouracil as adjuvant chemotherapy in colon cancer. Gastroenterology 1994;106:899–906.
25. O'Connell M, Maillaird J, Kahn M, et al. Controlled trial of fluorouracil and low dose leucovorin given for 6 months as postoperative adjuvant therapy for colon cancer. J Clin Oncol 1997;15:246–250.
26. Wolmark N, Rockette H, Fisher B, et al. The benefit of leucovorin-modulated fluorouracil as postoperative adjuvant therapy for primary colon cancer: results from National Surgical Adjuvant Breast and Bowel Project Protocol C–03. J Clin Oncol 1993;11:1879–1887.
27. O'Connell MJ, Laurie JA, Kahn M, et al. Prospectively randomized trial of postoperative adjuvant chemotherapy in patients with high-risk colon cancer. J Clin Oncol 1998;16:295–300.
28. Haller D, Catalano P, MacDonald J, et al. Phase III study of fluorouracil, leucovorin and levamisole in high-risk stage II and III colon cancer: final report of Intergroup 0089. J Clin Oncol 2005;23:8671–8678.
29. Wolmark N, Rockette H, Mamounas E, et al. Clinical trial to assess the relative efficacy of fluorouracil and leucovorin, fluorouracil and levamisole, and fluorouracil, leucovorin and levamisole in patients with Dukes' B and C carcinoma of the colon: results from National Surgical Adjuvant Breast and Bowel Project C–04. J Clin Oncol 1999;17:3553–3559.
30. Porschen R, Bermann A, Loffler T, et al. Fluorouracil plus leucovorin as effective adjuvant chemotherapy in curatively resected stage III colon cancer: results of the trial adjCCA–01. J Clin Oncol 2001;19:1787–1794.
31. Van Cutsem E, Dicato M, Wils J, et al. Adjuvant treatment of colorectal cancer (current expert opinion derived from the Third International Conference: Perspectives in Colorectal Cancer, Dublin, 2001). Eur J Cancer 2002;38:1429–1436.
32. Van Cutsem E, Katja V. ESMO minimum clinical recommendations for diagnosis, adjuvant treatment and follow-up of colon cancer. Ann Oncol 2005;16(suppl 1):i16–i17.
33. Quasar Collaborative Group. Comparison of fluorouracil with additional levamisole, higher dose folinic acid, or both, as adjuvant chemotherapy for colorectal cancer: a randomized trial. Lancet 2000;355:1588–1596.
34. Andre T, Colin P, Louvet C, et al. Semimonthly versus monthly regimen of fluorouracil and leucovorin administered for 24 or 36 weeks as adjuvant therapy in stage II and III colon cancer: results of a randomized trial. J Clin Oncol 2003;21:2896–2903.
35. Andre T, Quinaux E, Louvet C, et al. Updated results at 6 years for the GERCOR C96.1 phase III study comparing LV5FU2 to monthly 5FU-leucovorin (mFufol) as adjuvant therapy for Dukes B2 and C colon cancer patients. J Clin Oncol 2005;23: abstract 3522.
36. Carrato A, Köhne C, Bedenne L, et al. Folinic acid modulated bolus 5-FU or infusional 5-FU for adjuvant treatment of patients of UICC stage III colon cancer: preliminary analysis of the PETACC-2 study. J Clin Oncol 2006;24:161S (abstract 3563).
37. Saini A, Norman A, Cunningham D, et al. Twelve weeks of protracted venous infusion of fluorouracil (5-FU) is as effective as 6 months of bolus 5-FU and folinic acid as adjuvant treatment in colorectal cancer. Br J Cancer 2003;88:1859–1865.
38. Sakamoto J, Ohashi Y, Hamada C, et al. Efficacy of oral adjuvant therapy after resection of colorectal cancer: 5-year results from three randomised trials. J Clin Oncol 2004;22:484–492.
39. Twelves C, Wong A, Nowacki M, et al. Capecitabine as adjuvant treatment for stage III colon cancer. N Engl J Med 2005;352(26):2696–2704.
40. Lembersky B, Wieand H, Petrelli N, et al. Oral uracil and tegafur plus leucovorin compared with intravenous fluorouracil and leucovorin in stage II and III carcinoma of the colon: results from National Surgical Adjuvant Breast and Bowel Project Protocol C–06. J Clin Oncol 2006;24(13):2059–2064.
41. Andre T, Boni C, Mounedji-Boudiaf L, et al. Oxaliplatin, fluorouracil and leucovorin as adjuvant treatment for colon cancer. N Engl J Med 2004;350:2343–2351.
42. De Gramont A, Boni C, Navarro M, et al. Oxaliplatin/5FU/LV in the adjuvant treatment of stage II and stage III colon cancer: efficacy results with a median follow-up of 4 years. J Clin Oncol 2005;23:16S.
43. Kuebler J, Wieand H, O'Connell M, et al. Oxaliplatin combined with weekly bolus fluorouracil and leucovorin as surgical adjuvant chemotherapy for stage II and III colon cancer: results from NSABP C-07. J Clin Oncol 2007;25:2156–2158.
44. Schmoll HJ, Cartwright T, Tabernero J, et al. Phase III trial of capecitabine plus oxaliplatin ad adjuvant therapy for stage III colon cancer: a planned safety analysis in 1,864 patients. J Clin Oncol 2007;25:102–109.
45. Saltz L, Niedzwiecki D, Hollis D, et al. Irinotecan fluorouracil plus leucovorin is not superior to fluorouracil plus leucovorin alone as adjuvant treatment for stage III colon cancer: results of CALGB 89803. J Clin Oncol 2007;25:3456–3461.
46. Rothenberg M, Meropol N, Poplin E, et al. Mortality associated with irinotecan plus bolus fluorouracil/leucovorin: summary findings of an independent panel. J Clin Oncol 2001;19:3801–3807.
47. Ychou M, Raoul JL, Douillard JY, et al. A phase III randomized trial of

LV5FU2 + CPT-11 vs. LV5FU2 alone in adjuvant high risk colon cancer (FNCLCC Accord02/FFCD9802). *J Clin Oncol* 2005;23. abstract 3502.

48. Van Cutsem E, Labianca D, Hossfeld D, et al. Randomized phase III trial comparing infused irinotecan/5-fluorouracil (5-FU)/folinic acid (IF) versus 5-FU/FA (F) in stage III colon cancer patients (Petacc3). *J Clin Oncol* 2005;23:16S (abstract 8).

49. Riethmuller G, Schneider-Gadicke E, Schlimok G, et al. Randomised trial of monoclonal antibody for adjuvant therapy of resected Dukes' C colorectal carcinoma. German Cancer Aid 17-1A Study Group. *Lancet* 1994;343:1177–1183.

50. Punt C, Nagy A, Douillard JY, et al. Edrecolomab alone or in combination with fluorouracil and folinic acid in the adjuvant treatment of stage III colon cancer: a randomised study. *Lancet* 2002;360:671–677.

51. Nordlinger B, Rougier P, Arnaud JC, et al. Adjuvant regional chemotherapy and systemic chemotherapy versus systemic chemotherapy alone in patients with stage II–III colorectal cancer: a multicentre randomised controlled phase III trial. *Lancet Oncol* 2005;6(7):459–468.

52. International Multicentre Pooled Analysis of B2 Colon Cancer Trials (IMPACT B2) investigators: efficacy of adjuvant fluorouracil and folinic acid in B2 colon cancer. *J Clin Oncol* 1999;17:1356–1363.

53. Mamounas E, Wieand S, Wolmark N, et al. Comparative efficacy of adjuvant chemotherapy in patients with Dukes' B versus Dukes' C colon cancer: results from four National Surgical Adjuvant Breast and Bowel Project adjuvant studies (C-01, C-02, C-03, and C-04). *J Clin Oncol* 1999;17(5):1349–1355.

54. Figueredo A, Charette M, Maroun J, et al. Adjuvant therapy for stage II colon cancer: a systematic review from the Cancer Care Ontario Program in evidence-based care's gastrointestinal cancer disease site group. *J Clin Oncol* 2004;22:3395–3407.

55. Buyse M, Piedbois P. Should Dukes' B patients receive adjuvant therapy? A statistical perspective. *Semin Oncol* 2001;28:20–24.

56. Benson A, Schrag D, Somerfield M, et al. American Society of Clinical Oncology recommendations on adjuvant chemotherapy for stage II colon cancer. *J Clin Oncol* 2004;22(16):3408–3419.

57. Gray R, Barnwell J, Hills R, et al., for the Quasar Collaborative Group. QUASAR: a randomized study of adjuvant chemotherapy vs observation including 3238 patients. *J Clin Oncol* 2004;22: abstract 3501.

58. Grothey A, Sargent D. FOLFOX for stage II colon cancer? A commentary on the recent FDA approval of oxaliplatin for adjuvant therapy of stage III colon cancer. *J Clin Oncol* 2005;23:3311–3313.

59. Gill S, Loprinzi CL, Sargent DJ, et al. Pooled analysis of fluorouracil-based adjuvant therapy for stage II and III colon cancer: who benefits and by how much? *J Clin Oncol* 2004;22(10):1797–1806.

60. Sargent D, Wieand S, Benedetti J, et al. Disease-free survival vs overall survival as a primary endpoint for adjuvant colon cancer studies: individual patient data from 20898 patients on 18 randomised trials. *J Clin Oncol* 2005;23:8664–8670.

61. Chua Y, Sargent D, Cunningham D. Definition of disease-free survival: this is my truth—show me yours. *Ann Oncol* 2005;16:1719–1721.

CHAPTER 44 ■ RECTAL CANCER: MANAGEMENT OF LOCOREGIONAL DISEASE

MORTON S. KAHLENBERG, DENNIS L. ROUSSEAU, JR., JON STRASSER, ADAM RABEN, AND NICHOLAS PETRELLI

The evolution of the multidisciplinary management of rectal cancer has resulted in impressive local control rates, overall survival rates, and enhancements in quality of life. Surgical resection represents the focal point of the multidisciplinary management of patients with rectal cancer. Several anatomic factors make complete surgical extirpation of rectal cancer challenging. The absence of a serosal barrier and the rectum's close proximity to vital pelvic structures facilitates early tumor extension into the perirectal tissues and contiguous organs. The location of the mesorectum within the confines of the pelvis complicates the adequate removal of all mesenteric nodes at risk for regional spread. The relationship between tumor location and sphincters and the priority to maintain continence through sphincter preservation and other quality-of-life issues adds to the challenge of the surgical management of rectal cancer. Treatment decisions have become more complex as a result of an increased array of surgical options and the excellent response of rectal cancer to chemotherapy and radiation. This chapter focuses on the locoregional management of rectal cancer. Radical resections (RADs) including sphincter preservation procedures and less radical procedures including transanal excision (TAE) and transanal endoscopic microsurgery (TEMS) are addressed. The roles of total mesorectal excision (TME), surgical margins, en bloc resection, and pelvic exenteration are discussed. The choice of surgical approach is dependent upon accurate pretreatment staging as well as the role that chemotherapy and radiation play in the neoadjuvant and adjuvant settings. This chapter will provide a brief overview of the approach to the pretreatment evaluation of the patient with rectal cancer, and the roles of neoadjuvant and adjuvant chemoradiation in rectal cancer management will be addressed.

PRETREATMENT EVALUATION AND STAGING

The pretreatment evaluation and staging are essential in determining the surgical approach to rectal cancer and the order of the various treatment modalities (radiation, chemotherapy, and surgery). The determination of the extent of local involvement and the presence or absence of systemic disease is critical. Clinical determination of the local extent of disease (T and N stage) includes physical examination consisting of digital rectal examination. For experienced practitioners, digital rectal examination is fairly accurate in assessing the depth of rectal wall penetration but not the nodal status. Waizer et al. (1)

reported that digital examinations performed by experienced practitioners accurately predicted the degree of rectal wall invasion 82.8% of the time. Computed tomography (CT) has been part of the standard preoperative staging for rectal cancer. It is very good for assessing the involvement of adjacent organs by locally advanced tumors but has limited accuracy in determining the T stage of tumors or the presence of nodal metastases. Several studies indicate that the accuracy of CT for T stage is 33% to 77% and 22% to 73% for nodal staging (2–7).

Endorectal ultrasound (EUS) is the most accurate preoperative staging tool for rectal cancer. Several studies have shown that the overall accuracy for T stage is 67% to 93% and for N stage is 61% to 88% (8–20). A very large study by Garcia-Aguilar et al. (21) reviewed the EUS experience in 1,184 patients with rectal tumors. Pathologic correlation with T stage was available in 545 patients and N stage in 238 patients. Ultrasound accuracy for T stage was 69%; 18% of tumors were overstaged and 13% understaged. With regard to nodal status, ultrasound accuracy was 64%. Thirty-two percent of the ultrasound N0 group were understaged and 48% of the N1 group were overstaged. Marusch et al. (22) reviewed the accuracy of EUS in determining the T-stage correlation in 422 rectal cancer resections. The overall accuracy was only 50.8% for T1 tumors and 58.6% for T2 lesions. The rate of understaging was 12.8% for the entire group (T1 to T4). Overstaging of the primary tumor is often attributed to peritumoral inflammation and hypervascularity, whereas understaging may be due to microscopic tumor invasion and technical problems with bulky tumors or lesions near the anal canal or valves of Houston (16,20,23,24). Lymph node overstaging may be due to reactive changes, whereas understaging can be due to the fact that nodal size may not correlate with the presence of metastases (20,25,26).

Magnetic resonance imaging (MRI) with endorectal coil may offer accuracy in T and N staging that rivals EUS. Bianchi et al. (27) reported that the diagnostic accuracy for phased array coil MRI was equal to EUS for T stage and nodal involvement. Kim et al. (28) recently reported impressive results with their use of MRI with phased array coils. The diagnostic accuracy of MRI with phased array coil was 97% for T1, 89% for T2, and 91% for T3 tumors, and the accuracy for the detection of nodal metastases was 95%.

The determination of the presence or absence of systemic disease includes conventional chest x-ray (CXR) to rule out pulmonary metastases. Abnormalities noted on CXR should be further investigated with a chest CT. Abdominal CT provides valuable information with regard to the presence of metastatic hepatic disease, extrapelvic adenopathy, and the presence of peritoneal disease. Triple phase CT and MRI are used to fully delineate hepatic abnormalities that may be identified on initial abdominal-pelvic CT. Positron emission tomography (PET) scans play a valuable role in determining the presence of metastases and should be considered when there are equivocal findings on CT and/or MRI.

MANAGEMENT OF LOCOREGIONAL RECTAL CANCER

The goals of locoregional therapy for rectal cancer are complete tumor extirpation in a manner that maximizes survival and minimizes the risk of local recurrence yet preserves bowel continuity and the function of the anal sphincter, urinary bladder, and sexual organs. Due to the anatomic constraints of the pelvis, it is frequently difficult to attain all of these goals, and optimal treatment commonly requires a multidisciplinary approach. This approach involves a combination of chemoradiation therapy, surgery, and adjuvant chemotherapy. Adequate staging prior to institution of treatment is crucial to selecting optimal oncologic therapy for each patient. Treatment decisions must also include a careful risk/benefit discussion of aggressive cancer treatment with its associated morbidities of impaired bowel function, the need for permanent stoma, urinary and sexual dysfunction, and altered lifestyle.

In the past, rectal cancer was a surgical disease treated with resection alone, without attention to appropriate anatomic dissection and without knowledge of the modes of locoregional spread. This approach resulted in local recurrence rates around 30% and 5-year survival rates from 27% to 42% (29–32). In the past 20 years, the mechanism of locoregional spread has been elucidated, highlighting the importance of the mesorectum in rectal cancer resection. With the development of the technique of TME as a component of rectal cancer resection, there were marked improvements in both local recurrence rates as well as survival, with local recurrence rates dropping to below 10%, and 5-year survival rates improving to 70% or better (33,34). The recent advances in surgical technique and application of adjuvant and neoadjuvant therapy in the treatment of rectal cancer have made the management of this disease a true multidisciplinary endeavor. These recent advances in surgical technique, adjuvant therapy, and neoadjuvant therapy will be discussed.

The Mesorectum

The embryologic origin of the mesorectum is mesenchymal cells arranged in lamellae of rectal adventitia filled with fatty tissue during embryogenesis. The outer lamellae of the adventitia form the visceral fascia of the mesorectum. This visceral fascia envelopes the rectum and mesorectum (35,36). Parietal endopelvic fascia lines the pelvic walls, covering the piriformis, coccygeal, and levator ani muscles, the presacral venous plexus, the anterior surface of the sacrum and coccyx, and the anococcygeal ligament. The posterior visceral and parietal fascial layers are separated by an avascular plane of loose areolar tissue. This plane extends down to the anal sphincter. At the level of S4, the rectosacral fascia or ligament is encountered. This is a thickening of fibers between the visceral and parietal fascia that must be divided sharply to prevent traction injury and violation of the mesorectum or tearing of the presacral venous plexus. On the anterior surface, Denonvilliers' fascia separates the rectum/mesorectum from the prostate and seminal vesicles in men and the posterior vaginal wall in women. Posterior to Denonvilliers' fascia is the visceral fascia of the mesorectum. Dissection in the anterior plane can be performed anterior or posterior to Denonvilliers' fascia depending on the location of the rectal tumor (37,38). Laterally, condensations of the visceral fascia known as the lateral ligaments are encountered. These ligaments connect to the parietal fascia and contain the middle rectal artery and autonomic nerves passing to the mesorectum/rectum. Division of the lateral ligaments in the appropriate plane prevents unnecessary injury to the pelvic autonomic nerve plexus (PANP) in the lateral pelvic sidewall.

Sympathetic and Parasympathetic Pelvic Nerves

The autonomic nervous system anatomy in the pelvis was described by Havenga et al. (39). Sympathetic nerve fibers enter the pelvis as the right and left hypogastric nerves, which originate from the superior hypogastric plexus located at the pelvic brim near the bifurcation of the aorta and vena cava. The nerves run in the areolar tissue plane between the visceral and parietal fascia of the mesorectum. Havenga et al. (39) demonstrated that the hypogastric nerves actually penetrated the visceral fascia for a short course near the pelvic brim. Other reports demonstrated that the nerves were posterior to the visceral fascia but closely associated with it (40–42). Given the close relationship between the hypogastric nerves and the visceral fascia of the mesorectum at this level, careful dissection in the areolar plane near the pelvic brim is required to identify and spare these nerves.

The parasympathetic nerve fibers (nervi erigentes) of the pelvis originate from the S2–S4 nerve roots. Their course runs under the parietal fascia over the piriformis muscle to the lateral pelvic sidewall. There, the parasympathetic fibers and the sympathetic fibers from the hypogastric nerves join to form the inferior hypogastric plexus or PANP. Rectal innervation from the PANP courses through the lateral ligaments to the rectum and mesorectum. Genitourinary branches of the PANP continue anteriorly under the parietal fascia to the bladder and to the prostate/seminal vesicles in men or the uterus/vagina in women (39). Excessive lateral dissection near the pelvic sidewall at the level of the lateral ligaments can injure the PANP and result in urinary and/or sexual dysfunction.

With a complete understanding of the relationships of the visceral fascia of the rectum/mesorectum, the parietal fascia of the pelvis, and the autonomic innervation of the pelvis, TME with autonomic nerve preservation (ANP) can be performed to mobilize the rectum and mesorectum for resection. Sharp dissection in the appropriate anatomic planes down to the level of the levators will facilitate maximal mobilization of the rectum for optimal sphincter preservation and distal margins and will minimize local recurrence and the sequelae of autonomic nerve dysfunction.

Technique of Total Mesorectal Excision and Complete Rectal Mobilization for Rectal Cancer

The modern methods of rectal cancer resection are based on complete mobilization of the rectum and mesorectum in the pelvis along appropriate anatomic planes with attention to preservation of the pelvic autonomic nervous system when possible. With adequate mobilization, resection margins can be optimized, chance of sphincter preservation can be maximized, and risk of local recurrence will be minimized.

Utilizing a low midline incision taken down to the pubis, the abdomen is explored for evidence of unsuspected metastatic disease. Retraction is established, and the sigmoid colon is exposed. The sigmoid and descending colon are mobilized lateral to medial, and the splenic flexure is taken down if a low pelvic reconstruction is anticipated. The left ureter and gonadal vessels are identified and are left in the retroperitoneum. With the sigmoid colon mobilized to midline, the peritoneum in the pelvis is opened along the visualized mesorectum circumferentially with cautery. Medially, the peritoneum is divided along the course of the superior rectal artery and vein to the level of the inferior mesenteric artery (IMA). If there is no palpable adenopathy at the level of the IMA, the vascular pedicle can be divided with preservation of the left colic branch and the bowel can be divided at the proximal sigmoid colon. If there is palpable adenopathy at the level of the IMA, the vascular pedicle should be divided at the level of the aorta, taking the left colic branch. The bowel in this case should be divided at the level of the distal descending colon. In this circumstance, the splenic flexure should always be mobilized if reconstruction is planned, and often the inferior mesenteric vein will need to be ligated at the inferior border of the pancreas to allow adequate mobilization of the descending colon for tension-free reconstruction. After division of the bowel and mesenteric vessels, the colon is packed in the left upper quadrant and attention is turned to the pelvic dissection.

Complete mobilization of the rectum and mesorectum begins with the posterior dissection. The rectosigmoid colon is lifted, and the retrorectal space is entered at the level of the pelvic brim immediately posterior to the superior rectal vessels. The areolar plane between the visceral mesorectal fascia and the parietal pelvic fascia is identified and divided sharply with cautery. The right and left hypogastric nerves course posterolaterally along the pelvic brim and are often attached to and lifted with the mesorectal fascia. These nerves should be identified and carefully dissected free of the visceral mesorectal fascia, and the dissection plane then continued medially to these nerves. Dissection posteriorly continues in the areolar plane to the level of S4 where the rectosacral fascia is encountered. This fascia is divided sharply with cautery or scissors to gain mobilization of the distal 5 cm of the rectal wall. Blunt dissection in this area can result in anterior tearing of the mesorectum with possible increased local recurrence rates or posterior tearing of the presacral venous plexus, resulting in difficult-to-control hemorrhage. Posterior dissection is complete with visualization of the levator ani musculature.

The anterior dissection in women begins with opening the peritoneum of the Pouch of Douglas. The uterus is lifted and the posterior wall of the vagina is identified. In women who have had a hysterectomy, identification of the posterior wall of the vagina can be facilitated by an assistant placing two fingers or a flat malleable retractor into the vagina from the perineum. Anterior dissection along the posterior wall of the vagina is performed sharply with scissors or cautery down to the level of the levators. In men, the dissection begins at the anterior cul-de-sac, identified by lifting the bladder superiorly with a retractor. Opening the anterior cul-de-sac will expose the seminal vesicles and the anterior surface of Denonvilliers' fascia. For anterior tumors, continued dissection anterior to Denonvilliers' fascia is performed with cautery or scissors down to the level of the levators. For other tumor location, similar dissection is performed posterior to this fascia.

After completion of the anterior and posterior dissections, the lateral sidewall dissection is completed. The lateral ligaments are identified and divided. At this location, the PANP should be identified and preserved if possible. If adequate lateral margin is possible, the lateral ligaments should be divided at the level of the visceral fascia of the mesorectum to minimize potential injury to the PANP. Division can be accomplished

with cautery, clips, or stapling devices. With completion of the lateral sidewall dissection, the entire mesorectum and rectum are mobilized. At this point, if sphincter preservation is possible the rectum can be divided and the specimen removed. If sphincter preservation is not possible, the perineal portion of an abdominoperineal resection (APR) is undertaken to remove the specimen.

Extended Lymphadenectomy

In addition to TME, extended lymph node resection with ligation of the IMA at its junction with the aorta, and extended pelvic dissection and lymph node retrieval laterally along the pelvic sidewall have been advocated to improve local recurrence and survival. The issue of high ligation of the IMA is with regard to where the vascular pedicle is divided. Traditional ligation of the vascular pedicle is performed just distal to the origin of the left colic artery. However, anatomic studies have revealed that as many as 10 lymph nodes could be found between the origin of the left colic vessel and the origin of the IMA (43). In addition, pathology reviews reported that the lymph nodes between the origin of the IMA and the left colic branch were positive in 11% to 22% of cases (44,45). Therefore, high ligation of the IMA was proposed as a method to improve resection and survival. However, subsequent reports failed to support the superiority of high ligation, and it is not routinely practiced for oncologic reasons (46–48).

Lateral pelvic lymph nodes have been reported to be involved in rectal cancer in 9% to 14% of patients (49–51). Extended lateral lymph node dissection has been proposed by several Japanese groups to provide decreased local recurrence and improved survival (52). However, reported rates of local control have been variable, and overall survival rates are similar to those reported for TME alone. In addition, this extended lymphadenectomy is consistently associated with high rates of urinary and sexual dysfunction (53–55). With the routine use of neoadjuvant and adjuvant therapy in Western medicine, there is no current role for prophylactic lateral lymph node dissection in the treatment of rectal cancer.

Rectal Cancer Resection

The goal of resection in rectal cancer is complete tumor removal with negative circumferential (radial) and distal margins with *en bloc* resection of involved pelvic organs if necessary. Complete mobilization of the mesorectum down to the level of the levator ani complex using techniques describe above is crucial to attaining this goal and minimizing local recurrence rates. Secondary goals in rectal cancer resection include preserving the anal sphincter, re-establishing bowel continuity, preserving bladder and sexual function, and restoring the reservoir function of the rectum when indicated. Maximal achievement of these secondary goals is dependent on adequate knowledge of the appropriate planes of dissection in the pelvis and complete mobilization of the rectum and mesorectum.

Sphincter Preservation Procedures

The anal sphincter complex cannot be preserved in cases in which the cancer directly invades the external sphincter/levator ani complex and in cases where a negative distal margin cannot be achieved with a continent sphincter. In all other cases, the possibility of sphincter preservation and re-establishment of bowel continuity remains an option. However, the final decision can only be made intra-operatively, after complete rectal/mesorectal mobilization is performed and the tumor mobilized.

Only then can the distal margin and radial clearance be assessed and the likelihood of re-establishing bowel continuity be evaluated.

Low Anterior Resection

The hallmarks of low anterior resection for rectal cancer are complete mobilization of the rectum/mesorectum with division of the lateral ligaments and an extraperitoneal pelvic anastomosis. Tumors of the upper and middle rectum are treated most commonly with this procedure. Lower rectal lesions may be amenable to low anterior resection with a very low anastomosis depending on the size and location of the tumor, the ability to completely mobilize the rectum, and the ability to divide the rectum distal to the lesion with negative margins from an abdominal approach.

For lesions of the upper and middle rectum, the rectum is completely mobilized to the pelvic floor using the TME techniques described earlier. After mobilization, the rectum is divided with a transanastomotic (TA) stapling device, using a bowel clamp on the proximal margin (Fig. 44.1). There is some debate as to the extent of distal dissection/resection for upper rectal lesions. Distal margin length is rarely an issue for these lesions. Heald (33) advocates total mesorectal resection down to the pelvic floor for virtually all rectal cancers. Some researchers advocate complete mobilization of the rectum to the pelvic floor with division of the rectum 5 cm beyond the lower margin of the tumor (34,56,57). Although this may result in incomplete resection of the entire mesorectum for upper rectal lesions, it does not compromise oncologic outcome, as pathologic studies have demonstrated no distal spread of cancer in the mesorectum beyond 5 cm (50,57). A key component to the oncologic outcome of the 5-cm margin is that the mesorectum must be divided at right angles to the wall of the rectum to ensure adequate mesorectal resection. There is a tendency to cone down to the bowel wall distal to the lesion, which can potentially leave distal disease in an incompletely resected mesorectum. If there is any question regarding the margin, frozen section analysis is performed. After assurance of adequate distal margins, bowel continuity is restored using a side-to-end anastomosis, hand sewn or stapled (Fig. 44.2), or an end-to-end stapled anastomosis using an end-to-end anastomosis (EEA) stapling device (Fig. 44.3). For lesions in the upper and middle rectum, there is a sufficient distal rectal remnant for reservoir function, so reservoir construction in the proximal bowel with J-pouch or coloplasty is not required. Proximal diversion with a loop ileostomy is not required with upper and middle rectal reconstruction; however, in the setting of neoadjuvant chemoradiation, liberal use of proximal diversion is encouraged.

Tumors in the distal rectum can also be resected with low anterior resection and a very low rectal anastomosis. The rectum is mobilized to the pelvic floor with complete mobilization of the tumor. A distal margin of 2 cm is the goal of the resection. The rectum is divided just above the pelvic floor with a TA stapling device leaving only a small cuff of rectum above the anal canal. The specimen is opened and the distal margin assessed. If the margin is <2 cm, frozen section analysis is performed to ensure a negative margin. If the margin is positive or close, resection of the remainder of the rectum and coloanal reconstruction may be required. After confirming adequate distal margins, bowel continuity is restored with an end-to-end stapled anastomosis with an EEA stapling device. With very low rectal anastomoses, there is no significant rectal remnant to function as a reservoir. Reconstruction with a J-pouch or coloplasty should be considered for improved functional outcome (see below). We encourage proximal diversion of all low rectal reconstructions, especially in the setting of neoadjuvant chemoradiation and/or J-pouch or coloplasty reconstruction.

Proctectomy with Coloanal Anastomosis

For lesions of the distal rectum that do not involve the levator ani complex but cannot be resected to negative distal margins from an abdominal approach, proctectomy with coloanal reconstruction can allow sphincter preservation in selected patients. After complete mobilization of the rectum to the pelvic floor using the principles of TME, the distal margin is assessed. If there is insufficient room in the pelvis to divide the rectum with a negative distal margin, division of the rectum from a perineal approach via the anal canal is undertaken. For this approach, the anal canal is everted with several heavy sutures. Cautery is used to open the mucosa just above the dentate line

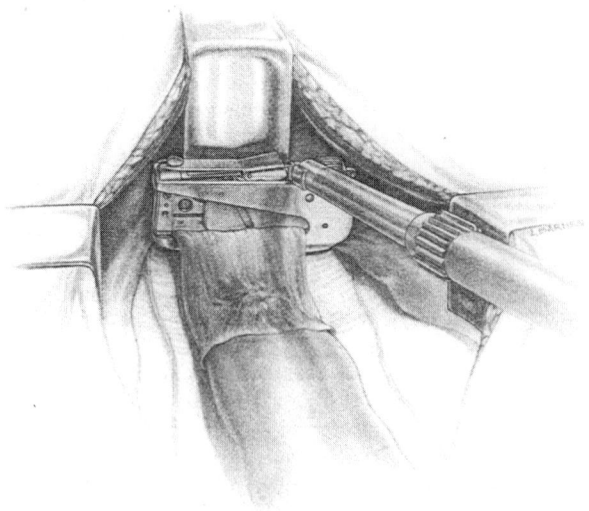

A

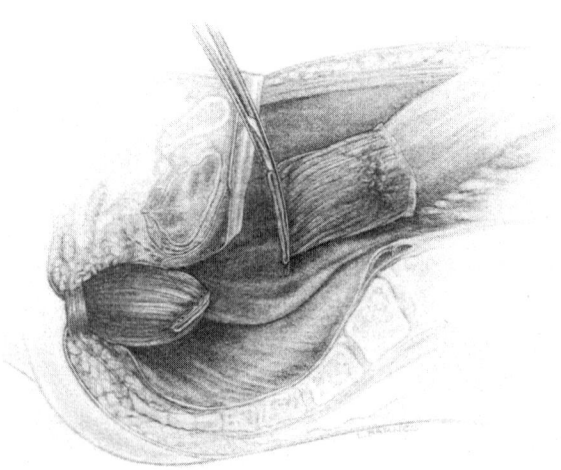

B

FIGURE 44.1. Division of the rectum for low anterior resection (LAR). **A.** Placement of a transanastomotic (TA) stapling device across the distal rectum to close the distal pouch after the rectum and tumor have been mobilized. **B.** Division of the distal rectum with a bowel clamp on the proximal margin. Reprinted with permission from Corman ML. *Colon and Rectal Surgery*, 5th ed. Philadelphia: Lippincott Williams & Wilkins; 2005.

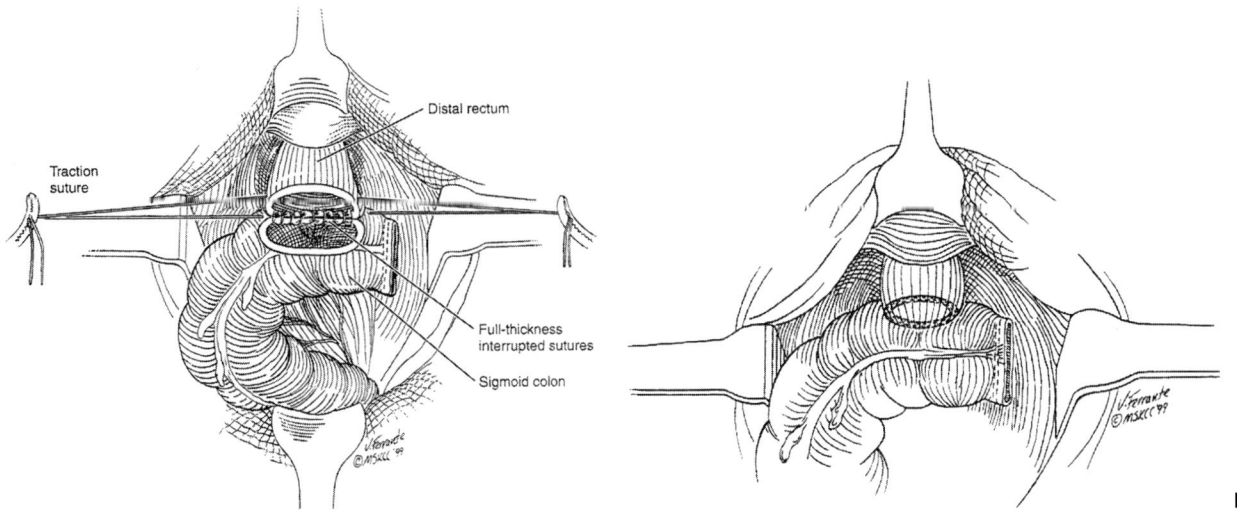

FIGURE 44.2. Side-to-end reconstruction after low anterior resection (LAR). **A.** A sutured side-to-end anastomosis after LAR. **B.** A stapled side-to-end anastomosis after LAR. The anvil of the end to end anastomosis (EEA) stapler is placed through the side of the colon at least 2 cm from the open end of the colon. After anvil placement, the end of the colon is closed with a (TA) stapler. The anastomosis is completed by placing the EEA stapler into the rectal pouch, connecting the stapler and anvil in the standard fashion, and firing the stapler. Reprinted with permission from Cohen, AM. Operations for colorectal cancer: low anterior resection. In: Zuidema GD, Yeo CJ, eds. *Surgery of the Alimentary Tract*, Vol IV. 5th ed. Philadelphia: W.B. Saunders; 2002;245–260.

down through the internal sphincter. Dissection is then performed in the intersphincteric plane up to the pelvis in a circumferential fashion, completely freeing the rectum. The specimen is sent to pathology for both distal and radial margin frozen section. If the margins are positive, APR is performed. If margins are adequate, bowel continuity is restored with a hand-sewn anastomosis at the level of the dentate line (Fig. 44.4). Reconstruction can be done with a straight coloanal anastomosis or with reservoir construction with a J-pouch or coloplasty. Proximal diversion with a loop ileostomy is then performed.

Pouch Reconstruction

Very low rectal anastomoses and coloanal anastomoses can significantly alter defecation patterns in the postoperative period. Frequency, urgency, soiling, and incontinence are all increased (58). The sensations of frequency and urgency are likely due to loss of the rectal reservoir with resection (59,60). Frequency of stool has been correlated to length of residual rectum, with increasing stool frequency associated with shorter rectal rem-

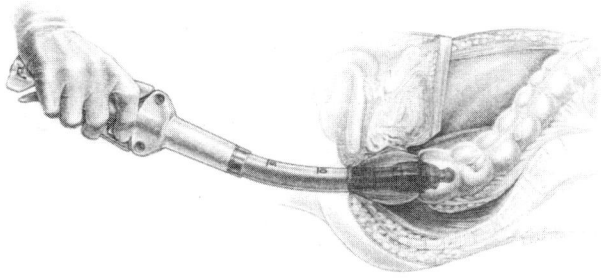

FIGURE 44.3. End-to-end stapled anastomosis after low anterior resection (LAR). Reprinted with permission from Corman ML. *Colon and Rectal Surgery*, 5th ed. Philadelphia: Lippincott Williams & Wilkins; 2005.

nants (61). Continence is also affected by low pelvic or coloanal anastomoses. Sphincter resting pressures are significantly reduced with coloanal anastomoses (62). Continence can also be affected by the use of transanal stapling devices and reduction in anal sensation (63,64). Over time, frequency, urgency, and continence can improve, and the improvement is likely due to dilation of the colon above the anastomosis to allow better reservoir function (65,66).

Efforts to improve functional outcome of low anastomoses focused on construction of a pouch in the colon just proximal to the anastomosis to improve the reservoir function of the neorectum. The two methods of pouch construction are J-pouch and coloplasty. Formation of either pouch construction requires complete mobilization of the left colon with takedown of the splenic flexure, ligation of the IMA at its origin, and division of the inferior mesenteric vein at the inferior boarder of the pancreas to allow sufficient length for a tension-free anastomosis in the pelvis. Formation of the J-pouch begins with folding the end of the colon back on itself for a length of 5 to 7 cm. A colotomy is made in the anterior wall of the folded colon at the site of planned anastomosis, and a gastrointestinal anastomosis (GIA) stapler is placed into the opening and across the posterior wall. The stapler is fired, creating the pouch with an ideal size of 5 to 7 cm (67). The anastomosis is then completed using a hand-sewn or stapled technique (Fig. 44.5). The coloplasty pouch is formed in the manner of a Heinecke–Mikulicz strictureplasty. At 4 to 6 cm proximal to the end of the colon, an 8- to 10-cm longitudinal colotomy is made. The colotomy is then closed in a transverse fashion, creating the pouch (Fig. 44.6). The anastomosis is completed at the distal end of the colon using a hand-sewn or stapled technique.

Colonic J-pouch reconstruction was first reported in 1986 by Lazorthes et al. (68) and Parc et al. (69). Both reports found improvements in function with the construction of a colonic reservoir as reflected by decreased frequency of stool, decreased urgency, and decreased incontinence. Several randomized trials comparing J-pouch to straight anastomosis have also been performed, demonstrating improved function with pouch reconstruction. Ortiz et al. (70) and Ho and Seow-Choen (71) demonstrated significant improvements in stool frequency at 12 months with J-pouch reconstruction.

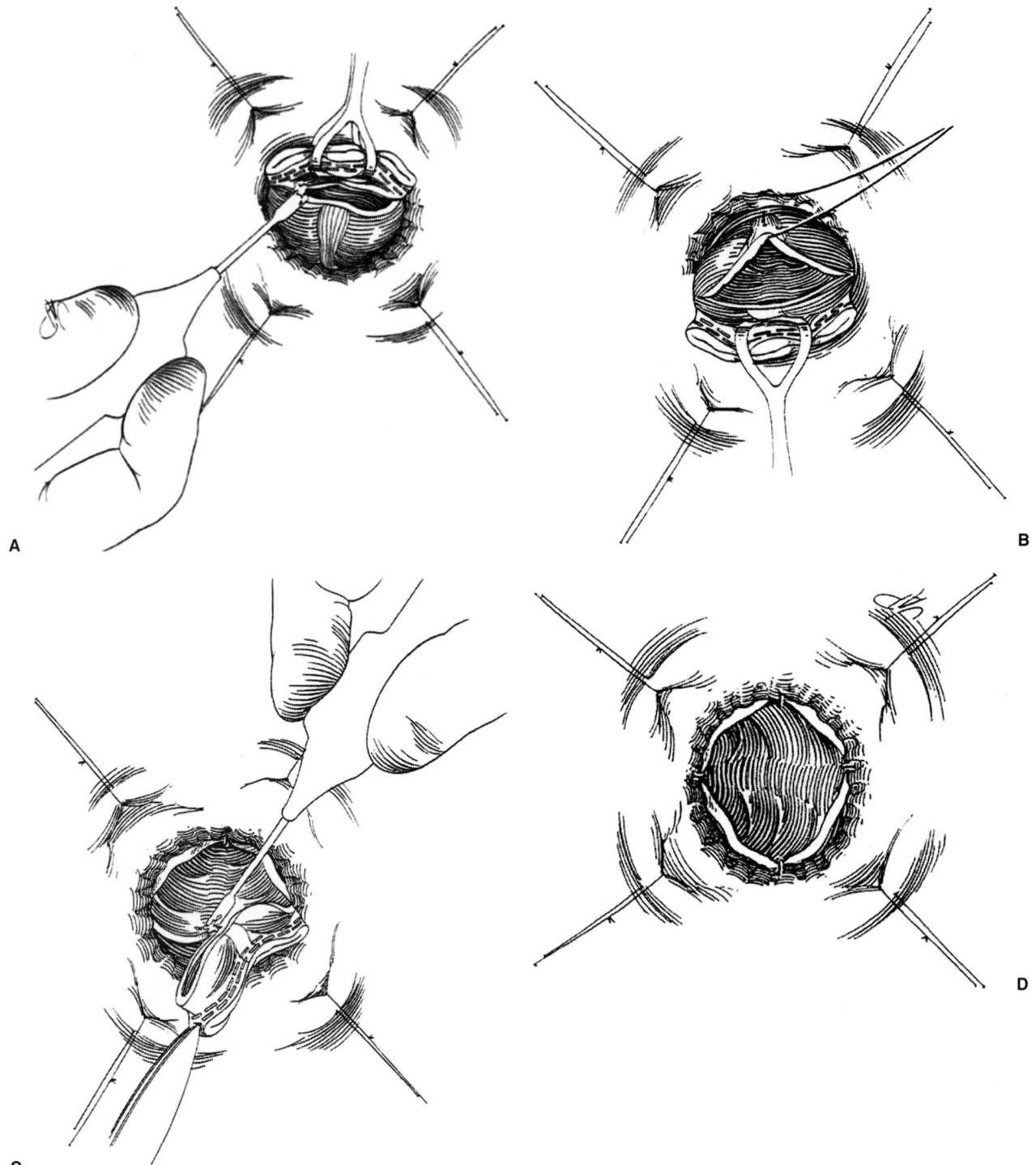

FIGURE 44.4. Construction of a hand-sewn coloanal anastomosis. **A.** The end of the colon is gently delivered through the anal canal with a Babcock clamp passed through the anus. Care is taken not to twist the bowel during delivery. The anterior wall of the bowel is then opened with cautery. **B.** An anterior suture is placed incorporating the anoderm, internal anal sphincter, and the full thickness of the colon wall. **C.** The staple line is further removed to the lateral aspect of the colon, and lateral sutures are placed in the anastomosis. The remainder of the staple line is removed, and a posterior suture is placed, finishing the four quadrant sutures. **D.** After placing the four quadrant sutures, two to three additional sutures are placed between the quadrant sutures to complete the anastomosis. Reprinted with permission from Milsom JW, Ludwig KA. Surgical management for rectal cancer. In: Wanebo HJ, ed. *Surgery for Gastrointestinal Cancer: A Multidisciplinary Approach*. Philadelphia: Lippincott-Raven; 1997;639–665.

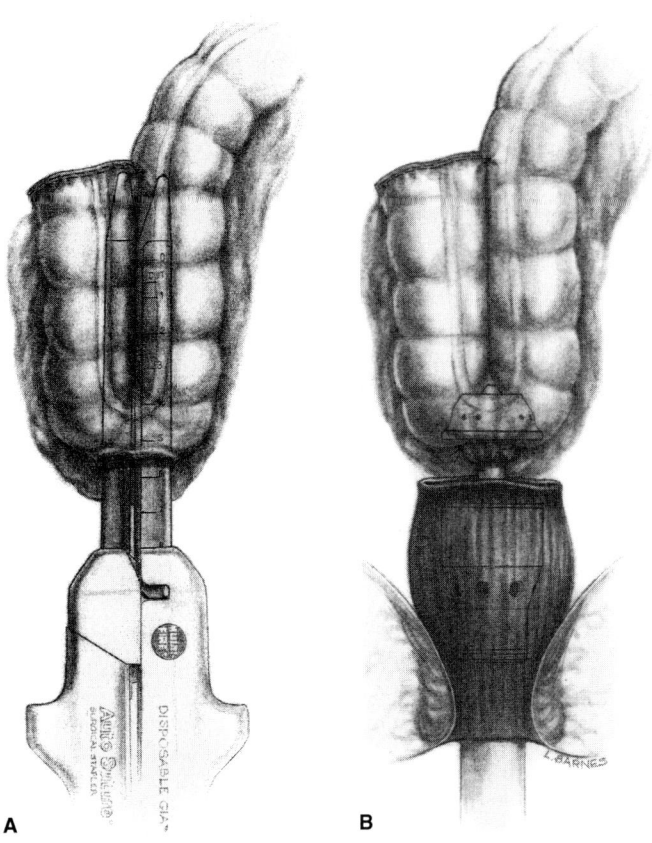

FIGURE 44.5. Formation of a colonic J-pouch. **A.** The J-pouch is formed by folding the end of the colon and securing the fold with sutures. An enterotomy is made in the anterior wall of the most distal extent of the colon. A gastrointestinal anastomosis (GIA) stapler is placed through the enterotomy across the common wall of the folded colon and is fired, creating a 5- to 7-cm pouch. **B.** A purse string suture is placed around the enterotomy in the anterior wall, and the anvil of an end to end anastomosis (EEA) stapler is secured. The anastomosis is completed with the EEA stapler inserted into the rectal pouch. Reprinted with permission from Corman ML. *Colon and Rectal Surgery,* 5th ed. Philadelphia: Lippincott Williams & Wilkins; 2005.

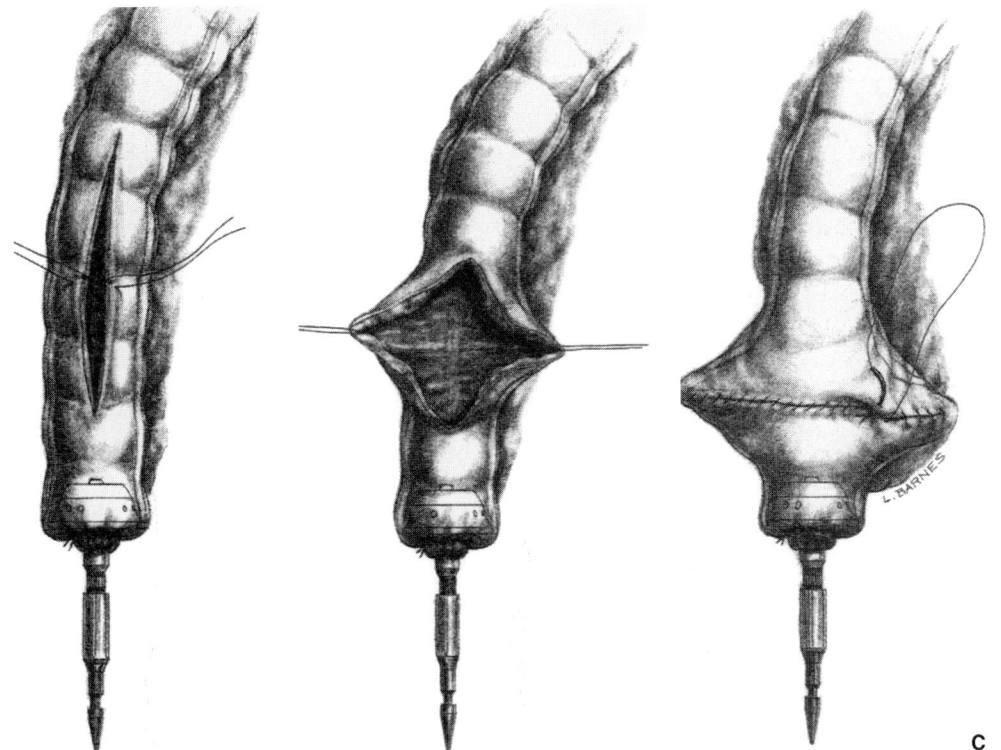

FIGURE 44.6. Formation of a colonic reservoir using the coloplasty technique. **A.** An 8- to 10-cm longitudinal colotomy is made between the teniae starting 4 to 6 cm from the stapled end. **B.** Traction sutures are placed in the colotomy to facilitate transverse closure in a Heinecke–Mikulicz fashion. **C.** The colotomy is closed in two layers. Bowel continuity is established with a standard stapled or hand-sewn anastomosis. Reprinted with permission from Corman ML. *Colon and Rectal Surgery*, 5th ed. Philadelphia: Lippincott Williams & Wilkins; 2005.

Seow-Choen and Goh (72) found significant improvement in both frequency of stool and continence at 12 months after reconstruction. Hallbook et al. (73) showed J-pouch reconstruction was significantly better for frequency, urgency, and continence at 12 months. Long-term studies comparing J-pouch reconstruction to straight anastomosis report durable improvements in stool frequency at 24 months and 60 months with the J-pouch (74,75). Improvements in urgency and continence are no longer evident at 24 months (74–76). An additional technical benefit of J-pouch reconstruction is an apparent lower rate of anastomotic leak, likely a result of improved perfusion of the J-pouch at the anastomosis site (73,77,78).

For patients who cannot undergo J-pouch reconstruction due to fatty colon, diverticular disease, small pelvis, or inadequate colon length to reach the distal pelvis with a J-pouch, coloplasty pouch formation can be utilized (79,80). Functional outcomes with coloplasty appear similar to those of J-pouch reconstruction. A prospective randomized trial comparing coloplasty to J-pouch reconstruction has completed accrual and is in the follow-up phase (58).

APR

For patients with low rectal tumors directly invading the levator ani complex or tumors that cannot be resected with negative circumferential and/or distal margins with preservation of the anal sphincter complex, APR with permanent end colostomy is required. APR and sphincter-saving procedures appear to have similar oncologic outcomes when comparing tumors of similar stage, pathologic features, and distance from the anal verge (81–85). The abdominal portion of the procedure is performed similar to that of low anterior resection, with complete mobilization of the rectum using the principles of TME. After mobilization of the rectum and confirmation of the need

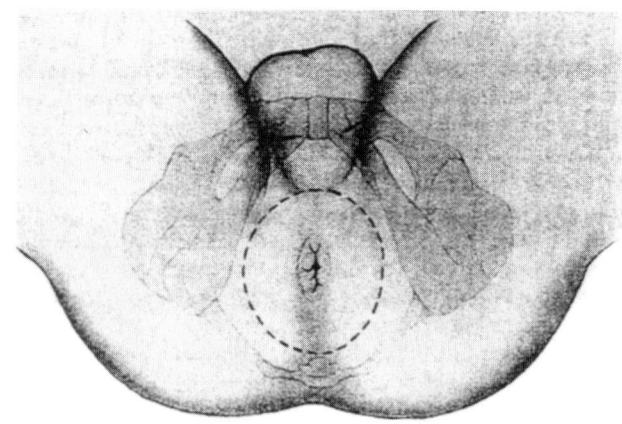

FIGURE 44.7. Incision for the perineal dissection for abdominoperineal resection (APR) in a man. Reprinted with permission from Enker WE, Martz J. Abdominoperineal resection of the rectum for cancer. In: Zuidema GD, Yeo CJ, eds. *Surgery of the Alimentary Tract*, Vol IV. 5th ed. Philadelphia: W.B. Saunders; 2002;261–268.

for sphincter resection, the perineal portion of the operation is performed. With the patient positioned in the lithotomy position in stirrups, an elliptical incision is made from the midpoint of the perineal body anteriorly to the level of the coccyx posteriorly encompassing the anus and 2 to 3 cm of skin measured for the anal verge (Fig. 44.7). In women with low-lying tumors involving the anterior surface of the rectum, posterior vaginectomy should be performed for adequate circumferential margins (Fig. 44.8). Cautery dissection is used to open the posterior and lateral tissues to the level of the pelvic floor. The inferior hemorrhoidal arteries are encountered in the ischiorectal space and should be ligated. The coccyx is then palpated, and the

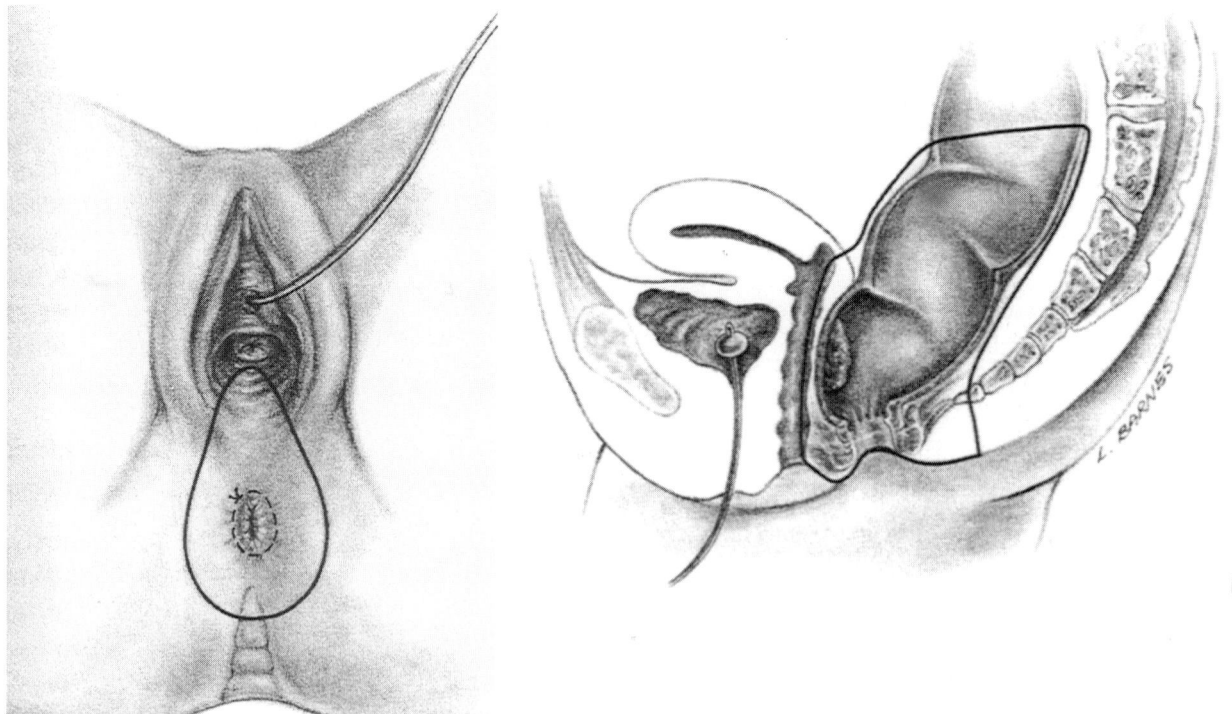

FIGURE 44.8. Incision for the perineal dissection for abdominoperineal resection (APR) in a woman with an anterior tumor. **A.** Perineal incision including the posterior vaginal wall. **B.** Sagittal view showing the extent of the resection. Reprinted with permission from Corman ML. *Colon and Rectal Surgery*, 5th ed. Philadelphia: Lippincott Williams & Wilkins; 2005.

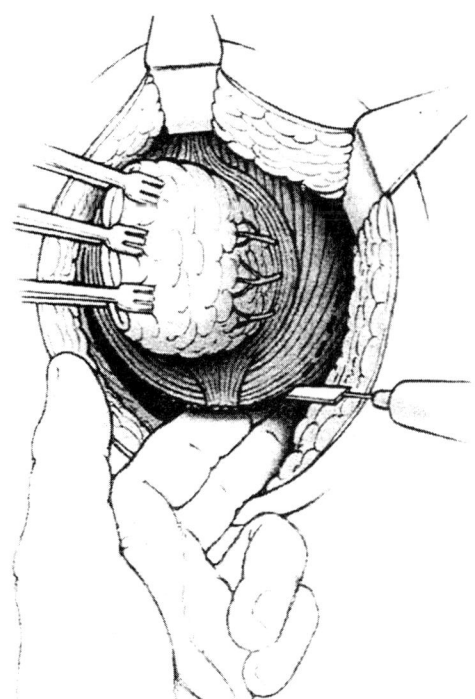

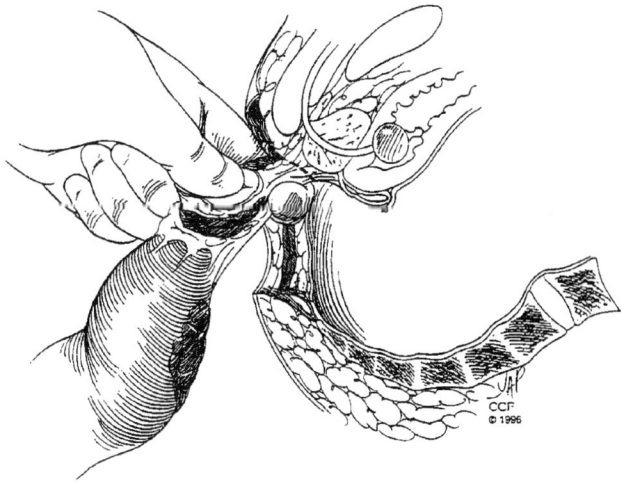

FIGURE 44.10. Completion of the anterior division of the levator ani muscles after delivery of the specimen to the perineum. Reprinted with permission from Milsom JW, Ludwig KA. Surgical management for rectal cancer. In: Wanebo HJ, ed. *Surgery for Gastrointestinal Cancer: A Multidisciplinary Approach*. Philadelphia: Lippincott-Raven; 1997; 639–665.

FIGURE 44.9. Division of the levator ani muscles from a posterior to anterior approach with a finger inside the pelvis as a guide. The muscles should be divided as widely as possible. Reprinted with permission from Enker WE, Martz J. Abdominoperineal resection of the rectum for cancer. In: Zuidema GD, Yeo CJ, eds. *Surgery of the Alimentary Tract*, Vol IV. 5th ed. Philadelphia: W.B. Saunders; 2002;261–268.

anococcygeal ligament is divided anterior to the tip of the coccyx. Dissection in this posterior plane is continued superiorly until the posterior pelvic floor is opened. This dissection can be facilitated by the abdominal surgeon placing a hand in the deep posterior pelvis for guidance. Next, the lateral levator ani complex is divided on both sides from a posterior to anterior approach (Fig. 44.9). The specimen is then delivered through the perineal wound, and the anterior dissection is completed. In men, careful palpation of the prostate and prostatic urethra during the anterior dissection is critical to maintaining the correct anatomic plane and preventing prostatic and/or urethral injury (Fig. 44.10). In women, the appropriate plane is along the posterior wall of the vagina. This plane may be scarred secondary to complications of childbirth and may necessitate resection of a small portion of the vaginal wall at the introitus. With anterior or circumferential tumors, larger resection of the posterior vaginal wall is required. The posterior wall of the vagina is resected between clamps. The cut edge is highly vascular and often requires suture ligation of bleeding vessels after the specimen is delivered. After margin analysis to assure complete resection, the perineum is irrigated and drains are placed in the pelvis. The skin is closed with sutures or staples. For women with posterior vaginal wall resection, the posterior wall can be closed primarily with the perineal wound in cases with small defects.

The perineal wound remains a major source of postoperative complications after APR. Wound complications can occur in 20% to 60% of cases (85–87). For patients with large tissue defects, prior pelvic irradiation, or extensive vaginal resection with APR, perineal reconstruction with a myocutaneous flap can be used to facilitate reconstruction and decrease wound morbidity. The rectus abdominis musculocutaneous (RAM) flap has been used in this situation with excellent results, providing a well vascularized, mobile flap to fill the soft tissue

defect, repair the vaginal defect if necessary, and decrease the incidence of perineal wound complications (85–89). Early involvement of the plastic surgery reconstruction team in operative planning prior to APR is critical to facilitate optimal perineal closure and improve outcome.

Urinary and Sexual Dysfunction After TME

The prevalence of urinary dysfunction after TME with attention to preservation of the autonomic nerve plexi is markedly improved as compared to that after conventional rectal surgery. The incidence of urinary dysfunction after conventional rectal resection ranges from 8% to 70% (90–93). With TME techniques with attention to preservation of the autonomic nerves in the pelvis, this incidence has been significantly improved. Urinary dysfunction in recent reports using TME techniques with ANP have ranged from 0% to 6.6% (39,93,94). In patients with urinary dysfunction immediately after surgery, function appears to improve with time (39,93).

Sexual dysfunction after conventional rectal surgery was a common occurrence, with incidence rates reported from 37% to 68% of patients (95–98). TME with ANP led to marked improvements in outcome for sexual function. With TME and ANP, the ability to have intercourse was preserved in 86% of patients younger than 60 years and in 67% of patients older than 60 years or undergoing APR. Orgasm could be achieved in 87% of men and 91% of women (39). In a small prospective study, TME with ANP was demonstrated to cause no impairment in sexual function (99). Masui et al. (100) demonstrated that the degree of sexual function impairment in 134 sexually active men depended on the degree of ANP with TME. Patients were grouped into three categories: bilateral complete nerve preservation, unilateral complete nerve preservation, and pelvic nerve plexus preservation only. For patients with bilateral complete nerve preservation, erection was preserved for 93%, erection sufficient for vaginal insertion was preserved in 90%, ejaculation was preserved in 83%, and orgasm was preserved in 94%. For patients with unilateral complete nerve preservation, the results were 82%, 53%, 47%, and 65% for the respective categories. For patients with pelvic plexus only preservation, the results were 61%, 26%, 0%, and 22%, respectively. Although preservation of sexual function is an important goal, it should not compromise the oncologic outcome. In many cases, complete ANP may not be possible secondary to tumor size, location, and anatomic constraints in the pelvis. In all cases of pelvic surgery, the patient must be counseled regarding the risks of sexual and urinary dysfunction that can occur. Postoperative sexual function should also be evaluated and followed, as patients seldom discuss or receive treatment for sexual dysfunction after rectal cancer therapy (101).

TAE

Although transabdominal resection using TME principles remains the gold standard for surgical therapy for rectal cancer, this approach can result in significant morbidity to the patient with regard to urinary dysfunction, sexual dysfunction, altered bowel function, risk of anastomotic leak, continence, and need for permanent stoma. The transabdominal approach also represents a significant physiological stress that would not be tolerated in patients with significant medical comorbidities. Efforts to minimize morbidity, offer treatment to patients with severe comorbidities, and treat patients who refused standard resection focused on local resection of rectal cancer using a transanal approach. With reasonable local control rates in these populations, the local excision approach was applied to patients who were otherwise fit and willing to undergo transabdominal resection. The question of whether local excision is an oncologic equivalent to transabdominal resection based on TME principles in appropriately selected patients is still under scrutiny.

Appropriate patient selection is the key to optimizing outcomes from a local resection approach. Because local excision does not address lymph node spread, patient selection hinges on identification of patients with no lymph node metastases. The diagnostic accuracy of predicting nodal involvement with preoperative imaging has been discussed elsewhere. In addition, there are multiple clinical and pathologic tumor characteristics that are associated with lymph node metastases in rectal cancer. Depth of invasion into the rectal wall is a significant predictor for presence of nodal disease, with an incidence of nodal metastases in T1 lesions from 0% to 13%, T2 lesions 12% to 28%, T3 lesions 33% to 66%, and T4 lesions 53% to 79% (102–106). Additional predictors reported include tumor differentiation and presence of lymphovascular invasion, mucinous features, and tumor ulceration (107). Given that T1 lesions have the lowest incidence of lymph node involvement and should be the optimal targets for local excision, studies have focused on these lesions to identify the incidence and predictors of nodal spread. Kikuchi et al. (108) divided T1 lesions by depth of invasion into the submucosa with slight invasion of the muscularis mucosa termed sm1, intermediate invasion termed sm2, and invasion extending to the inner surface of the muscularis propria termed sm3. In their series, there was no incidence of lymph node involvement for sm1 lesions but a 25% incidence of lymph node involvement for sm3 lesions. Nascimbeni et al. (109) reviewed data on 359 patients with resected T1 lesions of the colon or rectum and found a 13% overall incidence of lymph node metastases, with deep invasion into the submucosa (23% incidence of nodal disease), lymphovascular invasion (32% incidence of nodal disease), and location of the tumor in the distal one third of the rectum (34% incidence of nodal disease) as predictors of nodal involvement on multivariate analysis. Tumor grade was not significant on multivariate analysis. As demonstrated above, even T1 lesions have a marked variability in the incidence of lymph node metastases that would predict oncologic failure of local excision alone.

Other factors to be considered for local excision include tumor size, with lesions larger than 3 to 4 cm having a higher rate of local recurrence (110–112). Technical aspects of resection from a transanal approach often exclude tumors with involvement of >40% of the circumference of the rectal wall and tumors >10 cm from the anal verge. Based on tumor factors with regard to nodal spread and technical limitations of TAE, current recommendations for consideration for TAE of rectal cancer include tumor–node–metastasis (TNM) stage T1 or T2 N0 tumors with low grade histology, no evidence of lymphovascular invasion, size smaller than 4 cm, involvement of <40% of the rectal wall circumference, and position <10 cm from the anal verge.

The technical aspects of TAE are straightforward. All patients receive preoperative bowel prep and IV antibiotics. General or regional anesthesia can be used as long as complete paralysis of the anal sphincter can be accomplished. The patient is positioned in lithotomy for posterior lesions or in the prone-jackknife position for anterior lesions. After adequate anal dilation and establishment of retraction, the lesion is identified and a 1- to 2-cm margin is demarcated with cautery. A full-thickness excision with cautery is then performed down to perirectal fat. Care must be taken with anterior lesions to prevent injury to the prostate or posterior vaginal wall. The excised specimen is then carefully oriented and sent to pathology for margin analysis. Any close margin should be checked with frozen section, and if possible, additional margin should be taken to obtain a 1-cm margin around the lesion. After margins are verified, the defect in the rectal wall is closed with absorbable sutures. Patients are generally discharged within 24 to 48 hours after the procedure. Reported complications range from 0% to 22%, with bleeding, local sepsis, urinary infection or retention, anal incontinence, and rectovaginal fistula being the most common (106,107).

The results of TAE vary in numerous reports of single-institution results as there are no randomized controlled trial data to examine. Many of the early experiences with TAE alone were reviewed by Sengupta and Tjandra in 2001 (107). In this study, 22 trials with a total of 958 patients were examined, and local recurrence rates by T stage were reported. The overall local recurrence rate was 14%; for T1 lesions there was a 10% local recurrence rate (range 0% to 24%), for T2 lesions a 25% local recurrence rate (range 0% to 50%), and for T3 lesions a 38% local recurrence rate (range 0% to 100%) (106). These local recurrence rates were higher than would be expected with standard transabdominal resection based on TME principles. Mellgren et al. (104) compared local excision to RAD in a retrospective review in which neither group of patients received adjuvant chemoradiation. The groups compared included patients with 108 local excisions with 4.4 years of follow-up and 153 RADs with 4.8 years of follow-up. The groups differed significantly in distance of the lesion from the anal verge (lower in the local excision group), tumor size (smaller in the local excision group), and T stage (36% T2 for local excision vs 78% T2 for RAD). The results of the comparison showed a higher rate of local recurrence after local excision as compared to RAD (T1 = 18% vs 0%, T2 = 47% vs 6%) as well as a higher rate of overall recurrence (T1 = 21% vs 9%, T2 = 47% vs 16%). Although there was no difference in the 5-year cancer-specific mortality between the two groups, there was a significantly lower 5-year overall survival rate for T2 lesions treated with local excision as compared to RAD (65% vs 81%). The results of this comparison clearly suggest that T2 rectal cancers treated with local excision alone have inferior outcomes as compared to radical surgery. The results are less clear for T1 lesions from this study.

However, studies comparing local excision alone to standard resection alone for T1 lesions also suggest an inferior outcome for local excision alone. Nascimbeni et al. (113) compared 70 patients with T1 lesions who underwent resection to 74 patients with T1 lesions who underwent RAD. With a median follow-up of 8.1 years, there was no significant difference in local recurrence or distant metastasis, but there was a significant improvement in overall and cancer-free survival for the RAD group. Bentrem et al. (114) compared the results of 319 consecutive patients with T1 lesions treated with TAE ($n = 151$) versus RAD ($n = 168$). Adjuvant radiation therapy was used in 11% of the TAE group for either a close margin or the presence of lymphovascular invasion. No systemic chemotherapy was given in this group as part of initial therapy. Adjuvant radiation therapy was utilized in 10% of the RAD group, with 17% receiving adjuvant systemic chemotherapy for positive lymph nodes. These authors reported no difference in disease specific and overall survival, but significant differences in overall recurrence rates (23% TAE vs 6% RAD), local recurrence rates (15% TAE vs 3% RAD), and distant recurrence rates (12% TAE vs 3% RAD), all favoring RAD for superior outcome. The authors noted that with optimal salvage therapy, <50% of the patients with recurrence after TAE can be cured, and that based on salvage results and longer follow-up, they expect the disease-specific survival to be inferior for patients treated with TAE. Taken as a whole, these data would suggest that TAE alone for T1 lesions is inferior to RAD (114).

The addition of adjuvant radiation therapy or chemoradiation therapy to local excision has been demonstrated to improve survival and reduce local recurrence in multiple single-institution series (106). Variations in patient selection, surgical technique, and adjuvant therapy delivered between the numerous trials make more specific conclusions difficult. Multi-institutional phase II trial data also support improved outcomes for local excision with adjuvant chemoradiation for higher risk lesions. The Cancer and Leukemia Group B evaluated the results of local excision alone for T1 lesions ($n = 59$) and local excision with adjuvant chemoradiation therapy for T2 lesions ($n = 51$). With a median follow-up of 4 years, the T1 group had an estimated 6-year overall survival rate of 87% and disease-free survival of 83%. The T2 group rates were 85% and 71%, respectively (115). The Radiation Therapy Oncology Group Protocol 89–02 reported results of 65 patients treated with local excision who were then assigned adjuvant chemoradiation based on high risk features of the tumor after excision. In this study, 14 patients were assigned to observation alone because of the absence of any high risk features. Eighteen patients were assigned to receive adjuvant chemoradiation due to high risk features including stage T2 or T3, high grade histology, lymphovascular invasion, size >3 cm, or elevated carcinoembryonic antigen (CEA). Thirty-three patients (group 1) were assigned to adjuvant chemoradiation with higher dose radiotherapy than group 2 due to both the presence of high risk features as well as margins of resection <3 mm. With a median follow-up of 6.1 years, there was no difference in overall survival or disease-free survival between the treatment groups (116).

The use of neoadjuvant chemoradiation with local excision for locally advanced rectal cancers has also been evaluated in single-institution reports. In patients who achieved complete clinical responses or significant downstaging after neoadjuvant treatment, local excision appears to have similar local recurrence rates and overall survival rates as compared to RAD (117–122). There is also the suggestion that, in a subset of patients who achieve complete clinical responses to neoadjuvant therapy, surgery may not be required (123). These studies are limited by small numbers of patients and lack of long-term follow-up. However, these results must be viewed in the context of reported lymph node involvement in resected specimens of patients with locally advanced rectal cancer treated with neoadjuvant chemoradiation who achieved downstaging. For locally advanced disease downstaged to pT2-T0, residual mesorectal lymph node involvement was found in 14% to 17% of cases (124,125). For cases downstaged to pT0, residual nodal disease was found in 2% to 12% of cases (124–130). Although initial reports of neoadjuvant therapy with downstaging and local excision are promising, the long-term consequences of residual nodal disease are not yet known. In the absence of randomized controlled trial data comparing neoadjuvant therapy with local excision with standard surgical resection, local excision for locally advanced rectal cancers downstaged with neoadjuvant therapy must be approached with caution.

The lack of randomized controlled clinical trials for rectal cancer comparing TAE with or without adjuvant or neoadjuvant therapy to standard transabdominal resection using TME principles with or without adjuvant or neoadjuvant therapy requires caution in the recommendation of TAE for the treatment of rectal cancer. Although numerous reports suggest that, in highly selected patients, results for TAE and standard resection are equivalent, this equivalence is by no means certain. With salvage rates for recurrence after local excision reported to be around 50%, a significant number of patients treated with local excision will have lost the opportunity for cure (131). In addition, salvage surgery often requires a far more radical operation than would have been required at first presentation had the lesion been resected with standard surgery (132). Patients who are otherwise fit to undergo standard transabdominal resection who elect a transanal approach must be counseled regarding the known and unknown risks of such an approach. In the future, a better understanding of tumor biology, molecular markers, and patient selection, along with data from randomized trials, will facilitate the selection of appropriate patients for TAE with no compromise in oncologic outcome.

TEMS

Because TAE of rectal tumors is limited to lesions within 8 to 10 cm of the anal verge, for technical reasons efforts have been directed at improving the scope of transanal resection to include middle and upper third rectal lesions. TEMS has been successful at expanding the reach of the transanal approach for middle and upper rectal tumors. Originally described in the 1980s, the procedure uses a 4-cm-diameter rectoscope with stereoscopic magnification, CO_2 insufflation, and endoscopic instruments to improve lesion visualization and expand the transanal resection limit to as far as 24 cm from the anal verge (133–135). In expert hands, the technique may also have applications for lesions high in the rectum that may result in intraperitoneal perforation with full thickness resection (136). The outcomes using TEMS for both benign and malignant rectal lesions have recently been reviewed, and results are comparable to those of other methods of resection with the benefit of the decreased morbidity of the transanal approach (137). Small randomized trials comparing TEMS with transabdominal resection and TEMS with laparoscopic resection in early rectal cancers report comparable results in oncologic outcomes with decreased morbidity with the TEMS approach (138,139). Functional outcomes with the technique are also good (140–143). The role of TEMS in the treatment of rectal cancer is currently similar to that of TAE, with the benefit of expanding the cohort of patients who can be considered for TAE due to the ability to reach beyond the 8- to 10-cm limit from the anal verge.

Laparoscopic Resection and Rectal Cancer

The application of laparoscopic techniques to rectal cancer resection with adherence to the principles of TME has been reported in numerous series in the literature. The majority of these reports have been reviewed in a study by Bärlehner et al. (144), in which the results for 1,818 patients worldwide who had undergone laparoscopic resection for rectal malignancy were compiled. In this report, anterior resection was the most common laparoscopic procedure for 68% of the cases.

Mortality rates were low with the majority of series reporting 0% postoperative mortality. Rates of conversion to open procedures varied from 0% to 50%; however, in the larger series ($n \geq 100$), the conversion rates ranged from 1% to 23%, likely reflecting the learning curve of laparoscopic rectal resection. Morbidity rates ranged from 0% to 55%, with the larger series reporting ranges from 7% to 38%. The incidence of anastomotic leak varied from 0% to 27% overall, with the larger series reporting leak rates of 1% to 17%. With follow-ups of ≤ 53 months for all series, the overall oncologic outcomes appear similar to those published for standard resection. These authors concluded that, based on the reviewed literature, laparoscopic resection for rectal cancer does not increase morbidity and mortality and does not appear to compromise oncologic outcome, although much of the outcome data are not yet mature (144).

Short-term outcome results are available from two randomized controlled trials comparing laparoscopic resection to conventional resection for rectal cancer. The U.K. Medical Research Council (MRC) trial of conventional versus laparoscopic-assisted surgery in colorectal cancer (CLASICC) recently reported its short-term results for rectal cancer resection in 374 patients (132 open resection, 242 laparoscopic resection) (145). The conversion rate was 34% and was associated with a significant learning curve as seen in the reduction of conversions from 38% in year 1 to 16% in year 6. TME was performed in 10% more patients in the laparoscopic group. Operative time was shorter for open procedures; hospital stay was shorter for laparoscopic procedures. There was no difference in complication rates for open (14%) versus laparoscopic (18%) rectal resections. Time to resumption of regular diet and time to first bowel movement were also similar. On pathology review, there was no difference in the incidence of positive circumferential resection margins (14% open vs 16% laparoscopic). However, in patients undergoing anterior resection, the authors noted an increase in the incidence of positive circumferential margins in the laparoscopic group (12% vs 6%), which, although not statistically significant, did present a cause for concern. Oncologic outcome data are not yet mature.

Zhou et al. (146) reported the results of a randomized controlled trial of 171 patients who underwent laparoscopic ($n = 82$) versus open ($n = 89$) TME with anal sphincter preservation for low rectal cancer. The mortality rate was 0% in both groups, and there were no conversions from laparoscopic to open resection. The morbidity rate (12.4% open vs 6.1% laparoscopic) was significantly higher for the open resection group as was the operative blood loss, time to first bowel movement, and length of hospital stay. There were no positive resection margins in either group. Follow-up data were not sufficiently mature to comment on oncologic outcomes.

Functional outcomes comparing laparoscopic to conventional rectal cancer resection with regard to defecation are not well documented in the literature. There have been reports raising the concern of a higher incidence of bladder and sexual dysfunction after laparoscopic mesorectal excision (147). Patient assessment of bladder and sexual dysfunction after rectal cancer resection in the CLASICC trial revealed similar bladder function for laparoscopic or open resection. However, for men there was a trend for worse overall sexual function and erectile function in the laparoscopic group (148). Certainly, more attention will need to be paid to functional outcomes of laparoscopic TME in rectal cancer to assure equivalence to open resection.

From the available data, both from clinical series as well as randomized trials, several conclusions can be drawn. First, in expert hands the morbidity of laparoscopic resection for rectal cancer appears to be similar to that of open resection with regard to immediate postoperative complications. Mortality rates are also similar. Second, patients appear to benefit with shorter hospital stays and earlier resumption of bowel function with a laparoscopic approach. Third, functional outcomes with regard to defecation, bladder function, and sexual function need to be more carefully assessed after laparoscopic resection to ensure that morbidity rates in these areas are not significantly different than the rates for open resection. Finally, oncologic outcome data need to mature from the randomized studies before definitive conclusions can be reached on the role of laparoscopic resection in rectal cancer, although the available data suggest similar outcomes for the laparoscopic and open approaches.

ROLE OF CHEMOTHERAPY AND RADIATION

Adjuvant Therapies for Rectal Cancer

Surgical treatment is necessary in nearly all patients with rectal cancer, and adjuvant therapies are necessary for those patients at high enough risk of both local and systemic relapse. Several retrospective trials have helped to identify patients appropriate for adjuvant chemoradiotherapy (1–7,149–155). Surgery-alone series have identified patients with high pelvic recurrence rates. For patients with T1-2N0 rectal cancers, local failure rates are <10%. For patients with T3N0 disease, recurrence rates increase to 15% to 35%, and for nonmetastatic node-positive disease, recurrence rates can be as high as 45% to 65%. More than half of recurrences have been shown to occur locally (149). Survival tends to be inversely related to recurrence rates; patients with T1-2N0 rectal cancer have an approximate 80% 5-year survival with surgery alone, whereas patients with T3N0 or node-positive disease have 5-year survival rates <25% (156). It has been these failures and decrements in survival that have led investigators to consider adjuvant therapies in these patients. Adjuvant treatment is generally recommended for patients with local recurrence risks exceeding 20%.

The use of adjuvant radiation therapy in the postoperative management of rectal cancer was established in the late 1970s and early 1980s, and in the 1990s was recommended by a National Institutes of Health (NIH) Consensus Conference as the standard of care (150,151,157). A meta-analysis of adjuvant radiotherapy (both preoperative and postoperative) demonstrated no survival benefit but reduced local failures by 46% and 37%, respectively (158). Since the NIH's recommendations, the addition of adjuvant chemotherapy (both concurrently with radiation and after radiation) has also been established and continues to evolve (159,160). The significant progress made in rectal cancer is largely based on the integration of chemotherapy and radiation and the improvements in adjuvant chemotherapy.

Neoadjuvant Versus Adjuvant Treatment

The timing of concurrent chemotherapy and radiation in the management of rectal cancer has been controversial, and only recently have there been data potentially supporting neoadjuvant therapy in favor of adjuvant therapy. The primary rationale to delivering treatment in the adjuvant setting is the more accurate assessment of pathology. In the postoperative setting, there is an accurate assessment of both the thickness of wall invasion and the status of the pelvic lymph nodes, allowing stage I patients to be spared adjuvant treatment. In the preoperative setting, this information is typically determined by EUS of the tumor and interpretation of CT images. EUS has been shown to have an accuracy of approximately 70% to 80% for both T and N status and has been shown to overstage malignancies approximately 10% to 20% of the time (161–163). In the German Rectal Cancer Group trial, which randomized EUS stage T3–T4 or node-positive patients to neoadjuvant to adjuvant therapy, 18% of patients in the adjuvant arm were found to be overstaged (164). A second reason for adjuvant treatment is the preponderance of data from numerous published trials and clinical experience using this technique, particularly in the United States.

Over the last decade, many institutions (particularly in Europe) have published trials using neoadjuvant treatment with excellent results, comparable to trials using adjuvant treatment. This has led to several trials comparing neoadjuvant to adjuvant treatment. The use of neoadjuvant treatment has generated a lot of interest for several reasons. One of the major benefits is the ability to use neoadjuvant treatment in patients who might otherwise not be candidates for sphincter preservation (so that rates of sphincter preservation can be improved). Patients with clinical responses to neoadjuvant treatment may also be easier to operate on due to tumor regression. Another rationale for neoadjuvant therapy is the potential reduction in toxicity compared with adjuvant treatment. Typically after low anterior resection (LAR) or APR, small bowel falls into the pelvis, directly into the radiation portal, leading to potentially increased toxicity. In the neoadjuvant setting, the small bowel typically remains out of the pelvis, allowing for better shielding of this normal tissue. In addition, in patients treated with APR, because of the need to treat the perineal scar, the adjuvant treatment fields are significantly larger than the neoadjuvant fields, leading to increased bowel and cutaneous toxicity. Finally, from a radiobiologic standpoint, neoadjuvant therapy has the benefit of improved oxygenation of the tumor. In the adjuvant setting, because of surgical interruption of blood flow in the tumor bed, there are likely areas of hypoxia, which are typically less sensitive to radiation. In the neoadjuvant setting, the tumor and surrounding tissues are theoretically less hypoxic as the blood supplies are intact; theoretically, this should be more sensitive to radiation.

Adjuvant Trials Using Radiation Therapy

Several trials have shown local benefit with radiation therapy alone with acceptable toxicity (165–167). One additional trial from the Danish Cancer Society also demonstrated that adjuvant radiotherapy improved the probability of survival without local failure in Dukes B and C patients; however, this trial was closed early due to unacceptable toxicity (168). The National Surgical Adjuvant Breast and Bowel Project (NSABP) R-01 trial randomized 555 patients between 1977 and 1986 with Dukes B and C rectal cancer (analogous to deep wall penetration or node-positive patients in the TNM staging system) to observation; postoperative adjuvant chemotherapy with 5-fluorouracil (5-FU), semustine, and vincristine (MOF); or postoperative radiation therapy with 46 to 47 Gy in 26 to 27 fractions (167). No patients received concurrent chemoradiation. The results of this trial demonstrated a significant reduction in local failure with the addition of radiation therapy (25% vs 16%), but no overall survival or disease-free survival benefit. Patients who received chemotherapy had no improvement in local failure (24%); however, there was a significant improvement in disease-free survival (42% vs 30%, $p = .006$) and overall survival ($p = .05$).

A study from The Netherlands also prospectively evaluated postoperative radiation therapy for rectal cancer (166). One hundred seventy-two patients who had undergone surgical resection for rectal adenocarcinoma were randomized to observation or postoperative radiation to 50 Gy in 5 weeks. Local recurrences were reduced in patients who received postoperative treatment; however, this finding was not significant. There

was also no disease-free or overall survival benefit to adjuvant radiation therapy.

The MRC also evaluated adjuvant radiation therapy after surgical resection in patients with Dukes B or C rectal cancer (165). Four hundred sixty nine patients between 1984 and 1989 were randomized to observation or adjuvant radiation therapy to 40 Gy in 20 fractions over four weeks. Local failures were reduced with radiation therapy (34% vs 21%, $p = 0.001$), however, 5 year overall survival was unchanged (41% vs 39%, p = 0.18).

The results of the NSABP, Netherlands, and MRC trials were in agreement that radiation therapy did improve local control; however, as an adjuvant therapy alone, it did not improve overall survival. The NSABP trial did suggest a benefit to chemotherapy; however, it was not until the Gastrointestinal Tumor Study Group (GITSG) 7175 trial that combination therapies were evaluated (169,170). To evaluate the efficacy of concurrent chemoradiotherapy, 227 patients who had undergone a curative resection with Dukes B2 or C rectal cancer were randomized to observation, postoperative radiation with 40 to 48 Gy in 4 to 5 weeks, postoperative chemotherapy with 5-FU and semustine (methyl-CCNU), or a combination of radiation therapy and chemotherapy. With a median follow-up of 80 months, the overall recurrence rates were 55% for patients receiving no adjuvant treatment, 46% for postoperative chemotherapy, 48% for postoperative radiation, and 33% for the combination of adjuvant radiation and chemotherapy. Combination treatment significantly prolonged time to recurrence as well. Although an overall survival benefit was not initially seen, 6 years after the closure of the study a significant disease-free survival (70% vs 46%, $p = .009$) and overall survival (58% vs 45%, $p = .005$) were improved with the combination of chemotherapy and radiation therapy compared to surgery alone. There was no improvement in survival with combination chemoradiotherapy when compared to adjuvant chemotherapy or radiation therapy alone. The superiority of the combined-modality regimen was likely attributable to the effects of radiation therapy and chemotherapy in controlling local and distant recurrences, respectively (169).

A second trial conducted by the Mayo Clinic/North Central Cancer Treatment Group (NCCTG) was performed to further compare postoperative chemoradiotherapy and postoperative radiotherapy (159). The strategy in this trial was to use a regimen that optimized the contribution of chemotherapy, decrease local recurrences, and attempt to improve survival. Two hundred four patients with T3–T4 or N1–N2 rectal cancer were randomized to postoperative radiation therapy alone (45 to 50 Gy in 5 weeks) or to radiation plus 5-FU. Patients received a cycle of 5-FU plus semustine (methyl-CCNU) before and after concurrent chemoradiation. During concurrent therapy, patients received a 3-day bolus of 5-FU at the beginning and end of radiation. With a median follow-up of 7 years, overall recurrences were reduced 34% with the combination of chemoradiotherapy, and local recurrences were reduced 46% (25% vs 14%, $p = .0016$). Distant metastases were reduced by 37% ($p = .011$), and there was a 29% reduction in deaths. Major toxicities included diarrhea and dermatitis which occurred in similar proportions of patients. Patients who received concurrent chemotherapy had higher rates of nausea and hematologic toxicities Approximately 7% of patients in each treatment arm had severe late toxicity. This trial confirmed the results of the GITSG trial (170).

The Norwegian Radium Hospital conducted a two-arm trial comparing surgery alone to surgery with postoperative chemoradiotherapy (171). One hundred forty-four patients with Dukes B and C rectal cancer were randomized to surgery alone or surgery combined with postoperative chemoradiotherapy (46 Gy over 5 weeks) and bolus 5–FU before six of the radiotherapy fractions. Adjuvant therapy in this trial reduced local recurrences by 60% (30% vs 12%, $p = .01$), and increased 5-year recurrence-free and overall survival by 39% (46% vs 64%, $p = .01$) and 28% (50% vs 64%, $p = .05$), respectively. Toxicity was again reasonable, with no significant differences between the arms of the trial.

With the proven clinical success of concurrent adjuvant chemoradiotherapy in both the Mayo Clinic/NCCTG and GITSG trials, ensuing efforts were aimed at improving the postoperative chemotherapy regimen to further impact overall survival (159,169,170). Based on in vitro data that 5-FU enhances cytoxicity when used in combination with radiation, the NCCTG evaluated the use of standard bolus infusion of 5-FU with continuous infusion of 5-FU during radiation therapy (172,173). Previous comparisons of continuous infusion and bolus 5-FU in the metastatic setting showed no differences in outcomes with respect to survival (174). From a theoretical standpoint, continuous infusion 5-FU allows chemotherapy to be present during all radiation fractions, possibly increasing tumor cytotoxicity which potentially could influence local control and survival. O'Connell and others (173) reported on their experience with an altered chemotherapy regimen during radiation therapy. This trial used a 2 × 2 randomization to determine whether continuous infusion 5-FU during radiotherapy could improve the efficacy over bolus 5-FU, and whether the omission of semustine from this regimen would reduce the toxicity of chemotherapy without reducing efficacy. Six hundred sixty patients with TNM stage II or III rectal cancer were randomized to either continuous venous infusion of 5-FU (225 mg/m^2 every 24 hours) or bolus 5-FU (500 mg/m^2 on the first 3 and last 3 days of radiation). Patients were also randomized to receive either semustine and bolus 5-FU or bolus 5-FU before and after chemoradiation. With a median follow-up of 46 months, 4-year overall survival was significantly improved with continuous infusion 5-FU (70% vs 60%, $p = .005$), and the risk of any recurrence was reduced (37% vs 47%, $p = .01$). Continuous infusion 5-FU with concurrent radiation also reduced the risk of distant metastases from 40% to 31% ($p = .03$), possibly due to the higher doses of chemotherapy used in the continuous infusion arm. The addition of semustine to 5-FU had no beneficial effect on patient outcome.

The above trials have set the standard of care in the United States for the last decade, with respect to the utility of chemotherapy and radiation therapy in the management of TNM stages II and III rectal cancer. Concurrent chemoradiotherapy with continuous infusion 5-FU preceded and followed by additional chemotherapy has been clearly shown to be superior to chemotherapy or radiation therapy alone.

Neoadjuvant Trials Using Radiation Therapy

Early negative trials of preoperative radiation led to the adoption of adjuvant therapy in the United States (175–179). These trials used relatively low doses of radiation and potentially outdated techniques. Two early trials did demonstrate positive outcomes. One British trial randomized patients to surgery alone or to preoperative treatment of 5 Gy × 3 over 5 days preceding surgery (180). This trial failed to demonstrate any survival benefit; however, there did appear to be a reduction in local failures with low-dose hypofractionated radiotherapy. Kligerman and others (181) randomized patients to surgery alone or to preoperative radiotherapy of 45 Gy over 5 weeks. Although this trial actually suggested a survival benefit, patients treated with surgery alone had more liver metastases at operation than were expected compared with the patients treated preoperatively.

The push for preoperative treatment for rectal cancer was driven largely by successes of several trials conducted in Europe (164,182–188). These trials challenged the treatment standards practiced in the United States. The European Organization

for Research and Treatment of Cancer (EORTC) conducted a trial comparing surgery alone to preoperative radiotherapy (34.5 Gy in 15 fractions) in patients with T2–4Nx rectal cancer (182). As with trials using postoperative radiotherapy, this trial demonstrated a reduction in local recurrence (30% vs 15%, $p = .003$), with no difference in survival.

Swedish investigators conducted several trials evaluating preoperative therapy. In an initial trial, 849 patients with resectable rectal cancer were randomized to surgery alone or preoperative radiation (25 Gy delivered 5 to 7 days prior to surgery) (183). Radiation fields encompassed both pelvic and para-aortic lymph node groups (to L2). With a median follow-up of 53 months, local recurrences were significantly lower in the arm treated with preoperative radiation (25% vs 11%, $p = .001$), and time to local failure and distant metastasis was prolonged. As in the U.S. trials, the addition of radiotherapy to surgery had no impact on overall survival. Significantly, however, preoperative radiotherapy in this cohort imparted a much higher rate of postoperative morbidity and mortality (8% vs 2%, $p < .01$). The increase in toxicity was initially blamed on the fractionation schedule; however, comparison to other U.S. studies suggested that the larger field size, which included the para-aortic lymph nodes, was more likely to be the cause of increased toxicity. The Swedes eventually amended this protocol to irradiate just the pelvis, and follow-up of these patients demonstrated no significant difference in morbidity or mortality compared with those who received no radiation.

A second Swedish trial compared neoadjuvant radiation (25.5 Gy in 5 days just prior to surgery) with adjuvant radiation in a more conventional scheme (60 Gy in 8 weeks) in 471 patients with resectable rectal cancer (Dukes B or C) (185–187). Local recurrence rates were statistically significantly lower after preoperative than after postoperative radiotherapy (12% vs 21%; $p = .02$); however, there was no significant difference in survival. Review of toxicity data in the initial results of the trial suggested increased morbidity, particularly small bowel obstructions in those patients treated with postoperative radiotherapy, compared with patients who had preoperative treatment or surgery alone. One hypothesis for the potential increase in morbidity was the increased bowel in the postoperative fields. However, with longer follow-up, there appeared to be no significant difference in postoperative mortality. Although no chemotherapy was used in this trial, interestingly, local recurrence rates in the preoperative arm were similar to local recurrence rates in the GITSG 7175 and Mayo Clinic/NCCTG trials, which used longer courses of adjuvant radiotherapy and chemotherapy (159,169,170).

Building on the success of the previous trial, and using smaller radiation portals to reduce morbidity in the initial Swedish trial, the Swedes repeated their initial randomization (183–185,187). They randomized 1,168 patients with resectable rectal cancer to surgery alone or to neoadjuvant radiotherapy with 25 Gy in 5 fractions in the week prior to surgery, without chemotherapy. As in the prior trial, local recurrence was reduced from 27% to 11% with radiation therapy ($p < .001$). This recurrence rate again paralleled results in postoperative adjuvant trials. In addition, there was a significant improvement in disease-free survival (65% vs 74%, $p = .002$) and overall survival (48% vs 58%, $p = .004$) with preoperative treatment. On subset analysis, this benefit was seen in all stages, including in stage I patients, in which many argue that postoperative treatment is unnecessary. This trial clearly questions the validity of this argument and the basis for using postoperative treatment to minimize overtreatment of early stage patients.

The introduction of TME has demonstrated reduced local recurrences and improved disease-free survivals in patients with Dukes stages A, B, and C (186,189–193). Heald and Ryall (190) demonstrated a 5-year overall survival of 87%, with disease-free survivals by Dukes stage to be 94% for stage

A and 87% for stage B. More impressively, the local recurrence in this series at 4 years was 2.6%. Other series have demonstrated recurrence rates between 5% and 10%; this range of rates is similar to that in patients treated without TME with adjuvant chemoradiotherapy, such as in the GITSG or Mayo Clinic/NCCTG study (189,191–193). Dutch investigators have looked at the benefit of adding radiation therapy to the treatment of patients undergoing TME (186). They hypothesized that, because both preoperative therapy and TME have been shown to reduce local recurrences, the combination would reduce recurrence rates further. In a multicenter, randomized trial, 1,861 patients with resectable rectal cancer were randomized to either TME or preoperative radiotherapy (25 Gy in 5 days 1 week prior to surgery) and TME. The 2-year overall survival was similar in both groups (82% vs 81.8%); however, local recurrence was significantly reduced from 8.2% to 2.4% with preoperative radiotherapy. Although the follow-up to date is short, this result represents some of the lowest recurrence rates, and again demonstrates a role for additional therapy such as preoperative radiotherapy or postoperative chemoradiotherapy.

Adjuvant Versus Neoadjuvant Trials Using Chemoradiation Therapy

Through the early 1990s, there was no clear answer on whether preoperative or postoperative therapy is superior. The bias in the United States until recently has been to use postoperative chemoradiotherapy, whereas in Europe many institutions have adopted various preoperative strategies including hypofractionated radiotherapy or standard fractionated concurrent chemoradiotherapy. The NSABP attempted to compare these treatments in the R-03 trial (194,195). This trial was to accrue 900 patients randomized to preoperative or postoperative chemotherapy and radiotherapy (50.4 Gy in 5.5 weeks). Due to poor accrual, the trial closed in 1999 (after accruing 237 patients). In the preoperative group, 23% had a clinical response, and 10% had a complete pathological response. Preoperative therapy compared to postoperative therapy was found to improve the rate of sphincter-sparing surgery (44% vs 34%); however, disease-free survival at 1 year was similar (83% vs 78%). Postoperative complications were similar between the two groups (25 vs 22%; preoperative vs postoperative); however, grade 4/5 toxicity was greater in the preoperative arm (34 vs 23%; $p = .07$), with the largest difference in grade 4 diarrhea (24% vs 12%), which was most pronounced during the radiation.

One of the most important trials to evaluate the controversy of neoadjuvant therapy versus adjuvant therapy was conducted by the Germans (164,188). This trial compared equivalent preoperative and postoperative regimens of chemoradiotherapy in the setting of TME. Patients with locally advanced operable rectal cancer (ultrasound T3–T4 or node positive) were randomized to pre- or postoperative chemoradiotherapy to the tumor and regional lymph nodes. Patients received 50.4 Gy in 5.5 weeks with 5-FU (1000 mg/m^2/d) during the first and fifth weeks of radiotherapy as a continuous infusion and four additional cycles of adjuvant bolus 5-FU chemotherapy. In both arms, the timing between chemoradiotherapy and surgery was 4 to 6 weeks. Eight hundred twenty-three patients were randomized. Overall survival at 5 years was 76% in the preoperative arm and 74% in the postoperative arm ($p = .8$). The 5-year cumulative incidence of local recurrence was 6% for patients assigned to preoperative treatment and 13% in the postoperative treatment group ($p = .006$). The rate of sphincter-preserving surgery was nearly doubled from 20% with postoperative treatment to 39% with preoperative treatment. Acute grade 3 or 4 toxic effects were lower in the preoperative arm

(27% vs 40%, $p = .001$), and long-term toxic effects were also reduced in the preoperative arm (14% vs 24%, $p = .01$). This included reduced rates of anastomotic leaks, fistula tract formation, delayed wound healing, and postoperative bleeding rates. This trial is important in that the treatments were identical in the preoperative and postoperative setting, with the exception of an allowed boost in the postoperative setting. This trial is the only study that allows a true direct comparison between the sequence of surgery and chemoradiotherapy. Although follow-up is relatively short, this trial already demonstrates a reduction in local recurrence by 50% with preoperative chemoradiotherapy and a significant reduction in acute and long-term toxicity. The increase in toxicity in the postoperative setting likely represents irradiation of more bowel, due to anatomic positional changes of the bowel after surgery. Although no survival benefit has yet been seen, the ability to improve local control and increase the ability to spare the sphincter has led to a significant shift in the standard of care in the United States toward preoperative therapy. One caveat to this shift, however, is that treatment in the preoperative setting potentially leads to overtreatment in patients who are overstaged. In the German trial, this occurred in 18% of patients randomized to the postoperative arm.

Radiation Techniques

Radiation treatment, whether given in the neoadjuvant or adjuvant setting, remains fairly similar with respect to treatment portals and dose, with some modifications for those patients treated with APR. Treatment planning can be done under fluoroscopy with the use of rectal contrast, or with three-dimensional CT-based planning systems. Patients are given oral contrast 30 to 45 minutes prior to simulation to help to identify small bowel. A marker is also placed at the anal verge, typically using a small rectal catheter and solder wire. This facilitates the use of rectal contrast in patients undergoing fluoroscopic simulation. In patients treated with APR, the perineal scar should also be marked with solder wire. Standard external beam radiation fields include treatment to the primary tumor and regional lymphatics with a four field approach using anterior posterior/posterior anterior (AP/PA) and opposed lateral portals. Patients are typically treated prone on a belly board that allows small bowel to shift up in the pelvis out of the field.

Radiation Fields

Radiation field shaping is performed with blocking or multileaf collimation. For patients being treated preoperatively, the inferior border is at least 3 to 5 cm distal to the tumor (determined by digital palpation, measurements from colonoscopy and visualization on planning imaging). For patients being treated postoperatively, the inferior border should again be at least 3 to 5 cm distal to the anastomosis site (as determined from operative reports or fluoroscope of CT planning images). This is typically at the inferior edge of the obturator foramen, or can be lower if necessary (i.e., invasion of the anus). If it is possible, irradiation of the sphincter should be minimized to lessen late anal toxicity. For patients receiving postoperative radiation after APR, the inferior edge of the field must also include the perineal scar. For all patients, the superior border is typically placed between the sacral promontory and L4–5 interspace. The posterior border should include the entire sacrum (to allow for coverage of the sacral plexus nodes), and typically includes a margin of 1 cm. Many radiation oncologists will shield the posterior inferior portion of the lateral field to block the gluteal folds and perineum; however, in patients treated with APR, the perineal scar must be treated. The anterior border is typically placed at approximately the posterior edge of the pubic symphysis, but the field should be designed to treat the entire rectum and perirectal soft tissue. In the setting of T4 disease with invasion of the vagina, cervix, prostate, or bladder, the anterior border should be placed anteriorly to the pubic symphysis to allow coverage of the external iliac lymph nodes, as the risk of drainage to this nodal group increases with involvement of these anterior structures. For anal or lower vaginal involvement, coverage of the inguinal nodes is also recommended. The lateral borders of the AP/PA portals should allow adequate coverage or the pelvic lymph nodes, typically 1.5 to 2 cm lateral to the edge of the pelvic brim. The femoral heads can be shielded with custom blocks.

Boosts to the pelvis are typically delivered with a three-field approach with a PA and opposed lateral portals, or with lateral fields alone. These fields typically allow full coverage of the rectal tumor or anastomotic site. The superior borders are typically lowered to the middle portion of the sacroiliac-joint. The inferior border can also be raised; however, it should at a minimum allow 2 to 3 cm of margin on the inferior edge of the tumor or anastomosis. The posterior border is typically unchanged from the initial course of radiation. The anterior border is usually moved posteriorly to allow coverage of the tumor or anastomosis site by 2 to 3 cm, while allowing additional shielding of small bowel. The lateral border on the PA field is typically placed at the internal edge of the pelvic brim.

Radiation Dose

The dose to the extended tumor bed nodal field, for either preoperative or postoperative radiation, should be 50 Gy in 5 to 6 weeks of daily treatment in 1.8- to 2.0-Gy fractions with concurrent chemotherapy. This dose is considered the standard of care in the United States; however, in Europe some institutions will deliver 25 Gy preoperatively in five daily fractions of 5 Gy. At our institution, we typically deliver 45 Gy to the entire pelvis, with a boost to reduced fields to a total dose of 50.4 to 54 Gy in 1.8-Gy fractions per day with concurrent continuous infusion 5-FU. When doses >50.4 Gy are prescribed, we shield small bowel. If this is not possible due to the location of small bowel (usually in the postoperative setting), we limit the total dose to 50.4 Gy.

Future Directions

The multidisciplinary use of surgery, chemotherapy, and radiation therapy in rectal cancer has clearly established a benchmark by which future therapies will be evaluated. In the realm of radiation therapy, strategies to minimize normal tissue toxicities have become an important target to improve treatment-related side effects and to potentially allow dose escalation. Pelvic radiotherapy has been associated with an increased risk of femoral neck fractures (196). Intensity-modulated radiation therapy (IMRT), which allows enhanced beam shaping through variable radiation influences, allows potential sparing of radiosensitive structures, particularly the small bowel and femoral heads. Although long-term outcomes with this technology are not yet available, it has been used clinically in rectal cancer (169,197–199). The use of radioprotectors, such as amifostine, has also demonstrated the ability of chemical modifiers to protect normal tissues without compromising tumor control in other clinical situations (169,200–204). The Radiation Therapy Oncology Group (RTOG) 0315 protocol is currently evaluating the efficacy of somatostatin in reducing acute bowel toxicity. As treatments become more intensive, both strategies of improved dose conformality and radioprotectors allow the selective sparing of normal tissues. The issue of anal toxicity is also of importance. Long-term bowel dysfunction is common in patients treated with trimodality therapy, and efforts to reduce this problem need to be addressed.

In the realm of chemotherapy, a new class of targeted agents has become prevalent. Agents such as cetuximab and bevacizumab have been used successfully in metastatic colorectal cancer with improved outcomes compared with historical controls (205,206). These agents offer a novel approach in cancer management that will likely be the beginning of an era of targeted therapies. The integration of these targeted therapies to surgery, chemotherapy, and radiation therapy will hopefully improve on our current outcomes.

SPECIAL CONSIDERATIONS

TME: Effects on Outcome

Resection of the entire mesorectum (TME) has been touted to be the key component in the reduction of local recurrence rates in rectal cancer. The importance of TME is based on the fact that the mesorectum can serve as the site of nodal or occult micrometastatic disease that is within the pelvis when the mesorectum is partially mobilized and resected. The goal of TME is the resection of the rectum along with its blood vessels and lymph nodes. Resecting an intact mesorectal fascial envelope and obtaining a negative circumferential margin are essential for minimizing local recurrences. The progressive narrowing of the pelvis makes the resection of the distal extent of the mesorectum a technical challenge.

Pathologic analysis of resected specimens supports the use of TME. The presence of non-nodal tumor deposits in the distal mesorectum of patients with rectal cancer was noted in 1982 (207). Reynolds et al. showed tumor deposits in the mesorectum as far distal as 5 cm from the primary tumor (208) with serial transverse sectioning in 5-mm increments on 50 TME specimens to assess for the presence and location of mesorectal involvement (209). Although there were no nodal or mesorectal deposits in six T2N0 specimens, 28 of 44 T3 specimens (64%) had nodal or mesorectal deposits. Five of 21 T3N0 patients (24%) had non-nodal metastatic mesorectal deposits; 27% (12/44) had deposits distal to the inferior edge of the primary tumor, and 11% (5/44) were > 2 cm away. A similar study by Tocchi et al. (210) examining 53 TME specimens found nodal metastases and non-nodal deposits distal to the primary tumor in 33% and 44% of specimens, respectively. Ratto et al. (211) reported on the presence of mesorectal tumor involvement in 77 patients who underwent TME. Microscopic non-nodal tumor discontiguous from the primary tumor was noted in 44% of the patients. This finding suggests that pelvic recurrence may in part be due to the inadequate clearance of mesorectal tissue that may harbor metastatic disease.

The technique of TME was introduced by Heald in England in 1979 and has been described in this chapter (33). In 1986, Heald and Ryall (190) reported on 112 consecutive cases of TME at the time of anterior resection for rectal cancers with a 5-year local recurrence rate of 2.7%, a 5-year tumor-free survival rate of 82%, and an overall 5-year survival rate of 88%. These results were far superior to those in previous reports on the management of rectal cancer and served to strengthen the importance of TME in the surgical management of rectal cancer.

Historically, local recurrence rates after conventional surgery (non-TME) have averaged 30% with 5-year survival rates ranging from 27% to 42%. Several studies have addressed the role of TME in reducing local recurrence rates. In today's era of multimodality management of rectal cancer, it is important to note that, in order to determine fully the impact of

TME, studies can not offer chemoradiation to large numbers of patients.

Heald's first report and impressive local recurrence rate was met with criticisms and concerns focusing on selection bias and patient mix. Heald et al. (212) updated the initial series and reported on 519 rectal cancer resections. The average follow-up was 8.3 years, and all patients had tumors within 15 cm from the anal verge. Only 9% of these patients received radiation, and 6% received postoperative chemotherapy. The local recurrence rate at 5 years for patients undergoing sphincter preservation was 5%, and the 5-year cancer-specific survival rate was 80%.

Following the publication of Heald's results, there have been many reports in the literature touting the superiority of TME alone for local control and overall survival. These retrospective studies from single and multiple institutions compared the outcomes of surgery in the era of TME with the outcomes from conventional, non-TME surgery practiced prior to the introduction of TME. In 1996, Arbman et al. (213) compared 211 rectal cancer patients who underwent traditional non-TME resections from 1984 through 1986 to 230 patients who underwent TME from 1990 through 1992. There were no differences in terms of stage, complications, operative mortality, or the numbers of patients who received adjuvant chemoradiation. There was a 6% local recurrence rate after TME; this rate was significantly lower than the 14% rate with traditional surgery. Bokey et al. (81) examined 596 rectal cancer patients undergoing surgery alone from 1971 through 1991. All patients underwent surgery for curative intent. Standard surgical technique was adopted in 1979, and TME was routinely used beginning in 1984. The local recurrence rate significantly decreased from 13% during 1971 through 1985 to 7% during 1985 through 1991 ($p = .03$). On multivariate analysis, non-TME surgery was associated with a hazard ratio of 2 for developing local recurrence (81). Kockerling et al. (214) evaluated 1,581 curative resections performed in Germany between 1985 and 1991. TME was introduced as standard of care in 1985. These patients were compared with patients who underwent resection between 1974 and 1984. No patient received adjuvant therapy, and the mean follow-up period was 13.1 years. There was a significant decrease in local recurrence rate (39.4% to 9.8%) and a significantly improved overall survival rate (50% to 71%) in the group that underwent TME (214).

Havenga et al. (215) addressed the role of TME in rectal cancer surgery with a multinational review comparing "standardized" surgery (254 TME patients Memorial Sloan Kettering Cancer Center [MSKCC], 204 TME patients [Basingstoke], 233 D3 lymphadenectomy patients [Tokyo National Cancer Center]) to "conventional" surgery (366 patients [Norway], 354 patients [Netherlands Comprehensive Cancer Center West]) in potentially curative TNM stage II and/or III rectal cancer. There were significant benefits in local recurrence (4% to 9% vs 32% to 35%), 5-year cancer-specific survival (75% to 80% vs 52%), and overall survival (62% to 75% vs 42% to 44%) in the patients who underwent TME (215).

The results in the aforementioned studies were noted at single institutions by surgeons with significant experience in performing TME. Even in the hands of these surgeons, there has been some morbidity associated with this procedure. Although mortality is acceptably low at <3%, the rate of distal anastomotic leakage following TME is 3% to 13% (207,213, 216,217). As a result, routine creation of a diverting proximal stoma has been advocated.

Two large prospective European studies were undertaken to evaluate TME and its acceptance in larger surgical communities. In 1993, Norway initiated the Norwegian Rectal Cancer Project to improve the outcomes from rectal cancer as local recurrence rates were >25%. A national rectal cancer registry was created, and the organized training of surgeons in the technique of TME was conducted. In 2002, Wibe et al. (218) reported on the prospective analysis of 1,794 patients who underwent curative resections from 1993 through 1997. Surgery was performed at 55 different hospitals, and the use of TME increased throughout the study from 78% to 92% (1,395 TME patients, 229 non-TME patients). At a median follow-up of 30 months, the local recurrence rate was 6% for TME versus 12% for non-TME. Four-year overall survival was 73% for TME versus 60% for non-TME. Operative mortality was 3%, and the anastomotic leak rate was 10%, with no difference between TME and non-TME patients. This study showed that TME could be taught to a significant number of surgeons with minimal complications. In response to the mounting data in support of TME and European data suggesting a survival benefit with preoperative radiation therapy, the Dutch Colorectal Cancer Group initiated a prospective randomized trial in 1996 comparing preoperative radiation therapy followed by TME (RT+TME) to TME alone for rectal cancer (219). All participating surgeons were trained by certified instructors to perform TME. Radiation was given as a hypofractionated 5 Gy/d over 5 days. Patients (1,861) were enrolled from 1996 through 1999, and 1,805 patients were eligible for analysis (897 RT+TME, 908 TME alone). Based on the final pathology, 89% of the patients underwent a curative resection. There were no differences in age, sex, tumor location, type of resection, or TNM stage between the two groups. The 2-year local recurrence rates were 2.4% for RT+TME versus 8.2% for TME alone ($p <.001$). The 2-year overall survival was no different between the RT+TME and TME alone groups (82% vs 81.8%, respectively), and there was no difference in distant recurrence rates (14.8% for RT+TME vs 16.8% for TME alone).

A parallel report to the Dutch study compared the complications and acute side effects between the two treatment groups (220). RT+TME versus TME alone were similar with regard to operative mortality (3.5% vs 2.6%), overall morbidity (48% vs 41%), bleeding (13% both groups), and anastomotic leak rate (11% vs 12%), respectively. The rate of perineal wound-healing problems after APR was higher in the RT + TME group (29% vs 18%, $p = .008$). The Dutch trial confirmed that TME could be instituted at a national level with reasonable outcomes and complication rates.

In conclusion, TME has resulted in dramatic reductions in local recurrence rates and improvements in overall survival with minimal increases in morbidity.

MARGINS

Distal Margin

The importance of achieving negative margins has long been appreciated. The goal of sphincter preservation and technical advances in anastomosis resulted in the resurrection of the question of what is the minimal acceptable distal margin that is required for complete oncologic resection. The long held belief that a 5-cm distal margin was essential to achieve local control was initially championed by Goligher et al. (221). In his study of 1,500 rectal cancers, distal spread ≥ 2 cm beyond the tumor occurred in 2% of patients. Interestingly, this led to the suggestion that 5 cm was the appropriate safe distal margin. Dukes (222) and Grinnell (223) reported distal spread >2 cm to be rare. Pollett and Nicholls (224) reported that a 2-cm distal margin did not compromise survival or local recurrence. In their retrospective review of 334 patients undergoing restorative resections for rectal adenocarcinoma, they divided patients into three groups with regard to distal resection margin: ≤ 2 cm (55 patients), 2 to 5 cm (177 patients), or ≥ 5 cm (102 patients). There were no differences in overall 5-year survival (69.1%,

68.4%, 69.6%), cancer-specific death rates (25.5%, 23.2%, 21.6%), or local recurrence (7.3%, 6.2%, 7.8%), respectively (224). An analysis of the distal margins in the NSABP trials showed that local recurrence as the first site of treatment failure was slightly higher in patients with <2-cm margins (22%) as opposed to patients with ≥3-cm margins (12%). Importantly, overall survival was not significantly different if distal resection margins were <2 cm, 2 to 2.9 cm, or ≥3 cm (225). Distal spread may be related to the degree of tumor differentiation and other tumor-specific prognostic factors, suggesting that a single rule of distance for distal margins may not be applicable to all patients. In the studies by Dukes (223) and Grinnell (224), distal spread >2 cm was noted primarily in patients with poorly differentiated tumors. Williams et al. (226), Shirouzu et al. (227), Andreola et al. (228), and Ueno et al. (229) assessed 50 specimens from patients who underwent APR, and identified distal spread of >1 cm in 12 specimens. All were poorly differentiated primaries. Several other anatomic studies of resected specimens revealed that distal spread of >1 cm was rare and appeared to be limited to tumors with poor differentiation. Based on these studies and multiple other case series in the literature, the adequacy of a 2-cm distal margin was established.

The effects of neoadjuvant chemoradiation on the degree of distal intramural spread remain to be fully elucidated, but the recognized downsizing of tumors secondary to chemoradiation may also result in a decrease in distal spread allowing for decreases in distal margins. Mezhir et al. (230) examined the extent of distal spread in 20 patients who underwent neoadjuvant chemoradiation followed by rectal resection with TME. Eleven patients had distal spread, and the mean distance from the primary tumor was 0.5 cm. Only one patient had distal spread beyond 1 cm from the tumor. These findings suggest that margins <2 cm may be appropriate in patients who have undergone neoadjuvant chemoradiation (230). For patients treated with neoadjuvant chemoradiation therapy, negative margins of ≤1 cm do not appear to affect oncologic outcome (230,231,232).

Based on these results, general recommendations can be made for the extent of distal margins for rectal cancer resection. For lesions in the upper rectum, a 5-cm distal margin including 5 cm of distal mesorectum is an adequate oncologic procedure. For lesions in the middle/lower rectum, TME with a distal margin of 2 cm should be the goal although negative margins <2 cm may be adequate. For distal, locally advanced lesions or distal tumors with poor differentiation where 2 cm margins may not be possible, neoadjuvant chemoradiation therapy should be considered.

Circumferential Radial Margin

The importance of TME in minimizing local recurrences has been described. A frequently overlooked component of rectal cancer resection is the need to achieve negative circumferential radial margins (CRM). A properly performed TME will provide for adequate radial margins in the posterior aspect of the rectal dissection, but care must be taken to ensure the adequacy of radial margins in all aspects of the circumference of the rectum. Adam et al. (233) reviewed 141 potentially curative surgical resections for rectal cancer at the General Infirmary at Leeds. The circumferential margin was positive in 25% of patients. At a median follow-up of 5.3 years, the overall local recurrence rate was 23% (32/141). The 5-year local recurrence rate for patients with negative radial margins was 10%; this rate was significantly better than the 78% local recurrence rate for patients with positive radial margins (p <.001).

Hall et al. (234) examined the circumferential margin status of 152 patients undergoing potentially curative TME. The rate of a "positive" circumferential margin (defined as margins <1 mm) was 13%. Although the margin status did not correlate with local recurrence, it was associated with the risk of distant recurrence (24% for negative vs 50% for positive). Wibe et al. (218) reviewed the circumferential margins of 686 patients enrolled in the Norwegian Rectal Cancer Study who underwent potentially curative TME without radiation therapy. The local recurrence rate at a median follow-up of 29 months was 7%; 5% for negative circumferential margins but 22% for positive margins (<1 mm). On multivariate analysis, a positive circumferential margin correlated with an increased risk of local recurrence, distant metastases, and mortality.

Nagtegaal et al. (235) evaluated 656 patients in the Dutch Trial who underwent rectal resection and TME but no adjuvant treatment to assess the relationship of circumferential margin to recurrence and survival. A positive margin (≤1 mm) was seen in 18.3% of specimens. Tumors with a higher TNM stage, located <5 cm from the anal verge, and requiring APR had a higher rate of positive margins. After a median follow-up of 3 years, the overall local and distant recurrence rates were significantly higher in patients with positive radial margins. A positive radial margin was also associated with a 68% 2-year survival, which was significantly lower than the 90% 2-year survival rate for patients with negative radial margins (p <.001). Marr et al. (236) retrospectively reviewed 608 patients who underwent rectal cancer resections in Leeds Hospital from 1986 through 1997. The impact of TME on CRM status was evaluated by comparing groups who underwent APR before and after 1994 when TME was introduced at Leeds. CRM involvement in those patients undergoing APR before 1994 was 28%, and CRM involvement was 31% in patients who underwent APR with formal TME after 1994. Thus, CRM involvement did not diminish with TME, suggesting the need to ensure completeness of circumferential resection along with TME.

PELVIC EXENTERATION

Rectal cancer patients who present with locally advanced disease in the form of contiguous organ involvement are candidates for RAD if there is no evidence of systemic disease and if the patient can withstand the rigors of an extensive operative procedure. Chemoradiation plays an important role in the management of locally advanced disease as discussed in this chapter, and this must be considered when en bloc resections and pelvic exenteration is considered. Careful preoperative staging, including CT imaging, MRI, and PET scans, is required. MRI provides additional anatomic details and improves the visualization of tumor and adjoining tissue planes compared to CT (237). The four main types of pelvic exenteration are anterior, posterior, supralevator, and total exenteration. Anterior and posterior pelvic exenterations pertain to performing this procedure in women. The designation is based on the presence of internal genitalia as a barrier to further tumor extension.

Pelvic exenterations include the en bloc resection of the rectum, prostate, bladder, vagina, uterus, ovaries, and cervix and are associated with significant morbidity. Morbidity rates of 50% to 70% have been reported in recent series from centers with higher procedure volumes (238,239). Morbidity is primarily septic in origin. Intestinal fistulae, obstruction, and wound complications are also noted.

Much of the literature addressing the outcomes of pelvic exenteration for rectal cancer include heterogeneous populations with marked differences in organ involvement, nodal status, adjuvant therapies, the success of resections (R0, R1, or R2), and whether the procedures were performed for primary or recurrent disease. In those series that distinguish R0 versus R1 and R2 dissections, the average 5-year survival for R0 resection is 38% compared to 5% for R1 and R2 resections (239–242).

Thus, careful patient selection through accurate staging is required to ensure reasonable outcomes.

FUTURE DIRECTIONS

The evolution of the multidisciplinary approach to the management of rectal cancer has resulted in significant improvements in recurrence and overall survival rates. Significant enhancements in sphincter preservation and quality of life have also been realized. The challenge is to further improve these endpoints through the multidisciplinary approach. Molecular targeted therapies such as bevacizumab and cetuximab represent key components of present and future treatment paradigms. Novel radiation techniques such as IMRT and novel surgical techniques may also further improve the care of the rectal cancer patient.

References

1. Waizer A, Zitron S, Ben-Baruch D. Comparative study for preoperative staging of rectal cancer. *Dis Colon Rectum.* 1989;32:53–56.
2. Rifkin MD, Ehrlich SM, Marks G. Staging of rectal carcinoma: prospective comparison of endorectal US and CT. *Radiology.* 1989;170:319–322.
3. Balthazar EJ, Megibow AJ, Hulnick D. Carcinoma of the colon: detection and preoperative staging by CT. *AJR Am J Roentgenol.* 1988;150:301–306.
4. Thompson WM, Halvorsen RA, Foster WL. Preoperative and postoperative CT staging of rectosigmoid carcinoma. *AJR Am J Roentgenol.* 1986;146:703–710.
5. Holdsworth PJ, Johnston D, Chalmers AG. Endoluminal ultrasound and computed tomography in the staging of rectal cancer. *Br J S.* 1988;75:1019–1022.
6. Guinet C, Buy JN, Ghossain MA. Comparison of magnetic resonance imaging and computed tomography in the preoperative staging of rectal cancer. *Arch Surg.* 1990;125:385–388.
7. Shank B, Dershaw DD, Caravelli J. A prospective study of the accuracy of preoperative computed tomographic staging of patients with biopsy-proven rectal carcinoma. *Dis Colon Rectum.* 1990;33:285–290.
8. Beynon J. An evaluation of the role of rectal endosonography in rectal cancer. *Ann R Coll Surg Engl.* 1989;71:131–139.
9. Feifel G, Hildebrandt U, Dhom G. Assessment of depth of invasion in rectal cancer by endosonography. *Endoscopy.* 1987;19:64–67.
10. Yamashita Y, Machi J, Shirouzu K. Evaluation of endorectal ultrasound for the assessment of wall invasion of rectal cancer: report of a case. *Dis Colon Rectum.* 1988;31:617–623.
11. Waizer A, Zitron S, Ben-Baruch D. Comparative study for preoperative staging of rectal cancer. *Dis Colon Rectum.* 1989;32:53–56.
12. Glaser F, Schlag P, Herfarth C. Endorectal ultrasonography for the assessment of invasion of rectal tumours and lymph node involvement. *Br J Surg.* 1990;77:883–887.
13. Hildebrandt U, Klein T, Feifel G. Endosonography of pararectal lymph nodes: in vitro and in vivo evaluation. *Dis Colon Rectum.* 1990;33:863–868.
14. Orrom WJ, Wong WD, Rothenberger DA. Endorectal ultrasound in the preoperative staging of rectal tumors: a learning experience. *Dis Colon Rectum.* 1990;33:654–659.
15. Tio TL, Coene PP, van Delden OM. Colorectal carcinoma: preoperative TNM classification with endosonography. *Radiology.* 1991;179:165–170.
16. Katsura Y, Yamada K, Ishizawa T. Endorectal ultrasonography for the assessment of wall invasion and lymph node metastasis in rectal cancer. *Dis Colon Rectum.* 1992;35:362–368.
17. Herzog U, von Flue M, Tondelli P. How accurate is endorectal ultrasound in the preoperative staging of rectal cancer? *Dis Colon Rectum.* 1993;36:127–134.
18. Cho E, Nakajima M, Yasuda K. Endoscopic ultrasonography in the diagnosis of colorectal cancer invasion. *Gastrointest Endosc.* 1993;39:521–527.
19. Sailer M, Leppert R, Bussen D. Influence of tumor position on accuracy of endorectal ultrasound staging. *Dis Colon Rectum.* 1997;40:1180–1186.
20. Akasu T, Sugihara K, Moriya Y. Limitations and pitfalls of transrectal ultrasonography for staging of rectal cancer. *Dis Colon Rectum.* 1997;40(Suppl 10):S10–S15.
21. Garcia-Aguilar J, Pollack J, Lee S. Accuracy of endorectal ultrasonography in preoperative staging of rectal tumors. *Dis Colon Rectum.* 2002;45:10–15.
22. Marusch F, Koch A, Schmidt U. Routine use of transrectal ultrasound in rectal carcinoma: results of a prospective multicenter study. *Endoscopy.* 2002;34:385–390.
23. Hawes RH. New staging techniques: endoscopic ultrasound. *Cancer.* 1993;71(Suppl 12):4207–4213.
24. Hulsmans FJ, Tio TL, Fockens P. Assessment of tumor infiltration depth in rectal cancer with transrectal sonography: caution is necessary. *Radiology.* 1994;190:715–720.
25. Kruskal JB, Kane RA, Sentovich SM. Pitfalls and sources of error in staging rectal cancer with endorectal use. *Radiographics.* 1997;17:609–626.
26. Dworak O. Number and size of lymph nodes and node metastases in rectal carcinomas. *Surg Endosc.* 1989;3:96–99.
27. Bianchi PP, Ceriani C, Rottoli M, et al. Endoscopic ultrasonography and magnetic resonance in preoperative staging of rectal cancer: comparison with histologic findings. *J Gastrointest Surg.* 2005;9:1222–1228.
28. Kim CK, Kim SH, Chun HK, et al. Preoperative staging of rectal cancer: accuracy of 3-Tesla magnetic resonance imaging. *Eur Radiol.* 2006;17:1–9.
29. Glimelius B, Isacsson U, Jung B, et al. Radiotherapy in addition to radical surgery in rectal cancer. *Acta Oncol.* 1995;34:565–570.
30. Fisher B, Wolmark N, Rockette H, et al. Postoperative adjuvant chemotherapy or radiation therapy for rectal cancer: results from the NSABP protocol R-01. *J Natl Cancer Inst.* 1988;80:21–29.
31. Gastrointestinal Tumor Study Group (GITSG). Adjuvant therapy of colon cancer; results of a prospectively randomized trial. *N Engl J Med.* 1984;310:737–743.
32. Minsky BD. The role of adjuvant radiation therapy in the treatment of colorectal cancer. *Hematol Oncol Clin North Am.* 1997;11:679–697.
33. Heald RJ. A new approach to rectal cancer. *Br J Hosp Med.* 1979;22:277–281.
34. Enker WE, Martz J, Tepper JE, et al. Rectal cancer: management of locoregional disease. In: Kelson DP, Daly JM, Kern SE, et al., eds. *Gastrointestinal Oncology: Principles and Practice,* 1st ed. Philadelphia: Lippincott Williams & Wilkins; 2002:781–824.
35. Fritsch H. Development of the rectal fascia. *Anat Anz.* 1990;170:273–280.
36. Church JM, Raudkivi PJ, Hill GL. The surgical anatomy of the rectum—a review with particular relevance to the hazards of rectal mobilization. *Int J Colorectal Dis.* 1987;2:158–166.
37. Lindsey I, Guy RJ, Warren BF, et al. Anatomy of Denonvilliers' fascia and pelvic nerves, impotence, and implications for the colorectal surgeon. *Br J Surg.* 2000;87:1288–1299.
38. van Ophoven A, Roth S. The anatomy and embryological origins of the fascia of Denonvilliers; a medico-historical debate. *J Urol.* 1997;157:3–9.
39. Havenga K, Deruiter MC, Ender WE, et al. Anatomical basis of autonomic nerve-preserving total mesorectal excision in the management of rectal cancer. *Br J Surg.* 1996;83:384–388.
40. Bisset IP, Chau KY, Hill GL. Extrafascial excision of the rectum: surgical anatomy of the fascia propria. *Dis Colon Rectum.* 2000;43:903–910.
41. Takahashi T, Ueno M, Azekura K. Lateral ligament: its anatomy and clinical importance. *Semin Surg Oncol.* 2000;19:386–395.
42. Barabouti DG, Wong WD. Current management of rectal cancer: total mesorectal excision (nerve sparing) technique and clinical outcome. *Surg Oncol Clin N Am.* 2005;14:137–155.
43. Goligher JC. The blood-supply to the sigmoid colon and rectum with reference to the technique of rectal resection with restoration of continuity. *Br J Surg.* 1949;37:157–162.
44. Bacon HF, Dirbas F, Myers TB, et al. Extensive lymphadenectomy and high ligation of the inferior mesenteric artery for carcinoma of the left colon and rectum. *Dis Colon Rectum.* 1958;1:457–464.
45. Sugarbaker PH, Corlew S. Influence of surgical techniques on survival in patients with colorectal cancer: a review. *Dis Colon Rectum.* 1982;25:545–557.
46. Grinnel RS. Results of ligation of inferior mesenteric artery at the aorta in resections of carcinoma of the descending and sigmoid colon and rectum. *Surg Gynecol Obstet.* 1965;120:1031–1036.
47. Pezim ME, Nicholls RJ. Survival after high or low ligation of the inferior mesenteric artery during curative surgery for rectal cancer. *Ann Surg.* 1984;200:729–733.
48. Surtees P, Ritchie JK, Philips RKS. High versus low ligation of the inferior mesenteric artery in rectal cancer. *Br J Surg.* 1990;77:618–621.
49. Morikawa E, Yasutomi M, Shindou K. Distribution of metastatic lymph nodes in colorectal cancer by the modified clearing method. *Dis Colon Rectum.* 1994;37:219–223.
50. Hida JI, Yasutomi M, Fujimoto K, et al. Does lateral lymph node dissection improve survival in rectal carcinoma? Examination of node metastases by the clearing method. *J Am Coll Surg.* 1997;184:475–480.
51. Yamakoshi H, Ike H, Oki S, et al. Metastasis of rectal cancer to lymph nodes and tissues around the autonomic nerves spared for urinary and sexual function. *Dis Colon Rectum.* 1997;40:1079–1084.
52. Akasu T, Moriya Y. Abdominopelvic lymphadenectomy with autonomic nerve preservation for carcinoma of the rectum: Japanese experience. In: Wanebo HJ, ed. *Surgery for Gastrointestinal Cancer: A Multidisciplinary Approach,* 1st ed. Philadelphia: Lippincott-Raven; 1997:667–668.
53. Moriya Y, Sugihara K, Akasu T, et al. Importance of extended lymphadenectomy with lateral node dissection for advanced lower rectal cancer. *World J Surg.* 1997;21:728–732.
54. Masui H, Ike H, Yamaguchi S, et al. Male sexual function after autonomic nerve-preserving operation for rectal cancer. *Dis Colon Rectum.* 1996;39:1140–1145.
55. Sugihara K, Moriya Y, Akasu T, et al. Pelvic autonomic nerve preservation for rectal cancer: oncological and functional outcome. *Cancer.* 1996;78:1871–1880.

56. Enker WE. Potency, cure, and local control in the operative treatment of rectal cancer. *Arch Surg.* 1992;127:1396–1402.

57. Bissett I, Hill G. Extrafascial excision of the rectum for cancer: a technique for the avoidance of complications of rectal mobilization. *Semin Surg Oncol.* 2000;18:207–215.

58. Fazio V, Heriot A. Proctectomy with coloanal anastomosis. *Surg Oncol Clin N Am.* 2005;14:157–181.

59. Lane R, Parks A. Function of the anal sphincter following coloanal anastomosis. *Br J Surg.* 1977;64:596–599.

60. Williams N, Price R, Johnston D. The long term effect of sphincter preserving operations for rectal carcinoma on function of the anal sphincter in man. *Br J Surg.* 1980;67:203–208.

61. Matzel K, Stadelmaier U, Muehldorfer S, et al. Continence after colorectal reconstruction following resection: impact of level of anastomosis. *Int J Colorectal Dis.* 1997;12:82–87.

62. Molloy R, Moran K, Coulter J, et al. Mechanism of sphincter impairment following low anterior resection. *Dis Colon Rectum.* 1992;35:462–464.

63. Farouk R, Duthie G, Lee P, et al. Endosonographic evidence of injury to the internal anal sphincter after low anterior resection: long-term follow-up. *Dis Colon Rectum.* 1998;41:888–891.

64. Otto I, Ito K, Ye C, et al. Causes of rectal incontinence after sphincter-preserving operations for rectal cancer. *Dis Colon Rectum.* 1996;39:1423–1427.

65. Lewis W, Holdsworth P, Stephenson B, et al. Role of the rectum in the physiological and clinical results of coloanal and colorectal anastomosis after anterior resection for rectal cancer. *Br J Surg.* 1992;79:1082–1086.

66. McAnena O, Heald R, Lockhart-Mummery H. Operative and functional results of total mesorectal excision with ultralow anterior resection in the management of carcinoma of the lower one third of the rectum. *Surg Gynecol Obstet.* 1990;170:517–521.

67. Williams N, Seow-Choen F. Physiological and functional outcome following ultra-low anterior resection with colon pouch-anal anastomosis. *Br J Surg.* 1998;85:1029–1035.

68. Lazorthes F, Fages P, Chiotasso P, et al. Resection of the rectum with construction of a colonic reservoir and colo-anal anastomosis for carcinoma of the rectum. *Br J Surg.* 1986;73:136–138.

69. Parc R, Tiret E, Frileux P, et al. Resection and colo-anal anastomosis with colonic reservoir for rectal cancer. *Br J Surg.* 1986;73:139–141.

70. Ortiz H, De Miguel M, Armendariz P, et al. Coloanal anastomosis: are functional results better with a pouch? *Dis Colon Rectum.* 1995;38:375–377.

71. Ho YH, Seow-Choen F. Prospective randomized controlled study of clinical function and anorectal physiology after low anterior resection: comparison of straight and colonic J pouch anastomosis. *Br J Surg.* 1996;83:978–980.

72. Seow-Choen F, Goh H. Prospective randomized trial comparing J colonic pouch anal anastomosis and straight coloanal anastomosis. *Br J Surg.* 1995;82:608–610.

73. Hallbook O, Pahlman L, Krog M, et al. Randomized comparison of straight and colonic J pouch anastomosis after low anterior resection. *Ann Surg.* 1996;224:58–65.

74. Lazorthes F, Chiotasso P, Gamagami R, et al. Late clinical outcome in a randomized prospective comparison of colonic J pouch and straight coloanal anastomosis. *Br J Surg.* 1997;84:1449–1451.

75. Dehni N, Tiret E, Singland J, et al. Long-term functional outcome after low anterior resection: comparison of low colorectal anastomosis and colonic J-pouch-anal anastomosis. *Dis Colon Rectum.* 1998;41:817–823.

76. Joo J, Latulippe J, Alabaz O, et al. Long-term functional evaluation of straight coloanal anastomosis and colonic J-pouch. *Dis Colon Rectum.* 1998;41:740–746.

77. Berger A, Tiret E, Parc R, et al. Excision of the rectum with colonic J pouch-anal anastomosis for adenocarcinoma of the low and mid rectum. *World J Surg.* 1992;16:470–477.

78. Hallbook O, Johansson K, Sjodahl R. Laser Doppler blood flow measurement in rectal resection for carcinoma: comparison between the straight and colonic J pouch reconstruction. *Br J Surg.* 1996;83:389–392.

79. Fazio V, Mantyh C, Hull T. Colonic coloplasty: novel technique to enhance low colorectal or coloanal anastomosis. *Dis Colon Rectum.* 1000;43:1448–1450.

80. Harris G, Lavery I, Fazio V. Reasons for failure to construct the colonic J-pouch: what can be done to improve the size of the neorectal reservoir should it occur? *Dis Colon Rectum.* 2002;45:1304–1308.

81. Bokey E, Chapuis P, Dent O, et al. Factors affecting survival after excision of the rectum for cancer: a multivariate analysis. *Dis Colon Rectum.* 1997;40:3–10.

82. Jatzko G, Jagoditsch M, Lisborg P, et al. Long-term results of radical surgery for rectal cancer: multivariate analysis of prognostic factors influencing survival and local recurrence. *Eur J Surg Oncol.* 1999;25:284–291.

83. Dehni N, McFadden N, McNamara D, et al. Oncologic results following abdominoperineal resection for adenocarcinoma of the low rectum. *Dis Colon Rectum.* 2003;46:867–874.

84. Wibe A, Syse A, Andersen E, et al. Oncologic outcomes after total mesorectal excision for cure for cancer of the lower rectum: anterior vs abdominoperineal resection. *Dis Colon Rectum.* 2004;47:48–58.

85. Chessin D, Hartley J, Cohen A, et al. Rectus flap reconstruction decreases perineal wound complications after pelvic chemoradiation and surgery: a cohort study. *Ann Surg Oncol.* 2005;12:104–110.

86. Butler C, Rodriquez-Bigas M. Pelvic reconstruction after abdominoperineal resection: is it worthwhile? *Ann Surg Oncol.* 2005;12:91–94.

87. Bell S, Dehni N, Chaouat M, et al. Primary rectus abdominis myocutaneous flap for repair of perineal and vaginal defects after extended abdominoperineal resection. *Br J Surg.* 2005;92:482–486.

88. Kroll S, Pollock R, Jessup J, Ota D. Transpelvic rectus abdominis flap reconstruction of defects following abdominal-perineal resection. *Am Surg.* 1989;55:632–637.

89. Giampapa V, Keller A, Shaw W, Colen S. Pelvic floor reconstruction using the rectus abdominis muscle flap. *Ann Plast Surg.* 1984;13:56–59.

90. Gerstenberg T, Nielsen M, Clausen S, et al. Bladder function after abdominoperineal resection of the rectum for anorectal cancer. *Ann Surg.* 1979;191:81–86.

91. Neal D, Williams N, Johnston D. A prospective study of bladder function before and after sphincter-saving resections for low carcinoma of the rectum. *Br J Urol.* 1981;53:558–564.

92. Janu N, Bokey E, Chapuis P, et al. Bladder dysfunction following anterior resection for carcinoma of the rectum. *Dis Colon Rectum.* 1986;29:182–183.

93. Del Rio C, Sanchez-Santos R, Oreja V, et al. Long-term urinary dysfunction after rectal cancer surgery. *Colorectal Dis.* 2004;6:198–202.

94. Kneist W, Heintz A, Junginger T. Major urinary dysfunction after mesorectal excision for rectal carcinoma. *Br J Surg.* 2005;92:230–234.

95. Weinstein M, Roberts M. Sexual potency following surgery for rectal carcinoma: a follow-up of 44 patients. *Ann Surg.* 1977;185:295–300.

96. Balslev I, Harling H. Sexual dysfunction following operation for carcinoma of the rectum. *Dis Colon Rectum.* 1983;26:788.

97. Danzi M, Ferulano G, Abate S, et al. Male sexual function after abdominoperineal resection for rectal cancer. *Dis Colon Rectum.* 1983;26:665–668.

98. LaMonica G, Audisio R, Tamburini M, et al. Incidence of sexual dysfunction in male patients treated surgically for rectal malignancy. *Dis Colon Rectum.* 1985;28:937–940.

99. Pocard M, Zinzindohoue F, Haab F, et al. A prospective study of sexual and urinary function before and after total mesorectal excision with autonomic nerve preservation for rectal cancer. *Surgery.* 2002;131:368–372.

100. Masui H, Ike H, Yamaguchi S, et al. Male sexual function after autonomic nerve-preservation operation for rectal cancer. *Dis Colon Rectum.* 1996;39:1140–1145.

101. Hendren S, O'Conner B, Liu M, et al. Prevalence of male and female sexual dysfunction is high following surgery for rectal cancer. *Ann Surg.* 2005;242:212–223.

102. Brodsky J, Richard G, Cohen A, Minsky B. Variables correlated with the risk of lymph node metastases in early rectal cancer. *Cancer.* 1992;69:322–326.

103. Zenni G, Abraham K, Harford F, et al. Characteristics of rectal carcinoma that predict the presence of lymph node metastases: implications for patient selection for local therapy. *J Surg Oncol.* 1998;67:99–103.

104. Mellgren A, Sirivongs P, Rothenberger D, et al. Is local excision adequate therapy for early rectal cancer? *Dis Colon Rectum.* 2000;43:1064–1071.

105. Blumberg D, Paty PB, Guillem JG. All patients with small intramural rectal cancers are at risk for lymph node metastasis. *Dis Colon Rectum.* 1999; 42:881–885.

106. Nastro P, Beral D, Hartley J, Monson J. Local excision of rectal cancer: review of the literature. *Dig Surg.* 2005;22:6–15.

107. Sengupta S, Tjandra J. Local excision of rectal cancer: what is the evidence? *Dis Colon Rectum.* 2001;44:1345–1361.

108. Kikuchi R, Takano M, Takagi K, et al. Management of early invasive rectal cancer. Risk of recurrence and clinical guidelines. *Dis Colon Rectum.* 1995;38:1286–1295.

109. Nascimbeni R, Burgart L, Nivatvongs S. Risk of lymph node metastasis in T1 carcinoma of the colon and rectum. *Dis Colon Rectum.* 2002;45:200–206.

110. Blair S, Ellenhorn J. Transanal excision for low rectal cancers is curative in early-stage disease with favorable histology. *Am Surg.* 2000;66:817–820.

111. Chorost MI, Petrelli NJ, McKenna M. Local excision of rectal carcinoma. *Am Surg.* 2001;67:774–779.

112. Willet C, Compton C, Shellito P, Efird J. Selection factors for local excision or abdominoperineal resection of early stage rectal cancer. *Cancer.* 1994;73:2716–2720.

113. Nascimbeni R, Nivatvongs S, Larson D, et al. Long-term survival after local excision of T1 carcinoma of the rectum. *Dis Colon Rectum.* 2004;47:1773–1779.

114. Bentrem D, Okabe S, Wong D, et al. T1 adenocarcinoma of the rectum: transanal excision or radical surgery? *Ann Surg.* 2005;242:472–479.

115. Steele G, Herndon J, Bleday R, et al. Sphincter-sparing treatment for distal rectal adenocarcinoma. *Ann Surg Oncol.* 1999;6:433–441.

116. Russell A, Harris J, Rosenberg P, et al. Anal sphincter conservation for patients with adenocarcinoma of the distal rectum: long-term results of Radiation Therapy Oncology Group protocol 89-02. *Int J Radiat Oncol Biol Phys.* 2000;46:313–322.

117. Kim C, Yeatmen T, Coppola D, et al. Local excision of T2 and T3 rectal cancers after downstaging chemoradiation. *Ann Surg.* 2001;234:352–358.

118. Mohiuddin M, Marks G, Bannon J. High-dose preoperative radiation and full thickness local excision: a new option for selected T3 distal rectal cancers. *Int J Radiat Oncol Biol Phys.* 1994;30:845–849.

119. Mohiuddin M, Regine W, Marks G, Marks J. High-dose preoperative radiation and the challenge of sphincter-preserving surgery for cancer of the distal 2 cm of the rectum. *Int J Radiat Oncol Biol Phys.* 1998;40: 569–574.

120. Schell S, Zlotecki R, Mendenhall W, et al. Transanal excision of locally advanced rectal cancers downstaged using neoadjuvant chemoradiotherapy. *J Am Coll Surg.* 2002;194:584–590.

121. Bonnen M, Crane C, Vauthey J, et al. Long-term results using local excision after preoperative chemoradiation among selected T3 rectal cancer patients. *Int J Radiat Oncol Biol Phys.* 2004;60:1098–1105.

122. Bannon J, Marks G, Mohiuddin M, et al. Radical and local excisional methods of sphincter-sparing surgery after high-dose radiation for cancer of the distal 3 cm of the rectum. *Ann Surg Oncol.* 1995;2:221–227.

123. Habr-Gama A, Perez R, Nadalin W, et al. Operative versus nonoperative treatment for stage 0 distal rectal cancer following chemoradiation therapy: long-term results. *Ann Surg.* 2004;240:711–718.

124. Bedrosian I, Rodriguez-Bigas M, Feig B, et al. Predicting the node-negative mesorectum after preoperative chemoradiation for locally advanced rectal carcinoma. *J Gastrointest Surg.* 2004;8:56–63.

125. Stipa F, Zernecke A, Moore H, et al. Residual mesorectal lymph node involvement following neoadjuvant combined-modality therapy: rationale for radical resection? *Ann Surg Oncol.* 2004;11:187–191.

126. Read T, Andujar J, Caushaj P, et al. Neoadjuvant therapy for rectal cancer: histologic response of the primary tumor predicts nodal status. *Dis Colon Rectum.* 2004;47:825–831.

127. Tulchinsky H, Rabau M, Shacham-Shemueli E, et al. Can rectal cancers with pathologic T0 after neoadjuvant chemoradiation (ypT0) be treated by transanal excision alone? *Ann Surg Oncol.* 2006;13:1–6.

128. Onaitis M, Noone R, Fields R, et al. Complete response to neoadjuvant chemoradiation for rectal cancer does not influence survival. *Ann Surg Oncol.* 2001;8:801–806.

129. Zmora O, Dasilva G, Gurland B, et al. Does rectal wall tumor eradication with preoperative chemoradiation permit a change in the operative strategy? *Dis Colon Rectum.* 2004;47:1607–1612.

130. Bujko K, Nowacki M, Nasierowska-Guttmejer A, et al. Prediction of mesorectal nodal metastases after chemoradiation for rectal cancer: results of a randomized trial: implication for subsequent local excision. *Radiother Oncol.* 2005;76:234–240.

131. Kane JM, Petrelli NJ. Controversies in the surgical management of rectal cancer. *Semin Radiat Oncol.* 2003;13:403–418.

132. Weiser M, Landmann R, Wong W, et al. Surgical salvage of recurrent rectal cancer after transanal excision. *Dis Colon Rectum.* 2005;48:1169–1175.

133. Buess G, Theiss R, Gunther M, et al. Endoscopic operative procedure for the removal of rectal polyps. *Coloproctology.* 1984;184:254–261.

134. Buess G, Kipfmuller K, Ibald R, et al. Clinical results of transanal endoscopic microsurgery. *Surg Endosc.* 1988;2:245–250.

135. Buess G, Mentges B, Manncke K, et al. Technique and results of transanal endoscopic microsurgery in early rectal cancer. *Am J Surg.* 1992;163: 63–70.

136. Gavagan J, Whiteford M, Swanstrom L. Full-thickness intraperitoneal excision by transanal endoscopic microsurgery does not increase short-term complications. *Am J Surg.* 2004;187:630–634.

137. Middleton PF, Sutherland LM, Maddern GJ. Transanal endoscopic microsurgery: a systematic review. *Dis Colon Rectum.* 2005;48:270–284.

138. Winde G, Nottberg H, Keller R, et al. Surgical cure for early rectal carcinomas (T1). Transanal endoscopic microsurgery vs. anterior resection. *Dis Colon Rectum.* 1996;39:969–976.

139. Lezoche E, Guerrieri M, Paganini A, et al. Transanal endoscopic vs total mesorectal laparoscopic resections of T2-N0 low rectal cancers after neoadjuvant treatment. *Surg Endosc.* 2005;19:751–756.

140. Kreis M, Jehle E, Huag V, et al. Functional results after transanal endoscopic microsurgery. *Dis Colon Rectum.* 1996;39:1116–1121.

141. Kennedy M, Lobowski D, King D, et al. Transanal endoscopic microsurgery excision: is anorectal function compromised? *Dis Colon Rectum.* 2002;45:601–604.

142. Herman R, Richter P, Walega P, et al. Anorectal sphincter function and rectal barostat study in patients following transanal endoscopic microsurgery. *Int J Colorectal Dis.* 2001;6:370–376.

143. Cataldo P, O'Brien S, Osler T. Transanal endoscopic microsurgery: a prospective evaluation of functional results. *Dis Colon Rectum.* 2005;48: 1366–1371.

144. Bärlehner E, Benhidjeb T, Anders S, Schicke B. Laparoscopic resection for rectal cancer: outcomes in 194 patients and review of the literature. *Surg Endosc.* 2005;19:757–766.

145. Guillou P, Quirke P, Thorpe H, et al. Short-term endpoints of conventional versus laparoscopic-assisted surgery in patients with colorectal cancer (MRC CLASICC trial): multicentre, randomized controlled trial. *Lancet.* 2005;365:1718–1726.

146. Zhou Z, Hu M, Li Y, et al. Laparoscopic vs open total mesorectal excision with anal sphincter preservation for low rectal cancer. *Surg Endosc.* 2004;18:1211–1215.

147. Quah H, Janye D, Eu K, Seow-Choen F. Bladder and sexual dysfunction following laparoscopically assisted and conventional open mesorectal resection for cancer. *Br J Surg.* 2003;89:1551–1556.

148. Jayne D, Brown J, Thorpe H, et al. Bladder and sexual function following resection for rectal cancer in a randomized clinical trial of laparoscopic versus open technique. *Br J Surg.* 2005;92:1124–1132.

149. Cass AW, Million RR, Pfaff WW. Patterns of recurrence following surgery alone for adenocarcinoma of the colon and rectum. *Cancer.* 1976;37:2861–2865.

150. Gunderson LL, Martenson JA. Postoperative adjuvant irradiation with or without chemotherapy for rectal carcinoma. *Semin Radiat Oncol.* 1993; 3:55–63.

151. Gunderson LL, Sosin H. Areas of failure found at reoperation (second or symptomatic look) following "curative surgery" for adenocarcinoma of the rectum. Clinicopathologic correlation and implications for adjuvant therapy. *Cancer.* 1974;34:1278–1292.

152. Mendenhall WM, Million RR, Pfaff WW. Patterns of recurrence in adenocarcinoma of the rectum and rectosigmoid treated with surgery alone: implications in treatment planning with adjuvant radiation therapy. *Int J Radiat Oncol Biol Phys.* 1983;9:977–985.

153. Rich T, Gunderson LL, Lew R, Galdibini JJ, Cohen AM, Donaldson G. Patterns of recurrence of rectal cancer after potentially curative surgery. *Cancer.* 1983;52:1317–1329.

154. Walz BJ, Green MR, Lindstrom ER, Butcher HR Jr. Anatomical prognostic factors after abdominal perineal resection. *Int J Radiat Oncol Biol Phys.* 1981;7:477–484.

155. Minsky BD, Mies C, Recht A, Rich TA, Chaffey JT. Resectable adenocarcinoma of the rectosigmoid and rectum. I. Patterns of failure and survival. *Cancer.* 1988;61:1408–1416.

156. Thomas WH, Larson RA, Wright HK, Cleveland JC. Analysis of 830 patients with rectal adenocarcinoma. *Surg Gynecol Obstet.* 1969;129:10–14.

157. Gunderson LL. Indications for and results of combined modality treatment of colorectal cancer. *Acta Oncol.* 1999;38:7–21.

158. Adjuvant radiotherapy for rectal cancer: a systematic overview of 8,507 patients from 22 randomised trials. *Lancet.* 2001;358:1291–1304.

159. Krook JE, Moertel CG, Gunderson LL, et al. Effective surgical adjuvant therapy for high-risk rectal carcinoma. *N Engl J Med.* 1991;324:709–715.

160. Thomas PR, Lindblad AS. Adjuvant postoperative radiotherapy and chemotherapy in rectal carcinoma: a review of the Gastrointestinal Tumor Study Group experience. *Radiother Oncol.* 1988;13:245–252.

161. Knaebel HP, Koch M, Feise T, Benner A, Kienle P. Diagnostics of rectal cancer: endorectal ultrasound. *Recent Results Cancer Res.* 2005;165:46–57.

162. Bali C, Nousias V, Fatouros M, Stefanou D, Kappas AM. Assessment of local stage in rectal cancer using endorectal ultrasonography (EUS). *Tech Coloproctol.* 2004;8 Suppl 1:s170–s173.

163. Manger T, Stroh C. Accuracy of endorectal ultrasonography in the preoperative staging of rectal cancer. *Tech Coloproctol.* 2004;8 Suppl 1:s14–s15.

164. Sauer R, Becker H, Hohenberger W, et al. Preoperative versus postoperative chemoradiotherapy for rectal cancer. *N Engl J Med.* 2004;351:1731–1740.

165. Randomised trial of surgery alone versus surgery followed by radiotherapy for mobile cancer of the rectum. Medical Research Council Rectal Cancer Working Party. *Lancet.* 1996;348:1610–1614.

166. Treurniet-Donker AD, van Putten WL, Wereldsma JC, et al. Postoperative radiation therapy for rectal cancer. An interim analysis of a prospective, randomized multicenter trial in The Netherlands. *Cancer.* 1991;67:2042–2048.

167. Fisher B, Wolmark N, Rockette H, et al. Postoperative adjuvant chemotherapy or radiation therapy for rectal cancer: results from NSABP protocol R-01. *J Natl Cancer Inst.* 1988;80:21–29.

168. Balslev I, Pedersen M, Teglbjaerg PS, et al. Postoperative radiotherapy in Dukes' B and C carcinoma of the rectum and rectosigmoid. A randomized multicenter study. *Cancer.* 1986;58:22–28.

169. Prolongation of the disease-free interval in surgically treated rectal carcinoma. Gastrointestinal Tumor Study Group. *N Engl J Med.* 1985;312: 1465–1472.

170. Douglass HO Jr, Moertel CG, Mayer RJ, et al. Survival after postoperative combination treatment of rectal cancer. *N Engl J Med.* 1986;315:1294–1295.

171. Tveit KM, Guldvog I, Hagen S, et al. Randomized controlled trial of postoperative radiotherapy and short-term time-scheduled 5-fluorouracil against surgery alone in the treatment of Dukes B and C rectal cancer. *Br J Surg.* 1997;84:1130–1135.

172. McGinn CJ, Kinsella TJ. The clinical rationale for S-phase radiosensitization in human tumors. *Curr Probl Cancer.* 1993;17:273–321.

173. O'Connell MJ, Martenson JA, Wieand HS, et al. Improving adjuvant therapy for rectal cancer by combining protracted-infusion fluorouracil with radiation therapy after curative surgery. *N Engl J Med.* 1994;331:502–507.

174. Budd GT, Fleming TR, Bukowski RM, et al. 5-Fluorouracil and folinic acid in the treatment of metastatic colorectal cancer: a randomized comparison. A Southwest Oncology Group Study. *J Clin Oncol.* 1987;5:272–277.

175. The evaluation of low dose pre-operative x-ray therapy in the management of operable rectal cancer; results of a randomly controlled trial. *Br J Surg.* 1984;71:21–25.

176. Duncan W. Adjuvant radiotherapy in rectal cancer: the MRC trials. *Br J Surg.* 1985;72 Suppl:S59–S62.

177. Higgins GA, Humphrey EW, Dwight RW, Roswit B, Lee LE Jr, Keehn RJ. Preoperative radiation and surgery for cancer of the rectum. Veterans Administration Surgical Oncology Group Trial II. *Cancer.* 1986;58:352–359.

178. Rider WD, Palmer JA, Mahoney LJ, Robertson CT. Preoperative irradiation in operable cancer of the rectum: report of the Toronto trial. *Can J Surg.* 1977;20:335–338.

179. Roswit B, Higgins GA, Keehn RJ. Preoperative irradiation for carcinoma of the rectum and rectosigmoid colon: report of a National Veterans Administration randomized study. *Cancer.* 1975;35:1597–1602.

180. Goldberg PA, Nicholls RJ, Porter NH, Love S, Grimsey JE. Long-term results of a randomised trial of short-course low-dose adjuvant pre-operative radiotherapy for rectal cancer: reduction in local treatment failure. *Eur J Cancer.* 1994;30A:1602–1606.

181. Kligerman MM, Urdaneta N, Knowlton A, Vidone R, Hartman PV, Vera R. Preoperative irradiation of rectosigmoid carcinoma including its regional lymph nodes. *Am J Roentgenol Radium Ther Nucl Med.* 1972;114:498–503.

182. Gerard A, Buyse M, Nordlinger B, et al. Preoperative radiotherapy as adjuvant treatment in rectal cancer. Final results of a randomized study of the European Organization for Research and Treatment of Cancer (EORTC). *Ann Surg.* 1988;208:606–614.

183. Preoperative short-term radiation therapy in operable rectal carcinoma. A prospective randomized trial. Stockholm Rectal Cancer Study Group. *Cancer.* 1990;66:49–55.

184. Improved survival with preoperative radiotherapy in resectable rectal cancer. Swedish Rectal Cancer Trial. *N Engl J Med.* 1997;336:980–987.

185. Frykholm GJ, Glimelius B, Pahlman L. Preoperative or postoperative irradiation in adenocarcinoma of the rectum: final treatment results of a randomized trial and an evaluation of late secondary effects. *Dis Colon Rectum.* 1993;36:564–572.

186. Kapiteijn E, Marijnen CA, Nagtegaal ID, et al. Preoperative radiotherapy combined with total mesorectal excision for resectable rectal cancer. *N Engl J Med.* 2001;345:638–646.

187. Pahlman L, Glimelius B. Pre- or postoperative radiotherapy in rectal and rectosigmoid carcinoma. Report from a randomized multicenter trial. *Ann Surg.* 1990;211:187–195.

188. Sauer R, Fietkau R, Wittekind C, et al. Adjuvant versus neoadjuvant radiochemotherapy for locally advanced rectal cancer. A progress report of a phase-III randomized trial (protocol CAO/ARO/AIO-94). *Strahlenther Onkol.* 2001;177:173–181.

189. Arbman G, Nilsson E, Hallbook O, Sjodahl R. Local recurrence following total mesorectal excision for rectal cancer. *Br J Surg.* 1996;83:375–379.

190. Heald RJ, Ryall RD. Recurrence and survival after total mesorectal excision for rectal cancer. *Lancet.* 1986;1:1479–1482.

191. Law WL, Chu KW. Local recurrence following total mesorectal excision with double-stapling anastomosis for rectal cancers: analysis of risk factors. *World J Surg.* 2002;26:1272–1276.

192. Scott N, Jackson P, al-Jaberi T, Dixon MF, Quirke P, Finan PJ. Total mesorectal excision and local recurrence: a study of tumour spread in the mesorectum distal to rectal cancer. *Br J Surg.* 1995;82:1031–1033.

193. van Lingen CP, Zeebregts CJ, Gerritsen JJ, Mulder HJ, Mastboom WJ, Klaase JM. Local recurrence of rectal cancer after total mesorectal excision without preoperative radiotherapy. *Int J Gastrointest Cancer.* 2003;34:129–134.

194. Hyams DM, Mamounas EP, Petrelli N, et al. A clinical trial to evaluate the worth of preoperative multimodality therapy in patients with operable carcinoma of the rectum: a progress report of National Surgical Breast and Bowel Project Protocol R-03. *Dis Colon Rectum.* 1997;40:131–139.

195. Roh MS, Petrelli N, Wieand S, et al. A Phase III Randomized Trial of Preoperative Versus Postoperative Multimodality Therapy in Patients with Carcinoma of the Rectum (NSABP R-03). *ASCO Abstract #490.* 2001.

196. Baxter NN, Habermann EB, Tepper JE, Durham SB, Virnig BA. Risk of pelvic fractures in older women following pelvic irradiation. *JAMA.* 2005;294:2587–2593.

197. Chen YJ, Liu A, Tsai PT, et al. Organ sparing by conformal avoidance intensity-modulated radiation therapy for anal cancer: dosimetric evaluation of coverage of pelvis and inguinal/femoral nodes. *Int J Radiat Oncol Biol Phys.* 2005;63:274–281.

198. Duthoy W, De Gersem W, Vergote K, et al. Clinical implementation of intensity-modulated arc therapy (IMAT) for rectal cancer. *Int J Radiat Oncol Biol Phys.* 2004;60:794–806.

199. Milano MT, Jani AB, Farrey KJ, Rash C, Heimann R, Chmura SJ. Intensity-modulated radiation therapy (IMRT) in the treatment of anal cancer: toxicity and clinical outcome. *Int J Radiat Oncol Biol Phys.* 2005;63:354–361.

200. Kligerman MM, Liu T, Liu Y, Scheffler B, He S, Zhang Z. Interim analysis of a randomized trial of radiation therapy of rectal cancer with/without WR-2721. *Int J Radiat Oncol Biol Phys.* 1992;22:799–802.

201. Liu T, Liu Y, He S, Zhang Z, Kligerman MM. Use of radiation with or without WR-2721 in advanced rectal cancer. *Cancer.* 1992;69:2820–2825.

202. Myerson R. Rationale for a phase I/II radiation dose-escalation study with concurrent amifostine (Ethyol) and infusional 5-FU chemotherapy for preoperative treatment of unresectable or locally recurrent rectal carcinoma. *Semin Radiat Oncol.* 2002;12(1 Suppl 1):86–90.

203. Myerson R, Zobeiri I, Birnbaum E, et al. Early results from a phase I/II radiation dose-escalation study with concurrent amifostine and infusional 5-fluorouracil chemotherapy for preoperative treatment of unresectable or locally recurrent rectal carcinoma. *Semin Oncol.* 2002;29(6 Suppl 19):29–33.

204. Dunst J, Semlin S, Pigorsch S, Muller AC, Reese T. Intermittent use of

205. Emmanouilides C, Pegram M, Robinson R, Hecht R, Kabbinavar F, Isacoff W. Anti-VEGF antibody bevacizumab (Avastin) with 5FU/LV as third line treatment for colorectal cancer. *Tech Coloproctol.* 2004;8 Suppl 1:s50–s52.

206. Prewett MC, Hooper AT, Bassi R, Ellis LM, Waksal HW, Hicklin DJ. Enhanced antitumor activity of anti-epidermal growth factor receptor monoclonal antibody IMC-C225 in combination with irinotecan (CPT-11) against human colorectal tumor xenografts. *Clin Cancer Res.* 2002;8:994–1003.

207. Heald RJ, Husband EM, Ryall RD. The mesorectum in rectal cancer surgery—the clue to pelvic recurrence? *Br J Surg.* 1982;69:613–616.

208. Reynolds JV, Joyce WP, Dolan J, Sheahan K, et al. Pathologic evidence in support of total mesorectal excision in the management of rectal cancer. *Br J Surg.* 1996;83:384–388.

209. Reynolds JV, Joyce WP, Dolan J. Pathologic evidence in support of total mesorectal excision in the management of rectal cancer. *Br J Surg.* 1996;83:1112–1115.

210. Tocchi A, Mazzoni G, Lepre L. Total mesorectal excision and low rectal anastomosis for the treatment of rectal cancer and prevention of pelvic recurrences. *Arch Surg.* 2001;136:216–220.

211. Ratto C, Ricci R, Rossi C. Mesorectal microfoci adversely affect the prognosis of patients with rectal cancer. *Dis Colon Rectum.* 2002;45:733–742, discussion 742–743.

212. Heald RJ, Moran BJ, Ryall RD, et al. Rectal cancer-the Basingstoke experience of total mesorectal excision, 1978–1997. *Arch Surg.* 1998;133:894–899.

213. Arbman G, Nilsson E, Hallbook O. Local recurrence following total mesorectal excision for rectal cancer. *Br J Surg.* 1996;83:375–379.

214. Kockerling F, Reymond M, Altendor-Hofmann A, et al. Influence of surgery on metachronous distant metastases and survival in rectal cancer. *J Clin Oncol.* 1998;16:324–329.

215. Havenga K, Enker WE, Norstein J, et al. Improved survival and local control after total mesorectal excision or D3 lymphadenectomy in the treatment of primary rectal cancer: an international analysis of 1411 patients. *Eur J Surg Oncol.* 1999;25:368–374.

216. Arenas RB, Fichera A, Mhoon D. Total mesenteric excision in the surgical treatment of rectal cancer: a prospective study. *Arch Surg.* 1998;133:608–612.

217. Leong AF. Selective total mesorectal excision for rectal cancer. *Dis Colon Rectum.* 2000;43:1237–1240.

218. Wibe A, Moller B, Norstein J. A national strategic change in treatment policy for rectal cancer–implementation of total mesorectal excision as routine treatment in Norway: a national audit. *Dis Colon Rectum.* 2002;45:857–866.

219. Kapiteijn E, Marijnen CA, Nagtegaal ID. Preoperative radiotherapy combined with total mesorectal excision for resectable rectal cancer. *N Engl J Med.* 2001;345:638–646.

220. Marijnen CA, Kapiteijn E, van de Velde CJ. Acute side effects and complications after short-term preoperative radiotherapy combined with total mesorectal excision in primary rectal cancer: report of a multicenter randomized trial. *J Clin Oncol.* 2002;20:817–825.

221. Goligher J, Dukes C, Bussey H. Local recurrences after sphincter saving excisions for carcinoma of the rectum and rectosigmoid. *Br J Surg.* 1951;39:199–211.

222. Dukes C. The classification of cancer of the rectum. *J Pathol Bacteriol.* 1932;35:323–332.

223. Grinnell R. Distal intramural spread of carcinoma of the rectum and rectosigmoid. *Br J Surg.* 1951;39:199–211.

224. Pollett W, Nicholls R. The relationship between the extent of distal clearance and survival and local recurrence rates after curative anterior resection for carcinoma of the rectum. *Ann Surg.* 1983;198:159–163.

225. Wolmark N, Fischer B. An analysis of survival and treatment failure following abdominoperineal and sphincter saving resection in Dukes B and C rectal carcinoma. *Ann Surg.* 1986;204:480–487.

226. Williams N, Dixon M, Johnston D. Reappraisal of the 5 centimetre rule of distal excision for carcinoma of the rectum: a study of distal intramural spread and of patients' survival. *Br J Surg.* 1983;70:150–154.

227. Shirouzu K, Isomoto H, Kakegawa T. Distal spread of rectal cancer and optimal distal margin of resection for sphincter preserving surgery. *Cancer.* 1995;76:388–392.

228. Andreola S, Leo E, Belli F, et al. Distal intramural spread in adenocarcinoma of the lower third of the rectum treated with total rectal resection and coloanal anastomosis. *Dis Colon Rectum.* 1997;40:25–29.

229. Ueno H, Mochizuki H, Hashiguchi Y, et al. Preoperative parameters expanding the indication of sphincter preserving surgery in patients with advanced low rectal cancer. *Ann Surg.* 2004;239:34–42.

230. Mezhir J, Smith K, Fichera A, et al. Presence of distal intramural spread after preoperative combined-modality therapy for adenocarcinoma of the rectum: what is now the appropriate distal resection margin? *Surgery.* 2005;138:658–663.

231. Kuvshinoff B, Maghfoor I, Miedema B, et al. Distal margin requirements after preoperative chemoradiotherapy for distal rectal carcinomas: are ≤1 cm distal margins sufficient? *Ann Surg Oncol.* 2001;8:163–169.

232. Moore H, Riedel M, Minsky B, et al. Adequacy of 1-cm distal margin after restorative rectal cancer resection with sharp mesorectal excision

and preoperative combined-modality therapy. *Ann Surg Oncol.* 2003;10: 80–85.

233. Adam IJ, Mohamdee MO, Martin IG. Role of circumferential margin involvement in the local recurrence of rectal cancer. *Lancet.* 1994;344:707–711.

234. Hall NR, Finan PJ, Al-Jaberi T. Circumferential margin involvement after mesorectal excision of rectal cancer with curative intent: predictor of survival but not local recurrence? *Dis Colon Rectum.* 1998;41:979–983.

235. Nagtegaal ID, Marijnen CA, Kranenbarg EK. Circumferential margin involvement is still an important predictor of local recurrence in rectal carcinoma: not one millimeter but two millimeters is the limit. *Am J Surg Pathol.* 2002;26:350–357.

236. Marr R, Birbeck K, Garvican J, et al. The modern abdominoperineal excision: the next challenge after total mesorectal excision. *Ann Surg.* 2005;242:74–82.

237. Moore HG, Shoup M, Riedel E, et al. Colorectal cancer pelvic recurrences: determinants of respectability. *Dis Colon Rectum.* 2004;47:1599–1606.

238. Lopez MJ, Luna-Perez P. Composite pelvic exenteration: is it worthwhile? *Ann Surg Oncol.* 2004;11:27–33.

239. Oliveira Poletto AH, Lopes A, Carvalho AL, et al. Pelvic exenteration and sphincter preservation: an analysis of 96 cases. *J Surg Oncol.* 2004;86:122–127.

240. Ike H, Shimada H, Yamaguchi S, et al. Outcome of total pelvic exenteration for primary rectal cancer. *Dis Colon Rectum.* 2003;46:474–480.

241. Wiig JN, Poulsen JP, Larsen S, et al. Total pelvic exenteration with preoperative irradiation for advanced primary and recurrent rectal cancer. *Eur J Surg.* 2002;168:42–48.

242. Yamada K, Ishizawa T, Niwa K, et al. Pelvic exenteration and sacral resection for locally advanced primary and recurrent rectal cancer. *Dis Colon Rectum.* 2002;45:1078–1084.

CHAPTER 45 ■ SYSTEMIC THERAPY FOR METASTATIC COLORECTAL CANCER

LEONARD B. SALTZ

INTRODUCTION

The chemotherapy options available for metastatic colorectal cancer (CRC) patients have expanded dramatically since the 1990s. However, treatment for patients with metastatic disease should be approached with a balance of optimism and caution. Well-motivated patients with adequate performance status, bone marrow reserve, liver function, and renal function have a substantial potential to benefit from treatment, whereas patients with poor performance status and/or significant comorbidities should be considered for either less aggressive therapies or supportive care only. The therapeutic options for patients with metastatic CRC are reviewed in this chapter, and general treatment recommendations are given. The reader is cautioned that this is a rapidly evolving field and that many changes in practice can be anticipated in the near future.

CYTOTOXIC CHEMOTHERAPY

5-Fluorouracil

5-Fluorouracil (5-FU) was a rationally designed agent patented almost 50 years ago (1). Despite its venerability, this agent remains at the center of most CRC chemotherapy regimens. 5-FU is a prodrug that must be metabolized before it can become biologically active. The chemistry of this activation process has been well described, and the reader is referred elsewhere for a detailed description (2–5).

Of the biomodulation strategies explored with 5-FU, two in particular—leucovorin (LV) and protracted venous infusion (PVI)—have gained traction over the years. LV (folinic acid, citrovorum factor) is the reduced folate, 5-formyltetrahydrofolate. In the presence of reduced folates, the active metabolite of 5-FU binds more tightly to thymidylate synthase (TS), its primary target enzyme (6,7). Although this preclinical rationale for LV as a biomodulator of 5-FU is sound, the issue of clinical relevance, whether it improves the therapeutic index of 5-FU, remains unresolved.

Initial uncontrolled pilot trials of 5-FU plus LV showed high response rates (RRs) in comparison to historical controls of 5-FU alone. Substantial toxicity was also seen, however (8–11). Multiple treatment schedules were developed using a variety of 5-FU and LV doses, and these regimens, now not widely used, have been well described elsewhere (12–14). The Advanced Colorectal Cancer Meta-Analysis Project initially performed a meta-analysis of nine randomized studies that compared 5-FU/LV with 5-FU alone (15). An update of this meta-analysis was reported with longer follow-up and 10 additional trials (16). This analysis now contains 3,300 patients from 19 trials, some of which had multiple comparisons, and thus a total of 21 pairwise comparisons were analyzed. In 10 of the comparisons, the 5-FU doses were similar in both arms, with LV being added to one arm. In these comparisons, significant response and survival advantages were seen in the 5-FU/LV arms, albeit with more toxicity. An analysis of the 11 trials in which 5-FU/LV was compared to a higher dose of 5-FU failed to show benefits for 5-FU/LV over 5-FU alone. Taken as a whole, the evidence would suggest that LV adds little to the therapeutic index of 5-FU and that higher doses of 5-FU without LV would be a reasonable alternative. LV is so widely accepted, however, that it is unlikely that 5-FU–based regimens without LV will ever gain significant popularity.

Many trials have attempted to define the "optimal" schedule of LV administration. It would seem from available data that lower-dose LV has some advantages because it has been associated with less diarrhea, and once-weekly regimens have been associated with less neutropenia and stomatitis than daily ×5 regimens (17–19). Of note, relatively protracted LV infusion times of up to 3 hours are often used in various regimens. There are no clinical data to support the practice of prolonging these infusions, and shorter LV infusion times of 15 to 30 minutes would appear to be both clinically defensible and reasonable.

Preclinical evidence indicated that an increased duration of exposure to low-dose 5-FU could improve efficacy (20). Because the plasma half-life of 5-FU is in the range of 8 to 20 minutes, protracted infusional 5-FU schedules were explored. A PVI of 5-FU at a dose of 300 mg/m²/day was compared to bolus 5-FU (21). The PVI regimen yielded a substantially higher RR (30%) than the bolus regimen (7%); however, there was no difference in survival between the two treatment arms. The Eastern Cooperative Oncology Group (ECOG) performed a similar trial with similar results (22). In a meta-analysis of 1,219 patients in six trials comparing PVI 5-FU to bolus, RR was improved (22% vs. 14%, respectively, $P = 0.0002$) (23). A survival advantage of less than 1 month was seen for PVI 5-FU.

High-dose intermittent infusion schedules differ from PVI schedules in that patients receive 5-FU over 24 to 48 hours on a weekly or every other week schedule. An early pilot trial of 5-FU 2,600 mg/m² weekly over 24 hours with LV 500 mg/m² reported seven responses in 12 chemotherapy-naive patients and three responses out of 10 patients who were previously treated (24). A large randomized trial reported by Kohne et al. confirmed the activity of this regimen, with a major objective RR of 44% in 91 patients (25). This trial also had an interferon-α (IFN-α)–containing arm, which was found to have substantial toxicity but no benefit. A phase III confirmatory trial comparing weekly 5-FU 24-hour infusions of 2,600 mg/m², either alone or with 500 mg/m² of LV, to the Mayo Clinic bolus daily ×5 schedule of 5-FU was less encouraging, however. No overall survival (OS) differences were seen between the arms, and the RRs were 12% for the Mayo Clinic bolus schedule, 10% for the infusional 5-FU, and 17% for infusional 5-FU plus LV (P = NS). Progressionfree survival (PFS) was increased in the infusion plus LV arm (P = 0.029), but diarrhea was substantially increased (26).

Exploiting the different mechanisms of cytotoxicity of bolus and infusional 5-FU, de Gramont et al. piloted a regimen using both strategies simultaneously. This LV5FU2 regimen was administered as a 2-day treatment every other week. Patients receive LV 200 mg/m^2 over 2 hours, followed by a 5-FU bolus of 400 mg/m^2, followed by 5-FU 600 mg/m^2 by 22-hour infusion, with all drugs given on days 1 and 2, repeated every 14 days. In a randomized comparison of this LV5FU2 schedule to the Mayo Clinic bolus schedule, the RR was superior for LV5FU2 versus Mayo Clinic 5-FU (33% vs. 14%, P = 0.0004), as was the PFS (P = 0.0012) (27). OS for LV5FU2 was approximately 5 weeks longer than the Mayo Clinic group, a difference that trended toward, but just barely missed, statistical significance (P = 0.067). LV5FU2 patients experienced less overall toxicity than the patients on the Mayo Clinic arm.

Other biomodulation strategies that have been explored unsuccessfully include the use of methotrexate (13,28–33), trimetrexate (34–41), and IFN-α (42–49). These do not have a role in the current management of CRC, and the reader is referred elsewhere if further information on these agents is desired.

Capecitabine

Absorption of 5-FU from the gut is unreliable, and inactivation of orally absorbed 5-FU by dihydropyrimidine dehydrogenase in a first-pass clearance through the liver is highly variable between patients. Capecitabine is an orally available 5-FU precursor that is absorbed intact through the gut and then activated by a series of enzymatic alterations, the last of which is conversion by thymidine phosphorylase (TP) into 5-FU. Some evidence suggests that TP levels may be higher in tumor than in normal tissue, thus suggesting a preferential activation of capecitabine within the tumor (50). A phase II trial showed activity in CRC (51). The addition of LV did not appear to provide any benefit, and toxicity was increased. Randomized phase III trials showed that oral capecitabine was at least as effective as intravenous (IV) bolus 5-FU/LV, and the side effect profile of capecitabine was superior to the Mayo Clinic 5-FU schedule (52–54).

The major side effects of capecitabine in these trials were palmar-plantar erythrodysesthesia (hand–foot syndrome) and diarrhea. The hand–foot syndrome is frequently the dose-limiting side effect (55). Although the approved starting dose in the United States is 1,250 mg/m^2 twice daily, many clinicians, especially in North America, choose to initiate therapy at a lower dose and escalate in those rare circumstances when no toxicity is seen. A retrospective review of results from two large trials suggests that efficacy was not inferior in those patients who required dose reductions (56). Whether efficacy is maintained when patients are prospectively and routinely started at a lower dose of capecitabine has not been addressed. It should be noted that despite the claim that chronic oral capecitabine approximates the pharmacokinetics of a protracted infusion IV 5-FU schedule, no randomized comparison of capecitabine to infusional schedules of 5-FU/LV has been reported. The equivalence of capecitabine to infusional 5-FU, or lack thereof, is therefore not an issue that can be definitively answered at this time. Also, although some clinicians have expressed a preference for use of capecitabine as a salvage regimen after 5-FU–based regimens have failed, data do not support this approach (57).

UFT + Leucovorin

Uracil is a competitive inhibitor of DPD, the rate-limiting enzyme in 5-FU catabolism. UFT is a combination of uracil and the 5-FU prodrug tegafur (ftorafur) in a fixed molar ratio of 4:1. Tegafur is orally absorbed and is converted in the body to 5-FU. In its early development, tegafur was found to have some activity against CRC. A metabolite of this drug was found to be neurotoxic, however, and this toxicity limited the development of tegafur. By inhibiting DPD, uracil allows for small amounts of tegafur to produce 5-FU that persists in circulation, thereby reducing the amount of neurotoxic metabolite produced. The inhibition of DPD also reduces interpatient differences in DPD activity levels, making dosing more predictable (58).

UFT has been developed with oral LV on a three times daily schedule. Phase II showed acceptable tolerability, with activity comparable to what can be achieved with IV 5-FU bolus schedules (59,60). Two large randomized studies compared oral UFT plus LV to the IV Mayo Clinic 5-FU/LV schedule. Both trials showed equivalence in terms of RRs, time to tumor progression, and OS (61,62). The trials did not, however, fulfill the U.S. regulatory requirements for noninferiority of UFT/LV, and the issue of demonstration of the contribution of uracil to the activity of the compound was also not addressed adequately for regulatory approval. Therefore, this agent is not available in the United States.

Raltitrexed

Raltitrexed is a TS inhibitor that is not related to the fluoropyrimidines. Randomized trials have shown raltitrexed 3 mg/m^2 given once every 3 weeks to have similar activity to bolus 5-FU/LV (63–65). In one trial, however, survival for the raltitrexed arm versus the 5-FU/LV arm was statistically significantly worse (9.7 vs. 12.7 months, P = 0.01). TS levels may predict for response to this agent (66). Raltitrexed is not approved for use in the United States, but it is available in many other countries.

Irinotecan

Camptothecin was identified as an agent with preclinical antitumor activity as early as 1966. Its insolubility hindered early attempts at clinical development, until the identification of camptothecin's mechanism of action (inhibition of topoisomerase I) led to renewed efforts to develop soluble derivatives. Irinotecan, or CPT-11 (CPT is an abbreviation for camptothecin), was one such soluble derivative. CPT-11 possesses a bulky dipiperidino side chain joined to the camptothecin molecule by a carboxyl-ester bond. This side chain confers solubility but substantially decreases cytotoxic activity. Carboxylesterase, predominantly in the liver, cleaves the carboxylester bond to form the more active metabolite, 7-ethyl-10-hydroxycamptothecin (SN-38) (67). SN-38 has been shown to be as much as 1,000-fold more potent in inhibiting topoisomerase I than CPT-11 and is thus the predominant active form of the drug.

CPT-11 and SN-38 function via inhibition of the enzyme topoisomerase I (topo I). Topo I facilitates the uncoiling of DNA for replication and transcription. In binding to DNA, topo I causes reversible single-stranded DNA breaks. The topo I–DNA complex allows the intact strand to pass through the break, thereby relieving torsional stress in the coiled helix. Topo I then reseals the break. CPT-11 and SN-38 stabilize these single-stranded breaks. These stabilized breaks are reversible; however, the collision of replication forks with open single-stranded breaks result in double-stranded breaks, which result in irreversible DNA fragmentation.

In the initial phase I trials of CPT-11, some antitumor activity was observed in several CRC patients (68–72). Subsequently, there was a phase II trial in which a 22% RR was seen in a population of previously treated CRC patients (73). A confirmatory trial reported a 23% RR and 31% stable disease rate in 43 patients with 5-FU–refractory CRC (74). An analysis of three identical trials together using a weekly treatment for 4 weeks every 6 weeks in 5-FU–refractory CRC showed a RR of 13% (75). Using a once-every-21-day schedule of CPT-11 at a dose of 350 mg/m^2 an 18% RR was seen, both in the 48 chemotherapy-naive patients and in the 165 patients who had previously progressed through a 5-FU–based regimen (76). Trials in the front-line setting reported 32% and 26% RRs, respectively (77,78).

The first randomized trial to confirm the benefits of CPT-11 was a phase III comparison of CPT-11 once every 3 weeks at 350 mg/m^2 (300 mg/m^2 for patients age 70 and older) versus supportive care only in CRC patients who had progressed on 5-FU (79). The patients receiving CPT-11 had a 1-year survival that was 2.5 times greater than the control group (36% vs. 14%). Quality-of-life parameters for the CPT-11–treated patients, as measured by the EORTC QLQ-C30 questionnaire, were as good or better in all major indices than the control group. Another phase III trial compared CPT-11 to infusional 5-FU after front-line 5-FU failure and found the 1-year survival of the CPT-11 group to be 1.4 times better (76).

Diarrhea was the major dose-limiting toxicity in early trials. Two different diarrheal syndromes were identified: early onset and late onset. The early onset diarrhea, which occurs during or immediately after CPT-11 administration, is a cholinergic effect and is readily controlled by use of atropine (80). In those patients who experience this symptom (and who do not have a contraindication to atropine administration), 0.5 to 1 mg of atropine gives rapid resolution, and subsequent CPT-11 doses can then be given with atropine as a premedication. Late onset diarrhea is a far more significant clinical issue, and this has been managed by the use of intensive loperamide at the onset of late onset diarrhea.

A randomized comparison of weekly versus every-3-week CPT-11 showed similar efficacy; however, the once-every-3-week schedule showed less diarrhea in this trial (81). Subsequent studies have shown that changing the weekly schedule to a 2 week on, 1 week off schedule substantially reduces the risk of toxicity (82). A direct comparison of efficacy and safety on these two weekly schedules has not been done, however.

Camptothecin/5-Fluorouracil/Leucovorin Combinations

Building on the 4 week on, 2 week off CPT-11 schedule that had been selected for development in North America, Saltz et al. added a low dose (20 mg/m^2) of LV given weekly, in order to reduce the potential for LV-exacerbated diarrhea. The phase I trial of this schedule showed that the full single-agent dose of CPT-11 (125 mg/m^2) could be given with 500 mg/m^2 of 5-FU and 20 mg/m^2 LV (83).

In a large-scale randomized phase III trial, this combination of irinotecan, fluorouracil, and leucovorin (IFL) was compared to the Mayo Clinic schedule of 5-FU/LV (84). For regulatory reasons, a third arm using front-line single-agent CPT-11 was also included. This trial showed that IFL was superior to the Mayo Clinic 5-FU/LV arm in terms of RR, time to tumor progression, and OS. The CPT-11 alone arm appeared to be comparable in efficacy to the 5-FU/LV arm. Total toxicity incidence was similar in all arms of this trial. A greater amount of grades

3 and 4 diarrhea and vomiting were seen with IFL, whereas more dose-limiting neutropenia, neutropenic fever, and stomatitis were seen with 5-FU/LV. Treatment-related deaths occurred in 1% of patients in each arm of this trial.

Other investigators combined CPT-11 with infusional 5-FU (85). In France, an every other week (biweekly) 5-FU infusion for 2 consecutive days was developed, whereas in Germany investigators explored weekly 24-hour high-dose infusions of 5-FU combined with weekly CPT-11. A randomized phase III trial randomized patients to one of these 5-FU/LV schedules alone, or with CPT-11. RR, PFS, and OS were superior in the CPT-11–containing arm of this trial as well.

More recently, the biweekly schedule of LV5FU2 plus irinotecan has been studied with a simplified LV5FU2 infusion schedule, a regimen now widely known as FOLFIRI (FOL, folinic acid; F, 5-FU; IRI, irinotecan) (86). This regimen has now gained widespread acceptance as one of the preferred irinotecan/5-FU/LV administration schedules.

Oxaliplatin

The diaminocyclohexane (DACH) platinum compounds are a group of agents that demonstrated preclinical activity in some cisplatin-resistant cell lines and xenografts (87,88). One important member of this DACH platinum group is oxaliplatin, which demonstrated some preclinical activity against CRC (89). The size of the DACH carrier ligand results in bulkier platinum-DNA adducts than are created by cisplatin. This putatively results in greater resistance to repair mechanisms (90–92).

Phase I studies showed evidence of antitumor activity at tolerable doses, with nausea, vomiting, leucopenia, and thrombocytopenia being the major dose-limiting toxicities. Nephrotoxicity was not observed. Significant neurotoxicity, including pharyngolaryngeal dysesthesia, a sensation of choking without overt airway blockage, were also noted (93,94). A phase II trial of oxaliplatin monotherapy in previously untreated CRC showed a confirmed RR of 12% (95). A second in a similar population reported a 24% RR, with 13% grade 3 neurotoxicity (96). A trial of monotherapy in second-line treatment yielded a RR of 10% (97).

Although the single-agent activity was marginal, studies of oxaliplatin plus 5-FU/LV appeared far more promising. Based on a series of phase II trials by Levi et al. (98,99), Giachetti et al. from the same group reported a phase III trial of chronomodulated 5-FU/LV alone or with oxaliplatin (100). The group receiving oxaliplatin had a superior RR (53% vs. 16%, $P < 0.001$). PFS was also superior, just reaching statistical significance (8.7 vs. 7.4 months, $P = 0.048$). There were no differences in median OS (19.4 and 19.9 months, respectively).

FOLFOX is an acronym that denotes a series of biweekly, nonchronomodulated combinations of LV, 5-FU, and oxaliplatin (FOL, folinic acid [LV]; F, fluorouracil; OX, oxaliplatin) (27). Numerous permutations of this combination (i.e., FOLFOX 1, FOLFOX 2), involving modifications in doses and scheduling, have been evaluated. In a randomized comparison of LV5FU2 versus FOLFOX 4 in 420 previously untreated metastatic CRC patients, the FOLFOX 4 arm showed a significantly superior RR (51% vs. 22%, $P = 0.001$) and PFS (9.0 vs. 6.2 months, $P = 0.0003$) (101). The OS trended in favor of FOLFOX, but the difference was not statistically significant (16.2 vs. 14.7 months, $P = 0.12$). The number of patients experiencing grade 3–4 neutropenia was increased with FOLFOX 4 over LV5FU2 (42% vs. 5% of patients). Grade 3–4 diarrhea (12% vs. 5%) was also increased in the FOLFOX arm. Neurotoxicity, virtually absent in the LV5FU2 arm, was frequent in the FOLFOX arm, with 18% of patients experiencing grade 3 neurosensory toxicity.

The same FOLFOX 4 regimen was also studied in the second-line setting (102). Patients were randomized to FOLFOX 4, LV5FU2, or single-agent oxaliplatin. RRs were 10% for FOLFOX 4, 0% for LV5FU2, and 1% for oxaliplatin alone ($P <0.0001$ for FOLFOX vs. LV5FU2). Time to tumor progression was also superior for FOLFOX 4 (4.6 months) versus LV5FU2 (2.7 months) and oxaliplatin alone (1.6 months), while OS trended toward, but did not reach, statistical significance ($P = 0.07$) (103).

In FOLFOX 5, the oxaliplatin dose was increased from 85 to 100 mg/m^2; however, before FOLFOX 5 was ever tested clinically, FOLFOX 6 was developed. This regimen maintained the 100 mg/m^2 oxaliplatin dose but used a simplified 5-FU/LV schedule (104). Oxaliplatin 100 mg/m^2 was given over 2 hours, with LV 400 mg/m^2 given concurrently via a "T" connector. These are then followed by a 400 mg/m^2 bolus of 5-FU, and then a 46-hour infusion of 5-FU at 2,400 to 3,000 mg/m^2. More recently, the FOLFOX 7 regimen has been reported, using a 130 mg/m^2 dose of oxaliplatin every 14 days. The simplified LV and 5-FU administration of FOLFOX 6 is maintained, with deletion of the bolus 5-FU. In the FOLFOX 7 schedule, oxaliplatin is discontinued after 3 months and is planned for reintroduction after 12 weeks or sooner if clinical progression occurs. Although reintroduction of oxaliplatin was less frequent than had been intended in the protocol, the results of this trial showed the acceptability of a planned early stopping of oxaliplatin, with efficacy parameters being similar in both arms of the trial (105). This rationale of stopping oxaliplatin at an early time point, before the development of prohibitive neurotoxicity, with the potential for reintroduction at a later date, has now become widely accepted in standard practice, regardless of which FOLFOX schedule is used.

There has not been, and never will be, a randomized trial comparing FOLFOX 4 to FOLFOX 6. Most investigators have accepted that the LV5FU2 and simplified LV5FU2 schedules are comparable in efficacy and toxicity, and the simplified schedule has de facto replaced the original LV5FU2 in many practices. Most ongoing National Cancer Institute (NCI) cooperative group studies are using a modified FOLFOX 6 (mFOLFOX 6) that contains the simplified LV5FU2 doses from FOLFOX 6 with the lower 85 mg/m^2 starting dose of oxaliplatin from FOLFOX 4. Currently, this mFOLFOX 6 appears to be a reasonable schedule for routine clinical use.

One other practical modification that has often been made in the infusional 5-FU schedules of simplified LV5FU2 is to administer the infusion over a full 2 days (48 hours) as opposed to the original 46 hours in the published regimens. The current NCI cooperative protocols call for the dose to be given over 46 to 48 hours. The reason for this is one of medication safety. A 48-hour infusion has the advantage in that it can be written as two consecutive 24-hour infusions, thereby minimizing the risk that the total 2-day dose could be inadvertently written in a subsequent cycle as a daily dose, which would lead to a serious overdose. In the interest of minimizing such potentially catastrophic errors, a common and advisable practice is to avoid ever writing more than a 24-hour dose of a chemotherapy agent in the medication record. As such, a 46- to 48-hour infusion of 2,400 mg/m^2 is more safely written as 1,200 mg/m^2/day $\times$ 2 days. The 4% difference in infusion time is trivial, but the potential for improved safety is considerable.

A regimen of bolus 5-FU, oxaliplatin, and leucovorin (bFOL) has also been studied in a phase II trial (106); however, the results of a randomized phase II trial comparing this regimen to FOLFOX and to a capecitabine plus oxaliplatin combination do not support the routine use of the bFOL regimen in the metastatic setting (107).

Oxaliplatin versus Irinotecan in the First-Line Setting

First-line development of irinotecan and oxaliplatin occurred in parallel. It was not until after each had established a front-line role that head-to-head comparisons were performed. One of the more important trials to address the comparison of these two agents was the NCI intergroup study N9741. Although this study underwent many iterations, in its final form it was a three-arm study using the weekly bolus IFL regimen as the control arm, compared to FOLFOX 4 and to oxaliplatin plus irinotecan (IROX).

The results of N9741 showed superior outcome for the patients randomized to FOLFOX 4, as compared to those randomized to either IFL or IROX, in terms of RR, time to tumor progression, and OS (Table 45.1) (Table 45.2) (108). Toxicity for FOLFOX 4 was also superior for virtually all parameters, except, as would be expected, neurotoxicity. The results of the IROX arm did not differ significantly from those of the IFL arm in terms of toxicity, response, or time to tumor progression; however, survival was borderline significantly better in the IROX arm than the IFL arm ($P = 0.04$).

Although FOLFOX 4 was superior to IFL in both RR and time to tumor progression in this trial, interpretation of the OS results of N9741 is complicated by a number of issues. First, there were major imbalances between treatment arms in terms of availability of effective second-line therapy. Oxaliplatin was not commercially available in the United States during the course of N9741, and only a small percentage of patients on the IFL arm received second-line oxaliplatin. Furthermore, it is unknown what percentage of those who did receive oxaliplatin received it as part of the FOLFOX regimen versus as a single agent. The details of poststudy therapy were not recorded, and it was not yet known at the time of the trial that only FOLFOX, and not single-agent oxaliplatin, is active in the salvage setting (102). Second-line irinotecan, which has been shown to offer a survival benefit, was readily available to all patients who had received FOLFOX 4. To what degree these imbalances in second-line therapy may have influenced the survival results is not known. Another important point is that IFL uses bolus 5-FU, while FOLFOX 4 contains infusional LV5FU2. It is therefore not possible to isolate the irinotecan versus oxaliplatin comparison from the 5-FU bolus versus 5-FU infusion comparison in the relative efficacy of these regimens.

Tournigand et al. conducted a small phase III trial of FOLFOX 6 versus FOLFIRI in which the only variable was oxaliplatin versus irinotecan; identical simplified LV5FU2 schedules were used in each arm, and all patients were planned to cross over to the other regimen at time of progression (Table 45.3) (109). Although this study is underpowered, having a total of only 226 patients, the results are compelling, with first-line response, time to tumor progression, and OS being extremely similar in the two arms. Diarrhea and alopecia were somewhat more common with the irinotecan-based regimen; the oxaliplatin-based regimen had considerable neurotoxicity. A similar and somewhat larger trial of 360 patients that compared FOLFOX 4 to the equivalent FOLFIRI schedule also showed virtually no difference in efficacy, with more gastrointestinal toxicity and alopecia with FOLFIRI and more neurotoxicity and thrombocytopenia in the FOLFOX arm (110). A third trial using a bolus 5-FU schedule in both arms, as well as comparing irinotecan and oxaliplatin with identical 5-FU schedules and same access to effective second-line therapy, shows no difference in efficacy parameters between the two regimens (111). Another randomized trial using bolus 5-FU in each arm showed a better result for the group receiving first-line oxaliplatin; however, the oxaliplatin regimen initially had a higher dose of 5-FU, a factor that confounds interpretation of this trial (112).

TABLE 45.1

COMMONLY USED IRINOTECAN/FLUOROURACIL AND OXALIPLATIN FLUOROURACIL COMBINATION REGIMENS

Regimen	Reference	Schedule (all agents administered intravenously)
IFL	Saltz et al. (84)	Irinotecan 125 mg/m^2 over 90 minutes, followed by LV 20 mg/m^2 by brief infusion, followed by bolus 5-FU 500 mg/m^2, all treatments repeated weekly for 4 weeks, repeated every 6 weeks.
FOLFIRI	Douillard et al. (85)	Irinotecan 180 mg/m^2 over 2 hours; LV 200 mg/m^2 concurrently with irinotecan (given in same line through "Y" connector); followed by 5-FU bolus 400 mg/m^2, followed by 5-FU 600 mg/m^2 infusion over 22 hours. Irinotecan given day 1 only. Other meds given days 1 and 2. Cycle repeated every 14 days.
FOLFOX 4	de Gramont et al. (101)	Oxaliplatin 85 mg/m^2 over 2 hours; LV 200 mg/m^2 concurrently with oxaliplatin (given in same line through "Y" connector); followed by 5-FU bolus 400 mg/m^2, followed by 5-FU 600 mg/m^2 infusion over 22 hours. Oxaliplatin given day 1 only. Other meds given days 1 and 2. Cycle repeated every 14 days.
FOLFIRI (simplified)	Andre et al. (86)	Irinotecan 180 mg/m^2 over 2 hours; LV 400 mg/m^2 concurrently with irinotecan (can be given in same line through "Y" connector); followed by 5-FU bolus 400 mg/m^2, followed by 5-FU 2,400–3,000^a mg/m^2 infusion over 46–48 hours. Cycle repeated every 14 days.
FOLFOX 6	Tournigand et al. (109)	Oxaliplatin 100 mg/m^2 over 2 hours; LV 400 mg/m^2 concurrently with irinotecan (can be given in same line through "Y" connector); followed by 5-FU bolus 400 mg/m^2, followed by 5-FU 2,400–3,000^a mg/m^2 infusion over 46–48 hours. Cycle repeated every 14 days.
Modified FOLFOX 6 (mFOLFOX 6)	Widely used in current practice and in phase III trials, but not published	Oxaliplatin 85 mg/m^2 over 2 hours; LV 400 mg/m^2 concurrently with oxaliplatin (can be given in same line through "Y" connector); followed by 5-FU bolus 400 mg/m^2, followed by 5-FU 2,400 mg/m^2 infusion over 46–48 hours. Cycle repeated every 14 days.
FOLFOX 7	de Gramont et al. (105)	Oxaliplatin 130 mg/m^2 over 2 hours; LV 400 mg/m^2 concurrently with oxaliplatin (can be given through "Y" connector); followed by 5-FU 2,400 mg/m^2 infusion over 46–48 hours. Cycle repeats every 14 days. Oxaliplatin discontinued after 12 weeks and may be restarted after 12 additional weeks, or at progression.
FUFIRI	Douillard et al. (85)	Irinotecan 80 mg/m^2, then LV 500 mg/m^2, followed by 5-FU 2,300 mg/m^2; all drugs given weekly for 6 weeks, repeated every 7 weeks.
FUFOX	Grothey et al. (169)	Oxaliplatin 50 mg/m^2 over 2 hours, followed by LV 500 mg/m^2, followed by 5-FU 2,000 mg/m^2 over 24 hours, weekly for 5 weeks, repeated every 6 weeks.

Dose adjustments may be required. Listed doses are recommended starting doses for patients with normal renal, hepatic, and bone marrow function and good performance status.
^{a}Escalation above 2,400 mg/m^2/46–48 hours is rare.

TABLE 45.2

INTERGROUP TRIAL N9741: IRINOTECAN PLUS BOLUS 5-FU/LEUCOVORIN (IFL) VERSUS OXALIPLATIN PLUS INFUSIONAL 5-FU/LEUCOVORIN (FOLFOX-4) VERSUS IRINOTECAN PLUS OXALIPLATIN (IROX) IN FIRST-LINE METASTATIC COLORECTAL CANCER

	IFL (N = 264)	FOLFOX 4 (N = 267)	IROX (N = 264)	P value (IFL vs. FOLFOX)
Response rate	31%	45%	35%	0.03
Time to tumor progression	6.9 months	8.7 months	6.5 months	0.001
Overall survival	15.0 months	19.5 months	17.4 months	0.0001
Received potentially active second-line therapy	24% (oxaliplatin)	60% (irinotecan)	50% (fluorouracil)	Not given

Adapted from ref. 108.

TABLE 45.3

COMPARISON OF FIRST-LINE USE OF IRINOTECAN (FOLFIRI) VERSUS OXALIPLATIN (FOLFOX) IN CONJUNCTION WITH THE SAME BIWEEKLY INFUSIONAL 5-FU/LEUCOVORIN SCHEDULE

	Tournigand et al. (109)			Colucci et al. (110)		
	FOLFIRI (n = 109)	FOLFOX 6 (n = 111)	P value	FOLFIRI (n = 164)	FOLFOX 4 (n = 172)	P value
Response rate	56%	54%	0.68	31%	34%	0.6
Time to tumor progression (on first-line regimen)	8.5 months	8.1 months	0.65	7 months	7 months	NS
Time to tumor progression (after first- and second-line regimen)	14.4 months	11.5 months	0.65			
Overall survival (from initial randomization)	20.4 months	21.5 months	0.9	14 months	15 months	NS

5-FU, 5-fluoracil; NS, nonsignificant.

Thus, taken as a whole, the available data would indicate that irinotecan and oxaliplatin are equivalent in terms of activity in front-line metastatic regimens, whereas infusional 5-FU appears to have advantages over the bolus schedules. Current data support neither the routine use of the bolus IFL schedule, nor bolus 5-FU/LV with oxaliplatin. Routine use of IROX is also not supported by the currently available body of data. The choice of an irinotecan-based (i.e., FOLFIRI) versus an oxaliplatin-based (i.e., FOLFOX) combination in front-line management of good performance status patients can be considered a matter of patient preference, and discussion of the differing toxicity profiles is appropriate to help individuals decide. It would be highly desirable to have a more elegant means of individualizing therapy, such as the use of molecular prognostic indicators and/or pharmacogenomics; however, because no such approaches are validated at this time, they are not part of standard practice.

A number of investigators are evaluating the concurrent use of oxaliplatin, irinotecan, and 5-FU. Phase I and II trials have demonstrated high activity but substantial toxicity (113,114). A small randomized trial, thus far presented in abstract form only, showed a superior result for "FOLFOXIRI" as compared to FOLFIRI in front line. This result is intriguing and worthy of further investigation (115).

Oral Fluoropyrimidines in Combination Regimens

As discussed previously, evidence would suggest that the infusion schedules of 5-FU are more appropriate for combination therapies than bolus schedules. However, because the logistics of infusions are problematic for some, the question of whether oral fluoropyrimidines can replace infusions in combination regimens has been explored. Whether chronic oral administration of a fluoropyrimidine will prove to be therapeutically comparable to infusional schedules and be more or less acceptable to patients than the ambulatory infusion remains to be determined. Phase II data for these combinations suggest activity in the range of the infusional 5-FU–based combinations (116–118); however, randomized trials, currently ongoing, are necessary to determine whether these oral fluoropyrimidine-based combinations are acceptable alternatives to parenteral regimens. The first randomized comparison of a capecitabine/oxaliplatin combination versus a weekly

high-dose infusional 5-FU plus oxaliplatin (FUFOX) has been reported in abstract form and efficacy in terms of RR and PFS results appear to be comparable (119). A 1,600 patient trial of FOLFOX 4 versus capecitabine/oxaliplatin completed accrual in the spring of 2005, and data are expected to be available shortly.

Patient compliance and satisfaction with oral versus parenteral fluoropyrimidine *in the setting of a combination regimen* has not been well studied to date. The choice at hand is not whether patients would prefer to take their chemotherapy orally or by vein; IV medications are going to be given every 14 to 21 days anyway. Is it therefore better to have a 46- to 48-hour 5-FU infusion and then 12 days without chemotherapy, or to take multiple pills per day for 14 days, followed by a 7-day break, considering that the nausea from the parenteral chemotherapy may impact the ability and desirability of taking the oral chemotherapy? It should be recalled that oral components of chemotherapy require a highly motivated, reliable, and compliant patient because the responsibility of dosing and dose adjustment is shifted significantly to the patient.

Concurrent versus Sequential Therapy

Although most studies suggest a role for combination regimens in first-line treatment, some recent data, reported thus far in abstract form only, suggest that sequential administration of agents may be a viable alternative (120). The Fluorouracil, Oxaliplatin, CPT-11 Use and Sequencing (FOCUS) study randomized 2,135 first-line CRC patients to receive one of five treatment plans:

1. Biweekly bolus plus infusional 5-FU/LV (5FULV2), followed by change to single-agent irinotecan
2. 5FULV2, followed by addition of irinotecan (i.e., change to FOLFIRI) at time of progression
3. 5FULV2, followed by addition of oxaliplatin (i.e., change to FOLFOX)
4. First-line FOLFIRI
5. First-line FOLFOX

Although higher RRs and PFSs were seen in the front-line combination therapy arms (FOLFIRI and FOLFOX), there were not significant differences in survival between any of the five arms, although 5FULV2 followed by single-agent irinotecan appeared to trend toward inferiority compared to the other four arms.

Bevacizumab

Bevacizumab (bev) is a humanized monoclonal antibody that binds to vascular endothelial growth factor (VEGF), substantially reducing the availability of VEDF, and thereby preventing receptor activation (121,122). The initial trial with bev in CRC investigated two doses of bev in combination with the weekly Roswell Park schedule of 5-FU/LV (123). This small, three-arm, trial randomized 104 patients to bev 5 mg/kg or bev 10 mg/kg plus weekly 5-FU/LV or to 5-FU/LV alone. The 5-FU/LV + 5 mg/kg bev arm had the best outcome in terms of RR, time to tumor progression, and OS, and this arm was therefore selected for phase III development.

The initial plan for the phase III pivotal trial was a comparison of 5-FU/LV + placebo to 5-FU/LV + 5 mg/kg of bev. As this trial was about to be initiated, however, data from a randomized phase III trial showed a small but statistically significant survival advantage for the IFL regimen (irinotecan plus weekly bolus 5-FU/LV, IFL) compared with 5-FU/LV alone (84). Therefore, the IFL regimen was then believed to be the appropriate control arm for subsequent phase III trials. Because there were then no safety data, on the combination of bev plus IFL, a three-arm trial was designed that used IFL plus placebo as a control arm and compared that to IFL plus bev and to 5-FU/LV plus bev (124). As per study plan, a safety analysis was performed on all arms when enrollment reached 100 patients per arm and, because the IFL plus bev demonstrated acceptable safety, further enrollment on the 5-FU/LV arm was suspended at that time. No cross over to second-line bev in the IFL/placebo control arm was permitted. The IFL/bev cohort in this study demonstrated superior outcome compared to the IFL/placebo group in RR (45% vs. 35%, P <0.003), PFS (10.6 vs. 6.2 months, P <0.00001), and OS (20.3 vs. 15.6 months, P = 0.00003) (Table 45.4).

In a follow-up publication to the primary report, the results of the first 100 patients in each of the three arms of the study were reported to assess the outcome in the 5-FU/LV plus bev cohort. Although 100 patients per arm is too small to permit definitive conclusions, the activity of the 5-FU/LV plus bev arm appeared to be superior to 5-FU/LV alone and comparable to those of the IFL plus placebo arm, but with a superior toxicity profile. In another randomized phase II trial that was designed for those patients who were determined by their treating investigators to not be appropriate for irinotecan-based therapy, patients were given front-line 5-FU/LV (Roswell Park Schedule), with either placebo or 5 mg/kg of bev given every other week. Although this study also lacked sufficient power to assess for a survival advantage, the 5-FU/LV plus bev arm did show improved RR and time to tumor progression (125).

A combined analysis from the three separate trials that compared a 5-FU/LV arm with a 5-FU/LV plus bev arm was performed. This showed a statistically significant survival advantage for the patients who received 5-FU/LV plus bev (126). Given the favorable aspects of the biweekly infusional 5-FU used in the FOCUS trial discussed previously (120), this schedule of 5-FU would seem most appropriate for combination with bev in patients who are to receive a 5-FU/LV plus bev regimen.

Before the results of the phase III IFL plus bev versus IFL trial were known, the ECOG conducted a phase II trial (trial E2200) of IFL plus bev at 10 mg/kg in 92 previously untreated patients (127,128). At a median follow-up of 16.7 months, a 42% RR was noted. Preliminary safety data from 87 patients showed four bleeding events of ≥grade 2. Eleven thrombotic events were also reported. The 42% RR does not appear to be substantially different, and is certainly not superior to, the 45% RR seen with the 5 mg/kg dose in the pivotal phase III trial. At present, data do not support the use of the 10-mg/kg dose in first-line metastatic CRC.

The ECOG 3200 trial evaluated the use of bev in the second-line setting (129). It must be noted that this trial was performed only in patients who had not received bev in the first-line setting. Bev-naive patients who had failed irinotecan and fluorouracil were randomly assigned to one of three arms: FOLFOX plus bev 10 mg/kg, FOLFOX alone, or bev 10 mg/kg alone. The FOLFOX plus bev arm had a small but statistically superior survival advantage over FOLFOX alone (12.5 vs. 10.7 months, p = 0.0024), and grade 3/4 toxicities were not increased. The bev-alone arm had substantially inferior PFS and an investigator-adjudicated RR of 3%, suggesting that single-agent bev does not have meaningful activity in CRC and should not be used.

The safety of bev in combination with oxaliplatin-based regimens was further addressed by the TREE-2 study, a randomized phase II trial that compared three oxaliplatin-fluoropyrimidine regimens in first-line setting (107). In this trial, the addition of bev to FOLFOX, bFOL (oxaliplatin plus bolus 5-FU/LV), or cape/ox (oxaliplatin plus capecitabine) appeared to improve the overall response relative to historic controls from an earlier trial (TREE-1) with no significant additive toxicity.

Bevacizumab Toxicity

In the phase III IFL plus/minus bev trial, grade 3 hypertension was higher in the IFL plus bev arm than in the IFL plus placebo arm (11% vs. 2%) (124). Neither venous thrombotic events nor proteinuria were significantly different between the two arms. However, two rare but extremely serious toxicities were increased in the bev-containing arm: gastrointestinal (GI) perforations and arterial thrombotic events (ATEs).

The GI perforations were a somewhat diverse group of events that included a perforated gastric ulcer, small bowel

TABLE 45.4

IFL + PLACEBO VERSUS IFL PLUS BEVACIZUMAB VERSUS FL PLUS BEVACIZUMAB IN FIRST-LINE TREATMENT OF METASTATIC COLORECTAL CANCER

Treatment	Number of patients	Response rate	Progressionfree survival (months)	Overall survival (months)
IFL	411	35%	6.2	15.6
IFL + Bevacizumab	402	45%	10.6	20.3

I, irinotecan; F, fluorouracil; L, leucovorin.
Adapted from ref. 124.

perforations, and free air under the diaphragm without identified source. In the phase III IFL trial, six such events occurred on the bevacizumab-containing arm (one fatal) compared with none on the IFL-only arm. No specific risk factors for perforation were identified. Interestingly, in large cooperative group trials of bev in breast cancer and lung cancer, GI perforations were not significantly increased in the bev-containing arms. However, an unusually high GI perforation rate has recently halted accrual on a trial of bev in ovarian cancer patients. These perforations in ovarian patients demonstrate that there is not an association between the presence of a primary colonic tumor and a GI perforation. Some clinicians have raised the issue of possibly needing to remove an asymptomatic primary colorectal tumor in a patient with synchronous stage IV disease before using bev, fearing that the primary will put the patient at risk for perforation. Data do not support this fear, however, and palliative surgery for an asymptomatic primary tumor in a synchronous stage IV patient is not indicated, regardless of plans to use a bev-containing chemotherapy regimen.

ATEs are the other rare but serious event for which there is an increased risk with bev. Although no increased risk of this was detected in the pivotal phase III trial, a combined analysis of more than 1,700 patients from several trials showed a small but statistically significant increase in ATEs (defined here as either myocardial infarction, stroke, transient ischemic attack, or angina) in the population receiving bev plus chemotherapy versus chemotherapy alone. Patients with histories of ATEs in the past appeared to be at greater risk for increased bev-related arterial thrombotic complications. A further analysis of these events suggested that the risk was essentially linear over time, indicating that the risk of a new ATE is the same in earlier versus later months of bev treatment (130).

Cetuximab

The epidermal growth factor receptor (EGFR) is a transmembrane glycoprotein receptor of the HER family. When ligand binds to the receptor, either homodimerization with another EGFR or heterodimerization with another member of the HER family occurs. This stimulates phosphorylation of the intracellular tyrosine kinase domains, resulting in initiation of a signaling cascade that ultimately regulates cell proliferation and survival, as well as migration, adhesion, and differentiation (131–133). Cetuximab (cetux), previously known as C225, is a chimeric monoclonal immunoglobulin G_1 antibody that binds to the extracellular domain of the EGFR, blocking the binding site and preventing receptor activation (134).

Preclinical studies with cetuximab indicated minimal single-agent activity in most models but more robust activity when

given in combination with either chemotherapy or radiation. A multicenter phase II trial was performed in which patients who were determined by their treating investigator to have progressed on irinotecan were treated with cetuximab at the now standard dose of 400 mg/m² loading dose during week 1 over 2 hours, followed by weekly 250 mg/m² over 1 hour. Irinotecan was given on the same dose and schedule as had been previously failed, with maintenance of prior irinotecan dose reductions (135).

The RR in the 120 patients who were deemed to have failed prior irinotecan was 22.5%, as determined by an independent response assessment committee. Of the side effects specifically attributable to cetuximab, 3% of patients developed an allergic, anaphylactoid reaction requiring discontinuation of cetuximab therapy, and 75% of patients experienced an acnelike skin rash (12% grade 3), a rash now recognized to be characteristic of EGFR antagonists. Microscopically, although the rash clinically looks like acne, it can be seen that it is not acne, but rather a noncomedogenic process characterized by neutrophilic infiltration. Topical acne medications are ineffective and, because this rash is characterized by dryness and not oiliness, drying agents and retinoids appear to make it worse. An important observation from this trial, which has since been corroborated in multiple trials, is that the presence and severity of the rash appear to correlate with clinical activity.

The results of the cetuximab plus irinotecan combination trial raised the question of the activity of single-agent cetuximab in irinotecan-refractory CRC. A small phase II trial was therefore done in which 5 of 57 patients (9%) achieved a partial response, as determined by third-party review (136).

A randomized phase II confirmatory trial in 329 irinotecan-refractory CRC patients, which has become known as the "BOND" trial, compared cetuximab plus irinotecan to cetuximab monotherapy (137) (Table 45.5). The RRs of 22.9% for cetuximab plus irinotecan and 10.8% for cetuximab alone were virtually identical to the RRs that had been reported previously in the two prior U.S. phase II trials, confirming the activity of this agent in CRC. Time to tumor progression in the BOND trial was 4.1 months for the combination versus 1.5 months for single-agent cetuximab. Survival in the two arms was not significantly different; however, the study was neither designed nor powered to address the issue of a survival advantage for cetuximab, and cetuximab was given to all patients on both arms of the study.

A National Cancer Institute of Canada phase III comparing cetuximab monotherapy to best supportive care for chemotherapy-refractory CRC patients is ongoing.

First-line data for cetuximab are very scarce at this time. Only data from phase II trials have been reported thus far. Phase II pilot trials of cetuximab plus weekly bolus IFL,

TABLE 45.5

CETUXIMAB PLUS IRINOTECAN VERSUS CETUXIMAB ALONE IN IRINOTECAN-REFRACTORY COLORECTAL CANCER

	Number of patients	Response rate (95% CI)	Median time to progression (months)	Median overall survival (95% CI)
Cetuximab + Irinotecan	218	23% (18%–29%)[a]	4.1[b]	8.6 months (7.6–9.6)
Cetuximab	111	11% (6%–18%)	1.5	6.9 months (5.6–9.1)

CI, confidence interval.
[a]$p = 0.0074$.
[b]$p < 0.0001$.
Adapted from ref. 143.

weekly infusional 5-FU/LV (FUFIRI), and biweekly 5-FU/LV (FOLFIRI) have been reported (138–140). A 1,200 patient randomized trial of FUFIRI ± cetuximab in the front-line setting completed accrual as of November 2005, and the data are maturing.

First-line oxaliplatin-based regimens plus FOLFOX have also been studied in preliminary fashion. A preliminary report of a phase II first-line trial of FOLFOX 4 plus cetuximab shows substantial activity (141). Of 43 patients enrolled, third-party radiology review confirmed a 79% major objective RR. In addition, it was reported that 9 of the patients on study subsequently underwent an R0 resection of metastatic disease. A phase I/II trial of cetuximab plus 5-FU/LV (two dose cohorts) and weekly oxaliplatin 50 mg/m² (FUFOX) in first-line treatment has reported preliminary data from 38 of 49 enrolled patients (142). An overall RR of 55% was reported.

A trial of FOLFOX versus FOLFIRI ± cetuximab in a 2 × 2 design was initiated by the CALGB (CALGB trial 80203) in 2003; however, this trial was closed to accrual after the availability of the front-line bevacizumab made accrual to the chemotherapy-alone control arm inappropriate. Approximately 300 patients were accrued, and this has been restructured into a randomized phase II trial, which is scheduled to report in June 2006. This study will not have adequate power to assess survival, but it will be the first randomized front-line data regarding activity of cetuximab in the front line.

An assumption was made at the beginning of cetuximab's clinical development that EGFR expression would correlate with activity and that an absence of demonstrable EGFR on a tumor sample would mean that that tumor would be insensitive to cetuximab. Based on this untested hypothesis, the earlier cetuximab trials were restricted to those patients whose tumors demonstrated EGFR positivity by IHC. However, despite the preclinical data, virtually all clinical experience has shown that EGFR expression has no predictive value. None of the trials reported thus far have shown any correlation between degree of EGFR expression and clinical activity (135,136,143). Lenz et al. were the first to report responses in patients known to be EGFR negative by immunohistochemistry (144). Of 9 EGFR patients treated, two major objective responses were reported by the investigators, one of which was confirmed as a major response by third-party review and one of which was not.

Based on the available data, EGFR status was not used as an exclusion factor for patients being treated at Memorial Sloan-Kettering Cancer Center in New York. Subsequently, a retrospective review was conducted of all patients who had received nonresearch cetuximab-based therapy in the first 3 months of standard use of cetuximab at that center. Computerized pharmacy records were used to eliminate recall bias. Sixteen irinotecan-refractory, EGFR (−) CRC patients who had been treated were identified. Fourteen of these patients had received cetuximab in combination with irinotecan, and 2 had received cetuximab alone. Of the 16, 4 patients experienced major objective (RR 25%, 95% CI, 4%–46%) (145), thereby refuting the hypothesis that an EGFR (−) patient could not possibly respond to cetuximab. As a result of these aggregate clinical data, it has now become widely accepted that EGFR testing, as currently done, is of no clinical relevance for cetuximab usage, and the test should not be done on a routine basis.

Bevacizumab Plus Cetuximab

EGFR inhibition has been shown to downregulate VEGFR expression, suggesting a strong rationale for combined anti-EGFR and -VEGF strategies. A randomized phase II trial in patients with irinotecan-refractory CRC has been reported in abstract form (146). These preliminary data show a 20% RR and a 5.6-month median time to tumor progression for the two antibodies alone, and a 37% RR and a 7.9 month time to tumor progression for the two antibodies plus irinotecan, which appear to be better than historical controls from the initial North American and BOND studies (11% and 23% RR, 1.5 and 4 months TTP) (143,146). It should be noted, however, that this is a small trial with 41 and 40 patients, respectively, reported in each arm in this preliminary report. Ninety percent of the patients in this study had also previously received oxaliplatin, making the combination of antibodies an effective salvage regimen in the particular population studied. However, this study was conducted in patients who were naive to both cetuximab and bevacizumab. Because most patients now receive bevacizumab as part of their first-line regimen, the role of combination anti-EGFR plus anti-VEGF therapy in current practice should be extremely limited until further safety and efficacy results from ongoing trial are available.

Panitumumab

Panitumumab (ABX-EGF) is a fully humanized monoclonal antibody that, like cetuximab, targets the EGFR. Similar to the results seen with single-agent cetuximab, the results from phase II evaluations of panitumumab in CRC patients indicate a 10% RR, with nearly all patients experiencing some degree of acneiform rash (147). Because panitumumab is a fully humanized nature of this antibody, it will reduce the likelihood of anaphylactoid infusion reactions. One of the 148 patients treated experienced a dose-limiting allergic reaction. A randomized trial of panitumumab versus best supportive care in the salvage setting has recently been reported, which showed an 8% RR, with a clinically modest, although highly statistically significant PFS advantage over best supportive care alone (148). This study has been submitted as the basis for registration of the drug in CRC. A large randomized trial of FOLFOX/bevacizumab ± panitumumab in the front-line setting is actively accruing patients. Unfortunately, a trial of panitumumab plus irinotecan in the irinotecan-refractory setting has never been done, nor has there been a head-to-head comparison of panitumumab to cetuximab. Clinicians will therefore be challenged to decide to what degree panitumumab should be used in place of cetuximab without having any direct comparative data. Certainly, there is no reason to believe that panitumumab would have activity in cetuximab failures or vice versa.

OTHER ANTI–EPIDERMAL GROWTH FACTOR RECEPTOR AGENTS

Several other anti-EGFR antibodies are in clinical development. Among them are the fully humanized monoclonal antibodies matuzumab (EMD 72000) and nimotuzumab (r-h3). In a phase I trial of matuzumab that includes 11 patients with heavily pretreated CRC (149), two achieved major responses, with no grade 3 toxicities reported. These preliminary findings will have to be further explored in phase II and III trials. Nimotuzumab has shown evidence of clinical activity in pediatric glioma and in head and neck cancers in conjunction with radiation therapy. Studies in CRC are planned.

For reasons that are not at all clear, the limited experiences thus far with EGFR tyrosine kinase inhibitors gefitinib (ZD1839) and erlotinib (OSI-774) in CRC have been largely disappointing (150,151). One more recent single-agent trial of erlotinib in CRC has suggested some modest single-agent activity (152). The discrepancy between these results and earlier results is not yet understood. A single-center phase II trial of

FOLFOX 4 plus gefitinib reported a 77% objective RR in 30 evaluable patients (153). However, toxicity was prohibitive, with 54% grade 3/4 diarrhea and 52% grade 3/4 neutropenia reported.

Cyclo-Oxygenase 2 Inhibitors

Cyclo-oxygenase 2 (COX-2) catalyzes the synthesis of prostaglandins in the inflammatory response, and is frequently upregulated in malignant and premalignant tissues. Increasing COX-2 expression has been correlated with increased invasiveness, resistance to apoptosis, and increased angiogenesis (154). There is clear evidence that nonsteroidal anti-inflammatory drugs (NSAIDs) and selective COX-2 inhibitors can reduce the development of premalignant polyps. However, evidence that either NSAIDs or selective COX-2 inhibitors have activity in the treatment of CRC is lacking. Several randomized trials had been initiated to evaluate the contribution of COX-2 inhibitors with chemotherapy. Identification of cardiovascular toxicity with this class of agents and the withdrawal of several of these agents from the market has substantially decreased interest in this line of investigation. Routine use of COX-2 inhibitors with chemotherapy is not recommended at this time.

Gene Therapy

Because CRC may progress within a confined space such as the peritoneal cavity or within a solitary organ such as the liver, CRC is a reasonable potential target for gene therapy approaches (155) because regional administration of a gene vector may be practical. Trials of different gene therapy approaches, including virus-directed enzyme prodrug therapy, immunogenic manipulation, gene correction, and viral therapy have all been initiated. These innovative approaches remain highly investigational at this time.

Molecular Predictive Markers

With the availability of a number of active agents, it would be extremely useful to have the ability to scientifically select a particular drug or drug combination that would have an increased likelihood of efficacy or a decreased likelihood of toxicity. We are rapidly moving closer to such an approach.

One promising avenue of investigation has been the elucidation of markers of resistance to fluorouracil based on knowledge of its metabolic pathways. Studies have indicated that high levels of TS (156), dihydropyrimidine dehydrogenase (DPD) (157), or thymidine phosphorylase (TP) (158), as measured in a tumor specimen by reverse transcriptase-polymerase chain reaction, predict for failure to respond to an infusional 5-FU regimen. These observations are intriguing but need to be validated in large-scale prospective trials before being applied to routine practice. There is, at this time, insufficient evidence to support the routine use of these markers in standard practice.

Others have investigated genomic analysis as an indicator of response or toxicity. Although Innocenti et al. demonstrated that a particular genetic polymorphism of UGT1A1 can predict for toxicity to irinotecan (159), the routine applicability of such technology is not entirely clear (160). Although the concept of individualized treatment choices on the basis of molecularly selected approaches appears promising and would be highly desirable (161,162), most such approaches are not yet validated and should not be considered as part of standard care at this time.

DURATION OF THERAPY

The optimal duration of chemotherapy for palliation of metastatic disease has not been established. Prior to the improvements in chemotherapy options since the late 1990s, the question of duration of therapy was straightforward; therapy was necessarily of a limited duration because only one drug was available and it had only modest efficacy. Now with six or more active drugs and median survival times exceeding 2 years, the established practice of continuing chemotherapy until unacceptable toxicity, clinical deterioration, or disease progression needs to be reconsidered. In a trial in which 354 patients who were not progressing after 12 weeks of either fluorouracil- or raltitrexed-based chemotherapy where randomized to either continue chemotherapy until progression or to stop chemotherapy, followed by a planned restarting on the same chemotherapy at the time of progression, there was no evidence of a difference in the OS between the two groups, with an insignificant trend favoring the treatment break arm (163). The uninterrupted chemotherapy group has an insignificant longer time to tumor progression of 4.9 months versus 3.7 months ($P = 0.1$). Of note, 63% of patients receiving a treatment break did not restart the same chemotherapy at time of progression as planned. There was similar use of second-line chemotherapy in both arms. Serious adverse effects were lower in the group with the planned treatment break (6 vs. 17).

A critical factor to the viability of a planned treatment interruption strategy is the question of whether rechallenge after a planned interruption can reinduce a response. A pooled analysis was conducted on 613 patients involved in three randomized trials of first-line 5-FU–based therapy (164). All patients had a planned maximum treatment period of 6 months. Patients with responding or stable disease at the end of that period were observed off treatment with a plan for retreatment at the time of disease progression. Median time to rechallenge was 11.7 months. Seventeen percent of patients had an objective response to rechallenging. Median survival for the group was 14.8 months.

Planned discontinuation of therapy has also been evaluated in patients treated with irinotecan as second-line therapy (165). Patients were planned initially for 24 weeks of irinotecan therapy. Those who had not progressed by then were randomly assigned to continue or discontinue irinotecan at that time. Of the 333 patients who entered the trial, most discontinued before the end of the first 24 weeks secondary to either progression or unacceptable toxicity. In the 55 patients with responding or stable disease at 24 weeks who were randomized, PFS or OS and quality of life scores were similar in both arms.

MANAGEMENT OF SYNCHRONOUS PRIMARY AND METASTATIC DISEASE

Due to the relatively limited activity of chemotherapy that existed for CRC until recently, surgeons have favored palliative removal of the primary tumor in a patient presenting with synchronous incurable metastatic disease. More recent data, coupled with an appreciation for the activity of current chemotherapy, suggest that this practice is no longer appropriate in the majority of cases. The argument that the operation is "preparing the patient for chemotherapy" begs the question of what preparation is needed. Unless the patient has substantially active, acute bleeding from the tumor, or overt obstruction, palliative removal of the primary serves little if any purpose, and necessarily delays the start of systemic chemotherapy. Patients believed to be at acute risk for obstruction within the time period necessary to evaluate the efficacy of first-line chemotherapy may be considered for mechanical stenting using expandable endoscopically placed metal stents (166).

The complication rate from palliative bowel surgery is not trivial. Temple et al. used Surveillance, Epidemiology, and End Results medicare-linked data to determine whether surgery was performed within 90 days of diagnosis in patients presenting with synchronous metastatic disease (167). Of the 9,011 medicare-age patients with stage IV disease at presentation whose charts were reviewed, 72% were found to have undergone cancer-directed surgery with 4 months of diagnosis. Most notably, the perioperative mortality (death within 30 days of operation) was 10%, and this rose to 15% in patients older than 80 years. Among patients undergoing operation for colon cancer, 14% had a resection requiring an ostomy. For rectal cancer patients undergoing operation, 69% had resection with ostomy. Of the 28% of patients who did not undergo initial resection of the primary, only 32% ever underwent bowel surgery. Thus, removal of the primary, at least in the medicare-age population, is fraught with substantial morbidity and mortality.

Further data indicate that the risk of bowel complications after chemotherapy for patients with unresected primary CRC and synchronous metastasis is low. In a review of 10 years' experience in patients at the Royal Marsden Hospital in London, 82 patients received initial chemotherapy without surgery and 280 patients underwent surgery followed by chemotherapy. The incidences of peritonitis, fistula formation, and intestinal hemorrhage were not significantly different in the resected versus unresected patients in this nonrandomized, retrospective review (168). Intestinal obstruction occurred in 13% of both groups. Patients undergoing resection did have a lower incidence of requiring three or more blood transfusions (7.5% vs. 14.6%, $p = 0.048$), as well as lower rate of palliative abdominal radiotherapy (9.6% vs. 18.3%, $p = 0.03$).

Another single-institution experience over 12 years found that 66 patients had undergone initial resection and 23 did not. Two of the 23 patients (8.7%) who received initial surgery ultimately developed obstruction at the primary site and required diversion. None of the patients experienced tumor-related hemorrhage. It should be noted that virtually all retrospective data on the topic of palliative resection are derived from patients treated mostly in an age of single-agent fluorouracil treatments. Currently, available chemotherapy is far more active and would be expected to afford even greater local tumor control.

More recently, the issue of the risk of GI perforation has been invoked by some as justification for palliative resection of the primary before treatment of metastatic disease. This argument would not appear to be valid, as the primary colorectal tumor has rarely, if ever, been reported as the site of perforation, with most perforations occurring in the small intestines or large bowel in the absence of a residual primary. Of note, the highest rates of GI perforation have been reported in ovarian cancer patients, in whom no colorectal primary ever existed. Thus, concerns regarding bowel perforations due to bevacizumab would not seem to be relevant to the issue of palliative resection of synchronous primary disease.

References

1. Heidelberger C, Chaudhuri NK, Danneberg P, et al. Fluorinated pyrimidines: a new class of tumor inhibitory compounds. *Nature* 1957;179:663–666.
2. Bosch L, Habers E, Heidleberger C. Studies on fluorinated pyrimidines V. Effects on nucleic acid metabolism in vitro. *Cancer Res* 1958;18:335–343.
3. Sobrero A, Aschele C, Bertino JR. Fluorouracil in colorectal cancer—a tale of two drugs: implications for biochemical modulation. *J Clin Oncol* 1997;15:368–381.
4. Tanaka M, Kimura K, Yoshida S. Enhancement of the incorporation of 5-fluorodeoxyruidylate into DNA of HL-60 cells by metabolic modulations. *Cancer Res* 1983;43:5145–5150.
5. Grem JL. 5-Fluorouracil and its biomodulation in the management of colorectal cancer. In: Saltz LB, ed. *Colorectal Cancer: Multimodality Management*. Totowa, NJ: Humana Press; 2002:457–488.
6. Santi D, McHenry C, Sommer H. Mechanism of interaction of thymidylate synthetase with 5-fluorodeoxyuridylate. *Biochemistry* 1974;13:471–481.
7. Lockshin A, Danenberg PV. Biochemical factors affecting the tightness of 5-fluorodeoxyuridylate binding of human thymidylate synthetase. *Biochem Pharm* 1981;30:247–257.
8. Madajewicz S, et al. Phase I-II trial of high dose calcium leucovorin and 5-fluorouracil in advanced colorectal cancer. *Cancer Res* 1984;44:4667–4669.
9. Cunningham J, et al. 5-Fluorouracil and folinic acid: a phase I–II trial in gastrointestinal malignancy. *Invest New Drugs* 1984;2:391–395.
10. Bertrand M, et al. High dose continuous infusion folinic acid and bolus 5-fluorouracil in patients with advanced colorectal cancer: a phase II study. *J Clin Oncol* 1986;4:1058–1061.
11. Machover D, et al. Treatment of advanced colorectal and gastric carcinoma with 5-fluorouracil and high dose folinic acid. *J Clin Oncol* 1986;4:685–696.
12. Poon MA, et al. Biochemical modulation of fluorouracil: evidence of significant improvement of survival and quality of life in patients with advanced colorectal carcinoma. *J Clin Oncol* 1989;7:1407–1471.
13. Poon MA, et al. Biochemical modulation of fluorouracil with leucovorin: confirmatory evidence of improved therapeutic efficacy in advanced colorectal cancer. *J Clin Oncol* 1991;9:1967–1972.
14. Laufman L, et al. A randomized, double-blind trial of fluorouracil plus placebo versus fluorouracil plus oral leucovorin in patients with metastatic colorectal cancer. *J Clin Oncol* 1993;11(10):1888–1893.
15. Anonymous, A.C.C.M. Project. Modulation of fluorouracil by leucovorin in patients with advanced colorectal cancer: evidence in terms of response rate. Advanced Colorectal Cancer Meta-Analysis Project. *J Clin Oncol* 1992;10:896–903.
16. The Meta-Analysis Group in Cancer. Modulation of fluorouracil by leucovorin in patients with advanced colorectal cancer: an updated meta-analysis. *J Clin Oncol* 2004;22(18):3766–3775.
17. Buroker TR, et al. Randomized comparison of two schedules of fluorouracil and leucovorin in the treatment of advanced colorectal cancer. *J Clin Oncol* 1994;12:14–20.
18. Jager E, et al. Weekly high-dose leucovorin versus low-dose leucovorin combined with fluorouracil in advanced colorectal cancer: results of a randomized multicenter trial. *J Clin Oncol* 1996;14(8):2274–2279.
19. Leichman CG, et al. Phase II study of fluorouracil and its modulation in advanced colorectal cancer: a Southwest Oncology Group study. *J Clin Oncol* 1995;13:1303–1311.
20. Calbro-Jones PM, Byfield JE, Ward JF, Time–dose relationships for 5-fluorouracil cytotoxicity against human epithelial cancer cells in vitro. *Cancer Res* 1982;42:4413–4420.
21. Lokich JJ, et al. A prospective randomized comparison of continuous infusion fluorouracil with a conventional bolus schedule in metastatic colorectal carcinoma: a Mid-Atlantic Oncology Program Study. *J Clin Oncol* 1989;7:425–432.
22. O'Dwyer PJ, et al. Phase III trial of biochemical modulation of 5-fluorouracil by IV or oral leucovorin or by interferon in advanced colorectal cancer: an ECOG/CALGB phase III trial. *Proc Am Soc Clin Oncol* 1996;15:469.
23. Anonymous. Efficacy of intravenous continuous infusion of fluorouracil compared with bolus administration in advanced colorectal cancer. Meta-analysis Group in Cancer. *J Clin Oncol* 1998;16:301–308.
24. Ardalan B, et al. A phase II study of weekly 24-hour infusion with high dose fluorouracil with leucovorin in colorectal carcinoma. *J Clin Oncol* 1991;9:625–630.
25. Kohne CH, et al. Effective biomodulation by leucovorin of high-dose infusion fluorouracil given as a weekly 24-hour infusion: results of a randomized trial in patients with advanced colorectal cancer. *J Clin Oncol* 1998;16:418–426.
26. Kohne CH, et al. Randomized phase III study of high-dose fluorouracil given as a weekly 24-hour infusion with or without leucovorin versus bolus fluorouracil plus leucovorin in advanced colorectal cancer: European Organization of Research and Treatment of Cancer Gastrointestinal Group Study 40952. *J Clin Oncol* 2003;21(20):3711–3712.
27. de Gramont A, et al. Randomized trial comparing monthly low-dose leucovorin and fluorouracil bolus with bimonthly high-dose leucovorin and fluorouracil bolus plus continuous infusion for advanced colorectal cancer: a French Intergroup study. *J Clin Oncol* 1997;15:808–815.
28. Browman GB. Clinical application of the concept of methotrexate plus 5-FU sequence dependent "synergy": how good is the evidence? *Cancer Treat Rep* 1984;68:465–469.
29. Cadman E, Davis L, Heimer R. Enhanced 5-fluorouracil nucleotide formation following methotrexate: biochemical explanation for drug synergism. *Science* 1979;205:1135–1137.
30. Bertino JR, et al. Schedule-dependent antitumor effects of methotrexate and 5-fluorouracil. *Cancer Res* 1977;37:327–328.
31. Fernandes DJ, Bertino JR. Enhancement of 5-fluorodeoxyuridylate binding

to thymidylate synthase by dihydropteroylpolyglutamates. *Proc Natl Acad Sci U S A* 1980;77:5663–5667.

32. Anonymous. Meta-analysis of randomized trials testing the biochemical modulation of fluorouracil by methotrexate in metastatic colorectal cancer. *J Clin Oncol* 1994;12:960–969.

33. Grimelius B. Biochemical modulation of 5-fluorouracil: a randomized comparison of sequential methotrexate, 5-fluorouracil and leucovorin in patients with advanced symptomatic colorectal cancer. *Ann Oncol* 1993;4:235–240.

34. Romanini A, et al. Leucovorin enhances cytotoxicity of trimetrexate/fluorouracil, but not methotrexate/fluorouracil, in CCRF-CEM cells. *J Natl Cancer Inst* 2000;84:1033–1038.

35. Lin JT, Bertino JR. Update on trimetrexate, a folate antagonist with antineoplastic and antiprotozoal properties. *Cancer Invest* 1991;9:159–172.

36. Ajani JA, et al. A phase II study of trimetrexate therapy for metastatic colorectal carcinoma. *Cancer Invest* 1990;8:619–621.

37. Conti JA, et al. Trial of sequential trimetrexate, fluorouracil, and high-dose leucovorin in previously treated patients with gastrointestinal carcinoma. *J Clin Oncol* 1994;12:695–700.

38. Blanke CD, et al. Phase II study of trimetrexate, fluorouracil, and leucovorin for advanced colorectal cancer. *J Clin Oncol* 1997;15:915–920.

39. Blanke C, et al. A phase II trial of trimetrexate (TMTX), 5-fluorouracil (5-FU), and leucovorin (LCV) in patients (PTS) with previously treated unresectable or metastatic colorectal cancer (CRC) [abstract]. *Proc Am Soc Clin Oncol* 1999;18:246a.

40. Blanke CD, et al. A double-blind placebo-controlled randomized phase III trial of 5-fluorouracil and leucovorin, plus or minus trimetrexate, in previously untreated patients with advanced colorectal cancer. *Ann Oncol* 2002;13:87–91.

41. Punt CJ, et al. Integrated analysis of overall survival in two randomised studies comparing 5-fluorouracil/leucovorin with or without trimetrexate in advanced colorectal cancer. *Ann Oncol* 2002;13:92–94.

42. Wadler S, et al. Phase II trial of fluorouracil and recombinant interferon alfa-2a in patients with advanced colorectal carcinoma: an Eastern Cooperative Oncology Group Study. *J Clin Oncol* 1991;9:1806–1810.

43. Wadler S, et al. Fluorouracil and recombinant alfa-2a-interferon: An active regimen against advanced colorectal carcinoma. *J Clin Oncol* 1989;7:1769–1775.

44. Kemeny N, et al. Combination 5-fluorouracil and recombinant alpha interferon in advanced colorectal cancer: activity but significant toxicity. *Proc Am Soc Clin Oncol* 2000;9:109–114.

45. Hill M, et al. Royal Marsden phase III trial of fluorouracil with or without interferon alfa-2b in advanced colorectal cancer. *J Clin Oncol* 1995;13:1297–1302.

46. Greco FA, Figlin R, York M. Phase II randomized study to compare interferon alfa-2a in combination with fluorouracil versus fluorouracil alone in patients with advanced colorectal cancer. *J Clin Oncol* 1996;14:2674–2681.

47. Dufour P, Husseini F, Dreyfus B. 5-Fluorouracil versus 5-fluorouracil plus alpha interferon as treatment of metastatic colorectal cancer: a randomized study. *Ann Oncol* 1996;7:575–579.

48. Corfu-A SG. Phase III randomized study of two fluorouracil combinations with either interferon alfa-2a or leucovorin for advanced colorectal cancer. *J Clin Oncol* 1995;13:921–928.

49. Thirion P, et al. Alpha-interferon does not increase the efficacy of 5-fluorouracil in advanced colorectal cancer. *Br J Cancer* 2001;84:611–620.

50. Schuller J, et al. Preferential activation of capecitabine in tumor following oral administration to colorectal cancer patients. *Cancer Chemother Pharmacol* 2000;45:291–297.

51. Van Cutsem E, et al. Capecitabine, an oral fluoropyrimidine carbamate with substantial activity in advanced colorectal cancer: results of a randomized phase II study. *J Clin Oncol* 2000;18:1337–1345.

52. Van Cutsem E, et al. Oral capecitabine compared with intravenous fluorouracil plus leucovorin in patients with metastatic colorectal cancer: results of a large phase III study. *J Clin Oncol* 2001;19:4097–4106.

53. Hoff PM, et al. Comparison of oral capecitabine versus intravenous fluorouracil plus leucovorin as first-line treatment in 605 patients with metastatic colorectal cancer: results of a randomized phase III study. *J Clin Oncol* 2001;19:2282–2292.

54. Van Cutsem E, et al. Oral capecitabine vs intravenous 5-fluorouracil and leucovorin: integrated efficacy data and novel analyses from two large, randomised, phase III trials. *Br J Cancer* 2004;90:1190–1197.

55. Lassere Y, Hoff P. Management of hand foot syndrome in patients treated with capecitabine (Xeloda). *Eur J Oncol Nurs* 2004;8(suppl 1):S31–S40.

56. Cassidy J, et al. First-line oral capecitabine therapy in metastatic colorectal cancer: a favorable safety profile compared with intravenous 5-fluorouracil/leucovorin. *Ann Oncol,* 2002;13:566–575.

57. Hoff PM, et al. Phase II study of capecitabine in patients with fluorouracil-resistant metastatic colorectal carcinoma. *J Clin Oncol,* 2004;22:2078–2083.

58. Lu Z, Zhang RG, Diasio R. Dihydropyrimidine dehydrogenase activity in human liver: population characteristics and clinical implications in 5FU chemotherapy. *Clin Pharmacol* 1995;58:512–522.

59. Saltz LB, et al. A fixed-ratio combination of uracil and ftorafur (UFT) with low dose leucovorin: an active oral regimen for advanced colorectal cancer. *Cancer* 1995;75(3):782–785.

60. Pazdur R, et al. Phase II trials of uracil and tegafur plus oral leucovorin: an effective oral regimen in the treatment of metastatic colorectal cancer. *J Clin Oncol* 1994;12:2296–2300.

61. Douillard JY, et al. Multicenter phase III study of uracil/tegafur and oral leucovorin versus fluorouracil and leucovorin in patients with previously untreated metastatic colorectal cancer. *J Clin Oncol* 2002;20(17):3605–3616.

62. Carmichael J, et al. Randomized comparative study of tegafur/uracil and oral leucovorin versus parenteral fluorouracil and leucovorin in patients with previously untreated metastatic colorectal cancer. *J Clin Oncol* 2002;20(17):3617–3627.

63. Cocconi G, et al. Open, randomized, multicenter trial of raltitrexed versus fluorouracil plus high-dose leucovorin in patients with advanced colorectal cancer. Tomudex Colorectal Cancer Study Group. *J Clin Oncol* 1998;16(9):2943–2952.

64. Cunningham D, et al. Final results of a randomised trial comparing 'Tomudex' (raltitrexed) with 5-fluorouracil plus leucovorin in advanced colorectal cancer. "Tomudex" Colorectal Cancer Study Group. *Ann Oncol* 1996;7(9):961–965.

65. Cunningham D. Mature results from three large controlled studies with raltitrexed ('Tomudex'). *Br J Cancer* 1998;77(suppl 2):15–21.

66. Farrugia DC, et al. Thymidylate synthase expression in advanced colorectal cancer predicts for response to raltitrexed. *Clin Cancer Res* 2003;9(2):792–801.

67. Kawato Y, et al. Intracellular roles of SN-38, a metabolite of the camptothecin derivative CPT-11, in the antitumor effect of CPT-11. *Cancer Res* 1991;51(16):4187–4191.

68. Negoro S, et al. Phase I study of weekly intravenous infusions of CPT-11, a new derivative of camptothecin, in the treatment of advanced non-small-cell lung cancer. *J Natl Cancer Inst* 1991;83:1164–1168.

69. Ohe Y, et al. Phase I study and pharmacokinetics of CPT-11 with 5-day continuous infusion. *J Natl Cancer Inst* 1992;84(12):972–974.

70. Rothenberg ML, et al. Phase I and pharmacokinetic trial of weekly CPT-11. *J Clin Oncol* 1993;11:2194–2204.

71. Rowinsky EK, et al. Phase I and pharmacological study of the novel topoisomerase inhibitor 7-ethyl-10-[4-(1-piperidino)-1-piperidino]carbonyloxycamptothecin (CPT-11) administered as a ninety minute infusion every three weeks. *Cancer Res* 1994;54:427–436.

72. Abigerges D, et al. Phase I and pharmacologic studies of the camptothecin analogue irinotecan administered every three weeks in cancer patients. *J Clin Oncol* 1995;13:210–221.

73. Shimada Y, et al. Phase II study of CPT-11, a new camptothecin derivative, in metastatic colorectal cancer. *J Clin Oncol* 1993;11:909–913.

74. Rothenberg ML, et al. Phase II trial of Irinotecan in patients with progressive or rapidly recurrent colorectal cancer. *J Clin Oncol* 1996;14:1128–1135.

75. Von Hoff DD, et al. Irinotecan therapy for patients with previously treated metastatic colorectal cancer: overall results of FDA-reviewed pivotal U.S. clinical trials. *Proc Am Soc Clin Oncol* 1997;16:a803–a803.

76. Rougier P, et al. A phase II study of CPT-11 (irinotecan) in the treatment of advanced colorectal cancer in chemotherapy-naive patients and patients pretreated with 5-FU-based chemotherapy. *J Clin Oncol* 1997;15(2):808–815.

77. Conti JA, et al. Irinotecan is an active agent in untreated patients with metastatic colorectal cancer. *J Clin Oncol* 1996;14:709–715.

78. Pitot HC, Wender MJ, O'Connell M. A phase II trial of CPT-11 (irinotecan) in patients with metastatic colorectal carcinoma: a North Central Cancer Treatment Group (NCCTG) study. *Proc Am Soc Clin Oncol* 1994;13:a573-a573.

79. Cunningham D, et al., Randomised trial of irinotecan plus supportive care versus supportive care alone after fluorouracil failure for patients with metastatic colorectal cancer. *Lancet* 1998;352(9138):1413–1418.

80. Gandia D, et al. CPT-11 induced cholinergic effects in cancer patients. *J Clin Oncol* 1993;11:196–197.

81. Fuchs CS, et al. Phase III comparison of two irinotecan dosing regimens in second-line therapy of metastatic colorectal cancer. *J Clin Oncol* 2003;21(5):807–814.

82. Knight R, et al. Evaluation of age, gender, performance status (PS), and organ dysfunction as predictors of toxicity with first-line irinotecan (C), fluorouracil (F), leucovorin (L) therapy of metastatic colorectal cancer (MCRC). *Proc Am Soc Clin Oncol* 2001;19: abstract 534 (poster).

83. Saltz L, et al. A phase I clinical and pharmacologic trial of irinotecan, 5-fluorouracil, and leucovorin in patients with advanced solid tumors. *J Clin Oncol* 1996;14:2959–2967.

84. Saltz LB, et al. Irinotecan plus fluorouracil and leucovorin for metastatic colorectal cancer. Irinotecan Study Group. *N Engl J Med* 2000;343(13):905–914.

85. Douillard JY, et al. Irinotecan combined with fluorouracil compared with fluorouracil alone as first-line treatment for metastatic colorectal cancer: a multicentre randomised trial. *Lancet* 2000;355(9209):1041–1047.

86. Andre T, et al. CPT-11 (irinotecan) addition to bimonthly, high-dose leucovorin and bolus and continuous-infusion 5-fluorouracil (FOLFIRI) for pretreated metastatic colorectal cancer. GERCOR. *Eur J Cancer* 1999;35(9):1343–1347.

87. Burchenal JH, et al. Lack of cross-resistance between certain platinum

coordination compounds in mouse leukemia. *Cancer Res* 1977;37(9): 3455–3457.

88. Mathe G, et al. Antitumor activity of l-OHP in mice. *Cancer Lett* 1985;27(2):135–143.

89. Raymond E, et al. Activity of oxaliplatin against human tumor colony-forming units. *Clin Cancer Res* 1998;4(4):1021–1029.

90. Gibbons GR, et al. Role of carrier ligand in platinum resistance in L1210 cells. *Cancer Res* 1990;50(20):6497–6501.

91. Schmidt W, Chaney SG. Role of carrier ligand in platinum resistance of human carcinoma cell lines. *Cancer Res* 1993;53(4):799–805.

92. Scheeff ED, Briggs JM, Howell SB. Molecular modeling of the intrastrand guanine-guanine DNA adducts produced by cisplatin and oxaliplatin. *Mol Pharmacol*, 1999;56(3):633–643.

93. Extra JM, et al. Phase I study of oxaliplatin in patients with advanced cancer. *Cancer Chemother Pharmacol* 1990;25(4):299–303.

94. Raymond E, et al. Oxaliplatin: a review of preclinical and clinical studies. *Ann Oncol* 1998;9(10):1053–1071.

95. Diaz-Rubio E, et al. Oxaliplatin as single agent in previously untreated colorectal carcinoma patients: a phase II multicentric study. *Ann Oncol* 1998;9(1):105–108.

96. Becouarn Y, et al. Phase II trial of oxaliplatin as first-line chemotherapy in metastatic colorectal cancer patients. Digestive Group of French Federation of Cancer Centers. *J Clin Oncol* 1998;16(8):2739–2744.

97. Machover D, et al. Two consecutive phase II studies of oxaliplatin (L-OHP) for treatment of patients with advanced colorectal carcinoma who were resistant to previous treatment with fluoropyrimidines. *Ann Oncol* 1996;7(1):95–98.

98. Levi F, Zidani R, Misset JL. Randomised multicentre trial of chronotherapy with oxaliplatin, fluorouracil, and folinic acid in metastatic colorectal cancer. International Organization for Cancer Chronotherapy. *Lancet* 1997;350(9079):681–686.

99. Bertheault-Cvitkovic F, et al. Biweekly intensified ambulatory chronomodulated chemotherapy with oxaliplatin, fluorouracil, and leucovorin in patients with metastatic colorectal cancer. *J Clin Oncol* 1996;14(11):2950–2958.

100. Giacchetti S, et al. Phase III multicenter randomized trial of oxaliplatin added to chronomodulated fluorouracil-leucovorin as first-line treatment of metastatic colorectal cancer. *J Clin Oncol* 2000;18(1):136–147.

101. de Gramont A, et al. Leucovorin and fluorouracil with or without oxaliplatin as first-line treatment in advanced colorectal cancer. *J Clin Oncol* 2000;18(16):2938–2947.

102. Rothenberg ML, et al. Superiority of oxaliplatin and fluorouracil-leucovorin compared with either therapy alone in patients with progressive colorectal cancer after irinotecan and fluorouracil-leucovorin: interim results of a phase III trial. *J Clin Oncol* 2003;21(11):2059–2069.

103. Rothenberg ML, et al. Final results of a phase III trial of 5-FU/leucovorin versus oxaliplatin versus the combination in patients with metastatic colorectal cancer following irinotecan, 5-FU, and leucovorin [abstract]. *Proc Am Soc Clin Oncol* 2003;22:1011. Presentation in virtual meeting at http://www.asco.org/ac/1,1003,_12-002511-00_18-0023-00_19-002112,00.asphttp://www.asco.org/ac/1,1003,_12-002511-00_18-0023-00_19-002112,00.asp.

104. Maindrault-Goebel F, et al. Oxaliplatin added to the simplified bimonthly leucovorin and 5- fluorouracil regimen as second-line therapy for metastatic colorectal cancer (FOLFOX6). GERCOR 4. *Eur J Cancer* 1999;35(9):1338–1342.

105. de Gramont A, et al. OPTIMOX study: FOLFOX 7/LV5FU2 compared to FOLFOX 4 in patients with advanced colorectal cancer [abstract]. *Proc Am Soc Clin Oncol* 2004;22:3525. Virtual meeting at http://www.asco.org/ac/1,1003,_12-002511-00_18-0026-00_19-0010171,00.asphttp://www.asco.org/ac/1,1003,_12-002511-00_18-0026-00_19-0010171,00.asp.

106. Hochster H, et al. Oxaliplatin with weekly bolus fluorouracil and low-dose leucovorin as first-line therapy for patients with colorectal cancer. *J Clin Oncol* 2003;21(14):2703–2707.

107. Hochster H, et al. Safety and efficacy of bevacizumab (Bev) when added to oxaliplatin/fluoropyrimidine (O/F) regimens as first-line treatment of metastatic colorectal cancer (mCRC): TREE 1 & 2 studies [abstract]. *Proc Am Soc Clin Oncol* 2005;23:3515. Presentation at http://www.asco.org/ac/1,1003,_12-002511-00_18-0034-00_19-003814,00.asphttp://www.asco.org/ac/1,1003,_12-002511-00_18-0034-00_19-003814,00.asp.

108. Goldberg RM, et al. A randomized controlled trial of fluorouracil plus leucovorin, irinotecan, and oxaliplatin combinations in patients with previously untreated metastatic colorectal cancer. *J Clin Oncol* 2004;22(1):23–30.

109. Tournigand C, et al. FOLFIRI followed by FOLFOX6 or the reverse sequence in advanced colorectal cancer: a randomized GERCOR study. *J Clin Oncol* 2004;22(2):229–237.

110. Colucci G, et al. Phase III randomized trial of FOLFIRI vs FOLFOX4 in the treatment of advanced colorectal cancer: a multicenter study of the Grupo Oncologico Italia Meridionale. *J Clin Oncol* 2005;23(22):4866–4875.

111. Kalofonos HP, et al. Irinotecan or oxaliplatin combined with leucovorin and 5-flourouracil as first-line treatment in advanced colorectal cancer: a multicenter, randomized, phase II study. *Ann Oncol* 2005;16:869–877.

112. Comella P, et al. Oxaliplatin plus high-dose folinic acid and 5-fluorouracil i.v. bolus (OXAFAFU) versus irinotecan plus high dose folinic acid and 5-fluorouracil i.v. bolus (IRIFAFU) in patients with metastatic colorectal carcinoma: a Southern Italy Cooperative Oncology Group Trial. *Ann Oncol* 2005;16:878–886.

113. Souglakos J, et al. Triplet combination with irinotecan plus oxaliplatin plus continuous-infusion fluorouracil and leucovorin as first-line treatment in metastatic colorectal cancer: a multicenter phase II trial. *J Clin Oncol* 2002;20(11):2651–2657.

114. Falcone A, et al. Biweekly chemotherapy with oxaliplatin, irinotecan, infusional Fluorouracil, and leucovorin: a pilot study in patients with metastatic colorectal cancer. *J Clin Oncol* 2002;20(19):4006–4014.

115. Falcone A, Masi G, Murr R, et al. Biweekly irinotecan, oxaliplatin, and infusional 5FU/LV (FOLFOXIRI) versus FOLFIRI as first-line treatment of metastatic colorectal cancer (MCRC): results of a randomized, phase III trial by the Gruppo Oncologico Nord Ovest (GONO). 2006 Gastrointestinal Cancers Symposium; 2006; San Francisco, Calif.

116. Borner MM, et al. Phase II study of capecitabine and oxaliplatin in first- and second-line treatment of advanced or metastatic colorectal cancer. *J Clin Oncol* 2002;20(7):1759–1766.

117. Cassidy J, et al. XELOX (capecitabine plus oxaliplatin): active first-line therapy for patients with metastatic colorectal cancer. *J Clin Oncol* 2004;22(11):2084–2091.

118. Scheithauer W, et al. Randomized multicenter phase II trial of two different schedules of capecitabine plus oxaliplatin as first-line treatment in advanced colorectal cancer. *J Clin Oncol* 2003;21(7):1307–1312.

119. Arkenau H, et al. Infusional 5-fluorouracil/folinic acid plus oxaliplatin (FU-FOX) versus capecitabine plus oxaliplatin (CAPOX) as first line treatment of metastatic colorectal cancer (MCRC): results of the safety and efficacy analysis [abstract]. *Proc Am Soc Clin Oncol* 2005;23:3507. Virtual meeting presentation at http://www.asco.org/ac/1,1003,_12-002511-00_18-0034-00_19-002233-00_28-004,00.asphttp://www.asco.org/ac/1,1003,_12-002511-00_18-0034-00_19-002233-00_28-004,00.asp.

120. Seymour MT. Fluorouracil, oxaliplatin and CPT-11 (irinotecan), use and sequencing (MRC FOCUS): a 2135-patient randomized trial in advanced colorectal cancer (ACRC) [abstract]. *Proc Am Soc Clin Oncol* 2005;23:3518. Virtual meeting presentation at http://www.asco.org/ac/1,1003,_12-002511-00_18-0034-00_19-001999,00.asphttp://www.asco.org/ac/1,1003,_12-002511-00_18-0034-00_19-001999,00.asp.

121. Ferrara N, et al. Discovery and development of bevacizumab, an anti-VEGF antibody for treating cancer. *Nat Rev Drug Discov* 2004;3(5):391–400.

122. Ferrara N. Vascular endothelial growth factor: basic science and clinical progress. *Endocr Rev* 2004;25(4):581–611.

123. Kabbinavar F, et al. Phase II, randomized trial comparing bevacizumab plus fluorouracil (FU)/leucovorin (LV) with FU/LV alone in patients with metastatic colorectal cancer. *J Clin Oncol* 2003;21(1):60–65.

124. Hurwitz H, et al. Bevacizumab plus irinotecan, fluorouracil, and leucovorin for metastatic colorectal cancer. *N Engl J Med* 2004;350(23):2335–2342.

125. Kabbinavar FF, et al. Addition of bevacizumab to bolus fluorouracil and leucovorin in first-line metastatic colorectal cancer: results of a randomized phase II trial. *J Clin Oncol* 2005;23(16):3697–3705.

126. Kabbinavar FF, et al. Combined analysis of efficacy: the addition of bevacizumab to fluorouracil/leucovorin improves survival for patients with metastatic colorectal cancer. *J Clin Oncol* 2005;23(16):3706–3712.

127. Giantonio B, Levy DE, O'Dwyer P. Bevacizumab (anti-VEGF) plus IFL (irinotecan, fluorouracil, leucovorin) as front-line therapy for advanced colorectal cancer (advCRC): updated results from the Eastern Cooperative Oncology Group (ECOG) Study E2200. ASCO GI Symposium; 2004; San Francisco, Calif.

128. Sparano JA, et al. Evaluating antiangiogenesis agents in the clinic: the Eastern Cooperative Oncology Group Portfolio of Clinical Trials. *Clin Cancer Res* 2004;10(4):1206–1211.

129. Giantonio BJ, et al. High-dose bevacizumab improves survival when combined with FOLFOX4 in previously treated advanced colorectal cancer: Results from the Eastern Cooperative Oncology Group (ECOG) study E3200 [abstract]. *Proc Am Soc Clin Oncol* 2005;23:1s Abstract 2. Virtual meeting at http://www.asco.org/ac/1,1003,_12-002511-00_18-0034-00_19-004925,00.asphttp://www.asco.org/ac/1,1003,_12-002511-00_18-0034-00_19-004925,00.asp.

130. Skillings JA, et al. Arterial thromboembolic events (ATEs) in a pooled analysis of 5 randomized, controlled trials (RCTs) of bevacizumab (BV) with chemotherapy. *Proc Am Soc Clin Oncol* 2005.

131. Carpenter G, Cohen S. Epidermal growth factor. *J Biol Chem* 1990;265(14):7709–7712.

132. Real FX, et al. Expression of epidermal growth factor receptor in human cultured cells and tissues: relationship to cell lineage and stage of differentiation. *Cancer Res* 1986;46(9):4726–4731.

133. Ciardiello F, Tortora G. A novel approach in the treatment of cancer: targeting the epidermal growth factor receptor. *Clin Cancer Res* 2001;7(10):2958–2970.

134. Thomas SM, Grandis JR. Pharmacokinetic and pharmacodynamic properties of EGFR inhibitors under clinical investigation. *Cancer Treat Rev* 2004;30(3):255–268.

135. Saltz L, et al. Cetuximab (IMC-C225) plus irinotecan (CPT-11) is active in CPT-11-refractory colorectal cancer (CRC) that expresses epidermal

growth factor receptor (EGFR) [abstract]. *Proc Am Soc Clin Oncol* 2001;20:abstract 7.

136. Saltz LB, et al. Phase II trial of cetuximab in patients with refractory colorectal cancer that expresses the epidermal growth factor receptor. *J Clin Oncol* 2004;22(7):1201–1208.

137. Cunningham D, et al. Cetuximab monotherapy and cetuximab plus irinotecan in irinotecan-refractory metastatic colorectal cancer. *N Engl J Med* 2004;351(4):337–345.

138. Rosenberg AH, et al. Erbitux (IMC-C225) plus weekly irinotecan (CPT-11), fluorouracil (5FU) and leucovorin (LV) in colorectal cancer (CRC) that expresses the epidermal growth factor receptor (EGFr). Presented at the American Society of Clinical Oncology; 2002; Orlando, Fla.

139. Van Laethem JL., et al., Cetuximab (C225) in combination with bi-weekly irinotecan (CPT-11), infusional 5-fluorouracil (5-FU) and folinic acid (FA) in patients (pts) with metastatic colorectal cancer (CRC) expressing the epidermal growth factor receptor (EGFR): preliminary safety and efficacy results. *Proc Am Soc Clin Oncol* 2003;22.

140. Rougier P, Mayer RJ, Van Laethem J. Cetuximab + FOLFIRI as first-line treatment for metastatic colorectal CA. Presented at ASCO; 2004; Orlando, Fla.

141. Cervantes A, et al. Cetuximab plus oxaliplatin/5-fluorouracil (5-FU)/folinic acid (FA) (FOLFOX-4) for the epidermal growth factor receptor (EGFR)-expressing metastatic colorectal cancer (mCRC) in the first-line setting: a phase II study [abstract 642]. *Eur J Cancer Suppl* 2005;3(2):81.

142. Hohler T. Phase I/II study of cetuximab combined with 5-fluorouracil/leucovorin plus weekly oxaliplatin in first-line treatment of epidermal growth factor receptor-expressing metastatic colorectal cancer. Presented at European Society of Medical Oncology Congress; 2004; Vienna, Austria.

143. Cunningham D, HY, Siena S, et al. Cetuximab monotherapy and cetuximab plus irinotecan in irinotecan-refractory metastatic colorectal cancer. *N Engl J Med* 2004;351(4):337–345.

144. Lenz HJ, M.R., Gold PJ, et al. Activity of cetuximab in patients with colorectal cancer refractory to both irinotecan and oxaliplatin. Proceedings of the American Society of Clinical Oncology; 2004; New Orleans, La.

145. Chung KY, Shia J, Kemeny NE, et al. Cetuximab shows activity in colorectal cancer patients with tumors that do not express the epidermal growth factor receptor by immunohistochemistry. *J Clin Oncol* 2005;23:1803–1810.

146. Saltz LL, Kindler H. Interim report of randomized phase II trial of cetuximab/bevacizumab/irinotecan (CBI) versus cetuximab/irinotecan (CB) in irinotecan-refractory colorectal cancer. Presented at the ASCO GI Symposium; 2005; Hollywood, Fla.

147. Hecht J, Patnaik A, Malik I. ABX-EGF monotherapy in patients (pts) with metastatic colorectal cancer (mCRC): an updated analysis. *J Clin Oncol* 2004;22(14S):3511.

148. Peeters M, Van Cutsem E, Siena S, et al. A phase 3, multicenter, randomized controlled trial (RCT) of panitumumab plus best supportive care (BSC) vs BSC alone in patients (pts) with metastatic colorectal cancer (mCRC). Presented at American Association of Cancer Research; 2006; Washington, DC.

149. Vanhoefer U, et al. Phase I study of the humanized antiepidermal growth factor receptor monoclonal antibody EMD72000 in patients with advanced solid tumors that express the epidermal growth factor receptor. *J Clin Oncol* 2004;22(1):175–184.

150. Dorligschaw O, KT, Jordan K. ZD1839 (Iressa)-based treatment as last-line therapy in patients with advanced colorectal cancer (ACRC). Presented at ASCO; 2003.

151. Oza A, Townsley CA, Siu L. Phase II study of erlotinib(OSI-774) in patients with metastatic colorectal cancer. Presented at ASCO; 2003.

152. Keilholz U, et al. Erlotinib as 2nd and 3rd line monotherapy in patients with metastatic colorectal cancer: results of a multicenter two-cohort phase II trial [abstract]. *Proc Am Soc Clin Oncol* 2005;23:3575. Virtual meeting presentation at http://www.asco.org/ac/1,1003,_12-002511-00_18-0034-00_19-004880-00_28-002,00.asphttp://www.asco.org/ac/1,1003,_12-002511-00_18-0034-00_19-004880-00_28-002,00.asp.

153. Cho C, Fisher GA, Halsey J. A phase II study of gefitinib in combination with FOLFOX-4(IFOX) in patients with unresectable or metastatic colorectal cancer. Presented at ASCO; 2003.

154. Blanke CD. Celecoxib with chemotherapy in colorectal cancer. *Oncology (Huntingt)* 2002;16(4 suppl 3):17–21.

155. Menon AG, et al. Gene therapy strategies for colorectal cancer. In: Saltz LB, ed. *Colorectal Cancer: Multimodality Management*. Totowa, NJ: Humana Press; 2002:811–836.

156. Leichman CG, et al. Quantitation of intratumoral thymidylate synthase expression predicted for disseminated colorectal Cancer Response and resistance to protracted infusion 5-fluorouracil and weekly leucovorin. *J Clin Oncol* 1997;15:3223–3229.

157. Salonga D, et al. Colorectal tumors responding to 5-fluorouracil have low gene expression levels of dihydropyrimidine dehydrogenase, thymidylate synthase, and thymidine phosphorylase. *Clin Cancer Res* 2000;6(4):1322–1327.

158. Metzger R, et al. High basal level gene expression of thymidine phosphorylase (platelet-derived endothelial cell growth factor) in colorectal tumors is associated with nonresponse to 5-fluorouracil. *Clin Cancer Res* 1998;4(10):2371–2376.

159. Innocenti F, et al. Genetic variants in the UDP-glucuronosyltransferase 1A1 gene predict the risk of severe neutropenia of irinotecan. *J Clin Oncol* 2004;22(8):1382–1388.

160. McLeod HL, Watters J. Irinotecan pharmacogenetics: is it time to intervene? *J Clin Oncol* 2004:22(8):1356–1359.

161. McLeod HL. Individualized cancer therapy: molecular approaches to the prediction of tumor response. *Expert Rev Anticancer Ther* 2002;2(1):113–119.

162. Iqbal S, Lenz HJ. Targeted therapy and pharmacogenomic programs. *Cancer* 2003;97(8 suppl):2076–2082.

163. Maughan TS, et al. Comparison of intermittent and continuous palliative chemotherapy for advanced colorectal cancer: a multicentre randomised trial. *Lancet* 2003;361(9356):457–464.

164. Yeoh C, et al. Impact of 5-fluorouracil rechallenge on subsequent response and survival in advanced colorectal cancer: pooled analysis from three consecutive randomized controlled trials. *Clin Colorectal Cancer* 2003;3(2):102–107.

165. Lal R, et al. A randomized trial comparing defined-duration with continuous irinotecan until disease progression in fluoropyrimidine and thymidylate synthase inhibitor—resistant advanced colorectal cancer. *J Clin Oncol* 2004;22:3023–3031.

166. Baron TH. Expandable metal stents for the treatment of cancerous obstruction of the gastrointestinal tract. *N Engl J Med* 2001;344(22):1681–1687.

167. Temple LKF, et al. Use of surgery among elderly patients with stage IV colorectal cancer. *J Clin Oncol* 2004;22:3475–3484.

168. Tebbutt NC, et al. Intestinal complications after chemotherapy for patients with unresected primary colorectal cancer and synchronous metastases. *Gut* 2003;52(4):568–573.

169. Grothey A, et al. Phase III study of bolus 5-fluorouracil (5-FU)/folinic acid (FA) (Mayo) vs weekly high-dose 24h 5-FU infusion/FA + oxaliplatin (OXA) (FUFOX) in advanced colorectal cancer (ACRC). Presented at the American Society of Clinical Oncology Annual Meeting; 2002; Orlando, Fla.

CHAPTER 46 ■ COLORECTAL CANCER: SURGERY AND LOCAL ABLATION OF LIVER METASTESES

PHILIPPE TALEB AND BERNARD NORDLINGER

INTRODUCTION

The most frequent cause of death in patients with colorectal cancer (CRC) is liver metastases, which concern 20% of patients with stage II and 50% with stage III colon cancer. However, the presence of liver or lung metastases from CRC does not preclude curative treatment. If only a minority of patients with liver metastases is amenable to surgery, surgical resection remains the only treatment that can, to date, ensure longterm survival and cure in some patients. Recent progress, including new chemotherapeutic regimens, ablative techniques, and interventional radiology, may increase the number of patients that can be treated with a curative intent. Unfortunately, recurrences are still observed in most patients after resection of liver metastases. To reduce this risk, new therapeutic managements are tested using adjuvant intravenous and/or intraarterial chemotherapies, or curative treatments are provided, in the event of recurrence with either surgery or local ablative techniques.

RESECTION OF LIVER METASTASES: UPDATE

Without any treatment, the median survival of patients with CRC liver metastases rarely exceeds 1 year. In a large prospective study conducted from 1980 to 1990 and including 484 patients with untreated hepatic metastases from CRC, the median survival was 31% at 1 year, 7.9% at 2 years, 2.6% at 3 years, and 0.9% at 4 years. The volume of liver involvement, presence of extrahepatic disease, metastatic lymph nodes in the mesentery, carcinoembryonic antigen (CEA) level, and age of the patient all influenced the survival rate. Depending on the presence or absence of these criteria, median survival varied from 3.8 to 21 months (1). In the absence of any randomized trial, few retrospective studies have compared the survival of patients with potentially resectable metastases that were left untreated with survival of patients after resection of colorectal metastases (2,3). There were no 5-year survivors in untreated patients, whereas 25% to 30% of patients survived 5 years after complete resection of metastases. The benefit of surgical resection for liver metastases is now well recognized, and complete resection with intent to cure is, to date, the only treatment that can ensure a long-term survival. Liver transplantation has been abandoned for this indication because immunosuppression has been associated with relapse of cancer in all patients (4).

Preoperative Assessment

The decision to perform surgical resection for liver metastases and the extent of resection are based on the patient's condition, extent of the disease, and liver function. Surgery should be considered only with curative intent if liver metastases can be totally resected with tumorfree margins and sufficient postoperative remnant liver to avoid liver failure. Patients must not have nonresectable extrahepatic disease. The goals of preoperative assessment are to determine whether the patient's condition will permit hepatic resection (i.e., general anaesthesia, clamping maneuvers requiring a correct cardiovascular status). It should exclude the presence of nonresectable extrahepatic disease and delineate the anatomy of metastases. If remnant parenchyma is normal, 75% of the volume of the liver can be resected. However, many patients receive preoperative chemotherapy, which may alter liver parenchyma. Liver function can be assessed by the Child-Pugh classification, hepatic biochemical blood tests, and, in some cases, indocyanine green retention tests. The volume of the nontumorous parenchyma that will be left in place after hepatic resection should be evaluated by computed tomography (CT) scan volumetry.

Surgical Treatment

Intraoperative Assessment

The exact place of laparoscopy in liver surgery is not clearly determined (5). Surgery should begin with a careful exploration of the abdominal cavity to rule out peritoneal carcinosis or an unexpected bilobar involvement of the liver by metastases, which could be a contraindication for resection. The presence of metastatic lymph nodes in the porta hepatis and the coeliac region considerably worsens the prognosis but should not be considered as an absolute contraindication to resection if they can be completely removed because 5-year recurrencefree surviving patients have been reported in such cases (6). Intraoperative ultrasound (IOUS) should be performed in every case because it allows a precise mapping of the anatomical relations of the metastases to the main intraparenchymatous vascular pedicles and helps select the type of resection. IOUS can detect small intraparenchymatous lesions and thereby modify the extent of the initially planned operation (7). It may also be used to guide the fine-needle biopsy of doubtful lesions or to evaluate the degree of destruction of a metastasis treated by radiofrequency (RF) ablation.

Types of Liver Resection

If remnant liver parenchyma is normal, up to six of the eight anatomical segments can be resected without inducing postoperative liver failure. Liver resections can be divided in two groups: (a) anatomical resections removing one or several segments, and (b) atypical or wedge resections removing a portion of liver parenchyma surrounding a hepatic lesion. Resections removing three or more continuous segments are defined as major hepatic resections: right hepatectomy (segments V, VI, VII, and VIII); left hepatectomy (segments II, III, and IV); and extended right hepatectomy, also called right lobectomy (segments IV, V, VI, VII, and VIII) (8,9).

Surgical Strategy

The aim of carcinologic surgery for liver metastases is to remove or destroy with ablation procedures all metastatic sites with a free clearance margin. The type of liver resection depends on the size, number, and location of the metastases; their relation to the main vascular and biliary pedicles; and the volume of the liver parenchyma that can be left in place after surgery. Superficial small metastases can be resected with wedge resections. Larger lesions often require major resections. It should also be kept in mind that a large resection may preclude further surgery in the case of intrahepatic recurrence.

If synchronous metastases are discovered at the same time as the primary cancer, it is usually preferable to perform the bowel resection during a first procedure because combined resection of both primary and liver metastases is associated with an increased mortality and morbidity rate (intra-abdominal fluid infection, vascular clamping deleterious for the viability of digestive sutures) when hepatic resection is a major resection (6). Usually, surgical resection of the liver metastases is delayed for 2 to 4 months after bowel resection, allowing observation of the response of liver metastases to systemic chemotherapy, which is often administered during the interval, and constituting an important prognostic factor.

Results of Liver Resection for Colorectal Metastases

Complications of Surgery

In most recent studies, in-hospital mortality rates vary from 0% to 5% and are strongly influenced by perioperative blood loss, preoperative liver function, and extent of liver resection (Table 46.1). Reversible postoperative complications are ob-

served in 25% to 40% of patients. Morbidity after hepatic resection is usually due to transient liver failure, hemorrhage, subphrenic abcesses, or biliary fistula. The mean hospital stay after liver surgery ranges from 10 to 15 days in the absence of complications.

Long-Term Results

Liver resection of colorectal metastases is associated with 3- and 5-year survival rates close to 40% and 30%, respectively (Table 46.2). After resection, recurrences are observed in two-thirds of patients and involve the liver in 50% of cases. In a large retrospective survey, 5-year survival was 28% in 1,568 patients who had a resection of isolated colorectal liver metastases and 15% in 250 patients who had resected liver and extrahepatic metastases. None of the 77 patients who had a palliative resection survived for 5 years (18).

Several studies have assessed factors influencing survival. Gender and the site of the primary tumor do not seem to influence the outcome. The stage of the primary tumor is associated with 5-year survival rate of 70% in stage I or II CRCs and 33% in stage III (6). Prognosis seems better in cases of metachronous metastases and small lesions, and when there are less than four lesions but the involvement of one or both lobes does not influence the outcome. CEA level is strongly correlated to the recurrencefree survival. A free margin of ≥ 1 cm offers better chances of avoiding recurrence, but several series have shown that a smaller margin did not affect survival (19). The type of resection does not seem to influence the prognosis provided that a clear margin is obtained. Blood transfusions could be associated with an adverse outcome but may reflect the surgical difficulties for the resection of large and numerous lesions. In large retrospective series of 1,568 patients with resected liver metastases from carcinoma, a multivariate analysis showed that age, size of the largest metastasis, CEA level, stage of the primary tumor, diseasefree interval, number of liver nodules, and resection margin >1 cm or <1 cm were only independent prognosis factors (18).

Control of Extrahepatic Metastatic Sites

Preoperative chest radiograph combined with a CT scan is performed to detect lung metastases. Synchronous liver and lung metastases should not be considered a contraindication to hepatic resection, provided that both sites can be completely resected. The carcinologic principle for resection of lung metastases is similar to that for liver metastases. The primary tumor should have been totally resected with no evidence of local recurrence or other unresectable metastases. In one study, 239

TABLE 46.1

MORTALITY AND MORBIDITY RATES AFTER LIVER RESECTION FOR COLORECTAL LIVER METASTASES

Reference	Year	Patients (*n*)	Mortality (%)	Morbidity (%)
Nordlinger et al. (10)	1987	80	5	13
Doci et al. (11)	1991	100	5	39
AFC[a] (12)	1997	1,818	2	24
Sheele et al. (13)	1995	469	4	—
Jamison et al. (14)	1997	280	4	—
Fong et al. (15)	1999	1,001	3	—
Minagawa et al. (16)	2000	235	0	—

[a]AFC, Association Française de Chirurgie.

TABLE 46.2

OVERALL SURVIVAL AFTER SURGICAL RESECTION OF LIVER METASTASES
FROM COLORECTAL CANCER

Reference	Year	Patients (n)	Survival 3 Year (%)	5-Year (%)
Nordlinger et al. (10)	1987	80	40	25
AFC[a] (12)	1997	1,818	41	26
Gayowski et al. (17)	1994	204	—	32
Sheele et al. (13)	1995	469	41	33
Nordlinger et al. (18)	1996	1,569	41	26
Jamison et al. (14)	1997	280	—	27
Fong et al. (15)	1999	1,001	57	37
Minagawa et al. (16)	2000	235	51	38

[a]AFC, Association Française de Chirurgie.

patients were operated on for lung metastases of CRC, 43 (18%) had previously had synchronous liver metastases surgically resected. Seven patients (16%) underwent subsequent lung resection for recurrences, and the median survival from lung resection was 19 months (20). Similar results were reported by the Metastatic Lung Tumour Study Group of Japan, with 47 patients who underwent pulmonary and hepatic resection with 3-, 5-, and 8-year survivals of 36%, 31%, and 23%, respectively (21). Surgical resection of lung metastases can significantly prolong survival. Prognostic factors are similar to those associated with resection of liver metastases; age, gender, and type of resection have not not been shown to have an impact on survival. After resection of lung metastases, the lung is the first site of recurrence in 50% to 70% of cases, followed by locoregional recurrences at the site of the primary metastasis, and brain and liver metastases. Repeat lung resections can be considered in some cases because 5-year actuarial survival rates of 30% have been reported (22). Exploration of other sites of possible metastasis, such as brain by CT scan or bone by scintigraphy, is performed only if there is a clinical suspicion. Their presence is a contraindication to liver or lung resection because the prognosis depends on the evolution of these unresectable metastases.

Repeat Liver Resections for Recurrent Metastases

Recurrence limited to the liver following previous hepatic resection occurs in 25% to 50% of cases and may be amenable to repeat resection (23,24). Postoperative mortality and morbidity do not differ from those reported after a first resection, and mean survival approaches 2 years. In a recent series including 146 patients with intrahepatic recurrence following hepatectomy treated by repeat liver resection, the actuarial survival rates were 78% at 1 year, 30% at 3 years, and 16% at 5 and 10 years, comparable to that observed following primary liver resections (23). Hepatic recurrences should therefore be resected whenever technically feasible.

PROGRESS IN SURGERY OF LIVER METASTASES

Only 10% to 20% of patients with liver metastases fulfill standard selection criteria for direct resection. The trend is to be more aggressive and to increase the indications for surgical resection. Portal vein embolization, ablative techniques, and chemotherapy may be available to surgery patients who would have been considered unresectable some years ago.

Portal Vein Embolization

If the future remnant liver after liver resection is too small to provide sufficient postoperative liver function, preoperative selective portal vein embolization has been proposed to induce ipsilateral atrophy and controlateral hypertrophy of the remnant liver, thus preventing postoperative liver failure (25). In patients with noncirrhotic livers, preoperative portal vein embolization can be expected to induce a 40% to 60% increase in the size of the nonembolized portion. However, if liver metastases are present in the nonembolized portion of the liver, induced liver regeneration or hypertrophy is associated with an accelerated increase in the size of metastases (26). Following embolization, a liver resection judged primarily impossible, due to unsufficient volume of remnant liver, is feasible in 60% of cases, with mortality and morbidity rates comparable to those observed following liver resections without embolization. In a recent study, actuarial survival rates after hepatectomy with (n = 19) or without (n = 88) portal vein embolization were comparable: 81%, 67%, and 40% versus 88%, 61%, and 38% at 1, 3, and 5, years, respectively (25).

Chemotherapy

Systemic chemotherapy is used when liver metastases are not amenable to surgical resection. Clinical trials have shown that palliative chemotherapy is better for quality of life than symptomatic treatment alone, if administred before symptoms occur. Associations of 5-fluorouracil (5-FU) and folinic acid are associated with a tumor response rate close to 20% of cases. When associated with new drugs, such as oxaliplatin or CPT-11, response rates approach 50% (27). With active chemotherapy regimens (irinotecan or oxaliplatine + 5-FU/leucoverin) alone, survival rate is <5% at 5 years.

A phase III randomized trial evaluating the benefit of an antiangiogenic agent (bevacizumab) combined with chemotherapy using irinotecan shows that the rate of overall survival, progressionfree survival, and tumor response were improved in the combination therapy goup. The addition of antiangiogenic agents to chemotherapy is a new standard for the treatment of unresectable metastatic CRC (28).

Neoadjuvant Chemotherapy

After shrinkage of the tumors, neoadjuvant chemotherapy can be used to downstage previously unresectable metastases. Large lesions may also become accessible to ablative techniques, which are known to allow safe destruction of liver up to 3 to 5 cm in diameter, or resection. In one study, systemic chemotherapy permitted surgical resection of liver metastases in 16% of patients previously considered nonresectable because of the location, size, number of hepatic deposits, or association with extrahepatic disease. The cumulative 3- and 5-year survival rates were comparable to those observed after resection of resectable lesions (29).

New studies suggest the importance of neoadjuvant chemotherapy (30). The outcomes of patients referred for resection of synchronous colorectal liver metastases with or without previous neodjuvant chemotherapy were compared. Patient- and tumor-related variables were similar in both groups. Five-year survival was similar in both group (43% vs. 35%, $p = 0.4$), but the subgroup of patients with stable disease or disease responding to chemotherapy had a better survival when compared to patients who did not receive chemotherapy (85% vs. 35%, $p = 0.03$) (22).

In a retrospective analysis evaluating the outcome of patients with multiple bilobar hepatic metastases from CRC who had received or not received neoadjuvant chemotherapy before hepatectomy, patients with neoadjuvant chemotherapy had a better 3- and 5-year survival, 67% and 38.9% versus 51.8% and 20.7% (31).

Finally, a retrospective study suggests that tumor progression while on chemotherapy could be considered as a contraindication for liver resection for multiple metastases. A total of 131 patients who underwent liver resection for multiple metastases after systemic neoaduvant chemotherapy (5-FU, leucovorin, oxaliplatin, or irinotecan) were divided into three groups according to response to chemotherapy: patients with an objective response, patients with tumor stabilization, and patients with tumor progression. All patients had a liver resection with intent to cure. Patients with a tumor progression had a lower 5-year survival compared with those with objective response and stabilization (8% vs. 37% and 30%) (32). Response to neoadjuvant chemotherapy appears to be an important prognostic factor for survival of patients after resection of liver colorectal metastases.

The clear distinction between resectable and unresectable liver metastases is becoming obsolete with the emergence of new groups of patients: patients whose metastases become resectable after response to chemotherapy. In addition, patients with progression during chemotherapy may not be good candidates for liver resection.

Adjuvant Chemotherapy

Unfortunately, recurrences are still observed in many patients after resection of liver metastases despite progress in surgical technique and improved surgical skill. One way to reduce the risk of recurrence would be to improve selection of patients in whom surgery is considered. In this setting, simple prognostic scoring systems have been developed to evaluate the chances to cure patients after resection of liver metastases (15,18).

If these prognosis scoring systems are useful for the stratification of patients in randomized series, they should not be used to exclude candidates for surgical resection. Indeed, even in patients with a high risk of recurrence, no existing treatment other than surgery can result in long-time survivals, and the trend is to be more aggressive and to increase the indications for surgical resection of liver metastases.

The benefit of adjuvant chemotherapy after resection of colorectal metastases has not yet been clearly proven. Some studies have been published, mainly testing hepatic arterial infusion (HAI) of the drugs. HAI delivers high concentrations of cytotoxic drugs directly to malignant tissue. The technique is based on the understanding that metastases derive their blood supply largely from the hepatic artery, whereas healthy hepatocytes are supplied mainly by the portal vein. Intra-arterial therapy may result in a significant increase of exposure of tumor to the drug with reduced systemic side effects. HAI also has limitations, including the risks of extrahepatic progression, severe side effects such as biliary toxicity, and technical problems precluding the use of the intrahepatic catheter. Results from three randomized trials, which evaluated the potential benefit of hepatic arterial infusion as adjuvant treatment after resection of colorectal liver metastases, are available. A German multicenter trial failed to demonstrate any survival benefit of HAI with 5-FU and folinic acid without systemic treatment over surgery alone, with a significant toxicity in the patients receiving chemotherapy and an increased risk of death (33). A study from the Memorial Sloan-Kettering Cancer Center compared HAI + systemic 5-FU and folinic acid to systemic 5-FU and folinic acid only and concluded that combined treatment resulted in a decrease in the hepatic recurrence rate and an improved overall survival only at 2 years (86% vs. 72%, $P = 0.03$) (34). Another study, organized by the Eastern Cooperative Oncology Group, evaluated HAI with floxuridine and intravenous continuous infusion of 5-FU and concluded that HAI combined with intravenous 5-FU reduced the risk of recurrence when compared with surgery alone (46% vs. 25%, $P = 0.03$) but resulted in no benefit in overall survival (35). The message we can deduce from these studies is that HAI alone is not sufficient as adjuvant treatment for liver metastases. HAI associated with systemic chemotherapy can reduce the risk of recurrences after surgery at the expense of an increase in side effects. These studies are not sufficient to convince physicians that HAI administered after surgery should be the standard, but they do constitute an important step toward the validation of the principle of combined chemotherapy and surgery to treat liver metastases from CRCs.

Adjuvant systemic chemotherapy following hepatic resection has been evaluated in two phase III randomized trials. A French study organized by the Federation Francophone de Cancerologie Digestive and a European-Canadian study have compared systemic administration of 5-FU and folinic acid for 6 months after surgery versus surgery alone. Although there was no statistically significant difference between the groups, these studies show a trend toward a benefit for adjuvant chemotherapy (36,37). A meta-analysis of the two studies is in preparation. These regimens have some side effects with grade 3/4 toxicity in about one-fourth of the patients (neutropenia, thrombocytopenia, stomatitis, vomiting, diarrhea). Chemotherapeutic regimens are being investigated in phase III randomized trials, in particular, a combination of irinotecan and 5-FU/FA, following complete resection of hepatic metastases.

The beneficial effect of chemotherapy after complete surgical resection of colorectal metastases is likely but is not yet formally proven, and several questions remain unanswered. For example: Should the chemotherapy be administered intravenously or through the hepatic artery? Should it be given before surgery, after surgery, or both? Should the best regimen include oxaliplatin, irinotecan, or biological agents? Therefore, it is urgent that medical oncologists and surgeons participate in large prospective trials evaluating new regimens and new treatment modalities feasible in most institutions. Because of the difficulty in organizing such trials, it is likely that only multicenter trials, possibly with international cooperation, will help solve these questions. An international intergroup study organized by the European Organisation for Research and Treatment of Cancer has compared surgery with or without neoadjuvant and adjuvant oxaliplatin, 5-FU, and folinic acid in patients with resectable liver metastases. A total of 364 patients were entered in this large study, the results have been presented in abstract form. A significant advantage in progression free survival was noted for eligible patients randomized to receive preoperative FOLFOX chemotherapy.[37a]

Local Destruction

More recently, new methods of ablation of liver metastases, such as cryotherapy, RF ablation, and microwave and laser hyperthermia, have been developed. Among these techniques, RF has become the most widely used ablative technique for liver metastases from CRC (38–44).

Background and Basics of Radiofrequency Tissue Ablation

Technical Features. During the application of RF energy, a high-frequency alternating current (350–500 kHz) moves from the tip of an electrode into the tissue surrounding the electrode. RF current induces ionic agitation that in turn results in heating. As the temperature within the tissue becomes elevated beyond 60°C, cells begin to die, resulting in a region of necrosis surrounding the electrode (45). Different types of electrode design are available, including a water-cooled cluster of three parallel 19G electrodes (Tyco Healthcare Mansfield, MA), two expanding electrode designs (Radiotherapeutics and RITA Medical Systems, Mountain View, CA), and stiff electrode (Berchtold, Tuttlingen, Germany). A comparison, in an experimental model, between different types of electrode design showed no major difference concerning the volume of induced necrosis (46).

The thermal injury to the tumor is inversely related to blood flow in the tumor due to washout effect. Tissue perfusion has a direct impact on the volume of necrosis that can be induced (39,45). Occlusion of liver vessels, including the portal vein, hepatic artery, or both, has been shown to increase the volume of necrosis but requires laparotomy (39,47). Occlusion of the hepatic artery of the liver segment involved by tumor is also possible through a percutaneous approach using angiographic balloon or transhepatic portal balloon (48).

The area of necrosis induced by RF ablation should be 1 cm larger than the tumor, similar to the surgical margin obtained after surgical resection. Tumors <3 cm in their greatest diameter can be destroyed with one placement of the needle electrode, with an array diameter of 3.5 to 4 cm, when the electrode is positioned in the center of the tumor (43,49). For larger tumors, multiple placements and deployment of the electrode array may be necessary to completely destroy the tumor (43,50). However, for such larger tumors, completeness of tumor destruction may be more uncertain (51).

Radiofrequency Approach. RF ablation of liver tumors can be performed percutaneously, under laparoscopy, or during laparotomy. No study compares these three routes. The indications of these approaches are different, and their choice is individualized for each patient. The percutaneous approach is less invasive than laparotomy. It can be performed under general or local anesthesia as an outpatient procedure, carries a lower morbidity and complication rate, and is less expensive (38,42,43,45). However, lesions located in the dome of the liver near the diaphragm or close to the stomach or colon are not always accessible by percutaneous approach due to the risk of adjacent organ injury.

The laparoscopic approach requires a high level of skill. It is guided by laparoscopic ultrasound, allows a good evaluation of the number and location of liver tumors, and also allows a survey of the peritoneal cavity to exclude the presence of extrahepatic disease, which is not possible by percutaneous approach. Laparoscopic approach can be useful for tumors located centrally in the liver near major intrahepatic blood vessels because it allows more precise positioning of the RF needle (52). Laparoscopic approach can also be indicated when the tumor is adherent to structures that could be damaged by thermal ablation such as the colon, stomach, or duodenum (38,45).

Laparotomy is a more invasive approach but allows inspection of the peritoneal cavity to rule out extrahepatic disease. When combined with perioperative ultrasound, it can detect small liver lesions, which can be overlooked by preoperative imaging workup. RF ablation can also be combined with liver resection. For instance, resection of a large tumor in one lobe can be combined with RF ablation of small deposits in the opposite lobe (38,43,53).

Monitoring the Effectiveness of the Procedure and Follow-Up. Ultrasound has been used to assess the completeness of the procedure, but the hyperechogenic image seen during thermal ablation does not strictly correlate with the coagulative damage (38,39), and the image becomes heterogeneous within a few minutes. Both CT scan and magnetic resonance imaging (MRI) seem to be more reliable in this regard (38).

Contrast-enhanced CT scan is the preferred method for follow-up. A peripheral rim, which represents an inflammatory reaction to the thermally damaged cells, must resolve within 1 month. After this delay, persistent or new perilesional enhancement is considered to be residual or recurrent tumor, particularly when it increases in size on the follow-up scans (38). Comparable images are obtained with MRI. More recently, fluorodeoxyglucose positron emission tomography (FDG-PET) scan has been assessed for the follow-up of local ablative treatment (54). In this study, the positive predictive value and the negative predictive value of FDG-PET scan for the detection of local recurrence was 80% and 100%, respectively (54).

Mortality and Morbidity of Radiofrequency Ablation

Overall, RF ablation of livers tumors is well tolerated. Common side effects following the procedure include minimal right upper quadrant discomfort, transient fever and nausea, and usually asymptomatic right pleural effusion. Deterioration in liver function tests is also common, with complete recovery within 1 week (42). The morbidity rate varies from 2% to 10%, and the mortality rate is <1.5% (40,44,47,55–57). In a recent meta-analysis including 3,670 patients with hepatic malignancies treated by percutaneous, laparoscopic, or open RF ablation, the mortality and morbidity rates were 0.5% and 9%, respectively (55). The complication rate and mortality was comparable for the three RF ablation approaches. The causes of death were hepatic abscess, liver failure, cardiac complications, and peritoneal hemorrhage. Deaths related to colon perforation have been also reported (56,58). The more frequently encountered complications were hepatic abscesses, abdominal bleeding, biliary tract injuries, liver failure, and pulmonary complications (55,56,58). Several risk factors for complication can be identified. Portal vein thrombosis is more frequent in cirrhotic liver than in noncirrhotic liver, especially in the case of combined blood flow occlusion (34). Liver abscesses occurred more frequently in patients bearing a bilioenteric anastomosis than in other patients (56). Subcapsular tumors carry a higher risk of abdominal bleeding, especially by percutaneous approach. This complication could be prevented by careful cauterization of the electrode tract. Central tumor predisposes to biliary tract and central vessel damage, and there is consensus for considering tumors located <1 cm from the main biliary duct a contraindication to RF. Thermal damage to neighboring organs is found exclusively in the percutaneous approach. The best knowledge of complication risk should help lower the rate of complications of RF ablation. In many centers, RF ablation has now replaced cryoablation because of its lower rate of complications.

Radiofrequency Ablation of Liver Metastases

Indications. Only surgical resection can offer long-term survival rates in 25% to 30% of patients. Only 10% to 20% of patients with liver metastases fulfill criteria for resection and are amenable to surgery. The trend is to be more aggressive and to increase the indication for surgical resection in order to render a larger group of patients amenable to surgery (6). In this setting, RF has been developed in recent years for the treatment of liver metastases. Because its efficacy has not been tested in randomized trials, the use of RF ablation should currently be restricted to the treatment of unresectable liver deposits. The basic idea is to use it in patients with a limited number of intrahepatic deposits that are not totally resectable due to their location in the liver. Tumor ablation can be used alone or combined with liver resection, some metastases being resected and the others ablated (38,43,53). However, all metastatic disease has to be treated. Another potential indication of RF ablation is liver recurrence after hepatectomy (59).

Results. The results of RF ablation of colorectal liver metastases are difficult to evaluate. In many studies, several different types of tumors are included. Some patients have received chemotherapy and others have not, which can bias the interpretation of the primary effect of RF treatment. In addition, results on local tumor recurrence are often reported in different ways, either as the number of failures on a lesion basis or as a number of patients with local recurrence in relation to the total number of patients treated. It seems that for lesions up to 3 cm, RF is effective and can result in local tumor control in >90% of patients. For lesions >3 cm, local recurrence rate at the site treated is reported to be >30% (50,60–63). The risk of lesion recurrence was not related to the number of lesions ablated or to RF ablation approach (laparotomy, laparoscopy, or percutaneous) (43). The development of new hepatic tumors or extrahepatic disease is a crucial problem of RF ablation and occurs in 30% to 60% of patients (40,47,49,61,62). Thus, RF ablation may not be sufficient by itself and could require combination with chemotherapy.

If RF ablation is safe and effective to induce necrosis of liver metastases up to 3 cm in diameter, it must now be proven that this local effect is related to a survival benefit for the patient. This would require clinical trials comparing RF ablation to surgical resection, which is considered the gold standard treatment. In theory, two types of studies can be considered: (a) comparing RF ablation to surgical resection for resectable metastases, and (b) concerning patients with unresectable liver metastases for whom standard treatment is palliative chemotherapy. This trial organized by the European Organisation for Research and Treatment of Cancer compares chemotherapy alone in one arm to chemotherapy plus RF ablation of all metastases in the other arm. It is likely that in the near future, most patients with liver metastases will receive multimodality treatment, including surgical resection, RF ablation, and systemic chemotherapy.

More is known about RF ablation of hepatic malignancies. It is now clearly demonstrated that this new method of local ablation can safely and efficiently destroy small liver lesions. It has now a place in the management of hepatic malignancies. However, its impact on patient survival remains to be demonstrated in well-designed clinical trials, in which it is urgent that surgeons and medical oncologists enroll their patients.

CONCLUSION

The standard treatment for resectable hepatic metastases is complete surgical resection. Surgery is feasible in only 10%

to 20% of patients. The benefits of chemotherapy are being increasingly recognized, especially in facilitating the resection of initially unresectable liver metastases. In fact, recent progress in chemotherapy and the development of ablative techniques increases the number of operable patients with curative intent. It is likely that a combination of surgery and chemotherapy will be validated in the near future.

For resectable metastases, it is important to demonstrate with prospective randomized trials, whether pre- or postoperative chemotherapeutic regimens, that using new drugs decreases recurrence after surgical resection and improves survival. For nonresectable metastases, the benefits of new ablative techniques and neoadjuvant chemotherapy need to be formally demonstrated. The management of patients with hepatic metastases requires a multidisciplinary approach. Participation in randomized trials is of major importance to validate the different therapeutic strategies.

References

1. Stangl R, Altendorf-Hofmann A, Charnley RM, Scheele J. Factors influencing the natural history of colorectal liver metastases. *Lancet* 1994;343:1405–1410.
2. Wilson SM, Adson MA. Surgical treatment of hepatic metastases from colorectal cancer. *Arch Surg* 1976;111:330–333.
3. Wanebo HJ, Semoglou C, Attiyeh F, et al. Surgical management of patients with primary operable colorectal cancer and synchronous liver metastases. *Am J Surg* 1978;135:81–85.
4. Pichlmayr R. Is there a place for liver grafting for malignancy? *Transpl Proc* 1988;20:478–482.
5. Timothy GJ, Greig JD, Crosbie JL, Miles WFA, Garden OJ. Superior staging of liver tumors with laparoscopy and laparoscopic ultrasound. *Ann Surg* 1994;6:711–719.
6. Nordlinger B, Jaeck D, Guiguet M, Vaillant JC, Balladur P, Schaal JC. Surgical resection of hepatic metastases: multicentric retrospective study by the French Association of Surgery. In: Nordlinger B, Jaeck D, eds. *Treatment of Hepatic Metastases of Colorectal Cancer.* Paris: Springer-Verlag; 1992:129–146.
7. Zacherl J, Scheuba C, Imhof N, et al. Current value of intraoperative sonography during surgery for hepatic neoplasms. *World J Surg* 2002;26:550–554.
8. Bismuth H, Houssin D, Castaing D. Major and minor segmentectomies "réglées" in liver surgery. *World J Surg* 1982;6:10–24.
9. Starzl TE, Bell RH, Beart RW, Putnam CW. Hepatic trisegmentectomy and other liver resections. *Surg Gynecol Obstet* 1975;141:429–437.
10. Nordlinger B, Quilichini MA, Parc R, et al. Hepatic resection for colorectal liver metastases: influence on survival of preoperative factors and surgery for recurrences in 80 patients. *Ann Surg* 1987;205(3):256–263.
11. Doci R, Gennari L, Bignami P, et al. One hundred patients with hepatic metastases from colorectal cancer treated by resection: analysis of prognostic determinants. *Br J Surg* 1997;78(7):797–801.
12. Jaeck D, Bachellier P, Guiguet M, et al. Long-term survival following resection of colorectal hepatic metastases. Association Française de Chirurgie. *Br J Surg* 1997;84(7):977–980.
13. Scheele J, Stang R, Altendorf-Hofmann A, et al. Resection of colorectal metastases. *World J Surg* 1995;19(1):59–71.
14. Jamison RL, Donohue JH, Nagorney DM, et al. Hepatic resection for metastatic colorectal cancer results in cure for some patients. *Arch Surg* 1997;132(5):505–510; discussion 511.
15. Fong Y, Fortner J, Sun RL, Brennan MF, Blumgart LH. Clinical score for predicting recurrence after hepatic resection for metastatic colorectal cancer: analysis of 1001 consecutive cases. *Ann Surg* 1999;230:309–318.
16. Minagawa M, Makuuchi M, Torzilli G, et al. Extension of the frontiers of surgical indications in the treatment of liver metastases from colorectal cancer: long-term results. *Ann Surg* 2000;231(4):487–489.
17. Gayowski TJ, Iwatsuki S, Madariaga JR, et al. Experience in hepatic resection for metastatic colorectal cancer: analysis of clinical and pathological risk factors. *Surgery* 1994;116(4):703–710.
18. Nordlinger B, Guiguet M, Vaillant J-C, et al. Surgical resection of colorectal carcinoma metastases to the liver: a prognostic scoring system to improve case selection, based on 1568 patients. *Cancer* 1996;77:1254–1262.
19. Cady B, Jenkins RL, Steele GD, Jr, et al. Surgical margin in hepatic resection for colorectal metastasis: a critical and improvable determinant of outcome. *Ann Surg* 1998;227:566–571.
20. Regnard JF, Grunenwald D, Spaggiari L, et al. Surgical treatment of hepatic and pulmonary metastases from colorectal cancers. *Ann Thorac Surg* 1998;66(1):214–218.
21. Kobayashi K, Kawamura M, Ishihara T. Surgical treatment for both pulmonary and hepatic metastases from colorectal cancer. *J Thorac Cardiovasc Surg* 1999;118:1090–1096.

22. McAfee MK, Allen MS, Trastek F, et al. Colorectal lung metastases: results of surgical excision. *Ann Thorac Surg* 1992;53:780–786.
23. Lange JF, Leese T, Castaing D, Bismuth H. Repeat hepatectomy for recurrent malignant tumors of the liver. *Surg Gynecol Obstet* 1989;169:119–126.
24. Nordlinger B, Vaillant JC, Guiguet P, et al. Repeat liver resections for recurrent colorectal metastases: prolonged survivals. *J Clin Oncol* 1994;12:1491–1496.
25. Azoulay D, Castaing D, Smail A, et al. Resection of nonresectable liver metastases from colorectal cancer after percutaneous portal vein embolization. *Ann Surg* 2000;231:480–486.
26. Elias D, De Baere T, Roche A, Ducreux M, Leclere J, Lasser P. During liver regeneration following right portal embolization the growth rate of liver metastases is more rapid than that of the liver parenchyma. *Br J Surg* 1999;86:784–788.
27. Douillard JY, Cunningham D, Roth AD, et al. Irinotecan combined with fluorouracil compared with fluorouracil alone as first-line treatment for metastatic colorectal cancer: a multicentre randomized trial. *Lancet* 2000;355:1041–1047.
28. Hurwitz H, Fehrenbacher L, Novotny W, et al. Bevacizumab plus irinotecan, fluorouracil, and leucovorin for metastatic colorectal cancer. *N Engl J Med* 2004;350:2335–2342.
29. Bismuth H, Adam R, L,vi F, et al. Resection of nonresectable liver metastases from colorectal cancer after neoadjuvant chemotherapy. *Ann Surg* 1996;224:509–520.
30. Allen PJ, Kemeny N, Jarnagin W, et al. Importance of response to neoajuvant chemotherapy in patients undergoing resection of synchronous colorectal liver metastases. *J Gastrointest Surg* 2003;7:109–115.
31. Tanaka K, Adam R, Shimada H, et al. Role of neoadjuvant chemotherapy in the treatment of multiple colorectal metastases to the liver. *Br J Surg* 2003;90:963–969.
32. Adam R, Pascal G, Castaing D, et al. Tumor progression while on chemotherapy: a contraindication to liver resection for multiple colorectal metastases? *Ann Surg* 2004;240(6):1061–1064.
33. Lorenz M, Muller HH, Shramm H, et al. Randomized trial of surgery versus surgery followed by adjuvant hepatic arterial infusion with 5-fluorouracil and folinic acid for liver metastases of colorectal cancer. German Cooperative on Liver Metastases. *Ann Surg* 1998;228:756–762.
34. Kemeny N, Huang Y, Cohen A, et al. Hepatic arterial infusion of chemotherapy after resection of hepatic metastases from colorectal cancer. *N Engl J Med* 1999;341:2039–2048.
35. Kemeny MM, Sudeshna A, Gray B, et al. Combined modality treatment for resectable metastatic colorectal carcinoma to the liver: surgical resection of hepatic metastases in combination with continuous infusion of chemotherapy—an intergroup study. *J Clin Oncol* 2002;20:1499–1505.
36. Portier G, Rougier P, Milan C, et al. Adjuvant systemic chemotherapy (CT) using 5-fluorouracil (FU) and folinic acid (FA) after resection of liver metastases (LM) from colorectal (CRC) origin: results of an intergroup phase III study (trial FFCD-ACHBTH-AURC 9002). *J Clin Oncol* 2002, Proc. ASCO:#528
37. Langer B, Bleiberg H, Labianca R, et al. Fluorouracil (FU) plus l-leucovorin (l-LV) versus observation after potentially curative resection of liver or lung metastases from colorectal cancer (CRC): results of the ENG (EORTC/NCIC CTG/GIVIO) randomized trial. *J Clin Oncol* 2002, Proc. ASCO:#592.
37a. Nordlinger B, Sorbye H, Collette L, et al. Final results of the EORTC Intergroup randomized phase III study 40983 (EPOC) evaluating the benefit of perioperative FOLFOX4 chemotherapy for patients with potentially resectable colorectal cancer metastases. *J Clin Oncol* 2007, LBA5.
38. Ruers TJM. Tumour ablative procedures for colorectal livers metastases. *Eur J Cancer* 2003;1:189–199.
39. Erce C, Parks W. Interstitial ablative techniques for hepatic tumours. *Br J Surg* 2003;90:272–289.
40. Pawlik TM, Izzo F, Cohen DS, et al. Combined resection and radiofrequency ablation for advanced hepatic malignancies: results in 172 patients. *Ann Surg Oncol* 2003;10:1059–1069.
41. Mutsaerts EL, Van Coevorden F, Krause R, et al. Initial experience with radiofrequency ablation for hepatic tumours in the Netherlands. *Eur J Surg Oncol* 2003;29:731–734.
42. Garcea G, Lloyd TD, Aylott C, et al. The emergent role of focal liver ablation techniques in the treatment of primary and secondary liver tumours. *Eur J Cancer* 2003;39:2150–2164.
43. Curley SA. Radiofrequency ablation of malignant liver tumors. *Ann Surg Oncol* 2003;10:338–347.
44. Bleicher RJ, Allegra DP, Nora DT, et al. Radiofrequency ablation in 447 complex unresectable liver tumors: lessons learned. *Ann Surg Oncol* 2003;10:52–58.
45. Gillams AR. Radiofrequency ablation in the management of liver tumours. *Eur J Surg Oncol* 2003;29:9–16.
46. Denys AL, De Baere T, Kuoch V, et al. Radio-frequency tissue ablation of the liver: in vivo and ex vivo experiments with four different systems. *Eur Radiol* 2003;13:2346–2352.
47. Curley SA, Izzo F, Delrio P, et al. Radiofrequency ablation of unresectable primary and metastatic hepatic malignancies: results in 123 patients. *Ann Surg* 1999;230:1–8.
48. de Baere T, Bessoud B, Dromain C, et al. Percutaneous radiofrequency ablation of hepatic tumors during temporary venous occlusion. *AJR Am J Roentgenol* 2002;178:53–59.
49. Solbiati L, Livraghi T, Goldberg SN, et al. Percutaneous radio-frequency ablation of hepatic metastases from colorectal cancer: long-term results in 117 patients. *Radiology* 2001;221:159–166.
50. Livraghi T, Goldberg SN, Lazzaroni S, et al. Hepatocellular carcinoma: radio-frequency ablation of medium and large lesions. *Radiology* 2000;214:761–768.
51. Dodd GD III, Frank MS, Aribandi M, et al. Radiofrequency thermal ablation: computer analysis of the size of the thermal injury created by overlapping ablations. *AJR Am J Roentgenol* 2001;177:777–782.
52. Santambrogio R, Podda M, Zuin M, et al. Safety and efficacy of laparoscopic radiofrequency of hepatocellular carcinoma in patients with liver cirrhosis. *Surg Endosc* 2003;17:1826–1832.
53. Oshowo A, Gillams AR, Lees WR, Taylor I. Radiofrequency ablation extends the scope of surgery in colorectal liver metastases. *Eur J Surg Oncol* 2003;29:244–247.
54. Ruers TJ, Langenhoff BS, Neeleman N, et al. Value of positron emission tomography with [F-18] fluorodeoxyglucose in patients with colorectal liver metastases: a prospective study. *J Clin Oncol* 2002;20:388–395.
55. Mulier S, Mulier P, Ni Y, et al. Complications of radiofrequency coagulation of liver tumours. *Br J Surg* 2002;89:1206–1222.
56. de Baere T, Risse O, Kuoch V, et al. Adverse events during radiofrequency treatment of 582 hepatic tumors. *AJR Am J Roentgenol* 2003;181:695–700.
57. Qian J, Feng GS, Vogl T. Combined interventional therapies of hepatocellular carcinoma. *World J Gastroenterol* 2003;9:1885–1891.
58. Livraghi T, Solbiati L, Meloni MF, et al. Treatment of focal liver tumors with percutaneous radio-frequency ablation: complications encountered in a multicenter study. *Radiology* 2003;226:441–451.
59. Elias D, De Baere T, Smayra T, et al. Percutaneous radiofrequency thermoablation as an alternative to surgery for treatment of liver tumour recurrence after hepatectomy. *Br J Surg* 2002;89:752–756.
60. Wood TF, Rose DM, Chung M, et al. Radiofrequency ablation of 231 unresectable hepatic tumors: indications, limitations, and complications. *Ann Surg Oncol* 2000;7:593–600.
61. de Baere T, Elias D, Dromain C, et al. Radiofrequency ablation of 100 hepatic metastases with a mean follow-up of more than 1 year. *AJR Am J Roentgenol* 2000;175:1619–1625.
62. Gillams AR, Lees WR. Survival after percutaneous, image-guided, thermal ablation of hepatic metastases from colorectal cancer. *Dis Colon Rectum* 2000;43:656–661.
63. Bowles BJ, Machi J, Limm WM, et al. Safety and efficacy of radiofrequency thermal ablation in advanced liver tumors. *Arch Surg* 2001;136:864–869.

UNCOMMON CANCERS OF THE GASTROINTESTINAL TRACT

CHAPTER 47 ■ ANAL CANAL CANCER

CATHY ENG AND JAFFER AJANI

The treatment of squamous cell carcinoma (SCCA) of the anal canal is unique to gastrointestinal malignancies and depends solely on the efficacy of the combined modalities of chemotherapy and radiation therapy (XRT), reserving surgery for the management of residual or recurrent disease. This practice evolved from a systematic evaluation of a fortuitous observation in only three patients with SCCA of the anal canal, in which a treatment regimen intended as neoadjuvant chemoradiation prior to radical surgery proved sufficient of itself to completely eradicate their anal canal cancers (1). Additional studies have since confirmed the curability of SCCA of the anal canal with relatively low doses of radiation and chemotherapy. Although the current treatments have been largely successful, chemoradiation therapy may result in both acute and delayed treatment-related toxicities. However, the rarity of this cancer type has limited progress in the evaluation of its biological behavior and of proposals to further improve the treatment approach. The treatment concepts first developed in the 1970s have now been refined so that many patients are now not only cured but also retain anal sphincter function. Nevertheless, many questions are unanswered, and the optimum treatment schedules and chemotherapy agents, especially for larger or metastatic cancers, remain to be defined.

ANATOMY

The anal canal consists of the terminal 3 to 4 cm of the intestine, extending from the rectum to the junction with the perianal skin (Fig. 47.1). The posterior wall of the canal is generally approximately 1 cm longer than the anterior wall. The superior limit of the anal canal is more readily appreciated by palpation than visually and is the upper border of the anorectal muscle ring (2). The anorectal ring corresponds to the junction of the puborectalis part of the levator ani muscle with the external anal sphincter. The distal limit, or anal verge, is the level at which the walls of the canal come into contact in their normal resting state. The perianal area is the skin within the 5-cm radius of the anal verge. The anal margin has been defined in a variety of ways, including as a synonym for the anal verge, or as the perianal skin immediately adjacent to the distal limit of the anal canal. Some physicians apply the term anal margin to the whole extent of the perianal skin.

The perianal skin is similar histologically to hair-bearing skin elsewhere. At the anal verge, the pigmented perianal skin blends with the paler, modified squamous epithelium of the distal canal, lacking hair or cutaneous glands, and is known as the pecten. The modified squamous epithelium of the pecten merges, usually just below the pectinate or dentate line, which marks the level of the anal valves, with a reddened membranous transitional zone that includes features of rectal, urothelial, and squamous epithelia. The transitional zone extends proxi-

mally for approximately 2 cm, where it blends with the pink columnar-glandular mucosa of the rectum. This last histologic change bears a variable relationship to the palpable level of the upper border of the anorectal muscle ring.

There are three major lymphatic pathways from the anal tissue, with numerous lymphatic connections between the various levels of the canal and anal verge. Lymphatics from the uppermost part of the canal drain to the perirectal and superior hemorrhoidal nodes of the inferior mesenteric system. Those from the area around and above the dentate line flow to the internal pudendal, hypogastric, and obturator nodes of the internal iliac system. Lymphatics from the distal canal, anal verge, and perianal skin drain to the superficial inguinal nodes, and occasionally to the femoral nodes, of the external iliac system.

The arterial supply to the distal rectum and anal canal is from the superior, middle, and inferior hemorrhoidal vessels, arising from the inferior mesenteric, internal iliac, and internal pudendal arteries, respectively. The venous drainage follows the arterial inflow, and thus accesses the hepatic portal and systemic venous systems.

The external anal sphincter is a voluntary muscle that is innervated by the internal rectal nerve, a branch of the pudendal nerve derived from the second, third, and fourth sacral nerves (S2, S3, and S4, respectively). In addition to its motor function, the internal rectal nerve also transmits pain, touch, and other sensations from the anal canal below the dentate line and from the perianal skin. The internal anal sphincter is an involuntary muscle, innervated by parasympathetic fibers from S2, S3, and S4, and by sympathetic fibers from the hypogastric plexus.

INCIDENCE

Anal cancer remains one of the rarest malignancies of the gastrointestinal tract, affecting ≤1 per 100,000 persons (3), resulting in approximately 4,650 cases diagnosed and 690 deaths in 2007 (4). The majority of patients present with locally advanced disease and are treated with combined chemoradiation therapy with curative intent. The annual incidence is 1 per 100,000 in the heterosexual population but increases to 35 per 100,000 in men who have anal intercourse (5). Review of the Surveillance, Epidemiology, and End Results database between 1973 and 2000 indicates increasing incidence among both men and women, with black men having the highest incidence and worst prognosis relative to other races (6).

RISK FACTORS

Current literature suggests a strong link between cervical and anal cancer; it is believed that this is attributed to a history of

641

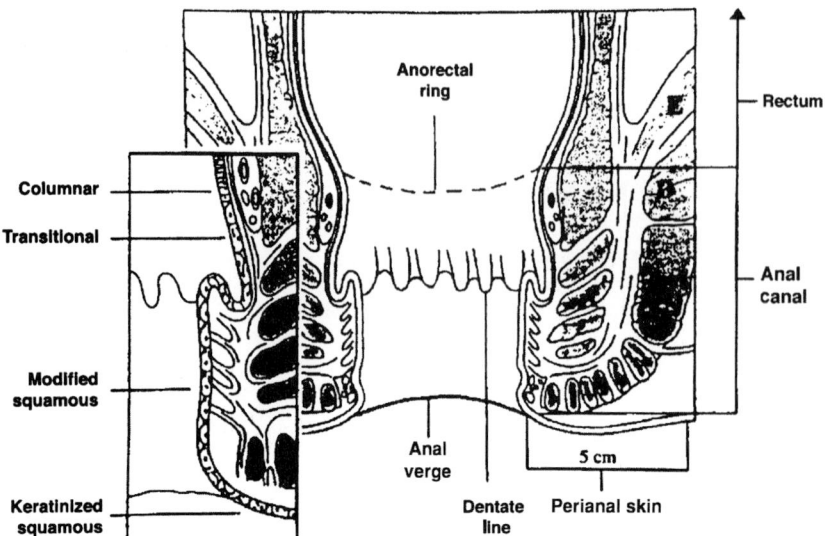

FIGURE 47.1. Anatomy of the anal canal. *Source:* Adapted from Skarin AT, ed. *Atlas of Diagnostic Oncology.* New York, NY: Gower Medical Publishing; 1991;3:43.

acquiring the human papillomavirus (HPV). It is believed that 20 million Americans ages 15 to 59 are currently infected with HPV or 1 in every 13 individuals, with 5.5 million new cases diagnosed per year. Approximately one-half of those individuals infected with HPV are adolescents, sexually active, and between the ages of 15 to 24 (7). As in cervical intraepithelial neoplasia, HPV infections may cause anal intraepithelial neoplasia (AIN). In addition to the relationship observed between HPV and intraepithelial neoplasia, HPV is also associated with the development of genital warts (condylomata acuminata), which can convert to SCCA after a prolonged latency period (5–40 years) (8,9). The prevalence of HPV appears to be bimodal with the greatest incidence occurring among individuals younger than 25 years of age, with a second peak after the age of 55 (10). In general, HPV infections are fairly common in young women, with the majority resolving spontaneously due to an effective immune response. However, persistent HPV infection may be the precursor for malignant transformation (9). More than 100 different subtypes of HPV exist; HPV subtypes 16, 18, 31, 33, 35, 39, 45, 51, 52, 56, 58, 59, 68, and 82 are considered to be the most carcinogenic, with subtypes 16 and 18 most frequently associated with anal cancer; and >70% of patients with invasive anal cancer are seropositive for subtype 16 (11). Controversy exists over whether having multiple subtypes of HPV in the same individual increases the persistence of HPV infection (12). At this time, the detection of HPV in patients with anal cancer does not appear to be a prognostic factor, but persistence of HPV infection may play a central role (13–15). The development of HPV is also linked to the less common anogenital cancers, including vulvar, vaginal, and penile cancers, as well as head and neck cancers of the oropharyngeal tract (16).

Other infectious diseases linked to the pathogenesis of anal cancer include herpes simplex virus (HSV), chlamydia trachomatis, gonorrhea, and other sexually transmitted diseases (17). In addition, an increased risk of developing anal cancer has been shown in men and women with a history of receptive anal intercourse prior to age 30 years; having had sexual intercourse with more than 10 partners; chronic immunosuppression; and/or having had a history of cervical, vulvar, or vaginal cancers (18).

The precise role of HIV infection as a causative agent in the development of anal carcinoma is still undefined. It has been observed that patients who are HIV positive are two to six times more likely than HIV-negative individuals to have anal HPV, regardless of sexual practices (19). In addition, HIV-positive patients are more likely to have persistent HPV infection and are two times more likely to progress from low-grade AIN to high-grade lesions, as compared with HIV-negative individuals. In fact, an inverse correlation with persistence of HPV infection and progression from low-grade to high-grade AIN has been shown to be related to the CD4 lymphocyte count (19).

Several reports suggest a direct correlation between HIV infection and anal cancer. In New York City between 1979 and 1985, the incidence of anal cancers increased 10-fold among men who were 20 to 49 years of age, coinciding with the appearance of AIDS (20). It has been estimated that men who are 25 to 44 years old are 60-fold more likely to die from anal cancer if they are HIV positive as compared to HIV-negative individuals (21). Melbye et al. showed that AIDS patients in the United States had a 64-fold higher relative risk of developing anal cancer as compared to the general population (22,23). In contrast to these data, prior studies have failed to demonstrate any direct association between AIDS and anal cancer. Data from analysis of single men in San Francisco during the 1980s demonstrated that the incidence of anal cancer increased during this time period but did not necessarily correlate with HIV status (24). It is clear, however, that HIV-positive patients are immunosuppressed and are predisposed to HPV infection and AIN, which have been shown to be involved in the development of anal cancer. Hence, anal carcinoma is considered an AIDS-associated malignancy and is not considered an AIDS-defining illness. Unexpectedly, the advances in the treatment of HIV patients with highly active antiretroviral therapy (HAART) has prolonged the survival of this patient population; yet, after the introduction of HAART, the prevalence of AIN has remained unchanged among HIV-positive men having sex with men (MSM) (25).

As in HIV-positive patients, a state of chronic immunosuppression (e.g., organ transplant patient) places the patients at high risk for developing HPV infection and subsequent development of AIN (26). It is reported that organ transplant patients have a 10-fold increase of developing carcinoma of the anal canal (27). Last, a history of tobacco use has been shown to increase the risk of anal cancer by a factor of two to five times, independent of sexual practice, and this risk appears to be greater in premenopausal than in postmenopausal women (28).

HISTOPATHOLOGY

Approximately 90% of primary cancers of the canal are of squamous cell histology (SCCA). The major subtypes are large cell keratinizing, large cell nonkeratinizing (transitional), and basaloid (29). The lack of prognostic differentiation for these various subtypes has largely led to a general category of SCCA of the anal canal. The remaining 10% of malignant anal canal cancers include adenocarcinoma of the anal glands, small and large cell cancers, and melanoma. Primary cancers of the perianal skin or anal margin are similar to cancers of the skin in other sites. The majority are SCCAs, with occasional basal cell cancers and melanomas.

PRESENTATION AND DIAGNOSIS

Most patients present with nonspecific symptoms. Bleeding, anal discharge, discomfort, itching, or pain is reported by approximately half of all patients with cancers of the canal; approximately 25% of patients are aware of a mass. Other patients may present with enlargement of their inguinal lymph nodes (30). Anal tumors are typically plaquelike or ulcerated and rarely pedunculated. Benign conditions, such as hemorrhoids, fibrous skin tags, redundant mucosa, and anal fissures, may make the diagnosis difficult. An incidental discovery of superficial cancer or high-grade dysplasia is sometimes identified after histologic examination of tissue removed during treatment for benign conditions such as hemorrhoids or chronic fissures. Gross fecal incontinence due to sphincter incompetence or fistula formation is uncommon and is seen in <5%. Extrapelvic metastases are a rare presenting indication of anal cancer and are diagnosed in <5% of patients at presentation (3); common sites include the liver, lungs, and bones. More than two-thirds of patients are diagnosed at a relatively early stage, before lymph node metastases or invasion of adjacent organs become clinically detectable (31).

DIAGNOSTIC WORKUP AND STAGING

Unless stated otherwise, the remainder of the chapter focuses primarily on SCCA. The features of greatest prognostic significance for diseasefree survival (DFS) are the size of the primary cancer, spread to regional lymph nodes, and extrapelvic sites. The probability of retaining anal function is determined principally by sphincter competence at presentation and the size of the primary cancer. Inguinal lymph node metastases are clinically detectable in approximately 15% of patients when the primary cancer is first diagnosed. In series managed by radical surgery, pelvic node metastases were found in approximately 30%, with approximately equal risk of involvement in the internal iliac and perirectal-superior hemorrhoidal node pathways (32,33).

The primary tumor and any clinically palpable inguinal nodes should be biopsied to establish the diagnosis. Abdominal and pelvic computed tomography (CT) scans or magnetic resonance imaging may disclose liver and nodal metastases, but small nodal metastases are not identified reliably by any currently available imaging technique, including transrectal ultrasound. A digital rectal examination, as well as anoscopy, proctosigmoidoscopy, or flexible sigmoidoscopy, should be done for a complete evaluation. A standard chest x-ray or CT scan of the chest is sufficient as a screen for pulmonary metastases. Localized skeletal symptoms should also be evaluated radiologically, but screening bone scans are not necessary in asymptomatic patients. Fluorine-18 2-fluoro-2-deoxy-D-glucose-positron emission tomography may also have a role in staging but is not advocated by all clinical investigators (34–36). Full blood count, kidney and liver function tests, and, if risk factors are present, HIV antibody tests, including CD4 count and viral load, should be performed. Unlike other gastrointestinal malignancies such as colorectal and pancreatic cancer, a tumor marker for SCCA of the anal canal has not been identified.

The current American Joint Committee on Cancer (AJCC) (37) and International Union Against Cancer (UICC) staging systems (38) are based on the size of the primary cancer and the presence or absence of regional lymph node or distant metastases (Table 47.1). Unlike other malignancies where the degree of tumor penetration is indicative of the T stage, the T stage of anal cancer is primarily based on the size of the tumor.

SURGERY AS THE PRIMARY MODALITY OF THERAPY

Prior to the discovery of combined chemoradiation therapy as a treatment modality with curative intent, the best treatment modality appeared to be an abdominoperineal resection (APR). As a single treatment modality, the estimated 5-year probability of survival is 40% to 70% (32). APR is a major surgical procedure involving en bloc resection of the rectum and the anal canal. The mesorectum is dissected from the posterior and lateral pelvic sidewalls distal to the aortic bifurcation, and the dissection includes the levator muscles and muscles of the pelvic floor. The final specimen includes the anorectum and mesorectum, together with the pelvic floor muscles, ischiorectal fat, and perianal skin. An end sigmoid colostomy is fashioned. Where necessary, the dissection is extended to include the posterior vaginal wall and, occasionally, other pelvic organs, such as the uterus, ovaries, prostate, or bladder, resulting in a pelvic exenteration. Despite the curative intent of surgery, the possibility of a permanent colostomy can be socially and emotionally distressing for patients. Some patients may be so overwhelmed with the possibility of an APR that they delay treatment, placing them at risk for further disease advancement.

With the widespread adoption of combined radiation and chemotherapy as the initial treatment for anal cancer, the role of surgery has changed. Local excision is now generally reserved for patients who have SCCA tumors up to 2 cm in diameter (T_1) and are superficial and well differentiated. The risk of nodal metastases is <10% for small, well-differentiated cancers that have not penetrated into the sphincter muscles. Local resection can also be considered for small cancers discovered at the time of surgery for benign anal conditions. Patients who fail local resection can be assessed for combined chemoradiation treatment if further local excision is not indicated.

The main role for APR is now reserved for surgical salvage of patients who have residual or recurrent cancer. An APR may also be indicated for patients who have contraindications to radiation or chemoradiation therapy. If residual cancer is suspected after completing chemoradiation and an adequate period has elapsed for the full treatment effects of XRT, it is advisable to confirm the presence of active cancer histologically with a tissue biopsy before proceeding with salvage surgery. The effectiveness of surgical salvage varies considerably, although several series have reported control rates of approximately 50% to 60% (39,40).

TABLE 47.1

TUMOR, NODE, METASTASIS (TNM) CLASSIFICATION

Subclass	Tumor (T)	Node (N)	Metastasis (M)
X	Cannot be assessed	Cannot be assessed	Cannot be assessed
1	<2 cm in dimension	Perirectal node involvement	Distant metastasis
2	>2 cm but <5 cm	Unilateral internal iliac and/or inguinal lymph node involvement	N/A
3	>5 cm in dimension	Perirectal and inguinal lymph nodes and/or bilateral internal iliac and/or inguinal lymph nodes	N/A

STAGE OF DISEASE

0	T_{is}	N_0	M_0
I	T_1	N_0	M_0
II	T_2	N_0	M_0
II	T_3	N_0	M_0
IIIA	T_1	N_1	M_0
	T_2	N_1	M_0
	T_3	N_1	M_0
	T_4	N_0	M_0
IIIB	T_4	N_1	M_0
	Any T	N_{2-3}	M_0
IV	Any T	Any N	M_1

Adapted from refs. 37 and 38.

SINGLE-AGENT RADIATION THERAPY

XRT is another option of preservation of the anal sphincter in lieu of surgery with evidence for long-term survival. When compared to APR, it has been reported that the overall survival (OS) is equivalent, with a complete response (CR) achieved in approximately 75% of patients (41,42). A large retrospective study completed by Deniaud-Alexandre et al. evaluated 305 patients treated with curative intent radiotherapy (RT) (43). The median dose of external beam radiation was 45 Gy. A radiation boost of 20 Gy was provided after a median delay of 37 days (median cumulative dose of 63 Gy) in 279 patients (92%). All palpable lymph nodes received a booster dose of 10 to 15 Gy. After a median follow-up of 103 months, a complete response was achieved in 79% to 96% of T_{1-3} tumors but in only 44% for T_4 tumors. Overall, XRT resulted in local regional control in only 68% of patients: T_{1-2} (78%–81%), T_3 (63%), and T_4 (33%). Tumor size ≥4 cm and a treatment delay of more than 38 days were both negative prognostic factors in patient outcome.

Uninterrupted courses of high-dose radiation, delivering 50 Gy in 4 weeks or 60 to 65 Gy in 6 weeks may control 80% or more of cancers up to approximately 4 cm in size and approximately 50% of larger tumors. Papillon et al. reported the success of the split-course regimen, in which an intensive course of small field external beam radiation is directed to the perineum (42 Gy in 10 fractions in 16 days), and followed 8 weeks later by 20 Gy interstitial radiation (44).

Radiation alone may be favored by some for the treatment of T_1 category cancers (≤2 cm) and may be curative (45). Although the use of radiation alone in these situations spares the patient side effects of chemotherapy, the higher doses required when radiation is used alone may increase the risk of normal tissue damage (46). Some surgeons may consider local excision of small cancers followed by adjuvant XRT (47).

TREATMENT OF ANAL CANAL CANCER WITH COMBINED RADIATION AND CHEMOTHERAPY: THE CLASSIC APPROACH

Clinical investigators proceeded to seek other options to enhance the efficacy of XRT. In 1974, Nigro et al. reported that treatment with concurrent radiation, 5-fluorouracil (5-FU), and mitomycin C (MMC) produced durable, complete regression of squamous cell cancers of the anal canal (1). After confirmation by numerous other clinicians, concurrent chemoradiation has replaced radical RT alone or surgery as the preferred initial treatment for most patients with anal canal cancer. Three major randomized trials have demonstrated that (a) delivering 5-FU and MMC concurrently with radiation gives outcomes superior to those of the same schedule of radiation alone (48,49) and (b) the combination of 5-FU and MMC with radiation is more effective than 5-FU with radiation (50).

In a trial by the United Kingdom Coordinating Committee for Cancer Research (UKCCCR), 577 patients with all stages of epidermoid cancer of the anal canal (75%) or anal margin (23%) were enrolled (48). Twenty percent were lymph node positive, and 2.5% had extrapelvic metastases. They were randomized to treatment with either radiation alone (45 Gy in 20–25 fractions in 4–5 weeks) or radiation with 5-FU (1,000 mg/m² per 24 hours for 96 hours or 750 mg/m² per 24 hours for 120 hours) by continuous intravenous (IV) infusion during the first and final weeks of radiation treatment, and MMC (12 mg/m²) by bolus injection on day 1 of the first course of 5-FU only. Patients with other comorbidities or those older than 80 were provided a reduced dose of 5-FU (750 mg/m², D1–D4) and MMC (10 mg/m², D1). Six weeks after the initial phase of treatment, patients received additional radiation without chemotherapy (15 Gy in six fractions by external beam

TABLE 47.2

THREE-YEAR RESULTS OF RANDOMIZED TRIALS OF RADIATION ALONE VERSUS RADIATION, 5-FLUOROURACIL, AND MITOMYCIN C

	UKCCCR (48)			EORTC (49)		
	XRT (%)	ChemoXRT(%)	p	XRT (%)	ChemoXRT (%)	p
LRC	39	61	<0.001	55	65	0.02
CPS	61	72	0.02	NS	NS	NS
OS	58	65	0.25	65	70	0.17

UKCCR, United Kingdom Coordinating Committee for Cancer Research; EORTC, European Organization for Research and Treatment of Cancer; XRT, radiation therapy; chemoXRT, chemoradiation therapy; LRC, locoregional control; CPS, cause-specific survival; NS, nonsignificant; OS, overall survival.

therapy or 25 Gy over 2 to 3 days by iridium-192 implant). For those patients whose tumor showed less than a clinical partial response (defined as shrinkage of <50%) at 6 weeks post treatment, radical surgery was performed rather than additional radiation. The definition of local failure in this trial included the presence of residual or recurrent cancer in the primary site or regional nodes, treatment-related morbidity requiring surgery, or inability to close a colostomy that was created prior to treatment. Surgery with colostomy was required for late treatment-induced toxicity in 10 patients (3.5%) in each study arm. Six patients (2%) in the combined modality group and two patients (0.7%) in the radiation alone group died of treatment-related morbidity. Local control and cause-specific survival rates were significantly improved and the need for colostomy decreased by combined modality treatment (Table 47.2). The OS rate was improved but was not statistically significant.

The European Organization for Research and Treatment of Cancer (EORTC) performed a similar study of only 103 patients with advanced cancers of the anal canal (49). Patients with extrapelvic metastases and those older than 76 years of age were ineligible. Eighty-five percent of those entered had stage T_{3-4} cancers, and 51% had abnormal nodes. Patients were randomized to pelvic radiation treatment (consisting of 45 Gy in 25 fractions over 5 weeks) alone or with 5-FU (750 mg/m^2 per 24 hours for 120 hours by continuous IV infusion) during weeks 1 and 5 of radiation. In the first week only, a bolus injection of MMC (15 mg/m^2) was given on the first day of the 5-FU infusion. Six weeks later, additional radiation was delivered by external beam or interstitial techniques (15 Gy if there had been complete clinical response to the initial course of treatment, 20 Gy if response had been partial). Inadequate response resulted in surgery in 5 patients on the radiation only arm. Acute and late toxicity rates were similar in each treatment group. One of 51 (2%) patients who received radiation and chemotherapy died of treatment-related toxicity. The local control and colostomyfree survival (CFS) rates were significantly better after combined modality but, as in the UK trial, the improvement in OS rates did not reach statistical significance (Table 47.2).

In North America, the Radiation Therapy Oncology Group (RTOG) and the Eastern Cooperative Oncology Group (ECOG) completed an Intergroup trial to study the contribution of MMC in the combined modality regimen (50). Two hundred and ninety-one patients with cancers of the anal canal of any T and N category (RTOG Staging System), without evidence of extrapelvic spread of cancer, were randomized to treatment with external beam pelvic radiation (45.0–50.4 Gy in 25–28 fractions over 5 weeks) with two courses of 5-FU (1,000 mg/m^2 per 24 hours by continuous IV infusion for 96 hours), with or without MMC (10 mg/m^2 by bolus injection on the first day of each 5-FU infusion), during weeks 1 and 5 of

radiation. The primary tumor site was biopsied 4 to 6 weeks after radiation. Biopsies were positive in 15% of those who received 5-FU only with radiation and in 8% of those treated with both 5-FU and MMC ($p = 0.14$). Patients with positive biopsies received additional radiation (9 Gy in five fractions in 1 week) concomitantly with a 96-hour infusion of 5-FU (1,000 mg/m^2 per 24 hours) and a short-term infusion of cisplatin (100 mg/m^2 over 6 hours) on the second day of the 5-FU infusion. Acute hematologic toxicity was more common after MMC, but otherwise the rates of acute and late toxicity were comparable in each group. One of 145 (0.7%) patients treated by 5-FU and radiation suffered fatal toxicity versus 4 of 146 (2.7%) who received 5-FU and MMC. The rates of locoregional control, CFS, and DFS were significantly better in those treated with radiation, 5-FU, and MMC, but OS rates at 4 years were similar (Table 47.3).

Five-year survival rates from nonrandomized series treated with 5-FU, MMC, and radiation are approximately 80% for cancers measuring up to 2 cm in size (T_1), 70% for 2- to 5-cm tumors (T_2), 45% to 55% for larger or deeply invasive cancers (T_{3-4}), and 65% to 75% overall. The corresponding local control rates (excluding the effects of salvage treatment) are approximately 90% to 100% (T_1), 65% to 75% (T_2), 40% to 55% (T_{3-4}), and 60% overall (Table 47.4).

TOXICITY OF CHEMORADIATION THERAPY

With standard-dose RT and concurrent chemotherapy with 5-FU and MMC, acute toxicity may include leukopenia, thrombocytopenia, proctitis, and perineal dermatitis.

TABLE 47.3

FOUR-YEAR RESULTS OF RANDOMIZED TRIAL OF RADIATION AND 5-FLUOROURACIL (5-FU) WITH AND WITHOUT MITOMYCIN C (MMC)

	5-FU/XRT (%)	5-FU/MMC/XRT (%)	p Value
LRC	66	84	<0.001
CFS	59	71	0.02
DFS	51	73	<0.001
OS	67	76	0.31

XRT, radiation therapy; LRC, locoregional control; CFS, colostomyfree survival; DFS, diseasefree survival; OS, overall survival. From ref. 50.

TABLE 47.4

SELECTED STUDIES OF COMBINED 5-FLUOROURACIL (5-FU), MITOMYCIN C (MMC), AND
RADIATION THERAPY (XRT)

Author	N	5-FU (mg/m²/d)	MMC (mg/m²/d)	XRT (Gy)	LRC	5-Year OS
Leichman et al. (98)	45	1,000, D1–4, and D29–32	15, D1	30	84%	80%
Sischy et al. (99)	79	1,000, D2–5, and D28–31	10, D2	40.8	84% (<3 cm)	3 years: 73%
Cummings et al. (45)	192	1,000, D1–4, and D43–46	10, D1	50	86%	Cause specific: 76%
Ferrigno et al. (100)	43	1,000, D1–4, and D27–30	10, D1 ± D30	45–55	79%	68%

LRC, locoregional control; OS, overall survival; D, day.

Hemolytic-uremic syndrome is a rare but serious severe adverse toxicity associated with MMC. The treatment advances for improving local control rates have resulted in an increase in the numbers of patients who retain anorectal function. Although sphincter function is chronically impaired in some patients (51,52). Few patients whose cancers have been eradicated require surgery for incontinence. Low-grade symptomatic morbidity of the perianal skin, anorectum, and other pelvic organs is usually managed conservatively.

RADIATION TECHNIQUES

The technical aspects of radiation treatment continue to be challenging due to difficulties associated with achieving homogeneous radiation distributions. It is likely that some treatment failures and complications are due to the irregular dose distributions caused by the curvatures and irregularities of the perineum and pelvis. The radiation techniques used depend largely on whether the primary cancer and the extent of regional lymph nodes are to be treated. Elective irradiation of clinically normal regional lymph nodes is an integral part of the treatment plan. Most centers prefer to prescribe a relatively homogeneous dose to the node groups at greatest risk (i.e., the inguinal, pararectal, and internal iliac). Although some centers extend the volume superiorly to the L5–S1 junction, others restrict the volume to the lower border of the sacroiliac joints, which approximates the bifurcation of the iliac arteries. The more extended volume includes the common iliac, upper pararectal, and lower sigmoid nodes. The common iliac nodes are considered metastatic sites rather than regional nodes under the AJCC/UICC staging system (37,38). Radiation is delivered most frequently by an anterior-posterior pair of parallel-opposed fields or by three- or four-field techniques. Potential disadvantages of the anterior-posterior pair and large multifield techniques include full-dose irradiation of the femoral head and neck, which lie behind the inguinal-femoral nodes, and irradiation of the bladder, bowel, and other contents of the pelvis. To reduce the risks of normal tissue damage, some centers prefer to restrict the width of anterior and posterior fields to the pelvic cavity, and treat the inguinal-femoral nodes by separate, direct anterior electron beams. Problems can also arise from this approach, due to unintended and unrecognized radiation field overlaps, particularly in the medial inguinal skin crease and adjacent tissues. Many radiation oncologists address the potential problem of damage to the pelvic organs by using a shrinking field schedule and by reducing the treatment volume to the immediate anal area after approximately 30 to 35 Gy over 3 to 4 weeks. High-energy linear accelerators (≥6 MeV) should be used and treatment should be given 5 days per week to all fields each day. Decreased acute and late toxicity can be obtained with administration of ≤2 Gy/day. Also, if a three-field technique

(a posterior and two lateral fields) is used, blocks can be placed to spare the posterior muscle and soft tissues behind the sacrum, as well as to reduce the amount of small bowel treated anteriorly. Treatment in the prone position allows further decrease in the amount of small bowel included in the field. Also, the development of conformal radiation techniques has permitted greater protection of uninvolved pelvic organs. However, these techniques, including conformal radiation, use radiation beams tangential to the perineum. The perineal skin and subdermal tissues are particularly susceptible to radiation damage, including telangiectasia, fibrosis, dryness, intermittent superficial ulceration, and necrosis. Low- and high-grade damage to the anal tissues and adjacent soft tissues and skin continue to pose a barrier to escalation of radiation dose.

Small-volume boost radiation is a common part of many treatment plans. Boost radiation to the primary cancer may be given by external beam or interstitial radiation techniques. External beam therapy is used most frequently, partly because of the bulk of many primary cancers and their location in the upper canal and anorectal region and partly because of the relative lack of familiarity of many radiation oncologists with interstitial radiation techniques. Fifteen to 20 Gy in 1 to 2 weeks is commonly prescribed as the boost dose if external radiation techniques are used.

Innovative methods such as intensity modulated XRT are currently being investigated to possibly further decrease the degree of gastrointestinal or skin toxicity but yet improve conformation of the radiation dose to the primary tumor site (53,54). RTOG investigators are currently evaluating this approach in an ongoing phase II study of 5-FU, MMC, and XRT with curative intent. The primary end point is evaluation of decreased gastrointestinal and genitourinary adverse events (grade II or greater) in the first 90 days after the start of treatment as compared to patients treated on the RT, 5-FU, and MMC arm on the recently completed clinical trial, Intergroup trial, RTOG 98-11 (55).

Radiation Dose Escalation and the Impact of Dose Delay

Efforts have been made to improve local control rates by intensifying radiation, chemotherapy, or both. Increases in total radiation dose, shortening of overall time of treatment delivery, and eliminating elective interruptions in radiation (split courses) have been advocated. When combined with 5-FU and MMC, radiation doses of as low as 30 Gy in 15 fractions in 3 weeks are capable of eradicating up to approximately 90% of anal cancers ≤3 cm. Higher doses, from 45 Gy in 45 fractions in 5 weeks to 54 Gy in 30 fractions in 6 weeks, often supplemented by further radiation after an interval of 6 to 8 weeks to a total of 60 to 65 Gy, have controlled from 65% to 75%

of primary tumors. The rationale for increasing the total radiation dose is based on a retrospective analysis of nonrandomized studies that suggest a positive dose control relationship (56).

Short interruptions in the delivery of radiation, either electively or as clinically necessary, may be necessary due to acute toxicities such as dermatitis and anoproctitis. However, extending the overall time of treatment may increase the risk of local failure (treatment delay >38 days vs. ≤38 days, $p = 0.0025$), which may be due to significant repopulation of the cancer (43,57). The extent to which prolongation of overall treatment time affects local control rates for anal cancers is not known, but the limited data available on potential tumor doubling times suggest that this is of the order of 5 days similar to cervical carcinoma (58). Yet, other studies suggest that patients may undergo a short dose delay ≤8 days without compromising local control (59). The introduction of conformal radiation treatment techniques has diminished the need for interruptions due to the acute toxicities, largely by reducing the area of radiation of the perineal skin.

ALTERNATIVES TO MITOMYCIN C

The cytotoxic drug that has been extensively studied in conjunction with 5-FU/XRT, other than MMC, is cisplatin (Table 47.5). Bleomycin was one of the first drugs to be studied. Bleomycin (5 mg by intramuscular injection 1 hour before radiation for the first 15 or 30 fractions) was given concurrently with radiation in nonrandomized series, but no benefit was discernible. Investigators have explored other strategies to intensify the treatment approach, including increasing the total chemotherapy dose, investigating induction chemotherapy before concurrent radiation, and adjuvant chemotherapy. The intent of the induction chemotherapy is intended to improve locoregional control, to reduce the incidence of late extrapelvic cancer growth, or both.

The Cancer and Leukemia Group B (CALGB) cooperative group has recently updated its results of the use of induction 5-FU/cisplatin in poor prognostic T_{3-4} and/or N_{2-3} positive disease (60). Forty-five patients were treated with induction infusional 5-FU (1,000 mg/m^2/day IV × 5 days) plus cisplatin (100 mg/m^2 IV × 1 day) on weeks 1 and 5, followed by 45 Gy XRT weeks 9 to 17 (a 19-day break was granted after 30.6 Gy) with concurrent infusional 5-FU (1,000 mg/m^2/day IV × 4 days) and MMC (10 mg/m^2 IV × 1 day) weeks 9 and 15. If residual disease was present, an additional 9 Gy XRT was given on week 19 with concurrent infusional 5-FU (800 mg/m^2/day IV × 5 days) plus cisplatin (100 mg/m^2 IV × 1 day). The primary grade 3/4 toxicities reported included neutropenia, anorexia, nausea, stomatitis, and infection. The investigators reported an impressive CR rate of 82% for this poor prognostic patient

population. After a median follow-up of 44 months, 61% are diseasefree and 50% of patients are both colostomy and disease free.

The promising early results of the CALGB trial served as the premise for a randomized Phase III Intergroup trial (RTOG 98-11) led by the Radiation Therapy Oncology Group (55). RTOG 98-11 is a randomized trial in North America in which patients with primary cancers >2 cm received either two courses of 5-FU and MMC or 5-FU and cisplatin concurrently with radiation (59.4 Gy in 33 fractions in 6.5 weeks). Induction 5-FU and cisplatin was given to patients randomized to the 5-FU, cisplatin, and radiation arm. Cisplatin was given in a dose of 75 mg/m^2 on the first day of each 4-day infusion of 5-FU. The doses of 5-FU and MMC are similar to those described previously. Between the years of 1998 and 2005, 650 patients were accrued. Patients with T_1N_0 or metastatic disease were excluded. The primary end point was DFS. Preliminary results indicate no difference in DFS ($p = 0.33$) or OS ($p = 0.13$) between the two arms. However, a slightly improved CFS was noted in the MMC arm (27% vs. 44%, HR = 1.63, $p = 0.04$). As expected, increased grade 3/4 hematologic toxicity was noted in the MMC arm ($p = 0.0013$), but overall grade 3/4 toxicities were fairly equivalent ($p = 0.12$). Final results are to be reported at a later date.

The EORTC is proceeding with a different chemotherapy approach and is currently conducting a phase II/III randomized trial of cisplatin/MMC/XRT versus 5-FU/MMC/XRT in patients with T_{2-4} or node-positive disease. The primary end point is response rate.

Other investigators are evaluating the role of the oral fluoropyrimidine, capecitabine, in lieu of IV 5-FU, as a radiation sensitizer in combination with XRT. EXTRA is a pilot phase II trial of capecitabine (825 mg/m^2 twice a day [BID] over days 1–5, 8–12, 15–19, 22–26, 29–33, and 36–40), MMC (12 mg/m^2, day 1 only), and XRT (30.6 Gy in 17 fractions, 19.8 Gy in 11 fractions). The primary end point is response. The trial has recently completed its accrual of 30 patients. Final results have not been reported to date.

At The University of Texas MD Anderson Cancer Center, investigators are currently conducting a phase II trial not only evaluating the role of capecitabine in place of IV 5-FU but also the role of oxaliplatin rather than cisplatin in the hopes of decreasing treatment-related toxicities without compromising efficacy (61).

MANAGEMENT OF REGIONAL LYMPH NODES

Regional metastases in lymph nodes can be managed successfully by the same chemoradiation schedule used to treat the primary anal canal tumor. As noted previously, nodal disease

TABLE 47.5

SELECTED STUDIES OF COMBINED 5-FLUOROURACIL (5-FU), CISPLATIN, AND RADIATION THERAPY (XRT)

Author	N	5-FU (mg/m^2/d)	Cisplatin (mg/m^2/d)	XRT (Gy)	CR	5-Year OS
Doci et al. (101)	35	750, D1–4	100, D1	36–38	94%	37 months: 94%
Martenson et al. (41)	19	1,000, D1–4, D43–46	75, D1 and D43	59.4 (split dose)	68%	NS
Hung et al. (102)	92	250, M–F, through all XRT	4, M–F, through all XRT	55	NS	85%

CR, complete response; OS, overall survival; D, day; NS, nonsignificant.

at presentation may originate in the perirectal, obturator, or hypogastric nodes in approximately 30% of patients, and inguinal node metastases in approximately 5% to 10%, of patients at presentation (62,63). Perirectal lymphadenopathy is less concerning because it is included in the radiation fields, but involvement of the inguinal lymph nodes may affect the radiation fields. Because the inguinal lymph nodes will be covered in the initial radiation fields, boost technique will often be required if the inguinal lymph nodes are ≥1 cm at presentation. A large retrospective series noted improved 5-year OS in synchronous versus metachronous inguinal lymph node metastases (54.4% vs. 41.4%) (64).

Sentinel lymph node biopsy continues to be investigated as a possible option in identifying nodal involvement (62). Rates of nodal detection range from 66% to 100%. Radical dissection of the inguinal-femoral nodes, either before or after high-dose radiation treatment, should be avoided if possible because of the risk of poor wound healing, chronic leg edema, seroma, and lymphocele; limited excisions are preferred and may be curative (65). Patients with nodal metastases are at increased risk of extrapelvic metastases. Five-year survival rates are approximately 20% less than in those patients who do not have demonstrable inguinal or pelvic node metastases (66). Elective irradiation of normal inguinal-femoral nodes reduces the rate of delayed recurrence to <5% and is associated with little morbidity.

CLINICAL ASSESSMENT OF RESPONSE TO THERAPY

Early in the development of combined modality therapy programs, many investigators advocated elective biopsy at approximately 6 weeks after combined radiation and chemotherapy as indicated by the pivotal phase III studies (49,50). However, there is evidence that anal epidermoid cancers may take up to 8 to 12 weeks to regress. Therefore, a patient's tumors should be carefully assessed for degree of response before submitting the patient to an APR. If there is clinical evidence of response, it is recommended that the patient be evaluated again in ≥4 weeks if there is slow regression (67). It has been noted that an early elective biopsy may place the patient at risk for radionecrosis. Hence, most investigators now recommend a biopsy only when residual or recurrent cancer is suspected clinically, reserving biopsy for those patients in whom an APR is likely to be pursued, but histological confirmation is desired before proceeding with such a radical procedure.

RECURRENT OR RESIDUAL DISEASE: SALVAGE SURGERY

As stated previously, surgery in the form of an APR is now reserved for patients with residual or recurrent disease. The effectiveness of surgical salvage is typically lower than that expected with combined modality chemoradiation therapy with OS rates reported at 30% to 55% (40,65,68,69).

MANAGEMENT OF EXTRAPELVIC METASTASES

Extrapelvic metastasis occurs in 10% to 20% of patients. In the two large randomized trials comparing the addition of two courses of 5-FU and MMC plus radiation to radiation alone, the risk of extrapelvic metastases was not significantly reduced by the addition of chemotherapy. In the EORTC trial, the crude rates of metastases were 21% (RT alone) and 17% (RT plus chemotherapy) (49). The corresponding rates in the UKCCCR study were 17% (RT alone) and 10% (RT plus chemotherapy) (48). Little literature exists in the treatment and outcome of a patient with metastatic SCCA of the anal canal. The majority of existing literature is based on small single institution studies. It has been reported that untreated patients with visceral metastases had a short median survival of 8 months (70).

Similar to the chemoradiation therapy that is provided for locally advanced disease, combination chemotherapy regimens have been the most commonly used approach, with median OS ranging from 12 to 36 months.

5-Fluorouracil and Cisplatin

The most frequently used and the most widely reported combination for metastatic anal cancer is 5-FU and cisplatin, resulting in partial response rates of up to 50% and complete responses of only 15% (3). Ajani et al. described partial responses in liver metastases in two patients treated with cisplatin and floxuridine administered intra-arterially, and in another patient managed by IV cisplatin and 5-FU (71). Faivre et al. reported that the combination of 5-FU/cisplatin resulted in a response rate of 66% and a prolonged median survival of 34.5 months (72), whereas Tanum et al. reported a much shorter median survival duration of approximately 12 months following treatment with 5-FU and cisplatin (73). Mahjoubi et al. reported a retrospective analysis of 20 patients who received prior therapy for the primary carcinoma (74). In this series, patients were treated with continuous infusion 5-FU and cisplatin for recurrent, advanced locoregional, or metastatic disease. Two patients achieved a complete response, and nine achieved a partial response, for an overall response rate of 55%. Final results have yet to be published. CR lasting more than 3 years has been reported in one patient treated with 5-FU and cisplatin for metastatic anal carcinoma (75).

Other Potential Chemotherapy Agents in Treating Extrapelvic Metastases

Wilking et al. administered a three-drug combination, consisting of bleomycin, vincristine, and high-dose methotrexate, to 15 patients (76). Three of 12 evaluable patients had a partial response, resulting in a disappointingly short duration of response of <3 months. The ECOG has recently reported the results of their small phase II study of MMC, Adriamycin, and cisplatin (MAP) followed by bleomycin and CCNU in patients with advanced SCCA of the anal canal (77). This study was initiated in 1983 and accrued only 20 patients. The investigators reported a PR of 60% (95% CI, 36%–81%), and no CRs were observed. The median survival was only 15 months. The predominant toxicity reported was grade 3 hematologic toxicity noted in more than one-third of the patients. Other chemotherapy regimens that have been anecdotally noted to be effective include those used in other SCCA malignancies such as carboplatin, irinotecan, and the taxanes. Molecularly targeted agents (e.g., cetuximab) that are now considered standard of care in other gastrointestinal malignancies are not considered standard of care at this time in anal canal cancers but are currently being investigated.

Surgical Resection of Extrapelvic Metastasis

In cases of isolated metastasis, aggressive treatment may also include hepatic resection with a favorable outcome (78). However, in a multicenter analysis of 35 patients who underwent hepatic resection (the majority were isolated liver metastasis), 23 of which were anal carcinoma patients, the median time to recurrence was brief at 9.2 months, and the 5-year DFS was 24.5% (79).

SURVEILLANCE GUIDELINES

Current surveillance guidelines following complete response with chemoradiation treatment with curative intent include physical examination, including inguinal lymph node exam every 3 to 6 months for up to 5 years, and anoscopy or proctoscopy. For patients with T_{3-4} or node-positive disease, an annual CT scan of the chest, abdomen, and pelvis is recommended for the first 3 years of surveillance. For salvage surgery patients, a full clinical examination, including inguinal lymph node evaluation, should be completed every 3 to 6 months for 5 years, as well as an annual CT scan of the chest, abdomen, and pelvis.

INNOVATIVE APPROACHES IN THE TREATMENT OF ANAL CANAL CANCERS

Induction Chemotherapy

As stated previously, the promising results of the CALGB study (60) resulted in the addition of two cycles of induction chemotherapy in the RTOG 98-11 cisplatin arm (55). The DFS and OS of both arms were equivalent despite the use of induction chemotherapy. However, prior to the results of RTOG 98-11, two phase II studies were designed and are currently underway. Both studies include two cycles of 5-FU, cisplatin, followed by chemoradiation therapy with 5-FU, cisplatin, cetuximab, and XRT in the HIV-negative and HIV-positive patient population and are led by investigators at the cooperative groups of ECOG (ECOG 3205) and the HIV consortium (AMC-045), respectively. AMC-045 will not only be the first prospective study of chemoradiation therapy in the HIV-positive patient population, but it will also be the first study to evaluate the role of molecular targeted therapy in the form of cetuximab, a chimeric monoclonal antibody against the epidermal growth factor receptor in the HIV-positive patient population. Cetuximab is a promising radiation sensitizer that is currently approved in the treatment of locoregionally advanced SCCA of the head and neck (80).

Adjuvant Chemotherapy

Phase II studies are currently underway in the United Kingdom to evaluate the role of adjuvant chemotherapy. The National Research Cancer Network, in collaboration with investigators at the University College of London, is currently conducting a phase III trial known as ACT II. In ACT II, patients are randomized to one of four arms: A: 5-FU/MMC/XRT; B: 5-FU/MMC/XRT, followed by two cycles of adjuvant 5-FU/cisplatin; C: 5-FU/cisplatin/XRT; or D: 5-FU/cisplatin/XRT, followed by two cycles of adjuvant 5-FU/cisplatin. To date, ACT II has accrued 94% of the expected 784 patients (81). The primary end point is response rate.

Anal Cytology and Screening

Given the increased risk of contracting HPV and the likelihood of persistent HPV (13) in the HIV-positive patient population, these patients are at high risk for AIN and the subsequent development of SCCA of the anal canal. Although Papanicolaou smears have been used as a screening tool in the prevention of cervical cancer, the use of anal cytology or anoscopy is not currently recommended as a standard screening modality in high-risk patients, such as the HIV-positive population. When investigators provided an anal cytology screening service, an impressive positive predictive value of 95.7% ± 2.1% was noted, and an anal cytologic abnormality was able to predict high-grade anal dysplasia of 55.9% ± 5.1% (82).

Human Papillomavirus Vaccine

The approval of the HPV vaccine, Gardasil (Merck & Co., Inc., Whitehouse Stations, NJ), may suggest a future role in the prevention of anal cancer. Gardasil protects against HPV types 6, 11, 16, and 18 (quadrivalent) and is currently indicated in the prevention of cervical cancer in girls and women ages 9 to 26, with a recommended vaccination at the age of 11 to 12 years old. Two prior phase III studies have demonstrated 100% efficacy in the prevention of persistent type-specific HPV infections and CIN 2/3, after a follow-up period of up to 5 years, among subjects who were adherent to the study protocol (83,84). Gardasil is given as three injections over 6 months. Common toxicities reported include pain, swelling, pruritus, and erythema at the injection site, as well as fever, nausea, and dizziness. No treatment-related deaths were noted. The duration of vaccinated immunity is unknown at this time. However, recent controversy has arisen regarding whether the vaccines should be mandated in adolescents and whether there are any unknown long-term effects of these vaccines (85). Currently, a study has been initiated in 4,000 men, including 500 MSM, evaluating it as a potential tool of prevention on the horizon. Preliminary results are expected in early 2008 (86). Despite the lack of current approval by the U.S. Food and Drug Administration, off-label use has been initiated due to the large number of requests in the HIV-positive patient population (86).

UNCOMMON ANAL CANAL CANCERS

Carcinoma of the Anal Margin

Regardless of histologic type, tumors of the anal margin are treated like epidermoid carcinomas of the skin. Generally, carcinoma of the anal margin has a more favorable prognosis than SCCA of the anal canal (87). Most investigators recommend wide local excision as treatment of $T_1N_0M_0$ anal margin tumors (67). Resection of these lesions should include a 1-cm margin of normal tissue, without sacrifice of anal continence. When the tumor involves >50% of the circumference of the anus, authorities have advocated performing an APR. In some instances, primarily in T_{2-4} or node-positive disease, treatment may involve radiation (88,89) or combined chemoradiation (90).

Most local recurrences are treated with repeat local excision. A more extensive surgical resection may be required for a recurrence that involves the deep muscles, perineural tissue, vascular system, or lymphatic system. Preoperative chemoradiation can be used to facilitate resection, unless the patient was recently irradiated. Overall, the survival rate for superficial anal margin tumors is favorable, exceeding 80%.

Adenocarcinomas of the Anal Canal

Adenocarcinomas of the anal canal are rare. Most arise from rectal glandular mucosa that extends below the upper limit of the anal canal. These adenocarcinomas are generally treated similarly to those confined to the rectum. Consequently, unlike the chemoradiation treatment of SCCA of the anal canal with curative intent, chemoradiation is used in the neoadjuvant or adjuvant setting, as in the treatment of rectal carcinoma. Overall, anal adenocarcinoma is more aggressive than SCCA of the anal canal and is at higher risk for local ($p = 0.004$) and distant recurrence ($p < 0.001$) (91). Men (0.37/100,000) are also more prone to develop anal adenocarcinoma when compared to women (0.25/100,000) (6). Anal adenocarcinomas are usually managed by APR and colostomy. Five-year survival rates after surgery alone are <50%, with local recurrence rates of approximately 25% (92). Beal et al. reported that combined chemoradiation therapy in the neoadjuvant or adjuvant setting resulted in a median OS of 26 months, local failure rate of 37%, and a 2-year actuarial survival of 62% (93). These tumors are much more aggressive and must be followed diligently for the development of metastatic disease. The expected 5-year survival rate for anal adenocarcinoma relative to SCCA in males (51% vs. 62%) versus females (48% vs. 67%) is significantly less (6).

Management of Melanomas of the Anal Canal

Primary melanoma of the anal canal is a rare pathological event and only represents 1% of all invasive tumors of the anal canal. Because of its rarity, it may be confused with hemorrhoids or a rectal polyp, causing a delay in diagnosis and therapy. Anal melanomas arise most frequently in the mid and upper canal, around the proximal pecten and transitional zone. Macroscopically, the tumors are polypoid and pigmented and arise near the dentate line (94). Microscopically, the tumor cells are arranged in nests and individual cells may be epithelioid or spindled and are characterized by immunostaining specific for the melanosome protein HMB-453.

Surgical therapy in the management of anal melanoma is uncertain and controversial, varying by stage of the disease. Treatment approaches may include wide local excision or an APR. Resection margins for wide local excision should include 2 cm of normal tissue surrounding the tumor, although this is sometimes not possible if continence is to be preserved. Memorial Sloan-Kettering reported on 71 cases with resectable melanoma of the anorectum over a 64-year period; the 5-year DFS rate in 43 patients treated by APR was only 40% in node-negative patients relative to 11% of patients with node-positive disease (95). Radiation may be helpful for palliation of bleeding or pain.

Overall, the prognosis of melanoma of the anal canal will often result in a 5-year survival rate of <20% despite an aggressive, multimodality approach and may be attributed to the fact that a high percentage of patients present with advanced stage disease (94). As in other melanomas, sentinel lymph node biopsy may be helpful in appropriately staging the patient (96). Patients with persistent local or advanced disease are generally treated with systemic therapy similar to that used for metastatic cutaneous melanoma. Response and survival rates remain poor.

Small and Large Cell Neuroendocrine Tumors of the Anal Canal

These rare cancers behave similarly to small cell carcinomas of the lung; they metastasize early and have a poor prognosis, with a median survival of 10.4 months (97). These tumors tend to be highly aggressive, often with lymph node, liver, and lung metastasis at presentation (29). The tumor cells can form sheets, nests, trabeculae and rosettes and are smaller than lymphocytes and contain minimal cytoplasm. Immunohistochemical (IHC) pathological markers that may be used include neurone-specific enolase, chromogranin A, synaptophysin, CD56, and Leu-7/CD57.

In contrast to small cell carcinoma, large cell neuroendocrine tumors are extremely rare. The cells appear round or polygonal with abundant cytoplasm, prominent nucleoli, and a coarse chromatin pattern. IHC for at least one of three neuroendocrine markers (neuron-specific enolase, chromogranin A, synaptophysin) in 10% of tumour cells is suggested as a minimum diagnostic criterion for large cell neuroendocrine carcinoma (97). The primary cancer is managed by surgery or radiation, with or without chemotherapy, with no consensus on which approach is more effective. Systemic chemotherapy similar to that used for small cell cancers arising elsewhere may be given for this variant but is of unpredictable value. Bernick et al. described the largest series of 16 cases, with no significant difference in OS between either small or large cell neuroendocrine carcinoma of the anal canal (97).

CONCLUSION

As demonstrated in this chapter, anal carcinoma is composed of many facets with the majority of patients presenting with SCCA of the anal canal. Despite the success of chemoradiation therapy in cure, the rarity of this tumor has hindered its progress regarding treatment advances in chemotherapy choices, the inclusion of molecular targeted therapy, radiation techniques, and revisions in treatment schedule. Additional studies are currently underway for screening and prevention in high-risk patients. Given the rarity of anal carcinoma, future progress depends on the willingness of physicians to enroll their patients in existing and future clinical trials.

References

1. Nigro ND, Vaitkevicius VK, Considine B, Jr. Combined therapy for cancer of the anal canal: a preliminary report. *Dis Colon Rectum* 1974;17(3):354–356.
2. Fenger C. Histology of the anal canal. *Am J Surg Pathol* 1988;12(1):41–55.
3. Cummings BJ. Metastatic anal cancer: the search for cure. *Onkologie* 2006;29(1–2):5–6.
4. Jemal A, Siegel R, Ward E, Murray T, Xu J, Thun MJ. Cancer statistics, 2007. *CA Cancer J Clin* 2007;57(1):43–66.
5. Clark MA, Hartley A, Geh JI. Cancer of the anal canal. *Lancet Oncol* 2004;5(3):149–157.
6. Johnson LG, Madeleine MM, Newcomer LM, Schwartz SM, Daling JR. Anal cancer incidence and survival: the surveillance, epidemiology, and end results experience, 1973–2000. *Cancer* 2004;101(2):281–288.
7. Centers for Disease Control and Prevention (CDC). *Human Papillomavirus: HPV Information for Clinicians* [brochure]. Atlanta, Ga: CDC; April 2007. Available at: http://www.cdc.gov/std/hpv/common-infection/CDC_HPV_ClinicianBro_HR.pdf. Accessed June 19, 2007.
8. Kagawa R, Yamaguchi T, Furuta R. Histological features of human papilloma virus 16 and its association with the development and progression of anal squamous cell carcinoma. *Surg Today* 2006;36(10):885–891.
9. Steenbergen RD, de Wilde J, Wilting SM, Brink AA, Snijders PJ, Meijer CJ. HPV-mediated transformation of the anogenital tract. *J Clin Virol* 2005;32(suppl 1):S25–S33.
10. Herrero R, Hildesheim A, Bratti C, et al. Population-based study of human papillomavirus infection and cervical neoplasia in rural Costa Rica. *J Natl Cancer Inst* 2000;92(6):464–474.
11. Tilston P. Anal human papillomavirus and anal cancer. *J Clin Pathol* 1997;50(8):625–634.
12. Woodman CB, Collins S, Winter H, et al. Natural history of cervical human papillomavirus infection in young women: a longitudinal cohort study. *Lancet* 2001;357(9271):1831–1836.
13. Hagensee ME, Cameron JE, Leigh JE, Clark RA. Human papillomavirus infection and disease in HIV-infected individuals. *Am J Med Sci* 2004;328(1):57–63.
14. Rihet S, Bellaich P, Lorenzato M, et al. Human papillomaviruses and DNA ploidy in anal condylomata acuminata. *Histol Histopathol* 2000;15(1):79–84.

15. Gervaz P, Hirschel B, Morel P. Molecular biology of squamous cell carcinoma of the anus. *Br J Surg* 2006;93(5):531–538.

16. Tran N, Rose BR, O'Brien CJ. Role of human papillomavirus in the etiology of head and neck cancer. *Head Neck* 2007;29(1):64–70.

17. Halperin DT. Heterosexual anal intercourse: prevalence, cultural factors, and HIV infection and other health risks, part I. *AIDS Patient Care STDS* 1999;13(12):717–730.

18. Eng C. Anal cancer: current and future methodology. *Cancer Invest* 2006;24(5):535–544.

19. Palefsky JM, Holly EA, Ralston ML, Jay N, Berry JM, Darragh TM. High incidence of anal high-grade squamous intra-epithelial lesions among HIV-positive and HIV-negative homosexual and bisexual men. *AIDS* 1998;12(5):495–503.

20. Biggar RJ, Burnett W, Mikl J, Nasca P. Cancer among New York men at risk of acquired immunodeficiency syndrome. *Int J Cancer* 1989;43(6):979–985.

21. Selik RM, Rabkin CS. Cancer death rates associated with human immunodeficiency virus infection in the United States. *J Natl Cancer Inst* 1998;90(17):1300–1302.

22. Melbye M, Cote TR, Kessler L, Gail M, Biggar RJ. High incidence of anal cancer among AIDS patients. The AIDS/Cancer Working Group. *Lancet* 1994;343(8898):636–639.

23. Frisch M, Biggar RJ, Engels EA, Goedert JJ. Association of cancer with AIDS-related immunosuppression in adults. *JAMA* 2001;285(13):1736–1745.

24. Koblin BA, Hessol NA, Zauber AG, et al. Increased incidence of cancer among homosexual men, New York City and San Francisco, 1978–1990. *Am J Epidemiol* 1996;144(10):916–923.

25. Palefsky JM, Holly EA, Efirdc JT, et al. Anal intraepithelial neoplasia in the highly active antiretroviral therapy era among HIV-positive men who have sex with men. *AIDS* 2005;19(13):1407–1414.

26. Busnach G, Piselli P, Arbustini E, et al. Immunosuppression and cancer: a comparison of risks in recipients of organ transplants and in HIV-positive individuals. *Transplant Proc* 2006;38(10):3533–3535.

27. Roka S, Rasoul-Rockenschaub S, Roka J, Kirnbauer R, Muhlbacher F, Salat A. Prevalence of anal HPV infection in solid-organ transplant patients prior to immunosuppression. *Transpl Int* 2004;17(7):366–369.

28. Frisch M, Glimelius B, Wohlfahrt J, Adami HO, Melbye M. Tobacco smoking as a risk factor in anal carcinoma: an antiestrogenic mechanism? *J Natl Cancer Inst* 1999;91(8):708–715.

29. Balachandra B, Marcus V, Jass JR. Poorly differentiated tumours of the anal canal: a diagnostic strategy for the surgical pathologist. *Histopathology* 2007;50(1):163–174.

30. Khatri VP, Chopra S. Clinical presentation, imaging, and staging of anal cancer. *Surg Oncol Clin N Am* 2004;13(2):295–308.

31. Maggard MA, Beanes SR, Ko CY. Anal canal cancer: a population-based reappraisal. *Dis Colon Rectum* 2003;46(11):1517–1523; discussion 23–24; author reply 24.

32. Boman BM, Moertel CG, O'Connell MJ, et al. Carcinoma of the anal canal: a clinical and pathologic study of 188 cases. *Cancer* 1984;54(1):114–125.

33. Golden GT, Horsley JS, III. Surgical management of epidermoid carcinoma of the anus. *Am J Surg* 1976;131(3):275–280.

34. Cotter SE, Grigsby PW, Siegel BA, et al. FDG-PET/CT in the evaluation of anal carcinoma. *Int J Radiat Oncol Biol Phys* 2006;65(3):720–725.

35. Nguyen BD, Ram PC, Roarke MC. F-18 FDG PET/CT imaging of anal canal squamous cell carcinoma. *Clin Nucl Med* 2007;32(3):234–236.

36. Nagle D, Henry D, Mastoris J, Chmielewski L, Rosenstock J. The utility of PET scanning in the clinical management of squamous cell carcinoma of the anal canal. Presented at: American Society of Clinical Oncology 2006; Orlando, Fla; 2006; Abstract #4152.

37. Greene F, Page D, Fleming I. *AJCC Cancer Staging Manual*. 6th ed. New York, NY: Springer; 2002.

38. Sobin L, Wittekind C. *UICC: TNM Classification of Malignant Tumors—Digestive System Tumors*. 6th ed. Hoboken, NJ: John Wiley & Sons; 2002.

39. Mullen JT, Rodriguez-Bigas MA, Chang GJ, et al. Results of surgical salvage after failed chemoradiation therapy for epidermoid carcinoma of the anal canal. *Ann Surg Oncol* 2007;14(2):478–483.

40. Papaconstantinou HT, Bullard KM, Rothenberger DA, Madoff RD. Salvage abdominoperineal resection after failed Nigro protocol: modest success, major morbidity. *Colorectal Dis* 2006;8(2):124–129.

41. Martenson JA, Lipsitz SR, Wagner H, Jr, et al. Initial results of a phase II trial of high dose radiation therapy, 5-fluorouracil, and cisplatin for patients with anal cancer (E4292): an Eastern Cooperative Oncology Group study. *Int J Radiat Oncol Biol Phys* 1996;35(4):745–749.

42. Svensson C, Goldman S, Friberg B. Radiation treatment of epidermoid cancer of the anus. *Int J Radiat Oncol Biol Phys* 1993;27(1):67–73.

43. Deniaud-Alexandre E, Touboul E, Tiret E, et al. Results of definitive irradiation in a series of 305 epidermoid carcinomas of the anal canal. *Int J Radiat Oncol Biol Phys* 2003;56(5):1259–1273.

44. Papillon J, Mayer M, Montbarbon JF, Gerard JP, Chassard JL, Bailly C. A new approach to the management of epidermoid carcinoma of the anal canal. *Cancer* 1983;51(10):1830–1837.

45. Cummings BJ, Keane TJ, O'Sullivan B, Wong CS, Catton CN. Epidermoid anal cancer: treatment by radiation alone or by radiation and 5-fluorouracil with and without mitomycin C. *Int J Radiat Oncol Biol Phys* 1991;21(5):1115–1125.

46. Newman G, Calverley DC, Acker BD, Manji M, Hay J, Flores AD. The management of carcinoma of the anal canal by external beam radiotherapy, experience in Vancouver 1971–1988. *Radiother Oncol* 1992;25(3):196–202.

47. Gerard JP, Chapet O, Romestaing P, Favrel V, Barbet N, Mornex F. [Local excision and adjuvant radiotherapy for rectal adenocarcinoma T1–2 N0.] *Gastroenterol Clin Biol* 2000;24(4):430–435.

48. Epidermoid anal cancer: results from the UKCCCR randomised trial of radiotherapy alone versus radiotherapy, 5-fluorouracil, and mitomycin. UKCCCR Anal Cancer Trial Working Party. UK Co-ordinating Committee on Cancer Research. *Lancet* 1996;348(9034):1049–1054.

49. Bartelink H, Roelofsen F, Eschwege F, et al. Concomitant radiotherapy and chemotherapy is superior to radiotherapy alone in the treatment of locally advanced anal cancer: results of a phase III randomized trial of the European Organization for Research and Treatment of Cancer Radiotherapy and Gastrointestinal Cooperative Groups. *J Clin Oncol* 1997;15(5):2040–2049.

50. Flam M, John M, Pajak TF, et al. Role of mitomycin in combination with fluorouracil and radiotherapy, and of salvage chemoradiation in the definitive nonsurgical treatment of epidermoid carcinoma of the anal canal: results of a phase III randomized intergroup study. *J Clin Oncol* 1996;14(9):2527–2539.

51. Vordermark D, Sailer M, Flentje M, Thiede A, Kolbl O. Curative-intent radiation therapy in anal carcinoma: quality of life and sphincter function. *Radiother Oncol* 1999;52(3):239–243.

52. Vordermark D, Sailer M, Flentje M, Thiede A, Kolbl O. Impaired sphincter function and good quality of life in anal carcinoma patients after radiotherapy: a paradox? *Front Radiat Ther Oncol* 2002;37:132–139.

53. Meyer J, Czito B, Yin FF, Willett C. Advanced radiation therapy technologies in the treatment of rectal and anal cancer: intensity-modulated photon therapy and proton therapy. *Clin Colorectal Cancer* 2007;6(5):348–356.

54. Milano MT, Jani AB, Farrey KJ, Rash C, Heimann R, Chmura SJ. Intensity-modulated radiation therapy (IMRT) in the treatment of anal cancer: toxicity and clinical outcome. *Int J Radiat Oncol Biol Phys* 2005;63(2):354–361.

55. Ajani J, Winter K, Gunderson L, et al. A phase III randomized study of 5-fluorouracil (5-FU), mitomycin, and radiotherapy versus 5-fluorouracil, cisplatin and radiotherapy in carcinoma of the anal canal. Presented at: American Society of Clinical Oncology 2006; Atlanta, Ga; 2006; Abstract #4009.

56. Rich TA, Ajani JA, Morrison WH, Ota D, Levin B. Chemoradiation therapy for anal cancer: radiation plus continuous infusion of 5-fluorouracil with or without cisplatin. *Radiother Oncol* 1993;27(3):209–215.

57. Graf R, Wust P, Hildebrandt B, et al. Impact of overall treatment time on local control of anal cancer treated with radiochemotherapy. *Oncology* 2003;65(1):14–22.

58. Wong J, Tsang RW, Cummings BJ, et al. Proliferation parameters in epidermoid carcinomas of the anal canal. *Radiother Oncol* 2000;56(3):349–353.

59. Meyer A, Meier Zu Eissen J, Karstens JH, Bremer M. Chemoradiotherapy in patients with anal cancer: impact of length of unplanned treatment interruption on outcome. *Acta Oncol* 2006;45(6):728–35.

60. Meropol N, Niedzwiecki D, Shank B. Combined-modality therapy of poor prognosis anal carcinoma: a phase II study of the Cancer and Leukemia Group B (CALGB). Presented at: ASCO GI 2005; San Francisco, Calif; 2005; Abstract #238.

61. Eng C, Crane C, Rosner G, et al. A phase II study of capecitabine plus oxaliplatin and radiation therapy, XELOX-XRT, in locally advanced squamous cell carcinoma of the anal canal: a preliminary toxicity analysis. Presented at: Gastrointestinal Cancer Symposium 2005; Hollywood, Fla; 2005; Abstract #216.

62. Damin DC, Rosito MA, Schwartsmann G. Sentinel lymph node in carcinoma of the anal canal: a review. *Eur J Surg Oncol* 2006;32(3):247–252.

63. Perera D, Pathma-Nathan N, Rabbitt P, Hewett P, Rieger N. Sentinel node biopsy for squamous-cell carcinoma of the anus and anal margin. *Dis Colon Rectum* 2003;46(8):1027–1029; discussion 30–31.

64. Gerard JP, Chapet O, Samiei F, et al. Management of inguinal lymph node metastases in patients with carcinoma of the anal canal: experience in a series of 270 patients treated in Lyon and review of the literature. *Cancer* 2001;92(1):77–84.

65. Akbari RP, Paty PB, Guillem JG, et al. Oncologic outcomes of salvage surgery for epidermoid carcinoma of the anus initially managed with combined modality therapy. *Dis Colon Rectum* 2004;47(7):1136–1144.

66. Swan MC, Furniss D, Cassell OC. Surgical management of metastatic inguinal lymphadenopathy. *BMJ* 2004;329(7477):1272–1276.

67. National Comprehensive Cancer Network (NCCN). *NCCN: Clinical Practice Guidelines in Oncology*. Jenkintown, Pa: NCCN; 2007. Available at: http://www.nccn.org/professionals/physician_gls/f_guidelines.asp?button=I+Agree#site. Accessed June 19, 2007.

68. Ferenschild FT, Vermaas M, Hofer SO, Verhoef C, Eggermont AM, de Wilt JH. Salvage abdominoperineal resection and perineal wound healing in local recurrent or persistent anal cancer. *World J Surg* 2005;29(11):1452–1457.

69. Renehan AG, Saunders MP, Schofield PF, O'Dwyer ST. Patterns of local disease failure and outcome after salvage surgery in patients with anal cancer. *Br J Surg* 2005;92(5):605–614.

70. Greenall MJ, Magill GB, Quan SH, DeCosse JJ. Recurrent epidermoid cancer of the anus. *Cancer* 1986;57(7):1437–1441.

71. Ajani JA, Carrasco CH, Jackson DE, Wallace S. Combination of cisplatin plus fluoropyrimidine chemotherapy effective against liver metastases from carcinoma of the anal canal. *Am J Med* 1989;87(2):221–224.

72. Faivre C, Rougier P, Ducreux M, et al. [5-Fluorouracil and cisplatinum combination chemotherapy for metastatic squamous-cell anal cancer.] *Bull Cancer* 1999;86(10):861–865.

73. Tanum G. Treatment of relapsing anal carcinoma. *Acta Oncol* 1993; 32(1):33–35.

74. Mahjoubi M, Sadek H, Francois E. Epidermoid anal canal carcinoma: activity of cisplatinum and continuous 5-fluorouracil in metastatic and/or local recurrent disease [abstract #114]. *Proc Am Soc Clin Oncol* 1990;9.

75. Jaiyesimi IA, Pazdur R. Cisplatin and 5-fluorouracil as salvage therapy for recurrent metastatic squamous cell carcinoma of the anal canal. *Am J Clin Oncol* 1993;16(6):536–540.

76. Wilking N, Petrelli N, Herrera L, Mittelman A. Phase II study of combination bleomycin, vincristine and high-dose methotrexate (BOM) with leucovorin rescue in advanced squamous cell carcinoma of the anal canal. *Cancer Chemother Pharmacol* 1985;15(3):300–302.

77. Jhawer M, Mani S, Lefkopoulou M, et al. Phase II study of mitomycin-C, Adriamycin, cisplatin (MAP) and bleomycin-CCNU in patients with advanced cancer of the anal canal: an Eastern Cooperative Oncology Group study E7282. *Invest New Drugs* 2006.

78. Tokar M, Bobilev D, Zalmanov S, Geffen DB, Walfisch S. Combined multimodal approach to the treatment of metastatic anal carcinoma: report of a case and review of the literature. *Onkologie* 2006;29(1–2):30–32.

79. Pawlik TM, Bauer TW, Reddy SK, et al. Hepatic resection for metastatic squamous cell carcinoma to the liver: a multi-center analysis. Presented at: 2007 Gastrointestinal Cancers Symposium 2007; Orlando, Fla; 2007; Abstract #192. Available at: http://www.asco.org/portal/site/ASCO/menuitem.34d60f5624ba07fd506fe310ee37a01dd/?vgnextoid=76f8201eb61a7010VgnVCM100000ed730ad1RCRD&vmview=abst_detail_view&confID=45&abstractID

80. Bonner JA, Harari PM, Giralt J, et al. Radiotherapy plus cetuximab for squamous-cell carcinoma of the head and neck. *N Engl J Med* 2006; 354(6):567–578.

81. UK Clinical Research Network. Study: ACT II: a second UK phase III anal cancer trial: a trial of chemoradiation and maintenance therapy for patients with anal cancer. 2007. Available at: http://pfsearch.ukcrn.org.uk/StudyDetail.aspx?TopicID=1&StudyID=691. Accessed June 19, 2007.

82. Cranston RD, Hart SD, Gornbein JA, Hirschowitz SL, Cortina R, Moe AA. The prevalence, and predictive value, of abnormal anal cytology to diagnose anal dysplasia in a population of HIV-positive men who have sex with men. *Int J STD AIDS* 2007;18(2):77–80.

83. Ferris DG. An update of clinical trial results with preventative HPV vaccines. Presented at: "Facing the Future: The Impact on HPV Vaccination on Adolescent Health" Symposium; Boston, Mass; March 24, 2006. Available at: http://www.medscape.com/viewarticle/533550_5. Accessed June 19, 2007.

84. Saslow D, Castle PE, Cox JT, et al. American Cancer Society guideline for human papillomavirus (HPV) vaccine use to prevent cervical cancer and its precursors. *CA Cancer J Clin* 2007;57(1):7–28.

85. Tanne JH. Texas governor is criticised for decision to vaccinate all girls against HPV. *BMJ* 2007;334(7589):332–333.

86. Tuller D. HPV vaccine may help prevent anal cancer. *International Herald Tribune* 2007. http://www.iht.com/articles/2007/01/31/healthscience/sncancer.php

87. Chawla AK, Willett CG. Squamous cell carcinoma of the anal canal and anal margin. *Hematol Oncol Clin North Am* 2001;15(2): 321–344, vi.

88. Chapet O, Gerard JP, Mornex F, et al. Prognostic factors of squamous cell carcinoma of the anal margin treated by radiotherapy: the Lyon experience. *Int J Colorectal Dis* 2007;22(2):191–199.

89. Peiffert D, Bey P, Pernot M, et al. Conservative treatment by irradiation of epidermoid carcinomas of the anal margin. *Int J Radiat Oncol Biol Phys* 1997;39(1):57–66.

90. Dwyer MK, Gebski VJ, Jayamohan J. The bottom line: outcomes after conservation treatment in anal cancer. *Australas Radiol* 2006;50(1): 46–51.

91. Papagikos M, Crane CH, Skibber J, et al. Chemoradiation for adenocarcinoma of the anus. *Int J Radiat Oncol Biol Phys* 2003;55(3):669–678.

92. Tarazi R, Nelson RL. Anal adenocarcinoma: a comprehensive review. *Semin Surg Oncol* 1994;10(3):235–240.

93. Beal KP, Wong D, Guillem JG, et al. Primary adenocarcinoma of the anus treated with combined modality therapy. *Dis Colon Rectum* 2003;46(10):1320–1324.

94. Rodrigues G, Kudva A, Kudva R. Primary anal malignant melanoma. *Internet J Surg* 2003;4:(1). Available at: http://www.ispub.com/ostia/index.php?xmlFilePath=journals/ijs/vol4n1/anal.xml. Accessed June 19, 2007.

95. Brady MS, Kavolius JP, Quan SH. Anorectal melanoma: a 64-year experience at Memorial Sloan-Kettering Cancer Center. *Dis Colon Rectum* 1995;38(2):146–151.

96. Sanli Y, Turkmen C, Kurul S, Tas F, Mudun A, Cantez S. Sentinel lymph node biopsy for the staging of anal melanoma: report of two cases. *Ann Nucl Med* 2006;20(9):629–631.

97. Bernick PE, Klimstra DS, Shia J, et al. Neuroendocrine carcinomas of the colon and rectum. *Dis Colon Rectum* 2004;47(2):163–169.

98. Leichman L, Nigro N, Vaitkevicius VK, et al. Cancer of the anal canal: model for preoperative adjuvant combined modality therapy. *Am J Med* 1985;78(2):211–215.

99. Sischy B, Doggett RL, Krall JM, et al. Definitive irradiation and chemotherapy for radiosensitization in management of anal carcinoma: interim report on Radiation Therapy Oncology Group study no. 8314. *J Natl Cancer Inst* 1989;81(11):850–856.

100. Ferrigno R, Nakamura RA, Dos Santos Novaes PE, et al. Radiochemotherapy in the conservative treatment of anal canal carcinoma: retrospective analysis of results and radiation dose effectiveness. *Int J Radiat Oncol Biol Phys* 2005;61(4):1136–1142.

101. Doci R, Zucali R, La Monica G, et al. Primary chemoradiation therapy with fluorouracil and cisplatin for cancer of the anus: results in 35 consecutive patients. *J Clin Oncol* 1996;14(12):3121–3125.

102. Hung A, Crane C, Delclos M, et al. Cisplatin-based combined modality therapy for anal carcinoma: a wider therapeutic index. *Cancer* 2003;97(5): 1195–1202.

CHAPTER 48 ■ NEUROENDOCRINE TUMORS OF THE GASTROINTESTINAL TRACT

MATTHEW H. KULKE AND CHANDRAJIT P. RAUT

INTRODUCTION

Neuroendocrine tumors are generally subcategorized as either carcinoid tumors or pancreatic endocrine tumors. Both tumor types are characterized by variable, but most often indolent, biological behavior, and have, in most cases, characteristic well-differentiated histologic features. Neuroendocrine tumors are typically composed of small cells containing regular, well-rounded nuclei, and are characterized histologically by positive reactions to silver stains and to neuroendocrine markers, including neuron-specific enolase, synaptophysin, and chromogranin (1). The cytoplasm of these cells contains numerous membrane-bound neurosecretory granules, which contain a variety of hormones and biogenic amines. The release of substances such as serotonin, gastrin, glucagon, and insulin into the systemic circulation results in the unique systemic syndromes associated with neuroendocrine tumors.

For patients with localized disease, surgical resection alone is often curative. Patients with metastatic disease, however, often present a therapeutic challenge. Although somatostatin analogs are highly effective in controlling symptoms of hormonal secretion, they are only rarely associated with tumor regression. Selected patients with hepatic metastases may benefit from surgical debulking, embolization, or other ablative therapies. The clinical benefit associated with the administration of systemic agents such as interferon-alpha (IFN-α) or cytotoxic chemotherapy is less clear, and the widespread use of such regimens has been limited by their relatively modest antitumor activity as well as concerns regarding their potential toxicity. The mixed clinical results seen with these agents in neuroendocrine tumors has led to great interest in the development of novel treatment approaches for patients with advanced disease.

PANCREATIC ENDOCRINE TUMORS

Incidence and Etiology

Pancreatic endocrine tumors are relatively rare, with an estimated incidence of <1 per 100,000 individuals (2). These tumors may arise either sporadically or, less commonly, in patients with multiple endocrine neoplasia type 1 (MEN 1). MEN 1 is most commonly diagnosed in patients with gastrinomas and insulinomas (3,4). MEN 1 is an autosomal dominant syndrome associated with mutations in the *MEN 1* tumor suppressor gene, and characterized by multiple neuroendocrine tumors involving the parathyroid and pituitary glands, as well as the pancreas. The protein encoded by *MEN 1*, menin, has been shown to localize to the nucleus and regulate gene transcription (5). *MEN 1* is located on chromosome 11q13, and loss of 11q13 has been demonstrated in both MEN 1-associated pancreatic neuroendocrine tumors and in >50% of sporadic pancreatic neuroendocrine tumors (6). Loss of heterozygosity in regions of chromosomes 22q, 9p, 6q, and 1 has also been observed in pancreatic neuroendocrine tumors, as have point mutations in the DPC4/Smad4 gene (7–11). In rare cases, pancreatic endocrine tumors may be associated with Von Hippel-Lindau disease (12).

Clinical Presentation

The clinical presentations of pancreatic endocrine tumors are diverse and are often related to symptoms of hormonal hypersecretion (Table 48.1). The best characterized of these syndromes are those associated with insulinoma, glucagonoma, VIPoma, and gastrinoma. Additional pancreatic neuroendocrine tumors include somatostatinomas and so-called "nonfunctioning" pancreatic neuroendocrine tumors, which are often associated with high serum levels of pancreatic polypeptide.

Insulinoma

Insulinomas have an estimated annual incidence of one to four cases per million persons (13). These tumors are most common in the fifth decade of life, but diagnoses have ranged from newborn up to the ninth decade (14). Between 8% and 10% of patients with insulinoma also have MEN 1 (13).

The clinical diagnosis of insulinoma is often related to symptoms of hypoglycemia. One of the first described patients with insulinoma is said to have "resembled an acute alcoholic—great motor activity, dancing and taking, squinting and frowning, apparently having hallucinations of sight and hearing, negatavistic, and difficult to control" (15). These symptoms are classic manifestations of hypoglycemia, which can cause both autonomic symptoms and central nervous system dysfunction. Hypoglycemic symptoms have been separated into two categories—adrenergic or neuroglycopenic. Adrenergic symptoms include nervousness, tremulousness, palpitations, anxiety, irritability, diaphoresis, hunger, and pallor, whereas neuroglycopenic symptoms include confusion, headache, personality changes, weakness, blurred vision, dizziness, amnesia, dysarthria, convulsions, and, in severe cases, loss of consciousness (14). The early symptoms of insulinoma can often be

TABLE 48.1

CLINICAL PRESENTATION OF PANCREATIC NEUROENDOCRINE TUMORS

Tumor	Symptoms or signs	Cell type	Incidence of metastases	Extrapancreatic location
Insulinoma	Hypoglycemia resulting in intermittent confusion, sweating, weakness, nausea; loss of consciousness may occur in severe cases	β cell	<15%	Rare
Glucagonoma	Rash (necrotizing migratory erythema), cachexia, diabetes, deep venous thrombosis	α cell	Majority	Rare
VIPoma, Verner-Morrison syndrome, WDHA syndrome	Profound secretory diarrhea, electrolyte disturbances	Non-β cell	Majority	10%
Gastrinoma, Zollinger-Ellison syndrome	Acid hypersecretion resulting in refractory peptic ulcer disease, abdominal pain, and diarrhea	Non-β cell	<50%	Frequently in duodenum
Somatostatinoma	Diabetes, diarrhea, cholelithiasis	δ cell	Majority	Rare
PPoma "nonfunctioning"	May be first diagnosed due to mass effect			

WDHA, watery diarrhea, hypokalemia, and achlorhydria.

nonspecific, and delays in diagnosis are common. The period from symptom onset to diagnosis may range from 2 weeks to 30 years (13). Indeed, in approximately half of cases, the diagnosis is not made until patients present in a hypoglycemic coma (16).

The combination of symptoms of hypoglycemia, inappropriately high insulin levels with associated documented blood glucose levels of <50 mg/dL, and symptom relief with administration of glucose, constitutes Whipple's triad, first described in 1935 and still useful in the diagnosis of insulinoma (17). The diagnosis of insulinoma can generally be confirmed with the detection of elevated fasting insulin and C-peptide levels in the plasma and the tolbutamide test (14,18).

Because of their association with hypoglycemia, insulinomas are typically small and are often detected before they grow to 2.5 cm (16). In 80% of cases, the tumor is detected without evidence of metastases. Because of their small size, standard imaging modalities such as computed tomography (CT), magnetic resonance imaging (MRI), and angiography are often unsuccessful in identifying the tumor (19,20). Nearly all insulinomas are found in the pancreas, and further imaging studies should focus on this area (14). Endoscopic ultrasound has been reported to be highly sensitive in the preoperative localization of insulinomas (21–23). Intraoperative localization techniques, which include both careful palpation of the pancreas and the use of intraoperative ultrasound, remain the most reliable way to localize insulinomas (19).

Dietary modification, together with the administration of diazoxide, is usually successful in the initial management of hypoglycemia due to an insulinoma (24). Isolated insulinomas are generally treated with enucleation; long-term survival following surgery in this patient population exceeds 90% (13). The role of surgical resection in patients with MEN 1 syndrome remains controversial because of the risk of additional tumors within the remaining pancreas and elsewhere. A more aggressive surgical approach, generally with subtotal pancreatectomy, may be undertaken in these patients due to the risk of multiple tumors and a higher rate of recurrence (25,26).

Gastrinomas and Zollinger-Ellison Syndrome

The gastrinoma syndrome, first described by Zollinger and Ellison, is characterized by gastric hypersecretion (27). Gastrin, which is normally secreted by the G cells in the gastric antrum, not only stimulates acid secretion in parietal cells but also acts as a trophic factor, causing parietal cell hyperplasia and an increase in maximal acid output. The profound acid hypersecretion associated with gastrinomas typically causes abdominal pain due to peptic ulcer disease, diarrhea, and reflux esophagitis (28).

Gastrinomas are slightly more common in males than in females, and the median age at presentation is between 40 and 50 years (28–30). The diagnosis of gastrinoma is often delayed due to the fact that most patients are initially diagnosed with benign peptic ulcer disease (28,29). A gastrinoma should be suspected in the setting of nonhealing peptic ulcers and a fasting gastrin level of >100 pg/mL (31). The diagnosis can be complicated by the fact that several other conditions can also cause moderate elevations of serum gastrin. The most common of these is concomitant therapy with proton pump inhibitors. In equivocal cases, the documentation of increased basal acid output and a positive secretin provocative test may be necessary to confirm the diagnosis (31–33).

Proton pump inhibitors are highly effective in controlling the symptoms associated with gastric hypersecretion (34,35). The localization and surgical resection of gastrinomas often presents a greater challenge. The overwhelming majority of gastrinomas is found in the "gastrinoma triangle," an area bounded by the cystic and common bile ducts, the duodenum, and the pancreas (36). Within this area, tumors are most commonly found in the duodenum or in surrounding lymph nodes, and less than half are found in the pancreas (29,30,37). Duodenal gastrinomas typically measure <1 cm, making them virtually impossible to detect with standard preoperative imaging studies. Although techniques such as endoscopic ultrasound and somatostatin scintigraphy appear to have some utility in the preoperative evaluation of patients with gastrinoma, intraoperative palpation and duodenotomy is often still required (29,30,38).

Surgical cure is possible in more than half of the patients with sporadic gastrinomas and localized disease (29). Many gastrinomas in patients with MEN 1 occur in the duodenum, and many of these tumors are not identifiable with preoperative imaging studies. Surgical exploration may therefore be necessary for tumor localization (30,39). In the approximate 25% of patients with Zollinger-Ellison syndrome and MEN 1, surgical resection remains controversial (40). In this patient population, a multiplicity of tumors makes curative resection difficult (41). In cases where an isolated lesion is seen with preoperative imaging studies, however, an attempt at resection may still be warranted (32,42,43). Even after extensive duodenal exploration in such cases, curative resection in patients with MEN 1 may still not be feasible (44). In patients with unresectable or metastatic disease, treatment with somatostatin analogs has been associated with improved control of serum gastrin levels and, in some cases, with tumor stabilization or regression (45).

Glucagonomas

Glucagonomas are among the rarest of the pancreatic endocrine tumors and typically present in the seventh decade of life. Approximately 80% of cases are sporadic, and 20% are associated with MEN 1 (46,47). Although glucagonomas may be associated with diabetes mellitus, clinically significant hyperglycemia occurs in only half of such patients. Patients with glucagonomas are frequently intially diagnosed by a dermatologist, after presenting with necrolytic migratory erythema (Fig. 48.1). This rash, characterized by raised erythematous patches beginning in the perineum and subsequently involving the trunk and extremeties, is found in more than two-thirds of all patients. The etiology of the rash is uncertain; possible causes include amino acid deficiency and zinc deficiency (48,49).

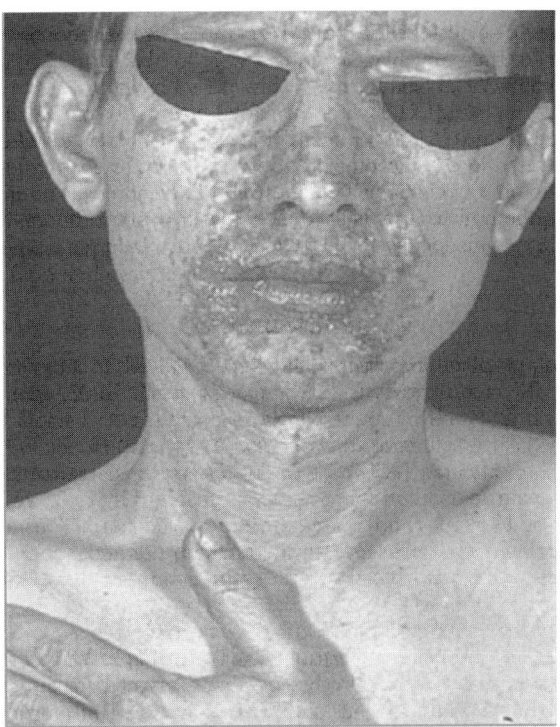

FIGURE 48.1. Necrolytic migratory erythema associated with glucagonoma syndrome (See also color Figure 48.1).

Plasma glucagon levels, which are <50 pg/mL in normal patients, often exceed 1,000 pg/mL in patients with glucagonomas (50). Somatostatin analogs are generally successful in the initial management of patients with the glucagonoma syndrome (51,52). Patients who are refractory to somatostatin analogs may benefit from the intravenous (IV) infusion of amino acids (46,51). CT is often the only localization study required in patients with glucagonomas, in part because the majority of patients initially present with clearly visible metastatic disease (46,47,53). Surgical resection may be performed with curative intent in the rare patient with localized disease. More often surgery is performed to diminish systemic symptoms in patients with metastases. Perioperative anticoagulation is often considered in such patients due to a high incidence of deep venous thrombosis.

VIPomas

Pancreatic endocrine tumors associated with profound diarrhea, hypokalemia, and achlorhydria were first described by Verner and Morrison in 1958 (54). This syndrome was subsequently found to be due to the ectopic secretion of vasoactive intestinal peptide (VIP) and has been aptly named "pancreatic cholera" (55,56). Like the cholera toxin, VIP causes intracellular elevation of cyclic AMP, resulting in intestinal smooth muscle relaxation, inhibition of electrolyte absorption and profound secretory diarrhea.

VIPomas most often present in the fifth decade of life and have a similar incidence in men and women (57). The diagnosis is generally based on the presence of elevated serum VIP levels, symptoms of diarrhea, and documentation of malignancy. Somatostatin analogs are highly effective in suppressing hormone secretion and in controlling the secretory diarrhea associated with the VIPoma syndrome (58,59). VIPomas are generally >1 cm in size and, in most cases, can be visualized with CT or MRI scan (60,61). Endoscopic ultrasonography or somatostatin scintigraphy may be helpful in localizing smaller tumors. Surgical resection is generally undertaken with curative intent in patients with localized disease, or for the purpose of cytoreduction in patients with metastases (59).

Somatostatinomas and PPomas

Two other types of pancreatic endocrine tumor have been somewhat less well characterized. The first of these, somatostatinomas, may be associated with diabetes, hypochlorhydria, and diarrhea. PPomas are pancreatic neuroendocrine tumors associated with high serum levels of pancreatic polypeptide. Secretion of pancreatic polypeptide is not associated with any clinical syndrome, and these tumors are therefore generally classified as "nonfunctioning" pancreatic endocrine tumors. They are usually first diagnosed when they grow large enough to cause symptoms from tumor bulk (62). Surgical resection is generally curative in patients with early stage disease; unfortunately, because of the clinically silent nature of these tumors, the majority of patients have metastatic disease at the time of diagnosis (63).

CARCINOID TUMORS

Incidence and Etiology

The incidence of carcinoid tumors has been estimated to be 1 to 2 per 100,000 population (64). Carcinoid tumors are more common than are pancreatic neuroendocrine tumors: By comparison, the incidence of carcinoid tumors is 8 to 11 times higher than that of insulinomas, and 7 to 26 times higher than that of gastrinomas (65–67). An early analysis of 2,837 cases

TABLE 48.2

PERCENTAGE OF CARCINOID TUMORS AT EACH SITE AS A PROPORTION OF
THE TOTAL NUMBER OF CARCINOID TUMORS IN EACH STUDY

Carcinoid site	End results study group (1950–1960) N = 1,867	Third national cancer survey (1969–1970) N = 970	SEER program (1973–1999) N = 10,878
Lungs and bronchi	10.2	14.1	27.9
Stomach	2.2	1.9	4.6
Duodenum	1.8	2.3	2.8
Jejunum	1.0	2.0	1.8
Ileum	10.8	13.8	14.9
Appendix	43.9	35.5	4.8
Cecum	2.7	3.0	4.1
Colon	4.7	3.9	8.6
Rectum	15.4	12.3	13.6

SEER, Surveillance, Epidemiology, and End Results.
Adapted from ref. 103.

in the United States using data from the End Results Group (1950–1969) and the Third National Cancer Survey (1969–1971) found that the appendix was the most common site of carcinoid tumors; appendiceal carcinoids were followed in frequency by carcinoids of the rectum, ileum, lungs, and stomach (Table 48.2) (68). A more recent analysis of 5,486 cases identified by the Surveillance, Epidemiology, and End Results (SEER) program of the National Cancer Institute between 1973 and 1991 found a relative increase in the proportion of carcinoids of the lung and stomach, and a decrease in the proportion of appendiceal carcinoids (64). However, these changes in relative incidence are likely due to variations in the detection and reporting of carcinoid tumors. Furthermore, because neuroendocrine tumors often pursue an indolent course, their true incidence may in fact be somewhat higher. The incidence of carcinoid tumors in autopsy series, for example, has been reported to be as high as 8 per 100,000 population, suggesting that a large proportion of patients with carcinoid tumors may in fact die of other, non–tumor-related causes (69).

There are no established environmental risk factors for carcinoid tumors, nor has a clear underlying genetic cause for carcinoid tumors been defined. A number of genetic aberrations have been observed in carcinoid tumors; these aberrations appear to differ, depending on site of origin. Although carcinoids are not generally part of the MEN 1 syndrome, mutations or deletions of the *MEN 1* gene may be involved in the tumorigenesis of some sporadic carcinoids. Carcinoid tumors arising in the lungs and stomach, for example, have been found to contain chromosomal loss at 11q in approximately one-third of cases (70–72). 11q deletions and MEN 1 mutations appear to be less common in carcinoid tumors arising from other sites. One recent study mapped LOH on chromosome 11 using array CGH, and showed that only one of nine midgut NETs had LOH at 11q13, whereas 3 of 9 had LOH at 11q23 (71).

In carcinoid tumors of the small intestine, loss of chromosome 18 has been identified in >50% of cases (73,74). Smad4/DPCr is a gene located on chromosome 18 and often mutates in colon and pancreatic adenocarcinomas; however, no mutations were observed in midgut carcinoids. Other major areas of chromosomal loss in midgut carcinoids include 9p (15%), 11q (13%), and 16q (12%) (10,73,75–77).

Clinical Presentation and Management of Localized Carcinoid Tumors

A commonly used classification scheme groups carcinoid tumors according to their presumed derivation from the embryonic gut: foregut (bronchial and gastric), midgut (small intestine and appendiceal), and hindgut (rectal). The clinical presentation and management of these tumors varies, depending on their site of origin (Table 48.3).

TABLE 48.3

CLINICAL PRESENTATION OF CARCINOID TUMORS

Tumor	Symptom
FOREGUT	
Bronchial carcinoids	Cough, hemoptysis, postobstructive pneumonia, Cushing syndrome; carcinoid syndrome rare
Gastric carcinoids	Usually asymptomatic and found incidentally
MIDGUT	
Small intestine carcinoids	Intermittent bowel obstruction or mesenteric ischemia; carcinoid syndrome common when metastatic
Appendiceal carcinoids	Usually found incidentally; may cause carcinoid syndrome when metastatic
HINDGUT	
Rectal carcinoids	Either found incidentally or discovered due to bleeding, pain, and constipation; rarely cause hormonal symptoms, even when metastatic

Bronchial Carcinoid Tumors

Bronchial carcinoids comprise approximately 2% of primary lung tumors (78,79). Typical carcinoids, also classified as well-differentiated pulmonary neuroendocrine tumors, usually present in the fifth decade of life (79–81). They are most often central in location, causing symptoms of cough, wheezing, hemoptysis, and recurrent postobstructive pneumonia (81,82). Typical pulmonary carcinoid tumors are only rarely associated with the classic carcinoid syndrome; they have, however, been associated with ectopic ACTH secretion, resulting in Cushing syndrome (81,83–85).

Approximately one-third of bronchial carcinoids demonstrate "atypical" histologic features (78,82,84,86). Atypical carcinoids are characterized by the presence of frequent mitoses or areas of necrosis. They tend to occur in older individuals, most commonly in the sixth decade of life and, unlike typical carcinoid tumors, are more common in smokers. They also tend to be larger in size than typical carcinoids and are more commonly peripheral in location (87,88).

Whereas typical carcinoid tumors are generally indolent, with metastases reported in <15% of cases, atypical carcinoids pursue an aggressive clinical course, metastasizing to mediastinal lymph nodes in 30% to 50% of cases (80,81,84,85). Accordingly, long-term survival rates for patients with typical carcinoid tumors following surgical resection generally exceed 85%, but are significantly less for patients who undergo resection for atypical carcinoids (78,82–86,88–91). Histology also influences the choice of surgical procedure: Conservative resection, consisting of wedge or segmental resection, is currently the preferred form of treatment for localized bronchial carcinoid tumors, whereas more aggressive procedures are often chosen for atypical carcinoids (85,88). The use of adjuvant therapy, generally with regimens similar to those used for small cell carcinoma, remains controversial but is at times considered following resection of atypical carcinoid tumors.

Gastric Carcinoid Tumors

Gastric carcinoid tumors comprise <1% of gastric neoplasms (68,92). Gastric carcinoid tumors can be subclassifed into three distinct groups: those associated with chronic atrophic gastritis (type 1), those associated with the Zollinger-Ellison syndrome (type 2), and sporadic gastric carcinoids (type 3) (Table 48.4). Both type 1 and type 2 gastric carcinoids are associated with hypergastrinemia. High levels of gastrin are believed to result in hyperplasia of the enterochromaffin cells in the stomach, ultimately leading to hyperplastic lesions and small, often multiple carcinoid tumors (92). These tumors generally pursue an indolent course and can be resected endoscopically, with sub-

sequent interval follow-up. Patients with larger or recurrent tumors may require more extensive surgical resection. In patients with chronic atrophic gastritis, antrectomy has been used to eliminate the source of gastric production and has been reported to result in tumor regression (93,94). In patients with Zollinger-Ellison syndrome, the use of somatostatin analogs has resulted in tumor regression (95).

Between 15% and 25% of gastric carcinoids are sporadic. In contrast to type I and type II carcinoids, these lesions develop in the absence of hypergastrinemia, are usually >1 cm in size, and tend to pursue an aggressive clinical course. Sporadic carcinoid tumors have been associated with an atypical carcinoid syndrome, which is manifested primarily by flushing and believed to be mediated by histamine. The majority of sporadic carcinoid tumors are metastatic at the time of presentation, and death due to disease is frequent. Because of the aggressive nature of these lesions, most are treated with total gastrectomy (96,97).

Small Intestine Carcinoid Tumors

Small bowel carcinoid tumors comprise approximately one-third of small bowel tumors in surgical series (98). Patients with small bowel carcinoids generally present in the sixth or seventh decade of life, most commonly with abdominal pain or small bowel obstruction; these symptoms are commonly misdiagnosed as "irritable bowel syndrome" (98–100). Approximately 5% to 7% will present with the carcinoid syndrome, at which time hepatic metastases are usually also present (101,102). The difficulty in diagnosing small bowel carcinoids is compounded by the fact that standard imaging techniques such as CT scan and small bowel barium contrast studies only rarely identify the primary tumor. When detected and surgically removed, they are most frequently located in the distal ileum and are often multicentric, occasionally appearing as dozens of lesions lining the small bowel (Fig. 48.2) (101). Tumor size is an unreliable predictor of metastatic disease, and metastases have been reported even from tumors measuring <0.5 cm (99). The 5-year survival rate is 60% for patients with localized disease and 73% for those with regional metastases, compared to 21% for patients with distant metastases (103).

Mesenteric fibrosis and associated ischemia, caused by a characteristic desmoplastic reaction, is often present in association with small bowel carcinoids. These tumors are also frequently associated with "buckling" or tethering of the intestine due to extensive mesenteric involvement (101,104). Resection of the small bowel primary tumor, together with associated mesenteric metastases, leads to significant reduction in tumor-related symptoms of pain and obstruction, and is therefore

TABLE 48.4

SUBTYPES OF GASTRIC CARCINOID TUMOR

	Hypergastrinemia	Gastric acid secretion	Typical size	Number of tumors	Clinical features
Type 1 (in setting of chronic atrophic gastritis type A)	Yes (as a result of achlorhydria)	Low	<1 cm	Multifocal	Rarely invasive; endoscopic removal often adequate
Type 2 (in setting of Zollinger-Ellison syndrome)	Yes (as a result of ectopic gastrin secretion)	High	<1 cm	Multifocal	Rarely invasive; may respond to somatostatin analogs
Sporadic	No	Normal	>1 cm	Solitary	Frequently invasive and metastatic

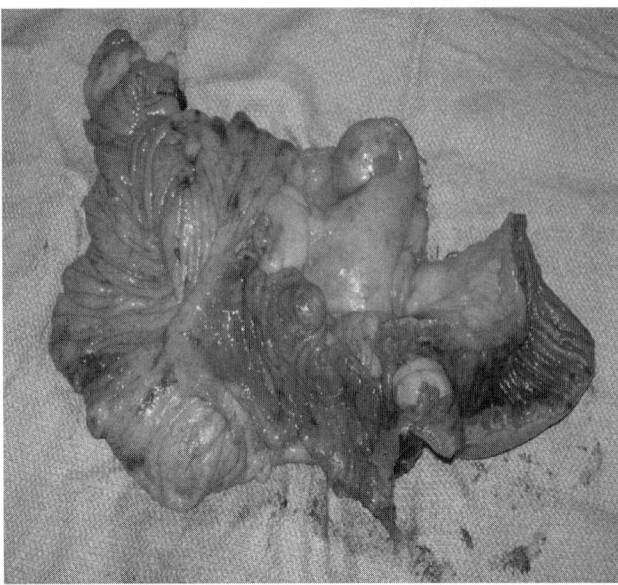

FIGURE 48.2. Multicentric carcinoids of the small intestine (See also color Figure 48.2).

recommended even in patients with known metastatic disease (100).

Appendiceal Carcinoid Tumors

Historically, carcinoid tumors have been considered the most common tumor of the appendix, accounting for >50% of all appendiceal malignancies and discovered in up to 7 of every 1,000 appendectomy specimens (105–107). In older surgical series, appendiceal carcinoids were most commonly discovered during incidental appendectomy for other reasons. The most common indication for appendectomy in a 1968 series of 137 appendiceal carcinoid tumors was benign pelvic disease (43%) or gallbladder disease (35%) (103). In recent series, however, the majority of appendiceal carcinoids are discovered during surgery for acute appendicitis (108). The carcinoid tumor itself is believed to be the cause of appendicitis in only a minority of these cases. Approximately two-thirds of appendiceal carcinoid tumors arise in the tip of the appendix, where they are unlikely to cause symptoms of obstruction. Less than 10% arise in the base, where they are more prone to obstruct the appendix, giving rise to acute appendicitis (107).

Patients with appendiceal carcinoid tumors generally present at a relatively young age: The mean age at presentation in the recent SEER database analysis was 49 years, and in older series, it is even younger (103,107). Although the early age at presentation may in part reflect the mean age at appendectomy, other explanations have also been proposed. Some investigators have speculated that the pattern of appendiceal carcinoid tumors parallels the biological behavior of subepithelial neuroendocrine cells, from which appendiceal carcinoid tumors are believed to arise. The density of these cells tends to peak in the third decade of life and subsequently decreases throughout the remainder of life (109–111).

Appendiceal carcinoids are more common in women than in men: In the SEER database, the male-to-female ratio was 0.82 (103). The higher incidence of appendiceal carcinoids in women, like the relatively young age at presentation, may be partially attributable to appendectomy patterns. Women are more likely to undergo incidental appendectomy as a result of gynecologic procedures. However, a female preponderance of appendiceal carcinoids has also been reported in children, an observation that cannot be explained by differences in appendectomy rates (112–114).

The clinical behavior of appendiceal carcinoid tumors can be predicted based on the size of the tumor. More than 95% of appendiceal carcinoid tumors are <2 cm in diameter (115,116). The incidence of metastatic disease in such patients is extraordinarily low, although rare cases have been reported in the literature (116–121). In contrast, approximately one-third of patients with appendiceal carcinoid tumors measuring >2 cm in diameter have either nodal or distant metastases (115). Other criteria such as invasion of the mesoappendix, perineural invasion, tumor location, and histologic pattern have not consistently correlated with the presence of metastatic disease.

The surgical management of appendiceal carcinoids derives from these historical data, and surgical recommendations are based on tumor size. Based on the low incidence of metastases in patients whose tumors measure <2 cm, simple appendectomy is believed to be sufficient in such cases. In contrast, the higher incidence of metastases in patients whose tumors measure >2 cm in diameter has led to the recommendation for complete right hemicolectomy. These recommendations are supported by data from surgical series, one of the largest of which was published by Moertel et al. (115). Among 122 patients undergoing simple appendectomy for tumors measuring <2 cm, none developed disease recurrence, whereas 1 of 12 patients undergoing simple appendectomy for a tumor measuring >2 cm developed a local recurrence. Whether right colectomy decreases the risk of future distant recurrence has not been formally evaluated, and simple appendectomy may at times be appropriate for larger tumors, particularly in older patients or patients with other comorbidities.

Rectal Carcinoid Tumors

Rectal carcinoid tumors comprise 1% to 2% of all rectal tumors, and are most common in the sixth decade of life (64). Approximately 50% are asymptomatic and found on routine endoscopy (122). Symptomatic patients usually present with rectal bleeding, pain, or constipation (122,123). The size of the primary lesion correlates closely with the probability of metastases, which occur in <5% of tumors measuring <1 cm but in the majority of lesions >2 cm (123,124).

Two-thirds of rectal carcinoid tumors are <1 cm and are successfully treated with local excision. The management of tumors measuring 1 to 2 cm is controversial. Although most tumors of this size can be managed with local excision, several authors have suggested that the presence of muscular invasion, symptoms at diagnosis, or ulceration are poor prognostic factors that warrant more extensive surgical procedures (122–124). Endosopic ultrasound, particularly in cases in which an endoscopic removal has been performed, may be helpful to ensure that all submucosal tumor has been removed.

Tumors measuring >2 cm have traditionally been managed with low anterior resection or abdominoperineal resection. The value of these procedures in the management of rectal carcinoids has been questioned, however, as they do not appear to result in a survival advantage when compared to retrospective series (125–127). An individualized approach, taking into account patient age and other comorbidities, may therefore be appropriate in deciding on a surgical approach to large rectal carcinoids.

MANAGEMENT OF PATIENTS WITH METASTATIC NEUROENDOCRINE TUMORS

Clinical Presentation of Metastatic Disease

The clinical course of patients with metastatic carcinoid and pancreatic neuroendocrine tumors is highly variable. Some patients with indolent tumors may remain symptom free for years, even without treatment. Others have symptomatic metastatic disease, either from tumor bulk or hormonal hypersecretion, and require therapy. Patients with functioning metastatic pancreatic neuroendocrine tumors will typically have symptoms related to the type of hormone secreted. In patients with metastatic carcinoid tumors, secretion of serotonin and other vasoactive substances causes the carcinoid syndrome, which is manifested by episodic flushing, wheezing, diarrhea, and eventual right-sided valvular heart disease (128). The carcinoid syndrome is associated primarily with midgut carcinoid tumors and occurs almost exclusively in the setting of metastatic, rather than localized, disease. A notable exception to this rule is ovarian carcinoid tumors, which due to their venous drainage directly into the systemic circulation may be associated with carcinoid syndrome in the absence of metastases.

The symptoms associated with the carcinoid syndrome are caused by secretory products released from the primary tumor or metastic lesions gaining direct access to systemic circulation and bypassing metabolism in the liver. Symptoms of carcinoid syndrome have traditionally been attributed to elevated levels of 5-HT (serotonin) (129). In one review of 748 patients with carcinoid syndrome, 92% had increased serum serotonin levels (130). In other studies, however, 12% to 26% of patients with elevated serotonin levels had no symptoms of carcinoid syndrome, suggesting that other vasoactive substances may also be involved (129). Classic carcinoid symptoms include flushing of the upper body, watery diarrhea, facial edema, sweating, wheezing, dyspnea, abdominal pain, and, in severe cases, hemodynamic instability. Patients with long-standing symptoms often have nasal telangectasia and permanent skin discoloration.

Episodes of carcinoid syndrome are usually intermittent and may last from a few minutes to several days (131). Common precipitating factors include stress or ingestion of alcohol. Pellagra is has been reported in 5% of cases of advanced carcinoid syndrome and can be prevented with the regular use of multivitamins or niacin supplementation.

Imaging of Metastatic Neuroendocrine Tumors

The predominant site of metastatic spread in patients with neuroendocrine tumors involving the GI tract is the liver (Fig. 48.3). Patients in whom metastatic disease is suspected should be evaluated with an abdominal CT scan to rule out liver metastases. Liver function tests are an unreliable indicator of tumor

involvement, and the serum alkaline phosphatase is frequently normal despite extensive liver involvement by carcinoid tumor. Carcinoid liver metastases are often hypervascular and may become isodense relative to the liver with the administration of IV contrast. CT scans should thus be performed both before and after the administration of IV contrast agents (132,133).

Somatostatin receptor scintigraphy provides a second useful imaging modality for the detection of metastatic disease in patients with neuroendocrine tumors. With the exception of insulinomas (of which only 50% express type 2 somatostatin receptors), >90% of neuroendocrine tumors, including nonfunctioning pancreatic tumors and carcinoids, contain high concentrations of somatostatin receptors and can be imaged with a radiolabeled form of the somatostatin analog octreotide (111-indium pentetreotide) (134–136). The uptake of radiolabeled octreotide is also predictive of clinical response to therapy with somatostatin analogs.

For neuroendocrine tumors, the sensitivity of planar pentetreotide scanning is better for extrahepatic than for hepatic lesions, presumably because of heterogeneous octreotide uptake in normal liver (137,138). In one series, octreotide scintigraphy detected 12 of 12 known extrahepatic lesions, but only 12 of 24 hepatic lesions (137). Greater sensitivity for hepatic lesions can be achieved by the use of single photon emission CT imaging (139,140).

Biochemical Monitoring in Patients With Metastatic Neuroendocrine Tumors

Serial measurement of the serotonin metabolite 5-hydroxyindoleacetic acid (HIAA) in 24-hour urine collections has been commonly used for monitoring of patients with metastatic carcinoid tumors. Although elevated urinary 5-HIAA levels are highly specific for carcinoid tumors, they are not particularly sensitive: In one study, only 73% of patients with metastatic carcinoid tumors had elevated levels (141). Furthermore, 5-HIAA levels are generally elevated in patients with primary midgut carcinoid tumors but are not useful in patients with either foregut (bronchial, gastric) or hindgut (rectal) carcinoid tumors, which only rarely secrete serotonin.

The clinical utility of urinary 5-HIAA levels can also be limited by false positives. The normal rate of 5-HIAA excretion ranges from 2 to 8 mg/day (10–42 μmol/day). Values of up to 30 mg/day (157 μmol/day) may be found in patients with malabsorption syndromes such as celiac and Whipple disease, as well as after the ingestion of large amounts of tryptophan-rich foods. Although some patients with the carcinoid syndrome have similar modest elevations, most have values for urinary 5-HIAA excretion >100 mg/day (523 μmol/day). In one study, urinary 5-HIAA excretion in patients with the carcinoid syndrome ranged from 99 to 2,070 mg/day (518–10,826 μmol/day) (142). Lower but still elevated values were seen in patients with metastatic carcinoid tumors but not carcinoid syndrome (50–260 mg/day [262–1,360 μmol/day]).

Plasma chromogranin A (CGA) is a more sensitive marker than urinary 5-HIAA in patients with carcinoid tumors, and can also be used as a marker in patients with both functional and nonfunctional pancreatic endocrine tumors (143–146). CGA should be used with caution as a marker of disease activity in patients treated with somatostatin analogs because these agents significantly reduce plasma CGA levels, a change that may be more reflective of changes in hormonal synthesis and release from tumor cells than an actual reduction in tumor mass (146). In patients on stable doses of somatostatin analogs, consistent increases in plasma CGA levels over time may reflect loss of secretory control and/or tumor growth. Plasma CGA levels have also been shown to have prognostic value: In one series of 71 patients with metastatic carcinoid tumors, CGA levels of

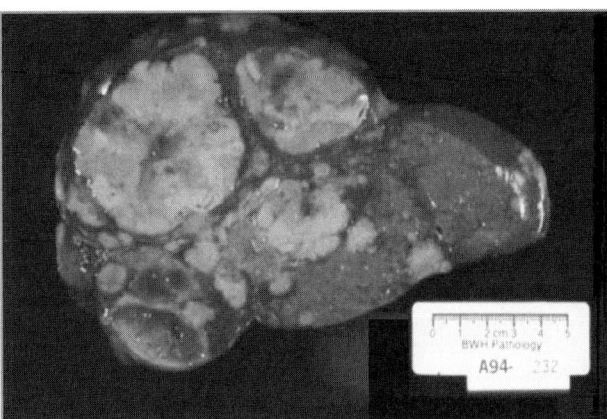

FIGURE 48.3. Carcinoid hepatic metastases (See also color Figure 48.3).

>5,000 μg/mL were independently associated with poor prognosis (147).

Surgical Options in Patients With Metastatic Disease

Hepatic Resection and Transplantation

Metastatic liver disease in some cases can be successfully treated with hepatic resection, providing both long-term symptomatic relief and prolonged survival times (148–151). In general, however, resection can only be undertaken in patients with a limited number of hepatic metastases and is most successful when undertaken with curative intent (152). Que et al. reported that nearly all patients with neuroendocrine tumor metastases to the liver undergoing hepatectomy had improvement in symptoms and that 4-year overall survival was 73% (150).

Liver transplantation for more common metastatic malignancies has commonly resulted in early tumor recurrences. The number of patients with liver-isolated metastatic neuroendocrine tumors in whom orthotopic liver transplantation (OLT) has been attempted remains small, and the role of OLT in such patients is unclear (151,153,154). Early series reported high rates of both perioperative mortality and tumor recurrence. Results from a more recent multicenter study from France are more encouraging and demonstrated a 5-year overall survival rate of 69% (151). Nevertheless, the impact of transplant on the natural history of patients with neuroendocrine tumors is difficult to assess due to their often indolent natural history. Furthermore, although long-term survival results are encouraging, liver transplantation as a viable treatment modality for metastatic carcinoid is limited by donor organ availability.

Management of Carcinoid Heart Disease

Carcinoid heart disease occurs in approximately two-thirds of patients with the carcinoid syndrome (155). Carcinoid heart lesions are characterized by plaquelike, fibrous endocardial thickening that classically involves the right side of the heart, and often causes retraction and fixation of the leaflets of the tricuspid and pulmonary valves (Fig. 48.4). Tricuspid regurgita-

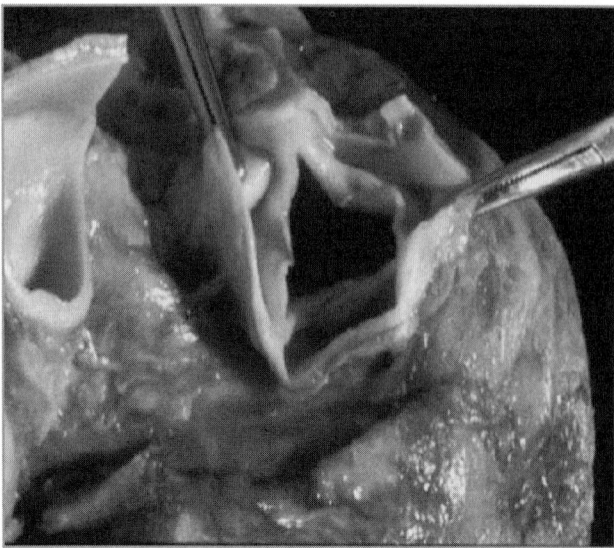

FIGURE 48.4. Carcinoid heart disease (See also color Figure 48.4).

tion is a nearly universal finding; tricuspid stenosis, pulmonary regurgitation, and pulmonary stenosis may also occur (156). Left-sided heart disease occurs in <10% of patients (157,158).

The preponderance of lesions in the right heart suggests that carcinoid heart disease is related to factors secreted by liver metastases into the hepatic vein. Among patients with carcinoid syndrome, patients with heart disease exhibit higher levels of serum serotonin and urinary 5-HIAA excretion than patients without heart disease (155,157–160). Other investigators have suggested that high atrial natriuretic peptide may also contribute to the pathogenesis of this disease. Whether these factors are directly responsible for the cardiac lesions, however, is unclear. Treatment with somatostatin analogs resulting in decreased serotonin secretion may not prevent the development of carcinoid heart disease and does not result in regression of cardiac lesions (158,159,161).

The indolent nature of metastatic carcinoid, combined with the availability of effective treatments for carcinoid syndrome, has led to interest in valve replacement surgery for selected patients. Right-sided heart failure in such patients may lead to significant morbidity and mortality. In early series, valvular replacement in patients with symptomatic carcinoid heart disease has been associated with relatively high perioperative morbidity (162,163). Surviving patients, however, appear to achieve significant symptomatic improvement, and more advanced techniques may facilitate the future use of valve replacement surgery in carcinoid patients (164).

Prevention and Management of Carcinoid Crisis

Carcinoid crisis is a life-threatening form of carcinoid syndrome triggered by specific events such as anesthesia, surgery, or chemotherapy, presumably stimulating release of an overwhelming amount of biologically active compounds, such as catecholamines. Specific symptoms include flushing, diarrhea, tachycardia, arrhythmias, hypertension or hypotension, bronchospasm, and altered mental status (165). Symptoms are generally refractory to fluid resuscitation and administration of vasopressors.

Carcinoid crisis may be precipitated by anesthesia, and intraoperative complications have been reported in 11% of patients who have carcinoid syndrome (166). Subcutaneous administration of 300 mcg of octreotide perioperatively reduces the incidence of carcinoid crisis, and intraperative octreotide should be readily available during any surgical procedure (167). During a carcinoid crisis, 300 mcg of octreotide may be given intravenously; a continous IV drip of octreotide at a rate of 50 to 150 mcg/hour may also be used (168).

Nonsurgical Hepatic-Directed Therapy

Hepatic Artery Embolization

Hepatic arterial embolization is commonly used as a palliative technique in patients with hepatic metastases who are not candidates for surgical resection. Hepatic artery embolization is based on the principle that tumors in the liver derive most of their blood supply from the hepatic artery, whereas healthy hepatocytes derive most of their blood supply from the portal vein. Embolization of the hepatic arterial blood supply can be performed with or without the concurrent injection of chemotherapy. The response rates associated with embolization, as measured either by decrease in hormonal secretion or by radiographic regression, are generally >50% (169–178). However, the duration of response can be brief, ranging from 4 to 24 months in uncontrolled series (170,173). In one of the largest series of 81 patients undergoing embolization or chemoembolization for carcinoid tumor, the median duration of response was 17 months, and the probability of progression-free survival at 1, 2, and 3 years was 75%, 35%, and 11%, respectively (173). Early studies reported a significant incidence of postembolization complications, which included renal failure, hepatic necrosis, and sepsis. Improved techniques have, in recent years, reduced the incidence of such complications, making embolization an important and generally safe treatment option for patients with neuroendocrine tumors (173).

Radiofrequency Ablation and Cryoablation

Other approaches to the treatment of hepatic metastases include the use of radiofrequency ablation (RFA) and cryoablation, either alone or in conjunction with surgical debulking. These approaches can be performed using a percutaneous or laparoscopic approach. Although they appear to be less morbid than either hepatic resection or hepatic artery embolization, their efficacy, particularly in patients with large volume hepatic disease, has not been well studied. Most published reports are small case studies of <40 patients (179–182). In the series with longest follow-up, 31 symptomatic patients

with metastatic carcinoid ($n = 20$), islet cell tumor ($n = 10$), or medullary thyroid cancer ($n = 1$) who were refractory to conventional therapy underwent resection, cryosurgery, and/or RFA (182). Symptoms were eliminated in 27 (87%), and 16 had progressive or recurrent disease with a median follow-up of 26 months.

Systemic Treatment of Metastatic Disease

Somatostatin Analogs and Interferon-α

The carcinoid syndrome, as well as other hormonal syndromes associated with neuroendocrine tumors, can often be well controlled with somatostatin analogs (Table 48.5). Somatostatin is a 14-amino acid peptide that inhibits the secretion of a broad range of hormones and acts by binding to somatostatin receptors, which are expressed on the majority of neuroendocrine tumors (183). In an initial study, the subcutaneous administration of the somatostatin analog octreotide, administered at a

TABLE 48.5

EFFICACY OF SOMATOSTATIN ANALOGS AND INTERFERON IN ADVANCED NEUROENDOCRINE TUMORS

Agent(s)	Patients (N)	Biochemical response rate (%)	Tumor response rate (%)	Reference
SOMATOSTATIN ANALOGS				
Octreotide	25	72	0	(184)
	22	63	0	(242)
	23	50	28	(243)
	34	NA	0	(196)
	55	37	2	(191)
	103	NA	0	(244)
Lanreotide	19	58	5	(245)
	39	42	0	(246)
Lanreotide SR	18	NA	0	(247)
INTERFERON-α (IFN-α)				
	27	39	20	(248)
	12	40	10	(249)
	20	55	0	(250)
	15	7	0	(251)
	111	42	15	(194)
	26	66	15	(252)
	14	50	0	(253)
	24	60	8	(254)
	12	8	16	(255)
	34	24	12	(256)
	22	58	18	(257)
	7	71	0	(258)
SOMATOSTATIN ANALOGS AND IFN-α				
	19	72	0	(191)
	21	69	5	(192)
RANDOMIZED STUDIES				
Lanreotide	27	NA	4	(190)
IFN	28	NA	3.7	
Lanreotide + IFN-α	29	NA	7.1	

NA, not applicable.

dosage of 150 ucg three times a day, improved the symptoms of carcinoid syndrome in 88% of patients (184). More recently, the use of a long-acting depot form of octreotide, which can be administered on a monthly basis, has largely obviated the need for patients to inject themselves on a daily basis. Long-acting octreotide is typically initiated at a dose of 20 mg intramuscularly after a brief trial of the short-acting formulation, with gradual escalation of the dose as needed for optimal control of symptoms (185). Patients may, in addition, use additional short-acting octreotide for breakthrough symptoms. Lanreotide, another somatostatin analog, appears to be similar to octreotide in its clinical efficacy (186–190). A randomized study of lanreotide SR versus octreotide in 33 patients with carcinoid syndrome demonstrated no significant differences in rates of symptom control and reduction of biochemical markers (188).

The addition of IFN-α to therapy with somatostatin analogs has been reported to be effective in controlling symptoms in patients with the carcinoid syndrome who may be resistant to somatostatin analogs alone (191,192). The ability of IFN-α to stimulate T-cell function and to control the secretion of tumor products led to its initial use in patients with the carcinoid syndrome (193). Therapy with low-dose IFN-α has been subsequently reported to result in biochemical responses in approximately 40% of patients with metastatic neuroendocrine tumors and is occasionally associated with tumor regression (194). In clinical trials, doses of IFN-α have ranged from 3 to 9 MU subcutaneously, administered from three to seven times per week. IFN-α is somewhat myelosuppressive, and the dose is often titrated in individual patients to achieve a total leukocyte count of 3,000/μL. The more widespread acceptance of IFN-α in the treatment of metastatic neuroendocrine tumors has been limited by studies challenging its efficacy as well as the potential for side effects, which may include myelosuppression, fatigue, depression, and alteration of thyroid function (195).

The direct antineoplastic effects of somatostatin analogs either with or without IFN remain uncertain, and the use of these agents in patients who are not symptomatic from symptoms of hormonal hypersecretion remains controversial (196). Radiologic evidence of tumor regression following treatment with these agents is rare. In a small study involving 21 patients with metastatic gastroenteropancreatic neuroendocrine tumors, a combined regimen of somatostain analogs and IFN-α appeared to significantly slow the rate of tumor progression in 67% of patients during follow-up (192). In a prospective study of 68 patients randomized to receive either octreotide alone or a combination of octreotide and IFN-α, there was no significant difference in overall survival, but patients treated with the combination regimen had a reduced risk of tumor progression, suggesting that the addition of IFN had a cytostatic effect (197). The comparable efficacy of lanreotide, IFN-α, or combined therapy was evaluated in a prospective randomized trial involving 80 therapy-naive patients with documented progressive metastatic neuroendocrine tumors (190). The rates of objective partial response (4%, 4%, and 7% for lanreotide, IFN, and combined therapy, respectively) were low in all three groups; however, treatment resulted in apparent disease stabilization in a higher proportion of patients (28%, 26%, and 18%, respectively).

Cytotoxic Chemotherapy

Studies of single-agent therapy with 5-fluorouracil (5-FU), streptozocin, or doxorubicin in patients with metastatic carcinoid tumors have shown that these agents are associated with only modest response rates (Table 48.6). Trials of combination chemotherapy in this disease have failed to demonstrate superiority to single-agent therapy; furthermore, many of these combination regimens have been associated with significant toxicity. In an initial trial, the Eastern Cooperative Oncology Group (ECOG) randomized 118 patients to receive streptozocin combined with either 5-FU or cyclophosphamide (198). Response rates, as measured either by tumor regression or a decrease in urinary 5-HIAA levels, were 33% in the strepotozicin/5-FU arm and 26% in the streptozocin/cyclophosphamide arm. There were no significant differences in survival between the two groups. In an attempt to decrease the toxicity associated with 5-FU and streptozocin, the ECOG in a subsequent trial increased the dosing interval between cycles of streptocin/5-FU and compared this regimen to doxorubicin alone (199). Although these regimens were somewhat better tolerated, the response rate for streptozocin and 5-FU dropped to 22%, as compared to only 21% for doxorubicin alone; again, there were no significant differences in survival. Most recently, streptozocin/5-FU was compared to 5-FU/doxorubicin in a randomized trial of 249 patients (200). The response rate associated with the two regimens was similar (16% vs. 15.9%). Although there was a slight survival benefit associated with streptozocin/5-FU (24.3 vs. 15.7 months) in this trial, more than one-third of the patients treated with streptozocin developed renal toxicity; this regimen is still only rarely used in the current treatment of patients with metastatic carcinoid tumors. A trial, from the Southwest Oncology Group, evaluated the four-drug combination of fluorouracil, doxorubicin, cyclophosphamide, and streptozocin in 56 patients (201). The response rate of 31% was not believed to be superior to that of fluorouracil and streptozocin.

Several studies suggest that pancreatic endocrine tumors are more responsive to chemotherapy than are carcinoid tumors (Table 48.7). In an initial randomized trial, Moertel et al. reported that the combination of streptozocin and doxorubicin was associated with a combined biochemical and radiologic response rate of 69% and a median overall survival time of 2.2 years (202). Two subsequent retrospective analyses of patients receiving this regimen questioned the high response rate reported in this initial trial, and reported objective radiologic response rates using modern response criteria of <10% (203,204). A larger retrospective analysis of 84 patients with either locally advanced or metastatic pancreatic endocrine tumors receiving a three-drug regimen of streptozocin, 5-FU, and doxorubicin showed that this regimen was associated with an overall response rate of 39% and a median survival duration of 37 months, suggesting that this combination is indeed active, although perhaps less active than Moertel's data initially suggested (205).

Dacarbazine (DTIC) has been evaluated as a potential alternative to streptozocin-based therapy in both carcinoid and pancreatic endocrine tumors. The ECOG performed a phase II study of DTIC in 50 patients with advanced pancreatic islet cell carcinoma and reported an objective response rate of 34% (206). A Southwest Oncology Group (SWOG) study reported that treatment with DTIC was associated with an objective radiologic response rate of 16% in 56 patients with metastatic carcinoid tumors (207). Toxicity was a concern in both studies: 88% of patients in the SWOG study reported nausea and/or vomiting, and there were two lethal toxicities in the ECOG study. In carcinoid patients receiving DTIC as a second-line therapy following treatment with combination chemotherapy, the overall response rate was 8% (200).

Temozolomide is a cytotoxic alkylating agent that was specifically developed as an oral and less toxic alternative to dacarbazine, and would therefore also be expected to have some efficacy against neuroendocrine tumors (208). In a phase II study, 30 patients with metastatic neuroendocrine tumors were treated with temozolomide, administered at a dose of 150 mg/m^2 for 7 days, followed by a 7-day rest, together with thalidomide administered at doses of 50 to 400 mg daily without interruption. The overall objective, radiologic response rate

TABLE 48.6

EFFICACY OF SELECTED CHEMOTHERAPY REGIMENS IN ADVANCED
CARCINOID TUMORS

Regimen	Patients (N)	Tumor response rate (%)	Reference
SINGLE-AGENT TRIALS			
Dacarbazine	15	13	(259)
	15	13	(260)
	56	16	(207)
	61	8.2	(200)
Streptozocin	6	17	(260)
Doxorubicin	33	21	(260)
Fluorouracil	19	26	(260)
Melphalan	7	0	(260)
Cisplatin	15	7	(261)
	10	10	(260)
Etoposide	17	12	(262)
Carboplatin	20	0	(263)
Actinomycin-D	17	6	(259)
Paclitaxel	24	8	(211)
Docetaxel	21	0	(212)
Gemcitabine[a]	10	0	(213)
PHASE II COMBINATION THERAPY TRIALS			
Streptozocin/5-FU/doxorubicin/ cyclophosphamide	56	31	(201)
Doxorubicin/5-FU/cisplatin	15	14	(264)
Darcarbazine/5-FU/leucovorin	9	11	(265)
Streptozocin/doxorubicin/IFN-α	11	0	(255)
5-FU/IFN-α	14	7	(266)

Randomized trials	Patients	Tumor response rate (%)	Median overall survival (months)	Reference
Streptozocin/cyclophosphamide	47	26	12.5	(198)
Streptozocin/5-FU	42	33	11.2	
Doxorubicin	81	21	11	(199)
Streptozocin/5-FU	80	22	14.7	
5-FU/doxorubicin	88	15.9	15.7	(200)
Streptozocin/5-FU	88	16	24.3	

5-FU, 5-fluorouracil; IFN, interferon.
[a]Included patients with both carcinoid and pancreatic endocrine tumors.

among patients receiving temozolomide and thalidomide in this study was 25%, a rate that is comparable to prior studies of both dacarbazine- and streptozocin-based chemotherapy in patients with neuroendocrine tumors.

Patients with poorly differentiated neuroendocrine tumors have been previously reported to be more responsive to cytotoxic chemotherapy than patients with well-differentiated tumors. In an initial study, a combination of cisplatin and etoposide commonly used for small cell lung cancer was associated with an overall tumor response rate of 67% in 18 patients with "anaplastic" neuroendocrine tumors (presumably analogous to poorly differentiated neuroendocrine tumors) but had little activity in more well-differentiated tumor subtypes (209). In a subsequent study of 36 patients with advanced neuroendocrine tumors, treatment with cisplatin and etoposide was associated with an overall radiologic response rate of 36% and a median

survival time of 19 months. All patients enrolled in this study had either poorly differentiated histology or a rapidly progressing clinical course, suggesting that few, if any of these patients had more classic, indolent carcinoid or pancreatic endocrine tumors (210).

Newer chemotherapeutic agents have, to date, proved relatively inactive in neuroendocrine tumors. High-dose paclitaxel, administered with granulocyte colony-stimulating factor, was evaluated in 24 patients with metastatic carcinoid and islet cell tumors (211). Significant hematologic toxicity was observed, and the objective radiologic response rate was only 8%. Treatment with docetaxel was associated with biochemical responses but no radiologic responses in a recent phase II trial of 21 patients with carcinoid tumors (212). No responses were observed in 19 neuroendocrine tumor patients treated with gemcitabine (213).

TABLE 48.7

EFFICACY OF SYSTEMIC CHEMOTHERAPY IN ADVANCED PANCREATIC
NEUROENDOCRINE TUMORS

Regimen	Patients (N)	Tumor response rate (%)	Median overall survival	Study
PROSPECTIVE STUDIES				
Chlorozotocin	33	30	18.0 months	(202)
Fluorouracil + streptozocin	33	45	16.8 months	
Doxorubicin + streptozocin	36	69	26.4 months	
Dacarbazine	50	34	19.3 months	(206)
RETROSPECTIVE STUDIES				
Doxorubicin + streptozocin	16	8	—	(203)
	16	8	20.2 months	(204)
Steptozocin + doxorubicin + fluorouracil	84	39	37 months	(205)

Novel Treatment Approaches for Metastatic Neuroendocrine Tumors

The modest efficacy of current systemic treatment regimens has led to interest in the development of novel therapeutic approaches for patients with advanced neuroendocrine tumors. Such approaches include the use of targeted radiotherapy, as well as regimens incorporating angiogenesis inhibitors and small molecule tyrosine kinase inhibitors.

Targeted Radiotherapy

Traditional external beam radiation therapy is beneficial in patients with neuroendocrine tumor metastases to bone but has little utility for more common visceral metastases. A more broadly applicable strategy includes the therapeutic use of radiolabeled somatostatin analogs (Table 48.8) (214–221). Scintigraphy with indium-111–labeled octreotide has been commonly used to localize previously undetected primary or metastatic neuroendocrine tumor lesions. At higher doses, indium-111–labeled octreotide has also been evaluated as a potential novel therapeutic; unfortunately, objective response rates with this agent have been low (222). More encouraging results have been obtained with octreotide coupled to yttrium-90, a high-energy beta particle emitter. In early phase II trials, objective radiologic responses have been noted in $\leq 23\%$ of patients with metastatic neuroendocrine tumors (218,223). The longer-term utility of this agent, however, appears to be limited by both renal and hematologic toxicity (224). Most recently, octreotide labeled with lutetium-177, a low-energy beta particle emitter, has been evaluated in a phase I study, with encouraging results. In one series, 131 patients with somatostatin receptor-positive advanced neuroendocrine tumors received 177Lu-octreotate administered every 6 to 10 weeks, to a final intended dose of 600 to 800 mCi (221). There were 35 objective responses (27%), 3 of which were complete.

Benefit has also been suggested for local tumor irradiation with 131-I-metaiodobenzylguanidine (131I-MIBG) (225,226). MIBG is a compound resembling norepinephrine that can be

TABLE 48.8

THERAPEUTIC EFFICACY OF RADIOLABELED AGENTS IN
NEUROENDOCRINE TUMORS

Agents	Patients (N)	Tumor response rate (%)	Reference
RADIOLABELED SOMATOSTATIN ANALOGS			
[111]In-pentreotide	9	0	(267)
^{90}Y-DOTA, Tyr[3]	30	23	(219)
	29	7	(268)
	41	24	(218)
	32	9	(222)
[177]Lu-Octreotate[a]	125	28	(221)
RADIOLABELED METAIODOBENZYLGUANIDINE (MIBG)			
^{131}I-MIBG	98	15	(226)
^{131}I-MIBG vs.	30	0	(269)
Unlabeled MIBG	20	0	

accumulated by neuroendocrine cells. One limitation of this strategy is that not all patients with metastatic carcinoid have evidence of MIBG uptake, limiting the number of patients potentially eligible for treatment. In one retrospective series, biochemical (5-HIAA) responses were observed in 37% of carcinoid patients treated with MIBG, and 15% had radiographic responses to therapy (226). Radiographic response did not, however, correlate with improved survival.

Targeted Therapies: Inhibition of Cell Signaling Pathways

A number of studies have also examined the expression of cellular growth factors and their receptors in neuroendocrine tumors. The expression of growth factors such as basic fibroblast growth factor (bFGF), transforming growth factor-alpha (TGF-α) and -beta (TGF-β) platelet-derived growth factor (PDGF), as well as growth factor receptors, including PDGF receptor (PDGFR), epidermal growth factor receptor (EGFR), and c-Kit, have all also been demonstrated in both GI and pulmonary carcinoids (76,227–233).

Disruption of these signaling pathways has resulted in inhibition of neuroendocrine cell growth in preclinical models, leading to a number of recent clinical trials with tyrosine kinase inhibitors and monoclonal antibodies targeting these pathways in patients with advanced neuroendocrine tumors. Imatnib mesylate inhibits receptor tyrosine kinases for BCR-Abl, PDGFR, stem cell factor, and KIT. Incubation of neuroendocrine tumor cells in the presence of imatinib mesylate resulted in inhibition of cell growth (233). In a preliminary report, however, the administration of imatinib mesylate to 15 patients with advanced neuroendocrine tumors did not result in any objective responses. Similarly, although exposure to gefitinib, a tyrosine kinase inhibitor targeting EGFR, resulted in growth inhibition of neuroendocrine cell lines, no responses were reported when gefitinib was administered to patients with neuroendocrine tumors in a phase II study (234,235).

Neuroendocrine tumors are highly vascular, and overexpression of vascular endothelial growth factor (VEGF) has been observed in both midgut carcinoid tumors and in pancreatic endocrine tumors (76). Similarly, expression of VEGF receptor subtypes 1 and 2 has been observed in the majority of carcinoid and pancreatic endocrine tumors, suggesting that binding of VEGF to its receptor may be involved in neuroendocrine tumorigenesis (236,237). Inhibition of the VEGF receptor with function-blocking antibodies disrupted tumor growth in a mouse model of pancreatic islet cell carcinogenesis, lending further preclinical support to this hypothesis (238).

Preliminary results of clinical trials of VEGF pathway inhibitors in patients with advanced neuroendocrine tumors have been encouraging, and suggest that inhibition of either VEGF or VEGFR has the potential to lead to inhibition of tumor growth and, in some cases, tumor regression. In one phase II trial of bevacizumab, 44 patients with advanced or metastatic carcinoid tumors were randomly assigned to receive either bevacizumab, a humanized monoclonal antibody targeting VEGF, or pegylated IFN-α 2b (239). In a preliminary report of 35 patients completing 18 weeks of therapy, 3 of 18 patients treated with bevacizumab experienced radiographic partial responses. Furthermore, after 18 weeks, 95% of patients treated with bevacizumab remained progressionfree compared to only 67% of patients treated with IFN.

Sunitinib, a multitargeted tyrosine kinase activity with activity against VEGFR, PDGFR, c-Kit, and RET, has also been shown to have activity in patients with advanced neuroendocrine tumors. A phase I study of sunitinib included four patients with neuroendocrine tumors; of these patients, one experienced an objective radiologic response and a second experienced a minor response with prolonged tumor stabilization

(240). These observations led to the development of a phase II study, in which 102 patients with advanced neuroendocrine tumors received repeated treatment cycles of sunitinib, administered at a dose of 50 mg daily for 4 weeks, followed by a 2-week break (241). In a preliminary analysis, 9 of 61 (15%) pancreatic neuroendocrine tumor patients and 1 of 41 (2%) carcinoid patients experienced a partial response. Stable disease was observed in 93% of the carcinoid patients and 74% of the pancreatic neuroendocrine tumor patients. The responders included 1 patient with a foregut carcinoid tumor, 1 patient with a gastrinoma, and 8 patients with nonfunctioning pancreatic neuroendocrine tumors. The median time to tumor progression was 42 weeks for carcinoid patients and 33 weeks for pancreatic neuroendocrine patients; for the entire cohort, the median time to progression was 40 weeks.

Future trials in patients with neuroendocrine tumors are likely to build on these promising observations, combining traditional cytotoxic agents with newer agents that target not only the VEGF pathway but also other molecular pathways important in neuroendocrine tumor growth and development.

References

1. Rindi G, Kloppel G. Endocrine tumors of the gut and pancreas tumor biology and classification. *Neuroendocrinology* 2004;80(suppl 1):12–15.
2. Oberg K, Eriksson B. Medical treatment of neuroendocrine gut and pancreatic tumors. *Acta Oncol* 1989;28:425–431.
3. Jensen RT. Management of the Zollinger-Ellison syndrome in patients with multiple endocrine neoplasia type 1. *J Intern Med* 1998;243:477–488.
4. Gibril F, Schumann M, Pace A, et al. Multiple endocrine neoplasia type 1 and Zollinger-Ellison syndrome: a prospective study of 107 cases and comparison with 1009 cases from the literature. *Medicine (Baltimore)* 2004;83:43–83.
5. Agarwal SK, Lee Burns A, Sukhodolets KE, et al. Molecular pathology of the *MEN1* gene. *Ann N Y Acad Sci* 2004;1014:189–198.
6. Hessman O, Lindberg D, Skogseid B, et al. Mutation of the multiple endocrine neoplasia type 1 gene in nonfamilial, malignant tumors of the endocrine pancreas. *Cancer Res* 1998;58:377–379.
7. Ebrahimi SA, Wang EH, Wu A, et al. Deletion of chromosome 1 predicts prognosis in pancreatic endocrine tumors. *Cancer Res* 1999;59:311–315.
8. Rigaud G, Missiaglia E, Moore PS, et al. High resolution allelotype of nonfunctional pancreatic endocrine tumors: identification of two molecular subgroups with clinical implications. *Cancer Res* 2001;61:285–292.
9. Bartsch D, Hahn SA, Danichevski KD, et al. Mutations of the DPC4/Smad4 gene in neuroendocrine pancreatic tumors. *Oncogene* 1999;18:2367–2371.
10. Lubomierski N, Kersting M, Bert T, et al. Tumor suppressor genes in the 9p21 gene cluster are selective targets of inactivation in neuroendocrine gastroenteropancreatic tumors. *Cancer Res* 2001;61:5905–5910.
11. Wild A, Langer P, Celik I, et al. Chromosome 22q in pancreatic endocrine tumors: identification of a homozygous deletion and potential prognostic associations of allelic deletions. *Eur J Endocrinol* 2002;147:507–513.
12. Marcos HB, Libutti SK, Alexander HR, et al. Neuroendocrine tumors of the pancreas in von Hippel-Lindau disease: spectrum of appearances at CT and MR imaging with histopathologic comparison. *Radiology* 2002;225:751–758.
13. Service F, McMahon M, O'Brien P, et al. Functioning insulinoma—incidence, recurrence, and long-term survival of patients: a 60-year study. *Mayo Clin Proc* 1991;66:711–719.
14. Hoff A, Gilbert J, Gagel R. Management of neuroendocrine cancers of the gastrointestinal tract: islet cell carcinoima of the pancreas and other neuroendocrine carcinomas. In: Abbruzzese J, Evans D, Willett C, et al., eds. *Gastrointestinal Oncology*. New York, NY: Oxford University Press; 2004:780–802.
15. Grant CS. Gastrointestinal endocrine tumours: insulinoma. *Bailliéres Clin Gastroenterol* 1996;10:645–671.
16. Dizon A, Kowakyk S, Hoogwerf B. Neuroglycopenic and other symptoms in patients with insulinomas. *Am J Med* 1999;106:307–310.
17. Whipple A, Franz V. Adenoma of islet cells with hyperinsulinism. *Am Surg* 1935;101:1299–1335.
18. Service F. Hypoglycemic disorders. *N Engl J Med* 1995;332:1144–1152.
19. Grant CS, van Heerden J, Charboneau JW, et al. Insulinoma: the value of intraoperative ultrasonography. *Arch Surg* 1988;123:843–848.
20. Pasieka J, McLeod M, Thompson N, et al. Surgical approach to insulinomas: assessing the need for preoperative localization. *Arch Surg* 1992;127:442–447.
21. Anderson M, Carpenter S, Thompson N, et al. Endoscopic ultrasound is highly accurate and directs management in patients with neuroendocrine tumors of the pancreas. *Am J Gastroenterol* 2000;95:2271–2277.

22. Menegaux F, Schmitt G, Mercadier M, et al. Pancreatic insulinomas. *Am J Surg* 1993;165:243–248.
23. Rosch T, Lightdale C, Botet J, et al. Localization of pancreatic endocrine tumors by endoscopic ultrasonography. *N Engl J Med* 1992;326:1721–1726.
24. Goode P, Farndon J, Anderson J, et al. Diazoxide in the management of patients with insulinoma. *World J Surg* 1986;10:586–592.
25. O'Riordain D, O'Brien T, van Heerden J, et al. Surgical management of insulinoma associated with multiple endocrine neoplasia type I. *World J Surg* 1994;18:488–493; discussion 493–494.
26. Demeure M, Klonoff D, Karam J, et al. Insulinomas associated with multiple endocrine neoplasia type I: the need for a different surgical approach. *Surgery* 1991;110:998–1004; discussion 1004–1005.
27. Zollinger R, Ellison E. Primary peptic ulcerations of the jejunum associates with islet cell tumors of pancrea. *Ann Surg* 1955;142:709–728.
28. Roy P, Venzon D, Shojamanesh H, et al. Zollinger-Ellison syndrome: clinical presentation in 261 patients. *Medicine (Baltimore)* 2000;79:379–411.
29. Norton J, Jensen R. Unresolved surgical issues in the management of patients with Zollinger-Ellison syndrome. *World J Surg* 1991;15:151–159.
30. Sugg S, Norton J, Fraker D, et al. A prospective study of intraoperative methods to diagnose and resect duodenal gastrinomas. *Ann Surg* 1993;218:138–144.
31. Jensen R. Gastrointestinal endocrine tumours: gastrinoma. *Baillieres Clin Gastroenterol* 1996;10:603–643.
32. Wolfe M, Jensen R. Zollinger-Ellison syndrome: current concepts in diagnosis and management. *N Engl J Med* 1987;317:1200–1209.
33. Frucht H, Howard J, Slaff J, et al. Secretin and calcium provocative tests in the Zollinger-Ellison syndrome: a prospective study. *Ann Intern Med* 1989;111:713–722.
34. Lambers C, Lind T, Moberg S, et al. Omeprazole in Zollinger-Ellison syndrome: effects of a single dose and of long-term treatment in patients resistant to histamine H_2-receptor antagonists. *N Engl J Med* 1984;310:758–761.
35. Frucht H, Maton P, Jensen R. Use of omeprazole in patients with Zollinger-Ellison syndrome. *Dig Dis Sci* 1991;36:394–404.
36. Stabile B, Morrow D, E Passaro J. The gastrinoma triangle: operative implications. *Am J Surg* 1984;147:25–31.
37. Fraker DL, Norton JA, Alexander HR, et al. Surgery in Zollinger-Ellison syndrome alters the natural history of gastrinoma. *Ann Surg* 1994;220:320–328; discussion 328–330.
38. deKerviler E, Cadiot G, Lebtahi R, et al. Somatostatin receptor scintigraphy in forty-eight patients with the Zollinger-Ellison syndrome. GRESZE: Groupe d'Etude du Syndrome de Zollinger-Ellison. *Eur J Nucl Med* 1994;21:1191–1197.
39. Norton J, Doppman J, Jensen R. Curative resection in Zollinger-Ellison syndrome: results of a 10-year prospective study. *Ann Surg* 1992;215:8–18.
40. Mignon M, Cadiot G. Diagnostic and therapeutic criteria in patients with Zollinger-Ellison syndrome and multiple endocrine neoplasia type 1. *J Intern Med* 1998;243:489–494.
41. MacFarlane M, Fraker D, Alexander H, et al. Prospective study of surgical resection of duodenal and pancreatic gastrinomas in multiple endocrine neoplasia type 1. *Surgery* 1995;118:973–979; discussion 979–980.
42. Sheppard B, Norton J, Doppman J, et al. Management of islet cell tumors in patients with multiple endocrine neoplasia: a prospective study. *Surgery* 1989;106:1108–1117; discussion 1117–1118.
43. Bartsch DK, Langer P, Wild A, et al. Pancreaticoduodenal endocrine tumors in multiple endocrine neoplasia type 1: surgery or surveillance? *Surgery* 2000;128:958–966.
44. Norton JA, Fraker DL, Alexander HR, et al. Surgery to cure the Zollinger-Ellison syndrome. *N Engl J Med* 1999;341:635–644.
45. Shojamanesh H, Gibril F, Louie A, et al. Prospective study of the antitumor efficacy of long-term octreotide treatment in patients with progressive metastatic gastrinoma. *Cancer* 2002;94:331–343.
46. Frankton S, Bloom SR. Gastrointestinal endocrine tumours: glucagonomas. *Baillieres Clin Gastroenterol* 1996;10:697–705.
47. Wermers R, Fatourechi V, Wynne A, et al. The glucagonoma syndrome: clinical and pathologic features in 21 patients. *Medicine (Baltimore)* 1996;75:53–63.
48. Horrobin D, Cunnane S. Interactions between zinc, essential fatty acids and prostaglandins: relevance to acrodermatitis enteropathica, total parenteral nutrition, the glucagonoma syndrome, diabetes, anorexia nervosa and sickle cell anaemia. *Med Hypotheses* 1980;6:277–296.
49. Roth E, Muhlbacher F, Karner J, et al. Free amino acid levels in muscle and liver of a patient with glucagonoma syndrome. *Metabolism* 1987;36:7–13.
50. Boden G. Insulinoma and glucagonoma. *Semin Oncol* 1987;14:253–262.
51. El Rassi Z, Partensky C, Valette PJ, et al. Necrolytic migratory erythema, first symptom of a malignant glucagonoma: treatment by long-acting somatostatin and surgical resection: report of three cases. *Eur J Surg Oncol* 1998;24:562–567.
52. Jockenhovel F, Lederbogen S, Olbricht T, et al. The long-acting somatostatin analogue octreotide alleviates symptoms by reducing posttranslational conversion of prepro-glucagon to glucagon in a patient with malignant glucagonoma, but does not prevent tumor growth. *Clin Investig* 1994; 72:127–133.
53. Edney JA, Hofmann S, Thompson JS, et al. Glucagonoma syndrome is an underdiagnosed clinical entity. *Am J Surg* 1990;160:625–628; discussion 628–629.
54. Verner J, Morrison A. Islet cell tumor and a syndrome of refractory watery diarrhea and hypokalemia. *Am J Med* 1958;25:374–380.
55. Kane M, O'Dorisio T, Krejs G. Production of secretory diarrhea by intravenous infusion of vasoactive intestinal polypeptide. *N Engl J Med* 1983;309:1482–1485.
56. Said S, Faloona G. Elevated plasma and tissue levels of vasoactive intestinal polypeptide in the watery-diarrhea syndrome due to pancreatic, bronchogenic and other tumors. *N Engl J Med* 1975;293:155–160.
57. Long R, Bryant M, Mitchell S, et al. Clinicopathological study of pancreatic and ganglioneuroblastoma tumors secreting vasoactive intestinal polypeptide (VIPomas). *Br Med J (Clin Res Ed)* 1981;282:1767–1771.
58. Kraenzlin M, Ch'ng J, Wood S, et al. Long-term treatment of a VIPoma with somatostatin analogue resulting in remission of symptoms and possible shrinkage of metastases. *Gastroenterology* 1985;88:185–187.
59. Debas H, Mulvihill S. Neuroendocrine gut neoplasms: important lessons from uncommon tumors. *Arch Surg* 1994;129:965–971; discussion 971–972.
60. Rothmund M, Stinner B, Arnold R. Endocrine pancreatic carcinoma. *Eur J Surg Oncol* 1991;17:191–199.
61. Park S, O'Dorisio M, O'Dorisio T. Vasoactive intestinal polypeptide-secreting tumours: biology and therapy. *Baillieres Clin Gastroenterol* 1996;10:673–696.
62. Cheslyn-Curtis S, Sitaram V, Williamson R. Management of nonfunctioning neuroendocrine tumours of the pancreas. *Br J Surg* 1993;80:625–627.
63. Matthews B, Heniford B, Reardon P, et al. Surgical experience with nonfunctioning neuroendocrine tumors of the pancreas. *Am Surg* 2000;66:1116–1122.
64. Modlin I, Sandor A. An analysis of 8305 cases of carcinoid tumors. *Cancer* 1997;79:813–829.
65. Watson RG, Johnston CF, O'Hare MM, et al. The frequency of gastrointestinal endocrine tumours in a well-defined population—Northern Ireland 1970–1985. *Q J Med* 1989;72:647–657.
66. Norheim I, Oberg K, Theodorsson-Norheim E, et al. Malignant carcinoid tumors: an analysis of 103 patients with regard to tumor localization, hormone production, and survival. *Ann Surg* 1987;206:115–125.
67. Eriksson B, Oberg K, Skogseid B. Neuroendocrine pancreatic tumors: clinical findings in a prospective study of 84 patients. *Acta Oncol* 1989;28:373–377.
68. Godwin J. Carcinoid tumors: an analysis of 2837 cases. *Cancer* 1975;36:560–569.
69. Berge T, Linnell F. Carcinoid tumors: frequency in a defined population during a 12-year period. *Acta Pathol Microbiol Scand [A]* 1976;84:322–330.
70. Petzmann S, Ullmann R, Klemen H, et al. Loss of heterozygosity on chromosome arm 11q in lung carcinoids. *Hum Pathol* 2001;32:333–338.
71. Petzmann S, Ullmann R, Halbwedl I, et al. Analysis of chromosome-11 aberrations in pulmonary and gastrointestinal carcinoids: an array comparative genomic hybridization-based study. *Virchows Arch* 2004;445:151–159.
72. Ullmann R, Petzmann S, Klemen H, et al. The position of pulmonary carcinoids within the spectrum of neuroendocrine tumors of the lung and other tissues. *Genes Chromosomes Cancer* 2002;34:78–85.
73. Lollgen RM, Hessman O, Szabo E, et al. Chromosome 18 deletions are common events in classical midgut carcinoid tumors. *Int J Cancer* 2001;92:812–815.
74. Wang GG, Yao JC, Worah S, et al. Comparison of genetic alterations in neuroendocrine tumors: frequent loss of chromosome 18 in ileal carcinoid tumors. *Mod Pathol* 2005;18:1079–1087.
75. Kytola S, Nord B, Elder EE, et al. Alterations of the SDHD gene locus in midgut carcinoids, Merkel cell carcinomas, pheochromocytomas, and abdominal paragangliomas. *Genes Chromosomes Cancer* 2002;34:325–332.
76. Terris B, Scoazec J, Rubbia L. Expression of vascular endothelial growth factor in digestive neuroendocrine tumors. *Histopathology* 1998;32:133–138.
77. Tonnies H, Toliat MR, Ramel C, et al. Analysis of sporadic neuroendocrine tumours of the enteropancreatic system by comparative genomic hybridisation. *Gut* 2001;48:536–541.
78. Harpole D, Feldman J, Buchanan S, et al. Bronchial carcinoid tumors: a retrospective analysis of 126 patients. *Ann Thorac Surg* 1992;54:50–55.
79. Vadasz P, Palffy G, Egervary M, et al. Diagnosis and treatment of bronchial carcinoid tumors: clinical and pathological review of 120 operated patients. *Eur J Cardiothorac Surg* 1993;7:8–11.
80. Torre M, Barberis M, Barbieri B, et al. Typical and atypical bronchial carcinoids. *Resp Med* 1989;83:305–308.
81. Okike N, Bernatz P, Woolner L. Carcinoid tumors of the lung. *Ann Thorac Surg* 1976;22:270–277.
82. Fink G, Krelbaum T, Yellin A, et al. Pulmonary carcinoid: presentation, diagnosis, and outcome in 142 cases in Israel and review of 640 cases from literature. *Chest* 2001;119:1647–1651.
83. Rea F, Binda R, Spreafico G, et al. Bronchial carcinoids: a review of 60 patients. *Ann Thorac Surg* 1989;47:412–414.

84. McCaughan B, Martini N, Bains M. Bronchial carcinoids: review of 124 cases. *J Thorac Cardiovasc Surg* 1985;89:8–17.

85. Chughtai T, Morin J, Sheiner N, et al. Bronchial carcinoid-twenty years' experience defines a selective surgical approach. *Surgery* 1997;122:801–808.

86. Skuladottir H, Hirsch F, Hansen H, et al. Pulmonary neuroendocrine tumors: incidence and prognosis of hislogical subtypes: a population-based study in Denmark. *Lung Cancer* 2002;37:127–135.

87. Smolle-Juttner F, Popper H, Klemen H, et al. Clinical features and therapy of "typical" and "atypical" bronchial carcinoid tumors (grade 1 and grade 2 neuroendocrine carcinoma). *Eur J Cardiothorac Surg* 1993;7:121–125.

88. Marty-Ane C, Costes V, Pujol J, et al. Carcinoid tumors of the lung: do atypical features require aggressive management? *Ann Thorac Surg* 1995;59:78–83.

89. Mezzetti M, Raveglia F, Panigalli T, et al. Assessment of outcomes in typical and atypical carcinoids according to latest WHO classification. *Ann Thorac Surg* 2003;76:1838–1842.

90. Fiala P, Petraskova K, Cernohorsky S, et al. Bronchial carcinoid tumors: long-term outcome after surgery. *Neoplasma* 2003;50:60–65.

91. Schrevens L, Vansteenkiste J, Deneffe G, et al. Clinical-Radiological presentation and outcome of surgically treated pulmonary carcinoid tumours: a long-term single institution expierence. *Lung Cancer* 2004;43:39–45.

92. Modlin I, Gilligan C, Lawton G, et al. Gastric carcinoids: the Yale experience. *Arch Surg* 1995;130:250–256.

93. Eckhauser F, Lloyd R, Thompson N, et al. Antrectomy for multicentric, argyrophil gastric carcinoids: a preliminary report. *Surgery* 1988;104:1046–1053.

94. Hirschowitz BI, Griffith J, Pellegrin D, et al. Rapid regression of enterochromaffinlike cell gastric carcinoids in pernicious anemia after antrectomy. *Gastroenterology* 1992;102:1409–1418.

95. Tomassetti P, Migliori M, Caletti G, et al. Treatment of type II gastric carcinoid tumors with somatostatin analogs. *N Engl J Med* 2000;343:551–554.

96. Rindi G, Luinetti O, Cornaggia M, et al. Three subtypes of gastric argyrophil carcinoid and the gastric neuroendocrine carcinoma: a clinicopathologic study. *Gastroenterology* 1993;104:994–1006.

97. Rindi G, Bordi C, Rappel S, et al. Gastric carcinoids and neuroendocrine carcinomas: pathogenesis, pathology, and behavior. *World J Surg* 1996;20:168–172.

98. Barclay T, Schapira D. Malignant tumors of the small intestine. *Cancer* 1983;51:878–881.

99. Makridis C, Oberg K, Juhlin C, et al. Surgical treatment of mid-gut carcinoid tumors. *World J Surg* 1990;14:377–385.

100. Hellman P, Lundstrom T, Ohrvall U, et al. Effect of surgery on the outcome of midgut carcinoid disease with lymph node and liver metastases. *World J Surg* 2002;26:991–997.

101. Moertel C, Sauer W, Dockerty M, et al. Life history of the carcinoid tumor of the small intestine. *Cancer* 1961;14:901–912.

102. Burke A, Thomas R, Elsayed A, et al. Carcinoids of the jejunum and ileum: an immunohistochemical and clinicopathologic study of 167 cases. *Cancer* 1997;79:1086–1093.

103. Modlin I, Lye K, Kidd M. A 5-decade analysis of 13,715 carcinoid tumors. *Cancer* 2003;97:934–959.

104. Eckhauser F, Argenta L, Strodel W, et al. Mesenteric angiopathy, intestinal gangrene, and midgut carcinoids. *Surgery* 1981;90:720–728.

105. Lyss A. Appendiceal malignancies. *Semin Oncol* 1988;15:129–137.

106. Collins D. 71,000 Appendectomy specimens: a final report summarizing 40 years of study. *Am J Proctol* 1963;14:365–381.

107. Moertel C, Dockerty M, Judd E. Carcinoid tumors of the vermiform appendix. *Cancer* 1968;21:270–278.

108. Roggo A, Wood W, Ottinger L. Carcinoid tumors of the appendix. *Ann Surg* 1993;217:385–390.

109. Lundqvist M, Wilander E. Subepithelial neuroendocrine cells and carcinoid tumors of the human small intestine and appendix: a comparative immunohistochemical study with regard to serotonin, neuron-specific enolase and S-100 protein reactivity. *J Pathol* 1986;148:141–147.

110. Lundqvist M, Wilander E. A study of the histopathogenesis of carcinoid tumors of the small intestine and appendix. *Cancer* 1987;60:201–206.

111. Shaw P. The topographical and age distribution of neuroendocrine cells in the normal human appendix. *J Pathol* 1991;164:235–239.

112. Moertel C, Weiland L, Telander R. Carcinoid tumor of the appendix in the first two decades of life. *J Pediatr Surg* 1990;25:1073–1075.

113. Jonsson T, Johannsson J, Hallgrimsson J. Carcinoid tumors of the appendix in children younger than 16 years. *Acta Chir Scand* 1989;155:113–116.

114. Parks S, Muir K, Alsheyyab M. Carcinoid tumors of the appendix in children: 1957–1985. *Br J Surg* 1993;80:502–504.

115. Moertel C, Weiland L, Nagorney D, et al. Carcinoid tumors of the appendix: treatment and prognosis. *N Engl J Med* 1987;317:1699–1701.

116. Anderson J, Wilson B. Carcinoid tumors of the appendix. *Br J Surg* 1985;72:545–546.

117. Syracuse D, Perzin K, Weidel P, et al. Carcinoid tumors of the appendix: mesoappendiceal extension and nodal metastases. *Ann Surg* 1979;190:58–63.

118. Bowman G, Rosenthal D. Carcinoid tumors of the appendix. *Am J Surg* 1983;146:700–703.

119. Thirlby R, Kasper C, Jones R. Metastatic carcinoid tumor of the appendix: report of a case and review of the literature. *Dis Colon Rectum* 1984;27:42–46.

120. MacGillivray D, Heaton R, Rushin J, et al. Distant metastases from a carcinoid tumor of the appendix less than one centimeter in size. *Surgery* 1992;111:466–471.

121. Pearlman D, Srinivasan K. Malignant carcinoid of the appendix: metastases from a small primary tumor which appeared as appendiceal intussusception. *N Y State J Med* 1971;71:1529–1531.

122. Jetmore A, Ray J, Gathright J, et al. Rectal carcinoids: the most frequent carcinoid tumor. *Dis Colon Rectum* 1992;35:717–725.

123. Soga J. Carcinoids of the rectum: tumors of the carcinoid family-urgut endocrinomas. *Acta Med Biol (Niigata)* 1982;29:157–201.

124. Naunheim K, Zeitels J, Kaplan E, et al. Rectal carcinoid tumors-treatment and prognosis. *Surgery* 1983;94:670–676.

125. Sauven P, Ridge J, Quan S, et al. Anorectal carcinoid tumors: is aggressive surgery warranted? *Ann Surg* 1990;211:67–71.

126. Burke M, Shepherd N, Mann C. Carcinoid tumors of the rectum and anus. *Br J Surg* 1987;74:358–361.

127. Koura A, Giacco G, Curley S, et al. Carcinoid tumors of the rectum: effect of size, histopathology, and surgical treatment on metastasis free survival. *Cancer* 1997;79:1294–1298.

128. Thorson A, Biorck G, Bjorkman G, et al. Malignant carcinoid of the small intestine with metastases to the liver, valvular disease on the right side of the heart (pulmonary stenosis and tricuspid regurgitation without septal defects), peripheral vasomotor symptoms, bronchoconstriction, and an unusual type of cyanosis. *Am Heart J* 1954;47:795–817.

129. Pernow B, Waldenstrom J. Determination of 5-hydroxytryptamine, 5-hydroxyindoleacetic acid, and histamine in 33 cases of carcinoid tumor. *Am J Med* 1957;23:16–25.

130. Soga J, Yakuwa Y. Somatostatinoma/inhibitory syndrome: a statistical evaluation of 173 reported cases as compared to other pancreatic endocrinomas. *J Exp Clin Cancer Res* 1999;18:13–22.

131. Schnirer I, Yao J, Ajani J. Carcinoid: a comprehensive review. *Acta Oncol* 2003;42:672–692.

132. Woodard P, Feldman J, Paine S, et al. Midgut carcinoid tumors: CT findings and biochemical profiles. *J Comput Assist Tomogr* 1995;19:400–405.

133. Sugimoto E, Lorelius L, Eriksson B, et al. Midgut carcinoid tumors: CT appearance. *Radiologica* 1995;36:367–371.

134. Lamberts S, Bakker W, Reubi J, et al. Somatostatin receptor imaging in the localization of endocrine tumors. *N Engl J Med* 1990;323:1246–1249.

135. Kvols LK, Brown ML, O'Connor MK, et al. Evaluation of a radiolabeled somatostatin analog (I-123 octreotide) in the detection and localization of carcinoid and islet cell tumors. *Radiology* 1993;187(1):129–133.

136. Kaltsas G, Korbonits M, Heintz E, et al. Comparison of somatostatin analog and meta-iodobenzylguanidine radionuclites in the diagnosis and localization of advanced neuroendocrine tumors. *J Clin Endocrinol Metab* 2001;86:895–902.

137. Krenning E, Kwekkeboom D, Bakker W, et al. Somatostatin receptory scintigraphy with [111In-DTPA-D-Phe1] - and [123-Tyr3]-octreotide: the Rotterdam experience with more than 1000 patients. *Eur J Nucl Med* 1993;20.

138. Schillaci O, Scopinaro F, Danieli R, et al. Single photon emission computerized tomography increases the sensitivity of indium-111-pentetreotide scintigraphy in detecting abdominal carcinoids. *Anticancer Res* 1997;17(3B):1753–1756.

139. Schillaci O, Corleto V, Annibale B. Single photon emission computed tomography procedure improves accuracy of somatostatin receptor scintigraphy in gasto-entero pancreatic tumours. *Ital J Gastroenterol Hepatol* 1999;31:(suppl 2).

140. Gibril F, Reynolds J, Doppman J, et al. Somatostatin receptor scintigraphy: its sensitivity compared to that of other imaging methods in detection of primary and metastatic gastrinomas: a prospective study. *Ann Intern Med* 1996;125:26–34.

141. Feldman J, O'Dirisio T. Role of neuropeptides and serotonin in the diagnosis of carcinoid tumors. *Am J Med* 1986;81(suppl 6B):41–48.

142. Meko JB, Norton JA. Management of patients with Zollinger-Ellison syndrome. *Ann Rev Med* 1995;46:395–411.

143. Seregni E, Ferrari L, Bajetta E, et al. Clinical significance of blood chromogranin A measurement in neuroendocrine tumours. *Ann Oncol* 2001; 12(suppl 2): S69–S72.

144. Tomassetti P, Migliori M, Simoni P, et al. Diagnostic value of plasma chromogranin A in neuroendocrine tumours. *Eur J Gastroenterol Hepatol* 2001; 13(1):55–58.

145. Stivanello M, Berruti A, Torta M, et al. Circulating chromogranin A in the assessment of patients with neuroendocrine tumours. A single institution experience. *Ann Oncol* 2001;12 suppl 2:S73–S77.

146. Oberg K, Kvols L, Caplin M, et al. Consensus report on the use of somatostatin analogs for the management of neuroendocrine tumors of the gastroenteropancreatic system. *Ann Oncol* 2004;15(6):966–973.

147. Janson ET, Holmberg L, Stridsberg M, et al. Carcinoid tumors: analysis of prognostic factors and survival in 301 patients from a referral center. *Ann Oncol* 1997;8(7):685–690.

148. Dousset B, Saint-Marc O, Pitre J, et al. Metastatic neuroendocrine tumors: medical treatment, surgical resection, or liver transplantation. *World J Surg* 1996;20:908–915.

149. McEntee G, Nagorney D, Kvols L, et al. Cytoreductive hepatic surgery for neuroendocrine tumors. *Surgery* 1990;108:1091–1096.

150. Que F, Nagorney D, Batts K, et al. Hepatic resection for metastatic neuroendocrine carcinomas. *Am J Surg* 1995;169:36–43.

151. LeTreut YP, Delpero JR, Dousset B, et al. Results of liver transplantation in the treatment of metastatic neuroendocrine tumors: A 31-case French multicentric report. *Ann Surg* 1997;225(4):355–364.

152. Cherner JA, Sawyers JL. Benefit of resection of metastatic gastrinoma in multiple endocrine neoplasia type I. *Gastroenterology* 1992;102(3):1049–1053.

153. Alsina AE, Bartus S, Hull D, et al. Liver transplant for metastatic neuroendocrine tumor. *J Clin Gastroenterol* 1990;12(5):533–537.

154. Lang H, Oldhafer K, Weimann A, et al. Liver transplantation for metastatic neuroendocrine tumors. *Ann Surg* 1997;225:347–354.

155. Lundin L, Norheim I, Landelius J, et al. Carcinoid heart disease: relationship of circulating vasoactive substances to ultrasound-detectable cardiac abnormalities. *Circulation* 1988;7:264–269.

156. Simula D, Edwards W, Tazelaar H, et al. Surgical pathology of carcinoid heart disease: a study of 139 valves from 75 patients spanning 20 years. *Mayo Clin Proc* 2002;77:139–147.

157. Robiolio P, Rigolin V, Wilson J, et al. Carcinoid heart disease: correlation of high serotonin levels with valvular abnormalities deteted by cardiac catherterization and echocardiography. *Circulation* 1995;77:264–269.

158. Pellikka P, Tajik A, Khandheria B, et al. Carcinoid heart disease: clinical and echocardiographic spectrum in 74 patients. *Circulation* 1993;87:1188–1196.

159. Moller J, Connolly H, Rubin J, et al. Factors associated with progression of carcinoid heart disease. *N Engl J Med* 2003;348:1005–1015.

160. Zuetenhorst J, Bonfrer J, Korse C, et al. Carcinoid heart disease: the role of urinary 5-hydroxyindoleacic acid excretion and plasma levels of atrial antriuretic peptide, transforming growth factor beta and fibroblast growth factor. *Cancer* 2003;97:1609–1615.

161. Denney WD, Kemp WE, Jr., Anthony LB, et al. Echocardiographic and biochemical evaluation of the development and progression of carcinoid heart disease. *J Am Coll Cardiol* 1998;32:1017–1022.

162. Robiolio P, Rigolin V, Harrison J, et al. Predictors of outcome of tricuspid valve replacement in carcinoid heart disease. *Am J Cardiol* 1995;75:485–488.

163. Connolly H, Nishimura R, Smith H, et al. Outcome of cardiac surgery for carcinoid heart disease. *J Am Coll Cardiol* 1995;25:410–416.

164. Voigt P, Braun J, Teng O, et al. Double bioprosthetic valve replacement in right sided carcinoid heart disease. *Ann Thorac Surg* 2005;79:2147–2149.

165. Basson MD, Ahlman H, Wangberg B, et al. Biology and management of the midgut carcinoid. *Am J Surg* 1993;165:288–297.

166. Woodside KJ, Townsend CM, Jr, Mark Evers B. Current management of gastrointestinal carcinoid tumors. *J Gastrointest Surg* 2004;8:742–756.

167. Dery R. Theoretical and clinical considerations in anaesthesia for secreting carcinoid tumors. *Can Anaesth Soc J* 1971;18:245–263.

168. Memon MA, Nelson H. Gastrointestinal carcinoid tumors: current management strategies. *Dis Colon Rectum* 1997;40:1101–1118.

169. Ajani JA, Carrasco CH, Charnsangavej C, et al. Islet cell tumors metastatic to the liver: effective palliation by sequential hepatic artery embolization. *Ann Intern Med* 1988;108(3):340–344.

170. Moertel C, Johnson C, McKusick M, et al. The management of patients with advanced carcinoid tumors and islet cell carcinoma. *Ann Intern Med* 1994;120:302–309.

171. Ruszniewski P, Rougier P, Roche A, et al. Hepatic arterial chemoembolization in patients with liver metastases of endocrine tumors. *Cancer* 1993;71:2624–2630.

172. Eriksson BK, Larsson EG, Skogseid BM, et al. Liver embolizations of patients with malignant neuroendocrine gastrointestinal tumors. *Cancer* 1998;83(11):2293–2301.

173. Gupta S, Yao J, Ahrar K, et al. Hepatic artery embolization and chemoembolization for treatment of patients with metastatic carcinoid tumors: the MD Anderson experience. *Cancer J* 2003;9:261–267.

174. Dominguez S, Denys A, Madeira I, et al. Hepatic arterial chemoembolization with streptozotocin in patients with metastatic digestive endocrine tumors. *Eur J Gastroenterol Hepatol* 2000;12(2):151–157.

175. Drougas JG, Anthony LB, Blair TK, et al. Hepatic artery chemoembolization for management of patients with advanced metastatic carcinoid tumors. *Am J Surg* 1998;175(5):408–412.

176. Diamandidou E, Ajani JA, Yang DJ, et al. Two-phase study of hepatic artery vascular occlusion with microencapsulated cisplatin in patients with liver metastases from neuroendocrine tumors. *AJR Am J Roentgenol* 1998;170(2):339–344.

177. Loewe C, Schindl M, Cejna M, et al. Permanent transarterial embolization of neuroendocrine metastases of the liver using cyanoacrylate and lipiodol: assessment of mid- and long-term results. *AJR Am J Roentgenol* 2003;180(5):1379–1384.

178. Brown K, Koh B, Brody L, et al. Particle embolization of hepatic neuroendocrine metastases for control of pain and hormonal symptoms. *J Vasc Interv Radiol* 1999;10.

179. Gulec SA, Mountcastle TS, Frey D, et al. Cytoreductive surgery in patients with advanced-stage carcinoid tumors. *Am Surg* 2002;68(8):667–671; discussion 71–72.

180. Hellman P, Ladjevardi S, Skogseid B, et al. Radiofrequency tissue ablation using cooled tip for liver metastases of endocrine tumors. *World J Surg* 2002;26(8):1052–1056.

181. Berber E, Flesher N, Siperstein AE. Laparoscopic radiofrequency ablation of neuroendocrine liver metastases. *World J Surg* 2002;26(8):985–990.

182. Chung MH, Pisegna J, Spirt M, et al. Hepatic cytoreduction followed by a novel long-acting somatostatin analog: a paradigm for intractable neuroendocrine tumors metastatic to the liver. *Surgery* 2001;130(6):954–962.

183. Reubi J, Kvols L, Waser B, et al. Detection of somatostatin receptors in surgical and percutaneous needle biopsy samples of carcinoids and islet cell carcinomas. *Cancer Res* 1990;50:5969–5977.

184. Kvols L, Moertel C, O'Connell M, et al. Treatment of the malignant carcinoid syndrome: evaluation of a long-acting somatostatin analog. *N Engl J Med* 1986;315:663–666.

185. Rubin J, Ajani J, Schirmer W, et al. Octreotide acetate long-acting formulation versus open-label subcutaneous octreotide acetate in malignant carcinoid syndrome. *J Clin Oncol* 1999;17:600–606.

186. Faiss S, Rath U, Mansmann U, et al. Ultra-high-dose lanreotide treatment in patients with metastatic neuroendocribe gastroenteropancreatic tumors. *Digestion* 1999;60.

187. Wymenga A, Eriksson B, Salmela P, et al. Efficacy and safety of prolonged-release lanreotide in patients with gastrointestinal neuroendocrine tumors and hormone-related symptoms. *J Clin Oncol* 1999;17.

188. O'Toole D, Ducreux M, Bommelaer G, et al. Treatment of carcinoid syndrome: A prospective crossover evaluation of lanreotide versus octreotide in terms of efficacy, patient acceptability, and tolerance. *Cancer* 2000;88.

189. Ducreux M, Ruszniewski P, Chayvialle J, et al. The antitumoral effect of the long-acting somatostatin analog lanreotide, interferon alpha, and their combination for therapy of metastatic neuroendocrine gastroenteropancreatic tumors—the International Laureotide and Interferon Alfa Study Group. *Am J Gastroenterol* 2000;95.

190. Faiss S, Pape U, Bohmig M, et al. Prospective, randomized multicenter trial on the antiproliferative effect of lanreotide, interferon alpha, and their combination for therapy of metastatic neuroendocrine gastroenteropancreatic tumors—the International Lanreotide and Interferon Alpha Study Group. *J Clin Oncol* 2003;21:2689–2696.

191. Janson E, Oberg K. Long term management of the carcinoid syndrome: treatment with octreotide alone and in combination with alpha-interferon. *Acta Oncol* 1993;32:225–229.

192. Frank M, Klose K, Wied M, et al. Combination therapy with octreotide and alpha-interferon: effect on tumor growth in metastatic endocrine gastroenteropancreatic tumors. *Am J Gastroenterol* 1999;94.

193. Oberg K, Funa K, Alm G. Effects of leukocyte interferon on clinical symptoms and hormone levels in patients with mid-gut carcinoid tumors and carcinoid syndrome. *N Engl J Med* 1983;309:129–133.

194. Oberg K, Eriksson B. The role of interferons in the management of carcinoid tumors. *Acta Oncol* 1991;30:519–522.

195. Valimaki M, Jarvinen H, Salmela P, et al. Is the treatment of metastatic carcinoid tumor with interferon not as successful as suggested? *Cancer* 1991;67:547–549.

196. Saltz L, Trochanowski B, Buckley M, et al. Octreotide as an antineoplastic agent in the treatment of functional and nonfunctional neuroendocrine tumors. *Cancer* 1993;72.

197. Kolby L, Persson G, Franzen S, et al. Randomized clinical trial of the effect of interferon alpha on survival in patients with disseminated midgut carcinoid tumours. *Br J Surg* 2003;90.

198. Moertel CG, Hanley JA. Combination chemotherapy trials in metastatic carcinoid tumor and the malignant carcinoid syndrome. *Cancer Clin Trials* 1979;2:327–334.

199. Engstrom P, Lavin P, Moertel C, et al. Streptozocin plus fluorouracil versus doxorubicin therapy for metastatic carcinoid tumor. *J Clin Oncol* 1984;2:1255–1259.

200. Sun W, Lipsitz S, Catalano P, et al. Phase II/III study of doxorubicin with fluorouracil compared with streptozocin with fluorouracil or dacarbazine in the treatment of advanced carcinoid tumors: Eastern Cooperative Oncology Group study E1281. *J Clin Oncol* 2005;23.

201. Bukowski R, Johnson K, Peterson R, et al. A phase II trial of combination chemotherapy in patients with metastatic carcinoid tumors. *Cancer* 1987;60:2891–2895.

202. Moertel C, Lefkopoulo M, Lipsitz S, et al. Streptozocin-doxorubicin, stretpzocin-fluorouracil, or chlorozotocin in the treatment of advanced islet-cell carcinoma. *N Engl J Med* 1992;326:519–523.

203. Cheng P, Saltz L. Failure to confirm major objective antitumor activity for streptozocin and doxorubicin in the treatment of patients with advanced islet cell carcinoma. *Cancer* 1999;86:944–948.

204. McCollum AD, Kulke MH, Ryan DP, et al. Lack of efficacy of streptozocin and doxorubicin in patients with advanced pancreatic endocrine tumors. *Am J Clin Oncol* 2004;27:485–488.

205. Kouvaraki M, Ajani J, Hoff P, et al. Fluorouracil, doxorubicin, and streptozocin in the treatment of patients with locally advanced and metastatic pancreatic endocrine carcinomas. *J Clin Oncol* 2004;22:4762–4771.

206. Ramanathan RK, Cnaan A, Hahn RG, et al. Phase II trial of dacarbazine (DTIC) in advanced pancreatic islet cell carcinoma: study of the Eastern Cooperative Oncology Group-E6282. *Ann Oncol* 2001;12:1139–1143.

207. Bukowski R, Tangen C, Peterson R, et al. Phase II trial of dimethyltri-azenoimidazole carboxamide in patients with metastatic carcinoid: a Southwest Oncology Group study. *Cancer* 1994;73:1505–1508.
208. Stevens MF, Hickman JA, Langdon SP, et al. Antitumor activity and pharmacokinetics in mice of 8-carbamoyl-3-methyl-imidazo[5,1-d]-1,2,3,5-tetrazin-4(3H)-one (CCRG 81045; M & B 39831), a novel drug with potential as an alternative to dacarbazine. *Cancer Res* 1987;47:5846–5852.
209. Moertel C, Kvols L, O'Connell M, et al. Treatment of neuroendocrine carcinomas with combined etoposide and cisplatin: evidence of major therapeutic activity in the anaplastic variants of these neoplasms. *Cancer* 1991;68:227–232.
210. Fjallskog ML, Granberg DP, Welin SL, et al. Treatment with cisplatin and etoposide in patients with neuroendocrine tumors. *Cancer* 2001;92(5):1101–1107.
211. Ansell S, Pitot H, Burch P, et al. A phase II study of high-dose paclitaxel in patients with advanced neuroendocrine tumors. *Cancer* 2001;91:1543–1548.
212. Kulke M, Fuchs C, Stuart K, et al. Phase II study of docetaxel in patients with metastatic carcinoid tumors. *Cancer Invest* 2004;22:353–359.
213. Kulke MH, Kim H, Clark JW, et al. A Phase II trial of gemcitabine for metastatic neuroendocrine tumors. *Cancer* 2004;101(5):934–939.
214. McCarthy K, Woltering E, Espenen G, et al. In situ radiotherapy with 111In-Pentreotide: initial observations and future directions. *Cancer J Sci Am* 1998;4:94–102.
215. Buscombe JR, Caplin ME, Hilson AJ. Long-term efficacy of high-activity 111in-pentetreotide therapy in patients with disseminated neuroendocrine tumors. *J Nucl Med* 2003;44(1):1–6.
216. Anthony LB, Woltering EA, Espenan GD, et al. Indium-111-pentetreotide prolongs survival in gastroenteropancreatic malignancies. *Semin Nucl Med* 2002;32(2):123–132.
217. Meyers MO, Anthony LB, McCarthy KE, et al. High-dose indium 111In pentetreotide radiotherapy for metastatic atypical carcinoid tumor. *South Med J* 2000;93(8):809–811.
218. Waldherr C, Pless M, Maecke H, et al. Tumor response and clinical benefit in neuroendocrine tumors after 7.4 GBq 90Y-DOTATOC. *J Nucl Med* 2002;43:610–616.
219. Paganelli G, Bodei L, Handkiewicz Junak D, et al. 90Y-DOTA-D-Phe1-Try3-octreotide in therapy of neuroendocrine malignancies. *Biopolymers* 2002;66(6):393–398.
220. Kwekkeboom DJ, Bakker WH, Kam BL, et al. Treatment of patients with gastro-entero-pancreatic (GEP) tumours with the novel radiolabelled somatostatin analogue [177Lu-DOTA(0),Tyr3]octreotate. *Eur J Nucl Med Mol Imaging* 2003;30(3):417–422.
221. Kwekkeboom DJ, Teunissen JJ, Bakker WH, et al. Radiolabeled somatostatin analog [177Lu-DOTA0,Tyr3]octreotate in patients with endocrine gastroenteropancreatic tumors. *J Clin Oncol* 2005;23(12):2754–2762.
222. DeJong M, Valkema R, Jamar F, et al. Somatostatin-receptor targeted radionucleotide therapy of tumors: preclinical and clinical findings. *Semin Nucl Med* 2002;32:133–140.
223. Virgolini I, Traub T, Novotny C, et al. Experience with indium-111 and yttrium-90-labeled somatostatin analogs. *Curr Pharm Des* 2002;8:1781–1807.
224. Jamar F, Barone R, Mathieu I, et al. 86Y-DOTA0-D-Phe1-Tyr3-octreotide (SMT487)—a phase I clinical study: pharmacokinetics, biodistribution, and renal protective effect of different regimens of amino acid co-infusion. *Eur J Nucl Med Mol Imaging* 2003;30:510–518.
225. Sywak M, Pasieka J, McEwan A, et al. 131I-meta-iodobenzylguanidine in the management of metastatic midgut carcinoid tumors. *World J Surg* 2004;28:1157–1162.
226. Safford SD, Coleman RE, Gockerman JP, et al. Iodine-131 metaiodobenzyl-guanidine treatment for metastatic carcinoid: Results in 98 patients. *Cancer* 2004;101(9):1987–1993.
227. Chaudhry A, Papanicolaou V, Oberg K, et al. Expression of platelet-derived growth factor and its receptors in neuroendocrine tumors of the digestive system. *Cancer Res* 1992;52:1006–1012.
228. Chaudhry A, Oberg K, Gobl A, et al. Expression of transforming growth factors beta 1, beta 2, beta 3 in neuroendocrine tumors of the digestive system. *AntiCancer Res* 1994;14:2085–2091.
229. Chaudhry A, Funa K, Oberg K. Expression of growth factor peptides and their receptors in neuroendocrine tumors of the digestive system. *Acta Oncol* 1993;32:107–114.
230. Ambs S, Bennett WP, Merriam WG, et al. Vascular endothelial growth factor and nitric oxide synthase expression in human lung cancer and the relation to p53. *Br J Cancer* 1998;78:233–239.
231. Nilsson O, Wangberg B, Kolby L, et al. Expression of transforming growth factor alpha and its receptor in human neuroendocrine tumours. *Int J Cancer* 1995;60:645–651.
232. Krishnamurthy S, Dayal Y. Immunohistochemical expression of transforming growth factor alpha and epidermal growth factor receptor in gastrointestinal carcinoids. *Am J Surg Pathol* 1997;21:327–333.
233. Lankat-Buttgereit B, Horsch D, Barth P, et al. Effects of the tyrosine kinase inhibitor imatinib on neuroendocrine tumor cell growth. *Digestion* 2005;71:131–140.
234. Hopfner M, Sutter AP, Gerst B, et al. A novel approach in the treatment of neuroendocrine gastrointestinal tumours: targeting the epidermal

growth factor receptor by gefitinib (ZD1839). *Br J Cancer* 2003;89:1766–1775.
235. Hobday TJ, Mahoney M, Erlichman C, et al. Preliminary results of a phase II trial of gefitinib in progressive metastatic neuroendocrine tumors (NET): a Phase II Consortium (P2C) study. 2005.
236. La Rosa S, Uccella S, Finzi G, et al. Localization of vascular endothelial growth factor and its receptors in digestive endocrine tumors: correlation with microvessel density and clinicopathologic features. *Hum Pathol* 2003;34:18–27.
237. Christofori G, Naik P, Hanahan D. Vascular endothelial growth factor and its receptors, flt-1 and flk-1, are expressed in normal pancreatic islets and throughout islet cell tumorigenesis. *Mol Endocrinol* 1995;9:1760–1770.
238. Casanovas O, Hicklin DJ, Bergers G, et al. Drug resistance by evasion of antiangiogenic targeting of VEGF signaling in late-stage pancreatic islet tumors. *Cancer Cell* 2005;8:299–309.
239. Yao J, Ng C, Hoff P, et al. Improved progression-free survival and rapid, sustained decrease in tumor perfusion among patients with advanced carcinoid treated with bevacizumab. *J Clin Oncol* 2005;23(No. 16S).
240. Faivre S, Delbaldo C, Vera K, et al. Safety, pharmacokinetic, and antitumor activity of SU11248, a novel oral multitarget tyrosine kinase inhibitor, in patients with cancer. *J Clin Oncol* 2006;24:25–35.
241. Kulke M, Lenz H, Meropol N, et al. A phase 2 study to evaluate the efficacy and safety of SU11248 in patients with unresectable neuroendocrine tumors. *Proc ASCO* 2005;A4008.
242. Kvols LK, Buck M, Moertel CG, et al. Treatment of metastatic islet cell carcinoma with a somatostatin analogue (SMS 201-995). *Ann Intern Med* 1987;107:162–168.
243. Oberg K, Norheim I, Theodorsson E. Treatment of malignant midgut carcinoid tumours with a long-acting somatostatin analogue octreotide. *Acta Oncol* 1991;30:503–507.
244. Arnold R, Trautmann ME, Creutzfeldt W, et al. Somatostatin analogue octreotide and inhibition of tumour growth in metastatic endocrine gastroenteropancreatic tumours. *Gut* 1996;38:430–438.
245. Eriksson B, Renstrup J, Imam H, et al. High-dose treatment with lanreotide of patients with advanced neuroendocrine gastrointestinal tumors: clinical and biological effects. *Ann Oncol* 1997;8:1041–1044.
246. Ruszniewski P, Ducreux M, Chayvialle J, et al. Treatment of the carcinoid syndrome with the long-acting somatostatin analogue lanreotide: a prospective study in 39 patients. *Gut* 1996;39:279–283.
247. Tomassetti P, Migliori M, Gullo L. Slow-release lanreotide treatment in endocrine gastrointestinal tumors. *Am J Gastroenterol* 1998;93:1468–1471.
248. Moertel CG, Rubin J, Kvols LK. Therapy of metastatic carcinoid tumor and the malignant carcinoid syndrome with recombinant leukocyte A interferon. *J Clin Oncol* 1989;7:865–868.
249. Hanssen LE, Schrumpf E, Kolbenstvedt AN, et al. Treatment of malignant metastatic midgut carcinoid tumours with recombinant human alpha2b interferon with or without prior hepatic artery embolization. *Scand J Gastroenterol* 1989;24:787–795.
250. Oberg K, Alm G, Magnusson A, et al. Treatment of malignant carcinoid tumors with recombinant interferon alfa-2b: development of neutralizing interferon antibodies and possible loss of antitumor activity. *J Natl Cancer Inst* 1989;81:531–535.
251. Creutzfeldt W, Bartsch HH, Jacubaschke U, et al. Treatment of gastrointestinal endocrine tumours with interferon-alpha and octreotide. *Acta Oncol* 1991;30:529–535.
252. Schober C, Schmoll E, Schmoll HJ, et al. Antitumour effect and symptomatic control with interferon alpha 2b in patients with endocrine active tumours. *Eur J Cancer* 1992;28A(10):1664–1666.
253. Joensuu H, Kumpulainen E, Grohn P. Treatment of metastatic carcinoid tumour with recombinant interferon alfa. *Eur J Cancer* 1992;28A:1650–1653.
254. Biesma B, Willemse PH, Mulder NH, et al. Recombinant interferon alpha-2b in patients with metastatic apudomas: effect on tumours and tumour markers. *Br J Cancer* 1992;66:850–855.
255. Janson ET, Ronnblom L, Ahlstrom H, et al. Treatment with alpha-interferon versus alpha-interferon in combination with streptozocin and doxorubicin in patients with malignant carcinoid tumors: a randomized trial. *Ann Oncol* 1992;3:635–638.
256. Bajetta E, Zilembo N, Di Bartolomeo M, et al. Treatment of metastatic carcinoids and other neuroendocrine tumors with recombinant interferon-alpha-2a. A study by the Italian Trials in Medical Oncology Group. *Cancer* 1993;72(10):3099–3105.
257. DiBartolomeo M, Bajetta E, Zilembo N, et al. Treatment of carcinoid syndrome with recombinant interferon alpha-2a. *Acta Oncol* 1993;32:235–238.
258. Doberauer C, Niederle N, Kloke O, et al. [Treatment of metastasized carcinoid tumor of the ileum and cecum with recombinant alpha-2b interferon.] *Onkologie* 1987;10:340–344.
259. vanHazel G, Rubin J, Moertel C. Treatment of metastatic carcinoid tumor with dactinomycin or dacarbazine. *Cancer Treat Rep* 1983;67:583–585.
260. Moertel CG. Treatment of the carcinoid tumor and the malignant carcinoid syndrome. *J Clin Oncol* 1983;1(11):727–740.
261. Moertel CG, Rubin J, O'Connell MJ. Phase II study of cisplatin therapy in patients with metastatic carcinoid tumor and the malignant carcinoid syndrome. *Cancer Treat Rep* 1986;70:1459–1460.

262. Kelsen DP, Buckner J, Einzig A, et al. Phase II trial of cisplatin and etoposide in adenocarcinomas of the upper gastrointestinal tract. *Cancer Treat Rep* 1987;71:329–330.

263. Saltz L, Lauwers G, Wiseberg J, et al. A phase II trial of carboplatin in patients with advanced APUD tumors. *Cancer* 1993;72:619–622.

264. Rougier P, Oliveria J, Ducreux M, et al. Metastatic carcinoid and islet cell tumours of the pancreas: a phase II trial of the efficacy of combination chemotherapy with 5-fluorouracil, doxorubicin and cisplatin. *Eur J Cancer* 1991;27:1380–1382.

265. Ollivier S, Fonck M, Becouarn Y, et al. Darcarbazine, fluorouracil, and leucovorin in patients with advanced neuroendocrine tumors: a phase II trial. *Am J Clin Oncol* 1998;21:237–240.

266. Saltz L, Kemeny N, Schwartz G, et al. A phase II trial of alpha-interferon and 5-fluorouracil in patients with advanced carcinoid and islet cell tumors. *Cancer* 1994;74:958–961.

267. Modlin I, Cornelius E, Zoghbi S, et al. Phase I-II Trial of Radiolabeled Pentetreotide Therapy (abstract). In: *Proc Am Soc Clin Oncol*; 1999; 1999. p. 716.

268. Otte A, Herrmann R, Heppeler A, et al. Yttrium-90 DOTATOC: first clinical results. *Eur J Nucl Med* 1999;26:1439–1447.

269. Taal BG, Hoefnagel C, Boot H, et al. Improved effect of 131I-MIBG treatment by predosing with non-radiolabeled MIBG in carcinoid patients, and studies in xenografted mice. *Ann Oncol* 2000;11:1437–1443.

CHAPTER 49 ■ LYMPHOMAS OF THE GASTROINTESTINAL TRACT

ANDREW D. ZELENETZ

The non-Hodgkin lymphomas (NHLs) are a broad spectrum of lymphoid malignancies arising from B cells, T cells, and natural killer (NK) cells, as shown in Table 49.1 (1). Gastrointestinal tract (GIT) involvement is seen either as part of a systemic disease (e.g., diffuse large B cell lymphoma [DLBCL], mantle cell lymphoma [MCL], follicular lymphoma [FL], or Burkitt lymphoma [BL]) or as an entity with primary GIT involvement (e.g., mucosa-associated lymphoid tissue [MALT] lymphoma of the stomach or bowel, immunoproliferative small bowel disease [IPSID], or enteropathy-associated T-cell lymphoma [EATL]). Over the past 10 to 15 years there has been a dramatic change in the management of the systematic lymphoma with common GIT involvement particularly involving the stomach with a move away from surgical management. Randomized studies in DLBCL and MALT involving the stomach have demonstrated that gastrectomy (either total or subtotal) does not improve outcome. This chapter will review the biology and management of those lymphomas that primarily involve the GIT and will discuss management issues associated with systemic lymphomas with frequent GIT involvement.

GASTRIC MALT LYMPHOMA

MALT lymphoma is the prototype of a localized indolent B cell lymphoma. MALT lymphomas can involve a wide variety of mucosal sites including the stomach, small bowel, and colon; however, involvement is often organ confined. MALT lymphomas can arise at a variety of sites outside the GIT including salivary glands, respiratory tract, ocular adnexa, thyroid, liver, breast, or genitourinary tract; however, discussion of the non-GIT MALT lymphoma is beyond the scope of this chapter.

Pathology

MALT lymphomas arise from sites normally devoid of lymphoid tissue that become colonized with lymphoid cells as a consequence of chronic inflammation, infection, or autoimmune reactions (2). In gastric MALT lymphoma, the tumors are frequently multifocal, and the gross appearance can range from that of chronic gastritis to the presence of distinct masses. The histologic features of MALT lymphoma have been well described (3–5). Morphologically, the tumor cells may have the appearance of centrocytes or small lymphoid cells, or they may be monocytoid. The presence of somatic hypermutation in the rearranged immunoglobulin heavy chain (IgH) gene indicates an origin from a postgerminal center B cell (6). The pattern of somatic mutation in gastric MALT lymphoma suggests that antigen stimulation is involved in tumor development (6,7). Specimens need to be examined carefully for transformed large

cells as transformation to aggressive lymphoma can be seen at presentation; furthermore, the presence of >10% of large cells in the biopsy is associated with shorter survival (8). The type of biopsy specimen, endoscopic biopsy versus gastrectomy, has been reported to influence histologic categorization (8). Biopsies obtained with endoscopy resulted in significantly fewer diagnoses of a high-grade large cell component compared to gastrectomy specimens. An important histologic finding is the presence of lymphoepithelial lesions (LELs) formed by the invasion of individual glands by aggregates of lymphoma cells (2). The presence of LELs is associated with longer survival compared to tumors having >10% high-grade cells (8). The immunophenotype of MALT lymphoma is not highly distinctive and is the same as marginal zone B cells: CD20+, CD21+, CD35+, IgM+, IgD–, CD5–, cyclin D1– (9); given the similarity to the marginal zone immunophenotype, the MALT lymphomas are categorized as a subset of the marginal zone lymphoma in the World Health Organization (WHO) Lymphoma Classification (1).

The evaluation of post-treatment biopsies can be challenging; chronic lymphoid infiltration is commonly observed even when tumor has been eradicated. Several sets of criteria have been proposed to aid in post-treatment evaluation (Tables 49.3 through 49.5). A histologic score has been published to aid in the diagnosis of gastric MALT lymphoma and to distinguish active disease from post-treatment effect (10); the widespread application of this scoring system is limited by difficulty in applying the criteria. Two additional sets of criteria have been proposed (11,12). The Groupe d'Etude des Lymphomas Agressifs (GELA) criteria in Table 49.5 have proven to be reproducible with a high degree of inter-observer concordance. Molecular assays for residual disease with either the clonotypic polymerase chain reaction (PCR) or PCR for the IgH gene rearrangement (IgH PCR) assays are not useful in the identification of clinically significant disease; in both of these assays a significant proportion of the population demonstrate persistence of clonal B cells despite the absence of histologic or clinical evidence of disease (13,14).

Association With *Helicobacter pylori*

Gastric MALT lymphoma is strongly associated with *H. pylori* infection, and infection is felt to have an etiologic role in infected patients though chronic antigen stimulation. *In vitro* studies have demonstrated that infiltrating T cells respond to *H. pylori* in an antigen-specific manner. These *H. pylori*-activated T cells provide a stimulus for B-cell proliferation. As the tumor evolves, the B-cell lymphoma proliferation becomes independent of T-cell help (2,15). Eradication of the *H. pylori* infection with antibiotic treatment can result in clinical regression of

TABLE 49.1

WHO CLASSIFICATION OF THE NON-HODGKIN'S LYMPHOMAS

B-Cell Neoplasms
  Precursor B-cell neoplasm
    Precursor B-lymphoblastic leukemia/lymphoma (precursor B-cell acute lymphoblastic leukemia)
  Mature (peripheral) B-cell neoplasms*
    B-cell chronic lymphocytic leukemia/small lymphocytic lymphoma
    B-cell prolymphocytic leukemia
    Lymphoplasmacytic lymphoma
    Splenic marginal zone B-cell lymphoma (± villous lymphocytes)
    Hairy cell leukemia
    Plasma cell myeloma/plasmacytoma
    Extranodal marginal zone B-cell lymphoma of MALT type including **Gastric, Small Intestine, Colonic**
    Nodal marginal zone B-cell lymphoma (± monocytoid B cells)
    Follicular lymphoma
    Mantle cell lymphoma
    Diffuse large B-cell lymphoma
      Mediastinal large B-cell lymphoma
      Primary effusion lymphoma
  Burkitt's lymphoma/Burkitt cell leukemia

T-Cell and NK-Cell Neoplasms
  Precursor T-cell neoplasm
    Precursor T-lymphoblastic lymphoma/leukemia (precursor T-cell acute lymphoblastic leukemia)
  Mature (peripheral) T-cell neoplasms
    T-cell prolymphocytic leukemia
    T-cell granular lymphocytic leukemia
    Aggressive NK-cell leukemia
    Adult T-cell lymphoma/leukemia (HTLV1+)
    Extranodal NK/T-cell lymphoma, nasal type
    Enteropathy-type T-cell lymphoma
    Hepatosplenic gamma-delta T-cell lymphoma
    Subcutaneous panniculitis-like T-cell lymphoma
    Mycosis fungoides/Sézary syndrome
    Anaplastic large-cell lymphoma, T/null cell, primary cutaneous type
    Peripheral T-cell lymphoma, not otherwise characterized
    Angioimmunoblastic T-cell lymphoma
    Anaplastic large-cell lymphoma, T/null cell, primary systemic type

WHO, World Health Organization; HTLV1+, human T-cell leukemia virus; MALT, mucosa-associated lymphoid tissue; NK, natural killer.
Adapted from Jaffe ES, Harris NL, Diebold J, et al. World Health Organization classification of lymphomas: a work in progress. *Ann Oncol.* 1998;9 Suppl 5:S25–S30 (Ref. 1).
*B-cell and T-cell/NK-cell neoplasms are grouped according to major clinical presentations (predominantly disseminated/leukemic, primary extranodal, predominantly nodal). Entities shown in **bold** present primarily in the gastrointestinal tract and those in *italics* often have gastrointestinal tract disease.

TABLE 49.2

STAGING STUDIES IN MALT LYMPHOMA

Ophthalmologic examination
Otorhinolaryngologic investigation
  –Sonography or magnetic resonance imaging of the salivary glands and lacrimal glands
Gastroscopy
  –Multiple biopsies
  –Endosonography of the upper GIT (to determine TNM stage)
Enteroclysis
Colonoscopy
Computed tomography of thorax and abdomen
Bone marrow biopsy

MALT, mucosa-associated lymphoid tissue; GIT, gastrointestinal tract; TNM, tumor–node–metastasis.
Adapted from Raderer M, Wohrer S, Streubel B, et al. Assessment of disease dissemination in gastric compared with extragastric mucosa-associated lymphoid tissue lymphoma using extensive staging: a single-center experience. *J Clin Oncol.* 2006;24:3136–3141 (Ref. 26).

clinical stage IE gastric MALT lymphoma in approximately 70% of patients. Large, deeply invasive tumors and those that have undergone high-grade transformation typically do not respond to antibiotic therapy (2,10,16). Despite the numerous studies demonstrating that clinical remissions can be induced by antibiotics in the majority of localized cases, molecular testing reveals persistence of disease in at least 50% of cases (17). Late relapses occur, which are sometimes self-limited, and careful clinical monitoring is essential. Some patients fail to respond to or recur following antibiotic therapy; this can be seen particularly in patients with specific chromosomal translocations (Fig. 49.1). The most common of these translocations is the t(11;18) translocation resulting in a unique fusion protein involving API2 and MALT1 (18–20). Patients with antibiotic-resistant disease can be effectively managed with involved field radiation therapy (IFRT), with excellent long-term disease control (21). Molecular studies using tumor-specific clonotypic PCR have demonstrated that, even after radiation therapy, tumor B cells persist in blind gastric biopsies despite absence of clinical relapse; these findings suggest that the radiation altered the microenvironment in a manner that no longer favored lymphoma growth (14).

TABLE 49.3

HISTOLOGIC SCORE FOR DIAGNOSIS AND POST-TREATMENT EVALUATION OF GASTRIC MALT LYMPHOMA AS PROPOSED BY WOTHERSPOON ET AL.

Score	Description
0	Healthy: Scattered plasma cells in LP
1	Chronic active gastritis: Small lymphoid clusters in LP; no LELs
2	Chronic active gastritis with lymphoid follicles: Prominent lymphoid follicles with surrounding mantle zone and plasma cells; no LELs
3	Suspicious lymphoid infiltrate, probably reactive: Diffuse infiltration of LP with lymphoid follicles surrounded by small lymphocytes; may involve epithelium
4	Suspicious lymphoid infiltrate, probably lymphoma: Diffuse infiltration of LP and epithelium with lymphoid follicles surrounded by CCL cells
5	Low-grade MALT lymphoma: Dense diffuse infiltrate of CCL cells in lamina propria with prominent LELs

MALT, mucosa-associated lymphoid tissue; LP, lamina propria; LEL, lymphoepithelial lesion; CCL, centrocyte-like.
Adapted from Wotherspoon AC, et al. Regression of primary low-grade B-cell gastric lymphoma of mucosa-associated lymphoid tissue type after eradication of *Helicobacter pylori*. *Lancet*. 1993;342:575–577 (Ref. 10) and Bertoni F, Zucca E. State-of-the-art therapeutics: marginal-zone lymphoma. *J Clin Oncol*. 2005;23:6415–6420 (Ref. 227).

TABLE 49.4

CRITERIA FOR DIAGNOSIS OF GASTRIC MALT LYMPHOMA AND POST-TREATMENT EVALUATION AS PROPOSED BY NEUBAUER ET AL.

Diagnosis	Description
Gastric MALT lymphoma	Unequivocal evidence of lymphoepithelial destruction and replacement of gastric glands by uniform centrocyte-like cells
Complete Regression	No remnant lymphoma cells, "empty" tunica propria with small basal clusters of lymphocytes and scattered plasma cells
Partial Regression	Partial depletion of atypical lymphoid cells from the tunica propria or focal lymphoepithelial destruction

MALT, mucosa-associated lymphoid tissue.
Adapted from Neubauer A, Thiede C, Morgner A, et al. Cure of *Helicobacter pylori* infection and duration of remission of low-grade gastric mucosa-associated lymphoid tissue lymphoma. *J Natl Cancer Inst*. 1997;89:1350–1355 (Ref. 12).

TABLE 49.5

GELA HISTOLOGICAL GRADING SYSTEM FOR POST-TREATMENT EVALUATION OF GASTRIC MALT LYMPHOMA

Score	Histologic Appearance
CR (complete histological remission)	LP stroma is normal or empty although fibrosis may be present; the LP is devoid of lymphoid cells or there are scattered plasma cells and small lymphoid cells; LELs are absent
pMRD (probable minimal residual disease)	LP stroma is normal or empty although fibrosis may be present; aggregates of lymphoid cells are present in the LP/MM and/or SM; LELs are absent
rRD (responding residual disease)	LP stroma is focally empty, fibrosis may be present; there are dense aggregates of lymphoid cells either diffusely or nodularly in the LP; LELs are focal or absent
NC (no change)	LP stroma is similar to diagnostic specimen and dense, diffuse, or nodular lymphoid infiltrates are present; LELs are generally present although may be absent

GELA, Groupe d'Etude des Lymphomes Agressifs; MM, muscularis mucosa; LP, lamina propria; SM, submucosa; LEL, lymphoepithelial lesions.
Adapted from Copie-Bergman C, Gaulard P, Lavergne-Slove A, et al. Proposal for a new histological grading system for post-treatment evaluation of gastric MALT lymphoma. *Gut*. 2003;52:1656 (Ref. 11).

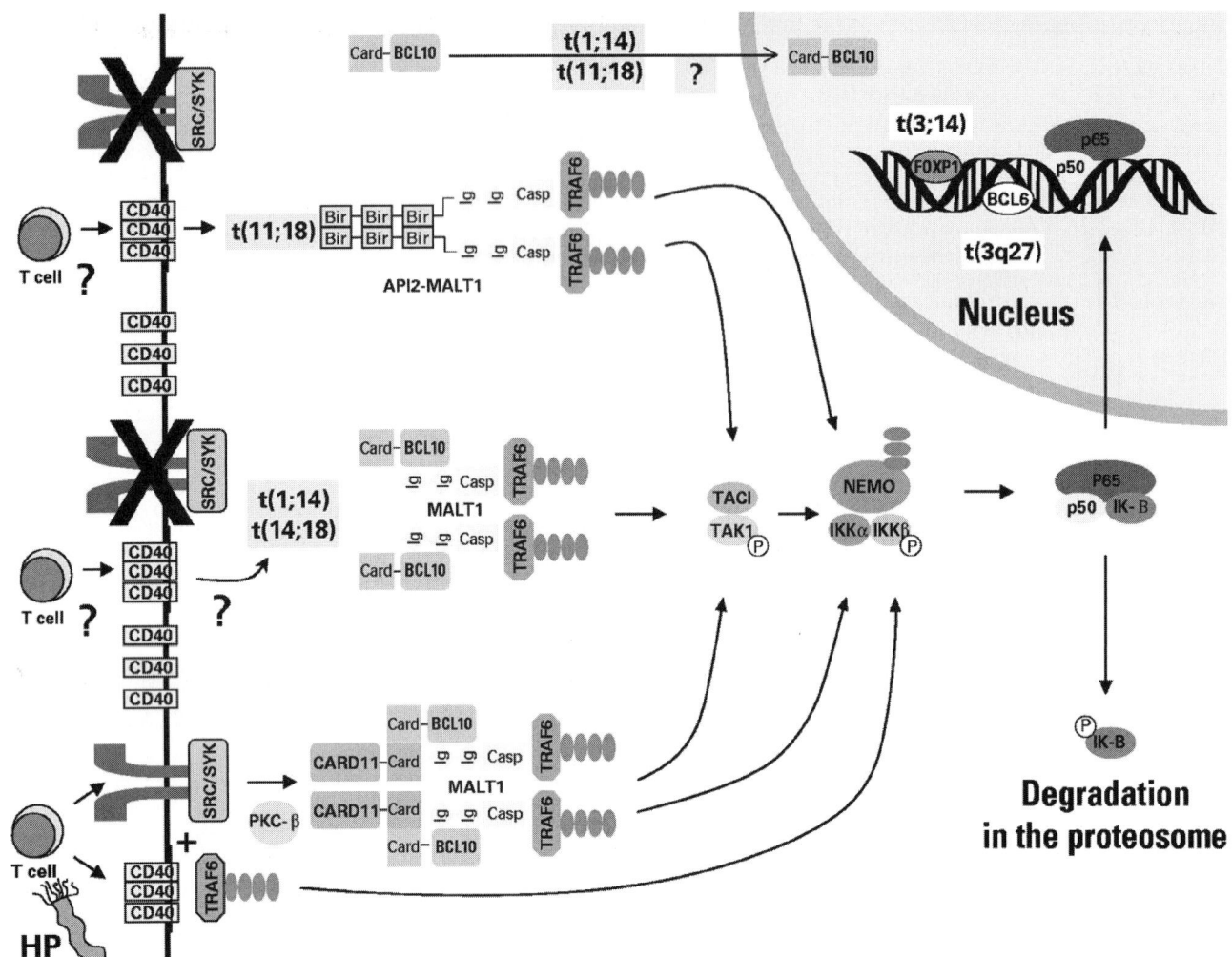

FIGURE 49.1. Molecular pathways in gastric mucosa-associated lymphoid tissue (MALT) lymphoma. T cells specific for *Helicobacter pylori* signal the B cell via CD40 and the immunoglobulin receptor (IGR). BCL10 interacts with CARD11 and MALT1-activating tumor necrosis factor (TNF) receptor activating factor 6 (TRAF6) promoting phosphorylation of IκB and thereby activation of NF-κB. The needs for IGR or CD40 activation is lost (or significantly diminished) with the t(1;14) translocation resulting in BCL10 overexpression or t(14;18) resulting in MALT1 overexpression. Similarly, the novel fusion protein API2-MALT1 produced as a consequence of the t(11;18) translocation bypasses the need for signaling via the IGR and CD40 and can interact with TRAF6 to activate NF-κB. Reprinted with permission from Farinha P, Gascoyne RD. Molecular pathogenesis of mucosa-associated lymphoid tissue lymphoma. *J Clin Oncol.* 2005;23:6370–6378 (See also color Figure 49.1).

Clinical Evaluation of MALT Lymphoma

Gastric MALT lymphoma most often presents as organ-confined disease, although it can frequently be multifocal. Molecular evaluation of gastrectomy specimens has revealed that disease is distributed throughout the gastric mucosa (22). This finding explains the high risk of late recurrence in patients treated with partial gastrectomy. However, retrospective studies of patients with gastric MALT lymphoma have reported that up to one-third of patients with gastric MALT lymphoma present with disseminated disease at diagnosis (23,24). Therefore, careful staging to exclude dissemination to other MALT sites is important. A prospective study of extensive staging in MALT lymphoma has been performed (25). The staging evaluation included ophthalmologic examination; otolaryngologic investigation; gastroscopy with multiple biopsies; endosonography of the upper GIT; enteroclysis; colonoscopy; computed tomography of the chest, abdomen, and pelvis; and bone marrow biopsy. Eight of 35 patients (23%) had simultaneous involvement of two MALT sites; among 11 cases of low-grade gastric MALT lymphoma, two cases with extragastric involvement were identified (one case of colon and one case of lung involvement). In a follow up series, the same authors reported 15 of 61 (25%) of gastric MALT lymphomas had multiorgan involvement (26). Lung and colon were the most common second sites in these patients with gastric MALT lymphoma. Among the nongastric MALT lymphomas, the risk of multiorgan involvement was 46% (37 of 79), with 9 of the 37 cases involving the stomach as the second site. When multiorgan involvement is identified, it is impossible to definitively determine the initial site of involvement; rather, the initial site is based on the clinical presentation. However, in some cases of simultaneous gastric and intestinal disease, DNA sequencing of the rearranged IgH variable gene has demonstrated a common clonal origin for the gastric and intestinal disease; the pattern of somatic mutations observed suggested that the primary disease arose in the stomach (7). Bone marrow involvement was uncommon, being identified in only 3 of 140 patients with MALT lymphoma; 2 patients were among the 61 with gastric MALT lymphoma. The presence of the t(11;18) translocation was significantly associated with the risk of dissemination among the patients with gastric MALT lymphoma; trisomy 18 was associated with dissemination of the nongastric MALT lymphomas. It is interesting that survival was not different for the patients with localized versus multifocal disease. The simultaneous presence of MALT lymphoma at multiple sites is also suggested by patients who have clonally identical relapse at distant sites after definitive local therapy; two reports of late recurrence of gastric lymphoma have been described with involvement of the lung, small bowel, and gall bladder (27,28). These data support the need for a thorough and careful staging evaluation of MALT lymphoma (Table 49.2).

Staging and Endoscopic Ultrasound

In gastric MALT lymphoma, evaluation of the local extent of the disease is achieved by upper gastroscopy. However, endoscopic ultrasound (EUS) has demonstrated more extensive disease when compared to conventional gastroscopy. Using EUS, four patterns of involvement of the stomach have been recognized: superficial spreading; infiltrating; mass-forming; and mixed type (29,30). The superficial spreading and the infiltrating patterns were strongly associated with low-grade MALT lymphoma, and the mass-forming pattern was associated with high-grade MALT or DLBCL.

The Ann Arbor staging system (31,32) has been modified for primary gastric lymphoma (33). The modification shown in Table 49.6 includes subdividing (CS IE) into IE1 (involving the mucosa and/or submucosa) and IE2 (in which disease extends beyond the submucosa). CS IIE disease is subdivided into IIE1 (involving perigastric lymph nodes) and IIE2 (involving lymph nodes beyond region nodes). The modified Ann Arbor staging system cannot distinguish the superficial spreading from infiltrating forms of gastric lymphoma.

The Tumor–Node–Metastasis (TNM) classification for gastric cancer staging has been applied to the staging of gastric lymphoma (Table 49.7) (34,35). T1 disease describes mucosal and submucosal involvement and is further subdivided into T1m (involving the mucosa only), T1sm (with extension to the

TABLE 49.6

MODIFIED ANN ARBOR STAGING SYSTEM FOR PRIMARY GASTRIC LYMPHOMA

Stage	Description
I$_E$	Localized disease without lymph node involvement
I$_{E1}$	Stage I confined to mucosa and submucosa
I$_{E2}$	Stage I extending beyond the submucosa (into muscularis propria)
II$_E$	Localized disease with lymph node involvement
II$_{E1}$	Regional lymph nodes involved
II$_{E2}$	Infiltration of lymph nodes beyond regional area
III$_E$	Localized disease but with lymph nodes involved on both sides of diaphragm
IV$_E$	Diffuse or disseminated involvement of non-GIT organs

GIT, gastrointestinal tract.

TABLE 49.7

TNM STAGING OF GASTRIC CANCER

T Stage	
1	Mucosal and submucosal invasion
—1m	Disease limited to the mucosa
—1sm	Involvement of the submucosa
2	Muscularis propria invasion
3	Invasion into the serosal layer
4	Invasion of adjacent structures
N Stage	
0	No adenopathy
1	Regional adenopathy
M Stage*	
0	No distant metastatic disease
1	Distant metastatic disease

TNM, tumor–node–metastasis.
Adapted from The new TNM classification in gastroenterology, 1997. *Endoscopy*. 1998;30:643–649 (Ref. 34).
*M stage is not generally used in staging of gastric mucosa-associated lymphoid tissue (MALT) lymphoma.

submucosa), T2 (involving the muscularis propria), and T3 disease invading into the serosal layer. Regional nodal disease is designated N1, and the absence of regional nodes N0. Conventional radial EUS assesses T stage with a precision and sensitivity of 85% to 90% and N stage with a sensitivity of 40% to 90%. Miniprobes have been compared to conventional radial EUS probes and have been found to have similar determination of T stage and N stage (T1 53% vs 60%, T2 33% vs 20%, N1 53% vs 60% for miniprobe vs conventional probe) (36).

Unfortunately, the utility of EUS is limited somewhat by inter-observer variability (37). A multicenter study was conducted in which black and white thermal images were assessed by other observers to determine the T and N stage. At diagnosis there was only moderate inter-observer agreement in the designation of T1m disease and only fair agreement for patients with T1sm and T2 disease. At diagnosis there was substantial inter-observer agreement in the designation of N stage. High degree of inter-observer variability can potentially have important clinical consequences, as T stage is associated with response to therapy.

Diagnosis of *H. pylori* Infection

H. pylori is a ubiquitous organism colonizing half of the global human population (38). However, this organism has also been strongly associated with a number of disease states including gastritis, gastric and duodenal ulcers, gastric adenocarcinoma, and gastric MALT lymphoma. Eradication of the *H. pylori* infection can result in clinical remission of MALT lymphoma (see response of gastric malt lymphoma to eradication of H. pylori). This would suggest that an accurate diagnosis of *H. pylori* is imperative. However, some researchers have advocated that all patients with localized gastric MALT lymphoma be treated with an empiric course of therapy aimed at *H. pylori* eradication in part because of the difficulty in establishing a definitive diagnosis of infection. Empiric therapy is a reasonable strategy; however, the emergence of clarithromycin-resistant strains of *H. pylori* has complicated the interpretation of the results. Failure to respond may be the result of a failure to eradicate the infection or an inherent resistance to treatment because of molecular evolution of the clone (see Figure 49.1). In the first case, the appropriate treatment might be alternative therapy directed at *H. pylori*; in the second, antitumor therapy with radiation or systemic treatment may be indicated. Thus, efforts should be undertaken to achieve an accurate diagnosis of *H. pylori* infection.

H. pylori can be detected by both noninvasive and invasive means. Invasive tests include endoscopy, with biopsy of the affected region with histopathologic examination of stained specimens to demonstrate the presence of the bacterium, rapid urease test, biopsy PCR, and culture of the bacterium. Upper GI endoscopy with biopsy and histologic examination has been the gold standard for the diagnosis of *H. pylori* infection, but this is costly and invasive. Fecal and saliva samples can be evaluated for *H. pylori* antigens using enzyme immunoassays or by PCR, although fecal testing has had greater reliability than saliva testing has had. Utility of PCR is limited by substances in the sample that inhibit the PCR; these substances can be addressed with pre-PCR treatment resulting in high specificity and sensitivity (39–41). The stool antigen test has also yielded high specificities (83% to 100%) and sensitivities (91% to 98%) in various regions of the world (41).

The gold standard among the noninvasive diagnostic methods has been the urea breath test (UBT), in which a patient is administered a dose of ^{13}C-urea and the $^{13}CO_2$ produced as a consequence of metabolism by the urease expressed by *H. pylori* is measured in the patient's exhaled breath (42). Using biopsy as the gold standard, reported sensitivity and specificity of the UBT is 91.8% to 98.9% and 98.4% to 100%, respectively (43–45). However, the clinical utility of this test is limited by cost and the need for specialized equipment.

More recently, a number of studies have evaluated the accuracy of the fecal antigen tests with the UBT. A number of fecal antigen immunoassays are available. The sensitivity of these assays have been reported to be 73.4% to 100%; the specificities 92.5% to 100% (43–46). Most series have concluded that the UBT and fecal antigen tests yield similar results. Given the high diagnostic accuracy of these noninvasive tests, the choice of test between these two options should be made on the basis of cost and local facilities.

Clarithromycin is a macrolide that has become part of standard therapy for *H. pylori* (47). However, clarithromycin-resistant *H. pylori* has been emerging (48,49), with higher rates of resistance in the developing countries (25% to 50%) than in the United States (5% to 10%) and Europe (10%). The emer-gance of macrolide resistance led to the development of methods for the rapid detection of macrolide-resistant *H. pylori* in paraffin embedded or fresh samples (49–51). This method uses the fluorescence in situ hybridization (FISH) method to detect clarithromycin resistance due to mutations in the 2143 and 2144 positions of the 23S ribosomal RNA (rRNA) gene. This test can be used in populations at high risk for macrolide resistance prior to therapy to clarify the cause of treatment failure in patients with persistence of infection after standard therapy (51).

Response of Gastric MALT Lymphoma to Eradication of *H. pylori*

Numerous series have validated the original observation by Wotherspoon et al. (10) that histologic remission could be achieved by the eradication of *H. pylori* infection; however, these data are limited by relatively few patients and relatively short follow-up for a disease with a long natural history. Various regimens have been used for *H. pylori* eradication including dual and triple therapy. The most common regimens include a proton pump inhibitor(PPI) with amoxicillin 1 g orally twice daily and clarithromycin 500 mg orally twice daily or metronidazole 250 mg orally four times daily for 14 days (though some series treat for only 7 days). Second-line therapy has generally included colloidal bismuth 120 mg, tetracycline 500 mg, and metronidazole 250 mg all taken orally four times daily in addition to a PPI for 14 days. Several of the larger series with extended follow-up are summarized in Table 49.8. In most series, there is very prompt resolution of presenting symptoms including dyspepsia as well as nausea and vomiting. The complete response rate ranged from 50% to 95%, with higher response rates in series restricted to CS IE. *H. pylori* eradication is successful in >94% of patients when second-line therapy is included, although two courses of therapy were needed in 4% to 16% of cases. Delayed tumor response is a common feature of antibiotic therapy, with responses occurring at a median time to response of 3 to 4.6 months with a range of 1 to 45 months.

EUS has been used to help predict those patients with gastric MALT lymphoma that will respond to antibiotic therapy. EUS based on pretreatment patterns of involvement has been

TABLE 49.8

GASTRIC MALT LYMPHOMA RESPONSE TO HELICOBACTER PYLORI ERADICATION

N	Stage I$_E$	Stage II$_E$	*H. pylori* Therapy Duration Days	*H. pylori* Eradication 1/2	Tumor CR (%)	CR @ 12 Months	Median Time to CR (Months)	Range	Failure*	Reference
26	26	0	14	21/4	15 (58)	NR	NR	3 to >9	2/15	228
28	23	5	14	27/1	14 (50)	NR	NR	3 to 45	NR	73
19	19	0	14	NR	18 (95)	NR	4.6	2 to 19	1/17†	229
90	90	0	7	88¹	56 (62)	56 (62)‡	NR	NR	4/54	230
120	120	0	14	116/4	96 (80)	84 (88)	<3	1 to 28	3/96§	231
90	72	13	14	78/7	85 (94)	79 (92)	3	1 to 24	8/77	232
100	73	27	NR	NR	55 (75)	NR	NR	NR	NR	76
38	38	0	7	34/4	29 (76)	NR	NR	NR	2/29	75

This analysis includes only patients positive for *H. pylori*. Primary and secondary *H. pylori* therapy were not distinguished. CR, complete reports; NR, not reported.
*Reported as relapsed of CR/evaluable patients (differences from total CR reflect patients lost to follow-up).
†Patient died of gastric carcinoma.
‡CR was defined as resolution of all disease at 12 months.
§Sixteen patients had histologic evidence of recurrence that cleared spontaneously on further follow-up.

TABLE 49.9

RELATIONSHIP OF T STAGE TO RESPONSE OF GASTRIC MALT LYMPHOMA AFTER ERADICATION OF
HELICOBACTER PYLORI

T1m	CR (%)	T1sm	CR (%)	T2	CR (%)	T3	CR (%)	Reference
14*	12 (85.7)*			6	0 (0)	3	0 (0)	52
28	26 (92.9)	13[†]	3 (23)[†]					54
7	7 (100)	6	0 (0)	0	NA	0	NA	55
9	7 (77.8)	8	1 (12.5)	4	0 (0)	1	0 (0)	56

T1m, CR, complete reports; T1sm, T2, T3, NA, not applicable; MALT, mucosa-associated lymphoid tissue.
*Ann Arbor (CS IE1) and are therefore a combination of T1m and T1sm.
[†]≥T1sm.

evaluated in a number of small studies with limited follow-up
(52–56). The initial pattern of gastric involvement determined
by EUS was related to pathologic lymphoma response following eradication of *H. pylori* infection (Table 49.9). High rates
of histologic remission were seen only in patients with T1m
disease; T1sm or greater disease was associated with a low rate
of complete response. EUS has not proven to be as accurate as
biopsy in the determination of response; therefore, gastroscopy
with biopsy is adequate for routine follow-up of gastric lymphoma (57,58).

Given the current data, it is possible to select patients with
gastric MALT lymphoma associated with *H. pylori* infection
for primary treatment with antibiotics. Fully staged patients
with CS IE1 have the highest likelihood of response. With EUS
demonstrating disease confined to the mucosa, T1m should definitely be treated with antibiotics. However, as some patients
with T1sm disease respond, using antibiotics in these patients
is appropriate. Patients should have an upper endoscopy with
biopsy every 3 to 6 months until remission, and then every
6 to 12 months for monitoring. Given the long time to treatment response, in the absence of symptoms or clear evidence of
disease progression, monitoring disease with serial gastroscopy
and biopsy is appropriate. Patients with autoimmune disease or
tumor bearing the t(11;14) translocation have a low rate of response, and either should be referred for alternative treatment
or monitored very closely after therapy with *H. pylori* eradication. A note of caution about considering these patients cured
after antibiotic therapy is warranted based on a report of a large
series of 86 patients who achieved a complete remission after *H.
pylori* eradication in which 37% of patients recurred between
14 and 307 months; the high recurrence rate suggests the need
for lifelong surveillance (59).

Eradication of MALT by Anti-*H. pylori* Therapy

In a large study of an unselected population with presentation
of ulcer-like symptoms referred for gastroscopy, gastric MALT
was seen in 70 of 151 patients with *H. pylori* infection whereas
it was observed in only 5 of 49 patients without *H. pylori* infection (60). Thirty-eight of the MALT- and *H. pylori*-positive
patients were treated with antibiotic therapy and underwent
repeat gastroscopy 6 months later. Twenty-one patients had
eradiation of the *H. pylori* and MALT. Twelve patients had
persistence of both the *H. pylori* and MALT. Four patients
had persistent MALT despite eradiation of the infection, and
one had resolution of MALT with persistence of infection.
MALT was persistent in a control group of 20 patients not
treated for *H. pylori*. Thus, treatment of *H. pylori* infection

presenting with concurrent MALT could prevent the development of gastric MALT lymphoma.

Gastric MALT Associated With Autoimmune Disease

Retrospective analyses have suggested that the presence of autoimmune disease is a predictor for poor response in early-stage
gastric MALT lymphoma to *H. pylori* eradication (61,62). The
impact of autoimmune disease was examined in a series of 22
patients with gastric MALT lymphoma, CS IE1, with *H. pylori* infection including 6 patients with autoimmune disease:
Sjögren syndrome (3); polymyalgia rheumatica (1); autoimmune thyroiditis with psoriasis (1); and autoimmune thyroiditis (1) (61). All patients had successful eradication of the *H.
pylori* infection; none of the 6 patients with autoimmune disease had a tumor response, whereas 15 of 16 control patients
entered a complete response. In a follow-up study, the investigators examined 26 patients with concurrent Sjögren syndrome
and MALT lymphoma (paraotid 14, orbit 2, submandibular 1,
gastric 9) for translocation of the MALT1 gene (62). Six of the
nine gastric MALT lymphomas bore the t(11;18) translocation,
and one bore the t(14;18) rearrangement involving the MALT1
gene. This incidence of t(11;18) was higher than was seen in
unselected series from the same institution (30%) (62). Alter-
nation of the MALT1 gene has been associated with decreased
response to antibiotics, potentially explaining the lack of response seen in patients with concurrent autoimmune disease
and gastric MALT lymphoma. Although these data potentially
suffer from selection bias as a consequence of the retrospective
nature of these series, the data suggest an altered biology in patients with autoimmune disease. Prospective trials evaluating
the impact of autoimmunity on the outcome of gastric MALT
lymphoma are necessary.

High-Grade Gastric MALT Lymphoma

The series reviewed above included patients with the diagnosis of low-grade gastric MALT lymphoma characterized by
diffuse infiltration by small- to medium-sized lymphoid cells.
Some cases of gastric MALT lymphoma are distinguished by the
presence of large transformed cells in clusters or sheets; these
cases are often referred to as high-grade gastric MALT lymphoma. They are distinguished from DLBCL of the stomach
by the persistence of LELs and cells with low-grade morphology (1). Early series based on very limited numbers of cases
suggested that these were *H. pylori* independent and not responsive to antibiotics (2,10,16). However, antibiotic therapy

has been prospectively evaluated in the management of high-grade gastric MALT lymphoma in 16 patients with *H. pylori*-associated CS IE disease (63). In 15 patients, *H. pylori* infection was successfully eradicated, and 63% of the patients achieved a clinical complete remission (10 of 16, 63%) at a median of 3.9 months (1.5 to 17.7 months). At a median follow-up of 44 months, all the responding patients were alive and disease free. Patients with tumors penetrating into the muscularis propria had a poorer response (29%, 2 of 7) than did patients with mucosal or submucosal disease (100%, 4 of 4). Long-term follow-up updating the patients with high-grade MALT lymphoma were reported to have a persistent high rate of complete remission with *H. pylori* eradication of 58% (14 of 24); among the complete responders, no recurrences were observed after a median of 5 years of follow-up (64). Similar results have been reported in responses from 2 of 4 patients with high-grade gastric MALT lymphoma (65). In a third series of eight patients with high-grade gastric MALT lymphoma, seven patients had a complete remission after antibiotics; however, three patients received postremission therapy with surgical resection (1) and chemotherapy (2). Of five patients treated with antibiotics alone, four had ongoing complete remissions ranging from 6 to 66 months (median 13.5 months). Based on these limited data, patients with superficial high-grade gastric MALT lymphoma associated with *H. pylori* infection are candidates for eradication therapy. Patients need to be monitored closely, and if there is evidence of progression patients need to be referred for chemotherapy or radiation.

Influence of Regional Nodal on Response to *H. pylori* Eradication Therapy

Lymph node involvement rather than depth of invasion has been found to be the dominant factor in predicting outcome in gastric MALT lymphoma (66,67). Among 34 patients with *H. pylori*-associated localized gastric MALT lymphoma, CS IE and IIE, the complete remission rate was tied to lymph node involvement, being 56% (19 of 34) in patients with nodal involvement and 79% in patients without perigastric nodal involvement. Although depth of involvement was also associated with outcome, in the multivariate analysis only the presence or absence of nodal involvement predicted outcome. In another series of 48 patients, the response to antibiotics was found to be related to perigastric lymph node involvement as assessed by EUS rather than the pattern of tumor involvement in the stomach or to the histologic grade (67). Seventy-six percent of patients achieved a complete remission in the absence of peri-

gastric lymph node involvement compared to 33% when EUS demonstrated lymph nodes ($p = .025$). Thus, nodal involvement determined by EUS is a predictor of poor outcome with *H. pylori* eradication therapy alone.

Role of Specific Translocation in Predicting Response

Cytogenetic abnormalities are relatively common in MALT lymphoma (68). A series of 252 primary MALT lymphomas were analyzed for translocations t(11;18)(q21;q21), t(14;18)(q32;q21), and t(1;14)(p22;q32), and for trisomies 3 and 18. These cytogenetic abnormalities were mutually exclusive and were found at a frequency of 14%, 11%, and 1.6%, respectively. Numeric abnormalities including trisomy 3 and/or 18 occurred in 42%. The cytogenetic abnormalities varied by primary site of MALT lymphoma: t(11;18)(q21;q21) was principally found in pulmonary and gastric lymphomas; t(14;18)(q32;q21) was most common in ocular adnexa/orbit, skin, and salivary gland lymphomas. Trisomies 3 and 18 each occurred most frequently in intestinal and salivary gland MALT lymphomas (68).

As shown in Table 49.10, 6% to 50% of cases of *H. pylori*-associated gastric MALT lymphoma did not respond to antibiotics. This finding may indicate an alternative etiology in these cases or evolution to antigen independence. The t(11;18)(q21;q21) translocation encodes a novel fusion protein between API2 and MALT1 that is most often seen in gastric MALT lymphoma (see Helicobacter pylori and Figure 49.1). A strong correlation has been observed between the presence of the API2-MALT1 transcript and resistance to treatment with antibiotics (18,19). A series of 111 patients with *H. pylori*-associated gastric MALT lymphoma were analyzed for the t(11;18) translocation, and the results were correlated to stage and response (19). Forty-three percent of the cases achieved a complete response, and 97% of these patients had CS IE disease. The API2-MALT1 fusion transcript was seen infrequently in responding cases (4%), whereas it was seen in 67% of the nonresponders including 60% of the patients with CS IE disease that failed to respond to *H. pylori* eradication.

The translocation can be detected by FISH (69). The assay uses two color probes, one derived from the API2 gene on chromosome 11 and the second derived from the MALT1 gene on chromosome 18 that can be applied to both interphase nuclei as well as metaphase chromosomes. The assay can be used on both fresh and archival tissue. Alternatively, the unique fusion transcript between the API2 and MALT1 genes can be

TABLE 49.10

OUTCOME OF ANTIBIOTIC THERAPY IN *HELICOBACTER PYLORI*–NEGATIVE GASTRIC MALT LYMPHOMA

Location	*H. pylori* +	Lymphoma CR (%)	*H. pylori* –	Lymphoma CR (%)	Reference
US	28	14 (50)	6	0 (0)	73
France	34	19 (56)	10	0 (0)	66
Taiwan/UK	NR	NR	5	0 (0)	20
Taiwan	32	24 (75)	2	0 (0)	64
Austria	NR	NR	6	4 (67)	74
Japan	73	55 (75)*	7	2 (29)	76
Japan	38	29 (76)	9	1 (11)	75

MALT, mucosa-associated lymphoid tissue; CR, complete response; PR, partial response.
*The lymphoma responses in this study were reported as CR/PR.

TABLE 49.11

INVOLVED FIELD RADIATION THERAPY FOR GASTRIC MALT LYMPHOMA

	CS				Dose (Gy)	CR	EFS	Follow-up (in months)	
N	I_E	II_E	Perf	Hem	Med (range)	(%)	(%)	Med (range)	Reference
51	51*		0	0	30 (22.5 to 43.5)	100	94	63 (19 to 117)	14,21
13	13*		0	0	25 (20 to 35)	100	100	55 (26 to 126)	78,233
6	6	0	0	0	30.6 (30 to 39)	100	100	12 (5 to 65)	79
3	3	0	0	0	39 (36 to 49)	100	100	42 (24 to 72)	81

CS, clinical stage; CR, complete response; EFS, event free survival; MALT, mucosa associated lymphoid tissue.
*Distribution of CS I_E and II_E not stated

detected by reverse transcriptase–PCR (RT–PCR) (70). The assay uses internal API2 and MALT1 primers, and amplification results in a variable length product because the breakpoints on chromosome 18 occur at three locations; the breakpoint on chromosome 11 is consistent occurring between exons 7 and 8. This assay requires fresh tissue but is more sensitive for rare transcripts than is the FISH technique.

A small series from Japan reports that trisomy 3 also predicts for a poor response to antibiotics; however, the patient numbers are very small and further validation is necessary in larger series (55).

Gastric MALT Lymphoma without *H. pylori*

Incidence of *H. pylori*-negative gastric MALT lymphoma varies geographically, ranging from ≤ 10% in Italy to 39% in Japan (71,72). The role of antibiotic therapy in *H. pylori*-negative gastric MALT lymphoma has not been fully clarified. A number of series have reported the response to a course of antibiotics appropriate for *H. pylori* in patients negative for *H. pylori* (Table 49.10) (20,64,66,73–75). The designation of "*H. pylori*-negative" always included histology but also included UBT, fecal antigen testing, serology, and culture in the various series. Only one small series of six patients reported a significant response rate in *H. pylori*-negative patients with complete response in four patients (26). However, several other series patients without evidence of *H. pylori* infection have consistently shown either no or minimal response to antibiotics, suggesting that occult infection was not the underlying etiology in these cases. Across multiple series, response to antibiotics appropriate for *H. pylori* has been reported in 16% of cases (7 of 45). The presence of the t(11;18) translocation and expression of BCL10 have been reported to occur frequently in *H. pylori*-negative cases (20,76). In addition, gastric MALT lymphoma without *H. pylori* was more strongly associated with disease that was infiltrative and/or involved regional nodes, both depth of invasion and nodal involvement were associated with a poor response to antibiotics (20,64,66,73,75,76). Thus, in light of the current data, in the absence of *H. pylori* infection antibiotics should be used only in highly selected cases of T1mN0 disease where there is no nuclear expression of BCL10 or the presence of t(11;18). However, even with these caveats, response to antibiotics alone would be atypical, and patients should be monitored closely with serial gastroscopy with or without EUS.

IFRT for Gastric MALT Lymphoma

About 20% to 35% of cases of gastric MALT lymphoma will not respond to *H. pylori* eradication, will not have an *H. pylori*

infection, or will relapse. For these patients, alternative therapy is necessary. Despite resistance to treatment and relapse, most of these patients still have local (CS IE) or regional (CS IIE1) disease, leading a number of groups to evaluate the role of IFRT for the treatment of these lymphomas (21,77–81). The target volume includes the whole stomach and the perigastric and celiac lymph nodes. Most centers use 1.5- to 1.8-Gy fractions with a total dose of 30 to 36 Gy. Patients are simulated and treated in the supine position on an empty stomach. Oral barium is used during the simulation to define the location of the stomach, and intravenous contrast may be administered to identify the outline of the kidneys. The goal is to limit the total dose to the kidney to <20 Gy and to the liver to <25 Gy. A variety of techniques can successfully meet these requirements, including opposing anterior–posterior and posterior–anterior (AP-PA) fields as well as intensity-modulated radiation therapy (IMRT). In general, radiation therapy is well tolerated (though nausea, grade 1 to 2, that was responsive to anti-emetics is common). As summarized in Table 49.11, IFRT for gastric MALT lymphoma is highly effective. All patients achieved a complete remission, and only 1 patient of the 73 reported a recurrence.

The potential risks associated with gastric radiation include perforation or bleeding as well as damage to adjacent organs, particularly the kidney. The perforation risk appears to be very low. In the reviewed series, there were no cases of perforation or hemorrhage associated with radiation of gastric MALT lymphoma (Table 49.11). Acute or late renal toxicity was not noted in these series. Among 13 patients, the Prince Margaret group reported an in-field pancreatic cancer and an out-of-field lung cancer following radiation therapy. However, the histologic appearance of the postradiation gastric biopsies consistently showed chronic gastritis that in some cases persisted for years. Given the limited number of patients, the limited follow-up in these series, and the known risk for gastric MALT lymphoma patients to develop gastric cancer, annual gastroscopy is warranted.

Reduced Role for Surgery in Gastric Lymphoma

The multicentric nature of gastric MALT lymphoma limits the utility of partial gastrectomy in the management of gastric MALT lymphoma; thus, the definitive resection is total gastrectomy. The quality of life of patients treated surgically (with total gastrectomy or partial gastrectomy) or nonsurgically for gastric lymphoma has been studied (82). Patients who had undergone total gastrectomy had poorer emotional function, more diarrhea, and more food-related problems than did patients who had other treatment approaches. This finding has prompted a reassessment in the surgical community regarding the role of surgery in the management of gastric lymphoma in general and gastric MALT lymphoma in particular. Unfortunately, there are few prospective clinical trial data; rather, most of the available data are derived from retrospective studies, which are limited by unknown biases in the selection of surgical versus nonsurgical management. One prospective randomized trial examined surgery and chemotherapy ($n = 52$) in comparison to chemotherapy alone ($n = 49$) in high-grade MALT lymphoma (83). The chemotherapy was CEOP-B (consisting of cyclophosphamide, epirubicin, vincristine, prednisone, and bleomycin). There was no difference in the complete remission rates (94% and 96%), 5-year event-free survival (EFS) (70% and 67%), and overall survival (OS) (78% and 76%) in the two treatment groups. A retrospective review of 79 patients with GIT lymphoma has been reported (84). This series included 26 patients for whom surgery was part of the management of lymphoma and 53 cases treated entirely nonsurgically. No differences were seen in the patients treated with surgery plus systemic therapy compared to patients managed with systemic therapy alone. Fifteen patients needed urgent surgical intervention. Another retrospective series from the Royal Marsden Hospital reported on the outcome 37 patients with gastric lymphoma (MALT in 15; DLBCL in 20; other histologies in 2); 24 were managed with chemotherapy alone and 13 with surgery followed by chemotherapy (85). Again, there was no difference in the long-term outcome of the patients managed with surgery followed by chemotherapy versus the patients managed with chemotherapy only. In the chemotherapy-treated group there were four episodes of hemorrhage (one patient underwent elective gastrectomy for recurrent hemorrhage), whereas there were no recorded episodes of bleeding in the combined treatment group. In a review of the experience in Lyon, the outcome treatment in patients with localized gastric MALT lymphoma resistant to *H. pylori* eradication (or treated prior to 1993) was evaluated (86). Patients treated with surgery ($n = 21$), chemotherapy ($n = 19$), and combined modality therapy ($n = 9$) all had the same OS. Together, these data suggest that, in most cases, surgical resection (particularly in the case of gastric lymphoma) is redundant with systemic therapy. In the absence of significant risks from perforation and hemorrhage associated with IFRT, immunotherapy, and chemotherapy, the role of surgical resection of gastric MALT lymphoma has diminished and has largely been relegated to management of the rare emergent situation. However, at other bowel sites of MALT lymphoma—including the small bowel, colon, and rectum—segmental resection of the involved area remains an

important component of therapy (87) and may be curative in CS IE disease.

Systemic Therapy for Gastric MALT Lymphoma

The diminished role of surgical therapy in gastric lymphoma has occurred in the context of improving systemic therapy. In general, the chemotherapeutic management of gastric MALT lymphoma has paralleled the management of indolent low-grade lymphoma. Guidelines for the treatment of indolent lymphoma have been published (88,89); an exhaustive review of these options is beyond the scope of this chapter. Instead, this section will focus on studies for treatment of gastric MALT lymphoma.

Immunotherapy With Rituximab

Rituximab is a chimeric monoclonal antibody with a murine variable domain (targeting human CD20) and a human IgG1 domain (90). The antibody is active in mediation of antibody-dependent cell-mediated toxicity (ADCC), complement fixation, and is able to directly induce apoptosis (90–92). The pivotal trial of single-agent rituximab for relapsed and refractory indolent lymphoma demonstrated an overall (complete and partial) response rate of 48% with a time-to-treatment failure of approximately 12 months (93). However, the pivotal trial was dominated by patients with FL. Several studies have examined the activity of single-agent rituximab in MALT lymphoma. There is a strong rationale for the use of this agent, as the MALT lymphomas strongly express CD20 and the indolent nature of the disease is similar to that of FL. However, the frequent involvement of extranodal sites is an important reason to independently confirm the activity of this agent in MALT lymphoma.

Three studies have examined the activity of rituximab in MALT lymphoma (94–96). The results are summarized in Table 49.12. As a single agent, rituximab is administered at a dose of 375 mg/m² weekly for four consecutive weeks. Infusion reactions, particularly rigor, fever, hypotension, angioedema, and skin rash, were most often observed after the first dose and were mild to moderate in severity. Symptoms generally resolved with temporary interruption of the infusion. Among the three series, only one case of hemorrhage was reported in a patient

TABLE 49.12

ACTIVITY OF RITUXIMAB IN MALT LYMPHOMA

Gastric* N	Nongastric* N	ORR N (%)	CR N (%)	PR N (%)	TTTF Median in Months	Ref	Notes
6	3	5 (55)	3 (33)	2 (22)	NA	95	Retrospective, heterogeneous patient population
15	20	25 (73)	15 (44)	10 (29)	14.2	94	No difference in ORR between gastric and non-gastric MALT lymphoma; Chemotherapy naïve patients with higher CR and longer TTTF
27	0	20 (77)	12 (46)	8 (31)	NR @ 33M	96	Presence of t(11;18) did not influence ORR

MALT, mucosa associated lymphoid tissue; ORR, overall response rate; CR, complete response; PR, partial response; TTTF, time to treatment failure; NA, not available; NR, not reached @ 33M, not reached at 33 months median follow-up.
*A number of patients had disease of multiple sites; they are recorded as their site of presentation.

with bulky gastric lymphoma (94). The overall response rate ranged from 55% to 77%, and the complete remission rate was 33% to 46%. The time-to-treatment failure was 14.2 months in one prospective series (94) and was not reached at a median follow-up of 33 months in the other retrospective series (96). Chemotherapy-naïve versus previously chemotherapy-treated patients were noted to have a statistically significantly higher complete response (CR) rate (48% vs 36%; $p = .03$) and time-to-treatment failure (22 months vs 12 months); furthermore, the original site of disease did not influence response as the overall response rate (ORR) and time-to-treatment failure were similar for gastric and nongastric MALT lymphomas (94). In a retrospective series of patients with gastric MALT lymphoma, the presence of rearrangement of the MALT1 gene was not associated with response to rituximab in contrast to its predictive value in response to *H. pylori* eradication (96). In patients with t(11;18) translocation minimal residual disease (MRD) has been detected by PCR in a very small series ($N = 3$); careful long-term monitoring is necessary to understand the significance of this MRD (97).

Chemotherapy for Gastric MALT Lymphoma

Few series have focused on specific chemotherapeutic regimens for gastric MALT lymphoma. Patients with disease resistant to *H. pylori* eradication, a relapse after eradication, or systemic disease are generally managed like patients with indolent lymphoma (88). Rituximab in combination with cyclophosphamide, doxorubicin, vincristine, and prednisone (R-CHOP) or its variant (with mitoxantrone substituted for doxorubicin; R-CNOP) are common regimens used for the treatment of indolent lymphoma. The activity of these regimens has been evaluated in a retrospective study of 26 patients with relapsed MALT lymphoma (98). Fifteen patients were treated with R-CHOP, and 11 with R-CNOP. Seven of the 26 patients had gastric MALT lymphoma. Patients had been treated with a range of prior therapies including surgery (6), radiation therapy (12), *H. pylori* eradication (6), and various chemotherapy regimens (15); a number of patients had received multiple prior regimens. The response rate was 100%, with 20 (77%) complete responses including 5 (71%) of those with gastric lymphoma. At a median follow-up of 19 months (range 10 to 45 months), only four patients had relapsed 12 to 19 months post-therapy. The follow-up of this study is short but it indicates that R-CHOP and R-CNOP are active regimens for treatment of relapsed gastric MALT lymphoma. Responses did not appear to be affected by the presence of rearrangement of the MALT1 gene.

The purine analogs—fludarabine, pentostatin, and cladribine—have documented single-agent activity in indolent lymphoma. A phase II study in 26 patients with extranodal marginal zone lymphoma (19 gastric and 7 nongastric) were treated with cladribine as a single agent (99). This trial included only chemotherapy-naïve patients; those with *H. pylori*-associated gastric MALT lymphoma had to have documentation of failure to respond to *H. pylori* eradication therapy. The overall response rate was 84%, and there was a trend to high complete responses in the gastric MALT lymphoma compared to the nongastric MALT lymphoma. At a median follow-up of 32 months, four patients had disease progression 13 to 22 months after therapy. In a subsequent analysis of the patients with gastric MALT lymphoma, it was found that response to cladribine occurred without respect to rearrangement of the MALT1 gene (100).

Oral alkylating agents have been a mainstay of the management of indolent lymphoma for decades. A retrospective analysis of chlorambucil therapy in 21 patients with gastric MALT lymphoma has been reported (101). The overall response was 72%; presence of the t(11;18) translocation was strongly as-

sociated with both a poor response (42% vs 89%) and a high rate of treatment failure (92% vs 11%). Thus, chlorambucil alone is not recommended for the palliative therapy of gastric MALT lymphoma with the t(11;18) translocation; cladribine or rituximab seems to be a better option for single-agent therapy.

Clinical Significance of Molecular Responses in Gastric MALT Lymphoma

There are several highly sensitive PCR-based assay techniques available to monitor responses in gastric MALT lymphoma that detect clonal markers within the tumor cells. During B-cell ontogeny the Ig heavy and light chains are rearranged, creating a clonal signature for the cells. The IgH variable chain gene can be detected in DNA from either fresh or paraffin-embedded tissue (102); this technique will detect a dominant B-cell clone but is not highly sensitive (~1:1000). This method can be used for detection of a clonal B-cell population at diagnosis as well as for monitoring response to therapy. The sensitivity of this technique can be enhanced by using primers derived from clonally unique sequences that arise during the process of rearranging the IgH locus, bringing together the variable gene (V), diversity (D), and joining (J) segments of DNA termed clonotypic PCR or allele-specific oligonucleotide–PCR (ASO–PCR) (103,104); this assay has enhanced sensitivity to ~1:100,000. Clonotypic PCR requires sequencing of the clonally rearranged IgH VDJ segment, limiting the utility of this assay to the monitoring of treatment response rather than to diagnosis. In some cases, other clonal markers can be identified in gastric MALT lymphoma, the most common of which is the t(11;18) translocation (see association with helico bacter pylori). This translocation creates a unique fusion transcript between the API2 and MALT1 genes that can be detected in an RT–PCR (70). During the diagnostic evaluation, this assay may have an important role in predicting sensitivity to *H. pylori* eradication (see above). If a tumor expresses the API2-MALT1 fusion transcript, this RT–PCR assay can be used for monitoring response to therapy.

The difficulty in establishing a definitive diagnosis of gastric MALT lymphoma and distinguishing it from benign gastritis or ulcer disease is discussed above. IgH PCR has been used to provide complementary information at the time of diagnosis to improve diagnostic accuracy (105,106). The IgH PCR has been positive in 54% to 69% of cases having histologic scores of 4 or 5 and in 3% to 4% of cases having histologic scores of 0 to 3 (Table 49.3). These data suggest that IgH PCR can aid in the diagnosis of lymphoma, but a combination of diagnostic tools is superior to a single test.

An important application of molecular testing is for the detection of MRD after the completion of therapy to establish whether the tumor clone had been eradicated. However, to have significant clinical utility, molecular detection needs to be able to predict clinical behavior. A number of investigators have examined post-treatment tumor biopsies to determine whether the detection of MRD by molecular means is indicative of clinical course. In a large series, the German MALT Lymphoma Study Group examined IgH PCR following the eradication of *H. pylori* in gastric MALT lymphoma. Seventy-nine percent (77 of 97) of patients obtained a CR; after a median duration of observation of 33 months (range 0 to 65 months), 69 patients remained in remission. Sixty-four percent (49 of 77) CR patients had monoclonal disease detected by IgH PCR and were therefore informative in follow-up samples. Forty-four of these patients had adequate follow-up specimens to evaluate MRD. MRD was detected in 20 of 44 patients for a median of 20.5 months (range 0 to 50 months); only 4 patients with MRD developed clinical relapse. The clonal cells were in basal lymphoid aggregates as determined by microdissection. Another study, although smaller, had extended follow-up. Twenty-two of 24 patients had histologic regression following antibiotic therapy. Eighteen of 22 had an informative IgH PCR at baseline, and 16 had long-term follow-up samples. IgH PCR identified the original clone either consistently or intermittently in 12 patients, but only 1 patient had clinical relapse despite persistence of the clone for a median of 66 months (range 20 to 113 months). Translocation of MALT1 was not detected in this series of patients. Taken together, these data demonstrate that, despite sustained clinical and histologic remissions, the B-cell clone persists for long durations following *H. pylori* eradication and does not predict clinical relapse.

Patients with persistent disease following *H. pylori* eradication can be managed with IFRT as described above. Twenty-four patients with pathologic CR following IFRT were evaluated by clonotypic PCR (14). Only one patient had clinical recurrence, and the median follow-up was 63 months (range 19 to 117 months). Informative clonotypic primers were prepared for 71% (17 of 24) patients. Only one patient had a persistently negative clonotypic PCR; eight patients were persistently positive (including the lone patient who recurred), and the remaining eight patients had intermittently positive and negative clonotypic PCR. These data suggest that clonal persistence was observed following IFRT and does not predict for early relapse.

Given the organ-confined nature of gastric MALT lymphoma, most investigators have studied residual disease in serial gastric biopsies. However, monitoring of MRD by IgH or clonotypic PCR in other forms of NHL is generally done by assessment of the peripheral blood. One study examined whether the B-cell clone from localized gastric lymphoma (6 MALT, 1 DLBCL with MALT, 1 BL) could be detected in peripheral blood by either real-time ASO–PCR or an RT–PCR for the fusion transcript (107). Circulating tumor cells could be detected by real-time ASO–PCR at diagnosis in 2 of 4 patients with gastric MALT lymphoma and in the patient with BL. The fusion transcript was detected in the peripheral blood of 4 of 5 gastric MALT lymphoma patients tested at diagnosis. Additional data are needed to confirm these findings and to determine whether circulating tumor cells in localized gastric MALT lymphoma is found generally or is restricted to patients with the t(11;18) translocation. Molecular evaluation for the API2-MALT1 fusion transcript introduces a significant biological selection; conclusions drawn apply to patients with t(11;18) and not necessarily to the population of patients with gastric MALT lymphoma.

Summary of Therapeutic Recommendations for Gastric MALT Lymphoma

The bulk of the evidence strongly supports the use of *H. pylori* eradication as the first line of therapy in infected patients with gastric MALT lymphoma. However, in gastric MALT lymphoma patients with disease resistant to eradication therapy, failure subsequent to eradication therapy (without relapse of the *H. pylori* infection) or in patients who do not have disease associated with *H. pylori* infection, it is impossible to establish a standard of care, as we lack adequately prospective trials. The data reviewed suggest that, in contrast to the previously prevailing opinion, gastrectomy (both partial and total) has a very limited role in the management of these patients. Patients who recur locally are candidates for IFRT and can expect prolonged disease-free outcome. For patients with systemic disease, a wide variety of options for therapy exist, ranging from single agents (such as cladribine or rituximab) to multiagent therapy (such

as R-CHOP or R-CNOP). The optimal choice of therapy will need to include consideration of a number of factors including the patient's age, extent of disease, prior therapies, and comorbid conditions. Furthermore, this is a long-term chronic illness, and many of the trials have short follow-up. Additional long-term information is necessary regarding the clinical significance of the MRD detected by sensitive PCR techniques following antibiotic therapy, radiation therapy, and chemotherapy; it will be critical to determine if the presence of clonal cells contributes to a potential for late relapse. Finally, the role of MALT1 rearrangement in the response to biological and chemotherapy needs to be more fully evaluated, particularly in prospective series.

MALT LYMPHOMA OF THE COLON AND RECTUM

Presentation and Pathogenesis of Colonic and Rectal MALT Lymphoma

Unlike the stomach, the small bowel and colon have Peyer's patches, which are physiologic islands of lymphoid tissue in the bowel mucosa. MALT lymphomas of the bowel arise from Peyer's patches. MALT lymphoma of the colon and rectum represent only a small proportion of cases of MALT lymphomas (108–110). Colonic MALT lymphomas can have a wide range of presentations: diffuse polyps with the gross appearance of lymphomatous polyposis (LP) (111); discoloration of the mucosa (112); and ulcerations and nodular mass lesions (108,113,114). Colonic MALT lymphomas may present with abdominal pain and/or GI bleeding or are identified as incidental findings on routine colonoscopy (87).

The pathogenesis of colonic and rectal MALT lymphoma remains unclear. Although there is no proven association with infection, there have been anecdotal reports of regression of colonic and rectal MALT lymphoma with therapy appropriate for *H. pylori* (115–117). However, regression has not been confirmed in a large series examining the treatment of nongastric MALT with *H. pylori* eradication (118). Thirty-five of 77 patients with nongastric MALT lymphoma were found to have *H. pylori* and underwent eradication therapy with triple therapy (clarithromycin, metronidazole, pantoprazole); 16 patients were treated this way as the primary form of therapy. One patient with simultaneous colonic and parotid disease had a response in the colon (the parotid had been removed at diagnosis); this patient subsequently recurred 5 months later in a submandibular gland. Despite eradication of the *H. pylori* infection, none of the other 15 patients had regression of the nongastric MALT lymphoma with the triple therapy. This finding suggests that *H. pylori* was not an etiologic factor in these cases (118). Nonetheless, the anecdotal response to antibiotics in some cases raises the possibility that an as yet unidentified organism or organisms are responsible for some of these colonic and rectal cases.

Therapeutic Approaches to Colonic and Rectal MALT Lymphoma

In contrast to gastric MALT lymphoma, surgical resection of disease localized to the bowel remains the mainstay of therapy (84). Segmental resection with dissection of regional nodes is the most frequent approach. Laparoscopy-assisted procedures have also been used in some cases (119). A case of spontaneous perforation of colonic MALT lymphoma has been reported, and emergency surgical intervention was performed

(120); however, it is likely that the risk of perforation is very small as it has not been reported in other series. Localized rectal lymphoma is also generally managed with surgical or endoscopy resection, with curative results (114).

An alternative to surgical management is the use of systemic therapy; however, there are few series evaluating the activity of chemotherapy in nongastric MALT lymphoma. A retrospective study from Italy examined the outcome of 31 patients with nongastric MALT lymphoma treated with fludarabine and mitoxantrone or with cyclophosphamide, vincristine, and prednisone (121). Both regimens were active, although there was a trend in favor of the fludarabine and mitoxantrone regimen for superior relapse-free survival; much larger trials would be necessary to validate this conclusion. A limitation of these data is that none of the nongastric MALT lymphomas in this series were at other sites in the GIT; thus, application of these findings to bowel MALT lymphoma is by extrapolation.

A small percentage of cases of colon MALT lymphoma present with multiple organ involvement including stomach, small bowel, thyroid, and/or lymph node (113). Involvement of the rectum is uncommon; however, multisite or multiorgan involvement has been observed in 20% of cases (114). Thus, careful staging of patients with colonic or rectal MALT lymphoma is essential (Table 49.2). Patients with multiorgan involvement have CS IV disease and are managed like patients with systemic disease (88).

MALT OF THE SMALL INTESTINE AND IMMUNOPROLIFERATIVE SMALL INTESTINE DISEASE

MALT lymphoma arising in the small bowel often takes the form of immunoproliferative small intestine disease (IPSID), also known as alpha-chain disease because of the characteristic expression of monotypic truncated Ig α-chain without associated light-chain expression (122,123). Recent studies have demonstrated an association with *Campylobacter jejuni* infection explaining the longstanding observation of antibiotic responsiveness in some cases of IPSID (123).

Epidemiology and Clinical Presentation of IPSID

IPSID had a striking geographical distribution with most cases reported from the Middle East and North Africa, although it is also present in India where it may be underdiagnosed (124,125). IPSID presents in children and young adults (ages 10 to 35 years, mean age 25 to 30 years) with an equal distribution of men and women; it involves the proximal small bowel with resulting malabsorption causing intermittent diarrhea, colicky abdominal pain, and weight loss occurring in 70% to 100% of patients (122,126–128). Other less common presenting symptoms include nausea and vomiting. On examination, adenopathy is uncommon, abdominal masses are more commonly see in advanced rather than early disease (30% vs 10%), and clubbing is seen in 20% to 60% of cases (122). Common laboratory findings include α-heavy-chain protein (in 40% to 100% of cases), low serum Igs and albumin, elevated alkaline phosphatase (intestinal isozyme), sugar and fat malabsorption (in 60% to 80% of cases), hypocalcemia and hypomagnesemia, moderate anemia, and parasitic infection (122). Radiographic features of early-stage disease include edema and "postage-stamp appearance" of duodenal folds; in advanced disease, there are multiple filling defects, ulceration strictures, and mesenteric lymph nodes by computed tomography scan (122).

Pathology and Molecular Features

The tumor is characterized by the infiltration of the small bowel mucosa by small centrocyte-like and plasma cells with the formation of LELs as is seen in gastric MALT lymphoma (129). The cells are of B-cell origin with expression of CD20 with monotypic light-chain expression confirming the monoclonal nature of the disease. Evolution to more aggressive disease with increased infiltration by large cells is seen in some cases; transformation is associated with increased expression of BCL6 and p53 (130). The rate of transformation to aggressive lymphoma has not been reported.

A hallmark of IPSID is the expression of a truncated α-heavy-chain protein, which is most sensitively detected by immunoelectrophoresis into gel containing anti-Fab α serum. The monomeric unit ranges between 29 and 35 kd (131). Protein sequence analysis has demonstrated that the variable chain sequence and the first constant domain is deleted from the α-chain (132). There are two noncontiguous deletions involving the heavy-chain variable gene (V_H) and joining segment (J_H) and a second involving the switch and C_H1 gene segment (133,134). Individual cases of IPSID have been found to have clonal cytogenetic abnormalities, although the t(11;18) translocation has consistently been found to be absent (135).

Pathogenesis

The geographic and ethnic clustering of cases of IPSID suggests possible genetic and/or environmental factors in the development of the disease. Genetic predisposition is suggested by a strong association with particular human leukocyte antigens: AW19, A9, and B12 (136,137). Further support for a genetic disposition comes from reports of IPSID occurring in family members living apart (136). However, a role for environmental factors cannot be excluded by these observations.

The observation that patients with early-stage disease frequently respond to antibiotic therapy suggests an infectious etiology in IPSID (138). Despite this observation, multiple attempts to identify an etiologic agent were unsuccessful. A molecular screening approach using PCR to amplify the 16S ribosomal DNA (rDNA) genes from most phyla of the bacterial superkingdom identified *C. jejuni* as being present in the index case. The involvement of *C. jejuni* in the index case was confirmed by a FISH assay developed to detect the organism in bowel mucosa. The general involvement of *C. jejuni* in IPSID was established by identifying the organism in 3 of 6 archival cases by the FISH technique. The organism was identified in one additional patient with immunohistochemistry using a *C. jejuni* specific antibody. This observation needs to be validated in larger series and does not exclude other infectious agents as the cause of the disease in some individuals.

Diagnostic Evaluation

Imaging with barium is the standard for radiographic evaluation of the small bowel. Characteristic findings are suggestive of the diagnosis of MALT lymphoma of the small bowel including a sprue-like radiologic pattern of the noninvolved gut. The involved gut has the appearance of other forms of small intestinal lymphoma (139,140).

Diagnosis by sonoenteroclysis is a promising technique for the diagnosis of small bowel disorders. This technique involves the sonographic examination of the bowel wall, lumen, bowel distention, and peristalsis after the infusion of an isotonic nonabsorbable electrolyte solution containing polyethylene glycol.

TABLE 49.13

TREATMENT OPTIONS AND RESPONSE IN IPSID

Stage of Disease	Treatment	Overall Response	Reference
1. Early bowel wall involvement, no visible tumor	1. Tetracycline 1 g/d ×6 months 2. Metronidazole plus ampicillin/tetracycline	CR 30% to 70% lasting months to years 5-year DFS 43%	126,142–144
2. Advanced disease with bowel wall tumor formation with or without mesenteric lymph node involvement	Anthracycline-based combination chemotherapy ± tetracycline	CR 50% to 60%; 3-year DFS 60% to 70%	138,145,146
3. Advanced bulky tumor with mechanical complications	Corrective surgery, palliative radiation therapy, combination chemotherapy	Palliation lasting months to <1 y	126,142,143

IPSID, immunoproliferative small intestinal disease; CR, complete response; DFS, disease free survival.
Modified from Al-Saleem T, Al-Mondhiry H. Immunoproliferative small intestinal disease (IPSID): a model for mature B-cell neoplasms. *Blood.* 2005;105:2274–2280 (Ref. 234).

Forty-five patients with suspected small bowel pathology underwent comparison of sonoenteroclysis with barium enteroclysis (141). Ten patients had both a normal bowel study and sonographic study. Among the 35 patients with small bowel pathology, there was generally good agreement between the techniques, although the sonoenteroclysis was able to demonstrate the presence of nodes and was more sensitive to changes in bowel wall thickness and stratification of layers of the bowel wall. The advantages of the sonographic technique include reduced radiation exposure, improved bowel wall imaging, and low cost.

Therapy of IPSID

Recommendations for therapy have been summarized (122) and are shown in Table 49.13. Treatment is dependent on extent of disease. Disease confined to the wall of the small bowel can be treated with antibiotics with expectation of high rates of response, CR 30% to 70%, and 5-year disease-free survival (DFS) of 43% (126,142–144). In advanced disease with visible tumor with or without mesenteric lymph node involvement, combination chemotherapy has been used with anthracycline-based regimens (such as CHOP) with 3-year DFS of 60% to 70% (138,145,146). The role of rituximab in IPSID has not been reported. Patients presenting with advanced disease with mechanical obstruction of the gut can be palliated by surgical intervention or radiation therapy; anthracycline-based chemotherapy may also provide palliative benefit (126,142,143).

Non-IPSID Small Bowel MALT

MALT lymphoma involving the small bowel occurs without the clinical characteristics and infectious associations of IPSID. These cases are similar to those of the colon. The patients need to be staged carefully to rule out multifocal or multiorgan disease. Patients with localized CS IE disease are candidates for resection, and those with more advanced disease are managed like patients with other indolent lymphomas (88).

EATL

Lymphoma of the bowel associated with enteropathy was first described in 1962 (147). A number of case series have confirmed the association with celiac disease or gluten-sensitive enteropathy (148–153). The most common malignancy associated with enteropathy is T-cell lymphoma involving the small bowel, particularly the jejunum. It is a rare disorder accounting for <1% of NHL (154).

Pathology

On gross examination there is small bowel or, rarely, colonic ulceration; the presence of a mass lesion is variable (155–157). The tumors may present with ulcerated plaques, strictures, and in some cases perforation. The tumor cells infiltrating the bowel cytologically range from small to large in size. There is often villous atrophy in the surrounding bowel, consistent with the histologic appearance of celiac disease (155). The tumor cells express the T-cell antigens CD3 and CD7 and the mucosal homing receptor CD103; the pattern suggests an origin from intraepithelial T cells (158). In addition, the cells have a cytotoxic phenotype with nearly universal expression of T cell–restricted intracellular antigen (TIA-1) in most cells and expression of granzyme B in a fraction of the tumor cells (159). Although Epstein–Barr virus (EBV) has generally not been associated with EATL (160), in up to 36% of cases EBV genome can be detected (161–163).

Immunophenotypic variants have been described that express the NK antigen CD56; these variants do not appear to be associated with pre-existing celiac disease, but can have the histologic appearance of enteropathy in surrounding bowel (164–166). The etiologic relationship of these NK lymphomas to the more conventional EATL is unknown. The lack of a strong association with pre-existing celiac disease suggests distinct pathogenesis.

Pathogenesis of EATL

Conventional cytogenetics has been largely unrevealing in EATL. However, comparative genomic hybridization (CGH) has revealed abnormalities in 87% of cases (167). Recurrent abnormalities included gains of chromosome 9q in 58% of cases, with less common gains at 7q (24%), 5q (18%), and 1q (16%). Recurrent losses were reported on chromosomes 8p (24%), 13q (24%), and 9p (18%). EATL was further examined using a battery of microsatellite markers (168). This study confirmed the frequent gain of 9q34 in 40% of cases. Other amplifications included 5q33.3–34 and 7q31 and losses at 6p24, 7p21, and 17q23–25. The abnormalities described fell into two mutually exclusive groups: one characterized by

9q34 amplifications; and a second characterized by allelic imbalances at 3q27. Further characterization demonstrated loss of heterozygosity (LOH) at 9p21 in 36% of cases of EATL; this region includes several potential tumor suppressor genes including p14/ARF, p15/INK4b, and p16/INK4a (169). All cases with LOH at 9q21 did not express p16 by immunohistochemistry.

Human leukocyte antigen (HLA) typing of patients with EATL demonstrated that 93% of the patients have the DQA1*501, DQB1*201 genotype that is characteristic of celiac disease (170). However, heterozygotes for DRB1*03,04 were more common in EATL patients (16 of 40, 40%) than in patients with celiac disease without lymphoma (3 of 151, 2%, $p < 10^{-6}$). These data confirm the association between celiac disease and EATL and are consistent with the hypothesis that a small subgroup of patients with celiac disease is at risk for EATL.

Given the poor prognosis of EATL, prevention strategies should be developed. The centerpiece of treatment of celiac disease is adherence to a gluten-free diet. However, serial histologic examination of 158 patients with celiac disease demonstrates that the characteristic histopathologic findings are slow to resolve (171). Histology was graded according to the Marsh classification (172). Histologic remission was seen in 65% of patients at 2 years and 89.9% after 5 years. Patients with more advanced disease, Marsh IIIC with total villous atrophy, had the slowest recovery with 50% at 2 years and 90% at >5 years. Seven percent of the patients had refractory celiac disease and five patients (3.2%) developed EATL; of note, EATL did not develop in any patient with a histologic remission. These data suggest that refractory celiac disease is a major risk factor for the development of lymphoma (171). Aberrant clonal intraepithelial T lymphocytes (IELs) have been identified in 84% of patients with refractory celiac disease (173–175). The aberrant IELs were clonal as judged by T-cell receptor γ rearrangement in 76% of the patients, and 10% developed EATL; refractory celiac disease represents a step in the pathogenesis of EATL derived from aberrant IES.

Clinical Presentation and Treatment

The diagnosis of celiac disease precedes the diagnosis of lymphoma in two-thirds of the cases and is concurrent in one-third. Common presenting symptoms for patients with EATL are abdominal pain, weight loss, and malabsorption. Malnutrition from long-term refractory celiac disease is common.

Development of EATL as a complication of refractory celiac disease is a poor prognostic event with few patients achieving long-term DFS. There are no prospective trials of chemotherapy for the treatment of this disease. A retrospective series of 31 patients treated between 1979 and 1996 has been reported (176). Twenty-four patients were managed with chemotherapy and seven with surgery. The ability to deliver a full course of chemotherapy was limited by the poor performance status associated with malnutrition. Complications of therapy include GI bleeding, bowel perforation, and development of enterocolic fistulae. The overall response rate to chemotherapy was 58% (CR 42%, partial response [PR] 17%). The 1- and 5-year actuarial survival was 38.7% and 19.7%; the EFS at 1 and 5 years was 19.4% and 3.2%. A second, single-center retrospective series has been reported for 10 patients with EATL (177). The outcome and range of complications were similar as in the larger but older treatment series. Thus, there is no standard approach to the treatment of EATL. Administration of chemotherapy is limited by the poor nutritional status of patients, and complication of therapy can be profound. Nonetheless, there are occasional patients who achieve long-term DFS.

Non-T-Cell Lymphoma Associated With Enteropathy

T-cell lymphoma associated with enteropathy has been well described. Investigators in Sweden undertook a population-based cohort study of 11,650 patients with celiac disease comparing lymphoma incidence in this population with that in the general population (178). As expected, the standardized incidence ratio (SIR) for T-cell lymphoma was 51. However, there was an increased risk in B-cell lymphoma with an SIR of 2.2 (95% confidence interval [CI], 1.2-3.6). In fact, the incidence of B-cell lymphoma exceeded that of T-cell lymphoma. The B-cell lymphomas seen in association with enteropathy were more likely to occur in women and in patients with autoimmune disease; these risk factors were not seen in patients with EATL. Thus, celiac disease is associated with an increased risk of lymphomagenesis of both B- and T-cell lymphomas. The etiology of these B-cell lymphomas is uncertain, although the chronic inflammation and an interaction with an underlying autoimmune defect may contribute to the pathogenesis.

LYMPHOMAS THAT FREQUENTLY INVOLVE THE GI TRACT

MCL

MCL is a systemic disease that became more widely recognized and diagnosed in the mid-1990s as a consequence of the identification of the overexpression of cyclin D1 caused by the characteristic t(11;14) chromosomal translocation. It represents about 6% of the cases of NHL (154). Early studies demonstrated that conventional chemotherapy resulted in modest periods of DFS and median survival of 3 to 5 years. MCL has an unusual propensity to involve the GIT.

Pathology

MCL morphologically is composed of small to medium sized lymphoid cells that can be arranged in nodules or diffusely. In the blastoid variant, the cells are larger and have a more primitive appearance. These tumors express CD20, CD5, and FMC7 and generally do not express CD23; these latter two markers distinguish MCL from small lymphocytic lymphoma of chronic lymophcytic leukemia (CLL) type (179,180). There is characteristic overexpression of cyclin D1 as consequence of the t(11;14) translocation that results in the juxtaposition of the BCL1/PRAD1/CYCLIN D1 locus on chromosome 11 with the IgH gene on chromosome 14 (181–184). It became possible to reliably and reproducibly diagnose MCL following the development of immunohistochemical reagents able to identify cyclin D1 in paraffin-embedded tissue sections (185).

The role of cyclin D1 expression in the definitive diagnosis of MCL is controversial. There are some cases of lymphoma that have the typical phenotype by flow cytometry (CD20+, CD5+, CD23–) that fail to express cyclin D1. A series from Japan suggests that these tumors have a natural history identical to that of other small lymphocytic lymphoma (186,187), whereas another study suggests that the outcome is no different (188). However, in many trials, expression of cyclin D1 has been considered necessary for inclusion on trials for MCL.

Clinical Presentation of MCL

Much of our knowledge of the natural history of MCL has been derived from retrospective studies. The disease has a striking male predominance for unknown reasons. Although most patients have an aggressive clinical course, a small portion of patients can have an indolent course (189) but these patients have been difficult to identify prospectively. Presentation as early-stage disease (CS I or II) is very uncommon, and information regarding management is either retrospective or anecdotal. Bone marrow, peripheral blood, and GIT involvement is common.

MCL Presentation in the GIT

A prominent clinical feature of MCL is the frequent involvement of the GIT. LP has been a well-defined entity representing NHL involvement of the colon in the form of innumerable polyps (190). Pathological study of LP has revealed that most cases represent MCL, although some cases are FL and some are MALT lymphoma. These polyps can be present throughout the bowel including: gastric; duodenal; small bowel; ileocecal; and sigmoid colon (191,192). In the Japanese series, FL was the most common cause of LP (191), although this finding is in contrast to those in most series. However, this presentation represents only a minor of cases with MCL of the bowel.

Early reports underestimated the frequency of bowel involvement because GIT evaluation was most often undertaken in patients with symptoms (193). A prospective evaluation of the GIT with endoscopy of both the upper and lower tracts was undertaken in 71 patients with newly diagnosed MCL. In this series, only 26% of patients presented with symptoms referable to the GIT. However, 88% of patients have histologic evidence of colon involvement. and 43% had upper tract involvement. Thirty-one patients had a visually normal colonoscopy; however, 84% of patients had microscopic evidence of disease. Macroscopic abnormalities of the colonic disease were seen in 49% of the cases; virtually all patients had microscopic evidence of disease (93%). In the upper tract, 22 patients had a normal examination although 45% had microscopic bowel involvement. Macroscopic upper tract abnormalities were seen in 62% of the patients; however, 33% of these patients had biopsies that did not show MCL. Similar results have been reported in a smaller prospective trial of upper and lower endoscopy for evaluation of MCL; microscopic disease was identified in the stomach of 77% patients and in the colon of 77% of patients (194). In these series, two-thirds of cases with normal mucosa by endoscopy had microscopic involvement. Thus, evaluation of the upper and lower tracts should be routinely performed in the staging of MCL with biopsies of both normal mucosa (for macroscopically negative cases) and abnormal areas (for macroscopically benign findings vs active lymphoma).

Treatment

GI presentation does not influence the choice of treatment, as MCL is almost invariably a systemic disease. Unlike other lymphomas involving the GIT, CS IE or IIE disease is uncommon. Early retrospective studies demonstrated that MCL is responsive to chemotherapy, but remission durations are brief and median OS is about 3 years (195–200). More recently, prospective trials have tried to determine if the natural history can be altered by intensification of therapy and addition of immunotherapy.

Single-agent rituximab has been shown to have modest activity in MCL with an ORR of 33% to 38% in newly diagnosed and relapsed patients; response was not influenced by prior treatment (201,202). The median duration of response was 0.7 to 1.2 years. A randomized trial of extended dosing of rituximab compared to standard did not show any benefit in outcome (EFS, response duration [RD], OS) between the prolonged therapy group and the observation group (203).

Intensified chemotherapy has been examined at the MD Anderson Cancer Center with alternating regimens of hyperCVAD (fractionated cyclophosphamide, vincristine, doxorubicin, dexamethasone) with MA (methotrexate, cytarabine) followed by high-dose therapy and autologous stem cell transplant (HDT/ASCT) (204). The 5-year EFS and OS among 33 patients was 43% and 77%, respectively (205). In 97 patients, addition of rituximab to the alternating hyperCVAD/MA regimens resulted in CR/CRu rate after 6 cycles of 87% with an estimated 3-year EFS and OS of 67% and 81%, respectively (206). Despite these encouraging results, the survival curve has no plateau and there is a steady relapsed rate over time suggesting that the R-hyperCVAD/R-MA regimen alone was not curative. The toxicity of the regimen was significant with five deaths on study (5%) and four patients subsequently developing myelodysplasia syndrome (MDS) with three deaths.

A regimen of rituximab and CHOP has also been evaluated in newly diagnosed MCL (207,208). These trials, one of which was randomized, have not demonstrated an improvement in progress-free survival or OS despite a higher overall and complete response rate with the addition of rituximab.

HDT/ASCT has demonstrated disappointing results for patients with relapsed and refractory disease (209). However, a retrospective analysis of the data on HDT/ASCT in MCL extracted from The European Group for Blood and Marrow Transplantation (EBMT) and the Autologous Blood and Marrow Transplant Registry (ABMTR) demonstrated that patients who underwent the procedure in first remission (CR1) had a far better outcome than those who underwent the procedure in second or greater remission (210). The European MCL network undertook a randomized phase III study to evaluate the role of consolidation of the first remission with HDT/ASCT (211). One hundred twenty-two patients were randomized: 60 to HDT/ASCT and 62 to interferon-α. Patients receiving consolidation with HDT/ASCT versus interferon-α had a superior median progression-free survival (PFS) (36 months vs 17 months, $p = .0108$). Despite a trend in improvement in OS, this result was not statistically significant; however, the survival analysis was complicated by the crossover design. Despite the improvement in PFS with HDT/ASCT in first remission, there is no plateau on the survival curve to suggest a group of patients being cured with this therapy.

Evaluation of Response of GI MCL

Because bowel involvement is so common in MCL (193), special consideration has to be made to evaluate the GIT after treatment. The most common technique is repeat upper and lower endoscopy. Evaluation must include blind biopsies, especially in cases that had pretreatment microscopic only involvement of the bowel. ^{18}F-fluorodeoxyglucose positron emission tomography (FDG PET) has emerged as a useful tool in the evaluation of lymphoma (212). A report from the University of Pennsylvania demonstrated that FDG PET was able to identify involvement of the small bowel by MCL in two cases where there was no clinical suspicion of disease (213). The same investigators have evaluated the use of FDG PET in determining the response of lymphomas involving the GIT, including four cases of MCL. Residual positivity of FDG PET after completion of therapy was associated with a poor outcome; 6 of 6 patients with residual FDG avidity had disease progression; in contrast, only 1 in 13 of the patients with a negative scan had disease recurrence. This test is obviously limited to tumors that can be detected, which typically corresponds with lesions with $\sim 10^8$ cells; thus, it would have no role in the evaluation of microscopic disease.

Summary

A detailed discussion of the management of relapsed and refractory disease is beyond the scope of this chapter. Management of MCL remains unsettled, as curative approaches with acceptable long-term toxicity have not emerged. Although GI involvement is common, this involvement does not influence treatment decisions. A wide range of investigative approaches is being explored, and patients with MCL should be managed on appropriate clinical trials when available.

FL

FL is the prototypical indolent lymphoma and accounts for approximately 20% of the diagnoses of NHLs in North America and Europe, although it is less common in other parts of the world (214). At initial presentation more than half of patients are in their seventh decade of life. The frequency is similar in men and women and is more common in whites than blacks. The tumor has a characteristic histologic appearance; about 90% of cases a have a chromosomal translocation t(14;18) resulting in the overexpression of the BCL2 anti-apoptotic protein. The large majority of patients present with Ann Arbor stage III and IV disease, although about 20% may present with limited stage disease. Limited stage patients may enjoy prolonged DFS following treatment with radiation therapy. However, patients with advanced stage disease are generally incurable with conventional chemotherapy. Therefore, advanced stage disease is often a chronic illness characterized by a relapsing and remitting course with treatment. Median OS for advanced stage disease is approximately 10 years.

Pathology

FL is characterized by effacement of normal nodal architecture by nodules of tumor cells and interfollicular areas consisting largely of non-neoplastic cells. The follicles can be composed of both small and large cells, and tumors are graded based on the relative number of large cells present within the follicles. The WHO classification of FL adopted the counting method described by Mann and Berard (215) for grading based on the number of centroblasts (CB) per high powered field (HPF): grade 1, 0 to 5 CB/HPF; grade 2, 6 to 15 CB/HPF; and grade 3, >15 CB/HPF. An HPF is defined as 0.159 mm^2, which results from an ocular with a 18-mm^2 field of view at a ×10 magnification and a ×40 objective; 10 fields are counted and averaged. Corrections are made for oculars with different fields of view: with a 10-mm field of view ocular, 10 fields are counted and the result is divided by 12; with a 22-mm field of view ocular, 10 fields are counted and divided by 15 (1,123).

Ninety percent of cases of FL have a t(14;18) translocation that juxtaposes the BCL2 gene on chromosome 18 with the IgH locus on chromosome 14 resulting in the overexpression of the anti-apoptotic protein BCL2 (216). The typical immunophenotype is expressing CD20, CD20, BCL2 while being negative for CD5 and cyclin D1.

GI Involvement

Primary FL of the GIT is uncommon and accounts for approximately 4% of GI lymphomas (217). Investigators at Memorial Sloan Kettering Cancer Center reported the clinical and pathologic features of 26 patients with primary GI FL (218). Ann Arbor stage was CS IE in 16 (62%) patients and CS IIE in 10 (38%) patients with an equal number of men and women. The median age was 54.5 years (range 26 to 81 years). The most common presenting symptom was abdominal pain (50%), although other symptoms included nausea and vomiting, GI bleeding, and epigastric burning. The most common endoscopic appearance was that of mucosal surface nodularity seen in 71% of patients. The majority of cases (22 of 26, 85%) involved small bowel, four involved colorectum alone, and two involved the ileocecal valve. Within the small bowel, the duodenum was the most commonly involved site (10 cases). Transmural involvement by FL was identified in 11 of the 16 patients who underwent surgical resection; five patients showed in-

volvement of mucosa and submucosa only. FL grade included: grade 1 in 13; grade 2 in 10; grade 3 in 3. Initial treatment modalities included surgery plus chemotherapy (nine cases), surgery alone (seven cases), chemotherapy alone (four cases), observation alone (four cases), and chemotherapy and abdominal radiation (one case). One case presented with rectal polyps and was treated with polypectomy. A complete response was observed in 15 of 22 cases that received treatment, and of the 15 cases, five recurred 27 to 60 months after the initial diagnosis. Recurrence and progression were associated with histologic transformation to diffuse large cell lymphoma in one case. None of the 26 patients died of lymphoma. One patient died of a concomitant pancreatic carcinoma. Of the remaining 25 patients, 14 were disease free and 11 were alive with disease at a mean follow-up of 43 months. The estimated 5-year DFS was 62%, and median DFS was 69 months. The estimated 5-year relapse-free survival was 54%, and the median relapse-free survival was 63 months.

Another series from Japan also noted the propensity for FL involving the GIT to occur in the duodenum. Eight cases of FL were identified from 222 cases of GI lymphoma; five of these involved the duodenum. The patients were all alive at a median follow-up of 27 months (2 to 50 months).

As mentioned above, LP is not invariably associated with MCL. In two series, a significant number of cases were FL (191,192). Therefore, in the evaluation of LP, FL, MALT lymphoma, and FL all have to be in the differential diagnosis.

Treatment

A wide range of treatment options are active in this disease including immunotherapy, chemotherapy, radiation therapy, radioimmunotherapy, and combinations of these various approaches. The optimal treatment approach is often best individualized to fit the patient's disease, comorbidities, and treatment history, which will focus on the uncommon presentation of CS IE and IIE FL of the GIT. Therapeutic options for primary GIT lymphoma are the same as those for patients with systemic disease. No trials have focused on the management of GI FL. The retrospective studies above have indicated that FL involvement of the GIT has a very indolent course and that observation may be most appropriate in selected cases in which the disease can be readily monitored. Observation is particularly appropriate in cases of duodenal FL, CS IE, as they have a very indolent course. A detailed discussion of the management of systemic FL is beyond the scope of this chapter, but the reader can consult National Comprehensive Cancer Network (NCCN) guidelines (88).

DLBCL

DLBCL is the most common form of lymphoma worldwide (154). DLBCL commonly involves the GIT after MALT lymphoma representing 40% of gastric lymphomas and 69% of lymphomas of the small and large bowel (219,220). The management of DLBCL of the GIT has evolved over the past 10 to 15 years with predominantly nonsurgical therapy. Surgery has become a means of managing complications of therapy.

Diminished Role of Surgery

One series examined the rate of surgical complication in patients with DLBCL receiving chemotherapy as primary therapy for gastric lymphoma (221). Seventy-three cases were retrospectively identified, and 18 (25%) developed 'surgical' complications. Surgical complication was defined as bleeding, gastric outlet obstruction, or gastric perforation. Hemorrhage was seen in eight patients (11%), but only one patient required gastrectomy. Gastric outlet was seen in eight patients (11%); 3 of the 8 required surgery. No cases of perforation were seen. Only six (8%) of the patients underwent surgery, four to address surgical complications and two for resistant or refractory disease. The median survival was 90 months. No patient died of a surgical complication. These results illustrate the diminished role for gastrectomy as a primary therapy for lymphoma. Another large series was undertaken; PPIs were administered uniformly to patients undergoing chemotherapy for gastric lymphoma (222). In this single-arm design it is impossible to evaluate the role of the PPI, but the rate of complications in the 82 patients (51 with DLBCL) was extremely low: 1 perforation; 0 hemorrhages.

A comparison of chemotherapy alone versus surgery followed by chemotherapy has been reported for 58 patients treated with chemotherapy alone and for 48 patients with sequential surgery and chemotherapy (223). Among the 48 surgery patients, total gastrectomy was performed in 27 patients, and partial gastrectomy in the remainder. At a median follow-up of 59 months (3 to 128 months) the 5-year EFS and OS for the chemotherapy alone versus sequential groups were 90.5% versus 91.1% and 85.9% versus 91.6%, respectively. The interpretation of this study is limited by the nonrandomized comparison and the lack of uniformity in the chemotherapy administered to both treatment groups. However, it is reasonable to conclude that, as a chemotherapy approach provided the same outcome as the sequential approach, surgery did not contribute to the long-term lymphoma control in these patients.

A randomized trial compared the efficacy and toxicity of surgery, surgery and radiation, surgery and chemotherapy, or chemotherapy alone for primary gastric DLBCL (224). Five hundred ninety-nine patients were randomized, the radiation dose was 40 Gy, and the chemotherapy was CHOP. The 10-year EFS was 28% for surgery, 23% for surgery and radiation, 82% for surgery and chemotherapy, and 92% for chemotherapy alone. Late toxicity was more frequent in patients undergoing surgery. This study also supports the conclusion that surgery does not add to a full course of chemotherapy alone.

CHOP chemotherapy alone had a CR rate of 86%, and at a median follow-up of 39 months, 34 of 37 patients were alive and disease free (225). The same investigators treated a cohort of 15 patients with rituximab and CHOP with a CR rate of 87%. Fourteen of the patients remained alive and disease free at a median of 15 months post-treatment (4 to 42 months). Although it was safe to administer the R-CHOP combination, only a randomized trial can demonstrate the benefit of this approach. Given the excellent results with CHOP, demonstrating superiority of R-CHOP would require an enormous trial.

Another common approach to the treatment of DLBCL is the use of combined modality therapy with chemotherapy followed by IFRT (226). Patients with DLBCL of the stomach were treated with CHOP for four cycles followed by IFRT to a dose of 40 Gy. The ORR after CHOP was 94% with 82% in CR. The CR rate rose to 92% after the completion of the radiation therapy. At a median follow-up of 30 months, the 2-year PFS and OS were 92% and 92%. In this trial, the radiation dose was relatively high and may have contributed to a risk for long-term toxicity. Treatment to doses of 30 to 36 Gy is effective and potentially less toxic.

DLBCL presenting at other bowel sites is generally managed with chemotherapy alone. The risk of perforation and hemorrhage exist. Anecdotal cases suggest that there may be a role for surgery in selected cases prior to the start of systemic therapy. However, no comparative data are available.

Summary

DLBCL localized to the bowel can be effectively managed with chemotherapy alone. The optimal therapy is not defined, although in the United States the most common regimen would be R-CHOP. The excellent results with full-course chemotherapy alone make this a reasonable treatment option, although in cases where limiting the chemotherapy would be beneficial (e.g., in patients with cardiac comorbidity), combined modality would be appropriate.

CONCLUSIONS

Lymphomatous involvement of the GIT is the most common extranodal site of involvement. Among GI organs, the most common site of involvement is the stomach. There are several lymphoma entities that present primary in the GIT including gastric MALT lymphoma and intestinal MALT lymphoma, IPSID, and EATL. In MCL, GI involvement is common, but patients have systemic disease on presentation. Patients with FL and DLBCL may present with CS IE or CS IIE disease. In the past, MALT lymphoma, FL, and DLBCL involving the stomach were frequently managed with surgery. There has been a dramatic shift away from surgical management as the risks of complications requiring surgical intervention are uncommon in patients primarily managed with chemotherapy and/or radiation. The reduction in surgical management has dramatically reduced the long-term morbidity associated with total gastrectomy. However, in some cases of CS IE disease outside the stomach, surgery remains a potentially important and curative option in selected cases, particularly in CS IE intestinal MALT lymphomas.

References

1. Jaffe ES, Harris NL, Diebold J, et al. World Health Organization Classification of lymphomas: a work in progress. *Ann Oncol.* 1998;9 Suppl 5:S25–S30.
2. Isaacson PG. Mucosa-associated lymphoid tissue lymphoma. *Semin Hematol.* 1999;36:139–147.
3. Isaacson PG, Spencer J. Malignant lymphoma of mucosa-associated lymphoid tissue. *Histopathology.* 1987;11:445–462.
4. Isaacson P, Wright DH. Malignant lymphoma of mucosa-associated lymphoid tissue. A distinctive type of B-cell lymphoma. *Cancer.* 1983;52:1410–1416.
5. Isaacson PG. Gastric MALT lymphoma: from concept to cure. *Ann Oncol.* 1999;10:637–645.
6. Qin Y, Greiner A, Trunk MJ, et al. Somatic hypermutation in low-grade mucosa-associated lymphoid tissue-type B-cell lymphoma. *Blood.* 1995;86:3528–3534.
7. Du MQ, Xu CF, Diss TC, et al. Intestinal dissemination of gastric mucosa-associated lymphoid tissue lymphoma. *Blood.* 1996;88:4445–4451.
8. Ferreri AJ, Freschi M, Dell'Oro S, et al. Prognostic significance of the histopathologic recognition of low- and high-grade components in stage I-II B-cell gastric lymphomas. *Am J Surg Pathol.* 2001;25:95–102.
9. Spencer J, Finn T, Pulford KA, et al. The human gut contains a novel population of B lymphocytes which resemble marginal zone cells. *Clin Exp Immunol.* 1985;62:607–612.
10. Wotherspoon AC, Doglioni C, Diss TC et al., Regression of primary low-grade B-cell lymphoma of mucosa-associated lymphoid tissue type after eradication of *Helicobacter pylori. Lancet.* 1993;342:575–577.
11. Copie-Bergman C, Gaulard P, Lavergne-Slove A, et al. Proposal for a new histological grading system for post-treatment evaluation of gastric MALT lymphoma. *Gut.* 2003;52:1656.
12. Neubauer A, Thiede C, Morgner A, et al. Cure of *Helicobacter pylori* infection and duration of remission of low-grade gastric mucosa-associated lymphoid tissue lymphoma. *J Natl Cancer Inst.* 1997;89:1350–1355.
13. Bertoni F, Conconi A, Capella C, et al. Molecular follow-up in gastric mucosa-associated lymphoid tissue lymphomas: early analysis of the LY03 cooperative trial. *Blood.* 2002;99:2541–2544.
14. Noy A, Yahalom J, Zaretsky L, et al. Gastric mucosa-associated lymphoid tissue lymphoma detected by clonotypic polymerase chain reaction despite continuous pathologic remission induced by involved-field radiotherapy. *J Clin Oncol.* 2005;23:3768–3772.
15. Hussell T, Isaacson PG, Crabtree JE, et al. The response of cells from low-grade B-cell gastric lymphomas of mucosa-associated lymphoid tissue to *Helicobacter pylori. Lancet.* 1993;342:571–574.
16. Wotherspoon AC, Doglioni C, de Boni M, et al. Antibiotic treatment for low-grade gastric MALT lymphoma. *Lancet.* 1994;343:1503.

17. Zucca E, Cavalli F. Are antibiotics the treatment of choice for gastric lymphoma? *Curr Hematol Rep.* 2004;3:11–66.
18. Liu H, Ruskon-Fourmestraux A, Lavergne-Slove A, et al. Resistance of t(11;18) positive gastric mucosa-associated lymphoid tissue lymphoma to *Helicobacter pylori* eradication therapy. *Lancet.* 2001;357:39–40.
19. Liu H, Ye H, Ruskone-Fourmestraux A, et al. T(11;18) is a marker for all stage gastric MALT lymphomas that will not respond to *H. pylori* eradication. *Gastroenterology.* 2002;122:1286–1294.
20. Ye H, Liu H, Raderer M, et al. High incidence of t(11;18)(q21;q21) in *Helicobacter pylori*-negative gastric MALT lymphoma. *Blood.* 2003;101:2547–2550.
21. Schechter NR, Portlock CS, Yahalom J. Treatment of mucosa-associated lymphoid tissue lymphoma of the stomach with radiation alone. *J Clin Oncol.* 1998;16:1916–1921.
22. Wotherspoon AC, Doglioni C, Isaacson PG. Low-grade gastric B-cell lymphoma of mucosa-associated lymphoid tissue (MALT): a multifocal disease. *Histopathology.* 1992;20:29–34.
23. Thieblemont C, Berger F, Dumontet C, et al. Mucosa-associated lymphoid tissue lymphoma is a disseminated disease in one third of 158 patients analyzed. *Blood.* 2000;95:802–806.
24. Zucca E, Bertoni F, Roggero E, et al. The gastric marginal zone B-cell lymphoma of MALT type. *Blood.* 2000;96:410–419.
25. Raderer M, Vorbeck F, Formanek M, et al. Importance of extensive staging in patients with mucosa-associated lymphoid tissue (MALT)-type lymphoma. *Br J Cancer.* 2000;83:454–457.
26. Raderer M, Wohrer S, Streubel B, et al. Assessment of disease dissemination in gastric compared with extragastric mucosa-associated lymphoid tissue lymphoma using extensive staging: a single-center experience. *J Clin Oncol.* 2006;24:3136–3141.
27. Kawamata N, Miki T, Fukuda T, et al. Determination of a common clonal origin of gastric and pulmonary mucosa-associated lymphoid tissue lymphomas presenting five years apart. *Intern Med.* 1995;34:220–223.
28. Stephen MR, Farquharson MA, Sharp RA, et al. Sequential malt lymphomas of the stomach, small intestine, and gall bladder. *J Clin Pathol.* 1998;51:77–79.
29. Suekane H, Iida M, Yao T, et al. Endoscopic ultrasonography in primary gastric lymphoma: correlation with endoscopic and histologic findings. *Gastrointest Endosc.* 1993;39:139–145.
30. Palazzo L, Roseau G, Ruskone-Fourmestraux A, et al. Endoscopic ultrasonography in the local staging of primary gastric lymphoma. *Endoscopy.* 1993;25:502–508.
31. Lister TA, Crowther D, Sutcliffe SB, et al. Report of a committee convened to discuss the evaluation and staging of patients with Hodgkin's disease: Cotswolds meeting. *J Clin Oncol.* 1989;7:1630–1636.
32. Musshoff K. Clinical staging classification of non-Hodgkin's lymphomas [in German]. *Strahlentherapie.* 1977;153:218–221.
33. Radaszkiewicz T, Dragosics B, Bauer P. Gastrointestinal malignant lymphomas of the mucosa-associated lymphoid tissue: factors relevant to prognosis. *Gastroenterology.* 1992;102:1628–1638.
34. The new TNM classification in gastroenterology (1997). *Endoscopy.* 1998;30:643–649.
35. Varas MJ, Fabra R, Abad R, et al. Endoscopic staging of low-grade gastric MALT lymphoma. *Rev Esp Enferm Dig.* 2006;98:189–195.
36. Lugering N, Menzel J, Kucharzik T, et al. Impact of miniprobes compared to conventional endosonography in the staging of low-grade gastric malt lymphoma. *Endoscopy.* 2001;33:832–837.
37. Fusaroli P, Buscarini E, Peyre S, et al. Interobserver agreement in staging gastric malt lymphoma by EUS. *Gastrointest Endosc.* 2002;55:662–668.
38. Algood HM, Cover TL. *Helicobacter pylori* persistence: an overview of interactions between *H. pylori* and host immune defenses. *Clin Microbiol Rev.* 2006;19:597–613.
39. Kabir S. Detection of *Helicobacter pylori* DNA in feces and saliva by polymerase chain reaction: a review. *Helicobacter.* 2004;9:115–123.
40. Kabir S. Clinic-based testing for *Helicobacter pylori* infection by enzyme immunoassay of faeces, urine and saliva. *Aliment Pharmacol Ther.* 2003;17:1345–1354.
41. Kabir S. Detection of *Helicobacter pylori* in faeces by culture, PCR and enzyme immunoassay. *J Med Microbiol.* 2001;50:1021–1029.
42. Thijs JC, van Zwet AA, Thijs WJ, et al. Diagnostic tests for *Helicobacter pylori*: a prospective evaluation of their accuracy, without selecting a single test as the gold standard. *Am J Gastroenterol.* 1996;91:2125–2129.
43. Kato S, Nakayama K, Minoura T, et al. Comparison between the 13C-urea breath test and stool antigen test for the diagnosis of childhood *Helicobacter pylori* infection. *J Gastroenterol.* 2004;39:1045–1050.
44. Manes G, Zanetti MV, Piccirillo MM, et al. Accuracy of a new monoclonal stool antigen test in post-eradication assessment of *Helicobacter pylori* infection: comparison with the polyclonal stool antigen test and urea breath test. *Dig Liver Dis.* 2005;37:751–755.
45. Perri F, Quitadamo M, Ricciardi R, et al. Comparison of a monoclonal antigen stool test (Hp StAR) with the 13C-urea breath test in monitoring *Helicobacter pylori* eradication therapy. *World J Gastroenterol.* 2005;11:5878–5881.
46. Hooton C, Keohane J, Clair J, et al. Comparison of three stool antigen assays with the 13C-urea breath test for the primary diagnosis of *Helicobacter pylori* infection and monitoring treatment outcome. *Eur J Gastroenterol Hepatol.* 2006;18:595–599.
47. Graham DY. Clarithromycin for treatment of *Helicobacter pylori* infections. *Eur J Gastroenterol Hepatol.* 1995;7 Suppl 1:S55–S58.
48. Graham DY, Qureshi WA. Antibiotic-resistant *H. pylori* infection and its treatment. *Curr Pharm Des.* 2000;6:1537–1544.
49. Juttner S, Vieth M, Miehlke S, et al. Reliable detection of macrolide-resistant *Helicobacter pylori* via fluorescence in situ hybridization in formalin-fixed tissue. *Mod Pathol.* 2004;17:684–689.
50. Can F, Yilmaz Z, Demirbilek M, et al. Diagnosis of *Helicobacter pylori* infection and determination of clarithromycin resistance by fluorescence in situ hybridization from formalin-fixed, paraffin-embedded gastric biopsy specimens. *Can J Microbiol.* 2005;51:569–573.
51. Yilmaz O, Demiray E. Clinical role and importance of fluorescence in situ hybridization method in diagnosis of *H. pylori* infection and determination of clarithromycin resistance in *H. pylori* eradication therapy. *World J Gastroenterol.* 2007;13:671–675.
52. Sackmann M, Morgner A, Rudolph B, et al. Regression of gastric MALT lymphoma after eradication of *Helicobacter pylori* is predicted by endosonographic staging. MALT Lymphoma Study Group. *Gastroenterology.* 1997;113:1087–1090.
53. Pavlick AC, Gerdes H, Portlock CS. Endoscopic ultrasound in the evaluation of gastric small lymphocytic mucosa-associated lymphoid tumors. *J Clin Oncol.* 1997;15:1761–1766.
54. Nakamura S, Matsumoto T, Suekane H, et al. Predictive value of endoscopic ultrasonography for regression of gastric low grade and high grade MALT lymphomas after eradication of *Helicobacter pylori*. *Gut.* 2001;48:454–460.
55. Taji S, Nomura K, Matsumoto Y, et al. Trisomy 3 may predict a poor response of gastric MALT lymphoma to *Helicobacter pylori* eradication therapy. *World J Gastroenterol.* 2005;11:89–93.
56. El-Zahabi LM, Jamali FR, El H, II, et al. The value of EUS in predicting the response of gastric mucosa-associated lymphoid tissue lymphoma to *Helicobacter pylori* eradication. *Gastrointest Endosc.* 2007;65:89–96.
57. Puspok A, Raderer M, Chott A, et al. Endoscopic ultrasound in the follow up and response assessment of patients with primary gastric lymphoma. *Gut.* 2002;51:691–694.
58. Di Raimondo F, Caruso L, Bonanno G, et al. Is endoscopic ultrasound clinically useful for follow-up of gastric lymphoma? *Ann Oncol.* 2007;18:351–356.
59. Raderer M, Streubel B, Woehrer S, et al. High relapse rate in patients with MALT lymphoma warrants lifelong follow-up. *Clin Cancer Res.* 2005;11:3349–3352.
60. Cammarota G, Tursi A, Montalto M, et al. Prevention and treatment of low-grade B-cell primary gastric lymphoma by anti-*H. pylori* therapy. *J Clin Gastroenterol.* 1995;21:118–122.
61. Raderer M, Osterreicher C, Machold K, et al. Impaired response of gastric MALT-lymphoma to *Helicobacter pylori* eradication in patients with autoimmune disease. *Ann Oncol.* 2001;12:937–939.
62. Streubel B, Huber D, Wohrer S, et al. Frequency of chromosomal aberrations involving MALT1 in mucosa-associated lymphoid tissue lymphoma in patients with Sjögren's syndrome. *Clin Cancer Res.* 2004;10:476–480.
63. Chen LT, Lin JT, Shyu RY, et al. Prospective study of *Helicobacter pylori* eradication therapy in stage I(E) high-grade mucosa-associated lymphoid tissue lymphoma of the stomach. *J Clin Oncol.* 2001;19:4245–4251.
64. Chen LT, Lin JT, Tai JJ, et al. Long-term results of anti-*Helicobacter pylori* therapy in early-stage gastric high-grade transformed MALT lymphoma. *J Natl Cancer Inst.* 2005;97:1345–1353.
65. Hiyama T, Haruma K, Kitadai Y, et al. *Helicobacter pylori* eradication therapy for high-grade mucosa-associated lymphoid tissue lymphomas of the stomach with analysis of p53 and K-ras alteration and microsatellite instability. *Int J Oncol.* 2001;18:1207–1212.
66. Ruskone-Fourmestraux A, Lavergne A, Aegerter PH, et al. Predictive factors for regression of gastric MALT lymphoma after anti-*Helicobacter pylori* treatment. *Gut.* 2001;48:297–303.
67. Levy M, Copie-Bergman C, Traulle C, et al. Conservative treatment of primary gastric low-grade B-cell lymphoma of mucosa-associated lymphoid tissue: predictive factors of response and outcome. *Am J Gastroenterol.* 2002;97:292–297.
68. Streubel B, Simonitsch-Klupp I, Mullauer L, et al. Variable frequencies of MALT lymphoma-associated genetic aberrations in MALT lymphomas of different sites. *Leukemia.* 2004;18:1722–1726.
69. Dierlamm J, Baens M, Stefanova-Ouzounova M, et al. Detection of t(11;18)(q21;q21) by interphase fluorescence in situ hybridization using API2 and MLT specific probes. *Blood.* 2000;96:2215–2218.
70. Baens M, Maes B, Steyls A, et al. The product of the t(11;18), an API2-MLT fusion, marks nearly half of gastric MALT type lymphomas without large cell proliferation. *Am J Pathol.* 2000;156:1433–1439.
71. Doglioni C, Wotherspoon AC, Moschini A, et al. High incidence of primary gastric lymphoma in northeastern Italy. *Lancet.* 1992;339:834–835.
72. Nakamura S, Yao T, Aoyagi K, et al. *Helicobacter pylori* and primary gastric lymphoma. A histopathologic and immunohistochemical analysis of 237 patients. *Cancer.* 1997;79:3–11.
73. Steinbach G, Ford R, Glober G, et al. Antibiotic treatment of gastric lymphoma of mucosa-associated lymphoid tissue. An uncontrolled trial. *Ann Intern Med.* 1999;131:88–95.

74. Raderer M, Streubel B, Wohrer S, et al. Successful antibiotic treatment of Helicobacter pylori negative gastric mucosa associated lymphoid tissue lymphomas. Gut. 2006;55:616–618.

75. Akamatsu T, Mochizuki T, Okiyama Y, et al. Comparison of localized gastric mucosa-associated lymphoid tissue (MALT) lymphoma with and without Helicobacter pylori infection. Helicobacter. 2006;11:86–95.

76. Nakamura S, Matsumoto T, Ye H, et al. Helicobacter pylori-negative gastric mucosa-associated lymphoid tissue lymphoma: a clinicopathologic and molecular study with reference to antibiotic treatment. Cancer. 2006;107:2770–2778.

77. Schechter NR, Yahalom J. Low-grade MALT lymphoma of the stomach: a review of treatment options. Int J Radiat Oncol Biol Phys. 2000;46:1093–1103.

78. Tsang RW, Gospodarowicz MK, Pintilie M, et al. Stage I and II MALT lymphoma: results of treatment with radiotherapy. Int J Radiat Oncol Biol Phys. 2001;50:1258–1264.

79. Park HC, Park W, Hahn JS, et al. Low grade MALT lymphoma of the stomach: treatment outcome with radiotherapy alone. Yonsei Med J. 2002;43:601–606.

80. Tsang RW, Gospodarowicz MK, Pintilie M, et al. Localized mucosa-associated lymphoid tissue lymphoma treated with radiation therapy has excellent clinical outcome. J Clin Oncol. 2003;21:4157–4164.

81. Sugimoto M, Kajimura M, Shirai N, et al. Outcome of radiotherapy for gastric mucosa-associated lymphoid tissue lymphoma refractory to Helicobacter pylori eradication therapy. Intern Med. 2006;45:405–409.

82. Hjermstad MJ, Hollender A, Warloe T, et al. Quality of life after total or partial gastrectomy for primary gastric lymphoma. Acta Oncol. 2006;45:202–209.

83. Aviles A, Neri N, Nambo MJ, et al. Surgery and chemotherapy versus chemotherapy as treatment of high-grade MALT gastric lymphoma. Med Oncol. 2006;23:295–300.

84. Radman I, Kovacevic-Metelko J, Aurer I, et al. Surgical resection in the treatment of primary gastrointestinal non-Hodgkin's lymphoma: retrospective study. Croat Med J. 2002;43:555–560.

85. Popescu RA, Wotherspoon AC, Cunningham D, et al. Surgery plus chemotherapy or chemotherapy alone for primary intermediate- and high-grade gastric non-Hodgkin's lymphoma: the Royal Marsden Hospital experience. Eur J Cancer. 1999;35:928–934.

86. Thieblemont C, Dumontet C, Bouafia F, et al. Outcome in relation to treatment modalities in 48 patients with localized gastric MALT lymphoma: a retrospective study of patients treated during 1976–2001. Leuk Lymphoma. 2003;44:257–262.

87. Zinzani PL, Magagnoli M, Pagliani G, et al. Primary intestinal lymphoma: clinical and therapeutic features of 32 patients. Haematologica. 1997;82:305–308.

88. Zelenetz AD, Advani RH, Buadi F, et al. Non-Hodgkin's lymphoma. Clinical practice guidelines in oncology. J Natl Compr Canc Netw. 2006;4:258–310.

89. Zelenetz AD, Hoppe RT. NCCN: non-Hodgkin's lymphoma. Cancer Control. 2001;8(6 Suppl 2):102–113.

90. Reff ME, Carner K, Chambers KS, et al. Depletion of B cells in vivo by a chimeric mouse human monoclonal antibody to CD20. Blood. 1994;83:435–445.

91. Maloney DG, Liles TM, Czerwinski DK, et al. Phase I clinical trial using escalating single-dose infusion of chimeric anti-CD20 monoclonal antibody (IDEC-C2B8) in patients with recurrent B-cell lymphoma. Blood. 1994;84:2457–2466.

92. Shan D, Ledbetter JA, Press OW. Signaling events involved in anti-CD20-induced apoptosis of malignant human B cells. Cancer Immunol Immunother. 2000;48:673–683.

93. McLaughlin P, Grillo-Lopez AJ, Link BK, et al. Rituximab chimeric anti-CD20 monoclonal antibody therapy for relapsed indolent lymphoma: half of patients respond to a four-dose treatment program. J Clin Oncol. 1998;16:2825–2833.

94. Conconi A, Martinelli G, Thieblemont C, et al. Clinical activity of rituximab in extranodal marginal zone B-cell lymphoma of MALT type. Blood. 2003;102:2741–2745.

95. Raderer M, Jager G, Brugger S, et al. Rituximab for treatment of advanced extranodal marginal zone B cell lymphoma of the mucosa-associated lymphoid tissue lymphoma. Oncology. 2003;65:306–310.

96. Martinelli G, Laszlo D, Ferreri AJ, et al. Clinical activity of rituximab in gastric marginal zone non-Hodgkin's lymphoma resistant to or not eligible for anti-Helicobacter pylori therapy. J Clin Oncol. 2005;23:1979–1983.

97. Salar A, Bellosillo B, Serrano S, et al. Persistent residual disease in t(11;18)(q21;q21) positive gastric mucosa-associated lymphoid tissue lymphoma treated with chemotherapy or rituximab. J Clin Oncol. 2005;23:7361–7362, author reply 7362–7363.

98. Raderer M, Wohrer S, Streubel B, et al. Activity of rituximab plus cyclophosphamide, doxorubicin/mitoxantrone, vincristine and prednisone in patients with relapsed MALT lymphoma. Oncology. 2006;70:411–417.

99. Jager G, Neumeister P, Brezinschek R, et al. Treatment of extranodal marginal zone B-cell lymphoma of mucosa-associated lymphoid tissue type with cladribine: a phase II study. J Clin Oncol. 2002;20:3872–3877.

100. Streubel B, Ye H, Du MQ, et al. Translocation t(11;18)(q21;q21) is not predictive of response to chemotherapy with 2CdA in patients with gastric MALT lymphoma. Oncology. 2004;66:476–480.

101. Levy M, Copie-Bergman C, Gameiro C, et al. Prognostic value of translocation t(11;18) in tumoral response of low-grade gastric lymphoma of mucosa-associated lymphoid tissue type to oral chemotherapy. J Clin Oncol. 2005;23:5061–5066.

102. Wan JH, Trainor KJ, Brisco MJ, et al. Monoclonality in B cell lymphoma detected in paraffin wax embedded sections using the polymerase chain reaction. J Clin Pathol. 1990;43:888–890.

103. Billadeau D, Quam L, Thomas W, et al. Detection and quantitation of malignant cells in the peripheral blood of multiple myeloma patients. Blood. 1992;80:1818–1824.

104. Noy A, Verma R, Glenn M, et al. Clonotypic polymerase chain reaction confirms minimal residual disease in CLL nodular PR: results from a sequential treatment CLL protocol. Blood. 2001;97:1929–1936.

105. Savio A, Franzin G, Wotherspoon AC, et al. Diagnosis and posttreatment follow-up of Helicobacter pylori-positive gastric lymphoma of mucosa-associated lymphoid tissue: histology, polymerase chain reaction, or both? Blood. 1996;87:1255–1260.

106. Aiello A, Giardini R, Tondini C, et al. PCR-based clonality analysis: a reliable method for the diagnosis and follow-up monitoring of conservatively treated gastric B-cell MALT lymphomas? Histopathology. 1999;34:326–330.

107. Schreuder MI, Hoeve MA, Groothuis L, et al. Monitoring gastric lymphoma in peripheral blood by quantitative IgH allele-specific oligonucleotide real-time PCR and API2-MALT1 PCR. Br J Haematol. 2005;131:619–623.

108. Isaacson PG. Gastrointestinal lymphomas of T- and B-cell types. Mod Pathol. 1999;12:151–158.

109. Harris NL, Jaffe ES, Diebold J, et al. World Health Organization classification of neoplastic diseases of the hematopoietic and lymphoid tissues: report of the Clinical Advisory Committee meeting-Airlie House, Virginia, November 1997. J Clin Oncol. 1999;17:3835–3849.

110. Nathwani BN, Anderson JR, Armitage JO, et al. Marginal zone B-cell lymphoma: a clinical comparison of nodal and mucosa-associated lymphoid tissue types. Non-Hodgkin's Lymphoma Classification Project. J Clin Oncol. 1999;17:2486–2492.

111. Chim CS, Shek TW, Chung LP, et al. Unusual abdominal tumors: case 3. Multiple lymphomatous polyposis in lymphoma of colon. J Clin Oncol. 2003;21:953–955.

112. Lee YG, Lee S, Han SW, et al. A case of multiple mucosa-associated lymphoid tissue (MALT) lymphoma of the colon identified as simple mucosal discoloration. J Korean Med Sci. 2005;20:325–328.

113. Yoshino T, Ichimura K, Mannami T, et al. Multiple organ mucosa-associated lymphoid tissue lymphomas often involve the intestine. Cancer. 2001;91:346–353.

114. Ahlawat S, Kanber Y, Charabaty-Pishvaian A, et al. Primary mucosa-associated lymphoid tissue (MALT) lymphoma occurring in the rectum: a case report and review of the literature. South Med J. 2006;99:1378–1384.

115. Inoue F, Chiba T. Regression of MALT lymphoma of the rectum after anti-H. pylori therapy in a patient negative for H. pylori. Gastroenterology. 1999;117:514–515.

116. Raderer M, Pfeffel F, Pohl G, et al. Regression of colonic low grade B cell lymphoma of the mucosa associated lymphoid tissue type after eradication of Helicobacter pylori. Gut. 2000;46:133–135.

117. Nakase H, Okazaki K, Ohana M, et al. The possible involvement of microorganisms other than Helicobacter pylori in the development of rectal MALT lymphoma in H. pylori-negative patients. Endoscopy. 2002;34:343–346.

118. Grunberger B, Wohrer S, Streubel B, et al. Antibiotic treatment is not effective in patients infected with Helicobacter pylori suffering from extragastric MALT lymphoma. J Clin Oncol. 2006;24:1370–1375.

119. Takada M, Ichihara T, Fukumoto S, et al. Laparoscopy-assisted colon resection for mucosa-associated lymphoid tissue (MALT) lymphoma in the cecum. Hepatogastroenterology. 2003;50:1003–1005.

120. Chim CS, Shek TW, Chung LP, et al. Gut perforation in MALT lymphoma of colon. Haematologica. 2002;87:EIM15.

121. Zinzani PL, Stefoni V, Musuraca G, et al. Fludarabine-containing chemotherapy as frontline treatment of nongastrointestinal mucosa-associated lymphoid tissue lymphoma. Cancer. 2004;100:2190–2194.

122. Salem PA, Estephan FF. Immunoproliferative small intestinal disease: current concepts. Cancer J. 2005;11:374–382.

123. Lecuit M, Abachin E, Martin A, et al. Immunoproliferative small intestinal disease associated with Campylobacter jejuni. N Engl J Med. 2004;350:239–248.

124. Azar HA. Cancer in Lebanon and the Near East. Cancer. 1962;15:66–78.

125. Ghoshal UC, Chetri K, Banerjee PK, et al. Is immunoproliferative small intestinal disease uncommon in India? Trop Gastroenterol. 2001;22:14–17.

126. Al-Bahrani ZR, Al-Mondhiry H, Bakir F, et al. Clinical and pathologic subtypes of primary intestinal lymphoma. Experience with 132 patients over a 14-year period. Cancer. 1983;52:1666–1672.

127. Rambaud JC. Small intestinal lymphomas and alpha-chain disease. Clin Gastroenterol. 1983;12:743–766.

128. Gilinsky NH, Novis BH, Wright JP, et al. Immunoproliferative small-intestinal disease: clinical features and outcome in 30 cases. Medicine (Baltimore). 1987;66:438–446.

129. Isaacson PG, Dogan A, Price SK, et al. Immunoproliferative small-intestinal disease. An immunohistochemical study. *Am J Surg Pathol.* 1989;13:1023–1033.

130. Vaiphei K, Kumari N, Sinha SK, et al. Roles of syndecan-1, bcl6 and p53 in diagnosis and prognostication of immunoproliferative small intestinal disease. *World J Gastroenterol.* 2006;12:3602–3608.

131. Rambaud JC, Halphen M, Galian A, et al. Immunoproliferative small intestinal disease (IPSID): relationships with alpha-chain disease and "Mediterranean" lymphomas. *Springer Semin Immunopathol.* 1990;12:239–250.

132. Seligmann M, Mihaesco E, Preud'homme JL, et al. Heavy chain diseases: current findings and concepts. *Immunol Rev.* 1979;48:145–167.

133. Bentaboulet M, Mihaesco E, Gendron MC, et al. Genomic alterations in a case of alpha heavy chain disease leading to the generation of composite exons from the JH region. *Eur J Immunol.* 1989;19:2093–2098.

134. Cogne M, Preud'homme JL. Gene deletions force nonsecretory alpha-chain disease plasma cells to produce membrane-form alpha-chain only. *J Immunol.* 1990;145:2455–2458.

135. Ye H, Liu H, Attygalle A, et al. Variable frequencies of t(11;18)(q21;q21) in MALT lymphomas of different sites: significant association with CagA strains of H. pylori in gastric MALT lymphoma. *Blood.* 2003;102:1012–1018.

136. Banihashemi A, Nasr K, Hedayatee H, et al. Familial lymphoma including a report of familial primary upper small intestinal lymphoma. *Blut.* 1973;26:363–368.

137. Nikbin B, Banisadre M, Ala F, et al. HLA AW19, B12 in immunoproliferative small intestinal disease. *Gut.* 1979;20:226–228.

138. Ben-Ayed F, Halphen M, Najjar l, et al. Treatment of alpha chain disease. Results of a prospective study in 21 Tunisian patients by the Tunisian-French intestinal Lymphoma Study Group. *Cancer.* 1989;63:1251–1256.

139. Ramos L, Marcos J, Illanas M, et al. Radiological characteristics of primary intestinal lymphoma of the "Mediterranean" type: observations on twelve cases. *Radiology.* 1978;126:379–385.

140. Vessal K, Dutz W, Kohout E, et al. Immunoproliferative small intestinal disease with duodenojejunal lymphoma: radiologic changes. *AJR Am J Roentgenol.* 1980;135:491–497.

141. Nagi B, Rana SS, Kochhar R, et al. Sonoenteroclysis: a new technique for the diagnosis of small bowel diseases. *Abdom Imaging.* 2006;31:417–424.

142. Al-Mondhiry H. Primary lymphomas of the small intestine: east-west contrast. *Am J Hematol.* 1986;22:89–105.

143. Khojasteh A, Haghighi P. Immunoproliferative small intestinal disease: portrait of a potentially preventable cancer from the Third World. *Am J Med.* 1990;89:483–490.

144. Akbulut H, Soykan I, Yakaryilmaz F, et al. Five-year results of the treatment of 23 patients with immunoproliferative small intestinal disease: a Turkish experience. *Cancer.* 1997;80:8–14.

145. Salimi M, Spinelli JJ. Chemotherapy of Mediterranean abdominal lymphoma. Retrospective comparison of chemotherapy protocols in Iranian patients. *Am J Clin Oncol.* 1996;19:18–22.

146. Celik AF, Pamuk GE, Pamuk ON, et al. Should we suppress the antigenic stimulus in IPSID for lifelong? *Am J Gastroenterol.* 2000;95:3318–3320.

147. Gough KR, Read AE, Naish JM. Intestinal reticulosis as a complication of idiopathic steatorrhoea. *Gut.* 1962;3:232–239.

148. Egan LJ, Walsh SV, Stevens FM, et al. Celiac-associated lymphoma. A single institution experience of 30 cases in the combination chemotherapy era. *J Clin Gastroenterol.* 1995;21:123–129.

149. Holmes GK, Stokes PL, Sorahan TM, et al. Coeliac disease, gluten-free diet, and malignancy. *Gut.* 1976;17:612–619.

150. Isaacson P, Wright DH. Intestinal lymphoma associated with malabsorption. *Lancet.* 1978;1:67–70.

151. Mathus-Vliegen EM, Van Halteren H, Tytgat GN. Malignant lymphoma in coeliac disease: various manifestations with distinct symptomatology and prognosis? *J Intern Med.* 1994;236:43–49.

152. Pricolo VE, Mangi AA, Aswad B, et al. Gastrointestinal malignancies in patients with celiac sprue. *Am J Surg.* 1998;176:344–347.

153. Swinson CM, Slavin G, Coles EC, et al. Coeliac disease and malignancy. *Lancet.* 1983;1:111–115.

154. A clinical evaluation of the International Lymphoma Study Group classification of non-Hodgkin's lymphoma. The Non-Hodgkin's Lymphoma Classification Project. *Blood.* 1997;89:3909–3918.

155. Chott A, Dragosics B, Radaszkiewicz T. Peripheral T-cell lymphomas of the intestine. *Am J Pathol.* 1992;141:1361–1371.

156. Domizio P, Owen RA, Shepherd NA, et al. Primary lymphoma of the small intestine. A clinicopathological study of 119 cases. *Am J Surg Pathol.* 1993;17:429–442.

157. Hsiao CH, Kao HL, Lin MC, et al. Ulcerative colon T-cell lymphoma: an unusual entity mimicking Crohn's disease and may be associated with fulminant hemophagocytosis. *Hepatogastroenterology.* 2002;49:950–954.

158. Spencer J, Cerf-Bensussan N, Jarry A, et al. Enteropathy-associated T cell lymphoma (malignant histiocytosis of the intestine) is recognized by a monoclonal antibody (HML-1) that defines a membrane molecule on human mucosal lymphocytes. *Am J Pathol.* 1988;132:1–5.

159. de Bruin PC, Connolly CE, Oudejans JJ, et al. Enteropathy-associated T-cell lymphomas have a cytotoxic T-cell phenotype. *Histopathology.* 1997;31:313–317.

160. Ilyas M, Niedobitek G, Agathanggelou A, et al. Non-Hodgkin's lymphoma, coeliac disease, and Epstein-Barr virus: a study of 13 cases of enteropathy-associated T- and B-cell lymphoma. *J Pathol.* 1995;177:115–122.

161. Pan L, Diss TC, Peng H, et al. Epstein-Barr virus (EBV) in enteropathy-associated T-cell lymphoma (EATL). *J Pathol.* 1993;170:137–143.

162. de Bruin PC, Jiwa NM, Oudejans JJ, et al. Epstein-Barr virus in primary gastrointestinal T cell lymphomas. Association with gluten-sensitive enteropathy, pathological features, and immunophenotype. *Am J Pathol.* 1995;146:861–867.

163. Quintanilla-Martinez L, Lome-Maldonado C, Ott G, et al. Primary intestinal non-Hodgkin's lymphoma and Epstein-Barr virus: high frequency of EBV-infection in T-cell lymphomas of Mexican origin. *Leuk Lymphoma.* 1998;30:111–121.

164. Chim CS, Au WY, Shek TW, et al. Primary CD56 positive lymphomas of the gastrointestinal tract. *Cancer.* 2001;91:525–533.

165. Chuang SS, Jung YC. Natural killer cell lymphoma of small intestine with features of enteropathy but lack of association with celiac disease. *Hum Pathol.* 2004;35:639–642.

166. Inagaki N, Asaoka D, Mori KL, et al. Enteropathy-type T-cell lymphoma expressing NK-cell intraepithelial lymphocyte (NK-IEL) phenotype. *Leuk Lymphoma.* 2004;45:1471–1474.

167. Zettl A, Ott G, Makulik A, et al. Chromosomal gains at 9q characterize enteropathy-type T-cell lymphoma. *Am J Pathol.* 2002;161:1635–1645.

168. Baumgartner AK, Zettl A, Chott A, et al. High frequency of genetic aberrations in enteropathy-type T-cell lymphoma. *Lab Invest.* 2003;83:1509–1516.

169. Obermann EC, Diss TC, Hamoudi RA, et al. Loss of heterozygosity at chromosome 9p21 is a frequent finding in enteropathy-type T-cell lymphoma. *J Pathol.* 2004;202:252–262.

170. Howell WM, Leung ST, Jones DB, et al. HLA-DRB, -DQA, and -DQB polymorphism in celiac disease and enteropathy-associated T-cell lymphoma. Common features and additional risk factors for malignancy. *Hum Immunol.* 1995;43:29–37.

171. Wahab PJ, Meijer JW, Mulder CJ. Histologic follow-up of people with celiac disease on a gluten-free diet: slow and incomplete recovery. *Am J Clin Pathol.* 2002;118:459–463.

172. Marsh MN. The immunopathology of the small intestinal reaction in gluten-sensitivity. *Immunol Invest.* 1989;18:509–531.

173. Cellier C, Delabesse E, Helmer C, et al. Refractory sprue, coeliac disease, and enteropathy-associated T-cell lymphoma. French Coeliac Disease Study Group. *Lancet.* 2000;356:203–208.

174. Daum S, Hummel M, Weiss D, et al. Refractory sprue syndrome with clonal intraepithelial lymphocytes evolving into overt enteropathy-type intestinal T-cell lymphoma. *Digestion.* 2000;62:60–65.

175. Daum S, Weiss D, Hummel M, et al. Frequency of clonal intraepithelial T lymphocyte proliferations in enteropathy-type intestinal T cell lymphoma, coeliac disease, and refractory sprue. *Gut.* 2001;49:804–812.

176. Gale J, Simmonds PD, Mead GM, et al. Enteropathy-type intestinal T-cell lymphoma: clinical features and treatment of 31 patients in a single center. *J Clin Oncol.* 2000;18:795–803.

177. Novakovic BJ, Novakovic S, Frkovic-Grazio S. A single-center report on clinical features and treatment response in patients with intestinal T cell non-Hodgkin's lymphomas. *Oncol Rep.* 2006;16:191–195.

178. Smedby KE, Akerman M, Hildebrand H, et al. Malignant lymphomas in coeliac disease: evidence of increased risks for lymphoma types other than enteropathy-type T cell lymphoma. *Gut.* 2005;54:54–59.

179. Banks PM, Chan J, Cleary ML, et al. Mantle cell lymphoma. A proposal for unification of morphologic, immunologic, and molecular data. *Am J Surg Pathol.* 1992;16:637–640.

180. Plank L, Hansmann ML, Lennert K. Centrocytic lymphoma. *Am J Surg Pathol.* 1993;17:638–639, author reply 641.

181. Tsujimoto Y, Yunis J, Onorato-Showe L, et al. Molecular cloning of the chromosomal breakpoint of B-cell lymphomas and leukemias with the t(11;14) chromosome translocation. *Science.* 1984;224:1403–1406.

182. Motokura T, Bloom T, Kim HG, et al. A novel cyclin encoded by a bcl1-linked candidate oncogene. *Nature.* 1991;350:512–515.

183. Williams ME, Meeker TC, Swerdlow SH. Rearrangement of the chromosome 11 bcl-1 locus in centrocytic lymphoma: analysis with multiple breakpoint probes. *Blood.* 1991;78:493–498.

184. Coignet LJ, Schuuring E, Kibbelaar RE, et al. Detection of 11q13 rearrangements in hematologic neoplasias by double-color fluorescence in situ hybridization. *Blood.* 1996;87:1512–1519.

185. Yang WI, Zukerberg LR, Motokura T, et al. Cyclin D1 (Bcl-1, PRAD1) protein expression in low-grade B-cell lymphomas and reactive hyperplasia. *Am J Pathol.* 1994;145:86–96.

186. Yatabe Y, Nakamura S, Seto M, et al. Clinicopathologic study of PRAD1/cyclin D1 overexpressing lymphoma with special reference to mantle cell lymphoma. A distinct molecular pathologic entity. *Am J Surg Pathol.* 1996;20:1110–1122.

187. Yatabe Y, Suzuki R, Tobinai K, et al. Significance of cyclin D1 overexpression for the diagnosis of mantle cell lymphoma: a clinicopathologic comparison of cyclin D1-positive MCL and cyclin D1-negative MCL-like B-cell lymphoma. *Blood.* 2000;95:2253–2261.

188. Rosenwald A, Wright G, Wiestner A, et al. The proliferation gene expression signature is a quantitative integrator of oncogenic events that predicts survival in mantle cell lymphoma. *Cancer Cell.* 2003;3:185–197.

189. Bookman MA, Lardelli P, Jaffe ES, et al. Lymphocytic lymphoma of intermediate differentiation: morphologic, immunophenotypic, and prognostic factors. *J Natl Cancer Inst.* 1990;82:742–748.

190. Cornes JS. Multiple lymphomatous polyposis of the gastrointestinal tract. *Cancer.* 1961;14:249–257.

191. Moynihan MJ, Bast MA, Chan WC, et al. Lymphomatous polyposis. A neoplasm of either follicular mantle or germinal center cell origin. *Am J Surg Pathol.* 1996;20:442–452.

192. Kodama T, Ohshima K, Nomura K, et al. Lymphomatous polyposis of the gastrointestinal tract, including mantle cell lymphoma, follicular lymphoma and mucosa-associated lymphoid tissue lymphoma. *Histopathology.* 2005;47:467–478.

193. Romaguera JE, Medeiros LJ, Hagemeister FB, et al. Frequency of gastrointestinal involvement and its clinical significance in mantle cell lymphoma. *Cancer.* 2003;97:586–591.

194. Salar A, Juanpere N, Bellosillo B, et al. Gastrointestinal involvement in mantle cell lymphoma: a prospective clinic, endoscopic, and pathologic study. *Am J Surg Pathol.* 2006;30:1274–1280.

195. Teodorovic I, Pittaluga S, Kluin-Nelemans JC, et al. Efficacy of four different regimens in 64 mantle-cell lymphoma cases: clinicopathologic comparison with 498 other non-Hodgkin's lymphoma subtypes. European Organization for the Research and Treatment of Cancer Lymphoma Cooperative Group. *J Clin Oncol.* 1995;13:2819–2826.

196. Pittaluga S, Bijnens L, Teodorovic I, et al. Clinical analysis of 670 cases in two trials of the European Organization for the Research and Treatment of Cancer Lymphoma Cooperative Group subtyped according to the Revised European-American Classification of Lymphoid Neoplasms: a comparison with the Working Formulation. *Blood.* 1996;87:4358–4367.

197. Argatoff LH, Connors JM, Klasa RJ, et al. Mantle cell lymphoma: a clinicopathologic study of 80 cases. *Blood.* 1997;89:2067–2078.

198. Bosch F, Lopez-Guillermo A, Campo E, et al. Mantle cell lymphoma: presenting features, response to therapy, and prognostic factors. *Cancer.* 1998;82:567–575.

199. Hiddemann W, Unterhalt M, Herrmann R, et al. Mantle-cell lymphomas have more widespread disease and a slower response to chemotherapy compared with follicle-center lymphomas: results of a prospective comparative analysis of the German Low-Grade Lymphoma Study Group. *J Clin Oncol.* 1998;16:1922–1930.

200. Oinonen R, Franssila K, Teerenhovi L, et al. Mantle cell lymphoma: clinical features, treatment and prognosis of 94 patients. *Eur J Cancer.* 1998;34:329–336.

201. Coiffier B, Haioun C, Ketterer N, et al. Rituximab (anti-CD20 monoclonal antibody) for the treatment of patients with relapsing or refractory aggressive lymphoma: a multicenter phase II study. *Blood.* 1998;92:1927–1932.

202. Foran JM, Rohatiner AZ, Cunningham D, et al. European phase II study of rituximab (chimeric anti-CD20 monoclonal antibody) for patients with newly diagnosed mantle-cell lymphoma and previously treated mantle-cell lymphoma, immunocytoma, and small B-cell lymphocytic lymphoma. *J Clin Oncol.* 2000;18:317–324.

203. Ghielmini M, Schmitz SF, Cogliatti S, et al. Effect of single-agent rituximab given at the standard schedule or as prolonged treatment in patients with mantle cell lymphoma: a study of the Swiss Group for Clinical Cancer Research (SAKK). *J Clin Oncol.* 2005;23:705–711.

204. Khouri IF, Romaguera J, Kantarjian H, et al. Hyper-CVAD and high-dose methotrexate/cytarabine followed by stem-cell transplantation: an active regimen for aggressive mantle-cell lymphoma. *J Clin Oncol.* 1998;16:3803–3809.

205. Khouri IF, Lee MS, Saliba RM, et al. Nonablative allogeneic stem-cell transplantation for advanced/recurrent mantle-cell lymphoma. *J Clin Oncol.* 2003;21:4407–4412.

206. Romaguera JE, Fayad L, Rodriguez MA, et al. High rate of durable remissions after treatment of newly diagnosed aggressive mantle-cell lymphoma with rituximab plus hyper-CVAD alternating with rituximab plus high-dose methotrexate and cytarabine. *J Clin Oncol.* 2005;23:7013–7023.

207. Howard OM, Gribben JG, Neuberg DS, et al. Rituximab and CHOP induction therapy for newly diagnosed mantle-cell lymphoma: molecular complete responses are not predictive of progression-free survival. *J Clin Oncol.* 2002;20:1288–1294.

208. Lenz G, Dreyling M, Hoster E, et al. Immunochemotherapy with rituximab and cyclophosphamide, doxorubicin, vincristine, and prednisone significantly improves response and time to treatment failure, but not long-term outcome in patients with previously untreated mantle cell lymphoma: results of a prospective randomized trial of the German Low Grade Lymphoma Study Group (GLSG). *J Clin Oncol.* 2005;23:1984–1992.

209. Freedman AS, Neuberg D, Gribben JG, et al. High-dose chemoradiotherapy and anti-B-cell monoclonal antibody-purged autologous bone marrow transplantation in mantle-cell lymphoma: no evidence for long-term remission. *J Clin Oncol.* 1998;16:13–18.

210. Vandenberghe E, Ruiz de Elvira C, Loberiza FR, et al. Outcome of autologous transplantation for mantle cell lymphoma: a study by the European Blood and Bone Marrow Transplant and Autologous Blood and Marrow Transplant Registries. *Br J Haematol.* 2003;120:793–800.

211. Dreyling M, Lenz G, Hoster E, et al. Early consolidation by myeloablative radiochemotherapy followed by autologous stem cell transplantation in first remission significantly prolongs progression-free survival in mantle-cell lymphoma: results of a prospective randomized trial of the European MCL Network. *Blood.* 2005;105:2677–2684.

212. Schoder H, Meta J, Yap C, et al. Effect of whole-body (18)F-FDG PET imaging on clinical staging and management of patients with malignant lymphoma. *J Nucl Med.* 2001;42:1139–1143.

213. Sam JW, Levine MS, Farner MC, et al. Detection of small bowel involvement by mantle cell lymphoma on F-18 FDG positron emission tomography. *Clin Nucl Med.* 2002;27:330–333.

214. Armitage JO, Weisenburger DD. New approach to classifying non-Hodgkin's lymphomas: clinical features of the major histologic subtypes. Non-Hodgkin's Lymphoma Classification Project. *J Clin Oncol.* 1998;16:2780–2795.

215. Mann RB, Berard CW. Criteria for the cytologic subclassification of follicular lymphomas: a proposed alternative method. *Hematol Oncol.* 1983;1:187–192.

216. Zelenetz AD, Chu G, Galili N, et al. Enhanced detection of the t(14;18) translocation in malignant lymphoma using pulsed-field gel electrophoresis. *Blood.* 1991;78:1552–1560.

217. Yoshino T, Miyake K, Ichimura K, et al. Increased incidence of follicular lymphoma in the duodenum. *Am J Surg Pathol.* 2000;24:688–693.

218. Shia J, Teruya-Feldstein J, Pan D, et al. Primary follicular lymphoma of the gastrointestinal tract: a clinical and pathologic study of 26 cases. *Am J Surg Pathol.* 2002;26:216–224.

219. Hatano B, Ohshima K, Tsuchiya T, et al. Clinicopathological features of gastric B-cell lymphoma: a series of 317 cases. *Pathol Int.* 2002;52:677–682.

220. Kohno S, Ohshima K, Yoneda S, et al. Clinicopathological analysis of 143 primary malignant lymphomas in the small and large intestines based on the new WHO classification. *Histopathology.* 2003;43:135–143.

221. Spectre G, Libster D, Grisariu S, et al. Bleeding, obstruction, and perforation in a series of patients with aggressive gastric lymphoma treated with primary chemotherapy. *Ann Surg Oncol.* 2006;13:1372–1378.

222. Wohrer S, Bartsch R, Hejna M, et al. Routine application of the proton-pump inhibitor pantoprazole in patients with gastric lymphoma undergoing chemotherapy. *Scand J Gastroenterol.* 2005;40:1222–1225.

223. Binn M, Ruskone-Fourmestraux A, Lepage E, et al. Surgical resection plus chemotherapy versus chemotherapy alone: comparison of two strategies to treat diffuse large B-cell gastric lymphoma. *Ann Oncol.* 2003;14:1751–1757.

224. Aviles A, Nambo MJ, Neri N, et al. The role of surgery in primary gastric lymphoma: results of a controlled clinical trial. *Ann Surg.* 2004;240:44–50.

225. Raderer M, Chott A, Drach J, et al. Chemotherapy for management of localised high-grade gastric B-cell lymphoma: how much is necessary? *Ann Oncol.* 2002;13:1094–1098.

226. Park YH, Lee SH, Kim WS, et al. CHOP followed by involved field radiotherapy for localized primary gastric diffuse large B-cell lymphoma: results of a multi center phase II study and quality of life evaluation. *Leuk Lymphoma.* 2006;47:1253–1259.

227. Bertoni F, Zucca E. State-of-the-art therapeutics: marginal-zone lymphoma. *J Clin Oncol.* 2005;23:6415–6420.

228. Roggero E, Zucca E, Pinotti G, et al. Eradication of *Helicobacter pylori* infection in primary low-grade gastric lymphoma of mucosa-associated lymphoid tissue. *Ann Intern Med.* 1995;122:767–769.

229. Montalban C, Santon A, Boixeda D, et al. Treatment of low grade gastric mucosa-associated lymphoid tissue lymphoma in stage I with *Helicobacter pylori* eradication. Long-term results after sequential histologic and molecular follow-up. *Haematologica.* 2001;86:609–617.

230. Fischbach W, Goebeler-Kolve ME, Dragosics B, et al. Long term outcome of patients with gastric marginal zone B cell lymphoma of mucosa associated lymphoid tissue (MALT) following exclusive *Helicobacter pylori* eradication therapy: experience from a large prospective series. *Gut.* 2004;53:34–37.

231. Wundisch T, Thiede C, Morgner A, et al. Long-term follow-up of gastric MALT lymphoma after *Helicobacter pylori* eradication. *J Clin Oncol.* 2005;23:8018–8024.

232. Hong SS, Jung HY, Choi KD, et al. A prospective analysis of low-grade gastric malt lymphoma after Helicobacter pylori eradication. *Helicobacter.* 2006;11:569–573.

233. Tsang RW, Gospodarowicz MK. Radiation therapy for localized low-grade non-Hodgkin's lymphomas. *Hematol Oncol.* 2005;23:10–17.

234. Al-Saleem T, Al-Mondhiry H. Immunoproliferative small intestinal disease (IPSID): a model for mature B-cell neoplasms. *Blood.* 2005;105:2274–2280.

CHAPTER 50 ■ GASTROINTESTINAL STROMAL TUMORS

GEORGE D. DEMETRI AND BRIAN P. RUBIN

Mesenchymal tumors of the gastrointestinal (GI) tract comprise a widely diverse group of neoplasms, completely separate from carcinomas or neuroendocrine tumors. This diverse grouping of tumors includes histopathological subtypes (e.g., leiomyosarcoma, leiomyoma, neurofibroma, schwannoma, desmoid fibromatosis, benign and malignant vascular tumors, glomus tumor, and other rare subtypes of sarcoma) that also can occur outside the GI tract; importantly, though, the most common subtype of mesenchymal tumor of this organ system is the subtype known as *gastrointestinal stromal tumor* (GIST) that occurs exclusively within the abdomen, retroperitoneum, and pelvis (1). Even before the advent of molecular-targeted therapy for this disease, much had been written about GIST, yet, until recently, these tumors defied precise histogenetic classification. Prognostication has also always been problematic. Recent advances in understanding the molecular pathogenesis of GISTs has led to fascinating new insights into the histogenesis and molecular lesions, which are fundamental to the biology and clinical behavior of GISTs. Based on these exciting developments in the molecular biology of GISTs, new approaches to therapy have been developed to target the molecular aberrancies that are causative for GISTs, and this disease is now a proof of concept for the rational investigation of "smart drugs," which target specific pathways that are selectively activated in cancer cells. This chapter focuses on the pathological and clinical characteristics of GISTs, with an emphasis on the recent therapeutic developments in this rapidly evolving field.

CLINICAL ASPECTS

GISTs can occur at any age, although they are more common in adults, with a peak incidence in the fifth and sixth decades of life (2–5). Although numbers vary slightly from study to study, it appears that males and females are affected equally (2,3,5). Although it is not possible to know the exact incidence of GISTs in the population, these tumors are not common. A population-based retrospective study in Sweden estimated the incidence at approximately 14.5 cases per 1 million (6). In the United States, the incidence of newly diagnosed GIST has been estimated to be at least 5,000 cases per year. GIST was clearly underdiagnosed prior to the year 2000, when newer diagnostic methods (e.g., immunohistochemical staining for the KIT protein antigen, CD117) made the characterization of GIST more accurate. This incidence figure for GIST is important considering that it is commonly reported that approximately 10,000 new cases of sarcomas overall present annually in the United States. Once GIST is included in these figures, the incidence of sarcomas is certainly greater than previously reported. It is also important to note that GIST is not reported separately in large databases such as the Surveillance, Epidemiology, and End

Results system of the National Cancer Institute. Also, many gastroenterologists and even pathologists are increasingly finding incidental small lesions that are true GISTs (7). Such "micro-GISTs" exhibit many of the same mutations that larger, more aggressive GISTs harbor (8), although lesions <1 cm in size clearly have only a trivial risk to behave in a malignant fashion.

GISTs occur along the entire length of the GI tract but with different frequencies at different anatomical locations (Table 50.1) (9). Importantly, GISTs from different GI sites of origin also exhibit different incidences of the underlying type of molecular mechanism: In other words, the specific activating pathway (usually through a specific activating mutation in a signaling kinase such as the *KIT* proto-oncogene) appears to correlate with the site of origin of the primary GIST (10). GISTs are extremely rare in the esophagus. Most mesenchymal tumors of the esophagus are leiomyomas, although increasingly small GIST lesions are detected incidentally on upper endoscopy (8,11–13). GISTs occur most commonly in the stomach, followed by the small intestine, and are rare in the colon and rectum. GISTs may also rarely arise in the omentum, mesentery, and peritoneum, and are known collectively as extragastrointestinal GISTs.

Most small GIST lesions are asymptomatic. When large lesions are present, or if the tumor is highly infiltrative into vascular or neural structures, initial symptoms may include abdominal fullness, pain, nausea, dyspepsia, acute abdominal crisis with perforation, or evidence of GI bleeding, such as melena, hematemesis, and anemia (14,15). Large tumors may be palpable, especially when located in the stomach. Small, incidental GISTs may be diagnosed at the time of surgery for unrelated reasons and generally pursue a more benign course (8,16).

There are no known etiologic factors that predispose to the development of GISTs besides rare germline genetic conditions. There is an increased incidence of GISTs in patients with neurofibromatosis (17), the significance of which is discussed in the Future Studies section (18). In addition, GISTs are one of the tumors associated with Carney's triad, a sporadic tumor syndrome that usually presents in childhood and is characterized by the combination of epithelioid leiomyoblastomas (GISTs), functioning extra-adrenal paragangliomas, and pulmonary chondromatous hamartomas (19). Rare familial GIST syndromes have also been described with a high penetrance of the disease and germline activation of the kinase-encoding *KIT* or PDGRA proto-oncogenes (20–24).

PATHOLOGY AND HISTOGENESIS

Grossly, GISTs are usually well-demarcated (although unencapsulated) nodules that arise from the wall of the GI tract or,

Esophagus	Rare (most stromal tumors in this location are leiomyomas)
Stomach	Most common site
Small intestine	Next most common site
Colon	Uncommon
Rectum	Uncommon
Omentum/mesentery	Rare

much less commonly, from the omentum, mesentery, or peritoneal surface. They vary in size from barely discernible nodules that present as incidental findings at autopsy or surgery for unrelated reasons to enormous masses measuring ≥30 cm (7,8,25–27). The histopathological grading of GISTs is misleading because the majority of these tumors are bland spindle cells with a rather monotonous and overall "low-grade" appearance (Fig. 50.1); approximately one-third to one-half of GIST lesions may have an epithelioid morphology or a mixture of epithelioid and spindle cells. Given the fact that even tiny GIST lesions harbor the activating mutations that are causative for GIST, it is critical to note that any GIST has the potential for malignant behavior: It is only a matter of likelihood and risk of such malignant behavior in the clinic (8). The lesions formerly called "benign GISTs" are now referred to more accurately as very low or low-risk GIST; these tend to be small, whereas more aggressively malignant lesions are more often large (>5 cm). Ulceration of the overlying mucosa is not uncommon, and cystic degeneration and necrosis can be seen in larger lesions (27). Many malignant GISTs have already metastasized at initial presentation; they present as multiple nodules, often dispersed throughout the peritoneal cavity or with liver metastases. Lesions of the more aggressively malignant GIST subtypes may also be characterized by gross invasion of adjacent organs (27). Distant metastases to extraabdominal soft tissues are rare but reported in GISTs. Importantly, the pattern of metastatic spread in GISTs is quite different from other soft tissue sarcomas. The risk of pulmonary metastases with GISTs is significantly lower than for other pathological subtypes of sarcomas. The biological reason(s)

for these observed differences in the pattern of metastases between GIST and other mesenchymal cell malignancies remains obscure.

Before the use of modern pathological techniques, the vast majority of GISTs were believed to exhibit a smooth muscle phenotype. Such nonepithelial tumors of the GI tract were classified by various names, including *leiomyomas*, *bizarre leiomyomas*, *leiomyoblastomas*, or *leiomyosarcomas* (4,15,28–30). The evidence cited to support the smooth muscle phenotype was that the tumors usually arose from the muscular wall of the GI tract, frequently adopted a fascicular architecture, and possessed fibrillar cytoplasm. However, GISTs had some peculiar features that suggested they might not be true smooth muscle tumors. They frequently exhibited a palisaded morphologic appearance reminiscent of neural tumors, such as schwannomas. In addition, a subset of GISTs had an epithelioid appearance with atypical nuclei, at least focally, that were difficult to reconcile with a smooth muscle phenotype. These unusual histologic features were often dismissed as representing degenerative changes.

However, once the cellular microanatomy of GIST cells were studies with electron microscopy, investigators failed to find evidence to support the putative smooth muscle phenotype of GISTs (31–37). In contrast to leiomyomas and leiomyosarcomas at other sites, actin filaments with focal densities were not abundant, and basal lamina was present only focally in most GISTs (31). In addition, GIST demonstrated ultrastructural features not usually associated with smooth muscle tumors, such as interdigitating processes. Many tumors were said to exhibit "incomplete smooth muscle differentiation" or "undifferentiated" phenotypes. In addition, subsets of GISTs were found to have unusual neuroaxonal characteristics with dense core granules (Fig. 50.2) and synapselike structures; these tumors became known as the so-called gastric autonomic neural tumors (GANTs), with other groups preferring the term *plexosarcomas* (32,35,36,38,39).

As immunohistochemical techniques came into widespread use and immunophenotypic data on GISTs became available, the results seemed to echo what was found with electron microscopy (2,3,35,37,40–49). Results of different studies varied considerably, with anywhere from 25% to 100% of tumors showing immunoreactivity for muscle-specific actin (2,40,41,44–49), 31% to 74% displaying immunoreactivity for smooth muscle actin (3,45,47,49), and 0% to 50% binding antibodies to desmin (2,3,35,37,40,44–47,49). In addition,

FIGURE 50.1. Hematoxylin-and-eosin section of a typical low-grade spindle cell gastrointestinal stromal tumor. (See also color Fig. 50.1.)

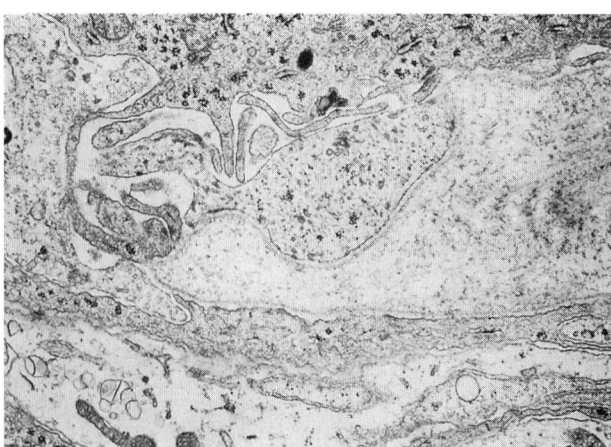

FIGURE 50.2. Gastrointestinal stromal tumor with a bulbous, synapselike structure containing dense core granules. (See also color Fig. 50.2.) *Source:* Courtesy of Dr. Christopher Fletcher, Brigham & Women's Hospital, Boston, MA.

TABLE 50.2

HISTOLOGIC DIFFERENTIAL DIAGNOSIS OF GASTROINTESTINAL STROMAL TUMOR

Leiomyoma
Leiomyosarcoma
Schwannoma
Neurofibroma
Malignant peripheral nerve sheath tumor
Solitary fibrous tumor
Endometrial stromal sarcoma
Desmoid fibromatosis
Sarcomatoid carcinoma
Dedifferentiated liposarcoma (with inadequate sampling)

some tumors revealed a neural phenotype with immunoreactivity to S-100 protein (2,3,35,37,40,41,44–47,49) and neuron-specific enolase (3,40). Still other GISTs were biphenotypic, expressing neural and partial smooth muscle phenotypes. Some GISTs failed to express any line of differentiation and were immunoreactive for vimentin only; these tumors were said to have a null phenotype (3,40).

Due to the bewildering array of histologic, ultrastructural, and immunohistochemical features, the noncommittal term of *GIST* was popularized with the recognition that the histogenesis, although certainly mesenchymal (stromal) in nature, was unclear (35). The widespread acceptance of the term *GIST* for a loose collection of nonepithelial tumors of the GI tract served to simplify the classification of these bewildering stromal tumors. However, the diversity of histopathological phenotypes and lack of consistent diagnostic criteria created a situation in which many different histogenetic tumor types were grouped into an excessively broad diagnostic category of *GISTs*, thereby creating a clinically indistinct and biologically heterogeneous tumor category (Table 50.2). Thus, tumors once diagnosed as *GIST* might include not only what would today be recognized as *true* GISTs but also could represent less common subtypes with different underlying biological behavior, such as true smooth muscle tumors (leiomyoma and leiomyosarcoma), true neural tumors (neurofibroma, schwannoma, and malignant peripheral nerve sheath tumor), desmoid fibromatosis, and others. More important, unusual epithelial tumors with a mesenchymal appearance, such as sarcomatoid carcinomas, were also occasionally misclassified as GISTs. This situation has persisted until relatively recently when our understanding of GISTs has been radically altered due to the convergence of several lines of investigation (discussed in Molecular Genetics of Gastrointestinal Stromal Tumors section).

BEHAVIOR, PROGNOSTIC FACTORS, AND GRADING OF GASTROINTESTINAL STROMAL TUMORS

There is a fascinating discordance in the experience base and the literature of pathologists, gastroenterologists, and oncologists. For many gastroenterologists, it has been widely taught that GISTs often follow a relatively indolent course. They have a tendency for local recurrence followed by metastasis only in an unusual subset of cases. This appears to be a matter of referral selection bias because many gastroenterologists care for patients with smaller lesions of lower risk. In the oncology literature, GIST is known as a consistently aggressive malignancy, with high rates of death due to recurrent and metastatic

disease (50,51). Although it is difficult to obtain absolute percentages due to a lack of consistent definitions about grading and diagnosis of GISTs, approximately 50% of low-grade lesions eventually recur. Of the low-grade tumors that do recur, 60% also metastasize (usually to other intra-abdominal sites, liver, or both) (52). Virtually all high-grade GISTs recur, and >80% of those tumors that recur eventually metastasize (52). Survival seems to be site dependent. In one large study, the overall 10-year survival was 48%; however, site-specific 10-year survival was 74% for gastric tumors and 17% for small bowel tumors (2). In a separate study, the median survival was 25 months for low-grade tumors and 98 months for high-grade lesions (52).

Most GISTs are low-grade neoplasms, and yet all GISTs appear to harbor the biological ability to pursue an aggressive, metastatic course in individual patients; however, it has been difficult to determine exactly *which* tumors at the low-grade end of the GIST spectrum will behave aggressively (15). Of particular concern, it has been noted by several pathologists that lesions that lack any "histologic criteria for malignancy" will nonetheless occasionally metastasize (26,30). A smaller number of GISTs are obviously malignant and exhibit features that divulge their propensity for aggressive behavior (as noted later in this section). The pathology literature prior to the year 2000 is confusing with many reports of so-called "benign" GISTs. However, experts now exhibit a consensus that GISTs of histologic low grade (aside from those that are discovered incidentally and are very small [<1 cm in maximal dimension]) are virtually all low-grade malignant and should be treated and undergo clinical surveillance as such (53,54). However, very long-term follow-up (on the order of 20–30 years) is hardly ever reported in the literature and would seem to be necessary to establish that a GIST is truly benign (55). Attempts to predict prognosis have focused on various clinical and histopathological features, and these are reviewed later in this section (Table 50.3) (53,54).

Tumor location is one of the most important factors. In a mammoth study of 1,004 GISTs, tumors that arose in the stomach had a better prognosis than those that occurred in the small bowel; colon or rectum; and peritoneum, omentum, or mesentery; in fact, tumors that had origin in the colon and peritoneum, omentum, or mesentery appeared to exhibit a particularly bad prognosis (9). Esophageal tumors were reported to have the best prognosis, but in retrospect these tumors were most likely esophageal leiomyomas and not true GISTs because no attempt was made to distinguish between GISTs and smooth muscle tumors, and GISTs only rarely occur primarily in the

TABLE 50.3

PROPOSED GUIDELINES FOR DEFINING RISK OF AGGRESSIVE BEHAVIOR IN GASTROINTESTINAL STROMAL TUMORS

	Size	Mitotic count
Very low risk	<2 cm	<5 per 50 HPFs
Low risk	2–5 cm	<5 per 50 HPFs
Intermediate risk	<5 cm	6–10 per 50 HPFs
	5–10 cm	<5 per 50 HPFs
High risk	>5 cm	>5 per 50 HPFs
	>10 cm	Any mitotic rate
	Any size	>10 per 50 HPFs

HPF, high-power field.

esophagus. These data are also supported by several smaller studies, which confirm the major conclusion that extragastric GISTs, in general, have a worse prognosis than gastric GISTs (5,42,44,56–59).

Tumor stage is also an important prognostic factor, although the contributions to tumor "stage" are somewhat different in GIST compared to carcinomas of the GI tract (e.g., GISTs virtually never spread to locoregional lymph nodes, so that is not a useful component of the staging system for prognostication). In addition, invasion of adjacent organs is an adverse factor, as is the presence of metastatic disease at diagnosis, both of which are associated with a worse prognosis (14,27,56). As noted previously, the pattern of metastatic spread of GISTs is characteristic and quite different from other soft tissue sarcomas. Metastatic disease is usually confined to the liver and peritoneal cavity, and rarely to the lungs (25–27,29,46,52,60,61). Individual GISTs have been documented to metastasize to virtually all organs and soft tissues; however, these metastases are the exception and not the rule (25,27,52). It is unusual for GISTs to metastasize to lymph nodes, and, in the authors' experience, lymph node metastases from purported GISTs should prompt a reappraisal of the diagnosis (26,27,29,46). The authors have frequently observed that metastatic omental or mesenteric implants that grossly resemble lymph node metastases are frequently misdiagnosed as such. Great care should be taken to identify residual lymph node tissue to determine that a tumor has indeed metastasized to a lymph node. In addition, "drop metastases" with invasion of nodal tissue may well explain incidental nodal involvement more than lymphatic spread of tumor, which does not seem to be characteristic of GISTs. The molecular mechanisms responsible for this unique pattern of spread have not been identified in GIST compared to other GI tract malignancies or other sarcomas.

The effect of age on prognosis has also been examined, and older age is associated with a worse prognosis (9,46). It has been suggested that the better prognosis associated with GISTs in the pediatric and young adult population might be attributable to their association with Carney's triad (62). Prolonged survival has been observed in patients with Carney's triad, even in the face of metastatic disease (63,64). The biological basis for this is unclear. However, it supports the hypothesis that the GISTs in Carney's triad may be fundamentally distinct from sporadic GISTs in adults, which is also consistent with the fact that the GIST lesions in children tend to lack defined mutations in the *KIT* or *PDGFRA* kinase genes, and yet KIT signaling is uncontrollably active in these cells (65). Further studies, including correlations with in-depth molecular analysis of signaling pathways in this clinicopathological syndrome, are necessary to elucidate the differences between pediatric (syndromic) GIST and the sporadic GISTs of adults.

In general, GISTs are not very mitotically active compared with many other sarcomas. However, the mitotic count has been widely accepted as the best prognostic indicator (1,5,9,14,25,27,29,46,52,56,58,59,66–69). Mitotic rates in the range of >1 to 5 mitoses per 10 high-power fields (HPFs) have been associated with a higher incidence of recurrences and metastases (9,26,29,46,47,56,70). Emory et al. showed that the utility of mitotic index in predicting prognosis is site dependent; although it is useful in gastric GISTs, it is not useful in stratifying those that occur in the small bowel (9). In addition, tumors without demonstrable mitotic activity have been known to recur, metastasize, or both (9,26). The presence of atypical mitoses has also been suggested as useful in predicting prognosis (56). In our own experience, atypical mitoses and significant mitotic activity (>10 mitoses per 10 HPFs) are uncommon in GISTs; their presence should prompt a reassessment of the diagnosis of GIST.

Tumor size has also been associated with aggressive behavior (16,26,29,52–54,56,58,59,66). Tumors <5 cm are gener-

ally indolent; however, some do behave aggressively (9,52). Small GISTs discovered incidentally at operation for other reasons are associated with a good prognosis. In one study, none of 19 tumors discovered incidentally behaved aggressively (16).

Although unequivocal necrosis in GISTs is slightly unusual, when present, it is usually associated with malignant behavior (71). However, many GISTs have degenerative changes and undergo cystification that should not be confused with true necrosis. The presence of infiltration by neutrophils is a good indicator of true necrosis in contrast to ischemic degeneration, which does not have necrosis associated with neutrophils. However, the presence of necrosis does not absolutely predict aggressive behavior because there are rare reports of clinically indolent tumors that had unequivocal tumor necrosis (5).

Cytologic atypia, increased cellularity, nuclear pleomorphism, or a combination of the three, have all been associated by various authors with a worse prognosis; however, many GISTs that behave aggressively exhibit boring uniform cytology without cytologic atypia, overwhelming cellularity, or nuclear pleomorphism (5,16,29,30,52,59,66,72). It is also accepted that some clinically indolent GISTs can have focal nuclear atypia (26). In addition, these features are notoriously subjective and difficult to measure, making them less useful than truly subjective criteria, such as tumor size.

Other histologic parameters that have been suggested to have prognostic importance are the presence of epithelioid cytomorphology and infiltration of the GI mucosa by tumor. Although epithelioid cytomorphology has been a particularly controversial topic, recent studies indicate that those GISTs with epithelioid cytomorphology tend to behave less aggressively than those lesions composed exclusively of spindle cells (3,26,58,59,73). Many GISTs fail to involve the mucosal layers of the GI tract; however, when mucosal infiltration is present, it is strongly indicative of aggressive behavior similar to that seen with invasion of adjacent organs.

Various groups have attempted to correlate prognosis in GISTs with various nuclear characteristics (70,71,74–76). Ploidy, obtained from flow or image cytometric analysis, has yielded mixed results. Most studies have shown that aneuploidy tends to portend a poor prognosis; however, ploidy loses its predictive value in multivariate analysis when mitotic count and the presence or absence of metastatic disease at diagnosis is taken into account (56). There is also an indication that aneuploidy of the G_2M peak may offer independent prognostic value beyond that predicted by mitotic index in comparison with that offered by aneuploidy of the G_0G_1 peak (56). Furthermore, several benign tumors have shown aneuploid and tetraploid peaks, whereas some malignant tumors have revealed a diploid or hypodiploid pattern. Studies of morphometric indices in GISTs have generally failed to identify any measurements of prognostic value. In a similar vein, immunohistochemistry for proliferating cell nuclear antigen (PCNA) and interphase nucleolar organizer regions have failed to consistently yield useful prognostic information. Some studies have indicated a statistically significant relationship between PCNA index and prognosis (57,70,72,77); however, when analyzed in multivariate analysis, PCNA index loses its predictive value over mitotic rate (78). Ki-67 labeling index may be of some use, but only a few studies have looked at Ki-67 or Mib-1 labeling index. In one study (72), Ki-67 index >10% was the most significant predictor of overall survival, whereas Ki-67 index >22% correlated with a bad prognosis in a separate study (71). However, Emory et al. found that mitotic index was more reliable at predicting prognosis than Ki-67 index (79). Differences in these results may be related to methodologic differences (80).

Due to the relative lack of any reliable single prognostic factor that can be used to predict prognosis in all GISTs, some have advocated a multiparametric approach that can be used to stratify GISTs for treatment and surveillance purposes (3,81).

Unfortunately, due to the relative rarity of GISTs, none of these approaches has been evaluated prospectively in a carefully controlled trial. Currently, in the absence of metastasis that automatically classifies a GIST as malignant, consensus guidelines have been issued that stratify GIST according to size and mitotic activity into four risk categories (very low risk, low risk, intermediate risk, high risk) (Table 50.3). From the previous discussion, it should be obvious that these are merely practical recommendations that would imperfectly predict biological behavior in any individual case. Further research is definitely required to improve our ability to predict the clinical risks of relapse and death from primary early stage, nonmetastatic GISTs.

MOLECULAR GENETICS OF GASTROINTESTINAL STROMAL TUMORS

With the coming of age of molecular biological techniques, researchers and now clinical pathologists have begun to define the molecular genetic characteristics of GISTs in the hope that such a fundamental understanding of the disease might yield advances in diagnosis, prognosis, and therapy (Table 50.4). Cytogenetic analysis of a relatively small number of GISTs has shown that their cytogenetic profile is unique and serves to distinguish them from other mesenchymal tumors (82–86). GISTs characteristically have a relatively simple karyotype and frequently exhibit losses of chromosomes 14, 1p, and 22. Comparative genomic hybridization has also demonstrated consistent losses of chromosome 14q (87,88), whereas loss of heterozygosity (LOH) studies have detected loss of chromosomal material at 1p12 to 13, 1p36, and 9p (89). The contribution of these chromosomal losses to GIST tumorigenesis is not known at this time; however, loss of chromosomal material generally indicates the presence of a tumor-suppressor gene that has been lost. Further studies are necessary to determine which, if any, specific tumor-suppressor genes are involved in the pathogenesis of GISTs. However, there does seem to be a multistep process of malignancy at work in GIST, as for other malignancies such as carcinomas. The more aggressive GISTs have more molecular genetic lesions that have accumulated, and the linkage between these mutations and the behavior of the disease holds great promise as a field of research to understand mechanisms of neoplastic transformation in general.

Since 1998, it has been realized that mutations in the *KIT* (also referred to as c-*kit*) proto-oncogene, which encodes the KIT receptor tyrosine kinase, are causally related to the pathogenesis of GIST (90). This critically important insight was preceded by decades of prior work in two apparently unrelated lines of research: (a) studies into the anatomy, physiology, and development of the interstitial cells of Cajal (ICC); and (b) the role of KIT in normal cellular functions and oncogenesis. Given the monumental significance of these findings, they are discussed separately.

TABLE 50.4

MOLECULAR ABERRATIONS IN GASTROINTESTINAL STROMAL TUMORS

Activating *KIT* gene mutations
Monosomy chromosome 14
Monosomy chromosome 22
Loss of heterozygosity at 1p12–13
Loss of heterozygosity at 1p36

THE INTERSTITIAL CELLS OF CAJAL

ICC is a network of unusual cells found along the entire length of the GI tract (91,92) (Fig. 50.3). ICC is interposed between Auerbach's nerve plexus and the smooth muscle cells of the wall of the gut. The morphology and ultrastructural characteristics of ICC are extraordinary. They not only have features such as caveolae and thin filaments in common with smooth muscle cells, but they also possess long processes suggestive of neural cells that are capable of conducting electrical activity (93–98). The unique morphology and anatomical niche of ICC have suggested multiple functions, all of which are supported by experimental work.

ICC serve as pacemaker cells to control the autonomic function of the GI tract muscles. Ultrastructurally, they have similarities with cardiac pacemaker cells; they have few contractile filaments, and they are rich in cytoplasmic organelles that are involved in the generation of spontaneous electrical activity (93). If the circular and longitudinal layers of the muscular wall of the GI tract are dissected free from each other, ICC segregate with the longitudinal layer and the longitudinal layer retains electrical rhythmicity, whereas the circular layer is inactive (99). When ICC are isolated in short-term culture, they have inherent autorhythmicity and excitability, features that would be expected of pacemaker cells (100,101). Gap junctions are found at points of contact between ICC and smooth muscle cells, and are believed to couple electrical activity to muscle contraction (93,98,102). In addition, ICC may play a role in neurotransmission. The ICC are in intimate contact with the axons of enteric neurons and are known to respond to various neurotransmitters (103–106).

Several classes of ICC exist, differing with respect to morphology, ultrastructural properties, and anatomical location throughout the GI tract (107). For instance, there are ICC within the circular smooth muscle of the human fundus that are elongated with oval nuclei and with few cell processes, whereas ICC at other locations are described as spindle shaped or stellate, some with numerous cell processes (93,94). Different classes of ICC develop at different times and are known to have different functions (108).

Elegant developmental biology work has confirmed that *KIT* gene expression during embryogenesis is important for the formation of the ICC. The *KIT* gene, allelic with the mouse W locus, encodes the KIT transmembrane protein, which is an RTK of the type III RTK family (109–112). This family of

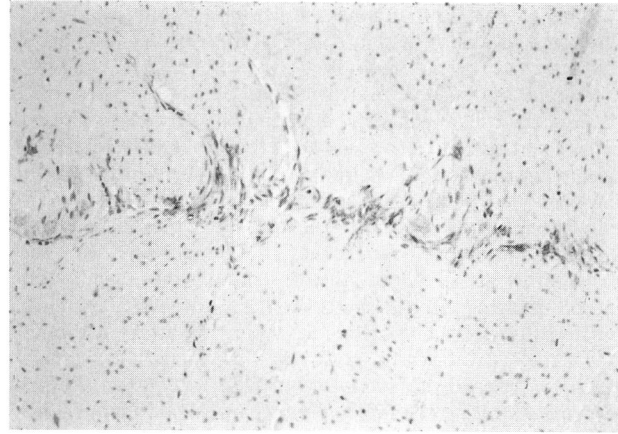

FIGURE 50.3. KIT immunostaining highlights the interstitial cells of Cajal in a section of small bowel. (See also color Fig. 50.3.)

RTKs is defined by common structural motifs, which include five immunoglobulinlike domains and a split kinase domain (113). Other members of this family include the platelet-derived growth factor receptor and macrophage colony-stimulating factor receptor (M-CSF receptor, also known as *FMS* or *CSF1* receptor). The ligand for KIT is steel factor, also known as stem cell factor (SCF); the gene for SCF is allelic with the *steel* locus in mice (114–117). Binding of SCF by KIT results in autophosphorylation of tyrosine residues within the intracellular domain of KIT, and activation of intracellular signaling cascades. KIT is involved not only in the formation of the ICC but is also important in melanogenesis, gametogenesis, and hematopoiesis (118–123).

Although complete loss of KIT protein during development is fatal, there are *KIT* mutations that do not completely abolish tyrosine kinase activity and that are compatible with life (118,124). One such mutation, W^v, produces progeny with markedly reduced numbers of ICC (122,125). The electrical activity in the gut is also abnormal and normal, slow-wave activity is not seen in the small intestinal muscles of mice possessing a W^v mutation (122,125). The ICC express KIT as shown by immunohistochemistry (106,108,122,126,127). Administration of neutralizing antibodies directed against KIT protein in newborn mice is able to reduce the number of ICC, and these mice have abnormal contractile patterns in their intestinal musculature (121,122).

Mutations within the gene encoding SCF also affect formation of the ICC (125). Although complete loss of SCF by deletion of the steel locus is lethal, steel mutants that retain activity are viable (128–130). Normally, SCF exists as a membrane-bound protein. One steel mutation, denoted Sl^d, encodes a truncated form of steel factor that is missing the intracellular and transmembrane portions and is thus soluble (130–132). Sl^d mutants have abnormal ICC networks and possess abnormal intestinal electrical activity (125).

ROLE OF *KIT* IN TUMORIGENESIS

Aside from its important role in development, *KIT* is also involved in tumorigenesis. The viral homolog of *KIT*, known as v-*kit*, was originally identified as the transforming gene of the Hardy-Zuckerman-4 strain of feline sarcoma virus (109). In addition, *KIT* expression is frequently elevated in chronic and acute myeloid leukemia, as well as small cell lung carcinoma cell lines, and is thus implicated in participating in the oncogenic process in these cancers (133–140). Importantly, expression of KIT alone does not appear to be the critical issue because KIT expression is noted in Ewing sarcomas without any detectable aberrant signaling activity from KIT (J.A. Fletcher, personal communication, February 2007) and without demonstrable activity of kinase inhibitors such as imatinib (141,142).

A model for GIST molecular pathogenesis existed, with an important distinction, in hematopoietic neoplasms: Specifically, direct evidence for KIT involvement in human cancer has been found in mast cell tumors. Experiments with a human mast cell leukemia cell line, HMC-1, revealed constitutive phosphorylation of KIT, even in the absence of exogenously added SCF ligand (143). Further analysis demonstrated that constitutive activation of KIT was not due to an autocrine mechanism whereby the HMC-1 cells produced their own SCF, but was due to the presence of activating mutations within the *KIT* gene. Two different mutations were identified: a glycine (Gly) for valine (Val) substitution in codon 560 in the juxtamembrane domain and a Val for aspartic acid (Asp) in codon 816 in the phosphotransferase domain. Introduction of *KIT* genes, harboring either or both of these mutations into a human embryonic kidney cell line resulted in ligand-independent con-

stitutively activated KIT proteins. Due to a relatively greater amount of phosphorylation of the codon 816 mutant construct, it was concluded that the mutation at codon 816 played a major role in constitutive activation of the KIT protein in HMC-1 cells, whereas the mutation at codon 560 played a minor role. Subsequent studies showed that the two different mutations confer ligand-independent activation by two different mechanisms. On binding of SCF, wild-type KIT dimerizes and results in the activation of KIT tyrosine kinase activity. The Gly for Val mutation at codon 560 was shown to undergo ligand-independent dimerization, whereas the Val for Asp codon 816 mutation was active in the absence of dimerization (144). Moreover, subcutaneous injections into nude mice of Ba/F3 cells expressing either of the two mutant *KIT* constructs resulted in the production of large tumors at the injection sites (144). More recent studies indicate that the Val for Asp codon 816 may actually undergo dimerization, but that the mechanism involves a novel and previously undefined method of association that does not use the extracellular SCF binding domain (145). Additional studies have reported other mutations in the *KIT* gene in rodent and human mast cell tumors (143,146–150). Furthermore, activating *KIT* mutations have also been detected in a minority of seminomas and dysgerminomas (151).

ROLE OF KIT IN THE PATHOGENESIS OF GASTROINTESTINAL STROMAL TUMORS

A breakthrough in understanding the histogenesis and pathogenesis of GISTs resulted from the elegantly reasoned hypothesis that there might be tumors within the GI tract that were related to the ICC. To address this question, Hirota et al., who had done much of the work elucidating the relationship between *KIT* mutation and mast cell tumors, looked at KIT protein expression by immunohistochemistry in a small number of "true" GI smooth muscle tumors, a single GI schwannoma, and many GISTs (90). Whereas no immunoreactivity was identified in the smooth muscle tumors or the schwannoma, 94% of GISTs expressed KIT. They surmised that if GISTs expressed KIT, then GISTs might also possess activating mutations in the *KIT* gene (similar to what was found in mast cell tumors). The entire cDNA sequence of six GISTs was determined, and *KIT* mutations were identified in the juxtamembrane region in five of six tumors. Interestingly, the mutations (in-frame deletions and point mutations) were clustered in an 11 amino acid stretch (lysine 550 to Val 560) in the juxtamembrane domain. When constructs containing the different *KIT* mutations were expressed in a human embryonic kidney cell line, they were found to confer ligand-independent activation of the KIT tyrosine kinase, just as had been seen in the mast cell tumors. In addition, the mutations were assayed for proliferative activity in the interleukin-3 (IL-3)–dependent Ba/F3 murine lymphoid cell line. The mutant constructs conferred IL-3– and SCF-independent proliferative abilities on Ba/F3 cells. When Ba/F3 cell lines containing the mutant constructs were injected subcutaneously into nude mice, tumors grew at the injection sites. These elegant studies implicated mutational activation of the *KIT* gene in the pathogenesis of GISTs. Further definitive proof to support a fundamental role for *KIT* mutation in GIST pathogenesis was demonstrated by the identification of a family with a germ-line mutation in the *KIT* gene in which affected family members had GISTs (152). Consistent with this hypothesis was the finding that the germ-line mutation seen in the familial GISTs (deletion of either Val 559 or 560) was

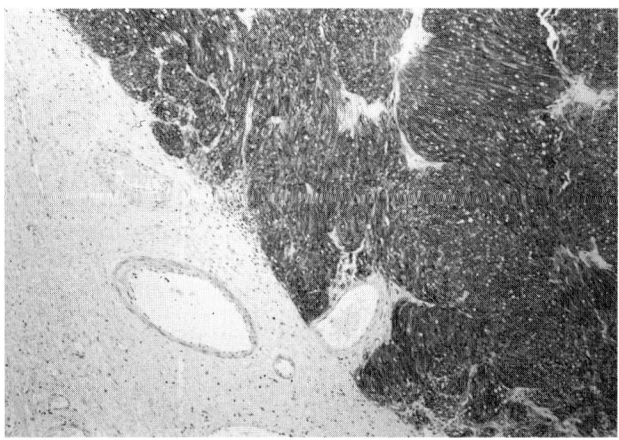

FIGURE 50.4. Strong and diffuse KIT immunoreactivity in a gastrointestinal stromal tumor. (See also color Fig. 50.4.)

in the same transmembrane region that was seen in the sporadic GISTs. Unaffected family members did not carry the *KIT* mutation.

The realization that GISTs are phenotypically related to the ICC provides an elegant framework within which to understand many of the previously most perplexing aspects of GISTs (31–36,126,127,153) (Figs. 50.4 and 50.5). Ultrastructurally, GISTs display a wide array of cellular differentiation features, even within single cases. Typically, ultrastructural characteristics of GISTs include prominent interdigitating, filopodialike cytoplasmic projections, incomplete myoid differentiation with subplasmalemmal actin filament bundles and occasional condensations, numerous large mitochondria, abundant smooth endoplasmic reticulum, prominent Golgi zones, microtubules, caveolae, incomplete external lamina, close apposition of cells with desmosomelike and rare gap junctions, and synapselike contacts. As pointed out by Kindblom et al., these ultrastructural features are all seen in ICC (126).

Immunohistochemically, approximately 90% of all GISTs are immunoreactive for antibodies to KIT (CD117) and vimentin. GIST cells display variable immunoreactivity antibodies recognizing CD34, P-glycoprotein 9.5 (PGP9.5), α-smooth muscle actin, and the embryonic form of smooth muscle myosin heavy chain (Smemb) (126,127,154,155). True GISTs are virtually always negative for antibodies to desmin, muscle-specific

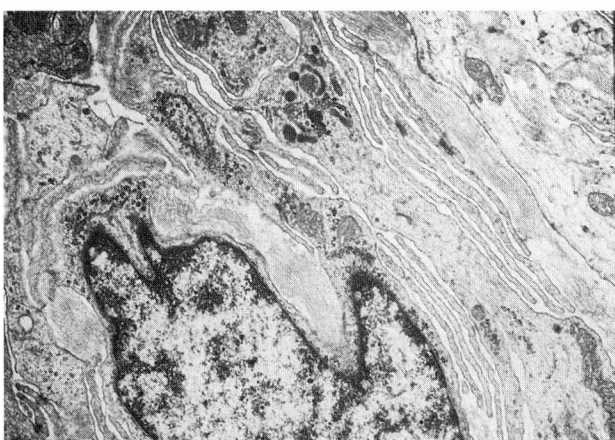

FIGURE 50.5. Gastrointestinal stromal tumor showing numerous interdigitating processes. (See also color Fig. 50.5.) *Source:* Courtesy of Dr. Christopher Fletcher, Brigham & Women's Hospital, Boston, MA.

actin, S-100 protein, neurofilament, and chromogranin. Attempts to determine the immunophenotype of ICC have shown that they are almost always positive for KIT and vimentin, and are usually positive for CD34 and Smemb, but do not show immunoreactivity for muscle-specific actin, desmin, PGP9.5, neuron-specific enolase, or S-100 protein (126,127,155). The immunohistochemical findings would therefore support a relationship between GISTs and ICC, although minor discrepancies, such as the presence of PGP9.5 staining in some GISTs, which is not seen in ICC, still need to be explained. Variations in immunophenotype with respect to CD34 staining are seen in ICC within normal bowel wall, which may reflect differences inherent to various classes of ICC (126). It may not be surprising therefore that differences in immunohistochemical staining and ultrastructure are seen in GISTs; this may merely be a reflection of the normal diversity seen in different classes of ICC. These findings also provide a rational framework for the understanding of GANTs (which most likely represent GISTs at one extreme end of the ICC spectrum with a neuroaxonal phenotype); they are characterized ultrastructurally by the presence of synapselike structures and dense core granules. Based on this perspective, and the lack of compelling evidence that they behave any differently than other GISTs, GANTs are now regarded simply as one variant of GISTs and not classified separately. Although some investigators had proposed that the name *GIST* be changed to *gastrointestinal pacemaker cell tumor*, or *ICC tumor*, to reflect the relationship between GISTs and ICC, no consensus was ever reached to adopt these propositions (126,127). Currently, GIST is the nomenclature that is most widely used by groups worldwide.

Importantly, other mesenchymal tumors, including true smooth muscle tumors (leiomyomas and leiomyosarcomas), neural tumors (schwannomas and malignant peripheral nerve sheath tumors), desmoid fibromatoses, as well as others, can also occur in the GI tract. These are generally not immunoreactive with anti-CD117 (KIT) antibodies and show ultrastructural features specific to their tumor type (126,154). However, immunohistochemistry depends on individual laboratory techniques, as well as tissue preservation, and results of immunostaining can potentially be misleading (156). Nonetheless, true KIT immunopositivity is limited in distribution (157), and this is a useful diagnostic marker. To a great extent, current diagnostic pathology methods allow mesenchymal tumors of the GI tract to be classified according to their line of differentiation; this is important because they are likely to exhibit different biological behaviors, and, more important, will have different sensitivities with regard to molecular-targeted therapy.

With the discovery that some GISTs possess activating mutations in the *KIT* gene, several groups have asked whether the presence or absence of *KIT* mutations might have prognostic importance, independent of kinase-inhibiting therapeutics (158–160). In early studies, exon 11 mutations were identified in 9 of 46 (21%) (161), 13 of 35 (37%) (159), 13 of 43 (30%) (158), and 71 of 124 (57%) (160) of GISTs in four separate published studies. Exon 11–*KIT* mutations were associated with a worse prognosis in three of the studies and were independent prognostic factors for overall and cause-specific survival in multivariate analysis in one study (156–160). However, exon 11–*KIT* mutations were also observed in low-grade (so-called "benign") GISTs, and not all malignant GISTs harbored exon 11–*KIT* mutations (158–160). Although the previously mentioned studies restricted their analysis of the *KIT* gene to exons 11 and 17, early studies at Brigham and Women's Hospital and the Dana-Farber Cancer Institute indicated that a far greater percentage of GISTs possess mutations in the *KIT* gene. The higher prevalence of *KIT* mutations in GIST has now been confirmed in many larger studies (163). Differences in the earlier detection of mutations are likely due to technical factors and to the sensitivity of the methodology used to find the mutations outside the exon 11 and 17 hot spots. The Boston studies initially found that *KIT* mutations can reside in exons that were not examined in earlier studies. These studies support the notion that virtually all GISTs have activating mutations within the *KIT* gene or another RTK pathway, such as the analogous kinase platelet-derived growth factor receptor-alpha (PDGFRA) (164). Even in GIST with no detectable mutations in KIT or PDGFRA, constitutive activation of the KIT signaling pathway is noted, indicating that activation of the KIT-RTK signaling pathways is central to the pathogenesis of GISTs (165). Importantly, at initial presentation, each patient with GIST has a homogeneous tumor with only a single form of KIT or *PDGFRA* mutation (if any mutation is present). It has been noted that mutations of exon 9 are associated with less favorable prognosis, and these are also correlated with small intestinal primaries (166). Other elements of prognostic importance independent of kinase-inhibitor therapeutic interventions require further study.

The other genetic changes mentioned previously, including loss of chromosomes 1p, 14, and 22, most likely represent secondary changes, which contribute to tumor progression. Interestingly, a recent study has shown that LOH at chromosome 1p36 may also have prognostic significance (89). Tumors that had LOH at 1p36 had significantly shorter survival than those tumors that did not, even when subjected to multivariate analysis.

CURRENT MOLECULAR-TARGETED SYSTEMIC THERAPY OF GASTROINTESTINAL STROMAL TUMORS

Prior to the year 2000, the only therapy of proven efficacy for GIST was surgical resection. Optimal surgical resection by a skilled sarcoma surgeon familiar with the clinical and biological potential of GIST is likely to be an important determinant of clinical outcomes, along with the underlying biology of the disease in any individual patient. Lymph node dissection is not recommended given the lack of lymphatic spread by these tumors. Margins of resection need to be carefully studied by the pathologist on an appropriately processed specimen to ensure that the tumor has been removed as completely as possible. In addition, local invasion into mucosa or surrounding tissues may carry important prognostic information, and the pathologist must be able to evaluate this aspect of the surgical resection sample by appropriate and expert processing and sampling. Conventional cytotoxic chemotherapeutic agents used for other types of sarcomas (e.g., doxorubicin or ifosfamide) had no demonstrable antineoplastic efficacy against the disease in GIST patients. Few studies of therapies for soft tissue sarcomas stratified to allow separate analysis of patients with GISTs prior to 2000. Recent studies have retrospectively confirmed that GISTs are exceptionally chemoresistant at presentation with expected response rates to chemotherapy of <5% (162,167). The biological reason(s) for this endogenous chemoresistance remains unclear, but it is likely that the uncontrolled kinase signaling through KIT or PDGFRA provides a powerful antiapoptotic signal that keeps GIST cells alive despite the most intensive cytotoxic insults. Given the lack of efficacy of conventional cytotoxic chemotherapy, there is no role for any systemic cytotoxic chemotherapy in the adjuvant setting after resection of GIST. Similarly, there are no definitive data to support the use of radiation therapy in the management of GIST. Thus, GIST represented a disease for which new treatment approaches were desperately needed and for which the promise of molecular-targeted therapy has been delivered to a great extent, as are discussed later.

To improve the otherwise limited therapeutic options for patients with GIST, the new molecular understanding of GIST pathogenesis has now been rapidly translated into novel therapeutic approaches based on selective and multitargeted small molecule tyrosine kinase inhibitor drugs. As noted previously, by 1999, there were intriguing data to support the hypothesis that the constitutively active signaling via the mutated KIT-RTK was responsible for the pathogenesis of a majority of GISTs. A corollary of this finding was that the inhibition of these dysregulated tyrosine kinase signals may be therapeutically useful for patients with GIST. The question in 1998 became how best to block that aberrant signal. A small molecule selective inhibitor of the KIT (as well as c-*abl* and the platelet-derived growth factor receptor, but no other RTKs) proved to be the initial shot across the bow of this disease. This drug, initially known as STI-571 and now known by the generic name imatinib mesylate (also known as Gleevec in North America or Glivec elsewhere in the world), had been studied extensively in the laboratories of Drs. Brian Druker (168) and Michael Heinrich (169) of the Oregon Cancer Center, Drs. David Tuveson and Jonathan Fletcher of Harvard Medical School (170), and investigators at Novartis Pharmaceuticals in Switzerland (170). In 1999, imatinib had already demonstrated dramatic clinical activity in the therapy of advanced chronic myelogenous leukemia associated with constitutive activation of the tyrosine kinase activity from the BCR-ABL fusion oncoprotein (172). In addition, preclinical studies in KIT-expressing hematopoietic cells had shown that imatinib could inhibit the signaling through KIT (173). Preclinical studies in which human GIST cells were exposed to imatinib demonstrated that proliferation of the tumor cells was dramatically decreased along with the inhibition of the KIT-RTK phosphorylation (170). On the basis of this compelling scientific rationale and strongly supportive preclinical data, a pilot study was designed to administer imatinib to a single patient with far advanced, unresectable GIST. This initial patient from Finland experienced a dramatic and durable response to this molecular-targeted therapy, documented by conventional magnetic resonance imaging, positron emission tomography scanning, and serial biopsies of the disease (174). An example of a dramatic metabolic response in a patient with metastatic GIST, as measured by 18FDG PET, is shown in Figs. 50.6 and 50.7. Armed with these highly encouraging data, a large-scale multicenter clinical trial was subsequently designed and conducted to test the efficacy of imatinib in patients with metastatic GIST (175). The results of this trial and its long-term follow-up have completely validated the concept that targeting the fundamental pathophysiological molecular lesion of this disease would lead to clinical benefits for patients: Overall, approximately two-thirds of the patients with far advanced metastatic GIST achieved major objective responses, and an additional 20% of patients experienced prolonged stabilization of the GIST lesions. The long-term follow-up confirmed the survival benefits for this population of patients, with median survival of nearly 5 years (58 months) for patients who would have been expected to die from their metastatic GIST in less than 6 months from the initial study entry (176). The impact of imatinib has been substantial, and careful correlative scientific studies in association with this trial have documented important differences in the impact of this agent based on the molecular form of the mutation driving the GIST. Specifically, GIST with exon 11 *KIT* mutations obtain the most benefit from imatinib, with superior rates of objective response, disease control, and survival, with exon 9 *KIT* mutants and those patients with no detectable *KIT* mutations faring less well (163).

The activity of imatinib in patients with advanced GIST has also been confirmed with remarkable concordance in a phase II

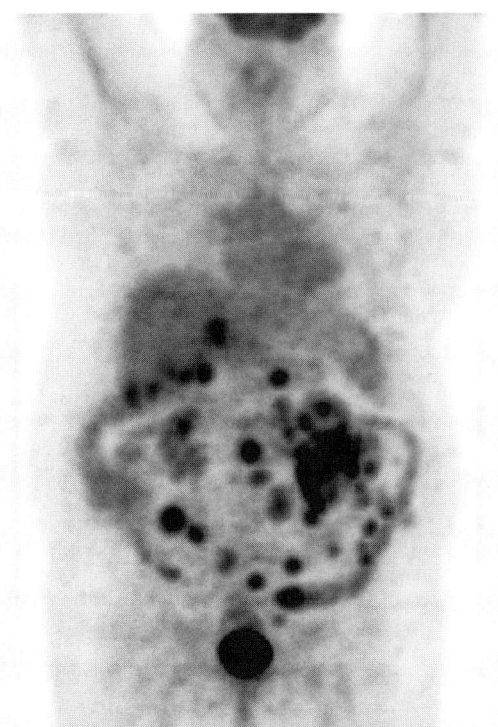

FIGURE 50.6. ^{18}FDG-PET scan showing significant activity in liver and mesenteric metastases prior to initiation of imatinib. *Source:* Courtesy of Dr. Annick Van den Abbeele and Leonid Syrkin, Dana-Farber Cancer Institute, Boston, MA.

European trial (177), as well as large-scale phase 3 trials testing different doses of imatinib (178,179). Intriguing hints suggest that certain molecular subsets might benefit differently from more intensively dosed imatinib, although this remains to be confirmed in larger analyses (180).

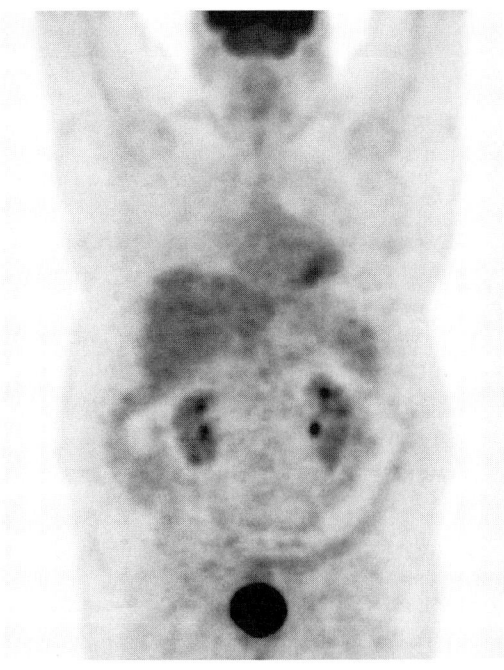

FIGURE 50.7. After 6 months on imatinib, there is near-complete resolution of abnormal metabolic uptake throughout the abdomen. *Source:* Courtesy of Dr. Annick Van den Abbeele and Leonid Syrkin, Dana-Farber Cancer Institute, Boston, MA.

MANAGING RESISTANCE TO IMATINIB

The initial results from the selective kinase inhibitor, imatinib, have been truly dramatic. However, resistance to this single agent has emerged in the majority of patients over time with continued follow-up and therapy. Managing imatinib-resistant GIST requires a multidisciplinary team for optimal results. Even the recognition of resistance can present challenges because novel radiographic patterns of clonally resistant disease are associated with GIST on imatinib therapy (181). Some patients might be noncompliant with drug dosing, and increasing vigilance and encouragement can truly be lifesaving for such patients. A subset of patients might benefit from dose escalation (to 800 mg daily), which has shown the ability to stabilize disease or even induce response in approximately 20% of patients following progression on conventional dose imatinib delivered at 400 mg daily (182). Surgical resection might also play a role in managing disease with limited clonal sites of resistance, in addition to continuing the kinase inhibitor to maintain control over the majority of clones, which retain sensitivity to the drug (183). However, for many patients, the imatinib-resistant GIST progresses despite all other attempts; research from many laboratories and teams worldwide has confirmed that the molecular basis for resistance to imatinib is usually due to the emergence of secondary resistance mutations in the etiologic kinase (184). For example, one GIST with an initial exon 11 *KIT* mutation might, after 2 years, begin to progress despite adequate continued dosing with imatinib; if this resistant lesion were genotyped, an exon 17 *KIT* mutation might be found in addition to the previous exon 11 *KIT* mutation (exon 17 *KIT* mutations are notoriously resistant to imatinib). New kinase inhibitors to manage such resistant disease were needed because GIST appeared to still be "addicted" to the aberrant signaling through the doubly mutated KIT kinase. Laboratory studies had indicated that the multitargeted kinase inhibitor sunitinib malate (initially referred to as SU11248 from Sugen and now known as Sutent from Pfizer) could inhibit double-mutant variants of KIT that were imatinib resistant (J. Fletcher, personal communication, September 2001). This was sufficient rationale to begin a phase I/II trial of the SU11248 kinase inhibitor for GIST patients following failure of imatinib. Initial data proved promising (185), and a large-scale international phase 3 trial has provided definitive evidence of the clinical benefit of sunitinib to extend control of advanced GIST following failure of prior imatinib therapy (186).

FUTURE PROSPECTS AND ONGOING RESEARCH STUDIES

Pathologists are now able to define GISTs more precisely than ever before: specifically as tumors that differentiate along the lines of ICC and exhibit immunoreactivity with anti-KIT (CD117) antibodies, and even now molecular genetics techniques can subset these diseases into specific subtypes based on the site of mutation within a given signaling kinase. Within this new classification framework, it will be important to reassess various clinical and pathological parameters of potential prognostic significance in "pure" cohorts of molecularly defined GISTs. It will also be important to dissect and understand the KIT (or PDGFRA)-RTK pathway from the standpoint of downstream effector targets. These pathways will almost certainly encompass novel targets, which might be amenable to possible therapeutic intervention. The various proteins involved in the downstream pathways of KIT signaling are increasingly understood and several novel targets have emerged

(187). There is some biological evidence to support the notion that proteins within the RAS-GAP pathway might interact either directly or indirectly with KIT, and therefore may contribute to oncogenesis of GISTs. Patients with type 1 neurofibromatosis (NF-1) harbor inactivating mutations in the *NF-1* (*GAP*) gene, resulting in proteins that are unable to oppose the actions of RAS, thus serving to functionally activate RAS. Patients with NF-1 have a higher incidence (perhaps as high as 200-fold) of GISTs than in the unaffected population (17,158–160), and the GIST lesions in neurofibromatosis patients have no detectable mutations in either *KIT* or *PDGFRA* (188). This suggests that NF-1 may interact with KIT because mutations in both genes predispose to GIST formation; however, involvement of NF-1 in the pathogenesis of sporadic, non–NF-1–related GISTs has not been demonstrated. Although other proteins are known to associate with KIT, none have been implicated directly in the formation of GISTs. Activating mutations of other members of the KIT pathway that lie downstream of KIT might be found in GISTs that lack activating mutations in KIT.

The precise mechanism(s) by which *KIT* mutation leads to ligand-independent KIT activation is not apparent at this point, although at least in some cases the mutated KIT proteins dimerize or oligomerize in the absence of ligand (144,145). Different mutations will likely confer different degrees of activation, which, in turn, may translate into differences in tumor aggressiveness. The molecular mechanisms should also help explain the differential activity of various drugs against different structural variants of the KIT or PDGFRA oncoproteins in GIST.

Based on the involvement of *KIT*-activating mutations in GIST pathogenesis, it is now clear that antagonists of the KIT-RTK pathway are definitely useful in the treatment of unresectable or metastatic GISTs. It was initially predicted that anti-KIT oncologic therapies would likely be toxic, particularly to bone marrow cells, because KIT signal transduction pathways regulate proliferation, differentiation, migration, and survival of hematopoietic stem cells, mast cells, melanocytes, and germ cells (118–120,123). However, selective and even multitargeted agents that inhibit the aberrant RTK activity of mutated KIT have proven to be adequately well tolerated by humans because much of the KIT function in hematopoiesis may be functionally redundant with other signaling pathways. Therefore, understanding of KIT oncogenic mechanisms might enable the development of highly specific therapies that target particular KIT oncogenic pathways and minimize toxicity to KIT-redundant nonneoplastic cell lineages.

However, the appearance of multiple resistance mutations in individual patients is worrisome. Because patients have developed so many different resistant variants, drug therapy that simply targets mutant KIT variants may eventually fail by missing some subset of resistant clones. Targeting all mutational variants of KIT and PDGFRA with an entirely different mechanism might be able to ameliorate this difficult clinical scenario. Mutant kinases do not fold in the normal configuration, and they are therefore more dependent on chaperone proteins (e.g., heat shock protein-90 [HSP-90]) to protect them in the posttranslational state until they can reach their cellular localization within the plasma membrane and begin signaling. Inhibition of HSP-90 has been shown to decrease the levels of mutant KIT selectively, and therefore is a promising new line of attack on GIST resistant to small molecule kinase inhibitors (189). This strategy has already shown promise in an early phase I clinical trial of a novel water-soluble HSP-90 inhibitor known as IPI-504 (190).

SUMMARY

GISTs have presented pathologists with a challenging histogenetic puzzle since their original description decades ago, and they have presented medical oncologists, surgeons, and gastroenterologists with even more difficult management problems prior to the introduction of effective molecular-targeted therapy in the clinic. Recent developments that have revealed the oncogenic role of KIT (or PDGFRA) kinase activation in GISTs provide support for a histogenetic relationship between the ICC and GISTs. These findings have also resulted in the routine use of anti-KIT (CD117) antibodies in the identification and classification of GISTs, permitting more reliable distinction from other mesenchymal and neural crest tumors of the GI tract. It is hoped that further analysis of kinase-driven oncogenic mechanisms in homogeneous cohorts of GISTs will translate into the ability to predict more reliably the clinical behavior of GISTs. In addition, it is likely that such improved understanding of GIST pathogenesis and molecular biology will rapidly lead to even further advances in the design of highly selective and clinically effective treatment strategies.

ACKNOWLEDGMENTS

The authors want to acknowledge the extraordinary mentorship of Dr. Christopher Fletcher, who has taught us both so much about this field. In addition, Drs. Jonathan Fletcher, Michael Heinrich, and Christopher Corless have been instrumental as we have defined our approach to the scientific basis and management of GISTs. GDD wants to acknowledge the support of the Virginia and Daniel K. Ludwig Trust for Cancer Research and the Semonian Family/Leslie's Links Foundation, as well as the Rotenberg and Zeckhauser families for supporting the work of the Sarcoma Center at the Dana-Farber Cancer Institute.

References

1. Rubin BP, Fletcher JA, Fletcher CD. Molecular insights into the histogenesis and pathogenesis of gastrointestinal stromal tumors. *Int J Surg Pathol* 2000;8(1):5–10.
2. Ueyama T, Guo KJ, Hashimoto H, et al. A clinicopathologic and immunohistochemical study of gastrointestinal stromal tumors. *Cancer* 1992;69:947–955.
3. Newman PL, Wadden C, Fletcher CD. Gastrointestinal stromal tumours: correlation of immunophenotype with clinicopathological features. *J Pathol* 1991;164:107–117.
4. Stout AP. Bizarre smooth muscle tumors of the stomach. *Cancer* 1962;15:400–409.
5. Brainard JA, Goldblum JR. Stromal tumors of the jejunum and ileum: a clinicopathologic study of 39 cases. *Am J Surg Pathol* 1997;21:407–416.
6. Nilsson B, Bumming P, Meis-Kindblom JM, et al. Gastrointestinal stromal tumors: the incidence, prevalence, clinical course, and prognostication in the preimatinib mesylate era—a population-based study in western Sweden. *Cancer* 2005;15;103(4):821–829.
7. Kawanowa K, Sakuma Y, Sakurai S, et al. High incidence of microscopic gastrointestinal stromal tumors in the stomach. *Hum Pathol* 2006;37(12):1527–1535.
8. Corless CL, McGreevey L, Haley A, Town A, Heinrich MC. *KIT* mutations are common in incidental gastrointestinal stromal tumors one centimeter or less in size. *Am J Pathol* 2002;160:1567–1572.
9. Emory TS, Sobin LH, Lukes L, et al. Prognosis of gastrointestinal smooth-muscle (stromal) tumors: dependence on anatomic site. *Am J Surg Pathol* 1999;23:82–87.
10. Penzel R, Aulmann S, Moock M, Schwarzbach M, Rieker RJ, Mechtersheimer G. The location of KIT and PDGFRA gene mutations in gastrointestinal stromal tumours is site and phenotype associated. *J Clin Pathol* 2005;58:634–639.
11. Seremetis MG, Lyons WS, DeGuzman VC. Leiomyomata of the esophagus: an analysis of 838 cases. *Cancer* 1976;38:2166–2177.
12. Lewin KJ, Appelman HD. Mesenchymal tumors and tumor-like proliferations of the esophagus. In: Lewin KJ, Appelman HD, eds. *Tumors of the Esophagus and Stomach.* Vol 18. Washington, DC: Armed Forces Institute of Pathology; 1996:154–155.
13. Appelman HD. Stromal tumors of the esophagus, stomach and duodenum. In: Appelman HD, ed. *Pathology of the Esophagus, Stomach and Duodenum: Contemporary Issues in Surgical Pathology.* New York, NY: Churchill Livingstone; 1984.

14. Akwari OE, Dozois RR, Weiland LH, et al. Leiomyosarcoma of the small and large bowel. *Cancer* 1978;42:1375–1384.
15. Appelman H, Helwig EB. Cellular leiomyomas of the stomach in 49 patients. *Arch Pathol Lab Med* 1977;101:373–377.
16. Cooper PN, Quirke P, Hardy GJ, et al. A flow cytometric, clinical, and histological study of stromal neoplasms of the gastrointestinal tract. *Am J Surg Pathol* 1992;16:163–170.
17. Kindblom LG, Remotti HE, Angervall L, et al. Gastrointestinal pacemaker cell tumor—a manifestation of neurofibromatosis type I (NFI). *Mod Pathol* 1999;12:77A.
18. Tuveson DA, Fletcher JA. Signal transduction pathways in sarcoma as targets for therapeutic intervention. *Curr Opin Oncol* 2001;13(4):249–255.
19. Carney JA, Sheps SG, Go VLW, et al. The triad of gastric leiomyosarcoma, functioning extra-adrenal paraganglioma and pulmonary chondroma. *N Engl J Med* 1977;296:1517–1518.
20. Nishida T, Hirota S, Taniguchi M, et al. Familial gastrointestinal stromal tumours with germline mutation of the KIT gene. *Nat Genet* 1998;19:323–324.
21. Hirota S, Nishida T, Isozaki K, et al. Familial gastrointestinal stromal tumors associated with dysphagia and novel type germline mutation of KIT gene. *Gastroenterology* 2002;122:1493–1499.
22. Antonescu C, Viale A, Sarran L, et al. Gene expression in gastrointestinal stromal tumors is distinguished by KIT genotype and anatomic site. *Clin Cancer Res* 2004;10:3282–3290.
23. Li FP, Fletcher JA, Heinrich MC, et al. Familial gastrointestinal stromal tumor syndrome: phenotypic and molecular features in a kindred. *J Clin Oncol* 2005;23(12):2735–2743.
24. Tarn C, Merkel E, Canutescu AA, et al. Analysis of KIT mutations in sporadic and familial gastrointestinal stromal tumors: therapeutic implications through molecular modeling. *Clin Cancer Res* 2005;11(10):3668–3677.
25. Lavin P, Hajdu SI, Foote FWJ. Gastric and extragastric leiomyoblastomas. *Cancer* 1972;29:305–311.
26. Appelman HD, Helwig EB. Gastric epithelioid leiomyoma and leiomyosarcoma (leiomyoblastoma). *Cancer* 1976;38:708–728.
27. Shiu MH, Farr GH, Papachristou DN, et al. Myosarcomas of the stomach: natural history, prognostic factors and management. *Cancer* 1982;49:177–187.
28. Martin JF, Bazin P, Feroldi J, et al. Tumeurs myoides intra-murales de l'estomac—considerations microscopiques a propos de 6 cas. *Ann Anat Pathol* 1960;5:484–497.
29. Ranchod M, Kempson RL. Smooth muscle tumors of the gastrointestinal tract and retroperitoneum: a pathologic analysis of 100 cases. *Cancer* 1977;39:255–262.
30. Golden T, Stout AP. Smooth muscle tumors of the gastrointestinal tract and retroperitoneal tissues. *Surg Gynecol Obstet* 1941;73:784–810.
31. Welsh RA, Meyer AT. Ultrastructure of gastric leiomyoma. *Arch Pathol* 1969;87:71–81.
32. Mackay B, Ro J, Floyd C, et al. Ultrastructural observations on smooth muscle tumors. *Ultrastruct Pathol* 1987;11:593–607.
33. Knapp RH, Wick MR, Goellner JR. Leiomyoblastomas and their relationship to other smooth-muscle tumors of the gastrointestinal tract: an electron-microscopic study. *Am J Surg Pathol* 1984;8:449–461.
34. Kay S, Still WJ. A comparative electron microscopic study of a leiomyosarcoma and bizarre leiomyoma (leiomyoblastoma) of the stomach. *Am J Clin Pathol* 1969;52:403–413.
35. Mazur MT, Clark HB. Gastric stromal tumors: reappraisal of histogenesis. *Am J Surg Pathol* 1983;7:507–519.
36. Weiss RA, Mackay B. Malignant smooth muscle tumors of the gastrointestinal tract: an ultrastructural study of 20 cases. *Ultrastruct Pathol* 1981;2:231–240.
37. Hjermstad BM, Sobin LH, Helwig EB. Stromal tumors of the gastrointestinal tract: myogenic or neurogenic? *Am J Surg Pathol* 1987;11:383–386.
38. Herrera GA, Pinto de Moraes H, Grizzle WE, et al. Malignant small bowel neoplasm of enteric plexus derivation (plexosarcoma): light and electron microscopic study confirming the origin of the neoplasm. *Dig Dis Sci* 1984;29:275–284.
39. Herrera GA, Cerezo L, Jones JE, et al. Gastrointestinal autonomic nerve tumors: "plexosarcomas." *Arch Pathol Lab Med* 1989;113:846–853.
40. Hurlimann J, Gardiol D. Gastrointestinal stromal tumours: an immunohistochemical study of 165 cases. *Histopathology* 1991;19:311–320.
41. Miettinen M. Gastrointestinal stromal tumors: an immunohistochemical study of cellular differentiation. *Am J Clin Pathol* 1988;89:601–610.
42. Ricci A Jr, Ciccarelli O, Cartun RW, et al. A clinicopathologic and immunohistochemical study of 16 patients with small intestinal leiomyosarcoma: limited utility of immunophenotyping. *Cancer* 1987;60:1790–1799.
43. Saul SH, Rast ML, Brooks JJ. The immunohistochemistry of gastrointestinal stromal tumors: evidence supporting an origin from smooth muscle. *Am J Surg Pathol* 1987;11:464–473.
44. Pike AM, Lloyd RV, Appelman HD. Cell markers in gastrointestinal stromal tumors. *Hum Pathol* 1988;19:830–834.
45. Franquemont DW, Frierson HF Jr. Muscle differentiation and clinicopathologic features of gastrointestinal stromal tumors. *Am J Surg Pathol* 1992;16:947–954.
46. Lee JS, Nascimento AG, Farnell MB, et al. Epithelioid gastric stromal tumors (leiomyoblastomas): a study of fifty-five cases. *Surgery* 1995;118:653–660; discussion 660–661.
47. Ma CK, Amin MB, Kintanar E, et al. Immunohistologic characterization of gastrointestinal stromal tumors: a study of 82 cases compared with 11 cases of leiomyomas. *Mod Pathol* 1993;6:139–144.
48. Mikhael AI, Bacchi CE, Zarbo RJ, et al. CD34 expression in stromal tumors of the gastrointestinal tract. *Appl Immunohistochem* 1994;2:89–93.
49. Monihan JM, Carr NJ, Sobin LH. CD34 immunoexpression in stromal tumours of the gastrointestinal tract and in mesenteric fibromatoses. *Histopathology* 1994;25:469–473.
50. DeMatteo RP, Lewis JJ, Leung D, Mudan SS, Woodruff JM, Brennan MF. Two hundred gastrointestinal stromal tumors: recurrence patterns and prognostic factors for survival. *Ann Surg* 2000;231(1):51–58.
51. Singer S, Rubin BP, Lux ML, et al. Prognostic value of KIT mutation type, mitotic activity, and histologic subtype in gastrointestinal stromal tumors. *J Clin Oncol* 2002;20(18):3898–3905.
52. Evans HL. Smooth muscle tumors of the gastrointestinal tract: a study of 56 cases followed for a minimum of 10 years. *Cancer* 1985;56:2242–2250.
53. Fletcher CD, Berman JJ, Corless C, et al. Diagnosis of gastrointestinal stromal tumors: a consensus approach. *Hum Pathol* 2002;33(5):459–465.
54. Fletcher CD. Clinicopathologic correlations in gastrointestinal stromal tumors. *Hum Pathol* 2002;33(5):455.
55. Van Steenbergen W, Kojima T, Geboes K, et al. Gastric leiomyoblastoma with metastases to the liver: a 36-year follow-up study. *Gastroenterology* 1985;89:875–881.
56. Cunningham RE, Federspiel BH, McCarthy WF, et al. Predicting prognosis of gastrointestinal smooth muscle tumors: role of clinical and histologic evaluation, flow cytometry, and image cytometry. *Am J Surg Pathol* 1993;17:588–594.
57. Franquemont DW, Frierson HF Jr. Proliferating cell nuclear antigen immunoreactivity and prognosis of gastrointestinal stromal tumors. *Mod Pathol* 1995;8:473–477.
58. Goldblum JR, Appelman HD. Stromal tumors of the duodenum: a histologic and immunohistochemical study of 20 cases. *Am J Surg Pathol* 1995;19:71–80.
59. Tworek JA, Appelman HD, Singleton TP, et al. Stromal tumors of the jejunum and ileum. *Mod Pathol* 1997;10:200–209.
60. Tworek JA, Goldblum JR, Weiss SW, et al. Stromal tumors of the anorectum: a clinicopathologic study of 22 cases. *Am J Surg Pathol* 1999;23:946–954.
61. Tworek JA, Goldblum JR, Weiss SW, et al. Stromal tumors of the abdominal colon: a clinicopathologic study of 20 cases. *Am J Surg Pathol* 1999;23:937–945.
62. de Saint Aubain Somerhausen N, Fletcher CDM. Gastrointestinal stromal tumours: an update. *Sarcoma* 1998;2:133–141.
63. Carney JA. The triad of gastric epithelioid leiomyosarcoma, pulmonary chondroma, and functioning extra-adrenal paraganglioma: a five-year review. *Medicine (Baltimore)* 1983;62:159–169.
64. Persson S, Kindblom LG, Angervall L, et al. Metastasizing gastric epithelioid leiomyosarcomas (leiomyoblastomas) in young individuals with long-term survival. *Cancer* 1992;70:721–732.
65. Knop S, Schupp M, Wardelmann E, et al. A new case of Carney triad: gastrointestinal stromal tumours and leiomyoma of the oesophagus do not show activating mutations of KIT and platelet-derived growth factor receptor. *J Clin Pathol* 2006;59:1097–1099.
66. Appelman HD, Helwig EB. Sarcomas of the stomach. *Am J Clin Pathol* 1977;67:2–10.
67. el-Naggar AK, Ro JY, McLemore D, et al. Gastrointestinal stromal tumors: DNA flow-cytometric study of 58 patients with at least five years of follow-up. *Mod Pathol* 1989;2:511–515.
68. Franquemont DW. Differentiation and risk assessment of gastrointestinal stromal tumors. *Am J Clin Pathol* 1995;103:41–47.
69. Ng EH, Pollock RE, Munsell MF, et al. Prognostic factors influencing survival in gastrointestinal leiomyosarcomas: implications for surgical management and staging. *Ann Surg* 1992;215:68–77.
70. Amin MB, Ma CK, Linden MD, et al. Prognostic value of proliferating cell nuclear antigen index in gastric stromal tumors: correlation with mitotic count and clinical outcome. *Am J Clin Pathol* 1993;100:428–432.
71. Carillo R, Candia A, Rodriguez-Peralto JL. Prognostic significance of DNA ploidy and proliferative index (MIB-1 index) in gastrointestinal stromal tumors. *Hum Pathol* 1997;28:160–165.
72. Rudolph P, Gloeckner K, Parwaresch R, et al. Immunophenotype, proliferation, DNA ploidy, and biological behavior of gastrointestinal stromal tumors: a multivariate clinicopathologic study. *Hum Pathol* 1998;29:791–800.
73. Lasota J, Stachura J, Miettinen M. GISTs with PDGFRA exon 14 mutations represented a subset of clinically favorable gastric tumors with epithelioid morphology. *Lab Invest* 2006;86:94–100.
74. Lerma E, Oliva E, Tugues D, et al. Stromal tumours of the gastrointestinal tract: a clinicopathological and ploidy analysis of 33 cases. *Virchows Arch* 1994;424:19–24.
75. Federspiel BH, Sobin LH, Helwig EB, et al. Morphometry and cytophotometric assessment of DNA in smooth-muscle tumors (leiomyomas and leiomyosarcomas) of the gastrointestinal tract. *Anal Quant Cytol Histol* 1987;9:105–114.
76. Flint A, Appelman HD, Beckwith AL. DNA analysis of gastric stromal neoplasms: correlation with pathologic features. *Surg Pathol* 1989;2:117–124.

77. Yu CC, Fletcher CD, Newman PL, et al. A comparison of proliferating cell nuclear antigen (PCNA) immunostaining, nucleolar organizer region (AgNOR) staining, and histological grading in gastrointestinal stromal tumours. *J Pathol* 1992;166:147–152.

78. Sbaschnig RJ, Cunningham RE, Sobin LH, et al. Proliferating-cell nuclear antigen immunocytochemistry in the evaluation of gastrointestinal smooth-muscle tumors. *Mod Pathol* 1994;7:780–783.

79. Emory TS, Derringer GA, Sobin LH, et al. Ki-67 (MIB-1) immunohistochemistry as a prognostic factor in gastrointestinal smooth-muscle tumors. *J Surg Pathol* 1997;2:239–242.

80. Emory TS, O'Leary TJ. Prognosis and surveillance of gastrointestinal stromal/smooth muscle tumors. *Ann Chir Gynaecol* 1998;87:306–310.

81. Suster S. Gastrointestinal stromal tumors. *Semin Diagn Pathol* 1996;13:297–313.

82. Bergmann I, Gunawan B, Hermanns B, et al. Cytogenetic and morphologic characteristics of gastrointestinal stromal tumors: recurrent rearrangement of chromosome 1 and losses of chromosomes 14 and 22 as common anomalies. *Verh Dtsch Ges Pathol* 1998;82:275–278.

83. Boghosian L, Dal Cin P, Turc-Carel C, et al. Three possible cytogenetic subgroups of leiomyosarcoma. *Cancer Genet Cytogenet* 1989;43:39–49.

84. Dal Cin P, Boghosian L, Sandberg AA. Cytogenetic findings in leiomyosarcoma of the small bowel. *Cancer Genet Cytogenet* 1988;30:285–288.

85. Marci V, Casorzo L, Sarotto I, et al. Gastrointestinal stromal tumor, uncommitted type, with monosomies 14 and 22 as the only chromosomal abnormalities. *Cancer Genet Cytogenet* 1998;102:135–138.

86. Mark J, Wedell B, Dahlenfors R, et al. Cytogenetic observations in a human gastric leiomyosarcoma. *Cancer Genet Cytogenet* 1989;37:215–220.

87. el-Rifai W, Sarlomo-Rikala M, Andersson LC, et al. DNA copy number changes in gastrointestinal stromal tumors—a distinct genetic entity. *Ann Chir Gynaecol* 1998;87:287–290.

88. el-Rifai W, Sarlomo-Rikala M, Miettinen M, et al. DNA copy number losses in chromosome 14: an early change in gastrointestinal stromal tumors. *Cancer Res* 1996;56:3230–3233.

89. O'Leary T, Ernst S, Przygodzki R, et al. Loss of heterozygosity at 1p36 predicts poor prognosis in gastrointestinal stromal/smooth muscle tumors. *Lab Invest* 1999;79:1461–1467.

90. Hirota S, Isozaki K, Moriyama Y, et al. Gain-of-function mutations of c-*kit* in human gastrointestinal stromal tumors. *Science* 1998;279:577–580.

91. Thuneberg L. Interstitial cells of Cajal. In: Wood JD, ed. *Handbook of Physiology: The Gastrointestinal System.* Bethesda, Md: American Physiological Society; 1989:349–386.

92. Cajal SR. Sur les ganglions et plexus nerveux de l'intestin. *CR Soc Biol (Paris)* 1893;45:217–223.

93. Faussone-Pellegrini M-S, Cortesini C, Romagnoli P. Sull'ultra-strutta della tunica muscolare della prozione cardiale dell'esofago e dello stomaco umano con particolara riferimento alle cossiddette cellule inerstiziali di Cajal. *Arch Ital Anat Embriol* 1977;82:157–177.

94. Faussone-Pellegrini M-S, Pantalone D, Cortesini C. An ultrastructural study of the interstitial cells of Cajal of the human stomach. *J Submicrosc Cytol Pathol* 1989;21:149–460.

95. Rumessen JJ, Mikkelsen HB, Qvortup K, et al. Ultrastructure of interstitial cells of Cajal associated with deep muscular plexus of human small intestine. *Gastroenterology* 1992;102:56–68.

96. Rumessen JJ, Peters S, Thuneberg L. Light and electron microscopical studies of interstitial cells of Cajal and muscle cells at the submucosal border of human colon. *Lab Invest* 1993;68:481–495.

97. Rumessen JJ, Mikelsen HB, Qvortrup K, et al. Ultrastructure of interstitial cells of Cajal in circular muscle of human small intestine. *Gastroenterology* 1993;104:343–350.

98. Thuneberg L. Interstitial cells of Cajal: intestinal pacemaker cells? In: Beck F, Hild W, van Limborgh J, et al., eds. *Advances in Anatomy: Embryology and Cell Biology.* New York, NY: Springer-Verlag; 1982:1–130.

99. Bortoff A. Myogenic control of intestinal motility. *Physiol Rev* 1976;56:418–434.

100. Don Koh S, Sanders KM, Ward SM. Spontaneous electrical rhythmicity in cultured interstitial cells of Cajal from the murine small intestine. *J Physiol* 1998;513:203–213.

101. Langton P, Ward SM, Carl A, et al. Spontaneous electrical activity of interstitial cells of Cajal isolated from canine proximal colon. *Proc Natl Acad Sci U S A* 1989;86:7280–7284.

102. Imaizumi M, Hama K. An electron microscopic study on the interstitial cells of the gizzard in the love bird (*Uronloncha domestica*). *Z Zellforsch Mikrosk Anat* 1969;97:351–357.

103. Publicover NG, Hammond EM, Sanders KM. Amplification of nitric oxide signaling by interstitial cells isolated from canine colon. *Proc Natl Acad Sci U S A* 1993;90:2087–2091.

104. Publicover NG, Hammond EM, Sanders KM. Calcium oscillations in freshly dispersed and cultured interstitial cells from canine colon. *Am J Physiol* 1992;262:C589–C597.

105. Daniel EE, Posey-Daniel V. Neuromuscular structures in opossum esophagus: role of interstitial cells of Cajal. *Am J Physiol* 1984;246:G305–G315.

106. Burns AJ, Lomax AEJ, Torihashi S, et al. Interstitial cells of Cajal mediate inhibitory neurotransmission in the stomach. *Proc Natl Acad Sci U S A* 1996;93:12008–12013.

107. Burns AJ, Herbert TM, Ward SM, et al. Interstitial cells of Cajal in the guinea-pig gastrointestinal tract as revealed by c-Kit immunohistochemistry. *Cell Tissue Res* 1997;290:11–20.

108. Torihashi S, Ward SM, Sanders KM. Development of c-Kit-positive cells and the onset of electrical rhythmicity in murine small intestine. *Gastroenterology* 1997;112:144–155.

109. Besmer P, Murphy JE, George PC, et al. A new acute transforming feline retrovirus and relationship of its oncogene v-*kit* with the protein kinase gene family. *Nature* 1986;320:415–421.

110. Chabot B, Stephenson DA, Chapman VM, et al. The proto-oncogene c-kit encoding a transmembrane tyrosine kinase receptor maps to the mouse W locus. *Nature* 1988;335:88–89.

111. Geissler EN, Ryan MA, Housman DE. The dominant-white spotting (W) locus of the mouse encodes the c-kit proto-oncogene. *Cell* 1988;55:185–192.

112. Yarden Y, Kuang W, Yang-Feng T, et al. Human proto-oncogene c-*kit*: a new cell surface receptor tyrosine kinase for an unidentified ligand. *EMBO J* 1987;6:3341–3351.

113. Yarden Y, Ullrich A. Growth factor receptor tyrosine kinases. *Ann Rev Biochem* 1988;57:443–448.

114. Williams DE, Eisenman J, Baird A, et al. Identification of a ligand for the c-*kit* proto-oncogene. *Cell* 1990;63:167–174.

115. Zsebo KM, Williams DA, Geissler EN, et al. Stem cell factor is encoded at the *Sl* locus of the mouse and is the ligand for the c-*kit* tyrosine kinase receptor. *Cell* 1990;63:213–224.

116. Flanagan JG, Leder P. The kit ligand: a cell surface molecule altered in steel mutant fibroblasts. *Cell* 1990;63:185–194.

117. Huang E, Nocka K, Beier DR, et al. The hematopoietic growth factor KL is encoded by the *Sl* locus and is the ligand of the c-*kit* receptor, the gene product of the W locus. *Cell* 1990;63:225–233.

118. Russell ES. Hereditary anemia of the mouse: a review for geneticists. *Adv Genet* 1979;20:357–459.

119. Kitamura Y, Go S, Hatanaka K. Decrease of mast cells in W/Wv mice and their increase by bone marrow transplantation. *Blood* 1978;52:447–452.

120. Kitamura Y, Go S. Decreased production of mast cells in Sl/Sl d anemic mice. *Blood* 1979;53:492–497.

121. Maeda H, Yamagata A, Nishikawa S, et al. Requirement of c-*kit* for development of intestinal pacemaker system. *Development* 1992;116:369–375.

122. Huizinga JD, Thuneberg L, Kluppel M, et al. W/kit gene required for interstitial cells of Cajal and for intestinal pacemaker activity. *Nature* 1995;373:347–349.

123. Isozaki K, Hirota S, Nakama A, et al. Disturbed intestinal movement, bile reflux to the stomach, and deficiency of c-kit-expressing cells in Ws/Ws mutant rats. *Gastroenterology* 1995;109:456–464.

124. Nocka K, Tan JC, Chiu E, et al. Molecular bases of dominant negative and loss of function mutations at the murine c-kit/white spotting locus: W37, Wv, W41 and W. *EMBO J* 1990;9:1805–1813.

125. Ward SM, Burns AJ, Torihashi S, et al. Impaired development of interstitial cells and intestinal electrical rhythmicity in steel mutants. *Am J Physiol* 1995;269:C1577–C1585.

126. Kindblom LG, Remotti HE, Aldenborg F, et al. Gastrointestinal pacemaker cell tumor (GIPACT): gastrointestinal stromal tumors show phenotypic characteristics of the interstitial cells of Cajal [see comments]. *Am J Pathol* 1998;152:1259–1269.

127. Sircar K, Hewlett BR, Huizinga JD, et al. Interstitial cells of Cajal as precursors of gastrointestinal stromal tumors. *Am J Surg Pathol* 1999;23:377–389.

128. Zsebo KM, Williams DA, Geissler EN, et al. Stem cell factor is encoded at the S1 locus of the mouse and is the ligand for the c-kit tyrosine kinase receptor. *Cell* 1990;63(1):185–194.

129. Flanagan JG, Leder P. The kit ligand: a cell surface molecule altered in steel mutant fibroblasts. *Cell* 1990;63(1):185–194.

130. Brannan CI, Lyman SD, Williams DE, et al. Steel-Dickie mutation encodes a c-kit ligand lacking transmembrane and cytoplasmic domains. *Proc Natl Acad Sci U S A* 1991;88(11):4671–4674.

131. Broudy VC. Stem cell factor and hematopoiesis. *Blood* 1997;90:1345–1364.

132. Flanagan JG, Chan DC, Leder P. Transmembrane form of the kit ligand growth factor is determined by alternative splicing and is missing in the S1 d mutant. *Cell* 1991;64(5):1025–1035.

133. Sekido Y, Obata Y, Ueda R, et al. Preferential expression of c-*kit* protooncogene transcripts in small cell lung cancer. *Cancer Res* 1991;51:2416–2419.

134. Krystal GW, DeBerry CS, Linnekin D, et al. Lck associates with and is activated by Kit in a small cell lung cancer cell line: inhibition of SCF-mediated growth by the Src family kinase inhibitor PP1. *Cancer Res* 1998;58:4660–4666.

135. Krystal GW, Hines SJ, Organ CP. Autocrine growth of small cell lung cancer mediated by coexpression of c-kit and stem cell factor. *Cancer Res* 1996;56:370–376.

136. Hibi K, Takahashi T, Sekido Y, et al. Coexpression of the stem cell factor and the c-kit genes in small-cell lung cancer. *Oncogene* 1991;6:2291–2296.

137. Buhring HJ, Herbst R, Kostka G, et al. Modulation of p145c-kit function in cells of patients with acute myeloblastic leukemia. *Cancer Res* 1993;53:4424–4431.

138. Wang C, Curtis JE, Geissler EN, et al. The expression of the proto-oncogene C-kit in the blast cells of acute myeloblastic leukemia. *Leukemia* 1989;3:699–702.

139. Ratajczak MZ, Luger SM, Gewirtz AM. The c-kit proto-oncogene in normal and malignant human hematopoiesis. *Int J Cell Cloning* 1992;10:205–214.

140. Ratajczak MZ, Luger SM, DeRiel K, et al. Role of the KIT protooncogene in normal and malignant human hematopoiesis. *Proc Natl Acad Sci U S A* 1992;89:1710–1714.

141. Te Kronnie G, Timeus F, Rinaldi A, et al. Imatinib mesylate (STI571) interference with growth of neuroectodermal tumour cell lines does not critically involve c-Kit inhibition. *Int J Mol Med* 2004;14(3):373–382.

142. Hotfilder M, Lanvers C, Jurgens H, Boos J, Vormoor J. c-KIT-expressing Ewing tumour cells are insensitive to imatinib mesylate (STI571). *Cancer Chemother Pharmacol* 2002;50(2):167–169.

143. Furitsu T, Tsujimura T, Tono T, et al. Identification of mutations in the coding sequence of the proto-oncogene c-*kit* in a human mast cell leukemia cell line causing ligand-independent activation of c-kit product. *J Clin Invest* 1993;92:1736–1744.

144. Kitayama H, Kanakura Y, Furitsu T, et al. Constitutively activating mutations of c-kit receptor tyrosine kinase confer factor-independent growth and tumorigenicity of factor-dependent hematopoietic cell lines. *Blood* 1995;85:790–798.

145. Tsujimura T, Hashimoto K, Kitayama H, et al. Activating mutation in the catalytic domain of c-*kit* elicits hematopoietic transformation by receptor self-association not at the ligand-induced dimerization site. *Blood* 1999;93:1319–1329.

146. Tsujimura T, Furitsu T, Morimoto M, et al. Ligand-independent activation of c-*kit* receptor tyrosine kinase in a murine mastocytoma cell line P-815 generated by a point mutation. *Blood* 1994;83:2619–2626.

147. Tsujimura T, Furitsu T, Morimoto M, et al. Substitution of an aspartic acid results in constitutive activation of c-*kit* receptor tyrosine kinase in a rat tumor mast cell line RBL-2H3. *Int Arch Allergy Immunol* 1995;106:377–385.

148. Tsujimura T, Morimoto M, Hashimoto K, et al. Constitutive activation of c-*kit* in FMA3 murine mastocytoma cells caused by deletion of seven amino acids at the juxtamembrane domain. *Blood* 1996;87:273–283.

149. Longley BJ, Tyrrell L, Lu SZ, et al. Somatic c-*KIT* activating mutation in urticaria pigmentosa and aggressive mastocytosis: establishment of clonality in a human mast cell neoplasm. *Nat Genet* 1996;12:312–314.

150. Nagata H, Worobec AS, Oh CK, et al. Identification of a point mutation in the catalytic domain of the protooncogene c-*kit* in peripheral blood mononuclear cells of patients who have mastocytosis with an associated hematologic disorder. *Proc Natl Acad Sci U S A* 1995;92:10560–10564.

151. Tian Q, Frierson HF Jr, Krystal GW, et al. Activating c-*kit* gene mutations in human germ cell tumors. *Am J Pathol* 1994;154:1643–1647.

152. Nishida T, Hirota S, Taniguchi M, et al. Familial gastrointestinal stromal tumours with germline mutation of the KIT gene [letter]. *Nat Genet* 1998;19:323–324.

153. Yagihashi S, Kimura M, Kurotaki H, et al. Gastric submucosal tumours of neurogenic origin with neuroaxonal and Schwann cell elements. *J Pathol* 1987;153:41–50.

154. Sarlomo-Rikala M, Kovatich AJ, Barusevicius A, et al. CD117: a sensitive marker for gastrointestinal stromal tumors that is more specific than CD34. *Mod Pathol* 1998;11:728–734.

155. Sakurai S, Fukasawa T, Chong J-M, et al. Embryonic form of smooth muscle myosin heavy chain (SMemb/MHC-B) in gastrointestinal stromal tumor and interstitial cells of Cajal. *Am J Pathol* 1999;154:23–28.

156. Fletcher CDM, Fletcher JA. Testing for KIT (CD117) in gastrointestinal stromal tumors: another HercepTest? *Am J Clin Pathol* 2002;118:163–164.

157. Hornick JL, Fletcher CDM. Immunohistochemical staining for KIT (CD117) in soft tissue sarcomas is very limited in distribution. *Am J Clin Pathol* 2002;117(2):188–193.

158. Lasota J, Jasinski M, Sarlomo-Rikala M, Miettinen M. Mutations in exon 11 of c-Kit occur preferentially in malignant *versus* benign gastrointestinal stromal tumors and do not occur in leiomyomas or leiomyosarcomas. *Am J Pathol* 1999;154:53–60.

159. Ernst SI, Hubbs AE, Przygodzki RM, et al. KIT mutation portends poor prognosis in gastrointestinal stromal/smooth muscle tumors. *Lab Invest* 1998;78:1633–1636.

160. Taniguchi M, Nishida T, Hirota S, et al. Effect of c-*kit* mutation on prognosis of gastrointestinal stromal tumors. *Cancer Res* 1999;59:4297–4300.

161. Moskaluk CA, Tian Q, Marshall CR, et al. Mutations of c-kit JM domain are found in a minority of human gastrointestinal stromal tumors. *Oncogene* 1999;18:1897–1902.

162. Goss GA, Merriam P, Manola J, et al. Clinical and pathological characteristics of gastrointestinal stromal tumors (GIST). *Proc Am Soc Clin Oncol* 2000;19:559a.

163. Heinrich MC, Corless CL, Demetri GD, et al. Kinase mutations and imatinib response in patients with metastatic gastrointestinal stromal tumor. *J Clin Oncol* 2003;21(23):4342–4349.

164. Heinrich MC, Corless CL, Duensing A, et al. *PDGFRA* activating mutations in gastrointestinal stromal tumors. *Science* 2003;299(5607):708–710.

165. Rubin BP, Singer S, Tsao C, et al. KIT activation is a ubiquitous feature of gastrointestinal stromal tumors. *Clin Cancer Res* 2001;61(22):8118–8121.

166. Corless CL, Fletcher JA, Heinrich MC. Biology of gastrointestinal stromal tumors. *J Clin Oncol* 2004;22(18):3813–3825.

167. Edmonson J, Marks R, Bucker J, et al. Contrast of response to d-map + sargramostim between patients with advanced malignant gastrointestinal stromal tumors and patients with other advanced leiomyosarcomas. *Proc Am Soc Clin Oncol* 1999;18:2088.

168. Druker BJ, Tamura S, Buchdunger E, et al. Effects of a selective inhibitor of the Abl tyrosine kinase on the growth of Bcr-Abl positive cells. *Nat Med* 1996;2(5):561–566.

169. Heinrich MC, Griffith DJ, Druker BJ, et al. Inhibition of c-kit receptor tyrosine kinase activity by STI571, a selective tyrosine kinase inhibitor. *Blood* 2000;96:925–932.

170. Tuveson DA, Willis NA, Jacks T, et al. STI571 inactivation of the gastrointestinal stromal tumor c-KIT oncoprotein: biological and clinical implications. *Oncogene* 2001;20(36):5054–5058.

171. Buchdunger E, Cioffi CL, Law N, et al. Abl protein-tyrosine kinase inhibitor STI571 inhibits in vitro signal transduction mediated by c-Kit and platelet-derived growth factor receptors. *J Pharm Exp Ther* 2000;295:139–145.

172. Druker BJ, Talpaz M, Resta D, et al. Clinical efficacy and safety of an abl specific tyrosine kinase inhibitor as targeted therapy for chronic myelogenous leukemia. *Blood* 1999;94(suppl 1):368a (abstract 1639).

173. Heinrich M, Zigler A, Griffith D, et al. Selective pharmacological inhibition of wild type and mutant c-kit receptor tyrosine kinase activity in hematopoietic cells. *Blood* 1999;94(suppl 1):62a (abstract 265).

174. Joensuu H, Roberts PJ, Sarlomo-Rikala M, et al. Effect of the tyrosine kinase inhibitor STI571 in a patient with a metastatic gastrointestinal stromal tumor. *N Engl J Med* 2001;344:1052–1056.

175. Demetri GD, Von Mehren M, Blanke CD, et al. Efficacy and safety of imatinib mesylate in advanced gastrointestinal stromal tumors. *N Engl J Med* 2002;347(7):472–480.

176. Blanke CD, Demetri GD, Von Mehren M, et al. Long-term follow-up of a phase II randomized trial in advanced gastrointestinal stromal tumor (GIST) patients (pts) treated with imatinib mesylate. *Proc ASCO* 2006;24(18S):9528.

177. Verweij J, van Oosterom A, Blay JY, et al. Imatinib mesylate (STI-571 Glivec, Gleevec) is an active agent for gastrointestinal stromal tumours, but does not yield responses in other soft-tissue sarcomas that are unselected for a molecular target: results from an EORTC Soft Tissue and Bone Sarcoma Group phase II study. *Eur J Cancer* 2003;39(14):2006–2011.

178. Verweij J, Casali PG, Zalcberg J, et al. Progression-free survival in gastrointestinal stromal tumours with high-dose imatinib: randomised trial. *Lancet* 2004;364(9440):1127–1134.

179. Rankin C, Von Mehren M, Blanke C, et al. Dose effect of imatinib (IM) in patients (pts) with metastatic GIST3/4Phase III Sarcoma Group Study S0033. *Proc ASCO* 2004;23:9005.

180. Debiec-Rychter M, Sciot R, Le Cesne A, et al. KIT mutations and dose selection for imatinib in patients with advanced gastrointestinal stromal tumours. *Eur J Cancer* 2006;42(8):1093–1103.

181. Desai J, Shankar S, Heinrich MC, et al. Clonal evolution of resistance to imatinib (IM) in patients (pts) with gastrointestinal stromal tumor (GIST): molecular and radiologic evaluation of new lesions. *Clin Cancer Res* In press.

182. Zalcberg JR, Verweij J, Casali PG, et al. Outcome of patients with advanced gastro-intestinal stromal tumours crossing over to a daily imatinib dose of 800 mg after progression on 400 mg. *Eur J Cancer* 2005;41(12):1751–1757.

183. Raut CP, Posner M, Desai J, et al. Surgical management of advanced gastrointestinal stromal tumors after treatment with targeted systemic therapy using kinase inhibitors. *J Clin Oncol* 2006;24(15):2325–2331.

184. Heinrich MC, Corless CL, Blanke CD, et al. Molecular correlates of imatinib resistance in gastrointestinal stromal tumors. *J Clin Oncol* 2006;24(29):4764–4774.

185. Demetri GD, Desai J, Fletcher JA, et al. SU11248, a multi-targeted tyrosine kinase inhibitor, can overcome imatinib (IM) resistance caused by diverse genomic mechanisms in patients (pts) with metastatic gastrointestinal stromal tumor (GIST). *Proc ASCO* 2004;23:3001.

186. Demetri GD, van Oosterom AT, Garrett CR, et al. Efficacy and safety of sunitinib in patients with advanced gastrointestinal stromal tumour after failure of imatinib: a randomised controlled trial. *Lancet* 2006;368(9544):1329–1338.

187. Duensing A, Medeiros F, McConarty B, et al. Mechanisms of oncogenic KIT signal transduction in primary gastrointestinal stromal tumors (GISTs). *Oncogene* 2004;23(22):3999–4006.

188. Miettinen M, Fetsch JF, Sobin LH, Lasota J. Gastrointestinal stromal tumors in patients with neurofibromatosis 1: a clinicopathologic and molecular genetic study of 45 cases. *Am J Surg Pathol* 2006;30(1):90–96.

189. Bauer S, Yu LK, Demetri GD, Fletcher JA. Heat shock protein 90 inhibition in imatinib-resistant gastrointestinal stromal tumor. *Cancer Res* 2006;66(18):9153–9161.

190. Demetri GD, George S, Van Den Abbeele A, et al. Inhibition of heat shock protein 90 (Hsp90) with the novel agent IPI-504 to overcome resistance to tyrosine kinase inhibitors (TKIs) in metastatic GIST: results of a phase I trial. Proceedings of the 2007 ASCO/ASTRO/SSO GI Cancer Symposium; abstract 12.

CHAPTER 51 ■ SMALL BOWEL CANCERS

KIMBERLY MOORE DALAL AND YUMAN FONG

INTRODUCTION

Small bowel cancers are relatively rare lesions, accounting for 2% of all gastrointestinal (GI) malignancies. Although most tumors are asymptomatic, some malignant masses only cause signs and symptoms after they have metastasized. Their rarity and insidious nature often lead to difficulty in diagnosis and discovery of disease at a late stage, resulting in a poor outcome.

EPIDEMIOLOGY AND ETIOLOGY

Although 40% to 50% of all small bowel cancers are adenocarcinomas, 75% to 80% of these neoplasms are located in the duodenum and proximal jejunum. The U.S. incidence of small bowel adenocarcinomas is 0.46 per 100,000 and 0.33 per 100,000 for men and women, respectively. The second most common small bowel cancer is a carcinoid tumor, accounting for 35% of all small intestinal cancers; 90% are found in the ileum. Originating from the enterochromaffin cell, the annual U.S. incidence of carcinoids is 0.33 and 0.26 per 100,000 men and women, respectively. Lymphomas comprise the third major group of small intestinal tumors; these neoplasms may originate from the small intestine or may represent disseminated disease. In industrialized nations, 15% to 30% of small bowel cancers are classified as non-Hodgkin lymphomas (NHLs). Extranodal immunoproliferative B-cell lymphoma has been described in Arab and Jewish Middle Eastern populations (aka, "Mediterranean lymphoma"), North Africa, and South African blacks. Small bowel sarcomas account for 10% of small bowel cancers.

The risk of small intestinal cancers correlates positively with colorectal cancer, although the incidence is one-fiftieth of colorectal cancer in Western nations. This risk is attributed to high consumption of animal protein and fat.

Adenomatous polyps tend to occur in the periampullary region and proximal jejunum, close to the entrance of bile and pancreatic secretions into the small intestine. The adenoma-carcinoma sequence seen in colorectal cancer is also seen in small bowel cancers (1). The risk of adenocarcinoma increases in relation to increasing polyp size, villous features, and extent of epithelial dysplasia.

Several explanations may account for the low prevalence of carcinoma in the small intestine, an organ that comprises 75% of the length of the GI tract and 90% of the mucosal surface area. These include the presence of secretary immunoglobulin, intramural lymphoid tissue, rapid transit time of enteric contents that limits exposure of the mucosal surface to ingested carcinogens, high concentrations of pancreatic and biliary secretions, and lower concentrations of bacteria compared with the colon.

CLINICAL PRESENTATION

The nonspecificity of symptoms and lack of physical signs explain the 6- to 8-month delay in diagnosis of small bowel cancers (2). For patients with malignant small bowel tumors, late or inaccurate diagnosis contributes to a 50% rate of metastasis at presentation (3,4).

Clinical features present at the time of diagnosis may include weight loss, malnutrition, anorexia, abdominal pain, nausea, vomiting, bleeding, or jaundice. More than 50% of patients present emergently with obstruction or bleeding. Perforation occurs in 10% of patients, particularly in those with lymphomas. Jaundice can occur with periampullary tumors or in patients with advanced liver metastases.

After a complete history, a palpable abdominal mass may be discovered in 25% of patients on physical examination. Rectal examination may reveal occult fecal blood.

DIAGNOSTIC TESTS

Laboratory Tests

Laboratory tests should include a complete blood count, serum electrolytes, and liver function tests. Although no clear role for serum carcinoembryogenic antigen (CEA) has been demonstrated, the majority of small bowel adenocarcinomas are positive for CEA immunohistochemically (5). Patients with suspected small bowel carcinoids should undergo measurement of 24-hour urinary excretion of 5-hydroxyindoleacetic acid (5-HIAA), the end product of serotonin metabolism; this test has 75% sensitivity and 100% specificity (6). Most patients with carcinoid syndrome have values >100 mg/day (523 μm/day); lower levels (50–260 mg/day) may be seen in patients with metastatic carcinoid without the carcinoid syndrome. 5-HIAA levels correlate well with tumor mass (7). If 5-HIAA levels are nondiagnostic, measurements of urinary 5-hydroxytryptamine (5-HT, serotonin), serum 5-HT, serum chromogranin A, neuron-specific enolase, substance P, and neuropeptide K should be undertaken (see Chapter 48 for a complete review of carcinoid tumors).

Radiologic Studies

Abdominal plain films may reveal air-fluid levels or dilated bowel loops suggesting obstruction, or free air demonstrating perforation, but in general these films are not helpful.

An upper gastrointestinal (UGI) series with small bowel follow-through (SBFT) with orally administered water-insoluble contrast is the traditional approach and has a sensitivity of 50% for small bowel tumors; they may show a mass lesion (Fig. 51.1), mucosal defect, or intussusception (Fig. 51.2).

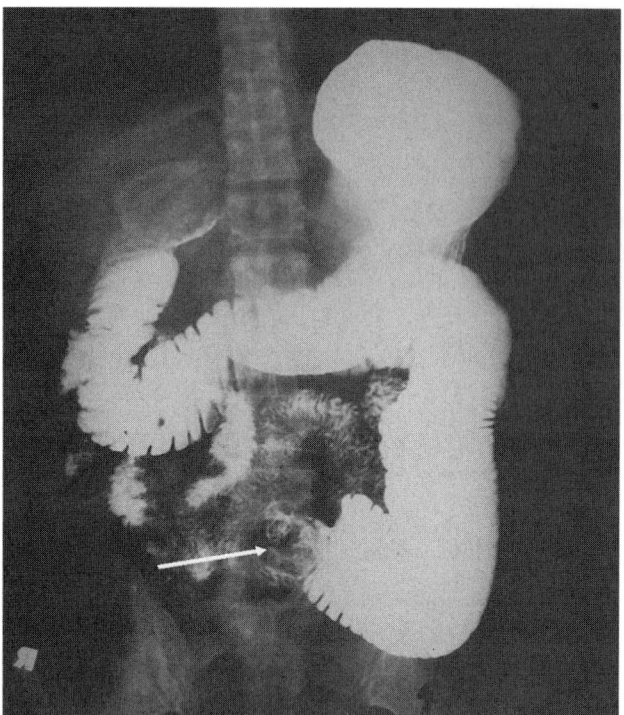

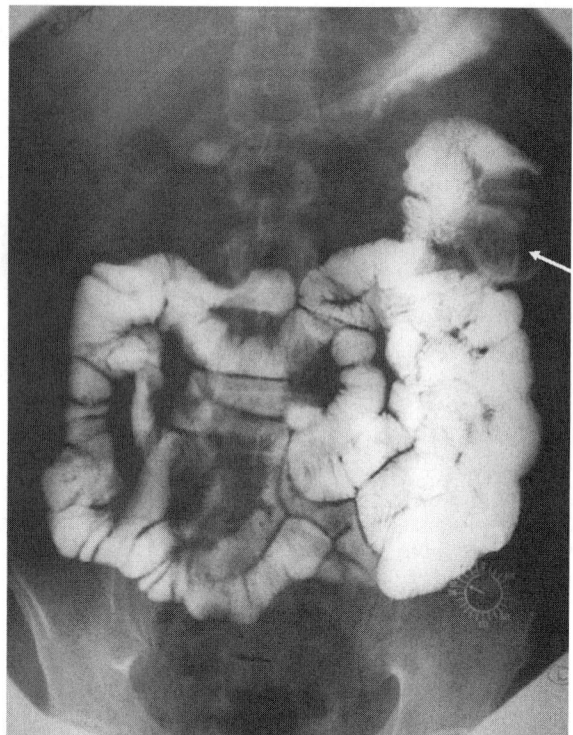

FIGURE 51.1. An upper gastrointestinal (UGI) series with small bowel follow-through (SBFT) of a 37-year-old female with familial adenomatous polyposis status post-proctocolectomy who presented with vomiting. UGI/SBFT demonstrates a mass in the jejunum (*arrow*); pathology after resection revealed a primary jejunal adenocarcinoma. *Source:* Courtesy of Marc Gollub, MD, Director of CT and Gastrointestinal Radiology, Memorial Sloan-Kettering Cancer Center, New York, NY.

FIGURE 51.2. An upper gastrointestinal (UGI) series with small bowel follow-through (SBFT) of a 41-year-old male with a history of melanoma who presented with crampy abdominal pain. UGI/SBFT reveals intussusception of metastatic melanoma (*arrow*). *Source:* Courtesy of Marc Gollub, MD, Director of CT and Gastrointestinal Radiology, Memorial Sloan-Kettering Cancer Center, New York, NY.

Enteroclysis is a double-contrast study in which a nasoenteric tube is advanced into the small bowel to a position above the suspected small bowel abnormality; this study is superior to UGI/SBFT for detecting small bowel tumors, with a sensitivity of 90% (8) except for flat infiltrating lesions, and is the diagnostic study of choice for small bowel tumors. Enteroclysis may be performed in conjunction with CT (9) and combines the benefits of cross-sectional imaging with barium contrast studies (Fig. 51.3). Only 50% to 60% of small bowel neoplasms are detected using UGI/SBFT or enteroclysis (4,10,11). Although enteroclysis may not allow visualization of a small carcinoid, mesenteric metastasis causing mass effect and angulation of bowel loops may suggest a possible diagnosis of carcinoid.

More commonly, patients will undergo abdominal and pelvic computed tomography (CT) for abdominal symptoms. CT has a sensitivity of 80% to 97% (4,10,11) and can evaluate proximal jejunal lesions often missed in contrast studies. CT may demonstrate a gastrointestinal stromal tumor (GIST) as a heterogeneous mass with focal areas of necrosis. In addition, CT can reveal the extraluminal extent of disease, as well as the lymphatic or intra-abdominal spread of disease. Magnetic resonance imaging is more costly than CT and in general is not more helpful in evaluating small bowel tumors. Finally, CT with intravenous and oral contrast is the procedure of choice for staging for carcinoid tumors and has an 87% sensitivity for identifying the primary tumor, mesenteric stranding and desmoplastic reaction, liver metastases, or mesenteric lymph node involvement (11) (Fig. 51.4).

UGI endoscopy and small bowel "push" enteroscopy are most helpful in delineating duodenal or proximal jejunal lesions, especially when radiographic evaluation has been un-

revealing. One may obtain tissue diagnosis via endoscopic biopsy and provide therapy in selected instances (12). Push enteroscopy, which uses a pediatric colonoscope and allows visualization of the proximal 60 cm of jejunum, can establish the diagnosis in 50% of patients with obscure GI bleeding (13). In addition, extended small bowel enteroscopy using a 120-degree, forward-viewing, 2,560-mm balloon-tipped endoscope can allow visualization of 70% of the small bowel mucosa. Capsule endoscopy is a relatively new technique that allows visualization of the entire small bowel and can aid in evaluation of bleeding lesions (14). The risk of this procedure, however, is of complete obstruction; therefore, gastroenterologists request a UGI/SBFT to evaluate the presence of a near-obstructing intestinal lesion before administering the capsule. To further evaluate bleeding lesions, tagged red blood cell scans can detect bleeding at a rate of 0.1 mL/minute but cannot accurately identify bleeding sites. Angiography requires a bleeding rate of 0.5 mL/minute, can localize the bleeding site, and may demonstrate tumor blush in carcinoid and leiomyosarcoma.

Radionuclide imaging using indium-111 octreotide localizes carcinoids as carcinoid tumor cells contain somatostatin receptors. Octreotide imaging has a >90% sensitivity for identifying carcinoid tumors in patients with carcinoid syndrome and is superior to metaiodobenzylguanidine (MIBG) scintigraphy (15). Iodine-131 or -121 MIBG scans can identify primary or metastatic carcinoids in 50% to 60% of patients (16). Rarely, a patient will benefit from selective venous sampling if other localization studies prove unsuccessful.

Laparoscopy or laparotomy is the most sensitive diagnostic modality in diagnosing a patient with a small bowel tumor. Laparoscopy with intraoperative endoscopy should be

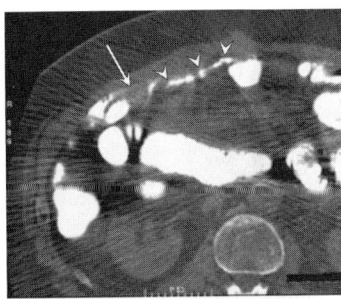

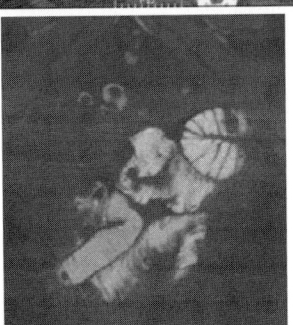

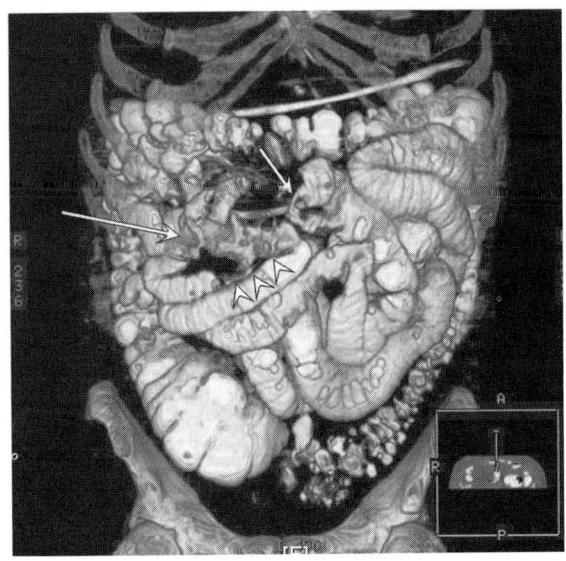

FIGURE 51.3. Computed tomography enteroclysis of a patient with metastatic pancreatic cancer to the peritoneum with multifocal small bowel obstruction (*arrows*). Three-dimensional images are rendered from this study. *Source:* Courtesy of Marc Gollub, MD, Director of CT and Gastrointestinal Radiology, Memorial Sloan-Kettering Cancer Center, New York, NY.

considered in a patient with occult GI bleeding, unexplained weight loss, or vague abdominal pain and an unrevealing workup. Laparoscopy also allows for tissue samples in order to make a diagnosis.

ADENOCARCINOMA

Adenocarcinomas comprise the most common type of malignant small bowel tumors. Forty percent are located in the duodenum and decrease in frequency as one progresses distally along the small intestine. The incidence of small bowel adenocarcinomas in the United States is rising in African Americans (17,18). Risk factors include adenomatous polyps,

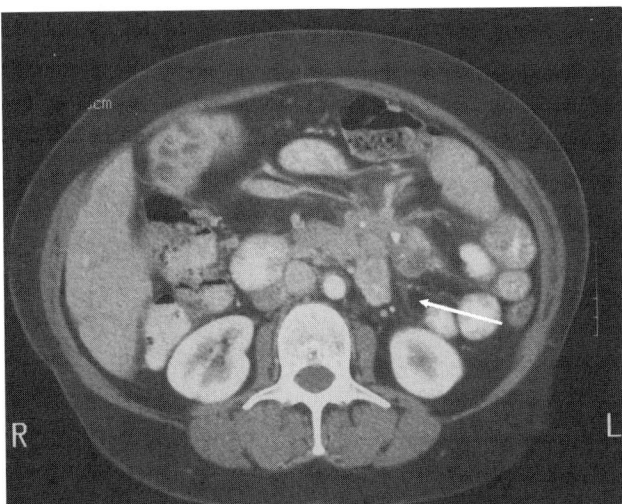

FIGURE 51.4. Computed tomography with intravenous and oral contrast is the procedure of choice for staging for carcinoid tumors and has a 87% sensitivity for identifying the primary tumor, mesenteric stranding and desmoplastic reaction with lymph node involvement (*arrow*), and liver metastases. The lymph nodes reveal characteristic calcifications. *Source:* Courtesy of Marc Gollub, MD, Director of CT and Gastrointestinal Radiology, Memorial Sloan-Kettering Cancer Center, New York, NY.

familial adenomatous polyposis, hereditary nonpolyposis colorectal cancer, and Crohn disease (19). The most commonly used staging system is the tumor, node, metastasis (TNM) system of the American Joint Commission on Cancer (20) (Table 51.1). Treatment is dictated by location. Before proceeding with aggressive resection, one must exclude hepatic or peritoneal metastases or extensive locoregional invasion that may preclude complete excision. Lymph node involvement does not preclude an attempt at curative resection; examination of ≥15 lymph nodes improves the prognostic discrimination of nodal staging (21).

Ampulla and Duodenum

Ampullary carcinoma is an uncommon malignancy, accounting for 6% of periampullary tumors (22), with an incidence of 5.7 cases per 1 million people (23). Ampullary tumors have a more favorable prognosis (24–28) compared with pancreatic or bile duct tumors, with median survival rates ranging from 30 to 50 months (29,30) and 5-year survival rates of 30% to 50% (31,32) in resected patients. In 1963, Whipple mused that the improved prognosis of ampullary cancers was due to its fungating nature, better differentiation, and decreased tendency toward lymphovascular invasion (33).

The ampulla is comprised of the junction of the pancreatic and common bile ducts that forms a 3-mm common intramucosal channel. Anatomical variability of this area is found in half of the population. Invasive carcinoma obliterates the site of origin and the defining anatomical landmarks (Fig. 51.5). Adjacent to some carcinomas are precursor neoplasia or dysplasia of the duodenal mucosa or ductal system. Ampullary cancers cause an early jaundice that results in earlier detection of disease compared with pancreatic tumors.

Adenocarcinomas of the duodenal ampulla represent a variety of tumors that have features of ductal or intestinal origin. Ampullary tumors are biologically more similar to intestinal than pancreatic cancers. In one study, 70% of cases had intestinal rather than pancreaticobiliary morphology (34). Moreover, the frequent finding of ampullary tumors in patients with familial adenomatous polyposis suggests similar genetic alterations and mechanisms of carcinogenesis in colonic and ampullary neoplasms. In addition, adenocarcinoma of the duodenum may

TABLE 51.1

2002 TUMOR, NODE, METASTASIS STAGING OF SMALL INTESTINE

PRIMARY TUMOR (T)

TX	Primary tumor cannot be assessed
T0	No evidence of primary tumor
Tis	Carcinoma in situ
T1	Tumor invades lamina propria or submucosa
T2	Tumor invades muscularis propria
T3	Tumor invades through the muscularis propria into the subserosa or into the nonperitonealized perimuscular tissue (mesentery or retroperitoneum) with extension 2 cm or less[a]
T4	Tumor perforates the visceral peritoneum or directly invades other organs or structures (includes other loops of the small intestine, mesentery, or retroperitoneum >2 cm, and the abdominal wall by way of the serosa; for the duodenum only, includes invasion of the pancreas)

Note: The nonperitonealized perimuscular tissue is for jejunum and ileum, part of the mesentery and, for duodenum in areas where serosa is lacking, part of the retroperitoneum.

REGIONAL LYMPH NODES (N)

NX	Regional lymph nodes cannot be assessed
N0	No regional lymph node metastasis
N1	Regional lymph node metastasis

DISTANT METASTASIS (M)

MX	Distant metastasis cannot be assessed
M0	No distant metastasis
M1	Distant metastasis

STAGE GROUPING

Stage 0	Tis	N0	M0
Stage I	T1	N0	M0
	T2	N0	M0
Stage II	T3	N0	M0
	T4	N0	M0
Stage III	Any T	N1	M0
Stage IV	Any T	Any N	M1

[a]Lymphomas, carcinoid tumors, and visceral sarcomas are not included.
Used with the permission of the American Joint Committee on Cancer (AJCC), Chicago, Illinois. The original source for this material is the *AJCC Cancer Staging Manual, Sixth Edition* (2002), published by Springer-New York, www.springeronline.com.

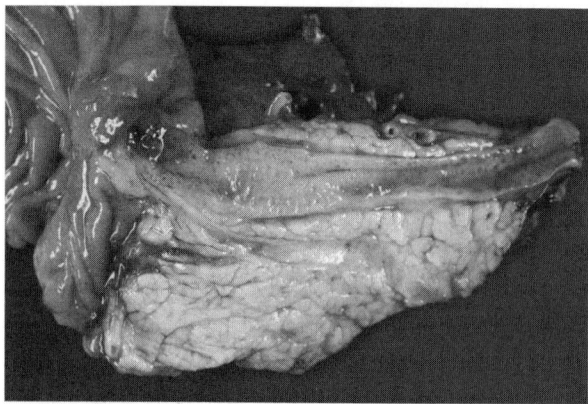

FIGURE 51.5. Gross photograph of an ampullary adenocarcinoma that demonstrates the longitudinal course of the pancreatic duct ending at the ampulla, which is obliterated by the adenocarcinoma. *Source:* Courtesy of Jinru Shia, MD, Gastrointestinal Pathology, Memorial Sloan-Kettering Cancer Center, New York, NY (See also color Figure 51.5).

be characterized by mutations of the APC/B-catenin pathway (35). Finally, K-ras mutations occur early in ampullary carcinomas with a pattern and incidence (37%) similar to colon cancer (36). DPC4 tumor-suppressor gene is inactivated in more than half of pancreatic adenocarcinomas; yet, complete loss of DPC4 was identified in only 34% of ampullary invasive carcinomas (37).

Duodenal adenocarcinoma progression mirrors that of colon cancer; mural penetration, nodal involvement, distant metastasis, and perineural invasion are associated with poor prognosis (5,38,39). Seventy to 80% of small adenocarcinomas are resectable at diagnosis; 35% have metastasized to regional lymph nodes and 20% to 25% to distant sites (40).

Standard surgical management of ampullary carcinoma is pancreaticoduodenectomy (34). The first radical resection for ampullary carcinoma was performed by Halsted in 1898; he performed a partial duodenectomy and reimplanted the common bile duct and pancreatic duct in the duodenum (41). Yet, perioperative morbidity rates can approach 50% (42). Roggin et al. (43) looked at 140 consecutive patients with nonfamilial ampullary neoplasms from a single institutional database.

Their group demonstrated that preoperative biopsy and frozen section had diagnostic accuracy rates of 79% and 84%, respectively (43). Moreover, patients with invasive cancer treated by ampullectomy had a decreased recurrencefree survival as well as disease-specific survival compared with those treated with pancreaticoduodenectomy. Although the morbidity rate of 66% was significantly higher in those patients who underwent pancreaticoduodenectomy, when ampullectomy is considered for periampullary neoplasms with benign disease or high-grade dysplasia, frozen section should be performed to rule out adenocarcinoma. If positive, pancreaticoduodenectomy should be performed if the patient can tolerate such a procedure in light of comorbidities. If the final pathology reveals an occult adenocarcinoma, strong consideration should be given to an interval pancreaticoduodenectomy.

For duodenal adenocarcinoma located on the antimesenteric side or more distal to the ampulla in the second portion of the duodenum, segmental resection followed by duodenojejunostomy may be performed. For duodenal adenocarcinoma located in the third or fourth portion of the duodenum that arises to the left of the superior mesenteric artery, a segmental resection provides a survival benefit equal to that of a pancreaticoduodenectomy with a decreased associated morbidity and mortality (38). For unresectable tumors, palliation of symptoms can be accomplished by gastrojejunostomy for gastric outlet obstruction, biliary bypass for obstructive jaundice, and celiac plexus nerve block for pain.

Five-year diseasefree survival (DFS) rates for adenocarcinoma of the duodenum or ampulla exceed that of pancreatic adenocarcinoma; long-term survival for resected duodenal adenocarcinoma is 50% to 60%, similar to those with colorectal carcinoma (3,4,38,44–47). Howe et al. examined factors predictive of survival in ampullary carcinoma (34) in a review of 123 patients from the Memorial Sloan-Kettering Cancer Center (MSKCC) single-institution prospective database. Of these patients, 101 tumors (82%) were resected. Factors significantly associated with improved survival were resection (P <0.01), and in resected tumors, negative nodes (P = 0.04) and margins (P = 0.02) independently predicted improved survival. When all patients with periampullary carcinoma who presented to MSKCC were examined, overall survival and rates of resection were highest in ampullary carcinomas. However, among resected patients, those with duodenal cancers had the best survival, followed by those with ampullary cancers (Fig. 51.6). In one series of 67 patients with nonampullary duodenal adenocarcinoma, the 5-year survival was 54%, stratified by stages I, 100%; II, 52%; III, 45%; and IV, 0% (46). One study also found a similarity in outcome to gastric antral adenocarcinoma in patients with nodal disease in which ≥15 lymph nodes were resected (21).

Jejunum and Ileum

Tumors in the jejunum and ileum present with obstruction, abdominal pain, and weight loss. On UGI/SBFT or enteroclysis, these adenocarcinomas appear as "apple core" lesions with ulcerated mucosa (Fig. 51.7). Intraoperatively, they often appear to involve the serosa, invade into adjacent structures, and be associated with lymphadenopathy.

Adenocarcinoma of the jejunum or ileum is treated for curative intent with wide en bloc resection of the mass and a 6-in. margin on each side. One should include the wedge of investing mesentery down to the origin of the arterial supply, surrounding tissues at risk for contiguous spread, and regional lymph nodes because of the high incidence of local nodal metastases. Moreover, wide resection provides surgical clearance of disease and important staging information. However, if advanced jejunal adenocarcinoma is associated with extensive lymph

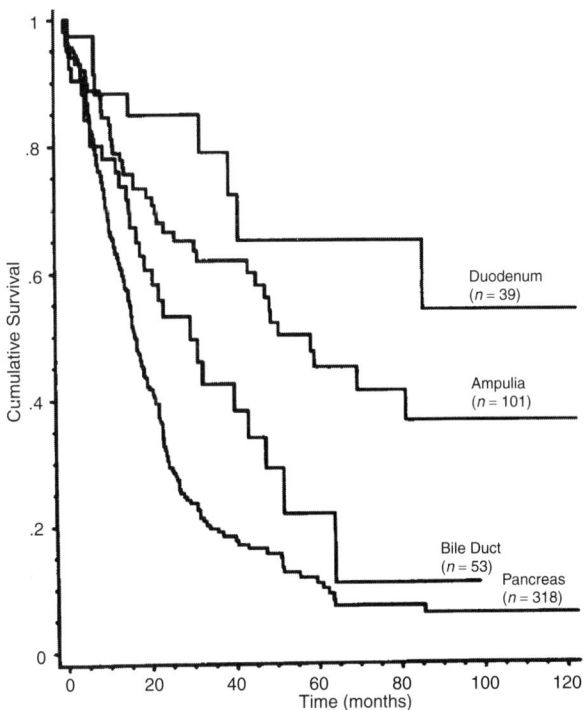

FIGURE 51.6. Survival in patients with resected periampullary carcinomas. Among resected patients with periampullary carcinomas, those with duodenal cancers had the best survival, followed by those with ampullary cancers (P <0.01). *Source:* Reprinted with permission from Lippincott-Raven Publishers. Howe JR, Klimstra DS, Moccia RD, Conlon KC, Brennan MF. Factors predictive of survival in ampullary carcinoma. *Ann Surg* 1998;228(1):87–94, Figure 5.

node involvement, a radical resection of all clinically involved nodes should not be performed, not only because this will compromise the blood supply to the entire small bowel but also because of the poor long-term survival of these patients. Reconstruction can be accomplished with a primary end-to-end

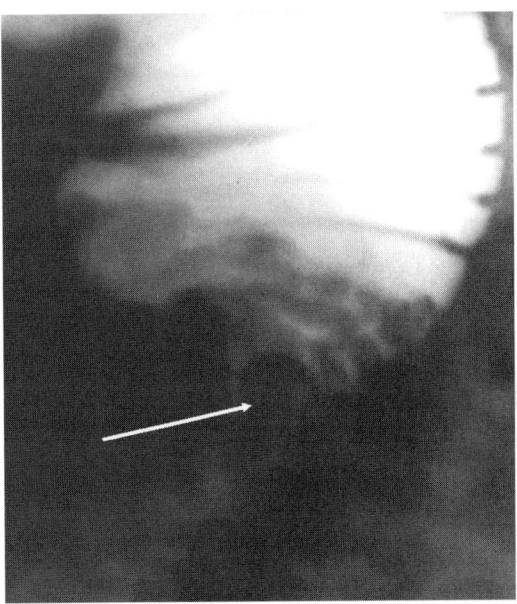

FIGURE 51.7. An upper gastrointestinal series with small bowel follow-through of a primary jejunal adenocarcinoma (*arrow*). *Source:* Courtesy of Marc Gollub, MD, Director of CT and Gastrointestinal Radiology, Memorial Sloan-Kettering Cancer Center, New York, NY.

or end-to-side anastomosis. For tumors at the terminal ileum, a right hemicolectomy with primary anastomosis should be performed. Even in the setting of advanced disease, resection with anastomosis should be performed for palliation of bleeding or obstruction.

Because most jejunal and ileal tumors present at advanced stage, their prognosis is worse than periampullary tumors; <50% of tumors in these locations are confined to the bowel wall, and 25% have stage IV disease. For patients with completely resected jejunal or ileal adenocarcinoma, the 5-year DFS is 60% to 70% for patients with negative nodes, but only 12% to 14% for those with nodal metastases (47).

Adjuvant Therapy

Although the role of adjuvant chemotherapy and radiation for small bowel adenocarcinoma is not well defined, most clinicians advocate postoperative treatment following pancreaticoduodenectomy or intestinal resection because of their demonstrated value in pancreatic cancer and colorectal cancer, with more modest benefit in gastric cancer. There has been substantial progress in the treatment of colorectal cancer, as described in Chapter 45, and somewhat less progress in the treatment of gastric cancer, as described in Chapter 23. The chemotherapy data for small bowel adenocarcinoma described in this section is reported from earlier studies. Currently, medical oncologists have considerably newer, more effective regimens in colorectal cancer or alternatively in gastric cancer, as a model for small bowel carcinomas. However, there are no studies in small bowel tumors that have yet been reported involving substantial numbers of patients treated with newer regimens such as FOLFOX and FOLFIRI, with or without the use of biological agents such as bevacizumab, or using gastric cancer as a model in regimens such as docetaxel, cisplatin, fluorouracil or epirubicin, cisplatin, and fluorouracil. These are being employed by some medical oncologists in advanced, incurable small bowel adenocarcinomas. The next discussion reviews earlier data involving older regimens.

Although a large retrospective review of 217 patients with small bowel adenocarcinoma, 59 of which were treated with adjuvant chemotherapy, did not show survival benefit on multivariate analysis (40), there has been a 20% increase in the use of adjuvant chemotherapy in the United States (48). Case reports of small bowel adenocarcinoma with extensive lymph nodes metastases have shown response to methotrexate/5-fluorouracil (5-FU) sequential therapy after 10 months. After recurrence, combination therapy with radiation, hyperthermia, and cisplatin have effectively reduced nodal swelling and preserved quality of life (49). Protracted venous infusion of 5-FU—based chemotherapy resulted in an overall response rate of 37.5% and a median overall survival of 13 months (50) in 8 patients with advanced small bowel adenocarcinoma. One Eastern Cooperative Oncology Group multi-institutional study demonstrated an 18.4% response rate with a median survival of 8 months in 36 evaluable patients with metastatic small bowel adenocarcinoma treated with 5-FU, doxorubicin, and mitomycin C (51); the response rate was 18.4%, with a median survival time of 8 months. Fishman et al. demonstrated a higher overall response rate in gemcitabine and irinotecan combinations (30%–40%) compared to older 5-FU—based regimens (13%) (52).

Preoperative chemoradiation was studied in 4 patients with duodenal carcinoma without distant metastases who received 5,040 cGy concurrently with 5-FU and mitomycin C 4 to 6 weeks before undergoing pancreaticoduodenectomy. All 4 patients had a complete pathological response after chemoradiation and were alive without recurrence with follow-up ranging from 12 to 90 months (53).

CARCINOID (see Chapter 48 for a more detailed description)

The annual incidence of small bowel carcinoid is 0.28 per 100,000, resulting in 600 new cases yearly in the United States. Most carcinoid tumors are asymptomatic and are found incidentally or at autopsy. Carcinoids originate from the Kulchitsky cell, an enterochromaffin cell. The small intestine is the most common location for carcinoids. Due to the distribution of these cells, most carcinoids are located in the appendix and ileum, are submucosal, and are yellow-orange in color.

Moertel et al. studied 183 consecutive patients with a surgical diagnosis and treatment of small bowel carcinoid (54). With a median follow-up of 15 years, this study showed a male predominance and a median age of diagnosis of 60 years. Although most patients presented with regional nodal metastasis at diagnosis, resection with curative intent was possible. The frequency of intestinal carcinoids increased as one moved distally from the duodenum; nearly 40% of the carcinoids were located within 2 feet of the ileocecal valve. Small bowel carcinoids tended to be larger than those in the appendix or rectum but were <2 cm in diameter. Thirty-five percent were multicentric. Metastasis correlated with increasing size, with almost all tumors >2 cm in size showing spread.

Patients may present with periodic abdominal pain, consistent with intermittent bowel obstruction. If present, symptoms are often vague. An abdominal mass is observed in only 20% of patients. Therefore, the diagnosis is usually made late, with metastatic disease present in half of the patients. When symptomatic, carcinoids present with obstruction or carcinoid syndrome. The intestinal obstruction may result from kinking of the bowel due to the intense desmoplastic reaction in the adjacent mesentery, which is attributed to local serotonin release, and may lead to intestinal ischemia and gangrene. Intestinal obstruction may also result from intussusception.

As the disease progresses into the mesenteric and celiac lymph nodes, encasement of the small mesenteric artery may occur; this, coupled with an unusual type of regional vascular thickening, may lead to ischemia, small bowel infarction, and death. Peritoneal implantation may occur, but metastatic spread is usually located in the liver. Because liver metastases grow slowly, the liver adapts to its presence. Classically, a patient with large metastatic masses may have a grossly enlarged liver with normal liver function tests. The next frequent site of distant metastases is bone; often asymptomatic, they may occur without radiographically detectable lesions. Interestingly, the bones of the orbit and the eye itself are sites of metastatic predilection, as are the female breast and ovary.

The treatment of choice is resection, dictated by site, size, and mesenteric nodal involvement. Seventy percent of patients have lymph node metastases. Small duodenal lesions may be enucleated or locally excised; carcinoids >2 cm or malignant appearing may require pancreaticoduodenectomy. Tumors of the jejunum and ileum may be resected en bloc with a large wedge of mesentery, with care to include the affected mesenteric lymph nodes. Resection may prove challenging due to the associated fibrosis and foreshortening of the mesentery. Wide excision is recommended even in the presence of distant metastasis in order to prevent fibrosing mesenteritis. Because 40% of patients with mid-gut carcinoids have a second GI primary, the entire small bowel and colon should be examined prior to surgical resection.

Small bowel carcinoids have a slow rate of local spread and metastasis. The overall 5-year survival is 60%. For patients with small tumors without lymphatic spread, 5-year survival is almost 100%. For patients in whom all visible malignant disease is resected, the median time to metastatic disease is 16 years (54). Fifty percent of patients with unresectable disease lived 5 years or longer; for those patients with hepatic metastases, the median survival was nearly 30% survival at 5 years (54).

Carcinoid Syndrome

First described in 1955, carcinoid syndrome is present in 10% of patients with carcinoid tumors and is a manifestation of late stage disease. Carcinoids of the small intestine produce serotonin, which is measured in urine excretion of 5-HIAA (55). When released from the tumors into the portal circulation, the liver inactivates 5-HIAA on first pass; therefore, the carcinoid syndrome, manifested by elevated urinary 5-HIAA, occurs only with hepatic metastases or with other metastatic tumors that bypass the portal circulation (e.g., teratomas of the ovary or testis). The occurrence and severity of the syndrome are directly related to tumor bulk in the liver. Two-thirds of patients have an enlarged liver or abdominal mass.

The carcinoid syndrome consists of diarrhea and flushing of the face, neck, and upper trunk lasting from seconds to minutes. In African Americans, conjunctival injection may be the sole manifestation of flushing. Other symptoms of the syndrome include bronchospasm, hypotension, tachycardia, coma, and even death. Pigmented dermatitis, mucositis, and central nervous system manifestations of niacin deficiency (or pellagra) have been reported in patients with carcinoid syndrome, due to the preferential use of tryptophan for serotonin synthesis away from nicotinic acid synthesis. Nicotinamide supplementation alleviates these symptoms. With time, patients with carcinoid syndrome develop endocardial and valvular fibrosis leading to tricuspid valve insufficiency, pulmonary valve stenosis, and subsequent right heart failure. Many substances, including serotonin and substance P, have been proposed to play a role in carcinoid-related cardiac effects.

Although management of liver metastases is controversial, some patients may derive benefit from surgical intervention. If there are no contraindications to surgery and curative resection is possible, an attempt at surgical extirpation should be undertaken because it can provide symptomatic relief and prolong DFS (56,57). The duration of symptom relief is often less than 12 months, and no survival benefit has been consistently demonstrated. If liver metastases are not amenable to surgical resection, radiofrequency ablation should be attempted to prevent the development of carcinoid syndrome. Octreotide may be used to reduce symptoms of carcinoid syndrome; this has been shown to be effective in reducing symptoms in 30% of patients for 2 years. For patients with the carcinoid syndrome, symptomatic relief may be obtained by debulking the liver with or without hepatic arterial embolization (57,58). Of note, general anesthesia can induce a life-threatening carcinoid crisis, which is manifested by hemodynamic instability; this is treated effectively with intravenous somatostatin intraoperatively, which should also be administered preoperatively to decrease the chance of developing carcinoid crisis.

Chemotherapy using doxorubicin, 5-FU, and streptozocin has shown response rates of 20% to 30%. Radiotherapy, however, is not effective. Median survival is 15 years for resected metastatic disease and 3 years for those with metastatic disease and carcinoid syndrome.

LYMPHOMA

Lymphomas comprise 15% of malignant small bowel tumors and are multifocal in 15% of patients. These tumors occur most commonly in the fifth to sixth decade of life with a slight male predominance. These lesions arise from lymphoid tissue in the intestinal wall and are most often in the ileum where the greatest concentration of lymphoid tissue exists. Most primary tumors are non-Hodgkin B-cell lymphomas with intermediate to high-grade features. Patients at risk for development of small bowel lymphomas include those with inflammatory conditions, such as celiac sprue or Crohn disease, or those who are immunosuppressed, with posttransplant lymphoproliferative disease, AIDS, systemic lupus erythematosus, or agammaglobinemia. (See Chapter 49 for a more detailed description of GI lymphomas.)

Primary follicular lymphoma is the most common type of NHL in the United States (59), and the GI tract is the most common site of extranodal primary NHL. The cytogenetic hallmark is t(14;18)(q32;21), with rearrangement of the BCL2 gene seen in up to 90% of cases (60). A rare entity, follicular lymphoma, accounts for 1% to 3.6% of GI lymphomas. Shia et al. (61) reported a series of 26 cases of GI follicular lymphoma from a single institution. With a median age of 55 years, abdominal pain was the most common presenting symptom that seemed to be related to bowel thickening and obstruction. The majority of cases (85%) involved small bowel, and the duodenum was the most commonly involved site. The most common histologic grade was grade 1. In this study, all cases were positive for DC20 and BCL2 and negative for CD3, CD5, CD23, CD43, and cyclin D1; most were positive for CD10. Four of 4 cases showed the t(14;18) rearrangement. Complete response was observed in 15 of 22 cases that received treatment, including surgery with or without chemotherapy, with 1 case receiving radiation. Recurrence and progression were associated with histologic transformation to diffuse large cell lymphoma. None of the patients died of lymphoma. Five-year DFS was 62%, with median DFS of 69 months.

Patients with small bowel lymphoma present with abdominal pain, weight loss, fatigue, and malaise. Interestingly, fever, night sweats, and lymphadenopathy are absent. One-third of patients present with an abdominal mass. One-fourth present with intussusception, obstruction, bleeding, or perforation.

A variant of small bowel lymphoma found in underdeveloped countries, Mediterranean lymphoma, presents with diarrhea, steatorrhea, and colicky abdominal pain. The entire small bowel is involved. Prognosis is poor due to progressive malnutrition and transformation to a disseminated and aggressive form of disease.

The diagnosis of small bowel lymphoma is usually made by UGI/SBFT, enteroclysis, or abdominal/pelvic CT scan. Although contrast studies can demonstrate thickened mucosa, ulceration, or submucosal nodules, CT may reveal thickened bowel, bulky mesenteric lymph nodes, or a mass (Fig. 51.8).

Localized small bowel lymphoma (stage IE or IIE) is treated by segmental bowel resection and wide resection of the associated mesentery in order to clear the high frequency of lymph node metastases. Thorough staging includes liver biopsy as well as periaortic and mesenteric lymph node sampling. Because of extensive submucosal infiltration, frozen section should be performed to confirm microscopically tumorfree margins. Only 30% of patients are cured by resection. Debulking may be beneficial in widespread disease as long as nutritional absorption is not compromised.

Chemotherapy is often offered because lymphoma is a systemic disease. For patients with a high risk of relapse after resection, especially those with regional nodal involvement or high-grade tumors, chemotherapy is warranted. In advanced disease (stage IIIE or IVE), treatment consists of multiagent chemotherapy and radiation.

Five-year survival for small lymphoma ranges from 45% for stage IE disease to 19% for stage IIE disease (62). Relapses commonly occur 5 to 10 years after resection, especially in patients with nodal involvement, high-grade histology, and extension beyond the bowel wall. For disseminated disease, survival is less than 1 year.

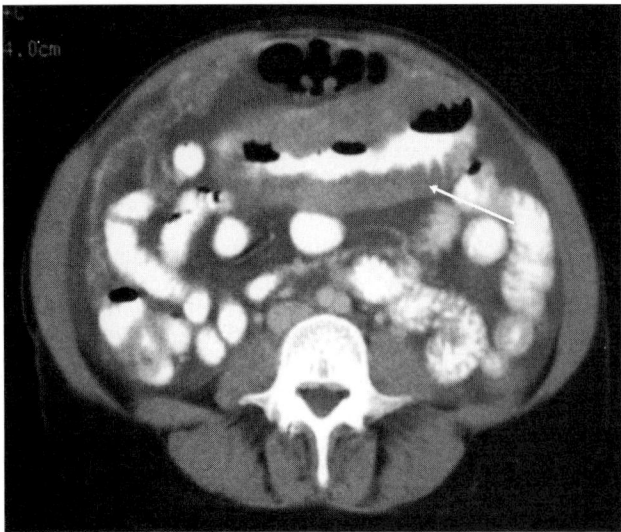

FIGURE 51.8. In patients with gastrointestinal lymphoma, computed tomography may reveal thickened bowel (*arrow*), bulky mesenteric lymph nodes, or a mass. *Source:* Courtesy of Marc Gollub, MD, Director of CT and Gastrointestinal Radiology, Memorial Sloan-Kettering Cancer Center, New York, NY.

GASTROINTESTINAL STROMAL TUMOR (see Chapter 49 for a more detailed description)

GISTs comprise 10% to 20% of all malignant small bowel tumors. GISTs are believed to originate from ICC, the intesti-nal pacemaker cell, or a common progenitor. Expression of KIT, a transmembrane tyrosine kinase receptor, detected by immunohistochemical staining with monoclonal antibodies reactive with CD117, is the gold standard for diagnosis. Gain of function mutations in the *c-kit* proto-oncogene that encodes KIT are found in GISTs, resulting in unopposed tyrosine kinase activation and subsequent malignant cell growth.

Found throughout the small bowel, GISTs are most often identified in the jejunum and ileum. They arise in the submucosa and can be recognized by their round and smooth appearance. When symptomatic, these lesions are quite large; 50% of patients present with an abdominal mass. The most common symptoms are obstruction, abdominal pain, weight loss, and bleeding, as these tumors can be extremely vascular.

Small bowel contrast studies reveal extraluminal masses. CT scans demonstrate large extraluminal masses with central necrosis and calcification.

A range of malignant potential exists. Large tumors (>5 cm), with high mitotic counts (>5/50 high-powered fields) have a greater risk of malignant behavior than do small tumors with low mitotic rates (63) (Table 51.2).

The treatment of choice for nonmetastatic GISTs is segmental resection and primary anastomosis with tumorfree margins. Because these tumors infrequently metastasize to regional lymph nodes, an extensive mesenteric lymphadenectomy is not indicated. For patients who undergo complete resection, 5-year disease-specific survival is 54% at a median follow-up of 24 months (64).

In widely metastatic disease, local resection may alleviate obstruction or bleeding. The treatment of metastatic and unresectable GISTs has been revolutionized by imatinib, an inhibitor of the activated *c-kit* tyrosine kinase (65). Representing the first "targeted therapeutic" agent active against solid tumors, imatinib treatment is first-line therapy for metastatic and unresectable GISTs; clinical trials have demonstrated a

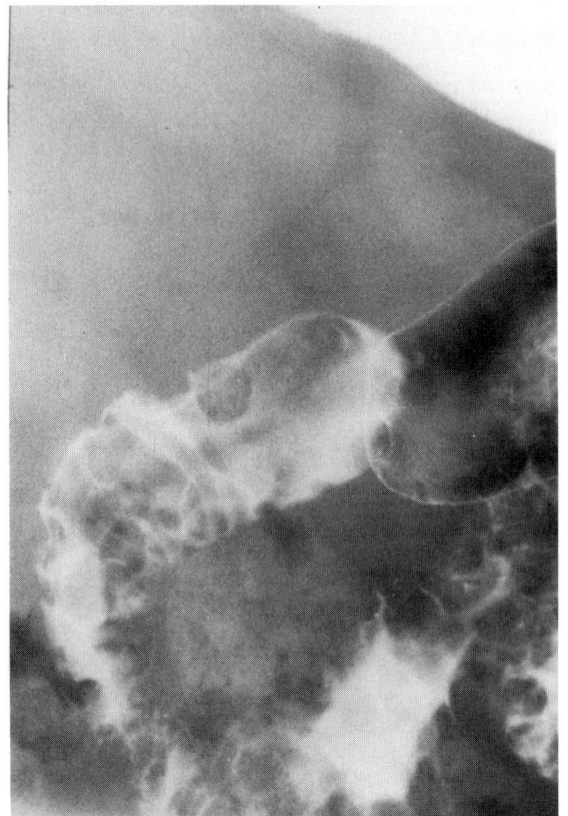

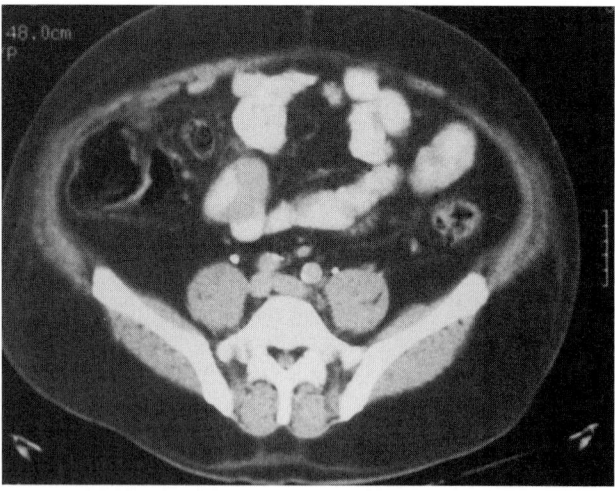

FIGURE 51.9. An upper gastrointestinal series with small bowel follow-through (**A**) and computed tomography (**B**) demonstrate multiple metastases to small bowel from malignant melanoma. *Source:* Courtesy of Marc Gollub, MD, Director of CT and Gastrointestinal Radiology, Memorial Sloan-Kettering Cancer Center, New York, NY.

TABLE 51.2

RISK OF AGGRESSIVE BEHAVIOR IN GASTROINTESTINAL STROMAL TUMORS

	Size	Mitotic count
Very low risk	<2 cm	<5 per 50 HPF
Low risk	2–5 cm	<5 per 50 HPF
Intermediate risk	<5 cm	6–10 per 50 HPF
	5–10 cm	<5 per 50 HPF
High risk	>5 cm	>5 per 50 HPF
	>10 cm	Any mitotic rate
	Any size	>10 per 50 HPF

HPF, high-powered fields.
From Fletcher CD, Berman JJ, Corless C, Gorstein F. Diagnosis of gastrointestinal stromal tumors: a consensus approach. *Int J Surg Pathol* 2002;10(2):87. Reprinted by permission of Sage Publications, Inc.

partial response rate of 60% with minimal toxicity. Current trials by American College of Surgeons Oncology Group evaluating higher doses, and adjuvant therapy are currently underway.

SARCOMA

Five-year disease-specific survival for other small bowel sarcomas is 39% with a median survival of 34 months (66). Tumor grade is an important determinant of survival. Low-grade lesions (<10 mitosis/50 high-power fields) have an 80% DFS at 8 years compared to a mean DFS of less than 18 months for high-grade lesions (67). In multivariate analysis, tumor size <5 cm, leiomyosarcoma histology, and localized disease are significant favorable prognostic factors for disease-specific survival (66).

METASTASES

The small bowel may be the site of distant metastases from melanoma (Figs. 51.2 and 51.9), breast, lung, gastric, colon, renal tumors, sarcomas, and pancreas (Fig. 51.3) via direct extension or hematogenous spread. Because surgical treatment of these tumors is palliative, a limited resection or bypass is indicated. In patients with metastatic melanoma, aggressive resection may improve quality of life and DFS (68).

References

1. Park S, Kim SW, Kim SH, et al. Loss of heterozygosity in ampulla of Vater neoplasms during adenoma-carcinoma sequence. *Anticancer Res* 2003;23(3C):2955–2959.
2. Ciresi DL, Scholten SD. The continuing clinical dilemma of primary tumors of the small intestine. *Am Surg* 1995;61:698–702.
3. Cunningham JD, Aleali R, Aleali M, et al. Malignant small bowel neoplasms: histopathologic determinants of recurrence and survival. *Ann Surg* 1997;225:300–306.
4. North JH, Pack M. Malignant tumors of the small intestine: a review of 144 cases. *Am Surg* 2000;66:46–51.
5. Talamonti MS, Goetz LH, Rao S, et al. Primary cancers of the small bowel: analysis of prognostic factors and results of surgical management. *Arch Surg* 2002;137:564–571.
6. Feldman JM. Urinary serotonin in the diagnosis of carcinoid syndrome. *Clin Chem* 1986;32:840–844.
7. Kema IP, de Vriese EG, Slooff MJ, et al. Serotonin, catecholamines, histamine, and their metabolites in urine, platelets, and tumor tissue of patients with carcinoid tumors. *Clin Chem* 1994;40:86–95.
8. Bessette JR, Maglinte DD, Kelvin FM, et al. Primary malignant tumors of the small bowel: a comparison of the small-bowel enema and conventional follow-through examination. *AJR Am J Roentgenol* 1989;153:741–744.
9. Boudiaf M, Jaff A, Soyer P, et al. Small-bowel diseases: prospective evaluation of multi-detector row helical CT enteroclysis in 107 consecutive patients. *Radiology* 2004;233:338–344.
10. Minardi AJ Jr, Zibari GB, Aultman DF, et al. Small-bowel tumors. *J Am Coll Surg* 1998;186:664–688.
11. Dudiak KM, Johnson CD, Stephens DH. Primary tumors of the small intestine: CT evaluation. *AJR Am J Roentgenol* 1989;152:995–998.
12. Ashley SW, Wells SA Jr. Tumors of the small intestine. *Semin Oncol* 1988; 15:116–128.
13. Lewis BS, Kornbluth A, Waye JD. Small bowel tumors: yield of enteroscopy. *Gut* 1991;32:763–765.
14. Schwartz GD, Barkin JS. Small bowel tumors. *Gastrointest Endosc Clin N Am* 2006;16(2):267–275.
15. Lamberts SW, Bakker WH, Reubi JC, et al. Somatostatin-receptor imaging in the localization of endocrine tumors. *N Engl J Med* 1990;323:1246–1249.
16. Bomanji J, Mather S, Moyes J, Ellison D. A scintigraphic comparison of iodine-123-metaiodobenzylguanidine and an iodine-labeled somatostatin analog (Tyr-3-octreotide) in metastatic carcinoid tumors. *J Nucl Med* 1992; 33:1121–1124.
17. Haselkorn T, Whittemore AS, Lilienfeld DE. Incidence of small bowel cancer in the United States and worldwide: geographic, temporal, and racial differences. *Cancer Causes Control* 2005;16(7):781–787.
18. Verma D, Stroehlein JR. Adenocarcinoma of the small bowel: a 60-yr perspective derived from M.D. Anderson Cancer Center Tumor Registry. *Am J Gastroenterol* 2006;101(7):1647–1654.
19. Canavan C, Abrams KR, Mayberry J. Meta-analysis: colorectal and small bowel cancer risk in patients with Crohn's disease. *Aliment Pharmacol Ther* 2006;23(8):1097–1104.
20. Evans DB, et al. Small intestine. In: Greene FL, Page DL, Fleming ID, et al., eds. *AJCC Cancer Staging Manual.* 6th ed. New York, NY: Springer; 2002:108.
21. Sarela AI, Brennan MF, Karpeh MS, et al. Adenocarcinoma of the duodenum: importance of accurate lymph node staging and similarity in outcome to gastric cancer. *Ann Surg Oncol* 2004;11(4):380–386.
22. Brennan MF. Surgical management of peripancreatic cancer. In: Karakousis CP, Copeland EM, III, Bland KI, ed. *Atlas of Surgical Oncology.* Philadelphia, Pa: WB Saunders; 1995:473–485.
23. Neoptolemus JP, Talbot IC, Carr-Locke DL, Shaw DE. Treatment and outcome in 52 consecutive cases of ampullary carcinoma. *Br J Surg* 1987;74: 957–961.
24. Warren KW, Choe DS, Plaza J, et al. Results of radical resection for periampullary cancer. *Ann Surg* 1975;181:534–540.
25. Cohen JR, Kutcha N, Geller N, et al. Pancreaticoduodenectomy: a 40 year experience. *Ann Surg* 1982;195:608–617.
26. Lerut JP, Gianello PR, Otte JB, et al. Pancreaticoduodenal resection: surgical experience and evaluation of risk factors in 103 patients. *Ann Surg* 1984;199:432–437.
27. Michelassi F, Erroi F, Dawson PJ, Pietrabissa A. Experience with 647 consecutive tumors of the duodenum, ampulla, head of the pancreas, and distal common bile duct. *Ann Surg* 1989;210:544–556.
28. Chan C, Herrera MF, de la Garza L, Quintanilla-Martinez L. Clinical behavior and prognostic factors of periampullary adenocarcinoma. *Ann Surg* 1995;211:447–458.
29. Monson JR, Donohue JH, McEntee GP, McIlrath DC. Radical resection for carcinoma of the ampulla of Vater. *Arch Surg* 1991;126:353–357.
30. Talamini MA, Moesinger RC, Pitt HA, et al. Adenocarcinoma of the ampullar of Vater: a 28-year experience. *Ann Surg* 1997;225:590–600.
31. Allema JH, Reinders ME, van Gulik TM, van Leeuwen DJ. Results of pancreaticoduodenectomy for ampullary carcinoma and analysis of prognostic factors for survival. *Surgery* 1995;117:247–253.
32. Cameron JL, Crist DW, Sitzmann JV, Hruban RH. Factors influencing survival after pancreaticoduodenectomy for pancreatic cancer. *Am J Surg* 1991; 161:120–124.
33. Whipple AO. A reminiscence: pancreaticoduodenectomy. *Rev Surg* 1963; 20:221–225.
34. Howe JR, Klimstra DS, Moccia RD, et al. Factors predictive of survival in ampullary carcinoma. *Ann Surg* 1998;228(1):87–94.
35. Wheeler JM, Warren BF, Mortensen NJ, Kim HC. An insight into the genetic pathway of adenocarcinoma of the small intestine. *Gut* 2002;50:218–223.
36. Howe JR, Klimstra DS, Cordon-Cardo C, et al. K-ras mutations in adenomas and carcinomas of the ampulla of Vater. *Clin Cancer Res* 1997;3:129–134.
37. McCarthy DM, Hruban RH, Argani P, Howe JR. Role of the DPC4 tumor suppressor gene in adenocarcinoma of the ampulla of Vater: analysis of 140 cases. *Mod Pathol* 2003;16(3):272–278.
38. Lowell JA, Rossi RL, Munson JL, et al. Primary adenocarcinoma of third and fourth portions of the duodenum: favorable prognosis after resection. *Arch Surg* 1992;127:557–560.
39. Abrahams NA, Halverson A, Fazio VW, et al. Adenocarcinoma of the small bowel: a study of 37 cases with emphasis on histologic prognostic factors. *Dis Colon Rectum* 2002;45:1496–1502.

40. Dabaja BS, Suki D, Pro B, et al. Adenocarcinoma of the small bowel: presentation, prognostic factors, and outcome of 217 patients. *Cancer* 2004; 101:518–526.

41. Halsted WS. Contributions to the surgery of the bile duct passages, especially of the common bile duct. *Boston Med Surg J* 1899;141:645–654.

42. Sohn TA, Yeo CJ, Cameron JL, Koniaris L. Resected adenocarcinoma of the pancreas—6161 patients: results, outcomes, and prognostic indicators. *J Gastrointest Surg* 2000;4:567–579.

43. Roggin KK, Yeh JJ, Ferrone CR, Riedel E. Limitations of ampullectomy in the treatment of nonfamilial ampullary neoplasms. *Ann Surg Oncol* 2005; 14(12):971–980.

44. Rose DM, Hochwald SN, Klimstra DS, et al. Primary duodenal adenocarcinoma: a ten-year experience with 79 patients. *J Am Coll Surg* 1996;183: 89–96.

45. Sohn TA, Lillemoe KD, Cameron JL, Pitt HA. Adenocarcinoma of the duodenum: factors influencing long-term survival. *J Gastrointest Surg* 1998;2: 79–87.

46. Barnes G Jr, Romero L, Hess KR, et al. Primary adenocarcinoma of the duodenum: management and survival in 67 patients. *Ann Surg Oncol* 1994;1: 73–78.

47. Ouriel K, Adams JT. Adenocarcinoma of the small intestine. *Am J Surg* 1984; 147:66–71.

48. Howe JR, Karnell LH, Menck HR, et al. Adenocarcinoma of the small bowel: review of the National Cancer Data Base 1985–1995. *Cancer* 1999; 86:2693–2706.

49. Onoder H, Nishitai R, Shimizu K, et al. Small intestinal cancer with extensive lymph node metastases showing complete remission by methotrexate/5-fluorouracil sequential therapy: report of a case. *Surg Today* 1997;27(1): 60–63.

50. Crawley C, Ross P, Norman A, et al. The Royal Marsden experience of a small bowel adenocarcinoma treated with protracted venous infusion 5-fluorouracil. *Br J Cancer* 1998;78(4):508–510.

51. Gibson MK, Holcroft CA, Kvols LK, et al. D. Phase II study of 5-fluorouracil, doxorubicin, and mitomycin C for metastatic small bowel adenocarcinoma. *Oncologist* 2005;10(2):132–137.

52. Fishman PN, Pond GR, Moore MJ, Oza A. National history and chemotherapy effectiveness for advanced adenocarcinoma of the small bowel: a retrospective review of 113 cases. *Am J Clin Oncol* 2006;29(3):225–231.

53. Coia L, Hoffman J, Scher R, Weese. Preoperative chemoradiation for adenocarcinoma of the pancreas and duodenum. *Int J Radiat Oncol Biol Phys* 1994;30(1):161–167.

54. Moertel CG, Sauer WG, Dockerty MG, et al. Life history of the carcinoid tumor of the small intestine. *Cancer* 1961;4:901–912.

55. Bean WB, Olch D, Weinberg HB. The syndrome of carcinoid and acquired valve lesions of the right side of the heart. *Circulation* 1955;12(1):1–6.

56. Sarmiento JM, Heywood G, Rubin J, et al. Surgical treatment of neuroendocrine metastases to the liver: a plea for resection to increase survival. *J Am Coll Surg* 2003;197(1):29–37.

57. Sartori P, Mussi C, Angelini C, et al. Palliative management strategies of advanced gastrointestinal carcinoid neoplasms. *Langenbecks Arch Surg* 2005; 390(5):391–396.

58. Wangberg B, Westberg G, Tylen U, Tisell L. Survival of patients with disseminated midgut carcinoid tumors after aggressive tumor reduction. *World J Surg* 1996;20:892–899.

59. Jones SE, Fuks Z, Bull M, Kadin ME. Non-Hodgkin's lymphomas. IV. Clinicopathologic correlation in 405 cases. *Cancer* 1973;31:806–823.

60. Freeman HJ, Anderson ME, Gascoyne RD. Clinical, pathological, and molecular genetic findings in small intestinal follicle center cell lymphoma. *Can J Gastroenterol* 1997;11:31–34.

61. Shia J, Teruya-Feldstein J, Pan D, Hege A. Primary follicular lymphoma of the gastrointestinal tract—a clinical and pathologic study of 26 cases. *Am J Surg Pathol* 2002;26(2):216–224.

62. Domizio P, Owen RA, Shepherd NA, et al. Primary lymphoma of the small intestine: a clinicopathological study of 119 patients. *Am J Surg Pathol* 1993; 17:429–434.

63. Fletcher CD, Berman JJ, Corless C, Gorstein F. Diagnosis of gastrointestinal stromal tumors: a consensus approach. *Int J Surg Pathol* 2002;10(2): 81–89.

64. DeMatteo RP, Lewis JJ, Leung J, et al. Two hundred gastrointestinal stromal tumors: recurrence patterns and prognostic factors for survival. *Ann Surg* 2000;231(1):51–58.

65. Gold JS, DeMatteo RP. Combined surgical and molecular therapy: the gastrointestinal stromal tumor model. *Ann Surg* 2006;244(2):176–184.

66. Howe JR, Karnell LH, Scott-Conner C. Small bowel sarcoma: analysis of survival from the National Cancer Data Base. *Ann Surg Oncol* 2001;8:496–508.

67. Dougherty MJ, Compton C, Talbert M, et al. Sarcomas of the gastrointestinal tract: separation into favorable and unfavorable prognostic groups by mitotic count. *Ann Surg* 1991;214:569.

68. Elsayed AM, Albahra M, Nzeako UC, et al. Malignant melanoma in the small intestine: a study of 103 patients. *Am J Gastroenterol* 1996;91: 1001–1006.

CHAPTER 52 ■ CANCER OF UNKNOWN PRIMARY SITE

JOHN D. HAINSWORTH AND F. ANTHONY GRECO

Cancer of unknown primary site accounts for approximately 2% of all cancer diagnoses. Despite the fact that this syndrome is not rare, relatively little attention has been given to this group of patients, and systematic study has lagged behind other areas of clinical oncology. The patient with carcinoma of unknown primary site is often stereotyped as an elderly, debilitated individual with metastases at multiple visceral sites. Because early attempts at empiric systemic therapy yielded low response rates and had little effect on survival, there exists widespread pessimism regarding treatment and prognosis of these patients. The heterogeneity of this patient group also makes the design of therapeutic trials difficult; it is well recognized that cancers with different biologies from different primary sites are represented.

Many patients with carcinoma of unknown primary site are initially suspected of having tumors of gastrointestinal origin. Adenocarcinoma accounts for approximately 70% of all unknown primary diagnoses, with an additional 20% of patients having poorly differentiated carcinoma or poorly differentiated adenocarcinoma. Often, metastases are present in intra-abdominal locations, frequently involving the liver, peritoneal surface, and retroperitoneal lymph nodes. Histologically, many adenocarcinomas have various features suggestive of gastrointestinal primaries, including positive staining for mucin, suggestive glandular formation, or signet ring features. Historically, autopsy series (performed prior to the routine use of computed tomography [CT] scanning) documented various abdominal sites (pancreas, stomach, liver, biliary tree, colon) collectively as the most common sites of identifiable primaries (1,2).

This chapter examines the spectrum of unknown primary cancer, with particular emphasis on subsites raising issues related to the management of gastrointestinal malignancies. The predominant focus is on adenocarcinoma and poorly differentiated adenocarcinoma, the most common histologic presentations of unknown primary cancer. Brief sections also discuss poorly differentiated carcinoma and neuroendocrine carcinoma of unknown primary site. The current clinical and pathological evaluations, as well as the recommended treatment for each subtype, are discussed.

ADENOCARCINOMA OF UNKNOWN PRIMARY SITE

Clinical Characteristics

The typical patient with adenocarcinoma of unknown primary site develops symptoms at a metastatic site, but routine history, physical examination, chest radiography, and laboratory studies fail to identify the primary site. Biopsy of a metastatic lesion establishes the diagnosis. In most patients, metastases are present at more than one visceral site; frequent metastatic sites include the liver, lungs, lymph nodes, and bones. The incidence of adenocarcinoma of unknown primary site increases with age.

The clinical course of patients with adenocarcinoma of unknown primary site is usually dominated by symptoms related to the sites of metastases. During the clinical course, the primary site becomes obvious in only 15% to 20% of patients (3). Many patients have widespread metastases and poor performance status at the time of diagnosis; outlook for most of these patients is poor, with median survival of 6 months. However, subsets of patients with much more favorable outlooks are contained within this large group, and optimal initial evaluation enables the identification of these treatable subsets. In addition, empiric chemotherapy incorporating newer agents has produced higher response rates and probably improved survival of patients with good performance status.

Pathology

The light microscopic diagnosis of adenocarcinoma is usually made without difficulty based on the formation of glandular structures of neoplastic cells. Features of adenocarcinoma can be reliably recognized by examining small tissue samples or even by cytology; therefore, fine-needle aspiration biopsy is a reliable diagnostic test in this subset of unknown primary cancer patients. Unfortunately, most adenocarcinomas share common histologic features so examination of tissue from a metastatic site cannot lead to reliable diagnosis of the primary. Several histologic features are especially common in patients with various gastrointestinal primaries; these include well-differentiated glandular structure, signet ring formations, and evidence of mucin production. However, even these features are not specific enough to define a primary site.

Immunoperoxidase stains are also of limited utility in identifying the site of origin of most adenocarcinomas. Positive staining for prostate-specific antigen (PSA) is an exception, reliably identifying the prostate as a site of origin. Immunoperoxidase staining for estrogen receptor and/or progesterone receptor suggest metastatic breast cancer in women with metastatic adenocarcinoma. Other immunoperoxidase stains, particularly the differential expression of cytokeratin 7 versus cytokeratin 20, have been evaluated (4–6). In particular, the staining combination of positive cytokeratin 20/negative CK 7 occurs in approximately 80% of colon cancers (4). Although not specific to colon cancer (e.g., 15% of gastric cancers have similar staining), colonoscopy should be considered in the evaluation of patients with this staining pattern.

The diagnosis of poorly differentiated carcinoma implies the loss of some of the distinctive features of adenocarcinoma and provides the pathologist with even fewer clues as to the site of tumor origin. This diagnosis should be interpreted with caution because some of these patients may have unrecognized tumor types (e.g., poorly differentiated neuroendocrine carcinoma) with specific treatment implications. The diagnosis of poorly differentiated adenocarcinoma is usually made when only minimal glandular formation is seen in histologic examination. However, the diagnosis is sometimes made based on positive mucin staining, even when no glandular features are present on histologic examination. It is clear that adenocarcinoma, poorly differentiated adenocarcinoma, and poorly differentiated carcinoma are diagnoses representing parts of a spectrum of tumor differentiation rather than specific, sharply demarcated entities. Different pathologists may use slightly different criteria for making each of these three diagnoses. Therefore, additional immunoperoxidase staining is appropriate in most patients with the initial diagnosis of poorly differentiated adenocarcinoma to identify specific subtypes. At present, evaluation and treatment of patients with poorly differentiated adenocarcinoma should follow guidelines outlined for poorly differentiated carcinoma.

The identification of increasing numbers of oncoproteins that define the malignant phenotype and are prognostically important has become a primary focus in the characterization of tumors. Some of these substances (e.g., epidermal growth factor, vascular endothelial growth factor, HER-2) are now targets for novel therapeutic agents. A substantial percentage of unknown primary cancers are known to overexpress p53, Bcl-2, Cmyc, RAS, and EGFR (7,8). However, the value of these markers in predicting prognosis or determining therapy is currently undefined.

The development of molecular pathology techniques enabling genetic profiling of specific cancer types may greatly modify the approach to patients with adenocarcinoma of unknown primary site in the future. Characteristic gene expression profiles have already been identified for many solid tumor types. A number of studies have recently shown that accurate classification of solid tumor types can be made based on specific expression of a limited number of genes (9,10). With reduced numbers of genes involved, quantitative polymerase chain reaction techniques can be used rather than microarray, enabling testing in formalin-fixed, paraffinized tissue (11).

More recently, several different DNA microarray platforms have been tested for their ability to successfully identify cancer types. Using a platform containing 79 gene markers, Tothill et al. identified specimens (primary or metastatic) from 14 known tumor types with 89% accuracy (12). Several gastrointestinal primary sites were included in this evaluation. In addition, a small group of specimens from patients with carcinoma of unknown primary site were tested. In 11 of 13 cases, the primary site was predicted with high confidence; in most cases, the predicted primary site was compatible with clinical features of the patient.

At present, several studies are ongoing to validate the ability of various microarray platforms to reliably identify primary sites in patients with carcinoma of unknown primary site. If predicted primary sites reliably correlate with suggestive clinical features, response to treatment, and observed tumor biology, these procedures will become vital diagnostic tools and will greatly reduce the number of patients with the final diagnosis of carcinoma of unknown primary site.

Diagnostic Evaluation

If a primary site is not evident in a patient with metastatic cancer after a basic evaluation (history, physical examination, complete blood counts, biochemistry profile, urinalysis, and chest radiography), several additional tests should be performed. All men should have a serum PSA determination, and women with clinical presentation compatible with metastatic breast cancer should undergo mammography because specific palliative therapy is available for patients with advanced prostate or breast cancer. CT of the abdomen should be performed in all patients because primary sites are identified in 10% to 35% of patients, and additional metastatic sites are often recognized (13,14). Positron emission tomography (PET) identifies a primary site in up to 30% of patients and is therefore a useful diagnostic procedure (15,16). Additional signs or symptoms should be evaluated with appropriate radiologic studies.

In patients who have no primary site identified after the previous diagnostic procedures are completed, further evaluation is extremely unlikely to demonstrate a primary site. In general, extensive radiologic evaluation of asymptomatic areas and routine gastrointestinal endoscopy should be avoided. However, the yield of endoscopy may be somewhat higher in patients with intra-abdominal presentations (e.g., predominant liver metastases, peritoneal carcinomatosis), particularly if histologic features are suggestive of a gastrointestinal primary site. In this relatively select group of patients, endoscopic evaluation of the gastrointestinal tract should be considered.

Commonly used serum tumor markers, including carcinoembryonic antigen, cancer antigen (CA) 19-9, CA 15-3, CA 125, human chorionic gonadotropin, and alpha-fetoprotein are frequently elevated in patients with carcinoma of unknown primary site. However, these markers are nonspecific and are rarely useful in defining a primary site (17,18). However, elevated serum tumor markers are frequently useful in monitoring response to therapy.

TREATMENT

Within the large and heterogeneous group of patients with adenocarcinoma of unknown primary site, several subsets with favorable prognosis can be identified based on clinical features. Specific treatment guidelines are available for these patients. In this chapter, special attention is given to those subsets with a gastrointestinal presentation.

Peritoneal Carcinomatosis

Adenocarcinoma with predominant or exclusive involvement of the peritoneal surface is more common in women than in men. Most women presenting with this syndrome have an easily identifiable primary tumor in the ovary, although occasionally cancer arising in the breast or gastrointestinal tract can present in this manner. Women who develop peritoneal carcinomatosis in the absence of an identifiable primary site should always be approached as if they had ovarian cancer. This syndrome can develop in women with normal ovaries or a history of previous oophorectomy, and occurs with increased incidence in women with BRCA-1 mutations (19,20). Many women with this syndrome have histologic features typical of ovarian carcinoma, such as papillary configuration or psammoma bodies. Serum CA 125 levels are usually elevated. When histologic features suggest ovarian carcinoma, this syndrome has been termed "peritoneal papillary serous carcinoma" or "multifocal extraovarian serous carcinoma."

Women with this syndrome often respond well to the chemotherapy regimens effective in the treatment of advanced ovarian carcinoma (Table 52.1). Initial response rates are high, and long-term remissions occur in 15% to 20% of patients (21–26). Recent reports have documented the activity of platinum/paclitaxel regimens, as used in patients with advanced

TABLE 52.1

RESULTS OF PLATINUM-BASED THERAPY FOR WOMEN WITH
ADENOCARCINOMA INVOLVING THE PERITONEUM

Author (ref)	Chemotherapy regimen	Number of patients	Response rate	5-Year survival rate
Strnad et al. (21)	Cisplatin based	18	39%	28% (3-year)
Ransom et al. (23)	Cisplatin based	33	NA	20%
Fromm et al. (24)	Cisplatin/cyclophosphamide	44	64%	22%
Bloss et al. (25)	Cisplatin/cyclophosphamide ± doxorubicin	33	64%	15%
Piver et al. (26)	Cisplatin/cyclophosphamide/ doxorubicin or cisplatin/ paclitaxel	46	66%	NA

NA, not applicable.

ovarian carcinoma (27). Most long-term remissions have been observed in patients who undergo successful surgical cytoreduction prior to the administration of chemotherapy.

The peritoneal epithelium is now accepted as a site of origin for some of the women with these carcinomas. The contiguity of the peritoneal and ovarian epithelial surfaces may explain the similar biology of these two tumor types. In fact, these tumors are now believed to be similar enough that women with peritoneal papillary serous carcinoma are routinely included in clinical trials for stage III ovarian carcinoma. At present, optimal management for women with this syndrome should include initial maximal surgical cytoreduction followed by taxane/platinum chemotherapy (27,28). For women with minimal residual disease after surgical cytoreduction, intraperitoneal chemotherapy may also play a role in treatment (29).

Most men presenting with peritoneal carcinomatosis do not have tumors that are highly responsive to chemotherapy. Presumably, most men with this syndrome have occult tumors of gastrointestinal primary origin. Occasional men have been reported with papillary adenocarcinoma and elevated serum CA125 levels (30). In these men, a trial of a taxane/platinum-based regimen, as used for ovarian cancer, seems reasonable. For other men presenting with peritoneal carcinomatosis, a trial of empiric chemotherapy for adenocarcinoma of unknown primary site should be considered. In addition, women with this syndrome who do not respond promptly to a taxane/platinum-based regimen are likely to have occult gastrointestinal primary sites, and a second-line empiric regimen effective in the treatment of gastrointestinal malignancies should be considered. Primary peritoneal mesothelioma is also a diagnostic consideration in these patients and is discussed in detail in Chapter 53.

Adenocarcinoma Presenting as a Single Metastatic Lesion

Occasionally, only a single metastatic lesion can be identified after a complete staging evaluation. Such single lesions have been described in a wide variety of sites, including lymph nodes, liver, brain, lung, adrenal gland, bone, and subcutaneous tissue. The possibility of a primary tumor in an unusual site (rather than a metastasis) should always be considered in such situations, but this possibility can usually be excluded on the basis of clinical or pathological features.

In most of these patients, other metastatic sites are recognized within a relatively short time. However, some patients have prolonged disease-free intervals following effective local

therapy of a single metastatic lesion. Prior to initiating local treatment, a PET scan is useful to rule out the presence of other unsuspected metastatic sites (31). If no other metastases are detectable, definitive local therapy of the solitary lesion should proceed. In most instances, surgical resection is preferable if technically feasible. Occasional patients with long-term survival following definitive treatment of a single "metastatic" lesion have been described (32). The role of systemic chemotherapy in addition to definitive local therapy is undefined; however, patients with poorly differentiated adenocarcinoma may benefit from empiric platinum-based therapy.

The most common gastrointestinal presentation with a single lesion involves a single liver lesion. Distinction between a primary hepatoma or hepatobiliary carcinoma versus a metastatic lesion is sometimes problematic. However, histologic features and/or specialized immunohistochemical staining are usually successful in identifying hepatobiliary origin. Immunoperoxidase staining patterns typical for hepatobiliary tumors include positive alpha-fetoprotein, polyclonal but not monoclonal carcinoembryonic antigen, and loss of reticulin staining. In patients who are surgical candidates, hepatic resection should be considered. In patients who are not surgical candidates but have tumor diameter ≤5 cm, radiofrequency ablation can provide excellent local control (see Chapter 33 for a detailed discussion of ablative techniques) (33). Other local therapies (e.g., stereotactic radiation, chemoembolization) may also be useful in selected patients. Patients with inadequate local control after attempted local therapy or those who develop additional metastases should be considered for empiric chemotherapy.

Women With Axillary Lymph Node Metastases

Metastatic breast cancer should be suspected in women who have axillary lymph node involvement with adenocarcinoma. Initial lymph node biopsy should include measurement of estrogen/progesterone receptors and HER-2 oncoprotein; elevated levels provide strong evidence for the diagnosis of breast cancer (34). Breast MRI scanning and PET scanning may identify a breast primary site even when mammography is normal (35,36). Women with metastases isolated to ipsilateral lymph nodes after complete evaluation should be managed according to guidelines for stage II breast cancer, whereas women with additional metastatic sites should receive treatment effective for metastatic breast cancer. Gastrointestinal tumor origin is usually not a clinical suspicion in this patient group; further discussion of management of these patients can be found elsewhere.

Men With Skeletal Metastases

Metastatic prostate carcinoma should be suspected in men with adenocarcinoma predominantly involving bone, particularly if the metastases are blastic. Elevated serum levels of PSA or tumor staining with PSA provides confirmatory evidence of prostate cancer. Treatment of these patients should follow guidelines for advanced prostate cancer. Occasionally, patients have been reported with clinical presentations atypical for prostate cancer, in whom the diagnosis was supported only by elevation of serum PSA (37,38). Most of these patients had adenopathy (retroperitoneal, mediastinal) or lung metastases; other intra-abdominal presentations are extremely rare.

Empiric Chemotherapy for Adenocarcinoma of Unknown Primary Site

Most patients with adenocarcinoma of unknown primary site do not fit into any of the specific clinical subgroups with favorable prognosis. During the 1980s, many of the empiric chemotherapy regimens evaluated in these patients were relatively ineffective 5-fluorouracil (5-FU) or doxorubicin-based regimens then employed for the treatment of advanced gastrointestinal primary tumors. These regimens, predictably, produced low response rates and had no convincing impact on patient survival. Results with many such regimens (e.g., single-agent 5-FU, doxorubicin/mitomycin, fluorouracil/doxorubicin/mitomycin [FAM]) were similar, with response rates in the 10% to 30% range, and median survivals from 4 to 8 months (39–51).

During the 1990s, several novel agents, including the taxanes, the topoisomerase I inhibitors, gemcitabine, vinorelbine, and oxaliplatin, have improved the treatment of a variety of advanced solid tumors. Although some of these agents have been investigated in the empiric treatment of adenocarcinoma of unknown primary site, only the taxanes have been thoroughly evaluated. Table 52.2 provides a summary of empiric

chemotherapy results using combinations containing newer agents. Most regimens contain a taxane and a platinum agent, although a few studies have incorporated gemcitabine and/or irinotecan (52–62). Results with these newer regimens suggest increased efficacy in the empiric treatment of adenocarcinoma of unknown primary site. Response rates are higher than those reported with previous empiric regimens and range from 25% to 55%. The median survivals also seem superior to previous regimens and are usually at least 9 months. When reported, 2-year survivals with these newer regimens are usually in the 20% to 25% range. Unfortunately, no randomized, comparative trials have been performed, and the optimum regimen remains undefined.

The relatively limited experience with newer chemotherapeutic agents and the absence of experience with any of the targeted agents creates a difficult situation for empiric treatment of patients who are clinically suspected of having a gastrointestinal primary site. For cancers of most gastrointestinal primary sites (with the possible exception of gastric cancer), regimens other than taxane/platinum combinations are used in standard treatment. To date, there has been no evaluation of the FOLFOX or FOLFIRI regimens, with or without bevacizumab, in patients with adenocarcinoma of unknown primary site. However, in patients who have a strong clinical suspicion of a GI primary site, empiric use of these regimens seems reasonable and appropriate. As regimens for gastrointestinal cancers continue to improve, the importance of selecting the "correct" regimen will increase.

Experience with second-line empiric chemotherapy is limited in patients with adenocarcinoma of unknown primary site. Single-agent gemcitabine, or the combination of gemcitabine/irinotecan, have modest activity following taxane/platinum combinations, but both give objective response rates of ≤15% (62,63). More recently, the combination of bevacizumab and erlotinib became the first regimen containing targeted agents to be evaluated in patients with carcinoma of unknown primary site (64). In a group of 51 patients previously treated with chemotherapy, the combination of bevacizumab (10 mg/kg IV every 2 weeks) and erlotinib (150 mg orally daily) produced objective response or disease stabilization in 67% when reevaluated at 2 months. The median survival in this group was 7.4 months, with 33% of patients alive at 1 year. These results compare favorably to other regimens tested as second-line

TABLE 52.2

EMPIRIC FIRST-LINE TREATMENT FOR ADENOCARCINOMA OF UNKNOWN PRIMARY SITES—RESULTS WITH NEWER CHEMOTHERAPY REGIMENS

Regimen (ref)	Number of patients	Response rate	Median survival (months)	2-Year survival rate
TAXANE/PLATINUM BASED				
PC (53)	77	39%	13	20%
PCE (52,56)	71	48%	11	20%
PCG (57)	113	25%	9	23%
PCE/GI (60)	132	30%	9	16%
DC (54,55)	92	43%	10	24%
OTHER REGIMENS				
GC (58)	40	55%	8	NA
IC (58)	40	38%	6	NA
DG (59)	35	40%	10	7%

P, paclitaxel; C, carboplatin or cisplatin; E, etoposide; G, gemcitabine; I, irinotecan; D, docetaxel; NA, not applicable.

treatment and are actually comparable to first-line survival results. Continued evaluation of regimens containing targeted agents is necessary in patients with adenocarcinoma of unknown primary site.

At present, all patients with good performance status should be considered for a trial of empiric chemotherapy. Based on existing clinical trial data, a taxane/platinum combination is appropriate for most patients. For patients who are strongly suspected of having a gastrointestinal primary site, empiric therapy with other highly effective GI regimens (e.g., FOLFOX + bevacizumab) is also reasonable. Additional clinical trials are urgently needed to better address these questions. Patients with poor performance status are much less likely to benefit from chemotherapy, and in some of these patients, optimal management may include supportive measures only.

POORLY DIFFERENTIATED CARCINOMA OF UNKNOWN PRIMARY SITE

Patients with poorly differentiated carcinoma account for approximately 20% of all patients with unknown primary site; an additional 10% of patients have poorly differentiated adenocarcinoma. This group of patients is also a heterogeneous group; some patients have neoplasms that are extremely responsive to chemotherapy, and some have the potential for long-term survival. Appropriate clinical and pathological evaluations are therefore critical in patients with poorly differentiated carcinoma so optimal therapy can be administered.

Pathological Evaluation

The pathological evaluation of a poorly differentiated carcinoma requires specialized pathological testing in addition to light microscopic examination. Additional tests are critical because some responsive tumors of well-defined types (e.g., germ cell tumor, lymphoma) are occasionally difficult to identify by histologic features alone.

Immunoperoxidase staining is currently the most widely available adjunctive tool for the classification of neoplasms. In contrast to most other specialized pathological techniques, immunoperoxidase staining can be performed on formalin-fixed, paraffinized tissue, which broadens its applicability. However, specific diagnoses cannot be made on the basis of immunoperoxidase staining alone because none of these reagents are directed at tumor-specific antigens. Therefore, results must be interpreted in conjunction with the light microscopic appearance. At times, clinical features can also be used to support a diagnosis. Clinical information (e.g., gender, age, location of metastases, symptoms) may help the pathologist narrow the differential diagnosis, thereby reducing the number of special stains required to reach a diagnosis.

In the evaluation of poorly differentiated carcinoma, several questions can usually be answered by immunoperoxidase staining. First, and most important, these stains can reliably distinguish lymphoma from carcinoma (65). Second, staining for chromogranin and/or synaptophysin can suggest a neuroendocrine carcinoma (e.g., small cell lung cancer, carcinoid tumor, islet cell tumor) (66). Third, staining for PSA strongly suggests prostate carcinoma in a male with metastatic poorly differentiated adenocarcinoma (67). Finally, certain staining characteristics can suggest amelanotic melanoma (staining for S-100 protein, HMB-45 antigen, vimentin) or sarcoma (staining for desmin, vimentin, or factor VIII antigen) (68,69).

Electron microscopy also plays a role in the pathological evaluation of poorly differentiated tumors because specific ultrastructural features are sometimes present. Because it is less widely available and requires special tissue fixation at the time of biopsy or rebiopsy, electron microscopy should be reserved for the study of neoplasms whose lineage is unclear after routine light microscopy and immunoperoxidase staining. Like immunoperoxidase staining, electron microscopy is extremely reliable in distinguishing lymphoma from carcinoma and is probably superior in the identification of poorly differentiated sarcoma. Other specific structures, such as neurosecretory granules (neuroendocrine tumors) or premelanosomes (melanoma), are also seen in some poorly differentiated neoplasms and allow specific diagnoses to be made. However, in the majority of patients found to have poorly differentiated carcinoma by histologic examination, electron microscopy confirms the diagnosis of carcinoma but does not result in a more specific diagnosis.

Occasionally, the identification of tumor-specific chromosomal abnormalities can lead to a diagnosis in the evaluation of poorly differentiated neoplasms. In the evaluation of poorly differentiated carcinoma, the ability to prospectively identify patients with germ cell tumors is of great importance. Most germ cell tumors have a distinctive and diagnostic i(12p) chromosomal abnormality (70). By detecting the presence of the i(12p) abnormality, germ cell tumors have been diagnosed in a group of young men with poorly differentiated carcinoma and clinical features of extragonadal germ cell tumor (i.e., mediastinal and/or retroperitoneal masses) (71). Patients who have extragonadal germ cell tumor diagnosed in this manner have treatment outcome similar to other patients with histologically typical extragonadal germ cell tumors.

Diagnostic Evaluation

The initial diagnostic evaluation of patients with poorly differentiated carcinoma is similar to that previously described for patients with adenocarcinoma of unknown primary site. A thorough history, physical examination, routine laboratory testing, and chest radiograph should be obtained in all patients. CT of the chest and abdomen, as well as a PET scan, should also be performed. Serum levels of human chorionic gonadotropin (HCG) and alpha-fetoprotein (AFP) should be obtained in all patients; significant elevations of these markers suggest the diagnosis of germ cell tumor.

Treatment

When specialized pathological studies identify a treatable neoplasm, therapy should be administered following guidelines established for the specific tumor identified. Examples of such tumor types occasionally identified in this group of patients include anaplastic lymphoma, Ewing tumor, neuroendocrine carcinoma, germ cell carcinoma, and undifferentiated sarcomas.

Young men with clinical features strongly suggestive of extragonadal germ cell tumor (predominant location in the mediastinum or retroperitoneum; marked elevations of HCG or AFP) should be treated according to guidelines established for extragonadal germ cell tumor. In some of these patients, the detection of an i(12p) chromosomal abnormality allows for a specific diagnosis. Even when this test is negative or cannot be obtained, empiric therapy for poor risk germ cell tumor should be administered to this group of patients.

Treatment of patients with poorly differentiated carcinoma of unknown primary site who do not have characteristics of extragonadal germ cell tumor is controversial. Most investigators have documented a higher response rate to empiric chemotherapy in this group of patients versus those with adenocarcinoma of unknown primary site (72–75). Other clinical features associated with a higher response rate and better treatment outcome included tumor location in lymph nodes, fewer metastatic sites, younger age, and female gender. Patients with liver and/or bone metastases did relatively poorly. In one large retrospective series, treatment with cisplatin-based regimens effective for germ cell tumors produced a 26% complete response rate, with 14% of patients alive and disease free more than 8 years later (72,76). However, this group of patients with poorly differentiated carcinoma was a selected group with a young median age (39 years) and frequent clinical features of extragonadal germ cell tumor. Other investigators have not documented a cohort of long-term survivors in the group of patients with poorly differentiated carcinoma (74).

At present, a trial of combination chemotherapy should be considered for most patients with poorly differentiated carcinoma or poorly differentiated adenocarcinoma of unknown primary site. For patients who do not have features of extragonadal germ cell tumor, the taxane/platinum combinations evaluated in adenocarcinoma of unknown primary site are relatively well tolerated and seem a reasonable choice. For patients with intra-abdominal metastases and clinical features strongly suggestive of a gastrointestinal primary site, empiric treatment with an accepted gastrointestinal regimen (e.g., FOLFOX plus bevacizumab, FOLFIRI) also seems reasonable but has not been specifically evaluated.

NEUROENDOCRINE CARCINOMA OF UNKNOWN PRIMARY SITE

A broad spectrum of neuroendocrine neoplasia is now recognized, in part due to improved pathological methods for making this diagnosis. Most adult neuroendocrine tumors have indolent biologies and typical histologic features (e.g., carcinoid tumors, islet cell tumors, paragangliomas, pheochromocytomas). Many of these histologic types originate in the abdomen or gastrointestinal tract (see Chapter 48 for a detailed discussion of gastrointestinal neuroendocrine tumors). A second group of neuroendocrine tumors, typified by a "small cell" anaplastic appearance on histologic examination, are high-grade tumors with aggressive biology. Small cell lung cancer is the most common cancer in this subgroup, but small cell neuroendocrine carcinomas can arise from a variety of gastrointestinal sites (77). Finally, a third group of neuroendocrine tumors has high-grade biology and no distinctive neuroendocrine features by light microscopy. In this group, the initial diagnosis is usually "poorly differentiated carcinoma" or "poorly differentiated adenocarcinoma." Neuroendocrine features are recognized only when immunoperoxidase staining or electron microscopy is performed. Neuroendocrine tumors of unknown primary site occur in each of these three categories, and should be considered separately in terms of diagnostic evaluation and treatment.

Low-Grade Neuroendocrine Carcinoma

Metastatic carcinoid or islet cell tumors are occasionally found at metastatic sites without an obvious primary site. In this situation, the metastatic tumor almost always involves the liver, but occasionally bone involvement predominates. Some of these patients have clinical syndromes produced by tumor secretion of bioactive substances. Because these tumor types usually originate in the gastrointestinal tract, a thorough evaluation including upper and lower GI endoscopy as well as an ^{111}In-DTPA-octreotide scan (Octreoscan) should be performed. Primary sites in the intestine and pancreas can be identified with

these studies; in other patients, these primary sites are identified during the clinical course.

Carcinoid or islet cell tumors of unknown primary site usually exhibit an indolent biology, and management should follow guidelines established for metastatic tumors of these types with known primary sites. Appropriate management may include local therapy (resection of isolated metastases, radiofrequency ablation, hepatic artery chemoembolization), treatment with somatostatin analogs, palliative chemotherapy, or symptomatic management. Intensive, platinum-based chemotherapy has not been useful in this group of patients.

Small Cell Carcinoma

Patients with small cell anaplastic carcinoma at a metastatic site usually have a bronchogenic primary. CT of the chest and fiber-optic bronchoscopy should be performed in these patients because they often identify the primary site. However, a large number of extrapulmonary primary sites have also been identified (e.g., esophagus, colon, rectum, bladder, prostate, ovary, cervix), and patients with localizing symptoms should have appropriate diagnostic studies performed.

Patients who have no primary site detected after complete evaluation should receive a trial of empiric chemotherapy. Most patients in this group have tumors with a high mitotic rate and aggressive biology. Unlike the low-grade neuroendocrine tumors described previously, these tumors are initially highly sensitive to chemotherapy. Although the "optimal" chemotherapy regimen is not defined, combination regimens effective in the treatment of small cell lung cancer are recommended.

Poorly Differentiated Neuroendocrine Carcinoma

Neuroendocrine features are identified in approximately 10% to 15% of patients with the initial diagnosis of poorly differentiated carcinoma of unknown primary site. Such patients have widely varying clinical presentations, but all have high-grade, rapidly progressive neoplasms. Most patients have multiple metastases, although a small subset has disease limited to a single site. Syndromes associated with tumor secretion of bioactive substances are rare in these patients.

The origin of these poorly differentiated neuroendocrine tumors remains unclear, but it is likely that the group is heterogeneous. Some patients may have small cell lung cancer with an "occult" primary site. However, this diagnosis is unlikely in most of these patients because many have no smoking history, and no evidence of metastatic tumor in the chest. Some of these tumors are probably undifferentiated variants of well-recognized neuroendocrine tumors, particularly carcinoid tumors. In the undifferentiated form, the clinical and pathological characteristics no longer resemble the characteristics of the more common well-differentiated tumors. Anaplastic carcinoids with known primary sites have been described; these carcinoid variants have demonstrated sensitivity to cisplatin-based chemotherapy (77,78).

Like other high-grade neuroendocrine carcinomas, poorly differentiated neuroendocrine carcinomas are highly sensitive to combination chemotherapy. In a retrospective series of 43 patients treated with combination chemotherapy effective in the treatment of small cell lung cancer, an overall response rate of 71% was obtained, with 28% complete responses (79). More recently, a group of 48 patients with poorly differentiated neuroendocrine carcinoma of unknown primary site were treated in a prospective study with the combination of paclitaxel, carboplatin, and etoposide (80). In this large group of

TABLE 52.3

CARCINOMA OF UNKNOWN PRIMARY SITE: EVALUATION AND TREATMENT OF SPECIFIC SUBSETS

Histopathology	Clinical evaluation (in addition to history, physical exam, routine laboratory, chest radiography)	Special pathological studies	Specific subsets for therapy	Therapy
Adenocarcinoma (well differentiated or moderately differentiated)	CT scan of abdomen, chest PET scan Men: serum PSA Women: mammograms Additional studies to evaluate signs, symptoms	Men: PSA stain Women: ER, PR stain	1) Women, peritoneal carcinomatosis 2) Solitary metastatic lesion 3) Women, axillary node involvement 4) Men, blastic bone metastases, or high serum PSA or tumor PSA staining	Treat as stage III ovarian cancer Definitive local therapy Treat as primary breast cancer Treat as stage IV prostate cancer
Poorly differentiated carcinoma	PET scan CT abdomen, chest Serum HCG, AFP Additional studies to evaluate signs, symptoms	Immunoperoxidase staining, electron microscopy, cytogenetic studies	1) Features of EGCT 2) Other patients	Treat as nonseminomatous EGCT Empiric platinum or paclitaxel/platinum regimen
Neuroendocrine carcinoma	CT scan of abdomen, chest Additional studies to evaluate signs, symptoms	Immunoperoxidase staining	1) Low grade 2) Small cell carcinoma or poorly differentiated	Treat as advanced carcinoid tumor Empiric platinum/etoposide or platinum/etoposide/paclitaxel

CT, computed tomography; PET, positron emission tomography; PSA, prostate-specific antigen; ER, estrogen receptor; PR, progesterone receptor; HCG, human chorionic gonadotropin; AFP, α-fetoprotein; EGCT, extragonadal germ cell tumor.

patients, the overall response rate to this three-drug regimen was 55%, with 13% complete responders. The median survival for this group of patients was 14.5 months, and 14% of patients had 5-year survival.

Appropriate evaluation and accurate diagnosis of patients with poorly differentiated neuroendocrine carcinoma is therefore important because effective treatment is available. Liver metastases and other intra-abdominal metastatic sites are frequent, and the possibility of a poorly differentiated neuroendocrine carcinoma should be considered in patients with poorly differentiated carcinoma. Recognition of neuroendocrine carcinoma in these patients may make a difference in the selection of empiric therapy because the regimens recommended for neuroendocrine carcinoma differ from those used for gastrointestinal adenocarcinomas. All patients with poorly differentiated neuroendocrine carcinoma of unknown primary site should receive a trial of therapy, using a platinum/etoposide-based regimen. The occasional patient with a single metastatic site may also benefit from local therapy with either surgical excision or radiation therapy.

SUMMARY AND FUTURE DIRECTIONS

The recognition of treatable subsets within the heterogeneous population of patients with carcinoma of unknown primary site has improved the management and treatment of these patients. Table 52.3 provides a summary of the recognized subsets, and outlines the recommended evaluation and treatment. Empiric chemotherapy for patients who do not fit into any defined subset has also improved. At present, taxane/platinum-based chemotherapy regimens have been the most thoroughly evaluated and produce median survivals of 9 to 11 months, with 2-year survivals of 20% to 25%. All patients with adequate performance status should be considered for a trial of empiric chemotherapy.

During the next several years, clinical research regarding carcinoma of unknown primary site will focus on three specific areas. First, the use of molecular profiling of tumors to identify a primary site will be of major importance. Several potential DNA microarray platforms are currently being tested in carcinomas of unknown primary; validation of these diagnostic techniques will enable specific treatment based on the identified primary site and will greatly narrow the spectrum of patients with unknown primary tumors. Second, further evaluation of empiric chemotherapy regimens is required. Several highly active combination regimens frequently employed in the treatment of gastrointestinal primary tumors (e.g., FOLFOX, FOLFIRI, IFL) are untested in patients with carcinoma of unknown primary site. Randomized, comparative trials of promising regimens are also now indicated. Finally, various targeted agents have been successfully introduced in the treatment of many common solid tumors. It is likely that these agents will also benefit patients with unknown primary site. Further evaluation of targeted agents, either alone or in combination with chemotherapy, is a priority in improving treatment for patients with carcinoma of unknown primary site. It is likely that treatment of these patients will continue to improve in parallel with improvements in the treatment of other relatively resistant epithelial tumors.

References

1. Nystrom JS, Weiner JM, Heffelfinger-Juttner J, et al. Metastatic and histologic presentations in unknown primary cancer. *Semin Oncol* 1977;4:53–58.
2. Mayordomo JI, Guerra JM, Guijarro C, et al. Neoplasms of unknown primary site. A clinicopathological study of autopsied patients. *Tumori* 1993; 79:321–324.
3. Shildt RA, Kennedy PS, Chen TT, et al. Management of patients with metastatic adenocarcinoma of unknown origin: a Southwest Oncology Group study. *Cancer Treat Rep* 1983;67:77–79.
4. Tot T. Adenocarcinomas metastatic to the liver: the value of cytokeratins 20 and 7 in the search for unknown primary tumors. *Cancer* 1999;85:171–174.
5. Brown RW, Campagna LB, Dunn JK, Cagle PT. Immunohistochemical identification of tumor markers in metastatic adenocarcinoma: a diagnostic adjunct in the determination of primary site. *Am J Clin Pathol* 1997;107:12–15.
6. Lagendijk JH, Mullink H, VanDiest PJ, et al. Tracing the origin of adenocarcinomas with unknown primary using immunohistochemistry: differential diagnosis between colonic and ovarian carcinomas as primary sites. *Hum Pathol* 1998;29:491–495.
7. Briasoulis E, Tsakos M, Fountzilas G, et al. Bcl2 and p53 protein expression in metastatic carcinoma of unknown primary origin: biological and clinical implications. A Hellenic Cooperative Oncology Group study. *Anticancer Res* 1998;18:1907–1914.
8. Pavlidis N, Briasoulis E, Baj M, et al. Overexpression of C-myc, Ras and C-erB-2 oncoproteins in carcinoma of unknown primary origin. *Anticancer Res* 1995;15:2563–2568.
9. Shedden KA, Taylor JM, Giordano TJ, et al. Accurate molecular classification of human cancers based on gene expression using a simple classifier with a pathological tree-based framework. *Am J Pathol* 2003;163:1985–1995.
10. Bloom G, Yang IV, Boulware D, et al. Multi-platform multi-side, microarray-based human tumor classification. *Am J Pathol* 2004;164:9–16.
11. Cronin M, Pho M, Dutta D, et al. Measurement of gene expression in archival paraffin-embedded tissues: development and performance of a 92-gene reverse transcriptase-polymerase chain reaction assay. *Am J Pathol* 2004; 164:35–42.
12. Tothill RW, Kowalczyk A, Rischin D, et al. An expression-based site of origin diagnostic method designed for clinical application to cancer of unknown origin. *Cancer Res* 2005;65:4031–4040.
13. Karsell PR, Sheedy PF, O'Connell MJ. Computerized tomography in search of cancer of unknown origin. *JAMA* 1982;248:340–343.
14. McMillan JH, Levine E, Stephens RH. Computed tomography in the evaluation of metastatic adenocarcinoma from an unknown primary site. *Radiology* 1982;143:143–146.
15. Kole AC, Nieweg OE, Pruim J, et al. Detection of unknown occult primary tumors using positron emission tomography. *Cancer* 1998;82:1160–1166.
16. Bohuslavski KH, Klutmann S, Kroger S, et al. FDG PET detection of unknown primary tumors. *J Nucl Med* 2000;41:816–822.
17. Currow DC, Findlay M, Cox K, Harnett PR. Elevated germ cell markers in carcinoma of unknown primary site do not predict response to platinum-based chemotherapy. *Eur J Cancer* 1996;32A:2357–2359.
18. Pavlidis N, Kalef-Ezra J, Briasoulis E, et al. Evaluation of six tumor markers in patients with carcinoma of unknown primary. *Med Pediatr Oncol* 1994;22:162–167.
19. Tobacman JK, Greene MH, Tucker MA, et al. Intra-abdominal carcinomatosis after prophylactic oophorectomy in ovarian cancer-prone families. *Lancet* 1982;2:795–796.
20. Schorge JO, Muto MG, Welch WR, et al. Molecular evidence for multifocal papillary serous carcinoma of the peritoneum in patients with germ-line BRCA1 mutations. *J Natl Cancer Inst* 1998;90:841–845.
21. Strnad CM, Grosh WW, Baxter J, et al. Peritoneal carcinomatosis of unknown primary site in women. *Ann Intern Med* 1989;111:213–217.
22. Dalrymple JC, Bannatyne P, Russell P, et al. Extraovarian peritoneal serous papillary carcinoma: a clinicopathologic study of 31 cases. *Cancer* 1989;64: 110–115.
23. Ransom DT, Patel SR, Kenney GL, et al. Papillary serous carcinoma of the peritoneum: a review of 33 cases treated with cisplatin-based chemotherapy. *Cancer* 1990;66:1091–1094.
24. Fromm GL, Gershenson DM, Silva EG. Papillary serous carcinoma of the peritoneum. *Obstet Gynecol* 1990;75:75–79.
25. Bloss JD, Liao SY, Buller RE, et al. Extraovarian peritoneal serous papillary carcinoma: a case-control retrospective comparison to papillary adenocarcinoma of the ovary. *Gynecol Oncol* 1993;50:347–351.
26. Piver MS, Eltabbakh GH, Hempling RE, et al. Two sequential studies for primary peritoneal carcinoma: induction with weekly cisplatin followed by either cisplatin/doxorubicin/cyclophosphamide or paclitaxel/cisplatin. *Gynecol Oncol* 1997;67:141–146.
27. McGuire WP, Hoskins WJ, Brady MF, et al. Cyclophosphamide and cisplatin compared with paclitaxel and cisplatin in patients with stage III and stage IV ovarian cancer. *N Engl J Med* 1996;334:1–6.
28. Vasey PA, Jayson GC, Gordon A, et al. Phase III randomized trial of docetaxel-carboplatin versus paclitaxel-carboplatin as first-line chemotherapy for ovarian carcinoma. *J Natl Cancer Inst* 2004;96:1682–1691.
29. Armstrong DK, Bundy B, Wenzel L, et al. Intraperitoneal cisplatin and paclitaxel in ovarian cancer. *N Engl J Med* 2006;354:34–43.
30. Shah IA, Jayram L, Gani OS, et al. Papillary serous carcinoma of the peritoneum in a man: a case report. *Cancer* 1998;82:860–866.
31. Rades D, Kuhnel G, Wildfang I, et al. Localised disease in cancer of unknown primary (CUP): the value of positron emission tomography (PET) for individual therapeutic management. *Ann Oncol* 2001;12:1605–1609.
32. Nguyen LN, Maor MH, Oswald MJ. Brain metastases as the only manifestation of an undetected primary tumor. *Cancer* 1998;83:2181–2184.

33. Bleicher RJ, Allegra DP, Nora DT, et al. Radiofrequency ablation in 447 complex unresectable liver tumors: lessons learned. *Ann Surg Oncol* 2003;10:52–62.

34. Bhatia SK, Saclarides TJ, Witt TR, et al. Hormone receptor studies in axillary metastases from occult breast cancers. *Cancer* 1987;59:1170–1172.

35. Henry-Tillman RS, Harms SE, Westbrook KC, et al. Role of breast magnetic resonance imaging in determining breast as a source of unknown metastatic lymphadenopathy. *Am J Surg* 1999;178:496–503.

36. Block EF, Meyer MA. Positron emission tomography in diagnosis of occult adenocarcinoma of the breast. *Am Surg* 1998;64:906–908.

37. Gentile PS, Carloss HW, Huant T-Y, et al. Disseminated prostatic carcinoma simulating primary lung cancer. *Cancer* 1988;62:711–715.

38. Tell DT, Khoury JM, Taylor HG, Veasey SP. Atypical metastasis from prostate cancer: clinical utility of the immunoperoxidase technique for prostate specific antigen. *JAMA* 1985;253:3574–3575.

39. Johnson RO, Castro R, Ansfield FJ. Response of primary unknown cancers to treatment with 5-fluorouracil. *Cancer Chemother Rep* 1964;38:63–64.

40. Moertel CG, Reitemeier RJ, Schutt AJ, Hahn RG. Treatment of the patient with adenocarcinoma of unknown origin. *Cancer* 1972;30:1469–1472.

41. Falkson CI, Cohen GL. Mitomycin C, epirubicin and cisplatin versus mitomycin C alone as therapy for carcinoma of unknown primary origin. *Oncology* 1998;33:116–121.

42. Eagan RT, Therneau TM, Rubin J, et al. Lack of value for cisplatin added to mitomycin/doxorubicin combination chemotherapy for carcinoma of unknown primary site. *Am J Clin Oncol* 1987;10:82–85.

43. Kambhus SA, Kelsen D, Niedzwiecki D, Ochoa M Jr. Phase II trial of mitomycin C, vindesine, and Adriamycin and predictive variables in the treatment of patients with adenocarcinoma of unknown primary site [abstract]. *Proc Am Assoc Cancer Res* 1986;27:185.

44. Milliken ST, Tattersall MH, Woods RL, et al. Metastatic adenocarcinoma of unknown primary site: a randomized study of two combination chemotherapy regimens. *Eur J Cancer Clin Oncol* 1987;23:1645–1648.

45. Woods RL, Fox RM, Tattersall MHN, et al. Metastatic adenocarcinomas of unknown primary: a randomized study of two combination chemotherapy regimens. *N Engl J Med* 1980;303:87–88.

46. Goldberg RM, Smith FP, Ueno W, et al. Fluorouracil, Adriamycin, mitomycin in the treatment of adenocarcinoma of unknown primary. *J Clin Oncol* 1986;4:395–399.

47. Sulkes A, Uziely B, Isaacson R, et al. Combination chemotherapy in metastatic tumors of unknown origin. *Int J Med Sci* 1988;24:604–610.

48. Treat J, Falchuk SC, Tremblay C, et al. Phase II trial of methotrexate-FAM (m-FAM) in adenocarcinoma of unknown primary. *Eur J Clin Oncol* 1989;25:1053–1055.

49. Van der Gaast AVD, Verweij J, Planting ASTH, Stoter G. 5-Fluorouracil, doxorubicin, and mitomycin C (FAM) combination chemotherapy for metastatic adenocarcinoma of unknown primary. *Eur J Cancer Clin Oncol* 1988;24:765–768.

50. Lenzi R, Abbruzzese J, Amato R, et al. Cisplatin, 5-fluorouracil and folinic acid for the treatment of carcinoma of unknown primary: a phase II study [abstract]. *Proc Am Soc Clin Oncol* 1991;10:301.

51. Karapetis CS, Yip D, Virik K, et al. The treatment of carcinoma of unknown primary with epirubicin, cisplatin, and 5-fluorouracil (ECF) [abstract]. *Proc Am Soc Clin Oncol* 1999;18:642a.

52. Hainsworth JD, Erland JB, Kalman LA, et al. Carcinoma of unknown primary site: treatment with one-hour paclitaxel, carboplatin, and extended-schedule etoposide. *J Clin Oncol* 1997;15:2385–2393.

53. Briasoulis E, Kalofonos H, Bafaloukos D, et al. Carboplatin plus paclitaxel in unknown primary carcinoma: a phase II Hellenic Cooperative Oncology Group study. *J Clin Oncol* 2000;18:3101–3107.

54. Greco FA, Erland JB, Morrissey LH, et al. Carcinoma of unknown primary site: phase II trials with docetaxel plus cisplatin or carboplatin. *Ann Oncol* 2000;11:211–215.

55. Mukai H, Watanabe T, Ando M, et al. A safety and efficacy trial of docetaxel and cisplatin in patients with cancer of unknown primary [abstract]. *Proc Am Soc Clin Oncol* 2003;22:286.

56. Greco FA, Burris HA, Erland JB, et al. Carcinoma of unknown primary site: long-term follow-up after treatment with paclitaxel, carboplatin, and etoposide. *Cancer* 2000;89:2655–2660.

57. Greco FA, Burris HA, Litchy S, et al. Gemcitabine, carboplatin and paclitaxel for patients with carcinoma of unknown primary site: a Minnie Pearl Cancer Research Network study. *J Clin Oncol* 2002;20:1651–1656.

58. Culine S, Lortholary A, Voigt JJ, et al. Cisplatin in combination with either gemcitabine or irinotecan in carcinomas of unknown primary site: results of a randomized phase II study—trial for the French Study Group in Carcinomas of Unknown Primary (GEFCAPI 01). *J Clin Oncol* 2003;21:3479–3482.

59. Pouessel D, Culine S, Becht C, et al. Gemcitabine and docetaxel as front-line chemotherapy in patients with carcinoma of an unknown primary site. *Cancer* 2004;100:1257–1261.

60. Greco FA, Rodriguez GI, Shaffer DW, et al. Carcinoma of unknown primary site: sequential treatment with paclitaxel/carboplatin/etoposide and gemcitabine/irinotecan: a Minnie Pearl Cancer Research Network phase II trial. *Oncologist* 2004;9:644–652.

61. Greco FA, Gray J, Burris HA, et al. Taxane-based chemotherapy for patients with carcinoma of unknown primary site. *Cancer J* 2001;7:203–212.

62. Hainsworth JD, Spigel DR, Raefsky EL, et al. Combination chemotherapy with gemcitabine and irinotecan in patients with previously treated carcinoma of an unknown primary site: a Minnie Pearl Cancer Research Network phase II trial. *Cancer* 2005;104:1992–1997.

63. Hainsworth JD, Burris HA, Calvert SW, et al. Gemcitabine in the second-line therapy of patients with carcinoma of unknown primary site: a phase II trial of the Minnie Pearl Cancer Research Network. *Cancer Invest* 2001;19:335–339.

64. Hainsworth JD, Spigel DR, Farley CL, et al. Phase II trial of bevacizumab and erlotinib in carcinomas of unknown primary site: The Minnie Pearl Cancer Research Network. *J Clin Oncol* 2007;25:1747–1752.

65. Warnke RA, Gatter KC, Falini B, et al. Diagnosis of human lymphoma with monoclonal antileukocyte antibodies. *N Engl J Med* 1983;209:1275–1281.

66. O'Connor DT, Burton D, Deftos LJ. Immunoreactive human chromogranin A in diverse polypeptide hormone-producing human tumors and normal endocrine tissues. *J Clin Endocrinol Metab* 1983;57:1084–1086.

67. Allhof EP, Proppe KH, Chapman CM. Evaluation of prostate-specific acid phosphatase and prostate-specific antigen. *J Urol* 1983;129:316–319.

68. Kahn HJ, Marks A, Thom H, Baumal R. Role of antibody to S-100 protein in diagnostic pathology. *Am J Clin Pathol* 1983;79:341–347.

69. Osborn M, Weber K. Biology of disease: tumor diagnosis by intermediate filament type: a novel tool for surgical pathology. *Lab Invest* 1983;48:372–394.

70. Bosl GJ, Ilson DH, Rodriguez E, et al. Clinical relevance of the i(12p) marker chromosome in germ cell tumors. *J Natl Cancer Inst* 1994;86:349–355.

71. Motzer RJ, Rodriguez E, Reuter VE, et al. Molecular and cytogenetic studies in the diagnosis of patients with midline carcinomas of unknown primary site. *J Clin Oncol* 1995;13:274–272.

72. Hainsworth JD, Johnson DH, Greco FA. Cisplatin-based combination chemotherapy in the treatment of poorly differentiated carcinoma and poorly differentiated adenocarcinoma of unknown primary site: results of a 12-year experience. *J Clin Oncol* 1992;10:912–922.

73. van der Gaast A, Verweij J, Henzen-Logmans SC, et al. Carcinoma of unknown primary: identification of a treatable subset. *Ann Oncol* 1991;1:119–121.

74. Lenzi R, Hess KR, Abbruzzese MC, et al. Poorly differentiated carcinoma and poorly differentiated adenocarcinoma of unknown origin: favorable subsets of patients with unknown primary carcinoma? *J Clin Oncol* 1997;15:2056–2062.

75. Pavlidis N, Kosmidis P, Skarlos D, et al. Subsets of tumors responsive to cisplatin or carboplatin combinations in patients with carcinoma of unknown primary site: a Hellenic Cooperative Oncology Group study. *Ann Oncol* 1992;3:631–634.

76. Greco FA, Thomas M, Hainsworth JD. Poorly differentiated carcinoma (PDC) or adenocarcinoma (PDA) of unknown primary site: long-term follow-up after cisplatin-based chemotherapy [abstract]. *Proc Am Soc Clin Oncol* 1997;16:274a.

77. Brenner B, Tang LH, Klimstra DS, Kelsen DP. Small-cell carcinomas of the gastrointestinal tract: a review. *J Clin Oncol* 2004;22:2730–2739.

78. Moertel CG, Evols LF, O'Connell MJ, Rubin J. Treatment of neuroendocrine carcinomas with etoposide and cisplatin: evidence of major therapeutic activity in anaplastic variants of these neoplasms. *Cancer* 1991;68:227–232.

79. Hainsworth JD, Johnson DH, Greco FA. Poorly differentiated neuroendocrine carcinoma of unknown primary site: a newly recognized clinicopathologic entity. *Ann Intern Med* 1988;109:364–372.

80. Hainsworth JD, Spigel DR, Litchy S, Greco FA. Treatment of advanced poorly differentiated neuroendocrine carcinoma with paclitaxel, carboplatin, and etoposide: a phase II trial of the Minnie Pearl Cancer Research Network. *J Clin Oncol* 2006;24:3548–3554.

CHAPTER 53 ■ MALIGNANT PERITONEAL MESOTHELIOMA

SAM G. PAPPAS AND DAVID L. BARTLETT

INTRODUCTION

Mesotheliomas are neoplasms arising from the lining of the pleural, pericardial, and peritoneal cavities. Malignant peritoneal mesothelioma (MPM) is a rare neoplasm arising from serosal cells lining the abdominal and pelvic peritoneum. The appropriate management of MPM remains a difficult therapeutic challenge. This underscores the importance of increased awareness of MPM, prompt diagnosis, and judicious surgical management. Previously, these tumors were regarded as a preterminal condition, where the majority of surgeries did not prolong survival and were performed mainly with palliative intent. More recently, aggressive surgical approaches, including cytoreductive radical tumor debulking combined with intraperitoneal hyperthermic chemoperfusion (IPHC), are associated with prolonged survival in selected patients with MPM.

Little is known about the natural history of MPM. The median age at diagnosis is 60 years, and there is a male-to-female ratio of 3:1. The age range in which the tumor has been reported is 2 to 92 years, however, the greater majority occur between 45 and 64 years of age (1). The geographic distribution of mesothelioma around the world does not appear to be uniform, and incidence rates in some countries continue to rise. The proportion of peritoneal mesotheliomas seen in the United States appears to be increasing. Peritoneal mesotheliomas now account for up to one-third of all malignant mesotheliomas (1–3). The incidence of MPM among all malignant mesotheliomas is approximately 15% but varies greatly among different studies. The annual rate of mesothelioma in Australia is reported as 15.8 to 28.9 per 1 million population age 20 years and older and appears to be on the rise (4). This is in contrast to the rate in the United States, which is about 2.2 cases per 1 million population and appears to be declining (5). This may be in part due to varying timing of asbestos exposure and the long latency period (20–40 years) between maximal asbestos exposure and disease presentation.

The most common presenting symptoms of MPM are increasing abdominal girth from ascites, pain, and weight loss. Patients generally present clinically as either the "pain-predominant" type or the "ascites-predominant" clinical type, and some patients present with concomitant pain and abdominal distension (6). The presence of symptoms as compared to patients with MPM diagnosed incidentally has been reported as a negative prognostic indicator. There are no uniformly accepted staging systems for MPM. This disease is generally confined to the abdominal cavity and will eventually spread to one or both pleural cavities late in the disease course. However, most patients die without evidence of distant metastases. The most important prognostic indicator in patients with MPM may be the biological phenotype of the tumor. Progressive tumor growth eventually leads to incapacitating ascites, abdominal organ and intestinal encasement, and repeated bowel obstructions. When left untreated, the median survival is a dismal 5 to 12 months (7).

RISK FACTORS

Epidemiologic studies have linked chronic peritoneal irritation (mainly from asbestos fibers) as the primary cause of MPM. Many other risk factors have also been implicated in the eventual development of MPM and include: radiotherapy for conditions such as Hodgkin disease (8,9), thorotrast exposure (10), recurrent peritonitis (11), familial Mediterranean fever (12), Simian virus 40 (SV40) (11–13), and endometriosis. It is interesting to note the long latency of MPM from time of environmental exposure to the onset of disease, which can often exceed 20 years. This finding would suggest that multiple somatic genetic mutational events need to occur prior to the eventual development of the malignant phenotype (7). No specific chromosomal alteration is known to occur in MPM. However, recent studies have begun to elucidate the molecular events that eventually lead to the malignant phenotype. For example, loss of a copy of chromosome 22 is the single most consistent numerical change seen in malignant mesothelioma (7).

Chronic asbestos exposure is believed to be a major risk factor for development of MPM (14). Although not uniformly accepted, up to 70% of MPM cases are believed to be associated with chronic exposure to asbestos (15–17). Occupational exposure to asbestos fibers in industrial and building trades is a common factor associated with most cases of MPM. In some series, it appears that the incidence and epidemiology of MPM may differ between men and women. The incidence rates of various countries parallels exposure to asbestos, and the peak incidences appear to follow the expected long latency period of MPM. For example, maximal exposure rates in Australia and Britain, which occurred during the 1960s and 1970s, would predict that peak incidence rates can be anticipated from 2010 to 2020 (15–17). How fiber inhalation leads to peritoneal seeding is unclear, but there are reports where inhaled asbestos fibers reach the peritoneal cavity (17). The precise mechanism by which asbestos exposure leads to the development of MPM remains to be fully elucidated (18).

Previous radiation exposure to the peritoneal cavity has been postulated as a causative factor for MPM. The presence of ascites or pleural effusion in a previously normal radiated abdomen should alert the physician to the possible development of MPM (8). It is unlikely that SV40 acts alone in MPM oncogenesis. More likely is the concept that MPM develops as a result of multiple factors cooperating to affect MPM oncogenesis. In this sense, many cocarcinogens (e.g., asbestos, SV40) can come together and lead to MPM (19). In some areas of Turkey, MPM appears to be inherited with an autosomal pattern of genetic inheritance (20). Whether genetic factors acting alone or in combination with environmental exposures result in MPM is unknown.

PRESENTATION AND DIAGNOSIS

Most patients presenting with MPM have had numerous non-specific symptoms that often result in a delay in diagnosis. Among other complaints, patients can present with abdominal pain, increasing abdominal distension, anorexia, malaise, and increasing abdominal girth from ascites (4). Rarely, patients may present with weight loss, a palpable mass, dysphagia, incomplete bowel obstruction, new onset inguinal hernia, deep vein thrombosis, or even a fever of unknown origin (4,6,8,21–23). Ascites is a nonspecific sign that occurs in roughly 90% of patients with MPM. It is not uncommon for many patients with MPM to be explored without a preoperative diagnosis. The symptoms of patients with MPM are often nonspecific and can overlap with a spectrum of diseases.

There are a variety of rare and unusual presentations of MPM that have been reported in the literature. They have been described in hernia sacs and hydroceles, and they may sometimes mimic gynecologic malignancies. These tumors can also present as isolated umbilical, small bowel, or retroperitoneal tumors. Some unusual presentations have been reported where MPM has an ectopic hormone-producing function. There are reports of patients with excess secretion of antidiuretic hormone (24), growth hormone (25,26), corticotrophin (27), and insulinlike substances (25).

The diagnosis of MPM is often elusive because it is an uncommon disease and the symptoms and clinical presentation are varied and nonspecific. A high index of suspicion, coupled with the presence of nonspecific findings and a significant history of asbestos exposure or findings of ascites, will suggest the diagnosis in the majority of cases. Diagnostic paracentesis of ascitic fluid is rarely helpful in providing the physician with an accurate diagnosis. Often, the aspirate will yield cells that are indeterminate in nature or that contains cells that resemble "mesothelial hyperplasia" (28). Paracentesis will infrequently yield a definitive diagnosis. Most patients will undergo an imaging study for nonspecific complaints such as an abdominal ultrasound (US) or an abdominal CT scan. Findings on US are nonspecific and may demonstrate an intra-abdominal mass, omental caking, or presence of ascites. The endoscopic appearance of MPM may be indistinguishable from other primary peritoneal neoplasms or metastases from other primaries. In addition to these findings, CT scan may display a wide spectrum of findings. Thickening of the mesentery and peritoneum and the presence of ascites should alert the physician to the possibility of MPM. Although some CT scan findings can predict surgical outcomes, CT scan rarely establishes a preoperative diagnosis but in some cases may help guide the physician for a CT-guided biopsy (1).

The majority of tumors involving the surface of the peritoneal cavity are due to primary or metastatic serous epithelial tumors (14). This may make the distinction between an MPM and a primary serous epithelial malignancy particularly challenging based on morphologic characteristics alone. The diagnosis is often aided with immunohistochemistry staining for mesothelial markers that increase the accuracy of a diagnosis preoperatively. Based on histologic features and combined with immunophenotyping, the correct diagnosis of MPM can be made in many of the patients prior to surgical exploration. This may represent an opportunity to select those patients who will be the best candidates for surgical exploration from those patients who have highly aggressive phenotype who may not

benefit from primary surgical debulking up front. Furthermore, there may be some variants of MPM that behave less aggressively than other variants and carry a significantly better prognosis. One such variant arising in younger women has been reported and may have a better prognosis than other MPM patients (21,22). These may be the optimal candidates for an aggressive approach with cytoreductive tumor debulking and IPHC. In some instances, obtaining a definitive diagnosis may require a multimodality approach, including clinicians, radiologists, and pathologists with special immunohistochemical stains and sometimes the aid of electron microscopy to secure an appropriate diagnosis (6).

The optimal technique of diagnosis should be some form of surgical biopsy. This approach avoids delay and potential misdiagnosis, and can be performed using various techniques. One technique that may be used is laparoscopic-guided biopsy, which is often required and can provide the surgeon with an assessment of the tumor burden prior to exploratory laparotomy (29). The laparoscopic appearance of MPM may be indistinguishable from other primary peritoneal neoplasms or metastases from other primaries. Knowledge of the absence of solid organ involvement including the liver may alert the surgeon that the tumor may represent an MPM, and careful examination of the entire abdomen and pelvis, including the mesentery and adnexa, should be made. Multiple laparoscopic-guided biopsies combined with peritoneal cytology might reveal lesions that are potentially mesothelial neoplasms and can be confirmed as MPM by immunocytochemistry. However, there is a measurable concern for port site tumor seeding, which may facilitate tumor dissemination (30–32). Laparoscopic intraperitoneal chemoperfusion is a newer treatment modality that may also provide a means of relief of debilitating ascites in patients who are not candidates for more radical surgical approaches. In a recent study of 14 patients with varying tumor histologies, all patients were relieved of their disabling ascites with acceptable morbidity (33).

PATHOLOGY AND STAGING

Multiple different pathological subtypes of mesothelioma have been identified and are broadly divided into multicystic, epithelioid, epithelial, biphasic, sarcomatous, and deciduoid (7). Patients with deciduoid, sarcomatous, or biphasic morphology tend to have a worse prognosis among the group. A broad spectrum of heterogeneous pathological subtypes has been reported with varying degrees of malignant potential (Fig. 53.1). This makes the interpretation of which therapeutic approaches are optimal for each different subtype difficult. Furthermore, the natural history of pleural mesothelioma is distinct from that of MPM and makes the extrapolation of phenotype characterization and selection for treatment strategies inappropriate.

There are a few benign tumors of the peritoneal cavity that may mimic MPM at presentation and are worth mentioning. Multicystic mesothelioma, also known as multilocular peritoneal inclusion cyst, is a benign inclusion cyst formed by multiple cysts arranged in grapelike clusters (7). Adenomatoid mesotheliomas are benign epithelial lesions of the genital system that may present with an abdominal or pelvic mass. Well-differentiated papillary mesothelioma is another benign proliferation that is commonly found in young women. There have been reports of malignant degeneration after prolonged observation of the lesions (7). These tumors histologically appear to be formed by papillary structures covered by cytologically benign mesothelial cells. In some instances, the differentiation between ovarian cancer and mesothelioma cannot be made until after removal of the surgical specimen along with the ovaries.

It is unclear what the exact histologic subtype has been for many of the patients reported in the recent literature. This

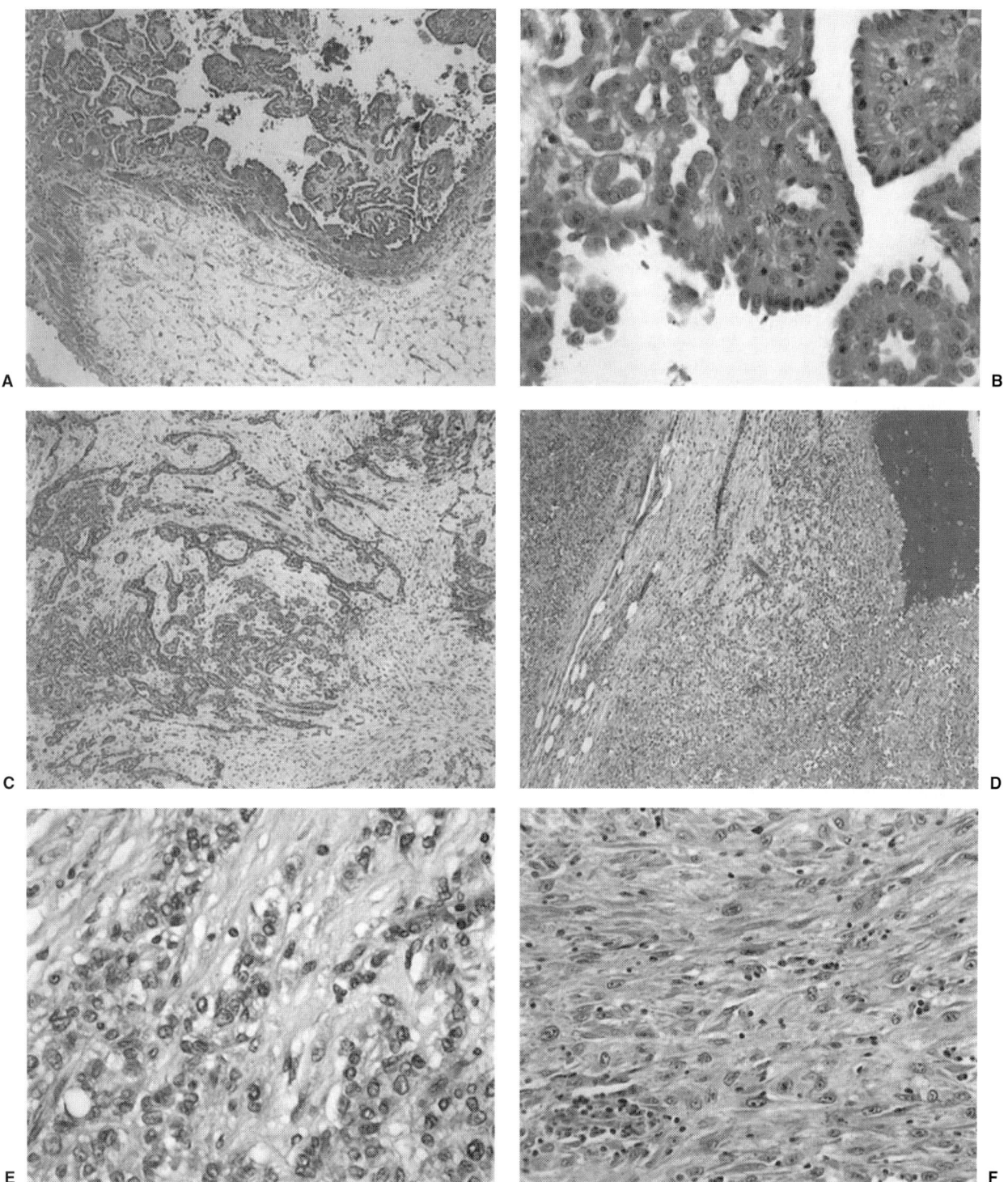

FIGURE 53.1. Histopathology of peritoneal mesothelioma. A, B: Low-grade, tubulopapillary type, without deep tissue invasion or desmoplasia. C: Low-grade, tubulopapillary type, with deep invasion and desmoplasias. D, E: High-grade, epithelioid type, with deep invasion and desmoplasia. F: High-grade, sarcomatoid type. [A, C, and D, 100×; B and E, 600×; F, 400×]. Permission for reprint pending from Feldman et al. (See also color Figure 53.1A-F)

will become increasingly important in identifying which patients will be best candidates for the aggressive surgical approaches to the treatment of MPM. Better understanding of the histologic features that separate the benign from frankly malignant tumors may help stratify patients for the appropriate surgical intervention. The presence of deep invasion in examined specimens may have stronger prognostic significance than histologic subtype (34). Histomorphologic parameters have been found to carry prognostic significance in predicting survival in patients with MPM (34a). Some patients with benign-appearing neoplasms may require only surgical excision and observation, whereas others with highly aggressive tumors may be spared the morbidity of aggressive surgery and IPHC.

No uniform consensus exists on the appropriate staging of MPM. As the treatment strategies expand and the availability of numerous combinations of systemic and regional approaches to treatment widens, a need for a uniform staging system will become more apparent. This will help select and stratify patients into various treatment strategies based on their stage, and help better define optimal candidates for current treatment approaches. These strategies will likely continue to be refined, and various prognostic indicators will likely be defined to help stratify patients into optimal treatment plans.

SURGICAL THERAPY

In the past, most systemic chemotherapeutic regimens failed to demonstrate a significant effect in the palliation of symptoms or extension of survival in patients with MPM. The lack of significant locoregional effect of previous chemotherapy led to renewing the interest in regional approaches to peritoneal surface malignancies, including peritonectomy procedures, IPHC, and early postoperative intraperitoneal chemotherapy. This approach has several advantages to conventional systemic chemotherapy. The peritoneal plasma barrier appears to provide favorable pharmacokinetics for dose-intensive regional therapy. Higher drug concentrations come into direct contact with tumor cells with concurrent reduced plasma concentrations and lower systemic toxicity (6). In many cases, exponential levels of drug can be delivered to the peritoneal cavity without achieving toxic systemic levels. The activity of multiple antitumor agents appears to be enhanced by the addition of heat to 42°C by augmenting their cytotoxicity and increasing their penetration into tissues (14). Theoretically, cytoreductive surgery (CRS) is performed to treat macroscopic disease, and IPHC is used to treat the microscopic disease left behind at the end of the tumor debulking. The combination of CRS and IPHC may act as a dose intensification device, which would result in improved outcomes.

The evolution of combined multimodality therapy for the treatment of MPM occurred primarily as a result of three sequential series of patients treated at the Dana-Farber Cancer Institute and Joint Center for Radiation Therapy (35). In the initial trial, conducted from 1980 to 1982, 1 of 9 patients treated with surgery plus intravenous chemotherapy of cyclophosphamide, doxorubicin, and dimethyltriazenoimidazole carboxamide before and after whole abdominal radiotherapy, survived longer than 10 years. In the second phase I trial from 1982 to 1985, 6 of 13 patients had a tumor debulking of all lesions >1 cm in size followed by intraperitoneal doxorubicin (6–50 mg/m^2) and cisplatin (66–100 mg/m^2) for a total of 8 to 12 treatments. At second-look laparotomy, all 6 patients had an objective decrease of ≤50% of their tumor burden. The complete planned treatment regimen was received by 4 patients in this study, which included tumor debulking, intraperitoneal chemotherapy, and whole abdominal radiotherapy. Patients remained disease free for at least 36 months (range 36–61 months) after diagnosis. In the third phase I trial, patients were treated with surgical debulking followed by an intraperitoneal dwell of cisplatin and doxorubicin every 2 weeks for 20 weeks. Those patients at second-look laparotomy found to have no residual tumor received whole abdominal radiotherapy, and those patients found to have residual disease were treated with intravenous chemotherapy followed by radiotherapy (7). Thirteen patients responded to therapy, and there were seven partial and six complete responses. Three patients with partial responses relapsed, and at the time of reporting, all 6 patients with complete responses remained in remission for a median of 25 months. These treatment regimens were well tolerated in most patients, with only mild to moderate hematologic toxicities been reported along with mild symptomatic toxicities of nausea and vomiting.

A recent change has occurred in the management of peritoneal mesotheliomas for what was previously believed to be a disease in which options were limited. Previously, patients were typically offered surgical interventions for palliation of symptoms. As late as 2000, 5-year survival rates for MPM were believed to be zero. More recently, several authors reported the success of aggressive surgical approaches, including CRS with IPHC for the treatment of MPM in combination with early postoperative intraperitoneal chemotherapy. These procedures are sometimes followed by second-look operations to ensure that early recurrence has not occurred and to give further information on how to guide postoperative therapy.

The importance of identifying those patients who will be the best candidates for such a radical approach should not be underestimated. In patients with known or suspected MPM, CT offers the possibility of selecting those patients who would be optimal candidates for cytoreductive surgery. In those patients who would be considered suboptimal candidates for surgical debulking by CT criteria, other modalities of treatment should be considered. Sugarbaker et al. discovered a correlation between objective preoperative CT scan findings and the completeness of cytoreduction (CC) (36). The extent of CRS performed largely depends on the distribution and amount of dissemination within the peritoneal cavity. Their data showed that the size of the tumor mass in the epigastric region and the appearance of the small bowel and its mesentery are reliable predictors of response to CRS. More specifically, patients with tumors in the epigastrium >5 cm in size and class III small bowel findings have a 100% probability of suboptimal cytoreduction. This is in contrast to patients without these findings, where a complete cytoreduction can be anticipated with a 94% probability (Table 53.1). These data strongly support the

TABLE 53.1

INTERPRETIVE COMPUTED TOMOGRAPHY (CT) CLASSIFICATION OF SMALL BOWEL AND MESENTERY

Class	Presence of ascites	Small bowel and mesentery involvement	Loss of mesenteric vessel clarity	CT interpretation
0	No	No	No	Normal Appearance
I	Yes	No	No	Ascites only
II	Yes	Thickening, enhancing	No	Solid tumor present
III	Yes	Nodular thickening, segmental obstruction	Yes	Loss of normal architecture

Reprint permission pending approval.

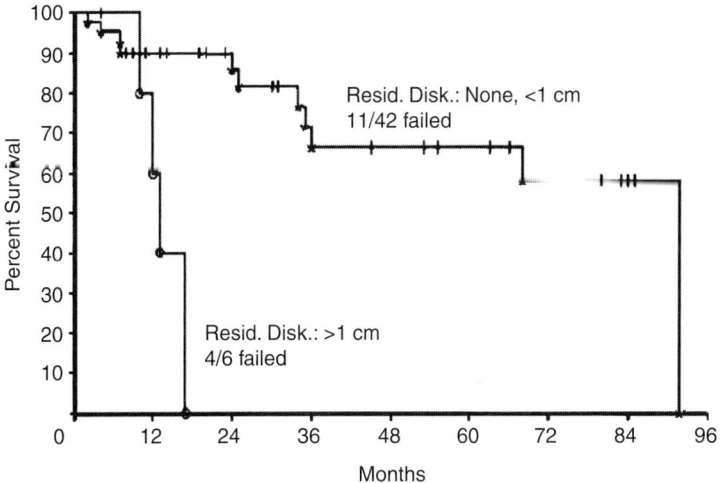

FIGURE 53.2. Completeness of cytoreduction (CC) as an important prognostic indicator. Significant effect in overall survival based on CC. Permission for reprint pending from Feldman et al.

value of preoperative CT scanning in selecting optimal candidates for surgical consideration. All patients evaluated for CRS need appropriate cardiopulmonary evaluation and clearance and optimization of preoperative morbid state. The degree of stress caused by the surgical procedure is substantial and should also be considered when evaluating a patient for such an approach.

CYTOREDUCTIVE SURGERY AND INTRAPERITONEAL HYPERTHERMIC CHEMOTHERAPY

Many authors recently reported their favorable institutional results with combined multimodality therapy for MPM, including CRS and HIIC. The observable trend among all studies is the significant increase in survival when patients are offered these approaches. These studies have demonstrated a marked prolongation in median survival in this group of patients as compared to historical controls with roughly half of patients alive after 5 years. This marks the proposal of a new standard therapy in the management of malignant peritoneal mesothelioma (37). As experience with these patients continues to expand, treatment strategies will continue to evolve and the best candidates for aggressive surgical approaches will be defined.

Sugarbaker et al. described their surgical approach to patients with MPM. In brief, patients undergo exploratory laparotomy and four quadrant peritonectomy ± regional organ resections as indicated by degree of tumor burden. The basic concept is to reduce the entire tumor burden down to <5 cm nodules in size. All areas of the peritoneal cavity need to be explored, including the lesser sac and hepatoduodenal ligament to optimize the surface contact with the chemoperfusate. The greater and lesser omenta are frequently removed during this exploration.

CC has been consistently found to be independently associated with better survival in multivariate analysis from many published series (34,38,39) (Fig. 53.2). In a recent series, those patients who had an adequate cytoreduction based on a CC score at the end of surgery had a significantly better survival. Five-year survival rate for those patients who had an adequate CC score as compared to those who did not had survivals of 59% versus 19%, respectively (40). Complete cytoreduction may be particularly more challenging in the MPM population

in that these patients may have more of an aggressive phenotype as compared to patients with carcinomatosis from colorectal or appendiceal origin. More specifically, the small bowel visceral surface can often harbor a significant amount of tumor burden (an area that is commonly spared in patients with appendiceal carcinomatosis) (Fig. 53.3). Following complete cytoreduction and aggressive tumor debulking, the abdominal cavity is connected to an extracorporeal circuit for the instillation of heated chemoperfusion. Several different regimens have been reported, all with apparent similar success. The various treatment regimens offered to this particular group of patients will likely continue to expand and evolve.

SYSTEMIC CHEMOTHERAPY

MPM is largely a locoregional disease that is most often confined to the peritoneal cavity for the majority, or all, of the disease course. This is the reason for the acceptance of aggressive combined locoregional approaches as the preferred primary treatment approach. Recent reports from several institutions of combined cytoreductive surgery and intraperitoneal chemotherapy, with or without early postoperative intraperitoneal chemotherapy and radiotherapy, have been evaluated in cohorts of patients with promising results. However, not all patients with MPM are candidates for such aggressive combined modality approaches, and the morbidities associated with these approaches are not insignificant. In addition, not all patients receive a complete cytoreduction, and additional postoperative therapies are needed to further improve survival in those with suboptimal surgical results.

It is difficult to know the exact role of systemic chemotherapy in the treatment of patients with MPM (41). Evaluation of efficacy of chemotherapeutic regimens is hampered by the lack of standardized objective measures of response. These tumors spread diffusely and often have minimal findings on imaging studies that are markers for disease response. Furthermore, data regarding the role of systemic chemotherapy in the treatment of mesothelioma of peritoneal origin are particularly scarce. Numerous single agent regimens and combination regimens have been tested over the past several decades with modest results. It is sometimes useful to discuss the role of chemotherapy in the management of malignant mesothelioma of any site of origin and then extrapolate the data to the patients with MPM (41).

Most cytotoxic agents tested in small heterogeneous populations have been found to have disappointing response rates. A recent meta-analysis has been published of all prospective

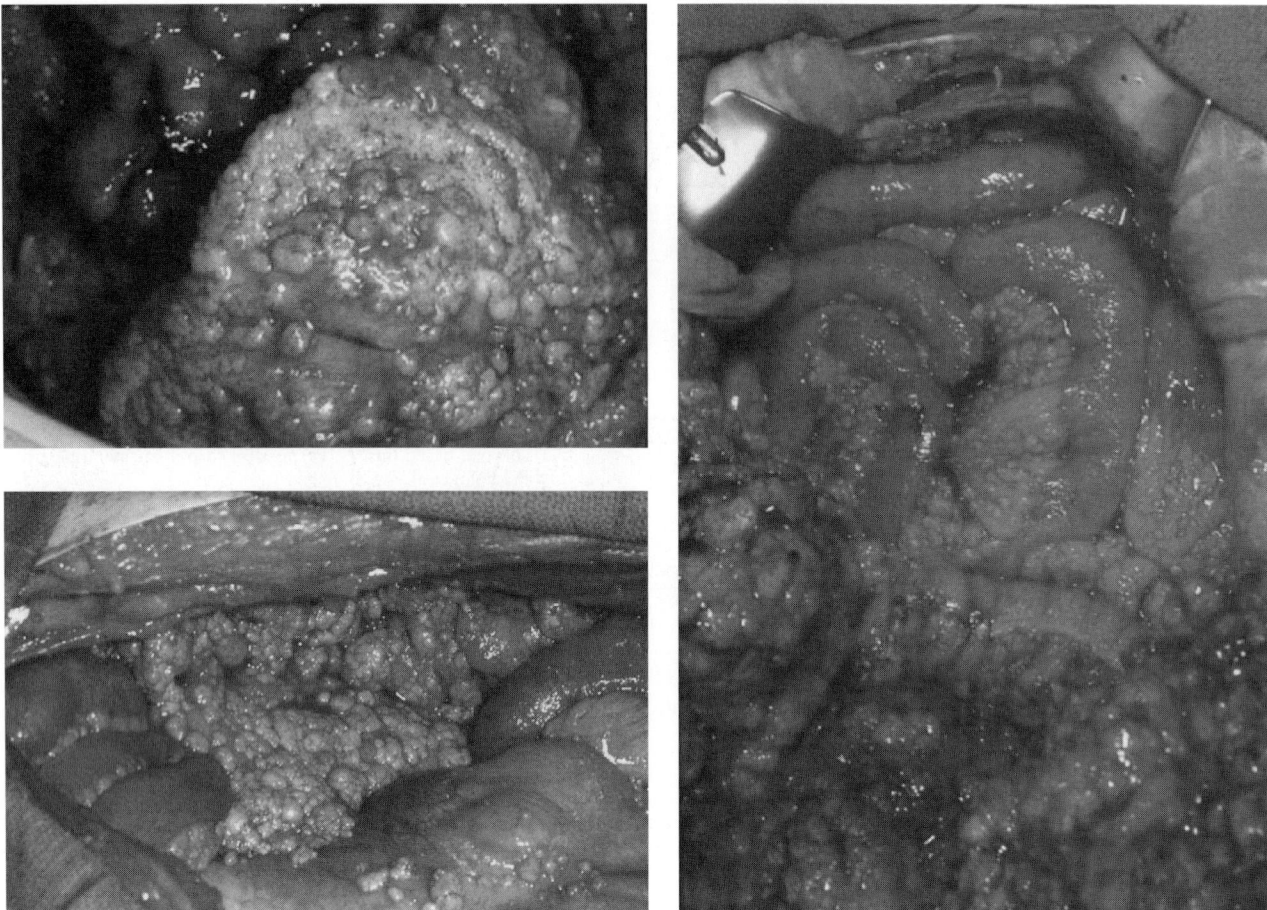

FIGURE 53.3. Malignant peritoneal mesothelioma involving the visceral surface of the intestine diffusely. Reprint permission pending (See also color Figure 53.3).

clinical trials in the literature from 1965 to 2001 regarding the value of systemic chemotherapy in treatment of mesothelioma of both pleural and peritoneal origin (42). This review included more than 2,300 patients included in 80 single-arm and 3 randomized phase II trials. Briefly, this meta-analysis suggested that single-agent cisplatin and combined cisplatin and doxorubicin are the most active agents in the treatment of malignant mesothelioma. Response rates observed for patients treated with cisplatin (23%) were significantly greater (*p* <0.001) than those observed for patients treated with doxorubicin (11%) or treatment regimens not including any of these two drugs. These results have not been validated by a randomized trial, and this meta-analysis was based on response rates and not survival or quality of life.

Newer agents have shown great promise in the management of this traditionally chemoresistant disease. The antifolates, in particular, deserve special attention in that they appear to be the most active agents against malignant mesothelioma. Pemetrexed disodium is a novel antifolate with broad activity against multiple tumor types (43). Early clinical results with pemetrexed combined with platinum-containing compounds have demonstrated response rates in phase I and II trials of up to 45%. Pemetrexed has been evaluated in the largest trial ever conducted in malignant mesothelioma (44). This phase III study compared response rates in chemotherapy-naive patients not eligible for curative resection to receive combined pemetrexed and cisplatin versus cisplatin alone. The response rate in patients with the combined regimen was significantly

higher than patients treated with cisplatin alone (41% vs. 17%, *p* <0.0001). Finally, preliminary data from a German study (45) and from the pemetrexed expanded access program (46) evaluating the antitumor activity of pemetrexed in patients with peritoneal mesothelioma suggest response rates in the ranges observed for pleural disease. There are also some preliminary data suggesting that the pharmacokinetic profile of pemetrexed may be suitable for intraperitoneal delivery, which will likely increase the interest in incorporating this drug into combined multimodality locoregional approaches (47).

Gemcitabine is a pyrimidine analog with in vitro activity against mesothelioma cell lines that appears to have synergistic effects with platinum-containing compounds (41). Response rates with single-agent gemcitabine pooled from three clinical trials are 12% (range: 0%–31%). More impressive are pooled rates from three clinic trials with gemcitabine combined with cisplatin, where a 16% to 48% response rate was observed (48–50). Currently no randomized trials exist to clarify the exact role of combination gemcitabine and cisplatin in the treatment of malignant peritoneal mesothelioma. Many other targeted therapies, including molecularly targeted therapies, are under current evaluation. For now, it appears that pemetrexed and cisplatin combined may be optimal therapy for patients who are not considered candidates for curative surgery. Improving our understanding of the underlying molecular basis of this disease will be an essential tool in helping us discover newer more rationally developed treatment strategies for MPM.

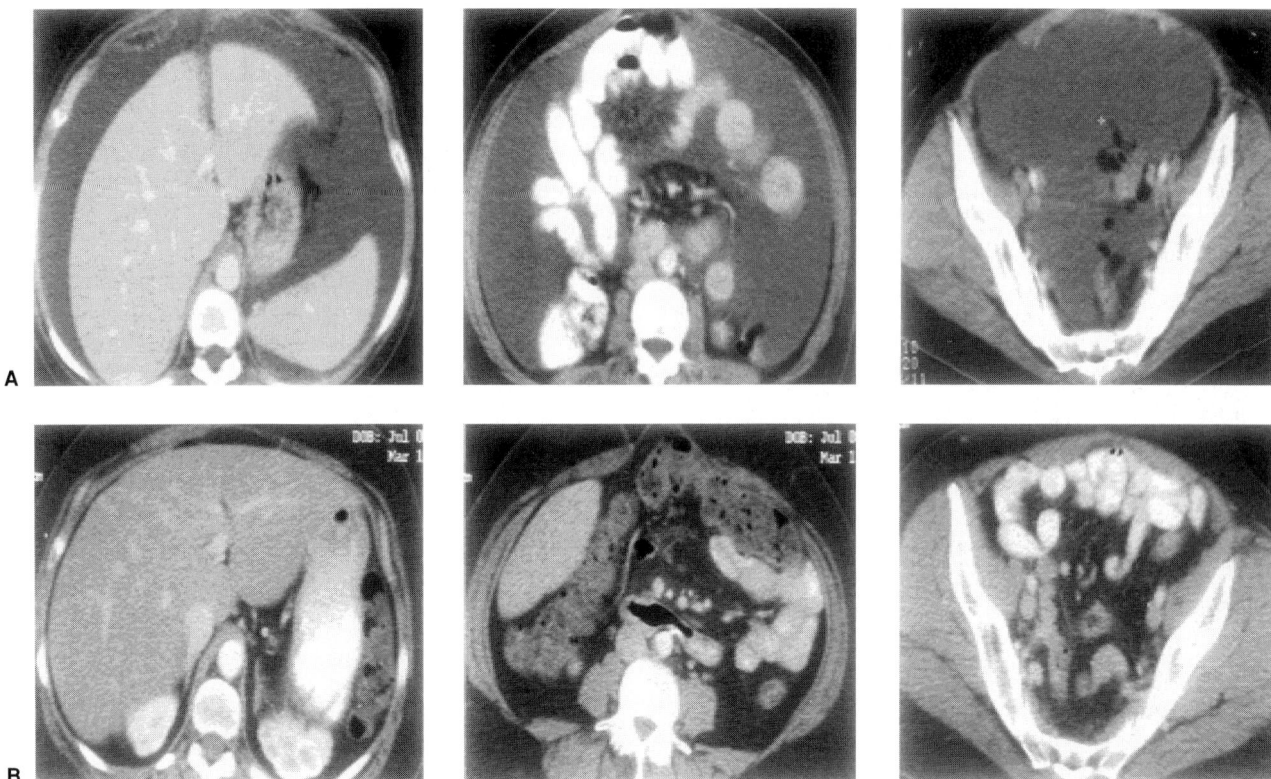

FIGURE 53.4. Axial computed tomography scans showing complete resolution of ascites in a patient following cytoreductive surgery (CRS) and intraperitoneal hyperthermic chemoperfusion (IPHC). **A:** Pre-CRS and -IPHC. **B:** 54 months post-CRS and -IPHC. Permission reprint pending from Feldman et al.

NOVEL TREATMENTS

Several recent reports of peritoneal directed regional therapies and molecularly targeted therapies are on the horizon in the management of MPM. Chemoimmunotherapy strategies, including cisplatin and interferon 2a therapy or cytotoxic T cells, intraperitoneal sulmarin, and gene therapy, have been reported (51–53). In addition, several molecularly targeted therapies against vascular endothelial growth factor, platelet-derived growth factor, and epidermal growth factor have been investigated (54). A National Cancer Institute–sponsored phase II trial of cisplatin/gemcitabine with or without bevacizumab in patients with malignant mesothelioma has been launched. Many other targeted therapies are currently under investigation. Interest in this area will continue to expand as knowledge of the molecular events that lead to malignant transformation is better understood. Recent advances in serum proteomics and genetic profiling have revealed two proteins (osteopontin and serum mesothelin-related protein or SMRP) as potential targets for early detection and treatment of patients with MPM (55).

OUTCOMES

Reports prior to 1999 using combined tumor debulking along with systemic chemotherapy demonstrated median survivals of roughly 12 months (2,3,56–60). Survival results from several institutions published since 1999 have supported the rationale that an aggressive surgical approach including CRS combined with IPHC has affected improved outcomes (28,34,38–40, 61–64). When surgery is combined with hyperthermic chemo-perfusion, median survivals approach 5 years and subsequent reports continue to show improvement.

Favorable outcomes to cytoreductive surgery and IPHC have been reported by several authors. Feldman et al. from the National Cancer Institute reported several consecutive trials of MPM treatment plans (34). Their most recent report that included intraoperative IPHC with cisplatin followed by postoperative 5-fourauracil and paclitaxel dwell reported a median overall survival of 92 months in 49 patients. Brigand et al. reported 15 patients undergoing CRS and IPHC with mitomycin C and cisplatin for 90 minutes (38). Their overall median survival was 46.7 months. One-, 3-, and 5-year survival rates were reported as 71.5%, 49%, and 36.8%, respectively. In a recently published trial of 49 patients receiving either cisplatin/mitomycin C or cisplatin and doxorubicin, the overall median survival has not been reached at the completion of the study and the progressionfree survival was 40 months. Another important outcome that appears to be particularly responsive to CRS and IPHC is the palliation of ascites (Fig. 53.4). Most series report the majority of their patients have relief of their symptoms and apparent resolution of ascites.

In a series of 100 consecutive patients treated with peritoneal mesothelioma, the overall median survival was 50 months (range: 1–143 months), with 1-, 3-, and 5-year survival rates of 77%, 53%, and 44%, respectively (40) (Fig. 53.5). Not all patients included in this analysis had the complete regimen being offered at this institution. In the group of 65 patients who underwent cytoreduction with cisplatin and doxorubicin followed by early postoperative intraperitoneal paclitaxel, the median survival was 79 months (range: 1–143 months).

Few data are available regarding the treatment-associated morbidity and mortality of CRS and IPHC in patients with peritoneal mesothelioma. It is likely that the morbidity and

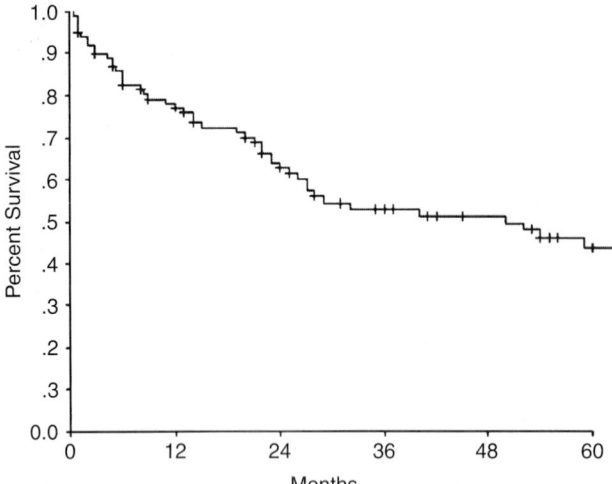

FIGURE 53.5. Overall survival of 100 patients with malignant peritoneal mesothelioma undergoing cytoreductive surgery and perioperative intraperitoneal hyperthermic chemoperfusion at the Washington Hospital Center, Washington, DC. Reprint permission pending.

mortality associated with treatment of patients with MPM will parallel the results in patients treated with CRS and IPHC for other diagnosis. In most large published series, the procedure-related morbidity ranges from 20% to 30%, and the mortality varies between 1% and 20%. In the largest published series of patients undergoing CRS and IPHC for peritoneal mesothelioma, the procedure-related mortality was reported as 5% (5 of 100 patients) (40). Their grade III and grade IV morbidity rates were 24% and 11%, respectively. The most common procedure-related morbidity was pleural effusion and occurred in 5% of patients. These values may appear acceptable in light of the acceptable rates for other GI malignancies, but the values also reflect a significant expertise in this area among institutions reporting such low rates of morbidity and mortality. There is a steep learning curve in mastering these techniques and applying them to this patient population. With better patient selection, the procedure-related morbidities will likely decrease even further.

CONCLUSION

MPM is a locally aggressive malignancy that often presents late in its course, making it particularly difficult to treat. Many issues in the optimal management of MPM remain to be fully resolved. As the awareness of this unique clinical entity increases, a greater proportion of patients who are candidates for surgery will likely present for treatment. A high index of suspicion in patients with a prior history of asbestos exposure or in patients presenting with the findings of ascites in the appropriate clinical scenario will aid in the diagnosis of MPM. Surgeons will gain increasing experience, and the indications and various treatment options will likely become more refined. Identifying more accurate prognostic indicators will allow for better patient selection and optimal timing of surgical intervention. The optimal temperatures and the precise techniques to deliver the chemoperfusate are areas in need of standardization.

Tumor debulking for palliation of symptoms followed by systemic chemotherapy is no longer the preferred approach to treating these patients. Complete cytoreductive surgery combined with heated intraperitoneal chemotherapy is the current treatment of choice for most patients who have resectable MPM. CC appears to consistently be regarded as an important

independent prognostic indicator in many published series. The precise role of systemic chemotherapy in the management of these patients remains to be fully elucidated. Furthermore, the development of preoperative tools to aid in the appropriate selection of MPM patients for comprehensive multimodality approaches is needed. Knowledgeable selection of the appropriate patients who are candidates for these approaches minimizes the treatment-related morbidity and mortality and will likely improve long-term outcomes. Those patients who are not candidates for CRS and IPHC, or who have suboptimal resections, should be offered additional systemic therapy as part of multi-institutional cooperative trials. Newer agents are available or under current investigation for patients who are at high risk for locoregional recurrence.

References

1. Asensio JA, Goldblatt P, Thomford NR. Primary malignant peritoneal mesothelioma: a report of seven cases and a review of the literature. *Arch Surg* 1990;125(11):1477–1481.
2. Sridhar KS, Doria R, Raub WA Jr, Thurer RJ, Saldana M. New strategies are needed in diffuse malignant mesothelioma. *Cancer* 1992;70(12):2969–2979.
3. Antman K, Shemin R, Ryan L, et al. Malignant mesothelioma: prognostic variables in a registry of 180 patients, the Dana-Farber Cancer Institute and Brigham and Women's Hospital experience over two decades, 1965–1985. *J Clin Oncol* 1988;6(1):147–153.
4. Clark JR, Ross WB. An unusual case of ascites: pitfalls in diagnosis of malignant peritoneal mesothelioma. *Aust N Z J Surg* 2000;70(5):384–388.
5. Piazza D, Caruso F, Scaringi S, Ferrara M, Latteri F, Dell'Erba D. Primary diffuse malignant peritoneal mesothelioma: case report and update of therapy. *J Surg Oncol* 2000;75(1):55–58.
6. Mohamed F, Sugarbaker PH. Peritoneal mesothelioma. *Curr Treat Options Oncol* 2002;3(5):375–386.
7. Pass HI, Hahn SM, Vogelzang NJ, Carbone M. *Benign and Malignant Mesothelioma. Cancer Principle and Practice in Oncology.* 7th ed. Philadelphia, PA; Lippincott Williams & Wilkins; 2006:1687–1715.
8. Sato F, Yamazaki H, Ataka K, et al. Malignant peritoneal mesothelioma associated with deep vein thrombosis following radiotherapy for seminoma of the testis. *Intern Med* 2000;39(11):920–924.
9. Weissmann LB, Corson JM, Neugut AI, Antman KH. Malignant mesothelioma following treatment for Hodgkin's disease. *J Clin Oncol* 1996;14(7):2098–2100.
10. Stey C, Landolt-Weber U, Vetter W, Sauter C, Marincek B. Malignant peritoneal mesothelioma after Thorotrast exposure. *Am J Clin Oncol* 1995;18(4):313–317.
11. Attanoos RL, Gibbs AR. Pathology of malignant mesothelioma. *Histopathology* 1997;30(5):403–418.
12. Gentiloni N, Febbraro S, Barone C, et al. Peritoneal mesothelioma in recurrent familial peritonitis. *J Clin Gastroenterol* 1997;24(4):276–279.
13. Shivapurkar N, Wiethege T, Wistuba II, et al. Presence of simian virus 40 sequences in malignant mesotheliomas and mesothelial cell proliferations. *J Cell Biochem* 1999;76(2):181–188.
14. Bani-Hani KE, Gharaibeh KA. Malignant peritoneal mesothelioma. *J Surg Oncol* 2005;91(1):17–25.
15. D'Albuquerque LA, Padilla JM, Rodrigues AL, et al. [Diffuse primary malignant mesothelioma in abdominal cavity.] *Arq Gastroenterol* 1997;34(3):163–168.
16. Barbieri PG, Migliori M, Merler E. [The incidence of malignant mesothelioma (1977–1996) and asbestos exposure in the population of an area neighboring Lake Iseo, northern Italy.] *Med Lav* 1999;90(6):762–775.
17. Cocco P, Dosemeci M. Peritoneal cancer and occupational exposure to asbestos: results from the application of a job-exposure matrix. *Am J Ind Med* 1999;35(1):9–14.
18. Dodson RF, O'Sullivan MF, Huang J, Holiday DB, Hammar SP. Asbestos in extrapulmonary sites: omentum and mesentery. *Chest* 2000;117(2):486–493.
19. Bocchetta M, Di Resta I, Powers A, et al. Human mesothelial cells are unusually susceptible to simian virus 40-mediated transformation and asbestos cocarcinogenicity. *Proc Natl Acad Sci U S A* 2000;97(18):10214–10219.
20. Roushdy-Hammady I, Siegel J, Emri S, Testa JR, Carbone M. Genetic-susceptibility factor and malignant mesothelioma in the Cappadocian region of Turkey. *Lancet* 2001;357(9254):444–445.
21. Acherman YI, Welch LS, Bromley CM, Sugarbaker PH. Clinical presentation of peritoneal mesothelioma. *Tumori* 2003;89(3):269–273.
22. Ustundag Y, Can U, Benli S, Buyukasik Y, Ozbek N. Internal carotid artery occlusion in a patient with malignant peritoneal mesothelioma: is it a sign of malignancy-related thrombosis? *Am J Med Sci* 2000;319(4):265–267.

23. Tejido GR, Anta FM, Hernandez Hernandez JL, Bravo GJ, Gonzalez MJ. [Fever of unknown origin as the clinical presentation of malignant peritoneal mesothelioma.] *Ann Med Intern* 1997;14(11):573–575.

24. Perks WH, Crow JC, Green M. Mesothelioma associated with the syndrome of inappropriate secretion of antidiuretic hormone. *Am Rev Respir Dis* 1978;117(4):789–794.

25. Anderson N, Lokich JJ. Mesenchymal tumors associated with hypoglycemia: case report and review of the literature. *Cancer* 1979;44(2):785–790.

26. Sparagana M, Phillips G, Hoffman C, Kucera L. Ectopic growth hormone syndrome associated with lung cancer. *Metabolism* 1971;20(8):730–736.

27. Knight RA, Ratcliffe JG, Besser GM. Tumour ACTH concentrations in ectopic ACTH syndrome and in control tissues. *Proc R Soc Med* 1971;64(12):1266–1267.

28. Sugarbaker PH, Welch LS, Mohamed F, Glehen O. A review of peritoneal mesothelioma at the Washington Cancer Institute. *Surg Oncol Clin N Am* 2003;12(3):605–621, xi.

29. Van de WP, Blomme Y, Van OL. Laparoscopy and primary diffuse malignant peritoneal mesothelioma: a diagnostic challenge. *Acta Chir Belg* 2004;104(1):114–117.

30. Sugarbaker PH, Yan H, Grazi RV, Shmookler BM. Early localized peritoneal mesothelioma as an incidental finding at laparoscopy: report of a case and implications regarding natural history of the disease. *Cancer* 2000;89(6):1279–1284.

31. Orosz Z, Nagy P, Szentirmay Z, Zalatnai A, Hauser P. Epithelial mesothelioma with deciduoid features. *Virchows Arch* 1999;434(3):263–266.

32. Muensterer OJ, Averbach AM, Jacquet P, Otero SE, Sugarbaker PH. Malignant peritoneal mesothelioma: case-report demonstrating pitfalls of diagnostic laparoscopy. *Int Surg* 1997;82(3):240–243.

33. Valle M, Garofalo A, Federici O, Cavaliere F. Laparoscopic intraperitoneal antiblastic hyperthermic chemoperfusion in the treatment of refractory neoplastic ascites: preliminary results. *Suppl Tumori* 2005;3:122–133.

34. Feldman AL, Libutti SK, Pingpank JF, et al. Analysis of factors associated with outcome in patients with malignant peritoneal mesothelioma undergoing surgical debulking and intraperitoneal chemotherapy. *J Clin Oncol* 2003;21(24):4560–4567.

34a. Cerruto CA, Brun EA, Chang D, Sugarbaker PH. Prognostic significance of histomorphologic parameters in diffuse malignant peritoneal mesothelioma. *Arch Pathol Lab Med* 2006;130(11):1654–1661.

35. Taub RN, Keohan ML, Chabot JC, Fountain KS, Plitsas M. Peritoneal mesothelioma. *Curr Treat Options Oncol* 2000;1(4):303–312.

36. Yan TD, Haveric N, Carmignani CP, Chang D, Sugarbaker PH. Abdominal computed tomography scans in the selection of patients with malignant peritoneal mesothelioma for comprehensive treatment with cytoreductive surgery and perioperative intraperitoneal chemotherapy. *Cancer* 2005;103(4):839–849.

37. Sugarbaker PH, Yan TD, Stuart OA, Yoo D. Comprehensive management of diffuse malignant peritoneal mesothelioma. *Eur J Surg Oncol* 2006;32(6):686–691.

38. Brigand C, Monneuse O, Mohamed F, et al. Peritoneal mesothelioma treated by cytoreductive surgery and intraperitoneal hyperthermic chemotherapy: results of a prospective study. *Ann Surg Oncol* 2006;13(3):405–412.

39. Deraco M, Nonaka D, Baratti D, et al. Prognostic analysis of clinicopathologic factors in 49 patients with diffuse malignant peritoneal mesothelioma treated with cytoreductive surgery and intraperitoneal hyperthermic perfusion. *Ann Surg Oncol* 2006;13(2):229–237.

40. Yan TD, Sugarbaker PH. Cytoreduction and intraperitoneal chemotherapy for peritoneal mesothelioma—analysis of 100 consecutive patients from a prospective database. *Eur J Surg Oncol* 2006;32(6):686–691.

41. Garcia-Carbonero R, Paz-Ares L. Systemic chemotherapy in the management of malignant peritoneal mesothelioma. *Eur J Surg Oncol* 2006;32(6):676–681.

42. Berghmans T, Paesmans M, Lalami Y, et al. Activity of chemotherapy and immunotherapy on malignant mesothelioma: a systematic review of the literature with meta-analysis. *Lung Cancer* 2002;38(2):111–121.

43. Adjei AA. Pemetrexed (ALIMTA), a novel multitargeted antineoplastic agent. *Clin Cancer Res* 2004;10(12 pt 2):4276s–4280s.

44. Vogelzang NJ, Rusthoven JJ, Symanowski J, et al. Phase III study of pemetrexed in combination with cisplatin versus cisplatin alone in patients with malignant pleural mesothelioma. *J Clin Oncol* 2003;21(14):2636–2644.

45. Karunaharan T, Metzner D, Maher G, Plahl A, Wert N. Pemetrexed + cisplatin in patients with malignant peritoneal mesothelioma (abstract). *Proc Am Soc Clin Oncol* 2004;22:7201.

46. Bloss J, Wozniak A, Janne P, et al. Pemetrexed alone or in combination with cisplatin in the treatment of patients with peritoneal mesothelioma: Outcomes of an expanded access program (EAP) in patients with malignant mesothelioma [abstract]. *Proc Am Soc Clin Oncol* 2004;22:7198.

47. Pestieau SR, Stuart OA, Sugarbaker PH. Multi-targeted antifolate (MTA): pharmacokinetics of intraperitoneal administration in a rat model. *Eur J Surg Oncol* 2000;26(7):696–700.

48. Byrne MJ, Davidson JA, Musk AW, et al. Cisplatin and gemcitabine treatment for malignant mesothelioma: a phase II study. *J Clin Oncol* 1999;17(1):25–30.

49. van Haarst JM, Baas P, Manegold C, et al. Multicentre phase II study of gemcitabine and cisplatin in malignant pleural mesothelioma. *Br J Cancer* 2002;86(3):342–345.

50. Nowak AK, Byrne MJ, Williamson R, et al. A multicentre phase II study of cisplatin and gemcitabine for malignant mesothelioma. *Br J Cancer* 2002;87(5):491–496.

51. Soulie P, Ruffie P, Trandafir L, et al. Combined systemic chemoimmunotherapy in advanced diffuse malignant mesothelioma: report of a phase I-II study of weekly cisplatin/interferon alfa-2a. *J Clin Oncol* 1996;14(3):878–885.

52. Westermann AM, Dubbelman R, Moolenaar WH, Beijnen J, Rodenhuis S. Successful intraperitoneal suramin treatment of peritoneal mesothelioma. *Ann Oncol* 1997;8(8):801–802.

53. Hoff CM, Shockley TR. The potential of gene therapy in the peritoneal cavity. *Perit Dial Int* 1999;19(suppl 2):S202–S207.

54. Levine EA. Diffuse malignant mesothelioma of the peritoneum and pleura, analysis of markers. *Mod Pathol* 2004;17:476–481.

55. Ramos-Nino ME, Testa JR, Altomare DA, et al. Cellular and molecular parameters of mesothelioma. *J Cell Biochem* 2006;98(4):723–734.

56. Chailleux E, Dabouis G, Pioche D, et al. Prognostic factors in diffuse malignant pleural mesothelioma: a study of 167 patients. *Chest* 1988;93(1):159–162.

57. Markman M, Kelsen D. Efficacy of cisplatin-based intraperitoneal chemotherapy as treatment of malignant peritoneal mesothelioma. *J Cancer Res Clin Oncol* 1992;118(7):547–550.

58. Yates DH, Corrin B, Stidolph PN, Browne K. Malignant mesothelioma in south east England: clinicopathological experience of 272 cases. *Thorax* 1997;52(6):507–512.

59. Neumann V, Muller KM, Fischer M. [Peritoneal mesothelioma—incidence and etiology.] *Pathologe* 1999;20(3):169–176.

60. Eltabbakh GH, Piver MS, Hempling RE, Recio FO, Intengen ME. Clinical picture, response to therapy, and survival of women with diffuse malignant peritoneal mesothelioma. *J Surg Oncol* 1999;70(1):6–12.

61. Park BJ, Alexander HR, Libutti SK, et al. Treatment of primary peritoneal mesothelioma by continuous hyperthermic peritoneal perfusion (CHPP). *Ann Surg Oncol* 1999;6(6):582–590.

62. Loggie BW, Fleming RA, McQuellon RP, Russell GB, Geisinger KR, Levine EA. Prospective trial for the treatment of malignant peritoneal mesothelioma. *Am Surg* 2001;67(10):999–1003.

63. Kerrigan SA, Turnnir RT, Clement PB, Young RH, Churg A. Diffuse malignant epithelial mesotheliomas of the peritoneum in women: a clinicopathologic study of 25 patients. *Cancer* 2002;94(2):378–385.

64. Wagmiller JA, Koehan ML, Chabot JA, Fountain KS, Hesdorffer M, Taub RN. *Peritoneal Mesothelioma: The Columbia Experience. Malignant Mesothelioma. Advances in Pathogenesis, Diagnosis, and Translational Therapies.* New York, NY: Springer Verlag; 2005:723–731.

Note: Page numbers followed by *f* indicate figures; *t,* tables.